D1450102

Medical and Health Information Directory

Volume 2:
Publications, Libraries, and Other Information Services

Highlights

Volume 2 of the sixth edition of the *Medical and Health Information Directory (MHID)* is a comprehensive guide to medical and health-related publications, libraries, and other information services, including:

- Journals
- Newsletters
- Annuals and Review Serials
- Abstracting and Indexing Services
- Directories
- Publishers
- Audiovisual Producers and Services
- Computer-Readable Databases
- Libraries and Information Centers

Entries in Volume 2 are carefully selected from a wide array of resources to provide a convenient one-stop source of information on a broad range of subjects. Coverage spans the complete spectrum of activity in the medical and health care fields, including:

- basic biomedical sciences
- clinical medicine
- technological and socioeconomic aspects of health care

Features of This Edition

Completely revised and updated, the sixth edition of Volume 2 features:

▶ 10,800 descriptive listings arranged within nine separate chapters, each covering a specific type of publication or information service

▶ Some 1,000 entries new to this edition

▶ Coverage of publishers expanded to include nonperiodical print publishers of all types and brief descriptions for each publisher

▶ Thousands of changes to addresses, telephone numbers, personnel, and other important details

▶ One-stop access to all listings via the Master Name and Keyword Index

Alternate Formats

The information in Volume 2 is available for licensing on magnetic tape or diskette.

ISSN 0749-9973

1992-93

SIXTH EDITION
(In Three Volumes)

Medical and Health Information Directory

A Guide to More Than 49,000 Associations, Agencies,
Companies, Institutions, Research Centers, Hospitals, Clinics,
Treatment Centers, Educational Programs, Publications,
Audiovisuals, Databases, Libraries, and Information Services
in Clinical Medicine, Basic Biomedical Sciences, and the
Technological and Socioeconomic Aspects of Health Care

Volume 2:

Publications, Libraries, and Other Information Services

Karen Backus, Editor

Kimberly A. Burton, Associate Editor

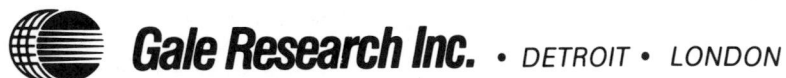 Gale Research Inc. • DETROIT • LONDON

Amy Lucas, *Senior Editor*
Karen Backus, *Editor*
Kimberly A. Burton, *Associate Editor*
Catherine A. Lada, *Assistant Editor*
Aided by: Beth A. Fhaner and Christine Tomassini

Victoria B. Cariappa, *Research Manager*
Lisa Lantz, *Editorial Associate*
Melissa E. Brown, Daniel L. Day, Brian Escamilla, L. Philip Naud,
Phyllis Shepherd, and Tracie A. Wade, *Editorial Assistants*

Mary Beth Trimper, *Production Director*
Shanna Heilveil, *Production Assistant*

Benita Spight, *Data Entry Supervisor*
Gwendolyn Tucker, *Data Entry Group Leader*
Civie Green and Frances Monroe, *Data Entry Associates*

Arthur Chartow, *Art Director*
Bernadette M. Gornie, *Graphic Designer*
C.J. Jonik and Yolanda Y. Latham, *Keyliners*

Theresa Rocklin, *Supervisor of Editorial Programming Services*
David Trotter, *Programmer*

∞™ The paper used in this publication meets the minimum requirements
of American National Standard for Information Sciences—Permanence
Paper for Printed Library Materials, ANSI Z39.48-1984.

✿ This book is printed on recycled paper that meets Environmental Protection Agency Standards.

ISSN 0749-9973
ISBN 0-8103-7524-9 (set)
ISBN 0-8103-7521-4 (v. 1)
ISBN 0-8103-7522-2 (v. 2)
ISBN 0-8103-7523-0 (v. 3)
Library of Congress Catalog Card Number 85-645724

Printed in the United States of America

Published simultaneously in the United Kingdom
by Gale Research International Limited
(An affiliated company of Gale Research Inc.)

Contents

Introduction

Volume 2 of the *Medical and Health Information Directory (MHID)*, now in its sixth edition, is a convenient one-stop source of contact and descriptive information on medical and health-related publications, libraries, and other information services. It directs health care professionals and the public alike to a wide variety of resources, including:

- Journals
- Newsletters
- Annuals and Review Serials
- Abstracting and Indexing Services
- Directories
- Publishers
- Audiovisual Producers and Services
- Computer-Readable Databases
- Libraries and Information Centers

Some 10,800 resources are profiled in Volume 2, including 1,000 new to this edition.

Comprehensive Coverage

Volume 2 covers domestic and foreign publications, libraries, and other information services related to the medical or health care fields. Entries represent a wide range of subject matter within the following broad areas:

- basic biomedical sciences
- clinical medicine
- technological and socioeconomic aspects of health care

Expanded Coverage of Publishers

The number of publishers covered in *MHID* has doubled since the previous edition with the inclusion of not only book publishers, but publishers that produce other types of nonperiodical print materials (i.e., reports, pamphlets, proceedings, etc.) on the medical and health care fields. In addition, brief descriptions have been added to each publisher's entry.

Arrangement and Indexing

Volume 2 consists of descriptive listings and a Master Name and Keyword Index.

▶ The **descriptive listings** are organized within nine separate chapters, according to type of publication or information service, as outlined on the "Contents" page.

▶ The **Master Name and Keyword Index** speeds access to Volume 2 entries through a single alphabetical listing of all publications, libraries, publishers, databases, and audiovisual services included in the book, as well as to significant keywords appearing in names or titles.

For additional information on the content, arrangement, and indexing of Volume 2, consult the "User's Guide" following this introduction.

Method of Compilation

The sixth edition of Volume 2 represents a complete revision and updating of all material presented in the fifth edition, incorporating thousands of changes to addresses, telephone numbers, personnel, and other key details.

Many sources were used to update this edition. Entries relevant to the medical and allied health fields were carefully selected from Gale Research Inc. directories and from federal government publications. Telephone inquiries, questionnaire mailings, and other written correspondence were also employed to gather data and/or verify information.

Companion Volumes Profile Organizations and Health Services

Volume 2's coverage of medical and health-related publications, libraries, and other information services is complemented by the companion volumes in the *MHID* set:

▶ Volume 1 covers more than 16,400 organizations, agencies, and institutions

▶ Volume 3 lists more than 24,500 health services, including clinics, treatment centers, care programs, and counseling/diagnostic services

Together, these volumes provide complete coverage of the medical and health care information and delivery system.

Volume 2 Information Offered in Alternate Formats

The information in Volume 2 is available for licensing on magnetic tape or diskette. Contact Customer Services at 800-877-GALE for details.

Comments Welcome

Every effort has been made to provide the most accurate, up-to-date information possible in this edition of Volume 2. Comments and suggestions for improvements are welcome. Please contact:

Medical and Health Information Directory
Gale Research Inc.
835 Penobscot Bldg.
Detroit, MI 48226-4094
Telephone: (313)961-2242
Toll-free: 800-347-GALE
Fax: (313)961-6815
Telex: 810-221-7086

Karen Backus

User's Guide

Volume 2 of the *Medical and Health Information Directory (MHID)* consists of a main body of **descriptive listings** grouped within separate chapters by type of publication or information service, and a **Master Name and Keyword Index**, which provides a convenient alphabetical listing of all publications, libraries, publishers, databases, and audiovisual services included in Volume 2. Each part is described below.

Descriptive Listings and Chapter Descriptions

Listings are numbered sequentially within nine separate chapters, as shown below. Details on the content, arrangement, sources, and indexing for each chapter are provided in the following descriptions.

1. Journals

- **Scope:** More than 1,700 English-language journals in the biomedical and health sciences.
- **Entries include:** Journal title, publisher name, address, telephone number (U.S. entries only), and in most cases, date first published, frequency of publication, and ISSN.
- **Arrangement:** Alphabetical by journal title.
- **Indexed by:** Journal title and significant keywords within titles.
- **Source:** The 1991 *List of Journals Indexed in Index Medicus* (published by the National Library of Medicine and available from the U.S. Government Printing Office), supplemented with original research by the *MHID* editorial staff.

2. Newsletters

- **Scope:** Some 1,400 medical and health-related newsletters published in the United States and Canada and readily available to the public.
- **Entries include:** Newsletter title, publisher name, address, telephone number, and a brief description, including newsletter scope, date first published, frequency of publication, and ISSN.
- **Arrangement:** Alphabetical by newsletter title.
- **Indexed by:** Newsletter title and significant keywords within titles.
- **Source:** *Newsletters in Print*, 6th Edition (published by Gale Research Inc.)

3. Annuals and Review Serials

- **Scope:** More than 370 English-language review publications in the biomedical and health sciences. These review serials are publications of special interest to the health professions because they evaluate and compress the journal literature for various medical specialties into a manageable and easily accessible form.
- **Entries include:** Publication title, publisher name, address, telephone number (U.S. entries only), and in most cases, date first published, frequency of publication, and ISSN.
- **Arrangement:** Alphabetical by publication title.
- **Indexed by:** Publication title and significant keywords within titles.
- **Source:** The 1991 *List of Journals Indexed in Index Medicus* (published by the National Library of Medicine and available from the U.S. Government Printing Office), supplemented with original research by the *MHID* editorial staff.

4. Abstracting and Indexing Services

- **Scope:** More than 280 English-language indexes and abstracting journals that summarize and/or reference the contents of multiple sources of published literature in the biomedical and health sciences.
- **Entries include:** Publication title, publisher name, address, telephone number (U.S. entries only), and in most cases, date first published, frequency of publication, and ISSN.

- **Arrangement:** Alphabetical by publication title.
- **Indexed by:** Publication title and significant keywords within titles.
- **Source:** Original research by the *MHID* editorial staff.

5. Directories

- **Scope:** Over 1,100 printed directories, lists, and guides that provide national, U.S. regional, or international coverage of a wide variety of medical and health-related subject areas.
- **Entries include:** Directory title, publisher name, address, telephone number (U.S. entries only), and a brief description, including directory scope, approximate number of pages, and frequency of publication.
- **Arrangement:** Alphabetical by directory title.
- **Indexed by:** Directory title and significant keywords within titles.
- **Source:** *Directories in Print*, 9th Edition (published by Gale Research Inc.)

6. Publishers

- **Scope:** Approximately 1,240 U.S. organizations, including major publishing companies, small presses, associations, government agencies, and others, that publish books and/or other types of nonperiodical print materials on medical and health-related topics.
- **Entries include:** Publisher name, address, telephone number, and a brief description of publishing activity.
- **Arrangement:** Alphabetical by publisher name.
- **Indexed by:** Publisher name and significant keywords within names.
- **Source:** *Publishers Directory*, 12th Edition (published by Gale Research Inc.)

7. Audiovisual Producers and Services

- **Scope:** Some 600 organizations, agencies, and institutions in the U.S. and Canada that produce and/or distribute medical and health-related audiovisual materials, and/or offer other audiovisual production services to clients in medical and allied health fields.
- **Entries include:** Organization name, address, telephone number, and a brief description of the products and services.
- **Arrangement:** Alphabetical by organization name.
- **Indexed by:** Organization name and significant keywords within names.
- **Source:** Original research by the *MHID* editorial staff.

8. Computer-Readable Databases

- **Scope:** Some 400 medical and health-related databases produced worldwide and publicly available in at least one of the following formats: online, CD-ROM, diskette, magnetic tape, or batch access.
- **Entries include:** Database name and acronym, producer name, address, telephone number, a general description of the contents of the database, alternate names by which the database is known, the main language in which the database is maintained and/or searched, and the subjects covered by the database.
- **Arrangement:** Alphabetical by database name.
- **Indexed by:** Database name and significant keywords within names.
- **Source:** *Computer-Readable Databases*, 8th Edition (published by Gale Research Inc.)

9. Libraries and Information Centers

- **Scope:** Nearly 3,670 U.S. and Canadian health sciences libraries and information centers maintained by businesses, nonprofit organizations, educational institutions, associations and societies, government agencies, and others.
- **Entries include:** Parent organization name, library name, address, telephone number, contact name, subject coverage of the collection, and quantitative data for holdings and subscriptions.
- **Arrangement:** U.S. entries appear first, followed by Canadian entries. Within each country, entries are alphabetical by state or province, then alphabetical by city names, and finally, alphabetical by parent organization name within cities.

- **Indexed by:** Parent organization name, specific library name, and significant keywords within names.
- **Source:** *Directory of Special Libraries and Information Centers*, 15th Edition (published by Gale Research Inc.)

Master Name and Keyword Index

The alphabetical **Master Name and Keyword Index** is a consolidated listing of all publications, libraries, publishers, databases, and audiovisual services included in Volume 2. All entries are indexed by the name or title listed and by principal keywords that are a part of that name or title. Index references are to book *entry numbers* rather than page numbers. Publication titles appear in italics.

Many of the entries in Volume 2 use a hierarchical organization name structure, with a parent organization and often intermediate subunits preceding the specific unit name. The Master Name and Keyword Index offers different methods for locating multiple-part organization names. All may be accessed via the parent organization name. These *general-to-specific* citations are identified by the presence of a • (bullet) separating parts of the name. In the same manner, some entries may also be referenced under the name of a significant intermediate unit. Additionally, some entries will be indexed in a *specific-to-general* format, beginning with the specific unit name, followed by intermediate units and the parent organization. Unit names are separated by a - (hyphen).

If several entries have the same parent organization, as is the case with many of the government and university groups listed in Volume 2, the related units appear as a group under the name of the parent organization. All Volume 2 chapter titles are also named in the index, with references to appropriate chapter numbers.

Indexing Sample

Following is a typical entry in Volume 2:

★800★   **MISSOURI BAPTIST MEDICAL CENTER**
SCHOOL OF NURSING LIBRARY
3015 N. Ballas Rd.
St. Louis, MO 63131   (314) 569-5193

The index provides the following citations to the above entry:

Missouri Baptist Medical Center • School of Nursing Library   **800**
Nursing Library; School of - Missouri Baptist Medical Center   **800**
School of Nursing Library - Missouri Baptist Medical Center   **800**

Medical and Health Information Directory

Volume 2:
Publications, Libraries, and Other Information Services

(1) Journals

Chapter 1 is arranged alphabetically by journal titles. For additional information, consult the User's Guide located at the front of this directory.

★1★   AANA JOURNAL
American Association of Nurse Anesthetists
216 W. Higgins Rd.
Park Ridge, IL 60068   Phone: (708) 692-7050
First Published: 1933. **Frequency:** Bimonthly. **ISSN:** 0094-6354.

★2★   ACADEMIC PSYCHIATRY
American Psychiatric Press, Inc.
1400 K St., NW
Washington, DC 20005   Phone: (202) 682-6420
Frequency: Quarterly. **ISSN:** 1042-9670.

★3★   ACTA ANAESTHESIOLOGICA SCANDINAVICA
Munksgaard International Publishers Ltd.
PO Box 2148
DK-1016 Copenhagen K, Denmark
First Published: 1957. **Frequency:** 8/yr. **ISSN:** 0001-5172.

★4★   ACTA ANATOMICA
S. Karger Publishers, Inc.
26 W. Avon Rd.
PO Box 529
Farmington, CT 06085   Phone: (203) 675-7834
First Published: 1945. **Frequency:** Monthly. **ISSN:** 0001-5180.

★5★   ACTA CARDIOLOGICA
Belgium Society for Cardiology
Avenue Circulair 138A
1180 Brussels, Belgium
First Published: 1946. **Frequency:** Bimonthly. **ISSN:** 0001-5385.

★6★   ACTA CHIRURGICA SCANDINAVICA
Almqvist & Wiksell Periodical Co.
PO Box 638
S-101 28 Stockholm, Sweden
First Published: 1869. **Frequency:** 10/yr. **ISSN:** 0001-5482.

★7★   ACTA CLINICA BELGICA
1400 Fr. Ave. E. Mounier 52
1200 Brussels, Belgium
First Published: 1974. **Frequency:** Semimonthly. **ISSN:** 0001-5512.

★8★   ACTA CYTOLOGICA
Science Printers and Publishers, Inc.
8342 Olive Blvd.
St. Louis, MO 63132   Phone: (314) 991-4440
First Published: 1957. **Frequency:** Bimonthly. **ISSN:** 0001-5547.

★9★   ACTA DERMATO-VENEREOLOGICA
Almqvist & Wiksell Periodical Co.
PO Box 638
S-101 28 Stockholm, Sweden
First Published: 1920. **Frequency:** 6/yr. **ISSN:** 0001-5555.

★10★   ACTA ENDOCRINOLOGICA
Rhodos International Publishing
Strandgade 36
DK-1401 Copenhagen, Denmark
First Published: 1948. **Frequency:** Monthly. **ISSN:** 0001-5598.

★11★   ACTA HAEMATOLOGICA
S. Karger Publishers, Inc.
26 W. Avon Rd.
PO Box 529
Farmington, CT 06085   Phone: (203) 675-7834
First Published: 1948. **Frequency:** 8/yr. **ISSN:** 0001-5792.

★12★   ACTA NEUROCHIRURGICA
Springer-Verlag New York, Inc.
175 5th Ave.
New York, NY 10010   Phone: (212) 460-1500
First Published: 1950. **Frequency:** 24/yr. **ISSN:** 0001-6268.

★13★   ACTA NEUROLOGICA SCANDINAVICA
Munksgaard International Publishers Ltd.
PO Box 2148
DK-1016 Copenhagen K, Denmark
First Published: 1961. **Frequency:** Monthly. **ISSN:** 0001-6314.

★14★   ACTA NEUROPATHOLOGICA
Springer-Verlag New York, Inc.
175 5th Ave.
New York, NY 10010   Phone: (212) 460-1500
First Published: 1961. **Frequency:** 12/yr. **ISSN:** 0001-6322.

**★15★   ACTA OBSTETRICA ET GYNECOLOGICA
SCANDINAVICA**
Scandinavian Association of Obstetricians and Gynecologists
Box 443
S-901 09 Umeaa, Sweden
First Published: 1921. **Frequency:** 8/yr. **ISSN:** 0001-6349.

★16★   ACTA ODONTOLOGICA SCANDINAVICA
Universitets Forlaget
PO Box 2959
0608 Oslo 1, Norway
First Published: 1942. **Frequency:** Bimonthly. **ISSN:** 0001-6357.

★17★ ACTA OPHTHALMOLOGICA
Scriptor Publisher ApS
Gasvaerksvej 15
DK-1656 Copenhagen K, Denmark
First Published: 1923. **Frequency:** Bimonthly. **ISSN:** 0001-639X.

★18★ ACTA ORTHOPAEDICA SCANDINAVICA
Munksgaard International Publishers Ltd.
PO Box 2148
DK-1016 Copenhagen K, Denmark
First Published: 1930. **Frequency:** Bimonthly. **ISSN:** 0001-6470.

★19★ ACTA OTO-LARYNGOLOGICA
Almqvist & Wiksell Periodical Co.
PO Box 638
S-101 28 Stockholm, Sweden
First Published: 1918. **Frequency:** Monthly. **ISSN:** 0001-6489.

★20★ ACTA PAEDIATRICA SCANDINAVICA
Almqvist & Wiksell Periodical Co.
PO Box 638
S-101 28 Stockholm, Sweden
First Published: 1921. **Frequency:** 6/yr. **ISSN:** 0001-656X.

★21★ ACTA PHYSIOLOGICA SCANDINAVICA
Blackwell Scientific Publications
3 Cambridge Center, Ste. 208
Cambridge, MA 02142   Phone: (617) 225-0401
First Published: 1940. **Frequency:** Monthly. **ISSN:** 0001-6772.

★22★ ACTA PSYCHIATRICA SCANDINAVICA
Munksgaard International Publishers Ltd.
PO Box 2148
DK-1016 Copenhagen K, Denmark
First Published: 1926. **Frequency:** Monthly. **ISSN:** 0001-690X.

★23★ ACTA RADIOLOGICA: SERIES 1: DIAGNOSIS
Munksgaard International Publishers Ltd.
PO Box 2148
DK-1016 Copenhagen, Denmark
First Published: 1921. **Frequency:** Bimonthly. **ISSN:** 0567-8056.

★24★ ACTA VETERINARIA SCANDINAVICA
Danske Dyrlaegeforening
Alhambravej 15
DK-1826 Copenhagen V, Denmark
Frequency: Quarterly. **ISSN:** 0044-605X.

★25★ ACTA VIROLOGICA
Academic Press, Inc.
1250 6th Ave.
San Diego, CA 92101   Phone: (619) 231-0926
First Published: 1957. **Frequency:** Bimonthly. **ISSN:** 0001-723X.

★26★ ACTIVITIES, ADAPTATION, AND AGING
The Haworth Press, Inc.
10 Alice St.
Binghamton, NY 13904   Phone: (800) 342-9678
First Published: 1991. **Frequency:** Quarterly.

★27★ ACUPUNCTURE AND ELECTRO-THERAPEUTICS RESEARCH
Pergamon Press, Inc.
Maxwell House, Fairview Park
Elmsford, NY 10523   Phone: (914) 592-7700
First Published: 1976. **Frequency:** Quarterly. **ISSN:** 0360-1293.

★28★ ACUTE CARE
S. Karger Publishers, Inc.
26 W. Avon Rd.
PO Box 529
Farmington, CT 06085   Phone: (203) 675-7834
First Published: 1964. **Frequency:** Quarterly. **ISSN:** 0254-0819.

★29★ ADDICTIVE BEHAVIORS
Pergamon Press, Inc.
Maxwell House, Fairview Park
Elmsford, NY 10523   Phone: (914) 592-7700
First Published: 1976. **Frequency:** 6/yr. **ISSN:** 0306-4603.

★30★ AESTHETIC PLASTIC SURGERY
Springer-Verlag New York, Inc.
175 5th Ave.
New York, NY 10010   Phone: (212) 460-1500
First Published: 1976. **Frequency:** Quarterly. **ISSN:** 0364-216X.

★31★ AFRICAN JOURNAL OF MEDICINE AND MEDICAL SCIENCES
Blackwell Scientific Publications
3 Cambridge Center, Ste. 208
Cambridge, MA 02142   Phone: (617) 225-0401
First Published: 1970. **Frequency:** Quarterly. **ISSN:** 0309-3913.

★32★ AGE AND AGEING
Oxford University Press
Oxford Journals
Pinkhill House, Southfield Rd.
Oxford OX8 1JJ, England
First Published: 1972. **Frequency:** Bimonthly. **ISSN:** 0002-0729.

★33★ AHME JOURNAL
Association for Hospital Medical Education
1101 Connecticut Ave. NW, Ste. 700
Washington, DC 20036   Phone: (202) 857-1196
First Published: 1972. **Frequency:** Quarterly. **ISSN:** 0090-7782.

★34★ AIDS
Current Science
20 N. 3rd St.
Philadelphia, PA 19106   Phone: (215) 514-2266
Frequency: Monthly. **ISSN:** 0269-9370.

★35★ AIDS AND PUBLIC POLICY JOURNAL
University Publishing Group
107 E. Church St.
Frederick, MD 21701   Phone: (800) 654-8188
First Published: 1986. **Frequency:** Quarterly. **ISSN:** 0887-3852.

★36★ AJNR: AMERICAN JOURNAL OF NEURORADIOLOGY
American Society of Neuroradiology
2210 Midwest Rd., Ste. 207
Oak Brook, IL 60521   Phone: (708) 574-0220
First Published: 1980. **Frequency:** Bimonthly. **ISSN:** 0195-6108.

★37★ AJR: AMERICAN JOURNAL OF ROENTGENOLOGY
American Roentgen Ray Society
c/o Paul R. Fullagar
1891 Preston White Dr.
Reston, VA 22091   Phone: (703) 648-8992
First Published: 1906. **Frequency:** Monthly. **ISSN:** 0361-803X.

★38★ ALABAMA MEDICINE
Medical Association of the State of Alabama
19 S. Jackson St.
PO Box 1900-C
Montgomery, AL 36104   Phone: (205) 263-6441
First Published: 1931. **Frequency:** Monthly. **ISSN:** 0738-4947.

★39★ ALASKA MEDICINE
Alaska State Medical Association
2401 E. 42nd Ave., No. 104
Anchorage, AK 99508   Phone: (907) 562-2662
First Published: 1959. **Frequency:** Bimonthly. **ISSN:** 0002-4538.

★40★ ALCOHOL
Pergamon Press, Inc.
Maxwell House, Fairview Park
Elmsford, NY 10523   Phone: (914) 592-7700
First Published: 1984. **Frequency:** Bimonthly. **ISSN:** 0741-8329.

★41★ ALCOHOL AND ALCOHOLISM
Pergamon Press, Inc.
Maxwell House, Fairview Park
Elmsford, NY 10523   Phone: (914) 592-7700
First Published: 1967. Frequency: 6/yr. ISSN: 0735-0414.

★42★ ALCOHOL HEALTH AND RESEARCH WORLD
U.S. National Institute on Alcohol Abuse and Alcoholism
1400 Eye St. NW, Ste. 600
Washington, DC 20005   Phone: (202) 842-7600
First Published: 1975. Frequency: Quarterly. ISSN: 0090-838X.

★43★ ALCOHOLISM: CLINICAL AND EXPERIMENTAL
      RESEARCH
Research Society on Alcoholism
4314 Medical Pkwy., Ste. 300
Austin, TX 78756   Phone: (512) 454-0022
First Published: 1977. Frequency: Bimonthly. ISSN: 0145-6008.

★44★ ALCOHOLISM TREATMENT QUARTERLY
The Haworth Press, Inc.
10 Alice St.
Binghamton, NY 13904   Phone: (800) 342-9678
First Published: 1983. Frequency: Quarterly. ISSN: 0734-7324.

★45★ ALIMENTARY PHARMACOLOGY AND THERAPEUTICS
Blackwell Scientific Publications
3 Cambridge Center, Ste. 208
Cambridge, MA 02142   Phone: (617) 225-0401
First Published: 1987. Frequency: 6/yr. ISSN: 0269-2183.

★46★ ALLERGY
Munksgaard International Publishers Ltd.
PO Box 2148
DK-1016 Copenhagen K, Denmark
First Published: 1948. Frequency: 8/yr. ISSN: 0105-4538.

★47★ AMERICAN ANIMAL HOSPITAL ASSOCIATION
      JOURNAL
PO Box 150899
Denver, CO 80215   Phone: (303) 279-2500
First Published: 1965. Frequency: Bimonthly. ISSN: 0587-2871.

★48★ AMERICAN ANNALS OF THE DEAF
Convention of American Instructors of the Deaf
800 Florida Ave., NE
Washington, DC 20002   Phone: (202) 651-5340
First Published: 1847. Frequency: Quarterly. ISSN: 0002-726X.

★49★ AMERICAN ASSOCIATION OF OCCUPATIONAL
      HEALTH NURSES JOURNAL
50 Lenox Pointe
Atlanta, GA 30324   Phone: (404) 262-1162
First Published: 1953. Frequency: Monthly. ISSN: 0891-0162.

★50★ AMERICAN FAMILY PHYSICIAN
American Academy of Family Physicians
8880 Ward Pkwy.
Kansas City, MO 64114   Phone: (816) 333-9700
First Published: 1950. Frequency: Monthly. ISSN: 0002-838X.

★51★ AMERICAN HEART JOURNAL
Mosby-Year Book, Inc.
11830 Westline Industrial Dr.
St. Louis, MO 63146   Phone: (800) 325-4117
First Published: 1925. Frequency: Monthly. ISSN: 0002-8703.

★52★ AMERICAN INDUSTRIAL HYGIENE ASSOCIATION
      JOURNAL
375 White Pond Dr.
Box 8390
Akron, OH 44320   Phone: (216) 873-2442
First Published: 1940. Frequency: Monthly. ISSN: 0002-8894.

★53★ THE AMERICAN JOURNAL OF ADDICTIONS
American Psychiatric Press, Inc.
1400 K St., NW
Washington, DC 20005   Phone: (202) 682-6420
First Published: 1992. Frequency: Quarterly.

★54★ AMERICAN JOURNAL OF ANATOMY
American Association of Anatomists
c/o Dr. Robert D. Yates
Tulane Medical Center
1430 Tulane Ave.
New Orleans, LA 70112   Phone: (504) 584-2727
First Published: 1901. Frequency: Monthly. ISSN: 0002-9106.

★55★ AMERICAN JOURNAL OF CARDIAC IMAGING
W. B. Saunders Co.
Curtis Center
Independence Sq. W.
Philadelphia, PA 19106   Phone: (407) 345-4200
First Published: 1987. Frequency: Quarterly. ISSN: 0887-7971.

★56★ AMERICAN JOURNAL OF CARDIOLOGY
Cahners Publishing Co., Inc.
249 W. 17th St.
New York, NY 10011   Phone: (212) 645-0067
First Published: 1958. Frequency: 22/yr. ISSN: 0002-9149.

★57★ AMERICAN JOURNAL OF CLINICAL HYPNOSIS
American Society of Clinical Hypnosis
2250 E. Devon Ave., Ste. 336
Des Plaines, IL 60018   Phone: (708) 297-3317
First Published: 1958. Frequency: Quarterly. ISSN: 0002-9157.

★58★ AMERICAN JOURNAL OF CLINICAL NUTRITION
American Society for Clinical Nutrition
9650 Rockville Pike
Bethesda, MD 20814   Phone: (301) 530-7110
First Published: 1952. Frequency: Monthly. ISSN: 0002-9165.

★59★ AMERICAN JOURNAL OF CLINICAL ONCOLOGY
Raven Press
1185 Avenue of the Americas
New York, NY 10036   Phone: (212) 930-9500
First Published: 1978. Frequency: Bimonthly. ISSN: 0277-3732.

★60★ AMERICAN JOURNAL OF CLINICAL PATHOLOGY
American Society of Clinical Pathologists
2100 W. Harrison
Chicago, IL 60612   Phone: (312) 738-1336
First Published: 1931. Frequency: Monthly. ISSN: 0002-9173.

★61★ AMERICAN JOURNAL OF DERMATOPATHOLOGY
Raven Press
1185 Avenue of the Americas
New York, NY 10036   Phone: (212) 930-9500
First Published: 1979. Frequency: Bimonthly. ISSN: 0193-1091.

★62★ AMERICAN JOURNAL OF DISEASES OF CHILDREN
American Medical Association
515 N. State St.
Chicago, IL 60610   Phone: (312) 464-5000
First Published: 1911. Frequency: Monthly. ISSN: 0002-922X.

★63★ AMERICAN JOURNAL OF DRUG AND ALCOHOL
      ABUSE
Marcel Dekker, Inc.
270 Madison Ave.
New York, NY 10016   Phone: (212) 696-9000
First Published: 1974. Frequency: Quarterly. ISSN: 0095-2990.

★64★ AMERICAN JOURNAL OF EEG TECHNOLOGY
American Society of Electroneurodiagnostic Technologists
6th at Quint
Carroll, IA 51401   Phone: (712) 792-2978
First Published: 1960. Frequency: Quarterly. ISSN: 0002-9238.

★65★   AMERICAN JOURNAL OF EMERGENCY MEDICINE
W.B. Saunders Co.
Curtis Center
Independence Sq. W.
Philadelphia, PA 19106   Phone: (215) 238-7800
First Published: 1983. **Frequency:** Bimonthly. **ISSN:** 0735-6757.

★66★   AMERICAN JOURNAL OF EPIDEMIOLOGY
Society for Epidemiologic Research
2007 E. Monument St.
Baltimore, MD 21205   Phone: (301) 955-3441
First Published: 1921. **Frequency:** Monthly. **ISSN:** 0002-9262.

★67★   AMERICAN JOURNAL OF FORENSIC MEDICINE AND PATHOLOGY
National Association of Medical Examiners
1402 S. Grand Blvd.
St. Louis, MO 63104   Phone: (314) 577-8298
First Published: 1980. **Frequency:** Quarterly. **ISSN:** 0195-7910.

★68★   AMERICAN JOURNAL OF GASTROENTEROLOGY
American College of Gastroenterology
4222 King St.
Alexandria, VA 22302   Phone: (703) 549-4440
First Published: 1934. **Frequency:** Monthly. **ISSN:** 0002-9270.

★69★   AMERICAN JOURNAL OF HEMATOLOGY
John Wiley & Sons, Inc.
605 3rd Ave.
New York, NY 10158   Phone: (212) 850-6000
First Published: 1976. **Frequency:** Monthly. **ISSN:** 0361-8609.

★70★   AMERICAN JOURNAL OF HOSPITAL PHARMACY
American Society of Hospital Pharmacists
4630 Montgomery Ave.
Bethesda, MD 20814   Phone: (301) 657-3000
First Published: 1945. **Frequency:** Monthly. **ISSN:** 0002-9289.

★71★   AMERICAN JOURNAL OF HUMAN GENETICS
American Society of Human Genetics
9650 Rockville Pike
Bethesda, MD 20814   Phone: (301) 571-1825
First Published: 1948. **Frequency:** Monthly. **ISSN:** 0002-9297.

★72★   AMERICAN JOURNAL OF HYPERTENSION
Elsevier Science Publishing Co., Inc.
655 Avenue of the Americas
New York, NY 10010   Phone: (212) 989-5800
Frequency: Monthly. **ISSN:** 0895-7061.

★73★   AMERICAN JOURNAL OF INDUSTRIAL MEDICINE
John Wiley & Sons, Inc.
605 3rd Ave.
New York, NY 10158   Phone: (212) 850-6000
First Published: 1980. **Frequency:** Monthly. **ISSN:** 0271-3586.

★74★   AMERICAN JOURNAL OF INFECTION CONTROL
Association for Practitioners in Infection Control
505 E. Hawley St.
Mundelein, IL 60060   Phone: (708) 949-6052
First Published: 1973. **Frequency:** Bimonthly. **ISSN:** 0196-6553.

★75★   AMERICAN JOURNAL OF KIDNEY DISEASES
National Kidney Foundation
30 E. 33rd St., Ste. 1100
New York, NY 10016   Phone: (212) 889-2210
First Published: 1981. **Frequency:** Monthly. **ISSN:** 0272-6386.

★76★   AMERICAN JOURNAL OF LAW AND MEDICINE
American Society of Law & Medicine
765 Commonwealth Ave., Ste. 1634
Boston, MA 02215   Phone: (617) 262-4990
First Published: 1975. **Frequency:** Quarterly. **ISSN:** 0098-8588.

★77★   AMERICAN JOURNAL OF MEDICAL GENETICS
John Wiley & Sons, Inc.
605 3rd Ave.
New York, NY 10158   Phone: (212) 850-6000
First Published: 1977. **Frequency:** Monthly. **ISSN:** 0148-7299.

★78★   AMERICAN JOURNAL OF THE MEDICAL SCIENCES
J.B. Lippincott Co.
E. Washington Sq.
Philadelphia, PA 19105   Phone: (215) 238-4200
First Published: 1820. **Frequency:** Monthly. **ISSN:** 0002-9629.

★79★   AMERICAN JOURNAL OF MEDICINE
Cahners Publishing Co., Inc.
249 W. 17th St.
New York, NY 10011   Phone: (212) 645-0067
First Published: 1946. **Frequency:** Monthly. **ISSN:** 0002-9343.

★80★   AMERICAN JOURNAL OF MENTAL RETARDATION
American Association on Mental Retardation
1719 Kalorama Rd., NW
Washington, DC 20009   Phone: (202) 387-1968
First Published: 1876. **Frequency:** Bimonthly. **ISSN:** 0895-8017.

★81★   AMERICAN JOURNAL OF NEPHROLOGY
S. Karger Publishers, Inc.
26 W. Avon Rd.
PO Box 529
Farmington, CT 06085   Phone: (203) 675-7834
First Published: 1981. **Frequency:** 6/yr. **ISSN:** 0250-8095.

★82★   AMERICAN JOURNAL OF NONINVASIVE CARDIOLOGY
S. Karger Publishers, Inc.
26 W. Avon Rd.
PO Box 529
Farmington, CT 06085   Phone: (203) 675-7834
First Published: 1987. **Frequency:** 6/yr. **ISSN:** 0258-4425.

★83★   AMERICAN JOURNAL OF NURSING
American Nurses' Association
2420 Pershing Rd.
Kansas City, MO 64108   Phone: (816) 474-5720
First Published: 1900. **Frequency:** Monthly. **ISSN:** 0002-936X.

★84★   AMERICAN JOURNAL OF OBSTETRICS AND GYNECOLOGY
American Gynecological and Obstetrical Society
c/o James R. Scott, M.D.
University of Utah
50 N. Medical Dr.
Salt Lake City, UT 84132   Phone: (801) 581-5501
First Published: 1920. **Frequency:** Monthly. **ISSN:** 0002-9378.

★85★   AMERICAN JOURNAL OF OCCUPATIONAL THERAPY
American Occupational Therapy Association
1383 Piccard Dr., Ste. 301
Rockville, MD 20850   Phone: (301) 948-9626
First Published: 1947. **Frequency:** Monthly. **ISSN:** 0272-9490.

★86★   AMERICAN JOURNAL OF OPHTHALMOLOGY
Ophthalmic Publishing Co.
435 N. Michigan Ave., Ste. 1415
Chicago, IL 60611   Phone: (312) 787-3853
First Published: 1884. **Frequency:** Monthly. **ISSN:** 0002-9394.

★87★   AMERICAN JOURNAL OF ORTHODONTICS AND DENTOFACIAL ORTHOPEDICS
American Association of Orthodontists
460 N. Lindbergh Blvd.
St. Louis, MO 63141   Phone: (314) 993-1700
First Published: 1915. **Frequency:** Monthly. **ISSN:** 0889-5406.

★88★ AMERICAN JOURNAL OF ORTHOPSYCHIATRY
American Orthopsychiatric Association
19 W. 44th St., Ste. 1616
New York, NY 10036   Phone: (212) 354-5770
First Published: 1930. **Frequency:** Quarterly. **ISSN:** 0002-9432.

★89★ AMERICAN JOURNAL OF OTOLARYNGOLOGY
W.B. Saunders Co.
Independence Sq., W.
Philadelphia, PA 19106   Phone: (215) 238-7800
First Published: 1979. **Frequency:** Quarterly. **ISSN:** 0196-0709.

★90★ AMERICAN JOURNAL OF OTOLOGY
B. C. Decker, Inc.
320 Walnut St., Ste. 400
Philadelphia, PA 19106   Phone: (215) 625-0004
First Published: 1979. **Frequency:** Bimonthly. **ISSN:** 0192-9763.

★91★ AMERICAN JOURNAL OF PATHOLOGY
American Association of Pathologists
9650 Rockville Pike
Bethesda, MD 20814   Phone: (301) 530-7130
First Published: 1901. **Frequency:** Monthly. **ISSN:** 0002-9440.

★92★ AMERICAN JOURNAL OF PEDIATRIC HEMATOLOGY/ONCOLOGY
American Society of Pediatric Hematology/Oncology
c/o Carl Pochedly, M.D.
Wyler Children's Hospital
5841 S. Maryland Ave.
Chicago, IL 60637   Phone: (312) 702-6808
First Published: 1979. **Frequency:** Quarterly. **ISSN:** 0192-8562.

★93★ AMERICAN JOURNAL OF PERINATOLOGY
Thieme Medical Publishers, Inc.
381 Park Ave., S., Ste. 1501
New York, NY 10016   Phone: (212) 683-5088
First Published: 1983. **Frequency:** Quarterly. **ISSN:** 0735-1631.

★94★ AMERICAN JOURNAL OF PHARMACEUTICAL EDUCATION
American Association of Colleges of Pharmacy
1426 Prince St.
Alexandria, VA 22314   Phone: (703) 739-2330
First Published: 1937. **Frequency:** Quarterly. **ISSN:** 0002-9459.

★95★ AMERICAN JOURNAL OF PHYSICAL MEDICINE AND REHABILITATION
Williams & Wilkins
428 E. Preston St.
Baltimore, MD 21202   Phone: (301) 528-4223
First Published: 1921. **Frequency:** Bimonthly. **ISSN:** 0894-9115.

★96★ AMERICAN JOURNAL OF PHYSIOLOGIC IMAGING
John Wiley & Sons, Inc.
605 3rd Ave.
New York, NY 10158   Phone: (212) 850-6000
First Published: 1986. **Frequency:** Quarterly. **ISSN:** 0885-8276.

★97★ AMERICAN JOURNAL OF PHYSIOLOGY
American Physiological Society
9650 Rockville Pike
Bethesda, MD 20814   Phone: (301) 530-7164
First Published: 1898. **Frequency:** Monthly. **ISSN:** 0002-9513.

★98★ AMERICAN JOURNAL OF PROCTOLOGY, GASTROENTEROLOGY AND COLON AND RECTAL SURGERY
International Academy of Proctology
c/o George Donnally, M.D.
1203 Hadley Rd.
Mooresville, IN 46158   Phone: (317) 831-9300
First Published: 1950. **Frequency:** Bimonthly. **ISSN:** 0162-6566.

★99★ AMERICAN JOURNAL OF PSYCHIATRY
American Psychiatric Association
1400 K St., NW
Washington, DC 20005   Phone: (202) 682-6240
First Published: 1844. **Frequency:** Monthly. **ISSN:** 0002-953X.

★100★ AMERICAN JOURNAL OF PSYCHOANALYSIS
Association for the Advancement of Psychoanalysis
329 E. 62nd St.
New York, NY 10021   Phone: (212) 838-8044
First Published: 1941. **Frequency:** Quarterly. **ISSN:** 0002-9548.

★101★ AMERICAN JOURNAL OF PSYCHOLOGY
University of Illinois Press
54 E. Gregory Dr.
Champaign, IL 61820   Phone: (217) 333-0950
First Published: 1887. **Frequency:** Quarterly. **ISSN:** 0002-9556.

★102★ AMERICAN JOURNAL OF PSYCHOTHERAPY
Association for the Advancement of Psychotherapy
114 E. 78th St.
New York, NY 10021   Phone: (212) 288-4466
First Published: 1946. **Frequency:** Quarterly. **ISSN:** 0002-9564.

★103★ AMERICAN JOURNAL OF PUBLIC HEALTH
American Public Health Association
1015 15th St., NW
Washington, DC 20005   Phone: (202) 789-5600
First Published: 1911. **Frequency:** Monthly. **ISSN:** 0090-0036.

★104★ AMERICAN JOURNAL OF SPORTS MEDICINE
American Orthopaedic Society for Sports Medicine
2250 E. Devon Ave., Ste. 115
Des Plaines, IL 60018   Phone: (708) 836-7000
First Published: 1972. **Frequency:** Bimonthly. **ISSN:** 0363-5465.

★105★ AMERICAN JOURNAL OF SURGERY
Cahners Publishing Co., Inc.
249 W. 17th St.
New York, NY 10011   Phone: (212) 645-0067
First Published: 1891. **Frequency:** Monthly. **ISSN:** 0002-9610.

★106★ AMERICAN JOURNAL OF SURGICAL PATHOLOGY
Raven Press
1185 Avenue of the Americas
New York, NY 10036   Phone: (212) 930-9500
First Published: 1977. **Frequency:** Monthly. **ISSN:** 0147-5185.

★107★ AMERICAN JOURNAL OF TROPICAL MEDICINE AND HYGIENE
American Society of Tropical Medicine and Hygiene
8000 Westpark Dr., Ste. 130
McLean, VA 22102   Phone: (703) 780-1745
First Published: 1921. **Frequency:** Monthly. **ISSN:** 0002-9637.

★108★ AMERICAN JOURNAL OF VETERINARY RESEARCH
American Veterinary Medical Association
930 N. Meacham Rd.
Schaumburg, IL 60196   Phone: (708) 605-8070
First Published: 1940. **Frequency:** Monthly. **ISSN:** 0002-9645.

★109★ AMERICAN KINESIOLOGY JOURNAL
American Kinesiotherapy Association
c/o David Ser
259-08, 148 Rd.
Rosedale, NY 11422   Phone: (718) 276-0721
First Published: 1947. **Frequency:** Quarterly.

★110★ AMERICAN PHARMACY
American Pharmaceutical Association
2215 Constitution Ave., NW
Washington, DC 20037   Phone: (202) 628-4410
First Published: 1912. **Frequency:** Monthly. **ISSN:** 0160-3450.

★111★   AMERICAN PSYCHOLOGIST
American Psychological Association
1200 17th St., NW
Washington, DC 20036   Phone: (202) 955-7600
First Published: 1946. **Frequency:** Monthly. **ISSN:** 0003-066X.

★112★   AMERICAN REHABILITATION
U.S. Rehabilitation Services Administration
U.S. Department of Education
Mary E. Switzer Bldg.
330 C St. SW, Rm. 3212
Washington, DC 20202   Phone: (202) 732-1296
First Published: 1975. **Frequency:** Quarterly. **ISSN:** 0362-4048.

★113★   AMERICAN REVIEW OF RESPIRATORY DISEASES
American Thoracic Society
1740 Broadway
New York, NY 10019   Phone: (212) 315-8700
First Published: 1917. **Frequency:** Monthly. **ISSN:** 0003-0805.

★114★   AMERICAN SCIENTIST
Sigma Xi, The Scientific Research Society
99 Alexander Dr.
PO Box 13975
Research Triangle Park, NC 27709   Phone: (919) 549-4691
First Published: 1886. **Frequency:** Bimonthly. **ISSN:** 0003-0996.

★115★   AMERICAN SURGEON
J.B. Lippincott Co.
E. Washington Sq.
Philadelphia, PA 19105   Phone: (215) 238-4200
First Published: 1935. **Frequency:** Monthly. **ISSN:** 0003-1348.

★116★   AMWA JOURNAL
American Medical Writers Association
9650 Rockville Pike
Bethesda, MD 20814   Phone: (301) 493-0003
First Published: 1972. **Frequency:** Quarterly.

★117★   ANAESTHESIA
Academic Press, Inc.
1250 6th Ave.
San Diego, CA 92101   Phone: (619) 231-0926
First Published: 1945. **Frequency:** Monthly. **ISSN:** 0003-2409.

★118★   ANAESTHESIA AND INTENSIVE CARE
Australian Society of Anaesthetists
PO Box 600
Edgecliff, NSW 2027, Australia
First Published: 1972. **Frequency:** Quarterly. **ISSN:** 0310-057X.

★119★   ANALYTICAL BIOCHEMISTRY
Academic Press, Inc.
1250 6th Ave.
San Diego, CA 92101   Phone: (619) 231-0926
First Published: 1960. **Frequency:** 16/yr. **ISSN:** 0003-2697.

★120★   ANALYTICAL AND QUANTITATIVE CYTOLOGY AND HISTOLOGY
Science Printers and Publishers, Inc.
8342 Olive St.
St. Louis, MO 63132   Phone: (314) 991-4440
First Published: 1979. **Frequency:** Bimonthly. **ISSN:** 0884-6812.

★121★   ANATOMICAL RECORD
American Association of Anatomists
c/o Dr. Robert D. Yates
Tulane Medical Center
1430 Tulane Ave.
New Orleans, LA 70112   Phone: (504) 584-2727
First Published: 1906. **Frequency:** Monthly. **ISSN:** 0003-276X.

★122★   ANATOMY AND EMBRYOLOGY
Springer-Verlag New York, Inc.
175 5th Ave.
New York, NY 10010   Phone: (212) 460-1500
First Published: 1892. **Frequency:** 12/yr. **ISSN:** 0340-2061.

★123★   ANESTHESIA AND ANALGESIA
International Anesthesia Research Society
2 Summit Park Dr., Ste. 140
Cleveland, OH 44131   Phone: (216) 624-1124
First Published: 1922. **Frequency:** Monthly. **ISSN:** 0003-2999.

★124★   ANESTHESIA PROGRESS
Elsevier Science Publishing Co., Inc.
655 Avenue of the Americas
New York, NY 10010   Phone: (212) 989-5800
Frequency: Bimonthly. **ISSN:** 0003-3006.

★125★   ANESTHESIOLOGY
American Society of Anesthesiologists
515 Busse Hwy.
Park Ridge, IL 60068   Phone: (708) 825-5586
First Published: 1940. **Frequency:** Monthly. **ISSN:** 0003-3022.

★126★   ANESTHESIOLOGY REVIEW
McMahon Publishing Co.
83 Peaceable St.
West Redding, CT 06896   Phone: (203) 544-9506
First Published: 1973. **Frequency:** Bimonthly. **ISSN:** 0093-4437.

★127★   ANGIOLOGY
Westminster Publications, Inc.
1044 Northern Blvd.
Roslyn, NY 11576   Phone: (516) 484-6880
First Published: 1950. **Frequency:** Monthly. **ISSN:** 0003-3197.

★128★   ANGLE ORTHODONTIST
Angle Orthodontists Research and Education Foundation, Inc.
100 W. Lawrence St., Ste. 406
Appleton, WI 54911   Phone: (414) 738-6938
First Published: 1931. **Frequency:** Quarterly. **ISSN:** 0003-3219.

★129★   ANNALS OF ALLERGY
American College of Allergists
800 E. Northwest Hwy., Ste. 1080
Palatine, IL 60067   Phone: (708) 359-7367
First Published: 1943. **Frequency:** Monthly. **ISSN:** 0003-4738.

★130★   ANNALS OF BIOMEDICAL ENGINEERING
Pergamon Press, Inc.
Maxwell House, Fairview Park
Elmsford, NY 10523   Phone: (914) 592-7700
First Published: 1979. **Frequency:** Bimonthly. **ISSN:** 0090-6964.

★131★   ANNALS OF CLINICAL BIOCHEMISTRY
Royal Society of Medicine Services Ltd.
1 Wimpole St.
London W1M 8AE, England   Phone: (617) 225-0401
Frequency: Bimonthly. **ISSN:** 0004-5632.

★132★   ANNALS OF CLINICAL AND LABORATORY SCIENCE
Association of Clinical Scientists
Department of Laboratory Medicine
University of Connecticut School of Medicine
Farmington, CT 06032   Phone: (203) 679-2328
First Published: 1971. **Frequency:** Bimonthly. **ISSN:** 0091-7370.

★133★   ANNALS OF CLINICAL PSYCHIATRY
Elsevier Science Publishing Co., Inc.
655 Avenue of the Americas
New York, NY 10010   Phone: (617) 989-5800
Frequency: Quarterly. **ISSN:** 1040-1237.

★134★ ANNALS OF CLINICAL RESEARCH
Finnish Medical Society Duodecim
Kalevankatu 11A
00100 Helsinki, Finland
First Published: 1969. **Frequency:** Bimonthly. **ISSN:** 0003-4762.

★135★ ANNALS OF EMERGENCY MEDICINE
American College of Emergency Physicians
PO Box 619911
Dallas, TX 75261   Phone: (214) 550-0911
First Published: 1972. **Frequency:** Monthly. **ISSN:** 0196-0644.

★136★ ANNALS OF EPIDEMIOLOGY
Elsevier Science Publishing Co., Inc.
655 Avenue of the Americas
New York, NY 10010   Phone: (212) 989-5800
Frequency: Bimonthly. **ISSN:** 1047-2797.

★137★ ANNALS OF HUMAN BIOLOGY
Society for the Study of Human Biology
c/o Dr. V. Reynolds
Department of Biological Anthropology
58 Banbury Rd.
Oxford OX2 6QS, England
First Published: 1974. **Frequency:** Bimonthly. **ISSN:** 0301-4460.

★138★ ANNALS OF HUMAN GENETICS
Cambridge University Press
40 W. 20th St.
New York, NY 10011   Phone: (212) 924-3900
First Published: 1925. **Frequency:** Quarterly. **ISSN:** 0003-4800.

★139★ ANNALS OF INTERNAL MEDICINE
American College of Physicians
6th St. at Race
Philadelphia, PA 19106   Phone: (215) 351-2400
First Published: 1922. **Frequency:** Semimonthly. **ISSN:** 0003-4819.

★140★ ANNALS OF NEUROLOGY
American Neurological Association
2221 University Ave. SE, Ste. 350
Minneapolis, MN 55414   Phone: (612) 378-3290
First Published: 1977. **Frequency:** Monthly. **ISSN:** 0364-5134.

★141★ ANNALS OF THE NEW YORK ACADEMY OF SCIENCES
2 E. 63rd St.
New York, NY 10021   Phone: (212) 838-0230
First Published: 1877. **Frequency:** Irregular. **ISSN:** 0077-8923.

★142★ ANNALS OF NUTRITION AND METABOLISM
S. Karger Publishers, Inc.
26 W. Avon Rd.
PO Box 529
Farmington, CT 06085   Phone: (203) 675-7834
First Published: 1959. **Frequency:** Bimonthly. **ISSN:** 0250-6807.

★143★ ANNALS OF OCCUPATIONAL HYGIENE
Pergamon Press, Inc.
Maxwell House, Fairview Park
Elmsford, NY 10523   Phone: (914) 592-7700
First Published: 1958. **Frequency:** 6/yr. **ISSN:** 0003-4878.

★144★ ANNALS OF OPHTHALMOLOGY
American Society of Contemporary Ophthalmology
233 E. Erie St., Ste. 710
Chicago, IL 60611   Phone: (312) 951-1400
First Published: 1969. **Frequency:** Monthly. **ISSN:** 0003-4886.

★145★ ANNALS OF OTOLOGY, RHINOLOGY AND LARYNGOLOGY
Annals Publishing Co.
4507 Laclede Ave.
St. Louis, MO 63108   Phone: (314) 367-4987
First Published: 1892. **Frequency:** Monthly. **ISSN:** 0003-4894.

★146★ ANNALS OF PLASTIC SURGERY
Little, Brown and Co.
34 Beacon St.
Boston, MA 02108   Phone: (617) 227-0730
First Published: 1978. **Frequency:** Monthly. **ISSN:** 0148-7043.

★147★ ANNALS OF THE RHEUMATIC DISEASES
British Medical Association
Box 560B
Kennebunkport, ME 04046
First Published: 1939. **Frequency:** Monthly. **ISSN:** 0003-4967.

★148★ ANNALS OF THE ROYAL COLLEGE OF SURGEONS OF ENGLAND
35/43 Lincoln's Inn Fields
London WC2A 3PN, England
First Published: 1947. **Frequency:** Bimonthly. **ISSN:** 0035-8843.

★149★ ANNALS OF SURGERY
American Surgical Association
c/o George F. Sheldon, M.D.
University of North Carolina at Chapel Hill
136 Burnett-Womack, Box CB 7245
Chapel Hill, NC 27599   Phone: (919) 966-4320
First Published: 1885. **Frequency:** Monthly. **ISSN:** 0003-4932.

★150★ ANNALS OF THORACIC SURGERY
Society of Thoracic Surgeons
401 N. Michigan Ave.
Chicago, IL 60611   Phone: (312) 644-6610
First Published: 1965. **Frequency:** Monthly. **ISSN:** 0003-4975.

★151★ ANNALS OF TROPICAL MEDICINE AND PARASITOLOGY
Academic Press, Inc.
1250 6th Ave.
San Diego, CA 92101   Phone: (619) 231-0926
First Published: 1907. **Frequency:** Bimonthly. **ISSN:** 0003-4983.

★152★ ANNALS OF TROPICAL PAEDIATRICS
Academic Press, Inc.
1250 6th Ave.
San Diego, CA 92101   Phone: (619) 231-0926
First Published: 1981. **Frequency:** Quarterly. **ISSN:** 0272-4939.

★153★ ANNALS OF VASCULAR SURGERY
Blackwell Scientific Publications
3 Cambridge Center, Ste. 208
Cambridge, MA 02142   Phone: (617) 225-0401
Frequency: Bimonthly. **ISSN:** 0890-5096.

★154★ ANTI-CANCER DRUGS
Rapid Communications of Oxford Ltd.
The Old Malthouse
Paradise St.
Oxford OX1 1LD, England
First Published: 1990. **Frequency:** Bimonthly. **ISSN:** 0959-4973.

★155★ ANTICANCER RESEARCH
c/o John G. Delinassios
5 Argyropoulou St.
Kato Patissia
GR-111 45 Athens, Greece
First Published: 1981. **Frequency:** Bimonthly. **ISSN:** 0250-7005.

★156★ ANTIMICROBIAL AGENTS AND CHEMOTHERAPY
American Society for Microbiology
1325 Massachusetts Ave. NW
Washington, DC 20005   Phone: (202) 737-3600
First Published: 1972. **Frequency:** Monthly. **ISSN:** 0066-4804.

★157★ ANTIVIRAL CHEMISTRY AND CHEMOTHERAPY
Blackwell Scientific Publications
3 Cambridge Center, Ste. 208
Cambridge, MA 02142   Phone: (617) 225-0401
Frequency: Bimonthly. **ISSN:** 0956-3202.

★158★   **ANTIVIRAL RESEARCH**
Elsevier Science Publishing Co., Inc.
655 Avenue of the Americas
New York, NY 10010   Phone: (212) 989-5800
First Published: 1981. **Frequency:** 12/yr. **ISSN:** 0166-3542.

★159★   **AORN JOURNAL**
Association of Operating Room Nurses
10170 E. Mississippi Ave.
Denver, CO 80231   Phone: (303) 755-6300
First Published: 1963. **Frequency:** Monthly. **ISSN:** 0001-2092.

★160★   **APMIS**
Munksgaard
Noerre Soegade 35
DK-1370 Copenhagen K, Denmark
First Published: 1926. **Frequency:** Monthly. **ISSN:** 0903-4641.

★161★   **APPETITE**
Academic Press, Inc.
1250 6th Ave.
San Diego, CA 92101   Phone: (619) 231-0926
First Published: 1980. **Frequency:** Bimonthly. **ISSN:** 0195-6663.

★162★   **APPLIED BIOCHEMISTRY AND BIOTECHNOLOGY**
Humana Press, Inc.
PO Box 2148
Clifton, NJ 07015   Phone: (201) 773-4389
First Published: 1976. **Frequency:** 15/yr. **ISSN:** 0273-2289.

★163★   **APPLIED AND ENVIRONMENTAL MICROBIOLOGY**
American Society for Microbiology
1325 Massachusetts Ave., NW
Washington, DC 20005   Phone: (202) 737-3600
First Published: 1953. **Frequency:** Monthly. **ISSN:** 0099-2240.

★164★   **APPLIED MICROBIOLOGY AND BIOTECHNOLOGY**
Springer-Verlag New York, Inc.
175 5th Ave.
New York, NY 10010   Phone: (212) 460-1500
First Published: 1975. **Frequency:** 12/yr. **ISSN:** 0175-7598.

★165★   **APPLIED PATHOLOGY**
S. Karger Publishers, Inc.
26 W. Avon Rd.
PO Box 529
Farmington, CT 06085   Phone: (203) 675-7834
First Published: 1983. **Frequency:** Bimonthly. **ISSN:** 0252-1172.

★166★   **APPLIED AND PREVENTIVE PSYCHOLOGY**
Cambridge University Press
40 W. 20th St.
New York, NY 10011   Phone: (212) 924-3900
First Published: 1992. **Frequency:** Quarterly. **ISSN:** 0962-1849.

★167★   **APPLIED RADIOLOGY**
Romaine Pierson Publishers, Inc.
80 Shore Rd.
Port Washington, NY 11050   Phone: (516) 883-6350
First Published: 1972. **Frequency:** Monthly. **ISSN:** 0160-9963.

★168★   **ARC**
Association for Retarded Citizens
2501 Ave. J, Box 6109
Arlington, TX 76006   Phone: (817) 640-0204
First Published: 1952. **Frequency:** Bimonthly. **ISSN:** 0199-9435.

★169★   **ARCHIVES OF ANDROLOGY**
Hemisphere Publishing Corporation
1900 Frost Rd., Ste. 101
Bristol, PA 19007   Phone: (215) 785-5800
First Published: 1978. **Frequency:** Bimonthly. **ISSN:** 0148-5016.

★170★   **ARCHIVES OF BIOCHEMISTRY AND BIOPHYSICS**
Academic Press, Inc.
1250 6th Ave.
San Diego, CA 92101   Phone: (619) 231-0926
First Published: 1942. **Frequency:** 16/yr. **ISSN:** 0003-9861.

★171★   **ARCHIVES OF CLINICAL NEUROPSYCHOLOGY**
Pergamon Press, Inc.
Maxwell House, Fairview Park
Elmsford, NY 10523   Phone: (914) 592-7700
First Published: 1986. **Frequency:** Quarterly. **ISSN:** 0887-6177.

★172★   **ARCHIVES OF DERMATOLOGICAL RESEARCH**
Springer-Verlag New York, Inc.
175 5th Ave.
New York, NY 10010   Phone: (212) 460-1500
First Published: 1869. **Frequency:** 8/yr. **ISSN:** 0340-3696.

★173★   **ARCHIVES OF DERMATOLOGY**
American Medical Association
515 N. State St.
Chicago, IL 60610   Phone: (312) 464-5000
First Published: 1920. **Frequency:** Monthly. **ISSN:** 0003-987X.

★174★   **ARCHIVES OF DISEASES IN CHILDHOOD**
British Medical Association
PO Box 560B
Kennebunkport, ME 04046
First Published: 1926. **Frequency:** Monthly. **ISSN:** 0003-9888.

★175★   **ARCHIVES OF EMERGENCY MEDICINE**
Blackwell Scientific Publications
3 Cambridge St., Ste. 208
Cambridge, MA 02142   Phone: (617) 225-0401
Frequency: 4/yr. **ISSN:** 0264-4924.

★176★   **ARCHIVES OF ENVIRONMENTAL CONTAMINATION AND TOXICOLOGY**
Springer-Verlag New York, Inc.
175 5th Ave.
New York, NY 10010   Phone: (212) 460-1500
First Published: 1972. **Frequency:** Bimonthly. **ISSN:** 0090-4341.

★177★   **ARCHIVES OF ENVIRONMENTAL HEALTH**
Heldreff Publications
4000 Albermarle St., NW
Washington, DC 20016   Phone: (202) 362-6445
First Published: 1950. **Frequency:** Bimonthly. **ISSN:** 0003-9896.

★178★   **ARCHIVES OF GENERAL PSYCHIATRY**
American Medical Association
515 N. State St.
Chicago, IL 60610   Phone: (312) 464-5000
First Published: 1959. **Frequency:** Monthly. **ISSN:** 0003-990X.

★179★   **ARCHIVES OF GERONTOLOGY AND GERIATRICS**
Elsevier Science Publishing Co., Inc.
655 Avenue of the Americas
New York, NY 10010   Phone: (212) 989-5800
Frequency: 6/yr. **ISSN:** 0167-4943.

★180★   **ARCHIVES OF GYNECOLOGY AND OBSTETRICS**
Springer-Verlag New York, Inc.
175 5th Ave.
New York, NY 10010   Phone: (212) 460-1500
First Published: 1870. **Frequency:** 8/yr. **ISSN:** 0932-0067.

★181★   **ARCHIVES OF INTERNAL MEDICINE**
American Medical Association
515 N. State St.
Chicago, IL 60610   Phone: (312) 464-5000
First Published: 1908. **Frequency:** Monthly. **ISSN:** 0003-9926.

★182★   ARCHIVES OF MICROBIOLOGY
Springer-Verlag New York, Inc.
175 5th Ave.
New York, NY 10010   Phone: (212) 460-1500
First Published: 1939. **Frequency:** 12/yr. **ISSN:** 0302-8933.

★183★   ARCHIVES OF NEUROLOGY
American Medical Association
515 N. State St.
Chicago, IL 60610   Phone: (312) 464-5000
First Published: 1959. **Frequency:** Monthly. **ISSN:** 0003-9942.

★184★   ARCHIVES OF OPHTHALMOLOGY
American Medical Association
515 N. State St.
Chicago, IL 60610   Phone: (312) 464-5000
First Published: 1869. **Frequency:** Monthly. **ISSN:** 0003-9950.

★185★   ARCHIVES OF ORAL BIOLOGY
Pergamon Press, Inc.
Maxwell House, Fairview Park
Elmsford, NY 10523   Phone: (914) 592-7700
First Published: 1959. **Frequency:** Monthly. **ISSN:** 0003-9969.

★186★   ARCHIVES OF ORTHOPAEDIC AND TRAUMATIC
   SURGERY
Springer-Verlag New York, Inc.
175 5th Ave.
New York, NY 10010   Phone: (212) 460-1500
First Published: 1903. **Frequency:** Bimonthly. **ISSN:** 0344-8444.

★187★   ARCHIVES OF OTOLARYNGOLOGY-HEAD AND NECK
   SURGERY
American Medical Association
515 N. State St.
Chicago, IL 60610   Phone: (312) 464-5000
First Published: 1925. **Frequency:** Monthly. **ISSN:** 0886-4470.

★188★   ARCHIVES OF OTO-RHINO-LARYNGOLOGY
Springer-Verlag New York, Inc.
175 5th Ave.
New York, NY 10010   Phone: (212) 460-1500
First Published: 1864. **Frequency:** 6/yr. **ISSN:** 0302-9530.

★189★   ARCHIVES OF PATHOLOGY AND LABORATORY
   MEDICINE
American Medical Association
515 N. State St.
Chicago, IL 60610   Phone: (312) 464-5000
First Published: 1926. **Frequency:** Monthly. **ISSN:** 0003-9985.

★190★   ARCHIVES OF PHYSICAL MEDICINE AND
   REHABILITATION
American Congress of Rehabilitation Medicine
130 S. Michigan Ave., Ste. 1310
Chicago, IL 60603   Phone: (312) 922-9368
First Published: 1921. **Frequency:** Monthly. **ISSN:** 0003-9993.

★191★   ARCHIVES OF PSYCHIATRIC NURSING
W. B. Saunders Co.
Curtis Center
Independence Sq. W.
Philadelphia, PA 19106   Phone: (215) 238-7800
First Published: 1987. **Frequency:** Bimonthly. **ISSN:** 0883-9417.

★192★   ARCHIVES OF SEXUAL BEHAVIOR
Plenum Publishing Corp.
233 Spring St.
New York, NY 10013   Phone: (212) 620-8000
First Published: 1971. **Frequency:** 6/yr. **ISSN:** 0004-0002.

★193★   ARCHIVES OF SURGERY
American Medical Association
515 N. State St.
Chicago, IL 60610   Phone: (312) 464-5000
First Published: 1920. **Frequency:** Monthly. **ISSN:** 0004-0010.

★194★   ARCHIVES OF TOXICOLOGY
Springer-Verlag New York, Inc.
175 5th Ave.
New York, NY 10010   Phone: (212) 460-1500
First Published: 1930. **Frequency:** 8/yr. **ISSN:** 0340-5761.

★195★   ARCHIVES OF VIROLOGY
Springer-Verlag New York, Inc.
175 5th Ave.
New York, NY 10010   Phone: (212) 460-1500
First Published: 1939. **Frequency:** 24/yr. **ISSN:** 0304-8608.

★196★   ARTERIOSCLEROSIS AND THROMBOSIS
American Heart Association
7320 Greenville Ave.
Dallas, TX 75231   Phone: (214) 706-1310
First Published: 1981. **Frequency:** Bimonthly. **ISSN:** 1049-8834.

★197★   ARTHRITIS CARE AND RESEARCH
Elsevier Science Publishing Co., Inc.
655 Avenue of the Americas
New York, NY 10010   Phone: (212) 989-5800
Frequency: Quarterly. **ISSN:** 0893-7524.

★198★   ARTHRITIS AND RHEUMATISM
American College of Rheumatology
17 Executive Park Dr. NE, Ste. 480
Atlanta, GA 30329   Phone: (404) 633-3777
First Published: 1958. **Frequency:** Monthly. **ISSN:** 0004-3591.

★199★   ARTHROSCOPY
Raven Press
1185 Avenue of the Americas
New York, NY 10036   Phone: (212) 930-9500
First Published: 1985. **Frequency:** Quarterly. **ISSN:** 0749-8063.

★200★   ARTIFICIAL ORGANS
International Society for Artificial Organs
8937 Euclid Ave.
Cleveland, OH 44106   Phone: (216) 421-0757
First Published: 1977. **Frequency:** Bimonthly. **ISSN:** 0160-564X.

★201★   ASDC JOURNAL OF DENTISTRY FOR CHILDREN
American Society of Dentistry for Children
211 E. Chicago Ave., Ste. 1430
Chicago, IL 60611   Phone: (312) 943-1244
First Published: 1933. **Frequency:** Bimonthly. **ISSN:** 0022-0353.

★202★   ASHA
American Speech-Language-Hearing Association
10801 Rockville Pike
Rockville, MD 20852   Phone: (301) 897-5700
First Published: 1959. **Frequency:** Monthly. **ISSN:** 0001-2475.

★203★   ASTHMA MANAGEMENT
Mary Ann Liebert, Inc.
1651 3rd Ave.
New York, NY 10128   Phone: (212) 289-2300
Frequency: Bimonthly. **ISSN:** 1050-5253.

★204★   ATHEROSCLEROSIS
Elsevier Science Publishing Co., Inc.
655 Avenue of the Americas
New York, NY 10010   Phone: (212) 989-5800
First Published: 1961. **Frequency:** 18/yr. **ISSN:** 0021-9150.

★205★   AUDECIBEL
National Hearing Aid Society
20361 Middlebelt Rd.
Livonia, MI 48152   Phone: (313) 478-2610
First Published: 1951. **Frequency:** Quarterly. **ISSN:** 0004-7473.

★206★   AUDIOLOGY
S. Karger Publishers, Inc.
26 W. Avon Rd.
PO Box 529
Farmington, CT 06085   Phone: (203) 675-7834
First Published: 1962. **Frequency:** Bimonthly. **ISSN:** 0020-6091.

★207★   AUSTRALASIAN JOURNAL OF DERMATOLOGY
Australasian College of Dermatologists
271 Bridge Rd.
Glebe, NSW 2037, Australia
First Published: 1951. **Frequency:** 3/yr. **ISSN:** 0004-8380.

★208★   AUSTRALASIAN RADIOLOGY
Royal Australasian College of Radiologists
37 Lower Fort St.
Millers Point, NSW 2000, Australia
First Published: 1957. **Frequency:** 4/yr. **ISSN:** 0004-8461.

★209★   AUSTRALIAN DENTAL JOURNAL
Australian Dental Association, Inc.
116 Pacific Hwy.
Box 441
North Sidney, NSW 2060, Australia
First Published: 1956. **Frequency:** Bimonthly. **ISSN:** 0045-0421.

★210★   AUSTRALIAN FAMILY PHYSICIAN
Royal Australian College of General Practitioners
70 Jolimont St., 4th Fl.
Jolimont, Victoria 3002, Australia
First Published: 1956. **Frequency:** Monthly. **ISSN:** 0300-8495.

★211★   AUSTRALIAN AND NEW ZEALAND JOURNAL OF MEDICINE
Royal Australasian College of Physicians
145 Macquarie St.
Sydney, NSW 2000, Australia
First Published: 1952. **Frequency:** Bimonthly. **ISSN:** 0004-8291.

★212★   AUSTRALIAN AND NEW ZEALAND JOURNAL OF OBSTETRICS AND GYNECOLOGY
Royal Australian College of Obstetricians and Gynecologists
254 Albert St.
Melbourne, Victoria 3002, Australia
First Published: 1961. **Frequency:** Quarterly. **ISSN:** 0004-8666.

★213★   AUSTRALIAN AND NEW ZEALAND JOURNAL OF PSYCHIATRY
Royal Australian and New Zealand College of Psychiatrists
PO Box 1239
Fremantle, Western Australia 6160, Australia
First Published: 1967. **Frequency:** Quarterly. **ISSN:** 0004-8674.

★214★   AUSTRALIAN AND NEW ZEALAND JOURNAL OF SURGERY
Blackwell Scientific Publications
3 Cambridge Center, Ste. 208
Cambridge, MA 02142   Phone: (617) 225-0401
First Published: 1931. **Frequency:** Monthly. **ISSN:** 0004-8682.

★215★   AVIAN DISEASES
American Association of Avian Pathologists
New Bolton Center
University of Pennsylvania
Kennett Square, PA 19348   Phone: (215) 444-5800
First Published: 1957. **Frequency:** Quarterly. **ISSN:** 0005-2086.

★216★   AVIATION, SPACE AND ENVIRONMENTAL MEDICINE
Aerospace Medical Association
320 S. Henry St.
Alexandria, VA 22314   Phone: (703) 739-2240
First Published: 1930. **Frequency:** Monthly. **ISSN:** 0095-6562.

★217★   BANGLADESH MEDICAL RESEARCH COUNCIL BULLETIN
Bangladesh Medical Research Council
Mahakali 12, Bangladesh
First Published: 1976. **Frequency:** Semiannual. **ISSN:** 0377-9238.

★218★   BASIC LIFE SCIENCES
Plenum Publishing Corp.
233 Spring St.
New York, NY 10013   Phone: (212) 620-8000
First Published: 1973. **Frequency:** Irregular. **ISSN:** 0090-5542.

★219★   BASIC RESEARCH IN CARDIOLOGY
Springer-Verlag New York, Inc.
175 5th Ave.
New York, NY 10010   Phone: (212) 460-1500
First Published: 1938. **Frequency:** Bimonthly. **ISSN:** 0300-8428.

★220★   BEHAVIOR GENETICS
Plenum Publishing Corp.
233 Spring St.
New York, NY 10013   Phone: (212) 620-8000
First Published: 1970. **Frequency:** Bimonthly. **ISSN:** 0001-8244.

★221★   BEHAVIORAL BRAIN RESEARCH
Elsevier Science Publishing Co., Inc.
655 Ave. of the Americas
New York, NY 10010   Phone: (212) 989-5800
First Published: 1980. **Frequency:** 18/yr. **ISSN:** 0166-4328.

★222★   BEHAVIORAL AND BRAIN SCIENCES
Cambridge University Press
40 W. 20th St.
New York, NY 10011   Phone: (212) 924-3900
Frequency: Quarterly. **ISSN:** 0140-525X.

★223★   BEHAVIORAL MEDICINE
Heldref Publications, Inc.
4000 Albemarle St. NW
Washington, DC 20016   Phone: (202) 362-6445
First Published: 1975. **Frequency:** Quarterly. **ISSN:** 0896-4289.

★224★   BEHAVIORAL AND NEURAL BIOLOGY
Academic Press, Inc.
1250 6th Ave.
San Diego, CA 92101   Phone: (619) 231-0926
First Published: 1968. **Frequency:** Bimonthly. **ISSN:** 0163-1047.

★225★   BEHAVIORAL NEUROSCIENCE
American Psychological Association
1200 17th St. NW
Washington, DC 20036   Phone: (202) 955-7600
First Published: 1983. **Frequency:** Bimonthly. **ISSN:** 0735-7044.

★226★   BINARY: COMPUTING IN MICROBIOLOGY
Academic Press, Inc.
1250 6th Ave.
San Diego, CA 92101   Phone: (619) 231-0926
First Published: 1989. **Frequency:** 6/yr. **ISSN:** 0266-304X.

★227★   BIOCHEMICAL AND BIOPHYSICAL RESEARCH COMMUNICATIONS
Academic Press, Inc.
1250 6th Ave.
San Diego, CA 92101   Phone: (619) 231-0926
First Published: 1959. **Frequency:** 24/yr. **ISSN:** 0006-291X.

★228★   BIOCHEMICAL GENETICS
Plenum Publishing Corp.
233 Spring St.
New York, NY 10013   Phone: (212) 620-8000
First Published: 1967. **Frequency:** Monthly. **ISSN:** 0006-2928.

★229★ BIOCHEMICAL JOURNAL
Biochemical Society
Box 32
Commerce Way, Colchester
Essex CO2 8HP, England
First Published: 1906. Frequency: Semimonthly. ISSN: 0264-6021.

★230★ BIOCHEMICAL MEDICINE AND METABOLIC
BIOLOGY
Academic Press, Inc.
1250 6th Ave.
San Diego, CA 92101   Phone: (619) 231-0926
First Published: 1967. Frequency: Bimonthly. ISSN: 0885-4505.

★231★ BIOCHEMICAL PHARMACOLOGY
Pergamon Press, Inc.
Maxwell House, Fairview Park
Elmsford, NY 10523   Phone: (914) 592-7700
First Published: 1958. Frequency: 24/yr. ISSN: 0006-2952.

★232★ BIOCHEMISTRY
American Chemical Society
1155 16th St. NW
Washington, DC 20036   Phone: (202) 872-4600
First Published: 1964. Frequency: Weekly. ISSN: 0006-2960.

★233★ BIOCHEMISTRY AND CELL BIOLOGY
The National Research Council of Canada
Montreal Rd. Laboratories
Ottawa, ON, Canada K1A 0R6   Phone: (613) 993-0362
First Published: 1929. Frequency: Monthly. ISSN: 0829-8211.

★234★ BIOCHIMICA ET BIOPHYSICA ACTA
Elsevier Science Publishing Co., Inc.
655 Avenue of the Americas
New York, NY 10010   Phone: (212) 989-5800
First Published: 1947. Frequency: 117/yr. ISSN: 0006-3002.

★235★ BIOELECTROMAGNETICS
Bioelectromagnetics Society
120 W. Church St., Ste. 4
Frederick, MD 21701   Phone: (301) 663-4252
First Published: 1980. Frequency: Quarterly. ISSN: 0197-8462.

★236★ BIOFEEDBACK AND SELF REGULATION
Plenum Publishing Corp.
233 Spring St.
New York, NY 10013   Phone: (212) 620-8000
First Published: 1975. Frequency: Quarterly. ISSN: 0363-3586.

★237★ BIOLOGICAL CONTROL
Academic Press, Inc.
1250 6th Ave.
San Diego, CA 92101   Phone: (619) 231-0926
First Published: 1991. Frequency: Quarterly. ISSN: 1049-9644.

★238★ BIOLOGICAL PSYCHIATRY
Society of Biological Psychiatry
2010 Wilshire Blvd., Ste. 607
Los Angeles, CA 90057   Phone: (213) 483-7863
First Published: 1969. Frequency: 16/yr. ISSN: 0006-3223.

★239★ BIOLOGICAL PSYCHOLOGY
Elsevier Science Publishing Co., Inc.
655 Avenue of the Americas
New York, NY 10010   Phone: (212) 989-5800
First Published: 1972. Frequency: 6/yr. ISSN: 0301-0511.

★240★ BIOLOGICAL SIGNALS
S. Karger Publishers, Inc.
26 W. Avon Rd.
PO Box 529
Farmington, CT 06085   Phone: (203) 675-7834
First Published: 1992. Frequency: Bimonthly. ISSN: 1016-0922.

★241★ BIOLOGICALS
Academic Press, Inc.
1250 6th Ave.
San Diego, CA 92101   Phone: (619) 231-0926
First Published: 1973. Frequency: Quarterly. ISSN: 0092-1157.

★242★ BIOLOGY OF THE NEONATE
S. Karger Publishers, Inc.
26 W. Avon Rd.
PO Box 529
Farmington, CT 06085   Phone: (203) 675-7834
First Published: 1959. Frequency: Monthly. ISSN: 0006-3126.

★243★ BIOLOGY OF REPRODUCTION
Society for the Study of Reproduction
309 W. Clark St.
Champaign, IL 61820   Phone: (217) 356-3182
First Published: 1969. Frequency: 13/yr. ISSN: 0006-3363.

★244★ BIOMATERIALS
Butterworth-Heinemann
80 Montvale Ave.
Stoneham, MA 02180   Phone: (617) 438-8464
Frequency: 9/yr. ISSN: 0142-9612.

★245★ BIOMATERIALS, ARTIFICIAL CELLS AND ARTIFICIAL
ORGANS
Marcel Dekker, Inc.
270 Madison Ave.
New York, NY 10016   Phone: (212) 696-9000
First Published: 1973. Frequency: 4/yr. ISSN: 0890-5533.

★246★ BIOMEDICAL AND ENVIRONMENTAL SCIENCES
Academic Press, Inc.
1250 6th Ave.
San Diego, CA 92101   Phone: (619) 231-0926
First Published: 1988. Frequency: Quarterly. ISSN: 0895-3988.

★247★ BIOMEDICAL INSTRUMENTATION AND
TECHNOLOGY
Association for the Advancement of Medical Instrumentation
3330 Washington Blvd., Ste. 400
Arlington, VA 22201   Phone: (703) 525-4890
First Published: 1967. Frequency: Bimonthly. ISSN: 0899-8205.

★248★ BIOMEDICAL MATERIALS AND ENGINEERING
Pergamon Press, Inc.
395 Saw Mill River Rd.
Elmsford, NY 10523   Phone: (914) 592-7700
Frequency: Quarterly. ISSN: 0959-2989.

★249★ BIOMEDICAL SCIENCES INSTRUMENTATION
Instrument Society of America
67 Alexander Dr.
PO Box 12277
Research Triangle Park, NC 27709   Phone: (919) 549-8411
First Published: 1963. Frequency: Annual. ISSN: 0067-8856.

★250★ BIOMEMBRANES
Plenum Publishing Corp.
233 Spring St.
New York, NY 10013   Phone: (212) 620-8000
First Published: 1971. Frequency: Irregular. ISSN: 0067-8864.

★251★ BIOMETRICS
Biometric Society
1429 Duke St., Ste. 401
Alexandria, VA 22314   Phone: (703) 836-8311
First Published: 1945. Frequency: Quarterly. ISSN: 0006-341X.

★252★ BIOORGANIC AND MEDICINAL CHEMISTRY
LETTERS
Pergamon Press, Inc.
395 Saw Mill River Rd.
Elmsford, NY 10523   Phone: (914) 592-7700
Frequency: Monthly. ISSN: 0960-894X.

★253★   BIOPHYSICAL CHEMISTRY
Elsevier Science Publishing Co., Inc.
655 Avenue of the Americas
New York, NY 10010   Phone: (212) 989-5800
First Published: 1974. **Frequency:** 9/yr. **ISSN:** 0301-4622.

★254★   BIOPHYSICAL JOURNAL
Biophysical Society
c/o Emily M. Gray
9650 Rockville Pike
Bethesda, MD 20814   Phone: (301) 530-7114
First Published: 1960. **Frequency:** Monthly. **ISSN:** 0006-3495.

★255★   BIORHEOLOGY
Pergamon Press, Inc.
Maxwell House, Fairview Park
Elmsford, NY 10523   Phone: (914) 592-7700
First Published: 1962. **Frequency:** Bimonthly. **ISSN:** 0006-355X.

★256★   BIOSCIENCE REPORTS
Plenum Publishing Corp.
233 Spring St.
New York, NY 10013   Phone: (212) 620-8000
First Published: 1981. **Frequency:** Bimonthly. **ISSN:** 0144-8463.

★257★   BIOTECHNOLOGY AND APPLIED BIOCHEMISTRY
Academic Press, Inc.
1250 6th Ave.
San Diego, CA 92101   Phone: (619) 231-0926
First Published: 1979. **Frequency:** Bimonthly. **ISSN:** 0885-4513.

★258★   BIRTH
Blackwell Scientific Publications
3 Cambridge Center, Ste. 208
Cambridge, MA 02142   Phone: (617) 225-0401
First Published: 1973. **Frequency:** 4/yr. **ISSN:** 0730-7659.

★259★   BIRTH DEFECTS ORIGINAL ARTICLE SERIES
March of Dimes Birth Defects Foundation
1275 Mamaroneck Ave.
White Plains, NY 10605   Phone: (914) 428-7100
Frequency: Irregular. **ISSN:** 0547-6844.

★260★   BLOOD
American Society of Hematology
c/o Slack, Inc.
6900 Grove Rd.
Thorofare, NJ 08086   Phone: (609) 845-0003
First Published: 1946. **Frequency:** Monthly. **ISSN:** 0006-4971.

★261★   BLOOD CELLS
Springer-Verlag New York, Inc.
175 5th Ave.
New York, NY 10010   Phone: (212) 460-1500
First Published: 1975. **Frequency:** 3/yr. **ISSN:** 0340-4684.

★262★   BLOOD COAGULATION AND FIBRINOLYSIS
Rapid Communications of Oxford Ltd.
The Old Malthouse
Paradise St.
Oxford OX1 1LD, England
First Published: 1990. **Frequency:** Bimonthly. **ISSN:** 0957-5235.

★263★   BLOOD PURIFICATION
S. Karger Publishers, Inc.
26 W. Avon Rd.
PO Box 529
Farmington, CT 06085   Phone: (203) 675-7834
Frequency: 6/yr. **ISSN:** 0253-5068.

★264★   BLOOD REVIEWS
Churchill Livingstone, Inc.
1560 Broadway
New York, NY 10036   Phone: (212) 819-5400
First Published: 1987. **Frequency:** Quarterly. **ISSN:** 0268-960X.

★265★   BLOOD VESSELS
S. Karger Publishers, Inc.
26 W. Avon Rd.
PO Box 529
Farmington, CT 06085   Phone: (203) 675-7834
First Published: 1964. **Frequency:** Bimonthly. **ISSN:** 0303-6847.

★266★   BLUT
Springer-Verlag New York, Inc.
175 5th Ave.
New York, NY 10010   Phone: (212) 460-1500
First Published: 1950. **Frequency:** 12/yr. **ISSN:** 0006-5242.

★267★   BONE
Pergamon Press, Inc.
Maxwell House, Fairview Park
Elmsford, NY 10523   Phone: (914) 592-7700
First Published: 1979. **Frequency:** Bimonthly. **ISSN:** 8756-3282.

★268★   BONE AND MINERAL
Elsevier Science Publishing Co., Inc.
655 Ave. of the Americas
New York, NY 10010   Phone: (212) 989-5800
First Published: 1986. **Frequency:** Bimonthly. **ISSN:** 0169-6009.

★269★   BRAIN
Oxford University Press
Walton St.
Oxford OX2 6DP, England
First Published: 1878. **Frequency:** 6/yr. **ISSN:** 0006-8950.

★270★   BRAIN, BEHAVIOR AND EVOLUTION
S. Karger Publishers, Inc.
26 W. Avon Rd.
PO Box 529
Farmington, CT 06085   Phone: (203) 675-7834
First Published: 1968. **Frequency:** Bimonthly. **ISSN:** 0006-8977.

★271★   BRAIN, BEHAVIOR, AND IMMUNITY
Academic Press, Inc.
1250 6th Ave.
San Diego, CA 92101   Phone: (619) 231-0926
First Published: 1986. **Frequency:** Quarterly. **ISSN:** 0889-1591.

★272★   BRAIN AND COGNITION
Academic Press, Inc.
1250 6th Ave.
San Diego, CA 92101   Phone: (619) 231-0926
First Published: 1982. **Frequency:** Bimonthly. **ISSN:** 0278-2626.

★273★   BRAIN DYSFUNCTION
S. Karger Publishers, Inc.
26 W. Avon Rd.
PO Box 529
Farmington, CT 06085   Phone: (203) 675-7834
First Published: 1988. **Frequency:** 6/yr. **ISSN:** 0259-1278.

★274★   BRAIN AND LANGUAGE
Academic Press, Inc.
1250 6th Ave.
San Diego, CA 92101   Phone: (619) 231-0926
First Published: 1974. **Frequency:** Bimonthly. **ISSN:** 0093-934X.

★275★   BRAIN RESEARCH
Elsevier Science Publishing Co., Inc.
655 Avenue of the Americas
New York, NY 10010   Phone: (212) 989-5800
First Published: 1966. **Frequency:** 87/yr. **ISSN:** 0006-8993.

★276★   BRAIN RESEARCH BULLETIN
Pergamon Press, Inc.
Maxwell House, Fairview Park
Elmsford, NY 10523   Phone: (914) 592-7700
First Published: 1976. **Frequency:** Monthly. **ISSN:** 0361-9230.

★277★ BRAIN TOPOGRAPHY
Human Sciences Press, Inc.
233 Spring St.
New York, NY 10013   Phone: (212) 620-8000
Frequency: Quarterly.

★278★ BREAST CANCER RESEARCH AND TREATMENT
Kluwer Academic Publishing Group
Distribution Center
Box 322
3300 AH Dordrecht, Netherlands
First Published: 1981. Frequency: Quarterly. ISSN: 0167-6806.

★279★ BREAST DISEASE
Elsevier Science Publishing Co., Inc.
655 Avenue of the Americas
New York, NY 10010   Phone: (212) 989-5800
Frequency: Quarterly. ISSN: 0888-6008.

★280★ BRITISH DENTAL JOURNAL
British Dental Association
64 Wimpole St.
London W1M 8AL, England
First Published: 1880. Frequency: Semimonthly. ISSN: 0007-0610.

★281★ BRITISH HEART JOURNAL
British Medical Association
PO Box 560B
Kennebunkport, ME 04046
First Published: 1939. Frequency: Monthly. ISSN: 0007-0769.

★282★ BRITISH JOURNAL OF ADDICTION
Society for the Study of Addiction to Alcohol and other Drugs
c/o Prof. M. Lader
Inst. of Psychiatry
Decrespigny Park
London SE5 8AF, England
First Published: 1903. Frequency: 12/yr. ISSN: 0952-0481.

★283★ BRITISH JOURNAL OF ANAESTHESIA
British Medical Association
PO Box 560B
Kennebunkport, ME 04046
First Published: 1923. Frequency: Monthly. ISSN: 0007-0912.

★284★ BRITISH JOURNAL OF AUDIOLOGY
Academic Press, Inc.
1250 6th Ave.
San Diego, CA 92101   Phone: (619) 231-0926
First Published: 1967. Frequency: 6/yr. ISSN: 0300-5364.

★285★ BRITISH JOURNAL OF CANCER
Macmillan Press, Ltd.
Houndmills
Basingstoke, Hants. RG21 2XS, England
First Published: 1947. Frequency: Monthly. ISSN: 0007-0920.

★286★ BRITISH JOURNAL OF CLINICAL PHARMACOLOGY
Blackwell Scientific Publications
3 Cambridge Center, Ste. 208
Cambridge, MA 02142   Phone: (617) 225-0401
First Published: 1974. Frequency: Monthly. ISSN: 0306-5251.

★287★ BRITISH JOURNAL OF CLINICAL PRACTICE
Medical Tribune, Ltd.
Tower House
Southampton St.
London WC2E 7LS, England
First Published: 1947. Frequency: Monthly. ISSN: 0007-0947.

★288★ BRITISH JOURNAL OF CLINICAL PSYCHOLOGY
British Psychological Society
St. Andrews House
48 Princess Rd., E.
Leicester LE1 7DR, England
First Published: 1981. Frequency: Quarterly. ISSN: 0144-6657.

★289★ BRITISH JOURNAL OF DERMATOLOGY
Blackwell Scientific Publications
3 Cambridge Center, Ste. 208
Cambridge, MA 02142   Phone: (617) 225-0401
First Published: 1886. Frequency: Monthly. ISSN: 0007-0963.

★290★ BRITISH JOURNAL OF DISORDERS OF
COMMUNICATION
Cole and Whurr Ltd.
19B Compton Terr.
London N1 2UN, England
First Published: 1966. Frequency: 3/yr. ISSN: 0007-098X.

★291★ BRITISH JOURNAL OF EXPERIMENTAL PATHOLOGY
Blackwell Scientific Publications
3 Cambridge Center, Ste. 208
Cambridge, MA 02142   Phone: (617) 225-0401
First Published: 1920. Frequency: Bimonthly. ISSN: 0007-1021.

★292★ BRITISH JOURNAL OF GENERAL PRACTICE
Royal College of General Practitioners
12 Queen St.
Edinburg EH2 HE, Scotland
First Published: 1958. Frequency: Monthly. ISSN: 0960-1643.

★293★ BRITISH JOURNAL OF HAEMATOLOGY
Blackwell Scientific Publications
3 Cambridge Center, Ste. 208
Cambridge, MA 02142   Phone: (617) 225-0401
First Published: 1955. Frequency: Monthly. ISSN: 0007-1048.

★294★ BRITISH JOURNAL OF HOSPITAL MEDICINE
Mark Allen Publishing, Ltd.
288 Croxted Rd.
London 2E24 9DA, England
First Published: 1966. Frequency: Monthly. ISSN: 0007-1064.

★295★ BRITISH JOURNAL OF INDUSTRIAL MEDICINE
British Medical Association
PO Box 560B
Kennebunkport, ME 04046
First Published: 1944. Frequency: Monthly. ISSN: 0007-1072.

★296★ BRITISH JOURNAL OF MEDICAL PSYCHOLOGY
British Psychological Society
St. Andrews House
48 Princes Rd., E.
Leicester LE1 7DR, England
First Published: 1920. Frequency: Quarterly. ISSN: 0007-1129.

★297★ BRITISH JOURNAL OF NUTRITION
Cambridge University Press
40 W. 20th St.
New York, NY 10011   Phone: (212) 924-3900
First Published: 1947. Frequency: Bimonthly. ISSN: 0007-1145.

★298★ BRITISH JOURNAL OF OBSTETRICS AND
GYNAECOLOGY
Blackwell Scientific Publications
3 Cambridge Center, Ste. 208
Cambridge, MA 02142   Phone: (617) 225-0401
First Published: 1902. Frequency: Monthly. ISSN: 0306-5456.

★299★ BRITISH JOURNAL OF OPHTHALMOLOGY
British Medical Association
PO Box 560B
Kennebunkport, ME 04046
First Published: 1917. Frequency: Monthly. ISSN: 0007-1161.

★300★ BRITISH JOURNAL OF ORAL AND MAXILLOFACIAL
SURGERY
Churchill Livingstone, Inc.
1560 Broadway
New York, NY 10036   Phone: (212) 819-5400
First Published: 1963. Frequency: Bimonthly. ISSN: 0266-4356.

★301★　BRITISH JOURNAL OF ORTHODONTICS
Churchill Livingstone, Inc.
1560 Broadway
New York, NY 10036　　　　　Phone: (212) 819-5400
First Published: 1974. **Frequency:** Quarterly. **ISSN:** 0301-228X.

★302★　BRITISH JOURNAL OF PHARMACOLOGY
Macmillan Press, Ltd.
Houndmills
Basingstoke, Hants. RG21 2XS, England
First Published: 1946. **Frequency:** Monthly. **ISSN:** 0007-1188.

★303★　BRITISH JOURNAL OF PLASTIC SURGERY
Churchill Livingstone, Inc.
1560 Broadway
New York, NY 10036　　　　　Phone: (212) 819-5400
First Published: 1948. **Frequency:** 6/yr. **ISSN:** 0007-1226.

★304★　BRITISH JOURNAL OF PSYCHIATRY
Royal College of Psychiatrists
17 Belgrave Sq.
London SW1X 8PG, England
First Published: 1853. **Frequency:** Monthly. **ISSN:** 0007-1250.

★305★　BRITISH JOURNAL OF PSYCHOLOGY
British Psychological Society
St. Andrews House
48 Princess Rd., E.
Leicester LE1 7DR, England
First Published: 1904. **Frequency:** Quarterly. **ISSN:** 0007-1269.

★306★　BRITISH JOURNAL OF RADIOLOGY
British Institute of Radiology
36 Portland Pl.
London W1N 4AT, England
First Published: 1896. **Frequency:** Monthly. **ISSN:** 0007-1285.

★307★　BRITISH JOURNAL OF RHEUMATOLOGY
Bailliere Tindall
24-28 Oval Rd.
London NW1 7DX, England
First Published: 1952. **Frequency:** Bimonthly. **ISSN:** 0263-7103.

★308★　BRITISH JOURNAL OF SPORTS MEDICINE
British Assn. of Sport and Medicine
c/o Dr. Wendy Dodds
66 W. Scholes
Queensbury, West Yorks. BD13 1NH, England
First Published: 1968. **Frequency:** Quarterly. **ISSN:** 0306-3674.

★309★　BRITISH JOURNAL OF SURGERY
Butterworth-Heinemann
80 Montvale Ave.
Stoneham, MA 02180　　　　　Phone: (617) 438-8464
First Published: 1913. **Frequency:** Monthly. **ISSN:** 0007-1323.

★310★　BRITISH JOURNAL OF UROLOGY
Churchill Livingstone, Inc.
1560 Broadway
New York, NY 10036　　　　　Phone: (212) 819-5400
First Published: 1929. **Frequency:** 12/yr. **ISSN:** 0007-1331.

★311★　BRITISH MEDICAL BULLETIN
Churchill Livingstone, Inc.
1560 Broadway
New York, NY 10036　　　　　Phone: (212) 819-5400
First Published: 1943. **Frequency:** Quarterly. **ISSN:** 0007-1420.

★312★　BRITISH MEDICAL JOURNAL
British Medical Association
PO Box 560B
Kennebunkport, ME 04046
First Published: 1832. **Frequency:** Weekly. **ISSN:** 0007-1447.

★313★　BRITISH VETERINARY JOURNAL
Bailliere Tindall
24-28 Oval Rd.
London NW1 7DX, England
First Published: 1875. **Frequency:** Bimonthly. **ISSN:** 0007-1935.

★314★　BULLETIN OF THE AMERICAN ACADEMY OF PSYCHIATRY AND THE LAW
1211 Cathedral St.
Baltimore, MD 21202　　　　　Phone: (301) 539-0379
First Published: 1973. **Frequency:** Quarterly. **ISSN:** 0091-634X.

★315★　BULLETIN OF THE AMERICAN COLLEGE OF SURGEONS
55 E. Erie St.
Chicago, IL 60611　　　　　Phone: (312) 664-4050
First Published: 1916. **Frequency:** Monthly. **ISSN:** 0002-8045.

★316★　BULLETIN OF ENVIRONMENTAL CONTAMINATION AND TOXICOLOGY
Springer-Verlag New York, Inc.
175 5th Ave.
New York, NY 10010　　　　　Phone: (212) 460-1500
First Published: 1966. **Frequency:** Monthly. **ISSN:** 0007-4861.

★317★　BULLETIN OF THE HISTORY OF MEDICINE
American Association for the History of Medicine
Boston University School of Medicine
80 E. Concord St.
Boston, MA 02118　　　　　Phone: (617) 638-4328
First Published: 1933. **Frequency:** Quarterly. **ISSN:** 0007-5140.

★318★　BULLETIN OF THE HOSPITAL FOR JOINT DISEASES ORTHOPAEDIC INSTITUTE
380 2nd Ave., 6th Fl.
New York, NY 10010　　　　　Phone: (212) 460-0121
First Published: 1940. **Frequency:** Semiannual. **ISSN:** 0018-5647.

★319★　BULLETIN OF THE MEDICAL LIBRARY ASSOCIATION
6 N. Michigan Ave., Ste. 300
Chicago, IL 60602　　　　　Phone: (312) 419-9094
First Published: 1911. **Frequency:** Quarterly. **ISSN:** 0025-7338.

★320★　BULLETIN OF THE MENNINGER CLINIC
Menninger Foundation
PO Box 829
Topeka, KS 66601　　　　　Phone: (913) 273-7500
First Published: 1936. **Frequency:** Bimonthly. **ISSN:** 0025-9284.

★321★　BULLETIN ON NARCOTICS
United Nations Publications
Rm. DC2-853
New York, NY 10017　　　　　Phone: (212) 754-8324
First Published: 1949. **Frequency:** Quarterly. **ISSN:** 0007-523X.

★322★　BULLETIN OF THE NEW YORK ACADEMY OF MEDICINE
2 E. 103rd St.
New York, NY 10029　　　　　Phone: (212) 876-8200
First Published: 1925. **Frequency:** 10/yr. **ISSN:** 0028-7091.

★323★　BULLETIN OF THE PAN AMERICAN HEALTH ORGANIZATION
525 23rd St. NW
Washington, DC 20037　　　　　Phone: (202) 861-3200
First Published: 1967. **Frequency:** Quarterly. **ISSN:** 0301-5750.

★324★　BULLETIN ON THE RHEUMATIC DISEASES
Arthritis Foundation
1314 Spring St. NW
Atlanta, GA 30309　　　　　Phone: (404) 872-7100
First Published: 1950. **Frequency:** Bimonthly. **ISSN:** 0007-5248.

★325★ BULLETIN OF THE WORLD HEALTH
ORGANIZATION
20 Ave. Appia
CH-1211 Geneva 27, Switzerland
First Published: 1947. Frequency: 6/yr. ISSN: 0043-9686.

★326★ BURNS, INCLUDING THERMAL INJURY
International Society for Burn Injuries
c/o John A. Boswick, Jr., M.D.
2005 Franklin St., Ste. 660
Denver, CO 80205   Phone: (303) 839-1694
First Published: 1974. Frequency: Bimonthly. ISSN: 0305-4179.

★327★ CA: A CANCER JOURNAL FOR CLINICIANS
American Cancer Society, Inc.
1599 Clifton Rd. NE
Atlanta, GA 30329   Phone: (404) 320-3333
First Published: 1950. Frequency: Bimonthly. ISSN: 0007-9235.

★328★ CALCIFIED TISSUE INTERNATIONAL
Springer-Verlag New York, Inc.
175 5th Ave.
New York, NY 10010   Phone: (212) 460-1500
First Published: 1967. Frequency: 12/yr. ISSN: 0171-767X.

★329★ CALIFORNIA FP
California Academy of Family Physicians
605 Market St.
San Francisco, CA 94105   Phone: (415) 541-0762
First Published: 1950. Frequency: Bimonthly. ISSN: 0410-2894.

★330★ CAMBRIDGE QUARTERLY OF HEALTHCARE ETHICS
Cambridge University Press
40 W. 20th St.
New York, NY 10011   Phone: (212) 924-3900
First Published: 1991. Frequency: Quarterly. ISSN: 0963-1801.

★331★ CANADIAN DENTAL ASSOCIATION JOURNAL
Canadian Dental Association
1815 Alta Vista Dr.
Ottawa, ON, Canada K1G 3Y6   Phone: (613) 523-1770
First Published: 1935. Frequency: Monthly. ISSN: 0709-8936.

★332★ CANADIAN JOURNAL OF ANAESTHESIA
Canadian Anaesthetists' Society
187 Gerrard St., E.
Toronto, ON, Canada M5A 2E5   Phone: (416) 923-1449
First Published: 1954. Frequency: 8/yr. ISSN: 0832-610X.

★333★ CANADIAN JOURNAL OF CARDIOLOGY
Canadian Cardiology Publications, Inc.
2160 Dunwin, Unit 1
Mississauga, ON, Canada L5L 1C7   Phone: (416) 828-3640
First Published: 1985. Frequency: 10/yr. ISSN: 0828-282X.

★334★ CANADIAN JOURNAL OF MEDICAL RADIATION
TECHNOLOGY
Canadian Association of Medical Radiation Technologists
294 Albert St., Ste. 601
Ottawa, ON, Canada K1P 6E6   Phone: (613) 234-0012
First Published: 1943. Frequency: Quarterly. ISSN: 0820-5930.

★335★ CANADIAN JOURNAL OF MEDICAL TECHNOLOGY
Canadian Society of Laboratory Technologists
Box 2830, Sta. A
Hamilton, ON, Canada L8N 3N5   Phone: (416) 528-8642
First Published: 1938. Frequency: Quarterly. ISSN: 0008-4158.

★336★ CANADIAN JOURNAL OF MICROBIOLOGY
National Research Council of Canada
Ottawa, ON, Canada K1A 0R6   Phone: (613) 993-9084
First Published: 1954. Frequency: Monthly. ISSN: 0008-4166.

★337★ CANADIAN JOURNAL OF NEUROLOGICAL SCIENCES
Canadian Congress of Neurological Sciences
PO Box 4220, Sta. C
Calgary, AB, Canada T2T 5N1   Phone: (403) 229-9575
First Published: 1974. Frequency: Quarterly. ISSN: 0317-1671.

★338★ CANADIAN JOURNAL OF OPHTHALMOLOGY
Canadian Ophthalmological Society
1525 Carling Ave., No. 601
Ottawa, ON, Canada K1Z 8R9   Phone: (613) 729-6779
First Published: 1966. Frequency: 7/yr. ISSN: 0008-4182.

★339★ CANADIAN JOURNAL OF PHYSIOLOGY AND
PHARMACOLOGY
National Research Council of Canada
Ottawa, ON, Canada K1A 0R6   Phone: (613) 993-9084
First Published: 1964. Frequency: Monthly. ISSN: 0008-4212.

★340★ CANADIAN JOURNAL OF PSYCHIATRY/REVUE
CANADIENNE DE PSYCHIATRIE
Canadian Psychiatric Association
294 Albert St., Ste. 204
Ottawa, ON, Canada K1P 6E6   Phone: (613) 234-2815
First Published: 1956. Frequency: 9/yr. ISSN: 0706-7437.

★341★ CANADIAN JOURNAL OF PSYCHOLOGY
Canadian Psychological Association
Rue Vincent Rd.
Old Chelsea, PQ, Canada J0X 2N0   Phone: (819) 827-3927
First Published: 1947. Frequency: Quarterly. ISSN: 0008-4255.

★342★ CANADIAN JOURNAL OF PUBLIC HEALTH/REVUE
CANADIENNE DE SANTE PUBLIQUE
Canadian Public Health Association
1565 Carling Ave., Ste. 400
Ottawa, ON, Canada K1Z 8N8   Phone: (613) 725-3769
First Published: 1910. Frequency: Bimonthly. ISSN: 0008-4263.

★343★ CANADIAN JOURNAL OF SURGERY
Canadian Medical Association
1867 Alta Vista Dr.
Box 8650
Ottawa, ON, Canada K1G 0G8   Phone: (613) 731-9331
First Published: 1957. Frequency: Bimonthly. ISSN: 0008-428X.

★344★ CANADIAN JOURNAL OF VETERINARY RESEARCH
Canadian Veterinary Medical Association
339 Booth St.
Ottawa, ON, Canada K1R 7K1   Phone: (613) 236-1162
First Published: 1937. Frequency: Quarterly. ISSN: 0830-9000.

★345★ CANADIAN MEDICAL ASSOCIATION JOURNAL
Canadian Medical Association
1867 Alta Vista Dr.
Box 8650
Ottawa, ON, Canada K1G 0G8   Phone: (613) 731-9331
First Published: 1911. Frequency: Semimonthly. ISSN: 0008-4409.

★346★ CANCER
American Cancer Society
1599 Clifton Rd. NE
Atlanta, GA 30329   Phone: (404) 320-3333
First Published: 1948. Frequency: Semimonthly. ISSN: 0008-543X.

★347★ CANCER BIOCHEMISTRY BIOPHYSICS
Gordon and Breach Science Publishers
PO Box 786, Cooper Sta.
New York, NY 10276   Phone: (212) 206-8900
First Published: 1975. Frequency: 8/yr. ISSN: 0305-7232.

★348★ CANCER CAUSES AND CONTROL
Rapid Communications of Oxford Ltd.
The Old Malthouse
Paradise St.
Oxford OX1 1LD, England
First Published: 1991. Frequency: Bimonthly. ISSN: 0957-5243.

★349★   CANCER CHEMOTHERAPY AND PHARMACOLOGY
Springer-Verlag New York, Inc.
175 5th Ave.
New York, NY 10010   Phone: (212) 460-1500
First Published: 1978. **Frequency:** 12/yr. **ISSN:** 0344-5704.

★350★   CANCER DETECTION AND PREVENTION
CRC Press, Inc.
2000 Corp. Blvd. NW
Boca Raton, FL 33431   Phone: (407) 994-0555
First Published: 1976. **Frequency:** Monthly. **ISSN:** 0361-090X.

★351★   CANCER EPIDEMIOLOGY BIOMARKERS AND PREVENTION
American Association for Cancer Research
620 Chestnut St., Ste. 816
Philadelphia, PA 19106   Phone: (215) 440-9300
Frequency: Bimonthly.

★352★   CANCER GENETICS AND CYTOGENETICS
Elsevier Science Publishing Co., Inc.
655 Ave. of the Americas
New York, NY 10010   Phone: (212) 989-5800
First Published: 1979. **Frequency:** 14/yr. **ISSN:** 0165-4608.

★353★   CANCER IMMUNOLOGY, IMMUNOTHERAPY
Springer-Verlag New York, Inc.
175 5th Ave.
New York, NY 10010   Phone: (212) 460-1500
First Published: 1976. **Frequency:** 12/yr. **ISSN:** 0340-7004.

★354★   CANCER INVESTIGATION
Marcel Dekker, Inc.
270 Madison Ave.
New York, NY 10016   Phone: (212) 696-9000
First Published: 1983. **Frequency:** 6/yr. **ISSN:** 0735-7907.

★355★   CANCER LETTERS
Elsevier Science Publishing Co., Inc.
655 Ave. of the Americas
New York, NY 10010   Phone: (212) 989-5800
First Published: 1975. **Frequency:** Monthly. **ISSN:** 0304-3835.

★356★   CANCER NURSING
Raven Press
1185 Avenue of the Americas
New York, NY 10036   Phone: (212) 930-9500
First Published: 1978. **Frequency:** Bimonthly. **ISSN:** 0162-220X.

★357★   CANCER PREVENTION
Williams & Wilkins
428 E. Preston St.
Baltimore, MD 21202   Phone: (301) 528-4000
First Published: 1990. **Frequency:** Quarterly. **ISSN:** 1043-8491.

★358★   CANCER RESEARCH
American Association for Cancer Research
Public Ledger Bldg.
6th and Chestnut Sts., Sta. 816
Philadelphia, PA 19106   Phone: (215) 440-9300
First Published: 1941. **Frequency:** Monthly. **ISSN:** 0008-5472.

★359★   CANCER SURVEYS
Oxford University Press
Walton St.
Oxford OX2 6DP, England
First Published: 1982. **Frequency:** Quarterly. **ISSN:** 0261-2429.

★360★   CANCER TREATMENT REPORTS
U.S. National Cancer Institute
Bethesda, MD 20892   Phone: (301) 496-6735
First Published: 1959. **Frequency:** Monthly. **ISSN:** 0361-5960.

★361★   CANCER TREATMENT REVIEWS
Academic Press, Inc.
1250 6th Ave.
San Diego, CA 92101   Phone: (619) 231-0926
First Published: 1974. **Frequency:** Quarterly. **ISSN:** 0305-7372.

★362★   CAP TODAY
College of American Pathologists
325 Waukegan Rd.
Northfield, IL 60093-2750   Phone: (708) 446-8800
First Published: 1947. **Frequency:** Monthly. **ISSN:** 0089-1525.

★363★   CARCINOGENESIS
IRL Press, Inc.
PO Box Q
McLean, VA 22101   Phone: (703) 437-3334
First Published: 1980. **Frequency:** Monthly. **ISSN:** 0143-3334.

★364★   CARDIOLOGY
S. Karger Publishers, Inc.
26 W. Avon Rd.
PO Box 529
Farmington, CT 06085   Phone: (203) 675-7834
First Published: 1937. **Frequency:** Bimonthly. **ISSN:** 0008-6312.

★365★   CARDIOLOGY IN THE ELDERLY
Current Science
20 N. 3rd St.
Philadelphia, PA 19106   Phone: (215) 514-2266
First Published: 1992. **Frequency:** Bimonthly. **ISSN:** 1058-3661.

★366★   CARDIOLOGY MANAGEMENT
MacMillan Professional Journals
1640 5th St.
Santa Monica, CA 90401   Phone: (213) 395-0234
First Published: 1973. **Frequency:** Monthly. **ISSN:** 0892-9327.

★367★   CARDIOVASCULAR AND INTERVENTIONAL RADIOLOGY
Springer-Verlag New York, Inc.
175 5th Ave.
New York, NY 10010   Phone: (212) 460-1500
First Published: 1977. **Frequency:** Bimonthly. **ISSN:** 0174-1551.

★368★   CARDIOVASCULAR PATHOLOGY
Elsevier Science Publishing Co., Inc.
655 Avenue of the Americas
New York, NY 10010   Phone: (212) 989-5800
Frequency: Quarterly. **ISSN:** 1054-8807.

★369★   CARDIOVASCULAR RESEARCH
British Medical Association
PO Box 560B
Kennebunkport, ME 04046   **Frequency:** Monthly. **ISSN:** 0008-6363.

★370★   CARIES RESEARCH
S. Karger Publishers, Inc.
26 W. Avon Rd.
PO Box 529
Farmington, CT 06085   Phone: (203) 675-7834
First Published: 1967. **Frequency:** Bimonthly. **ISSN:** 0008-6568.

★371★   CATHETERIZATION AND CARDIOVASCULAR DIAGNOSIS
John Wiley & Sons, Inc.
605 3rd Ave.
New York, NY 10158   Phone: (212) 850-6000
First Published: 1975. **Frequency:** 8/yr. **ISSN:** 0098-6569.

★372★   CELL
Cell Press
50 Church St.
Cambridge, MA 02138   Phone: (617) 661-7059
First Published: 1974. **Frequency:** 25/yr. **ISSN:** 0092-8674.

★373★ CELL BIOLOGY INTERNATIONAL REPORTS
Academic Press, Inc.
1250 6th Ave.
San Diego, CA 92101 Phone: (619) 231-0926
First Published: 1977. Frequency: Monthly. ISSN: 0309-1651.

★374★ CELL CALCIUM
Churchill Livingstone, Inc.
1560 Broadway
New York, NY 10036 Phone: (212) 819-5400
First Published: 1980. Frequency: 10/yr. ISSN: 0143-4160.

★375★ CELL DIFFERENTIATION AND DEVELOPMENT
Elsevier Science Publishing Co., Inc.
655 Avenue of the Americas
New York, NY 10010 Phone: (212) 989-5800
First Published: 1972. Frequency: 9/yr. ISSN: 0922-3371.

★376★ CELL GROWTH AND DIFFERENTIATION
American Association for Cancer Research
Public Ledger Bldg.
6th and Chestnuts, Ste. 816
Philadelphia, PA 19106 Phone: (215) 440-9300
First Published: 1990. Frequency: Monthly.

★377★ CELL MOTILITY AND THE CYTOSKELETON
John Wiley & Sons, Inc.
605 3rd Ave.
New York, NY 10158 Phone: (212) 850-6000
First Published: 1980. Frequency: Monthly. ISSN: 0886-1544.

★378★ CELL AND TISSUE KINETICS
Blackwell Scientific Publications
3 Cambridge Center, Ste. 208
Cambridge, MA 02142 Phone: (617) 225-0401
First Published: 1968. Frequency: Bimonthly. ISSN: 0008-8730.

★379★ CELL AND TISSUE RESEARCH
Springer-Verlag New York, Inc.
175 5th Ave.
New York, NY 10010 Phone: (212) 460-1500
Frequency: Monthly. ISSN: 0302-766X.

★380★ CELLULAR IMMUNOLOGY
Academic Press, Inc.
1250 6th Ave.
San Diego, CA 92101 Phone: (619) 231-0926
First Published: 1970. Frequency: 14/yr. ISSN: 0008-8749.

★381★ CELLULAR AND MOLECULAR BIOLOGY
Pergamon Press, Inc.
Maxwell House, Fairview Park
Elmsford, NY 10523 Phone: (914) 592-7700
First Published: 1956. Frequency: 8/yr. ISSN: 0145-5680.

★382★ CELLULAR AND MOLECULAR NEUROBIOLOGY
Plenum Publishing Corp.
233 Spring St.
New York, NY 10013 Phone: (212) 620-8000
First Published: 1981. Frequency: Quarterly. ISSN: 0272-4340.

★383★ CHEMICO-BIOLOGICAL INTERACTIONS
Elsevier Science Publishing Co., Inc.
655 Avenue of the Americas
New York, NY 10010 Phone: (212) 989-5800
First Published: 1969. Frequency: 12/yr. ISSN: 0009-2797.

★384★ CHEMOTHERAPY
S. Karger Publishers, Inc.
26 W. Avon Rd.
PO Box 529
Farmington, CT 06085 Phone: (203) 675-7834
First Published: 1960. Frequency: Bimonthly. ISSN: 0009-3157.

★385★ CHEST
American College of Chest Physicians
911 Busse Hwy.
Park Ridge, IL 60068 Phone: (312) 698-2200
First Published: 1935. Frequency: Monthly. ISSN: 0012-3692.

★386★ CHEST SURGERY CLINICS OF NORTH AMERICA
W.B. Saunders Co.
Curtis Center
Independence Sq., W.
Philadelphia, PA 19106 Phone: (215) 238-7800
Frequency: Quarterly.

★387★ CHILD AND ADOLESCENT PSYCHIATRIC CLINICS
W.B. Saunders Co.
Curtis Center
Independence Sq., W.
Philadelphia, PA 19106 Phone: (215) 238-7800
First Published: 1992. Frequency: Quarterly.

★388★ CHILD: CARE, HEALTH AND DEVELOPMENT
Blackwell Scientific Publications
3 Cambridge Center, Ste. 208
Cambridge, MA 02142 Phone: (617) 225-0401
First Published: 1975. Frequency: Bimonthly. ISSN: 0305-1862.

★389★ CHILD DEVELOPMENT
Society for Research in Child Development
University of Chicago Press
5720 S. Woodlawn Ave.
Chicago, IL 60637 Phone: (312) 702-7470
First Published: 1930. Frequency: Bimonthly. ISSN: 0009-3920.

★390★ CHILD NEPHROLOGY AND UROLOGY
S. Karger Publishers, Inc.
26 W. Avon Rd.
PO Box 529
Farmington, CT 06085
First Published: 1980. Frequency: Quarterly. ISSN: 1012-6694.

★391★ CHILD PSYCHIATRY AND HUMAN DEVELOPMENT
American Association of Psychiatric Services for Children
1200-C Scottsdale Rd., Ste. 225
Rochester, NY 14624 Phone: (716) 235-6910
First Published: 1970. Frequency: Quarterly. ISSN: 0009-398X.

★392★ CHILDBIRTH
Cahners Publishing Co.
475 Park Ave., S.
New York, NY 10016-6999 Phone: (212) 689-3600
Frequency: Annual.

★393★ CHILDREN TODAY
U.S. Department of Health and Human Services
Administration for Children and Families
200 Independence Ave. SW
Washington, DC 20201 Phone: (202) 245-6233
First Published: 1954. Frequency: Bimonthly. ISSN: 0361-4336.

★394★ CHILD'S NERVOUS SYSTEM
Springer-Verlag New York, Inc.
175 5th Ave.
New York, NY 10010 Phone: (212) 460-1500
First Published: 1972. Frequency: 8/yr. ISSN: 0256-7040.

★395★ CHIROPRACTIC SPORTS MEDICINE
Williams & Wilkins
428 E. Preston St.
Baltimore, MD 21202 Phone: (301) 528-4000
First Published: 1987. Frequency: Quarterly. ISSN: 0889-6976.

★396★ CIRCULATION
American Heart Association
7320 Greenville Ave.
Dallas, TX 75231 Phone: (214) 706-1310
First Published: 1950. Frequency: Monthly. ISSN: 0009-7322.

★397★   CIRCULATION RESEARCH
American Heart Association
7320 Greenville Ave.
Dallas, TX 75231   Phone: (214) 373-6300
First Published: 1953. **Frequency:** Monthly. **ISSN:** 0009-7330.

★398★   CIRCULATORY SHOCK
John Wiley & Sons, Inc.
605 3rd Ave.
New York, NY 10158   Phone: (212) 850-6000
First Published: 1974. **Frequency:** Monthly. **ISSN:** 0092-6213.

★399★   CLAO JOURNAL
Contact Lens Association of Ophthalmologists
c/o Edmund J. Perret, II
523 Decatur St., Ste. 1
New Orleans, LA 70130   Phone: (504) 581-4000
First Published: 1975. **Frequency:** Quarterly. **ISSN:** 0733-8902.

★400★   CLEFT PALATE JOURNAL
American Cleft Palate-Craniofacial Association
1218 Grandview Ave.
Pittsburgh, PA 15211   Phone: (412) 481-1376
First Published: 1964. **Frequency:** Quarterly. **ISSN:** 0009-8701.

★401★   CLEVELAND CLINIC JOURNAL OF MEDICINE
Cleveland Clinic Foundation
9500 Euclid Ave.
Cleveland, OH 44106   Phone: (216) 444-2662
First Published: 1932. **Frequency:** 8/yr. **ISSN:** 0891-1150.

★402★   CLINICA CHIMICA ACTA
Elsevier Science Publishing Co., Inc.
655 Avenue of the Americas
New York, NY 10010   Phone: (212) 989-5800
First Published: 1956. **Frequency:** 27/yr. **ISSN:** 0009-8981.

★403★   CLINICAL BIOCHEMISTRY
Pergamon Press, Inc.
Maxwell House, Fairview Park
Elmsford, NY 10523   Phone: (914) 592-7700
First Published: 1967. **Frequency:** Bimonthly. **ISSN:** 0009-9120.

★404★   CLINICAL BIOMECHANICS
Butterworth-Heinemann
80 Montvale Ave.
Stoneham, MA 02180   Phone: (617) 438-8464
Frequency: Quarterly. **ISSN:** 0268-0033.

★405★   CLINICAL CARDIOLOGY
Clinical Cardiology Publishing Co., Inc.
JBI Bldg.
Box 832
Mahwah, NJ 07430   Phone: (201) 529-0003
First Published: 1978. **Frequency:** Monthly. **ISSN:** 0160-9289.

★406★   CLINICAL CHEMISTRY
American Association for Clinical Chemistry
2029 K St. NW, 7th Fl.
Washington, DC 20006   Phone: (202) 857-0717
First Published: 1955. **Frequency:** Monthly. **ISSN:** 0009-9147.

★407★   CLINICAL ELECTROENCEPHALOGRAPHY
American Medical Electroencephalographic Association
850 Elm Grove Rd., Ste. 11
Elm Grove, WI 53122   Phone: (414) 797-7800
First Published: 1970. **Frequency:** Quarterly. **ISSN:** 0009-9155.

★408★   CLINICAL ENDOCRINOLOGY
Blackwell Scientific Publications
3 Cambridge Center, Ste. 208
Cambridge, MA 02142   Phone: (617) 225-0401
First Published: 1972. **Frequency:** Monthly. **ISSN:** 0300-0664.

★409★   CLINICAL AND EXPERIMENTAL ALLERGY
Blackwell Scientific Publications
3 Cambridge Center, Ste. 208
Cambridge, MA 02142   Phone: (617) 225-0401
Frequency: Monthly. **ISSN:** 0954-7894.

★410★   CLINICAL AND EXPERIMENTAL DERMATOLOGY
Blackwell Scientific Publications
3 Cambridge Center, Ste. 208
Cambridge, MA 02142   Phone: (617) 225-0401
First Published: 1976. **Frequency:** Bimonthly. **ISSN:** 0307-6938.

**★411★   CLINICAL AND EXPERIMENTAL HYPERTENSION,
    PART A: THEORY AND PRACTICE**
Marcel Dekker, Inc.
270 Madison Ave.
New York, NY 10016   Phone: (212) 696-9000
First Published: 1978. **Frequency:** 8/yr. **ISSN:** 0730-0077.

**★412★   CLINICAL AND EXPERIMENTAL HYPERTENSION,
    PART B: HYPERTENSION IN PREGNANCY**
Marcel Dekker, Inc.
270 Madison Ave.
New York, NY 10016   Phone: (212) 696-9000
First Published: 1982. **Frequency:** 3/yr. **ISSN:** 0730-0085.

★413★   CLINICAL AND EXPERIMENTAL IMMUNOLOGY
Blackwell Scientific Publications
3 Cambridge Center, Ste. 208
Cambridge, MA 02142   Phone: (617) 225-0401
First Published: 1966. **Frequency:** Monthly. **ISSN:** 0009-9104.

**★414★   CLINICAL AND EXPERIMENTAL PHARMACOLOGY
    AND PHYSIOLOGY**
Blackwell Scientific Publications
3 Cambridge Center, Ste. 208
Cambridge, MA 02142   Phone: (617) 225-0401
First Published: 1974. **Frequency:** Monthly. **ISSN:** 0305-1870.

★415★   CLINICAL GENETICS
Munksgaard
Noerre Soegade 35
DK-1370 Copenhagen K, Denmark
First Published: 1970. **Frequency:** Monthly. **ISSN:** 0009-9163.

★416★   CLINICAL IMAGING
Elsevier Science Publishing Co., Inc.
655 Avenue of the Americas
New York, NY 10010   Phone: (212) 989-5800
First Published: 1977. **Frequency:** Quarterly. **ISSN:** 0899-7071.

**★417★   CLINICAL IMMUNOLOGY AND
    IMMUNOPATHOLOGY**
Academic Press, Inc.
1250 6th Ave.
San Diego, CA 92101   Phone: (619) 231-0926
First Published: 1972. **Frequency:** Monthly. **ISSN:** 0090-1229.

**★418★   CLINICAL AND INVESTIGATIVE
    MEDICINE/MEDECINE CLINIQUE ET EXPERIMENTALE**
University of Toronto Press
10 St. Mary St., Ste. 7000
Toronto, ON, Canada M4Y 2WB   Phone: (416) 978-2239
First Published: 1978. **Frequency:** Quarterly. **ISSN:** 0147-958X.

★419★   CLINICAL JOURNAL OF PAIN
Raven Press
1185 Avenue of the Americas
New York, NY 10036   Phone: (212) 930-9500
First Published: 1985. **Frequency:** Quarterly. **ISSN:** 0749-8047.

★420★   CLINICAL JOURNAL OF SPORTS MEDICINE
Raven Press
1185 Avenue of the Americas
New York, NY 10036   Phone: (212) 930-9500
First Published: 1992. **Frequency:** Quarterly. **ISSN:** 1050-642X.

★421★ CLINICAL AND LABORATORY HAEMATOLOGY
Blackwell Scientific Publications
3 Cambridge Center, Ste. 208
Cambridge, MA 02142   Phone: (617) 225-0401
First Published: 1979. Frequency: Quarterly. ISSN: 0141-9854.

★422★ CLINICAL LABORATORY MANAGEMENT REVIEW
Clinical Laboratory Management Association
195 W. Lancaster Ave.
Paoli, PA 19301   Phone: (215) 647-8970
First Published: 1987. Frequency: Bimonthly. ISSN: 0888-7950.

★423★ CLINICAL LABORATORY SCIENCE
American Society for Medical Technology
2021 L St. NW, Ste. 400
Washington, DC 20036   Phone: (202) 785-3311
First Published: 1984. Frequency: Bimonthly. ISSN: 0894-959X.

★424★ CLINICAL MANAGEMENT IN PHYSICAL THERAPY
American Physical Therapy Association
1111 N. Fairfax St.
Alexandria, VA 22314   Phone: (703) 684-2782
First Published: 1981. Frequency: Bimonthly. ISSN: 0276-8038.

★425★ CLINICAL NEPHROLOGY
Dustri-Verlag, Dr. Karl Feistle
Bahnhofstr. 9
8024 Oberhaching-Deisenhofen, Germany
First Published: 1973. Frequency: Monthly. ISSN: 0301-0430.

★426★ CLINICAL NEUROLOGY AND NEUROSURGERY
Van Gorcum
PO Box 43
9400 AA Assen, Netherlands
First Published: 1975. Frequency: Quarterly. ISSN: 0303-8467.

★427★ CLINICAL NEUROPATHOLOGY
Dustri-Verlag, Dr. Karl Feistle
Bahnhofstr. 9
8024 Oberhaching-Deisenhofen, Germany
First Published: 1982. Frequency: Bimonthly. ISSN: 0722-5091.

★428★ CLINICAL NEUROPHARMACOLOGY
Raven Press
1185 Avenue of the Americas
New York, NY 10036   Phone: (212) 930-9500
First Published: 1976. Frequency: Quarterly. ISSN: 0362-5664.

★429★ CLINICAL NUCLEAR MEDICINE
J.B. Lippincott Co.
E. Washington Sq.
Philadelphia, PA 19105   Phone: (215) 238-4200
First Published: 1976. Frequency: Monthly. ISSN: 0363-9762.

★430★ CLINICAL NURSE SPECIALIST
Williams & Wilkins
428 E. Preston St.
Baltimore, MD 21202   Phone: (301) 528-4223
First Published: 1987. Frequency: Quarterly. ISSN: 0887-6274.

★431★ CLINICAL NUTRITION
Churchill Livingstone, Inc.
1560 Broadway
New York, NY 10036   Phone: (212) 819-5400
First Published: 1982. Frequency: Quarterly. ISSN: 0261-5614.

★432★ CLINICAL OBSTETRICS AND GYNECOLOGY
J.B. Lippincott Co.
E. Washington Sq.
Philadelphia, PA 19105   Phone: (215) 238-4200
First Published: 1958. Frequency: Quarterly. ISSN: 0009-9201.

★433★ CLINICAL ONCOLOGY
Springer-Verlag New York, Inc.
175 5th Ave.
New York, NY 10010   Phone: (212) 460-1500
First Published: 1991. Frequency: Quarterly. ISSN: 0936-6555.

★434★ CLINICAL ORTHOPAEDICS AND RELATED
   RESEARCH
J.B. Lippincott Co.
E. Washington Sq.
Philadelphia, PA 19105   Phone: (215) 238-4200
First Published: 1952. Frequency: Monthly. ISSN: 0009-921X.

★435★ CLINICAL OTOLARYNGOLOGY AND ALLIED
   SCIENCES
Blackwell Scientific Publications
3 Cambridge Center, Ste. 208
Cambridge, MA 02142   Phone: (617) 225-0401
First Published: 1976. Frequency: Bimonthly. ISSN: 0307-7772.

★436★ CLINICAL PEDIATRICS
J.B. Lippincott Co.
E. Washington Sq.
Philadelphia, PA 19105   Phone: (215) 238-4200
First Published: 1962. Frequency: Monthly. ISSN: 0009-9228.

★437★ CLINICAL PHARMACOLOGY AND THERAPEUTICS
Mosby-Year Book, Inc.
11830 Westline Industrial Dr.
St. Louis, MO 63146   Phone: (314) 872-8370
First Published: 1960. Frequency: Monthly. ISSN: 0009-9236.

★438★ CLINICAL PHARMACY
American Society of Hospital Pharmacists
4630 Montgomery Ave.
Bethesda, MD 20814   Phone: (301) 657-3000
First Published: 1982. Frequency: Monthly. ISSN: 0278-2677.

★439★ CLINICAL PHYSICS AND PHYSIOLOGICAL
   MEASUREMENT
American Institute of Physics
335 E. 45th St.
New York, NY 10017   Phone: (212) 661-9404
First Published: 1980. Frequency: Quarterly. ISSN: 0143-0815.

★440★ CLINICAL PHYSIOLOGY
Blackwell Scientific Publications
3 Cambridge Center, Ste. 208
Cambridge, MA 02142   Phone: (617) 225-0401
First Published: 1981. Frequency: Bimonthly. ISSN: 0144-5979.

★441★ CLINICAL PHYSIOLOGY AND BIOCHEMISTRY
S. Karger Publishers, Inc.
26 W. Avon Rd.
PO Box 529
Farmington, CT 06085   Phone: (203) 675-7834
First Published: 1982. Frequency: 6/yr. ISSN: 0252-1164.

★442★ CLINICAL PRACTICE OF GYNECOLOGY
Elsevier Science Publishing Co., Inc.
655 Avenue of the Americas
New York, NY 10010   Phone: (212) 989-5800
ISSN: 1043-3198.

★443★ CLINICAL PREVENTIVE DENTISTRY
J.B. Lippincott Co.
E. Washington Sq.
Philadelphia, PA 19105   Phone: (215) 238-4200
First Published: 1974. Frequency: Bimonthly. ISSN: 0163-9633.

★444★ CLINICAL RADIOLOGY
Blackwell Scientific Publications
3 Cambridge Center, Ste. 208
Cambridge, MA 02142   Phone: (617) 225-0401
Frequency: Monthly. ISSN: 0009-9260.

★445★ CLINICAL REHABILITATION
Cambridge University Press
40 W. 20th St.
New York, NY 10011   Phone: (212) 924-3900
Frequency: Quarterly. **ISSN:** 0269-2155.

★446★ CLINICAL REPRODUCTION AND FERTILITY
Blackwell Scientific Publications
3 Cambridge Center, Ste. 208
Cambridge, MA 02142   Phone: (617) 225-0401
First Published: 1982. **Frequency:** Bimonthly. **ISSN:** 0725-556X.

★447★ CLINICAL SCIENCE
Portland Press
Box 32
Commerce Way
Colchester, Essex CO2 8HP, England
First Published: 1909. **Frequency:** Monthly. **ISSN:** 0143-5221.

★448★ CLINICAL SYMPOSIA
CIBA Geigy Corp.
Medical Education Division
14 Henderson Dr.
West Caldwell, NJ 07006   Phone: (201) 575-6510
First Published: 1948. **Frequency:** 5/yr. **ISSN:** 0009-9295.

★449★ CLINICAL THERAPEUTICS
Elsevier Science Publishing Co., Inc.
655 Avenue of the Americas
New York, NY 10010   Phone: (212) 989-5800
First Published: 1978. **Frequency:** Bimonthly. **ISSN:** 0149-2918.

★450★ CLINICS IN APPLIED NUTRITION
Butterworth-Heinemann
80 Montvale Ave.
Stoneham, MA 02180   Phone: (617) 438-8464
Frequency: Quarterly. **ISSN:** 1053-0752.

★451★ CLINICS IN DERMATOLOGY
Elsevier Science Publishing Co., Inc.
655 Avenue of the Americas
New York, NY 10010   Phone: (212) 989-5800
Frequency: Quarterly. **ISSN:** 073X-081X.

★452★ CLINICS IN DEVELOPMENTAL MEDICINE
J.B. Lippincott Co.
E. Washington Sq.
Philadelphia, PA 19105   Phone: (215) 238-4200
First Published: 1959. **Frequency:** Irregular. **ISSN:** 0069-4835.

★453★ CLIO MEDICA
International Academy of the History of Medicine
Wellcome Institute for the History of Medicine
183 Euston Rd.
London NW1 2BP, England
First Published: 1966. **Frequency:** Semiannual. **ISSN:** 0045-7183.

★454★ COGNITIVE PSYCHOLOGY
Academic Press, Inc.
1250 6th Ave.
San Diego, CA 92101   Phone: (619) 231-0926
First Published: 1970. **Frequency:** Quarterly. **ISSN:** 0010-0285.

★455★ COLORADO MEDICINE
Colorado Medical Society
7800 E. Durado Pl.
Englewood, CO 80111   Phone: (303) 779-5455
First Published: 1903. **Frequency:** Monthly. **ISSN:** 0199-7343.

★456★ COMMUNITY DENTISTRY AND ORAL EPIDEMIOLOGY
Munksgaard
Noerre Soegade 35
DK-1370 Copenhagen K, Denmark
First Published: 1973. **Frequency:** Bimonthly. **ISSN:** 0301-5661.

★457★ COMMUNITY MENTAL HEALTH JOURNAL
National Council of Community Mental Health Centers
12300 Twinbrook Pkwy., No. 320
Rockville, MD 20852   Phone: (301) 984-6200
First Published: 1965. **Frequency:** Quarterly. **ISSN:** 0010-3853.

★458★ COMPARATIVE BIOCHEMISTRY AND PHYSIOLOGY, PART A: COMPARATIVE PHYSIOLOGY
Pergamon Press, Inc.
Maxwell House, Fairview Park
Elmsford, NY 10523   Phone: (914) 592-7700
First Published: 1961. **Frequency:** Monthly. **ISSN:** 0300-9629.

★459★ COMPARATIVE BIOCHEMISTRY AND PHYSIOLOGY, PART B: COMPARATIVE BIOCHEMISTRY
Pergamon Press, Inc.
Maxwell House, Fairview Park
Elmsford, NY 10523   Phone: (914) 592-7700
First Published: 1961. **Frequency:** Monthly. **ISSN:** 0305-0491.

★460★ COMPARATIVE BIOCHEMISTRY AND PHYSIOLOGY, PART C: COMPARATIVE PHARMACOLOGY AND TOXICOLOGY
Pergamon Press, Inc.
Maxwell House, Fairview Park
Elmsford, NY 10523   Phone: (914) 592-7700
First Published: 1975. **Frequency:** 9/yr. **ISSN:** 0742-8413.

★461★ COMPARATIVE IMMUNOLOGY, MICROBIOLOGY AND INFECTIOUS DISEASES
Pergamon Press, Inc.
Maxwell House, Fairview Park
Elmsford, NY 10523   Phone: (914) 592-7700
First Published: 1978. **Frequency:** Quarterly. **ISSN:** 0147-9571.

★462★ COMPARATIVE MEDICINE
Academic Press, Inc.
1250 6th Ave.
San Diego, CA 92101   Phone: (619) 231-0926
First Published: 1992. **Frequency:** Semiannual. **ISSN:** 1058-2401.

★463★ COMPREHENSIVE PSYCHIATRY
American Psychopathological Association
c/o Dr. Ellen Frank
Western Psychiatric Institute and Clinic
3811 O'Hara
Pittsburgh, PA 15213   Phone: (412) 624-2383
First Published: 1960. **Frequency:** Bimonthly. **ISSN:** 0010-440X.

★464★ COMPREHENSIVE THERAPY
American Society of Contemporary Medicine and Surgery
233 E. Erie St., Ste. 710
Chicago, IL 60611   Phone: (312) 951-1400
First Published: 1975. **Frequency:** Monthly. **ISSN:** 0098-8243.

★465★ COMPUTER METHODS AND PROGRAMS IN BIOMEDICINE
Elsevier Science Publishing Co., Inc.
655 Avenue of the Americas
New York, NY 10010   Phone: (212) 989-5800
First Published: 1970. **Frequency:** Monthly. **ISSN:** 0169-2607.

★466★ COMPUTERIZED MEDICAL IMAGING AND GRAPHICS
Pergamon Press, Inc.
Maxwell House, Fairview Park
Elmsford, NY 10523   Phone: (914) 592-7700
First Published: 1977. **Frequency:** Bimonthly. **ISSN:** 0895-6111.

★467★ COMPUTERS IN BIOLOGY AND MEDICINE
Pergamon Press, Inc.
Maxwell House, Fairview Park
Elmsford, NY 10523   Phone: (914) 592-7700
First Published: 1971. **Frequency:** Bimonthly. **ISSN:** 0010-4825.

★468★ COMPUTERS AND BIOMEDICAL RESEARCH
Academic Press, Inc.
1250 6th Ave.
San Diego, CA 92101   Phone: (619) 231-0926
First Published: 1969. **Frequency:** Bimonthly. **ISSN:** 0010-4809.

★469★ COMPUTERS AND MEDICINE
Medical Group News, Inc.
PO Box 36
Glencoe, IL 60022   Phone: (312) 441-6474
First Published: 1972. **Frequency:** Monthly. **ISSN:** 0163-0547.

★470★ COMPUTERS IN NURSING
J.B. Lippincott Co.
E. Washington Sq.
Philadelphia, PA 19105   Phone: (215) 238-4200
Frequency: Bimonthly. **ISSN:** 0736-8593.

★471★ CONNECTICUT MEDICINE
Connecticut State Medical Society
160 St. Ronan St.
New Haven, CT 06511   Phone: (203) 865-0587
First Published: 1937. **Frequency:** Monthly. **ISSN:** 0010-6178.

★472★ CONNECTIVE TISSUE RESEARCH
Gordon & Breach Science Publishers, Ltd.
PO Box 786, Cooper Sta.
New York, NY 10276   Phone: (212) 206-8900
First Published: 1972. **Frequency:** 2 vol./yr. **ISSN:** 0300-8207.

★473★ CONSULTANT
Cliggott Publishing Co.
55 Holly Hill Ln.
PO Box 4010
Greenwich, CT 06830   Phone: (203) 661-0600
First Published: 1961. **Frequency:** 12/yr. **ISSN:** 0010-7069.

★474★ CONTACT DERMATITIS
Munksgaard
Noerre Soegade 35
DK-1370 Copenhagen K, Denmark
First Published: 1975. **Frequency:** 10/yr. **ISSN:** 0105-1873.

★475★ CONTRACEPTION
Butterworth-Heinemann
80 Montvale Ave.
Stoneham, MA 02180   Phone: (617) 438-8464
First Published: 1970. **Frequency:** Monthly. **ISSN:** 0010-7824.

★476★ CONTROLLED CLINICAL TRIALS
Elsevier Science Publishing Co., Inc.
655 Avenue of the Americas
New York, NY 10010   Phone: (212) 989-5800
First Published: 1979. **Frequency:** Quarterly. **ISSN:** 0197-2456.

★477★ CORNEA
Raven Press
1185 Avenue of the Americas
New York, NY 10036   Phone: (212) 930-9500
First Published: 1982. **Frequency:** Quarterly. **ISSN:** 0277-3740.

★478★ CORNELL VETERINARIAN
Cornell Veterinarian, Inc.
Ithaca, NY 14853   Phone: (607) 253-3336
First Published: 1911. **Frequency:** Quarterly. **ISSN:** 0010-8901.

★479★ CORONARY ARTERY DISEASE
Current Science
20 N. 3rd St.
Philadelphia, PA 19106   Phone: (215) 514-2266
Frequency: Monthly. **ISSN:** 0954-6928.

★480★ CORTEX
Masson Italia Periodici
Via Statuto 2-4
20121 Milan, Italy
First Published: 1964. **Frequency:** Quarterly. **ISSN:** 0010-9452.

★481★ CRANIO: JOURNAL OF CRANIOMANDIBULAR PRACTICE
Williams & Wilkins
428 E. Preston St.
Baltimore, MD 21202   Phone: (301) 528-4223
First Published: 1982. **Frequency:** Quarterly. **ISSN:** 0734-5410.

★482★ CRITICAL CARE MEDICINE
Society of Critical Care Medicine
251 E. Imperial Hwy., Ste. 480
Fullerton, CA 92635   Phone: (714) 870-5243
First Published: 1973. **Frequency:** Monthly. **ISSN:** 0090-3493.

★483★ CRITICAL CARE NURSING QUARTERLY
Aspen Publishers, Inc.
200 Orchard Ridge Dr.
Gaithersburg, MD 20878   Phone: (301) 417-7500
First Published: 1978. **Frequency:** Quarterly. **ISSN:** 0160-2551.

★484★ CRNA: THE CLINICAL FORUM FOR NURSE ANESTHETISTS
W.B. Saunders Co.
Curtis Center
Independence Sq., W.
Philadelphia, PA 19106   Phone: (215) 238-7800
First Published: 1992. **Frequency:** Quarterly.

★485★ CRYOBIOLOGY
Society for Cryobiology
c/o Federation of American Societies for Experimental Biology
9650 Rockville Pike
Bethesda, MD 20814   Phone: (301) 530-7000
First Published: 1964. **Frequency:** Bimonthly. **ISSN:** 0011-2240.

★486★ CULTURE, MEDICINE AND PSYCHIATRY
D. Reidel Publishing Co.
190 Old Derby St.
Hingham, MA 02043   Phone: (617) 749-5042
First Published: 1977. **Frequency:** Quarterly. **ISSN:** 0165-005X.

★487★ CURRENT EYE RESEARCH
IRL Press
PO Box Q
McLean, VA 22101   Phone: (703) 437-3334
First Published: 1981. **Frequency:** Monthly. **ISSN:** 0271-3683.

★488★ CURRENT GENETICS
Springer-Verlag New York, Inc.
175 5th Ave.
New York, NY 10010   Phone: (212) 460-1500
First Published: 1980. **Frequency:** 12/yr. **ISSN:** 0172-8083.

★489★ CURRENT MICROBIOLOGY
Springer-Verlag New York, Inc.
175 5th Ave.
New York, NY 10010   Phone: (212) 460-1500
First Published: 1978. **Frequency:** 12/yr. **ISSN:** 0172-8083.

★490★ CURRENT TOPICS IN LEARNING DISABILITIES
Ablex Publishing Corp.
355 Chestnut St.
Norwood, NJ 07648   Phone: (201) 767-8450
First Published: 1984. **Frequency:** Irregular.

★491★ CUTIS
Cahners Publishing Co., Inc.
249 W. 17th St.
New York, NY 10011   Phone: (212) 645-0067
First Published: 1965. **Frequency:** Monthly. **ISSN:** 0011-4162.

★492★ CYTOGENETICS AND CELL GENETICS
S. Karger Publishers, Inc.
26 W. Avon Rd.
PO Box 529
Farmington, CT 06085   Phone: (203) 675-7834
First Published: 1962. **Frequency:** Monthly. **ISSN:** 0301-0171.

★493★ CYTOMETRY
John Wiley & Sons, Inc.
605 3rd Ave.
New York, NY 10158   Phone: (212) 850-6000
First Published: 1983. **Frequency:** 8/yr. **ISSN:** 0196-4763.

★494★ CYTOPATHOLOGY
Blackwell Scientific Publications
3 Cambridge Center, Ste. 208
Cambridge, MA 02142   Phone: (617) 225-0401
Frequency: Bimonthly. **ISSN:** 0012-1622.

★495★ DELAWARE MEDICAL JOURNAL
Medical Society of Delaware
1925 S. Lovering Ave.
Wilmington, DE 19806   Phone: (302) 658-7596
First Published: 1909. **Frequency:** Monthly. **ISSN:** 0011-7781.

★496★ DENTAL MANAGEMENT
Harcourt Brace Jovanovich, Inc.
7500 Old Oak Blvd.
Cleveland, OH 44130   Phone: (216) 243-8100
First Published: 1960. **Frequency:** Monthly. **ISSN:** 0011-8680.

★497★ DENTOMAXILLOFACIAL RADIOLOGY
Butterworth-Heinemann
80 Montvale Ave.
Stoneham, MA 02180   Phone: (617) 438-8404
Frequency: Quarterly. **ISSN:** 0250-832X.

★498★ DER CHIRURG
Springer-Verlag New York, Inc.
175 5th Ave.
New York, NY 10010   Phone: (212) 460-1500
First Published: 1928. **Frequency:** Monthly. **ISSN:** 0009-4722.

★499★ DERMATOLOGICA
S. Karger Publishers, Inc.
26 W. Avon Rd.
PO Box 529
Farmington, CT 06085   Phone: (203) 675-7834
First Published: 1893. **Frequency:** 8/yr. **ISSN:** 0011-9075.

★500★ DEUTSCHE MEDIZINISCHE WOCHENSCHRIFT
Georg Thieme Verlag
Ruedigerstr. 14
Postfach 10 48 53
D-7000 Stuttgart 10, Germany
First Published: 1875. **Frequency:** Weekly. **ISSN:** 0012-0472.

★501★ DEVELOPMENT
Company of Biologists, Ltd.
Box 32
Commerce Way
Colchester, Essex CO2 8HP, England
First Published: 1953. **Frequency:** 13/yr. **ISSN:** 0950-1991.

★502★ DEVELOPMENT AND PSYCHOPATHY
Cambridge University Press
40 W. 20th St.
New York, NY 10011   Phone: (212) 924-3900
Frequency: Quarterly. **ISSN:** 0954-5794.

★503★ DEVELOPMENTAL BIOLOGY
Academic Press, Inc.
1250 6th Ave.
San Diego, CA 92101   Phone: (619) 231-0926
First Published: 1959. **Frequency:** Monthly. **ISSN:** 0012-1606.

★504★ DEVELOPMENTAL AND COMPARATIVE IMMUNOLOGY
Pergamon Press, Inc.
Maxwell House, Fairview Park
Elmsford, NY 10523   Phone: (914) 592-7700
First Published: 1977. **Frequency:** Quarterly. **ISSN:** 0145-305X.

★505★ DEVELOPMENTAL GENETICS
John Wiley & Sons, Inc.
605 3rd Ave.
New York, NY 10158   Phone: (212) 850-6000
First Published: 1979. **Frequency:** Bimonthly. **ISSN:** 0192-253X.

★506★ DEVELOPMENTAL MEDICINE AND CHILD NEUROLOGY
J.B. Lippincott Co.
E. Washington Sq.
Philadelphia, PA 19105   Phone: (215) 238-4200
First Published: 1958. **Frequency:** Monthly. **ISSN:** 0012-1622.

★507★ DEVELOPMENTAL NEUROPSYCHOLOGY
Lawrence Erlbaum Associates, Inc.
365 Broadway
Hillsdale, NJ 07642   Phone: (201) 666-4110
Frequency: Quarterly.

★508★ DEVELOPMENTAL NEUROSCIENCE
S. Karger Publishers, Inc.
26 W. Avon Rd.
PO Box 529
Farmington, CT 06085   Phone: (203) 675-7834
First Published: 1979. **Frequency:** Bimonthly. **ISSN:** 0378-5866.

★509★ DEVELOPMENTAL PHARMACOLOGY AND THERAPEUTICS
S. Karger Publishers, Inc.
26 W. Avon Rd.
PO Box 529
Farmington, CT 06085   Phone: (203) 675-7834
First Published: 1980. **Frequency:** 8/yr. **ISSN:** 0379-8305.

★510★ DEVELOPMENTAL PSYCHOBIOLOGY
John Wiley & Sons, Inc.
605 3rd Ave.
New York, NY 10158   Phone: (212) 850-6000
First Published: 1967. **Frequency:** 8/yr. **ISSN:** 0012-1630.

★511★ DIABETES
American Diabetes Association
1660 Duke St.
PO Box 25757
Alexandria, VA 22313   Phone: (703) 549-1500
First Published: 1952. **Frequency:** Monthly. **ISSN:** 0012-1797.

★512★ DIABETES CARE
American Diabetes Association
1660 Duke St.
PO Box 25757
Alexandria, VA 22313   Phone: (703) 549-1500
First Published: 1978. **Frequency:** 10/yr. **ISSN:** 0149-5992.

★513★ DIABETES EDUCATOR JOURNAL
American Association of Diabetes Educators
500 N. Michigan Ave., Ste. 1400
Chicago, IL 60611   Phone: (312) 661-1700
First Published: 1975. **Frequency:** Bimonthly. **ISSN:** 0145-7217.

★514★ DIABETES RESEARCH AND CLINICAL PRACTICE
Elsevier Science Publishing Co., Inc.
655 Avenue of the Americas
New York, NY 10010   Phone: (212) 989-5800
Frequency: 9/yr. **ISSN:** 0168-8227.

★515★ DIABETIC MEDICINE
John Wiley & Sons, Inc.
605 3rd Ave.
New York, NY 10158   Phone: (212) 850-6000
First Published: 1984. Frequency: 10/yr. ISSN: 0742-3071.

★516★ DIABETOLOGIA
Springer-Verlag New York, Inc.
175 5th Ave.
New York, NY 10010   Phone: (212) 460-1500
First Published: 1965. Frequency: Monthly. ISSN: 0012-186X.

★517★ DIAGNOSTIC CYTOPATHOLOGY
John Wiley & Sons, Inc.
605 3rd Ave.
New York, NY 10158   Phone: (212) 850-6000
First Published: 1985. Frequency: Quarterly. ISSN: 8755-1039.

★518★ DIAGNOSTIC MICROBIOLOGY AND INFECTIOUS
DISEASE
Elsevier Science Publishing Co., Inc.
655 Avenue of the Americas
New York, NY 10010   Phone: (212) 989-5800
First Published: 1983. Frequency: 6/yr. ISSN: 0732-8893.

★519★ DIAGNOSTIC MOLECULAR PATHOLOGY
Raven Press
1185 Avenue of the Americas
New York, NY 10036   Phone: (212) 930-9500
First Published: 1992. Frequency: Quarterly. ISSN: 1052-9551.

★520★ DIAGNOSTIC ONCOLOGY
S. Karger Publishers, Inc.
26 W. Avon Rd.
PO Box 529
Farmington, CT 06085   Phone: (203) 675-7834
First Published: 1991. Frequency: Bimonthly. ISSN: 1013-8129.

★521★ DIAGNOSTICS AND CLINICAL TESTING
Nature Publishing Co.
65 Bleeker St.
New York, NY 10012   Phone: (212) 477-9600
First Published: 1963. Frequency: Monthly.

★522★ DIALYSIS AND TRANSPLANTATION
Creative Age Publications
7628 Densmore Ave.
Van Nuys, CA 91406   Phone: (818) 782-7328
First Published: 1972. Frequency: Monthly. ISSN: 0090-2934.

★523★ DICP: THE ANNALS OF PHARMACOTHERAPY
Harvey Whitney Books Co.
c/o Harvey A.K. Whitney, Jr.
PO Box 42696
Cincinnati, OH 45242   Phone: (513) 793-3555
First Published: 1967. Frequency: Monthly. ISSN: 1042-9611.

★524★ DIGESTION
S. Karger Publishers, Inc.
26 W. Avon Rd.
PO Box 529
Farmington, CT 06085   Phone: (203) 675-7834
First Published: 1968. Frequency: 12/yr. ISSN: 0012-2823.

★525★ DIGESTIVE DISEASES
S. Karger Publishers, Inc.
26 W. Avon Rd.
PO Box 529
Farmington, CT 06085   Phone: (212) 675-7834
Frequency: 6/yr. ISSN: 0257-2753.

★526★ DIGESTIVE DISEASES AND SCIENCES
Plenum Publishing Corp.
233 Spring St.
New York, NY 10013   Phone: (212) 620-8000
First Published: 1934. Frequency: Monthly. ISSN: 0163-2116.

★527★ DIGESTIVE SURGERY
S. Karger Publishers, Inc.
26 W. Avon Rd.
PO Box 529
Farmington, CT 06085   Phone: (203) 675-7834
Frequency: 6/yr. ISSN: 0253-4886.

★528★ DIMENSIONS IN HEALTH SERVICE
Canadian Hospital Association
17 York St., Ste. 100
Ottawa, ON, Canada K1N 9J6   Phone: (613) 238-8005
First Published: 1924. Frequency: 8/yr. ISSN: 0317-7645.

★529★ DISEASE MARKERS
John Wiley & Sons, Inc.
605 3rd Ave.
New York, NY 10158   Phone: (212) 850-6000
First Published: 1982. Frequency: Bimonthly. ISSN: 0278-0240.

★530★ DISEASES OF THE COLON AND RECTUM
American Society of Colon and Rectal Surgeons
800 E. Northwest Hwy., Ste. 1080
Palatine, IL 60067   Phone: (708) 359-9184
First Published: 1958. Frequency: Monthly. ISSN: 0012-3706.

★531★ DNA
Mary Ann Liebert, Inc.
1651 3rd Ave.
New York, NY 10128   Phone: (212) 289-2300
First Published: 1981. Frequency: 10/yr. ISSN: 0198-0238.

★532★ DRUG AND ALCOHOL DEPENDENCE
Elsevier Science Publishing Co., Inc.
655 Avenue of the Americas
New York, NY 10010   Phone: (212) 989-5800
First Published: 1975. Frequency: 6/yr. ISSN: 0376-8716.

★533★ DRUG AND CHEMICAL TOXICOLOGY
Marcel Dekker, Inc.
270 Madison Ave.
New York, NY 10016   Phone: (212) 696-9000
First Published: 1978. Frequency: 4/yr. ISSN: 0148-0545.

★534★ DRUG AND COSMETIC INDUSTRY
Harcourt Brace Jovanovich, Inc.
7500 Old Oak Blvd.
Cleveland, OH 44130   Phone: (216) 243-8100
First Published: 1914. Frequency: Monthly. ISSN: 0012-6527.

★535★ DRUG DEVELOPMENT RESEARCH
John Wiley & Sons, Inc.
605 3rd Ave.
New York, NY 10158   Phone: (212) 850-6000
First Published: 1981. Frequency: Monthly. ISSN: 0272-4391.

★536★ DREAMING: THE JOURNAL OF THE ASSOCIATION
FOR THE STUDY OF DREAMS
Human Sciences Press, Inc.
233 Spring St.
New York, NY 10013   Phone: (212) 620-8000
Frequency: Quarterly.

★537★ DRUG METABOLISM AND DISPOSITION
American Society for Pharmacology and Experimental Therapeutics
9650 Rockville Pike
Bethesda, MD 20814   Phone: (301) 530-7060
First Published: 1973. Frequency: Bimonthly. ISSN: 0090-9556.

★538★ DRUG TARGETING AND DELIVERY
Academic Press, Inc.
1250 6th Ave.
San Diego, CA 92101   Phone: (619) 231-0926
First Published: 1992. Frequency: Semiannual. ISSN: 1058-241X.

★539★ DRUG AND THERAPEUTICS BULLETIN
Consumers' Association
2 Marylebone St.
London NW1 4DX, England
First Published: 1963. Frequency: Biweekly. ISSN: 0012-6543.

★540★ DRUG THERAPY
Core Medical Journals
3131 Princeton Pike, Bldg. 2A
Lawrenceville, NJ 08648   Phone: (609) 896-9450
First Published: 1971. Frequency: Monthly. ISSN: 0001-7094.

★541★ DRUGS AND SOCIETY
The Haworth Press, Inc.
10 Alice St.
Binghamton, NY 13904   Phone: (800) 342-9678
Frequency: Quarterly.

★542★ DYSMORPHOLOGY AND CLINICAL GENETICS
Blackwell Scientific Publications
3 Cambridge Center, Ste. 208
Cambridge, MA 02142   Phone: (617) 225-0401
Frequency: Quarterly. ISSN: 0893-6633.

★543★ DYSPHAGIA
Springer-Verlag New York, Inc.
175 5th Ave.
New York, NY 10010   Phone: (212) 460-1500
First Published: 1986. Frequency: Quarterly. ISSN: 0179-051X.

★544★ EAR AND HEARING
Williams & Wilkins
428 E. Preston St.
Baltimore, MD 21202   Phone: (301) 528-4223
First Published: 1975. Frequency: Bimonthly. ISSN: 0196-0202.

★545★ EAR, NOSE, AND THROAT JOURNAL
Little, Brown, and Co.
34 Beacon St.
Boston, MA 02108   Phone: (617) 859-5500
First Published: 1922. Frequency: Monthly. ISSN: 0145-5613.

★546★ EARLY HUMAN DEVELOPMENT
Elsevier Science Publishing Co., Inc.
655 Avenue of the Americas
New York, NY 10010   Phone: (212) 989-5800
First Published: 1977. Frequency: 6/yr. ISSN: 0378-3782.

★547★ ECOTOXICOLOGY AND ENVIRONMENTAL SAFETY
Academic Press, Inc.
1250 6th Ave.
San Diego, CA 92101   Phone: (619) 231-0926
First Published: 1977. Frequency: Bimonthly. ISSN: 0147-6513.

**★548★ EINSTEIN QUARTERLY JOURNAL OF BIOLOGY AND
MEDICINE**
Springer-Verlag New York, Inc.
175 5th Ave.
New York, NY 10010   Phone: (212) 460-1500
First Published: 1982. Frequency: Quarterly. ISSN: 0724-6706.

**★549★ ELECTROENCEPHALOGRAPHY AND CLINICAL
NEUROPHYSIOLOGY**
Elsevier Science Publishing Co., Inc.
655 Avenue of the Americas
New York, NY 10010   Phone: (212) 989-5800
First Published: 1949. Frequency: 18/yr. ISSN: 0013-4694.

★550★ EMBO JOURNAL
IRL Press, Inc.
PO Box Q
McLean, VA 22101   Phone: (703) 437-3334
First Published: 1982. Frequency: 13/yr. ISSN: 0261-4189.

★551★ EMERGENCY
Hare Publications
PO Box 159
Carlsbad, CA 92008   Phone: (619) 438-2511
First Published: 1969. Frequency: Monthly. ISSN: 0162-5942.

★552★ EMERGENCY CARE QUARTERLY
Aspen Publishers, Inc.
200 Orchard Ridge Dr.
Gaithersburg, MD 20878   Phone: (301) 417-7500
First Published: 1985. Frequency: Quarterly. ISSN: 8755-8467.

★553★ EMERGENCY MEDICAL SERVICES
Creative Age Publications
7628 Densmore Ave.
Van Nuys, CA 91406   Phone: (818) 782-7328
First Published: 1972. Frequency: 11/yr. ISSN: 0094-6575.

★554★ EMERGENCY MEDICINE
Cahners Publishing Co.
249 W. 17th St.
New York, NY 10011   Phone: (212) 645-0067
First Published: 1969. Frequency: 21/yr. ISSN: 0013-6654.

★555★ ENDOCRINE PATHOLOGY
Blackwell Scientific Publications
3 Cambridge Center, Ste. 208
Cambridge, MA 02142   Phone: (617) 225-0401
Frequency: Quarterly. ISSN: 1046-3976.

★556★ ENDOCRINE RESEARCH
Marcel Dekker, Inc.
270 Madison Ave.
New York, NY 10016   Phone: (212) 696-9000
First Published: 1964. Frequency: Quarterly. ISSN: 0743-5800.

★557★ ENDOCRINOLOGY
Endocrine Society
9650 Rockville Pike
Bethesda, MD 20814   Phone: (301) 571-1802
First Published: 1917. Frequency: Monthly. ISSN: 0013-7227.

★558★ ENVIRONMENTAL HEALTH PERSPECTIVES
National Institute of Environmental Health Sciences
U.S. Department of Health and Human Services
PO Box 12233
Research Triangle Park, NC 27709   Phone: (919) 541-3406
First Published: 1972. Frequency: Bimonthly. ISSN: 0091-6765.

★559★ ENVIRONMENTAL AND MOLECULAR MUTAGENESIS
Environmental Mutagen Society
c/o Oak Ridge National Laboratory
PO Box 2008
Oak Ridge, TN 37831   Phone: (615) 574-7871
First Published: 1979. Frequency: 8/yr. ISSN: 0893-6692.

★560★ ENVIRONMENTAL RESEARCH
Academic Press, Inc.
1250 6th Ave.
San Diego, CA 92101   Phone: (619) 231-0926
First Published: 1967. Frequency: Bimonthly. ISSN: 0013-9351.

★561★ ENZYME
S. Karger Publishers, Inc.
26 W. Avon Rd.
PO Box 529
Farmington, CT 06085   Phone: (203) 675-7834
First Published: 1961. Frequency: 8/yr. ISSN: 0013-9432.

★562★ EPIDEMIOLOGY AND INFECTION
Cambridge University Press
40 W. 20th St.
New York, NY 10011   Phone: (212) 924-3900
First Published: 1901. Frequency: Bimonthly. ISSN: 0950-2688.

★563★ EPILEPSIA
Raven Press
1185 Avenue of the Americas
New York, NY 10036   Phone: (212) 930-9500
First Published: 1959. Frequency: Bimonthly. ISSN: 0013-9580.

★564★ EUROPEAN ARCHIVES OF PSYCHIATRY AND
NEUROLOGICAL SCIENCES
Springer-Verlag New York, Inc.
175 5th Ave.
New York, NY 10010   Phone: (212) 460-1500
First Published: 1868. Frequency: Bimonthly. ISSN: 0175-758X.

★565★ EUROPEAN HEART JOURNAL
Academic Press, Inc.
1250 6th Ave.
San Diego, CA 92101   Phone: (619) 231-0926
First Published: 1980. Frequency: Monthly. ISSN: 0195-668X.

★566★ EUROPEAN JOURNAL OF ANAESTHESIOLOGY
Blackwell Scientific Publications
3 Cambridge Center, Ste. 208
Cambridge, MA 02142   Phone: (617) 225-0401
Frequency: 6/yr. ISSN: 0265-0215.

★567★ EUROPEAN JOURNAL OF APPLIED PHYSIOLOGY
AND OCCUPATIONAL PHYSIOLOGY
Springer-Verlag New York, Inc.
175 5th Ave.
New York, NY 10010   Phone: (212) 460-1500
Frequency: 6/yr. ISSN: 0301-5548.

★568★ EUROPEAN JOURNAL OF BIOCHEMISTRY
Springer-Verlag New York, Inc.
175 5th Ave.
New York, NY 10010   Phone: (212) 460-1500
First Published: 1967. Frequency: 24/yr. ISSN: 0014-2956.

★569★ EUROPEAN JOURNAL OF CANCER CARE
Blackwell Scientific Publications
3 Cambridge Center, Ste. 208
Cambridge, MA 02142   Phone: (617) 225-0401
Frequency: 5/yr. ISSN: 0961-5423.

★570★ EUROPEAN JOURNAL OF CANCER AND CLINICAL
ONCOLOGY
Pergamon Press, Inc.
Maxwell House, Fairview Park
Elmsford, NY 10523   Phone: (914) 592-7700
First Published: 1965. Frequency: Monthly. ISSN: 0277-5379.

★571★ EUROPEAN JOURNAL OF CARDIOTHORACIC
SURGERY
Springer-Verlag New York, Inc.
175 5th Ave.
New York, NY 10010   Phone: (212) 460-1500
First Published: 1987. Frequency: Monthly. ISSN: 1010-7940.

★572★ EUROPEAN JOURNAL OF CHIROPRACTIC
Blackwell Scientific Publications
3 Cambridge Center, Ste. 208
Cambridge, MA 02142   Phone: (617) 225-0401
First Published: 1953. Frequency: Quarterly. ISSN: 0263-9114.

★573★ EUROPEAN JOURNAL OF CLINICAL INVESTIGATION
Blackwell Scientific Publications
3 Cambridge Center, Ste. 208
Cambridge, MA 02142   Phone: (617) 225-0401
First Published: 1971. Frequency: Bimonthly. ISSN: 0014-2972.

★574★ EUROPEAN JOURNAL OF CLINICAL
PHARMACOLOGY
Springer-Verlag New York, Inc.
175 5th Ave.
New York, NY 10010   Phone: (212) 460-1500
First Published: 1968. Frequency: Monthly. ISSN: 0031-6970.

★575★ EUROPEAN JOURNAL OF GASTROENTEROLOGY
AND HEPATOLOGY
Current Science
20 N. 3rd St.
Philadelphia, PA 19106   Phone: (215) 514-2266
Frequency: Monthly. ISSN: 0954-691X.

★576★ EUROPEAN JOURNAL OF HAEMATOLOGY
Munksgaard
Noerre Soegade 35
DK-1370 Copenhagen K, Denmark
First Published: 1964. Frequency: 10/yr. ISSN: 0902-4441.

★577★ EUROPEAN JOURNAL OF IMMUNOLOGY
VCH Publishers, Inc.
220 E. 23rd St.
New York, NY 10010
First Published: 1970. Frequency: Monthly. ISSN: 0014-2980.

★578★ EUROPEAN JOURNAL OF IMPLANT AND
REFRACTIVE SURGERY
Academic Press, Inc.
1250 6th Ave.
San Diego, CA 92101   Phone: (619) 231-0926
First Published: 1989. Frequency: Quarterly. ISSN: 0955-3681.

★579★ EUROPEAN JOURNAL OF NUCLEAR MEDICINE
Springer-Verlag New York, Inc.
175 5th Ave.
New York, NY 10010   Phone: (212) 460-1500
First Published: 1976. Frequency: Monthly. ISSN: 0340-6997.

★580★ EUROPEAN JOURNAL OF OBSTETRICS,
GYNECOLOGY, AND REPRODUCTIVE BIOLOGY
Elsevier Science Publishing Co., Inc.
655 Avenue of the Americas
New York, NY 10010   Phone: (212) 989-5800
Frequency: Monthly. ISSN: 0301-2115.

★581★ EUROPEAN JOURNAL OF ORTHODONTICS
Oxford University Press
Pinkhill House
Southfield Rd.
Eynsham, Oxford OX8 1JJ, England
First Published: 1979. Frequency: Quarterly. ISSN: 0141-5387.

★582★ EUROPEAN JOURNAL OF PEDIATRICS
Springer-Verlag New York, Inc.
175 5th Ave.
New York, NY 10010   Phone: (212) 460-1500
First Published: 1910. Frequency: 12/yr. ISSN: 0340-6199.

★583★ EUROPEAN JOURNAL OF PHARMACOLOGY
Elsevier Science Publishing Co., Inc.
655 Avenue of the Americas
New York, NY 10010   Phone: (212) 989-5800
First Published: 1967. Frequency: Weekly. ISSN: 0014-2999.

★584★ EUROPEAN JOURNAL OF PLASTIC SURGERY
Springer-Verlag New York, Inc.
175 5th Ave.
New York, NY 10010   Phone: (212) 460-1500
First Published: 1971. Frequency: 6/yr. ISSN: 0930-343X.

★585★ EUROPEAN JOURNAL OF RADIOLOGY
Elsevier Science Publishing Co., Inc.
655 Avenue of the Americas
New York, NY 10010   Phone: (212) 989-5800
First Published: 1980. Frequency: Quarterly. ISSN: 0720-048X.

★586★ EUROPEAN JOURNAL OF SURGICAL ONCOLOGY
Academic Press, Inc.
1250 6th Ave.
San Diego, CA 92101   Phone: (619) 231-0926
First Published: 1975. Frequency: 6/yr. ISSN: 0748-7983.

Medical and Health Information Directory, 1992-93

★587★ EUROPEAN JOURNAL OF VASCULAR SURGERY
Grune & Stratton, Inc.
6277 Sea Harbor Dr.
Orlando, FL 32886   Phone: (407) 345-4200
First Published: 1987. **Frequency:** Bimonthly. **ISSN:** 0950-821X.

★588★ EUROPEAN NEUROLOGY
S. Karger Publishers, Inc.
26 W. Avon Rd.
PO Box 529
Farmington, CT 06085   Phone: (203) 675-7834
First Published: 1968. **Frequency:** Bimonthly. **ISSN:** 0014-3022.

★589★ EUROPEAN RESPIRATORY JOURNAL
Munksgaard
Noerre Soegade 35
DK-1370 Copenhagen K, Denmark
First Published: 1924. **Frequency:** 10/yr. **ISSN:** 0903-1936.

★590★ EUROPEAN SURGICAL RESEARCH
S. Karger Publishers, Inc.
26 W. Avon Rd.
PO Box 529
Farmington, CT 06085   Phone: (203) 675-7834
First Published: 1969. **Frequency:** Bimonthly. **ISSN:** 0014-312X.

★591★ EUROPEAN UROLOGY
S. Karger Publishers, Inc.
26 W. Avon Rd.
PO Box 529
Farmington, CT 06085   Phone: (203) 675-7834
First Published: 1975. **Frequency:** 8/yr. **ISSN:** 0302-2838.

★592★ EVALUATION AND THE HEALTH PROFESSIONS
Sage Publications
2111 W. Hillcrest Dr.
Newbury Park, CA 91320   Phone: (805) 499-0721
First Published: 1978. **Frequency:** Quarterly. **ISSN:** 0163-2787.

★593★ EXCEPTIONAL CHILDREN
Council for Exceptional Children
1920 Association Dr.
Reston, VA 22091   Phone: (703) 620-3660
First Published: 1934. **Frequency:** Bimonthly. **ISSN:** 0014-4029.

★594★ EXPERIMENTAL AGING RESEARCH
Beech Hill Enterprises, Inc.
PO Box 136
Southwest Harbor, ME 04679   Phone: (207) 244-3931
First Published: 1975. **Frequency:** Quarterly. **ISSN:** 0361-073X.

★595★ EXPERIMENTAL BRAIN RESEARCH
Springer-Verlag New York, Inc.
175 5th Ave.
New York, NY 10010   Phone: (212) 460-1500
First Published: 1965. **Frequency:** 15/yr. **ISSN:** 0014-4819.

★596★ EXPERIMENTAL CELL RESEARCH
Academic Press, Inc.
1250 6th Ave.
San Diego, CA 92101   Phone: (619) 231-0926
First Published: 1950. **Frequency:** Monthly. **ISSN:** 0014-4827.

★597★ EXPERIMENTAL AND CLINICAL GASTROENTEROLOGY
Pergamon Press, Inc.
395 Saw Mill River Rd.
Elmsford, NY 10523   Phone: (914) 592-7700
Frequency: Quarterly. **ISSN:** 0353-9245.

★598★ EXPERIMENTAL AND CLINICAL IMMUNOGENETICS
S. Karger Publishers, Inc.
26 W. Avon Rd.
PO Box 529
Farmington, CT 06085   Phone: (203) 675-7834
First Published: 1984. **Frequency:** 4/yr. **ISSN:** 0254-9670.

★599★ EXPERIMENTAL EYE RESEARCH
Academic Press, Inc.
1250 6th Ave.
San Diego, CA 92101   Phone: (619) 231-0926
First Published: 1961. **Frequency:** Monthly. **ISSN:** 0014-4835.

★600★ EXPERIMENTAL GERONTOLOGY
Pergamon Press, Inc.
Maxwell House, Fairview Park
Elmsford, NY 10523   Phone: (914) 592-7700
First Published: 1965. **Frequency:** Bimonthly. **ISSN:** 0531-5565.

★601★ EXPERIMENTAL HEMATOLOGY
Springer-Verlag New York, Inc.
175 5th Ave.
New York, NY 10010   Phone: (212) 460-1500
First Published: 1973. **Frequency:** 11/yr. **ISSN:** 0301-472X.

★602★ EXPERIMENTAL LUNG RESEARCH
Hemisphere Publishing Corp.
1900 Frost Rd., Ste. 101
Bristol, PA 19007   Phone: (215) 785-5800
First Published: 1979. **Frequency:** Bimonthly. **ISSN:** 0190-2148.

★603★ EXPERIMENTAL AND MOLECULAR PATHOLOGY
Academic Press, Inc.
1250 6th Ave.
San Diego, CA 92101   Phone: (619) 231-0926
First Published: 1962. **Frequency:** Bimonthly. **ISSN:** 0014-4800.

★604★ EXPERIMENTAL NEUROLOGY
Academic Press, Inc.
1250 6th Ave.
San Diego, CA 92101   Phone: (619) 231-0926
First Published: 1959. **Frequency:** Monthly. **ISSN:** 0014-4886.

★605★ EXPERIMENTAL PARASITOLOGY
Academic Press, Inc.
1250 6th Ave.
San Diego, CA 92101   Phone: (619) 231-0926
First Published: 1952. **Frequency:** 8/yr. **ISSN:** 0014-4894.

★606★ EXPERIMENTAL PATHOLOGY
VEB Gustav Fischer Verlag
Villengang 2
Postfach 176
6900 Jena, Germany
First Published: 1967. **Frequency:** Irregular. **ISSN:** 0232-1513.

★607★ EXPERIMENTAL PHYSIOLOGY
Cambridge University Press
40 W. 20th St.
New York, NY 10011   Phone: (212) 924-3900
First Published: 1908. **Frequency:** Bimonthly.

★608★ FAHS REVIEW
Federation of American Health Systems
1405 N. Pierce, Ste. 311
Little Rock, AR 72207   Phone: (501) 661-9555
First Published: 1967. **Frequency:** Bimonthly. **ISSN:** 0148-9496.

★609★ FAMILY AND COMMUNITY HEALTH
Aspen Publishers, Inc.
200 Orchard Ridge Dr.
Gaithersburg, MD 20878   Phone: (301) 417-7500
First Published: 1978. **Frequency:** Quarterly. **ISSN:** 0160-6379.

★610★ FAMILY PLANNING PERSPECTIVES
Alan Guttmacher Institute
111 5th Ave.
New York, NY 10003   Phone: (212) 254-5656
First Published: 1969. **Frequency:** Bimonthly. **ISSN:** 0014-7354.

★611★ FAMILY PRACTICE RESEARCH JOURNAL
Human Sciences Press, Inc.
233 Spring St.
New York, NY 10013   Phone: (212) 620-8000
Frequency: Quarterly.

★612★ FAMILY PROCESS
Family Process, Inc.
841 Broadway, Ste. 504
New York, NY 10003   Phone: (212) 505-6517
First Published: 1962. **Frequency:** Quarterly. **ISSN:** 0014-7370.

★613★ FDA CONSUMER
U.S. Food and Drug Administration
Office of Public Affairs
5600 Fishers Ln.
Rockville, MD 20857   Phone: (301) 443-3220
First Published: 1967. **Frequency:** Monthly. **ISSN:** 0362-1332.

★614★ FDA DRUG BULLETIN
U.S. Food and Drug Administration
5600 Fishers Ln.
Rockville, MD 20857   Phone: (301) 443-3220
First Published: 1970. **Frequency:** Irregular. **ISSN:** 0361-4344.

★615★ FEBS LETTERS
Elsevier Science Publishing Co., Inc.
655 Avenue of the Americas
New York, NY 10010   Phone: (212) 989-5800
First Published: 1968. **Frequency:** 36/yr. **ISSN:** 0014-5793.

★616★ FEMALE PATIENT
PW Communications, Inc.
400 Plaza Dr.
Secaucus, NJ 07094   Phone: (201) 865-7500
First Published: 1976. **Frequency:** Monthly. **ISSN:** 0364-1198.

★617★ FERTILITY AND STERILITY
American Fertility Society
2140 11th Ave., S., Ste. 200
Birmingham, AL 35205   Phone: (205) 933-8494
First Published: 1949. **Frequency:** Monthly. **ISSN:** 0015-0282.

★618★ FETAL DIAGNOSIS AND THERAPY
S. Karger Publishers, Inc.
26 W. Avon Rd.
PO Box 529
Farmington, CT 06085   Phone: (203) 675-7834
First Published: 1986. **Frequency:** 4/yr. **ISSN:** 0257-2788.

★619★ FIBRINOLYSIS
Churchill Livingstone, Inc.
1560 Broadway
New York, NY 10036   Phone: (212) 819-5400
First Published: 1987. **Frequency:** Quarterly. **ISSN:** 0268-9499.

★620★ FOCUS ON CRITICAL CARE
American Association of Critical-Care Nurses
1 Civic Plaza
Newport Beach, CA 92660   Phone: (714) 644-9310
First Published: 1973. **Frequency:** Bimonthly. **ISSN:** 0736-3605.

★621★ FOLIA BIOLOGICA
Academic Press, Inc.
1250 6th Ave.
San Diego, CA 92101   Phone: (619) 231-0926
Frequency: Bimonthly. **ISSN:** 0015-5500.

★622★ FOLIA MICROBIOLOGICA
Academic Press, Inc.
1250 6th Ave.
San Diego, CA 92101   Phone: (619) 231-0926
Frequency: Bimonthly. **ISSN:** 0015-5632.

★623★ FOLIA PHONIATRICA
S. Karger Publishers, Inc.
26 W. Avon Rd.
PO Box 529
Farmington, CT 06085   Phone: (203) 675-7834
First Published: 1947. **Frequency:** Bimonthly. **ISSN:** 0015-5705.

★624★ FOOD AND CHEMICAL TOXICOLOGY
Pergamon Press, Inc.
Maxwell House, Fairview Park
Elmsford, NY 10523   Phone: (914) 592-7700
First Published: 1963. **Frequency:** Monthly. **ISSN:** 0278-6915.

★625★ FOOD AND NUTRITION
U.S. Department of Agriculture
Food and Nutrition Service
Alexandria, VA 22302   Phone: (202) 447-8046
First Published: 1971. **Frequency:** Quarterly. **ISSN:** 0046-4384.

★626★ THE FOOT
Churchill Livingstone, Inc.
1560 Broadway
New York, NY 10036   Phone: (212) 819-5400
First Published: 1991. **Frequency:** Quarterly. **ISSN:** 0958-2592.

★627★ FOOT AND ANKLE
American Orthopedic Foot and Ankle Society
222 S. Prospect Ave.
Park Ridge, IL 60068   Phone: (312) 698-1626
First Published: 1980. **Frequency:** Bimonthly. **ISSN:** 0198-0211.

★628★ FORENSIC REPORTS
Hemisphere Publishing Corp.
1900 Frost Rd., Ste. 101
Bristol, PA 19007   Phone: (212) 785-5800
First Published: 1987. **Frequency:** Quarterly. **ISSN:** 0888-692X.

★629★ FORENSIC SCIENCE INTERNATIONAL
Elsevier Science Publishing Co., Inc.
655 Avenue of the Americas
New York, NY 10010   Phone: (212) 989-5800
First Published: 1972. **Frequency:** 12/yr. **ISSN:** 0379-0738.

★630★ FREE RADICAL BIOLOGY AND MEDICINE
Pergamon Press, Inc.
Maxwell House, Fairview Park
Elmsford, NY 10523   Phone: (914) 592-7700
First Published: 1985. **Frequency:** 12/yr. **ISSN:** 0891-5849.

★631★ FRONTIERS OF HEALTH SERVICES MANAGEMENT
Health Administration Press
1021 E. Huron St.
Ann Arbor, MI 48104-9990   Phone: (313) 764-1380
First Published: 1984. **Frequency:** Quarterly. **ISSN:** 0748-8157.

★632★ FUNDAMENTAL AND APPLIED TOXICOLOGY
Academic Press, Inc.
1250 6th Ave.
San Diego, CA 92101   Phone: (619) 231-0926
First Published: 1980. **Frequency:** 8/yr. **ISSN:** 0272-0590.

★633★ GASTROENTEROLOGY
American Gastroenterological Association
6900 Grove Rd.
Thorofare, NJ 08086   Phone: (609) 848-1000
First Published: 1943. **Frequency:** Monthly. **ISSN:** 0016-5085.

★634★ GASTROENTEROLOGY NURSING
Williams & Wilkins
428 E. Preston St.
Baltimore, MD 21202   Phone: (301) 528-4000
Frequency: Quarterly. **ISSN:** 1042-895X.

★635★ GASTROINTESTINAL ENDOSCOPY
American Society for Gastrointestinal Endoscopy
13 Elm St.
PO Box 1565
Manchester, MA 01944   Phone: (508) 526-8330
First Published: 1953. **Frequency:** Bimonthly. **ISSN:** 0016-5107.

★636★ GASTROINTESTINAL RADIOLOGY
Springer-Verlag New York, Inc.
175 5th Ave.
New York, NY 10010   Phone: (212) 460-1500
First Published: 1976. **Frequency:** Quarterly. **ISSN:** 0364-2356.

★637★ GENE
Elsevier Science Publishing Co., Inc.
655 Avenue of the Americas
New York, NY 10010   Phone: (212) 989-5800
First Published: 1977. **Frequency:** 30/yr. **ISSN:** 0378-1119.

★638★ GENERAL AND COMPARATIVE ENDOCRINOLOGY
Academic Press, Inc.
1250 6th Ave.
San Diego, CA 92101   Phone: (619) 231-0926
First Published: 1961. **Frequency:** Monthly. **ISSN:** 0016-6480.

★639★ GENERAL HOSPITAL PSYCHIATRY
Elsevier Science Publishing Co., Inc.
655 Avenue of the Americas
New York, NY 10010   Phone: (212) 989-5800
First Published: 1979. **Frequency:** 6/yr. **ISSN:** 0163-8343.

★640★ GENERAL PHARMACOLOGY
Pergamon Press, Inc.
Maxwell House, Fairview Park
Elmsford, NY 10523   Phone: (914) 592-7700
First Published: 1970. **Frequency:** Bimonthly. **ISSN:** 0306-3623.

★641★ GENETIC EPIDEMIOLOGY
John Wiley & Sons, Inc.
605 3rd Ave.
New York, NY 10158   Phone: (212) 850-6000
Frequency: 6/yr. **ISSN:** 0741-0395.

★642★ GENETICAL RESEARCH
Cambridge University Press
20 W/ 20th St.
New York, NY 10011   Phone: (212) 924-3900
First Published: 1960. **Frequency:** Bimonthly. **ISSN:** 0016-6723.

★643★ GENETICS
Genetics Society of America
9650 Rockville Pike
Bethesda, MD 20814   Phone: (301) 571-1825
First Published: 1916. **Frequency:** Monthly. **ISSN:** 0016-6731.

★644★ GENITOURINARY MEDICINE
British Medical Association
PO Box 560B
Kennebunkport, ME 04046
Frequency: Bimonthly.

★645★ GENOME
Genetics Society of Canada
National Research Council of Canada
Ottawa, ON, Canada K1A 0R6   Phone: (613) 993-2054
First Published: 1959. **Frequency:** Bimonthly. **ISSN:** 0831-2796.

★646★ GENOMICS
Academic Press, Inc.
1250 6th Ave.
San Diego, CA 92101   Phone: (619) 231-0926
First Published: 1987. **Frequency:** Monthly. **ISSN:** 0888-7543.

★647★ GERIATRICS
Edgell Communications
1 E. 1st St.
Duluth, MN 55802   Phone: (216) 826-2839
First Published: 1946. **Frequency:** Monthly. **ISSN:** 0016-867X.

★648★ THE GERONTOLOGIST
Gerontological Society of America
1275 K St., NW, Ste. 350
Washington, DC 20005   Phone: (202) 842-1275
First Published: 1961. **Frequency:** Bimonthly. **ISSN:** 0016-9013.

★649★ GERONTOLOGY
S. Karger Publishers, Inc.
26 W. Avon Rd.
PO Box 529
Farmington, CT 06085   Phone: (203) 675-7834
First Published: 1957. **Frequency:** Bimonthly. **ISSN:** 0304-324X.

★650★ GERONTOLOGY AND GERIATRICS EDUCATION
The Haworth Press, Inc.
10 Alice St.
Binghamton, NY 13904   Phone: (800) 342-9678
First Published: 1981. **Frequency:** Quarterly. **ISSN:** 0270-1960.

★651★ GROUP PRACTICE JOURNAL
American Group Practice Association
1422 Duke St.
Alexandria, VA 22314   Phone: (703) 838-0033
First Published: 1951. **Frequency:** Bimonthly. **ISSN:** 0199-5103.

★652★ GROWTH REGULATION
Churchill Livingstone, Inc.
1560 Broadway
New York, NY 10036   Phone: (212) 819-5400
First Published: 1991. **Frequency:** Quarterly. **ISSN:** 0956-523X.

★653★ GULLET
Churchill Livingstone, Inc.
1560 Broadway
New York, NY 10036   Phone: (212) 819-5400
Frequency: August. **ISSN:** 0952-0643.

★654★ GUT
British Medical Association
PO Box 560B
Kennebunkport, ME 04046
First Published: 1960. **Frequency:** Monthly. **ISSN:** 0017-5749.

★655★ GYNAECOLOGICAL ENDOSCOPY
Blackwell Scientific Publications
3 Cambridge Center, Ste. 208
Cambridge, MA 02142   Phone: (617) 225-0401
First Published: 1992. **Frequency:** Quarterly. **ISSN:** 0962-1091.

★656★ GYNECOLOGIC AND OBSTETRIC INVESTIGATION
S. Karger Publishers, Inc.
26 W. Avon Rd.
PO Box 529
Farmington, CT 06085   Phone: (203) 675-7834
First Published: 1895. **Frequency:** 8/yr. **ISSN:** 0368-7346.

★657★ GYNECOLOGIC ONCOLOGY
Academic Press, Inc.
1250 6th Ave.
San Diego, CA 92101   Phone: (619) 231-0926
First Published: 1973. **Frequency:** Monthly. **ISSN:** 0090-8258.

★658★ HAEMOSTASIS
S. Karger Publishers, Inc.
26 W. Avon Rd.
PO Box 529
Farmington, CT 06085   Phone: (203) 675-7834
First Published: 1973. **Frequency:** Bimonthly. **ISSN:** 0301-0147.

★659★ HASTINGS CENTER REPORT
Hastings Center
255 Elm Rd.
Briarcliff Manor, NY 10510   Phone: (914) 478-0500
First Published: 1971. **Frequency:** Bimonthly. **ISSN:** 0093-0334.

★660★ HAWAII MEDICAL JOURNAL
Hawaii Medical Association
1360 S. Beretania St., 2nd Fl.
Honolulu, HI 96817   Phone: (808) 536-7702
First Published: 1941. **Frequency:** Monthly. **ISSN:** 0017-8594.

★661★ HEAD AND NECK SURGERY
John Wiley & Sons, Inc.
605 3rd Ave.
New York, NY 10158   Phone: (212) 850-6000
First Published: 1978. **Frequency:** Bimonthly. **ISSN:** 0148-6403.

★662★ HEAD TRAUMA REHABILITATION
Aspen Publishers, Inc.
200 Orchard Ridge Dr.
Gaithersburg, MD 20878   Phone: (301) 417-7500
First Published: 1986. **Frequency:** Quarterly.

★663★ HEADACHE
American Association for the Study of Headache
875 Kings Hwy., Ste. 200
West Deptford, NJ 08096   Phone: (609) 845-0322
First Published: 1961. **Frequency:** 10/yr. **ISSN:** 0017-8748.

★664★ HEADACHE QUARTERLY
International Universities Press, Inc.
59 Boston Post Rd.
PO Box 1524
Madison, CT 06443   Phone: (203) 245-4000
Frequency: Quarterly.

★665★ HEALTH
Family Media, Inc.
3 Park Ave.
New York, NY 10016   Phone: (212) 340-9200
First Published: 1969. **Frequency:** Monthly. **ISSN:** 0279-3547.

★666★ HEALTH AFFAIRS
People-to-People Health Foundation
Project HOPE Health Sciences Education Center
Millwood, VA 22646   Phone: (703) 837-2100
First Published: 1981. **Frequency:** Quarterly. **ISSN:** 0278-2715.

★667★ HEALTH CARE MANAGEMENT REVIEW
Aspen Publishers, Inc.
200 Orchard Ridge Dr.
Gaithersburg, MD 20878   Phone: (301) 417-7500
First Published: 1976. **Frequency:** Quarterly. **ISSN:** 0361-6274.

★668★ HEALTH CARE SUPERVISOR
Aspen Publishers, Inc.
200 Orchard Ridge Dr.
Gaithersburg, MD 20878   Phone: (301) 417-7500
First Published: 1982. **Frequency:** Quarterly. **ISSN:** 0731-3381.

★669★ HEALTH CARE FOR WOMEN INTERNATIONAL
Hemisphere Publishing Corp.
1900 Frost Rd., Ste. 101
Bristol, PA 19007-1598   Phone: (215) 785-5800
First Published: 1979. **Frequency:** Quarterly. **ISSN:** 0739-9332.

★670★ HEALTH COMMUNICATION
Lawrence Erlbaum Associates, Inc.
365 Broadway
Hillsdale, NJ 07642   Phone: (201) 666-4110
Frequency: Quarterly.

★671★ HEALTH ECONOMICS
John Wiley & Sons, Inc.
605 3rd Ave.
New York, NY 10158
First Published: 1992. **Frequency:** Quarterly. **ISSN:** 1057-9230.

★672★ HEALTH EDUCATION QUARTERLY
John Wiley & Sons, Inc.
605 3rd Ave.
New York, NY 10158   Phone: (212) 850-6000
First Published: 1973. **Frequency:** Quarterly. **ISSN:** 0195-8402.

★673★ HEALTH EDUCATION RESEARCH
IRL Press, Inc.
PO Box Q
McLean, VA 22101   Phone: (703) 437-3334
First Published: 1986. **Frequency:** 4/yr. **ISSN:** 0268-1153.

★674★ HEALTH FACILITIES MANAGEMENT
American Hospital Association
840 N. Lake Shore Dr.
Chicago, IL 60611   Phone: (312) 280-6000
Frequency: Monthly. **ISSN:** 0899-6210.

★675★ HEALTH AND HYGIENE
Blackwell Scientific Publications
3 Cambridge Center, Ste. 208
Cambridge, MA 02142   Phone: (617) 225-0401
First Published: 1977. **Frequency:** Quarterly. **ISSN:** 0140-2986.

★676★ HEALTH PHYSICS
Health Physics Society
8000 Westpark Dr., Ste. 130
McLean, VA 22102   Phone: (703) 790-1745
First Published: 1958. **Frequency:** Monthly. **ISSN:** 0017-9078.

★677★ HEALTH PROGRESS
Catholic Health Association of the U.S.
4455 Woodson Rd.
St. Louis, MO 63134   Phone: (314) 427-2500
First Published: 1920. **Frequency:** 11/yr. **ISSN:** 0882-1577.

★678★ HEALTH PSYCHOLOGY
American Psychological Association
1200 17th St., NW
Washington, DC 20036   Phone: (202) 955-7600
First Published: 1982. **Frequency:** Bimonthly. **ISSN:** 0278-6133.

★679★ HEALTH SERVICES RESEARCH
American College of Healthcare Executives
840 N. Lake Shore Dr., Ste. 1103W
Chicago, IL 60611   Phone: (312) 943-0544
First Published: 1965. **Frequency:** Bimonthly. **ISSN:** 0017-9124.

★680★ HEALTH AND SOCIAL WORK
National Association of Social Workers
7981 Eastern Ave.
Silver Spring, MD 20910   Phone: (301) 565-0333
First Published: 1976. **Frequency:** Quarterly. **ISSN:** 0360-7283.

★681★ HEALTHCARE FINANCIAL MANAGEMENT
Healthcare Financial Management Association
2 Westbrook Corporate Center, Ste. 700
Westchester, IL 60154   Phone: (708) 531-9600
First Published: 1947. **Frequency:** Monthly. **ISSN:** 0735-0732.

★682★ HEARING RESEARCH
Elsevier Science Publishing Co., Inc.
655 Avenue of the Americas
New York, NY 10010   Phone: (212) 989-5800
First Published: 1978. **Frequency:** 18/yr. **ISSN:** 0378-5955.

★683★   HEART AND LUNG
American Association of Critical Care Nurses
1 Civic Plaza
Newport Beach, CA 92660   Phone: (714) 644-9310
First Published: 1972. **Frequency:** Bimonthly. **ISSN:** 0147-9563.

★684★   HEART AND VESSELS
Springer-Verlag New York, Inc.
175 5th Ave.
New York, NY 10010   Phone: (212) 460-1500
First Published: 1985. **Frequency:** Quarterly. **ISSN:** 0910-8327.

★685★   HELVETICA PAEDIATRICA ACTA
Springer-Verlag New York, Inc.
175 5th Ave.
New York, NY 10010   Phone: (212) 460-1500
First Published: 1945. **Frequency:** Bimonthly. **ISSN:** 0018-022X.

★686★   HEMATOLOGICAL ONCOLOGY
John Wiley & Sons, Inc.
605 3rd Ave.
New York, NY 10158   Phone: (212) 850-6000
First Published: 1983. **Frequency:** Quarterly. **ISSN:** 0278-0232.

★687★   HEMOGLOBIN
Marcel Dekker, Inc.
270 Madison Ave.
New York, NY 10016   Phone: (212) 696-9000
First Published: 1977. **Frequency:** Bimonthly. **ISSN:** 0363-0269.

★688★   HENRY FORD HOSPITAL MEDICAL JOURNAL
Henry Ford Hospital
Editorial Office
411-413 New Center Pavilion
2921 W. Grand Blvd.
Detroit, MI 48202   Phone: (313) 876-2028
First Published: 1953. **Frequency:** Quarterly. **ISSN:** 0018-0416.

★689★   HEPATO-GASTROENTEROLOGY
Thieme Medical Publishers, Inc.
381 Park Ave., S.
New York, NY 10016   Phone: (212) 683-5088
First Published: 1954. **Frequency:** Bimonthly. **ISSN:** 0172-6390.

★690★   HEPATOLOGY
American Association for the Study of Liver Diseases
6900 Grove Rd.
Thorofare, NJ 08086   Phone: (609) 848-1000
First Published: 1980. **Frequency:** Bimonthly. **ISSN:** 0270-9139.

★691★   HEREDITAS
Mendelian Society
Institute of Genetics
S-223 62 Lund, Sweden
First Published: 1920. **Frequency:** Bimonthly. **ISSN:** 0018-0661.

★692★   HEREDITY
Longman Group, Ltd.
4th Ave.
Harlow, Essex CM19 5AA, England
First Published: 1947. **Frequency:** Bimonthly. **ISSN:** 0018-067X.

★693★   HILLSIDE JOURNAL OF CLINICAL PSYCHIATRY
Human Sciences Press, Inc.
233 Spring St.
New York, NY 10013   Phone: (212) 620-8000
First Published: 1979. **Frequency:** Semiannual. **ISSN:** 0193-5216.

★694★   HIPPOCAMPUS
Churchill Livingstone, Inc.
1560 Broadway
New York, NY 10036   Phone: (212) 819-5400
First Published: 1991. **Frequency:** Quarterly. **ISSN:** 1050-9631.

★695★   HIPPOCRATES NEWS
Hippocrates Health Institute
1443 Palmdale Ct.
W. Palm Beach, FL 33411   Phone: (305) 471-8876
First Published: 1987. **Frequency:** 3/yr. **ISSN:** 0893-0627.

★696★   HISTOCHEMICAL JOURNAL
Chapman & Hall, Ltd.
2-6 Boundary Row
London SE1, England
First Published: 1969. **Frequency:** Monthly. **ISSN:** 0018-2214.

★697★   HISTOCHEMISTRY
Springer-Verlag New York, Inc.
175 5th Ave.
New York, NY 10010   Phone: (212) 460-1500
First Published: 1958. **Frequency:** Monthly. **ISSN:** 0301-5564.

★698★   HISTOPATHOLOGY
Blackwell Scientific Publications
3 Cambridge Center, Ste. 208
Cambridge, MA 02142   Phone: (617) 225-0401
First Published: 1977. **Frequency:** Monthly. **ISSN:** 0309-0167.

★699★   HOLISTIC MEDICINE
American Holistic Medical Association
4101 Lake Boone Trail, Ste. 201
Raleigh, NC 27607-6518   Phone: (919) 787-5146
First Published: 1978. **Frequency:** Bimonthly. **ISSN:** 0898-6029.

★700★   HOLISTIC NURSING PRACTICE
Aspen Publishers, Inc.
200 Orchard Ridge Dr.
Gaithersburg, MD 20878   Phone: (301) 417-7500
First Published: 1979. **Frequency:** Quarterly. **ISSN:** 0164-0534.

★701★   HOME HEALTH CARE SERVICES QUARTERLY
The Haworth Press, Inc.
10 Alice St.
Binghampton, NY 13904   Phone: (800) 342-9678
Frequency: Quarterly.

★702★   HOMEOSTASIS IN HEALTH AND DISEASE
Pergamon Press, Inc.
395 Saw Mill River Rd.
Elmsford, NY 10523   Phone: (914) 592-7700
Frequency: Bimonthly. **ISSN:** 0960-7560.

★703★   HORMONE AND METABOLIC RESEARCH
Thieme Medical Publishers, Inc.
381 Park Ave., S.
New York, NY 10016   Phone: (212) 683-5088
First Published: 1969. **Frequency:** Monthly. **ISSN:** 0018-5043.

★704★   HORMONE RESEARCH
S. Karger Publishers, Inc.
26 W. Avon Rd.
PO Box 529
Farmington, CT 06085   Phone: (203) 675-7834
First Published: 1970. **Frequency:** 12/yr. **ISSN:** 0301-0163.

★705★   HORMONES AND BEHAVIOR
Academic Press, Inc.
1250 6th Ave.
San Diego, CA 92101   Phone: (619) 231-0926
First Published: 1969. **Frequency:** Quarterly. **ISSN:** 0018-506X.

★706★   HOSPITAL AND COMMUNITY PSYCHIATRY
American Psychiatric Association
1400 K St., NW
Washington, DC 20005   Phone: (202) 682-6000
First Published: 1950. **Frequency:** Monthly. **ISSN:** 0022-1597.

★707★ HOSPITAL AND HEALTH SERVICES
ADMINISTRATION
American College of Healthcare Executives
840 N. Lake Shore Dr., Ste. 1103, W.
Chicago, IL 60611   Phone: (312) 943-0544
First Published: 1956. Frequency: Quarterly. ISSN: 8750-3735.

★708★ HOSPITAL MATERIAL MANAGEMENT QUARTERLY
Aspen Publishers, Inc.
200 Orchard Ridge Dr.
Gaithersburg, MD 20878   Phone: (301) 417-7500
First Published: 1979. Frequency: Quarterly. ISSN: 0192-2262.

★709★ HOSPITAL MEDICINE
Hospital Publications, Inc.
500 Plaza Dr.
Secaucus, NJ 07094   Phone: (201) 864-4000
First Published: 1964. Frequency: 10/yr. ISSN: 0441-2745.

★710★ HOSPITAL PHARMACY
J.B. Lippincott Co.
E. Washington Sq.
Philadelphia, PA 19105   Phone: (215) 238-4200
First Published: 1966. Frequency: Monthly. ISSN: 0018-5787.

★711★ HOSPITAL PRACTICE
HP Publishing Co. Inc.
10 Astor Pl., 7th Fl.
New York, NY 10003   Phone: (212) 421-7320
First Published: 1966. Frequency: 18/yr. ISSN: 8750-2836.

★712★ HOSPITAL TOPICS
Heldref Publications
4000 Albemarle St., NW
Washington, DC 20016   Phone: (202) 362-6445
First Published: 1922. Frequency: Bimonthly. ISSN: 0018-5868.

★713★ HOSPITALS
American Hospital Association
840 N. Lake Shore Dr.
Chicago, IL 60611   Phone: (312) 280-6000
First Published: 1936. Frequency: Semimonthly. ISSN: 0018-5973.

★714★ HUMAN ANTIBODIES AND HYBRIDOMAS
Butterworth-Heinemann
80 Montvale Ave.
Stoneham, MA 02180   Phone: (617) 438-8464
Frequency: Quarterly. ISSN: 0956-960X.

★715★ HUMAN BIOLOGY
Wayne State University Press
5959 Woodward Ave.
Detroit, MI 48202   Phone: (313) 577-4626
First Published: 1929. Frequency: 6/yr. ISSN: 0018-7143.

★716★ HUMAN COMMUNICATION AND ITS DISORDERS
Ablex Publishing Corp.
355 Chestnut St.
Norwood, NJ 07648   Phone: (201) 767-8450
First Published: 1987. Frequency: Annual.

★717★ HUMAN DEVELOPMENT
S. Karger Publishers, Inc.
26 W. Avon Rd.
PO Box 529
Farmington, CT 06085   Phone: (203) 675-7834
First Published: 1958. Frequency: Bimonthly. ISSN: 0018-716X.

★718★ HUMAN AND EXPERIMENTAL TOXICOLOGY
Macmillan Press, Ltd.
Houndmills
Basingstoke, Hampshire RG21 2XS, England
First Published: 1981. Frequency: Bimonthly. ISSN: 0144-5952.

★719★ HUMAN GENETICS
Springer-Verlag New York, Inc.
175 5th Ave.
New York, NY 10010   Phone: (212) 460-1500
First Published: 1964. Frequency: 12/yr. ISSN: 0340-6717.

★720★ HUMAN HEREDITY
S. Karger Publishers, Inc.
26 W. Avon Rd.
PO Box 529
Farmington, CT 06085   Phone: (203) 675-7834
First Published: 1950. Frequency: Bimonthly. ISSN: 0001-5652.

★721★ HUMAN IMMUNOLOGY
American Society for Histocompatibility and Immunogenetics
PO Box 15804
Lenexa, KS 66215   Phone: (913) 541-0009
First Published: 1980. Frequency: Monthly. ISSN: 0198-8859.

★722★ HUMAN PATHOLOGY
W.B. Saunders Co.
Independence Sq., W.
Philadelphia, PA 19106   Phone: (215) 238-7800
First Published: 1970. Frequency: Monthly. ISSN: 0046-8177.

★723★ HUMAN PHYSIOLOGY
Plenum Publishing Corp.
233 Spring St.
New York, NY 10013   Phone: (212) 620-8000
First Published: 1975. Frequency: Bimonthly. ISSN: 0362-1197.

★724★ HUMAN PSYCHOPHARMACOLOGY: CLINICAL AND
EXPERIMENTAL
John Wiley & Sons, Inc.
605 3rd Ave.
New York, NY 10158   Phone: (212) 850-6000
First Published: 1986. Frequency: Quarterly. ISSN: 0885-6222.

★725★ HYBRIDOMA
Mary Ann Liebert, Inc.
1651 3rd Ave.
New York, NY 10128   Phone: (212) 289-2300
First Published: 1981. Frequency: Quarterly. ISSN: 0272-457X.

★726★ HYPERTENSION
American Heart Association, Inc.
7320 Greenville Ave.
Dallas, TX 75231   Phone: (214) 373-6300
First Published: 1979. Frequency: Monthly. ISSN: 0194-911X.

★727★ IEEE TRANSACTIONS ON BIOMEDICAL
ENGINEERING
Institute of Electrical and Electronics Engineers, Inc.
345 E. 47th St.
New York, NY 10017   Phone: (212) 705-7900
First Published: 1953. Frequency: Monthly. ISSN: 0018-9294.

★728★ ILLINOIS MEDICINE
Illinois State Medical Society
20 N. Michigan Ave., Ste. 700
Chicago, IL 60602   Phone: (312) 782-1654
First Published: 1899. Frequency: Semimonthly. ISSN: 0019-2120.

★729★ IMMUNOGENETICS
Springer-Verlag New York, Inc.
175 5th Ave.
New York, NY 10010   Phone: (212) 460-1500
First Published: 1974. Frequency: Monthly. ISSN: 0093-7711.

★730★ IMMUNOLOGIC RESEARCH
S. Karger Publishers, Inc.
26 W. Avon Rd.
PO Box 529
Farmington, CT 06085   Phone: (203) 675-7834
First Published: 1982. Frequency: Quarterly. ISSN: 0257-277X.

★731★ IMMUNOLOGY
Blackwell Scientific Publications
3 Cambridge Center, Ste. 208
Cambridge, MA 02142   Phone: (617) 225-0401
First Published: 1958. **Frequency:** Monthly. **ISSN:** 0019-2805.

★732★ IMMUNOLOGY LETTERS
Elsevier Science Publishing Co., Inc.
655 Avenue of the Americas
New York, NY 10010   Phone: (212) 989-5800
First Published: 1979. **Frequency:** Monthly. **ISSN:** 0165-2478.

★733★ IMMUNOMETHODS
Academic Press, Inc.
1250 6th Ave.
San Diego, CA 92101   Phone: (619) 231-0926
First Published: 1992. **Frequency:** 3/yr. **ISSN:** 1058-6687.

★734★ IMMUNOPHARMACOLOGY
Elsevier Science Publishing Co., Inc.
655 Avenue of the Americas
New York, NY 10010   Phone: (212) 989-5800
First Published: 1979. **Frequency:** 6/yr. **ISSN:** 0162-3109.

★735★ IMMUNOPHARMACOLOGY AND IMMUNOTOXICOLOGY
Marcel Dekker, Inc.
270 Madison Ave.
New York, NY 10016   Phone: (212) 696-9000
First Published: 1979. **Frequency:** Quarterly. **ISSN:** 0892-3973.

★736★ IN HEALTH
475 Gate Five Rd., Ste. 225
Sausalito, CA 94965
Frequency: Bimonthly.

★737★ IN VITRO CELLULAR AND DEVELOPMENTAL BIOLOGY
Tissue Culture Association, Inc.
19110 Montgomery Village Ave., Ste. 300
Gaithersburg, MD 20879   Phone: (301) 869-2900
First Published: 1965. **Frequency:** Monthly. **ISSN:** 0883-8364.

★738★ INDIAN HEART JOURNAL
Cardiological Society of India
Bombay Mutual Terr.
534 Sandhurst Bridge
Bombay 400007, India
First Published: 1949. **Frequency:** Bimonthly. **ISSN:** 0019-4832.

★739★ INDIAN JOURNAL OF BIOCHEMISTRY AND BIOPHYSICS
Council of Scientific and Industrial Research
Publications and Information Directorate
Hillside Rd.
New Delhi 110012, India
First Published: 1964. **Frequency:** Bimonthly. **ISSN:** 0301-1208.

★740★ INDIAN JOURNAL OF CANCER
Indian Cancer Society
Jerbai Wadia Rd.
Parel
Bombay 400012, India
First Published: 1963. **Frequency:** Quarterly. **ISSN:** 0019-509X.

★741★ INDIAN JOURNAL OF DERMATOLOGY
78 Lenin Saranee
Calcutta 700013, India
First Published: 1955. **Frequency:** Quarterly. **ISSN:** 0019-5154.

★742★ INDIAN JOURNAL OF EXPERIMENTAL BIOLOGY
Council of Scientific and Industrial Research
Publications and Information Directorate
Hillside Rd.
New Delhi 110012, India
First Published: 1963. **Frequency:** Monthly. **ISSN:** 0019-5189.

★743★ INDIAN JOURNAL OF GASTROENTEROLOGY
Bombay Mutual Terr.
534 Sandhurst Bridge
Bombay 400007, India
First Published: 1982. **Frequency:** Quarterly. **ISSN:** 0254-8860.

★744★ INDIAN JOURNAL OF LEPROSY
Indian Leprosy Association
Hind Kusht Nivaran Sangh
Red Cross Rd.
New Delhi 110001, India
First Published: 1929. **Frequency:** Quarterly. **ISSN:** 0254-9395.

★745★ INDIAN JOURNAL OF MEDICAL RESEARCH
Indian Council of Medical Research
Box 4508
Ansari Nagar
New Delhi 110029, India
First Published: 1913. **Frequency:** Monthly. **ISSN:** 0019-5340.

★746★ INDIAN JOURNAL OF MEDICAL SCIENCES
Indian Journal of Medical Sciences Trust
c/o J.C. Patel
Back Bay View
New Queen's Rd.
Bombay 4, India
First Published: 1947. **Frequency:** Monthly. **ISSN:** 0019-5359.

★747★ INDIAN JOURNAL OF OPHTHALMOLOGY
All India Ophthalmological Society
13 Cathedral Society
Madras 600086, India
First Published: 1953. **Frequency:** 4/yr. **ISSN:** 0301-4738.

★748★ INDIAN JOURNAL OF PATHOLOGY AND MICROBIOLOGY
Indian Association of Pathologists and Microbiologists
Nizam's Institute of Medical Sciences
Panjagutta
Hyderbaud 500 482, India
First Published: 1958. **Frequency:** Quarterly. **ISSN:** 0377-4929.

★749★ INDIAN JOURNAL OF PEDIATRICS
All India Institute of Medical Sciences
Dept. of Pediatrics
Old Operation Theatre Bldg.
D II-45 Ansari Nagar
New Delhi 110 029, India
First Published: 1933. **Frequency:** Bimonthly. **ISSN:** 0019-5456.

★750★ INDIAN JOURNAL OF PHYSIOLOGY AND PHARMACOLOGY
Association of Physiologists and Pharmacologists of India
All India Institute of Medical Sciences
Ansari Nagar
New Delhi 110029, India
First Published: 1957. **Frequency:** Quarterly. **ISSN:** 0019-5499.

★751★ INDIAN JOURNAL OF PUBLIC HEALTH
Indian Public Health Association
110 Chittaragjan Ave.
Calcutta 700073, India
First Published: 1956. **Frequency:** Quarterly. **ISSN:** 0019-557X.

★752★ INDIAN PEDIATRICS
Indian Academy of Pediatrics
Safdarjang Hospital
Box 4509
New Delhi 110016, India
First Published: 1964. **Frequency:** Monthly. **ISSN:** 0019-6061.

★753★ INDIANA MEDICINE
State Medical Association
3935 N. Meridian St.
Indianapolis, IN 46208   Phone: (317) 925-7545
First Published: 1908. **Frequency:** Monthly. **ISSN:** 0746-8288.

★754★ INDOOR ENVIRONMENT
S. Karger Publishers, Inc.
26 W. Avon Rd.
PO Box 529
Farmington, CT 06085   Phone: (203) 675-7834
First Published: 1992. **Frequency:** Bimonthly. **ISSN:** 1016-4901.

★755★ INFECTION
MMW Medizin Verlag
Neumarkter Str. 18
Postfach 801246
8000 Munich 80, Germany
First Published: 1973. **Frequency:** Bimonthly. **ISSN:** 0300-8126.

★756★ INFECTION CONTROL AND HOSPITAL EPIDEMIOLOGY
Slack, Inc.
6900 Grove Rd.
Thorofare, NJ 08086   Phone: (609) 848-1000
First Published: 1980. **Frequency:** Monthly. **ISSN:** 0899-823X.

★757★ INFECTION AND IMMUNITY
American Society for Microbiology
1325 Massachusetts Ave., NW
Washington, DC 20005   Phone: (202) 737-3600
First Published: 1970. **Frequency:** Monthly. **ISSN:** 0019-9567.

★758★ INFECTIOUS AGENTS AND DISEASE
Raven Press
1185 Avenue of the Americas
New York, NY 10036   Phone: (212) 930-9500
First Published: 1991. **Frequency:** Quarterly. **ISSN:** 1056-2044.

★759★ INFERTILITY AND REPRODUCTIVE MEDICINE CLINICS
W.B. Saunders Co.
Curtis Center
Independence Sq., W.
Philadelphia, PA 19106   Phone: (215) 238-7800
Frequency: Quarterly.

★760★ INFLAMMATION
Plenum Publishing Corp.
233 Spring St.
New York, NY 10013   Phone: (212) 620-8000
First Published: 1975. **Frequency:** Bimonthly. **ISSN:** 0360-3997.

★761★ INHALATION TOXICOLOGY
Hemisphere Publishing Corp.
1900 Frost Rd., Ste. 101
Bristol, PA 19007   Phone: (215) 785-5800
First Published: 1989. **ISSN:** 0895-8378.

★762★ INJURY: BRITISH JOURNAL OF ACCIDENT SURGERY
Butterworth-Heinemann
80 Montvale Ave.
Stoneham, MA 02180   Phone: (617) 438-8464
First Published: 1969. **Frequency:** Bimonthly. **ISSN:** 0020-1383.

★763★ INQUIRY: THE JOURNAL OF HEALTH CARE ORGANIZATION, PROVISION, AND FINANCING
Blue Cross and Blue Shield Association
676 N. St. Clair St.
Chicago, IL 60611   Phone: (312) 440-5575
First Published: 1963. **Frequency:** Quarterly. **ISSN:** 0046-9580.

★764★ INTEGRATIVE PSYCHIATRY
International Universities Press, Inc.
59 Boston Post Rd.
PO Box 1524
Madison, CT 06443   Phone: (203) 245-4000
Frequency: Quarterly.

★765★ INTENSIVE CARE MEDICINE
Springer-Verlag New York, Inc.
175 5th Ave.
New York, NY 10010   Phone: (212) 460-1500
First Published: 1974. **Frequency:** 8/yr. **ISSN:** 0342-4642.

★766★ INTENSIVE CARE NURSING
Churchill Livingstone, Inc.
1560 Broadway
New York, NY 10036   Phone: (212) 819-5400
First Published: 1985. **Frequency:** Quarterly. **ISSN:** 0266-612X.

★767★ INTERNATIONAL ANESTHESIOLOGY CLINICS
Little, Brown & Co.
34 Beacon St.
Boston, MA 02108   Phone: (617) 227-0730
First Published: 1963. **Frequency:** Quarterly. **ISSN:** 0020-5907.

★768★ INTERNATIONAL ARCHIVES OF ALLERGY AND APPLIED IMMUNOLOGY
S. Karger Publishers, Inc.
26 W. Avon Rd.
PO Box 529
Farmington, CT 06085   Phone: (203) 675-7834
First Published: 1950. **Frequency:** Monthly. **ISSN:** 0020-5915.

★769★ INTERNATIONAL ARCHIVES OF OCCUPATIONAL AND ENVIRONMENTAL HEALTH
Springer-Verlag New York, Inc.
175 5th Ave.
New York, NY 10010   Phone: (212) 460-1500
First Published: 1930. **Frequency:** 8/yr. **ISSN:** 0340-0131.

★770★ INTERNATIONAL CONTACT LENS CLINIC
Butterworth-Heinemann
80 Montvale Ave.
Stoneham, MA 02180   Phone: (617) 438-8464
Frequency: Bimonthly. **ISSN:** 0892-8967.

★771★ INTERNATIONAL DENTAL JOURNAL
Butterworth-Heinemann
80 Montvale Ave.
Stoneham, Surrey, 02180   Phone: (617) 438-8464
First Published: 1950. **Frequency:** Quarterly. **ISSN:** 0020-6539.

★772★ INTERNATIONAL DISABILITY STUDIES
Eular Publishers
Oberwilstrasse 23
PO Box 146
CH-4012 Basel, Switzerland
First Published: 1979. **Frequency:** Quarterly. **ISSN:** 0259-9147.

★773★ INTERNATIONAL ENDODONTIC JOURNAL
Blackwell Scientific Publications
3 Cambridge Center, Ste. 208
Cambridge, MA 02142   Phone: (617) 225-0401
First Published: 1981. **Frequency:** Bimonthly. **ISSN:** 0143-2885.

★774★ INTERNATIONAL AND FAMILY PLANNING PERSPECTIVES
The Alan Guttmacher Institute
111 5th Ave.
New York, NY 10003   Phone: (212) 254-5656
Frequency: Quarterly. **ISSN:** 0162-2749.

★775★ INTERNATIONAL JOURNAL OF THE ADDICTIONS
Marcel Dekker, Inc.
270 Madison Ave.
New York, NY 10016   Phone: (212) 696-9000
First Published: 1966. **Frequency:** 12/yr. **ISSN:** 0020-773X.

★776★   INTERNATIONAL JOURNAL OF AGING AND HUMAN DEVELOPMENT
Baywood Publishing Co., Inc.
27 Austin Ave.
Amityville, NY 11701   Phone: (516) 691-1270
First Published: 1973. **Frequency:** 8/yr. **ISSN:** 0091-4150.

★777★   INTERNATIONAL JOURNAL OF ANDROLOGY
Blackwell Scientific Publications
3 Cambridge Center, Ste. 208
Cambridge, MA 02142   Phone: (617) 225-0401
Frequency: Bimonthly. **ISSN:** 0105-6263.

★778★   INTERNATIONAL JOURNAL OF ARTIFICIAL ORGANS
Wichtig Editore s.r.l.
Viale Friuli 72-74
20135 Milan, Italy
First Published: 1978. **Frequency:** Monthly. **ISSN:** 0391-3988.

★779★   INTERNATIONAL JOURNAL OF BIOCHEMISTRY
Pergamon Press, Inc.
Maxwell House, Fairview Park
Elmsford, NY 10523   Phone: (914) 592-7700
First Published: 1970. **Frequency:** Monthly. **ISSN:** 0020-711X.

★780★   THE INTERNATIONAL JOURNAL OF BIOLOGICAL MARKERS
Wichtig Editor
PO Box 830350
Birmingham, AL 35283   Phone: (800) 633-4931
Frequency: Quarterly.

★781★   INTERNATIONAL JOURNAL OF BIO-MEDICAL COMPUTING
Elsevier Science Publishing Co. Inc.
655 Avenue of the Americas
New York, NY 10010   Phone: (212) 989-5800
First Published: 1970. **Frequency:** 8/yr. **ISSN:** 0020-7101.

★782★   INTERNATIONAL JOURNAL OF CANCER
John Wiley & Sons, Inc.
605 3rd Ave.
New York, NY 10158   Phone: (212) 850-6000
First Published: 1966. **Frequency:** Monthly. **ISSN:** 0020-7136.

★783★   INTERNATIONAL JOURNAL OF CARDIOLOGY
Elsevier Science Publishing Co., Inc.
655 Avenue of the Americas
New York, NY 10010   Phone: (212) 989-5800
First Published: 1973. **Frequency:** 12/yr. **ISSN:** 0167-5273.

★784★   INTERNATIONAL JOURNAL OF CELL CLONING
AlphaMed Press, Inc.
4100 S. Kettering Blvd.
Dayton, OH 45439   Phone: (513) 293-8508
First Published: 1983. **Frequency:** Bimonthly. **ISSN:** 0737-1454.

★785★   INTERNATIONAL JOURNAL OF CLINICAL AND EXPERIMENTAL HYPNOSIS
Society for Clinical and Experimental Hypnosis
128-A Kings Park Dr.
Liverpool, NY 13090   Phone: (315) 652-7299
First Published: 1953. **Frequency:** Quarterly. **ISSN:** 0020-7144.

★786★   INTERNATIONAL JOURNAL OF CLINICAL PHARMACOLOGY, THERAPY, AND TOXICOLOGY
Dustri Verlag, Dr. Karl Feistle
Bahnhofstrasse 9
D-8024 Deisenhofen, Germany
First Published: 1967. **Frequency:** Monthly. **ISSN:** 0174-4879.

★787★   INTERNATIONAL JOURNAL OF COLORECTAL DISEASE
Springer-Verlag New York, Inc.
175 5th Ave.
New York, NY 10010   Phone: (212) 460-1500
First Published: 1986. **Frequency:** 4/yr. **ISSN:** 0179-1958.

★788★   INTERNATIONAL JOURNAL OF DERMATOLOGY
International Society of Dermatology: Tropical, Geographic, and Ecologic
200 1st St., SW
Rochester, MN 55905   Phone: (507) 284-3736
First Published: 1962. **Frequency:** 10/yr. **ISSN:** 0011-9059.

★789★   INTERNATIONAL JOURNAL OF DEVELOPMENTAL NEUROSCIENCE
Pergamon Press, Inc.
Maxwell House, Fairview Park
Elmsford, NY 10523   Phone: (914) 592-7700
First Published: 1983. **Frequency:** Bimonthly. **ISSN:** 0736-5748.

★790★   INTERNATIONAL JOURNAL OF EATING DISORDERS
John Wiley & Sons, Inc.
605 3rd Ave.
New York, NY 10158   Phone: (212) 850-6000
Frequency: Bimonthly. **ISSN:** 0276-3478.

★791★   INTERNATIONAL JOURNAL OF EPIDEMIOLOGY
International Epidemiological Association
c/o Roger Detels, M.D.
School of Public Health, Rm. 71-269CHS
University of California
Los Angeles, CA 90024   Phone: (213) 206-2837
First Published: 1972. **Frequency:** Quarterly. **ISSN:** 0300-5771.

★792★   INTERNATIONAL JOURNAL OF EXPERIMENTAL PATHOLOGY
Blackwell Scientific Publications
3 Cambridge Center, Ste. 208
Cambridge, MA 02142   Phone: (617) 225-0401
Frequency: Bimonthly. **ISSN:** 0959-9673.

★793★   INTERNATIONAL JOURNAL OF FATIGUE
Butterworth-Heinemann
80 Montvale Ave.
Stoneham, MA 02180   Phone: (617) 438-8464
Frequency: Bimonthly. **ISSN:** 0142-1123.

★794★   INTERNATIONAL JOURNAL OF GERIATRIC PSYCHIATRY
John Wiley & Sons, Inc.
605 3rd Ave.
New York, NY 10158   Phone: (212) 850-6000
First Published: 1986. **Frequency:** Bimonthly. **ISSN:** 0885-6230.

★795★   INTERNATIONAL JOURNAL OF GROUP PSYCHOTHERAPY
American Group Psychotherapy Association
25 E. 21st St., 6th Fl.
New York, NY 10010   Phone: (212) 477-2677
First Published: 1951. **Frequency:** Quarterly. **ISSN:** 0020-7284.

★796★   INTERNATIONAL JOURNAL OF GYNECOLOGICAL CANCER
Blackwell Scientific Publications
3 Cambridge Center, Ste. 208
Cambridge, MA 02142   Phone: (617) 225-0401
Frequency: Bimonthly. **ISSN:** 1048-891X.

★797★   INTERNATIONAL JOURNAL OF GYNECOLOGICAL PATHOLOGY
Raven Press
1185 Avenue of the Americas
New York, NY 10036   Phone: (212) 930-9500
First Published: 1982. **Frequency:** Quarterly. **ISSN:** 0277-1691.

★798★ INTERNATIONAL JOURNAL OF GYNECOLOGY AND OBSTETRICS
Elsevier Science Publishing Co., Inc.
655 Avenue of the Americas
New York, NY 10010   Phone: (212) 989-5800
First Published: 1963. **Frequency:** Bimonthly. **ISSN:** 0020-7292.

★799★ INTERNATIONAL JOURNAL OF HEALTH CARE QUALITY
MCB Publications Ltd.
Representative Office
PO Box 10812
Birmingham, AL 35201
Frequency: Bimonthly. **ISSN:** 0952-6862.

★800★ INTERNATIONAL JOURNAL OF HEALTH SERVICES
Baywood Publishing Co., Inc.
27 Austin Ave.
Amityville, NY 11701   Phone: (516) 691-1270
First Published: 1970. **Frequency:** Quarterly. **ISSN:** 0020-7314.

★801★ INTERNATIONAL JOURNAL OF HEMATOLOGY
Elsevier Science Publishing Co., Inc.
655 Avenue of the Americas
New York, NY 10010   Phone: (212) 989-5800
Frequency: Bimonthly. **ISSN:** 0925-5710.

★802★ INTERNATIONAL JOURNAL OF IMMUNOPHARMACOLOGY
Pergamon Press, Inc.
Maxwell House, Fairview Park
Elmsford, NY 10523   Phone: (914) 592-7700
First Published: 1979. **Frequency:** 8/yr. **ISSN:** 0192-0561.

★803★ INTERNATIONAL JOURNAL OF LAW AND PSYCHIATRY
Pergamon Press, Inc.
Maxwell House, Fairview Park
Elmsford, NY 10523   Phone: (914) 592-7700
First Published: 1978. **Frequency:** Quarterly. **ISSN:** 0160-2527.

★804★ INTERNATIONAL JOURNAL OF LEPROSY AND OTHER MYCOBACTERIAL DISEASES
American Leprosy Missions International
1 Broadway
Elmwood Park, NJ 07407   Phone: (201) 794-8650
First Published: 1933. **Frequency:** Quarterly. **ISSN:** 0148-916X.

★805★ INTERNATIONAL JOURNAL OF NEUROLOGY
Fulton Society
Calle Buenos Aires 363
Montevideo, Uruguay
First Published: 1960. **Frequency:** Quarterly. **ISSN:** 0020-7446.

★806★ INTERNATIONAL JOURNAL OF NEUROSCIENCE
Gordon & Breach, Science Publishers, Inc.
270 8th Ave.
New York, NY 10011   Phone: (212) 206-8900
First Published: 1970. **Frequency:** 24/yr. **ISSN:** 0020-7454.

★807★ INTERNATIONAL JOURNAL OF NURSING STUDIES
Pergamon Press, Inc.
Maxwell House, Fairview Park
Elmsford, NY 10523   Phone: (914) 592-7700
First Published: 1965. **Frequency:** Quarterly. **ISSN:** 0020-7489.

★808★ INTERNATIONAL JOURNAL OF OBESITY
Macmillian Publishing Co.
866 3rd Ave.
New York, NY 10022   Phone: (212) 702-2000
First Published: 1977. **Frequency:** Bimonthly. **ISSN:** 0307-0565.

★809★ INTERNATIONAL JOURNAL OF OBSTETRIC ANESTHESIA
Churchill Livingstone, Inc.
1560 Broadway
New York, NY 10036   Phone: (212) 819-5400
First Published: 1991. **Frequency:** Quarterly. **ISSN:** 0959-289X.

★810★ INTERNATIONAL JOURNAL OF ORAL AND MAXILLOFACIAL SURGERY
Munksgaard
Noerre Soegade 35
DK-1370 Copenhagen K, Denmark
First Published: 1972. **Frequency:** Bimonthly. **ISSN:** 0901-5027.

★811★ INTERNATIONAL JOURNAL FOR PARASITOLOGY
Pergamon Press, Inc.
Maxwell House, Fairview Park
Elmsford, NY 10523   Phone: (914) 592-7700
First Published: 1971. **Frequency:** 8/yr. **ISSN:** 0020-7519.

★812★ INTERNATIONAL JOURNAL OF PEDIATRIC OTORHINOLARYNGOLOGY
Elsevier Science Publishing Co., Inc.
655 Avenue of the Americas
New York, NY 10010   Phone: (212) 989-5800
First Published: 1979. **Frequency:** 6/yr. **ISSN:** 0165-5876.

★813★ INTERNATIONAL JOURNAL OF PEPTIDE AND PROTEIN RESEARCH
Munksgaard
Noerre Soegade 35
DK-1370 Copenhagen K, Denmark
First Published: 1968. **Frequency:** Monthly. **ISSN:** 0367-8377.

★814★ INTERNATIONAL JOURNAL OF PERSONAL CONSTRUCT PSYCHOLOGY
Hemisphere Publishing Corp.
1900 Frost Rd., Ste. 101
Bristol, PA 19007   Phone: (215) 785-5800
ISSN: 0893-603X.

★815★ INTERNATIONAL JOURNAL OF PSYCHIATRY IN MEDICINE
Baywood Publishing Co., Inc.
27 Austin Ave.
Amityville, NY 11701   Phone: (516) 691-1270
First Published: 1970. **Frequency:** Quarterly. **ISSN:** 0091-2174.

★816★ INTERNATIONAL JOURNAL OF PSYCHO-ANALYSIS
Institute of Psychoanalysis
Routledge, 11
New Fetter Ln.
London EC4P 4EE, England
First Published: 1920. **Frequency:** Quarterly. **ISSN:** 0020-7578.

★817★ INTERNATIONAL JOURNAL OF PSYCHOSOMATICS
International Psychosomatics Institute
PO Box 1296
Philadelphia, PA 19105   Phone: (215) 525-5511
First Published: 1954. **Frequency:** Quarterly. **ISSN:** 0884-8297.

★818★ INTERNATIONAL JOURNAL OF RADIATION APPLICATIONS AND INSTRUMENTATION, PART B: NUCLEAR MEDICINE AND BIOLOGY
Pergamon Press, Inc.
Maxwell House, Fairview Park
Elmsford, NY 10523   Phone: (914) 592-7700
First Published: 1973. **Frequency:** Bimonthly. **ISSN:** 0883-2897.

★819★ INTERNATIONAL JOURNAL OF RADIATION BIOLOGY
Taylor & Francis, Ltd.
Rankine Rd.
Basingstoke, Hants. RG24 0PR, England
First Published: 1959. **Frequency:** Monthly. **ISSN:** 0020-7616.

★820★ INTERNATIONAL JOURNAL OF RADIATION ONCOLOGY, BIOLOGY, PHYSICS
Pergamon Press, Inc.
Maxwell House, Fairview Park
Elmsford, NY 10523   Phone: (914) 592-7700
First Published: 1976. **Frequency:** Monthly. **ISSN:** 0360-3016.

★821★ INTERNATIONAL JOURNAL OF REHABILITATION RESEARCH
Heidelberger Verlagsanstalt
Hans-Bunte Str. 18
D-6900 Heidelberg, Germany
First Published: 1977. **Frequency:** Quarterly. **ISSN:** 0342-5282.

★822★ INTERNATIONAL JOURNAL OF SOCIAL PSYCHIATRY
Avenue Publishing Co.
55 Woodstock Ave.
London NW11 9RG, England
First Published: 1955. **Frequency:** Quarterly. **ISSN:** 0020-7640.

★823★ INTERNATIONAL JOURNAL OF SPORTS MEDICINE
Thieme Medical Publishers, Inc.
381 Park Ave., S.
New York, NY 10016   Phone: (212) 683-5088
First Published: 1980. **Frequency:** Bimonthly. **ISSN:** 0172-4622.

★824★ INTERNATIONAL JOURNAL FOR VITAMIN AND NUTRITION RESEARCH
Verlag Hans Huber
Laenggasstrasse 76
CH-3000 Berne 9, Switzerland
First Published: 1930. **Frequency:** Quarterly. **ISSN:** 0300-9831.

★825★ INTERNATIONAL OPHTHALMOLOGY
Kluwer Academic Publishers
Box 17
3300 AA Dordrecht, Netherlands
First Published: 1978. **Frequency:** 6/yr. **ISSN:** 0165-5701.

★826★ INTERNATIONAL OPHTHALMOLOGY CLINICS
Little, Brown & Co.
34 Beacon St.
Boston, MA 02108   Phone: (617) 227-0730
First Published: 1961. **Frequency:** Quarterly. **ISSN:** 0020-8167.

★827★ INTERNATIONAL ORTHOPAEDICS
Springer-Verlag New York, Inc.
175 5th Ave.
New York, NY 10010   Phone: (212) 460-1500
First Published: 1977. **Frequency:** Quarterly. **ISSN:** 0341-2695.

★828★ INTERNATIONAL SURGERY
International College of Surgeons
1516 N. Lake Shore Dr.
Chicago, IL 60610   Phone: (312) 642-3555
First Published: 1937. **Frequency:** Quarterly. **ISSN:** 0020-8868.

★829★ INTERNATIONAL UROGYNECOLOGY JOURNAL
Springer-Verlag New York, Inc.
175 5th Ave.
New York, NY 10010   Phone: (212) 460-1500
First Published: 1991. **Frequency:** Quarterly. **ISSN:** 0937-9827.

★830★ INTERVIROLOGY
S. Karger Publishers, Inc.
26 W. Avon Rd.
PO Box 529
Farmington, CT 06085   Phone: (203) 675-7834
First Published: 1973. **Frequency:** Bimonthly. **ISSN:** 0300-5526.

★831★ INTRAVENOUS THERAPY NEWS
McMahon Publishing Co.
83 Peaceable St.
West Redding, CT 06896   Phone: (203) 544-9343
First Published: 1974. **Frequency:** Monthly.

★832★ INVASION AND METASTASIS
S. Karger Publishers, Inc.
26 W. Avon Rd.
PO Box 529
Farmington, CT 06085   Phone: (203) 675-7834
First Published: 1981. **Frequency:** Bimonthly. **ISSN:** 0251-1789.

★833★ INVESTIGATIONAL NEW DRUGS
Kluwer Academic Publishers
101 Philip Dr.
Norwell, MA 02061   Phone: (617) 871-6600
First Published: 1983. **Frequency:** Quarterly. **ISSN:** 0167-6997.

★834★ INVESTIGATIVE OPHTHALMOLOGY AND VISUAL SCIENCE
Association for Research in Vision and Ophthalmology
9650 Rockville Pike
Bethesda, MD 20814   Phone: (301) 530-1844
First Published: 1962. **Frequency:** Monthly. **ISSN:** 0146-0404.

★835★ INVESTIGATIVE RADIOLOGY
Association of University Radiologists
1891 Preston White Dr.
Reston, VA 22091   Phone: (703) 648-8900
First Published: 1966. **Frequency:** Monthly. **ISSN:** 0020-9996.

★836★ IOWA MEDICINE
Iowa Medical Society
1001 Grand Ave.
West Des Moines, IA 50265   Phone: (515) 223-1401
First Published: 1910. **Frequency:** Monthly. **ISSN:** 0746-8709.

★837★ IRISH JOURNAL OF MEDICAL SCIENCE
Royal Academy of Medicine in Ireland
6 Kildare St.
Dublin 2, Ireland
First Published: 1832. **Frequency:** Monthly. **ISSN:** 0021-1265.

★838★ IRISH MEDICAL JOURNAL
Irish Medical Organization
10 Fitzwilliam Pl.
Dublin 2, Ireland
First Published: 1937. **Frequency:** Quarterly. **ISSN:** 0332-3102.

★839★ ISRAEL JOURNAL OF MEDICAL SCIENCES
2 Etzel St.
French Hill
97853 Jerusalem, Israel
First Published: 1965. **Frequency:** Monthly. **ISSN:** 0021-2180.

★840★ ISRAEL JOURNAL OF PSYCHIATRY AND RELATED SCIENCES
Israel Science Publishers, Ltd.
Box 3115
91030 Jerusalem, Israel
First Published: 1963. **Frequency:** Quarterly. **ISSN:** 0333-7308.

★841★ ISSUES IN COMPREHENSIVE PEDIATRIC NURSING
Hemisphere Publishing Corp.
1900 Frost Rd., Ste. 101
Bristol, PA 19007   Phone: (215) 785-5800
First Published: 1976. **Frequency:** Bimonthly. **ISSN:** 0146-0862.

★842★ ISSUES IN MENTAL HEALTH NURSING
Hemisphere Publishing Corp.
1900 Frost Rd., Ste. 101
Bristol, PA 19007   Phone: (215) 785-5800
First Published: 1978. **Frequency:** Quarterly. **ISSN:** 0161-2840.

★843★ ITALIAN JOURNAL OF ORTHOPAEDICS AND TRAUMATOLOGY
Aulo Gaggi Editore
Via Andrea Costa 131/5
40134 Bologna, Italy
First Published: 1975. **Frequency:** Quarterly. **ISSN:** 0390-5489.

★844★   JAMA
American Medical Association
515 N. State St.
Chicago, IL 60610   Phone: (312) 464-5000
First Published: 1848. Frequency: Weekly. ISSN: 0098-7484.

★845★   JAPANESE HEART JOURNAL
Nankodo Co., Ltd.
3-42-6 Hongo
Bunkyo-ku
Tokyo 113, Japan
First Published: 1960. Frequency: Bimonthly. ISSN: 0021-4868.

★846★   JAPANESE JOURNAL OF MEDICAL SCIENCE AND
   BIOLOGY
National Institute of Health
2-10-35 Kamiosaki
Shinagawaku
Tokyo 141, Japan
First Published: 1948. Frequency: Bimonthly. ISSN: 0021-5112.

★847★   JAPANESE JOURNAL OF MEDICINE
Japanese Society of Internal Medicine
Nihon Maika Gakkai
Hongo Daiichi Bldg.
34-3, 3-Chome, Bunkyo-ku
Tokyo 113, Japan
First Published: 1962. Frequency: Quarterly. ISSN: 0021-5120.

★848★   JAPCA: THE INTERNATIONAL JOURNAL OF THE
   AIR AND WASTE MANAGEMENT ASSOCIATION
PO Box 2861
Pittsburgh, PA 15230   Phone: (412) 232-3444
First Published: 1951. Frequency: Monthly. ISSN: 0002-2470.

★849★   JCU: JOURNAL OF CLINICAL ULTRASOUND
John Wiley & Sons, Inc.
605 3rd Ave.
New York, NY 10158   Phone: (212) 850-6000
First Published: 1973. Frequency: 9/yr. ISSN: 0091-2751.

★850★   JEN: JOURNAL OF EMERGENCY NURSING
Mosby-Year Book, Inc.
11830 Westline Industrial Dr.
St. Louis, MO 63146   Phone: (314) 872-8370
First Published: 1975. Frequency: Bimonthly. ISSN: 0099-1767.

★851★   JMCI: JOURNAL OF MOLECULAR AND CELLULAR
   IMMUNOLOGY
Springer-Verlag New York, Inc.
175 5th Ave.
New York, NY 10010   Phone: (212) 460-1500
First Published: 1983. Frequency: Bimonthly. ISSN: 0724-6803.

★852★   JOGNN: JOURNAL OF OBSTETRIC, GYNECOLOGIC,
   AND NEONATAL NURSING
Nurses Association of the American College of Obstetricians and
   Gynecologists
409 12th St., SW
Washington, DC 20024   Phone: (202) 638-0026
First Published: 1972. Frequency: Bimonthly. ISSN: 0884-2175.

★853★   JOURNAL OF ABDOMINAL SURGERY
American Society of Abdominal Surgery
675 Main St.
Melrose, MA 02176   Phone: (617) 665-6102
First Published: 1959. Frequency: Monthly. ISSN: 0021-8421.

★854★   JOURNAL OF ABNORMAL CHILD PSYCHOLOGY
Plenum Publishing Corp.
233 Spring St.
New York, NY 10013   Phone: (212) 620-8000
First Published: 1973. Frequency: Bimonthly. ISSN: 0091-0627.

★855★   JOURNAL OF ABNORMAL PSYCHOLOGY
American Psychological Association
1200 17th St., NW
Washington, DC 20036   Phone: (202) 955-7600
First Published: 1906. Frequency: Quarterly. ISSN: 0021-843X.

★856★   JOURNAL OF ACQUIRED IMMUNE DEFICIENCY
   SYNDROMES
Raven Press
1185 Avenue of the Americas
New York, NY 10036   Phone: (212) 930-9500
First Published: 1988. Frequency: Bimonthly. ISSN: 0894-9255.

★857★   JOURNAL OF ADOLESCENCE
Academic Press, Inc.
1250 6th Ave.
San Diego, CA 92101   Phone: (619) 231-0926
Frequency: Quarterly. ISSN: 0140-1971.

★858★   JOURNAL OF ADOLESCENT CHEMICAL
   DEPENDENCY
The Haworth Press, Inc.
10 Alice St.
Binghamton, NY 13904   Phone: (800) 342-9678
First Published: 1990. Frequency: Quarterly. ISSN: 1279-1200.

★859★   JOURNAL OF ADOLESCENT HEALTH
Elsevier Science Publishing Co., Inc.
655 Avenue of the Americas
New York, NY 10010   Phone: (212) 989-5800
First Published: 1980. Frequency: 8/yr. ISSN: 1054-139X.

★860★   JOURNAL OF ADVANCED NURSING
Blackwell Scientific Publications
3 Cambridge Center, Ste. 208
Cambridge, MA 02142   Phone: (617) 225-0401
First Published: 1976. Frequency: Bimonthly. ISSN: 0309-2402.

★861★   JOURNAL OF ADVANCEMENT IN MEDICINE
Human Sciences Press, Inc.
233 Spring St.
New York, NY 10013   Phone: (212) 620-8000
Frequency: Quarterly.

★862★   JOURNAL OF AFFECTIVE DISORDERS
Elsevier Science Publishing Co., Inc.
655 Avenue of the Americas
New York, NY 10010   Phone: (212) 989-5800
First Published: 1979. Frequency: Monthly. ISSN: 0165-0327.

★863★   JOURNAL OF ALLERGY AND CLINICAL
   IMMUNOLOGY
American Academy of Allergy and Immunology
611 E. Wells St.
Milwaukee, WI 53202   Phone: (414) 272-6071
First Published: 1929. Frequency: Monthly. ISSN: 0091-6749.

★864★   JOURNAL OF ALLIED HEALTH
American Society of Allied Health Professions
1101 Connecticut Ave., NW, Ste. 700
Washington, DC 20036   Phone: (202) 857-1150
First Published: 1972. Frequency: Quarterly. ISSN: 0090-7421.

★865★   JOURNAL OF AMBULATORY CARE MANAGEMENT
Aspen Publishers, Inc.
200 Orchard Ridge Dr.
Gaithersburg, MD 20878   Phone: (301) 417-7500
First Published: 1978. Frequency: Quarterly. ISSN: 0148-9917.

★866★   JOURNAL OF THE AMERICAN ACADEMY OF CHILD
   AND ADOLESCENT PSYCHIATRY
3615 Wisconsin Ave., NW
Washington, DC 20016   Phone: (202) 966-7300
First Published: 1962. Frequency: Bimonthly. ISSN: 0890-8567.

★867★ JOURNAL OF THE AMERICAN ACADEMY OF DERMATOLOGY
1567 Maple Ave.
Evanston, IL 60201   Phone: (312) 869-3954
First Published: 1979. **Frequency:** Monthly. **ISSN:** 0190-9622.

★868★ JOURNAL OF THE AMERICAN ACADEMY OF PHYSICIAN ASSISTANTS
Mosby-Year Book, Inc.
11830 Westline Industrial Dr.
St. Louis, MO 63146   Phone: (314) 872-8370
First Published: 1988. **Frequency:** 10/yr.

★869★ JOURNAL OF THE AMERICAN ACADEMY OF PSYCHOANALYSIS
30 E. 40th St., Ste. 206
New York, NY 10016   Phone: (212) 679-4105
First Published: 1973. **Frequency:** Quarterly. **ISSN:** 0090-3604.

★870★ JOURNAL OF THE AMERICAN CHEMICAL SOCIETY
1155 16th St., NW
Washington, DC 20036   Phone: (202) 872-4600
First Published: 1879. **Frequency:** Biweekly. **ISSN:** 0002-7863.

★871★ JOURNAL OF THE AMERICAN COLLEGE OF CARDIOLOGY
9111 Old Georgetown Rd.
Bethesda, MD 20814   Phone: (301) 897-5400
Frequency: Monthly. **ISSN:** 0735-1097.

★872★ JOURNAL OF THE AMERICAN COLLEGE OF DENTISTS
7315 Wisconsin Ave., Ste. 352N
Bethesda, MD 20814   Phone: (301) 986-0555
First Published: 1934. **Frequency:** Quarterly. **ISSN:** 0002-7979.

★873★ JOURNAL OF AMERICAN COLLEGE HEALTH
American College Health Association
1300 Piccard Dr., Ste. 200
Rockville, MD 20850   Phone: (301) 963-1100
First Published: 1952. **Frequency:** Bimonthly. **ISSN:** 0744-8481.

★874★ JOURNAL OF THE AMERICAN COLLEGE OF NUTRITION
722 Robert E. Lee Dr.
Wilmington, NC 28412   Phone: (919) 452-1222
First Published: 1982. **Frequency:** 6/yr. **ISSN:** 0731-5724.

★875★ JOURNAL OF THE AMERICAN DENTAL ASSOCIATION
211 E. Chicago Ave.
Chicago, IL 60611   Phone: (312) 440-2500
First Published: 1913. **Frequency:** Monthly. **ISSN:** 0002-8177.

★876★ JOURNAL OF THE AMERICAN DIETETIC ASSOCIATION
216 W. Jackson Blvd., Ste. 800
Chicago, IL 60606-6995   Phone: (312) 899-4829
First Published: 1925. **Frequency:** Monthly. **ISSN:** 0002-8223.

★877★ JOURNAL OF THE AMERICAN GERIATRICS SOCIETY
770 Lexington Ave., Ste. 400
New York, NY 10021   Phone: (212) 308-1414
First Published: 1953. **Frequency:** Monthly. **ISSN:** 0002-8614.

★878★ JOURNAL OF THE AMERICAN MEDICAL RECORD ASSOCIATION
875 N. Michigan Ave., Ste. 1850
Chicago, IL 60611   Phone: (312) 787-2672
First Published: 1929. **Frequency:** Monthly. **ISSN:** 0273-9976.

★879★ JOURNAL OF THE AMERICAN MEDICAL WOMEN'S ASSOCIATION
801 N. Fairfax St., Ste. 400
Alexandria, VA 22314   Phone: (703) 838-0500
First Published: 1915. **Frequency:** Bimonthly. **ISSN:** 0098-8421.

★880★ JOURNAL OF THE AMERICAN OPTOMETRIC ASSOCIATION
243 N. Lindbergh Blvd.
St. Louis, MO 63141   Phone: (314) 991-4100
First Published: 1928. **Frequency:** Monthly. **ISSN:** 0003-0244.

★881★ JOURNAL OF THE AMERICAN OSTEOPATHIC ASSOCIATION
142 E. Ontario St.
Chicago, IL 60611   Phone: (312) 280-5800
First Published: 1901. **Frequency:** Monthly. **ISSN:** 0003-0287.

★882★ JOURNAL OF THE AMERICAN PODIATRIC MEDICAL ASSOCIATION
9312 Old Georgetown Rd.
Bethesda, MD 20814   Phone: (301) 571-9200
First Published: 1907. **Frequency:** Monthly. **ISSN:** 8750-7315.

★883★ JOURNAL OF THE AMERICAN PSYCHOANALYTIC ASSOCIATION
309 E. 49th St.
New York, NY 10022   Phone: (212) 752-0450
First Published: 1953. **Frequency:** Quarterly. **ISSN:** 0003-0651.

★884★ JOURNAL OF THE AMERICAN SOCIETY OF ECHOCARDIOGRAPHY
Mosby-Year Book, Inc.
11830 Westline Industrial Dr.
St. Louis, MO 63146   Phone: (314) 872-8370
First Published: 1988. **Frequency:** Bimonthly.

★885★ JOURNAL OF THE AMERICAN SOCIETY OF NEPHROLOGY
Williams & Wilkins
428 E. Preston St.
Baltimore, MD 21202   Phone: (301) 528-4000
First Published: 1990. **Frequency:** Monthly.

★886★ JOURNAL OF THE AMERICAN VETERINARY MEDICAL ASSOCIATION
930 N. Meacham Rd.
Schaumburg, IL 60196   Phone: (312) 605-8070
First Published: 1877. **Frequency:** Semimonthly. **ISSN:** 0003-1488.

★887★ JOURNAL OF ANALYTICAL PSYCHOLOGY
Academic Press, Inc.
1250 Sixth Ave.
San Diego, CA 92101   Phone: (619) 231-0926
First Published: 1955. **Frequency:** Quarterly. **ISSN:** 0021-8774.

★888★ JOURNAL OF ANALYTICAL TOXICOLOGY
Preston Publications, Inc.
7800 Merrimac Ave.
PO Box 48312
Niles, IL 60648   Phone: (708) 965-0566
First Published: 1977. **Frequency:** Bimonthly. **ISSN:** 0146-4760.

★889★ JOURNAL OF ANATOMY
Cambridge University Press
40 W. 20th St.
New York, NY 10011   Phone: (212) 924-3900
First Published: 1866. **Frequency:** 6/yr. **ISSN:** 0021-8782.

★890★ JOURNAL OF ANDROLOGY
J.B. Lippincott Co.
E. Washington Sq.
Philadelphia, PA 19105   Phone: (215) 238-4200
First Published: 1980. **Frequency:** Bimonthly. **ISSN:** 0196-3635.

★891★ JOURNAL OF ANTIMICROBIAL CHEMOTHERAPY
Academic Press, Inc.
1250 6th Ave.
San Diego, CA 92101   Phone: (619) 231-0926
First Published: 1975. **Frequency:** Monthly. **ISSN:** 0305-7453.

★892★ JOURNAL OF APPLIED BACTERIOLOGY
Blackwell Scientific Publications
3 Cambridge Center, Ste. 208
Cambridge, MA 02142   Phone: (617) 225-0401
First Published: 1938. **Frequency:** Monthly. **ISSN:** 0021-8847.

★893★ JOURNAL OF APPLIED CARDIOLOGY
Pergamon Press, Inc.
Maxwell House, Fairview Park
Elmsford, NY 10523   Phone: (914) 592-7700
First Published: 1986. **Frequency:** Bimonthly. **ISSN:** 0883-2935.

★894★ JOURNAL OF APPLIED PHYSIOLOGY
American Physiological Society
9650 Rockville Pike
Bethesda, MD 20814   Phone: (301) 530-7164
First Published: 1948. **Frequency:** Monthly. **ISSN:** 8750-7587.

★895★ JOURNAL OF APPLIED PSYCHOLOGY
American Psychological Association
1200 17th St., NW
Washington, DC 20036   Phone: (202) 955-7600
First Published: 1917. **Frequency:** Bimonthly. **ISSN:** 0021-9010.

★896★ JOURNAL OF APPLIED TOXICOLOGY
John Wiley & Sons, Inc.
605 3rd Ave.
New York, NY 10158   Phone: (212) 850-6000
First Published: 1970. **Frequency:** 10/yr. **ISSN:** 0260-437X.

★897★ JOURNAL OF THE ARKANSAS MEDICAL SOCIETY
PO Box 5776
Little Rock, AR 72215   Phone: (501) 224-8967
First Published: 1880. **Frequency:** Monthly. **ISSN:** 0004-1858.

★898★ JOURNAL OF ARTHROPLASTY
Churchill Livingstone, Inc.
1560 Broadway
New York, NY 10036   Phone: (212) 819-5400
First Published: 1986. **Frequency:** Quarterly. **ISSN:** 0883-5403.

★899★ JOURNAL OF ASTHMA
Association for the Care of Asthma
c/o Herbert C. Mansmann, Jr., M.D.
Jefferson Medical College
1025 Walnut St., Rm. 727
Philadelphia, PA 19107   Phone: (215) 955-8912
First Published: 1963. **Frequency:** Bimonthly. **ISSN:** 0277-0903.

★900★ JOURNAL OF AUDIOVISUAL MEDIA IN MEDICINE
Butterworth-Heinemann
80 Montvale Ave.
Stoneham, MA 02180   Phone: (617) 438-8464
First Published: 1951. **Frequency:** Quarterly. **ISSN:** 0140-511X.

★901★ JOURNAL OF AUTISM AND DEVELOPMENTAL DISORDERS
Plenum Publishing Corp.
233 Spring St.
New York, NY 10013   Phone: (212) 620-8000
First Published: 1971. **Frequency:** Quarterly. **ISSN:** 0162-3257.

★902★ JOURNAL OF AUTOIMMUNITY
Academic Press, Inc.
1250 6th Ave.
San Diego, CA 92101   Phone: (609) 231-0926
First Published: 1988. **Frequency:** Bimonthly. **ISSN:** 0896-8411.

★903★ JOURNAL OF THE AUTONOMIC NERVOUS SYSTEM
Elsevier Science Publishing Co., Inc.
655 Avenue of the Americas
New York, NY 10010   Phone: (212) 989-5800
First Published: 1979. **Frequency:** 12/yr. **ISSN:** 0165-1838.

★904★ JOURNAL OF BACK AND MUSCULOSKELETAL REHABILITATION
Butterworth-Heinemann
80 Montvale Ave.
Stoneham, MA 02180   Phone: (617) 438-8464
First Published: 1991. **Frequency:** Quarterly. **ISSN:** 1053-8127.

★905★ JOURNAL OF BACTERIOLOGY
American Society for Microbiology
1325 Massachusetts Ave., NW
Washington, DC 20005   Phone: (202) 737-3600
First Published: 1916. **Frequency:** Monthly. **ISSN:** 0021-9193.

★906★ JOURNAL OF BEHAVIOR THERAPY AND EXPERIMENTAL PSYCHIATRY
Pergamon Press, Inc.
Maxwell House, Fairview Park
Elmsford, NY 10523   Phone: (914) 592-7700
First Published: 1970. **Frequency:** Quarterly. **ISSN:** 0005-7916.

★907★ JOURNAL OF BEHAVIORAL EDUCATION
Human Sciences Press, Inc.
233 Spring St.
New York, NY 10013   Phone: (212) 620-8000
First Published: 1991. **Frequency:** Quarterly. **ISSN:** 1053-0819.

★908★ JOURNAL OF BEHAVIORAL MEDICINE
Plenum Publishing Corp.
233 Spring St.
New York, NY 10013   Phone: (212) 620-8000
First Published: 1978. **Frequency:** Bimonthly. **ISSN:** 0160-7715.

★909★ JOURNAL OF BIOCHEMICAL AND BIOPHYSICAL METHODS
Elsevier Science Publishing Co., Inc.
655 Avenue of the Americas
New York, NY 10010   Phone: (212) 989-5800
First Published: 1979. **Frequency:** 8/yr. **ISSN:** 0165-022X.

★910★ JOURNAL OF BIOCHEMISTRY
Japanese Biochemical Society
c/o Ishikawa Bldg. 3F
25-16 Hongo 5 Chome
Bunkyo-ku
Tokyo 113, Japan
First Published: 1922. **Frequency:** Monthly. **ISSN:** 0021-924X.

★911★ JOURNAL OF BIOCOMMUNICATION
170 Pomfret Rd.
Box 217
Brooklyn, CT 06234
First Published: 1974. **Frequency:** 4/yr. **ISSN:** 0094-2499.

★912★ JOURNAL OF BIOENERGETICS AND BIOMEMBRANES
Plenum Publishing Corp.
233 Spring St.
New York, NY 10013   Phone: (212) 620-8000
First Published: 1970. **Frequency:** Bimonthly. **ISSN:** 0145-479X.

★913★ JOURNAL OF BIOLOGICAL CHEMISTRY
American Society for Biochemistry and Molecular Biology, Inc.
9650 Rockville Pike
Bethesda, MD 20814   Phone: (301) 530-7145
First Published: 1905. **Frequency:** 36/yr. **ISSN:** 0021-9258.

★914★   JOURNAL OF BIOLOGICAL PHOTOGRAPHY
Biological Photographic Association, Inc.
115 Stoneridge Dr.
Chapel Hill, NC 27514   Phone: (919) 967-8247
First Published: 1933. **Frequency:** Quarterly. **ISSN:** 0274-497X.

**★915★   JOURNAL OF BIOLOGICAL REGULATORS AND
          HOMEOSTATIC AGENTS**
Wichtig Editor
PO Box 830350
Birmingham, AL 35283   Phone: (800) 633-4931
Frequency: Quarterly.

★916★   JOURNAL OF BIOLOGICAL RESPONSE MODIFIERS
Raven Press
1185 Avenue of the Americas
New York, NY 10036   Phone: (212) 930-9500
First Published: 1982. **Frequency:** Bimonthly. **ISSN:** 0732-6580.

★917★   JOURNAL OF BIOMEDICAL ENGINEERING
Butterworth-Heinemann
80 Montvale Ave.
Stoneham, MA 02180   Phone: (617) 438-8464
First Published: 1979. **Frequency:** Bimonthly. **ISSN:** 0141-5425.

★918★   JOURNAL OF BIOMEDICAL MATERIALS RESEARCH
John Wiley & Sons, Inc.
605 3rd Ave.
New York, NY 10158   Phone: (212) 850-6000
First Published: 1966. **Frequency:** Monthly. **ISSN:** 0021-9304.

★919★   JOURNAL OF BIOSOCIAL SCIENCE
Parkes Foundation
22 Newmarket Rd.
Cambridge CB5 8DT, England
First Published: 1969. **Frequency:** Quarterly. **ISSN:** 0021-9320.

★920★   JOURNAL OF BONE AND JOINT SURGERY
Journal of Bone and Joint Surgery, Inc.
10 Shattuck St.
Boston, MA 02115   Phone: (617) 734-2835
First Published: 1903. **Frequency:** 10/yr. **ISSN:** 0021-9355.

★921★   JOURNAL OF BURN CARE AND REHABILITATION
American Burn Association
c/o Andrew W. Munster, M.D.
Baltimore Regional Burn Center, Francis Scott Key Hospital
4940 Eastern Ave.
Baltimore, MD 21224   Phone: (301) 550-0886
First Published: 1980. **Frequency:** Bimonthly. **ISSN:** 0273-8481.

**★922★   JOURNAL OF THE CANADIAN ASSOCIATION OF
          RADIOLOGISTS**
Canadian Medical Association
PO Box 8650
Ottawa, ON, Canada K1G 0G8   Phone: (613) 731-9331
First Published: 1950. **Frequency:** Quarterly. **ISSN:** 0008-2902.

★923★   JOURNAL OF CANCER EDUCATION
Pergamon Press, Inc.
Maxwell House, Fairview Park
Elmsford, NY 10523   Phone: (914) 592-7700
First Published: 1986. **Frequency:** Quarterly. **ISSN:** 0885-8195.

**★924★   JOURNAL OF CANCER RESEARCH AND CLINICAL
          ONCOLOGY**
Springer-Verlag New York, Inc.
175 5th Ave.
New York, NY 10010   Phone: (212) 460-1500
First Published: 1903. **Frequency:** Bimonthly. **ISSN:** 0171-5216.

**★925★   JOURNAL OF CARDIOPULMONARY
          REHABILITATION**
J.B. Lippincott Co.
E. Washington Sq.
Philadelphia, PA 19105   Phone: (215) 238-4200
First Published: 1991. **Frequency:** Monthly. **ISSN:** 0883-9212.

**★926★   JOURNAL OF CARDIOTHORACIC AND VASCULAR
          ANESTHESIA**
W.B. Saunders Co.
Curtis Center
Independence Sq. W.
Philadelphia, PA 19106   Phone: (215) 238-7800
First Published: 1987. **Frequency:** Bimonthly. **ISSN:** 1053-0770.

★927★   JOURNAL OF CARDIOVASCULAR NURSING
Aspen Publishers, Inc.
200 Orchard Ridge Dr.
Gaithersburg, MD 20878   Phone: (301) 417-7500
First Published: 1986. **Frequency:** Quarterly. **ISSN:** 0889-4655.

★928★   JOURNAL OF CARDIOVASCULAR PHARMACOLOGY
Raven Press
1185 Avenue of the Americas
New York, NY 10036   Phone: (212) 575-0335
First Published: 1979. **Frequency:** Monthly. **ISSN:** 0160-2446.

★929★   JOURNAL OF CARDIOVASCULAR SURGERY
J.B. Lippincott Co.
E. Washington Sq.
Philadelphia, PA 19105   Phone: (215) 238-4200
First Published: 1960. **Frequency:** Bimonthly. **ISSN:** 0021-9509.

**★930★   JOURNAL OF CATARACT AND REFRACTIVE
          SURGERY**
American Society of Cataract and Refractive Surgery
3702 Pender Dr., Ste. 250
Fairfax, VA 22030   Phone: (703) 591-2220
First Published: 1974. **Frequency:** Bimonthly. **ISSN:** 0886-3350.

★931★   JOURNAL OF CELL BIOLOGY
American Society for Cell Biology
9650 Rockville Pike
Bethesda, MD 20814   Phone: (301) 530-7153
First Published: 1955. **Frequency:** 24/yr. **ISSN:** 0021-9525.

★932★   JOURNAL OF CELL SCIENCE
Company of Biologists, Ltd.
Box 32
Commerce Way
Colchester, Essex CO2 8HP, England
First Published: 1966. **Frequency:** 13/yr. **ISSN:** 0021-9533.

★933★   JOURNAL OF CELLULAR BIOCHEMISTRY
John Wiley & Sons, Inc.
605 3rd Ave.
New York, NY 10158   Phone: (212) 850-6000
First Published: 1972. **Frequency:** Monthly. **ISSN:** 0730-2312.

★934★   JOURNAL OF CELLULAR PHYSIOLOGY
John Wiley & Sons, Inc.
605 3rd Ave.
New York, NY 10158   Phone: (212) 850-6000
First Published: 1932. **Frequency:** Monthly. **ISSN:** 0021-9541.

**★935★   JOURNAL OF CEREBRAL BLOOD FLOW AND
          METABOLISM**
Raven Press
1185 Avenue of the Americas
New York, NY 10036   Phone: (212) 930-9500
First Published: 1981. **Frequency:** Bimonthly. **ISSN:** 0271-678X.

★936★ JOURNAL OF CHEMICAL DEPENDENCY
   TREATMENT
The Haworth Press, Inc.
10 Alice St.
Binghamton, NY 13904   Phone: (800) 342-9678
First Published: 1987. **Frequency:** Semiannual. **ISSN:** 0885-4734.

★937★ JOURNAL OF CHILD AND ADOLESCENT GROUP
   THERAPY
Human Sciences Press, Inc.
233 Spring St.
New York, NY 10013   Phone: (212) 620-8000
Frequency: Quarterly.

★938★ JOURNAL OF CHILD AND FAMILY STUDIES
Human Sciences Press, Inc.
233 Spring St.
New York, NY 10013   Phone: (212) 620-8000

★939★ JOURNAL OF CHILD NEUROLOGY
Mosby-Year Book, Inc.
11830 Westline Industrial Dr.
St. Louis, MO 63146   Phone: (314) 872-8370
First Published: 1986. **Frequency:** Quarterly.

★940★ JOURNAL OF CHIROPRACTIC
American Chiropractic Association
1701 Clarendon Blvd.
Arlington, VA 22209   Phone: (202) 276-8800
First Published: 1964. **Frequency:** Monthly. **ISSN:** 0744-9984.

★941★ THE JOURNAL OF THE CHRONIC FATIGUE
   SYNDROME
The Haworth Press, Inc.
10 Alice St.
Binghampton, NY 13904   Phone: (800) 342-9678
First Published: 1992. **Frequency:** Quarterly. **ISSN:** 1279-1200.

★942★ JOURNAL OF CLINICAL ANESTHESIA
Butterworth-Heinemann
80 Montvale Ave.
Stoneham, MA 02180   Phone: (617) 438-8464
Frequency: Bimonthly. **ISSN:** 0952-8180.

★943★ JOURNAL OF CLINICAL APHERESIS
John Wiley & Sons, Inc.
605 3rd Ave.
New York, NY 10158   Phone: (212) 850-6000
First Published: 1982. **Frequency:** 4/yr. **ISSN:** 0733-2459.

★944★ JOURNAL OF CLINICAL CHILD PSYCHOLOGY
Lawrence Erlbaum Associates, Inc.
365 Broadway
Hillsdale, NJ 07642   Phone: (201) 666-4110
Frequency: Quarterly.

★945★ JOURNAL OF CLINICAL ENDOCRINOLOGY AND
   METABOLISM
Endocrine Society
9650 Rockville Pike
Bethesda, MD 20814   Phone: (301) 571-1802
First Published: 1941. **Frequency:** Monthly. **ISSN:** 0021-972X.

★946★ JOURNAL OF CLINICAL EPIDEMIOLOGY
Pergamon Press, Inc.
Maxwell House, Fairview Park
Elmsford, NY 10523   Phone: (914) 592-7700
First Published: 1955. **Frequency:** Monthly. **ISSN:** 0895-4356.

★947★ JOURNAL OF CLINICAL AND EXPERIMENTAL
   GERONTOLOGY
Marcel Dekker, Inc.
270 Madison Ave.
New York, NY 10016   Phone: (212) 696-9000
First Published: 1979. **Frequency:** 4/yr. **ISSN:** 0192-1193.

★948★ JOURNAL OF CLINICAL GASTROENTEROLOGY
Raven Press
1185 Avenue of the Americas
New York, NY 10036   Phone: (212) 930-9500
First Published: 1979. **Frequency:** Bimonthly. **ISSN:** 0192-0790.

★949★ JOURNAL OF CLINICAL IMMUNOLOGY
Plenum Publishing Corp.
233 Spring St.
New York, NY 10013   Phone: (212) 620-8000
First Published: 1981. **Frequency:** Bimonthly. **ISSN:** 0271-9142.

★950★ JOURNAL OF CLINICAL INVESTIGATION
American Society for Clinical Investigation
6900 Grove Rd.
Thorofare, NJ 08086   Phone: (609) 848-1000
First Published: 1924. **Frequency:** Monthly. **ISSN:** 0021-9738.

★951★ JOURNAL OF CLINICAL LABORATORY ANALYSIS
John Wiley & Sons, Inc.
605 3rd Ave.
New York, NY 10158   Phone: (212) 850-6000
First Published: 1987. **Frequency:** Bimonthly. **ISSN:** 0887-8013.

★952★ JOURNAL OF CLINICAL AND LABORATORY
   IMMUNOLOGY
Teviot Scientific Publications, Ltd.
31 Montpelier Park
Edinburgh EH10 4LX, Scotland
First Published: 1978. **Frequency:** Monthly. **ISSN:** 0141-2760.

★953★ JOURNAL OF CLINICAL MICROBIOLOGY
American Society for Microbiology
1325 Massachusetts Ave., NW
Washington, DC 20005   Phone: (202) 737-3600
First Published: 1975. **Frequency:** Monthly. **ISSN:** 0095-1137.

★954★ JOURNAL OF CLINICAL MONITORING
Little, Brown & Company
34 Beacon St.
Boston, MA 02108   Phone: (617) 227-0730
First Published: 1985. **Frequency:** Quarterly. **ISSN:** 0748-1977.

★955★ JOURNAL OF CLINICAL NEURO-OPHTHALMOLOGY
Raven Press
1185 Avenue of the Americas
New York, NY 10036   Phone: (212) 930-9500
First Published: 1981. **Frequency:** Quarterly. **ISSN:** 0272-846X.

★956★ JOURNAL OF CLINICAL NEUROPHYSIOLOGY
American Electroencephalographic Society
1 Regency Dr.
PO Box 30
Bloomfield, CT 06002   Phone: (203) 243-3977
First Published: 1984. **Frequency:** Quarterly. **ISSN:** 0736-0258.

★957★ JOURNAL OF CLINICAL ONCOLOGY
American Society of Clinical Oncology
435 N. Michigan Ave., Ste. 1717
Chicago, IL 60611   Phone: (312) 644-0828
First Published: 1983. **Frequency:** Monthly. **ISSN:** 0732-183X.

★958★ JOURNAL OF CLINICAL PATHOLOGY
British Medical Association
PO Box 560B
Kennebunkport, ME 04046
First Published: 1947. **Frequency:** Monthly. **ISSN:** 0021-9746.

★959★ JOURNAL OF CLINICAL PERIODONTOLOGY
Munksgaard
Noerre Soegade 35
DK-1370 Copenhagen K, Denmark
First Published: 1974. **Frequency:** 10/yr. **ISSN:** 0303-6979.

★960★   JOURNAL OF CLINICAL PHARMACOLOGY
American College of Clinical Pharmacology
175 Strafford Ave., Ste. 1
Wayne, PA 19087   Phone: (215) 687-7711
First Published: 1961. **Frequency:** 12/yr. **ISSN:** 0091-2700.

**★961★   JOURNAL OF CLINICAL PHARMACY AND
    THERAPEUTICS**
Blackwell Scientific Publications
3 Cambridge Center, Ste. 208
Cambridge, MA 02142   Phone: (617) 225-0401
First Published: 1976. **Frequency:** Bimonthly. **ISSN:** 0269-4727.

★962★   JOURNAL OF CLINICAL PSYCHIATRY
American Academy of Clinical Psychiatrists
PO Box 3212
San Diego, CA 92103   Phone: (619) 298-4782
First Published: 1940. **Frequency:** Monthly. **ISSN:** 0160-6689.

★963★   JOURNAL OF CLINICAL PSYCHOLOGY
Clinical Psychology Publishing Co., Inc.
4 Conant Sq.
Brandon, VT 05733   Phone: (802) 247-6871
First Published: 1945. **Frequency:** Bimonthly. **ISSN:** 0021-9762.

★964★   JOURNAL OF CLINICAL PSYCHOPHARMACOLOGY
Williams & Wilkins
428 E. Preston St.
Baltimore, MD 21202   Phone: (301) 528-4223
First Published: 1981. **Frequency:** Bimonthly. **ISSN:** 0271-0749.

★965★   JOURNAL OF COMMUNICATION DISORDERS
Elsevier Science Publishing Co., Inc.
655 Avenue of the Americas
New York, NY 10010   Phone: (212) 989-5800
First Published: 1968. **Frequency:** Bimonthly. **ISSN:** 0021-9924.

★966★   JOURNAL OF COMMUNITY HEALTH
Human Sciences Press, Inc.
233 Spring St.
New York, NY 10013   Phone: (212) 620-8000
First Published: 1975. **Frequency:** Quarterly. **ISSN:** 0094-5145.

★967★   JOURNAL OF COMMUNITY HEALTH NURSING
Lawrence Erlbaum Associates, Inc.
365 Broadway
Hillsdale, NJ 07642   Phone: (201) 666-4110
First Published: 1984. **Frequency:** Quarterly. **ISSN:** 0737-0016.

★968★   JOURNAL OF COMPARATIVE NEUROLOGY
John Wiley & Sons, Inc.
605 3rd Ave.
New York, NY 10158   Phone: (212) 850-6000
First Published: 1891. **Frequency:** 48/yr. **ISSN:** 0021-9967.

★969★   JOURNAL OF COMPARATIVE PATHOLOGY
Academic Press, Inc.
1250 6th Ave.
San Diego, CA 92101   Phone: (619) 231-0926
First Published: 1888. **Frequency:** 8/yr. **ISSN:** 0021-9975.

**★970★   JOURNAL OF COMPARATIVE PHYSIOLOGY A:
    SENSORY, NEURAL, AND BEHAVIORAL PHYSIOLOGY**
Springer-Verlag New York, Inc.
175 5th Ave.
New York, NY 10010   Phone: (212) 460-1500
First Published: 1924. **Frequency:** 12/yr. **ISSN:** 0340-7594.

**★971★   JOURNAL OF COMPARATIVE PHYSIOLOGY B:
    BIOCHEMICAL, SYSTEMATIC, AND ENVIRONMENTAL
    PHYSIOLOGY**
Springer-Verlag New York, Inc.
175 5th Ave.
New York, NY 10010   Phone: (212) 460-1500
First Published: 1924. **Frequency:** 6/yr. **ISSN:** 0174-1578.

★972★   JOURNAL OF COMPARATIVE PSYCHOLOGY
American Psychological Association
1200 17th St., NW
Washington, DC 20036   Phone: (202) 955-7600
First Published: 1983. **Frequency:** Quarterly. **ISSN:** 0735-7036.

★973★   JOURNAL OF COMPUTER ASSISTED TOMOGRAPHY
Raven Press
1185 Avenue of the Americas
New York, NY 10036   Phone: (212) 930-9500
First Published: 1977. **Frequency:** Bimonthly. **ISSN:** 0363-8715.

**★974★   JOURNAL OF CONSULTING AND CLINICAL
    PSYCHOLOGY**
American Psychological Association
1200 17th St., NW
Washington, DC 20036   Phone: (202) 955-7600
First Published: 1968. **Frequency:** Bimonthly. **ISSN:** 0022-006X.

★975★   JOURNAL OF COUNSELING PSYCHOLOGY
American Psychological Association
1200 17th St., NW
Washington, DC 20036   Phone: (202) 955-7600
Frequency: Quarterly. **ISSN:** 0022-0167.

★976★   JOURNAL OF COUPLES THERAPY
The Haworth Press, Inc.
10 Alice St.
Binghamton, NY 13904   Phone: (800) 342-9678
Frequency: Quarterly.

**★977★   JOURNAL OF CRANIOFACIAL GENETICS AND
    DEVELOPMENTAL BIOLOGY**
John Wiley & Sons, Inc.
605 3rd Ave.
New York, NY 10158   Phone: (212) 850-6000
First Published: 1981. **Frequency:** Quarterly. **ISSN:** 0270-4145.

★978★   JOURNAL OF CRITICAL CARE
W.B. Saunders Co.
Curtis Center
Independence Sq. W.
Philadelphia, PA 19106   Phone: (215) 238-7800
First Published: 1986. **Frequency:** Quarterly. **ISSN:** 0883-9441.

★979★   JOURNAL OF CUTANEOUS PATHOLOGY
American Society of Dermatopathology
550 N. Broadway, Ste. 408
Baltimore, MD 21205   Phone: (301) 955-2332
First Published: 1974. **Frequency:** Bimonthly. **ISSN:** 0303-6987.

★980★   JOURNAL OF DENTAL EDUCATION
American Association of Dental Schools
1625 Massachusetts Ave., NW
Washington, DC 20036   Phone: (202) 667-9433
First Published: 1936. **Frequency:** Monthly. **ISSN:** 0022-0337.

★981★   JOURNAL OF DENTAL HYGIENE
American Dental Hygienists Association
444 N. Michigan Ave., Ste. 3400
Chicago, IL 60611   Phone: (312) 440-8900
First Published: 1927. **Frequency:** 9/yr.

★982★   JOURNAL OF DENTAL RESEARCH
American Association for Dental Research
1111 14th St., NW, Ste. 1000
Washington, DC 20005   Phone: (202) 898-1050
First Published: 1919. **Frequency:** 16/yr. **ISSN:** 0022-0345.

★983★   JOURNAL OF DENTISTRY
Butterworth-Heinemann
80 Montvale Ave.
Stoneham, MA 02180   Phone: (617) 438-8464
First Published: 1972. **Frequency:** Bimonthly. **ISSN:** 0300-5712.

★984★ JOURNAL OF DERMATOLOGIC SURGERY AND
ONCOLOGY
Journal of Dermatologic Surgery, Inc.
245 5th Ave.
New York, NY 10016   Phone: (212) 721-5175
First Published: 1975. Frequency: Monthly. ISSN: 0148-0812.

★985★ JOURNAL OF DEVELOPMENTAL AND BEHAVIORAL
PEDIATRICS
Williams & Wilkins
428 E. Preston St.
Baltimore, MD 21202   Phone: (301) 528-4223
First Published: 1980. Frequency: Bimonthly. ISSN: 0196-206X.

★986★ JOURNAL OF DEVELOPMENTAL PHYSIOLOGY
Oxford University Press
200 Madison Ave.
New York, NY 10016   Phone: (212) 679-7300
First Published: 1979. Frequency: Bimonthly. ISSN: 0141-9846.

★987★ JOURNAL OF DIABETES AND ITS COMPLICATIONS
Elsevier Science Publishing Co., Inc.
655 Avenue of the Americas
New York, NY 10010   Phone: (212) 989-5800
Frequency: Quarterly. ISSN: 1056-8727.

★988★ JOURNAL OF DRUG EDUCATION
Baywood Publishing Co., Inc.
26 Austin Ave.
Amityville, NY 11701   Phone: (516) 691-1270
First Published: 1971. Frequency: Quarterly. ISSN: 0047-2379.

★989★ JOURNAL OF EDUCATIONAL PSYCHOLOGY
American Psychological Association
1200 17 St., NW
Washington, DC 20036   Phone: (202) 955-7600
Frequency: Quarterly. ISSN: 0022-0683.

★990★ JOURNAL OF ELECTROCARDIOLOGY
Churchill Livingstone Inc.
1560 Broadway
New York, NY 10036   Phone: (212) 819-5440
First Published: 1968. Frequency: Quarterly. ISSN: 0022-0736.

★991★ JOURNAL OF ELECTROMYOGRAPHY AND
KINESIOLOGY
Raven Press
1185 Avenue of the Americas
New York, NY 10036   Phone: (212) 930-9500
First Published: 1992. Frequency: Quarterly. ISSN: 1050-6411.

★992★ JOURNAL OF ELECTRON MICROSCOPY TECHNIQUE
John Wiley & Sons, Inc.
605 3rd Ave.
New York, NY 10158   Phone: (212) 850-6000
First Published: 1984. Frequency: Monthly. ISSN: 0741-0581.

★993★ JOURNAL OF EMERGENCY MEDICINE
Pergamon Press, Inc.
Maxwell House, Fairview Park
Elmsford, NY 10523   Phone: (914) 592-7700
First Published: 1983. Frequency: Bimonthly. ISSN: 0736-4679.

★994★ JOURNAL OF EMERGENCY NURSING
Mosby-Year Book, Inc.
11830 Westline Industrial, Inc.
St. Louis, MO 63146   Phone: (314) 872-8370
First Published: 1975. Frequency: Bimonthly.

★995★ JOURNAL OF ENDOCRINOLOGY
Journal of Endocrinology, Ltd.
23 Richmond Hill
Bristol BS8 1EN, England
First Published: 1939. Frequency: Monthly. ISSN: 0022-0795.

★996★ JOURNAL OF ENDODONTICS
American Association of Endodontists
211 E. Chicago Ave.
Chicago, IL 60611   Phone: (312) 266-7255
First Published: 1975. Frequency: Monthly. ISSN: 0099-2399.

★997★ JOURNAL OF ENVIRONMENTAL HEALTH
National Environmental Health Association
720 S. Colorado Blvd., Ste. 970, S. Tower
Denver, CO 80222   Phone: (303) 756-9090
First Published: 1938. Frequency: Bimonthly. ISSN: 0022-0892.

★998★ JOURNAL OF ENVIRONMENTAL PATHOLOGY,
TOXICOLOGY AND ONCOLOGY
Chem-Orbital
Box 134
Park Forest, IL 60466   Phone: (312) 755-2080
First Published: 1981. Frequency: Bimonthly. ISSN: 0731-8898.

★999★ JOURNAL OF EPIDEMIOLOGY AND COMMUNITY
HEALTH
British Medical Association
PO Box 560B
Kennebunkport, ME 04046
First Published: 1947. Frequency: Quarterly. ISSN: 0143-005X.

★1000★ JOURNAL OF ET NURSING
International Association for Enterostomal Therapy
2081 Business Circle Dr., Ste. 290
Irvine, CA 92715   Phone: (714) 476-0268
First Published: 1974. Frequency: Bimonthly. ISSN: 0270-1170.

★1001★ JOURNAL OF ETHNOPHARMACOLOGY
Elsevier Science Publishing Co., Inc.
655 Avenue of the Americas
New York, NY 10010   Phone: (212) 989-5800
First Published: 1979. Frequency: 9/yr. ISSN: 0378-8741.

★1002★ JOURNAL OF THE EXPERIMENTAL ANALYSIS OF
BEHAVIOR
Society for the Experimental Analysis of Behavior
Psychology Department
Indiana University
Bloomington, IN 47405   Phone: (812) 336-5416
First Published: 1958. Frequency: Bimonthly. ISSN: 0022-5002.

★1003★ JOURNAL OF EXPERIMENTAL BIOLOGY
Company of Biologists, Ltd.
Box 32
Commerce Way
Colchester, Essex CO2 8HP, England
First Published: 1923. Frequency: 7/yr. ISSN: 0022-0949.

★1004★ JOURNAL OF EXPERIMENTAL CHILD
PSYCHOLOGY
Academic Press, Inc.
1250 6th Ave.
San Diego, CA 92101   Phone: (619) 231-0926
First Published: 1964. Frequency: Bimonthly. ISSN: 0022-0965.

★1005★ JOURNAL OF EXPERIMENTAL MEDICINE
Rockefeller University Press
222 E. 70th St.
New York, NY 10021   Phone: (212) 570-8572
First Published: 1896. Frequency: Monthly. ISSN: 0022-1007.

★1006★ JOURNAL OF EXPERIMENTAL PATHOLOGY
Mary Ann Liebert, Inc.
1651 3rd Ave.
New York, NY 10128   Phone: (212) 289-2300
First Published: 1983. Frequency: Quarterly. ISSN: 0730-8485.

★1007★ JOURNAL OF EXPERIMENTAL PSYCHOLOGY AND ANIMAL BEHAVIOR PROCESSES
American Psychological Association
1200 17th St., NW
Washington, DC 20036   Phone: (202) 955-7600
Frequency: Quarterly. ISSN: 0097-7403.

★1008★ JOURNAL OF EXPERIMENTAL PSYCHOLOGY: GENERAL
American Psychological Association
1200 17th St., NW
Washington, DC 20036   Phone: (202) 955-7600
First Published: 1975. Frequency: Quarterly. ISSN: 0096-3445.

★1009★ JOURNAL OF EXPERIMENTAL PSYCHOLOGY: HUMAN PERCEPTION AND PERFORMANCE
American Psychological Association
1200 17th St., NW
Washington, DC 20036   Phone: (202) 955-7600
First Published: 1975. Frequency: Quarterly. ISSN: 0096-1523.

★1010★ JOURNAL OF EXPERIMENTAL PSYCHOLOGY: LEARNING, MEMORY, AND COGNITION
American Psychological Association
1200 17th St., NW
Washington, DC 20036   Phone: (202) 955-7600
First Published: 1975. Frequency: Bimonthly. ISSN: 0278-7393.

★1011★ JOURNAL OF FAMILY PRACTICE
Appleton & Lange
25 Van Zant St.
East Norwalk, CT 06855   Phone: (203) 838-4400
First Published: 1974. Frequency: Monthly. ISSN: 0094-3509.

★1012★ JOURNAL OF THE FLORIDA MEDICAL ASSOCIATION
720 Riverside Ave.
Box 2411
Jacksonville, FL 32203   Phone: (904) 356-1571
First Published: 1914. Frequency: Monthly. ISSN: 0015-4148.

★1013★ JOURNAL OF FOOT SURGERY
Williams & Wilkins
428 E. Preston St.
Baltimore, MD 21202   Phone: (301) 528-4223
Frequency: Bimonthly. ISSN: 0449-2544.

★1014★ JOURNAL OF THE FORENSIC SCIENCE SOCIETY
Clarke House
18A Mount Parade
Harrogate, North Yorkshire HG1 1BX, England
First Published: 1960. Frequency: Bimonthly. ISSN: 0015-7368.

★1015★ JOURNAL OF FORENSIC SCIENCES
American Academy of Forensic Sciences
218 E. Cache La Poudre
Colorado Springs, CO 80901-0669   Phone: (719) 636-1100
First Published: 1956. Frequency: Bimonthly. ISSN: 0022-1198.

★1016★ JOURNAL OF GASTROENTEROLOGY AND HEPATOLOGY
Blackwell Scientific Publications
3 Cambridge Center, Ste. 208
Cambridge, MA 02142   Phone: (617) 225-0401
First Published: 1986. Frequency: Bimonthly. ISSN: 0815-9319.

★1017★ JOURNAL OF GASTROINTESTINAL MOTILITY
Blackwell Scientific Publications
3 Cambridge Center, Ste. 208
Cambridge, MA 02142   Phone: (617) 225-0401
Frequency: Quarterly. ISSN: 1043-4518.

★1018★ JOURNAL OF GAY AND LESBIAN PSYCHOTHERAPY
The Haworth Press, Inc.
10 Alice St.
Binghampton, NY 13904   Phone: (800) 342-9678
Frequency: Quarterly. ISSN: 8756-8225.

★1019★ JOURNAL OF GENERAL INTERNAL MEDICINE
Society of General Internal Medicine
700 13th St., NW, Ste. 250
Washington, DC 20005   Phone: (202) 393-1662
Frequency: Bimonthly. ISSN: 0884-8734.

★1020★ JOURNAL OF GENERAL MICROBIOLOGY
Society for General Microbiology
Harvest House
62 London Rd.
Reading, Berks RG1 5AS, England
First Published: 1947. Frequency: Monthly. ISSN: 0022-1287.

★1021★ JOURNAL OF GENERAL PHYSIOLOGY
Rockefeller University Press
222 E. 70th St.
New York, NY 10021   Phone: (212) 570-8572
First Published: 1918. Frequency: Monthly. ISSN: 0022-1295.

★1022★ JOURNAL OF GENERAL PSYCHOLOGY
Heldref Publications
4000 Albemarle St., NW
Washington, DC 20016   Phone: (202) 362-6445
First Published: 1927. Frequency: Quarterly. ISSN: 0022-1309.

★1023★ JOURNAL OF GENERAL VIROLOGY
Society for General Microbiology
Harvest House
62 London Rd.
Reading, Berks RG1 5AS, England
First Published: 1967. Frequency: Monthly. ISSN: 0022-1317.

★1024★ JOURNAL OF GENETIC COUNSELING
Human Sciences Press, Inc.
233 Spring St.
New York, NY 10013   Phone: (212) 620-8000

★1025★ JOURNAL OF GENETIC PSYCHOLOGY
Heldref Publications
4000 Albemarle St., NW
Washington, DC 20016   Phone: (202) 362-6445
First Published: 1891. Frequency: Quarterly. ISSN: 0022-1325.

★1026★ JOURNAL OF GERIATRIC PSYCHIATRY
International Universities Press, Inc.
59 Boston Post Rd.
PO Box 1524
Madison, CT 06443   Phone: (203) 245-4000
First Published: 1967. Frequency: Semiannual. ISSN: 0022-1414.

★1027★ JOURNAL OF GERIATRIC PSYCHIATRY AND NEUROLOGY
Mosby-Year Book, Inc.
11830 Westline Industrial Dr.
St. Louis, MO 63146   Phone: (314) 872-8370
First Published: 1988. Frequency: Quarterly.

★1028★ JOURNAL OF GERONTOLOGY
Gerontological Society of America
1275 K St., NW, Ste. 350
Washington, DC 20005   Phone: (202) 842-1275
First Published: 1946. Frequency: Bimonthly. ISSN: 0022-1422.

★1029★ JOURNAL OF GLAUCOMA
Raven Press
1185 Avenue of the Americas
New York, NY 10036   Phone: (212) 930-9500
First Published: 1992. Frequency: Quarterly. ISSN: 1057-0829.

★1030★ JOURNAL OF HAND SURGERY
American Society for Surgery of the Hand
3025 S. Parker Rd., Ste. 65
Aurora, CO 80014   Phone: (303) 755-4588
First Published: 1976. Frequency: Bimonthly. ISSN: 0363-5023.

★1031★ JOURNAL OF HAND SURGERY: BRITISH VOLUME
Churchill Livingstone, Inc.
1560 Broadway
New York, NY 10036   Phone: (212) 819-5400
First Published: 1969. Frequency: Quarterly. ISSN: 0072-968X.

★1032★ JOURNAL OF HEALTH AND SOCIAL BEHAVIOR
American Sociological Association
1722 N St., NW
Washington, DC 20036   Phone: (202) 833-3410
First Published: 1960. Frequency: Quarterly. ISSN: 0022-1465.

★1033★ JOURNAL OF HEART AND LUNG
TRANSPLANTATION
Mosby-Year Book, Inc.
11830 Westline Industrial Dr.
St. Louis, MO 63146   Phone: (314) 872-8370
First Published: 1982. Frequency: Bimonthly. ISSN: 0887-2570.

★1034★ JOURNAL OF HELMINTHOLOGY
Bureau of Hygiene and Tropical Diseases
Keppel St.
London WC1E 7HT, England
First Published: 1923. Frequency: Quarterly. ISSN: 0022-149X.

★1035★ JOURNAL OF HEPATOLOGY
Elsevier Science Publishing Co., Inc.
655 Avenue of the Americas
New York, NY 10010   Phone: (212) 989-5800
First Published: 1985. Frequency: Bimonthly. ISSN: 0168-8278.

★1036★ JOURNAL OF HEREDITY
American Genetic Association
PO Box 39
Buckeystown, MD 21717   Phone: (301) 695-9292
Frequency: Bimonthly. ISSN: 0022-1503.

★1037★ JOURNAL OF HISTOCHEMISTRY AND
CYTOCHEMISTRY
Histochemical Society
6900 Grove Rd.
Thorofare, NJ 08086   Phone: (609) 848-1000
First Published: 1953. Frequency: Monthly. ISSN: 0022-1554.

★1038★ JOURNAL OF THE HISTORY OF MEDICINE AND
ALLIED SCIENCES
333 Cedar St.
New Haven, CT 06510   Phone: (203) 785-4702
First Published: 1946. Frequency: Quarterly. ISSN: 0022-5045.

★1039★ JOURNAL OF HOME HEALTH CARE PRACTICE
Aspen Publishers, Inc.
200 Orchard Ridge Dr.
Gaithersburg, MD 20878   Phone: (301) 417-7500
Frequency: Quarterly.

★1040★ JOURNAL OF HOMOSEXUALITY
The Haworth Press, Inc.
10 Alice St.
Binghamton, NY 13904   Phone: (800) 342-9678
First Published: 1974. Frequency: Quarterly. ISSN: 0091-8369.

★1041★ JOURNAL OF HOSPITAL INFECTION
Academic Press, Inc.
1250 6th Ave.
San Diego, CA 92101   Phone: (619) 231-0926
First Published: 1980. Frequency: 8/yr. ISSN: 0195-6701.

★1042★ JOURNAL OF HUMAN LACTATION
Human Sciences Press, Inc.
233 Spring St.
New York, NY 10013   Phone: (212) 620-8000
Frequency: Quarterly.

★1043★ JOURNAL OF HUMAN NUTRITION AND DIETETICS
Blackwell Scientific Publications
3 Cambridge Center, Ste. 208
Cambridge, MA 02142   Phone: (617) 225-0401
Frequency: Bimonthly. ISSN: 0952-3871.

★1044★ JOURNAL OF HYPERTENSION
Current Science
20 N. 3rd St.
Philadelphia, PA 19106   Phone: (215) 514-2266
Frequency: Monthly. ISSN: 0263-6352.

★1045★ JOURNAL OF IMMUNOASSAY
Marcel Dekker, Inc.
270 Madison Ave.
New York, NY 10016   Phone: (212) 696-9000
First Published: 1980. Frequency: Quarterly. ISSN: 0197-1522.

★1046★ JOURNAL OF IMMUNOGENETICS
Blackwell Scientific Publications
3 Cambridge Center, Ste. 208
Cambridge, MA 02142   Phone: (617) 225-0401
First Published: 1974. Frequency: Bimonthly. ISSN: 0305-1811.

★1047★ JOURNAL OF IMMUNOLOGICAL METHODS
Elsevier Science Publishing Co., Inc.
655 Avenue of the Americas
New York, NY 10010   Phone: (212) 989-5800
First Published: 1971. Frequency: 20/yr. ISSN: 0022-1759.

★1048★ JOURNAL OF IMMUNOLOGY
American Association of Immunologists
9650 Rockville Pike
Bethesda, MD 20814   Phone: (301) 530-7178
First Published: 1916. Frequency: Semimonthly. ISSN: 0022-1767.

★1049★ JOURNAL OF IN VITRO FERTILIZATION AND
EMBRYO TRANSFER
Plenum Publishing Corp.
233 Spring St.
New York, NY 10013   Phone: (212) 620-8000
First Published: 1984. Frequency: Bimonthly. ISSN: 0740-7769.

★1050★ JOURNAL OF THE INDIAN MEDICAL ASSOCIATION
I.M.A. House
53 Creek Row
Calcutta 700014, India
First Published: 1931. Frequency: Monthly. ISSN: 0019-5847.

★1051★ JOURNAL OF INFECTION
Academic Press, Inc.
1250 6th Ave.
San Diego, CA 92101   Phone: (619) 231-0926
First Published: 1979. Frequency: Bimonthly. ISSN: 0163-4453.

★1052★ JOURNAL OF INFECTIOUS DISEASES
Infectious Diseases Society of America
c/o Vincent T. Andriole, M.D.
Yale University School of Medicine
333 Cedar St., 201 LCI
New Haven, CT 06510-8056   Phone: (203) 785-4141
First Published: 1904. Frequency: Monthly. ISSN: 0022-1899.

★1053★ JOURNAL OF INHERITED METABOLIC DISEASE
MTP Press, Ltd.
Falcon House
Queen Sq.
Lancaster LA1 1RN, England
First Published: 1978. Frequency: Bimonthly. ISSN: 0141-8955.

★1054★ JOURNAL OF INORGANIC BIOCHEMISTRY
Elsevier Science Publishing Co., Inc.
655 Avenue of the Americas
New York, NY 10010   Phone: (212) 989-5800
First Published: 1971. **Frequency:** 12/yr. **ISSN:** 0162-0134.

★1055★ JOURNAL OF INTELLECTUAL DISABILITY RESEARCH
Blackwell Scientific Publications
3 Cambridge Center, Ste. 208
Cambridge, MA 02142   Phone: (617) 225-0401
Frequency: Bimonthly. **ISSN:** 0964-2633.

★1056★ JOURNAL OF INTENSIVE CARE MEDICINE
Blackwell Scientific Publications
3 Cambridge Center, Ste. 208
Cambridge, MA 02142   Phone: (617) 225-0401
Frequency: Bimonthly. **ISSN:** 0885-0666.

★1057★ JOURNAL OF INTERFERON RESEARCH
Mary Ann Liebert, Inc.
1651 3rd Ave.
New York, NY 10128   Phone: (212) 289-2300
First Published: 1981. **Frequency:** Bimonthly. **ISSN:** 0197-8357.

★1058★ JOURNAL OF INTERNAL MEDICINE
Blackwell Scientific Publications
3 Cambridge Center, Ste. 208
Cambridge, MA 02142   Phone: (617) 225-0401
First Published: 1869. **Frequency:** Monthly. **ISSN:** 0954-6820.

★1059★ JOURNAL OF INTERNATIONAL MEDICAL RESEARCH
Cambridge University Press
40 W. 20th St.
New York, NY 10011   Phone: (212) 924-3900
First Published: 1972. **Frequency:** Bimonthly. **ISSN:** 0300-0605.

★1060★ JOURNAL OF INTERVENTIONAL RADIOLOGY
Churchill Livingstone, Inc.
1560 Broadway
New York, NY 10036   Phone: (212) 819-5400
First Published: 1986. **Frequency:** Quarterly. **ISSN:** 0268-0882.

★1061★ JOURNAL OF INTRAVENOUS NURSING
Intravenous Nurses Society
2 Brighton St.
Belmont, MA 02178   Phone: (617) 489-5205
First Published: 1978. **Frequency:** Bimonthly. **ISSN:** 0896-5846.

★1062★ JOURNAL OF INVESTIGATIVE DERMATOLOGY
Society for Investigative Dermatology
c/o David R. Bickers, M.D.
2074 Abington Rd.
University Hospitals of Cleveland
Cleveland, OH 44106   Phone: (216) 844-3682
First Published: 1938. **Frequency:** Monthly. **ISSN:** 0022-202X.

★1063★ JOURNAL OF THE KENTUCKY MEDICAL ASSOCIATION
3532 Ephraim McDowell Dr.
Louisville, KY 40205   Phone: (502) 459-9790
First Published: 1903. **Frequency:** Monthly. **ISSN:** 0023-0294.

★1064★ JOURNAL OF LABORATORY AND CLINICAL MEDICINE
Central Society for Clinical Research
c/o Dr. John P. Phair
Northwestern University Medical School
303 E. Chicago Ave.
Chicago, IL 60611   Phone: (312) 951-5610
First Published: 1915. **Frequency:** Monthly. **ISSN:** 0022-2143.

★1065★ JOURNAL OF LARYNGOLOGY AND OTOLOGY
Headley Brothers, Ltd.
Invicta Press
Ashford, Kent TN24 8HH, England
First Published: 1887. **Frequency:** Monthly. **ISSN:** 0022-2151.

★1066★ JOURNAL OF LAW AND ETHICS IN DENTISTRY
Mosby-Year Book, Inc.
11830 Westline Industrial Dr.
St. Louis, MO 63146   Phone: (314) 872-8370
First Published: 1988. **Frequency:** Annual.

★1067★ JOURNAL OF LEGAL MEDICINE
American College of Legal Medicine
5700 Old Orchard Rd., 1st Fl.
Skokie, IL 60077   Phone: (800) 433-9137
First Published: 1979. **Frequency:** Quarterly. **ISSN:** 0194-7648.

★1068★ JOURNAL OF LEUKOCYTE BIOLOGY
John Wiley & Sons, Inc.
605 3rd Ave.
New York, NY 10158   Phone: (212) 850-6000
First Published: 1967. **Frequency:** Monthly. **ISSN:** 0741-5400.

★1069★ JOURNAL OF LIPID RESEARCH
Federation of American Societies for Experimental Biology
9650 Rockville Pike
Bethesda, MD 20814   Phone: (302) 530-7000
First Published: 1959. **Frequency:** Monthly. **ISSN:** 0022-2275.

★1070★ JOURNAL OF LONG-TERM CARE ADMINISTRATION
American College of Health Care Administrators
325 S. Patrick St.
Alexandria, VA 22314   Phone: (703) 549-5822
First Published: 1972. **Frequency:** Quarterly. **ISSN:** 0093-4445.

★1071★ JOURNAL OF LONG-TERM EFFECTS OF MEDICAL IMPLANTS
CRC Press, Inc.
2000 Corporate Blvd., NW
Boca Raton, FL 33431   Phone: (407) 994-0555
Frequency: Quarterly.

★1072★ JOURNAL OF THE LOUISIANA STATE MEDICAL SOCIETY
1700 Josephine St.
New Orleans, LA 70113   Phone: (504) 561-1033
First Published: 1844. **Frequency:** Monthly. **ISSN:** 0024-6921.

★1073★ JOURNAL OF MANAGEMENT IN MEDICINE
MCB Publications Ltd.
Representative Office
PO Box 10812
Birmingham, AL 35201

★1074★ JOURNAL OF MANIPULATIVE AND PHYSIOLOGICAL THERAPEUTICS
Williams & Wilkins
428 E. Preston St.
Baltimore, MD 21202   Phone: (301) 528-4223
First Published: 1978. **Frequency:** Bimonthly. **ISSN:** 0161-4754.

★1075★ JOURNAL OF MANUAL MEDICINE
Springer-Verlag New York, Inc.
175 5th Ave.
New York, NY 10010   Phone: (212) 460-1500
First Published: 1983. **Frequency:** Quarterly. **ISSN:** 0254-9522.

★1076★ THE JOURNAL OF MATERNAL FETAL MEDICINE
John Wiley & Sons, Inc.
605 3rd Ave.
New York, NY 10158   Phone: (617) 850-6000
First Published: 1992. **Frequency:** Bimonthly. **ISSN:** 1057-0802.

★1077★ JOURNAL OF THE MEDICAL ASSOCIATION OF GEORGIA
938 Peachtree St., NE
Atlanta, GA 30309   Phone: (404) 876-7535
First Published: 1911. Frequency: Monthly. ISSN: 0025-7028.

★1078★ JOURNAL OF MEDICAL EDUCATION
Association of American Medical Colleges
1 DuPont Circle, NW
Washington, DC 20036   Phone: (202) 828-0400
First Published: 1926. Frequency: Monthly. ISSN: 0022-2577.

★1079★ JOURNAL OF MEDICAL ENGINEERING AND TECHNOLOGY
Taylor & Francis, Ltd.
Rankine Rd.
Basingstoke, Hants. RG24 0PR, England
First Published: 1965. Frequency: Bimonthly. ISSN: 0309-1902.

★1080★ JOURNAL OF MEDICAL ENTOMOLOGY
Entomological Society of America
9301 Annapolis Rd.
Lanham, MD 20706   Phone: (301) 731-4535
First Published: 1964. Frequency: Bimonthly. ISSN: 0022-2585.

★1081★ JOURNAL OF MEDICAL ETHICS
British Medical Association
PO Box 560B
Kennebunkport, ME 04046
First Published: 1975. Frequency: Quarterly. ISSN: 0306-6800.

★1082★ JOURNAL OF MEDICAL GENETICS
British Medical Association
PO Box 560B
Kennebunkport, ME 04046
First Published: 1964. Frequency: Monthly. ISSN: 0022-2593.

★1083★ JOURNAL OF MEDICAL HUMANITIES
Human Sciences Press, Inc.
233 Spring St.
New York, NY 10013   Phone: (212) 620-8000
First Published: 1976. Frequency: Quarterly. ISSN: 1041-3545.

★1084★ JOURNAL OF MEDICAL MICROBIOLOGY
Churchill Livingstone, Inc.
1560 Broadway
New York, NY 10036   Phone: (212) 819-5400
First Published: 1968. Frequency: Monthly. ISSN: 0022-2615.

★1085★ JOURNAL OF MEDICAL PRACTICE MANAGEMENT
Williams & Wilkins
428 E. Preston St.
Baltimore, MD 21202   Phone: (301) 528-4223
First Published: 1985. Frequency: Quarterly.

★1086★ JOURNAL OF MEDICAL PRIMATOLOGY
John Wiley & Sons, Inc.
605 3rd Ave.
New York, NY 10158   Phone: (212) 850-6000
First Published: 1972. Frequency: Bimonthly. ISSN: 0047-2565.

★1087★ JOURNAL OF MEDICAL SYSTEMS
Plenum Publishing Corp.
233 Spring St.
New York, NY 10013   Phone: (212) 620-8000
First Published: 1977. Frequency: Bimonthly. ISSN: 0148-5598.

★1088★ JOURNAL OF MEDICAL AND VETERINARY MYCOLOGY
Blackwell Scientific Publications
3 Cambridge Center, Ste. 208
Cambridge, MA 02142   Phone: (617) 225-0401
Frequency: Bimonthly. ISSN: 0268-1218.

★1089★ JOURNAL OF MEDICAL VIROLOGY
John Wiley & Sons, Inc.
605 3rd Ave.
New York, NY 10158   Phone: (212) 850-6000
First Published: 1977. Frequency: Monthly. ISSN: 0146-6615.

★1090★ JOURNAL OF MEDICINAL CHEMISTRY
American Chemical Society
1155 16th St., NW
Washington, DC 20036   Phone: (202) 872-4363
First Published: 1958. Frequency: Monthly. ISSN: 0022-2623.

★1091★ JOURNAL OF MEDICINE
PJD Publications, Ltd.
Box 966
Westbury, NY 11590   Phone: (516) 626-0650
First Published: 1970. Frequency: Bimonthly. ISSN: 0025-7850.

★1092★ JOURNAL OF MEDICINE AND PHILOSOPHY
D. Reidel Publishing Co.
101 Philip Dr.
Norwell, MA 02061   Phone: (617) 871-6300
First Published: 1976. Frequency: Bimonthly. ISSN: 0360-5310.

★1093★ JOURNAL OF MEMBRANE BIOLOGY
Springer-Verlag New York, Inc.
175 5th Ave.
New York, NY 10010   Phone: (212) 460-1500
First Published: 1969. Frequency: 18/yr. ISSN: 0022-2631.

★1094★ JOURNAL OF MENTAL DEFICIENCY RESEARCH
Blackwell Scientific Publications
3 Cambridge Center, Ste. 208
Cambridge, MA 02142   Phone: (617) 225-0401
First Published: 1957. Frequency: Quarterly. ISSN: 0022-264X.

★1095★ JOURNAL OF MENTAL HEALTH ADMINISTRATION
Association of Mental Health Administrators
840 N. Lake Shore Dr., Ste. 1103W
Chicago, IL 60611   Phone: (312) 943-2751
First Published: 1972. Frequency: Semiannual. ISSN: 0092-8623.

★1096★ JOURNAL OF MICROSCOPY
Blackwell Scientific Publications
3 Cambridge Center, Ste. 208
Cambridge, MA 02142   Phone: (617) 225-0401
First Published: 1878. Frequency: Monthly. ISSN: 0022-2720.

★1097★ JOURNAL OF THE MISSISSIPPI STATE MEDICAL ASSOCIATION
735 Riverside Dr.
Jackson, MS 39216   Phone: (601) 354-5433
First Published: 1960. Frequency: Monthly. ISSN: 0026-6396.

★1098★ JOURNAL OF MOLECULAR BIOLOGY
Academic Press, Inc.
1250 6th Ave.
San Diego, CA 92101   Phone: (619) 231-0926
First Published: 1959. Frequency: 24/yr. ISSN: 0022-2836.

★1099★ JOURNAL OF MOLECULAR AND CELLULAR CARDIOLOGY
Academic Press, Inc.
1250 6th Ave.
San Diego, CA 92101   Phone: (619) 231-0926
First Published: 1970. Frequency: Monthly. ISSN: 0022-2828.

★1100★ JOURNAL OF MOLECULAR EVOLUTION
Springer-Verlag New York, Inc.
175 5th Ave.
New York, NY 10010   Phone: (212) 460-1500
First Published: 1971. Frequency: Monthly. ISSN: 0022-2844.

★1101★ JOURNAL OF MOLECULAR NEUROSCIENCE
Birkhauser Boston
c/o Springer-Verlag New York, Inc.
PO Box 2485
Secaucus, NJ 07096-2491
Frequency: Quarterly. **ISSN:** 0895-8696.

★1102★ JOURNAL OF MORPHOLOGY
John Wiley & Sons, Inc.
605 3rd Ave.
New York, NY 10158   Phone: (212) 850-6000
First Published: 1887. **Frequency:** Monthly. **ISSN:** 0362-2525.

★1103★ JOURNAL OF MUSCLE RESEARCH AND CELL MOTILITY
Chapman and Hall, Ltd.
2-6 Boundary Row
London SE1, England
First Published: 1980. **Frequency:** Bimonthly. **ISSN:** 0142-4319.

★1104★ JOURNAL OF MUSCULOSKELETAL PAIN
The Haworth Press, Inc.
10 Alice St.
Binghampton, NY 13904   Phone: (800) 342-9678
First Published: 1992. **Frequency:** Quarterly.

★1105★ JOURNAL OF THE NATIONAL CANCER INSTITUTE
9030 Old Georgetown Rd.
Bldg. 82, Rm. 203
Bethesda, MD 20892   Phone: (301) 496-5491
First Published: 1940. **Frequency:** Monthly. **ISSN:** 0027-8874.

★1106★ JOURNAL OF THE NATIONAL MEDICAL ASSOCIATION
1012 10th St., NW
Washington, DC 20001   Phone: (202) 347-1895
First Published: 1908. **Frequency:** Monthly. **ISSN:** 0027-9684.

★1107★ JOURNAL OF NATURAL PRODUCTS
American Society of Pharmacognosy
c/o Dr. David I. Slatkin, Treasurer
School of Pharmacy, 512 Salk Hall
University of Pittsburgh
Pittsburgh, PA 15261   Phone: (308) 342-3080
First Published: 1938. **Frequency:** Bimonthly. **ISSN:** 0163-3864.

★1108★ JOURNAL OF NERVOUS AND MENTAL DISEASE
Williams & Wilkins
428 E. Preston St.
Baltimore, MD 21202   Phone: (301) 528-4223
First Published: 1874. **Frequency:** Monthly. **ISSN:** 0022-3018.

★1109★ JOURNAL OF NEURAL TRANSMISSION
Springer-Verlag New York, Inc.
175 5th Ave.
New York, NY 10010   Phone: (212) 460-1500
First Published: 1950. **Frequency:** Quarterly. **ISSN:** 0300-9564.

★1110★ JOURNAL OF NEUROBIOLOGY
John Wiley & Sons, Inc.
605 3rd Ave.
New York, NY 10158   Phone: (212) 850-6000
First Published: 1969. **Frequency:** 8/yr. **ISSN:** 0022-3034.

★1111★ JOURNAL OF NEUROCHEMISTRY
Raven Press
1185 Avenue of the Americas
New York, NY 10036   Phone: (212) 930-9500
First Published: 1956. **Frequency:** Monthly. **ISSN:** 0022-3042.

★1112★ JOURNAL OF NEUROCYTOLOGY
Chapman and Hall, Ltd.
2-6 Boundary Row
London SE1, England
First Published: 1972. **Frequency:** Bimonthly. **ISSN:** 0300-4864.

★1113★ JOURNAL OF NEUROIMAGING
Little, Brown, and Co.
34 Beacon St.
Boston, MA 02108   Phone: (617) 227-0730
First Published: 1991. **Frequency:** Quarterly. **ISSN:** 1051-2284.

★1114★ JOURNAL OF NEUROIMMUNOLOGY
Elsevier Science Publishing Co., Inc.
655 Avenue of the Americas
New York, NY 10010   Phone: (212) 989-5800
First Published: 1981. **Frequency:** 15/yr. **ISSN:** 0165-5728.

★1115★ JOURNAL NEUROLOGICAL AND ORTHOPAEDIC MEDICINE AND SURGERY
Springer-Verlag New York, Inc.
175 5th Ave.
New York, NY 10010   Phone: (212) 460-1500
First Published: 1991. **Frequency:** Quarterly. **ISSN:** 0890-6599.

★1116★ JOURNAL OF THE NEUROLOGICAL SCIENCES
Elsevier Science Publishing Co., Inc.
655 Avenue of the Americas
New York, NY 10010   Phone: (212) 989-5800
First Published: 1964. **Frequency:** 18/yr. **ISSN:** 0022-510X.

★1117★ JOURNAL OF NEUROLOGY
Springer-Verlag New York, Inc.
175 5th Ave.
New York, NY 10010   Phone: (212) 460-1500
First Published: 1891. **Frequency:** 8/yr. **ISSN:** 0340-5354.

★1118★ JOURNAL OF NEUROLOGY, NEUROSURGERY AND PSYCHIATRY
British Medical Association
PO Box 560B
Kennebunkport, ME 04046
First Published: 1926. **Frequency:** Monthly. **ISSN:** 0022-3050.

★1119★ JOURNAL OF NEURO-ONCOLOGY
Kluwer Academic Publishers
101 Philip Dr.
Norwell, MA 02061   Phone: (617) 871-6600
First Published: 1983. **Frequency:** Quarterly. **ISSN:** 0167-594X.

★1120★ JOURNAL OF NEUROPATHOLOGY AND EXPERIMENTAL NEUROLOGY
American Association of Neuropathologists
c/o Reid R. Heffner, Jr., M.D.
Dept. of Pathology, Buffalo Medical School
State University of New York
Buffalo, NY 14222   Phone: (716) 898-3510
First Published: 1942. **Frequency:** Bimonthly. **ISSN:** 0022-3069.

★1121★ JOURNAL OF NEUROPHYSIOLOGY
American Physiological Society
9650 Rockville Pike
Bethesda, MD 20814   Phone: (301) 530-7164
First Published: 1938. **Frequency:** Monthly. **ISSN:** 0022-3077.

★1122★ THE JOURNAL OF NEUROPSYCHIATRY AND CLINICAL NEUROSCIENCES
American Psychiatric Press, Inc.
1400 K St., NW
Washington, DC 20005   Phone: (202) 682-6420
Frequency: Quarterly. **ISSN:** 0895-0172.

★1123★ JOURNAL OF NEUROSCIENCE
Society for Neuroscience
11 Dupont Circle, Ste. 500
Washington, DC 20036   Phone: (202) 462-6688
First Published: 1981. **Frequency:** Monthly. **ISSN:** 0270-6474.

★1124★   JOURNAL OF NEUROSCIENCE METHODS
Elsevier Science Publishing Co., Inc.
655 Avenue of the Americas
New York, NY 10010   Phone: (212) 989-5800
First Published: 1979. Frequency: 15/yr. ISSN: 0165-0270.

★1125★   JOURNAL OF NEUROSCIENCE NURSING
American Association of Neuroscience Nurses
218 N. Jefferson St., Ste. 204
Chicago, IL 60606   Phone: (312) 993-0043
Frequency: Bimonthly. ISSN: 0888-0395.

★1126★   JOURNAL OF NEUROSCIENCE RESEARCH
John Wiley & Sons, Inc.
605 3rd Ave.
New York, NY 10158   Phone: (212) 850-6000
First Published: 1975. Frequency: Monthly. ISSN: 0360-4012.

★1127★   JOURNAL OF NEUROSURGERY
American Association of Neurological Surgeons
22 S. Washington St., Suite 100
Park Ridge, IL 60068   Phone: (708) 692-9500
First Published: 1944. Frequency: Monthly. ISSN: 0022-3085.

★1128★   JOURNAL OF NEUROTRAUMA
Mary Ann Liebert, Inc.
1651 3rd Ave.
New York, NY 10128   Phone: (212) 289-2300
First Published: 1984. Frequency: Quarterly. ISSN: 0897-7151.

★1129★   THE JOURNAL OF THE NEW YORK STATE NURSES
   ASSOCIATION
New York State Nurses Assoiation
2113 Western Ave.
Guilderland, NY 12084   Phone: (518) 456-5371
Frequency: Quarterly.

★1130★   JOURNAL OF THE NPHA
National Pharmaceutical Association
c/o Texas Southern University
College of Pharmacy
3100 Cleburne
Houston, TX 77004   Phone: (202) 806-6530
Frequency: 3/yr. ISSN: 0027-9897.

★1131★   JOURNAL OF NUCLEAR MEDICINE
Society of Nuclear Medicine
136 Madison Ave., 8th Fl.
New York, NY 10016   Phone: (212) 889-0717
First Published: 1960. Frequency: Monthly. ISSN: 0161-5505.

★1132★   JOURNAL OF NUCLEAR MEDICINE TECHNOLOGY
Soceity of Nuclear Medicine
136 Madison Ave., 8th Fl.
New York, NY 10016   Phone: (212) 889-0717
First Published: 1973. Frequency: Quarterly. ISSN: 0091-4916.

★1133★   JOURNAL OF NURSE-MIDWIFERY
American College of Nurse-Midwives
1522 K St., NW, Ste. 1000
Washington, DC 20005   Phone: (202) 289-0171
First Published: 1955. Frequency: Bimonthly. ISSN: 0091-2182.

★1134★   JOURNAL OF NURSING ADMINISTRATION
J.B. Lippincott Co.
E. Washington Sq.
Philadelphia, PA 19105   Phone: (215) 238-4200
First Published: 1971. Frequency: 11/yr. ISSN: 0002-0443.

★1135★   JOURNAL OF NURSING EDUCATION
Slack, Inc.
6900 Grove Rd.
Thorofare, NJ 08086   Phone: (609) 848-1000
First Published: 1962. Frequency: 9/yr. ISSN: 0022-3158.

★1136★   JOURNAL OF NURSING QUALITY ASSURANCE
Aspen Publishers, Inc.
200 Orchard Ridge Dr.
Gaithersburg, MD 20878   Phone: (301) 417-7500
First Published: 1986. Frequency: Quarterly. ISSN: 0889-4647.

★1137★   JOURNAL OF NURSING RESEARCH
Sage Publications, Inc.
2111 W. Hillcrest Dr.
Newbury Park, CA 91320   Phone: (805) 499-0721
First Published: 1979. Frequency: Bimonthly. ISSN: 1046-4972.

★1138★   JOURNAL OF NUTRITION
American Institute of Nutrition
9650 Rockville Pike
Bethesda, MD 20814   Phone: (301) 530-7050
First Published: 1928. Frequency: Monthly. ISSN: 0022-3166.

★1139★   JOURNAL OF NUTRITION EDUCATION
Society for Nutrition Education
1700 Broadway, Ste. 300
Oakland, CA 94612   Phone: (415) 444-7133
First Published: 1969. Frequency: Bimonthly. ISSN: 0022-3182.

★1140★   JOURNAL OF NUTRITIONAL BIOCHEMISTRY
Butterworth-Heinemann
80 Montvale Ave.
Stoneham, MA 02180   Phone: (617) 438-8464
First Published: 1990. Frequency: Monthly. ISSN: 0955-2863.

★1141★   JOURNAL OF OCCUPATIONAL MEDICINE
American College of Occupational Medicine
55 W. Seegers Rd.
Arlington Heights, IL 60005   Phone: (708) 228-6850
First Published: 1959. Frequency: Monthly. ISSN: 0096-1736.

★1142★   JOURNAL OF THE OKLAHOMA STATE MEDICAL
   ASSOCIATION
601 Northwest Expwy.
Oklahoma City, OK 73118   Phone: (405) 843-9571
First Published: 1908. Frequency: Monthly. ISSN: 0030-1876.

★1143★   JOURNAL OF THE OPTICAL SOCIETY OF AMERICA
   A, OPTICS AND IMAGE SCIENCE
2010 Massachusetts Ave., NW
Washington, DC 20036   Phone: (202) 223-8130
First Published: 1917. Frequency: Monthly. ISSN: 0740-3232.

★1144★   JOURNAL OF THE OPTICAL SOCIETY OF AMERICA
   B, OPTICAL PHYSICS
2010 Massachusetts Ave., NW
Washington, DC 20036   Phone: (202) 223-8130
First Published: 1917. Frequency: Monthly. ISSN: 0740-3224.

★1145★   JOURNAL OF ORAL AND MAXILLOFACIAL
   SURGERY
American Association of Oral and Maxillofacial Surgeons
9700 W. Bryn Mawr
Rosemont, IL 60018   Phone: (708) 678-6200
First Published: 1943. Frequency: Monthly. ISSN: 0278-2391.

★1146★   JOURNAL OF ORAL MEDICINE
American Academy of Oral Medicine
4143 Mischive
Houston, TX 77023   Phone: (713) 665-6029
First Published: 1945. Frequency: Quarterly. ISSN: 0022-3247.

★1147★   JOURNAL OF ORAL REHABILITATION
Blackwell Scientific Publications
3 Cambridge Center, Ste. 208
Cambridge, MA 02142   Phone: (617) 225-0401
First Published: 1974. Frequency: Bimonthly. ISSN: 0305-182X.

★1148★ JOURNAL OF ORTHOPAEDIC RESEARCH
Raven Press
1185 Avenue of the Americas
New York, NY 10036   Phone: (212) 930-9500
First Published: 1983. **Frequency:** Quarterly. **ISSN:** 0736-0266.

★1149★ JOURNAL OF ORTHOPAEDIC AND SPORTS PHYSICAL THERAPY
American Physical Therapy Association
1111 N. Fairfax St.
Alexandria, VA 22314   Phone: (703) 684-2782
First Published: 1979. **Frequency:** Monthly. **ISSN:** 0190-6011.

★1150★ THE JOURNAL OF ORTHOPAEDIC SURGICAL TECHNIQUES
Med Advanced Techniques Publishing House Ltd.
48 Aylestone Ave.
London NW6 7AA, England
ISSN: 0334-0236.

★1151★ JOURNAL OF ORTHOPAEDIC TRAUMA
Raven Press
1185 Avenue of the Americas
New York, NY 10036   Phone: (212) 930-9500
First Published: 1987. **Frequency:** Quarterly. **ISSN:** 0890-5339.

★1152★ JOURNAL OF OTOLARYNGOLOGY
Keith Health Care Communications
Sunnybrook Medical Centre
4953 Dundas St., W.
Toronto, ON, Canada H9A 1B6   Phone: (416) 239-1233
First Published: 1972. **Frequency:** Bimonthly. **ISSN:** 0381-6605.

★1153★ JOURNAL OF PAEDIATRIC DENTISTRY
Blackwell Scientific Publications
3 Cambridge Center, Ste. 208
Cambridge, MA 02142   Phone: (617) 225-0401
First Published: 1971. **Frequency:** Semiannual. **ISSN:** 0267-2073.

★1154★ JOURNAL OF PAIN AND SYMPTOM MANAGEMENT
Elsevier Science Publishing Co., Inc.
655 Avenue of the Americas
New York, NY 10010   Phone: (212) 989-5800
Frequency: 8/yr. **ISSN:** 0885-3924.

★1155★ JOURNAL OF PARASITOLOGY
American Society of Parasitologists
c/o Lillian F. Mayberry
University of Texas, El Paso, Dept. of Biological Sciences
500 W. University Ave.
El Paso, TX 79968   Phone: (915) 747-5844
First Published: 1914. **Frequency:** Bimonthly. **ISSN:** 0022-3395.

★1156★ JOURNAL OF PARENTERAL SCIENCE AND TECHNOLOGY
Parenteral Drug Association
1617 JFK Blvd., Ste. 640
Philadelphia, PA 19103   Phone: (215) 564-6466
First Published: 1947. **Frequency:** Bimonthly. **ISSN:** 0279-7976.

★1157★ JOURNAL OF PATHOLOGY
John Wiley & Sons, Inc.
605 3rd Ave.
New York, NY 10158   Phone: (212) 850-6000
First Published: 1892. **Frequency:** Monthly. **ISSN:** 0022-3417.

★1158★ JOURNAL OF PEDIATRIC AND CHILD HEALTH
Blackwell Scientific Publications
3 Cambridge Center, Ste. 208
Cambridge, MA 02142   Phone: (617) 225-0401
First Published: 1965. **Frequency:** Bimonthly. **ISSN:** 0004-993X.

★1159★ JOURNAL OF PEDIATRIC GASTROENTEROLOGY AND NUTRITION
Raven Press
1185 Avenue of the Americas
New York, NY 10036   Phone: (212) 930-9500
First Published: 1982. **Frequency:** Biweekly. **ISSN:** 0277-2116.

★1160★ JOURNAL OF PEDIATRIC HEALTH CARE
National Association of Pediatric Nurse Associates and Practitioners
1101 King's Hwy., N., Ste. 206
Cherry Hill, NJ 08034   Phone: (609) 667-1773
First Published: 1987. **Frequency:** Bimonthly. **ISSN:** 0740-1234.

★1161★ JOURNAL OF PEDIATRIC NURSING
W. B. Saunders Co.
Curtis Center
Independence Sq., W.
Philadelphia, PA 19106   Phone: (215) 238-7800
First Published: 1986. **Frequency:** Bimonthly. **ISSN:** 0882-5963.

★1162★ JOURNAL OF PEDIATRIC OPHTHALMOLOGY AND STRABISMUS
Slack, Inc.
6900 Grove Rd.
Thorofare, NJ 08086   Phone: (609) 848-1000
First Published: 1964. **Frequency:** Bimonthly. **ISSN:** 0191-3913.

★1163★ JOURNAL OF PEDIATRIC ORTHOPAEDICS
Raven Press
1185 Avenue of the Americas
New York, NY 10036   Phone: (212) 930-9500
First Published: 1981. **Frequency:** Biweekly. **ISSN:** 0271-6798.

★1164★ JOURNAL OF PEDIATRIC ORTHOPAEDICS, PART B
Raven Press
1185 Avenue of the Americas
New York, NY 10036   Phone: (212) 930-9500
First Published: 1992. **Frequency:** Bimonthly. **ISSN:** 0271-6798.

★1165★ JOURNAL OF PEDIATRIC PSYCHOLOGY
Society for Pediatric Psychology
c/o Gerald Koocher, M.D.
Dept. of Psychology, Children's Hospital
300 Longwood Ave.
Boston, MA 02115   Phone: (617) 735-6699
First Published: 1976. **Frequency:** Quarterly. **ISSN:** 0146-8693.

★1166★ JOURNAL OF PEDIATRIC SURGERY
American Academy of Pediatrics
141 Northwest Point Blvd.
PO Box 927
Orlando, FL 32886   Phone: (407) 345-4200
First Published: 1966. **Frequency:** Bimonthly. **ISSN:** 0022-3468.

★1167★ JOURNAL OF PEDIATRICS
Mosby-Year Book, Inc.
11830 Westline Industrial Dr.
St. Louis, MO 63146   Phone: (314) 872-8370
First Published: 1932. **Frequency:** Monthly. **ISSN:** 0022-3476.

★1168★ JOURNAL OF PERINATAL MEDICINE
Walter de Gruyter und Co.
200 Saw Mill Rd.
Hawthorne, NY 10532   Phone: (914) 747-0110
First Published: 1973. **Frequency:** Bimonthly. **ISSN:** 0300-5577.

★1169★ JOURNAL OF PERINATAL AND NEONATAL NURSING
Aspen Publishers, Inc.
200 Orchard Ridge Dr.
Gaithersburg, MD 20878   Phone: (301) 417-7500
First Published: 1987. **Frequency:** Quarterly. **ISSN:** 0893-2190.

★1170★ JOURNAL OF PERINATOLOGY
Appleton & Lange
25 Van Zant St.
East Norwalk, CT 06855   Phone: (203) 838-4400
Frequency: Quarterly. ISSN: 0743-8346.

★1171★ JOURNAL OF PERIODONTAL RESEARCH
Munksgaard
Noerre Soegade 35
DK-1370 Copenhagen K, Denmark
First Published: 1966. Frequency: Bimonthly. ISSN: 0022-3484.

★1172★ JOURNAL OF PERIODONTOLOGY
American Academy of Periodontology
211 E. Chicago Ave., Ste. 114
Chicago, IL 60611   Phone: (312) 787-5518
First Published: 1930. Frequency: Monthly. ISSN: 0022-3492.

★1173★ JOURNAL OF PERSONALITY
Duke University Press
6697 College Sta.
Durham, NC 27708   Phone: (919) 684-2173
First Published: 1932. Frequency: Quarterly. ISSN: 0022-3506.

★1174★ JOURNAL OF PERSONALITY ASSESSMENT
Society for Personality Assessment
866 Amelia Ct., NE
St. Petersburg, FL 33702   Phone: (813) 527-9863
First Published: 1970. Frequency: Quarterly. ISSN: 0022-3891.

★1175★ JOURNAL OF PERSONALITY AND SOCIAL
PSYCHOLOGY
American Psychological Association
1200 17th St., NW
Washington, DC 20036   Phone: (202) 955-7600
First Published: 1965. Frequency: Monthly. ISSN: 0022-3514.

★1176★ JOURNAL OF PHARMACEUTICAL MEDICINE
Blackwell Scientific Publications
3 Cambridge Center, Ste. 208
Cambridge, MA 02142   Phone: (617) 225-0401
Frequency: Quarterly. ISSN: 0958-0581.

★1177★ JOURNAL OF PHARMACEUTICAL SCIENCES
American Pharmaceutical Association
2215 Constitution Ave., NW
Washington, DC 20037   Phone: (202) 628-4410
First Published: 1961. Frequency: Monthly. ISSN: 0022-3549.

★1178★ JOURNAL OF PHARMACOKINETICS AND
BIOPHARMACEUTICS
Plenum Publishing Corp.
233 Spring St.
New York, NY 10013   Phone: (212) 620-8000
First Published: 1973. Frequency: Bimonthly. ISSN: 0090-466X.

★1179★ JOURNAL OF PHARMACOLOGICAL AND
TOXICOLOGICAL METHODS
Elsevier Science Publishing Co., Inc.
655 Avenue of the Americas
New York, NY 10010   Phone: (212) 989-5800
First Published: 1978. Frequency: 8/yr. ISSN: 1056-8719.

★1180★ JOURNAL OF PHARMACOLOGY AND
EXPERIMENTAL THERAPEUTICS
American Society for Pharmacology and Experimental Therapeutics
9650 Rockville Pike
Bethesda, MD 20814   Phone: (301) 530-7060
First Published: 1909. Frequency: Monthly. ISSN: 0022-3565.

★1181★ JOURNAL OF PHARMACY AND PHARMACOLOGY
Royal Pharmaceutical Society of Great Britain
1 Lambeth High St.
London SE1 7JN, England
First Published: 1949. Frequency: Monthly. ISSN: 0022-3573.

★1182★ JOURNAL OF PHYSIOLOGY
Cambridge University Press
40 W. 20th St.
New York, NY 10011   Phone: (212) 924-3900
First Published: 1878. Frequency: 13/yr. ISSN: 0022-3751.

★1183★ JOURNAL OF PINEAL RESEARCH
John Wiley & Sons, Inc.
605 3rd Ave.
New York, NY 10158   Phone: (212) 850-6000
Frequency: 6/yr. ISSN: 0742-3098.

★1184★ JOURNAL OF POST ANESTHESIA NURSING
American Society Post Anasthesia Nurses
11512 Allecingie Pkwy.
Richmond, VA 23235   Phone: (804) 379-5516
First Published: 1986. Frequency: Quarterly. ISSN: 0883-9433.

★1185★ JOURNAL OF PROFESSIONAL NURSING
American Association of Colleges of Nursing
1 Dupont Circle, NW, Ste. 530
Washington, DC 20036   Phone: (202) 463-6930
First Published: 1985. Frequency: Bimonthly. ISSN: 8755-7223.

★1186★ JOURNAL OF PROSTHETIC DENTISTRY
Mosby-Year Book, Inc.
11830 Westline Industrial Dr.
St. Louis, MO 63146   Phone: (314) 872-8370
First Published: 1951. Frequency: Monthly. ISSN: 0022-3913.

★1187★ JOURNAL OF PROSTHETICS AND ORTHOTICS
American Academy of Orthotists and Prosthetists
717 Pendleton St.
Alexandria, VA 22314   Phone: (703) 836-7116
First Published: 1970. Frequency: Quarterly. ISSN: 0735-0090.

★1188★ JOURNAL OF PROSTHODONTICS
W.B. Saunders Co.
Curtis Center
Independence Sq., W.
Philadelphia, PA 19106   Phone: (215) 238-7800
First Published: 1992. Frequency: Quarterly.

★1189★ JOURNAL OF PSYCHIATRIC RESEARCH
Pergamon Press, Inc.
Maxwell House, Fairview Park
Elmsford, NY 10523   Phone: (914) 592-7700
First Published: 1961. Frequency: Quarterly. ISSN: 0022-3956.

★1190★ JOURNAL OF PSYCHOACTIVE DRUGS
Haight-Asbury Publications
409 Clayton St., 2nd Fl.
San Francisco, CA 94117   Phone: (415) 626-2810
First Published: 1967. Frequency: Quarterly. ISSN: 0279-1072.

★1191★ JOURNAL OF PSYCHOLOGY
Heldref Publications
4000 Albemarle St., NW
Washington, DC 20016   Phone: (202) 362-6445
First Published: 1936. Frequency: Bimonthly. ISSN: 0022-3980.

★1192★ JOURNAL OF PSYCHOSOCIAL NURSING AND
MENTAL HEALTH SERVICES
Slack, Inc.
6900 Grove Rd.
Thorofare, NJ 08086   Phone: (609) 848-1000
First Published: 1962. Frequency: Monthly. ISSN: 0279-3695.

★1193★ JOURNAL OF PSYCHOSOMATIC OBSTETRICS AND
GYNAECOLOGY
Elsevier Science Publishing Co., Inc.
655 Avenue of the Americas
New York, NY 10010   Phone: (212) 989-5800
First Published: 1982. Frequency: Quarterly. ISSN: 0167-482X.

★1194★ JOURNAL OF PSYCHOSOMATIC RESEARCH
Pergamon Press, Inc.
Maxwell House, Fairview Park
Elmsford, NY 10523   Phone: (914) 592-7700
First Published: 1956. **Frequency:** Bimonthly. **ISSN:** 0022-3999.

★1195★ THE JOURNAL OF PSYCHOTHERAPY PRACTICE AND RESEARCH
American Psychiatric Press, Inc.
1400 K St., NW
Washington, DC 20005   Phone: (202) 682-6420
First Published: 1991. **Frequency:** Quarterly.

★1196★ JOURNAL OF PUBLIC HEALTH DENTISTRY
American Association of Public Health Dentistry
10619 Jousting Ln.
Richmond, VA 23235   Phone: (804) 272-8344
First Published: 1941. **Frequency:** Quarterly. **ISSN:** 0022-4006.

★1197★ JOURNAL OF PUBLIC HEALTH POLICY
Journal of Public Health Policy, Inc.
208 Meadowood Dr.
South Burlington, VT 05403   Phone: (802) 985-2901
First Published: 1980. **Frequency:** Quarterly. **ISSN:** 0197-5897.

★1198★ JOURNAL OF QUALITY ASSURANCE
The National Association of Quality Assurance Professionals
104 Wilmot Rd., Ste. 201
Deerfield, IL 60015   Phone: (708) 940-8800
Frequency: Bimonthly.

★1199★ JOURNAL OF RECEPTOR RESEARCH
Marcel Dekker, Inc.
270 Madison Ave.
New York, NY 10016   Phone: (212) 696-9000
First Published: 1980. **Frequency:** 6/yr. **ISSN:** 0197-5110.

★1200★ JOURNAL OF RECONSTRUCTIVE MICROSURGERY
Thieme Medical Publishers, Inc.
381 Park Ave., S., Ste. 1501
New York, NY 10016   Phone: (212) 683-5088
First Published: 1984. **Frequency:** Quarterly. **ISSN:** 0743-684X.

★1201★ JOURNAL OF REHABILITATION
National Rehabilitation Association
633 S. Washington St.
Alexandria, VA 22314   Phone: (703) 836-0850
First Published: 1935. **Frequency:** Quarterly. **ISSN:** 0022-4154.

★1202★ JOURNAL OF RELIGION IN DISABILITY AND REHABILITATION
The Haworth Press, Inc.
10 Alice St.
Binghampton, NY 13904   Phone: (800) 342-9678
First Published: 1992. **Frequency:** Quarterly.

★1203★ JOURNAL OF RENAL NUTRITION
W.B. Saunders Co.
Curtis Center
Independence Sq., W.
Philadelphia, PA 19106   Phone: (215) 238-7800
First Published: 1992. **Frequency:** Quarterly.

★1204★ JOURNAL OF REPRODUCTION AND FERTILITY
Journals of Reproduction and Fertility
22 Newmarket Rd.
Cambridge C85 8DT, England
First Published: 1960. **Frequency:** Bimonthly. **ISSN:** 0022-4251.

★1205★ JOURNAL OF REPRODUCTIVE IMMUNOLOGY
Elsevier Science Publishing Co., Inc.
655 Avenue of the Americas
New York, NY 10010   Phone: (212) 989-5800
First Published: 1981. **Frequency:** Bimonthly. **ISSN:** 0165-0378.

★1206★ JOURNAL OF REPRODUCTIVE MEDICINE
Journal of Reproductive Medicine, Inc.
8342 Olive St.
St. Louis, MO 63132   Phone: (314) 991-4440
First Published: 1969. **Frequency:** Monthly. **ISSN:** 0024-7758.

★1207★ JOURNAL OF REPRODUCTIVE TOXICOLOGY
Pergamon Press, Inc.
Maxwell House, Fairview Park
Elmsford, NY 10523   Phone: (914) 592-7700
Frequency: Quarterly.

★1208★ JOURNAL OF RHEUMATOLOGY
Journal of Rheumatology Publishing Co., Ltd.
920 Yonge St., Ste. 115
Toronto, ON, Canada M4W 3C7   Phone: (416) 967-5155
First Published: 1974. **Frequency:** Monthly. **ISSN:** 0315-162X.

★1209★ JOURNAL OF THE ROYAL COLLEGE OF SURGEONS OF EDINBURGH
Butterworth-Heinemann
80 Montvale Ave.
Stoneham, MA 02180   Phone: (617) 438-8464
First Published: 1955. **Frequency:** Bimonthly. **ISSN:** 0035-8835.

★1210★ JOURNAL OF THE ROYAL SOCIETY OF HEALTH
38-A St.
George's Dr.
London SW1V 4BH, England
First Published: 1876. **Frequency:** Bimonthly. **ISSN:** 0035-9238.

★1211★ JOURNAL OF THE ROYAL SOCIETY OF MEDICINE
Oxford University Press
200 Madison Ave.
New York, NY 10016   Phone: (212) 679-7300
First Published: 1907. **Frequency:** Monthly. **ISSN:** 0141-0768.

★1212★ JOURNAL OF SCHOOL HEALTH
American School Health Association
7263 State Rte. 43
PO Box 708
Kent, OH 44240   Phone: (216) 678-1601
First Published: 1930. **Frequency:** Monthly. **ISSN:** 0022-4391.

★1213★ JOURNAL OF SEX AND MARITAL THERAPY
Brunner/Mazel, Inc.
19 Union Sq., W.
New York, NY 10003   Phone: (212) 924-3344
First Published: 1974. **Frequency:** Quarterly. **ISSN:** 0092-623X.

★1214★ JOURNAL OF SHOULDER AND ELBOW SURGERY
Mosby-Year Book, Inc.
11830 Westline Industrial Dr.
St. Louis, MO 63146   Phone: (314) 872-8370
First Published: 1992. **Frequency:** Bimonthly.

★1215★ JOURNAL OF SLEEP RESEARCH
Blackwell Scientific Publications
3 Cambridge Center, Ste. 208
Cambridge, MA 02142   Phone: (617) 225-0401
First Published: 1992. **Frequency:** Quarterly. **ISSN:** 0962-1105.

★1216★ JOURNAL OF SOCIAL WORK AND HUMAN SEXUALITY
The Haworth Press, Inc.
10 Alice St.
Binghampton, NY 13904   Phone: (800) 342-9678
Frequency: Biannual.

★1217★ JOURNAL OF THE SOCIETY OF OBSTETRICIANS AND GYNECOLOGISTS OF CANADA
Ribsome Communications
55 Charles St., W., Ste. 3104
Toronto, ON, Canada M5S 2W9   Phone: (416) 323-1133
First Published: 1978. **Frequency:** 10/yr.

★1218★ JOURNAL OF THE SOCIETY OF OCCUPATIONAL
  MEDICINE
Butterworth-Heinemann
80 Montvale Ave.
Stoneham, MA 02180   Phone: (617) 438-8464
First Published: 1951. Frequency: Quarterly. ISSN: 0301-0023.

★1219★ JOURNAL OF THE SOUTH CAROLINA MEDICAL
  ASSOCIATION
PO Box 11188
Columbia, SC 29211   Phone: (803) 798-6207
First Published: 1905. Frequency: Monthly. ISSN: 0038-3139.

★1220★ JOURNAL OF SPEECH AND HEARING DISORDERS
American Speech-Language-Hearing Association
10801 Rockville Pike
Rockville, MD 20852   Phone: (301) 897-5700
First Published: 1936. Frequency: Quarterly. ISSN: 0022-4685.

★1221★ JOURNAL OF SPEECH AND HEARING RESEARCH
American Speech-Language-Hearing Association
10801 Rockville Pike
Rockville, MD 20852   Phone: (301) 897-5700
First Published: 1958. Frequency: Quarterly. ISSN: 0022-4685.

★1222★ JOURNAL OF SPINAL DISORDERS
Raven Press
1185 Avenue of the Americas
New York, NY 10036   Phone: (212) 930-9500
First Published: 1988. Frequency: Quarterly. ISSN: 0895-0385.

★1223★ JOURNAL OF SPORTS MEDICINE AND PHYSICAL
  FITNESS
J.B. Lippincott Co.
E. Washington Sq.
Philadelphia, PA 19105   Phone: (215) 238-4200
First Published: 1961. Frequency: Quarterly. ISSN: 0022-4707.

★1224★ JOURNAL OF STEROID BIOCHEMISTRY AND
  MOLECULAR BIOLOGY
Pergamon Press, Inc.
Maxwell House, Fairview Park
Elmsford, NY 10523   Phone: (914) 592-7700
First Published: 1970. Frequency: 18/yr. ISSN: 0022-4731.

★1225★ JOURNAL OF STRUCTURAL BIOLOGY
Academic Press, Inc.
1250 6th Ave.
San Diego, CA 92101   Phone: (619) 231-0926
First Published: 1957. Frequency: Bimonthly. ISSN: 0889-1605.

★1226★ JOURNAL OF STUDIES ON ALCOHOL
Alcohol Research Documentation, Inc.
PO Box 969
Piscataway, NJ 08855   Phone: (201) 932-2190
First Published: 1940. Frequency: Bimonthly. ISSN: 0096-882X.

★1227★ JOURNAL OF SUBSTANCE ABUSE
Ablex Publishing Corp.
355 Chestnut St.
Norwood, NJ 07648   Phone: (201) 767-8450
First Published: 1988. Frequency: Quarterly. ISSN: 0899-3289.

★1228★ JOURNAL OF SUBSTANCE ABUSE TREATMENT
Pergamon Press, Inc.
Maxwell House, Fairview Park
Elmsford, NY 10523   Phone: (914) 592-7700
First Published: 1984. Frequency: Quarterly. ISSN: 0740-5472.

★1229★ JOURNAL OF SURGICAL ONCOLOGY
John Wiley & Sons, Inc.
605 3rd St.
New York, NY 10158   Phone: (212) 850-6000
First Published: 1969. Frequency: Monthly. ISSN: 0022-4790.

★1230★ JOURNAL OF SURGICAL PRACTICE
McMahon Publishing Co.
83 Peaceable St.
West Redding, CT 06896
First Published: 1972. Frequency: Bimonthly. ISSN: 0161-9721.

★1231★ JOURNAL OF SURGICAL RESEARCH
Academic Press, Inc.
1250 6th Ave.
San Diego, CA 92101   Phone: (619) 231-0926
First Published: 1961. Frequency: Monthly. ISSN: 0022-4804.

★1232★ JOURNAL OF THE TENNESSEE MEDICAL
  ASSOCIATION
112 Louise Ave.
Nashville, TN 37203   Phone: (615) 327-1451
First Published: 1902. Frequency: Monthly. ISSN: 0040-3318.

★1233★ JOURNAL OF THORACIC AND CARDIOVASCULAR
  SURGERY
American Association for Thoracic Surgery
13 Elm St.
PO Box 1565
Manchester, MA 01944   Phone: (508) 526-8330
First Published: 1931. Frequency: Monthly. ISSN: 0022-5223.

★1234★ JOURNAL OF THORACIC IMAGING
Aspen Publishers, Inc.
200 Orchard Ridge Dr.
Gaithersburg, MD 20878   Phone: (301) 417-7550
First Published: 1985. Frequency: Quarterly.

★1235★ JOURNAL OF TOXICOLOGY: CLINICAL
  TOXICOLOGY
Marcel Dekker, Inc.
270 Madison Ave.
New York, NY 10016   Phone: (212) 696-9000
First Published: 1968. Frequency: Quarterly. ISSN: 0731-3810.

★1236★ JOURNAL OF TOXICOLOGY AND ENVIRONMENTAL
  HEALTH
Hemisphere Publishing Corporation
1900 Frost Rd., Ste. 101
Bristol, PA 19007   Phone: (212) 725-0772
First Published: 1975. Frequency: Monthly. ISSN: 0098-4108.

★1237★ JOURNAL OF TRAUMA
American Association for the Surgery of Trauma
c/o Cleon Goodwin, M. D.
New York Burn Center
525 E. 68th St., L-706
New York, NY 10021   Phone: (212) 746-5010
First Published: 1961. Frequency: Monthly. ISSN: 0022-5282.

★1238★ JOURNAL OF TROPICAL MEDICINE AND HYGIENE
Blackwell Scientific Publications
3 Cambridge Center, Ste. 208
Cambridge, MA 02142   Phone: (617) 225-0401
First Published: 1898. Frequency: Bimonthly. ISSN: 0022-5304.

★1239★ JOURNAL OF ULTRASOUND IN MEDICINE
American Institute of Ultrasound in Medicine
4405 East-West Hwy., Ste. 504
Bethesda, MD 20814   Phone: (301) 656-6117
First Published: 1982. Frequency: Monthly. ISSN: 0278-4297.

★1240★ JOURNAL OF UROLOGY
American Urological Association
1120 N. Charles St.
Baltimore, MD 21201   Phone: (301) 727-1100
First Published: 1917. Frequency: Monthly. ISSN: 0022-5347.

★1241★ JOURNAL OF VASCULAR MEDICINE AND BIOLOGY
Blackwell Scientific Publications
3 Cambridge Center, Ste. 208
Cambridge, MA 02142   Phone: (617) 225-0401
Frequency: Bimonthly. **ISSN:** 1042-5268.

★1242★ JOURNAL OF VASCULAR SURGERY
Mosby-Year Book, Inc.
11830 Westline Industrial Dr.
St. Louis, MO 63146   Phone: (314) 872-8370
First Published: 1984. **Frequency:** Monthly. **ISSN:** 0741-5214.

★1243★ JOURNAL OF VASCULAR TECHNOLOGY
Society of Vascular Technology
1101 Connecticut Ave., NW, Ste. 700
Washington, DC 20036   Phone: (202) 857-1149
First Published: 1977. **Frequency:** Bimonthly.

★1244★ JOURNAL OF VETERINARY PHARMACOLOGY AND THERAPEUTICS
Blackwell Scientific Publications
3 Cambridge Center, Ste. 208
Cambridge, MA 02142   Phone: (617) 225-0401
First Published: 1978. **Frequency:** Quarterly. **ISSN:** 0140-7783.

★1245★ JOURNAL OF VIROLOGICAL METHODS
Elsevier Science Publishing Co., Inc.
655 Avenue of the Americas
New York, NY 10010   Phone: (212) 989-5800
First Published: 1980. **Frequency:** 15/yr. **ISSN:** 0166-0934.

★1246★ JOURNAL OF VIROLOGY
American Society for Microbiology
1325 Massachusetts Ave., NW
Washington, DC 20005   Phone: (202) 737-3600
First Published: 1967. **Frequency:** Monthly. **ISSN:** 0022-538X.

★1247★ JOURNAL OF VOCATIONAL REHABILITATION
Butterworth-Heinemann
80 Montvale
Stoneham, MA 02180   Phone: (617) 438-8464
First Published: 1991. **Frequency:** Quarterly. **ISSN:** 1052-2263.

★1248★ JOURNAL OF WOMEN AND AGING
The Haworth Press, Inc.
10 Alice St.
Binghampton, NY 13904   Phone: (800) 342-9678
Frequency: Quarterly.

★1249★ JOURNAL OF WOMEN'S HEALTH
Mary Ann Liebert, Inc.
1651 3rd Ave.
New York, NY 10128   Phone: (212) 289-2300
First Published: 1992. **Frequency:** Quarterly.

★1250★ JPEN: JOURNAL OF PARENTERAL AND ENTERAL NUTRITION
American Society for Parenteral and Enteral Nutrition
8630 Fenton St., No. 412
Silver Spring, MD 20910-3803   Phone: (301) 587-6315
First Published: 1979. **Frequency:** Bimonthly. **ISSN:** 0148-6071.

★1251★ KANSAS MEDICINE
1300 Topeka Ave.
Topeka, KS 66612   Phone: (913) 235-2383
First Published: 1901. **Frequency:** Monthly. **ISSN:** 8755-0059.

★1252★ KIDNEY INTERNATIONAL
Springer-Verlag New York, Inc.
175 5th Ave.
New York, NY 10010   Phone: (212) 460-1500
First Published: 1972. **Frequency:** Monthly. **ISSN:** 0085-2538.

★1253★ LABORATORY ANIMAL SCIENCE
American Association for Laboratory Animal Science
70 Timber Creek Dr., Ste. 5
Cordova, TN 38018   Phone: (901) 754-8620
First Published: 1950. **Frequency:** Bimonthly. **ISSN:** 0023-6764.

★1254★ LABORATORY INVESTIGATION
Williams & Wilkins
428 E. Preston St.
Baltimore, MD 21202   Phone: (301) 528-4000
First Published: 1952. **Frequency:** Monthly. **ISSN:** 0023-6837.

★1255★ LABORATORY MEDICINE
American Society of Clinical Pathologists
2100 W. Harrison St.
Chicago, IL 60612   Phone: (312) 738-1336
First Published: 1965. **Frequency:** Monthly. **ISSN:** 0007-5027.

★1256★ LABORATORY AND RESEARCH METHODS IN BIOLOGY AND MEDICINE
John Wiley & Sons, Inc.
605 3rd Ave.
New York, NY 10158   Phone: (212) 850-6000
First Published: 1977. **Frequency:** Irregular. **ISSN:** 0160-8584.

★1257★ LANCET
Little, Brown and Co.
34 Beacon St.
Boston, MA 02108   Phone: (617) 227-0730
First Published: 1823. **Frequency:** Weekly. **ISSN:** 0140-6736.

★1258★ LARYNGOSCOPE
Triological Foundation, Inc.
9216 Clayton Rd.
St. Louis, MO 63124   Phone: (314) 997-5070
First Published: 1896. **Frequency:** Monthly. **ISSN:** 0023-852X.

★1259★ LASERS IN MEDICAL SCIENCE
Academic Press, Inc.
1250 6th Ave.
San Diego, CA 92101   Phone: (619) 231-0926
Frequency: Monthly. **ISSN:** 0268-8921.

★1260★ LASERS IN SURGERY AND MEDICINE
John Wiley & Sons, Inc.
605 3rd Ave.
New York, NY 10158   Phone: (212) 850-6000
First Published: 1980. **Frequency:** 6/yr. **ISSN:** 0196-8092.

★1261★ LEARNING DISABILITIES RESEARCH AND PRACTICE
Springer-Verlag New York, Inc.
175 5th Ave.
New York, NY 10010   Phone: (212) 460-1500
First Published: 1991. **Frequency:** Quarterly. **ISSN:** 0938-8982.

★1262★ LEGAL ASPECTS OF MEDICAL PRACTICE
American College of Legal Medicine
5700 Old Orchard Rd., 1st Fl.
Stokie, IL 60077   Phone: (800) 433-9137
First Published: 1972. **Frequency:** Monthly. **ISSN:** 0190-2350.

★1263★ LENS AND EYE TOXICITY RESEARCH
Marcel Dekker, Inc.
270 Madison Ave.
New York, NY 10016   Phone: (212) 696-9000
Frequency: Quarterly.

★1264★ LEPROSY REVIEW
British Leprosy Relief Association
Fairfax House
Causton Rd.
Colchester, Essex CO1 1PU, England
First Published: 1927. **Frequency:** Quarterly. **ISSN:** 0305-7518.

★1265★   LEUKEMIA
Williams & Wilkins
428 E. Preston St.
Baltimore, MD 21202   Phone: (301) 528-4000
First Published: 1987. Frequency: Monthly. ISSN: 0887-6924.

★1266★   LEUKEMIA RESEARCH
Pergamon Press, Inc.
Maxwell House, Fairview Park
Elmsford, NY 10523   Phone: (914) 592-7700
First Published: 1977. Frequency: Monthly. ISSN: 0145-2126.

★1267★   LIFE SCIENCES
Pergamon Press, Inc.
Maxwell House, Fairview Park
Elmsford, NY 10523   Phone: (914) 592-7700
First Published: 1962. Frequency: Weekly. ISSN: 0024-3205.

★1268★   LIPIDS
American Oil Chemists' Society
1608 Broadmoor Dr.
PO Box 3489
Champaign, IL 61821   Phone: (217) 359-2344
First Published: 1966. Frequency: Monthly. ISSN: 0024-4201.

★1269★   LITERATURE AND MEDICINE
Johns Hopkins University Press
Journals Publishing Division
701 W. 40th St., Ste. 275
Baltimore, MD 21211
First Published: 1982. Frequency: Annual. ISSN: 0278-9671.

★1270★   LITHIUM
Churchill Livingstone, Inc.
1560 Broadway
New York, NY 10036   Phone: (212) 819-5400
Frequency: Quarterly. ISSN: 0954-1381.

★1271★   LIVER
Munksgaard
Noerre Soegade 35
DK-1370 Copenhagen K, Denmark
First Published: 1981. Frequency: Bimonthly. ISSN: 0106-9543.

★1272★   LUNG
Springer-Verlag New York, Inc.
175 5th Ave.
New York, NY 10010   Phone: (212) 460-1500
First Published: 1903. Frequency: Bimonthly. ISSN: 0341-2040.

★1273★   LYMPHOKINE RESEARCH
Mary Ann Liebert, Inc.
1651 3rd Ave.
New York, NY 10128   Phone: (212) 289-2300
First Published: 1982. Frequency: Quarterly. ISSN: 0277-6766.

★1274★   MAGNESIUM AND TRACE ELEMENTS
S. Karger Publishers, Inc.
26 W. Avon Rd.
PO Box 529
Farmington, CT 06085   Phone: (203) 675-7834
First Published: 1982. Frequency: Bimonthly. ISSN: 0252-1156.

★1275★   MAGNETIC RESONANCE IMAGING
Pergamon Press, Inc.
Maxwell House, Fairview Park
Elmsford, NY 10523   Phone: (914) 592-7700
First Published: 1982. Frequency: Bimonthly. ISSN: 0730-725X.

★1276★   MAGNETIC RESONANCE IN MEDICINE
Academic Press, Inc.
1250 6th Ave.
San Diego, CA 92101   Phone: (619) 231-0926
First Published: 1984. Frequency: Monthly. ISSN: 0740-3194.

★1277★   MARYLAND MEDICAL JOURNAL
Medical and Chirurgical Faculty of the State of Maryland
1211 Cathedral St.
Baltimore, MD 21201   Phone: (301) 539-0872
First Published: 1952. Frequency: Monthly. ISSN: 0886-0572.

★1278★   MATERIALS MANAGEMENT IN HEALTH CARE
American Hospital Association
840 N. Lake Shore Dr.
Chicago, IL 60611   Phone: (312) 280-6000
Frequency: Monthly.

★1279★   MATERNAL/CHILD NURSING JOURNAL
University of Pittsburgh
School of Nursing, Parent-Child Nursing
437 Victoria Bldg.
3500 Victoria St.
Pittsburgh, PA 15261   Phone: (412) 624-4141
First Published: 1972. Frequency: Quarterly. ISSN: 0090-0702.

★1280★   MATRIX
Gustav Fischer New York, Inc.
220 E. 23rd St., Ste. 909
New York, NY 10010
Frequency: Bimonthly. ISSN: 0934-8832.

★1281★   MAYO CLINIC PROCEEDINGS
Mayo Foundation
Siebens Bldg., Rm. 660
Rochester, MN 55905   Phone: (507) 284-2154
First Published: 1926. Frequency: Monthly. ISSN: 0025-6196.

★1282★   MCN: AMERICAN JOURNAL OF MATERNAL CHILD
  NURSING
American Journal of Nursing Co.
555 W. 57th St.
New York, NY 10019   Phone: (212) 582-8820
First Published: 1976. Frequency: Bimonthly. ISSN: 0361-929X.

★1283★   MD COMPUTING
Springer-Verlag New York, Inc.
175 5th Ave.
New York, NY 10010   Phone: (212) 460-1500
First Published: 1983. Frequency: Bimonthly. ISSN: 0724-6811.

★1284★   MECHANISMS OF AGEING AND DEVELOPMENT
Elsevier Science Publishing Co., Inc.
655 Avenue of the Americas
New York, NY 10010   Phone: (212) 989-5800
First Published: 1972. Frequency: Monthly. ISSN: 0047-6374.

★1285★   MEDICAL ADVERTISING NEWS
Engel Communications
820 Bear Tavern Rd.
Mountainview Corporate Park, W.
Trenton, NJ 08628   Phone: (609) 530-0040
First Published: 1982. Frequency: 18/yr.

★1286★   MEDICAL ANTHROPOLOGY
Gordon & Breach, Science Publishers, Inc.
270 8th Ave.
New York, NY 10011   Phone: (212) 206-8900
First Published: 1977. Frequency: Quarterly. ISSN: 0145-9740.

★1287★   MEDICAL ASPECTS OF HUMAN SEXUALITY
Cahners Publishing Co.
Medical-Health Care Group
Division of Reed Publishing USA
249 W. 17th St.
New York, NY 10011   Phone: (212) 645-0067
First Published: 1967. Frequency: Monthly. ISSN: 0025-7001.

★1288★   MEDICAL AUDIT NEWS
Churchill Livingstone, Inc.
1560 Broadway
New York, NY 10036   Phone: (212) 819-5400
Frequency: Bimonthly. **ISSN:** 0959-2903.

**★1289★   MEDICAL AND BIOLOGICAL ENGINEERING AND
    COMPUTING**
International Federation for Medical and Biological Engineering
Peter Peregrinus, Ltd.
Southgate House
Box 8
Stevenage, Herts SG1 1HP, England
First Published: 1963. **Frequency:** Bimonthly. **ISSN:** 0140-0118.

★1290★   MEDICAL CARE
J.B. Lippincott Co.
E. Washington Sq.
Philadelphia, PA 19105   Phone: (215) 238-4200
First Published: 1967. **Frequency:** Monthly. **ISSN:** 0025-7079.

★1291★   MEDICAL DECISION MAKING
Hanley & Belfus, Inc.
210 S. 13th St.
Philadelphia, PA 19107   Phone: (215) 546-7293
First Published: 1980. **Frequency:** Quarterly. **ISSN:** 0272-989X.

★1292★   MEDICAL ECONOMICS
Medical Economics Co., Inc.
680 Kinderkamack Rd.
Oradell, NJ 07649   Phone: (201) 262-3030
First Published: 1923. **Frequency:** Biweekly. **ISSN:** 0025-7206.

★1293★   MEDICAL EDUCATION
Blackwell Scientific Publications
3 Cambridge Center, Ste. 208
Cambridge, MA 02142   Phone: (617) 225-0401
First Published: 1966. **Frequency:** Bimonthly. **ISSN:** 0308-0110.

★1294★   MEDICAL GROUP MANAGEMENT
Medical Group Management Association
1355 S. Colorado Blvd., Ste. 900
Denver, CO 80222   Phone: (303) 753-1111
First Published: 1953. **Frequency:** Bimonthly. **ISSN:** 0025-7257.

★1295★   MEDICAL HISTORY
Wellcome Institute for the History of Medicine
Box 560B
Kennebunkport, ME 04046
First Published: 1957. **Frequency:** Quarterly. **ISSN:** 0025-7273.

★1296★   MEDICAL HYPOTHESES
Churchill Livingstone, Inc.
1560 Broadway
New York, NY 10036   Phone: (212) 819-5400
First Published: 1975. **Frequency:** Monthly. **ISSN:** 0306-9877.

★1297★   MEDICAL JOURNAL OF AUSTRALIA
Australasian Medical Publishing Company
PO Box 116
Glebe, NSW 2037, Australia
First Published: 1914. **Frequency:** Biweekly. **ISSN:** 0025-729X.

★1298★   MEDICAL LABORATORY SCIENCES
Blackwell Scientific Publications
3 Cambridge Center, Ste. 208
Cambridge, MA 02142   Phone: (617) 225-0401
First Published: 1951. **Frequency:** Quarterly. **ISSN:** 0308-3616.

★1299★   MEDICAL LETTER ON DRUGS AND THERAPEUTICS
Medical Letter, Inc.
56 Harrison St.
New Rochelle, NY 10801   Phone: (914) 235-0500
First Published: 1959. **Frequency:** Biweekly. **ISSN:** 0025-732X.

★1300★   MEDICAL MARKETING AND MEDIA
CPS Communications, Inc.
7200 W. Camino Real, Ste. 215
Boca Raton, FL 33433   Phone: (407) 368-9301
First Published: 1966. **Frequency:** 14/yr. **ISSN:** 0025-7354.

★1301★   MEDICAL MICROBIOLOGY AND IMMUNOLOGY
Springer-Verlag New York, Inc.
175 5th Ave.
New York, NY 10010   Phone: (212) 460-1500
First Published: 1886. **Frequency:** Bimonthly. **ISSN:** 0300-8584.

**★1302★   MEDICAL ONCOLOGY AND TUMOR
    PHARMACOTHERAPY**
Pergamon Press, Inc.
Maxwell House, Fairview Park
Elmsford, NY 10523   Phone: (914) 592-7700
First Published: 1984. **Frequency:** Quarterly. **ISSN:** 0736-0118.

★1303★   MEDICAL AND PEDIATRIC ONCOLOGY
John Wiley & Sons, Inc.
605 3rd Ave.
New York, NY 10158   Phone: (212) 850-6000
First Published: 1975. **Frequency:** Bimonthly. **ISSN:** 0098-1532.

★1304★   MEDICAL PHYSICS
American Association of Physicists in Medicine
335 E. 45th St.
New York, NY 10017   Phone: (212) 661-9404
First Published: 1970. **Frequency:** Bimonthly. **ISSN:** 0094-2405.

★1305★   MEDICAL REFERENCE SERVICES QUARTERLY
The Haworth Press, Inc
10 Alice St.
Binghamton, NY 13904   Phone: (800) 342-9678
First Published: 1992. **Frequency:** Quarterly.

★1306★   MEDICAL STAFF LEADER
American Hospital Publishing, Inc.
211 E. Chicago Ave., Ste. 700
Chicago, IL 60611   Phone: (312) 440-6800
First Published: 1978. **Frequency:** Monthly.

★1307★   MEDICAL AND VETERINARY ENTOMOLOGY
Blackwell Scientific Publications
3 Cambridge Center, Ste. 208
Cambridge, MA 02142   Phone: (617) 225-0401
Frequency: Quarterly. **ISSN:** 0269-283X.

★1308★   MEDICINAL RESEARCH REVIEWS
John Wiley & Sons, Inc.
605 3rd Ave.
New York, NY 10158   Phone: (212) 850-6000
First Published: 1981. **Frequency:** Quarterly. **ISSN:** 0198-6325.

★1309★   MEDICINE
Williams & Wilkins
428 E. Preston St.
Baltimore, MD 21202   Phone: (301) 528-4223
First Published: 1922. **Frequency:** Bimonthly. **ISSN:** 0025-7974.

★1310★   MEDICINE, EXERCISE, NUTRITION, AND HEALTH
Blackwell Scientific Publications
3 Cambridge Center, Ste. 208
Cambridge, MA 02142   Phone: (617) 225-0401
First Published: 1992. **Frequency:** Bimonthly. **ISSN:** 1057-9354.

★1311★   MEDICINE AND LAW
Springer-Verlag New York, Inc.
175 5th Ave.
New York, NY 10010   Phone: (212) 460-1500
First Published: 1982. **Frequency:** Bimonthly. **ISSN:** 0723-1393.

★1312★ MEDICINE, SCIENCE AND THE LAW
Kluwer Publishing
1 Harlequin Ave.
Brentwood, Middlesex TW8 9EW, England
First Published: 1960. **Frequency:** Quarterly. **ISSN:** 0025-8024.

★1313★ MEDICINE AND SCIENCE IN SPORTS AND EXERCISE
American College of Sports Medicine
PO Box 1440
Indianapolis, IN 46206   Phone: (317) 637-9200
First Published: 1969. **Frequency:** Bimonthly. **ISSN:** 0195-9131.

★1314★ MEDICINE AND WAR
John Wiley & Sons, Inc.
605 3rd Ave.
New York, NY 10158   Phone: (212) 850-6000
First Published: 1965. **Frequency:** Quarterly. **ISSN:** 0748-8009.

★1315★ MEDICO-LEGAL BULLETIN
Department of Health
Medical Examiner Division
9 N. 14th St.
Richmond, VA 23219   Phone: (804) 786-3174
First Published: 1951. **Frequency:** Bimonthly. **ISSN:** 0025-8164.

★1316★ MEDICO-LEGAL JOURNAL
Dramrite Printers, Ltd.
129 Long Ln.
Southwark
London SE1 4PL, England
First Published: 1933. **Frequency:** Quarterly. **ISSN:** 0025-8172.

★1317★ MELANOMA RESEARCH
Rapid Communications of Oxford Ltd.
The Old Malthouse
Paradise St.
Oxford OX1 1LD, England
First Published: 1991. **Frequency:** Bimonthly. **ISSN:** 0960-8931.

★1318★ MEMBRANE BIOCHEMISTRY
Taylor & Francis, Inc.
1990 Frost Rd., Ste. 101
Bristol, PA 19007   Phone: (215) 785-5800
First Published: 1978. **Frequency:** Quarterly. **ISSN:** 0149-046X.

★1319★ METABOLISM: CLINICAL AND EXPERIMENTAL
W. B. Saunders Co.
Curtis Center
Independence Sq., W.
Philadelphia, PA 19106   Phone: (215) 238-7800
First Published: 1974. **Frequency:** Monthly. **ISSN:** 0026-0495.

★1320★ METHODS OF BIOCHEMICAL ANALYSIS
John Wiley & Sons, Inc.
605 3rd Ave.
New York, NY 10158   Phone: (212) 850-6000
First Published: 1954. **Frequency:** Irregular. **ISSN:** 0076-6941.

★1321★ METHODS IN CELL BIOLOGY
Academic Press, Inc.
1250 6th Ave.
San Diego, CA 92101   Phone: (619) 231-0926
First Published: 1964. **Frequency:** Irregular. **ISSN:** 0091-679X.

★1322★ METHODS IN ENZYMOLOGY
Academic Press, Inc.
1250 6th Ave.
San Diego, CA 92101   Phone: (619) 231-0926
First Published: 1955. **Frequency:** Irregular. **ISSN:** 0076-6879.

★1323★ MICHIGAN MEDICINE
Michigan State Medical Society
120 W. Saginaw St.
East Lansing, MI 48823   Phone: (517) 337-1351
First Published: 1902. **Frequency:** Monthly. **ISSN:** 0026-2293.

★1324★ MICROBIAL ECOLOGY
Springer-Verlag New York, Inc.
175 5th Ave.
New York, NY 10010   Phone: (212) 460-1500
Frequency: 6/yr. **ISSN:** 0095-3628.

★1325★ MICROBIAL PATHOGENESIS
Academic Press, Inc.
1250 6th Ave.
San Diego, CA 92101   Phone: (619) 231-0926
First Published: 1986. **Frequency:** Monthly. **ISSN:** 0882-4010.

★1326★ MICROBIOLOGICAL REVIEWS
American Society for Microbiology
1325 Massachusetts Ave., NW
Washington, DC 20005   Phone: (202) 737-3600
First Published: 1937. **Frequency:** Quarterly. **ISSN:** 0146-0749.

★1327★ MICROBIOLOGICAL SCIENCES
Blackwell Scientific Publications
3 Cambridge Center, Ste. 208
Cambridge, MA 02142   Phone: (617) 225-0401
First Published: 1984. **Frequency:** Monthly. **ISSN:** 0265-1351.

★1328★ MICROCHEMICAL JOURNAL
Academic Press, Inc.
1250 6th Ave.
San Diego, CA 92101   Phone: (619) 231-0926
Frequency: Bimonthly. **ISSN:** 0026-265X.

★1329★ MICROSURGERY
John Wiley & Sons, Inc.
605 3rd Ave.
New York, NY 10158   Phone: (212) 850-6000
First Published: 1979. **Frequency:** 4/yr. **ISSN:** 0738-1085.

★1330★ MICROVASCULAR RESEARCH
Academic Press, Inc.
1250 6th Ave.
San Diego, CA 92101   Phone: (619) 231-0926
First Published: 1968. **Frequency:** Bimonthly. **ISSN:** 0026-2862.

★1331★ MIDWIFERY
Churchill Livingstone, Inc.
1560 Broadway
New York, NY 10036   Phone: (212) 819-5400
First Published: 1984. **Frequency:** Quarterly. **ISSN:** 0266-6138.

★1332★ MILITARY MEDICINE
Association of Military Surgeons of the United States
9320 Old Georgetown Rd.
Bethesda, MD 20814   Phone: (301) 897-8800
First Published: 1891. **Frequency:** Monthly. **ISSN:** 0026-4075.

★1333★ MINERAL AND ELECTROLYTE METABOLISM
S. Karger Publishers, Inc.
26 W. Avon Rd.
PO Box 529
Farmington, CT 06085   Phone: (203) 675-7834
First Published: 1978. **Frequency:** Bimonthly. **ISSN:** 0378-0392.

★1334★ MINIMALLY INVASIVE THERAPY
Blackwell Scientific Publications
3 Cambridge Center, Ste. 208
Cambridge, MA 02142   Phone: (617) 225-0401
Frequency: Bimonthly. **ISSN:** 0961-625X.

★1335★ MINNESOTA MEDICINE
Minnesota Medical Association
2221 University Ave., SE, Ste. 400
Minneapolis, MN 55414   Phone: (612) 378-1875
First Published: 1918. **Frequency:** Monthly. **ISSN:** 0026-556X.

★1336★   MISSOURI MEDICINE
Missouri State Medical Association
113 Madison St.
PO Box 1028
Jefferson City, MO 65102   Phone: (314) 636-5151
First Published: 1904. Frequency: Monthly. ISSN: 0026-6620.

★1337★   MMWR CDC SURVEILLANCE SUMMARIES
U.S. Department of Health and Human Services
Centers for Disease Control
Epidemiology Program Office
1600 Clifton Rd., NE
Atlanta, GA 30333
First Published: 1950. Frequency: Weekly.

★1338★   MODERN CONCEPTS OF CARDIOVASCULAR
    DISEASE
American Heart Association
7320 Greenville Ave.
Dallas, TX 75231   Phone: (214) 373-6300
First Published: 1932. Frequency: Monthly. ISSN: 0026-7600.

★1339★   MODERN HEALTHCARE
Crain Communications, Inc.
740 Rush St.
Chicago, IL 60611   Phone: (312) 649-5341
First Published: 1974. Frequency: Monthly. ISSN: 0160-7480.

★1340★   MODERN MEDICINE
Harcourt Brace Jovanovich, Inc.
7500 Old Oak Blvd.
Cleveland, OH 44130   Phone: (216) 243-8100
First Published: 1932. Frequency: Monthly. ISSN: 0026-8070.

★1341★   MODERN PATHOLOGY
Williams & Wilkins
428 E. Preston St.
Baltimore, MD 21202   Phone: (301) 528-4223
First Published: 1988. Frequency: Bimonthly. ISSN: 0893-3952.

★1342★   MODERN PROBLEMS OF PHARMACOPSYCHIATRY
S. Karger Publishers, Inc.
26 W. Avon Rd.
PO Box 529
Farmington, CT 06085   Phone: (203) 675-7834
First Published: 1968. Frequency: Irregular. ISSN: 0077-0094.

★1343★   MODERN VETERINARY PRACTICE
American Veterinary Publications, Inc.
5782 Thornwood Dr.
Goleta, CA 93117   Phone: (805) 967-5988
First Published: 1920. Frequency: Monthly. ISSN: 0026-8542.

★1344★   MOLECULAR ASPECTS OF MEDICINE
Pergamon Press, Inc.
Maxwell House, Fairview Park
Elmsford, NY 10523   Phone: (914) 592-7700
First Published: 1975. Frequency: 6/yr. ISSN: 0098-2997.

★1345★   MOLECULAR BIOLOGY AND MEDICINE
Academic Press, Inc.
1250 6th Ave.
San Diego, CA 92101   Phone: (619) 231-0926
First Published: 1983. Frequency: Bimonthly. ISSN: 0735-1313.

★1346★   MOLECULAR AND CELLULAR BIOCHEMISTRY
Kluwer Academic Publishers
101 Philip Dr.
Norwell, MA 02061   Phone: (617) 871-6600
First Published: 1973. Frequency: 16/yr. ISSN: 0300-8177.

★1347★   MOLECULAR AND CELLULAR BIOLOGY
American Society for Microbiology
1325 Massachusetts Ave., NW
Washington, DC 20005   Phone: (202) 737-3600
First Published: 1981. Frequency: Monthly. ISSN: 0270-7306.

★1348★   MOLECULAR AND CELLULAR ENDOCRINOLOGY
Elsevier Science Publishing Co., Inc.
655 Avenue of the Americas
New York, NY 10010   Phone: (212) 989-5800
First Published: 1974. Frequency: 18/yr. ISSN: 0303-7207.

★1349★   MOLECULAR AND CELLULAR NEUROSCIENCES
Academic Press, Inc.
1250 6th Ave.
San Diego, CA 92101   Phone: (619) 231-0926
Frequency: Bimonthly. ISSN: 1044-7431.

★1350★   MOLECULAR AND CELLULAR PROBES
Academic Press, Inc.
1250 6th Ave.
San Diego, CA 92101   Phone: (619) 231-0926
First Published: 1986. Frequency: Bimonthly. ISSN: 0890-8508.

★1351★   MOLECULAR AND CHEMICAL NEUROPATHOLOGY
Humana Press, Inc.
PO Box 2148
Clifton, NJ 07015
First Published: 1983. Frequency: Bimonthly. ISSN: 1044-7393.

★1352★   MOLECULAR ENDOCRINOLOGY
Williams & Wilkins
428 E. Preston St.
Baltimore, MD 21202   Phone: (301) 528-4000
First Published: 1987. Frequency: Monthly. ISSN: 0888-8809.

★1353★   MOLECULAR AND GENERAL GENETICS
Springer-Verlag New York, Inc.
175 5th Ave.
New York, NY 10010   Phone: (212) 460-1500
First Published: 1908. Frequency: 18/yr. ISSN: 0026-8925.

★1354★   MOLECULAR IMMUNOLOGY
Pergamon Press, Inc.
Maxwell House, Fairview Park
Elmsford, NY 10523   Phone: (914) 592-7700
First Published: 1964. Frequency: Monthly. ISSN: 0161-5890.

★1355★   MOLECULAR PHARMACOLOGY
American Society for Pharmacology and Experimental Therapeutics
9650 Rockville Pike
Bethesda, MD 20814   Phone: (301) 530-7060
First Published: 1965. Frequency: Monthly. ISSN: 0026-895X.

★1356★   MOLECULAR TOXICOLOGY
Hemisphere Publishing Corp.
1900 Frost Rd., Ste. 107
Bristol, PA 19007   Phone: (215) 785-5800
First Published: 1986. Frequency: Quarterly. ISSN: 0883-9492.

★1357★   MOTHERS AND CHILDREN
American Public Health Association
1015 15th St., NW
Washington, DC 20005   Phone: (202) 789-5600
Frequency: 3/yr.

★1358★   MT. SINAI JOURNAL OF MEDICINE
Mt. Sinai Medical Center
Medical Publications Committee
19th E. 98th St.
Box 1094
New York, NY 10029   Phone: (212) 650-6108
First Published: 1934. Frequency: Bimonthly. ISSN: 0027-2507.

★1359★   MUSCLE AND NERVE
John Wiley & Sons, Inc.
605 3rd Ave.
New York, NY 10158   Phone: (212) 850-6000
First Published: 1979. Frequency: Monthly. ISSN: 0148-639X.

★1360★ MUTAGENESIS
IRL Press, Inc.
PO Box Q
McLean, VA 22101   Phone: (703) 437-3334
First Published: 1986. Frequency: Bimonthly. ISSN: 0267-8257.

★1361★ MUTATION RESEARCH
Elsevier Science Publishing Co., Inc.
655 Avenue of the Americas
New York, NY 10010   Phone: (212) 989-5800
First Published: 1964. Frequency: 54/yr. ISSN: 0027-5107.

★1362★ NARD JOURNAL
National Association of Retail Druggists
205 Daingerfield Rd.
Alexandria, VA 22314   Phone: (703) 683-8200
First Published: 1898. Frequency: Monthly. ISSN: 0027-5972.

★1363★ THE NATION'S HEALTH
American Public Health Association
1015 15th St., NW
Washington, DC 20005   Phone: (202) 789-5600
Frequency: 11/yr.

★1364★ NATURAL IMMUNITY AND CELL GROWTH
  REGULATION
S. Karger Publishers, Inc.
26 W. Avon Rd.
PO Box 529
Farmington, CT 06085   Phone: (203) 675-7834
First Published: 1981. Frequency: Bimonthly. ISSN: 0254-7600.

★1365★ NAVY MEDICINE
U.S. Navy
Bureau of Medicine and Surgery
Washington, DC 20372   Phone: (202) 653-1297
First Published: 1970. Frequency: Bimonthly. ISSN: 0364-6807.

★1366★ NEBRASKA MEDICAL JOURNAL
Nebraska Medical Association
1512 First National Bank Bldg.
Lincoln, NE 68508   Phone: (402) 474-4472
First Published: 1916. Frequency: Monthly. ISSN: 0091-6730.

★1367★ NEPHROLOGY, DIALYSIS, TRANSPLANTATION
Springer-Verlag New York, Inc.
174 5th Ave.
New York, NY 10010   Phone: (212) 460-1500
First Published: 1986. Frequency: Monthly. ISSN: 0931-0509.

★1368★ NEPHRON
S. Karger Publishers, Inc.
26 W. Avon Rd.
PO Box 529
Farmington, CT 06085   Phone: (203) 675-7834
First Published: 1964. Frequency: Monthly. ISSN: 0028-2766.

★1369★ NETHERLANDS JOURNAL OF MEDICINE
Bohn
Scheltema en Holkema
Postbus 13079
3507 LB Utrecht, Netherlands
First Published: 1969. Frequency: Bimonthly. ISSN: 0300-2977.

★1370★ NEUROBIOLOGY OF AGING
Pergamon Press, Inc.
Maxwell House, Fairview Park
Elmsford, NY 10523   Phone: (914) 592-7700
First Published: 1980. Frequency: 8/yr. ISSN: 0197-4580.

★1371★ NEUROCHEMICAL RESEARCH
Plenum Publishing Corp.
233 Spring St.
New York, NY 10013   Phone: (212) 620-8000
First Published: 1976. Frequency: Monthly. ISSN: 0364-3190.

★1372★ NEUROENDOCRINOLOGY
S. Karger Publishers, Inc.
26 W. Avon Rd.
PO Box 529
Farmington, CT 06085   Phone: (203) 675-7834
First Published: 1965. Frequency: Monthly. ISSN: 0028-3835.

★1373★ NEUROEPIDEMIOLOGY
S. Karger Publishers, Inc.
26 W. Avon Rd.
PO Box 529
Farmington, CT 06085   Phone: (203) 675-7834
First Published: 1982. Frequency: Bimonthly. ISSN: 0251-5350.

★1374★ NEUROFIBROMATOSIS
S. Karger Publishers, Inc.
26 W. Avon Rd.
PO Box 529
Farmington, CT 06085   Phone: (203) 675-7834
First Published: 1988. Frequency: 6/yr. ISSN: 1010-5662.

★1375★ NEUROIMAGE
Academic Press, Inc.
1250 6th Ave.
San Diego, CA 92101   Phone: (619) 231-0926
First Published: 1992. Frequency: Quarterly. ISSN: 1053-8119.

★1376★ NEUROIMAGING CLINICS OF NORTH AMERICA
W.B. Saunders Co.
Curtis Center
Independence Sq., W.
Philadelphia, PA 19106   Phone: (215) 238-7800
Frequency: Quarterly.

★1377★ NEUROLOGY
Edgell Communications
7500 Old Oak Blvd.
Cleveland, OH 44130   Phone: (216) 243-8100
First Published: 1977. Frequency: Monthly. ISSN: 0028-3878.

★1378★ NEUROLOGY AND URODYNAMICS
John Wiley & Sons, Inc.
605 3rd Ave.
New York, NY 10158   Phone: (212) 850-6000
First Published: 1982. Frequency: Bimonthly. ISSN: 0733-2467.

★1379★ NEURO-ORTHOPEDICS
Springer-Verlag New York, Inc.
175 5th Ave.
New York, NY 10010   Phone: (212) 460-1500
First Published: 1986. Frequency: 4/yr. ISSN: 0177-7955.

★1380★ NEUROPATHOLOGY AND APPLIED NEUROBIOLOGY
Blackwell Scientific Publications
3 Cambridge Center, Ste. 208
Cambridge, MA 02142   Phone: (617) 225-0401
First Published: 1975. Frequency: Bimonthly. ISSN: 0305-1846.

★1381★ NEUROPEPTIDES
Churchill Livingstone, Inc.
1560 Broadway
New York, NY 10036   Phone: (212) 819-5400
First Published: 1979. Frequency: Monthly. ISSN: 0143-4179.

★1382★ NEUROPHARMACOLOGY
Pergamon Press, Inc.
Maxwell House, Fairview Park
Elmsford, NY 10523   Phone: (915) 592-7700
First Published: 1962. Frequency: Monthly. ISSN: 0028-3908.

★1383★ NEUROPROTOCOLS
Academic Press, Inc.
1250 6th Ave.
San Diego, CA 92101   Phone: (619) 231-0926
First Published: 1992. Frequency: 3/yr. ISSN: 1058-6741.

★1384★ NEUROPSYCHIATRY, NEUROPSYCHOLOGY, AND BEHAVIORAL NEUROLOGY
Raven Press
1185 Avenue of the Americas
New York, NY 10036   Phone: (212) 930-9500
First Published: 1988. Frequency: Quarterly. ISSN: 0894-878X.

★1385★ NEUROPSYCHOBIOLOGY
S. Karger Publishers, Inc.
26 W. Avon Rd.
PO Box 529
Farmington, CT 06085   Phone: (203) 675-7834
First Published: 1975. Frequency: 8/yr. ISSN: 0302-282X.

★1386★ NEUROPSYCHOLOGIA
Pergamon Press, Inc.
Maxwell House, Fairview Park
Elmsford, NY 10523   Phone: (914) 592-7700
First Published: 1963. Frequency: 12/yr. ISSN: 0028-3932.

★1387★ NEURORADIOLOGY
Springer-Verlag New York, Inc.
175 5th Ave.
New York, NY 10010   Phone: (212) 460-1500
First Published: 1970. Frequency: Bimonthly. ISSN: 0028-3940.

★1388★ NEUROREHABILITATION
Butterworth-Heinemann
80 Montvale Ave.
Stoneham, MA 02180   Phone: (617) 438-8464
First Published: 1991. Frequency: Quarterly. ISSN: 1053-0752.

★1389★ NEUROREPORT
Rapid Communications of Oxford Ltd.
The Old Malthouse
Paradise St.
Oxford OX1 1LD, England
First Published: 1990. Frequency: Monthly. ISSN: 0959-4965.

★1390★ NEUROSCIENCE
Pergamon Press, Inc.
Maxwell House, Fairview Park
Elmsford, NY 10523   Phone: (914) 592-7700
First Published: 1976. Frequency: 18/yr. ISSN: 0306-4522.

★1391★ NEUROSCIENCE AND BEHAVIORAL PHYSIOLOGY
Federation of American Societies for Experimental Biology
9650 Rockville Pike
Bethesda, MD 20814   Phone: (301) 530-7000
First Published: 1967. Frequency: Bimonthly. ISSN: 0097-0549.

★1392★ NEUROSCIENCE LETTERS
Elsevier Science Publishing Co., Inc.
655 Avenue of the Americas
New York, NY 10010   Phone: (212) 989-5800
First Published: 1975. Frequency: 33/yr. ISSN: 0304-3940.

★1393★ NEUROSURGERY
Thomas G. Saul, M.D.
506 Oak St.
Cincinnati, OH 45219   Phone: (513) 872-2657
First Published: 1977. Frequency: Monthly. ISSN: 0148-396X.

★1394★ NEUROSURGERY QUARTERLY
Raven Press
1185 Avenue of the Americas
New York, NY 10036   Phone: (212) 930-9500
First Published: 1992. Frequency: Quarterly. ISSN: 1050-6438.

★1395★ NEUROSURGICAL CONSULTATIONS
Williams & Wilkins
428 E. Preston St.
Baltimore, MD 21202   Phone: (301) 528-4000
Frequency: Biweekly. ISSN: 1045-6694.

★1396★ NEUROTOXICOLOGY AND TERATOLOGY
Pergamon Press, Inc.
Maxwell House, Fairview Park
Elmsford, NY 10523   Phone: (914) 592-7700
First Published: 1979. Frequency: Bimonthly. ISSN: 0892-0362.

★1397★ NEW DIRECTIONS FOR CHILD DEVELOPMENT
Jossey-Bass, Inc.
350 Sansome St., 5th Fl.
San Francisco, CA 94104   Phone: (415) 433-1740
First Published: 1978. Frequency: Quarterly. ISSN: 0195-2269.

★1398★ NEW DIRECTIONS FOR MENTAL HEALTH SERVICES
Jossey-Bass, Inc.
350 Sansome St., 5th Fl.
San Francisco, CA 94104   Phone: (415) 433-1740
First Published: 1979. Frequency: Quarterly. ISSN: 0193-9416.

★1399★ NEW ENGLAND JOURNAL OF MEDICINE
Massachusetts Medical Society
1440 Main St.
Waltham, MA 02254   Phone: (617) 893-3800
First Published: 1812. Frequency: Weekly. ISSN: 0028-4793.

★1400★ NEW PHYSICIAN
American Medical Student Association
1890 Preston White Dr.
Reston, VA 22091   Phone: (703) 620-6600
First Published: 1952. Frequency: Monthly. ISSN: 0028-6451.

★1401★ NEW YORK JOURNAL OF DENTISTRY
New York Journal of Dentistry, Inc.
295 Madison Ave.
New York, NY 10017   Phone: (212) 889-8940
First Published: 1860. Frequency: 8/yr. ISSN: 0028-7296.

★1402★ NEW YORK STATE DENTAL JOURNAL
Dental Society of the State of New York
30 E. 42nd St.
New York, NY 10017   Phone: (212) 986-3937
First Published: 1933. Frequency: Monthly. ISSN: 0028-7571.

★1403★ NEW YORK STATE JOURNAL OF MEDICINE
Medical Society of the State of New York
420 Lakeville Rd.
Lake Success, NY 11042   Phone: (516) 488-6100
First Published: 1901. Frequency: Monthly. ISSN: 0028-7628.

★1404★ NEW ZEALAND MEDICAL JOURNAL
Souther Colour Print
PO Box 920
Dunedin, New Zealand
First Published: 1887. Frequency: Semimonthly. ISSN: 0028-8446.

★1405★ NMCD: NUTRITION, METABOLISM AND CARDIOVASCULAR
Springer-Verlag New York, Inc.
175 5th Ave.
New York, NY 10010   Phone: (212) 460-1500
First Published: 1991. Frequency: Quarterly. ISSN: 0939-4753.

★1406★ NORTH CAROLINA MEDICAL JOURNAL
North Carolina Medical Society
Rte. 1, Box 194
Bullock, NC 27507   Phone: (919) 684-5728
First Published: 1940. Frequency: Monthly. ISSN: 0029-2559.

★1407★ NUCLEAR MEDICINE COMMUNICATIONS
Chapman & Hall Ltd.
2-6 Boundary Row
London SE1, England
First Published: 1980. Frequency: 12/yr. ISSN: 0143-3636.

★1408★   NUCLEIC ACIDS RESEARCH
IRL Press, Inc.
PO Box Q
McLean, VA 22101   Phone: (703) 437-3334
First Published: 1974. Frequency: 24/yr. ISSN: 0305-1048.

★1409★   NURSE ANESTHESIA
Appleton & Lange
25 Van Zant St.
East Norwalk, CT 06855   Phone: (203) 838-4400
Frequency: Quarterly. ISSN: 0897-7437.

★1410★   NURSE EDUCATION TODAY
Churchill Livingstone, Inc.
1560 Broadway
New York, NY 10036   Phone: (212) 819-5400
First Published: 1981. Frequency: Bimonthly. ISSN: 0260-6917.

★1411★   NURSE PRACTITIONER
Vernon Publications, Inc.
3000 Northrop Way, Ste. 200
Bellevue, WA 98004   Phone: (206) 827-9900
First Published: 1975. Frequency: Monthly. ISSN: 0361-1817.

★1412★   NURSING ADMINISTRATION QUARTERLY
Aspen Publishers, Inc.
200 Orchard Ridge Dr.
Gaithersburg, MD 20878   Phone: (301) 417-7500
First Published: 1976. Frequency: Quarterly. ISSN: 0363-9568.

★1413★   NURSING FORUM
Nursing Publications, Inc.
PO Box 218
Hillsdale, NJ 07652   Phone: (201) 391-7845
First Published: 1961. Frequency: Quarterly. ISSN: 0029-6473.

★1414★   NURSING OUTLOOK
American Journal of Nursing Co.
555 W. 57th St.
New York, NY 10019   Phone: (212) 582-8820
First Published: 1953. Frequency: Bimonthly. ISSN: 0029-6554.

★1415★   NURSING RESEARCH
American Journal of Nursing Co.
555 W. 57th St.
New York, NY 10019   Phone: (212) 582-8820
First Published: 1952. Frequency: Bimonthly. ISSN: 0029-6562.

★1416★   NURSING SCIENCE QUARTERLY
Williams & Wilkins
428 E. Preston St.
Baltimore, MD 21202   Phone: (301) 528-4000
First Published: 1988. Frequency: Quarterly. ISSN: 0894-3184.

★1417★   NUTRITION AND CANCER
Lawrence Erlbaum Associates, Inc.
365 Broadway
Hillsdale, NJ 07642   Phone: (201) 666-4110
First Published: 1978. Frequency: Quarterly. ISSN: 0163-5581.

★1418★   NUTRITION IN CLINICAL PRACTICE
American Society for Parenteral and Enteral Nutrition
8630 Fenton St., No. 412
Silver Spring, MD 20910-3803
First Published: 1986. Frequency: Bimonthly. ISSN: 0884-5336.

★1419★   NUTRITION RESEARCH
Pergamon Press, Inc.
Maxwell House, Fairview Park
Elmsford, NY 10523   Phone: (914) 592-7700
First Published: 1981. Frequency: Monthly. ISSN: 0271-5317.

★1420★   NUTRITION REVIEWS
International Life Sciences Institute/Nutrition Foundation
1126 16th St., NW, No. 300
Washington, DC 20036   Phone: (202) 659-0074
First Published: 1942. Frequency: Monthly. ISSN: 0029-6643.

★1421★   NUTRITION TODAY
Williams & Wilkins
428 E. Preston St.
Baltimore, MD 21202   Phone: (301) 528-4223
First Published: 1966. Frequency: Bimonthly. ISSN: 0029-666X.

★1422★   OBESITY SURGERY
Rapid Communications of Oxford Ltd.
The Old Malthouse
Paradise St.
Oxford OX1 1LD, England
First Published: 1991. Frequency: Quarterly. ISSN: 0960-8923.

★1423★   OBSTETRICS AND GYNECOLOGY
American College of Obstetricians and Gynecologists
409 12th St., SW
Washington, DC 20024   Phone: (202) 638-5577
First Published: 1952. Frequency: 15/yr. ISSN: 0029-7844.

★1424★   OCCUPATIONAL HEALTH AND SAFETY
Stevens Publishing Corp.
Box 225 N. New Rd.
Waco, TX 76710
Frequency: 10/yr. ISSN: 0362-4064.

★1425★   OCCUPATIONAL THERAPY IN HEALTH CARE
The Haworth Press, Inc.
10 Alice St.
Binghampton, NY 13904   Phone: (800) 342-9678
First Published: 1984. Frequency: Quarterly.

★1426★   OCCUPATIONAL THERAPY IN MENTAL HEALTH
The Haworth Press, Inc.
10 Alice St.
Binghampton, NY 13904   Phone: (800) 342-9678
First Published: 1980. Frequency: Quarterly.

★1427★   OHIO STATE MEDICAL JOURNAL
Ohio State Medical Association
1500 Lakeshore Dr.
Columbus, OH 43204   Phone: (614) 228-6971
First Published: 1905. Frequency: Monthly. ISSN: 0030-1124.

★1428★   ONCOLOGY
S. Karger Publishers, Inc.
26 W. Avon Rd.
PO Box 529
Farmington, CT 06085   Phone: (203) 675-7834
First Published: 1948. Frequency: Bimonthly. ISSN: 0030-2414.

★1429★   OPERATIVE TECHNIQUES IN ORTHOPAEDICS
W.B. Saunders Co.
Curtis Center
Independence Sq., W.
Philadelphia, PA 19106   Phone: (215) 238-7800
Frequency: Quarterly.

★1430★   OPHTHALMIC AND PHYSIOLOGICAL OPTICS
Butterworth-Heinemann
80 Montvale Ave.
Stoneham, MA 02180   Phone: (617) 438-8464
First Published: 1980. Frequency: Quarterly. ISSN: 0275-5408.

★1431★   OPHTHALMIC RESEARCH
S. Karger Publishers, Inc.
26 W. Avon Rd.
PO Box 529
Farmington, CT 06085   Phone: (203) 675-7834
First Published: 1970. Frequency: Bimonthly. ISSN: 0030-3747.

★1432★ OPHTHALMIC SURGERY
Slack, Inc.
6900 Grove Rd.
Thorofare, NJ 08086   Phone: (609) 848-1000
First Published: 1968. Frequency: Monthly. ISSN: 0022-023X.

★1433★ OPHTHALMOLOGICA
S. Karger Publishers, Inc.
26 W. Avon Rd.
PO Box 529
Farmington, CT 06085   Phone: (203) 675-7834
First Published: 1899. Frequency: 8/yr. ISSN: 0030-3755.

★1434★ OPHTHALMOLOGY
American Academy of Ophthalmology
655 Beach St.
San Francisco, CA 94109   Phone: (415) 561-8500
First Published: 1978. Frequency: Monthly. ISSN: 0161-6420.

★1435★ OPTOMETRY CLINICS
Appleton & Lange
25 Van Zant St.
East Norwalk, CT 06855   Phone: (203) 838-4400
Frequency: Quarterly. ISSN: 1050-6918.

★1436★ OPTOMETRY AND VISION SCIENCE
American Academy of Optometry
5530 Wisconsin Ave., NW, Ste. 1149
Washington, DC 20815   Phone: (301) 652-0905
First Published: 1924. Frequency: Monthly. ISSN: 1040-5488.

★1437★ ORAL SURGERY, ORAL MEDICINE, ORAL PATHOLOGY
Mosby-Year Book, Inc.
11830 Westline Industrial Dr.
St. Louis, MO 63146   Phone: (314) 872-8370
First Published: 1948. Frequency: Monthly. ISSN: 0030-4220.

★1438★ ORL
S. Karger Publishers, Inc.
26 W. Avon Rd.
PO Box 529
Farmington, CT 06085   Phone: (203) 675-7834
First Published: 1938. Frequency: Bimonthly. ISSN: 0301-1569.

★1439★ ORTHOPAEDIC PHYSICAL THERAPY CLINICS
W.B. Saunders Co.
Curtis Center
Independence Sq., W.
Philadelphia, PA 19106   Phone: (215) 238-7800
First Published: 1992. Frequency: Quarterly.

★1440★ ORTHOPEDICS
Slack, Inc.
6900 Grove Rd.
Thorofare, NJ 08086   Phone: (609) 848-1000
First Published: 1978. Frequency: Monthly. ISSN: 0147-7447.

★1441★ OSTEOPATHIC ANNALS
Ronald Park Davis Publishing Co., Inc.
45 Whitney Rd.
Mahawah, NJ 07430
First Published: 1973. Frequency: Monthly. ISSN: 0092-9336.

★1442★ OSTEOPOROSIS INTERNATIONAL
Springer-Verlag New York, Inc.
175 5th Ave.
New York, NY 10010   Phone: (212) 460-1500
Frequency: Quarterly. ISSN: 0937-941X.

★1443★ OTOLARYNGOLOGY—HEAD AND NECK SURGERY
American Academy of Otolaryngology—Head and Neck Surgery
1 Prince St.
Alexandria, VA 22314   Phone: (703) 836-4444
First Published: 1896. Frequency: Monthly. ISSN: 0194-5998.

★1444★ PACE: PACING AND CLINICAL ELECTROPHYSIOLOGY
Futura Publishing Co.
2 Bedford Ridge Rd.
PO Box 330
Mt. Kisco, NY 10549   Phone: (800) 877-8761
First Published: 1978. Frequency: Monthly. ISSN: 0147-8389.

★1445★ PAEDIATRIC AND PERINATAL EPIDEMIOLOGY
Blackwell Scientific Publications
3 Cambridge Center, Ste. 208
Cambridge, MA 02142   Phone: (617) 225-0401
Frequency: Quarterly. ISSN: 0269-5022.

★1446★ PAIN
International Association for the Study of Pain
909 NE 43rd St., Ste. 306
Seattle, WA 98105   Phone: (206) 547-6409
First Published: 1975. Frequency: Monthly. ISSN: 0304-3959.

★1447★ PANCREAS
Raven Press
1185 Avenue of the Americas
New York, NY 10036   Phone: (212) 930-9500
First Published: 1986. Frequency: Bimonthly. ISSN: 0885-3177.

★1448★ PARAPLEGIA
Churchill Livingstone, Inc.
1560 Broadway
New York, NY 10036   Phone: (212) 819-5400
First Published: 1963. Frequency: 9/yr. ISSN: 0031-1758.

★1449★ PARASITE IMMUNOLOGY
Blackwell Scientific Publications
3 Cambridge Center, Ste. 208
Cambridge, MA 02142   Phone: (617) 225-0401
First Published: 1979. Frequency: Bimonthly. ISSN: 0141-9838.

★1450★ PARASITOLOGY
Cambridge University Press
40 W. 20th St.
New York, NY 10011   Phone: (212) 924-3900
First Published: 1908. Frequency: 6/yr. ISSN: 0031-1820.

★1451★ PATHOBIOLOGY
S. Karger Publishers, Inc.
26 W. Avon Rd.
PO Box 529
Farmington, CT 06085   Phone: (203) 675-7834
First Published: 1932. Frequency: Bimonthly. ISSN: 1015-2008.

★1452★ PATIENT CARE
Medical Economics Company, Inc.
690 Kinderkamack Rd.
Oradell, NJ 07649   Phone: (201) 262-3030
First Published: 1967. Frequency: 20/yr. ISSN: 0031-305X.

★1453★ PATIENT EDUCATION AND COUNSELING
Elsevier Science Publishing Co., Inc.
655 Avenue of the Americas
New York, NY 10010   Phone: (212) 989-5800
First Published: 1978. Frequency: Bimonthly. ISSN: 0738-3991.

★1454★ PAVLOVIAN JOURNAL OF BIOLOGICAL SCIENCE
J.B. Lippincott Co.
E. Washington Sq.
Philadelphia, PA 19105   Phone: (215) 238-4200
First Published: 1966. Frequency: Quarterly. ISSN: 0093-2213.

★1455★ PEDIATRIC ANNALS
Slack, Inc.
6900 Grove Rd.
Thorofare, NJ 08086   Phone: (609) 848-1000
First Published: 1972. Frequency: Monthly. ISSN: 0090-4481.

★1456★ **PEDIATRIC CARDIOLOGY**
Springer-Verlag New York, Inc.
175 5th Ave.
New York, NY 10010 Phone: (212) 460-1500
First Published: 1979. **Frequency:** Quarterly. **ISSN:** 0172-0643.

★1457★ **PEDIATRIC DERMATOLOGY**
Society for Pediatric Dermatology
c/o James E. Rasmussen, M.D.
University of Michigan Hospitals
1910 Taubman Health Care Center
Ann Arbor, MI 48109 Phone: (313) 936-4086
First Published: 1983. **Frequency:** Quarterly. **ISSN:** 0736-8046.

★1458★ **PEDIATRIC EMERGENCY CARE**
Williams & Wilkins
428 E. Preston St.
Baltimore, MD 21202 Phone: (301) 528-4000
First Published: 1985. **Frequency:** Quarterly. **ISSN:** 0749-5161.

★1459★ **PEDIATRIC HEMATOLOGY AND ONCOLOGY**
Hemisphere Publishing Corp.
1900 Frost Rd., Ste. 101
Bristol, PA 19007 Phone: (212) 785-5800
Frequency: Quarterly. **ISSN:** 0888-0018.

★1460★ **PEDIATRIC INFECTIOUS DISEASE JOURNAL**
Williams & Wilkins
428 E. Preston St.
Baltimore, MD 21202 Phone: (301) 528-4000
First Published: 1982. **Frequency:** Monthly. **ISSN:** 0891-3668.

★1461★ **PEDIATRIC NEPHROLOGY**
Springer-Verlag New York, Inc.
175 5th Ave.
New York, NY 10010 Phone: (212) 460-1500
First Published: 1987. **Frequency:** Bimonthly. **ISSN:** 0931-041X.

★1462★ **PEDIATRIC PATHOLOGY**
Hemisphere Publishing Corp.
1900 Frost Rd., Ste. 101
Bristol, PA 19007 Phone: (215) 785-5800
First Published: 1983. **Frequency:** Bimonthly. **ISSN:** 0277-0938.

★1463★ **PEDIATRIC PULMONOLOGY**
John Wiley & Sons, Inc.
605 3rd Ave.
New York, NY 10158 Phone: (212) 850-6000
First Published: 1985. **Frequency:** 8/yr. **ISSN:** 8755-6863.

★1464★ **PEDIATRIC RADIOLOGY**
Springer-Verlag New York, Inc.
175 5th Ave.
New York, NY 10010 Phone: (212) 460-1500
First Published: 1973. **Frequency:** 8/yr. **ISSN:** 0301-0449.

★1465★ **PEDIATRIC RESEARCH**
Williams & Wilkins
428 E. Preston St.
Baltimore, MD 21202 Phone: (301) 528-4000
First Published: 1967. **Frequency:** Monthly. **ISSN:** 0031-3998.

★1466★ **PEDIATRIC SURGERY INTERNATIONAL**
Springer-Verlag New York, Inc.
175 5th Ave.
New York, NY 10010 Phone: (212) 460-1500
Frequency: Bimonthly. **ISSN:** 0179-0358.

★1467★ **PEDIATRICIAN**
S. Karger Publishers, Inc.
26 W. Avon Rd.
PO Box 529
Farmington, CT 06085 Phone: (203) 675-7834
First Published: 1972. **Frequency:** Quarterly. **ISSN:** 0300-1245.

★1468★ **PEDIATRICS**
American Academy of Pediatrics
141 Northwest Point Blvd.
PO Box 927
Elk Grove Village, IL 60009 Phone: (708) 228-5005
First Published: 1948. **Frequency:** Monthly. **ISSN:** 0031-4005.

★1469★ **PENNSYLVANIA MEDICINE**
Pennsylvania Medical Society
Box 8820
Harrisburg, PA 17105 Phone: (717) 763-7151
First Published: 1897. **Frequency:** Monthly. **ISSN:** 0031-4595.

★1470★ **PEPTIDES**
Pergamon Press, Inc.
Maxwell House, Fairview Park
Elmsford, NY 10523 Phone: (914) 592-7700
First Published: 1980. **Frequency:** Bimonthly. **ISSN:** 0196-9781.

★1471★ **PERSPECTIVES IN BIOLOGY AND MEDICINE**
University of Chicago Press
5801 Ellis Ave.
Chicago, IL 60637 Phone: (312) 702-7700
First Published: 1957. **Frequency:** Quarterly. **ISSN:** 0031-5982.

★1472★ **PERSPECTIVES IN PSYCHIATRIC CARE**
Nursing Publications, Inc.
PO Box 218
Hillsdale, NJ 07642 Phone: (201) 391-7845
First Published: 1963. **Frequency:** Quarterly. **ISSN:** 0031-5990.

★1473★ **PFLUGERS ARCHIV: EUROPEAN JOURNAL OF PHYSIOLOGY**
Springer-Verlag New York, Inc.
175 5th Ave.
New York, NY 10010 Phone: (212) 460-1500
First Published: 1868. **Frequency:** Monthly. **ISSN:** 0031-6768.

★1474★ **PHARMACOEPIDEMIOLOGY AND DRUG SAFETY**
John Wiley & Sons, Inc.
605 3rd Ave.
New York, NY 10158 Phone: (617) 850-6000
First Published: 1992. **Frequency:** Bimonthly. **ISSN:** 1053-7569.

★1475★ **PHARMACOLOGICAL RESEARCH**
Academic Press, Inc.
1250 6th Ave.
San Diego, CA 92101 Phone: (619) 231-0926
First Published: 1969. **Frequency:** Bimonthly. **ISSN:** 0031-6989.

★1476★ **PHARMACOLOGY**
S. Karger Publishers, Inc.
26 W. Avon Rd.
PO Box 529
Farmington, CT 06085 Phone: (203) 675-7834
First Published: 1959. **Frequency:** Monthly. **ISSN:** 0031-7012.

★1477★ **PHARMACOLOGY, BIOCHEMISTRY AND BEHAVIOR**
Pergamon Press, Inc.
Maxwell House, Fairview Park
Elmsford, NY 10523 Phone: (914) 592-7700
First Published: 1973. **Frequency:** Monthly. **ISSN:** 0091-3057.

★1478★ **PHARMACOLOGY AND THERAPEUTICS**
Pergamon Press, Inc.
Maxwell House, Fairview Park
Elmsford, NY 10523 Phone: (914) 592-7700
First Published: 1975. **Frequency:** Monthly. **ISSN:** 0163-7258.

★1479★ **PHARMACOLOGY AND TOXICOLOGY**
Munksgaard
Noerre Soegade 35
DK-1370 Copenhagen K, Denmark
First Published: 1944. **Frequency:** 10/yr. **ISSN:** 0901-9928.

★1480★ PHARMACOTHERAPY
Pharmacotherapy Publications, Inc.
New England Medical Center
171 Harrison Ave.
PO Box 806
Boston, MA 02111   Phone: (617) 956-5390
First Published: 1981. **Frequency:** Bimonthly. **ISSN:** 0277-0008.

★1481★ PHOTOCHEMISTRY AND PHOTOBIOLOGY
American Society for Photobiology
8000 Westpark Dr., Ste. 130
McLean, VA 22102   Phone: (703) 790-1745
First Published: 1962. **Frequency:** Monthly. **ISSN:** 0031-8655.

★1482★ PHYSICAL MEDICINE AND REHABILITATION CLINICS
W.B. Saunders Co.
Curtis Center
Independence Sq., W.
Philadelphia, PA 19106   Phone: (215) 238-7800
Frequency: Quarterly.

★1483★ PHYSICAL AND OCCUPATIONAL THERAPY IN GERIATRICS
The Haworth Press, Inc.
10 Alice St.
Binghampton, NY 13904   Phone: (800) 342-9678
First Published: 1982. **Frequency:** Quarterly.

★1484★ PHYSICAL AND OCCUPATIONAL THERAPY IN PEDIATRICS
The Haworth Press, Inc.
10 Alice St.
Binghampton, NY 13904   Phone: (800) 342-9678
First Published: 1980. **Frequency:** Quarterly.

★1485★ PHYSICAL THERAPY
American Physical Therapy Association
1111 N. Fairfax St.
Alexandria, VA 22314   Phone: (703) 684-2782
First Published: 1921. **Frequency:** Monthly. **ISSN:** 0031-9023.

★1486★ PHYSICIAN ASSISTANT
American Academy of Physician Assistants
950 N. Washington St.
Alexandria, VA 22314   Phone: (703) 836-2272
First Published: 1976. **Frequency:** Monthly.

★1487★ THE PHYSICIAN AND SPORTSMEDICINE
McGraw-Hill Book Co.
1221 Avenue of the Americas
New York, NY 10020   Phone: (212) 512-2000
First Published: 1973. **Frequency:** Monthly. **ISSN:** 0091-3847.

★1488★ PHYSICIAN'S MANAGEMENT
Edgell Communications
7500 Old Oak Blvd.
Cleveland, OH 44130   Phone: (216) 243-8100
First Published: 1961. **Frequency:** Monthly. **ISSN:** 0031-9066.

★1489★ PHYSICS IN MEDICINE AND BIOLOGY
American Association of Physicists in Medicine
335 E. 45th St.
New York, NY 10017   Phone: (212) 661-9404
First Published: 1956. **Frequency:** Monthly. **ISSN:** 0031-9155.

★1490★ PHYSIOLOGIA BOHEMOSLOVACA
Academic Press, Inc.
1250 6th Ave.
San Diego, CA 92101   Phone: (619) 231-0926
First Published: 1952. **Frequency:** Bimonthly. **ISSN:** 0014-1291.

★1491★ PHYSIOLOGICAL CHEMISTRY AND PHYSICS AND MEDICAL NMR
Meridional Publications
7101 Winding Way
Wake Forest, NC 27587   Phone: (919) 556-2940
First Published: 1969. **Frequency:** Quarterly. **ISSN:** 0748-6642.

★1492★ PHYSIOLOGICAL RESEARCH
Academic Press, Inc.
1250 6th Ave.
San Diego, CA 92101   Phone: (619) 231-0926
Frequency: Bimonthly. **ISSN:** 0014-1291.

★1493★ PHYSIOLOGIST
American Physiological Society
9650 Rockville Pike
Bethesda, MD 20814   Phone: (301) 530-7164
First Published: 1958. **Frequency:** Bimonthly. **ISSN:** 0031-9376.

★1494★ PHYSIOLOGY AND BEHAVIOR
Pergamon Press, Inc.
Maxwell House, Fairview Park
Elmsford, NY 10523   Phone: (914) 592-7700
First Published: 1966. **Frequency:** Monthly. **ISSN:** 0031-9384.

★1495★ PHYSIOTHERAPY CANADA
Canadian Physiotherapy Association
890 Yonge St.
Toronto, ON, Canada M4W 3P4   Phone: (416) 924-5312
First Published: 1923. **Frequency:** Bimonthly. **ISSN:** 0300-0508.

★1496★ PIGMENT CELL RESEARCH
John Wiley & Sons, Inc.
605 3rd Ave.
New York, NY 10158   Phone: (212) 850-6000
First Published: 1987. **Frequency:** Bimonthly. **ISSN:** 0893-5785.

★1497★ PLACENTA
Bailliere Tindall
24-28 Oval Rd.
London MW1 7DX, England
First Published: 1980. **Frequency:** Bimonthly. **ISSN:** 0143-4004.

★1498★ PLASMID
Academic Press, Inc.
1250 6th Ave.
San Diego, CA 92101   Phone: (619) 231-0926
First Published: 1979. **Frequency:** 6/yr. **ISSN:** 0147-619X.

★1499★ PLASTIC AND RECONSTRUCTIVE SURGERY
American Society of Plastic & Reconstructive Surgeons
444 E. Algonquin Rd.
Arlington Heights, IL 60005   Phone: (708) 228-9900
First Published: 1946. **Frequency:** Monthly. **ISSN:** 0032-1052.

★1500★ PLATELETS
Churchill Livingstone, Inc.
1560 Broadway
New York, NY 10036   Phone: (212) 819-5400
Frequency: Quarterly. **ISSN:** 0953-7104.

★1501★ POSTGRADUATE MEDICAL JOURNAL
Macmillan Press, Ltd.
Houndmills
Basingstoke, Hants. RG21 2XS, England
First Published: 1924. **Frequency:** Monthly. **ISSN:** 0032-5473.

★1502★ POSTGRADUATE MEDICINE
McGraw-Hill Book Co.
1221 Avenue of the Americas
New York, NY 10020
First Published: 1947. **Frequency:** 16/yr. **ISSN:** 0032-5481.

★1503★ PRACTICAL CARDIOLOGY
Med Publishing, Inc.
Office Center at Princeton Meadows
Bldg. 1000
Plainsboro, NJ 08536   Phone: (609) 275-1900
First Published: 1975. Frequency: Monthly. ISSN: 0361-3372.

★1504★ PRACTITIONER
Morgan-Grampian, Ltd.
30 Calderwood St.
London SE18 6QH, England
First Published: 1868. Frequency: 20/yr. ISSN: 0032-6518.

★1505★ PRENATAL DIAGNOSIS
John Wiley & Sons, Inc.
605 3rd Ave.
New York, NY 10158   Phone: (212) 850-6000
First Published: 1981. Frequency: Monthly. ISSN: 0197-3851.

★1506★ PREPARATIVE BIOCHEMISTRY
Marcel Dekker, Inc.
270 Madison Ave.
New York, NY 10016   Phone: (212) 696-9000
First Published: 1971. Frequency: Quarterly. ISSN: 0032-7484.

★1507★ PREVENTIVE MEDICINE
American Health Foundation
320 E. 43rd St.
New York, NY 10017   Phone: (212) 953-1900
First Published: 1972. Frequency: Bimonthly. ISSN: 0091-7435.

★1508★ PRIMARY CARDIOLOGY
PW Communications, Inc.
400 Plaza Dr.
Secaucus, NJ 07094   Phone: (201) 865-7500
First Published: 1975. Frequency: Monthly. ISSN: 0363-5104.

★1509★ PRIVATE PRACTICE
Congress of County Medical Societies Publishing Co.
PO Box 1485
Shawnee, OK 74802
First Published: 1969. Frequency: Monthly. ISSN: 0032-891X.

★1510★ PROCEEDINGS OF THE NATIONAL ACADEMY OF
SCIENCES OF THE UNITED STATES OF AMERICA:
BIOLOGICAL SCIENCES
2101 Constitution Ave., NW
Washington, DC 20418   Phone: (202) 334-2000
First Published: 1915. Frequency: Semimonthly. ISSN: 0273-1134.

★1511★ PROCEEDINGS OF THE SOCIETY FOR
EXPERIMENTAL BIOLOGY AND MEDICINE
Society for Experimental Biology and Medicine
1300 New York Ave., Rm. A463A
New York, NY 10021
First Published: 1903. Frequency: 11/yr. ISSN: 0037-9727.

★1512★ PROFESSIONAL MEDICAL ASSISTANT
American Association of Medical Assistants
20 N. Wacker Dr., Ste. 1575
Chicago, IL 60606   Phone: (312) 889-1500
First Published: 1956. Frequency: Bimonthly. ISSN: 0033-0140.

★1513★ PROFESSIONAL PSYCHOLOGY RESEARCH AND
PRACTICE
American Psychological Association
1200 17th St., NW
Washington, DC 20036   Phone: (202) 955-7600
Frequency: Bimonthly.

★1514★ PROGRESS IN CARDIOVASCULAR DISEASES
W.B. Saunders Co.
Curtis Center
Independence Sq., W.
Philadelphia, PA 19106   Phone: (215) 238-7800
First Published: 1958. Frequency: Bimonthly. ISSN: 0033-0620.

★1515★ PROGRESS IN NEUROENDOCRINIMMUNOLOGY
Thieme Medical Publishers, Inc.
381 Park Ave., S., 4th Fl.
New York, NY 10016   Phone: (212) 683-5088
Frequency: Quarterly. ISSN: 1045-2001.

★1516★ PROSTAGLANDINS
Butterworth-Heinemann
80 Montvale Ave.
Stoneham, MA 02180   Phone: (617) 438-8464
First Published: 1972. Frequency: Monthly. ISSN: 0090-6980.

★1517★ PROSTAGLANDINS, LEUKOTRIENES AND
ESSENTIAL FATTY ACIDS
Churchill Livingstone, Inc.
1560 Broadway
New York, NY 10036   Phone: (212) 819-5400
First Published: 1978. Frequency: 15/yr. ISSN: 0952-3278.

★1518★ PROSTATE
John Wiley & Sons, Inc.
605 3rd Ave.
New York, NY 10158   Phone: (212) 850-6000
First Published: 1980. Frequency: 8/yr. ISSN: 0270-4137.

★1519★ PROTEINS: STRUCTURE, FUNCTION, AND
GENETICS
John Wiley & Sons, Inc.
605 3rd Ave.
New York, NY 10158   Phone: (212) 850-6000
First Published: 1987. Frequency: 8/yr. ISSN: 0887-3585.

★1520★ PROTOPLASMA
Springer-Verlag New York, Inc.
175 5th Ave.
New York, NY 10010   Phone: (212) 460-1500
First Published: 1926. Frequency: 18/yr. ISSN: 0033-183X.

★1521★ PROVIDER
American Health Care Association
1201 L St. NW
Washington, DC 20005   Phone: (202) 842-4444
First Published: 1975. Frequency: Monthly. ISSN: 0888-0352.

★1522★ PSYCHIATRIC NEWS
American Psychiatric Press, Inc.
1400 K St., NW
Washington, DC 20005   Phone: (202) 682-6240
First Published: 1966. Frequency: Biweekly. ISSN: 0033-2704.

★1523★ PSYCHIATRIC QUARTERLY
Human Sciences Press
233 Spring St.
New York, NY 10013   Phone: (212) 620-8000
First Published: 1927. Frequency: Quarterly. ISSN: 0033-2720.

★1524★ PSYCHIATRY
The Guilford Press
72 Spring St.
New York, NY 10012   Phone: (212) 431-9800
First Published: 1937. Frequency: Quarterly. ISSN: 0033-2747.

★1525★ PSYCHIATRY RESEARCH
Elsevier Science Publishing Co., Inc.
655 Avenue of the Americas
New York, NY 10010   Phone: (212) 989-5800
First Published: 1979. Frequency: Monthly. ISSN: 0165-1781.

★1526★ PSYCHOANALYSIS AND CONTEMPORARY
THOUGHT
International Universities Press, Inc.
59 Boston Post Rd.
PO Box 1524
Madison, CT 06443   Phone: (203) 245-4000
Frequency: Quarterly.

★1527★ PSYCHOANALYTIC QUARTERLY
Psychoanalytic Quarterly, Inc.
175 5th Ave., Rm. 210
New York, NY 10010   Phone: (212) 982-9358
First Published: 1932. **Frequency:** Quarterly. **ISSN:** 0033-2828.

★1528★ PSYCHOANALYTIC REVIEW
National Psychological Association for Psychoanalysis
150 W. 13th St.
New York, NY 10011   Phone: (212) 924-7440
First Published: 1913. **Frequency:** Quarterly. **ISSN:** 0033-2836.

★1529★ PSYCHOLOGICAL ASSESSMENT
American Psychological Association
1200 17th St., NW
Washington, DC 20036   Phone: (202) 955-7600
Frequency: Quarterly. **ISSN:** 1040-3590.

★1530★ PSYCHOLOGICAL BULLETIN
American Psychological Association
1200 17th St., NW
Washington, DC 20036   Phone: (202) 955-7600
First Published: 1904. **Frequency:** Bimonthly. **ISSN:** 0033-2909.

★1531★ PSYCHOLOGICAL MEDICINE
Cambridge University Press
40 W. 20th St.
New York, NY 10011   Phone: (212) 924-3900
First Published: 1970. **Frequency:** Quarterly. **ISSN:** 0033-2917.

★1532★ PSYCHOLOGICAL RESEARCH
Springer-Verlag New York, Inc.
175 5th Ave.
New York, NY 10010   Phone: (212) 460-1500
First Published: 1921. **Frequency:** Quarterly. **ISSN:** 0340-0727.

★1533★ PSYCHOLOGY AND AGING
American Psychological Association
1200 17th St., NW
Washington, DC 20036   Phone: (202) 955-7600
Frequency: Quarterly. **ISSN:** 0082-7974.

★1534★ PSYCHOLOGY OF WOMEN QUARTERLY
Cambridge University Press
40 W. 20th St.
New York, NY 10011   Phone: (212) 924-3900
Frequency: Quarterly. **ISSN:** 0361-6843.

★1535★ PSYCHONEUROENDOCRINOLOGY
Pergamon Press, Inc.
Maxwell House, Fairview Park
Elmsford, NY 10523   Phone: (914) 592-7700
First Published: 1976. **Frequency:** 6/yr. **ISSN:** 0306-4530.

★1536★ PSYCHO-ONCOLOGY
John Wiley & Sons, Inc.
605 3rd Ave.
New York, NY 10158   Phone: (617) 850-6000
First Published: 1992. **Frequency:** Quarterly. **ISSN:** 1057-9249.

★1537★ PSYCHOPATHOLOGY
S. Karger Publishers, Inc.
26 W. Avon Rd.
PO Box 529
Farmington, CT 06085   Phone: (203) 675-7834
First Published: 1968. **Frequency:** Bimonthly. **ISSN:** 0254-4962.

★1538★ PSYCHOPHARMACOLOGY
Springer-Verlag New York, Inc.
175 5th Ave.
New York, NY 10010   Phone: (212) 460-1500
First Published: 1959. **Frequency:** Monthly. **ISSN:** 0033-3158.

★1539★ PSYCHOPHARMACOLOGY BULLETIN
U.S. Public Health Service
Alcohol, Drug Abuse & Mental Health Administration
5600 Fishers Ln.
Rockville, MD 20852   Phone: (301) 496-4000
First Published: 1959. **Frequency:** Quarterly. **ISSN:** 0048-5764.

★1540★ PSYCHOPHYSIOLOGY
Society for Psychophysiological Research
J. Gatchel
Universtiy of Texas Southwestern Med Center
5323 Henry Hines Blvd.
Dallas, TX 75235   Phone: (214) 688-2031
First Published: 1964. **Frequency:** Bimonthly. **ISSN:** 0048-5772.

★1541★ PSYCHOSOCIAL REHABILITATION JOURNAL
IAPSRS/Boston University
730 Commonwealth Ave.
Boston, MA 02215   Phone: (617) 353-3549
Frequency: Quarterly.

★1542★ PSYCHOSOMATIC MEDICINE
American Psychosomatic Society
6728 Old McLean Village Dr.
McLean, VA 22101   Phone: (703) 556-9222
First Published: 1939. **Frequency:** Bimonthly. **ISSN:** 0033-3174.

★1543★ PSYCHOSOMATICS
Academy of Psychosomatic Medicine
5824 N. Magnolia
Chicago, IL 60660   Phone: (312) 784-2025
First Published: 1960. **Frequency:** Quarterly. **ISSN:** 0033-3182.

★1544★ PSYCHOTHERAPY AND PSYCHOSOMATICS
S. Karger Publishers, Inc.
26 W. Avon Rd.
PO Box 529
Farmington, CT 06085   Phone: (203) 675-7834
First Published: 1953. **Frequency:** 8/yr. **ISSN:** 0033-3190.

★1545★ PUBLIC HEALTH
Macmillan Press, Ltd.
Houndmills
Basingstoke, Hants. RG21 2XS, England
First Published: 1888. **Frequency:** Bimonthly. **ISSN:** 0033-3506.

★1546★ PUBLIC HEALTH NURSING
Blackwell Scientific Publications
3 Cambridge Center, Ste. 208
Cambridge, MA 02142   Phone: (617) 225-0401
Frequency: Quarterly. **ISSN:** 0737-1209.

★1547★ PUBLIC HEALTH REPORTS
U.S. Public Health Service
5600 Fishers Ln., Rm. 13C-26
Rockville, MD 20857   Phone: (301) 443-0762
First Published: 1878. **Frequency:** Bimonthly. **ISSN:** 0090-2818.

★1548★ PULMONARY PHARMACOLOGY
Churchill Livingstone, Inc.
1560 Broadway
New York, NY 10036   Phone: (212) 819-5400
Frequency: Quarterly. **ISSN:** 0952-0600.

★1549★ QUALITY ASSURANCE AND UTILIZATION REVIEW
American College of Utilization Review Physicians
1531 Tamiami Trail, Ste. 703
Venice, FL 34292   Phone: (813) 497-3340
First Published: 1986. **Frequency:** Quarterly. **ISSN:** 0885-713X.

★1550★ THE QUARTERLY JOURNAL OF EXPERIMENTAL PSYCHOLOGY
Lawrence Erlbaum Associates, Inc.
365 Broadway
Hillsdale, NJ 07642   Phone: (201) 666-4110
Frequency: Quarterly.

★1551★ QUARTERLY JOURNAL OF MEDICINE
Oxford University Press
200 Madison Ave.
New York, NY 10016   Phone: (212) 679-7300
First Published: 1907. **Frequency:** Monthly. **ISSN:** 0033-5622.

★1552★ RADIATION AND ENVIRONMENTAL BIOPHYSICS
Springer-Verlag New York, Inc.
175 5th Ave.
New York, NY 10010   Phone: (212) 460-1500
First Published: 1963. **Frequency:** Quarterly. **ISSN:** 0301-634X.

★1553★ RADIATION RESEARCH
Academic Press, Inc.
1250 6th Ave.
San Diego, CA 92101   Phone: (619) 231-0926
First Published: 1954. **Frequency:** Monthly. **ISSN:** 0033-7587.

★1554★ RADIOGRAPHY
College of Radiographers
14 Upper Wimpole St.
London W1M 8BN, England
First Published: 1935. **Frequency:** Bimonthly. **ISSN:** 0033-8281.

★1555★ RADIOLOGIC TECHNOLOGY
American Society of Radiologic Technologists
15000 Central Ave., SE
Albuquerque, NM 87123   Phone: (505) 298-4500
First Published: 1929. **Frequency:** Bimonthly. **ISSN:** 0033-8397.

★1556★ RADIOLOGY
Radiological Society of North America
1415 W. 22nd St., Tower B
Oak Brook, IL 60521   Phone: (708) 571-2670
First Published: 1915. **Frequency:** Monthly. **ISSN:** 0033-8419.

★1557★ RADIOTHERAPY AND ONCOLOGY
Elsevier Science Publishing Co., Inc.
655 Avenue of the Americas
New York, NY 10010   Phone: (212) 989-5800
Frequency: Monthly. **ISSN:** 0167-8140.

★1558★ RECOMBINANT DNA TECHNICAL BULLETIN
U.S. Department of Health and Human Services
National Institutes of Health
Bldg. 31, Rm. B1C34
Bethesda, MD 20892   Phone: (301) 496-9838
First Published: 1977. **Frequency:** Quarterly. **ISSN:** 0196-0229.

★1559★ RECONSTRUCTION SURGERY AND
  TRAUMATOLOGY
S. Karger Publishers, Inc.
26 W. Avon Rd.
PO Box 529
Farmington, CT 06085   Phone: (203) 675-7834
First Published: 1953. **Frequency:** Irregular. **ISSN:** 0080-0260.

★1560★ REGULATORY PEPTIDES
Elsevier Science Publishing Co., Inc.
655 Avenue of the Americas
New York, NY 10010   Phone: (212) 989-5800
First Published: 1980. **Frequency:** 15/yr. **ISSN:** 0167-0115.

★1561★ REGULATORY TOXICOLOGY AND PHARMACOLOGY
Academic Press, Inc.
1250 6th Ave.
San Diego, CA 92101   Phone: (619) 231-0926
First Published: 1981. **Frequency:** Quarterly. **ISSN:** 0273-2300.

★1562★ RENAL FAILURE
Marcel Dekker, Inc.
270 Madison Ave.
New York, NY 10016   Phone: (212) 696-9000
First Published: 1977. **Frequency:** Quarterly. **ISSN:** 0886-022X.

★1563★ RENAL PHYSIOLOGY
S. Karger Publishers, Inc.
26 W. Avon Rd.
PO Box 529
Farmington, CT 06085   Phone: (203) 675-7834
First Published: 1979. **Frequency:** Bimonthly. **ISSN:** 0378-5858.

★1564★ THE REPORTER ON UROLOGIC TECHNIQUES
Churchill Livingstone, Inc.
1560 Broadway
New York, NY 10036   Phone: (212) 819-5400
First Published: 1991. **Frequency:** 10/yr. **ISSN:** 1052-3987.

★1565★ REPRODUCTION, FERTILITY AND DEVELOPMENT
314 Albert St.
East Melbourne, Victoria 3002, Australia
First Published: 1948. **Frequency:** Quarterly. **ISSN:** 1031-3613.

★1566★ RESEARCH ON AGING
Sage Publications, Inc.
2111 W. Hillcrest Dr.
Newbury Park, CA 91320   Phone: (805) 499-0721
First Published: 1979. **Frequency:** Quarterly. **ISSN:** 0164-0275.

★1567★ RESEARCH COMMUNICATIONS IN CHEMICAL
  PATHOLOGY AND PHARMACOLOGY
PJD Publications, Ltd.
PO Box 966
Westbury, NY 11590   Phone: (516) 626-0650
First Published: 1970. **Frequency:** Monthly. **ISSN:** 0034-5164.

★1568★ RESEARCH IN DEVELOPMENTAL DISABILITIES
Pergamon Press, Inc.
Maxwell House, Fairview Park
Elmsford, NY 10523   Phone: (914) 592-7700
First Published: 1981. **Frequency:** Quarterly. **ISSN:** 0891-4222.

★1569★ RESEARCH IN EXPERIMENTAL MEDICINE
Springer-Verlag New York, Inc.
175 5th Ave.
New York, NY 10010   Phone: (212) 460-1500
First Published: 1971. **Frequency:** Bimonthly. **ISSN:** 0300-9130.

★1570★ RESEARCH IN MICROBIOLOGY
Elsevier Science Publishing Co., Inc.
655 Avenue of the Americas
New York, NY 10010   Phone: (212) 989-5800
First Published: 1886. **Frequency:** 9/yr.

★1571★ RESEARCH IN NURSING AND HEALTH
John Wiley & Sons, Inc.
605 3rd Ave.
New York, NY 10158   Phone: (212) 850-6000
First Published: 1978. **Frequency:** Bimonthly. **ISSN:** 0160-6891.

★1572★ RESEARCH IN VETERINARY SCIENCE
British Veterinary Association
7 Mansfield St.
London W1M 0AT, England
First Published: 1960. **Frequency:** Bimonthly. **ISSN:** 0034-5288.

★1573★ RESIDENT AND STAFF PHYSICIAN
Romaine Pierson Publishers, Inc.
80 Shore Rd.
Port Washington, NY 11050   Phone: (516) 883-6350
First Published: 1955. **Frequency:** Monthly. **ISSN:** 0034-5555.

★1574★ RESPIRATION
S. Karger Publishers, Inc.
26 W. Avon Rd.
PO Box 529
Farmington, CT 06085   Phone: (203) 675-7834
First Published: 1944. **Frequency:** Bimonthly. **ISSN:** 0025-7931.

★1575★   RESPIRATION PHYSIOLOGY
Elsevier Science Publishing Co., Inc.
655 Avenue of the Americas
New York, NY 10010   Phone: (212) 989-5800
First Published: 1965. **Frequency:** Monthly. **ISSN:** 0034-5687.

★1576★   RESPIRATORY MANAGEMENT
Choices Publishing Group
129 Washington St.
Hoboken, NJ 07030   Phone: (201) 792-1900
First Published: 1971. **Frequency:** Bimonthly. **ISSN:** 0892-9289.

★1577★   RESPIRATORY MEDICINE
Bailliere Tindall
24-28 Oval Rd.
London NW1 79X, England
First Published: 1907. **Frequency:** Quarterly. **ISSN:** 0007-0971.

★1578★   RESUSCITATION
Elsevier Science Publishing Co., Inc.
655 Avenue of the Americas
New York, NY 10010   Phone: (212) 989-5800
First Published: 1972. **Frequency:** Quarterly. **ISSN:** 0300-9572.

★1579★   RETINA
J.B. Lippincott Co.
E. Washington Sq.
Philadelphia, PA 19105   Phone: (215) 238-4200
First Published: 1981. **Frequency:** Quarterly. **ISSN:** 0275-004X.

★1580★   REVIEW OF SCIENTIFIC INSTRUMENTS
American Institute of Physics
355 E. 45th St.
New York, NY 10017   Phone: (212) 661-9404
First Published: 1930. **Frequency:** Monthly. **ISSN:** 0034-6748.

★1581★   RHEUMATOLOGY INTERNATIONAL
Springer-Verlag New York, Inc.
175 5th Ave.
New York, NY 10010   Phone: (212) 460-1500
First Published: 1981. **Frequency:** Bimonthly. **ISSN:** 0172-8172.

★1582★   RHINOLOGY JOURNAL
c/o Dept of O.R.L.
University Hospital Utrecht
Postbus 85500
3508 GA Utrecht, Netherlands
First Published: 1963. **Frequency:** Quarterly. **ISSN:** 0300-0729.

★1583★   RHODE ISLAND MEDICAL JOURNAL
Rhode Island Medical Society
106 Francis St.
Providence, RI 02903   Phone: (401) 331-3207
First Published: 1917. **Frequency:** Monthly. **ISSN:** 0363-7913.

★1584★   ROUX'S ARCHIVES OF DEVELOPMENTAL BIOLOGY
Springer-Verlag New York, Inc.
175 5th Ave.
New York, NY 10010   Phone: (212) 460-1500
First Published: 1894. **Frequency:** 8/yr. **ISSN:** 0930-035X.

★1585★   SCANDINAVIAN AUDIOLOGY
Almqvist & Wiksell Periodical Co.
Box 638
S-101 28 Stockholm, Sweden
First Published: 1952. **Frequency:** Quarterly. **ISSN:** 0105-0397.

★1586★   SCANDINAVIAN JOURNAL OF CLINICAL AND LABORATORY INVESTIGATION
Blackwell Scientific Publications
3 Cambridge Center, Ste. 208
Cambridge, MA 02142   Phone: (617) 225-0401
First Published: 1949. **Frequency:** 8/yr. **ISSN:** 0036-5513.

★1587★   SCANDINAVIAN JOURNAL OF DENTAL RESEARCH
Munksgaard
Noerre Soegade 35
DK-1370 Copenhagen K, Denmark
First Published: 1893. **Frequency:** Bimonthly. **ISSN:** 0029-845X.

★1588★   SCANDINAVIAN JOURNAL OF GASTROENTEROLOGY
200 Meacham Ave.
Elmont, NY 11003
First Published: 1966. **Frequency:** Monthly. **ISSN:** 0036-5521.

★1589★   SCANDINAVIAN JOURNAL OF IMMUNOLOGY
Blackwell Scientific Publications
3 Cambridge Center, Ste. 208
Cambridge, MA 02142   Phone: (617) 225-0401
First Published: 1972. **Frequency:** Monthly. **ISSN:** 0300-9475.

★1590★   SCANDINAVIAN JOURNAL OF INFECTIOUS DISEASES
Almqvist & Wiksell Periodical Co.
Box 638
S-101 28 Stockholm, Sweden
First Published: 1969. **Frequency:** Bimonthly. **ISSN:** 0036-5548.

★1591★   SCANDINAVIAN JOURNAL OF PLASTIC AND RECONSTRUCTIVE SURGERY AND HAND SURGERY
Almqvist & Wiksell Periodical Co.
Box 638
S-101 28 Stockholm, Sweden
First Published: 1967. **Frequency:** Quarterly. **ISSN:** 0036-5556.

★1592★   SCANDINAVIAN JOURNAL OF REHABILITATION MEDICINE
Almqvist & Wiksell Periodical Co.
Box 638
S-101 28 Stockholm, Sweden
First Published: 1969. **Frequency:** Quarterly. **ISSN:** 0036-5505.

★1593★   SCANDINAVIAN JOURNAL OF RHEUMATOLOGY
Almqvist & Wiksell Periodical Co.
Box 638
S-101 28 Stockholm, Sweden
Frequency: Bimonthly. **ISSN:** 0300-9742.

★1594★   SCANDINAVIAN JOURNAL OF SOCIAL MEDICINE
Almqvist & Wiksell Periodical Co.
Box 638
S-101 28 Stockholm, Sweden
First Published: 1973. **Frequency:** Quarterly. **ISSN:** 0300-8037.

★1595★   SCANDINAVIAN JOURNAL OF THORACIC AND CARDIOVASCULAR SURGERY
Almqvist & Wiksell Periodical Co.
Box 638
S-101 28 Stockholm, Sweden
First Published: 1967. **Frequency:** 3/yr. **ISSN:** 0036-5580.

★1596★   SCANDINAVIAN JOURNAL OF UROLOGY AND NEPHROLOGY
Almqvist & Wiksell Periodical Co.
Box 638
S-101 28 Stockholm, Sweden
First Published: 1967. **Frequency:** Quarterly. **ISSN:** 0036-5599.

★1597★   SCANDINAVIAN JOURNAL OF WORK, ENVIRONMENT AND HEALTH
Finnish Institute of Occupational Health
Topeliuksenkatu 41
SF-00250 Helsinki, Finland
First Published: 1975. **Frequency:** Bimonthly. **ISSN:** 0355-3140.

★1598★   SCANNING MICROSCOPY
PO Box 66507
AMF O'Hare, IL 60666   Phone: (312) 529-6677
First Published: 1987. **Frequency:** Quarterly.

★1599★   SCHIZOPHRENIA BULLETIN
U.S. Public Health Service
Alcohol, Drug Abuse and Mental Health Administration
Center for Studies of Schizophrenia
5600 Fishers Ln.
Rockville, MD 20857   Phone: (301) 496-4000
First Published: 1969. Frequency: Quarterly. ISSN: 0586-7614.

★1600★   SCIENCE
American Association for the Advancement of Science
1333 H St., NW
Washington, DC 20005   Phone: (202) 326-6400
First Published: 1880. Frequency: Weekly. ISSN: 0036-8075.

★1601★   TRENDS IN CARDIOVASCULAR MEDICINE
Elsevier Science Publishing Co., Inc.
655 Avenue of the Americas
New York, NY 10010   Phone: (212) 989-5800
Frequency: Bimonthly. ISSN: 1050-1738.

★1602★   TRENDS IN ENDOCRINOLOGY AND METABOLISM
Elsevier Science Publishing Co., Inc.
655 Avenue of the Americas
New York, NY 10010   Phone: (212) 989-5800
Frequency: 10/yr. ISSN: 1043-2760.

★1603★   SCIENTIFIC AMERICAN
Scientific American Books
41 Madison Ave.
New York, NY 10010   Phone: (212) 576-9400
First Published: 1845. Frequency: Monthly. ISSN: 0036-8733.

★1604★   SCOTTISH MEDICAL JOURNAL
Scottish Academic Press
33 Montgomery St.
Edinburgh EH7 5JX, Scotland
First Published: 1956. Frequency: Bimonthly. ISSN: 0036-9330.

★1605★   SECOND MESSENGERS AND PHOSPHOPROTEINS
Marcel Dekker Journals
270 Madison Ave.
New York, NY 10016   Phone: (212) 696-9000
First Published: 1975. Frequency: Bimonthly. ISSN: 0895-7479.

★1606★   SELECTIVE CANCER THERAPEUTICS
Mary Ann Liebert, Inc.
1651 3rd Ave.
New York, NY 10128   Phone: (212) 289-2300
First Published: 1983. Frequency: Quarterly. ISSN: 1043-0733.

★1607★   SERODIAGNOSIS AND IMMUNOTHERAPY IN
  INFECTIOUS DISEASE
Academic Press, Inc.
1250 6th Ave.
San Diego, CA 92101   Phone: (619) 231-0926
First Published: 1986. Frequency: Bimonthly. ISSN: 0888-0786.

★1608★   SEXUALITY AND DISABILITY
Human Sciences Press, Inc.
233 Spring St.
New York, NY 10013   Phone: (212) 620-8000
Frequency: Quarterly.

★1609★   SEXUALLY TRANSMITTED DISEASES
American Venereal Disease Association
PO Box 1753
Baltimore, MD 21203   Phone: (301) 955-3150
First Published: 1974. Frequency: Quarterly. ISSN: 0148-5717.

★1610★   SKELETAL RADIOLOGY
Springer-Verlag New York, Inc.
175 5th Ave.
New York, NY 10010   Phone: (212) 460-1500
First Published: 1976. Frequency: 8/yr. ISSN: 0364-2348.

★1611★   SKIN PHARMACOLOGY
S. Karger Publishers, Inc.
26 W. Avon Rd.
PO Box 529
Farmington, CT 06085   Phone: (203) 675-7834
First Published: 1988. Frequency: Quarterly. ISSN: 1011-0283.

★1612★   SKULL BASE SURGERY
Thieme Medical Publishers, Inc.
381 Park Ave., S., 4th Fl.
New York, NY 10016   Phone: (212) 683-5088
First Published: 1991. Frequency: Quarterly. ISSN: 1052-1453.

★1613★   SLEEP
Raven Press
1185 Avenue of the Americas
New York, NY 10036   Phone: (212) 930-9500
First Published: 1978. Frequency: Bimonthly. ISSN: 0161-8105.

★1614★   SMALL ANIMAL PRACTICE
Williams & Wilkins
428 E. Preston St.
Baltimore, MD 21202   Phone: (301) 528-4000
Frequency: Monthly. ISSN: 0894-3710.

★1615★   SOCIAL BIOLOGY
Society for the Study of Social Biology
c/o Valeda Slade
Population Council
One Dag Hammarskjold Plaza, 44th Fl.
New York, NY 10017   Phone: (212) 644-1614
First Published: 1954. Frequency: Quarterly. ISSN: 0037-766X.

★1616★   SOCIAL PSYCHIATRY AND PSYCHIATRIC
  EPIDEMIOLOGY
Springer-Verlag New York, Inc.
175 5th Ave.
New York, NY 10010   Phone: (212) 460-1500
First Published: 1966. Frequency: Bimonthly. ISSN: 0933-7954.

★1617★   SOCIAL SCIENCE AND MEDICINE
Pergamon Press, Inc.
Maxwell House, Fairview Park
Elmsford, NY 10523   Phone: (914) 592-7700
First Published: 1978. Frequency: 24/yr. ISSN: 0277-9536.

★1618★   SOCIAL WORK IN HEALTH CARE
The Haworth Press, Inc.
10 Alice St.
Binghamton, NY 13904   Phone: (800) 342-9678
First Published: 1975. Frequency: Quarterly. ISSN: 0098-1389.

★1619★   SOMATIC CELL AND MOLECULAR GENETICS
Plenum Publishing Corp.
233 Spring St.
New York, NY 10013   Phone: (212) 620-8000
First Published: 1975. Frequency: Bimonthly. ISSN: 0740-7750.

★1620★   SOMATOSENSORY AND MOTOR RESEARCH
The Guilford Press
72 Spring St.
New York, NY 10012   Phone: (212) 431-9800
First Published: 1983. Frequency: Quarterly. ISSN: 0889-0220.

★1621★   SOUTH AFRICAN JOURNAL OF SURGERY
Association of Surgeons of South Africa
Private Bag X1
Pinelands 7430, Republic of South Africa
First Published: 1963. Frequency: Quarterly. ISSN: 0038-2361.

★1622★   SOUTH DAKOTA JOURNAL OF MEDICINE
South Dakota State Medical Association
1323 S. Minnesota Ave.
Sioux Falls, SD 57105   Phone: (605) 336-1965
First Published: 1946. Frequency: Monthly. ISSN: 0038-3317.

★1623★   SOUTHEAST ASIAN JOURNAL OF TROPICAL
  MEDICINE AND PUBLIC HEALTH
Regional Tropical Medicine & Public Health Project
420-6 Rajvithi Rd.
Bangkok 10400, Thailand
First Published: 1970. **Frequency:** Quarterly. **ISSN:** 0038-3619.

★1624★   SOUTHERN MEDICAL JOURNAL
Southern Medical Association
35 Lakeshore Dr.
Box 190088
Birmingham, AL 35219   Phone: (205) 945-1840
First Published: 1906. **Frequency:** Monthly. **ISSN:** 0038-4348.

★1625★   THE SOVIET JOURNAL OF PSYCHOLOGY
International Universities Press, Inc.
59 Boston Post Rd.
PO Box 1524
Madison, CT 06443   Phone: (203) 245-4000
Frequency: Bimonthly.

★1626★   SPINAL NETWORK EXTRA
Spinal Network
PO Box 4162
Boulder, CO 80306   Phone: (800) 338-5412
Frequency: Quarterly.

★1627★   SPINE
J.B. Lippincott Co.
E. Washington Sq.
Philadelphia, PA 19105   Phone: (215) 238-4200
First Published: 1976. **Frequency:** 11/yr. **ISSN:** 0362-2436.

★1628★   STAIN TECHNOLOGY
Biological Stain Commission
Box 626
Rochester, NY 14642   Phone: (716) 275-3197
First Published: 1926. **Frequency:** Bimonthly. **ISSN:** 0038-9153.

★1629★   STATISTICS IN MEDICINE
John Wiley & Sons, Inc.
605 3rd Ave.
New York, NY 10158   Phone: (212) 850-6000
Frequency: Monthly. **ISSN:** 0277-6715.

★1630★   STEREOTACTIC AND FUNCTIONAL
  NEUROSURGERY
S. Karger Publishers, Inc.
26 W. Avon Rd.
PO Box 529
Farmington, CT 06085   Phone: (203) 675-7834
First Published: 1938. **Frequency:** 8/yr. **ISSN:** 1011-6125.

★1631★   STEROIDS
Butterworth-Heinemann
80 Montvale Ave.
Stoneham, MA 02180   Phone: (617) 438-8464
Frequency: Monthly. **ISSN:** 0039-128X.

★1632★   STRESS MEDICINE
John Wiley & Sons, Inc.
605 3rd Ave.
New York, NY 10158   Phone: (212) 850-6000
First Published: 1985. **Frequency:** Bimonthly. **ISSN:** 0748-8386.

★1633★   STROKE—A JOURNAL OF CEREBRAL CIRCULATION
American Heart Association, Inc.
7320 Greenville Ave.
Dallas, TX 75231   Phone: (214) 706-1310
First Published: 1970. **Frequency:** Monthly. **ISSN:** 0039-2499.

★1634★   STUDIES IN FAMILY PLANNING
Population Council
1 Dag Hammarskjold Plaza
New York, NY 10017   Phone: (212) 644-1300
First Published: 1963. **Frequency:** Bimonthly. **ISSN:** 0039-3665.

★1635★   SUICIDE AND LIFE-THREATENING BEHAVIOR
American Association of Suicidology
2459 S. Ash
Denver, CO 80222   Phone: (303) 692-0985
First Published: 1970. **Frequency:** Quarterly. **ISSN:** 0363-0234.

★1636★   SURGERY
Mosby-Year Book, Inc.
11830 Westline Industrial Dr.
St. Louis, MO 63146   Phone: (314) 872-8370
First Published: 1937. **Frequency:** Monthly. **ISSN:** 0039-6060.

★1637★   SURGERY, GYNECOLOGY AND OBSTETRICS
Franklin H. Martin Memorial Foundation
54 E. Erie St.
Chicago, IL 60611   Phone: (312) 787-9282
First Published: 1905. **Frequency:** Monthly. **ISSN:** 0039-6087.

★1638★   SURGICAL ENDOSCOPY
Springer-Verlag New York, Inc.
175 5th Ave.
New York, NY 10010   Phone: (212) 460-1500
First Published: 1987. **Frequency:** Quarterly. **ISSN:** 0930-2794.

★1639★   SURGICAL LAPAROSCOPY AND ENDOSCOPY
Raven Press
1185 Avenue of the Americas
New York, NY 10036   Phone: (212) 930-9500
First Published: 1992. **Frequency:** Quarterly. **ISSN:** 1051-7200.

★1640★   SURGICAL NEUROLOGY
Elsevier Science Publishing Co., Inc.
655 Avenue of the Americas
New York, NY 10010   Phone: (212) 989-5800
First Published: 1973. **Frequency:** Monthly. **ISSN:** 0090-3019.

★1641★   SURGICAL ONCOLOGY
Blackwell Scientific Publications
3 Cambridge Center, Ste. 208
Cambridge, MA 02142   Phone: (617) 225-0401
First Published: 1992. **Frequency:** Bimonthly. **ISSN:** 0960-7404.

★1642★   SURGICAL ONCOLOGY CLINICS
W.B. Saunders Co.
Curtis Center
Independence Sq., W.
Philadelphia, PA 19106   Phone: (215) 238-7800
First Published: 1992. **Frequency:** Quarterly.

★1643★   SURGICAL AND RADIOLOGIC ANATOMY
Springer-Verlag New York, Inc.
175 5th Ave.
New York, NY 10010   Phone: (212) 460-1500
First Published: 1978. **Frequency:** Quarterly. **ISSN:** 0930-312X.

★1644★   SURGICAL TECHNOLOGIST
Association of Surgical Technologists, Inc.
8307 Shaffer Pkwy.
Littleton, CO 80127   Phone: (303) 978-9010
First Published: 1972. **Frequency:** Bimonthly. **ISSN:** 0164-4238.

★1645★   SYNAPSE
John Wiley & Sons, Inc.
605 3rd Ave.
New York, NY 10158   Phone: (212) 850-6000
First Published: 1987. **Frequency:** Bimonthly. **ISSN:** 0885-8276.

★1646★   TEACHING AND LEARNING MEDICINE
Lawrence Erlbaum Associates, Inc.
365 Broadway
Hillsdale, NJ 07642   Phone: (201) 666-4110
Frequency: Quarterly.

★1647★ TECHNIQUES IN ORTHOPAEDICS
Aspen Publishers, Inc.
200 Orchard Ridge Dr.
Gaithersburg, MD 20878   Phone: (301) 417-7500
First Published: 1986. Frequency: Quarterly.

★1648★ TERATOGENESIS, CARCINOGENESIS, AND
  MUTAGENESIS
John Wiley & Sons, Inc.
605 3rd Ave.
New York, NY 10158   Phone: (212) 850-6000
First Published: 1980. Frequency: Bimonthly. ISSN: 0270-3211.

★1649★ TERATOLOGY
Teratology Society
9660 Rockville Pike
Bethesda, MD 20814   Phone: (301) 571-1841
First Published: 1968. Frequency: Monthly. ISSN: 0040-3709.

★1650★ TEXAS MEDICINE
Texas Medical Association
1801 N. Lamar Blvd.
Austin, TX 78701   Phone: (512) 477-6704
First Published: 1905. Frequency: Monthly. ISSN: 0040-4470.

★1651★ THEORETICAL AND APPLIED GENETICS
Springer-Verlag New York, Inc.
175 5th Ave.
New York, NY 10010   Phone: (212) 460-1500
First Published: 1929. Frequency: Monthly. ISSN: 0040-5752.

★1652★ THEORETICAL POPULATION BIOLOGY
Academic Press, Inc.
1250 6th Ave.
San Diego, CA 92101   Phone: (619) 231-0926
First Published: 1970. Frequency: Bimonthly. ISSN: 0040-5809.

★1653★ THEORETICAL SURGERY
Springer-Verlag New York, Inc.
175 5th Ave.
New York, NY 10010   Phone: (212) 460-1500
First Published: 1986. Frequency: Quarterly. ISSN: 0179-8669.

★1654★ THERAPEUTIC DRUG MONITORING
Raven Press
1185 Avenue of the Americas
New York, NY 10036   Phone: (212) 930-9500
First Published: 1979. Frequency: Quarterly. ISSN: 0163-4356.

★1655★ THERIOGENOLOGY
Butterworth-Heinemann
80 Montvale Ave.
Stoneham, MA 02180   Phone: (617) 438-8464
Frequency: Monthly. ISSN: 0093-691X.

★1656★ THORAX
British Medical Association
PO Box 560B
Kennebunkport, ME 04046
First Published: 1946. Frequency: Monthly. ISSN: 0040-6376.

★1657★ THROMBOSIS AND HAEMOSTASIS
F.K. Schattauer Verlag
Lenzhalde 3
Postfach 104545
7000 Stuttgart 1, Germany
First Published: 1957. Frequency: Bimonthly. ISSN: 0340-6245.

★1658★ THROMBOSIS RESEARCH
Pergamon Press, Inc.
Maxwell House, Fairview Park
Elmsford, NY 10523   Phone: (914) 592-7700
First Published: 1972. Frequency: 24/yr. ISSN: 0049-3848.

★1659★ TISSUE AND CELL
Churchill Livingstone, Inc.
1560 Broadway
New York, NY 10036   Phone: (212) 819-5400
Frequency: 6/yr. ISSN: 0041-3879.

★1660★ TOBACCO CONTROL
British Medical Association
PO Box 560B
Kennebunkport, ME 04046
Frequency: Quarterly. ISSN: 0964-4563.

★1661★ TOHOKU JOURNAL OF EXPERIMENTAL MEDICINE
Tohoku University Medical Press
2-1 Seiryomachi
Sendai 980, Japan
First Published: 1920. Frequency: Monthly. ISSN: 0040-8727.

★1662★ TOPICS IN CLINICAL NUTRITION
Aspen Publishers, Inc.
200 Orchard Ridge Dr.
Gaithersburg, MD 20878   Phone: (301) 417-7500
First Published: 1986. Frequency: Quarterly. ISSN: 0883-5691.

★1663★ TOPICS IN EMERGENCY MEDICINE
Aspen Publishers, Inc.
200 Orchard Ridge Dr.
Gaithersburg, MD 20878   Phone: (301) 417-7500
First Published: 1979. Frequency: Quarterly. ISSN: 0164-2340.

★1664★ TOPICS IN GERIATRIC REHABILITATION
Aspen Publishers, Inc.
200 Orchard Ridge Dr.
Gaithersburg, MD 20878   Phone: (301) 417-7500
First Published: 1985. Frequency: Quarterly.

★1665★ TOPICS IN HEALTH CARE FINANCING
Aspen Publishers, Inc.
200 Orchard Ridge Dr.
Gaithersburg, MD 20878   Phone: (301) 417-7500
First Published: 1974. Frequency: Quarterly. ISSN: 0095-3814.

★1666★ TOPICS IN HEALTH RECORD MANAGEMENT
Aspen Publishers, Inc.
200 Orchard Ridge Dr.
Gaithersburg, MD 20878   Phone: (301) 417-7500
First Published: 1980. Frequency: Quarterly. ISSN: 0270-5230.

★1667★ TOPICS IN HOSPITAL PHARMACY MANAGEMENT
Aspen Publishers, Inc.
200 Orchard Ridge Dr.
Gaithersburg, MD 20878   Phone: (301) 417-7500
First Published: 1981. Frequency: Quarterly. ISSN: 0271-1206.

★1668★ TOPICS IN LANGUAGE DISORDERS
Aspen Publishers, Inc.
200 Orchard Ridge Dr.
Gaithersburg, MD 20878   Phone: (301) 417-7500
First Published: 1980. Frequency: Quarterly. ISSN: 0271-8294.

★1669★ TOPICS IN MAGNETIC RESONANCE IMAGING
Aspen Publishers, Inc.
200 Orchard Ridge Dr.
Gaithersburg, MD 20878   Phone: (301) 417-7500
First Published: 1988. Frequency: Quarterly. ISSN: 0899-3459.

★1670★ TOXICOLOGIC PATHOLOGY
Society of Toxicologic Pathologists
PO Box 368
Lawrence, KS 66044   Phone: (908) 277-7409
First Published: 1973. Frequency: Quarterly. ISSN: 0192-6233.

★1671★ TOXICOLOGY
Elsevier Science Publishing Co., Inc.
655 Avenue of the Americas
New York, NY 10010   Phone: (212) 989-5800
First Published: 1973. **Frequency:** 15/yr. **ISSN:** 0300-483X.

★1672★ TOXICOLOGY AND APPLIED PHARMACOLOGY
Academic Press, Inc.
1250 6th Ave.
San Diego, CA 92101   Phone: (619) 231-0926
First Published: 1959. **Frequency:** 15/yr. **ISSN:** 0041-008X.

★1673★ TOXICOLOGY IN VITRO
Pergamon Press, Inc.
Maxwell House, Fairview Park
Elmsford, NY 10523   Phone: (914) 592-7700
First Published: 1987. **Frequency:** Bimonthly. **ISSN:** 0887-2333.

★1674★ TOXICOLOGY METHODS
Raven Press
1185 Avenue of the Americas
New York, NY 10036   Phone: (212) 930-9500
First Published: 1992. **Frequency:** Quarterly. **ISSN:** 1051-7235.

★1675★ TOXICON
Pergamon Press, Inc.
Maxwell House, Fairview Park
Elmsford, NY 10523   Phone: (914) 592-7700
First Published: 1962. **Frequency:** Monthly. **ISSN:** 0041-0101.

**★1676★ TRANSACTIONS OF THE ROYAL SOCIETY OF
    TROPICAL MEDICINE AND HYGIENE**
Manson House
26 Portland Pl.
London W1N 4EY, England
First Published: 1907. **Frequency:** Bimonthly. **ISSN:** 0035-9203.

★1677★ TRANSFUSION
American Association of Blood Banks
1117 N. 19th St., Ste. 600
Arlington, VA 22209   Phone: (703) 528-8200
First Published: 1961. **Frequency:** Bimonthly. **ISSN:** 0041-1132.

★1678★ TRANSFUSION MEDICINE
Blackwell Scientific Publications
3 Cambridge Center, Ste. 208
Cambridge, MA 02142   Phone: (617) 225-0401
Frequency: Quarterly. **ISSN:** 0958-7578.

★1679★ TRANSITIONS IN MENTAL RETARDATION
Ablex Publishing Corp.
355 Chestnut St.
Norwood, NJ 07648   Phone: (201) 767-8450
First Published: 1984. **Frequency:** Irregular.

★1680★ TRANSPLANTATION
Transplantation Society
c/o Ronald L. Ferguson, M.D.
Department of Surgery
1654 Ugham Dr.
Columbus, OH 43210   Phone: (416) 293-8545
First Published: 1963. **Frequency:** Monthly. **ISSN:** 0041-1337.

★1681★ TRANSPLANTATION PROCEEDINGS
Transplantation Society
c/o Ronald W. Ferguson, M.D.
Department of Surgery
1654 Ugham Dr.
Columbus, OH 43210   Phone: (416) 293-8545
First Published: 1969. **Frequency:** Bimonthly. **ISSN:** 0041-1345.

★1682★ TRAUMA QUARTERLY
Aspen Publishers, Inc.
200 Orchard Ridge Dr.
Gaithersburg, MD 20878   Phone: (301) 417-7500
First Published: 1984. **Frequency:** Quarterly. **ISSN:** 0743-6637.

★1683★ TROPICAL DOCTOR
Royal Society of Medicine
1 Wimpole St.
London W1M 8AE, England
First Published: 1971. **Frequency:** Quarterly. **ISSN:** 0049-4755.

★1684★ TRUSTEE
American Hospital Asociation
840 N. Lake Shore Dr.
Chicago, IL 60611   Phone: (312) 280-6000

★1685★ TUBERCLE
Churchill Livingstone, Inc.
1560 Broadway
New York, NY 10036   Phone: (212) 819-5400
First Published: 1919. **Frequency:** Quarterly. **ISSN:** 0041-3879.

★1686★ TUMOUR BIOLOGY
S. Karger Publishers, Inc.
26 W. Avon Rd.
PO Box 529
Farmington, CT 06085   Phone: (203) 675-7834
First Published: 1980. **Frequency:** Bimonthly. **ISSN:** 1010-4283.

★1687★ ULTRASONIC IMAGING
Academic Press, Inc.
1250 6th Ave.
San Diego, CA 92101   Phone: (619) 231-0926
First Published: 1979. **Frequency:** Quarterly. **ISSN:** 0161-7346.

★1688★ ULTRASOUND IN MEDICINE AND BIOLOGY
Pergamon Press, Inc.
Maxwell House, Fairview Park
Elmsford, NY 10523   Phone: (914) 592-7700
First Published: 1974. **Frequency:** 9/yr. **ISSN:** 0301-5629.

★1689★ ULTRASOUND QUARTERLY
Raven Press
1185 Avenue of the Americas
New York, NY 10036   Phone: (212) 930-9500
Frequency: Quarterly. **ISSN:** 0894-8771.

★1690★ ULTRASTRUCTURAL PATHOLOGY
Hemisphere Publishing Corp.
1900 Frost Rd., Ste.101
Bristol, PA 19007   Phone: (215) 785-5800
First Published: 1980. **Frequency:** Bimonthly. **ISSN:** 0191-3123.

★1691★ UNDERSEA BIOMEDICAL RESEARCH
Undersea and Hyperbaric Medical Society, Inc.
9650 Rockville Pike
Bethesda, MD 20814   Phone: (301) 571-1818
First Published: 1974. **Frequency:** 6/yr. **ISSN:** 0093-5387.

★1692★ UPSALA JOURNAL OF MEDICAL SCIENCES
Almqvist & Wiksell Periodical Company
Box 638
S-101 28 Stockholm, Sweden
First Published: 1865. **Frequency:** 3/yr. **ISSN:** 0300-9734.

★1693★ UROLOGIA INTERNATIONALIS
S. Karger Publishers, Inc.
26 W. Avon Rd.
PO Box 529
Farmington, CT 06085   Phone: (203) 675-7834
First Published: 1955. **Frequency:** Bimonthly. **ISSN:** 0042-1138.

★1694★ UROLOGIC NURSING
Mosby-Year, Inc.
11830 Westline Industrial Dr.
St. Louis, MO 63146   Phone: (314) 872-8370
First Published: 1980. **Frequency:** Quarterly.

★1695★ **UROLOGIC RADIOLOGY**
Springer-Verlag New York, Inc.
175 5th Ave.
New York, NY 10010   Phone: (212) 460-1500
First Published: 1979. **Frequency:** Quarterly. **ISSN:** 0171-1091.

★1696★ **UROLOGICAL RESEARCH**
Springer-Verlag New York, Inc.
175 5th Ave.
New York, NY 10010   Phone: (212) 460-1500
First Published: 1973. **Frequency:** Bimonthly. **ISSN:** 0300-5623.

★1697★ **UROLOGY**
Cahners Publishing Co.
Medical-Health Care Group
249 W. 17th St.
New York, NY 10011   Phone: (212) 645-0067
First Published: 1973. **Frequency:** Monthly. **ISSN:** 0090-4295.

★1698★ **VACCINE**
Butterwroth-Heinemann
80 Montvale
Stoneham, MA 02180   Phone: (617) 438-8464
Frequency: Monthly. **ISSN:** 0264-410X.

★1699★ **VACCINE RESEARCH**
Mary Ann Liebert, Inc.
1651 3rd Ave.
New York, NY 10128   Phone: (212) 289-2300
Frequency: Quarterly. **ISSN:** 1056-7909.

★1700★ **VASCULAR SURGERY**
Westminster Publications, Inc.
1044 Northern Blvd.
Roslyn, NY 11576   Phone: (516) 484-6880
First Published: 1967. **Frequency:** 9/yr. **ISSN:** 0042-2835.

★1701★ **VETERINARY ECONOMICS**
Veterinary Medicine Publishing Co.
9073 Lenexa Dr.
Lenexa, KS 66215   Phone: (913) 492-4300
First Published: 1960. **Frequency:** Monthly. **ISSN:** 0042-4862.

★1702★ **VETERINARY AND HUMAN TOXICOLOGY**
Kansas State University
Comparative Toxicology Laboratories
Veterinary and Human Toxicology
Manhattan, KS 66506   Phone: (913) 532-5679
First Published: 1958. **Frequency:** Bimonthly. **ISSN:** 0145-6296.

★1703★ **VETERINARY IMMUNOLOGY AND IMMUNOPATHOLOGY**
Elsevier Science Publishing Co., Inc.
655 Avenue of the Americas
New York, NY 10010   Phone: (212) 989-5800
First Published: 1979. **Frequency:** Monthly. **ISSN:** 0165-2427.

★1704★ **VETERINARY MICROBIOLOGY**
Elsevier Science Publishing Co., Inc.
655 Avenue of the Americas
New York, NY 10010   Phone: (212) 989-5800
First Published: 1976. **Frequency:** 16/yr. **ISSN:** 0378-1135.

★1705★ **VETERINARY PARASITOLOGY**
Elsevier Science Publishing Co., Inc.
655 Avenue of the Americas
New York, NY 10010   Phone: (212) 989-5800
First Published: 1975. **Frequency:** Monthly. **ISSN:** 0304-4017.

★1706★ **VETERINARY PATHOLOGY**
American College of Veterinary Pathologists
875 King Hwy., 2nd Fl.
West Deptford, NJ 08096   Phone: (609) 848-7748
First Published: 1964. **Frequency:** Bimonthly. **ISSN:** 0300-9858.

★1707★ **VETERINARY QUARTERLY**
Kluwer Academic Publishers
101 Philip Dr.
Assinippi Park
Norwell, MA 02061   Phone: (617) 871-6600
First Published: 1979. **Frequency:** Quarterly. **ISSN:** 0165-2176.

★1708★ **VETERINARY RECORD**
British Veterinary Association
7 Mansfield St.
London W1M 0AT, England
First Published: 1888. **Frequency:** Weekly. **ISSN:** 0042-4900.

★1709★ **VIRCHOWS ARCHIV. A: PATHOLOGICAL ANATOMY AND HISTOPATHOLOGY**
Springer-Verlag New York, Inc.
175 5th Ave.
New York, NY 10010   Phone: (212) 460-1500
First Published: 1847. **Frequency:** Monthly. **ISSN:** 0174-7398.

★1710★ **VIRCHOWS ARCHIV. B: CELL PATHOLOGY**
Springer-Verlag New York, Inc.
175 5th Ave.
New York, NY 10010   Phone: (212) 460-1500
First Published: 1968. **Frequency:** Bimonthly. **ISSN:** 0340-6075.

★1711★ **VIRGINIA MEDICAL QUARTERLY**
Medical Society of Virginia
4205 Dover Rd.
Richmond, VA 23221   Phone: (804) 353-2721
First Published: 1874. **Frequency:** Monthly. **ISSN:** 0146-3616.

★1712★ **VIROLOGY**
Academic Press, Inc.
1250 6th Ave.
San Diego, CA 92101   Phone: (619) 231-0926
First Published: 1955. **Frequency:** Monthly. **ISSN:** 0042-6822.

★1713★ **VISION RESEARCH**
Pergamon Press, Inc.
Maxwell House, Fairview Park
Elmsford, NY 10523   Phone: (914) 592-7700
First Published: 1961. **Frequency:** Monthly. **ISSN:** 0042-6989.

★1714★ **VISUAL NEUROSCIENCE**
Cambridge University Press
40 W. 20th St.
New York, NY 10011   Phone: (212) 924-3900
Frequency: Monthly. **ISSN:** 0952-5238.

★1715★ **VOLTA REVIEW**
Alexander Graham Bell Association for the Deaf, Inc.
3417 Volta Pl., NW
Washington, DC 20007   Phone: (202) 337-5220
First Published: 1899. **Frequency:** 7/yr. **ISSN:** 0042-8639.

★1716★ **VOX SANGUINIS**
S. Karger Publishers, Inc.
26 W. Avon Rd.
PO Box 529
Farmington, CT 06085   Phone: (203) 675-7834
First Published: 1956. **Frequency:** 8/yr. **ISSN:** 0042-9007.

★1717★ **WEST VIRGINIA MEDICAL JOURNAL**
West Virginia State Medical Association
4307 MacCorkle Ave.
Box 4106
Charleston, WV 25364   Phone: (304) 925-0342
First Published: 1906. **Frequency:** Monthly. **ISSN:** 0043-3284.

★1718★ **WESTERN JOURNAL OF MEDICINE**
California Medical Association
221 Main St.
San Francisco, CA 94103   Phone: (415) 882-5179
First Published: 1902. **Frequency:** Monthly. **ISSN:** 0093-0415.

★1719★   WISCONSIN MEDICAL JOURNAL
State Medical Society of Wisconsin
330 E. Lakeside St.
PO Box 1109
Madison, WI 53701   Phone: (608) 262-3266
First Published: 1903. **Frequency:** Monthly. **ISSN:** 0043-6542.

★1720★   WOMEN AND HEALTH
The Haworth Press, Inc.
10 Alice St.
Binghamton, NY 13904   Phone: (800) 342-9678
First Published: 1976. **Frequency:** Quarterly. **ISSN:** 0363-0242.

★1721★   WOMEN'S HEALTH ISSUES
Elsevier Science Publishing Co., Inc.
655 Avenue of the Americas
New York, NY 10010   Phone: (212) 989-5800
Frequency: Quarterly. **ISSN:** 1049-3867.

**★1722★   WORLD JOURNAL OF MICROBIOLOGY AND
            BIOTECHNOLOGY**
Rapid Communications of Oxford Ltd.
The Old Malthouse
Paradise St.
Oxford OX1 1LD, England
Frequency: Bimonthly. **ISSN:** 0959-3993.

★1723★   WORLD JOURNAL OF SURGERY
Springer-Verlag New York, Inc.
175 5th Ave.
New York, NY 10010   Phone: (212) 460-1500
First Published: 1977. **Frequency:** Bimonthly. **ISSN:** 0364-2313.

★1724★   WORLD JOURNAL OF UROLOGY
Springer-Verlag New York, Inc.
175 5th Ave.
New York, NY 10010   Phone: (212) 460-1500
First Published: 1983. **Frequency:** Quarterly. **ISSN:** 0724-4983.

★1725★   XENOBIOTICA
Taylor & Francis, Ltd.
Rankine Rd.
Basingstoke, Hants. RG24 0PR, England
First Published: 1971. **Frequency:** Monthly. **ISSN:** 0049-8254.

★1726★   YALE JOURNAL OF BIOLOGY AND MEDICINE
Yale University
333 Cedar St.
New Haven, CT 06510   Phone: (203) 785-4251
First Published: 1928. **Frequency:** Bimonthly. **ISSN:** 0044-0086.

(2) Newsletters

Newsletters listed below are alphabetical by titles. See the User's Guide located at the front of this directory for additional information.

★1727★   AAAD BULLETIN
American Athletic Association of the Deaf, Inc.
1313 Tanforan Dr.
Lexington, KY 40502   Phone: (606) 272-0537
Description: Provides news and information about sports for the deaf. Publicizes various sporting and social events, including the deaf olympic games and national basketball and softball tournaments. **First Published:** April 1947. **Frequency:** 6/yr.

★1728★   AABB NEWS BRIEFS
American Association of Blood Banks
1117 N. 19th St., Ste. 600
Arlington, VA 22209   Phone: (703) 528-8200
Description: Publishes scientific, technical, educational, and administrative news and information of interest to blood bank personnel. Covers blood-transmissible diseases, accreditation standards and inspection practices, and recent and expected changes in blood banking. Recurring features include Association news, publication briefs, news of research, a calendar of events, and a column titled Government and Legal Affairs Update. **Frequency:** 11/yr. **ISSN:** 8756-6095.

★1729★   AACP NEWS
American Association of Colleges of Pharmacy
1426 Prince St.
Alexandria, VA 22314-2815
Description: Discusses issues relating to pharmaceutical education. Carries legislative information, feature stories on award winners, and Association news. Recurring features include news of research, notices of continuing education and employment opportunities, and listings of publications. **First Published:** December 1972. **Frequency:** Monthly.

★1730★   AACPDM NEWS
American Academy for Cerebral Palsy and Developmental Medicine
PO Box 11086
Richmond, VA 23230   Phone: (804) 282-0036
Description: Concerned with research, treatment, and understanding of cerebral palsy and developmental disabilities and with acceptance of the handicaps caused by these conditions. Carries Academy news. **Frequency:** Biennially.

★1731★   AADPA COMMUNICATOR
American Academy of Dental Practice Administration
1063 Whipoorwill Ln.
Palatine, IL 60067   Phone: (708) 934-4404
Description: Serves as a medium of communication among dental organizations that are members of the Academy. Carries reports from meetings and seminars, news items, and relevant quotations. **First Published:** 1958. **Frequency:** 3/yr.

★1732★   AAHA PROVIDER NEWS
American Association of Homes for the Aging
1129 20th St. NW, Ste. 400
Washington, DC 20036-3489   Phone: (202) 296-5960
Description: Discusses topics concerning nonprofit homes and services for the aging, including legislative, regulatory, and judicial developments in long-term care and housing; issues in the field of gerontology; and new developments in alternative services for the aging. Publicizes Association events, services and growth, membership accomplishments, and professional opportunities. Recurring features include columns titled Job Mart, Health Issues, Employer Tips, Trends, and Housing Issues. **First Published:** April 1983. **Frequency:** 12/yr.

★1733★   AALAS BULLETIN
American Association for Laboratory Animal Science
70 Timber Creek Dr., Ste. 5
Cordova, TN 38018   Phone: (901) 754-8620
Description: Provides news and information on laboratory animal science. **First Published:** 1967. **Frequency:** 6/yr.

★1734★   AAO NEWS
Alberta Association of Optometrists
11830 Kingsway Ave., Ste. 902
Edmonton, AB, Canada T5G 0X5   Phone: (403) 451-6824
Description: Covers news of interest in the field of optometry in Canada. **First Published:** 1982. **Frequency:** Quarterly.

★1735★   AAOA NEWS
American Academy of Otolaryngic Allergy
8455 Colesville Rd., Ste. 745
Silver Spring, MD 20910-9998   Phone: (301) 588-1800
Description: Presents news of the Academy and pertinent socioeconomic and medical news. Recurring features include letters to the editor, news of members, a calendar of events, calls for papers, notices of publications available, and a column titled President's Message. **First Published:** 1982. **Frequency:** Quarterly.

★1736★   AAOA RECORD
Auxiliary to the American Osteopathic Association
142 E. Ontario St.
Chicago, IL 60611   Phone: (312) 280-5819
Description: Concerned with osteopathic medicine and related subjects such as safety projects, public health information, and osteopathic college scholarship awards. Recurring features include reports on the annual convention, a calendar of events, news of members, and an Association roster. **First Published:** 1941. **Frequency:** Quarterly.

★1737★   AAOHN NEWS
American Association of Occupational Health Nurses
50 Lenox Pointe
Atlanta, GA 30324-3176   Phone: (404) 262-1162
Description: Covers Association events as well as trends and legislation affecting occupational health nursing. Recurring features include news of

research, a calendar of events, reports of meetings, news of educational opportunities, job listings, notices of publications available, and a President's column. **Frequency:** Monthly.

★1738★ **AAOMS SURGICAL UPDATE**
American Association of Oral and Maxillofacial Surgeons
9700 W. Bryn Mawr Ave.
Rosemont, IL 60018   Phone: (708) 678-6200
Description: Provides "the dental profession and others with current information on the speciality of oral and maxillofacial surgery and patient care." **First Published:** 1985. **Frequency:** 3/yr.

★1739★ **AAOS REPORT**
American Academy of Orthopaedic Surgeons
222 N. Prospect Ave.
Park Ridge, IL 60068   Phone: (708) 823-7186
Description: Reports on Academy activities, as well as discussing socioeconomic developments and issues affecting orthopedic surgeons. Carries news of members, listings of new publications, news of members, notices of continuing education opportunities, and a calendar of events. **First Published:** August 1975. **Frequency:** Monthly.

★1740★ **AAP NEWS**
American Academy of Pediatrics
PO Box 927
Elk Grove, IL 60007   Phone: (800) 433-9016
Description: Reports Academy activities and developments in the child health field. Recurring features include letters to the editor, news of members, a calendar of events, and columns titled Washington Update, Focus on Practice, Health Alert, Course Calendar, and Chapter Newsline. **First Published:** January 1985. **Frequency:** Monthly.

★1741★ **AAPA NEWSLETTER**
American Association of Pathologists' Assistants, Inc.
c/o Leo J. Kelly
V.A. Medical Center
West Haven, CT 06516   Phone: (203) 932-5711
Description: Presents technical information and news of developments in anatomic pathology, including forensic pathology, histopathology, surgical pathology, and autopsy pathology. Recurring features include committee reports, case histories, a continuing medical education quiz, and notices of positions available. **First Published:** 1972. **Frequency:** Quarterly.

★1742★ **AAPSM NEWSLETTER**
American Academy of Podiatric Sports Medicine
1729 Glastonberry Rd.
Potomac, MD 20854   Phone: (301) 424-7440
Description: Features articles discussing injuries and treatments in the field of podiatry. Reports on Academy activities and meetings. Recurring features include news of research, editorials, and a calendar of events. **First Published:** June 1983. **Frequency:** Quarterly.

★1743★ **AARN NEWSLETTER**
Alberta Association of Registered Nurses
11620 168th St.
Edmonton, AB, Canada T5M 4A6   Phone: (403) 451-0043
Description: Lists and describes current nursing activities and events in Alberta. Contains articles of general public health concern and items discussing current developments in nursing practice, education, research, and administration. Includes career information and notices of career opportunities. Recurring features include letters to the editor, interviews, reports of meetings, news of educational opportunities and publications available, and a calendar of events. **First Published:** March 1948. **Frequency:** 11/yr. **ISSN:** 0001-0197.

★1744★ **AAROT NEWSLETTER**
Alberta Association of Registered Occupational Therapists
4245 97th St., No. 311
Edmonton, AB, Canada T6E 5Y7   Phone: (403) 436-8381
Description: Serves as an information exchange for member occupational therapists. Announces continuing education opportunities, offers news of various rehabilitation programs and related organizations, and carries articles on practical aspects of occupational therapy. Recurring features include job listings, book reviews, and a column titled President's Message. **First Published:** 1970. **Frequency:** 10/yr.

★1745★ **AARP BULLETIN**
American Association of Retired Persons
1909 K St. NW
Washington, DC 20049   Phone: (202) 662-4842
Description: Monitors issues and events affecting Americans aged 50 and over. Covers medical benefits and other services of interest. Recurring features include Association news, editorials, and columns titled As We See It, Bulletin Board, Washingtonwatch, Stateswatch, and Reader Forum. **First Published:** 1959. **Frequency:** 11/yr. **ISSN:** 0010-0200.

★1746★ **AAWH—QUARTERLY**
American Association for World Health
1729 20th St. NW, Ste. 400
Washington, DC 20036   Phone: (202) 466-5883
Description: Reports on health news throughout the world. Contains news of the Association, whose aim is to strengthen U.S. commitment to world health by informing Americans about the importance of international health issues. Recurring features include news of health legislation. **First Published:** 1981. **Frequency:** Quarterly.

★1747★ **AAZPA COMMUNIQUE**
American Association of Zoological Parks and Aquariums
Oglebay Park
Wheeling, WV 26003   Phone: (304) 242-2160
Description: Provides news and information on zoological parks and aquariums. **Frequency:** Monthly.

★1748★ **THE ABA NEWSLETTER**
Association for Behavior Analysis
Department of Psychology
Western Michigan University
Kalamazoo, MI 49008-5052   Phone: (616) 383-1629
Description: Covers Association activities, with reports of committees and special interest groups, and news from regional, state, and local associations for behavior analysis. Recurring features include convention details and overview, news of research, and positions-available notices. **First Published:** 1978. **Frequency:** 4/yr.

★1749★ **ABORTION RESEARCH NOTES**
Transnational Family Research Institute
8307 Whitman Dr.
Bethesda, MD 20817   Phone: (301) 469-6313
Description: Analyzes research and provides citations for abortion-related journal articles and books. Deals with legal, social, and psychological aspects of abortion, and abortion services and techniques. Studies abortion trends and legislation on country-by-country and international levels. **First Published:** 1972. **Frequency:** Periodic. **ISSN:** 0361-1116.

★1750★ **THE ABSTRACT**
National Tumors Registrars Association
505 E. Hawley St.
Mundelein, IL 60060   Phone: (708) 566-0833
Description: Provides educational and information articles on cancer research and data. Recurring features include news of educational opportunities, job listings, book reviews, and columns titled AJCC Staging Questions and ICD-O-II Coding Questions. **Frequency:** Quarterly.

★1751★ **ACA JOURNAL**
American Council on Alcoholism
5024 Campbell Blvd., Ste. H
Baltimore, MD 21236-5974   Phone: (301) 529-9200
Description: Educates the public on issues concerning alcoholism, emphasizing education, prevention, early diagnosis, and rehabilitation programs. Promotes a greater understanding of the alcoholic and alcoholic abuse individual. Contains results of research conducted on alcoholism. **First Published:** 1986. **Frequency:** Semiannually. **ISSN:** 088-5567.

★1752★ **ACA NEWS**
Alberta Council on Aging
10506 Jasper Ave., No. 501
Edmonton, AB, Canada T5J 2W9   Phone: (403) 423-7781
Description: Addresses issues affecting older persons, such as abuse or neglect of the elderly, seniors and substance abuse, and seniors and driving. Features winning entries from the Council's writing contests, profiles the activities of older persons, and reports on the committees and projects of the Council. Recurring features include letters to the editor, news of research, a calendar of events, reports of meetings, and columns titled

President's Corner, Yesterdays, New Horizons, and Senior Citizens Secretariat. **First Published:** 1967. **Frequency:** 6/yr. **ISSN:** 0826-497X.

★1753★ **ACADEMY OF MEDICINE, TORONTO—BULLETIN**
Academy of Medicine, Toronto
288 Bloor St., W.
Toronto, ON, Canada M5S 1V8   Phone: (416) 922-1134
Description: Provides news and developments in the field of medicine. Recurring features include letters to the editor, a calendar of events, book reviews, and the president's letter. **Frequency:** 4/yr.

★1754★ **ACADEMY REPORTER**
Academy of Pharmaceutical Research and Science
2215 Constitution Ave. NW
Washington, DC 20037   Phone: (202) 628-4410
Description: Reports on Academy news and developments in the pharmaceutical sciences. **First Published:** September 1965. **Frequency:** Quarterly. **ISSN:** 0199-6037.

★1755★ **THE ACAT NEWS**
American Center for the Alexander Technique, Inc.
Abraham Goodman House
129 W. 67th St.
New York, NY 10023   Phone: (212) 799-0468
Description: Contains news related to the Alexander Technique, an educational approach to gaining skill in bodily coordination, movement, and overall poise. Features news of the Center, news of members, and notices of publications available. **First Published:** 1985. **Frequency:** 3/yr.

★1756★ **ACCC COMPENDIA-BASED DRUG BULLETIN**
Association of Community Cancer Centers
11600 Nebel St., Ste. 201
Rockville, MD 20852   Phone: (301) 984-9496
Frequency: Quarterly.

★1757★ **ACCENT**
Maryland State Planning Council on Developmental Disabilities
300 W. Lexington St.
1 Market Center
PO Box 10
Baltimore, MD 21201   Phone: (301) 333-3688
Description: Provides a forum for a variety of issues affecting persons with disabilities. Contains news of the Council, its projects, programs, and activities. Recurring features include editorials, news of research, news of members, book reviews, a calendar of events, and notices of publications. **First Published:** 1977. **Frequency:** Bimonthly.

★1758★ **ACCH NETWORK**
Association for the Care of Children's Health
7910 Woodmont Ave., Ste. 300
Bethesda, MD 20814   Phone: (301) 654-6549
Description: Focuses on programs, policies, resources, and research that promote family-centered approaches to care for children with special needs and their families. Recurring features include resource reviews, a calendar of events, and columns on family resource libraries, pediatric AIDS/HIV, and support for infants with disabilities and life-threatening conditions. **First Published:** 1982. **Frequency:** Quarterly.

★1759★ **ACCREDITATION UPDATE**
Accreditation Council on Services for People With Developmental
    Disabilities
8100 Professional Pl., Ste. 204
Landover, MD 20785   Phone: (301) 459-3191
Description: Discusses the accreditation process for service agencies to promote the highest level of independence, productivity, community integration, and well-being of the families and the people with developmental disabilities . Reports the training and survey activities of The Accreditation Council's comprehensive national quality enhancement program as well as changes in and interpretation of its accreditation standards and policies. **First Published:** 1980. **Frequency:** Semiannually.

★1760★ **ACEP NEWS**
American College of Emergency Physicians
PO Box 619911
Dallas, TX 75261-9911   Phone: (214) 550-0911
Description: Informs emergency physicians of socioeconomic issues affecting the specialty of emergency medicine. Contains information on medical

practice management, pertinent federal and state legislation, and College activities and services. **First Published:** April 1969. **Frequency:** Monthly.

★1761★ **ACFD FORUM**
Association of Canadian Faculties of Dentistry
109-1815 Alta Vista Dr.
Ottawa, ON, Canada K1G 2Y6   Phone: (604) 738-7732
Description: Concerned with education and research in dentistry. Recurring features include letters to the editor, interviews, a calendar of events, reports of meetings, news of educational and employment opportunities, book reviews, and faculty reports. **First Published:** 1968. **Frequency:** Quarterly. **ISSN:** 0820-5949.

★1762★ **ACGP NEWSLETTER**
American College of General Practitioners in Osteopathic Medicine
    and Surgery
330 E. Algonquin Rd.
Arlington Heights, IL 60005   Phone: (800) 323-0794
Description: Reports news of the College, which works to advance standards of general osteopathic practice by increasing educational opportunities, enhance the understanding of the scope of general practice, and establish departments of general practice in hospitals. Recurring features include editorials, letters to the editor, news of members, and a calendar of events. **First Published:** January 1984. **Frequency:** Monthly.

★1763★ **ACHA ACTION**
American College Health Association
1300 Piccard Dr.
Rockville, MD 20850   Phone: (301) 963-1100
Description: Reports on the college and university health field, with legislative news and information on affiliated associations. Recurring features include a resource list, a calendar of events, and low-cost placement service listings. **Frequency:** 6/yr.

★1764★ **ACLS ALERT**
American Health Consultants, Inc.
3525 Piedmont Rd. NE
6 Piedmont Center, Ste. 400
Atlanta, GA 30305   Phone: (404) 351-4523

★1765★ **ACO NEWSLETTER**
American College of Orgonomy
PO Box 490
Princeton, NJ 08542   Phone: (201) 821-1144
Description: Discusses work at the College. Contains a calendar of events, progress reports, and notices of publications available.

★1766★ **ACOG NEWSLETTER**
American College of Obstetricians and Gynecologists
409 12th St. SW
Washington, DC 20024-2188   Phone: (202) 638-5577
Description: Reviews health policy issues, clinical research, national statistics, and other information pertaining to obstetrics and gynecology. Reports on College projects, staff, and meetings. Recurring features include columns titled Federal Roundup, Practice Perspectives, Fellows in the News, and New Resources. **First Published:** May 1952. **Frequency:** Monthly.

★1767★ **ACPA/CPF NEWSLETTER**
American Cleft Palate-Craniofacial Association
Cleft Palate Foundation
1218 Grandview Ave.
Pittsburgh, PA 15211   Phone: (412) 481-1376
Description: Provides Association news principally for members who are health care professionals devoted to the care of individuals with cleft lip, palate, and associated deformities of the mouth and face. Recurring features include minutes of meetings, information on conventions, symposia, elections, committee progress, and items of special interest. **First Published:** August 1976. **Frequency:** Quarterly.

★1768★ **ACPM NEWS**
American College of Preventive Medicine
1015 15th St. NW, Ste. 403
Washington, DC 20005   Phone: (202) 789-0003
Description: Discusses topics related to preventive medicine, public health, aerospace medicine, and occupational medicine. Carries information on continuing medical education, legislative activities, and programs of the College. Recurring features include news of members, news of research,

and a calendar of events. **First Published:** 1954. **Frequency:** Quarterly. **ISSN:** 0199-2481.

★1769★ ADA NEWSLETTER
Alberta Dental Association
8230 105th St., Ste. 101
Edmonton, AB, Canada T6E 5H9   Phone: (403) 432-1012
Description: Focuses on the meetings and professional concerns of Association members and provides general coverage of topics of concern to dentists practicing in Alberta. Recurring features include letters to the editor, a calendar of events, news of educational opportunities, and job listings. **First Published:** 1961. **Frequency:** 4-6/yr.

★1770★ ADAA REPORTER
Anxiety Disorders Association of America
6000 Executive Blvd.
Rockville, MD 20852-3801   Phone: (301) 231-9350
Description: Reports on new research, treatment advances, self-help techniques and programs, and Association activities. **First Published:** May 1990. **Frequency:** Quarterly.

★1771★ ADAMHA NEWS
Alcohol, Drug Abuse, and Mental Health Administration
U.S. Department of Health and Human Services
OCEA, Rm. 13C-05
5600 Fishers Ln.
Rockville, MD 20857   Phone: (301) 443-0746
Description: Publishes recent research findings conducted or supported by the National Institute on Alcohol Abuse and Alcoholism, National Institute on Drug Abuse, and the National Institute for Mental Health. Provides news on prevention and treatment of mental and substance abuse disorders from the Agency's Office for Substance Abuse Prevention and Office for Treatment Improvement. Includes staff news and articles on Agency researchers or key officials. **First Published:** 1974. **Frequency:** Bimonthly.

★1772★ ADARA NEWSLETTER
American Deafness and Rehabilitation Association
PO Box 251554
Little Rock, AR 72225-1554   Phone: (501) 663-7074
Description: Surveys news events, resources, legislation, and developments in services related to the deaf. Recurring features include notices of employment opportunities, news of the national Association and its local chapters, information on new publications, announcements of awards granted, and a calendar of events. **First Published:** September 1968. **Frequency:** Quarterly.

★1773★ THE ADDICTION LETTER
Manisses Communications Group, Inc.
Box 3357, Wayland Sq.
Providence, RI 02906-0357   Phone: (401) 831-6020
Description: Functions as a "resource exchange for professionals in preventing and treating alcoholism and drug abuse." Evaluates research and new techniques in addiction treatment. Recurring features include news of research, book reviews, and a calendar of events. **First Published:** 1985. **Frequency:** Monthly. **ISSN:** 8756-405X.

★1774★ ADOLESCENT MEDICINE
British Trading Co. Ltd.
821 Delaware Ave. SW
Washington, DC 20024   Phone: (202) 488-7533
Description: Covers the epidemiology, diagnosis, and therapy of diseases commonly suffered by adolescents. Provides news of national, state, and local programs, policies, and legislation promoting adolescent disease prevention and health promotion. Recurring features include interviews, news of research, reports of meetings, and book reviews. **First Published:** 1968. **Frequency:** Monthly. **ISSN:** 0044-6445.

★1775★ ADPA PROFESSIONAL
Alcohol and Drug Problems Association
1555 Wilson Blvd., Ste. 300
Arlington, VA 22209   Phone: (703) 875-8684
Description: Presents news items and discussions of public policy concerning drug and alcohol abuse. Recurring features include book reviews, announcements of educational opportunities, editorials, and a calendar of events. **Frequency:** Bimonthly.

★1776★ ADSA PULSE
American Dental Society of Anesthesiology
211 E. Chicago Ave., No. 948
Chicago, IL 60611   Phone: (312) 664-8270
Description: Features articles on developments in dental anesthesiology. Includes news of research, editorials, news of the Society and its members, and a calendar of events. **Frequency:** Bimonthly. **ISSN:** 0274-9793.

★1777★ ADULT DAY CARE LETTER
Health Resources Publishing
Brinley Professional Plaza, 3100 Hwy. 38
PO Box 1442
Wall Township, NJ 07719-1442   Phone: (201) 681-1133
Description: Provides crucial management information and serves as a link between adult day care programs across the country. Administrators and directors of adult day care programs. **First Published:** July 1985. **Frequency:** Monthly. **ISSN:** 0885-4572.

★1778★ ADVANCE
Association for Advancement of Psychology
PO Box 38129
Colorado Springs, CO 80937   Phone: (719) 520-0688
Description: Concerned with the advancement of psychology. Details the Association's work to represent the interests of professional, social, and scientific psychologists in the public policy arena. Recurring features include news of members, news of research, and a calendar of events. **Frequency:** Quarterly.

★1779★ ADVANCE
Foundation for Chiropractic Education and Research
1701 Clarendon Blvd.
Arlington, VA 22209-2712   Phone: (703) 276-7445
Description: Provides information on programs and projects related to the Foundation, including research sponsored by the Foundation. **First Published:** 1973. **Frequency:** Bimonthly.

★1780★ ADVANCES
Jonsson Comprehensive Cancer Center
University of California, Los Angeles
Louis Factor Health Sciences Bldg., 10-247
UCLA Center for the Health Sciences
Los Angeles, CA 90024   Phone: (213) 825-5268
Description: Serves as a professional newsletter on cancer, covering clinical and basic science research by members of the Jonsson Comprehensive Cancer Center at UCLA. Provides information on community cancer control programs, trends in cancer management and incidence, and related subjects. Recurring features include scientific articles; American Cancer Society programs; Center news; book reviews; notices of research awards; and announcements of meetings, conferences, courses, and ongoing patient clinical trials at UCLA. **First Published:** Spring 1990. **Frequency:** 3/yr.

★1781★ ADVENTURES IN MOVEMENT
Adventures in Movement for Handicapped Children
945 Danbury Rd.
Dayton, OH 45420   Phone: (513) 294-4611
Description: Publishes news of the organization, whose goal is "to help individuals with visual handicaps, hearing impairments, emotional or learning disabilities and orthopedic or coordination problems achieve their highest potential" through Specialized Movement Education (rhythmical exercise movements; locomotor movements using walks, skips, jumps, hops, and slides; and creative activities). **First Published:** 1958. **Frequency:** 3/yr.

★1782★ ADVOCACY UPDATE
Public Voice for Food and Health Policy
1001 Connecticut Ave. NW, Ste. 522
Washington, DC 20036   Phone: (202) 659-5930
Description: Directed toward consumers concerned about food safety and nutrition issues. Details progress made by the association in organizing public support for progressive legislation and policies responsive to consumers' needs in the marketplace. Recurring features include news of research and updates on legislation concerning food safety, nutrition, health, and the environment. **First Published:** 1983. **Frequency:** 11/yr.

★1783★ AER REPORT
Association for Education and Rehabilitation of the Blind and
Visually Impaired
206 N. Washington St., Ste. 320
Alexandria, VA 22314   Phone: (703) 548-1884
Description: Monitors legislative actions affecting the blind and visually
impaired. Announces services and technologies for blind persons. Recurring
features include news of research and reports on activities of the
Association and its members. **First Published:** 1984. **Frequency:** Bimonthly.

★1784★ AESTHETIC SURGERY
American Society for Aesthetic Plastic Surgery
3922 Atlantic Ave.
Long Beach, CA 90807   Phone: (310) 595-4275
Description: Reviews developments and the results of research in the field
of aesthetic plastic surgery. Reports on the use of new techniques. Includes
news of the Society. **First Published:** 1982. **Frequency:** 3/yr.

★1785★ AESTHETICS' WORLD TODAY
Aestheticians International Association, Inc.
4447 McKinney Ave.
Dallas, TX 75205   Phone: (214) 526-0752
Description: Promotes the advancement of education of aesthetics and
public awareness. Contains notices of educational seminars and classes
during annual regional, national, and international conventions. **First
Published:** August 1988. **Frequency:** Quarterly.

★1786★ AFB NEWS
Communications Dept.
American Foundation for the Blind
15 W. 16th St.
New York, NY 10011   Phone: (212) 620-2029
Description: Publishes articles for general readership about blindness and
low vision. Reports on the activities and staff of the Foundation. Recurring
features include news of research, letters to the editor, and columns titled
Regional Roundup, Briefings, and Features. **First Published:** 1966. **Frequency:** 4/yr.

★1787★ AFFILIATES IN TRAINING
American College of Cardiology
9111 Old Georgetown Rd.
Bethesda, MD 20814   Phone: (301) 897-5400
Description: Provides news of Association pertinent to the Affiliate-in-
Training category. Lists cardiology- and cardiovascular-related positions
available in private practice or teaching hospitals. Recurring features
include information on grants and workshops and a column titled
Washington Report. **First Published:** Fall 1984. **Frequency:** Bimonthly.

★1788★ AGBIOTECHNOLOGY NEWS
Freiberg Publishing
PO Box 7
Cedar Falls, IA 50613   Phone: (319) 277-3599
Description: Concerned with the business and technical aspects of agricultural
biotechnology. Offers news items, reviews of products, and research
and development updates. Recurring features include interviews, notices
of publications available and book reviews, a calendar of events, reports of
meetings, and news of educational opportunities. **First Published:** 1984.
Frequency: Bimonthly.

★1789★ AGD IMPACT
Academy of General Dentistry
211 E. Chicago Ave., Ste. 1200
Chicago, IL 60611   Phone: (312) 440-4300
Description: Seeks to keep Academy members abreast of issues, legislation,
and trends that may affect their practice, relationships in the profession,
and their position in the healthcare community. **First Published:** 1973.
Frequency: 11/yr. **ISSN:** 0194-729X.

★1790★ AGEING INTERNATIONAL
International Federation on Ageing
601 E St. NW
Washington, DC 20049   Phone: (202) 434-2430
Description: Reports on developments in service to the aged around the
world, with emphasis on innovations and expanded programs and options.
Covers education, employment, retirement, housing, health, social security,
social isolation, transportation, and other issues related to elderly
people. Recurring features include listings of new publications, news of

research, and a calendar of events. **First Published:** 1974. **Frequency:**
Quarterly. **ISSN:** 0163-5158.

★1791★ AGHE EXCHANGE NEWSLETTER
Association for Gerontology in Higher Education
1001 Connecticut Ave. NW, Ste. 410
Washington, DC 20036   Phone: (202) 429-9277
Description: Carries Association news, reports of gerontological programs,
items on legislative developments, and related material for persons at
member institutions interested in gerontology and higher education or
involved with other organizations concerned with the aging. Recurring
features include columns titled Principles & Practices, Program Planning,
Policy Page, Member Profiles, Research Reports, and In & Around AGHE.
Frequency: Quarterly. **ISSN:** 0890-278X.

★1792★ AGING ACTION ALERT
CD Publications
8204 Fenton St.
Silver Spring, MD 20910   Phone: (301) 588-6380
Description: Discusses issues affecting the elderly. Reviews the latest
developments in medical care, nutrition, drugs, education, housing, and
volunteer activities. Recurring features include news of research. **First
Published:** 1984. **Frequency:** Monthly.

★1793★ AGING RESEARCH & TRAINING NEWS
Business Publishers, Inc.
951 Pershing Dr.
Silver Spring, MD 20910   Phone: (301) 587-6300
Description: Reports on government and private sector funding sources for
aging research and training. Identifies grant and contract opportunities and
discusses guidelines, policy, related legislative and regulatory developments, and trends in services for the aged. **First Published:** 1977.
Frequency: Biweekly. **ISSN:** 0888-6830.

★1794★ AHA NEWS
American Hospital Publishing, Inc.
American Hospital Association
737 N. Michigan Ave., Ste. 700
Chicago, IL 60611   Phone: (312) 440-6800
Description: Highlights major news affecting hospitals and the healthcare
field. Reports on legislation and regulation, court cases, surveys, and
federal programs. Carries information on individual hospitals and allied
hospital associations. **First Published:** January 12, 1987. **Frequency:**
Weekly. **ISSN:** 0891-6608.

★1795★ AHCA NOTES
American Health Care Association
1201 L St. NW
Washington, DC 20005   Phone: (202) 842-4444
Description: Presents information on nursing homes and residential care
facilities. Covers legislation on prescription drug prices, nurse assistant
training, certification enforcement, Medicare/Medicaid and long term care
requirements, and legal activities. **Frequency:** 22/yr. **ISSN:** 0279-1692.

★1796★ AHI QUARTERLY
Animal Health Institute
119 Oronoco St.
PO Box 1417-D50
Alexandria, VA 22313-1480   Phone: (703) 684-0011
Description: Discusses developments of significance to animal health,
livestock, and veterinary industries. Includes legislative and regulatory
updates and news of research. **First Published:** 1981. **Frequency:** 4/yr.

★1797★ AHP PERSPECTIVE
Association for Humanistic Psychology
1772 Vallejo, Ste. 3
San Francisco, CA 94123   Phone: (415) 346-7929
Description: Focuses on the Association's programs, which apply "humanistic psychology principles to personal, professional and planetary transformation." Discusses growth therapies, holistic education, and social concerns. Recurring features include editorials, letters to the editor, news of
members, and a calendar of events. **First Published:** 1963. **Frequency:**
10/yr.

★1798★   AHPA PERSPECTIVE
Arthritis Health Professions Association
1314 Spring St. NW
Atlanta, GA 30309   Phone: (404) 872-7100
Description: Offers news and information on rheumatic disease and aids the Association in its goal of establishing a scientific base of knowledge for improving the quality and provision of health services to those suffering from it. Recurring features include news of research, practice, and trends; news of members; and news of Association events. **First Published:** 1965. **Frequency:** Quarterly.

★1799★   AICR NEWSLETTER
American Institute for Cancer Research
1759 R St. NW
Washington, DC 20009-2552   Phone: (202) 328-7744
Description: Examines the relationship between diet and cancer, recommending diet changes which may reduce cancer risks. Recurring features include health and nutrition information, news of research, and editorials. **First Published:** September 1983. **Frequency:** Quarterly.

★1800★   AIDS ALERT
American Health Consultants, Inc.
67 Peachtree Park Dr. NE
Atlanta, GA 30309-9990   Phone: (404) 262-2421
Description: Provides news and information on topics related to AIDS (Acquired Immune Deficiency Syndrome) and related conditions, including risks, hazards, costs, prevention, research, ethics, Center for Disease Control guidelines, and treatments. Recurring features include letters to the editor, interviews, news of research, notices of publications available, reports of meetings, and a calendar of events. **First Published:** January 1986. **Frequency:** Monthly. **ISSN:** 0887-0292.

★1801★   AIDS INFORMATION EXCHANGE
United States Conference of Mayors
1620 Eye St. NW
Washington, DC 20006   Phone: (202) 293-7330
Description: Covers local and community AIDS-related activities, policies, and government and school-based educational programs. Recurring features include a calendar of events, reports of meetings, and notices of publications available. **First Published:** June 1983. **Frequency:** Bimonthly.

★1802★   THE AIDS LETTER
Royal Society of Medicine
150 E. 58th St., 32nd Fl.
New York, NY 10155-0002   Phone: (212) 371-1150
Description: Disseminates information on recent advances which cover all aspects of AIDS (Acquired Immune Deficiency Syndrome) and HIV (the AIDS virus) in "an atmosphere free of commercial influence." Covers progress in research and immunization, the relationships between AIDS and drug abuse and sexuality and AIDS, and presents the responses of governments in countries around the world to AIDS. Contains articles on the reasons for and procedures involved in testing for the virus and dealing with AIDS in the workplace. Recurring features include news of research, reports of meetings, a calendar of events, and statistical updates. **First Published:** June 1987. **Frequency:** Bimonthly. **ISSN:** 0952-7427.

★1803★   AIDS POLICY AND LAW
Buraff Publications
Millin Publications, Inc.
1350 Connecticut Ave. NW
Washington, DC 20036   Phone: (202) 862-0926
Description: Reports on federal, state, and local news pertaining to the Acquired Immune Deficiency Syndrome (AIDS) virus. Discusses fair employment practices, litigation, legislation, regulation, policy guidelines, case studies, and interviews. Recurring features include news of research and summaries of state and federal legislation. **First Published:** January 29, 1986. **Frequency:** Biweekly. **ISSN:** 0887-1493.

★1804★   AIDS TARGETED INFORMATION NEWSLETTER
Williams & Wilkins
428 E. Preston St.
Baltimore, MD 21202
Description: Provides news and information on Acquired Immune Deficiency Syndrome (AIDS). **First Published:** 1987. **Frequency:** 4/yr.

★1805★   AIDS TREATMENT NEWS
ATN Publications
PO Box 411256
San Francisco, CA 94141   Phone: (415) 255-0588
Description: Presents news on the treatment of Acquired Immune Deficiency (AIDS). **First Published:** January 1987. **Frequency:** Semimonthly. **ISSN:** 1052-4207.

★1806★   AIDS UPDATE
Cancer Letter Inc.
PO Box 15189
Washington, DC 20003   Phone: (202) 543-7665
Description: Provides up-to-date information on HIV guidelines, research, and programs. Recurring features include calendar of events and news of research. **Frequency:** 48/yr. **ISSN:** 1042-4784.

★1807★   AIDS UPDATE
Lambda Legal Defense & Education Fund, Inc.
666 Broadway
New York, NY 10012-2317   Phone: (212) 995-8585
Description: Covers nationwide litigation, legislation, and advocacy grappling with legal problems occasioned by AIDS (Acquired Immune Deficiency Syndrome). Discusses AIDS-related aspects of confidentiality, criminal law, employment, and insurance. Features articles on public policy, access to care, and other HIV-related issues. **First Published:** December 1985. **Frequency:** 6/yr.

★1808★   AIDS WEEKLY
Charles W. Henderson
PO Box 5528
Atlanta, GA 30307-0528   Phone: (404) 377-8895
Description: Carries news, research, information on periodicals, and meetings on Acquired Immune Deficiency Syndrome (AIDS). Recurring features include news of research, reports of meetings, and a calendar of events. **First Published:** 1985. **Frequency:** Weekly. **ISSN:** 0884-903X.

★1809★   THE AIDS/HIV RECORD
Bio-Date Publishers
PO Box 66020
Washington, DC 20035   Phone: (202) 393-2437

★1810★   AIRWAVE
Manitoba Lung Association
629 McDermot Ave.
Winnipeg, MB, Canada R3A 1P6   Phone: (204) 774-5501
Description: Provides information concerning lung health. Focuses on asthma and chronic obstructive pulmonary disease. Recurring features include interviews, a calendar of events, book reviews, and a column titled Westman News. **Frequency:** 3/yr.

★1811★   ALAN GUTTMACHER INSTITUTE—WASHINGTON MEMO
Alan Guttmacher Institute
2010 Massachusetts Ave. NW
Washington, DC 20036   Phone: (202) 296-4012
Description: Covers legislative developments relating to family planning and reproductive health issues. Monitors federal appropriations for family planning and contraceptive research, congressional and court actions on abortion, international population assistance, teenage pregnancy, maternal health and pregnancy-related services, and other matters related to reproductive health and population issues in the U.S. and abroad. **First Published:** 1973. **Frequency:** Ca. 20/yr. **ISSN:** 0739-4179.

★1812★   AL-ANON/ALATEEN LONE MEMBER LETTER BOX
Al-Anon Family Group Headquarters, Inc.
Box 862, Midtown Sta.
New York, NY 10018-0862   Phone: (212) 302-7240
Description: Provides a forum for members of Al-Anon and Alateen who cannot regularly attend meetings to develop support correspondence with other Al-Anon and Alateen members. **Frequency:** Quarterly.

★1813★   AL-ANON IN INSTITUTIONS
Al-Anon Family Group Headquarters, Inc.
Box 862, Midtown Sta.
New York, NY 10018-0862   Phone: (212) 302-7240
Description: Relates experiences of members who introduce Al-Anon services to hospitals, treatment centers, correctional facilities, and other institutions. Recurring features include letters to the editor, news of

members, and columns titled Coordinator's Corner, Delegates Column, International Sharing, Alateen in Institutions, and Professionally Speaking. **First Published:** January 1974. **Frequency:** 3/yr. (March, July, and November). **ISSN:** 1054-142X.

★1814★ **AL-ANON SPEAKS OUT**
Al-Anon Family Group Headquarters, Inc.
Box 862, Midtown Sta.
New York, NY 10018-0862   Phone: (212) 302-7240
Description: Designed to inform professionals in the field of alcoholism and those in contact with families of alcoholics about the Al-Anon/Alateen program. Focuses on specific topics within the program and publications available through Al-Anon. **First Published:** 1978. **Frequency:** Semiannual (winter and summer). **ISSN:** 1054-1446.

★1815★ **ALASKA NURSE**
Alaska Nurses Association
237 E. 3rd Ave.
Anchorage, AL 99501
Description: Provides information on nursing and health. **First Published:** 1951. **Frequency:** Quarterly. **ISSN:** 0002-4546.

★1816★ **ALATEEN TALK**
Al-Anon Family Group Headquarters, Inc.
Box 862, Midtown Sta.
New York, NY 10018-0862   Phone: (212) 302-7240
Description: Publishes group information and personal sharings by Alateen members, who are adolescents whose lives have been adversely affected by someone else's drinking problem, usually a relative or friend. Recurring features include calendar of events. **First Published:** July 1964. **Frequency:** Bimonthly. **ISSN:** 1054-1411.

★1817★ **ALCOHOL AND DRUG ABUSE PULSE BEATS**
Insurance Field Company
PO Box 3006
Savannah, GA 31402-3006   Phone: (912) 355-4117
Description: Focuses on alcohol and drug abuse, providing information of current trends, legislative developments, and drug services and programs. Recurring features include columns titled Commentary, Top of the News, Prevention/Education, Intervention/Rehabilitation, and Enforcement/Corrections. **First Published:** January 1984. **Frequency:** Monthly.

★1818★ **ALCOHOL AND DRUG ABUSE REPORT**
National Association of State Alcohol and Drug Abuse Directors
444 N. Capitol St. NW, Ste. 642
Washington, DC 20001   Phone: (202) 783-6868
Description: Consists of alternating Special Report and Monthly Report issues. Summarizes federal and congressional issues related to alcohol and drug abuse in the Monthly Report; provides an in-depth analysis of national reports, papers, and concerns in the Special Report. Recurring features include news of research and of members. **First Published:** 1978. **Frequency:** Semimonthly.

★1819★ **ALCOHOL ISSUES INSIGHTS**
Beer Marketer's Insights, Inc.
51 Virginia Ave.
West Nyack, NY 10994   Phone: (914) 358-7751
Description: Provides information on issues concerning the use and misuse of alcohol. Covers such topics as misrepresentation in the media, minimum age requirements, advertising bans, deterrence of drunk driving, and the effects of tax increases on alcoholic beverage consumption. **First Published:** May 1984. **Frequency:** Monthly.

★1820★ **ALCOHOLISM AND DRUG ABUSE WEEKLY**
Manisses Communications Group, Inc.
Wayland Sq.
PO Box 3357
Providence, RI 02906-0359   Phone: (401) 831-6020
Description: Reports on state and private agencies on issues of importance to professionals in the field of alcohol and drug abuse. **First Published:** January 1989. **Frequency:** Weekly. **ISSN:** 1042-1394.

★1821★ **THE ALCOHOLISM REPORT**
National Council on Alcoholism and Drug Dependence
1511 K St. NW, Ste. 938
Washington, DC 20005   Phone: (202) 737-7342
Description: Reports on "national policy and funding developments in the field, covering the National Institute on Alcohol Abuse and Alcoholism as

well as activities elsewhere in the federal establishments and Congress." Discusses the effects of such decisions on alcohol and drug abuse programs. Recurring features include news of research, news of alcoholism professionals, and a calendar of events. **First Published:** 1972. **Frequency:** Monthly. **ISSN:** 0276-3613.

★1822★ **ALLEGHENY COUNTY PHARMACIST**
Allegheny County Pharmaceutical Association
111 Two Parkway Center
Pittsburgh, PA 15220   Phone: (412) 922-2440
Description: Covers various aspects of pharmacy and pharmaceuticals. **First Published:** 1947. **Frequency:** Monthly.

★1823★ **ALLERGY ALERT**
Allergy Foundation of Canada
PO Box 1904
Saskatoon, SK, Canada 57K 3S5   Phone: (306) 652-1608
Description: Covers topics of interest to allergic persons and their families. Recurring features include letters to the editor, news of research, book reviews, and columns titled Personal Glimpse, Food Facts, Product Reviews, Environmentally Yours, and Doctor Talk. **First Published:** 1981. **Frequency:** Quarterly.

★1824★ **ALLIED HEALTH EDUCATION NEWSLETTER**
American Medical Association
515 N. State St.
Chicago, IL 60601   Phone: (312) 464-4624
Description: Concerned with the accrediting activities engaged in by the Committee, which serves 2,850 allied health programs in 28 occupational areas. Recurring features include regulatory and legislative information. **Frequency:** Bimonthly.

★1825★ **ALPHA ACTION REPORTER**
Action League of Physically Handicapped Adults
1940 Oxford St. E., Ste. 8
London, ON, Canada N5V 2Z8   Phone: (519) 433-7221
Description: Provides information concerning issues that affect people with disabilities. **Frequency:** 6/yr.

★1826★ **ALPHA OMEGA INTERNATIONAL DENTAL FRATERNITY—LEADERSHIP NEWSLETTER**
Alpha Omega International Dental Fraternity
347 5th Ave.
New York, NY 10016   Phone: (212) 683-4155
Description: Provides news and information on dental education in the U.S. and Israel, on members' activities, and on the Alpha Omega Foundation. Carries announcements of awards to students and notices of seminars. Encourages fraternalism among dentists. **Frequency:** Quarterly.

★1827★ **ALS ASSOCIATION—LINK**
ALS Association
21021 Ventura Blvd., Ste. 321
Woodland Hills, CA 91364   Phone: (818) 991-2151
Description: Acts as a news service and forum for ideas and letters relating to Amyotrophic Lateral Sclerosis (ALS), a progressive, paralytic disease in which motor nerve cells cease functioning and often die. Highlights the latest research advancements, describes new publications, and evaluates fund-raising campaigns. Recurring features include letters to the editor, news of chapter events and activities, reports of meetings, notices of publications available, and book reviews. **First Published:** April 1987. **Frequency:** Bimonthly.

★1828★ **ALS NEWS**
Amyotrophic Lateral Sclerosis Society of Canada
250 Rogers Rd.
Toronto, ON, Canada M6E 1R1   Phone: (416) 656-5242
Description: Contains news of patients and research developments related to amyotrophic lateral sclerosis (ALS), a degenerative disorder that causes a progressive deterioration of the nerve cells that control muscle movement. Recurring features include interviews, a calendar of events, reports of meetings, and book reviews. **First Published:** 1978. **Frequency:** Quarterly.

★1829★ **ALS NEWSLETTER**
Amyotrophic Lateral Sclerosis Society of British Columbia
411 Dunsmuir St.
Vancouver, BC, Canada V6B 1X4   Phone: (604) 685-0737
Description: Provides medical information and news items on amyotroph-

ic lateral sclerosis (ALS), a degenerative disorder that causes a progressive deterioration of the nerve cells responsible for muscle movement. Reports on research projects and epidemiological studies. Recurring features include interviews, advice, fund raising efforts, a calendar of events, reports of meetings, medical articles, special events, honors, and awards. **First Published:** 1982. **Frequency:** Quarterly.

★1830★   ALTERNATIVE HEALTH THERAPIES
Science of Mind Church Counseling & Healing Center
PO Box 32236
Washington, DC 20007   Phone: (202) 333-6354
Description: Furnishes news on alternative forms of health therapies. Provides information on co-dependency, compulsive eating disorders, psychic consultations, self-esteem, self-nurturing, and spiritual prayer networks. Recurring features include a calendar of events and book reviews.

★1831★   ALTERNATIVES
Mountain Home Publishing
PO Box 829
Ingram, TX 78025   Phone: (512) 367-4492
Description: Gives laymen and health and medical professionals news and information on new discoveries occurring in the field of natural health care. Analyzes the uses of nutritional and health food products in the prevention and treatment of ailments. Also discusses natural alternatives to drugs and surgery and early detection of health problems. Recurring features include columns titled Kitchen Quicks and Mailbox, a question-and-answer column on health topics. **Frequency:** Monthly. **ISSN:** 0893-5025.

**★1832★   ALTERNATIVES FOR THE HEALTH CONSCIOUS
       INDIVIDUAL**
Mountain Home Publishing
PO Box 829
Ingram, TX 78025   Phone: (512) 367-4492
Description: Emphasizes natural therapies and self-help techniques to obtain optimal health without the use of drugs or surgery. Provides information regarding specific nutritional supplements, diets, exercises, and therapies for the prevention and/or treatment of various health conditions. Recurring features include letters to the editor and news of research. **First Published:** June 1985. **Frequency:** Monthly. **ISSN:** 0893-5025.

★1833★   ALZHEIMER FAMILY PROGRAM NEWSLETTER
Center for Aging
University of Alabama at Birmingham
933 19th St. S., Rm. 201
Birmingham, AL 35294-2041   Phone: (205) 934-2178
Description: Contains articles on coping with Alzheimer's Disease, strategies for care, and local resources. Recurring features include news of research and a calendar of events. **First Published:** 1980. **Frequency:** Monthly.

**★1834★   ALZHEIMER SOCIETY OF METROPOLITAN
       TORONTO—NEWSLETTER**
Alzheimer Society of Metropolitan Toronto
980 Yonge St., Ste. 301
Toronto, ON, Canada M4W 2J5   Phone: (416) 966-0700
Frequency: Quarterly.

★1835★   ALZHEIMER'S ASSOCIATION NEWSLETTER
Alzheimer's Association
919 N. Michigan Ave., Ste. 1000
Chicago, IL 60611-1676   Phone: (312) 335-8700
Description: Promotes the work of the Association, which is dedicated to supporting research into the causes, cure, and treatment of Alzheimer's disease, and to provide support and assistance. Recurring features include articles on research grants, chapter and member news, legal and financial issues, public policy, advocacy updates, and Association fundraising news. **First Published:** November 1981. **Frequency:** Quarterly.

★1836★   ALZHEIMER'S RESEARCH REVIEW
American Health Assistance Foundation
15825 Shady Grove Rd., Ste. 140
Rockville, MD 20850   Phone: (301) 948-3244
Description: Highlights the work of Alzheimer's disease researchers and provides tips for families dealing with Alzheimer's. Recurring features include news of research and columns titled From the President, Reader's

Exchange, and Ask the Experts. **First Published:** Spring 1986. **Frequency:** Quarterly.

★1837★   AMBULATORY ANESTHESIA NEWSLETTER
Society for Ambulatory Anesthesia
515 Busse Hwy.
Park Ridge, IL 60068   Phone: (312) 825-5586
Description: Reports on the educational and scientific work of the Society, which represents anesthesiologists who specialize in ambulatory anesthesia care in the U.S. Recurring features include editorials, letters to the editor, news of members, and a calendar of events. **First Published:** January 1986. **Frequency:** Quarterly.

**★1838★   AMBULATORY PEDIATRIC ASSOCIATION—
       NEWSLETTER**
Ambulatory Pediatric Association
6728 Old McLean Village
McLean, VA 22101   Phone: (703) 556-9222
Description: Publishes news of the members, activities, and concerns of the Association, "an organization devoted to promoting the health of children." Provides up-to-date information on efforts in affecting legislation concerned with child abuse, medical care for handicapped newborns, the nuclear arms freeze, and funding for pediatric care. Recurring features include a message from the president and announcements of available financial awards and fellowships. **Frequency:** 3/yr.

★1839★   AMCRA'S MANAGED CARE MONITOR
American Managed Care and Review Association
1227 25 St. NW, Ste. 610
Washington, DC 20037   Phone: (202) 728-0506
Description: Concerned with the delivery of better and more appropriate and economical medical care. Examines a specific topic in each issue, such as utilization review or technology assessment. Recurring features include a job bank section and columns titled From the Hill, Members in the News, and Legal Beat. **First Published:** 1970. **Frequency:** 8/yr.

★1840★   AMECD NEWSNOTES
Association for Measurement and Evaluation in Counseling and
    Development
Dept. of Counselor and Adult Education
East Carolina University
Greenville, NC 27858   Phone: (919) 757-4218
Description: Contains information about AMECD and other related divisions of the American Association for Counseling and Development. Carries articles on measurement, assessment, evaluation, and research in relation to guidance and counseling in human development. **First Published:** January 1965. **Frequency:** 4/yr.

**★1841★   AMERICAN ACADEMY OF ALLERGY AND
       IMMUNOLOGY—NEWS & NOTES**
American Academy of Allergy and Immunology
611 E. Wells St.
Milwaukee, WI 53202   Phone: (414) 272-6071
Description: Supports Academy efforts "to advance the knowledge and practice of allergy, foster the education of students and the public, encourage union and cooperation among those working in the field, and promote and stimulate research and the study of allergic disease." Recurring features include Academy news, a calendar of conferences and seminars, news of research, statistics, and obituaries. **First Published:** 1943. **Frequency:** Quarterly. **ISSN:** 0899-7489.

**★1842★   AMERICAN ACADEMY OF CHILD AND
       ADOLESCENT PSYCHIATRY—NEWSLETTER**
American Academy of Child and Adolescent Psychiatry
3615 Wisconsin Ave. NW
Washington, DC 20016   Phone: (202) 966-7300
Description: Publishes news of the Academy, child and adolescent psychiatrists, and AACAP members. Focuses on the practice of child and adolescent psychiatry. Recurring features include letters to the editor, legislative updates, news of research, statistics, and announcements of open positions. **First Published:** 1973. **Frequency:** 4/yr.

**★1843★   AMERICAN ACADEMY OF IMPLANT DENTISTRY—
       NEWSLETTER**
American Academy of Implant Dentistry
6900 Grove Rd.
Thorofare, NJ 08086   Phone: (609) 848-7027
Description: Covers current activities in the field of implant dentistry,

particularly the educational programs of the Academy. **First Published:** 1975. **Frequency:** Quarterly.

★1844★ AMERICAN ACADEMY OF OSTEOPATHY—
QUARTERLY NEWSLETTER
American Academy of Osteopathy
12 W. Locust St.
PO Box 750
Newark, OH 43055   Phone: (614) 349-8701
Description: Reports on the activities of the Academy and its members. **First Published:** 1937. **Frequency:** Quarterly.

★1845★ AMERICAN ACADEMY OF OTOLARYNGOLOGY-
HEAD AND NECK SURGERY—BULLETIN
American Academy of Otolaryngology-Head and Neck Surgery, Inc.
1 Prince St.
Alexandria, VA 22314   Phone: (703) 836-4444
Description: Reports governmental and socio-economic news of interest to otolaryngology-head and neck surgeons. Covers Academy activities, continuing education and job opportunities, and pertinent publications. Recurring features include news of members, editorials, letters to the editor, news of research, and a calendar of events. **First Published:** January 1982. **Frequency:** Monthly. **ISSN:** 0731-8359.

★1846★ AMERICAN ALLIANCE FOR HEALTH, PHYSICAL
EDUCATION, RECREATION, AND DANCE—UPDATE
American Alliance for Health, Physical Education, Recreation, and Dance
1900 Association Dr.
Reston, VA 22091-1599   Phone: (703) 476-3484
Description: Provides news and information on the Alliance. Discusses current issues and research in the areas of health, physical education, recreation, dance, fitness, and adapted physical education. Recurring features include news of research, a calendar of events, reports of meetings, news of educational opportunities, job listings, notices of publications available, and columns titled President's Message and District and State News. **First Published:** 1970. **Frequency:** 8/yr.

★1847★ AMERICAN ANOREXIA/BULIMIA ASSOCIATION—
NEWSLETTER
American Anorexia/Bulimia Association, Inc.
418 E. 76th St.
New York, NY 10021   Phone: (201) 734-1114
Description: Features articles on the symptoms, causes, and treatment of the eating disorders anorexia and bulimia. Carries news of research in the field, book reviews, and information about the services and activities of the Association. Recurring features include reprints of letters, news of conferences, notices of publications available, a calendar of events, and a column titled Therapist's Corner. **Frequency:** 4/yr.

★1848★ AMERICAN ART THERAPY ASSOCIATION—
NEWSLETTER
American Art Therapy Association, Inc.
1202 Allanson Rd.
Mundelein, IL 60060   Phone: (708) 949-6064
Description: Publishes news of developments and events in art therapy. Provides information on Association activities, related organizations, and available resources. Recurring features include legislative updates, editorials, letters to the editor, news of members, and a calendar of events. **First Published:** 1974. **Frequency:** Quarterly.

★1849★ AMERICAN ASSOCIATION OF CORRECTIONAL
PSYCHOLOGY—NEWSLETTER
American Association of Correctional Psychology
c/o Robert Smith, Ed.D.
West Virginia College of Graduate Studies
Institute, WV 25112   Phone: (304) 766-2000
Description: Provides information of interest to psychologists and other mental health professionals concerned with all aspects of the criminal justice system, including probation, parole, forensics, law enforcement, and adult and juvenile offenders in institutional and community programs. Includes news of the Association. **First Published:** 1969. **Frequency:** Quarterly.

★1850★ AMERICAN ASSOCIATION OF GYNECOLOGICAL
LAPAROSCOPISTS—NEWS SCOPE
American Association of Gynecological Laparoscopists
13021 E. Florence Ave.
Santa Fe Springs, CA 90670   Phone: (213) 946-8774
Description: Provides a forum for the exchange of information and ideas on the practice and ethics of gynecological laparoscopy. Carries new information on teaching practices and medical standards of the procedures. Recurring features include news of members, news of research, and editorials. **Frequency:** Annually.

★1851★ AMERICAN ASSOCIATION OF HOSPITAL
DENTISTS—INTERFACE
American Association of Hospital Dentists
211 E. Chicago Ave.
Chicago, IL 60611   Phone: (312) 440-2661
Description: Carries information about trends, legislation, policy changes, and issues that affect the practices of hospital dentists. Recurring features include Association news, news of research, a calendar of events, and columns titled Fellowships, Funding, Sources, In Brief, and What to Write For. **First Published:** August 1985. **Frequency:** Quarterly. **ISSN:** 0887-6304.

★1852★ AMERICAN ASSOCIATION ON MENTAL
RETARDATION—NEWS & NOTES
American Association on Mental Retardation
1719 Kalorama Rd. NW
Washington, DC 20009   Phone: (202) 387-1968
Description: Carries news on topics relating to the field of mental retardation and developmental disabilities. Reports on legislation, litigation, model programs, research, and news of the Association's state, regional, and national activities. Recurring features include letters to the editor, a calendar of events, reports of meetings, and news of educational opportunities. Also carries job listings, notices of publications available, and columns titled Viewpoint, Programs in Focus, International Viewpoint, and Legal and Social Issues. **First Published:** September 1987. **Frequency:** Bimonthly. **ISSN:** 0895-8033.

★1853★ AMERICAN ASSOCIATION OF ORTHODONTISTS—
BULLETIN
American Association of Orthodontists
460 N. Lindbergh Blvd.
St. Louis, MO 63141   Phone: (314) 993-1700
Description: Provides news and information on the Association. Recurring features include a calendar of events, reports of meetings, news of educational opportunities, and notices of publications available. **Frequency:** Bimonthly.

★1854★ AMERICAN ASSOCIATION OF SENIOR
PHYSICIANS—NEWSLETTER
American Association of Senior Physicians
515 N. State St., 14th Fl.
Chicago, IL 60610   Phone: (312) 464-2460
Description: Focuses on successful retirement for physicians. Supplies information on finances, social security, taxes, residence relocation, closing a medical practice, travel opportunities, estate considerations, and related subjects. **First Published:** 1976. **Frequency:** Bimonthly.

★1855★ AMERICAN ASSOCIATION OF SUICIDOLOGY—
NEWSLINK
American Association of Suicidology
2459 S. Ash
Denver, CO 80222   Phone: (303) 692-0985
Description: Serves to update Association members on advances in the study of suicide prevention and related self-destructive behaviors. Contains book reviews, news of the Association and its members, and a calendar of events. **First Published:** 1972. **Frequency:** Quarterly.

★1856★ AMERICAN ASSOCIATION OF TISSUE BANKS—
NEWSLETTER
American Association of Tissue Banks
1350 Beverly Rd., Ste. 220-A
McLean, VA 22101   Phone: (703) 827-9582
Description: Publishes news of the Association, whose purposes are "to promote scientific and technical knowledge concerning the recovery, processing, storage, transplantation, and evaluation of cells, tissues, and organs, and to make available through regional tissue bank programs safe, adequate, and economical materials for clinical and research purposes." Recurring features include a calendar of events and news of meetings,

members, and research. **First Published:** 1979. **Frequency:** Quarterly. **ISSN:** 0270-2673.

★1857★ AMERICAN ASSOCIATION OF WOMEN DENTISTS—CHRONICLE
American Association of Women Dentists
401 N. Michigan Ave.
Chicago, IL 60611-4267   Phone: (312) 644-6610
Description: Discusses Association news of interest to women dentists and women dental students. Includes short articles on scholarships, conferences, awards, and regional career and education opportunities. Also lists addresses and telephone numbers of officers, district chairs, and committees of the Association. Recurring features include news of research, book reviews, statistics, obituaries, and the column President's Message. **Frequency:** Bimonthly.

★1858★ AMERICAN BRAIN TUMOR ASSOCIATION—MESSAGE LINE
American Brain Tumor Association
3725 N. Talman Ave.
Chicago, IL 60618   Phone: (312) 286-5571
Description: Disseminates patient education information on brain tumors and brain tumor research. Also reports on the Association's efforts to raise funds for such research. Recurring features include notices of publications available. **First Published:** 1974. **Frequency:** 3/yr.

★1859★ AMERICAN COLLEGE OF APOTHECARIES—NEWSLETTER
American College of Apothecaries
205 Daingerfield Rd.
Alexandria, VA 22314   Phone: (703) 684-8603
Description: Presents national pharmacy news designed to assist Association members in their professional practices. Covers Association news, including items on membership, chapters, committees, elections, and conferences. Recurring features include book reviews and a necrology. **First Published:** 1940. **Frequency:** Monthly.

★1860★ AMERICAN COLLEGE OF DENTISTS—NEWS & VIEWS
American College of Dentists
7315 Wisconsin Ave., Ste. 352N
Bethesda, MD 20814   Phone: (301) 986-0555
Description: Presents accounts of College meetings, as well as remarks from the College's president. Publishes notices of scheduled events, spotlights individuals recognized or given awards by the College, and profiles convocation speakers. Recurring features include reports of meetings. **First Published:** 1973. **Frequency:** Quarterly.

★1861★ AMERICAN COLLEGE OF LEGAL MEDICINE—NEWSLETTER
American College of Legal Medicine
PO Box 3190
Maple Glen, PA 19002   Phone: (215) 646-6800
Description: Promotes advances in the field of medical jurisprudence. Presents information on the activities, programs, and members of the College. **First Published:** January 1970. **Frequency:** 4/yr.

★1862★ AMERICAN COLLEGE OF OSTEOPATHIC PEDIATRICIANS—NEWSLETTER
American College of Osteopathic Pediatricians
172 W. State St.
Trenton, NJ 06608   Phone: (609) 393-3350
Description: Concerned primarily with new regulations and sources of information in the field of osteopathic pediatrics. Recurring features include news of members, a calendar of events, and news of research. **Frequency:** Quarterly.

★1863★ AMERICAN COLLEGE OF PROSTHODONTISTS—NEWSLETTER
American College of Prosthodontists
2907 Deer Ledge
San Antonio, TX 78230   Phone: (512) 567-6450
Description: Publishes news of the College, which seeks to improve prosthodontic treatment for patients by encouraging educational activities designed to bring new ideas, techniques, and research into clinical practice. Provides news of members and College activities. Recurring features include editorials, news of research, letters to the editor, journal and book

reviews, a calendar of events, and president's and secretary's reports. **First Published:** 1971. **Frequency:** 4/yr. **ISSN:** 0736-346X.

★1864★ AMERICAN COLLEGE OF VETERINARY PATHOLOGISTS—NEWSLETTER
American College of Veterinary Pathologists
Department of Pathology
College of Vet. Med. Bio. Sci.
Colorado State University
Fort Collins, CO 80523   Phone: (303) 491-0599
Description: Covers developments in veterinary pathology and association news. Recurring features include a calendar of events, statistics, obituaries, calls for papers, and announcements of certification examinations. **First Published:** 1951. **Frequency:** 4/yr.

★1865★ AMERICAN DENTISTS FOR FOREIGN SERVICE—NEWSLETTER
American Dentists for Foreign Service, Inc.
619 Church Ave.
Brooklyn, NY 11218   Phone: (718) 436-8686
Description: Summarizes events of the Organization from the previous six months. Includes income, expenses, and support services reports, and correspondence letters.

★1866★ AMERICAN GERIATRICS SOCIETY—NEWSLETTER
American Geriatrics Society
770 Lexington Ave., Ste. 400
New York, NY 10021   Phone: (212) 308-1414
Description: Carries current information on legislative issues, meetings, symposia, seminars, and continuing education programs in geriatrics for physicians and others interested in health care for the elderly. Recurring features include a public policy update, news of the Society and its members, announcements of fellowships and scholarships available, and a calendar of events. **First Published:** April 1972. **Frequency:** Bimonthly.

★1867★ AMERICAN GROUP PRACTICE ASSOCIATION—EXECUTIVE NEWS SERVICE
American Group Practice Association
1422 Duke St.
Alexandria, VA 22314   Phone: (703) 838-0033
Description: Examines health policy and socio-economic and legislative and regulatory issues affecting physicians. Discusses Medicare, Medicaid, physician reimbursement, health maintenance organizations, and cost containment. Recurring features include editorials, news of research, news of members, a calendar of events, and columns titled In the News, Conferences, and Publications. **First Published:** February 1981. **Frequency:** 22/yr.

★1868★ AMERICAN GROUP PSYCHOTHERAPY ASSOCIATION—NEWSLETTER
American Group Psychotherapy Association
25 E. 21st St.
New York, NY 10010-6207   Phone: (212) 787-2618
Description: Presents psychotherapists and other mental health professionals with news of developments in the field of group psychotherapy. Recurring features include Association and committee reports, editorials, news of members, letters to the editor, news of research, notices of new publications, and a calendar of events. **First Published:** 1959. **Frequency:** 3/yr.

★1869★ AMERICAN HEARING RESEARCH FOUNDATION—NEWSLETTER
American Hearing Research Foundation
55 E. Washington St., Ste. 2022
Chicago, IL 60602   Phone: (312) 726-9670
Description: Reviews the latest developments in hearing research and education. Discusses the problems of the hearing impaired. **First Published:** January 1970. **Frequency:** 3/yr.

★1870★ AMERICAN HERB ASSOCIATION—QUARTERLY NEWSLETTER
American Herb Association
PO Box 1673
Nevada City, CA 95959
Description: Represents an international network of herbalists, both lay persons and professionals. Discusses herbal use in the areas of food and medicine, as well as herbal quality and related environmental problems. Recurring features include letters to the editor, interviews, news of

research, news of educational opportunities, and notices of publications available. Also includes book reviews, a calendar of events, and columns titled Legal Concerns, Foreign Correspondents, Herbal Clippings, and In the Leaves. **First Published:** Fall 1981. **Frequency:** Quarterly.

★1871★ AMERICAN HOSPITAL ASSOCIATION—OUTREACH
American Hospital Association
840 N. Lake Shore Dr.
Chicago, IL 60611   Phone: (312) 280-5921
Description: Analyzes the factors influencing market supply, demand, and competition. Recurring features include statistics, details on the latest accreditation standards, reviews of current literature, education and technical assistance updates, news of research, and resources. **First Published:** January 1980. **Frequency:** Bimonthly. **ISSN:** 0270-207X.

★1872★ AMERICAN INSTITUTE OF STRESS—NEWSLETTER
American Institute of Stress, Inc.
124 Park Ave.
Yonkers, NY 10703   Phone: (914) 963-1200
Description: Focuses on the Institute's concern for development of methods for the measurement and reduction of stress. Carries news of research, book reviews, listings of resource materials, and reports of meetings and conferences related to stress. **First Published:** September 1983. **Frequency:** Monthly. **ISSN:** 1047-2517.

★1873★ THE AMERICAN ISSUE
American Council on Alcohol Problems
3426 Bridgeland Dr.
Bridgeton, MO 63044   Phone: (314) 739-5944
Description: Focuses on alcoholism and the problems of alcohol addiction and its prevention. Contains news of state affiliates' activities, national developments in the treatment and prevention of alcoholism, and occasional items on abuse of other illicit drugs. **First Published:** 1895. **Frequency:** Monthly.

★1874★ AMERICAN OCCUPATIONAL THERAPY ASSOCIATION—FEDERAL REPORT
American Occupational Therapy Association
1383 Piccard Dr.
PO Box 1725
Rockville, MD 20850   Phone: (301) 948-9626
Description: Analyzes legislative and regulatory issues related to occupational therapy, primarily Medicare and Medicaid. Carries information on health care inflation, cost reimbursement for hospitals, the prospective payment system, taxes, physician competition, rehabilitation services, hospitals, home health agencies, skilled nursing facilities, and health planning. **First Published:** January 1973. **Frequency:** Bimonthly.

★1875★ AMERICAN ORTHODONTIC SOCIETY—NEWSLETTER
American Orthodontic Society
9550 Forest Lane, Ste. 215
Dallas, TX 75243   Phone: (214) 343-0805
Description: Publishes news of the Society, whose purpose is "to provide quality orthodontic education in order to allow general dentists and pedodontists to expand their horizons and provide more services to their patients." Mainly concerned with promoting educational programs and courses in orthodontia. **First Published:** 1975. **Frequency:** Quarterly.

★1876★ AMERICAN ORTHOPSYCHIATRIC ASSOCIATION—NEWSLETTER
American Orthopsychiatric Association
19 W. 44th St., Ste. 1616
New York, NY 10036   Phone: (212) 354-5770
Description: Intended for members of the Association, who are concerned with the early signs of mental and behavioral disorder and preventive psychiatry. Provides news notes and feature articles on the trends, issues, and events that concern mental health, as well as Association news. **Frequency:** Triennially.

★1877★ AMERICAN PARKINSON DISEASE ASSOCIATION—NEWSLETTER
American Parkinson Disease Association
60 Bay St., Ste. 401
Staten Island, NY 10301-2514   Phone: (718) 981-8001
Description: Provides updates on the symptoms and treatments of Parkinson's disease and on current research in the field. Also discusses patients' problems in coping with the disease and the support services available.

Recurring features include news of the Association and its members, book reviews, a calendar of events, and a column titled In Response to Reader's Questions. **First Published:** September 1979. **Frequency:** Quarterly.

★1878★ THE AMERICAN PSYCHOANALYST—NEWSLETTER
American Psychoanalytic Association
309 E. 49th St.
New York, NY 10022   Phone: (212) 752-0450
Description: Covers developments in psychoanalysis for those in the profession. Presents news of the Association, announces winners of grants and awards, and reports on conferences and other institutes. **First Published:** 1967. **Frequency:** Quarterly.

★1879★ AMERICAN PSYCHOLOGICAL ASSOCIATION—NETWORK
Office of Educational Affairs
1200 17th St. NW
Washington, DC 20036   Phone: (202) 955-7721
Description: Publishes articles discussing teaching practices, classroom activities, and computer software and other technological aids for psychology instructors. Recurring features include interviews, a calendar of events, news of research, book reviews, and a column titled For the Asking containing reprints of timely articles. **Frequency:** 3/yr.

★1880★ AMERICAN SOCIETY FOR ADOLESCENT PSYCHIATRY—NEWSLETTER
American Society for Adolescent Psychiatry
4330 East West Hwy., No 1117
Bethesda, MD 20814   Phone: (301) 718-6502
Description: Contains articles about adolescent psychiatry and Society news. Recurring features include news of research, a calendar of events, and book reviews. **First Published:** 1968. **Frequency:** 4/yr.

★1881★ AMERICAN SOCIETY OF ALLIED HEALTH PROFESSIONS—TRENDS
American Society of Allied Health Professions
1101 Connecticut Ave. NW, Ste. 700
Washington, DC 20036   Phone: (202) 857-1150
Description: Discusses the educational programs, grants and funding, and employment opportunities available to those employed in allied health professions. Examines the achievements of allied health professionals as well as the effects and implications of their work. Recurring features include Society news and legislative, organizational, and institutional updates. **Frequency:** Monthly.

★1882★ AMERICAN SOCIETY OF CLINICAL HYPNOSIS—NEWS LETTER
American Society of Clinical Hypnosis
2250 E. Devon Ave., Ste. 336
Des Plaines, IL 60018   Phone: (708) 297-3317
Description: Reflects the aims of the Society, which include promoting "the acceptance of hypnosis as an important tool of ethical clinical medicine and scientific research." Also seeks to provide members with assistance in increasing their knowledge of the basic techniques of psychiatry and in improving their communication with patients. Recurring features include notices of significant conferences, workshops, and meetings, and news of members. **First Published:** 1959. **Frequency:** 6/yr.

★1883★ AMERICAN SOCIETY FOR DENTAL AESTHETICS—NEWSLETTER
American Society for Dental Aesthetics
635 Madison Ave., 12th Floor
New York, NY 10022   Phone: (212) 371-4575
Description: Focuses on upcoming meetings and lectures of interest to ASDA members. Includes contributed items of a technical nature from members, discussing current projects, techniques, and products. Recurring features include interviews, news of research, a calendar of events, and columns titled But Paul You Can't Do That, Implants, Photography, The President Speaks, and Office Management. **First Published:** Spring 1972. **Frequency:** Biennially.

★1884★ AMERICAN SOCIETY FOR GERIATRIC DENTISTRY—NEWSLETTER
American Society for Geriatric Dentistry
211 East Chicago Ave.
Chicago, IL 60611   Phone: (212) 343-2100
Description: Publishes news of geriatric dentistry as well as the Society, its members and activities. Recurring features include legislative updates, a

calendar of events, news of members, book reviews, editorials, a message from the president, bibliographies, and biographies. **First Published:** January 1981. **Frequency:** Quarterly.

★1885★ AMERICAN SOCIETY OF HAND THERAPISTS— NEWSLETTER
American Society of Hand Therapists
1002 Vandora Springs Rd., Ste. 101
Garner, NC 27529   Phone: (919) 779-2748
Description: Promotes excellence in hand rehabilitation by publishing information to improve treatment techniques and standardize hand evaluation and care. Acts as a forum for communication among therapists. Recurring features include news of research and news of members. **First Published:** 1979. **Frequency:** Bimonthly.

★1886★ AMERICAN SOCIETY OF OPHTHALMIC REGISTERED NURSES—INSIGHT
American Society of Ophthalmic Registered Nurses
PO Box 193030
San Francisco, CA 94119   Phone: (415) 561-8513
Description: Designed to facilitate continuing education of registered nurses through the study, discussion, and exchange of knowledge, experience, and ideas in the field of ophthalmology. Features news of research and innovations in the field. **First Published:** 1977. **Frequency:** Bimonthly.

★1887★ AMFAR REPORT
American Foundation for AIDS Research
1515 Broadway, Ste. 3601
New York, NY 10036-8901   Phone: (212) 719-0033
Description: Covers news of the foundation, which is concerned with "developing an AIDS vaccine, improved treatments for AIDS, and, ultimately, a cure." Contains articles on such issues as fund raising, AIDS education, and medical advances. Recurring features include a calendar of events, news of members, and news of research. **Frequency:** 3/yr.

★1888★ AMHCA ADVOCATE
American Mental Health Counselors Association
5999 Stevenson Ave.
Alexandria, VA 22304   Phone: (703) 823-9800
Description: Publishes news of the programs, members, and activities of AMHCA. Provides updates on AMHCA efforts regarding credentialing of counselors, mental health-related legislation, and insurance coverage of the expenses of mental health counseling. Recurring features include news of meetings and conferences and a call for papers. **First Published:** 1980. **Frequency:** Monthly.

★1889★ AMI QUEBEC NEWSLETTER
Alliance for the Mentally Ill
PO Box 145
Cote-Des-Neiges
Montreal, PQ, Canada H35 2S5   Phone: (514) 486-1448
Description: Features new laws and events affecting the mentally ill. Includes notices and reports of meetings, lectures, and seminars. Provides news and schedules of AMI-Quebec. Recurring features include news of research and notices of publications available. **First Published:** 1979. **Frequency:** 4/yr.

★1890★ THE AMP
National Amputation Foundation
12-45 150th St.
Whitestone, NY 11357   Phone: (718) 767-0596
Description: Serves amputees, civilians, and veterans. Carries information on programs and events for amputees, profiles of personalities, and news of the activities of the Foundation. **First Published:** 1919. **Frequency:** Monthly.

★1891★ AMPLIFICATIONS
The Perkin-Elmer Corp.
761 Main Ave.
Norwalk, CT 06859-0251   Phone: (800) 762-4001
Description: Discusses polymerase chain reaction (PCR), a process through which deoxyribonucleic acid (DNA) is extracted from blood and cells for amplification of sequences. Includes news of research and developments and a queries column. **First Published:** 1989. **Frequency:** Quarterly.

★1892★ AMPLIFIER
American Psychological Association
c/o Dr. Roger Klein
SC-01 Forbes Quad.
University of Pittsburgh
Pittsburgh, PA 15260   Phone: (504) 865-5820
Description: Focuses on media psychology, which examines the influence of the media on people's attitude, behavior, and well-being and encourages use of the media in the prevention of physical and mental disorders. Recurring features include news of the Association and its members, film and book reviews, news of research, editorials, letters to the editor, and a calendar of events. **First Published:** 1982. **Frequency:** Quarterly.

★1893★ AMSA NEWS: LESBIAN AND GAY PEOPLE IN MEDICINE
Lesbian, Gay and Bisexual People in Medicine
American Medical Student Association
1890 Preston White Dr.
Reston, VA 22091   Phone: (703) 620-6600
Description: Addresses the problems facing gay and lesbian medical students, physicians, and patients and promotes the benefits of interaction and communication as a means of solving those problems. Publishes pertinent medical news and news of the Task Force and the American Medical Student Association. Recurring features include news of members, book reviews, a calendar of events, and essays describing personal experiences of members. **First Published:** September 1977. **Frequency:** 6/yr.

★1894★ AN OUNCE OF PREVENTION
Society of Prospective Medicine
PO Box 55110
Indianapolis, IN 46205-0110   Phone: (317) 549-3600
Description: Addresses the Society's concern for health promotion and the application of health risk assessment instrumentation. Recurring features include discussions of medical topics and research, Society updates, editorials, news of members, and a calendar of events. **First Published:** January 1976. **Frequency:** Quarterly. **ISSN:** 0733-1762.

★1895★ ANDREWS SCHOOL ASBESTOS ALERT
Andrews Publications, Inc.
PO Box 1000
Westtown, PA 19395   Phone: (215) 399-6600
Description: Alerts school districts to current legal proceedings, construction, and medical problems relating to exposure to asbestos in schools. Also monitors Environmental Protection Agency (EPA) and state government regulations. **First Published:** September 1984. **Frequency:** Monthly. **ISSN:** 0887-7866.

★1896★ ANIMAL CARE NEWSLETTER
Animal Care Program
Arizona State University
Tempe, AZ 85287-0608   Phone: (602) 965-4386
Description: Provides news and information on federal regulations and rules and regulations governing animal care and use in teaching research. **First Published:** 1986. **Frequency:** Quarterly.

★1897★ ANIMAL DEFENCE LEAGUE OF CANADA—NEWS BULLETIN
Animal Defence League of Canada
PO Box 3880, Sta. C
Ottawa, ON, Canada K1Y 4M5   Phone: (613) 233-6117
Description: Provides information on animal welfare and rights to increase public awareness and to educate, offer alternatives to, and reduce/eliminate "animal exploitation, cruelty, and suffering." Recurring features include a calendar of events, reports of meetings, updates on the League's activities, and news from the movement. **Frequency:** Biennially. **ISSN:** 0044-829X.

★1898★ ANIMAL PROTECTION DIVISION—ADVOCATE
Animal Protection Division
American Humane Association
63 Inverness Dr. E.
Englewood, CO 80112   Phone: (303) 792-9900
Description: Concerned with all aspects of animal protection, domestic and wild. Examines society's treatment of animals and programs demonstrating care and commitment to all forms of life. Reports on legislation, hearings, and lobbying efforts. Recurring features include reviews of films according to their treatment of animals, a listing of current animal-related legislation, and information on animal welfare and pet care and behavior. **Frequency:** Quarterly.

★1899★ THE ANIMAL RIGHTS REPORTER
Perceptions Press, Inc.
4200 Wisconsin Ave. NW, Ste. 106/345
Washington, DC 20016   Phone: (202) 331-3360
Description: Details protests, boycotts, infiltrations, legislative pressures, and regulatory developments concerning animal rights. Reports on animal rights groups and leaders, and their goals, tactics, and foibles. **First Published:** October 1988. **Frequency:** Semimonthly. **ISSN:** 0898-7599.

★1900★ ANIMALDOM
Pennsylvania SPCA
350 E. Erie Ave.
Philadelphia, PA 19134   Phone: (215) 426-6300
Description: Concerned with animal welfare. **First Published:** 1930. **Frequency:** Monthly.

★1901★ ANNUAL AMYLOID
Arthritis Center
Boston University
5th Floor Conte Bldg.
71 E. Newton St.
Boston, MA 02118   Phone: (617) 424-5154
Description: Discusses amyloid research. **First Published:** 1984. **Frequency:** Annual.

★1902★ ANNUAL SCIENTIFIC SESSION NEWS
American College of Cardiology
9111 Old Georgetown Rd.
Bethesda, MD 20814   Phone: (301) 897-5400
Description: Hightlights advances and news in the field of cardiology. Includes feature articles and coverage of meeting presentations. **First Published:** 1982. **Frequency:** 5/yr.

★1903★ ANR UPDATE
Americans for Nonsmokers' Rights
2530 San Pablo Ave., Ste. J
Berkeley, CA 94702   Phone: (415) 841-3032
Description: Contains news of efforts to restrict smoking and access to cigarettes through local, state, and federal legislation as well as private sector policy. Monitors activities of tobacco industry lobbyists and other special interest organizations. Recurring features include letters to the editor. **Frequency:** Quarterly.

★1904★ THE ANTIMICROBIC NEWSLETTER
Elsevier Science Publishing Company, Inc.
655 Avenue of the Americas
New York, NY 10017   Phone: (212) 989-3927
Description: Focuses on laboratory and clinical evaluations of newly formulated and established antimicrobics in order to aid in the delivery of rational therapy. Follows legislative and agency action concerning antimicrobics, and offers editorial comment to microbiology, infectious disease, and pharmacology audiences. **First Published:** 1984. **Frequency:** Monthly. **ISSN:** 0738-1751.

★1905★ ANTIVIRAL AGENTS BULLETIN
Biotechnology Information Institute
1700 Rockville Pike, Ste. 400
Rockville, MD 20852   Phone: (301) 942-1215
Description: Covers AIDS research and antiviral drug and vaccine development, including federal activities, information sources, patents and technology transfer, and recent literature abstracts. **First Published:** April 1988. **Frequency:** Monthly. **ISSN:** 0897-9871.

★1906★ AODRM NEWSLETTER
Academy of Oral Diagnosis, Radiology and Medicine
c/o James A. Cottone
University of Texas HSC
7703 Floyd Curl Dr.
San Antonio, TX 78284-7919   Phone: (512) 567-3333
Description: Covers Academy activites. Recurring features include a calendar of events, reports of meetings, and news of educational opportunities. **Frequency:** 3/yr.

★1907★ AOE NETWORK
American Health Information Management Association
919 N. Michigan Ave., Ste. 1400
Chicago, IL 60611   Phone: (312) 787-2672
Description: Reviews developments in the field of education for those teaching medical record management and technology. Reports on Association educational programs. Recurring features include Association news, notes on members, news of research, and a calendar of events. **Frequency:** Quarterly.

★1908★ AOHA
American Osteopathic Hospital Association
5301 Wisconsin Ave.
Washington, DC 20015
Description: Concerned with current legislation, court law, and federal regulations affecting osteopathic medicine, as well as with Association news. Recurring features include items on related organizations and personnel changes in member hospitals. **First Published:** January 1970. **Frequency:** Monthly.

★1909★ AOSA FORESIGHT
American Optometric Student Association
243 N. Lindbergh Blvd.
St. Louis, MO 63141   Phone: (314) 991-4100
Description: Reports news of AOSA and allied organizations and provides information concerning scholarships, grants, internships, and other educational issues related to the study of optometry. Recurring features include a calendar of events, news of research, editorials, and a President's Column. **Frequency:** Semiannual.

★1910★ APAGS NEWSLETTER
American Psychological Association
750 1st St. NE
Washington, DC 20002-4242   Phone: (202) 336-5500
First Published: 1989. **Frequency:** 2/yr.

★1911★ APLICOMMUNICATOR
Association for Population/Family Planning Libraries & Information Centers, International
2058 SW Olympic Club Terrace
Palm City, FL 34990
Description: Focuses on subjects related to population and family planning. Discusses organizations, associations, and networks involved in these issues throughout the world; and library and information center methodology. Includes news of members and chapters. **First Published:** April 1975. **Frequency:** Quarterly. **ISSN:** 0891-0847.

★1912★ APMA NEWS
American Podiatric Medical Association
9312 Old Georgetown Rd.
Bethesda, MD 20814-1621   Phone: (301) 571-9200
Description: Covers news of the Association as well as reporting on bylaws and on regulations that affect the profession. Recurring features include a calendar of events, statistics, news of research, and news of workshops. **First Published:** February 1974. **Frequency:** Monthly. **ISSN:** 8750-2585.

★1913★ APOTHECARY
Temple University School of Pharmacy
3307 N. Broad St.
Philadelphia, PA 19140   Phone: (215) 538-4782
Description: Provides news and information of interest to the alumni of Temple University School of Pharmacy. **First Published:** 1951. **Frequency:** 4/yr.

★1914★ APPLIED GENETICS NEWS
Business Communications Company, Inc.
25 Van Zant St.
Norwalk, CT 06855-1781   Phone: (203) 853-4266
Description: Concerned primarily with the application of genetic research to industry and technology. Evaluates ongoing research in the areas of aging, cancer, disease, and cell differentiation. Discusses research funding and finances. Analyzes new developments in venture capital and stock price movement. **First Published:** August 1980. **Frequency:** Monthly. **ISSN:** 0271-7107.

★1915★ APPM UPDATE
Academy of Pharmacy Practice and Management
American Pharmaceutical Association
2215 Constitution Ave. NW
Washington, DC 20037   Phone: (202) 628-4410
Description: Briefs members on Academy news and developments in pharmacy practice and management and in pharmacy as a profession. **First Published:** 1966. **Frequency:** Quarterly.

★1916★   ARDA ADVOCATE
Alberta Registered Dieticians Association
3704445 Calgary Trail S.
Edmonton, AB, Canada T6H 5X7   Phone: (403) 988-9898
Description: Provides information on association business, continuing education, upcoming events, and resources. Recurring features include letters to the editor, reports of meetings, news of educational opportunities, and notices of publications available. **First Published:** 1971. **Frequency:** 6/yr.

★1917★   ARIZONA CANCER CENTER—NEWSLETTER
Arizona Cancer Center
The University of Arizona
1515 N. Campbell Ave.
Tucson, AZ 85724   Phone: (602) 626-6044
Description: Consists of news and human interest stories on cancer research and treatment developments at the Center. **First Published:** 1977. **Frequency:** 3-4/yr.

★1918★   ARIZONA NURSE
Arizona Nurses Association
1850 E. Southern Ave., Ste. 1
Tempe, AZ 85282   Phone: (602) 831-0404
Description: Provides news and information of interest to nurses. **First Published:** 1947. **Frequency:** 4/yr. **ISSN:** 0004-1599.

★1919★   ARNN ACCESS
Association of Registered Nurses of Newfoundland
55 Military Rd.
PO Box 6116
St. John's, NF, Canada A1C 5X8   Phone: (709) 753-6040
Description: Presents information on nursing workshops, scholarships and grants, insurance, and training seminars. Acts as a vehicle for Association information, balloting, and reports of results of elections. Recurring features include news of research, a calendar of events, reports of meetings, news of educational opportunities, and feature articles by Association officers. **First Published:** 1981. **Frequency:** 4/yr.

★1920★   AROCC NEWSLETTER
Association for Research of Childhood Cancer, Inc.
PO Box 251
Buffalo, NY 14225-0251   Phone: (716) 684-8864
Description: Deals with pediatric cancer research news of interest to parents who have children with cancer. Association news includes information on community activities, fundraising projects, and membership. Recurring features include a list of reading material and obituaries. **First Published:** March 1972. **Frequency:** Bimonthly.

★1921★   ARTHRITIS FOUNDATION—CONNECTION
Minnesota Chapter
Arthritis Foundation
1730 Clifton Pl., No. A-1
Minneapolis, MN 55403   Phone: (612) 874-1201
Description: Describes education and fund raising efforts of the Association. Recurring features include profiles of volunteers, news of appointments, and President's and executive directors' letters. **First Published:** 1960. **Frequency:** 3/yr.

★1922★   ARTHRITIS NEWS
Arthritis Society
250 Bloor St. E., Ste. 401
Toronto, ON, Canada M4W 3P2   Phone: (416) 967-1414
Description: Features articles about the Society, voluntarism, rheumatological research, coping strategies, and patient education. Recurring features include interviews and practical advice for people with arthritis. **First Published:** December 1982. **Frequency:** Quarterly. **ISSN:** 0820-9006.

★1923★   ARTHRITIS TODAY
UAB Multipurpose Arthritis Center
University of Alabama at Birmingham
108 Basic Health Sciences Bldg.
Birmingham, AL 35294   Phone: (205) 934-0542
Description: Translates clinical and basic research on arthritis into relevant information that helps people with arthritis manage and control the disease. **Frequency:** Semiannual.

★1924★   ASA NEWSLETTER
American Society of Anesthesiologists
515 Busse Hwy.
Park Ridge, IL 60068-3189   Phone: (708) 825-5586
Description: Reports on the educational and scientific work of the organization, which represents anesthesiolgists in the U.S. Carries legislative updates, news of research, and historical items. Recurring features include editorials, letters to the editor and news of members. **First Published:** January 1938. **Frequency:** Monthly.

★1925★   ASBESTOS CONTROL REPORT
Business Publishers, Inc.
951 Pershing Dr.
Silver Spring, MD 20910-4464   Phone: (301) 587-6300
Description: Covers the industry ramifications of the Asbestos Hazard Emergency Response Act of 1986, with technical information on control techniques, worksite health and safety, federal standards, state and local regulations, waste disposal, insurance requirements, and contracts available and awarded. **First Published:** 1986. **Frequency:** Biweekly. **ISSN:** 0893-4533.

★1926★   ASBESTOS VICTIMS OF AMERICA—ADVISOR
Asbestos Victims of America
PO Box 559
Capitola, CA 95010   Phone: (408) 476-3646
Description: Provides nationwide public education regarding the hazards of asbestos and asbestos-related diseases, including asbestos abatement information and emergency asbestos damage information for disaster areas. Features articles on new medical treatment, legal/compensation issues, and health and safety procedures. Lists medical, legal, and financial resources for victims and reports on consumer products, construction materials, and other items containing asbestos. **First Published:** 1980. **Frequency:** Quarterly.

★1927★   ASC NEWSLETTER
Association of Systematics Collections
730 11th St. NW, 2nd Fl.
Washington, DC 20001   Phone: (202) 347-2850
Description: Discusses care, maintenance, management, and preservation of systematic biological collections. Carries news of wildlife permit regulations, and information on the Association and other museums and professional societies. Recurring features include book reviews, notices of employment opportunities, and a calendar of events. **First Published:** Summer 1973. **Frequency:** Bimonthly. **ISSN:** 0417-7889.

★1928★   ASC NEWSLETTER
Autism Society Canada
45 Sheppard Ave. E., Ste. 304
Toronto, ON, Canada M2N 5W9   Phone: (416) 924-4189
Description: Promotes the diagnosis, treatment, and education of autistic persons. Furnishes information on current research in autism done throughout the world. Discusses both experimental and successful educational programs geared toward autistic individuals. Highlights news of the Society and its activities. Recurring features include news of research, news of educational opportunities, book reviews, and a calendar of events. **First Published:** 1982. **Frequency:** Quarterly.

★1929★   ASDA NEWS
American Student Dental Association
211 E. Chicago Ave.
No. 840
Chicago, IL 60611   Phone: (312) 440-2795

★1930★   ASDC NEWSLETTER
American Society of Dentistry for Children
211 E. Chicago Ave., Ste. 1430
Chicago, IL 60611   Phone: (312) 943-1244
Description: Reviews developments in clinical research and applications for dental practices for children. Carries reports on Society activities and meetings, news of members, and a calendar of events. **First Published:** October 1981. **Frequency:** Bimonthly.

★1931★   ASET NEWSLETTER
American Society of Electroneurodiagnostic Technologists, Inc.
204 W. 7th
Carroll, IA 51401   Phone: (712) 792-2978
Description: Highlights the programs and activities of the Society, which is committed to the advancement of the science and technical standards of

electroencephalography (EEG) and neurodiagnostic medicine. Announces conferences, educational opportunities, chapter activities, and new publications in the field. **First Published:** 1976. **Frequency:** Quarterly. **ISSN:** 0886-5620.

★1932★   ASH SMOKING AND HEALTH REVIEW
Action on Smoking and Health
2013 H St. NW
Washington, DC 20006   Phone: (202) 659-4310
Description: Supports efforts to assert the rights of nonsmokers. Covers medical, legal, regulatory, commercial, institutional, and humorous news related to smoking. Recurring features include columns titled Ideas for Activists, News You Should Know, Research Reports, International Smoke Signals, and Now Available. **First Published:** 1981. **Frequency:** Bimonthly.

★1933★   ASHE TECHNICAL DOCUMENT SERIES
American Society for Hospital Engineering
American Hospital Association
840 N. Lake Shore Dr.
Chicago, IL 60611   Phone: (312) 280-6615
Description: Disseminates data on codes and standards, facilties management, design and construction, electrical safety, clinical engineering, and environmental safety "to promote and ensure better patient care and to maintain professional standards." **First Published:** April 1981. **Frequency:** Monthly.

★1934★   ASHP NEWSLETTER
American Society of Hospital Pharmacists
4630 Montgomery Ave.
Bethesda, MD 20814   Phone: (301) 657-3000
Description: Covers current developments in pharmacy and health care for institutional pharmacists. Recurring features include news of ASHP activities and reports of legislative and regulatory actions. **First Published:** 1968. **Frequency:** Monthly. **ISSN:** 0001-2483.

★1935★   ASPB NEWSLETTER
Alberta Society of Professional Biologists
370 Terrace Plaza
4445 Calgary Trail S.
Edmonton, AB, Canada T6H 5R7   Phone: (403) 434-5765
Description: Contains activities, viewpoints, and related information on the roles and obligations of the professional biologist. Recurring features include a calendar of events, reports of meetings, notices of publications available, articles on the effects of certification, and a column titled Viewpoint. **First Published:** August 1986. **Frequency:** Quarterly.

★1936★   ASPCA REPORT
American Society for the Prevention of Cruelty to Animals
441 E. 92nd St.
New York, NY 10128   Phone: (212) 876-7700
Description: Concerned with subjects related to "animal welfare, humane education, prevention of cruelty to animals, and over population." Recurring features include editorials, news of research, book, video, and computer program reviews, and a calendar of events. **First Published:** March 1977. **Frequency:** 3/yr.

★1937★   ASRA NEWSLETTER
American Society of Regional Anesthesia
PO Box 11086
Richmond, VA 23230   Phone: (804) 282-0010
Description: Carries news of the Society, its members, and its activities. Serves physicians, research Ph.D.s, and anesthesiologists. Recurring features include reports on conferences, meetings, awards, grants, lectures, and programs, and a question column on professional problems and techniques. **First Published:** 1974. **Frequency:** Quarterly.

★1938★   ASSEMBLYLINE
National Assembly of National Voluntary Health & Social Welfare
   Organizations, Inc.
1319 F St. NW, Ste. 601
Washington, DC 20004   Phone: (202) 347-2080
Description: Attempts to foster intercommunication and interaction among national voluntary health and social welfare agencies. Discusses topics relating to the impact of voluntarism on human needs, especially in regard to individual health and social welfare agencies. Recurring features include news of research. **Frequency:** Periodic.

★1939★   ASSOCIATION OF BIOTECHNOLOGY COMPANIES—DETAILS
Association of Biotechnology Companies
1666 Connecticut Ave. NW, Ste. 330
Washington, DC 20009-1039   Phone: (202) 234-3330
Description: Focuses on federal regulatory and legislative developments affecting the biotechnology industry. Furnishes information on trends in the field, biotechnology reports and documents, and Association activities. **First Published:** April 1985. **Frequency:** 6/yr.

★1940★   ASSOCIATION OF BIRTH DEFECT CHILDREN—NEWSLETTER
Association of Birth Defect Children Inc.
5400 Diplomat Circle, Ste. 270
Orlando, FL 32810   Phone: (407) 629-1466
Description: Publishes information on the prevention and rehabilitation of birth defects, including rehabilitation surgery, prosthesis devices, and handicapped services. Recommends books and articles on birth defects, reports current judicial decisions, and carries profiles of member children. Recurring features include columns titled Parent-to-Parent, A Different Perspective, and National Environmental Birth Defects Registry. **First Published:** April 1979. **Frequency:** Quarterly.

★1941★   ASSOCIATION FOR CHILD PSYCHOANALYSIS—NEWSLETTER
Association for Child Psychoanalysis
4524 Forest Park
St. Louis, MO 63108   Phone: (314) 361-4646
Description: Discusses child analysis methods, child psychoanalysis training, and the treatment and education of children throughout the world. Recurring features include news of members and the Association and announcements of research training programs, meetings, lectures, and committees concerned with child psychoanalysis. **First Published:** 1981. **Frequency:** Semiannually.

★1942★   ASSOCIATION FOR DEATH EDUCATION AND COUNSELING—THE FORUM
Association for Death Education & Counseling
638 Prospect Ave.
Hartford, CT 06105   Phone: (203) 232-4825
Description: Serves as a communication network for the Association, which promotes quality education and counseling in the areas of death, dying, and bereavement. Discusses developments and research in the field and reports on activities of the Forum and its members. Recurring features include editorials, letters to the editor, book reviews, and a calendar of events. **First Published:** Ca. 1975. **Frequency:** Bimonthly.

★1943★   ASSOCIATION FOR THE HISTORY OF CHIROPRACTIC—BULLETIN
Association for the History of Chiropractic, Inc.
4920 Frankford Ave.
Baltimore, MD 21206   Phone: (301) 488-6604
Description: Relates information on events and developments in the field of chiropractic history. Reviews Association activities. Recurring features include listings of educational opportunities and news of members. **First Published:** May 1980. **Frequency:** Periodic.

★1944★   ASSOCIATION OF MEDICAL REHABILITATION ADMINISTRATORS—NEWSLETTER
Association of Medical Rehabilitation Administrators
1733 Forest Hills Dr.
Vienna, WV 26105   Phone: (304) 485-5842
Description: Provides information on medical rehabilitation and related topics for directors and coordinators of rehabilitation centers or programs. Covers the activities of the Association and related medical associations. Recurring features include book reviews, news of research and of members, a calendar of events, and columns titled President's Message and From the Executive Director. **First Published:** 1956. **Frequency:** Semiannual.

★1945★   ASSOCIATION FOR PERSONS WITH SEVERE HANDICAPS—NEWSLETTER
Association for Persons With Severe Handicaps
11201 Greenwood Ave. N.
Seattle, WA 98133   Phone: (206) 523-8446
Description: Aims to disseminate information on all aspects of the education of persons with severe handicaps and to facilitate communications among readers. Covers services, programs, publications, equipment, legislation, and professional positions for those who work in this area of special education. Recurring features include announcements of confer-

ences and placements and reader requests. **First Published:** 1975. **Frequency:** Monthly.

★1946★ ASTHMA AND ALLERGY ADVOCATE
American Academy of Allergy and Immunology
611 E. Wells St.
Milwaukee, WI 53202   Phone: (414) 272-6071
Description: Informs patients of physicians and allergists about allergies. Contains information on asthma, allergy treatments and research, and seasonal, insect-related, and other allergies. **First Published:** Summer 1985. **Frequency:** Quarterly. **ISSN:** 0899-7470.

★1947★ ASTHMA UPDATE
123 Monticello Ave.
Annapolis, MD 21401   Phone: (301) 267-8329
Description: Presents medical information on asthma treatment, household air control measures, and exercise-induced asthma. **Frequency:** Quarterly. **ISSN:** 8756-4734.

★1948★ ATCC QUARTERLY NEWSLETTER
American Type Culture Collection
12301 Parklawn Dr.
Rockville, MD 20852   Phone: (301) 881-2600
Description: Publishes news of ATCC, which is a "resource for the acquisition, preservation, and distribution of authenticated microorganisms, viruses, cell cultures, and cloned DNA." Features new accessions to the collection, new products and uses, and research methods. Recurring features include statistics, news of research, a calendar of workshops, and a question and answer column. **First Published:** April 1981. **Frequency:** Quarterly. **ISSN:** 0894-9026.

★1949★ ATS NEWS
American Thoracic Society
1740 Broadway
New York, NY 10019   Phone: (212) 315-8808
Description: Provides information about the Society and its parent group, the American Lung Association. Contains articles on medical research related to respiratory diseases and a summary of health legislation. Recurring features include announcements of activities and courses for continuing medical education. **First Published:** August 1975. **Frequency:** Bimonthly.

★1950★ A2LA NEWS
American Association for Laboratory Accreditation
656 Quince Orchard Rd., Ste. 304
Gaithersburg, MD 20878-1409   Phone: (301) 670-1377
Description: Updates the latest accreditation actions. Provides information on improving the quality of test data. **First Published:** 1980. **Frequency:** 6/yr. **ISSN:** 1040-9157.

★1951★ AUL NEWSLETTER
Americans United for Life
343 S. Dearborn, Ste. 1804
Chicago, IL 60604   Phone: (312) 786-9494
Description: Discusses the legal aspects of and current court cases involving abortion, euthanasia, infanticide, in vitro fertilization, genetic engineering, and medical treatment for handicapped newborn infants. Carries announcements and ordering information for new publications. **Frequency:** Quarterly.

★1952★ AUTISM NEWSLINK
Autism Society Ontario
203-8108 Yonge St.
Thornhill, ON, Canada L4J 1W4   Phone: (416) 731-3629
Description: Covers Society activities. Contains information on autism. Recurring features include news of research, a calendar of events, reports of meetings, and book reviews. **First Published:** 1988. **Frequency:** Quarterly.

★1953★ AUTISM SOCIETY OF AMERICA—ADVOCATE
Autism Society of America
8601 Georgia Ave., Ste. 503
Silver Spring, MD 20910   Phone: (301) 565-0433
Description: Reports news of national significance concerning the welfare of children with severe communication and behavior disorders. Recurring features include abstracts of articles, book reviews, statistics, news of research, and a calendar of events. **First Published:** October 1968. **Frequency:** Quarterly. **ISSN:** 0047-9101.

★1954★ AVEA NEWSLETTER
American Veterinary Exhibitors Association
PO Box 6842
Santa Barbara, CA 93160   Phone: (805) 683-0489
Description: Reports on the Association's involvement in the area of veterinary exhibitions. Provides a forum to give firms exhibiting at veterinary conventions a voice in planning the time, place, programs, and facilities of such meetings. Also offers suggestions for more effective exhibits. Recurring features include letters to the editor, interviews, news of research, reports of meetings, notice of educational opportunities, job listings, book reviews, notices of publications available, and a calendar of events. Includes columns titled Budget Statement and President's Page. **Frequency:** Quarterly.

★1955★ AVENUES
National Support Group for Arthrogryposis Multiplex Congenita
c/o Mary Anne Schmidt
PO Box 5192
Sonora, CA 95370   Phone: (209) 928-3688
Description: Aimed at parents, relatives, friends and other supporters of people with Arthrogryposis Multiplex Congenita. **Frequency:** Semimonthly, January and July.

★1956★ AVMA NEWSLETTER
Alberta Veterinary Medical Association
8615-149th St., Ste. 100
Edmonton, AB, Canada T6A 0M2   Phone: (403) 465-4465
Description: Features letters to the editor, a calendar of events, reports of meetings, news of educational opportunities, and job listings. **First Published:** October 1990. **Frequency:** Bimonthly.

★1957★ AVSC NEWS
Association for Voluntary Surgical Contraception, Inc.
79 Madison Ave.
New York, NY 10016   Phone: (212) 561-8093
Description: Provides information on all aspects of voluntary sterilization: programs, research, legal issues, and new medical technologies. Discusses programs in the U.S. and developing countries. **First Published:** 1962. **Frequency:** 4/yr. **ISSN:** 0001-2904.

★1958★ AWARENESS
National Association for Parents of the Visually Impaired
2180 Linway Dr.
Beloit, WI 53511   Phone: (608) 362-4945
Description: Provides support for members and promotes public understanding of the needs and rights of the visually impaired child. Disseminates information about care, education, and treatment for visually impaired children and acts as a forum for the exchange of parental concerns. Recurring features include updates on Association programs, notices of publications available, and news of research and resources. **First Published:** Spring 1980. **Frequency:** Quarterly.

★1959★ BACK PAIN MONITOR
American Health Consultants, Inc.
PO Box 740056
Atlanta, GA 30374   Phone: (404) 262-7436
Description: Provides information on new back treatments, company-sponsored fitness programs, drugs, and rulings by the Occupational Safety and Health Administration (OSHA) concerning back problems and their prevention, treatment, rehabilitation, and compensation. **First Published:** October 1983. **Frequency:** Monthly. **ISSN:** 0746-9489.

★1960★ BACKTALK
Scoliosis Association, Inc.
PO Box 51353
Raleigh, NC 27609   Phone: (919) 846-2639
Description: Carries Association news and information on topics related to scoliosis. Serves patients, families, and the general public in helping to cope with the emotional and social problems that often accompany treatment. Recurring features include news of research, reviews of books not technically medical; information on chapter meetings; article reprints; and listings of publications, tapes, and films available. **First Published:** April 1976. **Frequency:** Periodic.

★1961★ THE BANDELETTE
International Association for Orthodontics
211 E. Chicago Ave., Ste. 915
Chicago, IL 60611　　　　　Phone: (312) 642-2602
Description: Provides information on the cause, control treatment, and prevention of malocclusion of the teeth and about dentistry in general. Also carries news of the activities of the Association. **First Published:** 1968. **Frequency:** Monthly (10/yr.).

★1962★ THE BANK ACCOUNT
Living Bank
PO Box 6725
Houston, TX 77265　　　　　Phone: (713) 528-2971
Description: Encourages the donation of organs for the purposes of transplantation, therapy, medical research, or anatomical study. Educates the public about donor registration and procedures, and presents news of the Living Bank's registry, referral, and promotional activities. **First Published:** Spring 1980. **Frequency:** 4/yr.

★1963★ BATTING THE BREEZE
Emphysema Anonymous, Inc.
PO Box 3224
Seminole, FL 34642　　　　　Phone: (813) 391-9977
Description: Provides medical and educational information for victims of emphysema and other respiratory diseases. Features messages of inspiration and humor centered on coping with emphysema. Recurring features include news of research, letters to the editor, and notices of publications available. **First Published:** 1965. **Frequency:** Bimonthly. **ISSN:** 0005-6367.

★1964★ THE BBI NEWSLETTER
Biomedical Business International, Inc.
1524 Brookhollow Dr.
Santa Ana, CA 92706　　　　　Phone: (714) 755-5757
Description: Reports on market information, analysis, and business projections. Provides information on new technologies, products, companies, competitors, market niches, and business opportunities. **First Published:** 1978. **Frequency:** Monthly. **ISSN:** 0739-4608.

★1965★ BCMA NEWS
British Columbia Medical Association
1665 W. Broadway, Ste. 115
Vancouver, BC, Canada V6J 5A4　　　　Phone: (604) 736-5551
Description: Provides news of Association political activities. Recurring features include letters to the editor, reports of meetings, and book reviews. **First Published:** 1969. **Frequency:** 6/yr.

★1966★ BCSMT OBJECTIVE
British Columbia Society of Medical Technologists
PO Box 715
New West, BC, Canada V3L 4Z3　　　Phone: (604) 520-1617
Description: Reports on the business of the Society, profiles individual technologists, and informs members of new issues in the field of medical technology. Concerned primarily with the continuing education of Society members. Recurring features include letters to the editor, interviews, news of research, a calendar of events, reports of meetings, news of educational opportunities, and notices of publications available. **First Published:** 1969. **Frequency:** 3/yr.

★1967★ BEGINNINGS
American Holistic Nurses' Association
4101 Lake Boone Trail, Ste. 201
Raleigh, NC 27607　　　　　Phone: (919) 787-5181
Description: Functions as the official newsletter of the Association, which seeks to "renew and enhance the art of nurturing and caring for the whole person." Offers educational information on holistic nursing and healing modalities, and provides news of the Association. Recurring features include editorials, news of research, letters to the editor, news of members, book reviews, a social and ethical column, and a calendar of events. **First Published:** March 1981. **Frequency:** 10/yr.

★1968★ BEHAVIOR THERAPIST
Association for Advancement of Behavior Therapy
15 W. 36th St.
New York, NY 10018　　　　　Phone: (212) 279-7970
Description: Concerned with behavior therapy/behavior modification, particularly the uses in medical, psychological, educational, and business settings. Contains news of the Association. Recurring features include book

reviews, film and tape reviews, news of research, and a calendar of events. **First Published:** 1978. **Frequency:** Monthly. **ISSN:** 0278-8403.

★1969★ BEHAVIOR TODAY
Atcom, Inc.
2315 Broadway
New York, NY 10024　　　　　Phone: (212) 873-5900
Description: Covers the latest developments in clinical research, legislation, marketing, and client care, in the mental health and social work professions. Recurring features include editorials, letters to the editor, book reviews, and a calendar of events. **First Published:** 1969. **Frequency:** Weekly. **ISSN:** 0005-7924.

★1970★ BEING WELL
Society for Professional Well-Being
21 W. Colony Pl., Ste. 150
Durham, NC 27705　　　　　Phone: (919) 489-9167
Description: Covers Society activities. Provides information on coping skills, networking, and stress reduction. Recurring features include letters to the editor, interviews, news of research, a calendar of events, reports of meetings, news of educational opportunities, job listings, book reviews, and notices of publications available. **First Published:** August 1988. **Frequency:** Quarterly.

★1971★ BEST OF HEALTH—NEWSLETTER
Best of Health
PO Box 40-1232
Brooklyn, NY 11240-1232　　　　Phone: (718) 756-2245
Description: Covers African American health issues. Contains news on nutrition and fitness. Recurring features include letters to the editor; interviews; a calendar of events; book reviews; notices of new products, videos, and audio cassettes available; and columns titled Kaye's Health Vine and Newsline. **First Published:** April 1987. **Frequency:** Quarterly. **ISSN:** 1055-3398.

★1972★ BETHPHAGE MESSENGER
Bethphage Mission, Inc.
Lind Center, Ste. A
4980 S. 118th St.
Omaha, NE 68137-2220　　　　Phone: (402) 896-3884
Description: Provides news and information on developmental disabilities. **First Published:** 1913. **Frequency:** Quarterly.

★1973★ BETTER HEARING INSTITUTE—COMMUNICATOR
Better Hearing Institute
PO Box 1840
Washington, DC 20013　　　　Phone: (703) 642-0580
Description: Highlights the activities of the Institute, which works for greater public understanding of hearing disorders through production of public service films, spot announcements, and programs of various kinds about enhancing communication and overcoming communicative problems. Recurring features include notices of awards. **First Published:** 1973. **Frequency:** Quarterly.

★1974★ BETWEEN FRIENDS
Beltone Electronics Corp.
4201 W. Victoria
Chicago, IL 60646　　　　　Phone: (312) 583-3600
Description: Provides health news and educational articles regarding hearing aids. Includes financial information and humorous items of interest. **First Published:** 1986. **Frequency:** Bimonthly.

★1975★ BIALYSTOKER STIMME
Bialystoker Center
228 E. Broadway
New York, NY 10002　　　　　Phone: (212) 475-7755
Description: Presents current and past news concerning the Center and nursing home. Features articles on Bialystok, Poland. Recurring features include letters to the editor, interviews, a calendar of events, reports of meetings, book reviews, notices of publications available, and obituaries. **First Published:** 1920. **Frequency:** Semiannual.

★1976★ BIBLIOTHERAPY FORUM—NEWSLETTER
Bibliotherapy Forum
American Library Association
50 E. Huron St.
Chicago, IL 19103　　　　　Phone: (312) 944-6780
Description: Promotes the use of reading for mental health and bibliother-

apy, the use of selective reading materials as therapeutic aids in medicine and psychiatry. Contains book reviews, descriptions of ongoing bibliotherapy programs, course announcements, and news of research. Publishes news of the Forum. **First Published:** 1976. **Frequency:** Quarterly. **ISSN:** 0740-9591.

★1977★   BIGEL INSTITUTE FOR HEALTH POLICY— NEWSLETTER
Bigel Institute for Health Policy
Brandeis University
Heller Graduate School
415 South St.
Waltham, MA 02254   Phone: (617) 736-3900
Description: Focuses on current substantive areas of research at the Institute. Discusses new grant awards and current publications. **First Published:** 1986. **Frequency:** Semiannually.

★1978★   BIO/CONNECTION
Michigan Biotechnology Institute
3900 Collins Rd.
PO Box 27609
Lansing, MI 48909   Phone: (517) 337-3181
Description: Discusses the work of the Institute. Profiles trends and leaders in the industrial and environmental biotechnology field. **First Published:** 1986. **Frequency:** 3/yr.

★1979★   BIOENGINEERING NEWS
Deborah J. Mysiewicz Publishers, Inc.
PO Box 2009
Oak Harbor, WA 98277   Phone: (206) 675-1370
Description: Covers developments in the bioengineering field, including news of recombinant DNA, genetic engineering, hybridomas, monoclonal antibodies, cell fusion, tissue culture, and fermentation and purification systems. Also carries items on laboratory equipment, law, patents, stocks, new companies, conferences, and other business and industry activities. Recurring features include news of research and a clinical trials column. **First Published:** August 1980. **Frequency:** Weekly. **ISSN:** 0275-4207.

★1980★   BIOFEEDBACK CLINICIAN
American Association of Biofeedback Clinicians
c/o Dr. Joseph Sargent
1913 Warner Court
Topeka, KS 66604   Phone: (913) 357-1156
Description: Reprints articles on biofeedback and offers miscellaneous items of interest to members, including listings of cassette presentations from Association conventions and notification of certification examinations. Recurring features include news of research, member news, and a calendar of events. **Frequency:** Quarterly.

★1981★   BIOLOGICAL THERAPIES IN DENTISTRY
Mosby-Year Book, Inc.
c/o Richard Wallace
545 Great Rd.
Littleton, MA 01460   Phone: (508) 486-8971
Description: Discusses the expanding role of therapeutic agents in dental practice. Covers developments in oral manifestations of systemic drugs, drug interactions, preventive dental medications, safety and toxicity of dental materials, agents for the control of plaque, sterilization and disinfection, antibiotics and peridontal therapy, and other issues related to dentistry. Recurring features include news of research. **First Published:** June 1985. **Frequency:** Bimonthly. **ISSN:** 0882-1852.

★1982★   BIOLOGICAL THERAPIES IN PSYCHIATRY
Mosby-Year Book, Inc.
c/o Richard Wallace
545 Great Rd.
Littleton, MA 01460   Phone: (508) 486-8971
Description: Reviews psychotropic drug issues directly affecting psychiatrists. Covers drug toxicity and physicians' liability, psychotropic drugs and cardiovascular function, dietary restrictions for patients, psychotropic drug use for a pregnant patient, new antidepressants, renal toxicity from lithium therapy, new indications for new drugs, and other issues related to psychiatry. **First Published:** January 1978. **Frequency:** Monthly. **ISSN:** 0199-2716.

★1983★   BIOMEDICAL SAFETY AND STANDARDS
Quest Publishing Co.
1351 Titan Way
Brea, CA 92621   Phone: (714) 738-6400
Description: Reports on biomedical safety and standards. Provides information on safety hazards, product recalls, product and facilities standards, legal actions, legislation and regulations, hospital safety, and biomedical equipment technician activities. Recurring features include news of research, employment opportunities, book reviews, and a calendar of events. **First Published:** 1971. **Frequency:** Semimonthly; monthly in January and August. **ISSN:** 0048-0282.

★1984★   BIOMEDICAL TECHNOLOGY AND HUMAN FACTORS ENGINEERING: AN ABSTRACT NEWSLETTER
National Technical Information Service
U.S. Department of Commerce
5285 Port Royal Rd.
Springfield, VA 22161   Phone: (703) 487-4630
Description: Carries abstracts of reports on biomedical facilities, instrumentation, and supplies. Also covers human factors engineering and man-machine relations; bionics and artificial intelligence; prosthetics and mechanical organs; life-support systems; space biology; and tissue preservation and storage. Recurring features include a form for ordering reports from NTIS. **Frequency:** Weekly. **ISSN:** 0163-1497.

★1985★   BIOMEDICAL TECHNOLOGY INFORMATION SERVICE
Quest Publishing Co.
1351 Titan Way
Brea, CA 92621   Phone: (714) 738-6400
Description: Monitors latest advances in medical technology, including developments in medical devices and electronics. Recurring features include new technology, computer applications, legislation and regulations, new inventions, and professional activities. Also includes book reviews, letters to the editor, and a calendar of events. **First Published:** 1974. **Frequency:** Semimonthly; Monthly in January and August. **ISSN:** 0147-2682.

★1986★   BIOMETRIC BULLETIN
Biometric Society
1429 Duke St., Ste. 401
Alexandria, VA 22314-3402   Phone: (703) 836-8311
Description: Describes member and Society activities in the field of biometry. Recurring features include letters to the editor, news of research, and a calendar of events. **First Published:** May 1984. **Frequency:** Quarterly. **ISSN:** 8750-0434.

★1987★   BIO-NOUVELLES
Societe de Biologie de Montreal
Case Postale 39, Succursale Outremont
Outremont, PQ, Canada H2V 4M6   Phone: (514) 277-9864
Description: Comments on issues related to biology and reports on society activities. Recurring features include a calendar of events and reports of meetings. **First Published:** 1970. **Frequency:** 6/yr. **ISSN:** 0319-3446.

★1988★   BIOTECH BUSINESS
Worldwide Videotex
Babson Park
PO Box 138
Boston, MA 02157   Phone: (617) 449-1603
Description: Provides news and information on biotechnology products, developments, and companies. Highlights marketing and investment opportunities. Reports on finances, management, company mergers, clinical drug trials, and scientific breakthroughs. **First Published:** January 1987. **Frequency:** Monthly. **ISSN:** 0899-5702.

★1989★   BIOTECHNOLOGY IN JAPAN NEWSSERVICE
Yoriko Kishimoto
467 Hamilton Ave., Ste. 2
Palo Alto, CA 94301   Phone: (415) 322-8441
Description: Tracks developments in the biotechnology sector in Japan, including biotechnological applications in pharmaceutical, chemical, agricultural, and other fields. Reports on developments at the research level, as well as at the scale-up, manufacturing, and marketing stages. **First Published:** July 1983. **Frequency:** 12/yr.

★1990★   BIOTECHNOLOGY NEWS
CTB International Publishing Co.
PO Box 218
Maplewood, NJ 07040-0218   Phone: (201) 763-6855
Description: Provides executives in the biotechnology industry with news and views on a variety of pertinent topics, including business deals, technical developments, financial performance, and government legislative and regulatory activity. Features reports on the practical use of biotechnology for the production of chemicals, fuels, foods, pharmaceutical products, crops, and the performance of services. Lists patents and meetings relating to the field of biotechnology. Recurring features include interviews and news of research. **First Published:** 1980. **Frequency:** 30/yr. **ISSN:** 0273-3226.

★1991★   BIOTECHNOLOGY NEWS WATCH
Energy and Business Newsletters
McGraw-Hill, Inc.
1221 Avenue of the Americas
New York, NY 10020   Phone: (212) 512-6410
Description: Provides business and technical news concerning companies involved in biotechnology sciences. Analyzes the business, legal, and industrial implications of biotechnology, in particular the latest developments in genetic engineering processes. **Frequency:** Semimonthly.

★1992★   BIOTECHNOLOGY NEWSLETTER
Biotechnology Program
Cornell University
130 Biotechnology Bldg.
Ithaca, NY 14853-2703   Phone: (607) 255-2300
Description: Covers activities of the Program and developments in biotechnology. Recurring features include interviews, news of research, a calendar of events, reports of meetings and symposia, news of educational opportunities, and reports from research facilities. **First Published:** February 1984. **Frequency:** Quarterly.

★1993★   BIOUPDATE
Biotechnology Center
University of Wisconsin at Madison
1710 University Ave.
Madison, WI 53705   Phone: (608) 262-2604
Description: Highlights programs and events within the Center and the UW-Madison biotech community. Recurring features include interviews, news of research, a calendar of events, reports of meetings, news of educational opportunities, job listings, and a column titled Briefs. **First Published:** May 1990. **Frequency:** Bimonthly.

★1994★   THE BLIND BOWLER
American Blind Bowling Association
67 Bame Ave.
Buffalo, NY 14215   Phone: (716) 836-1472
Description: Covers the bowling activities of the Association, with articles on blind bowling and announcements of tournaments and high score awards. Recurring features include news of members and Association officers. **First Published:** October 1953. **Frequency:** 3/yr.

★1995★   BLOOD BANK WEEK
American Association of Blood Banks
1117 N. 19th St., Ste. 600
Arlington, VA 22209   Phone: (703) 528-8200
Description: Reports on developments in the area of blood banking and transfusion medicine. Includes scientific, regulatory, legislative, and legal information. Recurring features include a calendar of events and notices of employment positions. **Frequency:** Weekly. **ISSN:** 0747-2420.

★1996★   BLUE VALLEY COMMUNITY ACTION—UPDATE
Blue Valley Community Action, Inc.
PO Box 273
Fairbury, NE 68352   Phone: (402) 729-2278
Description: Reports agency activities, legislative happenings, and current events pertaining to the area's low income and elderly people. Recurring features include profiles of volunteers and their activities. **First Published:** May 1977. **Frequency:** Quarterly.

★1997★   BMES BULLETIN
Biomedical Engineering Society
Box 2399
Culver City, CA 90231   Phone: (310) 618-9322
Description: Provides news and information on the Society; presents articles on bioengineering science. Recurring features include letters to the editor, news of research, a calendar of events, reports of meetings, news of educational opportunities, job listings, and columns titled Public Affairs, Student Chapter News, and Society News and Events.

★1998★   BNA'S MEDICARE REPORT
Bureau of National Affairs, Inc.
1231 25th St. NW
Washington, DC 20037   Phone: (202) 452-4200
Description: Covers legislative, regulatory, and legal developments affecting or pertaining to the Medicare program. Provides information on developments in the Medicaid program that could have implications for Medicare. **First Published:** May 18, 1990. **Frequency:** Biweekly. **ISSN:** 1049-7986.

★1999★   BOARDER CONNECTIONS
Los Ninos
9765 Marconi Dr., Ste. 105
San Ysidro, CA 92173   Phone: (619) 661-6912
Description: Covers Los Ninos development projects, such as nutrition, health, early childhood education, literacy, family, gardens, fund raising events, and development education programs for U.S. citizens. Presents fundraising news on a walkathon from Los Angeles-Tijuana. **First Published:** Spring 1989. **Frequency:** 3/yr.

★2000★   BODY BULLETIN
Rodale Press, Inc.
33 E. Minor St.
Emmaus, PA 18049   Phone: (215) 967-5171
Description: Touches on all aspects of health, including exercise, nutrition, stress control, disease prevention, and staying free of drugs. Treats "real issues that affect real people." Recurring features include book reviews, and news of research. **First Published:** 1982. **Frequency:** Monthly. **ISSN:** 0275-9101.

★2001★   BOSTON BIOMEDICAL RESEARCH INSTITUTE—MESSENGER
Boston Biomedical Research Institute
20 Staniford St.
Boston, MA 02114   Phone: (617) 742-2010
Description: Reports on the Institute's basic medical resarch programs. Discusses related issues and resource development topics. Recurring features include news of members and associates, and editorials. **First Published:** Spring 1983. **Frequency:** Periodic.

★2002★   BOWIE GASP
Bowie Group Against Smokers' Pollution
PO Box 863
Bowie, MD 20718   Phone: (301) 262-5867
Description: Promotes smoking restrictions through legislation, public education, and support for businesses with "no smoking" policies. Provides information on health updates and names establishments currently implementing "smoke-free" environment policies.

★2003★   BPA NEWS
Biological Photographic Association, Inc.
115 Stoneridge Dr.
Chapel Hill, NC 27514   Phone: (919) 967-8247
Description: Reports on the activities of the Association, whose members are concerned with advancing the techniques of biophotography. Recurring features include chapter updates, member news, a calendar of events, and job notices. **Frequency:** Bimonthly. **ISSN:** 0161-794X.

★2004★   BRAILLE EVANGELISM BULLETIN
Lutheran Braille Evangelism Association
1740 Eugene St.
White Bear Lake, MN 55110   Phone: (612) 426-0469
Description: Provides information concerning the large print, audio cassette, computer disk, and braille materials that the Association makes available to blind or visually impaired individuals. Recurring features include letters to the editor, a calendar of events, reports of meetings, and notices of publications available. **First Published:** 1952. **Frequency:** Quarterly.

★2005★ THE BRAILLE FORUM
American Council of the Blind
1155 15th St. NW, Ste. 720
Washington, DC 20005   Phone: (202) 467-5081
Description: Features articles on the Council's involvement in advocacy for blind and low-vision persons. Covers significant legislation and technical aids and carries human-interest stories. Recurring features include columns titled President's Message, High Tech Swap Shop, and Here and There. **First Published:** 1962. **Frequency:** Bimonthly.

★2006★ BRAILLE INSTITUTE—OUTLOOK
Braille Institute
741 N. Vermont Ave.
Los Angeles, CA 90029   Phone: (213) 663-1111
Description: Informs Institute students of services, opportunities, and products for the blind and reports on events at the several Institute centers. Recurring features include news of research and news of members. **First Published:** 1950. **Frequency:** Monthly.

★2007★ BRAIN WAVES
Brain Research Foundation
208 S. LaSalle St., Ste. 1426
Chicago, IL 60604   Phone: (312) 782-4311
Description: Informs of news and activities of the Foundation and of the Brain Research Institute, University of Chicago. Recurring features include interviews, news of research, a calendar of events, and news of educational opportunities. **First Published:** 1988. **Frequency:** 3/yr.

★2008★ BREASTFEEDING ABSTRACTS
La Leche League International, Inc.
9616 Minneapolis
Franklin Park, IL 60131-8209   Phone: (312) 455-7730
Description: Consists of abstracts from professional journals on the medical aspects of breastfeeding. **First Published:** Summer 1981. **Frequency:** Quarterly.

★2009★ BREATHLINE
American Society of Post Anesthesia Nurses
11512 Allecingie Pkwy.
Richmond, VA 23235   Phone: (804) 379-5516
Description: Publishes news of the Society, which is "an organization of licensed nurses engaged in the practice of post anesthesia patient care." Carries legislative updates, scientific articles, and state component society information. Discusses patient care standards, new drugs and treatments, and clinical issues relating to anesthesia and surgery. Recurring features include a calendar of events and columns titled Comment, Keeping Up, Resource Review, President's Message, Ambulatory Surgery, Manager's Minute, and Certification Corner. **First Published:** January 1981. **Frequency:** Bimonthly.

★2010★ BRITISH COLUMBIA DIETICIAN'S AND NUTRITIONISTS' ASSOCIATION—NEWSLETTER
British Columbia Dietician's and Nutritionists' Association
306-1037 W. Broadway
Vancouver, BC, Canada V6H 1E3   Phone: (604) 736-3790
Description: Contains news and announcements of activities of the Association. Recurring features include a calendar of events, reports of meetings, news of educational opportunities, book reviews, career opportunities, personnel movements, and a column titled Share the Wealth. **Frequency:** 9/yr.

★2011★ THE BRN REPORT
California Board of Registered Nursing
PO Box 944210
Sacramento, CA 94244-2100   Phone: (916) 322-3350
Description: Supplies information on various subjects of interest to registered nurses, particularly those in California. Recurring features include editorials, news of research, letters to the editor, news of members, and a calendar of events. **Frequency:** Quarterly.

★2012★ BROWARD COUNTY CHAPTER NEWSLETTER
International Association of Cancer Victims & Friends, Inc.
PO Box 175
Ft. Lauderdale, FL 33302   Phone: (305) 769-3549
Description: Provides news and information on health and emphasizes alternative therapies, practitioners, and clinics. **Frequency:** Monthly.

★2013★ THE BROWN UNIVERSITY CHILD AND ADOLESCENT BEHAVIOR LETTER
Manisses Communications Group, Inc.
Box 3357, Wayland Sq.
Providence, RI 02906   Phone: (401) 831-6020
Description: Reports on the problems of children and adolescents in growing up. Discusses clinical issues, news of research, public policy information, and book reviews. **First Published:** 1985. **Frequency:** Monthly.

★2014★ THE BROWN UNIVERSITY FAMILY THERAPY LETTER
Manisses Communications Group, Inc.
PO Box 3357
Providence, RI 02906-0757   Phone: (401) 831-6020
Description: Covers news and issues of interest to practicing family therapists, including new methods, techniques, research, assessment, and evaluation. Recurring features include news of research, book reviews, and columns titled Practice Management and Clinical Issues. **First Published:** 1989. **Frequency:** Monthly. **ISSN:** 1045-5051.

★2015★ BULLETIN OF PSYCHOLOGICAL TYPE
Association for Psychological Type
PO Box 5099
Gainesville, FL 32602-5099   Phone: (303) 794-5247
Description: Provides information on regional, national, and international events to keep professionals up-to-date in the study and application of psychological type theory and the Myers-Briggs Type Indicator. Contains announcements of training workshops; international, national, and regional conferences; and awards, along with articles on issues directly related to type theory. Recurring features include news of research, reports of meetings, news of educational opportunities, book reviews, and a calendar of events. **First Published:** Fall 1976. **Frequency:** Quarterly.

★2016★ BULLETIN ON THE RHEUMATIC DISEASES
Arthritis Foundation
1314 Spring St. NW
Atlanta, GA 30309   Phone: (404) 872-7100
Description: Contains concise discussions by distinguished authorities in each issue on some aspect of current developments in research and management in rheumatic diseases with seminal, annotated references. **First Published:** September 1950. **Frequency:** Bimonthly. **ISSN:** 0007-5248.

★2017★ CANADIAN AIDS NEWS
AIDS Education and Awareness Program
Canadian Public Health Association
1565 Carling Ave., Ste. 400
Ottawa, ON, Canada K1Z 8R1   Phone: (613) 725-3769
Description: Provides a forum for the exchange of current information regarding AIDS (Acquired Immune Deficiency Syndrome) education and information. Lists AIDS print and audiovisual resources. **First Published:** March 1987. **Frequency:** Bimonthly. **ISSN:** 1188-0325.

★2018★ CANADIAN ASSOCIATION OF ANATOMISTS— NEWSLETTER
Canadian Association of Anatomists
c/o Dept. of Anatomy
University of Western Ontario
London, ON, Canada N6A 5C1   Phone: (519) 679-2111
Description: Provides a review of Association activities. **First Published:** 1956. **Frequency:** Annual.

★2019★ CANADIAN ASSOCIATION OF CRITICAL CARE NURSES—NEWS AND VIEWS
Canadian Association of Critical Care Nurses
PO Box 8098
London, ON, Canada N6G 2B0   Phone: (519) 472-4150
Description: Provides updates on the members, chapters, and meetings of the Association, which represents critical care nurses from across Canada who practice in a variety of subspecialties. Offers information on upcoming conferences and workshops, notices of publications available, and columns titled Message From the President and From the Board Room. **First Published:** June 1986. **Frequency:** Quarterly.

★2020★ CANADIAN ASSOCIATION ON GERONTOLOGY—NEWSLETTER
Canadian Association on Gerontology
1565 Carling, Ste. 110
Ottawa, ON, Canada K1N 8R1 Phone: (613) 728-9347
Description: Provides local, national, and international coverage of news in the gerontology field, including new research information and resources. Presents reports concerning the business of the Association, notes from the executive, the committees, and the divisions. Recurring features include news from the provincial associations, the gerontology centers and programs, a column titled From the Hill, and a calendar of conferences and meetings. **First Published:** 1973. **Frequency:** Quarterly. **ISSN:** 0712-676X.

★2021★ CANADIAN ASSOCIATION OF PATHOLOGISTS—NEWSLETTER
Canadian Association of Pathologists
Dept. of Lab Medicine
Royal Alexandra Hospital
Edmonton, AB, Canada T5K 2J9 Phone: (403) 477-4366
Frequency: Bimonthly.

★2022★ CANADIAN ASSOCIATION OF PHYSICAL MEDICINE AND REHABILITATION NEWS
Canadian Association of Physical Medicine and Rehabilitation
c/o Department of PM & R
Parkwood Hospital
London, ON, Canada N6C 5J1 Phone: (519) 685-4029
Description: Provides a forum for information exchange for the Association. Recurring features include letters to the editor, a calendar of events, reports of meetings, job listings, archive and committee reports, and editorials. **First Published:** 1965. **Frequency:** 3-4/yr.

★2023★ CANADIAN ASSOCIATION OF SOCIAL WORK ADMINISTRATION IN HEALTH FACILITIES—NEWSLETTER
Canadian Association of Social Work Administration in Health Facilities
c/o Joan Dickenson
Burnaby Hospital
3935 Kincaid St.
Burnaby, BC, Canada V5G 2X6 Phone: (519) 432-5241
Description: Provides a forum for sharing information, ideas, and concerns among social work directors in health care institutions across Canada. Recurring features include a calendar of events and reports of meetings.

★2024★ CANADIAN HORTICULTURAL THERAPY ASSOCIATION—NEWSLETTER
Canadian Horticultural Therapy Association
PO Box 399
Hamilton, ON, Canada L8N 3H4 Phone: (416) 527-1158
Description: Covers aspects of professional horticultural therapy. Recurring features include reports of meetings, news of educational opportunities, book reviews, notices of publications available, and projects for disabled gardeners. **First Published:** Ca. 1980. **Frequency:** 4/yr.

★2025★ CANADIAN MEDICAL AND BIOLOGICAL ENGINEERING SOCIETY—NEWSLETTER
Canadian Medical and Biological Engineering Society
c/o 134-837 Eastvale Dr.
Gloucester, ON, Canada K1J 7T5 Phone: (613) 993-1686
Description: Disseminates Society news and information. Carries articles on biological, medical, and clinical engineering. Includes features related to the profession, cartoons, and anecdotes. Recurring features include letters to the editor, interviews, news of research, a calendar of events, and reports of meetings. Also includes news of educational opportunities, job listings, book reviews, and notices of publications available. **First Published:** 1964. **Frequency:** 4/yr. **ISSN:** 0384-1820.

★2026★ CANADIAN PAEDIATRIC SOCIETY—NEWS BULLETIN
Canadian Paediatric Society
401 Smyth Rd.
Ottawa, ON, Canada K1H 8L1 Phone: (613) 737-2728
Description: Serves as an information resource for pediatricians in Canada. Offers position papers on current issues, reviews of recent techniques, and news of pediatricians and pediatric appointments. Offers committee and liaison reports and information on upcoming meetings. **First Published:** February 1954. **Frequency:** Bimonthly.

★2027★ CANADIAN PHARMACEUTICAL ASSOCIATION—IMPACT
Canadian Pharmaceutical Association
1785 Alto Vista Dr.
Ottawa, ON, Canada K1G 3Y6 Phone: (616) 523-7877
Description: Tracks activities of the Association; provides information on the pharmaceutical industry. Recurring features include letters to the editor, news of research, a calendar of events, reports of meetings, and news of educational opportunities. **Frequency:** 5/yr.

★2028★ CANADIAN SOCIETY OF LABORATORY TECHNOLOGISTS—BULLETIN
Canadian Society of Laboratory Technologists
PO Box 2830, Sta. A
Hamilton, ON, Canada L8N 3N8 Phone: (416) 528-8642
Description: Contains information on continuing education, certification, public relations, and job opportunities. Reports on national and provincial activities of the Society, which is the certifying body and professional association for medical technologists in Canada. Recurring features include a calendar of events, reports on meetings, news of educational and employment opportunities, and notices of publications available. **First Published:** 1973. **Frequency:** Monthly. **ISSN:** 0381-5838.

★2029★ CANADIAN WHOLESALE DRUG ASSOCIATION NEWSLETTER
Canadian Wholesale Drug Association
1110 Sherbrooke St. W., Ste. 2206
Montreal, PQ, Canada H3A 1G8 Phone: (514) 842-8627
Description: Covers the Canadian wholesale drug industry and Association activities. Recurring features include letters to the editor, interviews, news of research, news of members, a calendar of events, reports of meetings, and news of educational opportunities. **First Published:** 1964. **Frequency:** Quarterly.

★2030★ THE CANCER CALENDAR
Northern California Cancer Center
1301 Shoreway Rd., No. 425
Belmont, CA 94002 Phone: (415) 591-4484
Description: Facilitates coordinated efforts against cancer in Northern California and Northwestern Nevada by disseminating information on continuing education programs and other events for health professionals in the region. Carries news of people, institutions, resources, and services concerning cancer care. **First Published:** October 1980. **Frequency:** 6/yr.

★2031★ THE CANCER CHALLENGE
Cancer Guidance Institute
1323 Forbes Ave.
Pittsburgh, PA 15219 Phone: (412) 261-2211
Description: Supports cancer patients and their families, promoting positive attitudes, education, and good medical care. Carries news of cancer research and personal stories from patients. Recurring features include book reviews, Institute news, and letters to the editor. **First Published:** Spring 1983. **Frequency:** Quarterly.

★2032★ CANCER COMMUNICATION
Patient Advocates for Advanced Cancer Treatments, Inc.
1143 Parmelee NW
Grand Rapids, MI 49504 Phone: (616) 453-1477
Description: Provides updated information regarding the detection, diagnosis, evaluation, and treatment of prostate cancer. Recurring features include letters to the editor, news of research, reports of meetings and conferences, reviews of journal publications, listing of support groups, and acknowledgement of contributions. **First Published:** April 1985. **Frequency:** 4/yr.

★2033★ THE CANCER LETTER
Cancer Letter Inc.
PO Box 15189
Washington, DC 20003 Phone: (202) 543-7665
Frequency: 48/yr. **ISSN:** 0096-3917.

★2034★ CANCER RESEARCH UPDATE
Eppley Institute for Research in Cancer and Allied Diseases
University of Nebraska at Omaha
Medical Center
600 S. 42nd St.
Omaha, NE 68198 Phone: (402) 559-4238
Description: Reports on the Institute's research, program, and faculty

activities; and provides news of other cancer research. **First Published:** 1984. **Frequency:** Quarterly.

★2035★ CANCER VICTORS JOURNAL
International Association of Cancer Victors and Friends
7740 W. Manchester Ave., No. 110
Playa Del Rey, CA 90293   Phone: (213) 822-5032
Description: Supports and follows the progress of independent research on cancer therapies. Disseminates information on "non-toxic" chemotherapies; provides education on nutrition in relation to cancer and regarding carcinogens in air, food, and water. Recurring features include meeting reports and notices of publications available. **First Published:** 1963. **Frequency:** Quarterly. **ISSN:** 0891-0766.

★2036★ CANDLELIGHTERS CHILDHOOD CANCER FOUNDATION—YOUTH NEWSLETTER
Candlelighters Childhood Cancer Foundation
1312 18th St. NW, Ste. 200
Washington, DC 20036   Phone: (202) 659-5136
Description: Publishes articles, stories, poems, and drawings for and by young people with cancer and their siblings and friends. Emphasizes coping with the disease while maintaining an otherwise normal lifestyle. Recurring features include profiles of teen patients, book and audiovisual reviews, letters, and news of young people who have recovered from cancer. **First Published:** September 1979. **Frequency:** Quarterly.

★2037★ CANINE LISTENER
Dogs for the Deaf
10175 Wheeler Rd.
Central Point, OR 97502   Phone: (503) 826-9220
Description: Highlights the organization's progress and needs in their work training hearing ear dogs for the deaf. Recurring features include editorials, letters to the editor, news of members, and testimonials from dog owners. **First Published:** 1977. **Frequency:** 4/yr.

★2038★ CARAL NEWSLETTER
California Abortion Rights Action League
300 Brannan St,. Ste. 501
San Francisco, CA 94118   Phone: (415) 546-7211
Description: Provides updates on legislation affecting abortion and family planning. Supports the right to safe, legal abortion, and addresses the concerns of those who are or who want to be involved in working for pro-choice legislation. Recurring features include news of legislation and a calendar of events. **First Published:** 1979. **Frequency:** Quarterly.

★2039★ CARDIAC ALERT
Phillips Publishing, Inc.
7811 Montrose Rd.
Potomac, MD 20854   Phone: (301) 340-2100
Description: Educates readers about heart disease and prevention. Discusses topics related to the heart such as surgery, rehabilitation, drugs, diet, and exercise. Recurring features include questions and answers and news of research. **First Published:** June 1979. **Frequency:** Monthly. **ISSN:** 0194-2557.

★2040★ CARDIOLOGY
American College of Cardiology
9111 Old Georgetown Rd.
Bethesda, MD 20814   Phone: (301) 897-5400
Description: Covers news and activities of the College, which is concerned with all aspects of cardiovascular disease and care. Reports on relevant legislation. Recurring features include news of endowments, symposia, and programs; chapter news; profiles; and a calendar of events. **First Published:** 1971. **Frequency:** Monthly.

★2041★ CARDIOPULMONARY NEWS AND INTERVIEWS
American College of Chest Physicians
3300 Dundee Rd.
Northbrook, IL 60062-2303   Phone: (312) 698-2200
Description: Disseminates information for those specializing in cardiopulmonary medicine and surgery, including scientific, socioeconomic, and fraternal news. Recurring features include interviews, reports of meetings, news of educational opportunities, and a calendar of events. Also includes a question-and-answer column offering legal counsel and columns titled News From ACCP, Education Update, and Members in the News. **First Published:** January 1987. **Frequency:** Quarterly.

★2042★ CAREERS IN INTERNAL MEDICINE
Association of Program Directors in Internal Medicine
700 13th St. NW, Ste. 250
Washington, DC 20005   Phone: (202) 393-1658
Description: Reflects the aims of the Association, which seeks to advance medical education through assisting accredited hospital internal medicine residency training programs. Profiles successful residency programs and summarizes developments in the field of internal medicine. **Frequency:** Quarterly.

★2043★ THE CAREGIVER
Duke Aging Center Alzheimer's Program
PO Box 3600
Duke Medical Center
Durham, NC 27710   Phone: (919) 684-2328
Description: Provides advice and suggestions for those dealing with victims of Alzheimer's disease. **First Published:** 1980. **Frequency:** 3/yr.

★2044★ CARING
Manitoba Association of Licensed Practical Nurses
615 Kernaghan Ave.
Winnipeg, MB, Canada R2C 2Z4   Phone: (204) 222-6743
Description: Contains educational articles, reports, and surveys pertinent to the nursing profession. Recurring features include letters to the editor, a calendar of events, reports of meetings, news of educational opportunities, board meeting highlights, and a licensed practical nurse (LPN) page. **First Published:** 1945. **Frequency:** Bimonthly.

★2045★ THE CARING CONNECTION
Phyllis A. Burns
3060 E. Bridge St., Ste. 342
Brighton, CO 80601-2724   Phone: (303) 659-4463
Description: Educates caregivers and handicapped persons about their rights and resources available to them. Provides information on research findings, travel accessibility, new products, programs and services for the handicapped and caregivers, and reading materials. Recurring features include helpful tips and inspirational items from readers. **First Published:** January 1984. **Frequency:** Monthly.

★2046★ CAROLINA TIPS
Carolina Biological Supply Co.
2700 York Rd.
Burlington, NC 27215   Phone: (919) 226-6000
Description: Contains articles of interest to science teachers from the elementary to college levels. **First Published:** 1938. **Frequency:** Monthly. **ISSN:** 0045-5865.

★2047★ CAT MEWS
Susan Behn
57 Whitehall Blvd., Ste. 7
Garden City, NY 11530   Phone: (516) 877-1337
Description: Provides in-depth information and veterinary advice on a single subject related to cats in each issue. Features articles dealing with systemics, specific diseases, nutrition, behavior, and age. **First Published:** January 1987. **Frequency:** Bimonthly. **ISSN:** 0889-3152.

★2048★ CATHOLIC HEALTH WORLD
Catholic Health Association of the United States
4455 Woodson Rd.
St. Louis, MO 63134   Phone: (314) 427-2500
Description: Focuses on Catholic health care facilities, and news of legislation that affects the quality of Catholic and general health care. Features articles on people and programs within the field. Recurring features include editorials, news of members, and letters to the editor. **First Published:** February 15, 1985. **Frequency:** Semimonthly. **ISSN:** 8756-4068.

★2049★ CAUSN NEWSLETTER
Canadian Association of University Schools of Nursing
151 Slater St., Ste. 1200
Ottawa, ON, Canada K1P 5N1   Phone: (613) 563-1236
Description: Reports Association news and events. Recurring features include a calendar of events, news of members, and job listings. **ISSN:** 0835-9660.

★2050★ CCBC NEWSLETTER
Council of Community Blood Centers
725 15th St. NW, Ste. 700
Washington, DC 20005-2109   Phone: (202) 393-5725
Description: Covers blood center management topics, pertinent federal and state government actions, legal issues, and developments in health care and medicine. Recurring features include news of members, notices of meetings and publications, and clinical abstracts. **First Published:** 1978. **Frequency:** Weekly.

★2051★ CCL FAMILY FOUNDATIONS
Couple to Couple League International, Inc.
PO Box 111184
Cincinnati, OH 45211   Phone: (513) 661-7612
Description: Concerned with natural family planning, its growth, social effects, health benefits, and advantages to couples and families. Carries practical help, supportive information, personal testimonies, and items on activities and developments in the movement and the League. Recurring features include news of research, letters to the editor, book reviews, news of members, and columns titled Natural Parenting, The Marriage Counselor, and Jottings. **First Published:** 1974. **Frequency:** Bimonthly.

★2052★ CCLV NEWS
Council of Citizens With Low Vision International
5707 Brockton Dr., No. 302
Indianapolis, IN 46220-5481   Phone: (800) 733-2258
Description: Offers a large-print format for individuals who may be legally blind, but still have some residual vision. Supports CCLV's dedication to the special needs of low vision people by publishing news of CCLV activities and projects. Carries information on computer products for the vision impaired, large print and braille publications and services, and legislative and regulatory developments of interest. Recurring features include letters to the editor, interviews, news of research, news of educational opportunities and job listings, book reviews, and a calendar of events. Also contains columns titled Random Access, Presidentially Speaking, F.Y.I., Chapters in Action, The Book Nook, Eye-Q, From the Field, and Frankly Speaking. **First Published:** 1984. **Frequency:** Quarterly.

★2053★ CDDR NEWS
Coalition for the Medical Rights of Women
25 Taylor St., No. 704
San Francisco, CA 94102   Phone: (415) 441-4434
Description: Focuses on women's medical rights, particularly reproductive rights, and other health issues. **First Published:** 1977. **Frequency:** 6/yr.

★2054★ CDF REPORTS
Children's Defense Fund
122 C St. NW
Washington, DC 20001   Phone: (202) 628-8787
Description: Highlights advocacy efforts in areas of child poverty, teen pregnancy prevention, child welfare, child health, child care and development, education, family services, and child mental health. Monitors policy and legislative developments at the federal, state, and local levels. Recurring features include news of research, successful programs, and congressional voting records. **First Published:** 1980. **Frequency:** Monthly. **ISSN:** 0276-6531.

★2055★ CDR REPORTS
Council for Disability Rights
208 S. La Salle, Ste. 1330
Chicago, IL 60604-1102   Phone: (312) 444-9484
Description: Presents news and commentary regarding the civil rights of persons with disabilities, and public policy affecting them. Provides updates on bills, legislation, services, and other governmental activities having an impact on people with disabilities. Also profiles other organizations that advocate for the rights of the disabled. Recurring features include letters to the editor, columns written by people with disabilities, and notices of publications and resources available. **First Published:** March 1983. **Frequency:** Monthly.

★2056★ CDRR NEWS
Committee to Defend Reproductive Rights
145 9th St.
San Francisco, CA 94103   Phone: (415) 431-8660
Description: Covers a wide range of reproductive rights issues, including such topics as abortion, access to contraceptive services, and sterilization abuse. Provides internal information on the Committee and news of related legislation. Recurring features include a calendar of events. **First Published:** September 1981. **Frequency:** Bimonthly.

★2057★ CELIAC NEWS
Canadian Celiac Association
6519B Mississauga Rd.
Mississauga, ON, Canada L5N 1A6   Phone: (416) 567-7195
Description: Deals with celiac disease, dermatitis, herpetiformis, and gluten-free diets. Recurring features include letters to the editor, news of research, a calendar of events, reports of meetings, and book reviews. **First Published:** 1981. **Frequency:** Quarterly. **ISSN:** 0833-1464.

★2058★ CENTER FOR BIOMEDICAL ETHICS—NEWSLETTER
Center for Biomedical Ethics
University of Minnesota
UMHC Box 33
420 Delaware St. SE
Minneapolis, MN 55455   Phone: (612) 625-4917
Description: Provides news and information relating to the Center and its research. Announces conferences. **First Published:** Winter 1986. **Frequency:** Quarterly.

★2059★ CENTER FOR HEALTH SERVICES—NEWSLETTER
Center for Health Services
Vanderbilt Medical Center
Sta. 17
Nashville, TN 37232   Phone: (615) 322-4773
Description: Focuses on the Center's community service work in the Kentucky, Tennessee, Virginia, West Virginia, and Alabama region. Carries the reports of staff members on their ongoing research and outreach projects. Also reports on projects of the Student Health Coalition, the Student Environmental Health Project, Maternal and Infant Health project, and Action Research. **Frequency:** Biennially.

★2060★ CENTER NEWS
Memorial Sloan-Kettering Cancer Center
1275 York Ave.
New York, NY 10021   Phone: (212) 639-3573
Description: Provides news of research and treatment advances and other Center news of activities. **Frequency:** Bimonthly.

★2061★ CENTER FOR REHABILITATION TECHNOLOGY—NEWS UPDATE
Center for Rehabilitation Technology
Georgia Institute of Technology
10th and Hemphill Sts.
Atlanta, GA 30332-0156   Phone: (404) 894-4960
Description: Informs the public on Center activities and products, upcoming conferences, and new technology in the market for persons with disabilities. **First Published:** December 1988. **Frequency:** Monthly.

★2062★ CENTER FOR SICKLE CELL DISEASE—NEWSLETTER
Center for Sickle Cell Disease
Howard University
2121 Georgia Ave. NW
Washington, DC 20059   Phone: (202) 806-7930
Description: Focuses on sickle cell disease. Reports on research, fundraising and community activities, and people in the field. Recurring features include news of the Center and its staff, letters from readers, profiles of sickle cell patients, reports of seminars and appointments, and notices of awards and continuing education opportunities. **First Published:** January 1973. **Frequency:** Quarterly.

★2063★ CENTER FOR THE STUDY OF DRUG DEVELOPMENT—NEWSLETTER
Center for the Study of Drug Development
Tufts University
136 Harrison Ave.
Boston, MA 02111   Phone: (617) 956-0070
Description: Provides information regarding the various aspects of drug development. Recurring features include announcements of conferences and publications and news of staff activities. **First Published:** 1976. **Frequency:** 3/yr.

★2064★ CENTRE FOR GERONTOLOGY—NEWSLETTER
Centre for Gerontology
University of Alberta
P-225 Biological Sciences Bldg.
Edmonton, AB, Canada T6G 2E9   Phone: (403) 492-4718
Description: Recurring features include news of research, a calendar of

97

events, and news of educational opportunities. **First Published:** 1982. **Frequency:** Quarterly.

★2065★ CFBS NEWSLETTER
Canadian Federation of Biological Societies
360 Booth St.
Ottawa, ON, Canada K1R 7K4   Phone: (613) 234-9555
Description: Follows the Federation's lobbying and other activities enacted on behalf of constituent biological societies. Offers scientific news from member societies, reports on meetings, and information on grant programs. **First Published:** Spring 1985. **Frequency:** Semiannually, spring and fall.

★2066★ CH NEWS
National AIDS Clearinghouse
Canadian Public Health Association
400-1565 Carling Ave.
Ottawa, ON, Canada K1Z 8R1   Phone: (613) 725-3796
Description: Promotes Acquired Immune Deficiency Syndrome (AIDS) awareness through education. Recurring features include notices of publications available. **Frequency:** 6/yr.

★2067★ CHAC INFO
Catholic Health Association of Canada
1247 Kilborn Pl.
Ottawa, ON, Canada K1H 6K9   Phone: (613) 731-7148
Description: Tracks the activities of the Association. Recurring features include a calendar of events, reports of meetings, news of educational opportunities and awards, and job listings. **First Published:** 1984. **Frequency:** Quarterly. **ISSN:** 0822-8426.

★2068★ THE CHALICE
Calix Society
7601 Wayzata Blvd.
Minneapolis, MN 55426   Phone: (612) 546-0544
Description: Directed toward Catholic and non-Catholic alcoholics who are maintaining their sobriety through affiliation with and participation in Alcoholics Anonymous. Emphasizes the virtue of total abstinence, through contributed stories regarding spiritual and physical recovery. Recurring features include obituaries, statistics, book announcements, news of research, and the column National Office News and Notes. **First Published:** 1956. **Frequency:** Bimonthly.

★2069★ CHANGE AND EXCHANGE
Health Care Material Management Society
13223 Black Mountain Rd., No. 1-432
San Diego, CA 92129   Phone: (619) 538-0863
Description: Provides information on Society membership activities, educational programs, certification, and local chapters. Recurring features include columns titled President's Message and Certification Tips. **First Published:** February 1987. **Frequency:** Bimonthly.

★2070★ CHANGING MEDICAL MARKETS
Theta Corp.
8 Old Indian Trail
Middlefield, CT 06455-1248   Phone: (203) 349-1054
Description: Covers marketing, new products and technologies, mergers and acquisitions, corporate actions, and product recalls. Reviews useful publications and reports on research papers in professional journals. Lists new products. Includes statistics and staff appointments of professionals in the field. **Frequency:** Monthly.

★2071★ CHARITY AND CHILDREN
Baptist Children's Homes of North Carolina, Inc.
PO Box 338
Thomasville, NC 27360   Phone: (919) 472-1000
Description: Presents news of interest to supporters of the Baptist Children's Homes of North Carolina. **First Published:** May 1887. **Frequency:** Monthly.

★2072★ CHEST SOUNDINGS
International Academy of Chest Physicians and Surgeons
American College of Chest Physicians
3300 Dundee Rd.
Northbrook, IL 60062   Phone: (708) 498-1400

★2073★ CHI NEWSLETTER
Children's Hospice International
901 N. Washington St., No. 700
Alexandria, VA 22314-1535   Phone: (703) 684-0330
Description: Covers aspects of pediatric hospice care from methodology to administration. Provides news and information on conferences and reference sources. Recurring features include editorials, news of research, book reviews, and a calendar of events. **First Published:** Fall 1983. **Frequency:** Quarterly.

★2074★ CHICAGO HERPETOLOGICAL SOCIETY—BULLETIN
Chicago Herpetological Society
2001 N. Clark St.
Chicago, IL 60614
Description: Concerned with the biology, captive care, and husbandry of reptiles and amphibians. Recurring features include editorials, news of research, letters to the editor, and book reviews. **First Published:** April 1966. **Frequency:** Monthly. **ISSN:** 0009-3464.

★2075★ CHICAGO NURSE
Chicago Nurses Association
180 N. Michigan Ave., Ste. 1510
Chicago, IL 60601   Phone: (312) 263-2708
Description: Contains general information and news relating to Association activities and health articles written by the membership. **Frequency:** 6/yr. **ISSN:** 0199-2066.

★2076★ CHILD HEALTH TALKS
National Black Child Development Institute
1023 15th St. NW, Ste. 600
Washington, DC 20005   Phone: (202) 387-1281
Description: Provides information and guidance to parents on health issues facing black children. **Frequency:** Quarterly.

★2077★ CHILD PROTECTION REPORT
Business Publishers, Inc.
951 Pershing Dr.
Silver Spring, MD 20910   Phone: (301) 587-6300
Description: Covers all child protection programs, child welfare, juvenile justice, and child abuse programs. Recurring features include news of research, a calendar of events, reports of meetings, and notices of publications available. **First Published:** 1974. **Frequency:** Biweekly. **ISSN:** 0147-1260.

★2078★ CHILDBIRTH WITHOUT PAIN EDUCATION ASSOCIATION—MEMO
Childbirth Without Pain Education Association
20134 Snowden
Detroit, MI 48235   Phone: (313) 341-3816
Description: Concerned with the Lamaze-Pavlov method of childbirth, obstetric care, parenting, and women. Recurring features include news of Association activities, book reviews, and a director's column. **First Published:** 1959. **Frequency:** Bimonthly.

★2079★ CHILDHAVEN—HAPPENINGS
Childhaven
316 Broadway
Seattle, WA 98122   Phone: (206) 624-6477
Description: Covers programs and events of the agency, which serves abused and underprivileged children in the Seattle area. Recurring features include case studies and columns titled From the Executive Director and Volunteer Spotlight.

★2080★ CHILDREN OF AGING PARENTS
Children of Aging Parents
Woodbourne Office Campus, Ste. 302A
1609 Woodbourne Rd.
Levittown, PA 19057   Phone: (215) 945-6900
Description: Contains articles and informational notices on the concerns and issues of elderly persons and those who care for them. Provides organizations, resources, and services to help caregivers of elderly. **First Published:** 1984. **Frequency:** Bimonthly.

★2081★ **CHILDREN IN HOSPITALS—NEWSLETTER**
Children in Hospitals
31 Wilshire Park
Needham, MA 02192   Phone: (617) 482-2915
Description: Centers on helping parents prepare themselves and their children for hospitalization. Concerned with the rights of hospitalized individuals, institutional and professional procedures and policies, existing agencies and services, and other issues. Covers efforts to initiate flexible visiting policies and to provide live-in hospital accommodations. Recurring features include book reviews and letters from parents. **First Published:** 1971. **Frequency:** Quarterly.

★2082★ **CHILDREN AND TEENS TODAY**
Atcom, Inc.
2315 Broadway, Ste. 300
New York, NY 10024-4397   Phone: (212) 873-5900
Description: Contains in-depth information on new therapeutic trends, techniques for helping victims of child abuse, and child and teen sexuality. **First Published:** 1979. **Frequency:** Monthly. **ISSN:** 0882-942X.

★2083★ **CHILDREN'S HOSPICE INTERNATIONAL NEWSLETTER**
Martha Blechar Gibbons
901 N. Washington St., No. 700
Alexandria, VA 22314   Phone: (703) 684-0330
Description: Examines issues and resources on children's hospice care. Recurring features include a calendar of events, book reviews, and notices of publications available. **First Published:** 1983. **Frequency:** Quarterly.

★2084★ **CHILDREN'S MAGAZINE**
Children's Hospital & Health Center
8001 Frost St.
San Diego, CA 92123   Phone: (619) 576-1700
Frequency: Quarterly.

★2085★ **CHILDREN'S RIGHTS OF NEW YORK—HOTLINE**
Children's Rights of New York, Inc.
15 Arbutus Ln.
Stony Brook, NY 11790-1408   Phone: (516) 751-7840
Description: Concerned with family problems, especially those involving children. Covers child custody, physical and emotional health, education, discipline, and pertinent legislation. Recurring features include interviews, news of research, and book reviews. **ISSN:** 0895-3171.

★2086★ **CHINESE AMERICAN MEDICAL SOCIETY—NEWSLETTER**
Chinese American Medical Society
281 Edgewood Ave.
Teaneck, NJ 07666   Phone: (212) 305-3569
Description: Publishes Society news for Chinese-American physicians. Recurring features include editorials, news of research, letters to the editor, news of members, job listings, and a calendar of events. **First Published:** 1985. **Frequency:** 3-4/yr.

★2087★ **CHIROPRACTORS' ASSOCIATION OF SASKATCHEWAN—THE BULLETIN**
Chiropractors' Association of Saskatchewan
3420A Hill Ave.
Regina, SK, Canada S4S 0W9   Phone: (306) 585-1411
Description: Features letters to the editor, interviews, news of research, a calendar of events, reports of meetings, news of educational opportunities, job listings, and notices of publications available. **Frequency:** 3/yr.

★2088★ **CHOOSE LIFE**
National Right to Life Committee, Inc.
419 7th St. NW, Ste. 500
Washington, DC 20004   Phone: (202) 626-8800
Description: Provides educational and religious information for religiously based pro-life groups and individuals. Recurring features include news of research, reports of meetings, news of educational opportunities, book reviews, notices of publications available, guest editorials, church bulletin inserts, suggested prayers, and legislative alerts. **First Published:** June 1988. **Frequency:** Bimonthly.

★2089★ **CHRONICLE**
Center for Health Research
1315 N. Kaiser Center Dr.
Portland, OR 97227-1042
Description: Covers Center activities. Recurring features include news of research. **Frequency:** Quarterly.

★2090★ **CICI'S CONTACT**
Cochlear Implant Club International
PO Box 464
Buffalo, NY 14223-0464   Phone: (716) 838-4662
Description: Reviews research and developments in cochlear implants and provides items on deafness and deaf persons. Contains profiles of patient experiences, news of members, and a calendar of events. **First Published:** Spring 1982. **Frequency:** 4/yr.

★2091★ **CLEAN INDOOR AIR NEWS**
Houston Group to Alleviate Smoking Pollution
PO Box 27227
Hoston, TX 77227   Phone: (713) 453-5798
Description: Acts as a forum for nonsmokers, and smokers who are trying to quit, to share information and discover new ways to enjoy clean indoor air at work and during leisure time. Provides information on meetings, "smoke-free" dining in the Houston area, legislation, and Environmental Protection Agency (EPA) reports on tobacco smoke and indoor air pollution. **Frequency:** Quarterly.

★2092★ **CLEARING THE AIR**
Georgians Against Smoking Pollution
PO Box 450981
Atlanta, GA 30345   Phone: (404) 296-9526
Description: Promotes smoking restrictions through legislation, public education, and support for businesses with "no smoking" policies. Recurring features include columns titled From the President's Desk, Announcement of Coming Events, and Dine-Out.

★2093★ **CLIMB FOR INDEPENDENCE**
Wheelchair Motorcycle Association
101 Torrey St.
Brockton, MA 02401   Phone: (617) 583-8614
Description: Advocates the adaptation of motorized vehicles for use by the handicapped. The preferred vehicle is a three-wheeled all-terrain cycle with hand controls, which is easily accessible from a wheelchair. Recurring features include news of research.

★2094★ **CLIN-ALERT**
Science Editors, Inc.
143 Marlton Pike
Metford, NJ 08055   Phone: (609) 654-6266
Description: Reports on adverse drug reactions, drug interactions, and related therapeutic hazards. Summarizes information from leading medical and pharmaceutical journals, reporting patient history, diagnosis, treatment, dosage, author's conclusion and warning, trade names of drugs, legal actions, if any, and dispositions. **First Published:** 1962. **Frequency:** Semimonthly. **ISSN:** 0069-4770.

★2095★ **CLINIC NEWS**
Center for Population Options
1025 Vermont Ave. NW, Ste. 210
Washington, DC 20005   Phone: (202) 347-5700
Description: Reports on news from school-barred and school-linked clinics around the country. Features articles on funding, provision of family planning, mental health, general health, HIV prevention and other types of services in a school setting. **Frequency:** Quarterly.

★2096★ **CLINICAL ABSTRACTS/CURRENT THERAPEUTIC FINDINGS**
Harvey Whitney Books Co.
Box 42696
Cincinnati, OH 45242   Phone: (513) 793-3555
Description: Provides abstracts of current international literature concerning drug therapy, interactions, and reactions. **First Published:** 1982. **Frequency:** Monthly. **ISSN:** 1043-3031.

★2097★   CLINICAL CANCER LETTER
Cancer Letter, Inc.
PO Box 15189
Washington, DC 20003   Phone: (202) 543-7665
Description: Reports on cancer research, drugs, and protocols activated by the National Biotherapy Study Group and National Cancer Institute's Division of Cancer Treatment. **Frequency:** Monthly. **ISSN:** 164-985X.

★2098★   CLINICAL CARDIOLOGY ALERT
American Health Consultants, Inc.
PO Box 740056
Atlanta, GA 30374   Phone: (404) 262-7436
Description: Concerned primarily with the origin, detection, and treatment of heart disease. Offers commentary on current medical research papers which have been published in national medical journals. "Does not provide advice regarding medical diagnosis or treatment of any individual case." **First Published:** 1982. **Frequency:** Monthly. **ISSN:** 0741-4218.

★2099★   CLINICAL CONSULT
American Society of Consultant Pharmacists
2300 9th St. S., Ste. 515
Arlington, VA 22204   Phone: (703) 920-8492
Description: Contains news of the Society, which seeks to improve consultant pharmacist services to nursing homes and other long-term care facilities. Provides a forum for the exchange of information about the profession, the advantages of certification, and professional standards. Reports on the results of lobbying efforts to promote legislation beneficial to the Society. Profiles different extended-care pharmacy operations. **First Published:** 1982. **Frequency:** Monthly.

★2100★   CLINICAL DENTAL BRIEFINGS
Goldman School of Graduate Dentistry
Boston University
100 E. Newton St.
Boston, MA 02118   Phone: (617) 638-4677
Description: Covers dental topics such as endodontic disease, corrosion in nonprecious metal castings, oral leukoplakia, dental treatments for asthmatic patients, pharmacological management, and methods of recapping needles. **Frequency:** Monthly. **ISSN:** 0893-665X.

★2101★   CLINICAL DIABETES
American Diabetes Association
1660 Duke St.
Alexandria, VA 22314   Phone: (703) 549-1500
Description: Provides scientific information on diabetes and its treatment. **Frequency:** Bimonthly.

★2102★   CLINICAL ENGINEERING INFORMATION SERVICE
Scientific Enterprises, Inc.
5104 Randolph Rd.
North Little Rock, AR 72116   Phone: (501) 771-1775
Description: Discusses management and technology in the field of clinical engineering. Reports on regulatory requirements, liability, cost analysis, and new technology. Recurring features include listings of employment opportunities. Contains FDA recalls and clinical engineering abstracts. **First Published:** January 1977. **Frequency:** Bimonthly. **ISSN:** 0277-0393.

★2103★   CLINICAL IMMUNOLOGY NEWSLETTER
Elsevier Science Publishing Company, Inc.
655 Avenue of the Americas
New York, NY 10010   Phone: (212) 633-3927
Description: Publishes original foot-noted articles on immunology, serodiagnosis, and immunopathology, covering such topics as monoclonal antibodies, AIDS, legionella, and interferon. Reports on new techniques in detection, current research, case studies, and meetings in the field. **First Published:** 1979. **Frequency:** Monthly. **ISSN:** 0197-1859.

★2104★   CLINICAL LAB LETTER
Quest Publishing Company
1351 Titan Way
Brea, CA 92621   Phone: (714) 738-6400
Description: Covers the latest advances in clinical laboratory technology, with special attention to safety and management in laboratories. Includes regular sections on government activities, safety hazards and product recalls, new diagnostic technology, professional activities of clinical lab personnel, information sources, business news, meetings and conventions, and educational opportunities. **First Published:** 1980. **Frequency:** Semimonthly; monthly in January and August. **ISSN:** 0197-8454.

★2105★   CLINICAL LASER MONTHLY
American Health Consultants, Inc.
67 Peachtree Park Dr. NE
Atlanta, GA 30309   Phone: (404) 262-7436
Description: Concerned with topics related to lasers in surgery and medicine in general. Considers safety, legal issues, reimbursement, cost containment, and new products and procedures. Recurring features include news of research and conferences, a calendar of events, guest columns, and laser practice reports. **First Published:** August 1983. **Frequency:** Monthly.

★2106★   CLINICAL MICROBIOLOGY NEWSLETTER
Elsevier Science Publishing Co., Inc.
655 Avenue of the Americas
New York, NY 10010   Phone: (212) 633-3927
Description: Informs clinical microbiologists, pathologists, and laboratory technologists of the most recent developments in diagnostic and antimicrobial therapy. Covers identification, diagnostic methods, and interpretation of laboratory test results. Recurring features include case reports, letters to the editor, and announcements of interest to microbiologists. **First Published:** 1978. **Frequency:** Semimonthly. **ISSN:** 0196-4399.

★2107★   CLINICAL ONCOLOGY ALERT
American Health Consultants, Inc.
PO Box 740056
Atlanta, GA 30374   Phone: (404) 262-7426
Description: Consists of abstracts from medical literature pertaining to the diagnosis and treatment of cancer. Includes editorial commentary on each abstract. **First Published:** January 1986. **Frequency:** Monthly. **ISSN:** 0886-7186.

★2108★   CMT NEWSLETTER
Charcot-Marie-Tooth Disease/Peroneal Muscular Atrophy International Association, Inc.
1 Springbank Dr.
St. Catharines, ON, Canada L2S 2K1   Phone: (416) 687-3630
Description: Provides information for patients, their families, and interested health care professionals on Charcot-Marie-Tooth (CMT) disease, a hereditary neuro-muscular condition that causes loss of feeling and/or movement from the knees down and the elbows down; breathing and other functons may also be affected. Recurring features include letters from people with CMT, interviews, two columns by doctors who answer questions about CMT, research news, a calendar of events, news of new aids for daily living, and up-to-date lists of new research papers printed around the world. **First Published:** August 1984. **Frequency:** Bimonthly. **ISSN:** 0831-6279.

★2109★   CNSW NEWSLETTER
Council of Nephrology Social Workers
National Kidney Foundation, Inc.
30 E. 33rd St.
New York, NY 10016   Phone: (212) 889-2210
Description: Serves as a source of practice information, program ideas, and discussion on current controversies for members who are in the field of nephrology. Carries regional and chapter news, legislative information, and news of research. Recurring features include editorials, book reviews, reports on meetings, and a calendar of events. **First Published:** April 1975. **Frequency:** Quarterly.

★2110★   CODING CLINIC FOR ICD-9-CM
American Hospital Association
840 N. Lake Shore Dr.
Chicago, IL 60611   Phone: (312) 280-6000
Description: Provides current information for hospitals and other health-related organizations on improving the accuracy and uniformity of coding. Gives advice on achieving consistency, maintaining integrity, and determining standards for medical coding. Discusses compiling reliable data for trend analysis, assigning codes for new technologies, supplementing the training of coders, and expanding the coder's knowledge of medical science. Recurring features include a column titled Ask the Editor. **First Published:** 1984. **Frequency:** Quarterly. **ISSN:** 0742-9800.

★2111★   COLLEGE OF DENTAL SURGEONS OF BRITISH COLUMBIA—BULLETIN
College of Dental Surgeons of British Columbia
1765 W. 8th Ave., Ste. 500
Vancouver, BC, Canada V6J 5C6   Phone: (604) 736-3621
Description: Gives information on current events, new techniques, continuing education programs, government issues, and various activities related

to the dental community. Recurring features include letters to the editor, reports of meetings, and job listings. **First Published:** 1940. **Frequency:** 5-6/yr. **ISSN:** 0831-7941.

★2112★ COLLEGE OF PHARMACISTS OF BRITISH COLUMBIA—BULLETIN
College of Pharmacists of British Columbia
1765 W. 8th Ave., Ste. 200
Vancouver, BC, Canada V6J 1V8   Phone: (604) 733-2440
Description: Focuses on developments pertaining to professional guidelines and related concerns for pharmacists. Reports on the meetings and decisions of the College and of the Council of the College of Pharmacists. Recurring features include information on continuing education opportunities and news briefs. **Frequency:** 10/yr.

★2113★ COLLEGE OF PHYSICIANS AND SURGEONS OF MANITOBA—NEWSLETTER
College of Physicians and Surgeons of Manitoba
494 St. James St.
Winnipeg, MB, Canada R3G 3J4   Phone: (204) 774-4344
Frequency: 6/yr.

★2114★ COLLEGE OF PSYCHOLOGISTS IN NEW BRUNSWICK—CONTACT
College of Psychologists of New Brunswick
PO Box 1194, Sta. A
Fredericton, NB, Canada E3B 1B0   Phone: (506) 459-1994
Description: Covers issues in clinical psychology. Recurring features include letters to the editor, interviews, news of research, a calendar of events, reports of meetings, news of educational opportunities, job listings, book reviews, and notices of publications available. **First Published:** 1984. **Frequency:** 5/yr.

★2115★ COMMON GROUND
National Catholic Rural Life Conference
4625 Beaver Ave.
Des Moines, IA 50310   Phone: (515) 270-2634
Description: Covers rural issues, environmental concerns, natural resources, faith issues, the world food situation, poverty, alternative energy, and land ownership. Recurring features include news of activities of the Conference and book reviews. **First Published:** July 1982. **Frequency:** 9/yr. **ISSN:** 0748-5114.

★2116★ COMMUNICATION OUTLOOK
Artificial Language Laboratory
405 Computer Center
Michigan State University
East Lansing, MI 48824-1042   Phone: (517) 353-0870
Description: Provides information on modern techniques and aids for persons who experience communication handicaps due to neurological or neuromuscular conditions. Reports on current research, centers, programs, and projects in the field. Recurring features include listings of new publications, questions and letters from readers, and a calendar of events. **First Published:** Spring 1978. **Frequency:** Quarterly. **ISSN:** 0161-4126.

★2117★ COMMUNITY CARE QUARTERLY
National Institute on Community-Based Long-Term Care
National Council on the Aging
600 Maryland Ave. SW
Washington, DC 20024   Phone: (202) 470-1200
Description: Reviews the latest developments in community-based long-term care, which enables older adults to live in a home or community setting as long as possible. Contains an update on public policy issues affecting senior housing and an article related to care for older adults. **First Published:** 1985. **Frequency:** Quarterly.

★2118★ COMMUNITY HEALTH SERVICES ASSOCIATION LTD.—FOCUS
Community Health Services Saskatoon Association Ltd.
455 2nd Ave. N.
Saskatoon, SK, Canada S7K 2C2   Phone: (306) 652-0300
Description: Profiles Association events and programs. Discusses health issues. Recurring features include news of research, a calendar of events, reports of meetings, news of educational opportunities, book reviews, and notices of publications available. **First Published:** 1964. **Frequency:** 4/yr.

★2119★ COMPANION ANIMAL NEWS
Morris Animal Foundation
45 Inverness Dr., E.
Englewood, CO 80112   Phone: (303) 790-2345
Description: Contains reports on research funded by the Foundation to study ways to cure animal diseases and maintain the health of pets. Recurring features include news of Foundation and volunteer activities and a calendar of events. **Frequency:** 3/yr.

★2120★ COMPARATIVE PATHOLOGY BULLETIN
Registry of Comparative Pathology
Armed Forces Institute of Pathology
Washington, DC 20306   Phone: (202) 576-2452
Description: Publishes descriptions of animal models of human disease. Analyzes models in terms of biologic features, comparison with human disease, and usefulness. Describes one or two models with references per issue, and includes other items of interest concerning the comparative aspects of disease. **First Published:** 1979. **Frequency:** Quarterly.

★2121★ COMPASSION CORPS
People for the Ethical Treatment of Animals
PO Box 42516
Washington, DC 20015   Phone: (301) 770-7444

★2122★ THE COMPASSIONATE SHOPPER
Beauty Without Cruelty USA
175 W. 12th St., Ste. 16G
New York, NY 10011-8275   Phone: (212) 989-8073
Description: Lists cosmetics, houshold, office, and construction products manufactured and tested without the suffering, confinement, or death of any animal. Provides information on various places where "animal-free tested products" can be purchased. Recurring features include news of research, news of educational opportunities, book reviews, and notices of publications available. **First Published:** Spring 1973. **Frequency:** 3/yr.

★2123★ COMPUTERS AND MEDICINE
Carol Brierly
PO Box 36
Glencoe, IL 60022   Phone: (708) 446-3100
Description: Contains news and ideas on using computers in the health field for diagnosis, treatment, education, and other purposes. Discusses the social and behavioral implications of computer technology, the utilization of artificial intelligence, and similar considerations. Recurring features include reviews of pertinent articles and books, news of research, and a calendar of events. **First Published:** November/December 1972. **Frequency:** Monthly. **ISSN:** 0163-0547.

★2124★ CONCENSUS NEWSLETTER
The Keystone Center
PO Box 606
Keystone, CO 80435   Phone: (303) 468-5822
Description: Reports on the activities of the Center, which provides mediation and facilitation services to resolve disputes concerning science, technology, energy, health, and the environment; and focuses on environmental quality and health, biotechnology and genetic resources, and natural resources. **Frequency:** 3/yr.

★2125★ CONCERN
Saskatchewan Registered Nurses' Association
2066 Retallack St.
Regina, SK, Canada S4T 2K2   Phone: (306) 757-4643
Description: Informs registered nurses (RNs) on the Association's activities; provides a forum for discussion. Recurring features include letters to the editor, interviews, news of research, calendar of events, reports of meetings, news of educational opportunities, job listings, book reviews, and notices of publications available. **First Published:** 1948. **Frequency:** Bimonthly. **ISSN:** 0319-8499.

★2126★ CONCERN FOR DYING—NEWSLETTER
Society for the Right to Die
250 W. 57th St.
New York, NY 10107   Phone: (212) 246-6962
Description: Supports the organization's concern to "protect patient autonomy in regard to treatment during terminal illness." Reports on developments in legislation, case law, public policy, and professional perspectives related to death, dying, and medical decision-making. Recurring features include letters to the editor and columns titled Action in the Courts and Bookshelf. **First Published:** January 1974. **Frequency:** 31/yr.

★2127★ CONCERN NEWS
Project Concern International
3550 Afton Rd.
PO Box 85323
San Diego, CA 92138   Phone: (619) 279-9690
Description: Highlights Project Concern's health development programs in the U.S. and abroad. Reports on training projects related to nutrition, family health, disease prevention, hygiene, and sanitation. Recurring features include news of fundraising and programmatic activities. **Frequency:** Quarterly.

★2128★ CONCERNED RELATIVES OF NURSING HOME PATIENTS—INSIGHT
Concerned Relatives of Nursing Home Patients
Nursing Home Advisory and Research Council, Inc.
PO Box 18820
Cleveland, OH 44118-0820   Phone: (216) 321-0403
Description: Reflects the goals of the organization, whose purpose is to improve the quality of nursing home care through better regulations and enforcement. Reports on subjects related to nursing homes, including regulations, enforcement, fraud, Medicaid discrimination, quality of care, information and Medicare, nursing home rates, and proposed legislation. Recurring features include news of research, letters to the editor, and columns titled From the School Marm's Desk, From the Nurse's Station, The Advocate's Tour, This and That, and Interviews. **First Published:** October 1976. **Frequency:** Bimonthly.

★2129★ CONCERRN
Saskatchewan Registered Nurses Association
2066 Retallack St.
Regina, SK, Canada S4T 2K2   Phone: (306) 757-4643
Description: Provides a forum for discussion of issues and concerns in the field of nursing. Carries Association news and notices, profiles members, discusses current and future nursing trends, and alerts nurses to technological changes in the field. Recurring features include letters to the editor, news of research, a calendar of events, reports of meetings, news of educational opportunities, job listings, book reviews, and notices of publications available. Also includes columns titled Pat on the Back, Ideas and Resources, Ask the Experts, and People and Pathways. **First Published:** 1971. **Frequency:** 6/yr. **ISSN:** 0319-8499.

★2130★ CONFERENCE CALL
Association of State and Territorial Directors of Public Health
    Education
Health Promotion
Vermont Department of Health
PO Box 70
Burlington, VT 05402   Phone: (802) 863-7330
Description: Disseminates information to directors of public health education in state and territorial departments of health to promote the quality of public health education practice and develop practice guidelines. Discusses topics relevant to public health education and Association activities and programs. **Frequency:** Quarterly.

★2131★ CONNECTICUT NURSING NEWS
Connecticut Nurses Association
377 Research Pkwy., Ste. 2D
Meriden, CT 06450   Phone: (203) 238-1207
Description: Focuses on the nursing profession. Aims to advance the nursing practice through promoting high standards of education while assuring quality health care. **First Published:** 1921. **Frequency:** 10/yr. **ISSN:** 0278-4092.

★2132★ CONNECTIVE ISSUES
National Marfan Foundation
382 Main St.
Port Washington, NY 11050-3121   Phone: (516) 883-8712
Description: Designed to disseminate accurate and timely information on Marfan syndrome, a heritable disease of the connective tissue affecting the skeleton, lungs, eyes, heart, and blood vessels. Recurring features include news of research, Foundation news, and notices of publications. **First Published:** 1984. **Frequency:** Quarterly. **ISSN:** 8756-9086.

★2133★ CONSULTANT'S NEWSLETTER
Society of Medical-Dental Management Consultants
6215 Larson
Kansas City, MO 64133   Phone: (816) 353-8488
Description: Discusses news of the Society, including notices and reports of meetings, group activities, and information regarding members. Also

covers management consulting for the health professional in such areas as taxes, medical design, retirement, medical economics, estate planning, and trends in medical and dental practices. **First Published:** 1968. **Frequency:** Monthly or Bimonthly.

★2134★ CONSUMER PHARMACIST
ELBA Medical Foundation Inc.
PO Box 1403
Metairie, LA 70001   Phone: (504) 833-3600
Description: Features letters to the editor, interviews, news of research, reports of meetings, book reviews, and columns titled Infobits, New Drugs, and OTC Preparations. **First Published:** 1980. **Frequency:** 6/yr.

★2135★ CONSUMER REPORTS ON HEALTH
Consumers Union
101 Truman Ave.
Yonkers, NY 70004   Phone: (914) 378-2000
Description: Presents information on health and medicine from a consumer's point of view. Recurring features include news of research. **First Published:** September 1989. **Frequency:** Monthly.

★2136★ CONSUMERS UNION NEWS DIGEST
Consumers Union of the United States, Inc.
101 Truman Ave.
Yonkers, NY 10703-1057
Description: Presents information on consumer interest issues such as home fuel savings, environmentalism, health care costs, financial planning, food and nutrition pensions, housing, insurance, product packaging, philanthropy, and safety products. **Frequency:** Semimonthly. **ISSN:** 1047-4048.

★2137★ CONTINENTAL ASSOCIATION OF FUNERAL AND MEMORIAL SOCIETIES—LEADER
Continental Association of Funeral and Memorial Societies
6900 Lost Lake Rd.
Egg Harbor, WI 54209-9231   Phone: (301) 913-0030
Description: Concerned with the funeral industry, activities of memorial societies, and legislation related to consumer rights in making funeral arrangements. Includes articles and bibliographies pertaining to funerals, death, and dying. **First Published:** 1980. **Frequency:** Quarterly.

★2138★ THE CONTINUUM
Saskatchewan Health-Care Association
1445 Park St.
Regina, SK, Canada S4N 4C5   Phone: (306) 347-5500
Description: Provides a forum for the discussion of issues and events in the health care community. Carries news of happenings in the safety and health field, including human interest pieces relating to the health care industry and Association news. Recurring features include news of research, legislation, a calendar of events, reports of meetings, news of educational opportunities, and a column titled Associate Members' Corner. **First Published:** March 1976. **Frequency:** Quarterly.

★2139★ CONTRACEPTIVE TECHNOLOGY UPDATE
American Health Consultants, Inc.
67 Peachtree Park Dr. NE
Atlanta, GA 30309   Phone: (404) 262-7436
Description: Provides information on all major methods of contraception, including new research, new products, case histories, and major conference coverage. Publishes studies on the effectiveness and hazards of different contraceptives, the effects of abortion, and contraceptive failure. Recurring features include news of research, a calendar of events, and columns titled Sources of Information, Journal Review, and Commentary. **First Published:** April 1980. **Frequency:** Monthly. **ISSN:** 0274-726X.

★2140★ COOPERATIVE CONNECTION
Nurse Healers-Professional Associates, Inc.
85 Hawthorne Rd.
Williamstown, MA 01267   Phone: (413) 458-9181
Description: Discusses holistic treatment, healing techniques, and other health issues. Promotes the sharing of healing experiences among health practitioners. Recurring features include news of research, book reviews, news of members, and a calendar of events. **First Published:** Ca. 1980. **Frequency:** Quarterly.

★2141★ CORHEALTH
American Correctional Health Services Association
11 W. Monument Ave., Ste. 510
PO Box 2307
Dayton, OH 45401   Phone: (513) 223-9630
Description: "Dedicated to improving correctional health services." Covers news of the Association and its chapters and affiliates, who administer and monitor efficiency of health care in correctional institutions. Concerned with the multidisciplinary approach to nursing, dentistry, medicine, surgery, and medical administration. Recurring features include editorials, news of members, statistics, publications available, calls for papers, abstracts, book reviews, and a calendar of events. First Published: Summer 1975. Frequency: Bimonthly.

★2142★ CORNELL ANIMAL HEALTH NEWSLETTER
Department CL
53 Park Pl., 8th Fl.
New York, NY 10007   Phone: (800) 525-0643
Description: Concerned with all aspects of animal health. First Published: 1983. Frequency: Monthly. ISSN: 0884-092X.

★2143★ CORONARY HEART DISEASE RESEARCH UPDATE
American Health Assistance Foundation
15825 Shady Grove Rd., Ste. 140
Rockville, MD 20850   Phone: (301) 948-3244
Description: Highlights work of coronary heart disease researchers and provides tips for preventing and dealing with the disease. Recurring features include news of research and columns titled From the President and Ask the Experts. First Published: 1986. Frequency: Quarterly.

★2144★ CORRESPONDENCE SOCIETY OF SURGEONS:
COLLECTED LETTERS
Laux Company, Inc.
63 Great Rd.
Maynard, MA 01754-2025   Phone: (508) 897-5552
Description: Provides a question-and-answer format related to medical surgery. Usually concentrates on one or two subjects and contains responses from medical experts from throughout the world. Includes references with each response. First Published: January 1978. Frequency: Monthly. ISSN: 0162-6477.

★2145★ COSMETIC SURGERY TODAY
John Munna
3280 Howell Mill Rd., Ste. 212
Atlanta, GA 30327   Phone: (404) 355-6994
Description: Discusses aspects of cosmetic plastic surgery. Recurring features include interviews. Frequency: Quarterly.

★2146★ COTH REPORT
Council of Teaching Hospitals
Association of American Medical Colleges
2450 North St. NW
Washington, DC 20037-1126   Phone: (202) 828-0490
Description: Provides news, commentary, and analysis particularly for health care executives and medical educators in teaching hospitals and medical schools. Reviews current federal and state legislation and general activities of the Association and its affiliates, and relates events of interest to teaching hospitals. Recurring features include a list of current officers of the Association. First Published: July 1967. Frequency: 6/yr. ISSN: 0146-2814.

★2147★ COURAGE
National MPS Society, Inc.
17 Kraemer St.
Hicksville, NY 11801   Phone: (516) 931-6338
Description: Provides information for families of children with mucopolysaccharidosis (MPS) and mucolipidosis, extremely rare genetic disorders caused by particular enzyme deficiencies. Facilitates the exchange of ideas between families on how to care for and cope with a chronically ill child. Provides the latest medical information about MPS and related disorders. Recurring features include news of research, interviews, letters to the editor, reports of conferences, and a calendar of events. First Published: 1975. Frequency: Quarterly.

★2148★ COURAGE NEWS
Courage Center
3915 Golden Valley Rd.
Golden Valley, MN 55422   Phone: (612) 588-0811
Description: Publishes news of the Center, a nonprofit organization providing rehabilitation and independent living services to people with physical disabilities and speech, hearing, and vision impairments. Recurring features include news of members and donations, information on Camp Courage, news of research, and columns titled The Best of Courage, Courage Information, and From the Executive Director. First Published: March 1952. Frequency: Quarterly.

★2149★ C-P UPDATE
Canadian Association of Cardio-Pulmonary Technologists
Box 848, Sta. A
Toronto, ON, Canada M5W 1G3   Phone: (416) 340-4086
Description: Reports on meetings, announces seminars, and contains product information of interest to cardiopulmonary technologists and individuals in related fields. Recurring features include a calendar of events, employment opportunities, books reviews, and examiniation notices. First Published: Ca. 1972. Frequency: Quarterly.

★2150★ CPHA HEALTH DIGEST
Canadian Public Health Association
1565 Carling Ave. Ste. 400
Ottawa, ON, Canada K1Z 8R1   Phone: (613) 725-3769
Description: Features updates on Association's activities and conference announcements. Recurring features include columns titled Executive Director's Page and Resolutions and Motions. Frequency: Quarterly. ISSN: 0703-5624.

★2151★ CRANIAL LETTER
Cranial Academy
1140 W. 8th St.
Meridian, ID 83642   Phone: (208) 888-1201
Description: Provides information about osteopathy in the cranio-sacral field for doctors of osteopathy, dentistry, and medicine. Carries news of reports, papers, seminars, courses offered by the Academy, and research projects. Recurring features include obituaries, a calendar of events, and columns titled President's Message, The Dental Corner, and Scientific Section. First Published: 1948. Frequency: Quarterly.

★2152★ CRIME VICTIMS DIGEST
Washington Crime News Services
3918 Prosperity Ave., Ste. 318
Fairfax, VA 22031   Phone: (703) 573-1600
Description: Reports on a variety of crime and victim related issues, including crime statistics and trends, police reports, terrorism, and legislative actions and their implications. Also contains examples of violent crimes as well as preventative suggestions to avoid victimization. Recurring features include reports of meetings, a calendar of events, and a column titled In the Courts. First Published: 1983. Frequency: Monthly. ISSN: 0884-5107.

★2153★ CROHN'S AND COLITIS FOUNDATION OF
AMERICA—FOUNDATION FOCUS
Crohn's & Colitis Foundation of America
444 Park Ave. S.
New York, NY 10016-7374   Phone: (212) 685-3440
Description: Covers the activities of the Foundation, which is dedicated to funding research to find a cure for Crohn's disease (ileitis) and ulcerative colitis and to improving the quality of life for people who suffer from these diseases. Focuses on research developments, medical treatment, and coping with chronic illness. Recurring features include insurance and pharmacology columns, IBD File, Mutual Help Network, and member news. Frequency: 3/yr. ISSN: 0897-6759.

★2154★ THE CRYER
California Children's Lobby
PO Box 448
Sacramento, CA 95812-0448   Phone: (916) 444-7477
Description: Covers child-related issues pending in the California legislature. Recurring features include statistics and editorials. Frequency: Monthly during the legislative session.

★2155★ CSA ALERTS
Clinical Systems Association
2265 Genesa Ln.
Vero Beach, FL 32963-3148   Phone: (407) 231-1686
Description: Discusses clinical systems. **First Published:** 1975. **Frequency:** Semimonthly.

★2156★ CUE-IN
American Red Cross
17th & D St. NW
Washington, DC 20006   Phone: (202) 639-3629
Description: Provides policy information on the activities of the American Red Cross. **First Published:** 1985. **Frequency:** Biweekly.

★2157★ CURRENT AWARENESS BULLETIN
Suicide Information and Education Centre
201-1615 10th Ave. SW
Calgary, AB, Canada T3C 0J7   Phone: (403) 245-3900
Description: Provides information on resources, notices of publications available, conferences, programs, books, and audiovisual materials on suicide and suicidal behaviors. **Frequency:** Quarterly. **ISSN:** 0823-8340.

★2158★ CVO UPDATE
College of Veterinarians of Ontario
340 Woodlawn Rd., W., Ste. 24-25
Guelph, ON, Canada N1H 2X1   Phone: (519) 824-5600
First Published: 1978. **Frequency:** 5/yr. **ISSN:** 0821-6320.

★2159★ CYSTIC FIBROSIS FOUNDATION—METRO NEWS
Cystic Fibrosis Foundation
Metropolitan Washington, DC Chapter
6931 Arlington Rd., Ste. T200
Bethesda, MD 20814   Phone: (301) 657-8444
Description: Represents the metropolitan Washington, D.C., chapter of the Foundation. Publicizes advances in cystic fibrosis research and education as well as news of the Foundation's patient, family service programs, and special events. Recurring features include news of research, news of members, a calendar of events, and a column titled Message From the President. **Frequency:** 2/yr.

★2160★ DAMIEN DUTTON CALL
Damien Dutton Society for Leprosy Aid, Inc.
616 Bedford Ave.
Bellmore, NY 11710   Phone: (516) 221-5909
Description: Covers the Society's efforts to "provide relief, research and recreation to victims of leprosy all over the world regardless of race, color or creed." Offers news about projects to aid leprosy victims worldwide to encourage further donation of funds for medical, social, research, and educational programs. Recurring features include letters to the editor, a calendar of events, reports of meetings, news of educational opportunities, and news of members. **First Published:** 1948. **Frequency:** 3/yr.

★2161★ DAV
Disabled American Veterans
807 Maine Ave. SW
Washington, DC 20024   Phone: (202) 554-3501
Description: Discusses issues affecting disabled veterans and their dependants and survivors. **First Published:** 1922. **Frequency:** Monthly. **ISSN:** 0885-6400.

★2162★ DAYCARE HEALTH
Mathanna Publications
PO Box 5351
Bellingham, WA 98227-9970   Phone: (206) 671-4350
Description: Provides information on health care issues in child day-care centers. Recurring features include news of research, news of educational opportunities, notices of publications available, and case studies. **First Published:** 1987. **Frequency:** 5/yr. **ISSN:** 0893-9020.

★2163★ DDR HEALTH POLICY AND BIOMEDICAL RESEARCH: THE BLUE SHEET
F-D-C Reports, Inc.
5550 Friendship Blvd., Ste. 1
Chevy Chase, MD 20815   Phone: (301) 657-9830
Description: Reviews health policy and biomedical research. Discusses Medicare/Medicaid, public health, health professions education and supply, and issues affecting the National Science Foundation and other federal research efforts and regulations. Recurring features include news of

research and a calendar of events. **First Published:** 1957. **Frequency:** Weekly. **ISSN:** 0162-3605.

★2164★ THE DEAF EPISCOPALIAN
Episcopal Conference of the Deaf
100 Wilson Pl.
Syracuse, NY 13214
Description: Discusses the activities of the Episcopal Conference as well as carrying news, reports, and informative articles that address issues of interest to deaf members of the Episcopal Church. Includes news on clergy, individual congregations, and congregation members. **First Published:** 1927. **Frequency:** Bimonthly.

★2165★ DEAFPRIDE ADVOCATE QUARTERLY
Deafpride
1350 Potomac Ave. SE
Washington, DC 20003   Phone: (202) 675-6700
Description: Reports on the organization's advocacy programs on behalf of deaf persons. Works for the rights of deaf people and their families and assists groups throughout the U.S. to deal with issues in their communities. Recurring features include updates on the programs, services, conferences, and educational projects of the organization. **Frequency:** Quarterly.

★2166★ DEFENCE MEDICAL ASSOCIATION OF CANADA— NEWSLETTER
Defence Medical Association of Canada
Box 2716, Sta. D
Ottawa, ON, Canada K1P 6H7   Phone: (613) 733-3323
First Published: 1989. **Frequency:** Monthly.

★2167★ DENTAL COMPUTER NEWSLETTER
Andent, Inc.
1000 North Ave.
Waukegan, IL 60085   Phone: (708) 223-5077
Description: Emphasizes "practical use of all brands of computers for the professional office." Provides news of the computer industry as well as computer-use tips, information on computer gadgets and systems, and system recommendations. Recurring features include editorials, news of research, letters to the editor, news of members, book reviews, and columns titled Education, Hardware, Software, Specials, and Report on Hardware/Software. **First Published:** October 1978. **Frequency:** Bimonthly. **ISSN:** 0738-9744.

★2168★ THE DENTAL LABORATORY CONFERENCE—NEWS AND VIEWS
The Dental Laboratory Conference
4222 King St.
Alexandria, VA 22302-1507   Phone: (215) 546-2313
Description: Presents news of the dental laboratory trade. **First Published:** 1976. **Frequency:** Quarterly.

★2169★ THE DENTIST'S PATIENT NEWSLETTER
Doctor's Press, Inc.
Pitney Rd.
PO Box 11177
Lancaster, PA 17605   Phone: (717) 393-1010
Description: Intended for distribution to dental patients. Carries patient-oriented articles on dental health topics such as the prevention of decay and gum disease, new treatments and technologies, diet, and dental care. Recurring features include cartoons and quizzes. **First Published:** 1983. **Frequency:** Quarterly.

★2170★ DERMASCOPE MAGAZINE
Aestheticians International Association, Inc.
4447 McKinney Ave.
Dallas, TX 75205   Phone: (214) 526-0752
Description: Features articles written by doctors, make up artists, and body therapists on subjects of skin care, make up, and body care. Recurring features include dates of conventions and seminars and columns titled Medical Update, National and International News and Book Review. **First Published:** 1978. **Frequency:** Bimonthly.

★2171★ DES ACTION VOICE
DES Action USA
1615 Broadway, No. 510
Oakland, CA 94612   Phone: (510) 465-4011
Description: Provides medical and legal information about the drug DES (Diethylstilbestrol) and those exposed to it. Contains accounts of personal

experiences, DES international outreach programs, and on lawsuits. Recurring features include abstracts, letters to the editor, news of research, member news, and a column titled Dear Doctor. **First Published:** 1979. **Frequency:** Quarterly.

★2172★ **DEVELOPMENTAL DISABILITIES SPECIAL INTEREST SECTION—NEWSLETTER**
Developmental Disabilities Special Interest Section
1383 Piccard Dr., Ste. 301
Rockville, MD 20850   Phone: (301) 770-2200
Description: Serves as an information exchange for occupational therapists interested in improving function and performance capacity of persons with developmental disabilities. Reports on the progress of various programs, current research, and pertinent legislation. Recurring features include bibliographies. **First Published:** Summer 1978. **Frequency:** Quarterly. **ISSN:** 0279-4098.

★2173★ **DEVICES AND DIAGNOSTICS LETTER**
Washington Business Information, Inc.
1117 N. 19th St.
Arlington, VA 22209-1978   Phone: (703) 247-3427
Description: Seeks to provide executives in the industry with information on regulatory developments regarding medical devices and in vitro diagnostic products. Reports on the Food and Drug Administration (FDA), the Health Care Financing Administration, and Congress. Discusses a variety of issues, including manufacturing practices, compliance and inspection programs, defect reporting, labeling and testing rules, and performance standards. Recurring features include news of research and reports of meetings. **First Published:** 1974. **Frequency:** Weekly. **ISSN:** 0098-7573.

★2174★ **DIABETES NEWSLETTER—THUMB AREA DIABETES ADVISORY COUNCIL**
Diabetes Research and Training Center
University of Michigan
University of Michigan Hospital
1331 E. Ann St., Room 5111
Ann Arbor, MI 48109-0580   Phone: (313) 763-5256

★2175★ **DIABETES '93**
American Diabetes Association
National Service Center
1660 Duke St.
Alexandria, VA 22314   Phone: (703) 549-1500
Description: Intended to provide practical assistance in coping with diabetes. Discusses basics such as medication, exercise, diet, self-testing, and other concerns. Recurring features include recipes, notices of publications available, letters to the editor, and columns titled News Beat and Clip and Save. **First Published:** May 1983. **Frequency:** Quarterly.

★2176★ **THE DIABETIC TRAVELER**
Traveling Healthy, Inc.
PO Box 8223 RW
Stamford, CT 06905   Phone: (203) 327-5832
Description: Contains ideas to help diabetics make safe and economical travel arrangements. Furnishes tips on such precautions as insulin adjustments over time zones, travel storage cases for diabetes supplies, how to carry medical history, foot care for the diabetic traveler, and coping with the common cold while traveling. Focuses on a specific destination or type of travel in each issue. **First Published:** Fall 1986. **Frequency:** Quarterly. **ISSN:** 0899-2398.

★2177★ **DIAGNOSTICS INTELLIGENCE**
CTB International Publishing, Inc.
PO Box 218
Maplewood, NJ 07040   Phone: (201) 763-6855
Description: Covers developments in diagnostics research, new product launches, regulatory affairs, patents, litigation, business opportunities, and finance. Features news of diseases, conditions, and drugs that create new markets for diagnostics. **First Published:** 1989. **Frequency:** 12/yr. **ISSN:** 1054-9609.

★2178★ **DICKINSON'S FDA**
Ferdic, Inc.
PO Box 848
Morgantown, WV 26507-0848   Phone: (304) 291-6690
Description: Monitors medical devices and veterinary and human drug issues. Provides news and analysis covering regulatory, legislative, legal,

and personnel developments and changes within the Food and Drug Administration that have an impact on health care products. Recurring features include news of research and interviews. **First Published:** June 1, 1985. **Frequency:** Bimonthly.

★2179★ **DIET CENTER—NEWSLETTER**
Diet Center, Inc.
76 W. Main
Rexburg, ID 83440   Phone: (208) 356-9381
Description: Promotes better health through sound nutrition. Contains articles on dietary goals and guidelines, anorexia, the cholesterol controversy, and other diet-related concerns. Recurring features include success stories of dieters and menu planners. **First Published:** January 1982. **Frequency:** Monthly.

★2180★ **DIN NEWSERVICE**
Do It Now Foundation
PO Box 27568
Tempe, AZ 85285-7568   Phone: (602) 257-0797
Description: Covers health and behavior. Focuses on drug and alcohol abuse and rehabilitation. **First Published:** May 1983. **Frequency:** 6/yr.

★2181★ **THE DIPLOMATE**
American Board of Professional Psychology
2100 E. Broadway, Ste. 313
Columbia, MO 65201-6082   Phone: (314) 875-1267
Description: Serves the aims of the Board, which conducts oral examinations and awards diplomas to advanced specialists in eight professional specialties: clinical psychology, industrial and organizational psychology, forensic psychology, counselingpsychology, clinical neuropsychology, school psychology, health psychology, and family phsychology. Recurring features include news of awards and educational opportunities. **First Published:** 1980. **Frequency:** Semianual.

★2182★ **DIRECT LINE NEWSLETTER**
American Medical Association Auxiliary
535 N. Dearborn St.
Chicago, IL 60610   Phone: (312) 645-4470
Description: Updates readers on programs aimed at improving public health and providing quality health care. Describes the community service activities of auxiliaries across the U.S. in such areas as venereal disease awareness, the prevention of child abuse, and services to the aging. Recurring features include information on the Shape Up for Life Campaign and on health fairs sponsored by the Association. **Frequency:** Bimonthly.

★2183★ **DIRECT RELIEF INTERNATIONAL—NEWSLETTER**
Direct Relief International
PO Box 30820
Santa Barbara, CA 93130-0820   Phone: (805) 687-3694
Description: Reports on DRI's programs and concern for world health and emergency needs. Recurring features include profiles of volunteers, listings of volunteer opportunities and needs, and recognition of special gifts. **First Published:** Ca. 1970. **Frequency:** 2-3/yr.

★2184★ **DIRECTIONS**
Live Free, Inc.
PO Box 1743
Harvey, IL 30426   Phone: (312) 928-5830
Description: Concerned with techniques for emergency survival and long-term self-sufficiency during and after war or other disasters. Covers survivalist philosophy, firearms and other survival equipment, networking with civil defense and other organizations, and alternative food and energy sources. Recurring features include editorials, letters to the editor, news of members, book reviews, and a calendar of events. **First Published:** July 1977. **Frequency:** Monthly.

★2185★ **DIRECTIONS**
Health Care Material Management Society
13223 Black Mountain Rd., No. 1-432
San Diego, CA 92129   Phone: (619) 538-0863
Description: Provides technical and managment information to promote the Society's goal of advancing the theory and practice of material management within the health care industry. Recurring features include publication of winning papers from an annual technical paper contest. **First Published:** Spring 1986. **Frequency:** Annual.

★2186★   DIRECTIONS IN APPLIED NUTRITION
Aspen Publishers, Inc.
1600 Research Blvd.
Rockville, MD 20850   Phone: (301) 251-5554
Description: Aimed at dietetic practitioners. **Frequency:** Monthly.

★2187★   DISABILITY ISSUES
Information Center for Individuals With Disabilities
27/43 Wormwood St.
Boston, MA 02210-1606   Phone: (617) 727-5540
Description: Addresses persons with disabilities, their relatives and friends, and service providers through articles on education, employment, transportation, housing, legislation, equipment, and entertainment. Recurring features include new product and meeting announcements and resources. **First Published:** January 1980. **Frequency:** 12/yr.

★2188★   DISCHARGE PLANNING UPDATE
Society for Hospital Social Work Directors
840 N. Lake Shore Dr.
Chicago, IL 60611   Phone: (312) 280-6000
Description: Devoted to issues of discharge planning, an interdisciplinary program designed to promote the cooperation of health care professionals, patients, and their families in order to minister to the patient's needs from hospital admittance through post-hospital care. Recurring features include columns titled Washington Report, Legal Qs & As, Research and Discharge Planning (R&DP), and Discharge Dilemmas. **First Published:** Fall 1980. **Frequency:** 6/yr.

★2189★   DISCOVER
Coriell Institute for Medical Research
401 Haddon Ave.
Camden, NJ 08103   Phone: (609) 757-4832
Description: Provides information on advances in basic biomedical research and cell culture storage techniques at the Institute. Includes interviews. **Frequency:** Quarterly.

★2190★   THE DLD TIMES
Division for Learning Disabilities
Council for Exceptional Children
1920 Association Dr.
Reston, VA 22091   Phone: (703) 620-3660
Description: Concerned with research, educational programs, and services for children, youth, and adults with learning disabilities. Recurring features include news of research, news of members, and columns titled LD Newsmakers, News from ERIC, For Your Calendar, and DLD Research Bulletin Board. **First Published:** 1983. **Frequency:** 3/yr.

★2191★   DR. SCHOLL'S FOOT HEALTH FORUM
Scholl, Inc.
303 E. Wacker Dr., 12th Fl.
Chicago, IL 60601-5212
Frequency: Semiannually.

★2192★   DOCTOR'S OFFICE LAB NEWS
Duwest Research/Scientific Newsletters
Rd. 4, Box 7
Stapleton Ct.
Middletown, NY 10940-9683   Phone: (914) 355-9144
Description: Describes new products for the doctor's/group office laboratory as well as government regulations affecting in-office laboratory use. Studies cost-effectiveness, accuracy, and quality of in-office lab testing. Recurring features include editorials, news of research, book reviews, and a calendar of events. **First Published:** January 1985. **Frequency:** 10/yr. **ISSN:** 8756-3754.

★2193★   DOUBLE FEATURE
Parents of Multiple Births Association of Canada, Inc.
4981 Hwy. No. 7 E., Unit 12A, Ste. 161
Markham, ON, Canada L3R 1N1   Phone: (416) 513-7506
Description: Offers articles by parents and health and education professionals on parenting issues of particular concern to parents of twins, triplets, or quadruplets. **First Published:** September 1977. **Frequency:** Quarterly. **ISSN:** 0824-278X.

★2194★   THE DOUBLE HELIX
National Foundation for Infectious Diseases
4733 Bethesda Ave., Ste. 750
Bethesda, MD 20814   Phone: (301) 656-0003
Description: Supplies news of the association's activities concerning public welfare and support of research, education, and prevention of infectious disease. Monitors legislation affecting the biomedical profession and covers scientific developments and announcements of interest to professionals in the immunology, epidemiology, parasitology, and pathology fields. Recurring features include announcements of fellowship winners, reports on meetings, biographies, and a calendar of events. **First Published:** 1976. **Frequency:** Bimonthly.

★2195★   DOWN SYNDROME NEWS
National Down Syndrome Congress
1800 Dempster St.
Park Ridge, IL 60068-1146   Phone: (708) 823-7550
Description: Provides information on educational, research, and service program updates. Carries referrals, presentation synopses, and news items on local, national, and international topics related to Down Syndrome. Recurring features include book and film reviews in Resources section, editorials, notices of coming events, letters, and columns titled Resources, Potpourri, and Good Press. **First Published:** 1975. **Frequency:** 10/yr. **ISSN:** 0161-0716.

★2196★   DREAM NETWORK JOURNAL
Helen Roberts Ossana
1337 Powerhouse Ln., No. 22
Moab, UT 84532   Phone: (801) 259-5936
Description: Intended for those interested in better understanding their dreams. Contains articles submitted by readers on their dreams and survey articles, focusing on "experiential dreamwork." Recurring features include book reviews, a calendar of events, news of research, letters to the editor, information on groups of interest, and "dream art and poetry." **First Published:** 1982. **Frequency:** Quarterly. **ISSN:** 1054-6707.

★2197★   DRG MONITOR
Hanley & Belfus, Inc.
210 S. 13th St.
Philadelphia, PA 19107   Phone: (215) 546-7293
Description: Analyzes the ramifications of new federal regulations governing the control of hospital costs and the costs of health care delivery in general. Recurring features include news of research and essays on critical issues. **First Published:** September 1983. **Frequency:** Monthly, September-June. **ISSN:** 0741-6512.

★2198★   DRUG ABUSE NEWSLETTER
Committees of Correspondence, Inc.
57 Conant St., Rm. 113
Danvers, MA 01923   Phone: (508) 774-2641
Description: Examines drug abuse issues. Focuses on the "detection and exposure of drug culture proponents who have been 'legitimized' in various sectors of our society." Recurring features include editorials, news of research, and book reviews. **First Published:** May 1980. **Frequency:** Quarterly.

★2199★   THE DRUG EDUCATOR
American Council for Drug Education
204 Monroe St., Ste. 110
Rockville, MD 20850   Phone: (301) 294-0600
Description: Describes the Council's projects, including conferences, publications, and promotion of research directed toward the understanding of the behavioral and psychological effects of marijuana, cocaine, and other psychoactive drugs. Contains summaries of scientific findings on the effects of these drugs, advice to parents in coping with their children's drug abuse, and information and commentary on "the harmful effects of illicit drug use." Recurring features include a form for ordering relevant publications, and columns titled Parent Power Line, Publications Update, and Youth Connection. **First Published:** 1979. **Frequency:** Quarterly. **ISSN:** 0897-7321.

★2200★   DRUG AND MARKET DEVELOPMENT— NEWSLETTER
Drug and Market Development
2170 Broadway, Ste. 1200
New York, NY 10024   Phone: (212) 873-8140
Description: Provides analyses of technological, clinical, and market developments in human therapeutics. Assesses important developments and evaluates their impact on the industry. Emphasizes new commercial

opportunities and their affect on existing therapies and markets. Recurring features include news of research, reports of meetings, and columns titled Cardiovascular, Cancer, Inflammation and Infection, Nervous System, Drug Development Technology, and Anesthesiology Strategy. **First Published:** June 1990. **Frequency:** Monthly. **ISSN:** 1053-1564.

★2201★ DRUG UTILIZATION REVIEW
American Health Consultants, Inc.
PO Box 740056
Atlanta, GA 30374   Phone: (404) 262-7436
Description: "Provides practical, how-to articles and examples to help hospital pharmacists and other staff monitor and guide therapy and contain costs." Describes hospital programs designed to monitor or guide drug use and review criteria. Recurring features include reviews of individual drugs, journal reviews, interviews, news of research, a calendar of events, and reports of meetings. Also includes a bimonthly 4-page supplement titled Drug Criteria Network. **First Published:** January 1985. **Frequency:** Monthly. **ISSN:** 0884-8998.

★2202★ DRUGS AND DRUG ABUSE EDUCATION NEWSLETTER
Substance Abuse News Service
PO Box 21133
Washington, DC 20009   Phone: (202) 783-2929
Description: Provides information on a variety of drugs such as tobacco, alcohol, cocaine, LSD, heroin, and marijuana, as well as on the side effects of prescription drugs. Discusses education of the public, results of research studies and nation-wide surveys, federal and state drug legislation, and law enforcement. Recurring features include a calendar of events, book reviews, news of research, and a column titled Briefly. **First Published:** 1969. **Frequency:** Monthly. **ISSN:** 0044-7226.

★2203★ DRUGS IN THE WORKPLACE
Business Research Publications, Inc.
817 Broadway
New York, NY 10003   Phone: (212) 673-4700
Description: Concentrates on scientific, legal, and governmental issues regarding alcohol and drug abuse in the workplace. Focuses on the Employee Assistance Program (EAP) and its role in substance abuse prevention, detection, and treatment. Also discusses drug-testing methods and the merits of various treatment programs. Recurring features include a section titled Recent Rulings (covering court and arbitration cases). **First Published:** November 1986. **Frequency:** Monthly. **ISSN:** 1040-4228.

★2204★ DWD NEWSLETTER
Dying With Dignity
175 St. Clair Ave., W.
Toronto, ON, Canada M4V 1P7   Phone: (416) 921-2329
Description: Contains information on voluntary euthanasia in Canada and elsewhere. Addresses the concerns of physicians, families, and individuals who are facing the issue of "the right to die." Monitors the activities and services of the organization and spotlights the actions of similar groups in North America. Recurring features include letters to the editor, reports of meetings, book reviews, notices of publications available, and a calendar of events. **First Published:** 1984. **Frequency:** Quarterly. **ISSN:** 0847-1797.

★2205★ DYSTONIA MEDICAL RESEARCH FOUNDATION— NEWSLETTER
Dystonia Medical Research Foundation
8383 Wilshire Blvd., No. 800
Beverly Hills, CA 90211   Phone: (213) 852-1630
Description: Updates medical and research aspects of dystonia, a group of disorders typified by irregular muscle tone and/or involuntary muscle contractions. Recurring features include news of the Foundation, its chapters and meetings; in-depth examination of dystonia; profiles of persons with dystonia; a listing of scientific advisory board members around the world; and news of research. **First Published:** 1977. **Frequency:** Quarterly.

★2206★ EARLY INTERVENTION
Illinois Early Childhood Intervention Clearinghouse
840 S. Spring St.
Springfield, IL 62704   Phone: (217) 785-1364
Description: Covers early childhood issues with an emphasis on special health needs or disability. Primarily focused on issues specific to Illinois residents, including legislation. Recurring features include a calendar of events, reports of meetings, book reviews, audiovisual reviews, and notices of publications available. **First Published:** November 1986. **Frequency:** Quarterly. **ISSN:** 1058-8396.

★2207★ EATING DISORDERS REVIEW
PM, Inc.
PO Box 10172
Van Nuys, CA 91410   Phone: (818) 873-4399
First Published: July/August 1990. **Frequency:** Bimonthly. **ISSN:** 1048-6984.

★2208★ EATWRITE
Stephanie Brandenburger
245 Concord Ave., No. 17
Cambridge, MA 02138   Phone: (617) 354-6039
Description: Provides original recipes accompanied by commentary and nutritional breakdowns. Promotes healthy eating habits. **First Published:** April 1991. **Frequency:** Bimonthly.

★2209★ EB REPORTER
Dystrophic Epidermolysis Bullosa Research Association
141 5th Ave., Ste. 7-S
New York, NY 10010   Phone: (212) 995-2220
Description: Serves the families and sufferers of epidermolysis bullosa (EB), an inherited skin disorder. Features articles on helpful hints, pen pals, and questions and answers. **First Published:** June 1989. **Frequency:** Semiannually.

★2210★ ECLIPSE
Shanti Project
525 Howard St.
San Francisco, CA 94105-3080   Phone: (415) 777-2273
Description: Promotes the work of the Project, which offers volunteer practical and emotional support services and on-going support to individuals and their loved ones who face a diagnosis of Acquired Immune Deficiency Syndrome (AIDS). Publishes articles about people with AIDS, news of Shanti programs/services, articles on volunteers and clients, interviews, plus features on staff, administrators, and honorary board members. **First Published:** 1974. **Frequency:** 6/yr.

★2211★ ECONOMIC TRENDS
American Hospital Association
840 N. Lake Shore Dr.
Chicago, IL 60611   Phone: (312) 280-6522
Description: Provides statistical analysis of community hospital finances, utilization, and staffing trends, based on data from the American Hospital Association National Hospital Panel Survey. Examines the implications of key trends. **First Published:** 1985. **Frequency:** Quarterly. **ISSN:** 0882-5807.

★2212★ EDUCATION OF THE HANDICAPPED
Capitol Publications, Inc.
1101 King St., Ste. 444
Alexandria, VA 22314   Phone: (703) 683-4100
Description: Carries news of federal legislation, programs, and funding for educating handicapped children. Covers federal and state litigation on the Individuals with Disability Education Act and other relevant laws. Provides news of research. **First Published:** December 12, 1975. **Frequency:** Biweekly.

★2213★ EFFICIENT VISION
Optometric Extention Program Foundation
2912 S. Daimler
Santa Ana, CA 92705   Phone: (714) 250-8070
Description: Serves as a forum for maintaining contact with patients. Provides news of interest regarding vision and developmental optometry for patients. **First Published:** 1928. **Frequency:** 3/yr.

★2214★ EL BOLETIN
National Hispanic Psychological Association
c/o Joe Carabajal
2415 W. Sixth St.
P.O. Box 451 Health
Brookline, MA 02146   Phone: (617) 266-6336
Description: Supports the work and professional advancement of Hispanic psychologists by encouraging cooperation and communication among them. Includes news and information on the Association and its work to influence local, state, and national policies in the interests of Hispanics. Recurring features include news of members, listings of educational opportunities, and news of research. **Frequency:** Quarterly.

★2215★ ELDERLY HEALTH SERVICES LETTER
Health Resources Publishing
Brinley Professional Plaza, 3100 Hwy. 38
PO Box 1442
Wall Township, NJ 07719-1442   Phone: (201) 681-1133
Description: Predicts future trends in hospital based health care services for the elderly. **First Published:** October 1986. **Frequency:** Monthly. **ISSN:** 0891-9275.

★2216★ ELECTROLYSIS WORLD
American Electrology Association
106 Oak Ridge Rd.
Trumbull, CT 06611   Phone: (203) 372-7119
Description: Emphasizes the Association's desire to unite electrologists for education, professional advancement, and the protection of public welfare. Reports on and discusses progress toward uniform legislative standards throughout the states and the coordination of efforts by individual affiliated associations toward the same end. Recurring features include reports on Association activities and events, news of research, and news of members. **First Published:** 1981. **Frequency:** Quarterly.

★2217★ ELLON BACH NEWSLETTER
Ellon Bach
644 Merrick Rd.
Lynbrook, NY 11563-2332   Phone: (516) 593-2206
Description: Acts as a forum "for the exchange of current ideas and research on the Bach Flower Remedies." Recurring features include editorials, letters, news of research, case studies, announcements and columns titled Remedy Usage and Highlight Remedy. **First Published:** March 1984. **Frequency:** 2/yr.

★2218★ EM RESIDENT
Society for Academic Emergency Medicine
900 W. Ottawa
Lansing, MI 48915   Phone: (517) 485-5484
Description: Focuses on the issues involved in emergency medicine graduate medical education such as residency electives, appropriate and inappropriate utilization of emergency room services, and educational opportunities. Carries news and activities information from emergency medicine professional associations, including the American College of Emergency Physicians, University Association for Emergency Medicine, and American Board of Emergency Medicine. Recurring features include Association news and a column titled President's Message. **First Published:** 1975. **Frequency:** Bimonthly.

★2219★ EMERGENCY DEPARTMENT MANAGEMENT
American Health Consultants, Inc.
3525 Piedmont Rd. NE
6 Piedmont Center, Ste. 400
Atlanta, GA 30305   Phone: (404) 351-4523

★2220★ EMERGENCY LEGAL BRIEFINGS
American Health Consultants, Inc.
3525 Piedmont Rd. NE
6 Piedmont Center, Ste. 400
Atlanta, GA 30305   Phone: (405) 351-4523

★2221★ EMERGENCY MEDICINE REPORTS
American Health Consultants, Inc.
3525 Piedmont Rd. NE
6 Piedmont Center, Ste. 400
Atlanta, GA 30305   Phone: (404) 262-7436
Description: Covers emergency medicine topics for emergency physicians. Focuses on one major topic per issue. **First Published:** 1980. **Frequency:** Biweekly. **ISSN:** 0746-2506.

★2222★ EMPLOYERS' HEALTH BENEFITS MANAGEMENT LETTER
American Business Publishing
Brinley Professional Plaza
3100 Hwy. 138
PO Box 1442
Wall Township, NJ 07719-1442   Phone: (908) 681-1133
Description: Monitors what employers are doing to adequately save on health care costs. Includes information on ways to cut health care costs and actions by lawmakers which will dramatically affect the future of health care programs, as well as actions taken by Blue Cross-Blue Shield and other health care agencies. **First Published:** August 1983. **Frequency:** Monthly. **ISSN:** 0740-9087.

★2223★ THE EMS LEADER
Cornell Communications
330 Garfield Ave.
Eau Claire, WI 54701   Phone: (715) 834-6046
Description: Provides management/leadership articles for owners, managers, and supervisors of ambulance services, Emergency Medical Services (EMS) educators, and other EMS agency personnel. Presents articles on the people of EMS, performance appraisals, motivation, public relations, and ideas from people in the field. Recurring features include columns titled Leadership Notes and National Scene. **First Published:** 1984. **Frequency:** 10/yr. **ISSN:** 0897-0297.

★2224★ THE ENDEAVOR
American Society for Deaf Children
814 Thayer Ave.
Silver Spring, MD 20910   Phone: (301) 585-5400
Description: Reflects the goals of the Association, which provides "information and support to families with children who are deaf or hard of hearing." Promotes equal educational opportunities for the deaf, the use of sign language within the family, and national recognition of the special needs of the hearing impaired. Reports on relevant legislation and proposed regulations. Recurring features include a calendar of events, book reviews, statistics, editorials, news of the Association, announcements of scholarship awards, information on organizations for the deaf, and news of activities and programs that are interpreted for the deaf. **Frequency:** Bimonthly.

★2225★ ENDOMETRIOSIS ASSOCIATION NEWSLETTER
International Endometriosis Association
8585 N. 76th Pl.
Milwaukee, WI 53223   Phone: (414) 355-2200
Description: Publishes news and concerns of the Association, a self-help organization devoted to "offering mutual support and help to those affected by endometriosis, educating the public and medical community about the disease, and promoting research related to endometriosis." Recurring features include medical updates, letters from women with endometriosis, news of members and chapters of the Association, book reviews, and columns titled In the Mail, News/Announcements, and Research Recap. **First Published:** 1980. **Frequency:** Bimonthly. **ISSN:** 0897-1870.

★2226★ THE ENVIRONMENTAL GUARDIAN
C.U.R.E. Formaldehyde Poisoning Association, Inc.
Waconia, MN 55387-9583   Phone: (612) 442-4665
Description: Serves to inform victims of formaldehyde poisoning of their medical and legal options. Provides information on nonformaldehyde products, state coordination officials, and special problems in children. Recurring features include news of members and news of research; book reviews; letters to the editor; victims' personal stories; interviews with medical and legal professionals; questionnaires; and columns titled Legal Ledger, Calendar, State Updates, and Media Events. **First Published:** June 1980. **Frequency:** Quarterly.

★2227★ ENVIRONMENTAL HEALTH AND SAFETY NEWS
Department of Environmental Health
University of Washington
School of Public Health
Seattle, WA 98195   Phone: (206) 543-4252
Description: Covers pollution, safety, and health in occupations. **First Published:** 1951. **Frequency:** Irregular.

★2228★ ENVIRONMENTAL NUTRITION
Environmental Nutrition, Inc.
2112 Broadway, No. 200
New York, NY 10023   Phone: (212) 362-0424
Description: Keeps readers abreast of new findings and breakthroughs in nutrition and diet. Discusses nutrition in connection with food additives, food fads and diets, pharmaceuticals and vitamins, and disease prevention. Recurring features include diet book reviews, editorials, letters to the editor, and resources. **First Published:** November 1977. **Frequency:** Monthly. **ISSN:** 0195-4024.

★2229★ ENVIRONS
Marine Biomedical Center
Marine Laboratory
Duke University
Beaufort, NC 28516   Phone: (919) 728-2111
Description: Focuses on issues related to environmental biomedicine, with particular emphasis on toxicology and pollution. Reports on seminars, conferences, and feasibility studies in progress. Recurring features include statistics, book reviews, and news of research. First Published: February 15, 1978. Frequency: 6/yr.

★2230★ EPI NOTES
Epidemiology Division
North Carolina Department of Environment, Health, and Natural Resources
PO Box 27687
Raleigh, NC 27611-7687   Phone: (919) 733-3421
Description: Contains excerpts from epidemiologic studies and related feature articles. Recurring features include news of conferences.

★2231★ EPIDEMIC
STRAIGHT, Inc.
3001 Gandy Blvd.
St. Petersburg, FL 33702-2032   Phone: (813) 577-6011
Description: Furnishes news on STRAIGHT, a drug treatment program that attempts to retrain adolescents in the values and rules of their culture and help them to unlearn the rules of behavior and values of the drug subculture. Includes news of therapy programs and of staff members. Frequency: Periodic.

★2232★ EPIDEMIOLOGY BULLETIN
Communicable Diseases Division
Oklahoma State Department of Health
1000 NE 10th St.
Oklahoma City, OK 73117-1299   Phone: (405) 271-4060
Description: Reports on communicable diseases, outbreaks, immunizations, and injuries. Frequency: Monthly.

★2233★ EPI-GRAM
Maine State Department of Human Services
State House, Sta. No. 11
Augusta, ME 04333   Phone: (207) 289-5301
Description: Concerned with public health issues. First Published: 1977. Frequency: Monthly.

★2234★ EPILEPSY USA
Epilepsy Foundation of America
4351 Garden City Dr.
Landover, MD 20785   Phone: (301) 459-3700
Frequency: 10/yr.

★2235★ ESTHETICS
American Academy of Esthetic Dentistry
211 E. Chicago Ave., Ste. 948
Chicago, IL 60611
Description: Presents news about this organization of dentists concerned with restorative procedures of natural teeth. Recurring features include news of research, member news, a calendar of events, information on the annual meeting, and a column titled A Letter From the President. First Published: 1980. Frequency: 3/yr.

★2236★ EUROPE DRUG AND DEVICE REPORT
Washington Business Information, Inc.
117 N. 19th St.
Arlington, VA 2209-1798   Phone: (703) 247-3434
Description: Covers rules and standards of the European Community, its member states, and other nations as they affect human and veterinary prescription and over-the-counter drugs, medical devices, and diagnostic products. First Published: 1991. Frequency: Biweekly. ISSN: 1056-179X.

★2237★ EXCEPTIONAL NEWS
Center for Persons With Disabilities
Utah State University
Logan, UT 84322-6845   Phone: (801) 750-1991
Description: Provides news of activities in the field of special education. Frequency: Quarterly.

★2238★ THE EXCHANGE
Nisonger Center for Mental Retardation and Developmental Disabilities
Ohio State University
1581 Dodd Dr.
Columbus, OH 43210-1296   Phone: (614) 292-8365
Description: Covers mental retardation and developmental disabilities. Includes new studies, conference announcements, new publications , Center courses and special projects, and information from other organizations. First Published: 1976. Frequency: Quarterly.

★2239★ THE EXCHANGE PROJECT
Exchange Project
Peace Development Fund
PO Box 270
Amherst, MA 01004   Phone: (413) 256-0216
Description: Promotes the exchange of information, ideas, and resources among peace and justice groups. Publicizes the activities of the Project, which offers training in organizational development to grassroots groups. Recurring features include fundraising tips. First Published: Fall 1984. Frequency: 3/yr.

★2240★ EXECUTIVE HEALTH'S GOOD HEALTH REPORT
Executive Health
PO Box 8880
Chapel Hill, NC 27515-8880   Phone: (919) 929-7519
Description: Features articles on personal health, nutrition, weight reduction, and exercise. Gives primary consideration to one health topic per issue. First Published: 1963. ISSN: 0882-2131.

★2241★ THE EXPLORER
National Association of Dental Assistants
900 S. Washington St., No. G13
Falls Church, VA 22046-4020   Phone: (703) 237-8616
Description: Reflects the Association's goal of improving the professional and personal lives of dental assistants and other staff. Provides information relating to the field of dentistry. First Published: 1974. Frequency: Monthly.

★2242★ EYE TO EYE
Eye-Bank for Sight Restoration, Inc.
210 E. 64th St.
New York, NY 10021   Phone: (212) 980-6700
Description: Focuses on corneal transplantation and provides information on corneal disease, legislative updates, and news of the organization's work collecting and distributing corneal tissue for transplants. Recurring features include news of research, stories about donors and recipients, and news of fundraising and other volunteer activities. First Published: Summer 1981. Frequency: Quarterly.

★2243★ EYE TO EYE
Steen-Hall Eye Institute
2611 Greenwood Rd.
Shreveport, LA 71103   Phone: (318) 631-2020
Description: Presents information concerning new ophthalmic developments and the Institute's public service activities. Recurring features include news of research, member news, a calendar of events, news of community projects and programs related to the eye, and human interest stories. First Published: January 1985. Frequency: Quarterly.

★2244★ EYE TO EYE
International Eye Foundation/Society of Eye Surgeons
7801 Norfolk Ave.
Bethesda, MD 20814   Phone: (301) 986-1830
Description: Describes the programs of and opportunities offered by the Foundation and the Society concerned with the prevention of blindness in the developing areas of the world. Discusses Foundation activities, including prevalence surveys, needs assessment, and the development and implementation of assistance (i.e., the training of ophthalmologists, physicians, nurses, technicians, and health workers in the delivery of eye care). First Published: 1972. Frequency: Semiannually.

★2245★ EYE INSIGHT
American Interprofessional Foundation
601 Driftwood Ln.
Northbrook, IL 60062   Phone: (708) 564-4641
Description: Reports on issues related to eye health care. Provides information on subjects such as devices for correcting vision, resource

material for the visually handicapped, and eye research. Offers tips for better care and preservation of sight. **First Published:** 1984. **Frequency:** Bimonthly.

★2246★   EYE INSTITUTE OF NEW JERSEY—UPDATE
Eye Institute of New Jersey
15 S. 9th St.
Newark, NJ 07107   Phone: (201) 268-8053
First Published: 1980. **Frequency:** Quarterly.

★2247★   THE EYE OPENER
American Narcolepsy Association
PO Box 26230
San Francisco, CA 94126-6230   Phone: (415) 788-4793
Description: Provides information on medications, research developments, political and regulatory affairs, and Association and government activities affecting people with narcolepsy. **First Published:** 1976. **Frequency:** Quarterly.

★2248★   EYEWITNESS
Contact Lens Society of America
190 Market St.
Lexington, KY 40507   Phone: (606) 233-1606
Description: Informs members of developments in the contact lens industry. Also reports on related educational information and technical papers. Recurring features include news of research, calendar of events, reports of meetings, and associate member listing. **Frequency:** Quarterly.

★2249★   FACETS
San Diego County Dental Society
3942 Hancock St.
San Diego, CA 92110-1562   Phone: (619) 223-5391
Description: Reports information on the Society, awards, externship programs, new applicants, and health guidelines. Recurring features include a calendar of events and columns titled New Applicants, Classified Advertising, and Continuing Education.

★2250★   FAMILY HEALTH INTERNATIONAL—NETWORK
PO Box 13950
Research Triangle Park, NC 27709   Phone: (919) 549-7040
Description: Covers research into new methods of family planning, maternal and child health care, and the transfer of technology in these areas. Focuses on the impact of this research on the developing countries and the population problem. Recurring features include resource references and information on AIDS. **First Published:** October 1979. **Frequency:** Quarterly. **ISSN:** 0270-3637.

★2251★   FAMILY SUPPORT BULLETIN
United Cerebral Palsy Associations, Inc.
1522 K St. NW, Ste. 112
Washington, DC 20005   Phone: (202) 842-1266
Frequency: Quarterly.

★2252★   FANS—NEWSLETTER
Fresh Air for Nonsmokers
PO Box 24052
Seattle, WA 98124   Phone: (206) 932-7011
Description: Promotes smoking restrictions through legislation, public education, and support for businesses with "no smoking" policies. Provides statistics on smoking and the tobacco industry.

★2253★   FDA MEDICAL BULLETIN
Dept. of Health and Human Services
Food and Drug Administration
5600 Fishers Ln.
Rockville, MD 20857   Phone: (301) 443-3220
Description: Reports on recent developments in drugs, biologics, medical and radiological devices, and food from the FDA's perspective. **First Published:** 1970. **Frequency:** 3/yr.

★2254★   FDA SURVEILLANCE INDEX FOR PESTICIDES
National Technical Information Service
U.S. Department of Commerce
5285 Port Royal Rd.
Springfield, VA 22161   Phone: (703) 487-4630
Description: Alerts readers to the potential health risks of dietary exposure to individual pesticides. Provides an evaluation that includes FDA monitoring results; chemical, biological, and toxicological data; and usage estimates. **Frequency:** Monthly.

★2255★   FEDERAL VETERINARIAN
National Association of Federal Veterinarians
1023 15th St. NW, No. 300
Washington, DC 20005   Phone: (202) 289-6334
Description: Reports developments in federal veterinary medicine and in personnel policy affecting veterinarians. **First Published:** 1920. **Frequency:** Monthly. **ISSN:** 0164-6257.

★2256★   FEDERATION OF AMERICAN HEALTH SYSTEMS
1111 19th St. NW, Ste. 402
Washington, DC 20036   Phone: (202) 833-3090
Description: Monitors "health legislation, regulatory and reimbursement matters, current developments in the health care industry, appointments in the health field," and related matters for investor-owned hospitals. Recurring features include state updates. **First Published:** 1968. **Frequency:** Biweekly.

★2257★   FEDERATION OF STATE MEDICAL BOARDS OF THE UNITED STATES—FEDERATION BULLETIN
Federation of State Medical Boards of the United States, Inc.
6000 Western Pl., Ste. 707
Fort Worth, TX 76107-4618   Phone: (817) 735-8445
Description: Contains medical and educational news significant to state medical boards, along with Federation news. Recurring features include reports of meetings, news of research, statistics, and a calendar of events. **First Published:** 1915. **Frequency:** Monthly.

★2258★   FELINE HEALTH TOPICS
Cornell Feline Health Center
College of Veterinary Medicine
Cornell University
Ithaca, NY 14853   Phone: (607) 253-3414
Description: Focuses on diseases of cats, examining particular diseases in depth in each issue. Provides news of disease outbreaks, recommendations for treatment, and news of research. Publishes news and activities of the Center, and social issues pertaining to veterinarians. **First Published:** October 1979. **Frequency:** Quarterly.

★2259★   FIELD EXTRACT
Merck Sharp & Dohme
West Point, PA 19486   Phone: (215) 661-5000
Description: Focuses on medical news and developments in the pharmaceutical industry. Recurring features include company and corporate news and personnel notes. **First Published:** 1965. **Frequency:** Weekly.

★2260★   FIGHTING BLINDNESS NEWS
RP Foundation Fighting Blindness
1401 Mt. Royal Ave.
Baltimore, MD 21217   Phone: (301) 225-9400
Description: Contains scientific research updates and feature articles on persons with retinitis pigmentosa (RP) and allied retinal degenerations. Relates affiliate and departmental news. Recurring features include information on relevant products, services, and legislation, member news, and a calendar of events. **First Published:** 1972. **Frequency:** 4/yr. **ISSN:** 0899-7756.

★2261★   THE FITNESS BULLETIN
The Fitness Institute
255 Yorkland
Willowdale, ON, Canada M2J 1S3   Phone: (416) 491-5830
Description: Provides news and information on health and fitness and instructive articles. **First Published:** January 1978. **Frequency:** Monthly.

★2262★   FLASHPOINT
Captive Audience Communications, Corp.
1564 Dixie Way
Melbourne, FL 32935   Phone: (904) 736-9163
Description: Addresses medical and social issues such as suicide, birth control, Acquired Immune Deficiency Syndrome (AIDS), abortion, and general health concerns. **Frequency:** Quarterly.

★2263★ THE FLYER
Smithsonian Institution
USDA-Systematic Entomology Laboratory
US National Museum NHB-168
Washington, DC 20560

★2264★ FOCAL POINT
Research and Training Center on Family Support and Children's
  Mental Health
Portland State University
PO Box 751
Portland, OR 97207-0751   Phone: (503) 725-4040
Description: Features information on support groups, organizations, strategies, and conferences to aid families that have children with emotional, mental, and/or behavioral disorders. Recurring features include news of research, reports of meetings, and notices of publications available. **First Published:** Fall 1986. **Frequency:** 3/yr.

**★2265★ FOCUS ON GERIATRIC CARE AND
  REHABILITATION**
Aspen Publishers, Inc.
1600 Research Blvd.
Rockville, MD 20850   Phone: (301) 251-5554
Description: Focuses on clinical topics in the geriatric field. **Frequency:** 10/yr.

**★2266★ FOCUS: LIBRARY SERVICE TO OLDER ADULTS,
  PEOPLE WITH DISABILITIES**
Michael G. Gunde
216 N. Frederick Ave.
Daytona Beach, FL 32114-3804   Phone: (904) 257-4259
Description: Discusses library programs for older adults and disabled persons and presents new programs and approaches for meeting their needs. Contains brief items highlighting activities in U.S. libraries. Recurring features include reviews of books, videotapes, and films and notices of meetings of interest to librarians. **First Published:** January 1983. **Frequency:** Monthly. **ISSN:** 0740-4956.

**★2267★ FOOD SCIENCE AND NUTRITION ADVISORY
  COUNCIL—NEWSLETTER**
Food Science and Nutrition Advisory Council
Dept. of Food Science and Nutrition
University of Minnesota
PO Box 8164
St. Paul, MN 55108   Phone: (612) 624-2787
Description: Informs the Council of Department programs, research, services, and staff news. Recurring features include columns titled Advisory Council News, Alumni News, and Grants & Awards. **First Published:** Spring 1975. **Frequency:** 3/yr., Fall, Winter, Spring.

**★2268★ FOUNDATION FOR BIOMEDICAL RESEARCH—
  NEWSLETTER**
Foundation for Biomedical Research
818 Connecticut Ave. NW, Ste. 303
Washington, DC 20006   Phone: (202) 457-0654
Description: Serves the Foundation's objective to "educate the public about the responsible use of laboratory animals in research to benefit animals and humans." Reports on biomedical advances, Foundation activities and publications, animal rights/welfare activities, and legislative developments concerning the use of animals in biomedical research. **First Published:** Spring 1984. **Frequency:** Ca. 6/yr.

★2269★ THE FRAT
National Fraternal Society of the Deaf
1300 W. Northwest Hwy.
Mt. Prospect, IL 60056   Phone: (708) 392-9282
Description: Provides news of this fraternal benefit insurance society, whose members are deaf persons and those involved in the field of deafness. Focuses on the life insurance program sponsored by the Society and carries general news items which may be of interest to the deaf. Recurring features include a calendar of events, reports of meetings, news of educational opportunities, member and division news, and columns titled Questions and Answers, Treasurer's Statement, and Tidbits From the Grand President. **First Published:** February 1904. **Frequency:** Bimonthly. **ISSN:** 0739-9243.

★2270★ A FRIEND INDEED
A Friend Indeed Publications, Inc.
3575 Boul. St. Laurent, Ste. 402
Montreal, PQ, Canada H2X 2T7   Phone: (514) 843-5730
Description: Deals with menopause and women's midlife issues. Recurring features include letters to the editor, news of research, a calendar of events, reports of meetings, book reviews, and notices of publications available. **First Published:** April 1984. **Frequency:** 10/yr. **ISSN:** 0824-1961.

★2271★ FRIENDS OF YOUTH—NEWSLETTER
Friends of Youth
2500 Lake Washington Blvd., N.
Renton, WA 98056   Phone: (206) 228-5775
Description: Carries news of this agency's programs, goals, needs, and activities on behalf of emotionally disturbed adolescents. Promotes services to youth including residential treatment, emergency youth shelter, counseling, foster homes, teen parent services, and drug abuse prevention services. **Frequency:** Quarterly.

★2272★ FROM THE COUCH
Mental Health Record Section
American Medical Record Association
919 Michigan Ave., Ste. 1400
Chicago, IL 60611   Phone: (312) 787-2672
Description: Covers aspects of the medical records industry that pertain to mental health records. **Frequency:** Quarterly.

★2273★ FROM THE STATE CAPITALS: PUBLIC HEALTH
Wakeman/Walworth, Inc.
300 N. Washington St., Ste. 204
Alexandria, VA 22314   Phone: (703) 549-8606
Description: Acts as a digest of state and municipal health care financing and cost containment measures. Coverage includes Medicaid legislation, mental health and developmental disabilty programs, abortion, and disease control. Also discusses regulation of hospitals and nursing homes. **First Published:** 1950. **Frequency:** Weekly. **ISSN:** 0734-1156.

★2274★ THE FRONT PAGE
Bugle Publishing
PO Box 27928
Raleigh, NC 27611   Phone: (919) 829-0181
Description: Provides news of interest to gay men and lesbians in North and South Carolina, southern Virginia, and eastern Tennessee. Recurring features include letters to the editor, interviews, news of research regarding AIDS, a calendar of events, reports of meetings, notices of publications available, and columns titled Back Page and News Briefs. **First Published:** October 1979. **Frequency:** Biweekly.

**★2275★ FRONTIERS IN IMMUNOASSAY AND
  BIOTECHNOLOGY**
Duwest Research/Scientific Newsletters
Rd. 4, Box 7
Stapelton Ct.
Middletown, NY 10940-9683   Phone: (914) 355-9144
Description: Provides information on the latest developments in the non-isotopic immunoassay field, including products, applications, and recent legislation and regulations. Recurring features include notices of recent publications, special reports and abstracts, and a calendar of events. **First Published:** 1976. **Frequency:** 10/yr. **ISSN:** 0270-0426.

★2276★ FSMB NEWSLETTER
Federation of State Medical Boards of the United States, Inc.
6000 Western Pl., Ste. 707
Ft. Worth, TX 76107-4618   Phone: (817) 735-8445
Description: Reports news of the Federation, which is the association of state medical examining and licensing boards. Reviews legislative developments affecting medical care and outlines Federation policies and activities. Recurring features include news of members and Federation leaders. **First Published:** 1981. **Frequency:** Quarterly.

★2277★ FYI
Fran Jurga
PO Box 7008
Gloucester, MA 01930   Phone: (508) 281-3222
Description: Reports on the farrier profession and veterinary medicine, including news of research on lameness problems in horses. Recurring features include a calendar of events, news of research, book reviews, and reports of meetings. **First Published:** January 1985. **Frequency:** 4/yr.

★2278★ GASK NEWSLETTER
Telecommunications for the Deaf, Inc.
8719 Colesville Rd., Ste. 300
Silver Spring, MD 20910   Phone: (301) 589-3786
Description: Serves the hearing-impaired and deaf community, and organizations and services concerned with communications with and among the same. Focuses on telecommunications for hearing-impaired users, including computer communications. Recurring features include news of research; news of members; notices of conventions, new products and resources; listings of TDI by-laws; an Odds and Ends section; and columns titled ASCLI Advisor and TDF Bytes. **Frequency:** Quarterly.

★2279★ THE GATHERED VIEW
Prader-Willi Syndrome Association
6490 Excelsior Blvd., E-102
St. Louis Park, MN 55436   Phone: (612) 933-0113
Description: Centered on education and learning problems for the mentally retarded. Focuses on information helpful to parents whose children have the disorder Prader-Willi Syndrome. Looks at medical needs, therapy, and dietary problems. Recurring features include exchanges of ideas among parents and others, reports on chapters throughout the U.S. and Canada, book reviews, news of research, and a president's message. **First Published:** July 1975. **Frequency:** Bimonthly.

★2280★ GAUCHER'S DISEASE—NEWSLETTER
National Gaucher Foundation
19241 Montgomery Village Ave., Ste. E-21
Gaithersburg, MD 20879   Phone: (301) 990-3800
Description: Carries information on the activities of the National Gaucher Foundation. Covers research and research funding, insurance accessibility, nutrition, treatment, and genetic engineering. Recurring features include legislative alerts, bibliographies, a question-and-answer section, news of new publications, and the column News Briefs. **First Published:** July 1981. **Frequency:** Bimonthly.

★2281★ GENERATIONS
National Ataxia Foundation
750 Twelve Oaks Center
15500 Wayzata Blvd.
Wayzata, MN 55391   Phone: (612) 473-7666
Description: Relates the activities of the Foundation and its chapters in their fight against the neurological disorder ataxia. Recurring features include news of research and a calendar of events. **First Published:** 1971. **Frequency:** Quarterly.

★2282★ GENERIC LINE
Scitec Services, Inc.
5324 Sinclair Rd.
Columbus, OH 43229-5002   Phone: (614) 433-0648
Description: Focuses on the pharmaceutical industry, emphasizing generic products. Discusses regulatory, legislative, technical, and business developments of interest to generic and small pharmaceutical manufacturers. Recurring features include reports on current research and actions of pharmaceutical companies. **First Published:** January 1984. **Frequency:** Semimonthly.

★2283★ GENETIC ENGINEERING LETTER
Environews, Inc.
8750 Georgia Ave., Ste. 124
Silver Spring, MD 20910   Phone: (301) 587-3398
Description: Focuses on legislative and regulatory news in biotechnology. Recurring features include news of research. **First Published:** 1981. **Frequency:** Semimonthly.

★2284★ GENETIC RESOURCE
New England Regional Genetics Group
PO Box 682
Gorham, ME 04038-0682   Phone: (207) 839-5324
Description: Provides information on topics of interest in genetics. **First Published:** September 1991. **Frequency:** Annually.

★2285★ GENETIC TECHNOLOGY NEWS
Technical Insights, Inc.
PO Box 1304
Fort Lee, NJ 07024-9967   Phone: (201) 568-4744
Description: Informs corporate development and research managers of advances in genetic engineering with applications in medical, agricultural, chemical, food, and other businesses. Covers areas such as recombinant DNA, monoclonal antibodies, and interferon. Recurring features include news of research, company reports, a calendar of events, and columns titled Patents and Market Forecasts. **First Published:** February 1981. **Frequency:** Monthly. **ISSN:** 0272-9032.

★2286★ GENETICS DIGEST
Foundation for Blood Research
PO Box 190
Scarborough, ME 04074-0190   Phone: (207) 883-4131
Description: Provides updates on selected advancements of human genetics. Summarizes and references articles from scientific and lay publications. Recurring features include news of research, reports of meetings, and book reviews. **First Published:** December 1983. **Frequency:** 5/yr.

★2287★ GENETICS IN PRACTICE
March of Dimes Birth Defects Foundation
1275 Mamaroneck Ave.
White Plains, NY 10605   Phone: (914) 997-4527
Description: Provides the clinical practitioner and social worker with abstracts of the developments in clinical genetics. Sample topics include the role of drugs as teratogens in pregnancy, advances in prenatal testing, findings on syndromes, and research in molecular genetics. Recurring features include news of medical conferences and symposia. **First Published:** 1984. **Frequency:** Quarterly.

★2288★ GERIATRIC CARE NEWS
DRS Geriatric Publishing Co.
7435 SE 71st St.
Mercer Island, WA 98040   Phone: (206) 232-9689
Description: Provides information of concern to geriatrics health care professionals. Recurring features include news of research and a calendar of events. **First Published:** 1974. **Frequency:** Monthly. **ISSN:** 1048-7514.

★2289★ GERI-SOURCE
Jefferson House Gerontology Resource Center
1 John H. Stewart Dr.
Newington, CT 06111   Phone: (203) 667-4453
Description: Publishes articles discussing the needs of and programs for the aged. Describes selected educational programs in gerontology, and provides an annotated bibliography of recent acquisitions to the Resource Center. Recurring features include news of research, book reviews, reports of meetings, and a calendar of events. **First Published:** 1982. **Frequency:** 3/yr.

★2290★ GEROFILES
Center for Gerontological Studies
University of Florida
3357 Turlington Hall
Gainesville, FL 32611   Phone: (904) 392-2116
Description: Carries information on the Center's research projects, faculty, and students. Reports on research and services of other organizations concerned with gerontology. Recurring features include book reviews and announcements of conferences in the field. **First Published:** Fall 1977. **Frequency:** Annually.

★2291★ THE GERONTARION
Gerontology Research Centre
University of Guelph
Guelph, ON, Canada N1H 3Z5   Phone: (519) 824-4120
Description: Provides a forum for the exchange of information and the dissemination of research findings of gerontological studies conducted under the auspices of the Gerontology Research Centre. Recurring features include news of research, a calendar of events, reports of meetings, news of educational opportunities, and notices of publications available. **First Published:** 1983. **Frequency:** 3/yr. **ISSN:** 8026-8215.

★2292★ GERONTOLOGY CENTRE NEWSLETTER
Gerontology Research Centre
Simon Fraser University
515 W. Hastings St.
Vancouver, BC, Canada V6B 5K3   Phone: (604) 291-5062
First Published: 1982. **Frequency:** Bimonthly.

★2293★ GERONTOLOGY NEWS
Gerontological Society of America
1275 K St. NW, Ste. 350
Washington, DC 20005-4006   Phone: (202) 842-1275
Description: Summarizes research results and recently released major

reports on aging. Discusses legislative actions and reports on Society events. Lists grants, fellowships, and job opportunities, and identifies relevant publications recently available. **First Published:** November 1978. **Frequency:** Monthly.

★2294★ GERONTOLOGY SPECIAL INTEREST SECTION— NEWSLETTER
Gerontology Special Interest Section
American Occupational Therapy Association
1383 Piccard Dr.
PO Box 1725
Rockville, MD 20850   Phone: (301) 948-9626
Description: Focuses on the clinical management of the elderly. Publishes articles relevant to occupational therapy practice, including such topics as assessment protocols, treatment approaches, and program administration. Recurring features include editorials, news of research, case reports, bibliographies, and notices of new equipment. **First Published:** Summer 1978. **Frequency:** Quarterly. **ISSN:** 0279-4101.

★2295★ GERONTOLOGY UPDATE
Office of Gerontological Studies
McMaster University
DC-229
1280 Main St. West
Hamilton, ON, Canada L8S 4K1   Phone: (416) 525-9140
Description: Provides information concerning activities in the field of aging within the community. Reports on current issues in research and education in gerontological studies. **First Published:** 1981. **Frequency:** Quarterly.

★2296★ GIFT OF SIGHT
Co-Optics of America
Rt. 7, Oneonta Plaza
PO Box 398
Oneonta, NY 13820   Phone: (607) 432-0557
Description: Carries timely articles about eye care, eye wear, and health. **First Published:** 1987. **Frequency:** 2/yr.

★2297★ GIG NEWSLETTER
Gluten Intolerance Group of North America
PO Box 23053
Seattle, WA 98102-0353   Phone: (206) 325-6980
Description: Provides medical journal abstracts concerning research on the digestive disease Celiac Sprue and the required gluten-free diet. Carries information on the gluten content of products, gluten-free recipes, and news of the Group. Recurring features include book reviews, letters to the editor, and a calendar of events. **First Published:** July 1974. **Frequency:** 4/yr. **ISSN:** 0890-507X.

★2298★ THE GIMP EXCHANGE
National Handicap Motorcyclist Association
35-24 84th St., No. F8
Jackson Heights, NY 11372   Phone: (718) 565-1243
Description: Written by and for handicapped persons who are interested in making motorcycle modifications that will enable them to ride motorcycles. Publishes interviews with handicapped motorcyclists which detail the complete what, how, and where of all modifications made and features products that address the special needs of handicapped motorcyclists. Recurring features include news of research. **First Published:** March 1986. **Frequency:** Quarterly.

★2299★ GLEAMS
Foundation for Glaucoma Research
490 Post St., Ste. 830
San Francisco, CA 94102   Phone: (415) 986-3162
Description: Examines the results of clinical and basic research on glaucoma. Seeks to increase public knowledge of the eye disease and discusses prevention of blindness from the disease. Reports on the activities of the Foundation. **First Published:** 1982. **Frequency:** Quarterly.

★2300★ GLOBAL MISSIONS
International Christian Leprosy Mission, Inc.
PO Box 23353
Portland, OR 97223   Phone: (503) 244-5935
Description: Presents articles concerned with leprosy relief, rehabilitation, and prevention. Includes news from the different overseas fields, notes on the Philippine Children's Mission Home for those whose parents have leprosy, and information on hospital and clinical work with leprosy

patients in India, assisted and sponsored by the Mission. **First Published:** 1943. **Frequency:** 3/yr.

★2301★ GRANTS AND YOU
Kirksville College of Osteopathic Medicine
800 West Jefferson
Kirksville, MO 63501   Phone: (816) 626-2121
Description: Announces funding sources available from foundations, associations, institutes, and programs for special projects. **First Published:** September 1979. **Frequency:** Monthly.

★2302★ GRAY PANTHER NETWORK
Gray Panther Project Fund
1424 16th St. NW, Ste. 602
Washington, DC 20036   Phone: (202) 387-3111
Description: Provides information on gerontology-related subjects, including health care, geriatric services, and consumer protection. Updates special events, meetings, and anniversaries. Recurring features include letters to the editor. **Frequency:** Quarterly.

★2303★ GROWING CHILD
Dunn & Hargitt, Inc.
22 N. Second St.
Lafayette, IN 47902   Phone: (317) 423-2624
Description: Supplies information on specific stages of children's growth and learning. Follows a child's development through each month from birth to six years to assist parents in guiding their child's growth. **First Published:** 1971. **Frequency:** Monthly. **ISSN:** 0193-8037.

★2304★ GROWING CHILD RESEARCH REVIEW
Dunn & Hargitt, Inc.
22 N. Second St.
Lafayette, IN 47902   Phone: (317) 423-2624
Description: Provides news, research findings, and specialists' viewpoints on topics relating to child development in the fields of education, mental health, psychology, sociology, and medicine. **First Published:** January 1983. **Frequency:** Monthly. **ISSN:** 0737-0318.

★2305★ GROWING PARENT
Dunn & Hargitt, Inc.
22 N. Second St.
Lafayette, IN 47902   Phone: (317) 423-2624
Description: Contains features on current parenting issues, including improving self-image, dealing with stress, and coping with the problems and pressures of parenting. **First Published:** 1972. **Frequency:** Monthly. **ISSN:** 0193-8037.

★2306★ THE GUARDIAN
National Association of Counsel for Children
1205 Oneida St.
Denver, CO 80220   Phone: (303) 322-2260
Description: Concerned with legal rights of children. Covers cases involving such issues as child abuse and neglect, custody rights, adoptions, and foster care. Reports on new legislation and social services. Recurring features include news of members, book reviews, and a calendar of events. **First Published:** 1979. **Frequency:** Quarterly.

★2307★ THE GUARDIAN
Pennsylvania Association for the Blind
2843 N. Front St.
Harrisburg, PA 17110-1284   Phone: (717) 234-3261
Description: Educates children about eye health and safety and blindness. Publishes news of Sergeant Seymour's Eye Safety Program and provides information on related subjects such as the Decade for Disabled Persons. Recurring features include short stories, puzzles, drawings, mystery message, eye safety rules, and a page of contributions from young readers titled Our Readers Write. **First Published:** September 1963. **Frequency:** 4/academic yr.

★2308★ GUIDE DOG NEWS
Guide Dogs for the Blind, Inc.
PO Box 151200
San Rafael, CA 94915-1200   Phone: (415) 499-4000
Description: Provides information on the Guide Dogs for the Blind school in San Rafael, California. Recurring features include news of present and former students, fund raising events, 4-H puppy raisers, a calendar of events, and a column on dog care by the staff veterinarian. **Frequency:** Quarterly.

★2309★   HALO NEWSLETTER
Homophile Association of London Ontario
649 Colborne St.
London, ON, Canada N6A 3Z2   Phone: (519) 433-3762
Description: Carries articles on topics affecting the gay and lesbian community. Covers health, politics, social events, "fag bashing" incidents, recreation, and Association news. Includes editorials, games, and trivia. Recurring features include letters to the editor, a calendar of events, reports of meetings, book reviews, news of educational opportunities, and news of research. **First Published:** 1974. **Frequency:** Monthly.

★2310★   HAND IN HAND
Saskatchewan Association of Certified Nursing Assistants
2310 Smith St.
Regina, SK, Canada S4P 2P6   Phone: (306) 525-1436
Description: Provides the Association members with information of topical interest. Recurring features include columns titled President's Ponderings, Committee Feedback, Auditors' Report, C.A.P.N.A. Corner, and Rules and Regulations.

★2311★   HANYS NEWS
Hospital Association of New York State
74 N. Pearl St.
Albany, NY 12207   Phone: (518) 434-7600
Description: Presents articles on health care issues. Recurring features include reports of meetings. **First Published:** 1976. **Frequency:** Weekly.

**★2312★   THE HARVARD MEDICAL SCHOOL HEALTH
    LETTER**
Department of Continuing Education
Harvard Medical School
164 Longwood Ave., 4th Fl.
Boston, MA 02115   Phone: (617) 432-1485
Description: Provides information on medicine and health to the general public, including background reviews, perspective on recent topics, and reports on new research and analysis. Advises on health maintenance and general wellness and coping with acute and chronic medical problems. Recurring features include a column titled Medical Forum. **First Published:** November 1975. **Frequency:** Monthly. **ISSN:** 0161-7486.

★2313★   HAZELDEN NEWS AND PROFESSIONAL UPDATE
Hazelden Foundation
PO Box 11
Center City, MN 55012   Phone: (612) 349-9400
Description: Reports on Hazelden activities and programs, and discusses developments and issues in chemical dependency treatment, prevention, and employee intervention. Carries notices of professional education opportunities, reviews of resources in the field, and a calendar of events. **First Published:** Winter 1990. **Frequency:** 3/yr.

★2314★   HEADLINES
Migraine Foundation
120 Carlton St., Ste. 210
Toronto, ON, Canada M5A 4K2   Phone: (416) 920-4916
Description: Supports migraine headache sufferers. Provides educational information. Recurring features include interviews, news of research, a calendar of events, reports of meetings, book reviews, notices of publications available, and a column titled QA. **First Published:** September 1990. **Frequency:** Quarterly.

★2315★   HEALTH ACTION LETTER
National Association of Employers on Health Care Action
PO Box 220
Key Biscayne, FL 33149-0220   Phone: (305) 361-2810
Description: Designed to educate and assist employers in the understanding and implementation of health care action programs. Provides health care corporations with news on cost-effective programs that can control rising health care costs for employers and organized systems that provide comprehensive health care services. Reports on Association-conducted research and federal legislation and regulatory activity that affects health care systems and employers. Recurring features include news of members, news of research, and a calendar of events. **First Published:** July 1, 1976. **Frequency:** Bimonthly.

**★2316★   HEALTH ADMINISTRATORS' ASSOCIATION OF
    BRITISH COLUMBIA—NEWSLETTER**
Health Administrators' Association of British Columbia
1867 W. Broadway, No. 203
Vancouver, BC, Canada V6J 4W1   Phone: (604) 734-6696
Frequency: Quarterly.

★2317★   HEALTH ALERT
Capital Consultants, Inc.
643 Pennsylvania Ave.
Washington, DC 20003   Phone: (202) 546-CAPS
Description: Reports on legislative developments in health care. **Frequency:** Monthly.

★2318★   HEALTH BREAK
Dartnell Marketing Publications
286 Congress St. at Russia Wharf, 6th Fl.
Boston, MA 02210   Phone: (617) 451-7551
Description: Contains short articles on health-related topics, including fitness, ear and eye care, prenatal medicine, disease, and lifestyle. Recurring features include columns titled Capsules, Question Corner, and Health and Fitness Briefs. **Frequency:** Monthly.

★2319★   HEALTH BUSINESS
Faulkner & Gray, Inc.
1133 15th St. NW
Washington, DC 20005   Phone: (202) 828-4148
Frequency: Weekly.

★2320★   HEALTH CARE: AN ABSTRACT NEWSLETTER
National Technical Information Service
U.S. Department of Commerce
5285 Port Royal Rd.
Springfield, VA 22161   Phone: (703) 487-4630
Description: Consists of abstracted reports covering planning methodology, health services, facilities utilization, and health needs. Also covers health care assessment, quality assurance, forecasting and measurement methods, and legislation and regulations. Recurring features include information on services available through NTIS and a form for ordering reports from NTIS. **Frequency:** Weekly. **ISSN:** 0017-9086.

★2321★   HEALTH CARE COMPETITION WEEK
Capitol Publications, Inc.
1101 King St., Ste. 444
Alexandria, VA 22314   Phone: (703) 683-4100
Description: Focuses on the concerns of health care providers regarding the new competitive environment. Looks at health care marketing and strategic planning and development from a how-to perspective and discusses trends in the field, HMOs (Health Maintenance Organizations), and PPOs (Preferred-Provider Organizations), and other alternative delivery services. Recurring features include articles by "highly regarded health care executives," reports of meetings, and a column titled The Keckley Report on Healthcare Market Research. **First Published:** August 1984. **Frequency:** 50/yr. **ISSN:** 0886-2095.

★2322★   HEALTH CARE NEWSLETTER
National Safety Council
444 N. Michigan Ave.
Chicago, IL 60611   Phone: (312) 527-4800
Description: Concerned with safety education and awareness for workers in the health care field, particularly in institutional settings. Counsels the use of safe work practices and products. Recurring features include discussions of the legal and financial aspects of accidents, and a column of letters from readers. **Frequency:** Bimonthly.

★2323★   HEALTH COMMERCE LINE
Scitec Services, Inc.
5324 Sinclair Rd.
Columbus, OH 43229-5002   Phone: (614) 433-0648
Description: Monitors events and changes occurring in the health care industry. Profiles detailed financial tables for health care companies, trends in production, employment expenditures, and utilization and insurance. **First Published:** September 1988. **Frequency:** Monthly.

★2324★ **HEALTH DAILY**
FDC Reports
5550 Friendship Blvd., Ste. 1
Chevy Chase, MD 20815   Phone: (301) 657-9830
Description: Tracks developments in health care policy, legislation and regulation, insurance, pharmaceuticals, delivery, manufacturing, technology and treatment, funding, and research. **First Published:** June 21, 1988. **Frequency:** Every business day. **ISSN:** 0277-0679.

★2325★ **HEALTH DEVICES ALERTS**
ECRI
5200 Butler Pike
Plymouth Meeting, PA 19462   Phone: (215) 825-6000
Description: Contains health equipment hazards and technical assessments derived from medical and technical literature, reporting networks, and governmental sources. Includes manufacturer, source of information, a brief description of the problem, and any resolution. **First Published:** 1977. **Frequency:** Weekly. **ISSN:** 0163-0458.

★2326★ **HEALTH EDUCATION REPORTS**
Feistritzer Publications
4401-A Connecticut Ave. NW, Ste. 212
Washington, DC 20008   Phone: (202) 362-3444
Description: Focuses on developments relating to public health and wellness programs and government health policy. Covers activities at Centers for Disease Control around the U.S. and subjects such as health promotion, disease prevention, and medical studies. Recurring features include interviews, news of educational opportunities, job listings, book reviews and notices of publications available, reports of meetings, and a calendar of events. **First Published:** 1978. **Frequency:** Biweekly.

★2327★ **HEALTH EXCHANGE**
Medical Group Management Association
104 Inverness Terrace E.
Englewood, CO 80112-5306   Phone: (303) 799-1111
Description: Contains general articles related to health and wellness on frequently discussed medical subjects. Includes exercise tips, diet recommendations, and lifestyle features. **First Published:** Fall 1983. **Frequency:** Quarterly. **ISSN:** 0742-8081.

★2328★ **HEALTH FACTS**
Center for Medical Consumers
237 Thompson St.
New York, NY 10012   Phone: (212) 674-7105
Description: Profiles and critiques current medical practices. Aims to provide information to help consumers make educated choices concerning their medical care. Recurring features include editorials, news of research, and columns titled Updates and Rx News. **First Published:** 1976. **Frequency:** Monthly. **ISSN:** 0738-811X.

★2329★ **HEALTH FUNDS DEVELOPMENT LETTER**
Health Resources Publishing
Brinley Professional Plaza, 3100 Hwy. 138
PO Box 1442
Wall Township, NJ 07719-1442   Phone: (908) 681-1133
Description: Provides concise information which is compiled, organized, and designed to assist research efforts of medical schools, hospitals, and community health projects/programs that need federal aid or foundation grants. **First Published:** December 1978. **Frequency:** Monthly. **ISSN:** 0193-7928.

★2330★ **HEALTH GRANTS AND CONTRACTS WEEKLY**
Capitol Publications, Inc.
1101 King St., Ste. 444
Alexandria, VA 22314   Phone: (703) 683-4100
Description: Covers funding announcements for federal health grants and contracts. Provides profiles of key funding agencies, updates on legislation and regulations, budget development, and early alerts to upcoming funding opportunities. **Frequency:** Weekly. **ISSN:** 0194-235Q.

★2331★ **HEALTH HAZARDS OF THE WORKPLACE REPORT**
Van Nostrand Reinhold
c/o Irene Hoffman
115 Fifth Ave.
New York, NY 10003   Phone: (212) 254-3232
Description: Provides reports concerning occupational health standards, services, and safety. **Frequency:** Monthly. **ISSN:** 1042-7473.

★2332★ **HEALTH LABOR RELATIONS REPORTS**
Interwood Publications
PO Box 20241
Cincinnati, OH 45220   Phone: (513) 221-3715
Description: Focuses on employee and labor relations in the health care field. Reports on court and National Labor Relations Board (NLRB) decisions in the areas of wrongful discharge, employment-at-will, discrimination, and union organizing. Also notifies readers of arbitration awards and contract settlements. **First Published:** November 1976. **Frequency:** Biweekly. **ISSN:** 0148-4761.

★2333★ **HEALTH LAW DIGEST**
National Health Lawyers Association
1620 I St. NW, Ste. 900
Washington, DC 20006   Phone: (202) 833-1100
Description: Carries approximately 100 synopses of court decisions in approximately 100 cases affecting the health care field. Recurring features include a list of publications of interest to members, and a list of job openings in the field, and a calendar of events. **First Published:** May 1973. **Frequency:** Monthly.

★2334★ **HEALTH LAW INSTITUTE—NEWSLETTER**
Health Law Institute
University of Alberta
461 Law Centre
Edmonton, AB, Canada T6G 2H5   Phone: (403) 492-8343
Description: Features articles concerning health law. **First Published:** September 1987. **Frequency:** 3/yr.

★2335★ **HEALTH LAWYERS NEWS REPORT**
National Health Lawyers Association
1620 I St. NW, Ste. 900
Washington, DC 20006   Phone: (202) 833-1100
Description: Presents "legislative, administrative, court, organization, labor relations and other health-related developments of importance to lawyers, administrators, and other health-care professionals." **First Published:** May 1973. **Frequency:** Monthly. **ISSN:** 0145-4129.

★2336★ **HEALTH LEGISLATION AND REGULATION**
Faulkner & Gray, Inc.
1133 15th St. NW, No. 450
Washington, DC 20005   Phone: (202) 828-4148
Description: Monitors the two largest federal medical aid programs, Medicare and Medicaid, and their effect on the health-care industry, including the drive for national health insurance. Provides information on important hearings, updates on actual and proposed legislation, and analyses of regulations. Recurring features include notices of conventions, grants, meetings, studies, and publications, and an editorial titled The Health Scene in Review. **First Published:** 1975. **Frequency:** Weekly.

★2337★ **THE HEALTH LETTER**
North America Syndicate
PO Box 90190
Collingswood, NJ 08108   Phone: (609) 869-3464
Description: Addresses health topics, with discussion of cause and effect, practical counsel, and information on normal variations. Carries news of research, briefings from current medical literature, and highlights of conferences and other events. **First Published:** January 1973. **Frequency:** Monthly.

★2338★ **HEALTH LETTER**
Public Citizen Health Research Group
2000 P St. NW, Ste. 700
Washington, DC 20036   Phone: (202) 872-0320
Description: Designed as a personal health guide for "reducing preventable illnesses and also avoiding needless and unnecessarily dangerous or overpriced medical care." Discusses specific diseases and treatments and other issues, including Medicare, health maintenance organizations (HMOs), government regulations, and getting a second medical opinion. **First Published:** March 1985. **Frequency:** Monthly. **ISSN:** 0882-598X.

★2339★ **HEALTH MANAGER'S UPDATE**
Faulkner & Gray, Inc.
1133 15th St. NW
Washington, DC 20005   Phone: (202) 828-4148
Description: Provides news of activities and legislation concerning health planning, national health insurance, antitrust proposals, quality assurance, certificates-of-need, privacy of medical records, Medicare, Medicaid, and

health maintenance organizations. Recurring features include news of new publications, seminars, and programs; interviews with national policy leaders; and an editorial titled The Health Scene This Week. **First Published:** 1973. **Frequency:** Biweekly.

★2340★ HEALTH MATTERS
Boynton Health Service
University of Minnesota
410 Church St. SE
Minneapolis, MN 55455　　　　Phone: (612) 624-2965
Description: Informs University students, faculty, and staff about the health services and educational programs provided by the Health Service. Promotes self-care techniques and healthy living styles. Recurring features include columns titled Help Yourself to Health and Welcome to Boynton Health Service. **First Published:** December 1989. **Frequency:** 3/yr.

★2341★ HEALTH NEWS
Faculty of Medicine
University of Toronto
Medical Sciences Bldg.
Toronto, ON, Canada M5S 1A8　　　Phone: (416) 978-5411
Description: Provides detailed articles on such topics as caffeine, foot problems, and bowel polyps. **First Published:** 1983. **Frequency:** Bimonthly. **ISSN:** 0821-3925.

★2342★ HEALTH NEWS DAILY
F-D-C Reports, Inc.
5550 Friendship Blvd., Ste. 1
Chevy Chase, MD 20815　　　　Phone: (301) 657-9830
Description: Covers developments affecting the pharmaceutical industry; medical devices and diagnostics; biomedical research; provider payment policies; and cost containment. Recurring features include columns titled Washington This Week, Legislative Round-Up, New Products, and People. **Frequency:** Daily. **ISSN:** 1042-2781.

★2343★ HEALTH AND NUTRITION UPDATE
Canadian Schizophrenia Foundation
7375 Kingsway
Burnaby, BC, Canada V3N 3B5　　　Phone: (604) 521-1728
Description: Provides information on the developments in the field of health and nutrition. Recurring features include letters to the editor, interviews, news of research, calendar of events, reports of meetings, and book reviews. **Frequency:** Quarterly. **ISSN:** 0831-8530.

★2344★ HEALTH/PAC BULLETIN
Health Policy Advisory Center
47 W. 14th St., 3rd Fl.
New York, NY 10011
Description: Monitors developments in the health care system, promoting the establishment of low-cost, high-quality health services for everyone. Analyzes current practices of hospitals and physicians. Recurring features include editorials, letters to the editor, book reviews, and columns titled Body English, Media Scan, Vital Signs, and Know News. **First Published:** June 1968. **Frequency:** 4/yr. **ISSN:** 0017-9051.

★2345★ HEALTH PLUS
Bureau of Business Practice
24 Rope Ferry Rd.
Waterford, CT 06386　　　　Phone: (203) 442-4365
Description: Focuses on employee health, fitness, and wellness. **Frequency:** Monthly.

★2346★ HEALTH POLICY WEEK
United Communications Group
11300 Rockville Pike, Ste. 1100
Rockville, MD 20852-3030　　　Phone: (301) 816-8950
Description: Monitors activities in Washington and the marketplace affecting the administration of health care institutions. Covers topics such as malpractice, Medicaid and Medicare, regulation of medical products, and actions of major medical organizations. Recurring features include research updates and a column titled News in Brief. **First Published:** March 1982. **Frequency:** Weekly. **ISSN:** 0732-7439.

★2347★ HEALTH PROFESSIONS REPORT
Whitaker Newsletters, Inc.
313 South Ave.
Fanwood, NJ 07023-0340　　　　Phone: (908) 889-6336
Description: Reports on the education and training of doctors, nurses, and

allied health professionals. Includes pending legislation, information on public and private funding sources, cost-cutting measures, curriculum ideas, recruiting efforts and admission policies, new medical breakthroughs, scientific research and advanced programs from America's leading medical training facilities. **Frequency:** 26/yr. **ISSN:** 0736-9077.

★2348★ HEALTH OF THE REP NEWSLETTER
United Association of Manufacturers' Representatives
PO Box 3407
Laguna Hills, CA 92654　　　　Phone: (714) 859-6363
Description: Provides manufacturers' representatives "the latest tips on how to stay healthy." Carries information on various diseases and a list of related publications. **First Published:** 1956. **Frequency:** Monthly.

★2349★ HEALTH RESOURCES
Kelly Communications
410 E. Water St.
Charlottesville, VA 22901　　　Phone: (804) 296-5676
Description: Concerned with the field of health education resources and materials. Reviews health education materials from over 300 sources and recommends brochures, posters, and audiovisual items best suited for internal wellness programs. Recurring features include complete ordering information, notices of publications available, a calendar of events, and health-oriented articles. **First Published:** April 1986. **Frequency:** Monthly.

★2350★ HEALTH SECURITY NEWS
Committee for National Health Insurance
1757 N St. NW
Washington, DC 20036　　　　Phone: (202) 223-9685
Description: Advocates a comprehensive national health insurance program. Reports on Committee programs, educational conferences, and events of interest. Recurring features include news of members and news of research. **First Published:** 1980. **Frequency:** Bimonthly.

★2351★ HEALTH SENSE
Kelly Communications
410 E. Water St.
Charlottesville, VA 22901　　　Phone: (804) 296-5676
Description: Focuses on practical self-care approaches to a healthy life. Covers all aspects of personal health, including education on nutrition, fitness, and safety habits and tips for prevention and treatment of diseases such as cancer, substance abuse, and heart desease. **First Published:** September 1987. **Frequency:** Bimonthly.

★2352★ HEALTH VICTORY BULLETIN
Arlin J. Brown Information Center, Inc.
PO Box 251
Fort Belvoir, VA 22060　　　　Phone: (703) 752-9511
Description: Presents information on alternative forms of medical treatments, and medical inquisitions. **Frequency:** 12/yr.

★2353★ HEALTH WATCH
Gray Panthers
National Office
1424 16th St. NW, Ste. 602
Washington, DC 20036　　　　Phone: (202) 387-3111
Description: Tracks health issues concerning senior citizens. Covers pending legislation and discussion of such topics as a national health system, long-term care, and Acquired Immune Deficiency Syndrome (AIDS). **First Published:** 1986. **Frequency:** Bimonthly.

★2354★ HEALTHACTION MANAGERS
Kelly Communications
410 E. Water St.
Charlottesville, VA 22901　　　Phone: (804) 296-5676
Description: Contains topics of interest to health promotion professionals, such as program evaluation, health risk statistics, health education, program selection, and management. Incorporates profiles of successful health programs, independent analyses, and evaluations of national program vendors. Recurring features include letters to the editor, book reviews and publication announcements, and research news. **First Published:** September 1987. **Frequency:** Semimonthly. **ISSN:** 0895-108X.

★2355★ HEALTHCARE COMMUNITY RELATIONS AND
MARKETING LETTER
Health Resources Publishing
Brinley Professional Plaza, 3100 Hwy. 138
PO Box 1442
Wall Township, NJ 07719-1442   Phone: (201) 681-1133
Description: Designed to keep professionals abreast of the newest market-
ing and public relations techniques and strategies within the field of health
care. First Published: July 1987. Frequency: Monthly. ISSN: 0894-9980.

★2356★ HEALTHCARE CONVENTION AND EXHIBITORS
ASSOCIATION—ACTION MEMO
Healthcare Convention & Exhibitors Association
5775 Peachtree-Dunwoody Rd., Ste. 500-G
Atlanta, GA 30342   Phone: (404) 252-3663
Description: Disseminates information to health care associations, exhibitors, and their Exhibitors Advisory Councils (EAC). Reports on EAC
accomplishments, highlighting innovative ideas and focusing on specific
problems and solutions pertaining to the effective display of health care
products. Seeks to facilitate improved communication among exhibitors
and associations. Recurring features include news of research, reports of
meetings, news of educational opportunities, news of members, and
notices of publications available. First Published: July 1985. Frequency:
3/yr.

★2357★ HEALTHCARE CONVENTION AND EXHIBITORS
ASSOCIATION—INSIGHT
Healthcare Convention & Exhibitors Association
5775 Peachtree-Dunwoody Rd., Ste. 500-G
Atlanta, GA 30342   Phone: (404) 252-3663
Description: Represents the Association, which seeks to secure a more
effective display of members' products at professional conventions and to
promote ethical convention practices. Contains items of interest to the
exhibit management profession, including articles on exhibition techniques and problem solving. Also includes news of Association ev-
ents/activities and news of members. Recurring features include news of
research, reports of meetings, notices of publications available, and a
column titled From the President. First Published: Winter 1986. Frequency: 4/yr.

★2358★ HEALTHCARE FINANCIAL BRIEFS
Arnold P. Silver
PO Box 35425
Phoenix, AZ 85069   Phone: (602) 242-9276
Description: Covers recent developments in health care economics, legisla-
tion, regulation, research, and analysis. Includes columns titled Economic
Briefs, Issue Briefs, and Analytical and Statistical Briefs. First Published:
1978. Frequency: Monthly.

★2359★ HEALTHCARE FUND RAISING NEWSLETTER
Health Resources Publishing
Brinley Professional Plaza, 3100 Hwy. 138
PO Box 1442
Wall Township, NJ 07719-1442   Phone: (201) 681-1133
Description: Reviews news of hospital building funds and capital cam-
paigns, annual giving campaign news, special events, and innovative ideas
for attracting hospital gifts. First Published: January 1979. Frequency:
Bimonthly. ISSN: 0193-9939.

★2360★ HEALTHCARE INFORMATION MANAGEMENT
Healthcare Information and Management Systems Society
American Hospital Association
840 N. Lake Shore Dr.
Chicago, IL 60611   Phone: (312) 280-6680
Description: Reports on health care information management systems,
including the latest management trends in information systems, management engineering, and telecommunications. Recurring features include
news of the Society and its members, book reviews, news of research, a
calendar of events, a list of job openings, letters to the editor, and columns
titled President's Message, Society News, and Directions. First Published:
1967. Frequency: Quarterly.

★2361★ HEALTHCARE INFORMATION AND MANAGEMENT
SYSTEMS SOCIETY—MONTHLY UPDATE
Healthcare Information and Management Systems Society
American Hospital Association
840 N. Lake Shore Dr.
Chicago, IL 60611   Phone: (312) 280-6680
Description: Reports on health care information management systems,

including the latest management trends in information systems, management engineering, and telecommunications. First Published: April 1990.
Frequency: Monthly.

★2362★ HEALTHCARE MANAGEMENT TEAM LETTER
Health Resources Publishing
Brinley Professional Plaza, 3100 Hwy. 38
PO Box 1442
Wall Township, NJ 07719-1442   Phone: (201) 681-1133
Description: Alerts management teams or department heads to information
that may help them in their roles as decisionmakers. First Published: May
1985. Frequency: Bimonthly. ISSN: 0891-9267.

★2363★ HEALTHCARE MARKETING ABSTRACTS
COR Research Inc.
PO Box 40959
Santa Barbara, CA 93140-0959   Phone: (805) 564-2177
Description: Contains summaries of articles on healthcare marketing
selected from more than 120 publications. First Published: 1986. Frequen-
cy: Monthly except July. ISSN: 0891-5016.

★2364★ HEALTHCARE PLANNING AND MARKETING
Society for Healthcare Planning and Marketing
American Hospital Association
840 N. Lake Shore Dr.
Chicago, IL 60611   Phone: (312) 280-6086
Description: Focuses on health care planning and marketing, providing
information on topics such as reimbursement reform, marketing strategies,
research projects, and relevant issues in the health care industry. Recurring
features include items on regional and national health care planning and
marketing activities, literature reviews, news of members, and listings of
upcoming educational programs. First Published: January 1980. Frequency: Bimonthly.

★2365★ HEALTHLINE
Mosby-Year Book
11830 Westline Industrial Dr.
St. Louis, MO 63141
Description: Features easy-to-read articles by physicians on general health
topics. First Published: 1981. Frequency: Monthly.

★2366★ HEALTHNET NEWSLETTER
General Videotex Corp.
3 Blackstone St.
Cambridge, MA 02139   Phone: (617) 491-3393
Description: Serves as an enhancement to the HealthNet database.
Dedicated to recent advances and issues in the medical field. Frequency:
Bimonthly.

★2367★ HEALTHSPAN
Law and Business, Inc.
Prentice-Hall, Inc.
910 Sylvan Ave.
Englewood Cliffs, NJ 07632   Phone: (201) 894-8538
Description: Covers legal, business, and regulatory events that are shaping
the nature of the health care industry. First Published: August 1984.
Frequency: 11/yr. ISSN: 0883-0452.

★2368★ HEALTHWATCHERS SYSTEM
6821 E. Thomas Rd.
Scottsdale, AZ 85251   Phone: (602) 946-5515
Description: Discusses the merits of various "natural health products"
(mainly dietary supplements) available through Nutripathic Formulas, Inc.
Also provides information on studies and research relating to health
problems brought on by vitamin deficiencies. Recurring features include
letters from students of the company's nutripathic program, an order form
for available products, interviews, book reviews, and notices of publications available. First Published: 1976. Frequency: 10/yr.

★2369★ HEALTHY HORIZONS
Now Foods
2000 Bloomingdale Rd., Ste. 250
Glendale Heights, IL 60139-2182   Phone: (708) 893-1330
First Published: 1975. Frequency: 4/yr.

★2370★   HEART EXPRESSED
American Heart Association—Florida Affiliate
1213 16th St. N.
St. Petersburg, FL 33705   Phone: (813) 894-7400
Description: Contains news of interest to Association staff and volunteers. Recurring features include news of research and a calendar of events.

★2371★   HEF NEWS
Health Education Foundation
600 New Hampshire Ave., Ste. 452
Washington, DC 20037   Phone: (202) 338-3501
Description: Presents current information and perspectives on behavior, lifestyles, and trends as they relate to health and well-being. Recurring features include commentary on current health topics. **First Published:** September 1977. **Frequency:** Quarterly.

★2372★   HEIR RAISING NEWS
Midwest Parentcraft Center
3921 N. Lincoln
Chicago, IL 60613   Phone: (312) 281-6638
Description: Educates expectant mothers and others in the Gamper Method of childbirth, which aims to instill in the mother self-determination and confidence in her ability to work with the physiological changes of her body during pregnancy, labor, and delivery. Provides information on Center prenatal and parenting classes and workshops. Recurring features include news of research, Center reports, and a calendar of events. **Frequency:** Quarterly.

★2373★   HELPER
Herpes Resource Center
American Social Health Association
PO Box 13827
Research Triangle Park, NC 27709   Phone: (919) 361-8400
Description: Covers the latest research and news on the herpes simplex virus. Recurring features include book reviews, statistics, and drug research updates. **First Published:** 1979. **Frequency:** Quarterly.

★2374★   HEMOPHILIA NEWSNOTES
National Hemophilia Foundation
110 Green St., Rm. 406
New York, NY 10012   Phone: (212) 219-8180
Description: Considers all aspects of the work of the Foundation and provides coverage of relevant medical and non-medical issues. Recurring features include news of research, a calendar of events, and columns titled President's Desk, Medical Corner, Board Actions, Chapter Exchange, and Committee Actions. **First Published:** 1972. **Frequency:** Quarterly.

★2375★   HERBALGRAM
American Botanical Council
PO Box 201660
Austin, TX 78720   Phone: (512) 331-8868
Description: Disseminates information on medicinal plants and herbal products and provides coverage of the latest news in the herb industry. Recurring features include lists of recent books and publications, notices of articles in the popular press, market reports, legal and regulatory updates, news of research, and a calendar of events. **First Published:** 1979. **Frequency:** Quarterly. **ISSN:** 0899-5648.

★2376★   HERS NEWSLETTER
Hysterectomy Educational Resources and Services Foundation
422 Bryn Mawr Ave.
Bala Cynwyd, PA 19004   Phone: (215) 667-7757
Description: Features articles on information and services concerning hysterectomy and castration. Covers health issues, and chronicles of individual experiences. Recurring features include news of research, book reviews and reviews of medical literature, and reports of meetings. **First Published:** Spring 1982. **Frequency:** Quarterly. **ISSN:** 0892-628X.

★2377★   HESCA FEEDBACK
Health Sciences Communications Association
6105 Lindell Blvd.
St. Louis, MO 63112   Phone: (314) 725-4722
Description: Disseminates information for the Association, which is concerned with applying instructional technology to health education. Contains briefs on new products, new technologies, services, and programs; articles on videodisc; visits to member institutions; and news of the activities of the Association. Recurring features include editorials, news of

members, book reviews, a calendar of events, and job placement notices. **First Published:** 1975. **Frequency:** 6/yr.

★2378★   HE-XTRA
Association for the Advancement of Health Education
1900 Association Dr.
Reston, VA 22091   Phone: (703) 476-3437
Description: Reflects the aims of the Association, which promotes the advancement of health education through program activities and federal legislation and the achievement of good health and well-being for all Americans. Reports on health education programs across the nation and discusses the responsibilities of those responsible for health education in schools, the community, hospitals and clinics, and industry. Recurring features include news of members, news of research, and Association updates. **Frequency:** 6/yr.

★2379★   THE HIP REPORT
Help for Incontinent People, Inc.
PO Box 544
Union, SC 29379   Phone: (803) 579-7900
Description: Furnishes information on the causes, prevention, diagnosis, treatments, and management alternatives of incontinence. Recurring features include Contains letters to the editor, news of research, reports of meetings, news of educational opportunities, book reviews, and notices of publications available. **First Published:** September 1982. **Frequency:** Quarterly.

★2380★   HIPPOCRATES HEALTH INSTITUTE—NEWSLETTER
Hippocrates Health Institute
1443 Palmdale Court
West Palm Beach, FL 33411-3319   Phone: (407) 471-8876
Description: Concerned with health, nutrition, attitude, consciousness raising, and other subjects relating to holistic lifestyles. Carries personal accounts from individuals who have healed themselves naturally through the program. Recurring features include information on teaching programs, products, publications, and research. **First Published:** 1963. **Frequency:** 3/yr.

★2381★   HIV/AIDS SURVEILLANCE REPORT
National Center for Infectious Diseases
Centers for Disease Control
1600 Clifton Rd. NE, Mailstop E49
Atlanta, GA 30333
Description: Provides an update on the number of AIDS cases reported to the Centers for Disease Control. **Frequency:** Monthly.

★2382★   HKI REPORT
Helen Keller International, Inc.
15 W. 16th St.
New York, NY 10011   Phone: (212) 807-5800
Description: Covers HKI programs for the prevention of blindness, education of blind children, and rehabilitation of blind adults in developing countries. Focuses on the prevention of vitamin A deficiency, a major cause of child blindness in third world countries. Recurring features include news of staff activities, board actions, and grants and gifts to HKI. **First Published:** 1977. **Frequency:** 3/yr.

★2383★   HMO MANAGERS LETTER
Group Health Association of America, Inc.
1129 20th St. NW, Ste. 600
Washington, DC 20036   Phone: (202) 778-3200
Description: Covers legislative, regulatory, and financial news in the health maintenance organization (HMO) industry. Recurring features include research news, industry briefs, news of coming events, and career classifieds. **Frequency:** 22/yr. **ISSN:** 1050-902X.

★2384★   HOLISTIC DENTAL ASSOCIATION—THE COMMUNICATOR
Holistic Dental Association
974 N. 21st St.
Newark, OH 43055-2922   Phone: (303) 259-6144
Description: Explores a holistic approach to dental care. Encourages the use of homeopathic medications, acupuncture, cranial techniques, nutrition, and physical therapy in addition to conventional treatments. Recurring features include news of research, information on Association activities, member notes, and a calendar of events. **Frequency:** Bimonthly.

★2385★   THE HOLISTIC DENTAL DIGEST
Once Daily, Inc.
263 West End Ave., No. 2A
New York, NY 10023   Phone: (212) 874-4212
Description: Deals with holistic dental practices. Discusses oral disorders, tooth decay, and vitamin therapy. **First Published:** 1979. **Frequency:** 6/yr.

★2386★   HOLISTIC MEDICINE
American Holistic Medical Association
4101 Lake Boone Trail, Ste. 201
Raleigh, NC 27607   Phone: (919) 787-5146
Description: Reviews developments in holistic medicine, and carries information on nutrition, exercise, spiritual attunement, and self-regulation. Recurring features include Association news, book reviews, announcements of meetings and workshops, notices of continuing education opportunities, and synopses of related articles in print. **First Published:** May 1978. **Frequency:** Quarterly. **ISSN:** 0898-6029.

★2387★   HOLOGRAM
Canadian Holistic Medical Association
167 Craighurst Ave.
Toronto, ON, Canada M4R 1K1   Phone: (416) 487-0882
Description: Provides news and information on holistic medicine. **First Published:** 1983. **Frequency:** 6/yr.

★2388★   HOLOS INSTITUTES OF HEALTH—NEWSLETTER
Holos Institutes of Health
1328 E. Evergreen
Springfield, MO 65803   Phone: (417) 865-5940
Description: Provides information on medical networks, primarily holistic. **First Published:** 1985. **Frequency:** Bimonthly.

★2389★   HOLOS PRACTICE REPORTS
Holos Institute of Health
1328 E. Evergreen
Springfield, MO 65803   Phone: (417) 865-5940
Description: Presents information on homeopathic remedies, health and fitness practices, holistic healing, and resources on medical treatments. Recurring features include book reviews. **Frequency:** Bimonthly.

★2390★   HOME HEALTH AGENCY INSIDER
American Federation of Home Health Agencies
1320 Fenwick Ln., Ste. 100
Silver Spring, MD 20910   Phone: (301) 588-1454
Description: Provides information on regulatory and legislative issues of concern to home health agencies. Discusses employment topics and the issues of providing care. Recurring features include current legislation, regulatory developments, and news of meetings. **First Published:** 1984. **Frequency:** Every 3 weeks.

★2391★   HOME HEALTH LINE
Karen Rak
PO Box 250
Port Republic, MD 20676   Phone: (410) 535-4103
Description: Reports on Medicare, Medicaid, and other federal coverage and payment for home health care, including hospice care, durable medical equipment, home infusion therapy, and the home health/home care industry as a business. **First Published:** 1975. **Frequency:** Weekly.

★2392★   HOMEOPATHY TODAY
National Center for Homoeopathy
1500 Massachusetts Ave. NW, No. 41
Washington, DC 20005   Phone: (202) 223-6182
Description: Presents articles concerning the history, philosophy, and practice of homoeopathy. Carries excerpts of books from the Center's library collection, news of research, book reviews, editorials, and Center news. Recurring features include letters to the editor, news of members, a calendar of events, and columns titled Gleanings From the Media, Homoeopathic History, Veterinary Homeopathy, and News From the Lay Groups. **First Published:** 1974. **Frequency:** Monthly. **ISSN:** 0886-1676.

★2393★   HOMEOSTASIS QUARTERLY
Hypoglycemia Foundation
Adrenal Metabolic Research Society
153 Pawling Ave.
Troy, NY 12180   Phone: (518) 272-7154
Description: Focuses on health problems arising from hypoglycemia, adrenal cortex disorders, diabetes, and from vitamin deficiencies and other deficiency states. Recurring features include references to other reading material on the subjects discussed and news of research. **First Published:** 1972. **Frequency:** Quarterly.

★2394★   HOPE HEALTH LETTER
The Hope Heart Institute
350 E. Michigan Ave., Ste. 301
Kalamazoo, MI 49007-3851   Phone: (616) 343-0770
Description: Offers brief, carefully researched articles focusing on factors affecting employee health and corporate health care cost containment. Emphasizes preventive measures and discusses health issues, including AIDS, smoking, self-care, safety, nutrition, weight loss, exercise, substance abuse, stress, and safe driving. **First Published:** November 1978. **Frequency:** Monthly; Spanish edition published quarterly. **ISSN:** 0891-3374.

★2395★   HOPE NEWS
Project HOPE
People-to-People Health Foundation, Inc.
Millwood, VA 22646   Phone: (703) 837-2100
Description: Carries news of Project HOPE's international and domestic programs, which promote better world health through the training of medical, dental, and allied health personnel in developing areas of the world. Contains reports on headquarters conferences and meetings, personnel briefs, fund-raising activities, and volunteer events. **First Published:** March 1961. **Frequency:** Quarterly.

★2396★   HORIZON
Bergen-Passaic Chapter
National Multiple Sclerosis Society
730 River Rd., 2nd Fl.
PO Box 348
New Milford, NJ 07646-3032   Phone: (201) 967-5599
Description: Serves the organization and its members. Recurring features include a calendar of events, news of research, book reviews, restaurant reviews, and profiles. **Frequency:** Quarterly.

★2397★   HOSPICE LETTER
Health Resources Publishing
Brinley Professional Plaza
3100 Hwy. 138
Wall Township, NJ 07719-1442   Phone: (908) 681-1133
Description: Briefs readers on developments in existing hospice care programs for the terminally ill around the country. Covers federal and state legislative and regulatory actions; types of hospice care delivery; funding; and updates on practices that work. **First Published:** April 1979. **Frequency:** Monthly. **ISSN:** 0913-6816.

★2398★   HOSPITAL ADMINISTRATION NEWSLETTER
National Research Bureau, Inc.
424 N. Third St.
Burlington, IA 52601   Phone: (319) 752-5415
Description: Provides up-to-date information on Medicare, health care, employee relations, cost reduction, and new developments in the health field. Recurring features include statistics and news of research. **Frequency:** Monthly.

★2399★   HOSPITAL ADMITTING MONTHLY
American Health Consultants, Inc.
67 Peachtree Park Dr. NE
Atlanta, GA 30305   Phone: (404) 262-7436
Description: Covers "the full spectrum of admissions management," including business office and patient account topics, cost containment, and legal advice for better management in admitting. Recurring features include news of research, letters to the editor, book reviews, a calendar of events, and columns titled Perspectives on Admitting, Legal Issues, and Readers Write. **First Published:** July 1982. **Frequency:** Monthly.

★2400★   HOSPITAL CAPITAL FORMATION & MANAGEMENT LETTER
Health Resources Publishing
Brinley Professional Plaza, 3100 Hwy. 38
PO Box 1442
Wall Township, NJ 07719-1442   Phone: (201) 681-1133
Description: Monitors all aspects of hospital capital, including federal and state regulatory actions and long-range outlooks. **First Published:** November 1982. **Frequency:** Monthly. **ISSN:** 0738-6370.

★2401★ HOSPITAL COST ACCOUNTING ADVISOR
Aspen Publishers, Inc.
1600 Research Blvd.
Rockville, MD 20850   Phone: (301) 251-5554
Frequency: Monthly.

★2402★ HOSPITAL COST MANAGEMENT AND ACCOUNTING
Aspen Publishers, Inc.
200 Orchard Ridge Dr., Ste. 200
Gaithersburg, MD 20878   Phone: (301) 417-7500
Description: Discusses negotiations and hospital costs of health maintenance organizations (HMOs) and preferred-provider organizations (PPOs). Deals with the quality of cost data and how financial managers should view the value of data collected. **Frequency:** Monthly. **ISSN:** 8756-7288.

★2403★ HOSPITAL EDITORS' IDEA EXCHANGE
William R. Brinton
PO Box 1806
Kansas City, MO 64141
Description: Provides advice on writing, editing, and producing hospital publications. Recurring features include The Forum, which provides short articles on what other editors are doing to improve their newsletters. **First Published:** January 1990. **Frequency:** Monthly. **ISSN:** 1046-1647.

★2404★ HOSPITAL EMPLOYEE HEALTH
American Health Consultants, Inc.
67 Peachtree Park Dr. NE
Atlanta, GA 30309   Phone: (404) 262-7436
Description: Provides information on how to protect hospital employees from work-related hazards. Discusses prevention, treatment, detection, and the degree of risk, as well as government regulations and employee's legal rights. Recurring features include columns titled Legal Commentary, Reader Questions, and Quest. **First Published:** January 1982. **Frequency:** Monthly. **ISSN:** 0744-6470.

★2405★ HOSPITAL ENTREPRENEUR'S NEWSLETTER
Aspen Publishers, Inc.
1600 Research Blvd.
Rockville, MD 20850   Phone: (301) 251-5554
Description: Covers strategies in hospital finance, law, management, marketing, and planning. **Frequency:** Monthly.

★2406★ HOSPITAL ETHICS
American Hospital Association
840 N. Lake Shore Dr.
Chicago, IL 60611   Phone: (312) 280-6232
Description: Reviews latest information in the field of hospital ethics. Reports on court opinions, discusses their implications, and suggests strategies for resolving specific ethical concerns. Recurring features include news of research, a calendar of events, reports on meetings, book reviews, and notices of publications available. Also includes columns titled Institutional Ethics, Organ Transplantation, Care of the Newborn, Care of the Dying, and Hospital Ethics Committees. **First Published:** March-April 1985. **Frequency:** Bimonthly. **ISSN:** 8756-8519.

★2407★ HOSPITAL FUND RAISING NEWSLETTER
Health Resources Publishing
PO Box 1442
Belmar, NJ 07719   Phone: (201) 681-1133
Description: Covers fund raising for hospitals. **First Published:** January 1979. **Frequency:** 6/yr. **ISSN:** 0193-9939.

★2408★ HOSPITAL HOME HEALTH
American Health Consultants, Inc.
PO Box 740056
Atlanta, GA 30374   Phone: (404) 262-7436
Description: Provides clinical, legal, and management information pertinent to hospital-based home health agencies. Also monitors government regulation and profiles successful or unique programs. **First Published:** 1983. **Frequency:** Monthly. **ISSN:** 0884-8521.

★2409★ HOSPITAL INFECTION CONTROL
American Health Consultants, Inc.
67 Peachtree Park Dr. NE
Atlanta, GA 30309   Phone: (404) 262-7436
Description: Publishes information on hospital-acquired infections and how to prevent infections in patients and hospital staff members. Recur-

ring features include news of research, book reviews, a calendar of events, new sources of information, a question-and-answer column, and reviews of articles in current medical journals. **First Published:** 1974. **Frequency:** Monthly. **ISSN:** 0098-180X.

★2410★ HOSPITAL LAW NEWSLETTER
Aspen Publishers, Inc.
1600 Research Blvd.
Rockville, MD 20850   Phone: (301) 251-5554
Description: Covers mergers, medical staff appointments, hospital-physician contracts, protection confidentiality, etc. **Frequency:** Monthly.

★2411★ HOSPITAL LITIGATION REPORTER
Strafford Publications, Inc.
1201 Peachtree St. NE, Ste. 1150
Atlanta, GA 30361   Phone: (404) 881-1141
Description: Provides a digest of case law on hospital litigation. Highlights medical malpractice, certificate of need applications, health planning, informed consent, negligence, and wrongful death. **First Published:** January 1990. **Frequency:** Monthly. **ISSN:** 1048-5201.

★2412★ HOSPITAL MANAGEMENT REVIEW
COR Research Inc.
PO Box 40959
Santa Barbara, CA 93140-0959   Phone: (805) 564-2177
Description: Contains summaries of articles on health care management selected from more than 120 publications. **First Published:** 1982. **Frequency:** Monthly except July. **ISSN:** 0737-903X.

★2413★ HOSPITAL MATERIALS MANAGEMENT NEWS
American Society for Hospital Materials Management
American Hospital Association
840 N. Lake Shore Dr.
Chicago, IL 60611   Phone: (312) 280-6137
Description: Provides information about hospital purchasing and materials management. Includes reviews of educational programs, current legal and legislative problems, and new materials management techniques. Recurring features include Society news, affiliated chapter reports, and news of members. **First Published:** 1957. **Frequency:** Quarterly. **ISSN:** 0749-6672.

★2414★ HOSPITAL PATIENT RELATIONS REPORT
Business Publishers, Inc.
951 Pershing Dr.
Silver Spring, MD 2091-4464   Phone: (301) 587-6300
Description: Advises hospitals on how to improve their patient and public relations programs. **First Published:** 1986. **Frequency:** Monthly. **ISSN:** 0899-8957.

★2415★ HOSPITAL PEER REVIEW
American Health Consultants, Inc.
PO Box 740056
Atlanta, GA 30374   Phone: (404) 262-7436
Description: Discusses hospital quality assurance and quality management, utilization review, discharge planning, ancillary services review, reimbursement, accreditation, and peer review organization (PRO) compliance. Recurring features include book reviews, a calendar of events, news briefs, and columns titled Legal Issues and Quality/Cost Connection. **First Published:** 1976. **Frequency:** Monthly.

★2416★ HOSPITAL RISK MANAGEMENT
American Health Consultants, Inc.
PO Box 740056
Atlanta, GA 30374   Phone: (404) 262-7436
Description: Analyzes specific legal cases and trends relevant to hospital liability. Discusses malpractice, liablity for patients, staff and visitor injury, injury prevention, biomedical engineering, and medical staff credentials. Also covers high-risk areas of hospitals, accreditation, Medicare reimbursement, physician liability, medical records, and claims management. Recurring features include interviews, statistics, news of research, guest columns, legal briefs, and commentaries. **First Published:** October 1979. **Frequency:** Monthly. **ISSN:** 0199-6312.

★2417★ HOSPITAL SAFETY INFORMATION SERVICE
Scientific Enterprises, Inc.
5104 Randolph Rd.
North Little Rock, AR 72116   Phone: (501) 771-1775
Description: Described as "the only newsletter that focuses on hospital safety for the patient, employee, and visitor." Presents suggestions on how

to meet various government agency safety standards as well as information on hazard communication, disaster preparation, risk management, and industrial hygiene. Recurring features include a calendar of events, notices of publications available, and columns titled FDA Recalls and Questions and Answers. **First Published:** March 1979. **Frequency:** Bimonthly. **ISSN:** 0276-2323.

★2418★ **HOSPITAL SUPERVISOR'S BULLETIN**
Bureau of Business Practice
24 Rope Ferry Rd.
Waterford, CT 06386   Phone: (203) 442-4365
Description: Offers management techniques for solving departmental problems such as absenteeism and tardiness, turnover, low productivity, and funding/personnel cutbacks. **First Published:** 1968. **Frequency:** Semimonthly. **ISSN:** 0018-585X.

★2419★ **HOSPITAL TECHNOLOGY ALERTS**
Ross Publication
PO Box 80
Boston, MA 02113   Phone: (617) 720-4556
Description: Intends to "provide the hospital materials manager or product safety coordinator with a convenient and systematic way of documenting any required corrective actions to medical devices." Description of each faulty device includes source of information, manufacturer, device name, model/serial number, lot/distribution, description of hazard, and recommended action. **First Published:** August 1982. **Frequency:** Monthly. **ISSN:** 0735-4479.

★2420★ **HOSPITAL TECHNOLOGY SERIES**
American Hospital Association
840 N. Lake Shore Dr.
Chicago, IL 60611   Phone: (312) 280-6084
Description: Focuses on technology used in clinical and management operations of a hospital. Divided into 4 sections: Executive Briefing, a summary of significant developments in technology affecting hospitals' strategic planning and decision-making; Technology Scanner, a summary of medical and technical journal articles translated into management language; Special Reports, which provides information on health care technology developments, issues, and trends; and Guideline Report, an in-depth analysis of diagnostic, therapeutic, computer, and related systems and technologies. **First Published:** August 1982. **Frequency:** Monthly. **ISSN:** 0735-4681.

★2421★ **HOT FLASH**
National Action Forum for Midlife and Older Women
PO Box 816
Stony Brook, NY 11790-0609
Description: Addresses the health and social concerns of both mid-life and older women. Recurring features include editorials, legislative items, abstracts, conference agenda, book reviews, news of research, and announcements and resources. **First Published:** Summer 1981. **Frequency:** Quarterly.

★2422★ **HOUSTON EAR RESEARCH FOUNDATION— NEWSLETTER**
Houston Ear Research Foundation
7737 SW Freeway, Ste. 630
Houston, TX 77074   Phone: (713) 771-9966
First Published: 1986. **Frequency:** Semiannually.

★2423★ **HUMAN PERFORMANCE ELEMENTS**
Human Performance Institute
University of Texas at Arlington
Box 19180
Arlington, TX 76019   Phone: (817) 273-2335
Description: Covers research and student projects conducted by the Institute, which studies the development and bounds of human physical performance. Recurring features include notices of publications available. **First Published:** Spring 1987. **Frequency:** Semiannually.

★2424★ **HUMAN SURVIVAL**
Negative Population Growth, Inc.
PO Box 1206, 210 The Plaza
Teaneck, NJ 07666-1206   Phone: (201) 837-3555
Description: Dedicated to the stabilization and reduction of the world's population by means of national and international programs. Concerned with all the ramifications of overpopulation—social, economic, health, and, particularly, environmental. Recurring features include demographic

study reports and news of legislative action affecting population control. **First Published:** 1974. **Frequency:** 3/yr.

★2425★ **HYGIENIC COMMUNITY NETWORK—NEWS**
Hygienic Community Network
PO Box 1132
Springfield, MD 65806
Description: Serves as a communication network for people who are committed to community living as an essential part of the Natural Hygiene lifestyle. Discusses information and issues of interest to people considering joining or forming cooperative communities for healthful living. Carries self-descriptions from individuals desiring contact with like-minded people. Recurring features include letters to the editor, news of members, book reviews, and a calendar of events. **First Published:** September 1980. **Frequency:** Bimonthly.

★2426★ **HYPNOTHERAPY IN REVIEW**
Academy of Scientific Hypnotherapy
PO Box 12041
San Diego, CA 92112-3041   Phone: (619) 427-6225
Description: Offers information of interest to professional hypnotherapists. Reports on the latest medical and psychological research. Recurring features include editorials, letters to the editor, news of the Academy and its members, book reviews, and a column titled Hypno-Briefs. **First Published:** 1977. **Frequency:** Periodic.

★2427★ **HYPNOTHERAPY TODAY**
American Association of Professional Hypnotherapists
PO Box 731
McLean, VA 22101   Phone: (703) 448-9623
Description: Serves as a forum for the exchange of information and experience among professionals who use hypnosis in clinical therapy and education. Features discussions of theories, methods, and ideas. Covers practice promotion and management as well. Recurring features include news of research, book reviews, news of members, and a calendar of events. **First Published:** 1981. **Frequency:** 4/yr. **ISSN:** 0882-8652.

★2428★ **IBCA SCOPE**
Institute on Black Chemical Abuse
2616 Nicollet Ave. S.
Minneapolis, MN 55408   Phone: (612) 871-7878
Description: Views alcohol and drug abuse from an African-American perspective. Recurring features include interviews, news of research, a calendar of events, reports of meetings, book reviews, and notices of publications available. **First Published:** 1979. **Frequency:** Quarterly. **ISSN:** 0895-8661.

★2429★ **IBFAN NEWS**
International Baby Food Action Network
Infant Formula Action Coalition
3255 Hennepin Ave. S., Ste. 220
Minneapolis, MN 55408   Phone: (612) 825-6837
Description: Covers issues related to the use of infant formula. Reports on government action towards implementing the World Health Organization's (WHO) Code of Breastmilk Substitutes, company violations of the WHO Code, and citizen efforts to promote breastfeeding. Aims to monitor infant foods marketing and apply pressure to infant foods corporations. Recurring features include news of companies and information about breastfeeding. **First Published:** 1979. **Frequency:** Quarterly.

★2430★ **ICA UPDATE**
Interstitial Cystitis Association, Inc.
Box 1553, Madison Sq. Sta.
New York, NY 10159   Phone: (212) 979-6057
Description: Highlights activities of the Association, a support and information network for patients with the bladder disease Interstitial Cystitis. Recurring features include announcements of upcoming events. **First Published:** 1985. **Frequency:** Quarterly.

★2431★ **THE ICARUS FILE**
Phoenix Society for Burn Survivors, Inc.
11 Rust Hill Rd.
Levittown, PA 19056   Phone: (215) 946-BURN
Description: Concerned with burn injuries, burn prevention, and the rehabilitation and medical care of burn victims. Discusses new medical techniques and products, and reprints pertinent articles. Recurring features include profiles of members, lists of area burn victim support coordinators, book reviews, news of research, statistics, and columns titled Director's

Corner and The Mail Box. **First Published:** Spring 1980. **Frequency:** Quarterly.

★2432★   ICEA SHARING
International Childbirth Education Association, Inc.
PO Box 20048
Minneapolis, MN 55420   Phone: (612) 854-8660
Description: Intended for childbirth educators. Offers articles, commentary, and surveys on parent education, perinatal nutrition, the mother/neonatal relationship, and labor and birth. Also monitors legislation affecting childbirth educators. Recurring features include Association news on projects, service, workshops, and conferences; also includes letters, guest editorials, news of research, and a calendar of events. **First Published:** 1974. **Frequency:** 3/yr.

★2433★   IFFLP BULLETIN
International Federation for Family Life Promotion
1511 K St. NW, Ste. 326
Washington, DC 20005   Phone: (202) 738-1037
Description: Supplies information on national family planning events and research. Includes articles on family planning, zonal development programs, and primary health care. Includes news of natural family planning meetings and conferences. Recurring features include news of research, news of members, book reviews, and a calendar of events. **First Published:** February 1984. **Frequency:** Semiannually.

★2434★   ILLINOIS CANCER UPDATE
Illinois Cancer Center
200 S. Michigan Ave., 17th Fl.
Chicago, IL 60604-2404   Phone: (312) 226-2379
Description: Supplies information on the programs, projects, activities, and people connected with the Council. Serves as a forum for the exchange of information about cancer among those involved in care and research. Focuses on new technology, and seminars presented for professionals. Recurring features include news of research, announcements of awards, and officers, staff, and committee chairpersons. **First Published:** Winter 1981. **Frequency:** Quarterly.

★2435★   IMAGERY TODAY
Brandon House, Inc.
PO Box 240
Bronx, NY 10471
Description: Dedicated to the study and stimulation of mental imagery, which conducts the central creative and expressive core of the individual. Facilitates information exchange relating to the imagery field from an interdisciplinary perspective. Explores how imagery is central to finding fulfilling expression of human potential. Recurring features include news of members, news of research, and notices of national and international meetings. **First Published:** 1983. **Frequency:** Semiannually. **ISSN:** 1041-8377.

★2436★   IMPLANT UPDATE
Academy for Implants and Transplants
PO Box 223
Springfield, VA 22150   Phone: (703) 451-0001
Description: Discusses developments in the field of implant and transplant dentistry, with the purpose of assisting dentists in general practice. Carries articles on techniques and procedures in implant and transplant dentistry. **Frequency:** Quarterly.

★2437★   IMPOTENCE WORLDWIDE
Impotence Institute International
119 S. Ruth St.
Maryville, TN 37801-5746   Phone: (615) 983-6064
Description: Disseminates information on the treatment and cure of chronic male impotence to members of Impotents Anonymous and I-Anon (organizations based on the Alcoholics Anonymous model), offering support to couples suffering from chronic impotence. Recurring features include news of research, book reviews, and columns titled The Institutes' Pulse, Professionally Speaking, Points to Ponder, Speak Out (letters to the editor), Read About Impotence, and In the News. **First Published:** 1985. **Frequency:** Quarterly.

★2438★   IMPRINTS
Birth & Life Bookstore
7001 Alonzo Ave. NW
PO Box 70625
Seattle, WA 98107   Phone: (206) 789-4444
Description: Publishes reviews of books on childbirth, child care, family planning, breastfeeding, and women's health issues. Reports on forthcoming books, new editions, and paperbacks. Contains an annotated list of books available from the Bookstore. Provides an order form and information on book and shipping costs. **First Published:** April 1980. **Frequency:** 3-4/yr.

★2439★   IN THE MAINSTREAM
Mainstream, Inc.
1030 15th St. NW, Ste. 1010
Washington, DC 20005   Phone: (202) 898-1400
Description: Publishes up-to-date information on issues affecting individuals with disabilities and their employers. "Reports on advances companies are making in the employment of disabled individuals, with particular focus on innovative solutions and the people who are using them." **First Published:** Fall 1976. **Frequency:** Bimonthly. **ISSN:** 0888-9724.

★2440★   IN SEARCH
Juvenile Diabetes Foundation-Toronto Chapter
49 The Donway W., Ste. 320
Don Mills, ON, Canada M2N 4Z9   Phone: (416) 510-1350
Description: Features information on the Foundation. Recurring features include news of research, a calendar of events, and notices of publications available. **First Published:** 1984. **Frequency:** Bimonthly.

★2441★   IN SEARCH OF IDENTITY
Missing Persons-International, Inc.
PO Box 46896
Los Angeles, CA 90046-896
Description: Concerned with adoption, parental and children's rights, runaways, abuse victims, M.I.A's and P.O.W's, families of murder victims, genealogy, heirs, grandparents, child support, missing/exploited children and adults, rape, abduction, abandonment, and catastrophic experiences. **First Published:** January 1960. **Frequency:** Monthly.

★2442★   IN TOUCH
Programs for the Blind and Physically Handicapped
Texas State Library
PO Box 12927
Austin, TX 78711   Phone: (512) 463-5458
Description: Reports on new services and publications available for blind, visually-impaired, and physically handicapped Texans. Also contains stories on topics of interest to persons with reading-related disabilities. Recurring features include an order form for new recorded books and columns titled Around the State, Volunteer Corner, Newsbriefs, and Reminders. **First Published:** Spring 1976. **Frequency:** Quarterly.

★2443★   IN TOUCH
Stroking Community Network
PO Box 307
Arlington, VT 05250
Description: Dedicated to promoting physical, mental, and spiritual healing through touch. Carries news and opinion on matters of interest to those who perform massage and other kinds of "bodywork," either professionally or avocationally. Recurring features include editorials, news of research, book reviews, and a calendar of events. **First Published:** 1987. **Frequency:** 3/yr.

★2444★   IN TOUCH FOR HEALTH
Touch for Health Foundation
1174 N. Lake Ave.
Pasadena, CA 91104   Phone: (818) 794-1181
Description: Disseminates information on research, methodology, and self-development programs in health enhancement, both mental and physical. Provides current information on self-care instructor training, workshops in holistic health care, seminars, and other Foundation activities. Recurring features include editorials, news of research, letters to the editor, news of members, book reviews, a calendar of events, and a column titled President's Message. **First Published:** 1983. **Frequency:** 6/yr.

★2445★ INDUSTRY UNIVERSITY COOPERATIVE RESEARCH CENTER—NEWSLETTER
Industry University Cooperative Research Center
University of Texas Health Science Center at San Antonio
7703 Floyd Curl Dr.
San Antonio, TX 78284-7823   Phone: (512) 567-2023
Description: Features activities of the Center's researchers and their projects. Introduces new members and profiles meetings sponsored/co-sponsored by the Center. **First Published:** Fall 1988. **Frequency:** Quarterly.

★2446★ INFECTIOUS DISEASE ALERT
American Health Consultants, Inc.
PO Box 740056
Atlanta, GA 30374   Phone: (404) 262-7436
Description: Focuses on infectious diseases, discussing causes and treatments as well as means of diagnosis. Designed to "stimulate thought and further investigation." Recurring features include news of research. **First Published:** 1981. **Frequency:** Semimonthly. **ISSN:** 0739-7348.

★2447★ INFECTIOUS DISEASES NEWSLETTER
Elsevier Science Publishing Co., Inc.
655 Avenue of the Americas
New York, NY 10010   Phone: (212) 633-3927
Description: Seeks to provide concise reports of the current state of knowledge and practice in infectious diseases. Recurring features include news of research, book reviews, and case studies. **First Published:** October 1981. **Frequency:** Monthly. **ISSN:** 0278-2316.

★2448★ INFO ALS
Amyotrophic Lateral Sclerosis Society of Canada
B101 - 90 Adelaide St., E.
Toronto, ON, Canada M5C 2R4   Phone: (416) 362-0269
Description: Contains abstracts of research on amyotrophic lateral sclerosis (ALS), a degenerative disorder that causes a progressive deterioration of the nerve cells responsible for muscle movement. Recurring features include research news and notices of available publications. **First Published:** 1980. **Frequency:** Annual.

★2449★ INFORMATION FROM HEATH
HEATH Resource Center
1 Dupont Circle, Ste. 800
Washington, DC 20036   Phone: (202) 939-9320
Description: Covers topics of concern such as technology and disability, legislation, court decisions, new resources, campus highlights, and "transition trends," all relating to education of the handicapped. Recurring features include interviews, news of research, book reviews, notices of publications available, and notices of educational opportunities. **First Published:** 1979. **Frequency:** Semiannually.

★2450★ INFORMED
MDT Publications
1145 Main St.
Springfield, MA 01103   Phone: (413) 732-4890
Description: Reports on corporate, regulatory, and international news concerning the pharmaceutical industry and drugs as related to medical research. Discusses trends in therapeutics as well as new uses for old drugs. Also includes statistics on sales and earnings in pharmaceutical corporations. Recurring features include book reviews, notices of meetings, personnel news, and announcements of Food and Drug Administration approvals. **First Published:** 1970. **Frequency:** Weekly. **ISSN:** 0730-6628.

★2451★ INJURY PREVENTION PROGRAMS
Darrell Heppner Risk Management Services, Inc.
PO Box 958
San Leandro, CA 94577   Phone: (510) 632-2200
Description: Publishes news about backs, back injury prevention, and general back education. Discusses back support systems, care, exercises, and programs. Recurring features include news of research and book reviews. **First Published:** 1985. **Frequency:** Periodic.

★2452★ INNER EAR
National Temporal Bone Banks Program
Deafness Research Foundation
c/o Massachusetts Eye & Ear Infirmary
243 Charles St.
Boston, MA 02114   Phone: (617) 573-3711
Description: Outlines the objectives of the organization, discussing the medical need and use of temporal bones for hearing-impaired persons.

Includes information about donations to the Bank. **Frequency:** Semiannually.

★2453★ INNOVATIONS
Pharmacia LKB Biotechnology, Inc.
800 Centennial Ave.
Piscataway, NJ 08854   Phone: (201) 457-8000
Description: Describes biomolecular engineering products available from Pharmacia LKB Biotechnology, Inc. Discusses techniques and innovations in the industry.

★2454★ INSIDE AL-ANON
Al-Anon Family Group Headquarters, Inc.
Box 862, Midtown Sta.
New York, NY 10018-0862   Phone: (212) 302-7240
Description: Presents news, policy, and commentary from volunteers, staff, and readers sharing experiences of individual and group growth through service. Features national Al-Anon news and personal stories. Recurring features include news of research, news of members, and a calendar of events. **First Published:** January 1979. **Frequency:** Bimonthly. **ISSN:** 1054-1438.

★2455★ INSIDE MS
National Multiple Sclerosis Society
205 E. 42nd St.
New York, NY 10017   Phone: (212) 986-3240
Description: Presents articles on topics of interest to persons with multiple sclerosis (MS) and their families. Recurring features include news of the Society's projects and programs, news of research, news of members, editorials, letters, reports of relevant legislation, and columns titled Up Front, Faces, Peer to Peer, Q&A About MS, and Book News. **First Published:** January 1983. **Frequency:** Quarterly. **ISSN:** 0739-9774.

★2456★ INSTITUTE ON AGING NEWSLETTER
Institute on Aging
University of Pennsylvania
3615 Chestnut St.
Philadelphia, PA 19104-6006   Phone: (215) 898-1939
Description: Contains articles on biomedical, clinical, social-behavioral, and scientific research subjects in geriatrics and gerontology. Spotlights interviews with University affiliated individuals who have aged successfully or experts in the field. Provides news of the Institute and its activities and programs. Recurring features include a calendar of events, reports of meetings, news of educational opportunities, notices of publications available, and columns titled Institute Update and Focus on the Community. **First Published:** November 1978. **Frequency:** 3/yr. **ISSN:** 1059-2431.

★2457★ INSTITUTE FOR HEALTH, HEALTH CARE POLICY, AND AGING RESEARCH—NEWSLETTER
Institute for Health, Health Care Policy, and Aging Research
Rutgers University
30 College Ave.
PO Box 5170
New Brunswick, NJ 08903-5170   Phone: (908) 932-8413
Description: Describes ongoing research projects and programs at the Institute. **First Published:** 1985. **Frequency:** 1-2/yr.

★2458★ INSTITUTE FOR POSITIVE WEIGHT MANAGEMENT—NEWSLETTER
Institute for Positive Weight Management
PO Box 1271
Boca Raton, FL 33429   Phone: (407) 750-7004
Description: Reflects the Institute's philosophy of weight management. Recurring features include columns titled The PWM Philosophy and You, Health Corner, Practical Tips, Research Corner, and Answer to Your Question. **First Published:** January 1990. **Frequency:** Quarterly.

★2459★ INTEGRATED RISK INFORMATION SYSTEM (IRIS)
National Technical Information Service
U.S. Department of Commerce
5285 Port Royal Rd.
Springfield, VA 22161   Phone: (703) 487-4630
Description: Provides information concerning the effects of chemicals on human health. Includes data on reference doses and carcinogen assessments. **Frequency:** Quarterly.

★2460★ INTENSIVE CARING UNLIMITED
Intensive Caring Unlimited
910 Bent Ln.
Philadelphia, PA 19118   Phone: (215) 233-4723
Description: Provides information and support for parents of high risk and premature babies. Deals with prematurity, hospitalization, developmental delays, high-risk pregnancy, and grieving, as well as other general parenting topics. Includes articles written by parents and professionals. Recurring features include news of research and book reviews. **First Published:** May 1983. **Frequency:** Bimonthly.

★2461★ INTERACTION NEWSLETTER
American Assembly for Men in Nursing
PO Box 31753
Independence, OH 44131
Description: Aimed at male nurses and male nursing students. **First Published:** Quarterly.

★2462★ INTERGOVERNMENTAL AIDS REPORT
Intergovernmental Health Policy Project
2021 K St. NW, Ste. 800
Washington, DC 20006   Phone: (202) 872-1445
Description: Features state legislative trends, policy research findings, and innovative programs and strategies. **Frequency:** 6/yr.

★2463★ INTERNAL MEDICINE ALERT
American Health Consultants, Inc.
PO Box 740056
Atlanta, GA 30374   Phone: (404) 262-7436
Description: Reviews medical literature pertaining to internal medicine. Includes brief comments at the conclusion of most reviews. Recurring features include news of research. **First Published:** 1978. **Frequency:** Semimonthly. **ISSN:** 0195-315X.

★2464★ INTERNATIONAL ACADEMY OF BEHAVIORAL MEDICINE, COUNSELING, AND PSYCHOTHERAPY— NEWSLETTER
International Academy of Behavioral Medicine, Counseling, and Psychotherapy
6750 Hillcrest Plaza, Ste. 304
Dallas, TX 75230   Phone: (214) 458-8334
Description: Publishes research articles in the field of behavioral medicine, "the systematic application of various principles of behavioral science to health care problems." Contains news of the Academy and its members. Recurring features include book reviews, letters to the editor, and a calendar of events. **First Published:** 1979. **Frequency:** Quarterly.

★2465★ INTERNATIONAL ACADEMY OF CHEST PHYSICIANS AND SURGEONS—BULLETIN
International Academy of Chest Physicians and Surgeons
American College of Chest Physicians
3300 Dundee Rd.
Northbrook, IL 60062   Phone: (708) 498-1400
Description: Informs members concerning chapters, meetings, and other members of the Academy and announces upcoming events of interest. Reports in general upon the Academy's ongoing efforts to further the continuing education of specialists in chest medicine and surgery. **First Published:** 1978. **Frequency:** 3-4/yr.

★2466★ INTERNATIONAL ASSOCIATION OF RADIOPHARMACOLOGY—NEWSLETTER
International Association of Radiopharmacology
c/o Professor L.I. Wiebe
3118 Dent-Pharm Centre
University of Alberta
Edmonton, AB, Canada T6G 2N8   Phone: (403) 492-5905
Description: Covers all aspects of radiopharmacology. **First Published:** 1980. **Frequency:** 3/yr.

★2467★ INTERNATIONAL ASSOCIATION FOR THE STUDY OF PAIN—NEWSLETTER
International Association for the Study of Pain
909 NE 43rd St., Ste. 306
Seattle, WA 98105   Phone: (206) 547-6409
Description: Reports on activities of the Association, whose members are engaged in research/management of pain syndromes. Recurring features include meeting minutes, lists of international conferences and congresses, and a section on new books by IASP members and other publications

available, and columns titled President's Message, Committee Corner, Chapter Activities, and Positions Available, plus a Technical/scientific column on issues and topics in pain research and management. **First Published:** 1975. **Frequency:** 6/yr. **ISSN:** 1017-0057.

★2468★ INTERNATIONAL COMMITTEE NEWSLETTER
Manitoba League of the Physically Handicapped
200-294 Portage Ave.
Winnipeg, MB, Canada R3C 0B9   Phone: (204) 943-6099
Description: Contains news of the Committee's international projects. Promotes disability rights. Attempts to link people interested in disability issues. Recurring features include news of members. **Frequency:** 4/yr.

★2469★ INTERNATIONAL DRUG AND DEVICE REGULATORY MONITOR
Newsletter Services, Inc.
1545 New York Ave. NE
Washington, DC 20002-1765   Phone: (202) 529-5700
Description: Reports on legal, medical, and scientific issues pertaining to the pharmaceutical, medical device, and biotechnology industries. Offers international coverage of pharmaceutical and medical device regulations that affect manufacturing, marketing, research and development, and legal entry into other markets. **First Published:** 1974. **Frequency:** Monthly. **ISSN:** 0888-6393.

★2470★ INTERNATIONAL DRUG THERAPY NEWSLETTER
Ayd Medical Communications
1130 E. Cold Spring Lane
Baltimore, MD 21239   Phone: (301) 433-9220
Description: Focuses on psychotropic drugs, discussing individual drugs, their effectiveness, and history. Examines illnesses and the drugs used to treat them, studies done on various drugs, their chemical make-up, and new developments and changes in drugs. Recurring features include book reviews and news of research. **First Published:** January 1966. **Frequency:** 10/yr. **ISSN:** 0020-6571.

★2471★ INTERNATIONAL FEDERATION ON AGEING— NETWORK NEWS
International Federation on Ageing
601 E St. NW
Washington, DC 20049   Phone: (202) 434-2430
Description: Tracks proposals and ongoing programs designed to benefit older women in various countries. Recurring features include a calendar of international conferences, book reviews, and columns titled Global Link Update and Update on Older Women's Health. **First Published:** Winter 1985. **Frequency:** Semiannually.

★2472★ INTERNATIONAL GUILD OF PROFESSIONAL ELECTROLOGISTS—NEWSLETTER
International Guild of Professional Electrologists
202 Boulevard, Ste. B
High Point, NC 27262   Phone: (516) 482-1311
Description: Reflects the aims of the Guild, which are to elevate the practice of electrolysis to a professional status. Recurring features include news of members, conference reports, discussions of policy and state licensing, items from related associations, notices of awards and useful publications, and the column PR: Professional Recognition. **First Published:** 1980. **Frequency:** 4/yr.

★2473★ INTERNATIONAL HEALTH SOCIETY—QUARTERLY BULLETIN
International Health Society
1001 E. Oxford Lane
Englewood, CO 80110   Phone: (303) 789-3003
Description: Follows the Society's efforts to improve the health of all people through international cooperation and the maintenance of high standards of medical care. Consists of two sections, Professional and General: the former comprises a contribution from an "outstanding professional;" the latter, organizational items and notices of continuing medical education. Recurring features include news of research, a calendar of events, meeting reports, and notices of publications available.

★2474★ INTERNATIONAL ORGANIZATION FOR MYCOPLASMOLOGY—NEWSLETTER
International Organization for Mycoplasmology
Department of Microbiology
School of Medicine
University of Alabama at Birmingham
Birmingham, AL 35294   Phone: (205) 934-9339
Description: Highlights "timely scientific topics" in the field of mycoplasmology, which is the study of microorganisms that cause disease in humans, plants, and farm animals. Publishes organizational and member news, meeting announcements, and disseminates news of research. Recurring features include notices of publications available and a calendar of events. Frequency: Quarterly.

★2475★ INTERNATIONAL PSYCHOLOGIST
International Council of Psychologists, Inc.
c/o Dr. Carleton Shay
2261 Talmadge St.
Los Angeles, CA 90027   Phone: (213) 666-1480
Description: Publishes news of the professional and scientific activities of the Council while promoting better understanding within the profession. Also contains official announcements and reports of the International Council. Recurring features include book reviews, a list of new members, a message from the president, and sections titled Convention Calendar and News of Members. First Published: 1959. Frequency: Quarterly. ISSN: 0047-116X.

★2476★ INTERNATIONAL REHABILITATION REVIEW
Rehabilitation International
25 E. 21st St.
New York, NY 10010   Phone: (212) 420-1500
Description: Contains news and articles on international, national, and local developments in the fields of disability prevention and rehabilitation. Provides regular coverage of United Nations agencies, discusses the elimination of architectural and attitudinal barriers to disabled persons, and examines new trends in service delivery. Recurring features include news of research, book reviews, and a calendar of events. First Published: 1949. Frequency: 3/yr.

★2477★ INTERNATIONAL RESCUER JOURNAL
International Rescue and Emergency Care Association
627 Thompson Way
Covington, VA 24426-2179   Phone: (612) 941-2926
Description: Supplies advice and instruction on handling personal injury situations and notices of meetings and classes on rescue methods and emergency care procedures for all levels of EMS (Emergency Medical Service). Notifies members of new EMS equipment and related problems or recalls. Recurring features include news of research, a calendar of events, and updates on Association activities. First Published: 1957. Frequency: Quarterly.

★2478★ INTERNATIONAL SOCIETY FOR DEVELOPMENTAL PSYCHOBIOLOGY—NEWSLETTER
International Society for Developmental Psychobiology
Department of Psychology
Barnard College
Columbia University
New York, NY 10027   Phone: (212) 854-2329
Description: Contains organizational news, announcements, job listings, and meeting information for members of the Society, which promotes research into "the relationship between behavioral and biological aspects of the developing organism." Frequency: 2-3/yr.

★2479★ INTERNATIONAL SOCIETY OF DIFFERENTIATION—NEWSLETTER
International Society of Differentiation
Department of Genetics and Cell Bilology
750 Biological Sciences Center
University of Minnesota
St. Paul, MN 55108   Phone: (612) 624-2285
Description: Announces upcoming Society meetings and publications concerned with biological differentiation, "the process leading to specializations of structure and function of cells, tissues and intact organisms." Recurring features include conference reports and notices about membership dues. First Published: August 1982. Frequency: Periodic.

★2480★ INTERNATIONAL TREMOR FOUNDATION—NEWSLETTER
International Tremor Foundation
360 W. Superior St.
Chicago, IL 60610   Phone: (312) 664-2344
Description: Contains essays by movement disorders neurologists and geneticists offering information on diagnoses, treatments, and research in essential tremor and other disorders having tremors as symptoms. Answers questions in layman's language and provides a glossary for technical terms. First Published: August 1988. Frequency: Quarterly.

★2481★ INTERNATIONAL VENTILATOR USERS NETWORK NEWS
International Polio Network
5100 Oakland Ave., No. 206
St. Louis, MO 63110   Phone: (314) 534-0457
Description: Serves as a communications network for polio survivors who use ventilators. First Published: 1987. Frequency: Semiannual.

★2482★ THE INTERNIST'S INTERCOM
American Society of Internal Medicine
1101 Vermont Ave. NW, Ste. 500
Washington, DC 20005   Phone: (202) 289-1700
Description: Reflects the Society's commitment "to study and respond to the social, economic and political forces affecting the cost, quality and availability of their services to patients." Provides news and information of interest to internists, covering regulatory and legislative actions, socioeconomic issues and trends, and Society activities and services. Recurring features include conference announcements and notices of publications available. First Published: January 1976. Frequency: Monthly. ISSN: 0164-6419.

★2483★ IPRS NEWSLETTER
International Confederation for Plastic and Reconstructive Surgery
30, boul. St.-Joseph Est., Ste. 220
Montreal, PQ, Canada H2T 1G9   Phone: (514) 842-3855
Description: Disseminates information on IPRS activities, emphasizing international topics in plastic and reconstructive surgery. Highlights scientific developments in the field such as new products, techniques, or "philosophical changes in treatment." Provides news of members and member activity, profiling individuals in features. Recurring features include editorials, news from national societies and national chapters, letters to the editor, news of research, reports of meetings, a calendar of events, and a column titled Meet Your Executive. Frequency: 2/yr.

★2484★ IRONIC BLOOD
Iron Overload Diseases Association, Inc.
244 Datura St., Ste. 911
West Palm Beach, FL 33401   Phone: (407) 659-5616
Description: Exposes the medical facts concerning the dangers of excess iron in the human body. Focuses on iron-overload diseases such as hemochromatosis, porphyria cutanea tarda, cirrhosis, diabetes, arthritis, arrhythmia, and anemia. Also reports on secondary iron loading resulting from liver disease, genetic characteristics, medication, and food. Recurring features include items on Association activities, comments from readers, articles on diagnosis and treatment, and columns titled News About You and IOD News. First Published: May 1981. Frequency: Bimonthly. ISSN: 0895-7762.

★2485★ IVUN NEWS
International Ventilator Users Network
Gazette International Networking Institute
5100 Oakland Ave., No. 206
St. Louis, MO 63110   Phone: (314) 534-0475
Description: Disseminates information on breathing techniques and equipment to help persons who use mechanical ventilation to live at home rather than in an institution. Discusses related issues such as adaptation and psychological adjustment, attendant care, funding sources, travel with ventilators, and sleep-disordered breathing. Recurring features include a calendar of events and news of relevant legislation. First Published: December 1986. Frequency: Semiannually.

★2486★ THE JAPAN MEDICAL REVIEW
Japan Publications, Inc.
150 Post St., Ste. 500
San Francisco, CA 94108   Phone: (415) 772-5555
Description: Reports on the Japanese health care market, taking the viewpoint of the health care executive. Covers legislative and regulatory developments, market activity, new product breakthroughs, and Ministry

of Health approvals in Japan. Recurring features include news of market research, a calendar of events, and columns titled Stock Market Trends, Manufacturer/Distributor Profile, and Ministry of Health Approvals. **First Published:** June 1986. **Frequency:** Monthly. **ISSN:** 0914-0255.

★2487★ JBI POINTS
Jewish Braille Institute of America, Inc.
110 E. 30th St.
New York, NY 10016   Phone: (212) 889-2525
Description: Provides news about the Institute, which serves the religious, cultural, educational, and communal needs of the Jewish blind and visually impaired in Israel and the U.S. Offers information on talking books, braille and large-print publications, and on the Institute's meetings and elections. Recurring features include letters to the editor. **Frequency:** Periodic.

★2488★ JCAHO PERSPECTIVES
Joint Commission on Accreditation of Healthcare Organizations
1 Renaissance Blvd.
Oakbrook Terrace, IL 60181   Phone: (708) 916-5600
Description: Identifies new and revised Joint Commission standards. Provides updates on revised policies and procedures concerning accreditation and survey processes. Reports on "Agenda for Change" initiatives. Recurring features include columns titled President's Column, On Site, Surveys-at-a-Glance, Interpretations, Briefs, and Accreditation Clinic. **First Published:** November 1952. **Frequency:** Bimonthly. **ISSN:** 0277-8327.

★2489★ JEWISH GUILD FOR THE BLIND—NEWSLETTER
Jewish Guild for the Blind
15 W. 65th St.
New York, NY 10023   Phone: (212) 769-6200
Description: Distributed to professionals in the health/service field and to supporters of the Guild, a service agency for blind senior citizens and visually handicapped people of all ages, races, and creeds. Furnishes information on Guild programs, patrons, personnel, and clients. Recurring features include news of research, reports of meetings, and news of programs designed to help the blind and visually impaired. **First Published:** 1967. **Frequency:** Quarterly.

★2490★ JIN SHIN DO ACUPRESSURE NEWSLETTER
Jin Shin Do Foundation
366 California Ave., No. 16
Palo Alto, CA 94306   Phone: (415) 328-1811
Description: Provides information on bodymind acupressure, news, and main contacts in the U.S., Canada, and Europe. Features a product catalog, a calendar of events, and reports of meetings.

★2491★ JOB SAFETY CONSULTANT
Business Research Publications, Inc.
817 Broadway
New York, NY 10003   Phone: (212) 673-4700
Description: Covers industrial safety and health, Occupational Safety and Health Administration (OSHA) and company safety strategies. Recurring features include columns titled Editor's Corner, Updates & Alerts, Safety in Action, Technical Tips, and Safety Talks. **First Published:** November 1972. **Frequency:** Monthly.

★2492★ JOB SAFETY AND HEALTH
Bureau of National Affairs, Inc.
1231 25th St. NW
Washington, DC 20037   Phone: (202) 452-4200
Description: Designed to help employers deal with occcupational safety and health regulations, standards, and practices, and to understand the effects of compliance on employee relations. Covers the establishment, management, evaluation, maintenance, and administration of health and safety programs. Includes reviews of regulations, policies, practices, and trends. Also carries information on recordkeeping, inspections, enforcement, employer defenses, and training. **First Published:** 1977. **Frequency:** Biweekly. **ISSN:** 0149-7510.

★2493★ JOB SAFETY AND HEALTH QUARTERLY
Occupational Safety and Health Administration
U.S. Department of Labor
200 Constitution Ave. NW, N 3647
Washington, DC 20210   Phone: (202) 523-8615
Description: Informs readers of changes, developments, and new rulings made by the Occupational Safety and Health Administration (OSHA). **First Published:** October 1989. **Frequency:** Quarterly.

★2494★ JOHN C. ROGERS MEDICAL MANAGEMENT ADVISORY
102 S. Maple Ave.
Ridgewood, NJ 07450   Phone: (201) 444-2144
Description: Contains tips and strategies for effective management of medical practices. Recurring features include a column titled Problem/Solution. **Frequency:** Quarterly.

★2495★ JOHNS HOPKINS CENTER FOR ALTERNATIVES TO ANIMAL TESTING—NEWSLETTER
Center for Alternatives to Animal Testing
Johns Hopkins School for Public Health
615 N. Wolfe St., Rm. 1604
Baltimore, MD 21205-2179   Phone: (410) 955-3343
Description: Covers Center research and activities. Recurring features include interviews, reports of meetings, news of educational opportunities, and a calendar of events. **First Published:** 1981. **Frequency:** Bimonthly.

★2496★ THE JOHNS HOPKINS MEDICAL LETTER—HEALTH AFTER 50
Medletter Associates Inc.
5 Water Oak
PO Box 420179
Palm Coast, FL 32035
Description: Covers physical and medical health issues of interest to persons over fifty years old. Recurring features include a column titled Our Readers Ask. **Frequency:** Monthly. **ISSN:** 1042-1882.

★2497★ JOTTINGS
Gospel Association for the Blind, Inc.
PO Box 62
Delray Beach, FL 33447   Phone: (305) 499-8900
Description: Publishes articles, particularly of a religious inspirational nature, on blindness and blind people. Recurring features include announcements of upcoming events and individual testimonies. **First Published:** 1955. **Frequency:** Monthly.

★2498★ JOURNAL OF THE BERGEN COUNTY DENTAL SOCIETY NEWSLETTER
Bergen County Dental Society
1606 Main St.
River Edge, NJ 07661   Phone: (201) 487-1073
Description: Provides information on legislation regarding dental hygienists, dental product approval by the American Dental Association (ADA), and setting standards in the profession. Recurring features include a calendar of events and reports of meetings.

★2499★ JOURNAL OF COUNSELING AND DEVELOPMENT
American Association for Counseling and Development
5999 Stevenson Ave.
Alexandria, VA 22304   Phone: (703) 823-9800
Description: Publishes archival and current news of the Association. Reports on advances in research and in techniques or innovations. **Frequency:** Bimonthly. **ISSN:** 0748-9633.

★2500★ KAPLAN CENTER NEWS
Rita & Stanley H. Kaplan Cancer Center
New York University
Medical Center
550 1st Ave.
New York, NY 10016
Description: Informs about the Center's activities and accomplishments of cancer research. **Frequency:** Semiannual.

★2501★ KEEPING AWAKE
Sleep/Wake Disorders Canada
Box 223, Sta. S
Toronto, ON, Canada M5M 4L7   Phone: (416) 398-1627
Description: Reports on the latest developments in research, treatment, and methods of coping with sleep/wake disorders. Chronicles recent events in the national office and within the individual chapters of the Association, providing an essential communication link between members. Recurring features include letters to the editor and columns titled President's Message, Meeting Notices, Canadian Neurological Coalition Report, and Treasurer's Report. **First Published:** Fall 1985. **Frequency:** Quarterly.

★2502★ KEYNOTES
USA Section/International College of Dentists
51 Monroe St., Ste. 1501
Rockville, FL 20850   Phone: (301) 251-8861
Description: Contains news of the activities and projects of the organization, which provides networking and educational opportunities for professionals in the dental field. Recurring features include a calendar of events, reports of meetings, news of educational opportunities, and a column titled the History Corner. **First Published:** 1989. **Frequency:** Semiannually.

★2503★ KIDNEY '91
National Kidney Foundation, Inc.
30 E. 33rd St.
New York, NY 10016   Phone: (212) 889-2210
Description: Provides readers with information on the work of the Foundation in the areas of research, legislation, education, and community and patient service. Recurring features include news of research, news of members, a calendar of events, and columns titled President's Letter, Chairman's Message, Legislative Update, and Medical News Report. **First Published:** December 1976. **Frequency:** Quarterly.

★2504★ LAB REPORT
S. Raymond Gambino, M.D.
155 Federal St., 16th Fl.
Boston, MA 02110   Phone: (617) 338-8860
Description: Presents information on developments in laboratory medicine. Discusses which tests are best, and why. Identifies outdated and ineffective tests, and identifies important new tests. Includes the latest, most practical information relevant to laboratory medicine. Recurring features include a column titled Diagnostic Bulletins. **First Published:** November 1979. **Frequency:** Monthly. **ISSN:** 1045-7313.

★2505★ LABOR OCCUPATIONAL HEALTH PROGRAM—MONITOR
Labor Occupational Health Program
University of California, Berkeley
2515 Channing Way
Berkeley, CA 94720   Phone: (510) 642-5507
Description: Discusses occupational health and safety from a trade union standpoint. Analyzes health hazards and relevant legal and legislative issues. Recurring features include columns titled Newswire, Clearinghouse (book and audiovisual reviews), Datebook, Around LOHP, and Women Working (women and occupational health). **First Published:** October 1974. **Frequency:** 4/yr.

★2506★ THE LANTERN
Perkins School for the Blind
175 N. Beacon St.
Watertown, MA 02172   Phone: (617) 924-3434
Description: Explores the School's programs and educational philosophy. Features articles on students, clients, and employees. Includes interviews, a calendar of events, and a column titled Message from the Director. **First Published:** 1933. **Frequency:** 2/yr. **ISSN:** 0023-8414.

★2507★ THE LATER YEARS
Dunn & Hargitt Investment Management
PO Box 1100
Lafayette, IN 47906   Phone: (317) 423-2624
Description: Provides information and advice to people responsible for the care of aging adults. Recurring features include news of research, interviews, and book reviews. **First Published:** May 1987. **Frequency:** Monthly. **ISSN:** 0892-6921.

★2508★ LAUGHTER WORKS—THE NEWSLETTER
Laughter Works
222 Selby Ranch Rd., No. 4
Sacramento, CA 95864-5832   Phone: (916) 484-7988
Description: Offers information on the application of humor and laughter in the business and health care fields. Recurring features include interviews, news of research, a calendar of events, reports of meetings, news of educational opportunities, and book reviews. **First Published:** 1987.

★2509★ THE LAWRENCE REVIEW OF NATURAL PRODUCTS
Facts and Comparisons
111 W. Port Plaza, Ste. 423
St. Louis, MO 63146-3098   Phone: (314) 878-2515
Description: Provides referenced information on the origins, uses, abuses, and toxicities of natural products. Discusses the chemical components and pharmacological uses of natural products. Examines natural products of social, economic, and medical importance. **First Published:** December 1980. **Frequency:** Monthly. **ISSN:** 0734-4961.

★2510★ LDA NEWSBRIEFS
Learning Disabilities Association of America
4156 Library Rd.
Pittsburgh, PA 15234   Phone: (412) 341-1515
Description: Concerned with the handicapped and children with learning disabilities. Discusses topics such as pertinent legislation, implications of the White House Conference on Handicapped Individuals, special education, summer camp programs, and media presentations. Recurring features include reports of the activities of local units, letters to the editor, a conference calendar, calls for papers, news of research, and book reviews. **First Published:** 1965. **Frequency:** Bimonthly. **ISSN:** 0739-909X.

★2511★ LDI HEALTH POLICY & RESEARCH QUARTERLY
Leonard David Institute of Health Economics
University of Pennsylvania
3641 Locust Walk
Philadelphia, PA 19104-6218   Phone: (215) 898-4750
Description: Reports on the study and teaching of medical, social, and economic issues that influence the organization, financing, management, and delivery of health care in the U.S. and worldwide. Recurring features include interviews, news of research affecting major health policy, a calendar of events, news of educational opportunities, and notices of publications available. **First Published:** Spring 1991. **Frequency:** Quarterly.

★2512★ THE LEAFLET
National Organization for the Reform of Marijuana Laws
1636 R St. NW, 3rd Fl.
Washington, DC 20009   Phone: (202) 483-5500
Description: Reports on the legal, health, industrial, and social aspects of marijuana use. Provides updates of legislative activities, the activities of NORML, and analyses of government studies and reports on the use and production of marijuana. Recurring features include news of research, a calendar of events, and notices of conferences. **First Published:** 1971. **Frequency:** Quarterly.

★2513★ THE LEAFLET
National Sudden Infant Death Syndrome Foundation, Inc.
10500 Little Patuxent Parkway. Ste. 420
Columbia, MD 21044   Phone: (301) 964-8000
Description: Promotes wider understanding of and research into sudden infant death syndrome. Reports on research advances and on activities of the Foundation and its chapters. **First Published:** October 1976. **Frequency:** 4/yr.

★2514★ LEPIDOPTERA RESEARCH FOUNDATION—NEWSLETTER
Lepidoptera Research Foundation
9620 Heather Rd.
Beverly Hills, CA 90210   Phone: (213) 274-1052
Description: Functions as a supplement to the technical publication The Journal of Research on the Lepidoptera. Reports on the Foundation's activities and carries calls for papers, notices of publications available, job listings, and announcements. **First Published:** 1981. **Frequency:** Semiannually.

★2515★ LET'S FACE IT—RESOURCES NEWSLETTER
Let's Face It
PO Box 711
Concord, MA 01742   Phone: (508) 371-3186
Description: Links people with facial disfigurement, their family, friends, and professionals with resources for recovery. **First Published:** Fall 1987. **Frequency:** 2/yr.

★2516★ LET'S TALK
Anamilo Club of Detroit
110 E. Warren
Detroit, MI 48201   Phone: (313) 833-0710
Description: Contains news of interest for the membership of the Club, which is devoted to teaching people who have undergone surgery for removal of the larynx to speak again. Recurring features include news of members, news of research, and a calendar of events. **Frequency:** Quarterly.

★2517★ LEUKEMIA SOCIETY OF AMERICA NEWSLINE
Leukemia Society of America, Inc.
733 Third Ave.
New York, NY 10017   Phone: (212) 573-8484
Description: Publicizes activities of the Society, including fundraising and Society-supported research. Provides information about advances in the research into leukemia and other related diseases. Profiles celebrities who aid the Society and other volunteers. Recurring features include news of research, news of members, book reviews, and columns titled President's Corner, Grantee Spotlight, and Volunteer Profiles. **First Published:** August 1983. **Frequency:** Quarterly.

★2518★ LEX VITAE
American United for Life
343 S. Dearborn, Ste. 1804
Chicago, IL 60604   Phone: (312) 263-5029
Description: Discusses legislation and current court cases involving abortion, euthanasia, infanticide, in vitro fertilization, and genetic engineering. **First Published:** 1977. **Frequency:** Quarterly.

★2519★ LEXINGTON/BLUEGRASS ALZHEIMER'S ASSOCIATION—NEWSLETTER
801 S. Limestone, Ste. E
Lexington, KY 40508   Phone: (606) 252-6282
Description: Discusses Alzheimer's Disease: the nature of the disease, research into cause and treatment, stress on the patient and his/her family, behavior problems, financial problems, and community resources for persons suffering from the disease. Recurring features include in-depth examinations of some aspect of the disease, news from support groups, a list of contributions to the Center, a calendar of events, and suggestions for caring for patients with Alzheimer's Disease. **First Published:** October 1982. **Frequency:** Quarterly.

★2520★ LFL REPORTS: THE NEWSLETTER OF LIBERTARIANS FOR LIFE
Libertarians for Life
13424 Hathaway Dr.
Wheaton, MD 20906   Phone: (301) 460-4141
Description: Concerned with the libertarian and pro-life movements, particularly the principles and policies of the group, who contend that "dependent children, born and unborn, have the right to be provided for and protected by their parents." Recurring features include the column titled From Doris, written by the national coordinator. **First Published:** August 1981. **Frequency:** Occasional. **ISSN:** 0882-116X.

★2521★ LIFE & BREATH
Saskatchewan Lung Association
1231-8th St. E.
Saskatoon, SK, Canada S7H 0S5   Phone: (306) 343-9511
Description: Provides updates on respiratory health and activities and Association activities. **First Published:** December 1919. **Frequency:** 4/yr.

★2522★ LIFE-GUARDIAN
Birthright International
PO Box 98361
Atlanta, GA 30359-2061   Phone: (404) 451-2273
Description: Provides information on programs operated by group members of the organization to help pregnant women find alternatives to abortion. Discusses issues involved with childbirth and parenting and offers assistance to groups wishing to form Birthright chapters. Recurring features include reports from chapters and group members. **First Published:** Autumn 1971. **Frequency:** Bimonthly.

★2523★ LIFE-LIFE
National Hydrocephalus Foundation
400 N. Michigan Ave., Ste. 1102
Chicago, IL 60611-4102   Phone: (312) 645-0701
Description: Serves as an information and support network for persons with hydrocephalus and their families. Covers medical developments and programs and services for patients with the condition. Recurring features include letters to the editor, notices of publications available, Foundation and member news, and a calendar of events. **First Published:** 1985. **Frequency:** 4/yr.

★2524★ LIFEDATE
Lutherans for Life
PO Box 819
Benton, AR 72015   Phone: (501) 794-2212
Description: Devoted to "guarding and upholding the dignity and worth of all human life." Concerned about the care of children, unwed mothers, handicapped persons, the poor, and the repressed, but focuses special attention on the lives of preborn and newborn children. Covers issues such as abortion, adoption, euthanasia, infanticide, church policies and policymaking, and counseling and research related to these issues. Recurring features include legislative updates, news briefs, fiction, book reviews, organization news, and inspirational items. **First Published:** 1981. **Frequency:** Quarterly.

★2525★ LIFELETTER
Ad Hoc Committee in Defense of Life
1187 National Press Bldg.
Washington, DC 20045   Phone: (202) 347-8686
Description: Disseminates information opposing abortion and euthanasia and monitors lobbying efforts for legislation against abortion and euthanasia. Seeks to have the Roe vs. Wade decision of 1973 repealed. **Frequency:** 12/yr.

★2526★ LIFELINE
Children's Liver Foundation
14245 Ventura Blvd., Ste. 201
Sherman Oaks, CA 91423   Phone: (818) 906-3021
Description: Designed to educate the public and health care professionals about liver disease in children. Reviews research projects on the prevention and cure of pediatric liver disease and its complications. Seeks to provide support for parents of afflicted children. **Frequency:** Quarterly.

★2527★ LIFELINE
Cooley's Anemia Foundation, Inc.
105 E. 22nd St., Ste. 911
New York, NY 10010   Phone: (212) 598-0911
Description: Provides a forum for the dissemination of information on Cooley's Anemia. Includes pertinent medical and legislative updates, as well as Foundation news on the local chapter and national level. Recurring features include Foundation events, editorials, news of research, news of members, a calendar of events, and columns titled President's Message, Legislative Update, and Chapter News From Across the Country. **First Published:** 1954. **Frequency:** Quarterly.

★2528★ LIFELINE
National Chronic Pain Outreach Association
7979 Old Georgetown Rd., Ste. 100
Bethesda, MD 20814-2429   Phone: (301) 652-4948
Description: Contains features, book reviews, and personal profiles on topics relating to chronic pain and its management. **First Published:** 1985. **Frequency:** Quarterly. **ISSN:** 1043-0776.

★2529★ LIFELINELETTER
Oley Foundation for Home Parenteral & Enteral Nutrition
Albany Medical Center
214 Hun Memorial, A-23
Albany, NY 12208   Phone: (518) 445-5079
Description: Explains the home use of specialized nutritional therapies: tube enteral nutrition, for those who cannot eat but have a functioning intestinal tract; and parenteral nutrition, for those who cannot absorb nutrients into their systems because of a damaged or removed intestinal tract. Fosters patient-to-patient communication for those on this specialized nutritional support therapy at home. Recurring features include guest articles by clinicians and patients, news of research, insurance and government policy information, letters to the editor, and columns titled Lifeline Profile and Kidstuff. **First Published:** July 1980. **Frequency:** Bimonthly.

★2530★ LINUS PAULING INSTITUTE OF SCIENCE AND MEDICINE—NEWSLETTER
Linus Pauling Institute of Science and Medicine
440 Page Mill Rd.
Palo Alto, CA 94306   Phone: (415) 327-4064
Description: Publishes news of the Institute and its research in the prevention and treatment of degenerative diseases, with particular emphasis on the relationship between cancer and diet. Focuses on research into the origin of cancer, identification of cancer-causing genes, herpes viruses, and changes involved in aging. Recurring features include profiles of

Institue personnel and visitors, news of research, book reviews, and obituaries. **First Published:** 1976. **Frequency:** Periodic.

★2531★ **THE LISTENER**
HEAR Center
301 E. Del Mar Blvd.
Pasadena, CA 91101   Phone: (818) 796-2016
Description: Informs readers of the activities of the HEAR Center, which employs the auditory-verbal approach to help those with communication problems due to hearing loss. Provides information on the latest technology, philosophies of treatment, and legislation that could affect the speech and hearing impaired. Recurring features include news of research, news of members, and a calendar of events. **First Published:** 1956. **Frequency:** Bimonthly.

★2532★ **LOCAL HEALTH OFFICERS NEWS**
U.S. Conference of Local Health Officers
1620 Eye St. NW
Washington, DC 20006   Phone: (202) 293-7330
Description: Contains news of city, county, and district health departments across the nation; organization activities; and pertinent legislative and governmental actions. Recurring features include notices of new publications and reports and of job opportunities for local health officers. **First Published:** 1963. **Frequency:** 6/yr.

★2533★ **LONG CANE NEWS**
American Foundation for the Blind
15 E. 16th St.
New York, NY 10011   Phone: (212) 620-2000
Description: Features news from training programs, conferences, research projects, and workshops in universities, clinics, schools, and professional association programs that assist blind and visually impaired individuals. Recurring features include letters to the editor, news of research, a calendar of events, reports of meetings, and job listings. **First Published:** March 1982. **Frequency:** Semiannually. **ISSN:** 0899-644X.

★2534★ **LONG TERM CARE MANAGEMENT**
Faulkner & Gray, Inc.
1133 15th St. NW
Washington, DC 20005   Phone: (202) 828-4148
Description: Contains news of governmental and private actions affecting the long term care field. Covers the entire spectrum of non-acute care institutions: nursing homes, hospices, home health, rehabilitative and long term psychiatric, life care, and extended care units. Also discusses management trends and techniques. Recurring features include news of research, book reviews, a calendar of events, industry financial information, and columns titled Data Processing, Personnel, Patient Care, Marketing, Legal, Revenue Sources, State News, Research, Technology, and Gerontology. **Frequency:** Semimonthly. **ISSN:** 0743-1422.

★2535★ **LOOKING FORWARD**
The Hope Heart Institute
350 E. Michigan Ave., Ste. 301
Kalamazoo, MI 49007-3851   Phone: (616) 343-0770
Description: Offers health tips for persons over age 50. Emphasizes preventive measures and discusses health issues such as nutrition, weight loss, exercise, self-care, medical care, safe driving, stress management, and family and lifestyle issues. **First Published:** 1988. **Frequency:** Quarterly. **ISSN:** 0896-7032.

★2536★ **LOOSE CONNECTIONS**
Ehlers-Danlos National Foundation
PO Box 1212
Southgate, MI 48195   Phone: (313) 282-0180
Description: Provides updated information about Ehlers-Danlos Syndrome (EDS), a hereditary connective tissue disorder. Recurring features include Personal stories, letters to the editor, interviews, news of research, reports of meetings, and notices of publications available. **First Published:** 1986. **Frequency:** Quarterly.

★2537★ **LOS ANGELES COLLEGE OF CHIROPRACTIC— NEWS AND ALUMNI REPORT**
Los Angeles College of Chiropractic
16200 E. Amber Valley Dr.
PO Box 1166
Whittier, CA 90609   Phone: (213) 947-8755
Description: Covers chiropractic and other forms of physical medicine. **First Published:** 1933. **Frequency:** 4/yr.

★2538★ **LPNABC NEWSLETTER**
The Licenced Practical Nurses Association of British Columbia
448 Watfield Ave.
Nanaimo, BC, Canada V9R 3P7
Description: Contains minutes of executive meetings, chapter reports, and news of events. **First Published:** 1965. **Frequency:** 3/yr.

★2539★ **LTC SOURCE UPDATE**
The Bennett Group
PO Box 7
Middlebury, VT 05673   Phone: (802) 388-9888
Description: Provides news of nursing home and other long-term care providers. Recurring features include news of research, a calendar of events, reports of meetings, news of educational opportunities, and book reviews. **First Published:** May 1990. **Frequency:** Bimonthly.

★2540★ **LUMINA**
Epilepsy Canada
1470 Peel St., Ste. 745
Montreal, PQ, Canada H3A 1T1   Phone: (514) 845-7855
Description: Allows for the exchange of information among member chapters. Offers articles on advances in epilepsy research, and follows the Epilepsy Canada's programs and activities on behalf of those with epilepsy. Recurring features include interviews, reports of meetings, and a calendar of events. **First Published:** March 1983. **Frequency:** Semiannually. **ISSN:** 1181-8212.

★2541★ **LUNG LINE LETTER**
National Jewish Center for Immunology and Respiratory Medicine
1400 Jackson St.
Denver, CO 80206   Phone: (303) 398-1080
Description: Covers issues discussed by the Center's registered nurses. Recurring features include news of research. **First Published:** Spring 1986. **Frequency:** Quarterly.

★2542★ **LUPUS NEWS**
Lupus Foundation of America
111 Pleasant St., No. 27
Watertown, MA 02172   Phone: (617) 924-3034
Description: Covers the diagnosis, treatment, and research of lupus erythematosus. Reports on the Lupus Foundation of America, Inc., its chapter news, and educational programs. Recurring features include statistics, book reviews, and columns titled Ask the Attorney, Ask the Doctor, and Letters to the Editor. **First Published:** Summer 1979. **Frequency:** Quarterly.

★2543★ **LUPUS TODAY**
The American Lupus Society
3914 Del Amo Blvd., Ste. 922
Torrance, CA 90503   Phone: (213) 542-8891
Description: Reports on current research both directly and indirectly related to the disease Lupus Erythematosus. Carries profiles of eminent lupus researchers, lupus patients, and individuals involved in lupus organizations. Contains announcements of Society meetings and programs. **First Published:** 1978. **Frequency:** Quarterly. **ISSN:** 0277-1748.

★2544★ **THE MA REPORT**
National Allergy and Asthma Network
3554 Chain Bridge Rd., Ste. 200
Fairfax, VA 22030   Phone: (703) 385-4403
Description: Presents educational, medical, and resource information on asthma and allergies. Recurring features include news of research, a calendar of events, news of educational opportunities, and notices of publications available. **First Published:** 1985.

★2545★ **THE MAC MAINLINE**
University of Michigan Multipurpose Arthritis and Musculoskeletal Diseases Center
3918 Taubman Center, Box 0358
Ann Arbor, MI 48109-0358   Phone: (313) 936-5562
Description: Provides information on workshops, conferences, and meetings dealing with arthritis, musculoskeletal diseases, internal medicine, and rheumatology. Recurring features include news of research, a calendar of events, reports of meetings, news of educational opportunities, and notices of publications available.

★2546★ MANITOBA LEAGUE OF THE PHYSICALLY HANDICAPPED—UPDATE
Manitoba League of the Physically Handicapped
294 Portage Ave., Ste. 200
Winnipeg, MB, Canada R3C 0B9   Phone: (204) 943-6099
Description: Reports on League activities, issues, and priorities. Provides a forum for events and other concerns of the disabled. **First Published:** 1976. **Frequency:** Quarterly.

★2547★ THE MARKER
Huntington's Disease Society of America, Inc.
140 W. 22nd St., 6th Fl.
New York, NY 10011-2420   Phone: (212) 242-1968
Description: Reports on research findings, legislative developments, patient care issues, and other matters relevant to Huntington's Disease. Recurring features include announcements of workshops and meetings, chapter activities, new publications issued, and other Society news. **First Published:** 1983. **Frequency:** 3/yr.

★2548★ MARKETING HEALTH CLASSES
LERN
1550 Hayes Dr.
Manhattan, KS 66502   Phone: (913) 539-5376
Description: Covers marketing, program and staff development, and management for health education programs. **First Published:** 1989. **Frequency:** Monthly.

★2549★ MAYO CLINIC HEALTH LETTER
Mayo Foundation for Medical Education and Research
200 First St. NW
Rochester, MN 55905   Phone: (507) 284-4587
Description: Discusses health-related issues such as diet and nutrition, advances in drugs, the benefits and risks of specific physical exercises, and medical ethics. Recurring features include in-depth medical essays. **First Published:** September 1983. **Frequency:** Monthly. **ISSN:** 0741-6245.

★2550★ MCGRAW-HILL'S BIOTECHNOLOGY NEWSWATCH
McGraw-Hill, Inc.
1221 Ave. of the Americas, 36th Fl.
New York, NY 10020   Phone: (212) 512-6751
Description: Features news of scientific, financial, commercial, and governmental developments in the biotechnology field. Covers genetic engineering, hybridoma technology, applied plant genetics, enzymology, and biomass conversion. Lists current literature, meetings, symposia, and courses. Recurring features include news of research, book reviews, a calendar of events, and columns titled Biobusiness, State of the Art, WordWatch, Five-Year Update, and European Patent Disclosures. **First Published:** September 1981. **Frequency:** Semimonthly. **ISSN:** 0275-3685.

★2551★ MDR WATCH
Washington Business Information, Inc.
1117 N. 19th St.
Arlington, VA 22209-1798   Phone: (703) 247-3424
Description: Monitors compliance with the Food and Drug Administration's medical device reporting (MDR) regulation. Provides charts of MDRs filed each month, listed under the following categories: manufacturer and product; company; product; top ten firms filing the most reports; and top ten products for which most reports were filed. Also includes an index of reported deaths by product. Recurring features include industry briefs and legislative updates. **First Published:** 1986. **Frequency:** Monthly. **ISSN:** 0890-7587.

★2552★ MDS NEWS
Massachusetts Dental Society
83 Speen St.
Natick, MA 01760-4125   Phone: (508) 651-7511
Description: Provides news on the Society's activities and articles on the dental profession. Recurring features include letters to the editor, reports of meetings, news of educational opportunities, job listings, and notices of publications available. **First Published:** 1963. **Frequency:** 6/yr. **ISSN:** 0738-4556.

★2553★ MED TECH MARKET LETTER
M. Daniel Tatkon
PO Box 581
Sheffield, MA 01257-6607   Phone: (413) 229-6607
Description: Offers investment analysis of medical high technology. **First Published:** January 1, 1983. **Frequency:** Biweekly. **ISSN:** 0730-6640.

★2554★ MED-COM
St. Patrick Hospital
500 W. Broadway
PO Box 4587
Missoula, MT 59806   Phone: (406) 543-7271

★2555★ MEDICAID FRAUD REPORT
National Association of Attorneys General
444 N. Capitol St., Ste. 403
Washington, DC 20001   Phone: (202) 628-0445
Description: "Focuses on state prosecution of Medicaid provider fraud." Covers legal cases involving hospitals, nursing homes, physicians, dentists, pharmacies, laboratories, and others who are eligible for reimbursement under the Medicaid program. Recurring features include columns titled State Activities and Legislation. **First Published:** June 1981. **Frequency:** 10/yr.

★2556★ MEDICAL ABSTRACTS NEWSLETTER
Communi-T Publications
PO Box 2170
Teaneck, NJ 07666   Phone: (201) 836-5030
Description: Publishes "easy-to-understand" abstracts with bibliographic citations of medical research articles selected from over 150 medical journals. Categorizes summaries under the headings: General Medicine, Heart Disease, Cancer, Pediatrics, Obstetrics-Gynecology, Sexual Medicine, Psychiatry, Sports Medicine, and Aging. **First Published:** June 1981. **Frequency:** Monthly. **ISSN:** 0730-7810.

★2557★ MEDICAL DEVICES, DIAGNOSTICS & INSTRUMENTATION REPORTS-THE GRAY SHEET
F-D-C Reports, Inc.
5550 Friendship Blvd., Ste. 1
Chevy Chase, MD 20815   Phone: (301) 657-9830
Description: Covers the medical device and diagnostics field, including FDA regulations; policies and congressional reform initiatives concerning pre-market approvals and 501(k) exemptions; new products; business start-ups and financial deals; international developments; and technology reimbursement. Recurring features include columns titled In Brief, Financings In Brief, Device Approvals, Recalls & FDA Seizures, and MDDI Stock Index. **First Published:** 1975. **Frequency:** Weekly.

★2558★ MEDICAL DEVICES BULLETIN
Center for Devices and Radiological Health
Food and Drug Administration (HFZ-30)
5600 Fishers Ln.
Rockville, MD 20857   Phone: (301) 443-5807
Description: Communicates semi-technical information on the Agency's medical devices programs to a primarily professional audience. Recurring features include a calendar of events, notices of publications available, and news of meetings. **First Published:** August 1983. **Frequency:** Monthly.

★2559★ MEDICAL ETHICS ADVISOR
American Health Consultants, Inc.
67 Peachtree Park Dr. NE, Ste. 220
Atlanta, GA 30309   Phone: (404) 351-4523
Description: Examines real-life ethical dilemmas in health care institutions such as hospitals and nursing homes. Provides comments from experts on how to approach the ethical, legal, and financial aspects of cases involving organ transplants, patient competency, terminating life support, Baby Doe and Granny Doe, and more. Recurring features include news of research, letters to the editor, book reviews, a calendar of events, and columns titled Reader Questions, Legal Questions, and Health View. **First Published:** February 1985. **Frequency:** Monthly.

★2560★ MEDICAL GROUP MANAGEMENT ASSOCIATION—WASHINGTON REPORT
Medical Group Management Association
104 Inverness Terrace E.
Englewood, CO 80112-5306   Phone: (303) 799-1111
Description: Covers current legislation and regulation concerning the health care industry. **First Published:** March 1983. **Frequency:** Monthly. **ISSN:** 0741-4293.

★2561★ THE MEDICAL HUMANIST
Department of Medical Education
University of Illinois at Chicago
Medical Education, M/C 591, Box 6998, 986 CME
Chicago, IL 60680   Phone: (312) 996-3590
Description: Provides a forum for essays on human values in the health-science industry. Promotes programs, activities, and events in the medical humanities and bioethic community. Recurring features include a calendar of events, reports of meetings, news of educational opportunities, book reviews, case commentaries, and opinions. **First Published:** January 1991. **Frequency:** 2/yr.

★2562★ MEDICAL INTELLIGENCE
Edward Rosenfeld
PO Box 20008
New York, NY 10025-1510   Phone: (212) 222-1123
Description: Covers developments in advanced medical technology, with emphasis on computers in medicine and medical applications of neural networks. **First Published:** January 1990. **Frequency:** Monthly.

★2563★ THE MEDICAL LETTER
1000 Main St.
New Rochelle, NY 10801   Phone: (914) 235-0500
Description: Appraises new drugs in terms of their effectiveness, toxicity, side effects, and possible alternative medications. Reviews other developments in medicine, including nondrug therapy and new diagnostic aids. **First Published:** January 23, 1959. **Frequency:** Biweekly. **ISSN:** 0025-732X.

★2564★ MEDICAL LETTER ON DRUGS AND THERAPEUTICS
Medical Letter, Inc.
1000 Main St.
New Rochelle, NY 10801   Phone: (914) 235-0500
Description: Contains information on the effectiveness of various drug treatments. **First Published:** 1959. **Frequency:** Biweekly. **ISSN:** 0025-732X.

★2565★ MEDICAL LIABILITY ADVISORY SERVICE
Business Publishers, Inc.
951 Pershing Dr.
Silver Spring, MD 20910-4464   Phone: (301) 587-6300
Description: Concerned with malpractice lawsuits involving health care providers, reporting pertinent legal decisions and legislation across the nation. Covers malpractice-related activities of insurance companies, medical societies, law associations, and government committees. Recurring features include a list of resource materials on malpractice and medical ethics. **First Published:** 1975. **Frequency:** Monthly. **ISSN:** 0199-1272.

★2566★ MEDICAL LIABILITY MONITOR
Carol Brierly
PO Box 36
Glencoe, IL 60022   Phone: (708) 446-3100

★2567★ MEDICAL MALPRACTICE LAW & STRATEGY
Leader Publications
New York Law Publishing Co.
111 8th Ave.
New York, NY 10011   Phone: (212) 714-8300
Description: Reports on legal developments, practice and strategy, verdicts, and settlements in the area of medical malpractice. **First Published:** November 1983. **Frequency:** Monthly. **ISSN:** 0747-8925.

★2568★ MEDICAL MALPRACTICE: VERDICTS,
  SETTLEMENTS & EXPERTS
M. Lee Smith, Publishers & Printers
Box 2678, Arcade Sta.
Nashville, TN 37219   Phone: (615) 242-7395
Description: Follows current cases and "important new rulings in state and federal courts," with docket numbers and counsel named for 200 cases in each issue. Also lists the names of experts testifying for both the plaintiff and the defense. Categorizes summaries by topic, e.g., cardiology, emergency medicine, and psychiatry. **First Published:** June 1985. **Frequency:** Monthly.

★2569★ MEDICAL MALPRACTICE-OB/GYN LITIGATION
REPORTER
Andrews Publications
PO Box 1000
Westtown, PA 19395   Phone: (215) 399-6600
Description: Presents summations as well as reprints of the complete texts of key decisions and pleadings in the area of medical malpractice, obstetrical- and gynecological-related litigation affecting physicians, surgeons, hospitals, and their insurers. Reports on such areas as surgical complications, birth injuries, resuscitation policies, errors in diagnosis, and misapplication of drugs, with particular emphasis on disputes involving standard of care and patient consent to medical procedures. **First Published:** April 1985. **Frequency:** Monthly. **ISSN:** 0882-8555.

★2570★ MEDICAL MISSION NEWS
Catholic Medical Mission Board
10 W. 17th St.
New York, NY 10011-5765   Phone: (212) 242-7757
Description: Publishes news of the Board and its work in assisting Catholic medical institutions in different areas of the world in giving care to the destitute sick. Recurring features include news of personnel placement and shipments of medicines, instruments, and supplies to various countries. **First Published:** 1931. **Frequency:** Quarterly.

★2571★ THE MEDICAL-MORAL NEWSLETTER
Ayd Medical Communications
1130 E. Cold Spring Lane
Baltimore, MD 21239   Phone: (301) 433-9220
Description: Provides in-depth coverage of timely topics in medical ethics. Discusses issues such as genetic experimentation, sex therapy, euthanasia, drug dependence, population control, organ transplants, and abortion. Recurring features include editorials and news of research. **First Published:** September 1964. **Frequency:** Monthly except July and August. **ISSN:** 0002-7397.

★2572★ MEDICAL REFORM
Medical Reform Group of Ontario
PO Box 366, Sta. J
Toronto, ON, Canada M4J 4Y8   Phone: (416) 588-9167
Description: Addresses issues pertaining to the reform of the health care system in Canada, including govermental policy and social conditions. Recurring features include reports of meetings, job listings, and book reviews. **First Published:** 1979. **Frequency:** 6/yr.

★2573★ MEDICAL REHABILITATION REVIEW
National Association of Rehabilitation Facilities
PO Box 17675
Washington, DC 20041   Phone: (703) 556-8848
Description: Monitors developments in the medical rehabilitation industry. Carries news of research, editorials, news of members, and a calendar of events. **Frequency:** Weekly.

★2574★ MEDICAL RESEARCH FUNDING BULLETIN
Science Support Center
PO Box 7507, FDR Sta.
New York, NY 10150   Phone: (212) 371-3398
Description: Provides information on grants and contracts available from government and private sources. Recurring features include a calendar of events, news of research, book reviews, and notices of publications available. **First Published:** 1973. **Frequency:** 36/yr.

★2575★ MEDICAL SCIENCES BULLETIN
Pharmaceutical Information Associates, Ltd.
2761 Trenton Rd.
Levittown, PA 19056   Phone: (215) 949-0490
Description: Reports on new drugs, their medical uses, and approvals and recommendations of the Food and Drug Administration (FDA). Discusses current medical research. **First Published:** September 1978. **Frequency:** Monthly. **ISSN:** 0199-4905.

★2576★ MEDICAL/SCIENTIFIC UPDATE
National Jewish Center for Immunology and Respiratory Medicine
1400 Jackson St.
Denver, CO 80206   Phone: (303) 398-1705
Description: Focuses on research and treatment of chronic respiratory diseases and immunological disorders such as asthma, allergies, COPD, ILD, sleep-related disorders, and autoimmune diseases. Carries research updates and reports on Center activities. **Frequency:** 10/yr.

★2577★   MEDICAL SOCIETY OF NOVA SCOTIA—INFORMED
Medical Society of Nova Scotia
5 Spectacle Lake Dr.
City of Lakes Business Parks
Dartmouth, NS, Canada B3B 1X7   Phone: (902) 468-1866
Description: Covers health-related issues in Nova Scotia, such as acquired
immunodeficiency syndrome (AIDS), poverty, nutrition, and health poli-
tics regarding The Royal Commission on Health Care. **First Published:**
April 11, 1986. **Frequency:** Bimonthly. **ISSN:** 1180-1840.

**★2578★   MEDICAL SOCIETY OF PRINCE EDWARD ISLAND—
    NEWSLETTER**
Medical Society of Prince Edward Island
559 North River Rd.
Charlottetown, PE, Canada C1E 1J7   Phone: (902) 368-7303
Description: Acts as an information tool for all members of the medical
profession in the province, including medical students, interns, and
residents. Topics of interest include anything affecting day-to-day practice,
including tariffs, continuing education, and reports of meetings, and
events. **Frequency:** Monthly.

★2579★   MEDICAL STAFF LEADER
American Hospital Publishing, Inc.
American Hospital Association
737 N. Michigan Ave., Ste. 700
Chicago, IL 60611   Phone: (312) 440-6800
Description: Devoted to specific and common concerns of medical staff
and hospital administration. Recurring features include articles on joint
ventures, ethics, legislation, malpractice, and medical by-laws. **First
Published:** 1971. **Frequency:** Monthly. **ISSN:** 1041-6510.

★2580★   MEDICAL TOYS AND BOOKS
Pediatric Projects, Inc.
PO Box 571555
Tarzana, CA 91357   Phone: (818) 705-3660
Description: Contains reviews of medically-oriented educational toys and
books that help infants, children, and adolescents understand and deal
with health care. **First Published:** January 1989. **Frequency:** Quarterly.
ISSN: 1040-7085.

★2581★   MEDICAL UPDATE
Medical Education and Research Foundation
Benjamin Franklin Literary & Medical Society
PO Box 567
Indianapolis, IN 46206   Phone: (317) 636-8881
Description: Publishes news of the Foundation and its concern with
"preventive medicine, safety procedures and techniques, health dangers
and proper dietary habits." Also "reports on current developments in areas
of medical research and explores the discovery of new medication and
treatment available today." Recurring features include tips for travelers.
First Published: July 1976. **Frequency:** Monthly.

★2582★   MEDICAL UTILIZATION REVIEW
Faulkner & Gray, Inc.
1133 15th St. NW
Washington, DC 20005   Phone: (202) 828-4148
Description: Monitors developments related to medical care utilization
review, both government and private. Includes coverage of congressional
action and that of federal agencies. Discusses Medicare and Medicaid
problems in relation to the Federal Peer Review Organization program.
First Published: 1973. **Frequency:** Semimonthly.

★2583★   MEDICAL WASTE NEWS
Business Publishers, Inc.
951 Pershing Dr.
Silver Spring, MD 20910   Phone: (301) 587-6300
Description: Covers regulation, legislation, and technology related to
medical waste. Reports on businesses involved in waste management and
Environmental Protection Agency (EPA) efforts to control waste levels.
First Published: 1989. **Frequency:** Biweekly. **ISSN:** 1048-4493.

★2584★   MEDICARE COMPLIANCE ALERT
United Communications Group
11300 Rockville Pike, Ste. 1100
Rockville, MD 20852-3030   Phone: (301) 816-8950
Description: Disseminates news and guidance for keeping health care
business arrangements within bounds of changing Medicare rules on
patient referrals, physician investments, limited partnerships, and other

joint ventures. Reports latest developments of "safe harbors" regulations,
legislation, and enforcement of civil money penalty laws. **Frequency:**
Semimonthly.

**★2585★   MEDICINE & BIOLOGY: AN ABSTRACT
    NEWSLETTER**
National Technical Information Service
U.S. Department of Commerce
5285 Port Royal Rd.
Springfield, VA 22161   Phone: (703) 487-4630
Description: Reports on public health and industrial medicine; biochemistry; clinical chemistry and medicine; pharmacology and pharmacological
chemistry; botany; and toxicology. Provides information on radiobiology,
electrophysiology, physiological psychology, and stress physiology. Covers
a wide range of other subjects related to medicine, biology, and allied
health sciences. **Frequency:** Weekly. **ISSN:** 0364-6432.

★2586★   MEDICINE & HEALTH REPORT
Faulkner & Gray, Inc.
1133 15th St. NW, Ste. 450
Washington, DC 20005   Phone: (202) 828-4148
Description: Discusses socioeconomic developments in Washington, D.C.,
that relate to health, medicine, hospitals, nursing, and dentistry. **First
Published:** 1947. **Frequency:** Weekly.

★2587★   MEDICOM DRUG INFORMATION NEWSLETTER
Professional Drug Systems, Inc.
530 Maryville Centre Dr., Ste. 250
St. Louis, MO 63141   Phone: (314) 275-8848
Description: Contains information on new drugs, drug information, and
drug interactions. **First Published:** 1983. **Frequency:** Bimonthly. **ISSN:**
0737-3139.

★2588★   MEETING GROUND
Courage Center
3915 Golden Valley Rd.
Golden Valley, MN 55422   Phone: (612) 520-0520
Description: Serves to establish communication between family members
and rehabilitation professionals who have an interest in the care of
children with disabilities. Recurring features include a calendar of events,
reports of meetings, news of educational opportunities, book reviews, and
articles by parents. **First Published:** 1972. **Frequency:** 4/yr. **ISSN:** 1047-
7993.

★2589★   THE MELANOMA LETTER
Skin Cancer Foundation
245 5th Ave., Ste. 2402
New York, NY 10016   Phone: (212) 725-5176
Description: Presents semi-technical articles on diagnoses and the latest
advance in the field of melanoma research and treatment. Includes
statistics, symptomatology, and psychological factors influencing treatment. Recurring features include editorials and news of research. **First
Published:** Fall 1982. **Frequency:** Quarterly.

★2590★   MEMBRANE & SEPARATION TECHNOLOGY NEWS
Business Communications Co., Inc.
25 Van Zant St.
Norwalk, CT 06855-1781   Phone: (203) 853-4266
Description: Examines the science, technology, and business opportunities
in microfiltration, reverse osmosis, ultrafiltration, cross filtration, electro-
dialysis, and specialty chromatography. Discusses commercial and energy
applications in pharmaceuticals, biotechnology, electronics, water, foods
and beverages, and pollution control. **First Published:** September 1982.
Frequency: Monthly. **ISSN:** 0720-8483.

★2591★   MEN IN NURSING
National Male Nurse Association
2309 State St., West Office
Saginaw, MI 48602   Phone: (517) 799-8208
Description: Provides information on nursing and health, particularly as it
affects male registered and licensed practical nurses. Recurring features
include book reviews, job opportunity notices, and letters to the editor.
First Published: March 1975. **Frequency:** Bimonthly.

★2592★ MENNONITE DISASTER SERVICE—NEWSLETTER
Mennonite Disaster Service
Mennonite Central Committee
21 S. 12th St.
PO Box 500
Akron, PA 17501   Phone: (717) 859-3889
Description: Reports news of the Service, and covers recent activities in volunteer disaster aid. Recurring features include notices of service opportunities and a calendar of events. **First Published:** 1971. **Frequency:** Quarterly.

★2593★ MEN'S HEALTH NEWSLETTER
Rodale Press, Inc.
33 E. Minor St.
Emmaus, PA 18049   Phone: (215) 967-5171
Description: Focuses on the physical and psychological health concerns of men. Discusses issues relevant to male health, exercise, appearance, sexuality, nutrition, and peak mental performance. Recurring features include columns titled Phil Dunphy on Men Fitness, Weird Men's Health, Men's Health Mail, and Ask Dr. Private Parts. **First Published:** July 1984. **Frequency:** Monthly. **ISSN:** 0747-8461.

★2594★ MENTAL HEALTH LAW NEWS
Interwood Publications
PO Box 20241
Cincinnati, OH 45220   Phone: (513) 221-3715
Description: Presents summaries of legal decisions in the field of mental health law. Monitors rulings in such areas as mental health malpractice, voluntary/involuntary commitment, patient rights, patient danger to the community, consent/appropriate treatment, and insanity defense. **First Published:** January 1986. **Frequency:** Monthly. **ISSN:** 0889-017X.

★2595★ MENTAL HEALTH LAW PROJECT ACTION LAW
Mental Health Law Project
1101 15th St. NW, No. 1212
Washington, DC 20005-5002   Phone: (202) 467-5730
Description: Reports on the advocacy and educational activities of the Project on behalf of people with mental disabilities. Covers programs in which the Project is active, including housing, disability benefits, children, elders, people of color, and rights in institutions. Provides notices of publications available.

★2596★ MENTAL HEALTH LAW REPORTER
Business Publishers, Inc.
951 Pershing Dr.
Silver Spring, MD 20910   Phone: (301) 587-6300
Description: Provides news and coverage of court cases pertaining to legal issues affecting mental health professionals. **First Published:** 1983. **Frequency:** Monthly. **ISSN:** 0741-5141.

★2597★ MENTAL HEALTH REPORT
Business Publishers, Inc.
951 Pershing Dr.
Silver Spring, MD 20910   Phone: (301) 587-6300
Description: Disseminates news pertaining to the activities of Congress, the courts, and federal agencies in the area of mental health. Publishes information on potential national health insurance plans, new laws and their ramifications, federal funding patterns, community mental health services and other social science programs, legislative and administrative trends on the state and local levels, and activities of national organizations concerned with mental health. **First Published:** February 1, 1977. **Frequency:** Biweekly. **ISSN:** 0191-6750.

★2598★ MENTAL HEALTH SPECIAL INTEREST SECTION—NEWSLETTER
Mental Health Special Interest Section
American Occupational Therapy Association
1383 Piccard Dr.
PO Box 1725
Rockville, MD 20850   Phone: (301) 948-9626
Description: Focuses on the clinical management of patients requiring mental health services. Publishes articles relevant to occupational therapy practice, including such topics as assessment protocols, treatment approaches, and program administration. **First Published:** Summer 1978. **Frequency:** Quarterly. **ISSN:** 0279-4136.

★2599★ THE MERIDIAN
Acupuncture Research Institute
313 W. Andrix St.
Monterey Park, CA 91754   Phone: (213) 722-7353
Description: Investigates aspects of acupuncture with a view to establishing its validity and application in the U.S. Emphasizes the integration of other healing methods with acupuncture, particularly homeopathy. Recurring features include news of research, book reviews, position and course announcements, and a section on homeopathic medicine. **First Published:** 1973. **Frequency:** 3/yr.

★2600★ THE MESSAGE LINE
American Brain Tumor Association
3725 N. Talman Ave.
Chicago, IL 60618   Phone: (312) 286-5571
Description: Provides information concerning research advances, services offered by the Association, feature articles, news of members, news of programs, and award recipients. **Frequency:** 3/yr.

★2601★ MHLP ACTION LINE
Mental Health Law Project
1101 15th St. NW, Ste. 1212
Washington, DC 20005   Phone: (202) 467-5730
Description: Describes activities of the Project, which tries to clarify, establish, and enforce the legal rights of mentally and developmentally disabled persons through test-case litigation, technical assistance to direct service advocates, and administrative and legislative policy advocacy at the federal and state level. Summarizes federal legislation, regulatory developments, and supreme court decisions. **First Published:** September 1989. **Frequency:** 5/yr.

★2602★ MICHIGAN ASSOCIATION OF SCHOOL NURSES—THE COMMUNICATOR
Michigan Association of School Nurses
4396 Underhill Dr.
Flint, MI 45506   Phone: (313) 736-8000
Description: Provides news of Association events and other information regarding school nursing. Includes news of conferences, reports of meetings, legislation news, notices of publications available, and president's and vice-president's columns. **Frequency:** 4-5/yr.

★2603★ MICHIGAN COMMUNITIES IN ACTION FOR DRUG-FREE YOUTH—NEWSLETTER
Michigan Communities in Action for Drug-Free Youth
925 E. Maple Rd., Ste. 103
Birmingham, MI 48009   Phone: (313) 642-6270
Description: Provides information on the organization, which has the goal of reaching Michigan families with a firm "No Drug Use" message through newsletters, conferences, regional director support, and formation of new groups. Advocates early intervention and good treatment and aftercare when children become drug dependent. Recurring features include a calendar of events, book reviews, notices of publications available, and columns titled Spotlight on Youth and From the Chairman.

★2604★ MICHIGAN DIABETES RESEARCH AND TRAINING CENTER—NEWSLETTER
Michigan Diabetes Research and Training Center
University of Michigan
1331 E. Ann St., Rm. 5111
Ann Arbor, MI 48109-0580   Phone: (313) 763-5256
Description: Provides information regarding the diabetes-related research, educational and clinical activities of University faculty and staff. Disseminates general diabetes information. Recurring features include news of research, a calendar of events, reports of meetings, news of educational opportunities, notices of publications available, and columns titled Research Highlights and Changes in Personnel. **First Published:** October 21, 1977. **Frequency:** Quarterly.

★2605★ MICHIGAN HANDICAPPED SPORTS & RECREATION ASSOCIATION—NEWSLETTER
Michigan Handicapped Sports & Recreation Association
238 Woodview Ct., Apt. 244
Rochester Hills, MI 48307-4191   Phone: (313) 853-0648
Description: Provides information concerning Association activities and events. Includes information on learn-to-ski clinics, beginner ski lessons, ski racing, camping, golfing, and other seasonal events. Discusses issues of concern to handicapped individuals, such as current legislation and services for disabled travellers. Features notices of publications available.

★2606★ MICHIGAN NURSE
Michigan Nurses Association
2310 Jolly Oak Rd.
Okemos, MI 48864   Phone: (517) 349-5640
Description: Publishes information of interest to nurses, including topics related to the profession, announcements of continuing education opportunities, and convention reports. Reports on Association programs, elections, and committee activities. **First Published:** September 1927. **Frequency:** 11/yr. **ISSN:** 0026-2366.

**★2607★ MILTON H. ERICKSON FOUNDATION—
NEWSLETTER**
Milton H. Erickson Foundation, Inc.
3606 N. 24th St.
Phoenix, AZ 85016   Phone: (602) 956-6196
Description: Promotes the work of the Foundation, which focuses on training physicians, dentists, psychologists, and masters' level mental health practitioners in techniques of hypnotherapy. Recurring features include editorials, news of research, a calendar of workshops, congresses, and training series, news of the Foundation and its members, and media and book reviews. **First Published:** Summer 1981. **Frequency:** 3/yr.

★2608★ MIND MATTERS
Florida Mental Health Institute
University of South Florida
13301 Bruce B. Downs Blvd.
Tampa, FL 33612-3899   Phone: (813) 974-4585
Description: Covers programs, events, research, and staff of the Institute. **First Published:** December 1988. **Frequency:** 2/yr.

★2609★ MIND SCIENCE FOUNDATION—NEWS
Mind Science Foundation
8301 Broadway, Ste. 100
San Antonio, TX 78209   Phone: (512) 821-6094
Description: Reflects the concerns of the Foundation, which is dedicated to "the study of the human mind using all scientific disciplines" and whose research specialists are from the fields of parapsychology, psychology, physics, and the neurosciences. Discusses specific topics such as "mind-made" health, creativity, self-esteem, ESP, and psychokinesis. Recurring features include updates on the Foundation's activities and news of research. **First Published:** 1977. **Frequency:** Quarterly.

★2610★ MINNESOTA NURSING ACCENT
Minnesota Nurses Association
1295 Bandana Blvd. N., No. 140
St. Paul, MN 55108   Phone: (612) 646-4807
Description: Focuses on news in the field of nursing. **First Published:** 1929. **Frequency:** 10/yr.

★2611★ MIRACLES IN PROGRESS
Rehabilitation Institute of Pittsburgh
6301 Northumberland St.
Pittsburgh, PA 15217   Phone: (412) 521-9000
Description: Publishes news of the Institute, which is "an accredited specialty hospital and rehabilitation center, a fully-licensed school, a training facility for professional and student rehabilitation specialists, and a research and development center for children and adults with severe disabilities." Promotes Institute programs for persons with injuries from accidents, brain damage, stroke, amputation, cerebral palsy, emotional disorders, learning disabilities, spina bifida, speech defects, and orthopedic and pain problems. Includes case histories. **First Published:** 1961. **Frequency:** Quarterly.

★2612★ MLA NEWS
Medical Library Association
6 N. Michigan Ave., No. 300
Chicago, IL 60602   Phone: (312) 419-9094
Description: Provides information about mission and planning activities of the Association, with news of health sciences libraries. Recurring features include articles on committee, chapter, and section programs; reports of continuing education and employment opportunities; and governmental relations, media, and international news. **First Published:** 1961. **Frequency:** Monthly, except June/July and November/December, which are combined issues. **ISSN:** 0541-5489.

★2613★ MNA ACCENT
Minnesota Nurses Association
1295 Bandana Blvd., No. 140
St. Paul, MN 55108   Phone: (612) 646-4807
Description: Provides news of developments and legal issues affecting the nursing field in Minnesota. Reports on arbitration, resolutions, and community activities involving nurses. Recurring features include interviews and reports of meetings. **First Published:** 1924. **Frequency:** 10/yr.

★2614★ MNABA NEWSLETTER
Minnesota Association for Behavior Analysis
1777 E. Oak St.
Brainerd, MN 56401   Phone: (218) 828-2317
Description: Publishes news of MNABA, its concerns, members, and activities. Recurring features include conference reports, a calendar of events, and job postings. **Frequency:** Ca. 4/yr.

★2615★ THE MOISTURE SEEKERS NEWSLETTER
Sjogren's Syndrome Foundation
382 Main St.
Port Washington, NY 11051   Phone: (516) 767-2866
Description: Educates patients and their families about Sjogren's Syndrome, a disorder marked by dryness of all mucous membranes resulting from deficient secretion of the glands. Allows patients to share information on coping with the syndrome and notifies them of opportunities to participate in clinical investigative programs. Recurring features include medical findings, reports of meetings conducted by the Foundation in which doctors speak on aspects of the disorder, and news of research. **First Published:** October 1984. **Frequency:** Monthly.

★2616★ MOMENTUM
Eastman Dental Center
625 Elmwood Ave.
Rochester, NY 14620   Phone: (716) 275-5064
Description: Contains news of interest to Center alumni. Recurring features include interviews, news of research, a calendar of events, and columns titled Kudos and Spreading the Word. **First Published:** 1974. **Frequency:** Quarterly.

★2617★ MOMENTUM
National Fitness Foundation
5150 E. Pacific Coast, Ste. 200
Long Beach, CA 90804   Phone: (213) 498-9570
Description: Furthers the Foundation's objective of increasing participation in exercise and sports activities by Americans of all ages. Monitors training programs conducted by the Foundation to train fitness and sports leaders to serve as fitness instructors for communities and industries. Recurring features include news of fitness research, articles on program development, and news of members. **Frequency:** Periodic.

★2618★ MONDAY MORNING REPORT
Alcohol Research Information Service
1106 E. Oakland Ave.
Lansing, MI 48906   Phone: (517) 485-9900
Description: Carries brief articles and news items on alcohol and other drug-related issues and problems. Covers such subjects as alcohol consumption among college students, drinking and driving, and alcohol in advertising and as a promotional tool. Reports on significant lawsuits and legislation. **First Published:** December 1976. **Frequency:** Semimonthly.

★2619★ THE MONDAY REPORT
Massachusetts Hospital Association
5 New England Executive Park
Burlington, MA 01915   Phone: (617) 272-8000
Description: Carries hospital-related news, quality of care concerns, finance and legal issues, research studies, policies, and seminar events. **First Published:** 1972. **Frequency:** Weekly.

★2620★ MRC RELAY
Multi Resource Centers, Inc.
1900 Chicago Ave.
Minneapolis, MN 55404   Phone: (612) 871-2402
Description: Carries information useful to members of the human services profession, community groups, business, and industry. Focuses on the programs, activities, and research of MRC, which provides service models in employment, training, vocational rehabilitation, mental health, and chemical dependency. **First Published:** September 1983. **Frequency:** Quarterly.

★2621★   MRI NEWSLETTER
Mental Research Institute
555 Middlefield Rd.
Palo Alto, CA 94301   Phone: (415) 321-3055
Description: Provides information on MRI research projects in the areas of human behavior, family therapy, communication, and child abuse and on problem resolution in corporate, educational, and political systems. Reports on workshops, conferences, and symposia sponsored by MRI or conducted by MRI Senior Research Fellows. Free reviews of books and articles published by the Institute and announcements of awards and grants. **First Published:** 1962. **Frequency:** Annually.

★2622★   MS CANADA
Multiple Sclerosis Society of Canada
250 Bloor St., E., Ste. 820
Toronto, ON, Canada M4W 3P9   Phone: (416) 922-6065
Description: Follows the activities and services of the Society and informs members of developments in multiple sclerosis research. Profiles noteworthy members, volunteers, and accomplishments by persons who have multiple sclerosis. Recurring features include interviews, book reviews and notices of publications available, reports of meetings, and chapter news. **First Published:** February 1974. **Frequency:** Quarterly. **ISSN:** 0315-1131.

★2623★   MUTUAL AID
EMS Management Institute
PO Box 102
Sterling, VA 22170   Phone: (703) 450-6097
Description: Covers a broad range of Emergency Medical Services (EMS) management issues, including planning, staffing, administering, and evaluating pre-hospital EMS systems. Supplies current information on federal initiatives, college programs, training for managers, and technical innovations. Recurring features include book reviews, news of research, and columns titled EMS Forum, The Professional Volunteer, Micro Bytes, and Job Mart. **First Published:** July 1981. **Frequency:** Bimonthly.

★2624★   NAACLS NEWS
National Accrediting Agency for Clinical Laboratory Sciences
8410 W. Bryn Mawr, Ste. 670
Chicago, IL 60631   Phone: (312) 714-8880
Description: Provides news of the activities of the Agency as well as issues related to laboratory scientists. **First Published:** June 1974. **Frequency:** 3/yr.

★2625★   NAACOG NEWSLETTER
NAACOG
409 12th St. SW
Washington, DC 20024-2191   Phone: (202) 638-0026
Description: Provides information on developments and activities regarding obstetrics, gynecology, and neonatal nursing. Includes news of Association events, education funding, a calendar of events, and columns titled From the President, Ask the Experts, Reliable Sources, Rx Facts, and Legislation Update. **First Published:** 1967. **Frequency:** Monthly. **ISSN:** 0889-0579.

★2626★   NAAFA NEWSLETTER
National Association to Advance Fat Acceptance, Inc.
PO Box 188620
Sacramento, CA 95818   Phone: (916) 443-0303
Description: Helps members fight discrimination on the basis of body weight in employment, education, medical care, insurance, social activities, media, public seating, and fashion. Carries commentary on the progress in the weight acceptance movement. Recurring features include research results, book reviews, items on Association activities, and a feature on lifestyles. **First Published:** October 1970. **Frequency:** Monthly.

★2627★   NABP NEWSLETTER
National Association of Boards of Pharmacy
1300 Higgins Rd., Ste. 103
Park Ridge, IL 60068   Phone: (708) 698-6227
Description: Reports on regulation and licensure in the pharmacy profession. Contains information on the NABP licensure exam, interstate reciprocity of licensure, court cases, and colleges of pharmacy. Provides news of the activities of the Association and other pharmacy associations. Recurring features include a column by the NABP's legal counsel, who examines legal problems confronting pharmacy regulatory boards. **First Published:** 1906. **Frequency:** 10/yr.

★2628★   NABR ALERT
National Association for Biomedical Research
818 Connecticut Ave. NW, Ste. 303
Washington, DC 20006   Phone: (202) 857-0540
Description: Provides news on legislative and regulatory issues concerning the use of laboratory animals in biomedical research, education, and testing. Follow-up information is provided in the Association's sister publication, NABR Update (see separate listing). **Frequency:** Periodic.

★2629★   NABR UPDATE
National Association for Biomedical Research
818 Connecticut Ave. NW, Ste. 303
Washington, DC 20006   Phone: (202) 857-0540
Description: Provides information on legislative and regulatory issues concerning the use of laboratory animals in biomedical research, testing, and education. Recurring features include news of members and items on the activities of organizations against animal research. **First Published:** November 1979. **Frequency:** Periodic.

★2630★   THE NACA NEWS
National Animal Control Association
PO Box 1600
Indianola, WA 98342   Phone: (206) 297-3293
Description: Focuses on the regulation and control of dogs, cats, and other domestic animals; municipal enforcement of animal complaints; and the humane aspects of animal control. Provides technical and assistance information to animal shelter professionals in both the humane and municipal sectors. Recurring features include columns titled Letter from the President and Training Opportunities. **First Published:** January 1979. **Frequency:** Bimonthly.

★2631★   NACDS LEGISLATIVE NEWSLETTER
National Association of Chain Drug Stores, Inc.
PO Box 1417-D49
Alexandria, VA 22313   Phone: (703) 549-3001
Description: Reports federal legislation affecting health care, prescription drugs, and retailing and business. Reviews recent regulations issued by the Drug Enforcement Administration, Department of Health and Human Services, and Occupational Safety and Health Administration. **Frequency:** Monthly.

★2632★   NADAP NEWS/REPORT
National Association on Drug Abuse Problems, Inc.
355 Lexington Ave.
New York, NY 10017   Phone: (212) 986-1170
Description: Promotes employment for recovered drug addicts and alcoholics; works to overcome stereotypes; and provides a transitional helping hand to those overcoming drug abuse problems. Offers a comprehensive approach to drug abuse prevention and intervention in the family, community, and workplace. Recurring features include announcements of conferences and awards, individual success stories, and a Company of the Month write-up. **First Published:** 1972. **Frequency:** Quarterly.

★2633★   NAFAC NEWS
National Association for Ambulatory Care
2333 Ponce de Leon Blvd., No. 511
Coral Gables, FL 33134-5418   Phone: (305) 441-2421
Description: Reports on issues current to the ambulatory care industry, including government activity, national developments, and trends in health care. Recurring features include editorials, news of research, letters to the editor, Association news, and stock watch column. **First Published:** August 1981. **Frequency:** Bimonthly.

★2634★   NAHC REPORT
National Association for Home Care
519 C St. NE
Washington, DC 20002   Phone: (202) 547-7424
Description: Reports on legislative, regulatory, judicial affairs, and research developments in the home care industry. **Frequency:** Weekly.

★2635★   NAMES NEWS
National Association of Medical Equipment Suppliers
625 Slaters Lane, Ste. 200
Alexandria, VA 22314   Phone: (703) 836-6263
Description: Informs members of developments in government agencies, state legislatures, and on Capitol Hill, as well as any other pertinent information that affects the medical equipment supply industry. **Frequency:** Monthly.

★2636★ NAOSMM NEWSLINE
National Association of Scientific Materials Managers
Grinnell College
Grinnell, IA 50112   Phone: (515) 269-3012
Description: Discusses "waste disposal, the relationship between exposure to chemicals and cancer, dealing with salespersons, the U.S. Occupational Safety and Health Administration (OSHA), and inventory control for stockrooms." Recurring features include Association news, an editorial, a president's message, and information on new members. **First Published:** June 1978. **Frequency:** Quarterly.

★2637★ NAPH NATIONAL NEWSLETTER
National Association of the Physically Handicapped, Inc.
124 Medina St.
Lodi, OH 44254-1106   Phone: (216) 948-2065
Description: Carries "news items about or of concern to the physically handicapped." Covers such subjects as legislation, employment, travel, and barrier-free architecture. Recurring features include items on local chapter events. **First Published:** 1958. **Frequency:** Quarterly. ISSN: 0741-1405.

★2638★ NAPM NEWS BULLETIN
National Association of Pharmaceutical Manufacturers
747 3rd Ave.
New York, NY 10017   Phone: (212) 838-3720
Description: Focuses on the regulatory, legal, and technical aspects of the generic pharmaceutical industry. Covers legislative developments and changes in government regulations. Recurring features include summaries of notices appearing in the Federal Register, notices of conferences and seminars, and news of members. **First Published:** 1960. **Frequency:** Monthly.

★2639★ NAPSAC NEWS
International Association of Parents and Professionals for Safe
   Alternatives in Childbirth
Rt. 1, Box 646
Marble Hill, MO 63764   Phone: (314) 238-2010
Description: Promotes the philosophy of natural childbirth and responsible patient self-determination and independence. Covers such topics as midwifery, home birth, breastfeeding, obstetrics, medical economics and politics, legal aspects of maternal and child health care, hospitals, and birth centers. Recurring features include book reviews, a calendar of events, editorials, news of research, letters from readers, statistics, and a column for parents. **First Published:** March 1976. **Frequency:** Quarterly. ISSN: 0192-1233.

★2640★ NAPT NEWSLETTER
National Association for Poetry Therapy
225 Williams St.
Huron, OH 44839-1688
Description: Discusses poetry and the arts in a variety of therapeutic capacities. Carries Association news and information (e.g., on certification training as a poetry therapist). Recurring features include book reviews and information on regional and national poetry therapy conferences, workshops, courses, and publications. **First Published:** August 1981. **Frequency:** 2/yr.

★2641★ NARAL NEWSLETTER
National Abortion Rights Action League
1101 14th St. NW
Washington, DC 20005   Phone: (202) 408-4600
Description: Monitors legislative news regarding the issue of abortion. Contains organizational news on various NARAL affiliates and covers action taken by NARAL to help keep abortion safe and legal. **First Published:** 1975. **Frequency:** Quarterly. ISSN: 0742-7506.

★2642★ NARD NEWSLETTER
National Association of Retail Druggists
205 Daingerfield Rd.
Alexandria, VA 22314   Phone: (703) 683-8200
Description: Reports on topics affecting independents, including developments within the pharmaceutical industry, regulatory and legislative activity, and pricing and import information. Recurring features include reports of meetings, news of educational opportunities, notices of publications available, and news of NARD activities and events. **Frequency:** Semimonthly, except January. ISSN: 0162-1602.

★2643★ NASNEWSLETTER
Health Information Publications, Inc.
92 S. Highland Ave.
Ossining, NY 10562   Phone: (914) 762-6498
Description: Covers recent activity regarding school nursing. **First Published:** 1985. **Frequency:** 5/yr. ISSN: 1047-4757.

★2644★ NAT-CENT NEWS
Helen Keller National Center for Deaf-Blind Youths and Adults
111 Middle Neck Rd.
Sands Point, NY 11050   Phone: (516) 944-8900
Description: Contains articles on legislation, services, aids and devices, and problems related to deaf-blindness. Covers Center activities. **Frequency:** 3/yr.

★2645★ NATIONAL ALOPECIA AREATA NEWSLETTER
National Alopecia Areata Foundation
714 C St., No. 216
San Rafael, CA 94901-3856   Phone: (415) 456-4644
Description: Provides information about Alopecia Areata. Presents articles about the medical, psychological, insurance information, and cosmetic aspects of the condition. Recurring features include news of research, news of members, a calendar of events, letters from patients on coping with Alopecia Areata, and columns titled Looking Good, Support Groups, and Penpal. **First Published:** 1981. **Frequency:** 5/yr.

★2646★ NATIONAL ASSOCIATION OF ADVISORS FOR THE
   HEALTH PROFESSIONS—ADVISOR
National Association of Advisors for the Health Professions, Inc.
College of Liberal Arts and Sciences
Arizona State University
Tempe, AZ 85287-1701   Phone: (602) 965-2365
Description: Intended for college and university faculty who advise undergraduate students on health careers. Focuses on manpower statistics, financial aid, admission procedures, curriculum, advising, recruitment, counseling practice, and ethics. Covers Association and legislative news and announcements from affiliated organizations. Recurring features include interviews, statistics, book reviews, news of research, editorials, opinion, and items on awards, meetings, and membership. **First Published:** June 1980. **Frequency:** Quarterly. ISSN: 0736-0436.

★2647★ NATIONAL ASSOCIATION OF AREA AGENCIES ON
   AGING—NETWORK NEWS
National Association of Area Agencies on Aging, Inc.
1112 16th St. NW, No. 100
Washington, DC 20036-4823   Phone: (202) 484-7520
Description: Monitors developments and programs concerned with the care and service for the elderly. Emphasizes community-based services that assist older people to remain independent in their homes. Recurring features include news of members, a calendar of events, and columns on legislative developments and private sector initiatives. **Frequency:** Monthly.

★2648★ NATIONAL ASSSOCIATION OF PHARMACEUTICAL
   MANUFACTURERS—NEWS BULLETIN
National Association of Pharmaceutical Manufacturers
747 3rd Ave.
New York, NY 10017   Phone: (212) 838-3702
Description: Gives information on the Food and Drug Administration's (FDA) reviews of pharmaceutical products. Offers news on Association's programs. Recurring features include reports of meetings, news of educational opportunities, and notices of publications available. **First Published:** 1960. **Frequency:** Monthly.

★2649★ NATIONAL ASSOCIATION FOR VISUALLY
   HANDICAPPED—IN FOCUS
National Association for Visually Handicapped
22 W. 21st St.
New York, NY 10010   Phone: (212) 889-3141
Description: Reaches visually handicapped children through stories, poems, and drawings contributed by young readers. Covers subjects of interest to youngsters, especially those related to their experiences and hopes for the future. Also includes puzzles, contests, and items of interest to parents and educators, such as new book and symposium announcements. **First Published:** December 1972. **Frequency:** 1-2/yr.

★2650★   THE NATIONAL BOARD EXAMINER
National Board of Medical Examiners
3930 Chestnut St.
Philadelphia, PA 19104   Phone: (215) 349-6400
Description: Presents reports on new medical evaluation programs, new directions in the research and development of examinations, and particular legislation as it affects the NBME. Recurring features include examination schedules, a listing of staff and committees, and news of the activities of the organization. **First Published:** 1923. **Frequency:** Quarterly.

★2651★   NATIONAL BRAILLE PRESS RELEASE
National Braille Press Inc.
88 St. Stephen St.
Boston, MA 02115   Phone: (617) 266-6160
Description: Covers the activities of the National Braille Press. **First Published:** 1980. **Frequency:** 2/yr.

★2652★   NATIONAL CANCER BULLETIN
National Foundation for Cancer Research
7315 Wisconsin Ave., Ste. 332W
Bethesda, MD 20814
Description: Reviews cancer research activities at the Foundation. Contains interviews with researchers and a column titled Important Cancer Research Terms. **Frequency:** Periodic.

★2653★   NATIONAL CHARACTER LABORATORY—
    NEWSLETTER
National Character Laboratory
4635 Leeds Ave.
El Paso, TX 79903   Phone: (915) 562-5046
Description: Carries news of educational activities pertaining to character development and behavioral improvement. Concerned with ethics and morality and the impact of family, church, school, and other influences. Encourages and coordinates character research and discusses its applications. Recurring features include news on professionals in the field. **First Published:** Fall 1971. **Frequency:** Quarterly.

★2654★   NATIONAL CLEARINGHOUSE ON MARITAL & DATE
    RAPE—NEWSLETTER
National Clearinghouse on Marital & Date Rape
2325 Oak St.
Berkeley, CA 94708   Phone: (415) 524-1582
Description: Edited by a consultant, speaker, and researcher of marital/date rape; functions as part of a campaign to protect women by changing current rape laws. Documents marital/date rape trials, court decisions, legislation, statutes, and related news. Reports on cohabitation and date rape, as well. Recurring features include statistics, court reports, letters, and lobbying updates. **First Published:** 1982. **Frequency:** Quarterly.

★2655★   NATIONAL COALITION AGAINST DOMESTIC
    VIOLENCE—VOICE
National Coalition Against Domestic Violence
PO Box 34103
Washington, DC 20043-4103   Phone: (202) 638-6388
Description: Acts as the voice of the Coalition, which is concerned with eliminating domestic violence. Disseminates information on member battered women's service organizations and shelters. Recurring features include updates on the Coalition's task forces, legislative reports, and news of research. **Frequency:** 3/yr.

★2656★   NATIONAL COMMITTEE FOR CLINICAL
    LABORATORY STANDARDS—UPDATE
National Committee for Clinical Laboratory Standards
771 E. Lancaster Ave.
Villanova, PA 19085   Phone: (215) 525-2435
Description: Reports on Committee projects, activities, and publications and carries items of interest to professionals in clinical laboratory medicine. Recurring features include a calendar of events and meetings reports. **First Published:** 1978. **Frequency:** Monthly.

★2657★   NATIONAL DISABLED LAW OFFICERS
    ASSOCIATION—NEWSLETTER
National Disabled Law Officers Association
75 New St.
Nutley, NJ 07110   Phone: (201) 667-9569
Description: Contains news of interest to disabled law officers, including the availability of benefits from federal, state, and local governments.

Reports on relevant legislation. Reprints newspaper articles about the Association and its members. **Frequency:** Periodic.

★2658★   NATIONAL ENVIRONMENTAL HEALTH
    ASSOCIATION—NEWSLETTER
National Environmental Health Association
720 S. Colorado Blvd., Ste. 970
South Tower
Denver, CO 80222   Phone: (303) 861-9090
Description: Publishes nonreviewed technical material from affiliated organizations. Contains organizational news. Recurring features include job listings, state chapter news, and news of members. **First Published:** 1987. **Frequency:** 4/yr.

★2659★   NATIONAL FEDERATION OF STATE HIGH SCHOOL
    ASSOCIATIONS—NATIONAL FEDERATION NEWS
National Federation of State High School Associations
11724 NW Plaza Circle
PO Box 20626
Kansas City, MO 64195-0626   Phone: (816) 464-5400
Description: Covers Federation news, national high school athletic/activities rules and regulations, sportsmanship, sports medicine and psychology, athletic administration, and chemical health. Recurring features include columns titled Around the Nation, Music and Speech, and Rules Changes and Interpretations. **First Published:** 1940. **Frequency:** 10/yr.

★2660★   NATIONAL FOUNDATION FOR FACIAL
    RECONSTRUCTION—NEWSLETTER
National Foundation for Facial Reconstruction, Inc.
317 E. 34th St.
New York, NY 10016   Phone: (212) 340-6656
Description: Carries news of the activities of the Foundation and their committees, which function to aid the rehabilitation of individuals suffering from facial disfigurement. Recurring features include case histories, news of research, and news of members. **First Published:** 1967. **Frequency:** 1-2/yr.

★2661★   NATIONAL GLAUCOMA RESEARCH REPORT
American Health Assistance Foundation
15825 Shady Grove Rd., Ste. 140
Rockville, MD 20850   Phone: (301) 948-3244
Description: Highlights the work of glaucoma researchers and provides tips for individuals with glaucoma. Recurring features include news of research and columns titled From the Presidents and Ask the Experts. **First Published:** 1986. **Frequency:** Quarterly.

★2662★   NATIONAL HEADACHE FOUNDATION—
    NEWSLETTER
National Headache Foundation
5252 N. Western Ave.
Chicago, IL 60625   Phone: (312) 878-8815
Description: Promotes the goals of the Foundation, which are to educate physicians and the public about headache causes and treatments, support and fund research on headaches, and sponsor public education programs. Recurring features include news of research, menus, book reviews, a question-and-answer section, and a calendar of events. **First Published:** 1970. **Frequency:** Quarterly.

★2663★   NATIONAL INFORMATION CENTER FOR CHILDREN
    AND YOUTH WITH HANDICAPS—NEWS DIGEST
National Information Center for Children and Youth With Handicaps
PO Box 1492
Washington, DC 20013   Phone: (703) 893-6061
Description: Addresses current issues affecting individuals concerned with handicapped children and youth. Focuses on a single topic in each issue. Serves as an information exchange for individuals working with the handicapped. **Frequency:** 3/yr.

★2664★   NATIONAL LIBRARY SERVICE FOR THE BLIND
    AND PHYSICALLY HANDICAPPED—UPDATE
National Library Service for the Blind and Physically Handicapped
Library of Congress
1291 Taylor St. NW
Washington, DC 20542   Phone: (202) 707-5100
Description: Reports on volunteer activities related to library services for the blind and physically handicapped, including braille and recorded book production and machine repair. Carries profiles of the work of specific

volunteer organizations and answers by braille instructors to questions about literary braille rules. Recurring features include lists of certified braillists. **Frequency:** Quarterly. **ISSN:** 0160-9203.

★2665★ NATIONAL LYMPHEDEMA NETWORK NEWSLETTER
National Lymphedema Network
2211 Post St., Ste. 404
San Francisco, CA 94115   Phone: (800) 541-3259
Description: Discusses the management of Lymphedema. Provides information on treatment centers and products available to alleviate the condition. **Frequency:** Quarterly.

**★2666★ NATIONAL MENTAL HEALTH ASSOCIATION—
FOCUS**
National Mental Health Association
1021 Prince St.
Alexandria, VA 22314-2971   Phone: (703) 684-7722
Description: Deals with all topics concerning mental health issues and mental illnesses, legislative issues, federal budgeting and other mental health organizations. Recurring features include book reviews, a calendar of events, resource lists, and columns titled An Executive View; Advocacy; Research; Resources; and Calendar. **First Published:** 1981. **Frequency:** 4/yr.

**★2667★ NATIONAL NEUROFIBROMATOSIS FOUNDATION—
LAY NEWSLETTER**
National Neurofibromatosis Foundation, Inc.
141 5th Ave., Ste. 7-S
New York, NY 10010   Phone: (212) 869-9034
Description: Focuses on the problems and treatment of neurofibromatosis (NF). Carries news of research, information on publications and resources, Foundation and chapter news, and reports on meetings and programs. **Frequency:** Quarterly.

**★2668★ NATIONAL NEUROFIBROMATOSIS FOUNDATION—
RESEARCH NEWSLETTER**
National Neurofibromatosis Foundation, Inc.
141 5th Ave., Ste. 7-S
New York, NY 10010   Phone: (212) 460-8980
Description: Provides news and information on research developments in the field of neurofibromatosis from a medical standpoint. **Frequency:** Quarterly.

**★2669★ NATIONAL ORGANIZATION FOR VICTIM
ASSISTANCE—NEWSLETTER**
National Organization for Victim Assistance
1757 Park Rd. NW
Washington, DC 20010   Phone: (202) 232-6682
Description: Carries feature articles, biographies, and legislative news regarding vicitims of crime and other traumatic events in an attempt to express the rights of victims to decency, compassion, and justice. Recurring features include news of research, book reviews, and training outlines that summarize state-of-the-art practices in victim services. **First Published:** 1980. **Frequency:** Monthly.

**★2670★ NATIONAL ORGANIZATION OF WORLD WAR
NURSES—NEWSLETTER**
National Organization of World War Nurses
569 S. Main St.
Red Lion, PA 17356   Phone: (717) 244-9132
Description: Contains announcements of organizational activities and other items of interest to members, including a list of new members, address changes, contributions, requests for information, and notices of relevant publications. **Frequency:** Quarterly.

**★2671★ NATIONAL PEDICULOSIS ASSOCIATION—
PROGRESS**
National Pediculosis Association
PO Box 149
Newton, MA 02161   Phone: (617) 449-6487
Description: Provides new information on the diagnosis, treatment, prevention, and management of pediculsosis (head lice), as well as other entomological diseases affecting children. **First Published:** 1984. **Frequency:** Quarterly (Winter, Spring, Summer, and Fall).

★2672★ NATIONAL PKU NEWS
Virginia Schuett
7760 Ridge Dr. NE
Seattle, WA 98115   Phone: (206) 525-8140
Description: Provides information on management of PKU (Phenylketonuria), a metabolism disorder. **First Published:** May 1989. **Frequency:** 3/yr.

★2673★ NATIONAL PSORIASIS FOUNDATION—BULLETIN
National Psoriasis Foundation
6443 SW Beaverton Hwy., Ste. 210
Portland, OR 97221   Phone: (503) 297-1545
Description: Discusses conventional and experimental treatments for psoriasis, and reports current research on this chronic skin disease. Serves as an educational forum providing information to the general public as well as to victims of the disease, family members, friends, and physicians. Recurring features include news of the Foundation and its staff, announcements of research awards, information on symposiums and meetings, and a question and answer column. **First Published:** 1968. **Frequency:** Bimonthly. **ISSN:** 1040-0060.

**★2674★ NATIONAL RENAL ADMINISTRATORS
ASSOCIATION—PRESIDENT'S LETTER**
National Renal Administrators Association
PO Box 610129
Port Huron, MI 48061-0129   Phone: (313) 987-3625
Frequency: Monthly.

**★2675★ THE NATIONAL REPORT ON COMPUTERS &
HEALTH**
United Communications Group
11300 Rockville Pike, Ste. 1100
Rockville, MD 20852-3030   Phone: (301) 816-8950
Description: Reports on data processing and clinical hospital information systems. Includes user comments on health care software. **First Published:** May 1980. **Frequency:** Biweekly. **ISSN:** 0273-4974.

★2676★ THE NATIONAL REPORT ON SUBSTANCE ABUSE
Buraff Publications
Millin Publications, Inc.
1350 Connecticut Ave. NW
Washington, DC 20036   Phone: (202) 862-0914
Description: Reviews federal, state, and local laws and regulations concerning alcohol and drug use, testing, and policies. Discusses significant court decisions. Contains information on the drug enforcement budgets at all levels of government. Examines employee assistance plans and other educational programs designed to help substance abusers. **First Published:** December 10, 1986. **Frequency:** Biweekly. **ISSN:** 0891-5709.

**★2677★ NATIONAL REYE'S SYNDROME FOUNDATION—IN
THE NEWS**
National Reye's Syndrome Foundation
PO Box 829
Bryan, OH 43506   Phone: (419) 636-2679
Description: Promotes awareness and early detection of Reye's Syndrome. Reports current research findings and items concerning aspects of Reye's Syndrome. Recurring features include news of the activities of the Foundation, chapter news, notices of meetings, and a message from the Foundation's president. **First Published:** 1974. **Frequency:** Semiannual.

★2678★ NATIONAL RIGHT TO LIFE NEWS
National Right to Life Committee
419 7th St., Ste. 500
Washington, DC 20004   Phone: (202) 626-8820
Description: Discusses pro-life issues, abortion, and euthanasia. Recurring features include letters to the editor, interviews, news of research, reports of meetings, job listings, book reviews, editorials, and a column titled From the President. **First Published:** 1973. **Frequency:** Semimonthly.

**★2679★ NATIONAL SOCIETY TO PREVENT BLINDNESS—
MEMBER NEWS**
National Society to Prevent Blindness
500 E. Remington Rd.
Schaumburg, IL 60173-4556   Phone: (708) 843-2020
Description: Discusses information on advances in the eye care field, especially regarding eye health and safety. **First Published:** 1951. **Frequency:** Quarterly.

**★2680★   NATIONAL TAY-SACHS AND ALLIED DISEASES
ASSOCIATION—BREAKTHROUGH**
National Tay-Sachs & Allied Diseases Association, Inc.
2001 Beacon St.
Brookline, MA 02146   Phone: (617) 277-4463
Description: Presents news of Association activities, continuing public
education programs, and of Tay-Sachs and similar genetic diseases.
Recurring features include items on carrier detection, medical research,
and relevant legislation, and listings of publications concerning Tay-Sachs
disease prevention. **Frequency:** Ca. 2/yr.

**★2681★   NATIONAL TUBEROUS SCLEROSIS ASSOCIATION—
PERSPECTIVE**
National Tuberous Sclerosis Association, Inc.
8000 Corporate Dr., Ste. 120
Landover, MD 20785   Phone: (301) 459-9888
Description: Focuses on the research, fundraising, and other efforts to help
those with tuberous sclerosis and their families. Recurring features include
items on Association activities, financial reports, personal accounts of
those coping with tuberous sclerosis, announcements of Parent/Medical
meetings and other events of interest, and questions and answers regarding
medical problems and coping with tuberous sclerosis. Also contains
columns titled State Activities, and Ask the Doctor. **First Published:** 1974.
Frequency: Quarterly.

**★2682★   NATIONAL WOMEN'S HEALTH NETWORK—
NETWORK NEWS**
National Women's Health Network
1325 G St. NW
Washington, DC 20005   Phone: (202) 347-1140
Description: Carries timely health information and medical alerts for
women. Emphasizes matters affecting reproductive rights and occupational and environmental health. Reports federal health policies and local
health actions affecting women, including the aged, the poor, minorities,
and others termed medically neglected. **Frequency:** Bimonthly. **ISSN:**
8755-867X.

★2683★   NATURAL NUTRITION NEWS
Now Foods
2000 Bloomingdale Rd., Ste. 250
Glendale Heights, IL 60139-2182   Phone: (708) 793-1330
Description: Provides methods of aiding healing and health through
natural alternative, including applied nutrition. **First Published:** Summer
1991.

★2684★   NBA BULLETIN
National Braille Association, Inc.
1290 University Ave.
Rochester, NY 14607   Phone: (716) 473-0900
Description: Offers updates on the activities of the Association, which
provides continuing education in the production of materials (braille, large
type, and tape) for visually impaired readers. Includes skills columns
designed to inform transcribers for the visually impaired of current
practices and code changes. Recurring features include reports of meetings
and conferences, notices of publications and services available to readers
and transcribers, and columns titled President's Message, Tech Talk, and
Sharpen Your Skills. **First Published:** Winter 1964. **Frequency:** Quarterly.
ISSN: 0550-5666.

★2685★   NCHRTM MEMO
National Clearing House of Rehabilitation Training Materials
816 W. 6th St.
Oklahoma State University
Stillwater, OK 74078-0433   Phone: (405) 624-7650
Description: Announces new acquisitions of mixed media materials of the
National Clearing House and provides brief descriptions. Provides annota-
tions of noteworthy products offered from other sources and notices of
additional products/services relating to the rehabilitation of persons with
disabilities. **First Published:** 1962. **Frequency:** Quarterly.

★2686★   NCI CANCER WEEKLY
Charles W. Henderson
PO Box 5528
Atlanta, GA 30307-0527   Phone: (404) 377-8895
Description: Covers a variety of topics related to cancer, including research
developments and meetings of cancer groups. Each issue contains inter-
views, a calendar of events, notices of educational opportunities, and book
reviews. **First Published:** April 1988. **Frequency:** Weekly.

★2687★   NCOA NETWORKS
National Council on the Aging
409 3rd St. SW
Washington, DC 20024   Phone: (202) 479-1200
Description: Highlights specific activities of the constituent units of the
Council, reports legislative and regulatory activity and judicial decisions
affecting older persons, and explores significant developments in the field
of aging. **First Published:** 1989. **Frequency:** Bimonthly. **ISSN:** 1045-9073.

★2688★   NEBRASKA SAFETY CENTER NEWSLETTER
Nebraska Safety Center
University of Nebraska at Kearney
W.C. UNK
Kearney, NE 68849   Phone: (308) 234-8256
Description: Recurring features include a calendar of events. **First Pub-
lished:** September 1978. **Frequency:** Quarterly.

★2689★   NEURODEVELOPMENTS
Center for Neurodevelopmental Studies, Inc.
8434 N. 39th Ave.
Phoenix, AZ 85051   Phone: (602) 433-1400
Description: Features news of the Center, research projects, and support
groups; and articles on neurological developments and disorders.

★2690★   NEUROLOGY ALERT
American Health Consultants, Inc.
PO Box 740056
Atlanta, GA 30374   Phone: (404) 262-7436
Description: Discusses diagnoses, causes, and treatments for such neurolog-
ical problems as strokes, intracranial aneurysms and hemorrhages, demen-
tia, and epilepsy. Examines current medical opinions and diagnostic
difficulties. Recurring features include news of research. **First Published:**
September 1982. **Frequency:** Monthly. **ISSN:** 0741-4234.

★2691★   NEUROSCIENCE NEWSLETTER
Society for Neuroscience
11 Dupont Circle, NW, Ste. 500
Washington, DC 20036   Phone: (202) 462-6688
Description: Covers developments in neuroscience, with attention to
research findings and funding, education, and interdisciplinary programs.
Carries summaries or text of talks, papers, and of the prepared testimony
of the Society's representative before congressional committees. Recurring
features include announcements of meetings and symposia, reports of
foreign neuroscience societies, and Society news. **First Published:** 1970.
Frequency: Bimonthly.

★2692★   NEW BEGINNINGS
La Leche League International, Inc.
PO Box 1209
Franklin Park, IL 60131-8209   Phone: (708) 455-7730
Description: Covers breastfeeding, childbirth and nutrition, and child care
in relation to breastfeeding. Recurring features include book reviews,
poems, medical and scientific information, and news of research pertain-
ing to breastfeeding. **First Published:** 1958. **Frequency:** Bimonthly.

**★2693★   NEW BRUNSWICK HEALTH RECORDS
ASSOCIATION—NEWSBREAK**
New Brunswick Health Records Association
c/o Moncton Hospital
135 MacBeath Ave.
Moncton, NB, Canada E1C 6Z8   Phone: (506) 857-5395
Description: Covers Association activities and developments in the health
care records field. Recurring features include news of research, a calendar
of events, reports of meetings, news of educational opportunities, and job
listings. **First Published:** 1966. **Frequency:** 4/yr.

★2694★   NEW CONNECTIONS
Patty Jackson
107 Ledgelawn Ave.
Bar Harbor, ME 04609
Description: Assists individuals with multiple sclerosis (MS) in meeting
other people with the same condition. Includes short biographies. **First
Published:** 1986. **Frequency:** Bimonthly.

★2695★ NEW DIRECTIONS
National Association of State Mental Retardation Program Directors
113 Oronoco St.
Alexandria, VA 22314   Phone: (703) 683-4202
Description: Monitors administrative, legislative, and judicial activities and other events affecting mental retardation programs. Discusses issues and developments in the field. **Frequency:** Monthly.

★2696★ NEW DIRECTIONS NEWSLETTER
National Jewish Center for Immunology and Respiratory Medicine
1400 Jackson St.
Denver, CO 80206   Phone: (303) 398-1083
Description: Provides updates on research and clinical progress at the Center. **First Published:** Summer 1970. **Frequency:** Quarterly.

★2697★ NEW DRUGS—DRUG NEWS
OCP Drug Information Centre
Faculty of Pharmacy
University of Toronto
19 Russell St.
Toronto, ON, Canada M5S 1A1   Phone: (800) 268-8058
Description: Evaluates new drugs and treatments. Lists new Canadian pharmaceutical products, including trade names, generic names, manufacturers, dosage forms, and indications. **First Published:** 1983. **Frequency:** Bimonthly.

★2698★ NEW ENGLAND REGIONAL GENETICS GROUP—REGIONAL NEWSLETTER
New England Regional Genetics Group
PO Box 682
Gorham, ME 04038-0682   Phone: (207) 839-5324
Description: Provides news concerning the regional genetic services network of New England. **First Published:** August 1985. **Frequency:** Quarterly.

★2699★ THE NEW FACTS OF LIFE
Canadian Public Health Association
400-1565 Carling Ave.
Ottawa, ON, Canada K1Z 8R1   Phone: (613) 725-3769
Description: Promotes Acquired Immune Deficiency Syndrome (AIDS) awareness through education. Focuses on programs, networks, and multi- and ethnocultural initiatives. Publishes information on publications, campaigns, conferences, and mass media efforts supporting AIDS prevention. **Frequency:** Quarterly. **ISSN:** 0841-9396.

★2700★ NEW JERSEY NETWORK ON ADOLESCENT PREGNANCY—EXCHANGES
New Jersey Network on Adolescent Programs
Center for Community Education
Rutgers University School of Social Work
73 Easton Ave.
New Brunswick, NJ 08903   Phone: (908) 932-8636
Description: Discusses unwanted pregnancy, teen parenting, birth control, and related issues. **First Published:** 1979. **Frequency:** Quarterly.

★2701★ NEW METHODS
Ronald S. Lippert, A.H.T.
PO Box 22605
San Francisco, CA 94122-0605   Phone: (415) 664-3469
Description: Examines common problems and concerns in the field of animal health technology. "Provides professionals with the best in network sources" as well as items on animal care and protection and medical breakthroughs. Recurring features include letters to the editor, interviews, notices of publications available, job listings, news of educational opportunities, and news of research. **First Published:** 1981. **Frequency:** Monthly. **ISSN:** 0277-3015.

★2702★ NEW SENSE BULLETIN
Interface Press
PO Box 42211
Los Angeles, CA 90042   Phone: (213) 223-2500
Description: Discusses findings and social implications in areas of psychology, consciousness, human potential, early learning, drugs, hypnosis, parapsychology, and similar subjects. Provides full bibliographic references to works cited. Recurring features include editorials, commentaries, news of research, a calendar of events, book reviews, and lists of resources. **First Published:** November 1975. **Frequency:** Monthly. **ISSN:** 1057-0705.

★2703★ NEW YORK SOCIETY FOR THE DEAF—CHRONICLE
New York Society for the Deaf
817 Broadway, 7th Fl.
New York, NY 10003   Phone: (212) 777-3900
Description: Publishes news of the Society, whose "total communication" policy encourages deaf persons to communicate by any means they find comfortable: sign language, fingerspelling, lipreading, speech, writing, mime, gestures, and body language. Promotes programs sponsored by the Society and highlights legislation affecting deaf and other handicapped persons. Recurring features include a calendar of events and news of research. **First Published:** 1952. **Frequency:** Quarterly.

★2704★ NEWFOUNDLAND MEDICAL ASSOCIATION—NEWSLETTER
Newfoundland Medical Association
164 MacDonald Dr.
St. John's, NF, Canada A1A 4B3   Phone: (709) 726-7424
Description: Contains information of interest to members of the Association. **Frequency:** 6/yr.

★2705★ NEWSLETTER TO DIPLOMATES
American Board of Neurological Surgery
6550 Fannin St., Ste. 2139
Houston, TX 77030   Phone: (713) 790-6015
Description: Describes the activities of the organization, a certification board established to investigate qualifications of, administer examinations to, and certify as diplomates medical doctors specializing in neurological surgery. Also promotes adequate training facilities and reports on the activities of Board committees. Recurring features include reports of meetings. **First Published:** 1981. **Frequency:** Annually.

★2706★ NEWSLETTER FROM THE SIERRA MADRE
Hesperian Foundation
PO Box 1692
Palo Alto, CA 94302   Phone: (415) 325-9017
Description: Discusses developments in the international rural self-care movement. Reports on Foundation activities and profiles health care workers and patients. Recurring features include articles on the politics of international health. **First Published:** 1965. **Frequency:** Semiannually.

★2707★ NEWSLETTER FOR PARENTS AND PATIENTS
Cleft Palate Foundation
1218 Grandview Ave.
Pittsburgh, PA 15211   Phone: (412) 481-1376
Description: Offers information and support for cleft palate patients and their families. Carries statements from patients, research updates, and information about cleft palate organizations and support groups. Recurring features include Foundation news and listings of resources available. **First Published:** 1977. **Frequency:** Quarterly.

★2708★ THE NEWSLETTER FOR PEOPLE WITH LACTOSE INTOLERANCE AND MILK ALLERGY
Commercial Writing Service
PO Box 3074
Iowa City, IA 52244
Description: Offers "research updates, product information, book reviews, recipes, and a reader's forum" on lactose intolerance. **First Published:** Winter 1987. **Frequency:** Quarterly.

★2709★ NEWSLETTER OF THE PROTEIN IDENTIFICATION RESOURCE
National Biomedical Research Foundation
3900 Reservoir Rd. NW
Washington, DC 20007   Phone: (202) 687-2121
Description: Covers databases, software, and other services used in protein identification research. Includes highlights of special projects, announcements of scientific meetings, and notices of publications available. **First Published:** January 1985. **Frequency:** 2-3/yr.

★2710★ NEWSOUNDS
Alexander Graham Bell Association for the Deaf, Inc.
3417 Volta Pl. NW
Washington, DC 20007   Phone: (202) 337-5220
Description: Carries news of interest to the hearing impaired. Provides coverage of legislative and social events of significance in the field and reports activities of the Association. Recurring features include newsbreaks, legislative news, news of research, news of members, and a calendar of events. **First Published:** 1976. **Frequency:** 10/yr. **ISSN:** 0147-4057.

★2711★ NFCR REPORTS
National Foundation for Cancer Research
7315 Wisconsin Ave., Ste. 332W
Bethesda, MD 20814   Phone: (301) 654-1250
Description: Reports on the Foundation's progress in conducting basic scientific research and investigation into the structure and function of normal and abnormal cells. Reflects the Foundation's belief that cancer is a disturbance of normal cellular function at the submolecular level. Also carries news from laboratories funded by the Foundation, both in the U.S. and abroad. **Frequency:** Quarterly.

★2712★ NFPRHA NEWS
National Family Planning & Reproductive Health Association
122 C St. NW, Ste. 380
Washington, DC 20001   Phone: (202) 628-3535
Description: Promotes the Association's concern with the maintenance and improvement of family planning and reproductive health care services. Discusses issues and news of interest to family planning professionals and Title X delegates. Recurring features include editorials, news of research, legislative updates, and news of the Association and its members. **First Published:** 1982. **Frequency:** Monthly.

★2713★ NHO NEWSLINE
National Hospice Organization
1901 N. Moore St., Ste. 901
Arlington, VA 22209   Phone: (703) 243-5900
Description: Advocates the importance of hospice care, a specialized health care program emphasizing the management of pain, fear, and loneliness associated with terminal illness while providing care and support for the family as well as the patient. Contains news and information about hospice programs in the United States. Recurring features include list of training programs and resources for hospice personnel, a calendar of events, and news of members. **First Published:** October 1979. **Frequency:** 20/yr.

★2714★ NIAGARA CENTRE FOR INDEPENDENT LIVING NEWSLETTER
CMT International
75 Lincoln St. W.
Welland, ON, Canada L3C 5J3   Phone: (416) 734-1060
Description: Provides information for disabled people in the Niagara Peninsula along with news reports of recent government decisions concerning the disabled. Recurring features include a column on aids for daily living, recent events, letters to the editor, calendar of events, announcements of trips, forums, peer support meetings, drug rehabilitation programs, and consumer monitoring of disability issues. **First Published:** February 1989. **Frequency:** Bimonthly. **ISSN:** 0847-3722.

★2715★ NIDA NOTES
National Institute on Drug Abuse
Alcohol, Drug Abuse, and Mental Health Administration
Room 10A-39
Rockville, MD 20857   Phone: (301) 443-1124
Description: Covers recent developments relating to drug abuse treatment and prevention research, epidemiology, and behavioral pharmacology. Seeks to "report on advances in the drug abuse field, identify resources, promote an exchange of information, and improve communications between clinicians, researchers, administrators, and policymakers." Recurring features include synopses of research advances and projects, NIDA news, news of legislative and regulatory developments, results of surveys and studies, clinical observations, and announcements of resources and educational opportunities available. **Frequency:** Bimonthly.

★2716★ NIDR RESEARCH DIGEST
National Institute of Dental Research
National Institute of Health
Bldg. 31, Rm. 2C35
Bethesda, MD 20892   Phone: (301) 496-4261
Description: Highlights recent dental research advances. **Frequency:** Irregular.

★2717★ THE NIGHTINGALE
National Association of Physician Nurses
900 S. Washington St., No. G13
Falls Church, VA 22046-4020   Phone: (703) 237-8616
Description: Presents items on "medical and personal subjects pertaining to office nurses and other staff." **First Published:** 1973. **Frequency:** Monthly.

★2718★ NKF FAMILY FOCUS
The National Kidney Foundation, Inc.
30 E. 33rd St.
New York, NY 10016   Phone: (212) 889-2210
Description: Provides news on kidney disease. Includes articles on nutrition, news of research, and columns titled From the Editor, Medical News Spotlight, Patient Services Update, Lifestyles, and Ask the Doctor, and Patient/Family Network. **First Published:** December 1989. **Frequency:** Quarterly.

★2719★ NKI REPORT
Nathan S. Kline Institute for Psychiatric Research
Bldg. 37
Orangeburg, NY 10962   Phone: (914) 365-2000
First Published: 1983. **Frequency:** Annual.

★2720★ NOCIRC—NEWSLETTER
National Organization of Circumcision Information Research Centers
PO Box 2512
San Anselmo, CA 94979-2512   Phone: (415) 488-9883
Description: Features letters to the editor, news of research, reports of meetings, book reviews, and notices of publications available. **First Published:** 1985.

★2721★ NOHA NEWS
Nutrition for Optimal Health Association
PO Box 380
Winnetka, IL 60093   Phone: (312) 491-0429
Description: Examines the links between good nutrition and health. Reports nutritional information and research findings culled from a wide range of scientific sources; includes a column written by the Professional Advisory Board. **First Published:** Fall 1976. **Frequency:** Quarterly.

★2722★ THE NONSMOKERS' VOICE
Group to Alleviate Smoking Pollution of Colorado
2885 Aurora Ave., No. 16
Boulder, CO 80303   Phone: (303) 444-9799
Description: Describes nonsmokers' rights issues, new medical research on secondhand smoke, legislative alerts, and the tactics of the tobacco industry. Recurring features include news of research, actions taken regarding environmental tobacco smoke, reports of meetings, and listings of smoke-free establishments. **First Published:** 1977. **Frequency:** Quarterly. **ISSN:** 0897-9626.

★2723★ NORTH AMERICAN ASSOCIATION OF JEWISH HOMES AND HOUSING FOR THE AGED—PERSPECTIVES
North American Association of Jewish Homes and Housing for the Aged
10830 N. Central Expressway, No. 150
Dallas, TX 75231-1022   Phone: (214) 696-9838
Description: Provides information on services to the aged, Jewish homes and housing for the aged, and events in the news concerning Jewish groups, persons, or institutions concerned for the elderly. Recurring features include a column titled Tintype, which profiles an outstanding executive in the field, and a column describing a particular facility or home. **First Published:** 1960. **Frequency:** Quarterly.

★2724★ NORTH AMERICAN SOCIETY OF ADLERIAN PSYCHOLOGY—NEWSLETTER
North American Society of Adlerian Psychology
65 E. Wacker Pl., Ste. 400
Chicago, IL 60601-7203   Phone: (312) 629-8801
Description: Relates news and events of the North American Society of Adlerian Psychology and regional news of affiliated associations. Recurring features include lists of courses and workshops offered by affiliated associations, reviews of new publications in the field, professional employment opportunities, a calendar of events, and a column titled President's Message. **Frequency:** Monthly.

★2725★ NORTH DAKOTA SOCIETY FOR MEDICAL TECHNOLOGY—NEWSLETTER
North Dakota Society for Medical Technology
Department of Pathology
University of North Dakota
Grand Forks, ND 58202   Phone: (701) 777-2561
Description: Discusses current topics in medical technology. Carries news of national, regional, and state medical technology events. Includes statistics and a feature article on a scientific topic. Recurring features

include news of members, a calendar of events, and a column titled President's Message. **First Published:** 1950. **Frequency:** Quarterly.

★2726★   **NORTHWEST ARCTIC NUNA**
Maniilaq Association
PO Box 256
Kotzebue, AK 99752   Phone: (907) 442-3311
Description: Reflects the aims of the Association, a health corporation promoting public health and social welfare in Alaskan Eskimo villages. Reports on Inupiaq Eskimo customs, arts, and language to promote understanding between natives and non-natives. Highlights programs of the Association and profiles members. **Frequency:** 8-10/yr.

★2727★   **NORTHWEST TERRITORIES REGISTERED NURSES' ASSOCIATION—NEWSLETTERIT2**
Northwest Territories Registered Nurses' Association
PO Box 2757
Yellowknife, NT, Canada X1A 2R1   Phone: (403) 873-2745
Description: Informs registered nurses of Association activities, provides a forum for discussion, and disseminates information of interest. Recurring features include notices of community education courses, a calendar of events, and reports of meetings. **First Published:** 1975. **Frequency:** 4/yr.

★2728★   **NOVA**
American Osteopathic College of Pathologists
c/o Joan Gross
12368 N.W. 13th Court
Pembroke Pines, FL 33026   Phone: (305) 432-9640
Description: Contains news and information relevant to osteopathic physicians. Discusses residency training programs and monitors developments in the field. Includes job and placement listings. **First Published:** 1980. **Frequency:** Quarterly.

★2729★   **NRAA JOURNAL**
National Renal Administrators Association
4046 Gratiot Ave.
Port Huron, MI 48060-1202   Phone: (313) 987-3625
Description: Serves as an educational and informational resource for administrative personnel involved in the End Stage Renal Disease (ESRD) Program. Discusses subjects related to the economics, management, and regulation of renal dialysis units. **First Published:** 1979. **Frequency:** Annually.

★2730★   **NSDA NEWSLETTER**
Nova Scotia Dietetic Association
Box 8841, Sta. A
Halifax, NS, Canada B3K 5M5   Phone: (902) 798-1177
Description: Contains committee reports, items of interest, and resources for NSDA members. Recurring features include columns titled Nutrition Trivia and Ideas Corner. **Frequency:** 7/yr. **ISSN:** 0827-7281.

★2731★   **NSNU NEWSLETTER**
Nova Scotia Nurses' Union
65 Queen St.
Dartmouth, NS, Canada B2Y 1G4   Phone: (902) 469-1422
Description: Provides news of Union activities and nursing issues in Nova Scotia. **First Published:** 1976. **Frequency:** 4/yr.

★2732★   **NSVMA COUNCIL MEETING MINUTES**
Nova Scotia Veterinary Medical Association
Agricultural Centre
Kentville, NS, Canada B4N 1J5   Phone: (902) 679-5740
Description: Provides minutes of council meetings of the Nova Scotia Veterinary Medical Association. Recurring features include job openings, a calendar of events, news of educational opportunities, and notices of available publications. **Frequency:** Approximately every 6 weeks.

★2733★   **NURSE-ENTREPRENEUR'S EXCHANGE**
David Norris
47 6th St.
Petaluma, CA 94952   Phone: (707) 763-6021
Description: Provides news and information of interest to nurse entrepreneurs. **First Published:** 1985. **Frequency:** Bimonthly. **ISSN:** 0889-2733.

★2734★   **NURSE TO NURSE**
Registered Nurses Association of Nova Scotia
120 Eileen Stubbs Ave., Ste. 104
Dartmouth, NS, Canada B3B 1Y1   Phone: (902) 423-6156
Description: Informs members of the activities and achievements of the Association. Provides a forum for the exchange of ideas, information, research, and concerns relevant to nursing practice. Recurring features include a calendar of events, letters to the editor, interviews, news of research, news of developments and innovation in nursing, reports of meetings, news of educational opportunities, and columns titled Entry to Practice, Continuing Education, Standards for Nursing Practice, and From the President. **First Published:** 1969. **Frequency:** Bimonthly. **ISSN:** 0319-4604.

★2735★   **NURSING ARCHIVES NEWSLETTER**
Nursing Archives
Department of Special Collections
Boston University
771 Commonwealth Ave.
Boston, MA 02215   Phone: (617) 353-3696
Description: Covers activities and information relating to the Nursing Archives. **First Published:** March 1981. **Frequency:** Irregular.

★2736★   **NURSING HOME LAW LETTER**
National Senior Citizens Law Center
1815 H St. NW, Ste. 700
Washington, DC 20006   Phone: (202) 887-5280
Description: Examines issues affecting nursing home residents. Discusses such issues as Medicaid discrimination, transfers, and use of personal needs allowance. **Frequency:** Quarterly.

★2737★   **NURSING NETWORK NEWS**
National Hemophilia Foundation
110 Green St., Rm. 406
New York, NY 10012   Phone: (212) 219-8180
Description: Provides information on care of patients with hemophilia and nursing issues concerning hemophilia. Includes articles, updates, abstracts, and reports of meetings. Publicizes the programs sponsored by the Foundation. **Frequency:** Semiannually.

★2738★   **NUTRITION ACTION HEALTHLETTER**
Center for Science in the Public Interest
1875 Connecticut Ave. NW, No. 300
Washington, DC 20009-5728   Phone: (202) 332-9110
Description: Covers food and nutrition, the food industry, and relevant government regulations and legislation. Focuses on the connections among diet, lifestyle, and disease. Includes nutritional comparisons of food products, reader questions and answers, and health-promoting recipes. **First Published:** 1974. **Frequency:** 10/yr. **ISSN:** 0199-5510.

★2739★   **NUTRITION FORUM**
PO Box 1747
Allentown, PA 18105   Phone: (215) 437-1795
Description: Covers nutrition news with emphasis on the investigation and exposure of nutrition fads, fallacies, and frauds. Includes book reviews. **First Published:** October 1984. **Frequency:** Bimonthly.

★2740★   **NUTRITION AND HEALTH**
Institute of Human Nutrition
Columbia University College of Physicians and Surgeons
701 W. 168th St.
New York, NY 10032
Description: Geared towards treating and preventing diseases. Covers a single topic each month. **Frequency:** Monthly.

★2741★   **NUTRITION HEALTH REVIEW**
Vegetus Publications
171 Madison Ave.
New York, NY 10016   Phone: (212) 679-3590
Description: Aims to educate the public about nutrition and health. Covers developments in areas including medical care, psychology, childraising, and geriatrics. Recurring features include news of research, editorials, letters to the editor, and book reviews. **First Published:** 1976. **Frequency:** Quarterly.

★2742★ NUTRITION AND THE M.D.
PM, Inc.
PO Box 10172
Van Nuys, CA 91410 Phone: (818) 873-4399
Description: Covers such topics as foodborne illness, the effects of infection on nutrient metabolism, environmental contamination, food allergies, and amino acid therapy. Reports on specific food coloring dyes, preservatives, and other additives, and examines various health and nutrition studies conducted by major health institutions. Recurring features include news of research, reprints from national medical journals, book reviews, a bibliography, and a question and answer column. **First Published:** 1974. **Frequency:** Monthly. **ISSN:** 0732-0167.

★2743★ NUTRITION NEWS
National Dairy Council
6300 N. River Rd.
Rosemont, IL 60018 Phone: (312) 696-1020
Description: Provides information on nutrition education and related subjects. Discusses current research; provides innovative teaching ideas; and includes a master that may be reproduced and made available as a handout to students and clients. **First Published:** 1937. **Frequency:** 3/yr. **ISSN:** 0369-6464.

★2744★ NUTRITION NEWS
Gurumantra S. Khalsa
4108 Watkins Dr.
Riverside, CA 92507 Phone: (714) 784-7500
Description: Disseminates current research on nutrition and wellness in non-technical, in-depth articles. Focuses on one topic per issue. **First Published:** 1976. **Frequency:** Monthly. **ISSN:** 8756-5919.

★2745★ NUTRITION NOTES
American Institute of Nutrition
9650 Rockville Pike
Bethesda, MD 20814-3990 Phone: (301) 530-7050
Description: Contains updates on nutrition legislation, public affairs, and public information policies. Reviews the results of nutritional research conducted by members of the Institute, which is comprised of nutrition scientists from universities, government, and industry. Recurring features include news of members, letters to the editor, job listings, notices of publications available, information on awards and fellowships, and news of scientific meetings. **First Published:** 1960. **Frequency:** Quarterly.

★2746★ NUTRITION RESEARCH NEWSLETTER
Lyda Associates
PO Box 700
Palisades, NY 10964 Phone: (914) 359-8282
Description: Summarizes more than 400 biomedical journals to provide abstracts and citations to literature in nutrition research and clinical nutrition research. Recurring features include listing of reviews. **First Published:** November 1982. **Frequency:** Monthly. **ISSN:** 0736-0037.

★2747★ NUTRITION WEEK
Community Nutrition Institute
2001 S St. NW
Washington, DC 20009 Phone: (202) 462-4700
Description: Reports on the Institute's activities in continuing "improvement and expansion of federal food assistance programs through development of the capabilities of community organizations, consumer groups, and state and local officials." Discusses prices, packaging, nutrition, and poverty and welfare issues. Recurring features include listings of employment opportunities and a calendar of events. **First Published:** August 1970. **Frequency:** 50/yr. **ISSN:** 0736-0096.

★2748★ NWDA EXECUTIVE NEWSLETTER
National Wholesale Druggists' Association
105 Oronoco St.
PO Box 238
Alexandria, VA 22314 Phone: (703) 684-6400
Description: Reports trends and changes in the wholesale drug industry. Covers promotions within member companies, instructional and promotional material available, and Association activities. **First Published:** 1945. **Frequency:** Biweekly.

★2749★ OAO NEWS
Ontario Association of Optometrists
290 Lawrence Ave. W.
Toronto, ON, Canada M5M 1B3 Phone: (416) 256-4411
Description: Carries information on Association activities and covers issues relating to the state of the optometry profession in Ontario. Recurring features include a calendar of events, reports of meetings, news of educational opportunities, and job listings. **Frequency:** 6/yr.

★2750★ OBESITY AND HEALTH
Healthy Living Institute
402 S. 14th St.
Hettinger, ND 58639 Phone: (701) 567-2646
Description: Publishes research information for professionals involved in health issues relating to obesity. Features articles considering various aspects of obesity, including causes, treatment, cultural, social, health, and psychological perspectives. Recurring features include book reviews, guest spots, editorials, treatment tips, features on weight loss fraud and size acceptance, and conference information. **First Published:** 1986. **Frequency:** Bimonthly. **ISSN:** 1044-1522.

★2751★ OB/GYN CLINICAL ALERT
American Health Consultants, Inc.
PO Box 740056
Atlanta, GA 30374 Phone: (404) 262-7436
Description: Reviews medical literature and research related to obstetrics and gynecology, providing commentary on each item. Covers diseases, treatments, drugs, general health, and professional trends. **First Published:** 1983. **Frequency:** Monthly. **ISSN:** 0743-8354.

★2752★ OCCUPATIONAL HEALTH AND SAFETY LETTER
Business Publishers, Inc.
951 Pershing Dr.
Silver Spring, MD 20910 Phone: (301) 587-6300
Description: Covers federal and state legislation, standards, regulations, research activities, and enforcement cases concerning safety and health in the workplace environment. Concerned particularly with the Occupational Safety and Health Act (OSHA) of 1970. Recurring features include information on the medical, economic, and technological aspects of occupational health, and a calendar of events. **First Published:** 1971. **Frequency:** Biweekly. **ISSN:** 0148-4079.

★2753★ OCCUPATIONAL SAFETY AND HEALTH REPORTER
Bureau of National Affairs, Inc.
1231 25th St. NW
Washington, DC 20037 Phone: (202) 452-4200
Description: Provides a notification and reference service covering federal and state regulation of occupational safety and health, standards, legislation, enforcement activities, research, and legal decisions. Recurring features include a calendar of meetings and seminars and the full text of selected administrative rulings, proposed standards, criteria documents, variance notices, and compliance manuals. **First Published:** May 6, 1971. **Frequency:** Weekly. **ISSN:** 0095-3237.

★2754★ OCP NEWSLETTER
Ontario College of Pharmacists
483 Huron St.
Toronto, ON, Canada M5R 2R4 Phone: (416) 962-4861
Description: Covers developments in pharmaceuticals and the pharmacist profession. Contains information on new laws and regulations, continuing education programs, and drugs. Reports on the activities of the Ontario College of Pharmacists. Recurring features include news of research, news of educational opportunities, reports of meetings, and a calendar of events. **First Published:** 1961. **Frequency:** Monthly.

★2755★ OF CURRENT INTEREST
Policy Center on Aging
Brandeis University
Heller Graduate School
Waltham, MA 02254-9110 Phone: (617) 736-3860
Description: Covers policies and news of interest on aging. Spotlights economic issues. **First Published:** 1981. **Frequency:** 1-2/yr.

★2756★ OHIO GASP, INC. NEWSLETTER
Ohio Group Against Smoking Pollution, Inc.
PO Box 8324
Akron, OH 44320 Phone: (216) 321-2320
Description: Promotes smoking restrictions through legislation, public

education, and support for businesses with "no smoking" policies. **Frequency:** Quarterly.

★2757★   OHIO VMA NEWSLETTER
Veterinary Medical Association
1350 W. Fifth Ave.
Columbus, OH 43212   Phone: (614) 486-7253
Description: Covers the activities of the Association. **First Published:** September 1970. **Frequency:** Monthly.

★2758★   OHIS NEWSLETTER
Oral Hearing Impaired Section
Alexander Graham Bell Association for the Deaf, Inc.
3417 Volta Place, NW
Washington, DC 20007   Phone: (202) 337-5220
Description: Supports the goal of OHIS to help those among the hearing-impaired who have chosen to communicate through speech and lip reading to "improve their educational, vocational, and social opportunities in the hearing environment." Recurring features include news of members, news of research, reports of conferences and conventions, chapter news, profiles, obituaries, statistics, and Chairman's Column. **First Published:** April 1972. **Frequency:** Quarterly.

★2759★   OLSEN'S BIOTECHNOLOGY REPORT
G.V. Olsen Associates
123 Picketts Ridge Rd.
W. Redding, CT 06896   Phone: (203) 938-4188
Description: Reports on developments in the field of biotechnology: genetic engineering research, scale-up, production, marketing, and licensing of plant, animal, and agricultural chemicals. Provides financial analysis of the biotechnology market and related investment activity. Recurring features include book reviews and notices of publications available. **First Published:** 1983. **Frequency:** Monthly. **ISSN:** 0889-616X.

★2760★   ON THE BEAM
Lowe's Syndrome Association
222 Lincoln St.
West Lafayette, IN 47906   Phone: (317) 743-3636
Description: Aims to foster communication between families affected by Lowe's Syndrome and other interested persons, to provide medical and educational information, and to report news of the Association and its members. Recurring features include letters from parents and pictures of their children, news of research, and listings of resources. **First Published:** Summer 1982. **Frequency:** 3/yr. **ISSN:** 0740-218X.

★2761★   ON THE RECORD
Association for Children With Retarded Mental Development, Inc.
162 Fifth Ave., 11th Fl.
New York, NY 10010   Phone: (212) 741-0100
Description: Informs Association members of developments in the human services field. Includes information on recent research in the field of developmental disabilities, updates on handicapped legislation developments, and news from direct care facilities. Features news of Association members and announcements of upcoming Association events. Recurring features include editorials, news of research, letters to the editor, news of members, book reviews, a calendar of events, and columns titled Spotlight On, Kudos, Moving Up, and On the Front Line. **First Published:** 1981. **Frequency:** Semiannually.

★2762★   ON THE SCENE
Pittsburgh Research Institute
5th Ave. Pl., Ste. 1711
Pittsburgh, PA 15222   Phone: (412) 255-7824
Description: Covers injury and trauma information, research, and policy affecting trauma center programs. Recurring features include notices of publications available and columns titled Legislative Update and Trauma Registry Corner. **First Published:** Summer 1989. **Frequency:** Quarterly.

★2763★   ON YOUR MARK
The Sugar Association, Inc.
1101 15th St. NW
Washington, DC 20005   Phone: (202) 785-1122
Description: Presents news and information on nutrition and fitness. Recurring features include letters to the editor, news of research, and notices of publications available. **First Published:** 1989.

★2764★   ONA NEWSLETTER
Ontario Nurses' Association
85 Grenville St., Ste. 600
Toronto, ON, Canada M5S 3A2   Phone: (416) 964-8833
Description: Highlights labor, education, and procedural issues affecting the nursing profession. **First Published:** 1974. **Frequency:** Monthly.

★2765★   ONCO-LOGIC
Patient Advocates for Advanced Cancer Treatments, Inc.
1143 Parmelee NW
Grand Rapids, MI 49504   Phone: (616) 453-1477
Description: Contains reviews of current publications of prostate cancer research. Recurring features include reports of meetings and lists of affiliated prostate cancer research physicians. **First Published:** 1991. **Frequency:** 4/yr.

★2766★   ONCOLOGY ISSUES
Association of Community Cancer Centers
11600 Nebel St., Ste. 201
Rockville, MD 20852   Phone: (301) 984-9496
Description: Provides information on community cancer programs for cancer care providers, including physicians, nurses, social workers, and other health professionals. Also carries news on legislation and new programs and concepts in cancer prevention. Recurring features include Association announcements regarding membership, workshops, and conferences. **First Published:** 1986. **Frequency:** Quarterly. **ISSN:** 1046-3356.

★2767★   ONCONEWS NEWSLETTER
Comprehensive Cancer Center
Columbia University
701 W. 168th St.
New York, NY 10032   Phone: (212) 305-6905
Description: Describes activities and programs of the Center, new treatments and research into cancer at the Columbia-Presbyterian Medical Center, and shared core resources available to researchers and clinicians. **First Published:** 1988. **Frequency:** 3/yr.

★2768★   ONE-IN-TEN
Technical Support Programme
Rehabilitation International
25 E. 21st St.
New York, NY 10010   Phone: (212) 420-1500
Description: Focuses on childhood disabilities, their prevention and rehabilitation. **First Published:** 1980. **Frequency:** Quarterly.

★2769★   ONTARIO ASSOCIATION OF DIRECTORS OF HEALTHCARE VOLUNTEER SERVICES—BULLETIN
Ontario Association of Directors of Healthcare Volunteer Services
150 Ferrand Dr.
Don Mills, ON, Canada M3C 1H6   Phone: (416) 429-2661
Description: Discusses issues relating to volunteer administration, primarily in the health care setting. Recurring features include reports of meetings, guest columnists, and health care film reviews. **First Published:** 1969. **Frequency:** 3/yr.

★2770★   ONTARIO HEALTH RECORD ASSOCIATION—NEWS & VIEWS
Ontario Health Record Association Secretariat
c/o P. Huelin
R.R. 1, 3924 Doane Rd. E.
Sharon, ON, Canada L0G 1V0   Phone: (416) 473-1411
Description: Publishes educational information for health record personnel in Ontario. **Frequency:** Quarterly.

★2771★   OPEN MINDS
Behavioral Health Industry News, Inc.
4465 Old Harrisburg Rd.
Gettysburg, PA 17325   Phone: (717) 334-1329
Description: Provides information on marketing, financial, and legal trends in the delivery of mental health and chemical dependency benefits and services. Recurring features include interviews, news of research, a calendar of events, job listings, book reviews, notices of publications available, and industry statistics. **First Published:** April 1988. **Frequency:** Monthly. **ISSN:** 1043-3880.

★2772★ OPPORTUNITY
Public Relations Department
National Industries for the Blind
524 Hamburg Tpke.
Wayne, NJ 07474-0969   Phone: (201) 595-9200
Description: Publishes news and feature articles on agencies for the blind and describes industries, agencies, and projects that employ blind workers. Recurring features include a personality profile, conference news, and news of programs and events of various associations for the blind. **Frequency:** Quarterly.

★2773★ OPTIONS
Center for Population Options
1025 Vermont Ave. NW, No. 210
Washington, DC 20005   Phone: (202) 347-5700
Description: Features information on improving the quality of life for adolescents by preventing too-early childbearing. Seeks to improve adolescent decision-making through life planning and sexuality education programs. Promotes access to comprehensive health care, including family planning through school- and community-based clinics. Educates on the prevention and spread among adolescents of HIV/AIDS and other sexually transmitted diseases. Recurring features include letters to the editor, interviews, news of research, a calendar of events, reports of meetings, book reviews, and notices of publications available. **First Published:** 1980. **Frequency:** Quarterly.

★2774★ THE OPTOMETRIST'S PATIENT NEWSLETTER
Doctor's Press, Inc.
Pitney Rd.
PO Box 11177
Lancaster, PA 17605   Phone: (717) 393-1010
Description: Carries patient-oriented articles on vision and eye health topics such as prevention and detection of eye disease, new vision products and technologies, and eye safety. **First Published:** 1988. **Frequency:** Quarterly.

★2775★ THE ORBIT
Hadley School for the Blind
700 Elm St.
Winnetka, IL 60093   Phone: (708) 446-8111
Description: Contains news on Hadley courses designed for serving blind students by correspondence at the national and international levels. Features articles on long-range plans, students and faculty members, school history, and programs for students and parents of blind children. Recurring features include news of educational opportunities and columns titled Honor Roll and From the President. **First Published:** 1974. **Frequency:** 2/yr.

★2776★ ORNITHOLOGICAL NEWSLETTER
American Ornithologists' Union
National Museum of Natural History
Smithsonian Institution
Washington, DC 20560   Phone: (202) 357-1970
Description: Provides information of interest to ornithologists. Recurring features include listings of available grants and awards, news of members, a calendar of events, activities of sponsoring societies, notices of employment opportunities, and notices of publications available. Members of sponsoring societies. **First Published:** October 1976. **Frequency:** Bimonthly. **ISSN:** 0274-564X.

★2777★ ORPHAN DISEASE UPDATE
National Organization for Rare Disorders
PO Box 8923
New Fairfield, CT 06812-1783   Phone: (203) 746-6518
Description: Disseminates information about rare disorders and orphan drugs, which are used to treat rare disorders but are not commercially attractive because they are not profitable. Evaluates the actions of government, industry, and volunteer agencies relevant to rare disorders and orphan drugs. Lists research projects being conducted and orphan drugs being manufactured. Recurring features include editorials, letters to the editor, news of voluntary agencies, and health-related congressional news. **First Published:** 1983. **Frequency:** 3/yr. **ISSN:** 0887-0306.

★2778★ ORTHOTICS AND PROSTHETICS TODAY
American Orthotic and Prosthetic Association
1650 King St., Ste. 500
Alexandria, VA 22314   Phone: (703) 836-7116
Description: Contains information on current activities and developments in the field of orthotics and prosthetics. **First Published:** 1989. **Frequency:** 2/yr.

★2779★ OSLA NEWSLETTER
Ontario Association of Speech-Language Pathologists and Audiologists
410 Jarvis St.
Toronto, ON, Canada M4Y 2G6   Phone: (416) 920-3676
Description: Informs speech-language pathologists and audiologists of relevant developments in Ontario. **Frequency:** Quarterly.

★2780★ OSTEOGENESIS IMPERFECTA FOUNDATION—BREAKTHROUGH
Osteogenesis Imperfecta Foundation, Inc.
5005 W. Laurel St., No. 210
Tampa, FL 33607-3836   Phone: (201) 489-9232
Description: Offers ways of coping with osteogenesis imperfecta. Covers chapter and area coordinator news, information on clinics, fund raising, education, new products, and treatment. Written by parents, patients, physicians, and researchers. Recurring features include news of research, book reviews, reports of meetings and conferences, an annual report, and columns titled Parents' Forum and In the Spotlight. **First Published:** 1970. **Frequency:** Quarterly.

★2781★ OSTEOPATHIC COLLEGE OF OPHTHALMOLOGY AND OTORHINOLARYNGOLOGY—NEWS LETTER
Osteopathic College of Ophthalmology and Otorhinolaryngology
Academy Office
405 Grand Ave.
Dayton, OH 45405   Phone: (513) 224-0138
Description: Presents articles related to health care, the osteopathic profession, and the specialized fields of eye, ear, nose, and throat medicine. **Frequency:** Quarterly.

★2782★ OTO REVIEW
House Ear Institute
2100 W. 3rd St., 5th Fl.
Los Angeles, CA 90057   Phone: (213) 483-4431
Description: Reports Institute and staff activities and provides information on other organizations and individuals involved in hearing research. Discusses subjects related to hearing impairment such as "nerve deafness," cochlear implants, hearing aids, audiology tests, and problems encountered by deaf children and their parents. Recurring features include news of members, news of research, a calendar of events and columns titled Question-and-Answer, Patient of the Month, and Personality Profile. **First Published:** 1968. **Frequency:** 3/yr.

★2783★ OUR PEACEFUL WORLD
Alex Jack
PO Box 10
Becket, MA 01223   Phone: (413) 623-2322
Description: Provides information on macrobiotics, a lifestyle based on a balanced diet consisting mostly of whole grains and vegetables that is held to promote health and well-being. **First Published:** 1989. **Frequency:** Quarterly.

★2784★ OUR VOICE NEWSLETTER
Our Voice
799 Broadway, Ste. 640
New York, NY 10003
Description: Addresses the needs of patients with spasmodic dysphonia, a neurological disorder that disables the vocal cords. Provides information on the disorder. Discusses therapies and coping strategies. Reports on current legislation, support groups, conferences, and research developments. Recurring features include letters to the editor, news of research, a calendar of events, and reports of meetings. **Frequency:** Semiannual.

★2785★ OUTLOOK ON AGING: FLORIDA
Center for Gerontological Studies
University of Florida
3357 Turlington Hall
Gainesville, FL 32611   Phone: (904) 392-2116
Description: Provides information on better living for the elderly. **Frequency:** Semiannual.

★2786★ OVULATION METHOD NEWSLETTER
Ovulation Method Teachers Association
PO Box 101780
Anchorage, AK 99510   Phone: (907) 344-8606
Description: Disseminates information on the ovulation method of birth control and natural family planning for the continuing education of teachers, health professionals, and the public. Includes notices of educational materials available, news of the Association's educational programs, and teaching tips. **Frequency:** Quarterly.

★2787★ THE P&L CONNECTION
Paul & Lisa, Inc.
PO Box 348
Westbrook, CT 06498   Phone: (203) 399-5338
Description: Promotes the organization's goals of increasing the awareness of sexual abuse and exploitation of children with the aim of eradicating it from our society. Describes the organization's streetwork-outreach program with child prostitutes. Provides informational articles, profiles of volunteer activities, and a calendar of events. Also carries columns titled From the Director's Chair, Bits-'n-Pieces, and A Short Walk with the Street Team. **First Published:** 1981. **Frequency:** 2-3/yr.

★2788★ P M NEWS
Phobia Clinic
White Plains Hospital Medical Center
Davis Ave. at Post Rd.
White Plains, NY 10601   Phone: (914) 681-1038
Description: Discusses the treatment of phobias. Carries items from readers on phobic reactions and recovery techniques. Recurring features include announcements of self-help group meetings, a list of telephone numbers of "Phobia Aides" who practice Contextual Therapy regarding phobias and panic, and a question-and-answer column by Manuel D. Zane, M.D. **First Published:** 1973. **Frequency:** Bimonthly.

★2789★ PACIFIC BASIN REHABILITATION RESEARCH AND TRAINING CENTER—NEWSLETTER
Pacific Basin Rehabilitation Research & Training Center
226 N. Kuakini St., Rm. 233,
Honolulu, HI 96817   Phone: (808) 537-5986
Description: Focuses on Center's research, training activities, and rehabilitation services. Recurring features include news of research, a calendar of events, and reports of meetings. **First Published:** January 1985. **Frequency:** Semiannual.

★2790★ PACIFIC HEALTH BULLETIN
PO Box 112
Pearl Harbor, HI 96860-5040   Phone: (808) 471-9505
Description: Deals primarily with preventive medicine and occupational health issues of interest to Navy personnel. Coverage includes environmental/ecology and medical topics. **Frequency:** Bimonthly.

★2791★ PARAPLEGIA NEWS
Paralyzed Veterans of America
5201 N. 19th Ave., Ste. 111
Phoenix, AZ 85015   Phone: (602) 246-9426
Description: Presents articles and briefs on wheelchair living, education, employment, housing, transportation, travel, spinal cord injury, research, legislation, new products, and sports and recreation for the wheelchair user. **First Published:** 1946. **Frequency:** Monthly. **ISSN:** 0031-1766.

★2792★ PARENT CARE
Gerontology Center
University of Kansas
4089 Dole Center
Lawrence, KS 66045   Phone: (913) 864-4130
Description: Provides information on research, programs, and educational materials for professionals and families involved in caring for the elderly. Acts as a clearinghouse for supportive materials addressing caregiver issues and concerns. Recurring features include book reviews, notices of publications available, and columns titled What Do You Think and Readers Respond. **First Published:** November 1985. **Frequency:** Bimonthly. **ISSN:** 0883-2843.

★2793★ PARENT CARE, INC. NEWSBRIEF
Parent Care, Inc.
9041 Colgate St.
Indianapolis, IN 46268-1210   Phone: (317) 872-9913
Description: Provides information on prematurity, special needs, chronic

illness, neonatal intensive care units, and parent support groups. Recurring features include news of research, a calendar of events, and book reviews. **First Published:** 1982. **Frequency:** Quarterly.

★2794★ PARENT NEWS
Center for Persons With Disabilities
Utah State University
Logan, UT 84322-6845   Phone: (801) 750-1991
Description: Provides news of interest concerning handicapped children. **Frequency:** Quarterly.

★2795★ PARENTS/FAMILY NEWSLETTER
Barbara Akin
3106 N. 42nd St.
Phoenix, AZ 85018   Phone: (602) 956-1459
Description: Provides news of developments regarding blind parents who raise sighted children. Includes information on helping children with homework, using home computers, infant care, dealing with blindness, and interviews with parents. **First Published:** 1984. **Frequency:** 6/yr.

★2796★ PARKINSON REPORT
National Parkinson Foundation
1501 NW 9th Ave.
Bob Hope Rd.
Miami, FL 33136   Phone: (305) 547-6666
Description: Carries news of the programs of the Foundation, which is involved in the diagnosis, treatment, care, and rehabilitation of victims of Parkinson's Disease. Provides research updates from around the country, human interest stories, and articles on drugs and medication, neuroscience, and physical medicine and rehabilitation. Recurring features include editorials; letters to the editor; news of fund raising events, gifts, meetings, and symposia; news of members; and columns titled Action Update and Message from the President. **First Published:** 1974. **Frequency:** Quarterly.

★2797★ PARKINSONIAN SPEAK-OUT
Robert Bernen
55 Merrick St.
Rumford, RI 02916-2520   Phone: (401) 435-3179
Description: Discusses the importance of active participation of therapy for Parkinson Disease patients. Recurring features include letters to the editor, interviews, reports of meetings, and book reviews. **First Published:** July 1987. **Frequency:** Monthly.

★2798★ PARKINSON'S DISEASE FOUNDATION— NEWSLETTER
Parkinson's Disease Foundation
650 W. 168th St.
New York, NY 10032   Phone: (212) 923-4700
Description: Educates the public about treatments, ongoing medical research, drug therapies, support groups, and educational programs for Parkinson's Disease. Contains news of fundraising events and publicity programs, helpful suggestions for patients, and success stories about persons with Parkinson's Disease. **First Published:** July 1979. **Frequency:** Quarterly.

★2799★ PART B NEWS
United Communications Group
11300 Rockville Pike, Ste. 1100
Rockville, MD 20852-3030   Phone: (301) 816-8950
Description: Provides explanation of rules of the Medicare Part B reimbursement program. Features news of developments on Part B law and federal regulations and funding changes, and gives advice and strategies regarding claims filing. **First Published:** May 1987. **Frequency:** Biweekly. **ISSN:** 0893-8121.

★2800★ PASSAGES
Center for Population Options
1025 Vermont Ave. NW, No. 210
Washington, DC 20005   Phone: (202) 347-5700
Description: Tracks world developments in the area of adolescent fertility. **First Published:** 1978. **Frequency:** Quarterly.

★2801★ PATHWAYS
Postgraduate Center for Mental Health
124 E. 28th St.
New York, NY 10016   Phone: (212) 689-7700
Description: Reports on the programs and developments of the four divisions of the Center: Therapeutic Services Division, Training Division,

Research Division, and Community Services and Education Division. Carries interviews, news of research, announcements of awards, editorials, news of members, and a calendar of events. **First Published:** 1983. **Frequency:** 2/yr.

★2802★ **PATHWAYS TO HEALTH**
A.R.E. Clinic, Inc.
4018 N. 40th St.
Phoenix, AZ 85018   Phone: (602) 955-0551
Description: Describes programs and services provided by the Clinic, which aims "to foster medical and scientific research and to provide holistic health care of body, mind and spirit." Carries a calendar of events and a section titled Medical Research Bulletin providing health tips and news of research. **First Published:** April 1979. **Frequency:** Quarterly.

★2803★ **PAWTRACKS**
Guide Dog Users, Inc.
c/o Kim Charlson
57 Grandview Ave.
Watertown, MA 02172   Phone: (617) 926-9198
Description: Reports on issues affecting visually impaired persons who use guide dogs. Covers "legislative affairs, electronic aids and appliances for the visually impaired, electronic aids used by guide dog users in mobility, education, public relations, employment skills, recreational facilities," plus activities of the association. **First Published:** 1972. **Frequency:** Quarterly.

★2804★ **THE PDF UPDATE**
Paget's Disease Foundation, Inc.
165 Cadman Plaza E
Brooklyn, NY 11201   Phone: (718) 596-1043
Description: Provides information about recent research on Paget's disease and news of the Foundation, its members, and activities. Informs Paget's sufferers of ways to obtain reduced-price medicines and qualified doctors who can treat the disease. **First Published:** 1978. **Frequency:** 3/yr.

★2805★ **PEDIATRIC DENTISTRY TODAY**
American Academy of Pediatric Dentistry
211 E. Chicago Ave., Ste. 1036
Chicago, IL 60611   Phone: (312) 351-8387
Description: Reports on the activities of the Academy, which seeks to advance the specialty of pediatric dentistry through practice, education, and research. Recurring features include news of research, profiles of members, and legislative updates. **First Published:** 1958. **Frequency:** 6/yr.

★2806★ **PEDIATRIC MENTAL HEALTH**
Pediatric Projects, Inc.
PO Box 571555
Tarzana, CA 91357   Phone: (818) 705-3660
Description: Serves as an information exchange concerning child hospitalization and surgery, therapeutic play programs in health centers, and emotional support for families of children with health problems. Examines current research findings. **First Published:** January 1982. **Frequency:** Bimonthly. **ISSN:** 0278-4998.

★2807★ **THE PEDIATRIC NURSE PRACTITIONER**
National Association of Pediatric Nurse Associates and Practitioners
1101 Kings Hwy., N., Ste. 206
Cherry Hill, NJ 08034   Phone: (609) 667-1773
Description: Reflects the aims of the Association, which seeks to improve the quality of infant, child, and adolescent health care by making health care services accessible and providing a forum for continuing the education of members. Includes information on legislative decisions, certification qualifications, and the health care industry in general. Provides listings of job opportunities. **Frequency:** Bimonthly.

★2808★ **PEDIATRIC REPORT'S CHILD HEALTH**
   NEWSLETTER
IGM Enterprises, Inc.
71 Hope St.
Box 155
Providence, RI 02906-2062
Description: Provides information on children's health. Discusses common and traditional questions in pediatric health care and reports current developments in pediatric medical literature through a review of more than 50 medical journals each month. **First Published:** February 1984. **Frequency:** Monthly except July.

★2809★ **PEDIATRICS FOR PARENTS**
Pediatrics for Parents, Inc.
358 Broadway, Ste. 105
PO Box 1069
Bangor, ME 04401   Phone: (207) 942-6212
Description: Provides information on children's health care and child safety. Carries original articles and abstracts on such topics as poison prevention, food labeling, and various childhood diseases and medical problems. Recurring features include letters to the editor, book reviews, and news of research. **First Published:** 1981. **Frequency:** Monthly. **ISSN:** 0730-6725.

★2810★ **PEOPLE CONCERNED FOR THE UNBORN CHILD—**
   NEWSLETTER
People Concerned for the Unborn Child
3050 Pioneer Ave.
Pittsburgh, PA 15226   Phone: (412) 531-9272
Description: Concerned with issues of importance to the right-to-life movement, including abortion, euthanasia, infanticide, fetal experimentation, and government birth control policies. Emphasizes state and federal legislation that affects these issues. Features organization news and information from allied groups. Recurring features include editorials, news of research, news of members, and a calendar of events. **First Published:** 1970. **Frequency:** Bimonthly.

★2811★ **PEOPLE-TO-PEOPLE NEWS & VIEWS**
People-to-People Committee for the Handicapped
PO Box 18131
Washington, DC 20036   Phone: (301) 774-7446
Description: Reports on international developments in services for the handicapped. Presents rehabilitation-oriented feature articles and serves as a forum for the exchange of ideas among those in the rehabilitation field. Recurring features include news of research, book reviews, reports of meetings, and a column titled People Here, People There. **First Published:** September 1959. **Frequency:** Quarterly.

★2812★ **PEOPLE WITH AIDS UPDATE**
Shanti Project
525 Howard St.
San Francisco, CA 94105-3080   Phone: (415) 777-2273
Description: Provides news of Project activities. **Frequency:** Monthly.

★2813★ **PEOPLENET**
PO Box 897
Levittown, NY 11756   Phone: (516) 579-4043
Description: Provides a forum for disabled people to meet one another. Carries articles on dating, friendship, and sexuality. Recurring features include poetry, book reviews, and personal classified ads. **First Published:** August 1987. **Frequency:** 3/yr.

★2814★ **PEOPLE'S MEDICAL SOCIETY—NEWSLETTER**
People's Medical Society
462 Walnut St.
Allenton, PA 18102   Phone: (215) 770-1670
Description: Promotes the Society's goals of giving people access to medical information previously not available outside the profession and of compelling our health care system to make reforms so that it can better serve everyone. Discusses policy issues affecting the quality and cost of health care, and profiles individuals who have fought "organized medicine." Recurring features include news about successful reform projects, editorials, letters to the editor, and a calendar of events. **First Published:** Winter 1983. **Frequency:** Bimonthly. **ISSN:** 0736-4873.

★2815★ **PEP EXCHANGE**
Parkinson's Educational Program
3900 Birch St., No. 105
Newport Beach, CA 92660   Phone: (714) 250-2975
Description: Carries items of interest to people with Parkinsonism, Parkinson's Syndrome, and Parkinson's disease, including news of current research, tips for daily living, and information about support groups. Alerts readers to new drugs, and provides information on new studies and how to volunteer for participation. Emphasizes acceptance of the illness. Recurring features include statistics, book reviews, editorials, and letters to the editor. **First Published:** January 1981. **Frequency:** Monthly.

★2816★ PERINATAL ADDICTION RESEARCH AND EDUCATION UPDATE
National Association for Perinatal Addiction Research and Education
11 E. Hubbard St., Ste. 200
Chicago, IL 60611   Phone: (312) 329-2512
Description: Provides information on NAPARE's research and education activities. Discusses treatment and childcare programs. Recurring features include news of research, a calendar of events, reports of meetings, and news of educational opportunities. **First Published:** 1988. **Frequency:** Quarterly.

★2817★ PERINATAL PRESS, INC.—NEWSLETTER
Perinatal Press, Inc.
PO Box 710698
San Diego, CA 92171   Phone: (619) 541-6875
Description: Presents abstracts and reviews of articles concerned with research and developments in perinatal and neonatal health care. Seeks to provide practical information for perinatal clinicians. Recurring features include editorials, letters to the editor, a calendar of events, and a column titled What Your Clients are Reading. **First Published:** 1977. **Frequency:** 6/yr. **ISSN:** 0160-7219.

★2818★ PERRIN & TREGGETT'S REVIEW
Thomas W. Perrin, Inc.
PO Box 190
Rutherford, NJ 07070   Phone: (201) 777-2277
Description: Focuses on the effects of alcoholism on the families of alcoholics. Discusses children of alcoholics, fetal alcohol syndrome, the genetics of alcoholism, families and alcoholism, child abuse and neglect, and eating disorders. Recurring features include information on chemical dependency and alcoholism treatment, editorials, news of research, letters to the editor, book reviews, and a list of resources for children of alcoholics. **First Published:** January 1983. **Frequency:** Irregular. **ISSN:** 0738-1395.

★2819★ PERSPECTIVES ON CATS
Cornell Feline Health Center
College of Veterinary Medicine
Cornell University
Ithaca, NY 14853   Phone: (607) 253-3414
Description: Publishes news of the Center, whose purpose is "to improve the health of cats everywhere, by developing methods to prevent or cure feline diseases, and by providing continuing education to veterinarians and cat owners." Articles about research at the Center and basic feline healthcare topics are written by faculty, staff, and students of the Center and the College of Veterinary Medicine. **First Published:** January 1980. **Frequency:** Quarterly.

★2820★ PERSPECTIVES ON DYSLEXIA
The Orton Dyslexia Society
Chester Bldg., Ste. 382
8600 LaSalle Rd.
Baltimore, MD 21204-6020   Phone: (410) 296-0232
Description: Presents articles of general interest about dyslexia, reports of Society and branch activities, and information about training programs. Recurring features include news of research, letters to the editor, news of members, and a calendar of events. **First Published:** 1975. **Frequency:** 4/yr.

★2821★ PET CARE UPDATE
Pet Care Clinics
7530 Mineral Point Rd.
Madison, WI 53717   Phone: (608) 833-6585
Description: Furnishes information on pet care and veterinary science, covering animal nutrition, diseases, and treatment. Details the Clinics' programs and services. Recurring features include news of research and columns titled Questions Our Patients Ask, Updates, Veterinary Technology, News From the World of Pet Care, and Meet Our Staff. **First Published:** Spring 1984. **Frequency:** Quarterly.

★2822★ PHARMACEUTICAL LITIGATION REPORTER
Andrews Publications
PO Box 1000
Westtown, PA 19395   Phone: (215) 399-6600
Description: "Designed for attorneys involved in litigation affecting the pharmaceutical industry and medical device manufacturers." Focuses on product liability suits, antitrust and unfair competition actions, patent and trademark infringement actions, and suits brought by and against various government agencies. Follows pretrial, trial and appellate proceedings and

offers complete texts of documents taken from the cases. **First Published:** July 1985. **Frequency:** Monthly. **ISSN:** 0887-7815.

★2823★ PHARMACIA LKB BIOTECHNOLOGY—ANALECTS
Pharmacia LKB Biotechnology, Inc.
800 Centennial Ave.
Piscataway, NJ 08854   Phone: (201) 457-8000
Description: Describes new products in the areas of molecular biology and biochemistry, discussing the products' characteristics and applications. Recurring features include news of research. **First Published:** November 1973. **Frequency:** 4/yr.

★2824★ PHARMACY NEWS
National Psoriasis Foundation
6443 SW Beaverton Hwy., Ste. 210
Portland, OR 97221   Phone: (503) 297-1545
Description: Provides consumer related articles and a comprehensive listing of over-the-counter (OTC) and prescription products for psoriasis.

★2825★ PHARMACY AND THERAPEUTICS FORUM
University of California at San Francisco
3rd Ave. & Parnassus
Box 0622
San Francisco, CA 94143-0622   Phone: (415) 476-4240
Description: Features excerpts of Pharmacy and Therapeutics Committee actions and articles on the pharmaceutical industry. **Frequency:** Bimonthly.

★2826★ PHARMACY TODAY
American Pharmaceutical Association
2215 Constitution Ave. NW
Washington, DC 20037   Phone: (202) 628-4410
Description: Covers news and information of interest to pharmacists and reports on federal and state legislation and regulation of pharmaceutical products and dispensing pharmacists. Covers developments at the Food and Drug Administration, in congressional and Association committees, and in Medicaid. **First Published:** 1962. **Frequency:** Biweekly. **ISSN:** 0098-2814.

★2827★ PHARMASCOPE
Transpharma, Inc.
13072 Camino Del Valle
Poway, CA 92064   Phone: (619) 487-3868
Description: Reports on investigational drugs and patents and recently approved drugs. Recurring features include news of research. **First Published:** 1961. **Frequency:** Monthly. **ISSN:** 0048-3648.

★2828★ PHARMCHEM NEWSLETTER
PharmChem Laboratories, Inc.
1505A O'Brien Dr.
Menlo Park, CA 94025   Phone: (415) 328-6200
Description: Disseminates factual information on drugs and related subjects. Focuses on the problem of drug abuse and addiction. **First Published:** 1972. **Frequency:** 4/yr. **ISSN:** 0146-3128.

★2829★ PHARMINDEX
Skyline Publishers, Inc.
PO Box 1029
Portland, OR 97207   Phone: (503) 235-0071
Description: Compiles information on new, changed, and forthcoming pharmaceutical products, including description, adverse reactions, warnings, cautions, pharmacology, and related products. Recurring features include reviews of continuing education programs and information on new and changed products, package sizes, drug prices, discontinued items, and investigational drugs. **First Published:** October 1958. **Frequency:** Monthly. **ISSN:** 0031-7152.

★2830★ THE PHOENIX
United Ostomy Association, Inc.
5284 Dawes St.
San Diego, CA 92109-1231   Phone: (619) 488-4854
Description: Reports on the committees and chapters of the Association, which is dedicated to the welfare and rehabilitation of ostomy patients (ostomy is a type of surgery performed to allow normal body wastes to be expelled through a surgical opening on the abdominal wall). Supplies tips for chapter and satellite group leaders and updates on legislation that affects ostomates. Recurring features include news of research, a calendar of events, meeting reports, and news of educational opportunities. **First**

Published: October 1, 1986. **Frequency:** Monthly, except March and August.

★2831★ **THE PHYSIATRIST**
American Academy of Physical Medicine and Rehabilitation
122 S. Michigan Ave., Ste. 1300
Chicago, IL 60603-6107   Phone: (312) 922-9366
Description: Seeks to foster better communication between members of the Academy and the profession. Presents news of the activities of the Academy's committees and its Board of Governors, and carries information pertaining to the practice of physical medicine and rehabilitation. Recurring features include news of research, editorials, news of members, a calendar of events, and reports from legislative, education, and policy specialists. **First Published:** March 1985. **Frequency:** 10/yr.

★2832★ **PHYSICAL DISABILITIES SPECIAL INTEREST SECTION—NEWSLETTER**
Physical Disabilities Special Interest Section
American Occupational Therapy Association
1383 Piccard Dr.
Rockville, MD 20850   Phone: (301) 948-9626
Description: Focuses on the clinical management of people with physical disabilities. Publishes articles relevant to occupational therapy practice, including such topics as assessment protocols, treatment approaches, and program administration. Recurring features include editorials, news of research, case reports, bibliographies, and notices of new equipment. **First Published:** Summer 1978. **Frequency:** Quarterly. **ISSN:** 0279-411X.

★2833★ **PHYSICIAN'S MARKETING AND MANAGEMENT**
American Health Consultants, Inc.
PO Box 740056
Atlanta, GA 30374
Description: Discusses medical practice issues of physician liability, insurance tracking, Acquired Immune Deficiency Syndrome (AIDS) transfer from doctors to patients, employee rights, Medicare concerns, and advertising medical practices. **Frequency:** Monthly. **ISSN:** 1042-2625.

★2834★ **THE PHYSICIAN'S PATIENT NEWSLETTER**
Doctor's Press, Inc.
Pitney Rd.
PO Box 11177
Lancaster, PA 17605   Phone: (717) 393-1010
Description: Carries brief, non-technical articles on a variety of general health topics. Deals with such subjects as nutrition, illness prevention and treatment, and exercise. Recurring features include items on the results of recent medical research and quizzes. **First Published:** 1983. **Frequency:** Quarterly.

★2835★ **THE PHYSIOLOGIST**
The American Physiological Society
9650 Rockville Pike
Bethesda, MD 20814   Phone: (301) 530-7070
Description: Contains articles on Society affairs and announcements, as well as articles on physiology not suitable for other Society publications. **First Published:** 1957. **Frequency:** 6/yr.

★2836★ **PLANETALK**
Program Planetree
2040 Webster St.
San Francisco, CA 94115   Phone: (415) 923-3680
Description: Provides health tips and news of the Program's members and staff. Recurring features include book reviews and a calendar of events. **First Published:** 1981. **Frequency:** Irregular. Biennially.

★2837★ **PLANNED PARENTHOOD OF MINNESOTA— NETWORK NEWS**
Planned Parenthood of Minnesota
1965 Ford Pkwy.
St. Paul, MN 55116   Phone: (612) 698-2401
Frequency: Quarterly.

★2838★ **PLEDGE FOR LIFE**
Pharmaceutical Manufacturers Association of Canada
1111 Prince of Wales Dr., Ste. 302
Ottawa, ON, Canada K2P 3T2
Description: Addresses matters concerning the program, including activities, policy information, and plans.

★2839★ **PMAC INSIGHT**
Pharmaceutical Manufacturers Association of Canada
1111 Prince of Wales Dr., Ste. 302
Ottawa, ON, Canada K2C 3T2   Phone: (613) 727-1380
Description: Provides information on the Association's objectives and activities. Also provides information on developments affecting Canada's research-based pharmaceutical industry. Recurring features include letters to the editor, interviews, news of research, and reports of meetings. **First Published:** January 1981. **Frequency:** Quarterly.

★2840★ **PMS ACCESS—NEWSLETTER**
PMS Access
Madison Pharmacy Associates, Inc.
PO Box 9326
Madison, WI 53715   Phone: (608) 833-4767
Description: Updates patients and health professionals on the latest developments in research into and treatment of premenstrual syndrome (PMS). Carries book reviews, information on PMS support groups, listings of workshops and symposia, and columns titled Dimensions in PMS, Ask the Expert, and PMS Cuisine. **First Published:** May 1985. **Frequency:** Bimonthly.

★2841★ **THE PODIATRIST'S PATIENT NEWSLETTER**
Doctor's Press, Inc.
Pitney Rd.
PO Box 11177
Lancaster, PA 17605   Phone: (717) 393-1010
Description: Intended for distribution to podiatrists' patients. Carries articles and items on topics related to foot health. **First Published:** 1983. **Frequency:** Quarterly.

★2842★ **POLIO NETWORK NEWS**
Gazette International Networking Institute
International Polio Network
5100 Oakland Ave., No. 206
St. Louis, MO 63110   Phone: (314) 534-0475
Description: Serves as a communications network for polio survivors, support groups, and health professionals. Highlights the late effects of postpolio syndrome, its cause, treatment, and latest research. Contains information on independent living and psychological support. Recurring features include news of research, a calendar of events, notices of publications available, a directory of clinics and health professionals, and notices of regional and national seminars. **First Published:** November 1985. **Frequency:** Quarterly.

★2843★ **POLITICAL STETHOSCOPE**
American Medical Political Action Committee
1101 Vermont Ave. NW
Washington, DC 20005   Phone: (202) 789-7400
Description: Focuses on physicians and spouses who are actively involved in the political process of running for office or working on election campaigns. Promotes AMPAC educational programs and activities. **Frequency:** Quarterly.

★2844★ **POPULATION TODAY**
Population Reference Bureau, Inc.
777 14th St. NW
Washington, DC 20005   Phone: (202) 785-4664
Description: Carries population-related news, including items on trends, demography (U.S. and worldwide), family planning, and ecology. Reviews news of the developing world and world political events, food production, and other population organizations. Includes book reviews and features articles on countries, cities, and states. **First Published:** August 1973. **Frequency:** Monthly. **ISSN:** 0749-2448.

★2845★ **PORPHYRIA NEWS**
American Porphyria Foundation
PO Box 1075
Santa Rosa Beach, FL 32459   Phone: (904) 654-4754
Description: Reviews current research and new treatments related to the disease porphyria, which causes an extreme sensitivity to light. Recurring features include historical notes and a calendar of events. **First Published:** 1983. **Frequency:** Quarterly.

★2846★ POYNTER CENTER NEWSLETTER
Poynter Center for the Study of Ethics in American Institutions
Indiana University
410 N. Park Ave.
Bloomington, IN 47405   Phone: (812) 855-0261
Description: Focuses on Center programs in American institutions, such as political institutions, legal system, science and technology, medicine, media, military, business, academia, and other areas. **First Published:** Fall 1986. **Frequency:** Semiannual.

★2847★ PRAIRIE ROSE
North Dakota Nurses Association
212 N. 4th St.
Bismarck, ND 58501   Phone: (701) 223-1385
Description: Covers nursing and health care issues in North Dakota. **First Published:** 1933. **Frequency:** Quarterly.

★2848★ PREHOSPITAL CARE REPORTS
American Health Consultants, Inc.
3525 Piedmont Rd., NE
6 Piedmont Center, Ste. 400
Atlanta, GA 30305   Phone: (404) 351-4523

★2849★ PRESCRIPTION AND OTC PHARMACEUTICALS— THE PINK SHEET
F-D-C Reports, Inc.
5550 Friendship Blvd., Ste. 1
Chevy Chase, MD 20815   Phone: (301) 657-9830
Description: Cover developments affecting the prescription and over-the-counter medicine industry, including regulatory policies and actions by the FDA, FTC, Congress, the courts, and other federal and state agencies. Tracks mergers and acquisitions, new products, drug reimbursement initiatives, research and development, biotechnology start-ups, international developments, manufacturing and distribution, and retail sales. Recurring features include columns titled In Brief, NDA Approvals, Recalls and FDA Seizures, Generic Drug Approvals, and F-D-C Stock Index. **First Published:** 1939. **Frequency:** Weekly.

★2850★ THE PRESS REPORT
American Health Consultants, Inc.
67 Peachtree Park Dr.
Atlanta, GA 30309   Phone: (404) 351-4523
Description: Covers practice marketing and management for dentists. **First Published:** 1984. **Frequency:** Monthly (except June and December).

★2851★ PRESSURE
Undersea and Hyperbaric Medical Society
9650 Rockville Pike
Bethesda, MD 20814   Phone: (301) 571-1818
Description: Provides a forum for professional scientific communication concerning life sciences and human factors aspects of the underseas environment. Recurring features include notices of forthcoming scientific meetings and physician training courses in the field of hyperbaric medicine, book reviews, and obituaries. **First Published:** 1972. **Frequency:** Bimonthly.

★2852★ PRIDE NEWSLETTER
National Parents' Resource Institute for Drug Education
50 Hurt Plaza, Ste. 210
Atlanta, GA 30303   Phone: (404) 577-4500
Description: Discusses the legal, pharmacological, psychological, social, cultural, and physiological effects of adolescent drug use. Gives overviews and updates of research and current events in the field. Recurring features include statistics and columns titled Pride Editorials, National Overview, Drug Overview, Scientific Overview, Book Look, Capital Comments, and Georgia Update. **First Published:** Summer 1978. **Frequency:** Quarterly.

★2853★ PRIMAL INSTITUTE—NEWSLETTER
Primal Institute
1950 Cotner Ave.
Los Angeles, CA 90025   Phone: (213) 478-0167
Description: Focuses on developments and research in primal therapy in regard to science, medicine, society, and culture. Emphasizes how health, child care, and human relationships relate to primal therapy. Recurring features include editorials, letters to the editor, book reviews, news of members, a calendar of events, and interviews. **First Published:** September 1978. **Frequency:** Bimonthly. **ISSN:** 0164-5056.

★2854★ PRIMARY CARE REPORTS
American Health Consultants, Inc.
3525 Piedmont Rd. NE
6 Piedmont Center, Ste. 400
Atlanta, GA 30305   Phone: (404) 351-4523
Description: Covers topics in clinical medicine for internists and family physicians. Focuses on one major topic per issue. **First Published:** 1985. **Frequency:** Monthly. **ISSN:** 0893-9837.

★2855★ PRIMUM NON NOCERE
World Federation of Doctors Who Respect Human Life
PO Box 508
Oak Park, IL 60303   Phone: (312) 848-3835
Description: Reflects the Federation's commitment to the "traditional Hippocratic medical position" through opposition to abortion, suicide, and direct euthanasia. Monitors developments in these areas. Recurring features include information on Federation educational programs and other activities, news of members, and a calendar of events. **First Published:** 1980. **Frequency:** Quarterly.

★2856★ PRINCE EDWARD ISLAND COUNCIL OF THE DISABLED—NEWSLETTER
Prince Edward Island Council of the Disabled, Inc.
PO Box 2128
Charlottetown, PE, Canada C1A 7N7   Phone: (902) 892-9149
Description: Provides an update on the activities and programs of the Council. Also reports on local and national issues concerning accessibility, housing, transportation, education, human rights, sport and recreation, and technical aids for persons with disabilities. Recurring features include news from the Board of Directors, reports from disability groups and associations, and a directory of disability groups of Prince Edward Island. **First Published:** October 1987. **Frequency:** 4/yr.

★2857★ PRIORITY PARENTING
Tamra B. Orr
PO Box 1793
Warsaw, IN 46581-1793   Phone: (219) 453-3864
Description: Offers commentary "geared for those parents who raise their children according to nature, not society." Explores such topics as home birth, prolonged breast-feeding, family beds, immunizations, home schooling, and related issues. Recurring features include book reviews, letters to the editor, notices of publications available, poems, and a section listing names and addresses of pen pals. **First Published:** May 1987. **Frequency:** Monthly.

★2858★ PRISM
New York State Institute for Basic Research in Developmental Disabilities
1050 Forest Hill Rd.
Staten Island, NY 10314-6399   Phone: (718) 494-5172
Description: Reports on Institute events and activities. Provides information on education, research, and services in the area of developmental disabilities. Recurring features include interviews, news of research, a calendar of events, and reports of meetings. **First Published:** 1987. **Frequency:** Quarterly.

★2859★ PROBE
Biotechnology Institute
Pennsylvania State University
519 Wartik Laboratory
University Park, PA 16802   Phone: (814) 863-3650
Description: Focuses on Institute research, programs, and seminars. **First Published:** December 1988. **Frequency:** 3/yr.

★2860★ PRO-CHOICE NEWS
Canadian Abortion Rights Action League
344 Bloor St. W., No. 306
Toronto, ON, Canada M5S 3A7   Phone: (416) 961-1507
Description: Provides news and commentary relating to the purpose of the League, which is "to ensure that no woman in Canada is denied access to safe legal abortion." Follows the League's actions to help establish comprehensive contraceptive and abortion services across Canada. Recurring features include news of research, notices of publications available, and columns titled Medical Update, Around the World, You Asked Us, You Told Us, President's Report, and Report From Parliament Hill. **First Published:** 1975. **Frequency:** 4/yr. **ISSN:** 0836-7221.

★2861★ PROGRESS
American Liver Foundation
1425 Pompton Ave.
Cedar Grove, NJ 07009   Phone: (201) 256-2550
Description: Reports on research awards and fellowships directed toward finding the causes, treatments, and cures for liver diseases. Includes updates on latest research advances, new or improved treatments, and patient-support programs. Gives information on the Foundation and its chapters. **First Published:** Spring 1980. **Frequency:** Quarterly.

★2862★ PROGRESS IN INFLAMMATORY BOWEL DISEASE
Crohn's & Colitis Foundation of America
444 Park Ave., S.
New York, NY 10016-7374   Phone: (212) 685-3440
Description: Publishes news of clinical, medical, and research developments in Crohn's disease (ileitis) and ulcerative colitis, which are painful, chronic digestive diseases. Maintains an up-to-date bibliography of medical journal articles in the field. Recurring features include book reviews and news of research. **First Published:** 1976. **Frequency:** 3/yr.

★2863★ PROJECT HOPE—ALUMNI BULLETIN
Project Hope
People-to-People Health Foundation, Inc.
Millwood, VA 22646   Phone: (703) 837-2100

★2864★ PRO-LIFE ACTION LEAGUE—ACTION NEWS
Pro-Life Action League
6160 N. Cicero Ave.
Chicago, IL 60646   Phone: (312) 777-2900
Description: Describes actions taken by the League and the results of media appearances by Scheidler, the League's director. Recurring features include editorials. **First Published:** 1980. **Frequency:** Quarterly.

★2865★ PROLIFE NEWS
Alliance for Life
B1-90 Garry St.
Winnipeg, MB, Canada R3C 4H1   Phone: (204) 942-4772
Description: Reports on developments in the areas of abortion, infanticide, and euthanasia in Canada. Recurring features include research news, interviews, reports of meetings, and book and video reviews. **First Published:** 1973. **Frequency:** Monthly. **ISSN:** 0715-4356.

★2866★ PROVENTIL ADVISOR
PACE, Inc.
PO Box 3010
Teaneck, NJ 07666
Description: Concerned with the importance of using medication to provide relief of asthma. Relates success stories of individuals with asthma; offers resource guides; answers questions on asthma; and provides guidelines of what to do when experiencing an asthma attack. **First Published:** 1991.

★2867★ PRT NEWSLETTER
Biostructures Participating Research Team
University City Science Center
Biostructures Institute
3401 Market St., Ste. 320
Philadelphia, PA 19104   Phone: (215) 386-1912
Description: Provides news on scientific reports concerning biostructures. Includes program announcements. **Frequency:** Annual.

★2868★ PSR REPORTS
Physicians for Social Responsibility, Inc.
1000 16th St. NW, Ste. 810
Washington, DC 20036   Phone: (202) 785-3777
Description: Dedicated to informing the public of the medical consequences of nuclear war and environmental catastrophes. Focuses on such topics as disarmament talks, nuclear weapons production, and the environment and public health. Recurring features include grassroots organizing news, announcements of symposia and other events, editorials, and legislative updates. **First Published:** January 1980. **Frequency:** 3/yr. **ISSN:** 0894-6264.

★2869★ PSYCH DISCOURSE
Association of Black Psychologists
PO Box 55999
Washington, DC 20040   Phone: (202) 722-0808
Description: Publishes news of the Association, whose aim is to "address the long neglected needs of Black professionals and begin to positively impact upon the mental health of the national Black community by means of planning, programs, services, training, and advocacy." Recurring features include editorials, news of research, letters to the editor, a calendar of events, and columns titled Social Actions, Chapter News, Publications, and Members in the News. **First Published:** 1970. **Frequency:** Bimonthly.

★2870★ PSYCHOHISTORY NEWS
International Psychohistorical Association
PO Box 314
New York, NY 10024   Phone: (718) 857-8075
Description: Includes news of Association events, abstracts of papers presented at the Association convention, conference announcements, events in the psychohistorical field, and lists of related publications. **First Published:** 1977. **Frequency:** Semiannually.

★2871★ PSYCHOLOGICAL SCIENCE AGENDA
Science Directorate
American Psychological Association
750 1st St. NE
Washington, DC 20002   Phone: (202) 955-7653
Description: Disseminates information on scientific psychology, including news on activities of the Association and congressional and federal advocacy efforts of the Directorate. Recurring features include reports of meetings, news of research, notices of publications available, interviews, and the columns titled Science Directorate News, On Behalf of Science, Science Briefs, Announcements, and Funding Opportunities. **Frequency:** Bimonthly. **ISSN:** 1040-404X.

★2872★ PSYCHOSOCIAL NEWS
National Hemophilia Foundation
110 Green St., Rm. 406
New York, NY 10012   Phone: (212) 219-8180
Description: Addresses the psychosocial aspects of hemophilia. Discusses social attitudes and stigmas regarding hemophiliacs and offers advice for coping with these problems. Recurring features include news of research, medical updates, and news of members. **Frequency:** Quarterly.

★2873★ PSYCHOTHERAPY BULLETIN
Division of Psychotherapy
American Psychological Association
3875 N. 44th St., Ste. 102
Phoenix, AZ 85018   Phone: (602) 956-8656
Description: Recurring features include letters to the editor, news of research, reports of meetings, news of educational opportunities, committee reports, legislative issues, and columns titled Washington Scene, Finance, Marketing, Professional Liability, Medical Psychology Update, and Substance Abuse. **First Published:** 1965. **Frequency:** Quarterly.

★2874★ PSYCHOTHERAPY TODAY
Atcom Inc.
2315 Broadway, No. 300
New York, NY 10024   Phone: (212) 873-5900
Description: Covers clinical developments in therapy, practice management and marketing, legal issues, and newest trends in mental health counseling. **Frequency:** Monthly.

★2875★ PUBLIC HEALTH FOUNDATION—NEWSLETTER
Public Health Foundation
1220 L St. NW
Washington, DC 20005   Phone: (202) 898-5600
Description: Serves to promote the aim of the Foundation, which is to strengthen health activities "in order to improve the health of all Americans." Reports on Public Health Foundation's projects, including workshops, grants to states, hotlines, and publications on timely health policy and health data issues. Recurring features include a calendar of events. **First Published:** May 1988. **Frequency:** Quarterly.

★2876★ PUBLIC HEALTH MACROVIEW
Public Health Foundation
1220 L St. NW
Washington, DC 20005   Phone: (202) 898-5600
Description: Provides information on expenditures and services of the nation's state health agencies and local health departments. Highlights state's progress toward meeting selected Healthy People 2000 objectives. Contains announcements of newly released publications and ordering information. **First Published:** January 1988. **Frequency:** 6/yr.

★2877★ PULSE
Canadian Health Care Guild
17410 107th Ave., No. 200
Edmonton, AB, Canada T5S 1E9　　　　Phone: (403) 483-8126
Description: Provides members with updates on opportunities for continuing professional education and employment as well as updates on union activities to promote effective and compassionate health care for patients. Recurring features include a calendar of events, meeting reports, articles, a financial column, and columns titled Pulse Beat, Just for the Health of It, and Let's Talk Labour. **First Published:** 1980. **Frequency:** Bimonthly. **ISSN:** 0706-2192.

★2878★ THE PUN
Parents United International, Inc.
232 E. Gish Rd., 1st Fl.
San Jose, CA 95112　　　　Phone: (408) 453-7611
Description: Publishes news of Parents United, a peer support group for people who were sexually abused as children or who are parents or relatives of sexually abused children. Devotes space to news of Daughters & Sons United (a children's peer support group) and Adults Molested as Children United, which are the guided components of Parents Unlimited International, Inc. Provides personal stories and chapter information. **First Published:** 1975. **Frequency:** Quarterly.

★2879★ PURE FACTS
Feingold Association of the United States
PO Box 6550
Alexandria, VA 22306　　　　Phone: (703) 768-3287
Description: Promotes the use of the dietary management program devised by Dr. Ben F. Feingold, which claims to alleviate overactivity, anxiety, aggression, sleep disturbances, and learning disabilities. Disseminates information on the Feingold program and on products that have been researched and found to be free of certain synthetic additives. Seeks to "generate public awareness of the potential role of food and synthetic additives in behavior, learning and health problems." Recurring features include news of local and national groups, news of members, and news of research. **Frequency:** 10/yr.

★2880★ QA SECTION CONNECTION NEWSLETTER
American Health Information Association
919 N. Michigan Ave., Ste. 1400
Chicago, IL 60611-1601　　　　Phone: (312) 787-2672
Description: Covers issues of quality assurance in medical record practice. **First Published:** 1983. **Frequency:** Bimonthly. **ISSN:** 1040-2950.

★2881★ QRC ADVISOR
Aspen Publishers, Inc.
1600 Research Blvd.
Rockville, MD 20850　　　　Phone: (301) 251-5554
Description: Offers advice on critical quality assurance, risk management, and cost control issues. **Frequency:** Monthly.

★2882★ QUALITY CARE ADVOCATE
National Citizens' Coalition for Nursing Home Reform
1424 16th St. NW, Ste. L-2
Washington, DC 20036　　　　Phone: (202) 797-0657
Description: Reports on current efforts at federal, state, and local levels to achieve better quality nursing homes in the U.S. Discusses current legislation and regulations, summarizes current litigation proceedings and past court cases related to nursing home care, and evaluates the effectiveness of various direct advocacy campaigns. Recurring features include news of research and notices of publications available. **First Published:** January 1986. **Frequency:** Bimonthly. **ISSN:** 0892-6174.

★2883★ QUALITY CONTROL REPORTS—THE GOLD SHEET
F-D-C Reports, Inc.
5550 Friendship Blvd., Ste. 1
Chevy Chase, MD 20815　　　　Phone: (301) 657-9830
Description: Covers changes in FDA policies regulating manufacturing practices for pharmaceutical companies and their suppliers. Contains information on production and quality techniques. **First Published:** 1967. **Frequency:** Monthly.

★2884★ QUICKENING
American College of Nurse-Midwives
1522 K St. NW, Ste. 1120
Washington, DC 20005　　　　Phone: (202) 347-5445
Description: Promotes the training and certification of nurse-midwives.

Recurring features include membership, board and convention news, announcements of relevant meetings and workshops, help-wanted items, and lists of significant publications. **First Published:** December 1970. **Frequency:** Bimonthly. **ISSN:** 0196-3805.

★2885★ RADIOASSAY-LIGAND ASSAY NEWS
Duwest Research/Scientific Newsletters
Rd. 4, Box 7
Stapleton Ct.
Middletown, NY 10940-9683　　　　Phone: (914) 355-9147
Description: Summarizes current news and developments in the field of radioimmunoassay and other ligand techniques. Contains information on quality control, government regulations, and new products and services, as well as scientific papers. Recurring features include a calendar of events, a bibliography, and information on educational materials relating to radio-immunoassay. **First Published:** August 1974. **Frequency:** 10/yr.

★2886★ RADIOLOGICAL HEALTH BULLETIN
Center for Devices and Radiological Health
Food and Drug Administration
5600 Fishers Lane
Rockville, MD 20857　　　　Phone: (301) 443-5860
Description: Reports on the Center's programs to eliminate "unnecessary human exposure to man-made radiation from medical, occupational, and consumer products." Recurring features include regulatory updates, listings of related publications, and a calendar of events. **First Published:** 1967. **Frequency:** Monthly.

★2887★ RADIOLOGY & IMAGING LETTER
Quest Publishing Co.
1351 Titan Way
Brea, CA 92621　　　　Phone: (714) 738-6400
Description: Provides information on new technology and procedures in radiology and imaging. Discusses new devices and products, safety hazards, government activities and legislation, and computer applications. Recurring features include news of research, a calendar of events, reports of meetings and events, news of educational opportunities, and notices of publications available. **Frequency:** Bimonthly. **ISSN:** 0741-160X.

★2888★ RATE CONTROLS
Rate Controls Publications, Inc.
PO Box 35425
Phoenix, AZ 85069　　　　Phone: (602) 242-9276
Description: Analyzes health care trends and developments. Provides an economic analysis service for health care management. Discusses statistics and financial trends in short stay hospitals. Includes editorials and columns titled Washington Issues and Hospital Market Basket Inflation. **First Published:** 1977. **Frequency:** Semimonthly.

★2889★ RDL NEWSLETTER
Foundation for Blood Research
PO Box 190
Scarborough, ME 04074　　　　Phone: (207) 883-4131
Description: Discusses projects of the Rheumatic Disease Laboratory (RDL), including new tests, existing tests, and on-going research activities. Serves as an educational newslettr designed to clarify laboratory issues such as ordering specific tests. **First Published:** January 1989. **Frequency:** Quarterly.

★2890★ REACHING OUT
Cornelia de Lange Syndrome Foundation
60 Dyer Ave.
Collinsville, CT 06022　　　　Phone: (203) 693-8353
Description: Provides updates on the medical aspects of Cornelia de Lange Syndrome, a rare birth defect resulting in low birth weight babies who continue to develop slowly, both mentally and physically. Aims to ensure early and accurate diagnosis of the syndrome and to enable families, friends, and professionals to make responsible decisions and plans for the affected child. Recurring features include letters to the editor, notices of publications available, meeting reports, news of research, and and a column titled Medical Column. **First Published:** July 1977. **Frequency:** Bimonthly.

★2891★ THE READING LIGHT: A NEWSLETTER
Handicapped Services
Mississippi Library Commission
5455 Executive Pl.
Jackson, MS 39206   Phone: (601) 354-7208
Description: Provides information on special services, aids, recent publications, and locally-produced talking books which are not available through the Library of Congress. Reviews new aids and appliances, pertinent activities and events, staff members, and related organizations. **First Published:** 1970. **Frequency:** Semiannually.

★2892★ RECEIVER
Deafness Research Foundation
9 E. 38th St.
New York, NY 10016   Phone: (212) 684-6556
Description: Provides news and information on the advances made in otologic research and sciences throughout the country. Recurring features include a calendar of events. **First Published:** 1963. **Frequency:** 4/yr.

★2893★ RECORDING FOR THE BLIND—NEWS
Recording for the Blind
20 Roszel Rd.
Princeton, NJ 08540   Phone: (609) 452-0606
Description: Reports news of the programs of Recording of the Blind, "a national, nonprofit organization that provides educational resources for those who cannot read standard print because of a visual, physical, or perceptual disability". Carries articles, features, and news about the 75,000 volume Master Tape Library, the accomplishments and achievements of those who use the recorded texts, and the volunteers who read, monitor, and prepare the tapes. Recurring features include columns titled News in Brief, Notes from the Units, and From the President. **First Published:** June 1956. **Frequency:** 3/yr.

★2894★ REFLECTIONS
American Council of the Blind Parents
c/o American Council of the Blind
1155 15th St. NW, Ste. 720
Washington, DC 20005   Phone: (202) 467-5081
Description: Offers support and a forum for the sharing of experiences among sighted parents of blind and visually impaired children and blind and visually impaired parents. Imparts cultural information about child development and monitors developments in technical and legislative arenas. Recurring features include news of research, member news, and letters to the editor. **Frequency:** Quarterly.

★2895★ REGULATORY WATCHDOG SERVICE
Washington Business Information, Inc.
1117 N. 19th St.
Arlington, VA 22209   Phone: (703) 247-3423
Description: Describes documents relating to health care, medical devices, and drugs available from the Consumer Product Safety Commission (CPSC), the Food and Drug Administration (FDA), Congress, and other agencies. Documents may be ordered through the Watchdog Service for a nominal reproduction fee. **First Published:** 1975. **Frequency:** Weekly. **ISSN:** 0275-0902.

★2896★ REHAB CONSULTANT
Paul M. Deutsch Press Inc.
2208 Hillcrest St.
Orlando, FL 32803   Phone: (407) 895-3600
Description: Covers developments in the rehabilitation professions, technological innovations, and legislation affecting disabled persons. Recurring features include news of research, book reviews, and columns titled Life Care Planning Resource Tips, Collateral Sources, and Rehab Technology. **First Published:** 1990. **Frequency:** Quarterly.

★2897★ REHAB REVIEW
California State Dept. of Rehabilitation
830 K St., Rm. 320
Sacramento, CA 95814   Phone: (916) 445-8638
Description: Discusses issues affecting persons with disabilities, including building access legislation and standards, medical and technological advances, and other special services for the disabled. Promotes the Department's programs. Recurring features include news of research, news of employee awards, and columns titled Director's Corner and Placement Pipeline. **First Published:** January 1981. **Frequency:** Bimonthly.

★2898★ REHABILITATION GAZETTE
Gazette International Networking Institute
5100 Oakland Ave., No. 206
St. Louis, MO 63108   Phone: (314) 534-0475
Description: Covers issues of interest to individuals with disabilities. Recurring features include a calendar of events and columns titled Potpourri and Friends Around the World. **First Published:** 1958. **Frequency:** Semiannual. **ISSN:** 0361-4166.

★2899★ REHABILITATION INTERNATIONAL NEWSLETTER
Rehabilitation International
25 E. 21st St.
New York, NY 10010   Phone: (212) 420-1500
Description: Provides news of organization events to member organizations and affiliates. **Frequency:** Periodic.

★2900★ REHABILITATION NEWSLETTER
National Institute for Rehabilitation Engineering
PO Box T
Hewitt, NJ 07421   Phone: (201) 853-6585
Description: Carries news of the Institute, which is a research, training, and service organization providing custom-designed tools and devices and intensive personal task-performance training to help handicapped persons become more self-sufficient. Recurring features include departmental and staff news and announcements of upcoming seminars. **Frequency:** Bimonthly.

★2901★ REHABILITATION REPORT
Hanley & Belfus Inc.
210 S. 13th St.
Philadelphia, PA 19107   Phone: (215) 546-7293
Description: Covers medical rehabilitation. **First Published:** 1986. **Frequency:** Monthly.

★2902★ REHOBOTH NEWSLETTER
Rehoboth Christian Association
PO Box 1089
Stony Plain, AB, Canada T0E 2G0   Phone: (403) 963-4044
Description: Serves the Association, which is a Christian organization for the mentally handicapped of Alberta. **First Published:** May 1975. **Frequency:** Quarterly.

★2903★ REIMBURSEMENT ADVISOR
Aspen Publishers, Inc.
200 Orchard Ridge Dr., Ste. 200
Gaithersburg, MD 20878   Phone: (301) 417-7500
Description: Provides information on health care spending and professionals. Deals with universal health insurance, physician payments, preventative services, and the industry's regulations. **Frequency:** Monthly. **ISSN:** 0884-2795.

★2904★ THE REIMBURSEMENT UPDATE
Dr. Fred R. Curtiss
355 Oak Trail Dr.
Double Oak, TX 75067   Phone: (817) 491-3593
Description: Supplies information updates on health care legislation, regulations, and other developments affecting reimbursement and financing of health care services. Recurring features include news of research. **First Published:** December 1984. **Frequency:** Quarterly.

★2905★ RELIGIOUS COALITION FOR ABORTION RIGHTS NEWSLETTER
Religious Coalition for Abortion Rights
100 Maryland Ave. NE, No. 307
Washington, DC 20002-5625   Phone: (202) 543-7032
Description: Focuses on reproductive rights and religious freedom. Carries news of national and state activities, legislative information, articles by pro-choice clergy, and conference information. Recurring features include interviews, news of research, a calendar of events, reports of meetings, book reviews, notices of publications available, and updates on the activities of the organization. **First Published:** 1973. **Frequency:** 3/yr.

★2906★ RENAL NURSING & TECHNOLOGY TODAY
Council of Nephrology Nurses & Technicians
National Kidney Foundation, Inc.
30 E. 33rd St.
New York, NY 10016   Phone: (212) 889-2210
Description: Reports on clinical topics of interest to renal nurses and

technicians. Provides news of events, programs, and other activities of the Council. Includes a calendar of events. **Frequency:** Quarterly.

★2907★ RENALIFE
American Association of Kidney Patients Inc.
111 S. Parker St., Ste. 405
Tampa, FL 33606   Phone: (813) 251-0725
Description: Gives news and information of interest to kidney patients, their families, and health care professionals. **First Published:** 1969. **Frequency:** Semiannual.

★2908★ REPORT ON DISABILITY PROGRAMS
Business Publishers, Inc.
951 Pershing Dr.
Silver Spring, MD 20910-4464   Phone: (301) 587-6300
Description: Reviews developments and issues affecting programs and services for people with disabilities. Reports on related administrative, legislative, and judicial actions, as well as on technological and managerial innovations. Recurring features include columns titled News Analysis, Around the States, Calendar of Events, and Publications and Resources. **First Published:** 1977. **Frequency:** Biweekly. **ISSN:** 0191-6734.

★2909★ REPORT, NYSNA'S OFFICIAL NEWSLETTER
New York State Nurses Association
2113 Western Ave.
Guilderland, NY 12084   Phone: (518) 456-5371
Frequency: Monthly.

★2910★ RESEARCH AT GALLAUDET
Gallaudet Research Institute
Gallaudet University
800 Florida Ave., NE
Washington, DC 20002   Phone: (202) 651-5400
Description: Details research conducted by the Institute, which involves issues related to deafness and hearing impairment, including intellectual and social development, education of the deaf, strides in communication technology, and the needs of special populations. Recurring features include news of meetings and notices of publications available. **Frequency:** Periodic.

★2911★ RESEARCH TO PREVENT BLINDNESS—PROGRESS REPORT
Research to Prevent Blindness
598 Madison Ave.
New York, NY 10022   Phone: (212) 752-4333
Description: Presents articles focusing on basic and applied research into the causes, prevention, and treatment of blinding eye diseases. Also reports on the foundation's financial support of such research through various grants. **Frequency:** Annual.

★2912★ RESEARCH PROFILES
Center for Gerontological Studies
University of Florida
3357 Turlington Hall
Gainesville, FL 32611   Phone: (904) 392-2116
Description: Discusses the Center's research in the area of gerontology. **First Published:** Fall 1987. **Frequency:** Semiannually.

★2913★ THE RESEARCH REPORTER
Worcester Foundation for Experimental Biology
222 Maple Ave.
Shrewsbury, MA 01545   Phone: (508) 842-9632
Description: Monitors current activities at the Foundation and relates ongoing research in the areas of neurobiology, cancer and cell biology, and endocrine-reproductive biology. Recurring features include items on grants and awards, personal profiles, meeting and conference reports, and a column titled Distillations. **Frequency:** 3/yr.

★2914★ RESEARCH RESOURCES REPORTER
Research Resources Information Center
National Institutes of Health
U.S. Department of Health and Human Services
1601 Research Blvd.
Rockville, MD 20850   Phone: (301) 251-4970
Description: Follows current biomedical research, especially that supported by the National Institutes of Health. Includes clinical and animal models as well as developments in biomedical research technology. Recurring features include letters to the editor, interviews, a calendar of meetings,

and columns titled Questions and Answers, Information Exchange, and Research Service. **First Published:** January 1977. **Frequency:** Monthly. **ISSN:** 0160-807X.

★2915★ RESIDENTIAL TREATMENT NEWS
American Association of Children's Residential Centers
440 First St. NW, Ste. 520
Washington, DC 20001   Phone: (202) 638-1604
Description: Serves as an in-house communication for the Association, which seeks to enhance residential treatment of emotionally disturbed children and adolescents. Provides information on federal legislative and regulatory activities and on the Association's programs. Recurring features include news of research, news of members, and a calendar of events. **First Published:** June 1979. **Frequency:** 6/yr.

★2916★ RESNA NEWS
RESNA
1101 Connecticut Ave. NW, Ste. 700
Washington, DC 20036   Phone: (202) 857-1199
Description: Monitors developments in rehabilitation technology. Covers topics such as the affect of federal health care policies on the industry, new products, and market trends. Recurring features include editorials, news of the Society and its members, book reviews, listings of job and educational opportunities, and a calendar of events. **First Published:** 1982. **Frequency:** Bimonthly. **ISSN:** 0882-2476.

★2917★ RESOLVE—NEWSLETTER
Resolve, Inc.
1310 Broadway
Somerville, MA 02144-1731   Phone: (617) 623-1156
Description: Serves to establish contact and support among members of the organization, which focuses on the problems of infertility. Provides information on medical conditions and treatments, and the emotional impact on persons involved. Recurring features include letters to the editor, news of research, book reviews, conference schedules, and requests for contact. **First Published:** Ca. 1975. **Frequency:** 4/yr. **ISSN:** 1042-0290.

★2918★ RESPITE NEWS
Texas Respite Resource Network
Box 7330
San Antonio, TX 78207-3198   Phone: (512) 228-2794
Description: Represents TRRN, "a model clearinghouse providing information and technical assistance for respite, or relief, services for citizens with developmental disabilities or chronic illnesses and their families." Recurring features include reprints of relevant articles from periodicals, a calendar of events, and a section of Newsbriefs, which provides notices of TRRN activities, notices of publications available, workshops and conferences, and general news items of interest. **First Published:** Winter 1987. **Frequency:** Quarterly.

★2919★ RESPONSE TO THE VICTIMIZATION OF WOMEN AND CHILDREN
Guilford Publications
72 Spring St.
New York, NY 10012   Phone: (212) 431-9800
Description: Concerned with issues and problems of violence against women and children, spouse abuse, child sexual abuse, elder abuse, sexual assault, and exploitation. Provides information on medical and social services, state and federal legislative developments and court actions. Recurring features include book reviews, resource listings, a calendar of events, letters to the editor, notices of workshops and seminars, funding alerts, and conference reports. **First Published:** October 1976. **Frequency:** Quarterly. **ISSN:** 0894-7597.

★2920★ RID—IN ACTION BULLETIN
Remove Intoxicated Drivers - USA, Inc.
PO Box 520
Schenectady, NY 12301   Phone: (518) 372-0034
Description: Provides information on RID campaigns and projects. **First Published:** May 1991. **Frequency:** Bimonthly.

★2921★ RID—USA NATIONAL NEWSLETTER
Remove Intoxicated Drivers - USA, Inc.
PO Box 520
Schenectady, NY 12301   Phone: (518) 372-0034
Description: Monitors enforcement of drunken driving laws and reports on legislative status of various bills throughout the country. Features articles on how different states handle drunk driving. Recurring features include

data analysis, news of chapter activities and projects, stories on victims and their families, book reviews, editorials, letters to the editor, and a calendar of events. **First Published:** 1978. **Frequency:** Quarterly.

★2922★ **RIGHT-TO-KNOW PLANNING REPORT**
Bureau of National Affairs, Inc.
1231 25th St. NW
Washington, DC 20037   Phone: (202) 452-4200
Description: Provides information on new community right-to-know issues and community emergency response programs. **First Published:** October 1, 1987. **Frequency:** Biweekly.

★2923★ **ROPE LINKS**
Pho Pi Phi Pharmacy Fraternity
c/o Robert M. Heyman
9280 Hamlin
Des Plaines, IL 60016   Phone: (312) 635-9391
Description: Carries news of this professional fraternity for pharmacists. Lists job opportunities and announces winners of society awards and scholarships. Examines developments and professional issues in the pharmaceutical industry. Recurring features include news of society activities, profiles of members, news of research, and a calendar of events. **Frequency:** 4/yr.

★2924★ **ROUNDS**
Office of Planning and Marketing
Georgetown University Hospital
2233 Wisconsin Ave. NW, Ste. 333
Washington, DC 20007   Phone: (202) 784-3102
Description: Informs the Washington, D.C. community of programs and services offered by the Hospital. Features articles on health and medical problems and on the Hospital's treatment programs. Recurring features include news of research and a calendar of events. **First Published:** Spring 1983. **Frequency:** Quarterly.

★2925★ **RPNAM UPDATE**
Registered Psychiatric Nurses Association of Manitoba
1854 Portage Ave.
Winnipeg, MB, Canada R3J 0G9   Phone: (204) 888-4841
Description: Provides a forum for communications among psychiatric nurses in Manitoba. Recurring features include letters to the editor, a calendar of events, research news, reports of meetings, notices of educational and employment opportunities, publication announcements, and a column titled Current Trends & Issues. **First Published:** 1967. **Frequency:** 2/yr.

★2926★ **RURAL HEALTH CARE**
National Rural Health Association
301 E. Armour Blvd., Ste. 420
Kansas City, MO 64111   Phone: (816) 756-3140
Description: Disseminates news and information of interest to rural health professionals to help establish a network of rural health advocates. Recurring features include interviews, news of research, a calendar of events, reports of meetings, news of educational opportunities, job listings, and notices of publications available. **First Published:** January 1985. **Frequency:** Monthly.

★2927★ **RUSH CANCER CENTER—REPORT**
Rush Cancer Center
Rush Presbyterian-St. Luke's Medical Center
1725 W. Harrison St., Ste. 817
Chicago, IL 60612   Phone: (312) 942-6028
Description: Informs health care professionals and supporters of the Center about the programs, services, and talents of Center employees. Contains basic science articles and articles on the the clinical programs, investigations, and services of the Center. Recurring features include a column titled Rush Cancer Center Profile, which highlights the career and work of different Center clinicians and information on meetings, seminars, and Center events. **First Published:** 1980. **Frequency:** Quarterly.

★2928★ **RX: LIVE WELL**
Wellness Communications, Inc.
6060 N. Central Expy., Ste. 608
Dallas, TX 75206   Phone: (214) 691-7690
Description: Designed as a direct mail piece for promoting health, which doctors, clinics, hospitals, and corporations may customize with their own masthead, personalized column, and photographs. Contains articles on topics such as nutrition, exercise, disease prevention, and stress manage-

ment. Recurring features include news of research. **First Published:** July 1983. **Frequency:** Quarterly.

★2929★ **THE RYAN ADVISORY**
Advisory Newsletter Group, Inc.
PO Drawer 90833
Washington, DC 20090   Phone: (301) 656-1995
Description: Focuses on trends in and ideas for health service governance and administration. Provides insight into national and Washington news in relation to health care. Covers topics such as strategic, educational, and volunteer programs, personnel management, strategic and facilities planning, and health care financing. Recurring features include editorials. **First Published:** May 1973. **Frequency:** Monthly.

★2930★ **SACNA NEWSLETTER**
Saskatchewan Association of Certified Nursing Assistants
2310 Smith St.
Regina, SK, Canada S4P 2P6   Phone: (306) 525-1436
Description: Serves the Association, keeping membership advised of chapter and provincial activities. **Frequency:** 4/yr.

★2931★ **SAFETY FORUM**
School & Community Safety Society of America
1900 Association Dr.
Reston, VA 22091   Phone: (703) 476-3430
Description: Covers Society activities as well as issues in school and community safety. Recurring features include news of research, reports of meetings, news of educational opportunities, and notices of publications available.

★2932★ **ST. ANTHONY'S HEALTHCARE RESOURCES ALERT**
St. Anthony Publishing
500 Montgomery St., Ste. 700
Alexandria, VA 22314   Phone: (800) 632-0123
Description: Provides information on medical records and reimbursement in the health care industry. **Frequency:** Monthly.

★2933★ **ST. ANTHONY'S PHYSICIAN RESOURCES ALERT**
St. Anthony Publishing
500 Montgomery St., Ste. 700
Alexandria, VA 22314   Phone: (800) 632-0123
Description: Provides information for physicians concerning coding and reimbursement. **Frequency:** Monthly.

★2934★ **ST. PATRICK HOSPITAL—MESSENGER**
St. Patrick Hospital
500 W. Broadway
PO Box 4587
Missoula, MT 59806   Phone: (406) 543-7271
Description: Covers health care topics, including new health technologies, exercise, and health issues for seniors. Contains occupational health news. **First Published:** 1985. **Frequency:** Monthly.

★2935★ **SALK INSTITUTE FOR BIOLOGICAL STUDIES— NEWSLETTERS**
Salk Institute for Biological Studies
PO Box 85800
San Diego, CA 92186-5800   Phone: (619) 453-4100
Description: Updates readers on activities of the Institute. **Frequency:** Periodic.

★2936★ **SALUBRITAS**
American Public Health Association
1015 15th St. NW, Ste. 300
Washington, DC 20005   Phone: (202) 789-5689
Description: Concerned with the delivery or support of public health services in developing countries. Covers planning, training, implementation, and evaluation of primary health-care services, including maternal and child health, family planning, nutrition, sanitation, and immunization. Recurring features include a readers' exchange, notices of conferences and training opportunities, and publications and materials available. **First Published:** 1977. **Frequency:** Quarterly. **ISSN:** 0191-5789.

★2937★   SAME-DAY SURGERY
American Health Consultants, Inc.
PO Box 740056
Atlanta, GA 30374   Phone: (404) 262-7436
Description: Focuses on the management, structure, and legal and medical aspects of ambulatory surgery. Carries expert opinions and recommendations on policies and procedures. **First Published:** 1977. **Frequency:** Monthly. **ISSN:** 0190-5066.

★2938★   SASKATCHEWAN ABILITIES COUNCIL—BULLETIN
Saskatchewan Abilities Council
2310 Louise Ave.
Saskatoon, SK, Canada S7J 2C7   Phone: (306) 374-4448
Description: Contains articles on issues, programs, and services concerning persons with a disability. Recurring features include interviews, a calendar of events, reports of meetings, and news of educational opportunities. **First Published:** 1971. **Frequency:** Quarterly. **ISSN:** 0929-4224.

★2939★   SASKATCHEWAN MEDICAL JOURNAL
Continuing Medical Education
University of Saskatchewan
Saskatoon, ON, Canada S7N 0W0   Phone: (306) 966-8864
Description: Presents articles on family medical practice. Recurring features include a calendar of events and letters to the editor. **First Published:** March 1990. **Frequency:** 4/yr.

★2940★   SATH NEWS
Society for the Advancement of Travel for the Handicapped
347 5th Ave., No. 610
New York, NY 10016   Phone: (212) 447-7284
Description: Provides an educational forum for the exchange of knowledge on how to better serve the handicapped traveler. Offers practical advice, health tips, information on carrier provisions (such as airlines facilities) and on other services in rail and bus terminals, hotels, and museums. Recurring features include items on available tours and awards granted for promotion of travel for the handicapped; book reviews; information on new products and on international games for the disabled; and other news relating to tourism and travel for handicapped people. **First Published:** 1978. **Frequency:** Quarterly.

★2941★   SCANNER
American Society of Radiologic Technologists
15000 Central Ave. SE
Albuquerque, NM 87123-4605   Phone: (505) 298-4500
Description: Reflects the aims of the Society, which seeks to "advance the science of radiologic technology, to establish and maintain high standards of education and training, to elevate the quality of patient care, and to improve the welfare and socioeconomics of radiologic technologists." Recurring features include news of research and news of members. **Frequency:** Bimonthly. **ISSN:** 01610-3863.

★2942★   SCEH NEWSLETTER
Society for Clinical and Experimental Hypnosis
128-A Kings Park Dr.
Liverpool, NY 13090   Phone: (315) 652-7299
Description: Provides research and clinical notes related to the field of hypnosis. Carries Society and international news, announcements of conferences and workshops, meeting reports, and notices of examinations and of awards. Recurring features include profiles of members and their activities, film and book reviews, obituaries, and information on published materials available in reprint or in journals in other fields. **First Published:** 1950. **Frequency:** Quarterly. **ISSN:** 0583-8975.

★2943★   SCENE
Braille Institute
741 N. Vermont Ave.
Los Angeles, CA 90029   Phone: (213) 663-1111
Description: Seeks to enhance public awareness about the abilities of blind or visually impaired people to enjoy full, productive, and independent lives as a result of the Institute's assistance. Promotes the Institute's educational training programs, recreational and counseling services, library and braille press services, and special events. **First Published:** 1974. **Frequency:** 3/yr.

★2944★   SCIENCE FOR THE HANDICAPPED GOOD NEWSLETTER
Science for the Handicapped Association
9613 Dallas Ave.
Silver Springs, MD 20901   Phone: (715) 832-5357
Description: Reflects the aims of the Association, which are to disseminate information about science career opportunities for the handicapped and to serve as a clearinghouse for those who are seeking information about teaching science to handicapped individuals. Identifies and describes programs, curricula, research, books, and journal articles of interest. Recurring features include editorials, news of research, news of members, book reviews, and a calendar of events. **First Published:** 1973. **Frequency:** 3/yr.

★2945★   SCIENCE/HEALTH ABSTRACT
Yuchi Pines Institute
Box 319
Ft. Mitchell, AL 36856   Phone: (205) 288-5495
Description: Provides news of interest regarding science and health. **First Published:** 1980. **Frequency:** 6/yr.

★2946★   SCLERODERMA INTERNATIONAL FOUNDATION— THE CONNECTOR
Scleroderma International Foundation
704 Gardner Center Rd.
New Castle, PA 16101   Phone: (412) 652-3109
Description: Serves as an information and support network for victims of scleroderma, a progressive skin disease. Reviews research into the cause, cure, and control of scleroderma. Recurring features include Foundation news, notes on members, and a calendar of events. **First Published:** 1971. **Frequency:** Quarterly.

★2947★   THE SCORE SHEET
Charleston Dog Training Club, Inc.
PO Box 1304
Charleston, SC 29402
Description: Discusses the activities of the Club. Covers such topics as finances, meetings, new members, training seminars for dogs, and the symptoms of medical problems. Recurring features include letters to the editor, a calendar of events, and news of members. **Frequency:** Monthly.

★2948★   THE SCRIPT
International Transactional Analysis Association
1772 Vallejo St.
San Francisco, CA 94123-5009   Phone: (415) 885-5992
Description: Communicates Association business and policy changes to members. Covers member activities, news of international developments in transactional analysis or group psychotherapy, and items of theoretical interest. Recurring features include letters to the editor, a calendar of events, and special features. **First Published:** September 1966. **Frequency:** 9/yr.

★2949★   SDA NEWSLETTER
Saskatchewan Dietetic Association
PO Box 3894
Regina, SK, Canada S4P 3R8   Phone: (306) 359-3040
Description: Provides news of upcoming events, provincial developments, job opportunities, new resources, and general information. Recurring features include letters to the editor, news of research, a calendar of events, news of educational opportunities, job listings, and notices of publications available. **Frequency:** 3/yr.

★2950★   SECOND OPINION
Second Opinion Publishing, Inc.
1350 Center Dr., Ste. 100
Dunwoody, GA 30338   Phone: (404) 668-0432
Description: Discusses alternative medical treatments and inexpensive cures. Provides "outspoken critiques" of the current system of established medicine and warnings of unpublished health risks. Recurring features include letters to the editor and news of research. **Frequency:** Monthly.

★2951★   SEEING CLEARLY
National Association for Visually Handicapped
22 W. 21st St.
New York, NY 10010   Phone: (212) 889-3141
Description: Offers poems, stories, humor, a crossword puzzle, and other items of interest to readers in large (18-point) print. **First Published:** 1975. **Frequency:** Annually.

★2952★   THE SEEING EYE GUIDE
The Seeing Eye, Inc.
PO Box 375
Morristown, NJ 07963-0375   Phone: (201) 539-4425
Description: Directed towards the regaining or enhancement of the quality of life made possible by the mobility and independence afforded by a Seeing Eye dog. Publishes news of graduates of the Seeing Eye program, and profiles of instructors, trustees, volunteers, staff, and 4-H puppy raisers. Recurring features include columns titled Canine Guidelines (on the care and training of dog guides), Graduate Profiles, and Highlights. **First Published:** January 1935. **Frequency:** Quarterly. **ISSN:** 0037-0819.

★2953★   SENIOR CARE PROFESSIONAL
CD Publications
8204 Fenton St.
Silver Spring, MD 20910   Phone: (301) 588-6380
Description: Offers practical advice for senior care professionals on how to work more effectively with families of the elderly. Recurring features include special sections designed for reproduction and distribution to friends and family of the aged. **First Published:** 1987. **Frequency:** Monthly.

★2954★   SENIOR UPDATE
St. Patrick Hospital
500 W. Broadway
PO Box 4587
Missoula, MT 59806   Phone: (406) 543-7271

★2955★   SENSORY INTEGRATION SPECIAL INTEREST
SECTION—NEWSLETTER
Sensory Integration Special Interest Section
American Occupational Therapy Association
1383 Picard Ave.
Rockville, MD 20850   Phone: (301) 948-9626
Description: Discusses theory, treatment, and therapy for sensory integration. Offers equipment ideas and case histories, and examines questions and special problems. Recurring features include bibliographies of relevant publications, news of research, and notices of meetings and conferences. **First Published:** Summer 1978. **Frequency:** Quarterly. **ISSN:** 0279-4128.

★2956★   SERVO
Association of Hospital Auxiliaries of the Province of Quebec
505, Maisonneuve W., Ste. 400
Montreal, PQ, Canada H3A 3C2   Phone: (514) 842-4861
Description: Provides news on the activities of the Association. Recurring features include President's message, a calendar of events, reports of meetings, and notices of publications available. **First Published:** 1953. **Frequency:** 3/yr.

★2957★   SHELTER NEWS
National Cat Protection Society
1528 W. 17th St.
Long Beach, CA 90813   Phone: (213) 436-3162
Description: Acts as an educational vehicle for the public promoting the need for cat protection. Promotes the use of controlled cat breeding and euthanasia for homeless cats. Reviews the status of legislation which will protect cats and afford them the same rights as other domestic animals. **Frequency:** Quarterly.

★2958★   SHELTER SENSE
Humane Society of the United States
2100 L St. NW
Washington, DC 20037   Phone: (202) 452-1100
Description: Aims to "reduce animal suffering and solve community animal-control problems." Supplies information on animal shelter operation, care of animals, pet adoptions, animal pickup in the field, spay/neuter and public education programs, relevant laws, and cooperation between humane societies and municipal animal-control agencies. Discusses professional qualifications of workers and officers and programs at local humane societies. Recurring features include editorials, news of research, news of relevant supplies and materials, job listings, and ready-to-copy PSAs. **First Published:** April 1978. **Frequency:** 10/yr. **ISSN:** 0734-3078.

★2959★   SH'MA
Sh'ma Inc.
PO Box 567
Port Washington, NY 11050   Phone: (516) 944-9791
Description: Covers issues of concern to the Jewish community. Recurring

features include letters to the editor and book reviews. **First Published:** November 1970. **Frequency:** Biweekly. **ISSN:** 0049-0385.

★2960★   SHOPTALK
American Humane Association
63 Inverness Dr. E.
Englewood, CO 80112   Phone: (303) 792-9900
Description: Covers animal control and sheltering issues. Reports on ideas, technologies, and procedures to enhance and expand shelter programs and animal care. **First Published:** June 1983. **Frequency:** Bimonthly.

★2961★   SIAMESE NEWS QUARTERLY
Siamese Cat Society of America, Inc.
304 SW 13th St.
Ft. Lauderdale, FL 33315   Phone: (305) 524-1747
Description: Discusses the Siamese cat and cats in general. Carries information about cat health, breeding, shows, and activities of the Society. Recurring features include book reviews and columns titled The Breeder Writers, Morris Animal Foundation (on research), and Q&A Vet Column. **First Published:** October 1942. **Frequency:** Quarterly.

★2962★   SIBLING INFORMATION NETWORK—NEWSLETTER
The A.J. Pappanikou Center
991 Main St.
East Hartford, CT 06108   Phone: (203) 282-7050
Description: Carries news of this organization "for those interested in the welfare of siblings of handicapped children." Contains professional information, material on program developments for handicapped children and their families, and accounts of personal experiences. Recurring features include reports and reviews on professional literature available and journal articles helpful to parents, professionals, and siblings of handicapped children; Network announcements; and news of members and staff. **First Published:** April 1981. **Frequency:** Quarterly.

★2963★   SICKLE CELL DISEASE FOUNDATION OF GREATER
NEW YORK—NEWSLETTER
Sickle Cell Disease Foundation of Greater New York
127 W. 127th St., Rm. 421
New York, NY 10027   Phone: (212) 865-1500
Description: Provides information on sickle cell anemia and the Foundation's programs and services. Recurring features include editorials, news of research, news of members, and a calendar of events. **First Published:** 1972. **Frequency:** Quarterly.

★2964★   SIECUS REPORT
Sex Information & Education Council of the U.S.
130 W. 42nd St.
New York, NY 10036   Phone: (212) 673-3850
Description: Covers all aspects of human sexuality, including AIDS, with articles by authorities in the field. Recurring features include reviews of books and audiovisual materials, editorials on specific issues, information on available resources, a calendar of events, research notes, specialized bibliographies, and reading lists for lay persons and professionals. **First Published:** 1965. **Frequency:** Bimonthly. **ISSN:** 0091-3995.

★2965★   SIGBIO NEWSLETTER
Special Interest Group on Biomedical Computing
Association for Computing Machinery
11 W. 42nd St.
New York, NY 10036   Phone: (213) 869-7440
Description: Provides information for individuals interested in the potential use of digital and analog computers in biomedical computing. Represents SIGBIO in its efforts to encourage and facilitate communication and exchange of information "concerning problem areas, computer routines, techniques, and activities between individuals and laboratories involved in biomedical research applications." Occasionally includes SIGBIO symposium proceedings. **Frequency:** Quarterly.

★2966★   SIGCAPH NEWSLETTER
Special Interest Group on Computing and the Physically
   Handicapped
Association for Computing Machinery
11 W. 42nd St.
New York, NY 10036   Phone: (212) 869-7440
Description: Supports the Group's concern to promote professional interests of computing personnel with the physically handicapped; promotes the "application of computing and information technology toward solutions of disability problems and to perform a public education function in support

157

of computing careers for suitably trained blind, deaf, or motor impaired persons." **First Published:** 1970. **Frequency:** Quarterly.

★2967★　SKIING WITH A DIFFERENCE
Alberta Association for Disabled Skiers
Percy Page Centre
11759 Groad Rd.
Edmonton, AB, Canada T25M 3K6
Description: Provides news of the various instruction programs offered by the Association on downhill, cross-country, and water skiing. Notifies readers of registration and program dates, instructors' clinics, social functions, and equipment for sale. Recurring features include a calendar of events, race results, and various committee reports. **Frequency:** Quarterly.

★2968★　SKYLINE NEWS
Greater New York Hospital Association
555 W. 57th St.
New York, NY 10019　　　　Phone: (212) 246-7100
Description: Focuses on legislative and regulatory developments affecting the financing and delivery of health care services in New York City. **First Published:** Biweekly.

★2969★　SOAP NEWSLETTER
Society for Obstetric Anesthesia and Perinatology
Department of Anesthesiology
Baylor College of Medicine
6550 Fannin, Ste. 1003
Houston, TX 77030　　　　Phone: (713) 798-5119
Description: Offers physicians and scientists interested in perinatal health care news and information commensurate with the Society's purpose, which is to improve the health care of pregnant women and their unborn children. Recurring features include news of research, news of members, and a calendar of events. **Frequency:** Quarterly.

★2970★　SOBERING THOUGHTS
Women for Sobriety
PO Box 618
Quakertown, PA 18951-0618　　　　Phone: (215) 536-8026
Description: Focuses on women recovering from alcoholism and chemical dependencies. Contains personal accounts of recovery and growth, and articles on life in a WFS group and on handling stress. Promotes a thirteen statement program that "encourages emotional and spiritual growth." Recurring features include editorials, news of research, letters to the editor, news of members, book reviews, and a calendar of events. **First Published:** 1976. **Frequency:** Monthly.

★2971★　SOCIETY OF CARDIOVASCULAR ANESTHESIOLOGISTS—NEWSLETTER
Society of Cardiovascular Anesthesiologists
PO Box 11086
Richmond, VA 23230　　　　Phone: (804) 282-0084
Description: Includes pro and con discussions of major issues within the cardiovascular anesthesiology field and reviews of related literature being published. Covers Society news, chapter reports, meeting programs and information, and lists new members. **First Published:** 1981. **Frequency:** 6/yr.

★2972★　SOCIETY FOR CRYOBIOLOGY—NEWS NOTES
Society for Cryobiology
Medical College of Georgia
Department of Pharmacology
Augusta, GA 30912-2300
Description: Provides members of the Society with current news of developments within the field of cryobiology. Contains member news and commentaries as well as announcements of Society events and activities. Recurring features include "extensive listings of publications relevant to low temperature biology"; news of recent products, services, and meetings; and a detailed profile of one prominent Society member. **First Published:** 1979. **Frequency:** Quarterly.

★2973★　SOCIETY OF MEDICAL FRIENDS OF WINE— BULLETIN
Society of Medical Friends of Wine
PO Box 218
Sausalito, CA 94965　　　　Phone: (415) 383-5057
Description: Gives news of the Society and its member physicians and surgeons who advocate the nutritional and therapeutic values of wine. Provides articles on various historical, cultural, and medicinal aspects of

wine. Recurring features include announcements of tours of vineyards, wine-tasting activities, dinners, meetings, book reviews, and news of research. **First Published:** 1956. **Frequency:** Semiannually.

★2974★　SOCIETY OF NUCLEAR MEDICINE—NEWSLINE
Society of Nuclear Medicine
136 Madison Ave.
New York, NY 10016-6760　　　　Phone: (212) 889-0717
Description: Provides socio-economic and regulatory news affecting the climate of nuclear medicine. **First Published:** 1985. **Frequency:** Monthly. **ISSN:** 0161-5505.

★2975★　SOCIETY FOR PEDIATRIC DERMATOLOGY— NEWSLETTER
Society for Pediatric Dermatology
Department of Dermatology
1100 W. Michigan St.
Indianapolis, IN 46223　　　　Phone: (317) 630-6691
Description: Carries literature reviews of current publications in the field of pediatric dermatology. Includes reviews in the areas of allergy and immunology, genetics and syndromes, infectious diseases, and diagnosis and treatment. **First Published:** 1976. **Frequency:** Quarterly.

★2976★　SOCIETY FOR PEDIATRIC PSYCHOLOGY— NEWSLETTER
c/o Lawrence J. Siegel, Ph.D.
Ferkauf Graduate School
Yeshiva University
1300 Morris Pack Ave.
Bronx, NY 10024　　　　Phone: (212) 430-4201
Description: Evaluates the results of research, the practice of pediatric psychology, and the application of psychology to medical and psychological problems of children, youths, and their families. Monitors developments in the training and professional practice of pediatric psychology. Recurring features include news of members, news of research, and updates on Society events. **Frequency:** 3/yr.

★2977★　SOCIETY FOR THE RIGHT TO DIE—NEWSLETTER
Society for the Right to Die
250 W. 57th St.
New York, NY 10107　　　　Phone: (212) 246-6973
Description: Discusses recent developments, court cases, medical policies, ethics and religion, and popular opinion of the right-to-die movement. Recurring features include news of members and the Society and book reviews. **First Published:** 1981. **Frequency:** 3/yr.

★2978★　SOCIETY FOR THE SCIENTIFIC STUDY OF SEX— THE SOCIETY NEWSLETTER
Society for the Scientific Study of Sex, Inc.
Graduate School of Education
3700 Walnut St.
University of Pennsylvania
Philadelphia, PA 19104-6216　　　　Phone: (319) 895-8407
Description: Reflects the aims of the Society, which "supports the study of sexuality as a valid area for research and promotes interdisciplinary cooperation among professionals committed to the scientific study of sexuality." Recurring features include news of members, a calendar of events, and columns titled A Few Words From..., and Briefly Noted, Announcements and Future Events. **First Published:** 1980. **Frequency:** Quarterly.

★2979★　SOCIETY OF VASCULAR TECHNOLOGY—SPECTRUM
Society of Vascular Technology
1101 Connecticut Ave. NW, Ste. 700
Washington, DC 20036-4303　　　　Phone: (202) 857-1149
Description: Disseminates news and information on noninvasive vascular technology (which is a highly technical and specialized method of monitoring the blood flow in arms and legs in order to better diagnose disease and blood clots). Carries articles on the Society's efforts to facilitate cooperation among noninvasive vascular technology facilties and other health professionals. Recurring features include news of members and of symposia, and notices of publications. **First Published:** 1982. **Frequency:** 4/yr.

★2980★ SOUNDING BOARD
Sanders-Brown Center on Aging
101 Sanders-Brown Bldg.
Lexington, KY 40536-0230 Phone: (606) 233-6040
Description: Presents activities and physiological, psychological, and sociological research in gerontology at the Center. Recurring features include information on area support and community service organizations for the aged, health and exercise tips, and a calendar of educational and gerontological opportunities. **First Published:** November 1976. **Frequency:** Quarterly.

★2981★ SOUTH DAKOTA DENTAL ASSOCIATION—NEWSLETTER
South Dakota Dental Association
PO Box 1194
Pierre, SD 57501 Phone: (605) 224-9133
Description: Provides updates on dental profession issues, small business, employer/employee relations, nutrition, and safe work place practices. Recurring features include letters to the editor, a calendar of events, reports of meetings, news of educational opportunities, and a column titled President's Corner. **First Published:** 1962. **Frequency:** Monthly.

★2982★ SOUTHERN CALIFORNIA COALITION ON BATTERED WOMEN—NEWSLETTER
Southern California Coalition on Battered Women
PO Box 5036
Santa Monica, CA 90405 Phone: (213) 392-9874
Description: Seeks to facilitate communications and networking among agencies and individuals concerned with domestic abuse. Reports on current legislation and announces employment opportunities. Recurring features include editorials, news of research, letters to the editor, news of members, book reviews, and a calendar of events. **First Published:** 1977. **Frequency:** 4/yr.

★2983★ SOUTHERN CONNECTION
Southern Medical Association Auxiliary
35 Lakeshore Dr.
PO Box 190088
Birmingham, AL 35219-0088 Phone: (205) 945-1840
Description: Acts as the official newsletter of the Auxiliary to the Southern Medical Association (SMA). Informs member spouses of physicians about upcoming events and meetings, news of SMAA projects, and member accomplishments. Recurring features include news of educational opportunities, listings of SMA and SMAA awards, memorials, and columns titled The President's Message and In The Spotlight. **First Published:** September 1981. **Frequency:** 3/yr.

★2984★ SOUTHERN MEDICINE
Southern Medical Association
35 Lakeshore Dr.
PO Box 190088
Birmingham, AL 35219-0088 Phone: (205) 945-1840
Description: Informs members about the programs and benefits offered by the Association and relates news of members' professional accomplishments. Features brief articles on topics of interest to physicians, such as practice management, professional liability and risk management, and continuing medical education. Recurring features include a calendar of events, reports of meetings, news of educational opportunities, and columns titled Message From the President and Message From the Executive Vice-President. **First Published:** 1972. **Frequency:** 3/yr.

★2985★ SPECIAL DELIVERY
Informed Homebirth/Informed Birth & Parenting
PO Box 3675
Ann Arbor, MI 48106 Phone: (313) 662-6857
Description: Provides information on midwifery, legislation, pregnancy, and labor and delivery. Recurring features include letters to the editor, interviews, news of research, a calendar of events, reports of meetings, news of educational opportunities, book reviews, and notices of publications available. **First Published:** 1978. **Frequency:** Quarterly.

★2986★ SPECIAL DELIVERY
Maternity Center Association
48 E. 92nd St.
New York, NY 10128 Phone: (212) 369-7300
Description: Contains information on the Association and its programs for childbearing families. Includes articles on all aspects of maternity care, maternal and infant health, and family life. **Frequency:** 2/yr.

★2987★ SPECTRUM
Massachusetts State Dept. of Public Health
150 Tremont St.
Boston, MA 02111 Phone: (617) 727-0049
Description: Carries news about the Department of Public Health and public health issues in Massachusetts. Includes information on health regulation and planning, environmental health, community health services, maternal and child health, preventive medicine, dental health, and emergency medical services. **First Published:** May 1980. **Frequency:** Quarterly.

★2988★ SPHA NEWSLETTER
Saskatchewan Pharmaceutical Association
2631 28th Ave., Ste. 301
Regina, SK, Canada S4S 6X3 Phone: (306) 584-2292
Description: Contains information of concern to pharmacists and other pharmaceutical professionals in Saskatchewan, Canada. **First Published:** 1980. **Frequency:** 5/yr.

★2989★ SPINA BIFIDA INSIGHTS
Spina Bifida Association of America
1700 Rockville Pike, Ste. 250
Rockville, MD 20852-1654 Phone: (301) 770-7222
Description: Concerned with developments in medicine, education, and legislation affecting the problems and needs of persons with spina bifida. Recurring features include information on conferences, seminars, and programs of interest; news of research; household tips and other practical advice; reports on funding and equal employment issues; and columns titled From the Executive Director, Chapter Chatter, A Matter of Opinion, News From National, New Products and Ideas, and Bits and Pieces. **Frequency:** Bimonthly.

★2990★ THE SPINAL CONNECTION
National Scoliosis Foundation
72 Mt. Auburn St.
Watertown, MA 02172 Phone: (617) 926-0397
Description: Serves as a clearinghouse of information for the Foundation, which promotes programs and activities leading to the elimination of the crippling effects of scoliosis and educates the public about all spinal curvatures. Reviews programs and screening and detection plans in elementary schools. Recurring features include news of research and news of the Foundation. **First Published:** 1985. **Frequency:** Biennially.

★2991★ SPINAL CORD INJURY LIFE
National Spinal Cord Injury Association
600 W. Cummings Park
Woburn, MA 01801 Phone: (617) 935-2722
Description: Educates medical professionals, persons with spinal cord injuries, their families, and the public about spinal cord injury. Reviews research in the field. Highlights Association advocacy, support, and research activities. Recurring features include news of members and a calendar of events. **Frequency:** Quarterly.

★2992★ SPINAL CORD SOCIETY—NEWSLETTER
Spinal Cord Society
R.R. 5, Box 22A
Fergus Falls, MN 56537-9805 Phone: (218) 739-5252
Description: Offers news of research pertaining to the cure of spinal cord injuries. Contains reprints of significant articles, information on studies and projects being enacted, and commentary. Recurring features include letters to the editor, chapter news, a listing of current research projects contracted by SCS, news of members, and columns titled Odds & Ends and Services. **First Published:** 1980. **Frequency:** Monthly.

★2993★ SPIRE
Spina Bifida Association of British Columbia
9460 140th St.
Surrey, BC, Canada V3V 5Z4 Phone: (604) 584-1361
Description: Contains Association news and information of interest to spina bifida patients and their caregivers. Recurring features include news of research, a calendar of events, reports of meetings, and news of educational opportunities. **First Published:** 1978. **Frequency:** Quarterly.

★2994★ SPORTS MEDICINE BULLETIN
American College of Sports Medicine
PO Box 1440
Indianapolis, IN 46206-1440 Phone: (317) 637-9200
Description: Publishes general news about sports medicine, clinical reports,

and information about the activities of the College. Recurring features include editorials, book reviews, a sports medicine calendar, news of members, news of research, and columns titled ACSM Insight, President's Column, and Viewpoint. **First Published:** March 1966. **Frequency:** Quarterly. **ISSN:** 0746-9306.

★2995★   **SPORTS MEDICINE DIGEST**
PM, Inc.
PO Box 10172
Van Nuys, CA 91404   Phone: (818) 873-4399
Description: Reports on various aspects of sports medicine, including drugs and athletic performance and accounts of diagnosis and treatment of specific sports-related injuries and conditions. Provides abstracts of current articles. Recurring features include letters to the editor, book reviews, a calendar of events, and columns titled Training Tips and Nutrition Update. **First Published:** 1979. **Frequency:** Monthly. **ISSN:** 0731-9770.

★2996★   **SPORTS-NUTRITION NEWS**
Healthmere Press, Inc.
PO Box 986
Evanston, IL 60204   Phone: (312) 251-3696
Description: Reports on the relationship between nutrition and exercise, focusing on sports and endurance. Recurring features include news of research, letters to the editor, book reviews, a calendar of events, and columns titled the Athlete's Kitchen and The Winner's Table. **First Published:** June 1982. **Frequency:** Bimonthly. **ISSN:** 0741-3696.

★2997★   **SS HEALTH CARE SYSTEM—ISSUES**
SSM Health Care System
477 N. Lindbergh Blvd.
St. Louis, MO 63141-7813   Phone: (314) 994-7910
Description: Analyzes current legislation and philosophies that affect decisions made by and on behalf of patients. Focuses on the ethical concerns of physicians, patients, families, and nurses when dealing with the medical decision-making process. **First Published:** July 1986. **Frequency:** Bimonthly. **ISSN:** 0888-9201.

★2998★   **SSM NETWORK**
SSM Health Care System
477 N. Lindbergh Blvd.
St. Louis, MO 63141   Phone: (314) 994-7800
Description: Reports on activities and programs within the SSM Health Care System. Covers all aspects of health care. Recurring features include news of members. **First Published:** December 1984. **Frequency:** Quarterly.

★2999★   **STATE ADM REPORTS**
Intergovernmental Health Policy Project
2021 K. St. NW, Ste. 800
Washington, DC 20006   Phone: (202) 872-1445
Description: Designed "to cover important research and policy developments affecting mental health, alcoholism and drug abuse programs in the 50 states." Provides information on state programs and federal and state legislation. **First Published:** Spring 1983. **Frequency:** 10/yr.

★3000★   **STATE HEALTH NOTES**
Intergovernmental Health Policy Project
2021 K St. NW, Ste. 800
Washington, DC 20006   Phone: (202) 872-1445
Description: Deals with "almost any health policy issue of concern to state governments": Medicaid, public health issues, health planning and insurance, licensure, staffing in the health-care field, and mental health. Recurring features include news of research, sections on trends and innovations and recent developments in state Medicaid programs, and announcements of conferences, reports, and publications. **First Published:** 1979. **Frequency:** 24/yr.

★3001★   **STAYING WELL NEWSLETTER**
Foundation for Chiropractic Education and Research
c/o Acme Printing Co.
66 Washington Ave.
Des Moines, IA 50314   Phone: (515) 282-7118
Description: Promotes chiropractic health and fitness. Carries a feature article and news briefs on such topics as living a better life after age 65, the effect of fitness on life insurance premiums, milk intolerance, and other health-related issues. Recurring features include news of chiropractic research and a column titled Ask Your Doctor. **First Published:** 1982. **Frequency:** Bimonthly.

★3002★   **STC NEWSLETTER**
Society of Toxicology of Canada
c/o Dr. D.J. Ecobichon
Department of Pharmacology & Therapeutics
McGill University
Montreal, PQ, Canada H3G 1Y6   Phone: (514) 398-3604
Description: Discusses current issues in the field of toxicology. **First Published:** Spring 1981. **Frequency:** 3/yr.

★3003★   **STD SPOTLIGHT**
Citizens Alliance for VD Awareness
PO Box 1073
Chicago, IL 60648   Phone: (312) 236-6339
Description: Features articles on venereal disease and AIDS (Acquired Immune Deficiency Syndrome), information and education programs, strategies, and political considerations. Recurring features include news of research, new products information, statistics, and a section of news items on STD and AIDS control. **First Published:** January 1976. **Frequency:** Quarterly.

★3004★   **STRATEGIES FOR HEALTHCARE EXCELLENCE**
COR Research Inc.
PO Box 40959
Santa Barbara, CA 93140-0959   Phone: (805) 564-2177
Description: Contains case studies detailing how health care organizations are achieving productivity and quality in the delivery of health care services. Recurring features include interviews, book reviews, and notices of publications available. **First Published:** 1988. **Frequency:** Monthly. **ISSN:** 1058-7829.

★3005★   **STRESS CLAIMS ADVISOR**
Genesis Publishing, Inc.
10455 Sorrento Valley Rd., Ste. 103
San Diego, CA 92121   Phone: (619) 453-0858
Description: Contains information on stress reduction and management. Recurring features include letters to the editor, interviews, news of research, a calendar of events, reports of meetings, news of educational opportunities, book reviews, notices of publications available, and columns titled Stress Reduction Tips, Stress Management Buyers Guide, and Stress Briefs. **Frequency:** Monthly. **ISSN:** 1056-5868.

★3006★   **STROKE CLUBS, INTERNATIONAL—BULLETIN**
Stroke Clubs, International
805 12th St.
Galveston, TX 77550   Phone: (713) 762-1022
Description: Relates news of interest to persons who have suffered strokes. Recurring features include letters to the editor, news of research, and book reviews.

★3007★   **THE STUDENT ADVOCATE**
National Alliance of Blind Students
1155 15th St. NW, Ste. 720
Washington, DC 20005   Phone: (202) 467-5081
Description: Discusses topics of interest and importance to blind and visually impaired students enrolled in post-secondary schools. A major concern is the full accessibility of colleges and universities to the handicapped. Publishes a message from the President and seminar news. **First Published:** 1985. **Frequency:** 3/yr.

★3008★   **SUBSTANCE ABUSE REPORT**
Business Research Publications, Inc.
817 Broadway
New York, NY 10003   Phone: (212) 673-4700
Description: Concentrates on regulatory news, trends, and developments in the field of drug and alcohol abuse. Discusses treatment methods and community facilities for handling substance abuse. Recurring features include news of upcoming conferences. **First Published:** 1970. **Frequency:** Biweekly. **ISSN:** 1040-4163.

★3009★   **SUN AND SKIN NEWS**
Skin Cancer Foundation
245 Fifth Ave., Ste. 2402
New York, NY 10016   Phone: (212) 725-5176
Description: Published to inform the general public about skin health and the prevention of skin cancer through effective protection from the sun. Recurring features include news of research and information on publications available from the Foundation. **First Published:** April 1984. **Frequency:** Quarterly.

★3010★ SUPPORT GROUP NEWSLETTER
ALS and Neuromuscular Research Foundation
California Pacific Medical Center
2351 Clay St., No. 416
San Francisco, CA 94115   Phone: (415) 923-3604
Description: Publishes news of the Foundation's support group for Amyotrophic Lateral Sclerosis (ALS) patients and their families in the San Francisco Bay area. Offers articles on medical and psychosocial aspects of ALS and on how to cope with related problems. Recurring features include profiles of ALS patients and their achievements and news of research. **Frequency:** Monthly.

★3011★ SWEEPSTAKES NEWS
International Arabian Breeders Sweepstakes
International Arabian Horse Association
PO Box 33696
Denver, CO 80233   Phone: (303) 450-4774
Description: Informs members of the IAHA on the activities of the Sweepstakes program, including the Sweepstakes Commission and the Sweepstakes Trust. Offers information on how to enroll horses in the Sweepstakes program as well as on entry classifications and fees; also lists annual Sweepstakes-sponsored competition winners and nominated sires. Recurring features include meeting reports. **First Published:** Ca. 1985. **Frequency:** Quarterly.

★3012★ SYNAPSE
American Association of Neuroscience Nurses
218 N. Jefferson St., No. 204
Chicago, IL 60606-1112   Phone: (312) 993-0043
Description: Publishes information about the neuroscience nursing community, including news of Association activities. **First Published:** 1973. **Frequency:** Bimonthly.

★3013★ SYNERGY
International Division
Association of Universities and Colleges of Canada
151 Slater St.
Ottawa, ON, Canada K1P 5N1   Phone: (613) 563-1236
Description: Provides information on international health, emphasizing Canadian initiatives. Serves to inform international health professionals and to provide awareness of Canadian expertise and activities related to improving health in developing countries. Recurring features include letters to the editor, news of research, discussion of issues, a calendar of events, reports of meetings, news of educational opportunities, and notices of publications available. **First Published:** April 1988. **Frequency:** 4/yr. **ISSN:** 0838-0368.

★3014★ TAKE A BREATHER
Lung Association - Metropolitan Toronto and York Region
573 King St. E., Ste. 201
Toronto, ON, Canada M5A 1M5   Phone: (416) 864-1112
Description: Covers Association issues; provides financial updates and volunteer news. Offers information on health and environmental concerns, especially air pollution. Recurring features include interviews, news of research, a calendar of events, reports of meetings, news of educational opportunities, book reviews, and notices of publications available. **First Published:** September 1990. **Frequency:** 4/yr.

★3015★ TAKING CARE
Center for Corporate Health Promotion
10467 White Granite Dr., No. 300
Oakton, VA 22124-2763   Phone: (703) 391-2400
Description: Contains articles on common health risks and problems. Emphasizes wellness, physical fitness, and preventive medicine. **First Published:** 1984. **Frequency:** Monthly.

★3016★ TECHNOLOGY FOR ANESTHESIA
ECRI
5200 Butler Pike
Plymouth Meeting, PA 19462   Phone: (215) 825-6000
Description: Addresses "problems and issues in health care technology of interest to clinical specialists in anesthesiology." Provides a summary of reported problems, hazards, and recalls. Recurring features include updates on medical devices and news of research. **First Published:** 1980. **Frequency:** Monthly. **ISSN:** 8756-8578.

★3017★ TECHNOLOGY FOR CARDIOLOGY
ECRI
5200 Butler Pike
Plymouth Meeting, PA 19462   Phone: (215) 825-6000
Description: Reports on ECRI comparative product evaluations and offers hazard reports on medical devices and device operation data. Recurring features include health care technology abstracts and news of research. **First Published:** 1980. **Frequency:** Monthly. **ISSN:** 8756-8586.

★3018★ TECHNOLOGY FOR CRITICAL-CARE NURSES
ECRI
5200 Butler Pike
Plymouth Meeting, PA 19462   Phone: (215) 825-6000
Description: Concerned with current problems in critical care nursing. Carries ECRI comparative product evaluations, issues analyses, and hazard reports on medical devices, as well as discussions of the principles of medical device operation. Recurring features include news of research and health care technology abstracts. **ISSN:** 1050-9620.

★3019★ TECHNOLOGY FOR EMERGENCY CARE NURSES
ECRI
5200 Butler Pike
Plymouth Meeting, PA 19462   Phone: (215) 825-6000
Description: Concerned with current problems in emergency nursing. Carries ECRI comparative product evaluations, issues analyses, and hazard reports on medical devices, as well as discussions on the principles of medical device operation. Recurring features include news of research and health care technology abstracts. **First Published:** 1980. **Frequency:** Bimonthly. **ISSN:** 1059-454X.

★3020★ TECHNOLOGY FOR HEALTH CARE SERIES
ECRI
5200 Butler Pike
Plymouth Meeting, PA 19462   Phone: (215) 825-6000
Description: Concerned with the safety, performance, reliability, and cost effectiveness of health care technology. Covers areas of anesthesia, cardiology, emergency medicine, imaging and radiology, laboratory medicine, materials management, nursing, respiratory therapy, and surgery. Reviews device test results and warns of hazards and deficiencies. Recurring features include news of research, Institute reports, and news of members. **Frequency:** Monthly.

★3021★ TECHNOLOGY FOR MATERIALS MANAGEMENT
ECRI
5200 Butler Pike
Plymouth Meeting, PA 19462   Phone: (215) 825-6000
Description: Focuses on medical devices and equipment in materials management. Reports ECRI comparative product evaluations and discusses the principles of device operation. Summarizes reported problems, hazards, and recalls involving medical devices. **First Published:** 1980. **Frequency:** Monthly. **ISSN:** 8756-8608.

★3022★ TECHNOLOGY FOR RESPIRATORY THERAPY
ECRI
5200 Butler Pike
Plymouth Meeting, PA 19462   Phone: (215) 825-6000
Description: Reviews medical device technology and summarizes reported problems, hazards, and recalls. Recurring features include news of research and health care technology abstracts. **First Published:** 1980. **Frequency:** Monthly. **ISSN:** 8756-8616.

★3023★ TECHNOLOGY FOR SURGERY
ECRI
5200 Butler Pike
Plymouth Meeting, PA 19462   Phone: (215) 825-6000
Description: Concerned with problems relating to surgical medical devices. Offers ECRI comparative product evaluations and summarizes reported problems, hazards, and recalls involving medical devices. Recurring features include health care technology abstracts and news of research. **First Published:** 1980. **Frequency:** Monthly. **ISSN:** 8756-8624.

★3024★ TEL-MED—NEWS
TEL-MED
952 S. Mount Vernon
PO Box 1768
Colton, CA 92324   Phone: (714) 825-6034
Description: Carries general organizational news for licensees of this health and medical telephone information service which operates throughout the

U.S., Canada, South America, and Saudi Arabia. Recurring features include news briefs, lists of new licensees, and a tape update column. **First Published:** February 1976. **Frequency:** 5/yr.

★3025★   TENNESSEE MEDICO-LEGAL REPORTER
Lewis L. Laska
901 Church St.
Nashville, TN 37203   Phone: (615) 255-6288
Description: Contains reports on cases involving or of interest to Tennessee healthcare providers. **First Published:** 1983. **Frequency:** Monthly.

★3026★   TERRAP TIMES
TSC Management Corp.
648 Mendo Ave., No. 5
Menlo Park, CA 94025   Phone: (415) 327-1312
Description: Discusses agoraphobia, phobias, anxiety, and panic attacks and their treatment. Recurring features include editorials, letters to the editor, news of research, and columns titled Turning Point, Success Story, Helpful Hints, Pen Pals, The Support Column, and Dr. Hardy's Message. **First Published:** 1965. **Frequency:** Bimonthly.

★3027★   TEXAS TALK
Association for Retarded Citizens/Texas
833 Houston St.
Austin, TX 78756   Phone: (512) 454-6694
Description: Covers Association activities. Contains discussions of issues affecting mentally retarded citizens. Recurring features include a calendar of events and news of meetings. **Frequency:** Bimonthly.

★3028★   THYROBULLETIN
Thyroid Foundation of Canada
PO Box 1597
Kingston, ON, Canada K7L 5C8   Phone: (613) 542-8330
Description: Contains news of the Foundation, which serves to increase awareness of thyroid disease, provide support to thyroid patients and their families, and advocate fundraising for thyroid disease research. Recurring features include letters to the editor, news of research, a calendar of events, reports of meetings, chapter news, and news of educational opportunities. **First Published:** March 1985. **Frequency:** Quarterly.

★3029★   TIBIA TRIBUNE
Southern Orthopaedic Association
PO Box 190088
Birmingham, AL 35219-0088   Phone: (205) 945-1848
Description: Disseminates news of Association activities and events, including announcements of conferences, workshops, annual meetings, and continuing education opportunities. Also provides news of members and a column titled Message From the President. Recurring features include reports of meetings and a calendar of events. **First Published:** Fall 1986. **Frequency:** Quarterly.

★3030★   THE TIMELY PERSPECTIVE
Lupus Foundation of America, Inc.
Northeast Indiana Chapter
5401 Keystone Dr., Ste. 202
Fort Wayne, IN 46825   Phone: (219) 482-8205
Description: Focuses on Lupus and individualized treatment of the disease. Carries news of the Foundation. Recurring features include a column titled Around the Area. **Frequency:** Bimonthly.

★3031★   TINNITUS TODAY
American Tinnitus Association
PO Box 5
Portland, OR 97207   Phone: (503) 248-9985
Description: Studies tinnitus, the presence of ringing in the ears, or head noises, which "can appear in a variety of forms such as buzzing, roaring, whistling, hissing, or high-pitched screeches." Recurring features include Association news, news of research, analysis of treatments, statistics, book reviews, and convention and meeting news. **First Published:** April 1975. **Frequency:** 4/yr. **ISSN:** 0897-6368.

★3032★   TIPSHEET
Minnesota Chapter
Arthritis Foundation
1730 Clifton Pl., No. A-1
Minneapolis, MN 55403   Phone: (612) 874-1201
Description: Provides tips for people with arthritis such as medical

information and coping suggestions. **First Published:** January 1988. **Frequency:** 6/yr.

★3033★   TO YOUR HEALTH
Cornell Communications
330 Garfield Ave.
Eau Claire, WI 54701   Phone: (715) 834-6046
Description: Provides information on health, safety, and drug/alcohol awareness to employees of business and industry. Includes topics on nutrition and fitness, emotional health issues, general health care, parenting tips, and first aid. **First Published:** 1986. **Frequency:** Bimonthly. **ISSN:** 0891-1304.

★3034★   TOGETHER
Association for Specialists in Group Work
American Association for Counseling & Development
5999 Stephenson Ave.
Alexandria, VA 22304   Phone: (703) 823-9800
Description: Publishes news of the members, activities, and concerns of the Association, a group of professional counselors concerned with the training, education, certification, licensing, and professional growth of counselors. Acts as an exchange of professional knowledge and expertise for group counselors, including family and marriage counselors. Recurring features include a calendar of events and a roster of Association officers and leaders. **First Published:** 1973. **Frequency:** 4/yr. **ISSN:** 0193-3922.

★3035★   TORCHBEARER NEWSLETTER
American Kidney Fund
6110 Executive Blvd., Ste. 1010
Rockville, MD 20852-3903   Phone: (301) 881-3052
Description: Supports the goals of the Kidney Fund, which are to alleviate the financial burdens caused by kidney disease, to improve the quality of life for kidney patients, and to promote kidney care nationwide. Recurring features include news of research and educational programs, information on patient family training and organ donation, and news of members. **First Published:** 1976. **Frequency:** Semiannually.

★3036★   TORONTO WOMEN'S HEALTH NETWORK—NEWSLETTER
Toronto Women's Health Network
c/o L. Spring
1884 Davenport Rd.
Toronto, ON, Canada M6N 4Y2   Phone: (416) 392-0898
Description: Serves as an information exchange on women's health issues and events. Includes reports of monthly meetings. **First Published:** April 1982. **Frequency:** 10/yr.

★3037★   TOUCHING
World Relief
PO Box WRC
Wheaton, IL 60189   Phone: (708) 665-0235
Description: Focuses on World Relief activities in more than 25 countries, including staff and donor profiles, news updates, prayer requests, and refugee resettlement reports. **First Published:** February 1983. **Frequency:** Quarterly.

★3038★   TOUGH STUFF
Osteogenesis Imperfecta Foundation, Inc.
5005 W. Laurel St., No. 210
Tampa, FL 33607-3836   Phone: (201) 489-9232
Description: Aimed at children with Osteogenesis Imperfecta. **Frequency:** Quarterly.

★3039★   TOURETTE SYNDROME ASSOCIATION—NEWSLETTER
Tourette Syndrome Association
42-40 Bell Blvd.
Bayside, NY 11361   Phone: (718) 224-2999
Description: Publishes information concerning research and treatment of the neurological disorder Tourette Syndrome. Includes reports of medical papers dealing with Tourette Syndrome and news of the Association's regional group activities. Recurring features include editorials, letters to the editor, news of members and of research, book reviews, and a calendar of events. **First Published:** January 1975. **Frequency:** Quarterly.

★3040★ THE TOURNIQUET
National Phlebotomy Association, Inc.
2623 Bladensburg Rd. NE
Washington, DC 20018   Phone: (202) 636-4515
Description: Details the Association's certification, accreditation, and
educational activities in relation to phlebotomy programs in the U.S.
Recurring features include news of research, listings of approved programs,
and notices of regional workshops and national certification examinations
conducted by the Association. Frequency: 3/yr.

★3041★ TRANSITION SUMMARY
National Information Center for Children and Youth With Handicaps
PO Box 1492
Washington, DC 20013   Phone: (703) 893-6061
Description: Serves as an information exchange for persons working on
transition issues. Addresses current issues in career education, vocational
education, vocational rehabilitation, and the transition of young people
with disabilities from school to work or other settings. Recurring features
include news of research. First Published: Spring 1985. Frequency:
Annually.

★3042★ TRANSPLANT ACTION
American Council on Transplantation
PO Box 2326
Ellicott City, MD 21043-0017
Description: Seeks to motivate the public to donate organs and tissues for
transplantation through the dissemination of information about the
logistical, financial, ethical, and other issues regarding transplantation.
Publicizes procurement programs and tissue banks and profiles transplan-
tation programs across the country. Recurring features include news of
members, programs, and research. Frequency: Bimonthly.

★3043★ TRAVELING HEALTHY
Traveling Healthy, Inc.
108-48 70th Rd.
Forest Hills, NY 11375
Description: Discusses health and medical issues of interest to travelers.
Offers tips for adapting to differing climates, time zones, foods, and
sanitation standards. Reports on the quality of medical facilities in other
countries. Primarily concerned with a certain global region in each issue.
First Published: 1988. Frequency: Bimonthly. ISSN: 0899-2169.

★3044★ THE TRIPLET CONNECTION—NEWSLETTER
Triplet Connection
PO Box 99571
Stockton, CA 95209   Phone: (209) 474-0885
Description: Provides information for families with, or who are expecting,
triplets, quadruplets, or quintuplets. First Published: 1983. Frequency:
Quarterly.

★3045★ TUFTS UNIVERSITY DIET & NUTRITION LETTER
Tufts University
203 Harrison Ave.
Boston, MA 02111   Phone: (617) 482-3530
Description: Addresses the medical and health aspects of nutrition and
dieting. Offers professional advice in nontechnical language about vitamins, sodium, cholesterol, dieting, and other nutrition-related topics.
Reports on relevant research, government actions, and industry developments. Recurring features include special reports and the column Ask the
Experts. First Published: March 1983. Frequency: Monthly. ISSN: 0747-
4105.

★3046★ TUNING IN: AAMT NEWSLETTER
American Association for Music Therapy
PO Box 80012
Valley Forge, PA 19484-0012   Phone: (215) 265-4006
Description: Concerned with developments in music therapy and related
topics, such as art and dance therapy, psychodrama, and psychotherapy.
Recurring features include editorials, news of members and of research,
book reviews, letters to the editor, and columns titled New and Notewor-
thy, Organizational Affairs, Upcoming Events, and Point-Counterpoint.
First Published: 1977. Frequency: Quarterly.

★3047★ THE TWELVE STEP RAG
Families Anonymous, Inc.
PO Box 528
Van Nuys, CA 91408   Phone: (818) 989-7841
Description: Contains information for friends and relatives concerned

about someone else's use of drugs, chemicals, and alcohol and behavioral
problems related to their use. Recurring features include sharing of
personal experiences and a column titled Chairman's Message. First
Published: February 1971. Frequency: Bimonthly.

★3048★ TWIN SERVICES REPORTER
Twin Services
PO Box 10066
Berkeley, CA 94709   Phone: (510) 524-0863
Description: Offers parenting advice and research updates on the care and
development of twins, triplets, quadruplets, and quintuplets, from prenatal
care through their adjustment as adults. Concerned with such issues as
preventing pre-term births, multiple-pregnancy management, breastfeed-
ing multiples, coping with toddlers, and the twin relationship. Recurring
features include letters to the editor, interviews, book reviews and notices
of publications available, and a calendar of events, as well as columns titled
Reminiscing: On Growing Up a Twin, What's Up at Twin Services, Twin
Tips, and Multiple Viewpoint. First Published: Fall 1983. Frequency:
Quarterly. ISSN: 0895-0784.

★3049★ TWINLAB NUTRITION UPDATE
Advanced Research Press, Inc.
Twin Laboratories, Inc.
2552 Regis Dr.
Davis, CA 95616   Phone: (916) 756-3311
Description: Features semi-technical articles on the effects of nutrition on
health and disease. Emphasizes the nutritional modulation of disease.
Recurring features include news of research, a calendar of events, current
controversies in nutrition, and a column titled Literature Update. First
Published: November 1985. Frequency: Quarterly.

★3050★ UAB ARTHRITIS TODAY
Multipurpose Arthritis Center
University of Alabama at Birmingham
Tinsley Harrison Tower, 429A
UAB Sta.
Birmingham, AL 35294   Phone: (205) 934-5306
Description: Provides information on the control and management of
arthritis. Recurring features include news of research, interviews, news of
educational opportunities, and columns titled My Little Jenny and Makin'
Lemonade. First Published: 1980. Frequency: 2/yr.

★3051★ UCLA CANCER TRIALS
Jonsson Comprehensive Cancer Center
University of California, Los Angeles
Louis Factor Health Sciences Bldg., 10-10-145
UCLA Center for the Health Sciences
Los Angeles, CA 90024-1781   Phone: (213) 206-2805
Description: Provides listing of selected clinical trials of community
interest. First Published: Spring 1990. Frequency: Quarterly.

★3052★ UMBILICUS
Birthways, Inc.
Box 12097
Berkeley, CA 94701-3097   Phone: (510) 540-4588
Description: Offers advertising, educational articles, and community news
intended to serve those individuals and couples seeking support during
pregancy, birth, and parenting. Recurring features include editorials, news
of members, letters to the editor, book reviews, a calendar of events, and
the columns titled The Childbearing Year, Health & Fitness, Community
News, and Birthway News. First Published: 1982. Frequency: Quarterly.

★3053★ UNA NEWSBULLETIN
United Nurses of Alberta
Principal Plaza, Ste. 760
10303 Jasper Ave.
Edmonton, AB, Canada T5J 3N6   Phone: (403) 425-1025
Description: Offers educational information for nurses regarding bargaining, organizing, labor legislation, health and safety, and grievance and
arbitration. Recurring features include letters to the editor, news of
research, a calendar of events, reports of meetings, news of educational
opportunities, and columns titled Health & Safety and Fight Back. First
Published: 1977. Frequency: Bimonthly.

★3054★ THE UNION SIGNAL
National Woman's Christian Temperance Union
1730 Chicago Ave.
Evanston, IL 60201   Phone: (708) 864-1396
Description: Stresses the biological and social damage to persons and to society from consumption of alcoholic beverages, tobacco, and narcotics. Carries news briefs and legislative and consumer information. Recurring features include reports from officers of the organization worldwide, inspirational items, poetry, announcements of available publications, excerpts from other publications, and columns titled Washington Letter and Youth Temperance Council. **First Published:** 1874. **Frequency:** Monthly. **ISSN:** 0041-7033.

**★3055★ UNITARIAN UNIVERSALIST WOMEN'S
FEDERATION—THE COMMUNICATOR**
Unitarian Universalist Women's Federation
25 Beacon St.
Boston, MA 02108   Phone: (617) 742-2100
Description: Carries Federation news and reports in the fields of equality for women, responsible abortion laws, child advocacy, violence against women, and women's spirituality. **First Published:** October 1976. **Frequency:** 6/yr.

★3056★ UNITED PARKINSON FOUNDATION—NEWSLETTER
United Parkinson Foundation
360 W. Superior St.
Chicago, IL 60610   Phone: (312) 664-2344
Description: Disseminates information on symptoms, medication and therapy for Parkinson's disease and related illnesses. Recurring features include news of patient services, educational programs, and relevant publications and news of research. **First Published:** September 1968. **Frequency:** Quarterly.

**★3057★ UNITED SCLERODERMA FOUNDATION—
NEWSLETTER**
United Scleroderma Foundation, Inc.
PO Box 350
Watsonville, CA 95077   Phone: (408) 728-2202
Description: Devoted solely to information concerning scleroderma, including research reports, forms of treatment, suggestions for care and management, and occasional surveys of readers. Recurring features include news of Foundation activities, notices of conferences and workshops, obituaries, chapter news, news of members, material submitted by physicians, and the column From the Mailbag. **First Published:** May 1977. **Frequency:** Quarterly.

★3058★ U.S. NATIONAL LIBRARY OF MEDICINE—NEWS
National Library of Medicine
National Institutes of Health
U.S. Department of Health and Human Services
8600 Rockville Pike
Bethesda, MD 20894   Phone: (301) 496-6308
Description: Reports on Library programs, policies, services, exhibits, and collections. Recurring features include notices of publications available, staff notes, and a list of references citing works that discuss the products and services of the Library. **First Published:** 1945. **Frequency:** Monthly; irregular bimonthly issues. **ISSN:** 0027-965X.

★3059★ U.S. NEWS AND NOTES
International College of Surgeons, U.S. Section
1516 N. Lake Shore Dr.
Chicago, IL 60610-1694   Phone: (312) 787-6274
Description: Carries general news items and technical information for surgeons. Recurring features include news of research, news of members, a calendar of events, and notes from the president. **First Published:** 1973. **Frequency:** Quarterly.

★3060★ U.S. REGULATORY REPORTER
Parexel International Corp.
195 West St.
Walthan, MA 02154-1116   Phone: (617) 487-9900
Description: Reports regulatory news from the FDA and other government agencies for companies in the drug, medical device, diagnostic, and biotechnology industries. Recurring features include analyses of FDA product approval standards and review processes and sections titled Congressional Monitor and Regulatory Review. **First Published:** June 1984. **Frequency:** Monthly. **ISSN:** 0749-5005.

★3061★ UNITED WAY LEADER
United Way Services
3100 Euclid Ave.
Cleveland, OH 44115-2577   Phone: (216) 881-3170
Description: Provides year-round news concerning the United Way's fundraising, allocations, and community problem-solving volunteer efforts. Highlights agencies and clients and reports new health and human services available to the community. Recurring features include calendar of events. **First Published:** Summer 1978. **Frequency:** Quarterly.

**★3062★ UNIVERSITY OF CALIFORNIA AT BERKELEY
WELLNESS LETTER**
Rodney M. Friedman
637 Broadway, 11th Fl.
New York, NY 10012   Phone: (212) 505-2255
Description: Gives latest medical findings and practical information on achieving a healthier lifestyle. **First Published:** October 1984. **Frequency:** Monthly. **ISSN:** 0748-9234.

**★3063★ UNIVERSITY CENTER ON AGING AND HEALTH—
NEWSLETTER**
University Center on Aging and Health
Case Western Reserve University
2009 Adelbert Rd.
Cleveland, OH 44106-7131   Phone: (216) 368-2692
Description: Contains descriptions of current research activities of gerontologists at the University and in the Northeast Ohio region. Features news items, articles, and a calendar of events and conferences. **First Published:** April 1979. **Frequency:** Quarterly.

**★3064★ THE UNIVERSITY OF TEXAS LIFETIME HEALTH
LETTER**
Health Science Center
University of Texas
1100 Holcombe Blvd.
PO Box 20036
Houston, TX 77225   Phone: (713) 792-4265
Description: Designed to promote proactive health, fitness, nutrition, and mental well-being for consumers. Recurring features include news of research and columns titled Ask the Doctor and Health Notes. **First Published:** February 1989. **Frequency:** Monthly. **ISSN:** 0142-203X.

★3065★ THE URINE NATION NEWS
Digit Press
PO Box 920066
Norcross, GA 30092
Description: Protests random drug testing and provides information concerning the percentage of false results. Examines "any and all unnecessary and/or unconstitutional government intrusion into Americans' lives." Discusses current legislation. **Frequency:** Monthly.

★3066★ UROGRAM
American Urological Association Allied
11512 Allecingie Pkwy.
Richmond, VA 23235   Phone: (816) 358-3317
Description: Informs members, including registered and licensed practical nurses, technicians, physician assistants, and those working in urology-related industries about the continuing education programs of the Association. Recurring features include chapter news, notices of regional and local seminars, and news of members. **Frequency:** Quarterly.

★3067★ VCC NEWSLETTER
Vermont Cancer Center
University of Vermont
1 S. Prospect St.
Burlington, VT 05401-3498   Phone: (802) 656-4414
Description: Reports on Center research and activities. Recurring features include book reviews and news of research, talks, papers presented, upcoming symposia and events, and grants awarded. **First Published:** 1978. **Frequency:** Periodic.

★3068★ VEGETARIAN JOURNAL
Vegetarian Resource Group
PO Box 1463
Baltimore, MD 21203   Phone: (410) 366-8343
Description: Focuses on the ethical and nutritional aspects of vegetarianism, as well as health, ecology, animal rights, and world hunger. Recurring features include restaurant reviews, recipes, a calendar of events, and

reviews of scientific and informational articles. **First Published:** October 1982. **Frequency:** Bimonthly. **ISSN:** 0885-7636.

★3069★   **VELLO KULBIN'S COMMENTARY**
Vello Kulbin
31731 Outer Hwy. 10
Redlands, CA 92373-7570
Description: Provides commentary on world and domestic events. Recurring features include news of research. **First Published:** April 1982. **Frequency:** Irregular.

★3070★   **VIP NEWSLETTER**
Blind Children's Fund
230 Central St.
Auburndale, MA 02166-2399   Phone: (617) 332-4014
Description: Contains articles of interest to parents and teachers of young blind and visually impaired children. Recurring features include editorials, news of members, letters to the editor, book reviews, and columns titled The Toy Box, Causes of Visual Impairment, and Agency Reports. **First Published:** January 1979. **Frequency:** Quarterly. **ISSN:** 0728-7091.

★3071★   **VIRGINIA SOCIETY OF ANESTHESIOLOGISTS—**
NEWSLETTER
Virginia Society of Anesthesiologists, Inc.
1910 Byrd Ave., Ste. 100
Box 11086
Richmond, VA 23230-1086   Phone: (804) 282-0062
Description: Carries Society news and other items of interest to anesthesiologists. Discusses bills, regulations, Congressional actions, and other legislation affecting anesthesiologists, particularly in Virginia. Recurring features include a calendar of events, announcements of research fellowships available, news of the American Board of Anesthesiology (ABA) and of the American Society of Anesthesiologists (ASA), and announcements concerning the ASA Distinguished Service Award. **First Published:** 1979. **Frequency:** Quarterly.

★3072★   **VISION RESOURCE UPDATE**
Vision Foundation, Inc.
818 Mt. Auburn St.
Watertown, MA 02172   Phone: (617) 926-4232
Frequency: 6/yr.

★3073★   **VITA**
International Association for Suicide Prevention
c/o Charlotte Ross
445 Virginia Ave.
San Mateo, CA 94402   Phone: (415) 342-5755
Description: Covers news of the suicide prevention field for concerned professional persons everywhere. Presents personal accounts of problem handling, reports from foreign chapters, and reprints of scientific papers. Recurring features include documentation, statistics, news of research, news of Association meetings, book reviews in original language, and a calendar of events. **First Published:** November 1965. **Frequency:** 2-3/yr.

★3074★   **VITAL SIGNS**
National Black Women's Health Project
1237 Gordon St. SW
Atlanta, GA 30310   Phone: (404) 753-0916
Description: Encourages mutual and self-help activism among women to bring about a reduction in health care problems prevalent among black women. Reports on research conducted on the health problems of black women and discusses black women's health issues. Recurring features include news of upcoming conferences and lectures sponsored by the Project. **First Published:** 1984. **Frequency:** Quarterly.

★3075★   **VITILIGO**
The National Vitiligo Foundation, Inc.
Texas American Bank Bldg.
PO Box 6337
Tyler, TX 75711   Phone: (214) 534-2925
Description: Dedicated to bringing hope and encouragement to persons afflicted with Vitiligo, a skin disorder. Features news of research and correspondence from patients. **First Published:** 1987. **Frequency:** 2/yr.

★3076★   **THE VIVA VITAL VIEWS**
Visually Impaired Veterans of America
c/o Charles L. Rhein
5016 Silk Oak Dr.
Sarasota, FL 34232-5410   Phone: (813) 371-2153
Description: Concerned with matters relating to the loss or impairment of eyesight of veterans and men and women in U.S. Armed Forces. Covers related laws, regulations, and information from the Veterans Administration. Includes news of research; information on resources, rights, and benefits; and announcements of meetings and conferences of interest. **First Published:** 1976. **Frequency:** Quarterly.

★3077★   **VOCATIONAL/DEVELOPMENTAL REHABILITATION**
REVIEW
National Association of Rehabilitation Facilities
PO Box 17675
Washington, DC 20041   Phone: (703) 648-9300
Description: Compiles legislation and regulation news for facilities that provide training, employment, and residential services to persons with mental or physical disabilities. Recurring features include reports of meetings, news of educational opportunities, and notices of publications available. **First Published:** 1982. **Frequency:** Weekly.

★3078★   **VOICE OF THE PHARMACIST—NEWSLETTER**
Voice of the Pharmacist, Inc.
American College of Apothecaries
205 Daingerfield Rd.
Alexandria, VA 22314   Phone: (703) 684-8603
Description: Examines current issues and opportunities affecting the retail, hospital, and consultant practices of pharmacy. Discusses controversial issues, often with commentary by pharmacists. Recurring features include editorials, news of research, and letters to the editor. **First Published:** 1957. **Frequency:** Quarterly.

★3079★   **THE VOLUNTEER LEADER**
American Hospital Publishing, Inc.
American Hospital Association
737 N. Michigan Ave., Ste. 700
Chicago, IL 60611   Phone: (312) 440-6800
Description: Discusses issues pertaining to hospital auxiliary leaders and directors of volunteer services departments. Covers in-service programs, community outreach services, personnel management, fundraising, organization and governance, and volunteer recruitment. Recurring features include news of research, a calendar of events, and columns titled Point of View, Programs in Action, and Notes and Quotes. **First Published:** January 1960. **Frequency:** Quarterly. **ISSN:** 0005-1861.

★3080★   **VOLUNTEER SERVICES ADMINISTRATION**
American Society of Directors of Volunteer Services
American Hospital Association
840 N. Lake Shore Dr.
Chicago, IL 60611   Phone: (312) 280-6110
Description: Provides a means of intercommunication for directors of volunteer services within health care institutions. Offers guidance on matters relating to health care volunteer services management in order to maintain professional standards and increase the competence of individual members. Recurring features include a calendar of events, news of Society and member activities, and notices of educational opportunities. **Frequency:** Bimonthly.

★3081★   **VOLUNTEERS' VOICE FOR COMMUNITY SAFETY &**
HEALTH
National Safety Council
444 N. Michigan Ave.
Chicago, IL 60611   Phone: (312) 527-4800
Description: Promotes safety awareness and the use of safe practices and products in the home. Carries consumer tips and suggestions on family conduct and emergency action. **Frequency:** Bimonthly.

★3082★   **WALKWAYS**
WalkWays Center
733 15th St. NW, No. 427
Washington, DC 20005   Phone: (205) 737-9555
Description: Provides information on walking, including news, health and fitness tips, networking, travel and tours, and foot care. Recurring features include book reviews, news of research, a calendar of events, interviews, and a column titled Walk at Your Own Pace. **First Published:** June 1985. **Frequency:** Bimonthly. **ISSN:** 0883-430X.

★3083★ WALTHER CANCER INSTITUTE, INC.—NEWSLETTER
Walther Cancer Institute, Inc.
3202 N. Meridian St.
Indianapolis, IN 46208   Phone: (317) 921-2040
Description: Provides update on Institute efforts in cancer research. **First Published:** 1986. **Frequency:** Quarterly.

★3084★ WASHINGTON DRUG LETTER
Washington Business Information, Inc.
1117 N. 19th St.
Arlington, VA 22209-1978   Phone: (703) 247-3426
Description: Focuses on regulation and legislation affecting prescription and proprietary drugs. Monitors Food & Drug Administration (FDA) actions and new drug applications, manufacturing procedures, advertising and labeling, compliance cases, research, and testing rules. **First Published:** 1969. **Frequency:** Weekly. **ISSN:** 0194-1291.

★3085★ WASHINGTON HEALTH RECORD
Faulkner & Grey, Inc.
1133 15th St. NW
Washington, DC 20005   Phone: (202) 828-4148
Description: Covers federal health regulations and legislation. Publishes the Department of Health and Human Services' final and proposed rulings, and announces the Department's hearings. Recurring features include listings of new publications and a calendar of conferences in the health industry throughout the country. **Frequency:** Weekly.

★3086★ WASHINGTON REPORT
American Association of Homes for the Aging
1129 20th St. NW, Ste. 400
Washington, DC 20036-3489   Phone: (202) 296-5960
Description: Covers Association activities regarding homes and services for the elderly. **First Published:** September 27, 1989. **Frequency:** Biweekly.

★3087★ WASHINGTON SOCIAL LEGISLATION BULLETIN
Social Legislation Information Service
440 First St. NW, Ste. 310
Washington, DC 20001   Phone: (202) 638-2952
Description: Concerned with federal social legislation and the activities of federal agencies affecting children, the elderly, the handicapped, and delinquents. Also concerned with health, education, welfare, housing, employment, and other social welfare conditions and issues. **First Published:** 1944. **Frequency:** Semimonthly. **ISSN:** 0149-2578.

★3088★ THE WEB
Illinois Head Injury Association, Inc.
8903 W. Burlington
Brookfield, IL 60513   Phone: (800) 284-IHIA
Description: Publicizes the activities of the Association, which seeks to reduce the unnecessary frustrations of head-injured individuals and their families. Provides information about available programs, prevention and treatment advice, support groups, and recreational and sports events for head-injured individuals. Recurring features include a calendar of events and reports of meetings. **Frequency:** Quarterly.

★3089★ THE WEBB REPORT
Pacific Resource Development Group
4044 58th St. NE
Seattle, WA 98105   Phone: (206) 782-7015
Description: Provides information on court cases and issues involving sexual harassment and guidelines concerning what is and what is not considered to be harassment and what to do about it. Recurring features include news of research and notices of publications available. **First Published:** January 1985. **Frequency:** Monthly.

★3090★ WEEKLY PHARMACY REPORTS—THE GREEN SHEET
F-D-C Reports, Inc.
5550 Friendship Blvd., Ste. 1
Chevy Chase, MD 20815   Phone: (301) 657-9830
Description: Provides information on the pharmacy profession and pharmaceutical distribution system. Covers new drug introductions, pharmaceutical pricing and deals, governmental actions, and national and state pharmacy association activities. **First Published:** 1951. **Frequency:** Weekly. **ISSN:** 0043-1893.

★3091★ WELLNESS ASSOCIATES—JOURNAL
Wellness Associates
12347 Dupont Rd.
Sebastopol, CA 95472   Phone: (707) 874-1466
Description: Devoted to wellness, focusing on "the linking of personal and planetary; and shifting prevailing dominator norms to norms recognizing our interdependence and enchance personal integrity, diversity, and partnership." **First Published:** 1981. **Frequency:** Quarterly.

★3092★ WELLNESS MANAGEMENT
National Wellness Institute, Inc.
1319 Fremont-S. Hall
Stevens Point, WI 54481   Phone: (715) 346-2172
Description: Serves as a forum for the National Wellness Association. Provides information on recent developments, resources, programming, events, and educational opportunities in the wellness and health promotion fields. **First Published:** June 1985. **Frequency:** Quarterly.

★3093★ THE WELLNESS NEWSLETTER
Dr. Carolyn Chambers Clark
3451 Central Ave.
St. Petersburg, FL 33713-8522
Description: Focuses on the wellness dimensions of fitness, nutrition, stress management, interpersonal relationships, and on wellness programs themselves. Discusses barriers to wellness and how to overcome them. Recurring features include news of research, announcements of workshops and free resources, and columns titled Book News and Reviews, Reader Queries, and From the Editor. **First Published:** January 1980. **Frequency:** Bimonthly. **ISSN:** 0740-8498.

★3094★ WESTERN CENTER NEWS
Northwest Regional Educational Laboratory
101 SW Main St., No. 500
Portland, OR 97204   Phone: (503) 248-6800
Description: Offers information on drug education and prevention from the Western and Pacific states. **Frequency:** Quarterly.

★3095★ WESTVIEWS
Western Dental Society
6242 Westchester Pkwy., Ste. 220
Los Angeles, CA 90045   Phone: (213) 641-5561
Description: Carries information on current issues in dentistry. Recurring features include letters to the editor, interviews, news of research, a calendar of events, reports of meetings, news of educational opportunities, and job listings. **Frequency:** 8/yr.

★3096★ WIDHH NEWSLETTER
Western Institute for the Deaf and Hard of Hearing
2125 W. 7th Ave.
Vancouver, BC, Canada V6K 1X9   Phone: (604) 736-7391
Description: Covers Institute activities. Recurring features include reports of meetings and news of educational opportunities. **Frequency:** Quarterly.

★3097★ WILDERNESS MEDICINE LETTER
Wilderness Medical Society
PO Box 397
Point Reyes Station, CA 94956   Phone: (415) 663-9107
Description: Keeps members informed of research and educational projects that increase scientific knowledge about human activities in wilderness environments. Includes articles on such topics as bites and stings, exotic infectious diseases, toxic plants, and desert survival. **First Published:** 1983. **Frequency:** Quarterly.

★3098★ WILDERNESS MEDICINE NEWSLETTER
1208 St. Francis Rd.
Bel Air, MD 21014   Phone: (301) 838-0462
Description: Discusses practices and ideas regarding medical care and treatment in remote environments. Provides information on bacteria and viruses, techniques, medication, and seminars. **First Published:** May 1988. **Frequency:** 6/yr.

★3099★ WIN NEWS
Women's International Network
187 Grant St.
Lexington, MA 02173   Phone: (617) 862-9431
Description: Acts as "a worldwide open communication system by, for, and about women of all backgrounds, beliefs, nationalities, and age-groups." Provides news and commentary on women and health, violence, the

environment, human rights, science, media, and the United Nations. Contains reports from North America, Latin America, Europe, Africa, the Middle East, Asia, and the Pacific. Recurring features include names/addresses of all report and contact persons, statistics, book reviews, news of conferences, a calendar of events, and a section on career opportunities in the international field. **First Published:** January 1975. **Frequency:** Quarterly. **ISSN:** 0145-7985.

★3100★   WISTAR INSTITUTE OF ANATOMY AND BIOLOGY—
NEWSLETTER
Wistar Institute of Anatomy and Biology
36th & Spruce Sts.
Philadelphia, PA 19104   Phone: (215) 898-3700
Description: Communicates non-scientific employee news. **First Published:** June 1987. **Frequency:** Bimonthly.

★3101★   WISTAR PROSPECTUS
Wistar Institute of Anatomy and Biology
36th & Spruce Sts.
Philadelphia, PA 19104   Phone: (215) 898-3700
First Published: October 1991. **Frequency:** Quarterly.

★3102★   WOMEN AND HEALTH ROUNDTABLE REPORT
Women & Health Roundtable
1000 Connecticut Ave. NW, Ste. 9
Washington, DC 20036   Phone: (301) 953-4215
Description: Reports on health issues relating to women. **Frequency:** 10/yr. **ISSN:** 0272-0515.

★3103★   WOMEN, INFANTS, AND CHILDREN NEWSLETTER
Center on Budget and Policy Priorities
777 N. Capitol St. NE, Ste. 705
Washington, DC 20002   Phone: (202) 408-1080
Description: Provides legislative and administrative updates on the Special Supplemental Food Program for Women, Infants and Children (WIC), and covers other maternal and child health issues. **First Published:** August 1981. **Frequency:** 9/yr.

★3104★   WOMEN'S STUDIES RESEARCH CENTER—
NEWSLETTER
Women's Studies Research Center
University of Wisconsin, Madison
209 N. Brooks St.
Madison, WI 53715   Phone: (608) 263-2053.
Description: Presents information on research conducted at the UW - Madison, and administered by the Women's Studies Research Center. Includes topics such as motherhood, childbirth, health issues, feminism and science, technology, and women's autobiographies. Recurring features include editorials, news of research, news of members, book reviews, and a calendar of events. **First Published:** September 1979. **Frequency:** Biennially.

★3105★   WORD & DEED
American Leprosy Missions International
1 A.L.M. Way
Greenville, SC 29601   Phone: (201) 794-8650
Description: Profiles the Mission's international field programs, which include medical treatment and rehabilitation of leprosy victims, training of medical personnel, public education about the disease, and reconstructive surgery and rehabilitation of persons with disabilities. Carries reports from different countries, fundraising news, information on films and publications by the Mission, and the Mission's annual report. **Frequency:** 10/yr.

★3106★   WORD FROM WASHINGTON
United Cerebral Palsy Associations, Inc.
1522 K St. NW, Ste. 112
Washington, DC 20005   Phone: (202) 842-1266
Description: Covers federal legislation, programs, and policy and regulatory actions affecting persons with developmental disabilities. Discusses Medicaid, child health, appropriations, special education, vocational rehabilitation, housing, Social Security, assistive technology, social services, and activities of concerned groups. Recurring features include announcements of grants and new publications. **First Published:** January 1969. **Frequency:** Bimonthly.

★3107★   WORK PROGRAMS SPECIAL INTEREST SECTION—
NEWSLETTER
Work Programs Special Interest Section
American Occupational Therapy Association
1383 Piccard Dr.
PO Box 1725
Rockville, MD 20850   Phone: (301) 948-9626
Description: Focuses on habilitation and rehabilitation of the worker in areas of physical disabilities, developmental disabilities, and mental health. **First Published:** January 1987. **Frequency:** Quarterly. **ISSN:** 1043-1470.

★3108★   WORKING TOGETHER
National Association of Anorexia Nervosa and Associated Disorders
PO Box 7
Highland Park, IL 60035   Phone: (708) 831-3438
Description: Publishes news of the Association, which is "dedicated to alleviating the problems of eating disorders." Features articles written by victims of anorexia nervosa and/or bulimia, therapists, and family members. Recurring features include editorials, letters to the editor, book reviews, news of members, a calendar of events, poetry, and news of Association chapters. **First Published:** 1981. **Frequency:** Quarterly.

★3109★   WORLD FEDERATION OF HEALTH AGENCIES FOR
THE ADVANCEMENT OF VOLUNTARY SURGICAL
CONTRACEPTION—COMMUNIQUE
World Federation of Health Agencies for the Advancement of
Voluntary Surgical Contraception
122 E. 42nd St.
New York, NY 10168   Phone: (212) 351-2536
Description: Covers all aspects of voluntary surgical contraception, including programs, research, legal issues, new technologies, medical guidelines, and counseling. Emphasizes voluntary sterilization issues in developing countries. Recurring features include news of research and news of members. **First Published:** 1980. **Frequency:** 2/yr. **ISSN:** 0001-2904.

★3110★   WORLD MEDICAL RELIEF—NEWSLETTER
World Medical Relief
11745 12th St.
Detroit, MI 48206   Phone: (313) 866-5322
Description: Chronicles activities of the agency, a nonsectarian philanthropic organization contributing medical supplies to the world's destitute sick. Recurring features include a calendar of events and notices of awards. **Frequency:** Periodic.

★3111★   WORLD NEIGHBORS IN ACTION
World Neighbors Inc.
4127 NW 122nd St.
Oklahoma City, OK 73120-8869   Phone: (405) 752-9700
Description: Serves as part of a worldwide, people-to-people movement for cooperative self-help projects in developing nations. Focuses on a specific concern in each issue, such as health and nutrition, family planning, community development, or agriculture and food production. Recurring features include suggestions for reducing program costs, practical information for putting programs into effect, and notices of pertinent reading materials and resources. **First Published:** March 6, 1964. **Frequency:** Quarterly.

★3112★   WORLDWIDE BIOTECH
Worldwide Videotex
Babson Pk.
PO Box 138
Boston, MA 02157   Phone: (617) 449-1603
Description: Focuses on developments of domestic biotechnology companies and international pharmaceutical companies. Covers joint ventures , European markets, and activities in Japan. **Frequency:** Monthly.

★3113★   WORLDWIDE SERIAL REPORTS: EPIDEMIOLOGY
Joint Publications Research Service
National Technical Information Service
Springfield, VA 22162   Phone: (703) 487-4650

★3114★   WYOMING NURSE
Wyoming Nurses' Association, Inc.
1603 Capitol Ave., Ste. 305
Cheyenne, WY 82001   Phone: (307) 635-3955
Description: Discusses issues affecting Association members. Recurring features include an editorial, reports of board of directors, meetings, and a

calendar of events. Also includes state and national convention reports, continuing education awards and programs, legislative news, economic and general welfare news, and lists of publications and audiovisual materials available. **Frequency:** 4/yr.

★3115★   YOUR HEALTH REPORT
General Learning Corp.
60 Revere Dr.
Northbrook, IL 60062-1563   Phone: (708) 205-3000
Description: Encourages good health habits among company employees and their families, community members, and managed care group members. **Frequency:** Quarterly.

★3116★   ZERO TO THREE
National Center for Clinical Infant Programs
2000 14th St. N., Ste. 350
Arlington, VA 22201   Phone: (703) 528-4300
Description: Focuses on infant health, mental health, and development. Carries clinical case studies, research reports, news of publications and conferences, information on relevant government initiatives, and descriptions of programs in the field. Recurring features include book reviews and news of the Center. **First Published:** September 1980. **Frequency:** 5/yr. **ISSN:** 0736-8083.

(3) Annuals and Review Serials

The following are arranged alphabetically by publication titles. For additional information, see the User's Guide located at the front of this directory.

★3117★ ADOLESCENT PSYCHIATRY
American Society for Adolescent Psychiatry
5530 Wisconsin Ave., NW, Ste. 1149
Washington, DC 20815   Phone: (301) 652-0646
First Published: 1971. Frequency: Annual. ISSN: 0065-2008.

★3118★ ADVANCES IN ALCOHOL AND SUBSTANCE ABUSE
The Haworth Press, Inc.
10 Alice St.
Binghamton, NY 13904   Phone: (800) 342-9678
First Published: 1981. Frequency: Quarterly. ISSN: 0270-3106.

★3119★ ADVANCES IN ANATOMY, EMBRYOLOGY AND
CELL BIOLOGY
Springer-Verlag New York, Inc.
175 5th Ave.
New York, NY 10010   Phone: (212) 460-1500
First Published: 1966. Frequency: Irregular. ISSN: 0301-5556.

★3120★ ADVANCES IN ANESTHESIA
Mosby-Year Book, Inc.
11830 Westline Industrial Dr.
St. Louis, MO 63146   Phone: (314) 872-8370
First Published: 1982. Frequency: Annual. ISSN: 0737-6146.

★3121★ ADVANCES IN APPLIED DEVELOPMENTAL
PSYCHOLOGY
Ablex Publishing Corp.
355 Chestnut St.
Norwood, NJ 07648   Phone: (201) 767-8450
First Published: 1985. Frequency: Irregular. ISSN: 0748-8572.

★3122★ ADVANCES IN APPLIED MICROBIOLOGY
Academic Press, Inc.
1250 6th Ave.
San Diego, CA 92101   Phone: (619) 231-0926
First Published: 1959. Frequency: Irregular. ISSN: 0065-2164.

★3123★ ADVANCES IN BEHAVIOR RESEARCH AND
THERAPY
Pergamon Press, Inc.
Maxwell House, Fairview Park
Elmsford, NY 10523   Phone: (914) 592-7700
First Published: 1978. Frequency: Quarterly. ISSN: 0146-6402.

★3124★ ADVANCES IN BIOCHEMICAL
PSYCHOPHARMACOLOGY
Raven Press
1185 Avenue of the Americas
New York, NY 10036   Phone: (212) 930-9500
First Published: 1969. Frequency: Irregular. ISSN: 0065-2229.

★3125★ ADVANCES IN BIOLOGICAL PSYCHIATRY
S. Karger Publishers, Inc.
26 W. Avon Rd.
PO Box 529
Farmington, CT 06085   Phone: (203) 675-7834
First Published: 1978. Frequency: Irregular. ISSN: 0378-7354.

★3126★ ADVANCES IN CANCER RESEARCH
Academic Press, Inc.
1250 6th Ave.
San Diego, CA 92101   Phone: (619) 231-0926
First Published: 1953. Frequency: Irregular. ISSN: 0065-230X.

★3127★ ADVANCES IN CARBOHYDRATE CHEMISTRY AND
BIOCHEMISTRY
Academic Press, Inc.
1250 6th Ave.
San Diego, CA 92101   Phone: (619) 231-0926
First Published: 1945. Frequency: Irregular. ISSN: 0065-2318.

★3128★ ADVANCES IN CARDIAC SURGERY
Mosby-Year Book, Inc.
11830 Westline Industrial Dr.
St. Louis, MO 63146   Phone: (314) 872-8370
First Published: 1988. Frequency: Annual. ISSN: 0889-5074.

★3129★ ADVANCES IN CARDIOLOGY
S. Karger Publishers, Inc.
26 W. Avon Rd.
PO Box 529
Farmington, CT 06085   Phone: (203) 675-7834
First Published: 1956. Frequency: Irregular. ISSN: 0065-2326.

★3130★ ADVANCES IN CARDIOVASCULAR PHYSICS
S. Karger Publishers, Inc.
26 W. Avon Rd.
PO Box 529
Farmington, CT 06085   Phone: (203) 675-7834
Frequency: Irregular. ISSN: 0378-6900.

★3131★ ADVANCES IN CELL CULTURE
Academic Press, Inc.
1250 6th Ave.
San Diego, CA 92101   Phone: (619) 231-0926
First Published: 1981. Frequency: Annual. ISSN: 0275-6358.

★3132★   ADVANCES IN CHILD DEVELOPMENT AND BEHAVIOR
Academic Press, Inc.
1250 6th Ave.
San Diego, CA 92101   Phone: (619) 231-0926
First Published: 1963. **Frequency:** Irregular. **ISSN:** 0065-2407.

★3133★   ADVANCES IN CLINICAL CHEMISTRY
Academic Press, Inc.
1250 6th Ave.
San Diego, CA 92101   Phone: (619) 231-0926
First Published: 1958. **Frequency:** Irregular. **ISSN:** 0065-2423.

★3134★   ADVANCES IN CLINICAL ENZYMOLOGY
S. Karger Publishers, Inc.
26 W. Avon Rd.
PO Box 529
Farmington, CT 06085   Phone: (203) 675-7834
First Published: 1979. **Frequency:** Irregular. **ISSN:** 0250-4197.

★3135★   ADVANCES IN CONTRACEPTION
Kluwer Academic Publishers
101 Philip Dr.
Assinippi Park
Norwell, MA 02061   Phone: (617) 871-6600
First Published: 1985. **Frequency:** Quarterly. **ISSN:** 0267-4874.

★3136★   ADVANCES IN DERMATOLOGY
Mosby-Year Book, Inc.
11830 Westline Industrial Dr.
St. Louis, MO 63146   Phone: (314) 872-8370
First Published: 1986. **Frequency:** Annual. **ISSN:** 0882-0880.

★3137★   ADVANCES IN DESCRIPTIVE PSYCHOLOGY
JAI Press, Inc.
55 Old Post Rd., No. 2
Box 1678
Greenwich, CT 06836   Phone: (203) 661-7602
First Published: 1981. **Frequency:** Annual. **ISSN:** 0276-9913.

★3138★   ADVANCES IN DEVELOPMENTAL AND BEHAVIORAL PEDIATRICS
JAI Press, Inc.
55 Old Post Rd., No. 2
Box 1678
Greenwich, CT 06836   Phone: (203) 661-7602
First Published: 1980. **Frequency:** Annual.

★3139★   ADVANCES IN DEVELOPMENTAL PSYCHOLOGY
Lawrence Erlbaum Associates, Inc.
365 Broadway
Hillsdale, NJ 07642   Phone: (201) 666-4110
First Published: 1981. **Frequency:** Irregular. **ISSN:** 0275-3049.

★3140★   ADVANCES IN DRUG RESEARCH
Academic Press, Inc.
1250 6th Ave.
San Diego, CA 92101   Phone: (619) 231-0926
First Published: 1964. **Frequency:** Irregular. **ISSN:** 0065-2490.

★3141★   ADVANCES IN ENDOCRINOLOGY AND METABOLISM
Mosby-Year Book, Inc.
11830 Westline Industrial Dr.
St. Louis, MO 63146   Phone: (314) 872-8370
First Published: 1990. **ISSN:** 1049-6734.

★3142★   ADVANCES IN ENZYME REGULATION
Pergamon Press, Inc.
Maxwell House, Fairview Park
Elmsford, NY 10523   Phone: (914) 592-7700
First Published: 1963. **Frequency:** Annual. **ISSN:** 0065-2571.

★3143★   ADVANCES IN ENZYMOLOGY AND RELATED AREAS OF MOLECULAR BIOLOGY
John Wiley & Sons, Inc.
605 3rd. Ave.
New York, NY 10158   Phone: (212) 850-6000
First Published: 1942. **Frequency:** Irregular. **ISSN:** 0065-258X.

★3144★   ADVANCES IN EXPERIMENTAL MEDICINE AND BIOLOGY
Plenum Publishing Corp.
233 Spring St.
New York, NY 10013   Phone: (212) 620-8000
First Published: 1967. **Frequency:** Irregular. **ISSN:** 0065-2598.

★3145★   ADVANCES IN FOOD AND NUTRITION RESEARCH
Academic Press, Inc.
1250 6th Ave.
San Diego, CA 92101   Phone: (619) 231-0926
First Published: 1948. **Frequency:** Irregular. **ISSN:** 0065-2628.

★3146★   ADVANCES IN GENETICS
Academic Press, Inc.
1250 6th Ave.
San Diego, CA 92101   Phone: (619) 231-0926
First Published: 1947. **Frequency:** Irregular. **ISSN:** 0065-2660.

★3147★   ADVANCES IN HUMAN FERTILITY AND REPRODUCTIVE ENDOCRINOLOGY
Raven Press
1185 Avenue of the Americas
New York, NY 10036   Phone: (212) 930-9500
First Published: 1982. **Frequency:** Annual.

★3148★   ADVANCES IN HUMAN GENETICS
Plenum Publishing Corp.
233 Spring St.
New York, NY 10013   Phone: (212) 620-8000
First Published: 1970. **Frequency:** Irregular. **ISSN:** 0065-275X.

★3149★   ADVANCES IN HUMAN PSYCHOPHARMACOLOGY
JAI Press, Inc.
55 Old Post Rd., No. 2
Box 1678
Greenwich, CT 06836   Phone: (203) 661-7602
First Published: 1980. **Frequency:** Annual. **ISSN:** 0272-068X.

★3150★   ADVANCES IN IMMUNOLOGY
Academic Press, Inc.
1250 6th Ave.
San Diego, CA 92101   Phone: (619) 231-0926
First Published: 1961. **Frequency:** Irregular. **ISSN:** 0065-2776.

★3151★   ADVANCES IN INFANCY RESEARCH
Ablex Publishing Corp.
355 Chestnut St.
Norwood, NJ 07648   Phone: (201) 767-8450
First Published: 1981. **Frequency:** Annual. **ISSN:** 0732-9598.

★3152★   ADVANCES IN INFLAMMATION RESEARCH
Raven Press
1185 Avenue of the Americas
New York, NY 10036   Phone: (212) 930-9500
First Published: 1979. **Frequency:** Irregular. **ISSN:** 0197-8322.

★3153★   ADVANCES IN INTERNAL MEDICINE
Mosby-Year Book, Inc.
11830 Westline Industrial Dr.
St. Louis, MO 63146   Phone: (314) 872-8370
First Published: 1954. **Frequency:** Annual. **ISSN:** 0065-2822.

★3154★ ADVANCES IN LEARNING AND BEHAVIORAL
DISABILITIES
JAI Press, Inc.
55 Old Post Rd., No. 2
Box 1678
Greenwich, CT 06836   Phone: (203) 661-7602
First Published: 1982. Frequency: Annual.

★3155★ ADVANCES IN LIPID RESEARCH
Academic Press, Inc.
1250 6th Ave.
San Diego, CA 92101   Phone: (619) 231-0926
First Published: 1963. Frequency: Irregular. ISSN: 0065-2849.

★3156★ ADVANCES IN NEPHROLOGY
Mosby-Year Book, Inc.
11830 Westline Industrial Dr.
St. Louis, MO 63146   Phone: (314) 872-8370
First Published: 1971. Frequency: Annual.

★3157★ ADVANCES IN NEUROLOGY
Raven Press
1185 Avenue of the Americas
New York, NY 10036   Phone: (212) 930-9500
First Published: 1973. Frequency: Irregular. ISSN: 0091-3952.

★3158★ ADVANCES IN NEUROSURGERY
Springer-Verlag New York, Inc.
175 5th Ave.
New York, NY 10010   Phone: (212) 460-1500
First Published: 1973. Frequency: Irregular. ISSN: 0302-2366.

★3159★ ADVANCES IN NURSING SCIENCE
Aspen Publishers, Inc.
200 Orchard Ridge Dr.
Gaithersburg, MD 20878   Phone: (301) 417-7500
First Published: 1978. Frequency: Quarterly. ISSN: 0161-9268.

★3160★ ADVANCES IN OPHTHALMIC PLASTIC AND
RECONSTRUCTIVE SURGERY
Pergamon Press, Inc.
Maxwell House, Fairview Park
Elmsford, NY 10523   Phone: (914) 592-7700
First Published: 1982. Frequency: Annual. ISSN: 0276-3508.

★3161★ ADVANCES IN ORTHOPAEDIC SURGERY
Williams & Wilkins
428 E. Preston St.
Baltimore, MD 21202   Phone: (301) 528-4223
First Published: 1977. Frequency: Bimonthly. ISSN: 0738-2278.

★3162★ ADVANCES IN OTOLARYNGOLOGY: HEAD AND
NECK SURGERY
Mosby-Year Book, Inc.
11830 Westline Industrial Dr.
St. Louis, MO 63146   Phone: (314) 872-8370
First Published: 1987. Frequency: Annual. ISSN: 0887-6916.

★3163★ ADVANCES IN OTO-RHINO-LARYNGOLOGY
S. Karger Publishers, Inc.
26 W. Avon Rd.
PO Box 529
Farmington, CT 06085   Phone: (203) 675-7834
First Published: 1953. Frequency: Irregular. ISSN: 0065-3071.

★3164★ ADVANCES IN PAIN RESEARCH AND THERAPY
Raven Press
1185 Avenue of the Americas
New York, NY 10036   Phone: (212) 930-9500
First Published: 1976. Frequency: Irregular. ISSN: 0146-0722.

★3165★ ADVANCES IN PARASITOLOGY
Academic Press, Inc.
1250 6th Ave.
San Diego, CA 92101   Phone: (619) 231-0926
First Published: 1963. Frequency: Annual. ISSN: 0065-308X.

★3166★ ADVANCES IN PEDIATRIC INFECTIOUS DISEASES
Mosby-Year Book, Inc.
11830 Westline Industrial Dr.
St. Louis, MO 63146   Phone: (314) 872-8370
First Published: 1986. Frequency: Annual. ISSN: 0884-9404.

★3167★ ADVANCES IN PEDIATRICS
Mosby-Year Book, Inc.
11830 Westline Industrial Dr.
St. Louis, MO 63146   Phone: (314) 872-8370
First Published: 1942. Frequency: Annual. ISSN: 0065-3101.

★3168★ ADVANCES IN PERSONALITY ASSESSMENT
Lawrence Erlbaum Associates, Inc.
365 Broadway
Hillsdale, NJ 07642   Phone: (201) 666-4110
First Published: 1982. Frequency: Irregular. ISSN: 0278-2367.

★3169★ ADVANCES IN PHARMACEUTICAL SCIENCES
Academic Press, Inc.
1250 6th Ave.
San Diego, CA 92101   Phone: (619) 231-0926
First Published: 1964. Frequency: Irregular. ISSN: 0065-3136.

★3170★ ADVANCES IN PHARMACOLOGY AND
CHEMOTHERAPY
Academic Press, Inc.
1250 6th Ave.
St. Louis, MO 92101   Phone: (619) 231-0926
First Published: 1962. Frequency: Irregular. ISSN: 0065-3144.

★3171★ ADVANCES IN PLASTIC AND RECONSTRUCTIVE
SURGERY
Mosby-Year Book, Inc.
11830 Westline Industrial Dr.
St. Louis, MO 63146   Phone: (314) 872-8370
First Published: 1984. Frequency: Annual. ISSN: 0748-5212.

★3172★ ADVANCES IN PROSTAGLANDIN, THROMBOXANE
AND LEUKOTRIENE RESEARCH
Raven Press
1185 Avenue of the Americas
New York, NY 10036   Phone: (212) 930-9500
First Published: 1976. Frequency: Irregular. ISSN: 0732-8141.

★3173★ ADVANCES IN PROTEIN CHEMISTRY
Academic Press, Inc.
1250 6th Ave.
San Diego, CA 92101   Phone: (619) 231-0926
First Published: 1944. Frequency: Annual. ISSN: 0065-3233.

★3174★ ADVANCES IN PSYCHOSOMATIC MEDICINE
S. Karger Publishers, Inc.
26 W. Avon Rd.
PO Box 529
Farmington, CT 06085   Phone: (203) 675-7834
First Published: 1960. Frequency: Irregular. ISSN: 0065-3268.

★3175★ ADVANCES IN RADIATION BIOLOGY
Academic Press, Inc.
1250 6th Ave.
San Diego, CA 92101   Phone: (619) 231-0926
First Published: 1964. Frequency: Irregular. ISSN: 0065-3292.

★3176★ ADVANCES IN SECOND MESSENGER AND
PHOSPHOPROTEIN RESEARCH
Raven Press
1185 Avenue of the Americas
New York, NY 10036   Phone: (212) 930-9500
First Published: 1972. Frequency: Irregular.

★3177★ ADVANCES IN SUBSTANCE ABUSE: BEHAVIORAL AND BIOLOGICAL RESEARCH
JAI Press, Inc.
55 Old Post Rd., No. 2
Box 1678
Greenwich, CT 06836   Phone: (203) 661-7602
First Published: 1980. **Frequency:** Annual. **ISSN:** 0272-1740.

★3178★ ADVANCES IN SURGERY
Mosby-Year Book, Inc.
11830 Westline Industrial Dr.
St. Louis, MO 63146   Phone: (314) 872-8370
First Published: 1966. **Frequency:** Annual. **ISSN:** 0065-3411.

★3179★ ADVANCES AND TECHNICAL STANDARDS IN NEUROSURGERY
Springer-Verlag New York, Inc.
175 5th Ave.
New York, NY 10010   Phone: (212) 460-1500
First Published: 1974. **Frequency:** Irregular. **ISSN:** 0095-4829.

★3180★ ADVANCES IN TRAUMA
Mosby-Year Book, Inc.
11830 Westline Industrial Dr.
St. Louis, MO 63146   Phone: (314) 872-8370
First Published: 1986. **Frequency:** Annual. **ISSN:** 0886-7755.

★3181★ ADVANCES IN UROLOGY
Mosby-Year Book, Inc.
11830 Westline Industrial Dr.
St. Louis, MO 63146   Phone: (314) 872-8370
First Published: 1988. **Frequency:** Annual. **ISSN:** 0894-4385.

★3182★ ADVANCES IN VETERINARY SCIENCE AND COMPARATIVE MEDICINE
Academic Press, Inc.
1250 6th Ave.
San Diego, CA 92101   Phone: (619) 231-0926
First Published: 1953. **Frequency:** Irregular. **ISSN:** 0065-3519.

★3183★ ADVANCES IN VIRAL ONCOLOGY
Raven Press
1185 Avenue of the Americas
New York, NY 10036   Phone: (212) 930-9500
First Published: 1982. **Frequency:** Irregular.

★3184★ ADVANCES IN VIRUS RESEARCH
Academic Press, Inc.
1250 6th Ave.
San Diego, CA 92101   Phone: (619) 231-0926
First Published: 1953. **Frequency:** Irregular. **ISSN:** 0065-3527.

★3185★ ADVERSE DRUG REACTIONS AND ACUTE POISONING REVIEWS
Oxford University Press, Inc.
200 Madison Ave.
New York, NY 10016   Phone: (212) 679-7300
First Published: 1982. **Frequency:** Quarterly. **ISSN:** 0260-647X.

★3186★ AMBULATORY MONITORING AND BLOOD PRESSURE VARIABILITY
Current Science
20 N. 3rd St.
Philadelphia, PA 19106   Phone: (215) 514-2266

★3187★ ANNUAL OF CARDIAC SURGERY
Current Science
20 N. 3rd St.
Philadelphia, PA 19106   Phone: (215) 514-2266
ISSN: 0952-0562.

★3188★ ANNUAL OF GASTROINTESTINAL ENDOSCOPY
Current Science
20 N. 3rd St.
Philadelphia, PA 19106   Phone: (215) 514-2266
ISSN: 0952-6293.

★3189★ ANNUAL OF OPTHALMIC LASER SURGERY
Current Science
20 N. 3rd St.
Philadelphia, PA 19106   Phone: (215) 514-2266
First Published: 1992.

★3190★ ANNUAL PROGRESS IN CHILD PSYCHIATRY AND CHILD DEVELOPMENT
Brunner/Mazel, Inc.
19 Union Sq., W.
New York, NY 10003   Phone: (212) 924-3344
First Published: 1968. **Frequency:** Annual. **ISSN:** 0066-4030.

★3191★ ANNUAL REPORTS IN MEDICINAL CHEMISTRY
Academic Press, Inc.
1250 6th Ave.
San Diego, CA 92101   Phone: (619) 231-0926
First Published: 1966. **Frequency:** Irregular. **ISSN:** 0065-7743.

★3192★ ANNUAL REVIEW OF ADDICTIONS RESEARCH AND TREATMENT
Pergamon Press Inc.
395 Saw Mill River Rd.
Elmsford, NY 10523   Phone: (914) 592-7700
ISSN: 0955-663X.

★3193★ ANNUAL REVIEW OF BIOCHEMISTRY
Annual Reviews, Inc.
4139 El Camino Way
PO Box 10139
Palo Alto, CA 94303   Phone: (415) 493-4400
First Published: 1932. **Frequency:** Annual. **ISSN:** 0066-4154.

★3194★ ANNUAL REVIEW OF BIOPHYSICS AND BIOMOLECULAR CHEMISTRY
Annual Reviews, Inc.
4139 El Camino Way
PO Box 10139
Palo Alto, CA 94303   Phone: (415) 493-4400
First Published: 1972. **Frequency:** Annual. **ISSN:** 0883-9182.

★3195★ ANNUAL REVIEW OF CELL BIOLOGY
Annual Reviews, Inc.
4139 El Camino Way
PO Box 10139
Palo Alto, CA 94303   Phone: (415) 493-4400
First Published: 1985. **Frequency:** Annual. **ISSN:** 0743-4634.

★3196★ ANNUAL REVIEW OF GENETICS
Annual Reviews, Inc.
4139 El Camino Way
PO Box 10139
Palo Alto, CA 94303   Phone: (415) 493-4400
First Published: 1967. **Frequency:** Annual. **ISSN:** 0066-4197.

★3197★ ANNUAL REVIEW OF GERONTOLOGY AND GERIATRICS
Springer Publishing Co.
536 Broadway
New York, NY 10012   Phone: (212) 431-4370
First Published: 1980. **Frequency:** Annual. **ISSN:** 0198-8794.

★3198★ ANNUAL REVIEW OF IMMUNOLOGY
Annual Reviews, Inc.
4139 El Camino Way
PO Box 10139
Palo Alto, CA 94303   Phone: (415) 493-4400
First Published: 1983. **Frequency:** Annual. **ISSN:** 0732-0582.

★3199★ ANNUAL REVIEW OF MEDICINE: SELECTED TOPICS IN THE CLINICAL SCIENCES
Annual Reviews, Inc.
4139 El Camino Way
PO Box 10139
Palo Alto, CA 94303   Phone: (415) 493-4400
First Published: 1950. **Frequency:** Annual. **ISSN:** 0066-4219.

★3200★   ANNUAL REVIEW OF MICROBIOLOGY
Annual Reviews, Inc.
4139 El Camino Way
PO Box 10139
Palo Alto, CA 94303   Phone: (415) 493-4400
First Published: 1947. Frequency: Annual. ISSN: 0066-4227.

★3201★   ANNUAL REVIEW OF NEUROSCIENCE
Annual Reviews, Inc.
4139 El Camino Way
PO Box 10139
Palo Alto, CA 94303   Phone: (415) 493-4400
First Published: 1977. Frequency: Annual. ISSN: 0147-006X.

★3202★   ANNUAL REVIEW OF NURSING RESEARCH
Springer Publishing Co.
536 Broadway
New York, NY 10012   Phone: (212) 431-4370
First Published: 1984. Frequency: Annual. ISSN: 0739-6686.

★3203★   ANNUAL REVIEW OF NUTRITION
Annual Reviews, Inc.
4139 El Camino Way
PO Box 10139
Palo Alto, CA 94303   Phone: (415) 493-4400
First Published: 1981. Frequency: Annual. ISSN: 0199-9885.

★3204★   ANNUAL REVIEW OF PHARMACOLOGY AND
   TOXICOLOGY
Annual Reviews, Inc.
4139 El Camino Way
PO Box 10139
Palo Alto, CA 94303   Phone: (415) 493-4400
First Published: 1961. Frequency: Annual. ISSN: 0362-1642.

★3205★   ANNUAL REVIEW OF PHYSIOLOGY
Annual Reviews, Inc.
4139 El Camino Way
PO Box 10139
Palo Alto, CA 94303   Phone: (415) 493-4400
First Published: 1939. Frequency: Annual. ISSN: 0066-4278.

★3206★   ANNUAL REVIEW OF PSYCHOLOGY
Annual Reviews, Inc.
4139 El Camino Way
PO Box 10139
Palo Alto, CA 94303   Phone: (415) 493-4400
First Published: 1950. Frequency: Annual. ISSN: 0066-4308.

★3207★   ANNUAL REVIEW OF PUBLIC HEALTH
Annual Reviews, Inc.
4139 El Camino Way
PO Box 10139
Palo Alto, CA 94303   Phone: (415) 493-4400
First Published: 1980. Frequency: Annual. ISSN: 0163-7525.

★3208★   ANNUAL REVIEW OF SOCIOLOGY
Annual Reviews, Inc.
4139 El Camino Way
PO Box 10139
Palo Alto, CA 94303   Phone: (415) 493-4400
First Published: 1975. Frequency: Annual. ISSN: 0360-0572.

★3209★   ANTIBIOTICS AND CHEMOTHERAPY
S. Karger Publishers, Inc.
26 W. Avon Rd.
PO Box 529
Farmington, CT 06085   Phone: (203) 675-7834
First Published: 1954. Frequency: Irregular. ISSN: 0066-4758.

★3210★   AUSTRALIAN CLINICAL REVIEW
Blackwell Scientific Publications Pty. Ltd.
PO Box 378
Carlton, Vic. 3053, Australia
First Published: 1981. Frequency: Quarterly. ISSN: 0726-3139.

★3211★   BAILLIERE'S CLINICAL ANESTHESIOLOGY
W.B. Saunders Co.
Curtis Center
Independence Sq., W.
Philadelphia, PA 19106   Phone: (215) 238-7800
First Published: 1983. Frequency: Quarterly. ISSN: 0950-3501.

★3212★   BIOMEDICAL SCIENCE AND TECHNOLOGY
Academic Press
1250 6th Ave.
San Diego, CA 92101   Phone: (619) 669-6412
First Published: 1991. Frequency: Quarterly. ISSN: 1051-2020.

★3213★   BIOTECHNOLOGY ADVANCES
Pergamon Press, Inc.
Maxwell House, Fairview Park
Elmsford, NY 10523   Phone: (914) 592-7700
First Published: 1983. Frequency: Quarterly. ISSN: 0734-9750.

★3214★   BREAST DISEASES—A YEAR BOOK QUARTERLY
Mosby-Year Book, Inc.
11830 Westline Industrial Dr.
St. Louis, MO 63146   Phone: (314) 872-8370
First Published: 1990. Frequency: Quarterly.

★3215★   CANCER AND METASTASIS REVIEWS
Kluwer Academic Publishers
101 Philip Dr.
Norwell, MA 02066
First Published: 1981. Frequency: Quarterly. ISSN: 0891-9992.

★3216★   CARDIOLOGY CLINICS
W.B. Saunders Co.
Curtis Center
Independence Sq., W.
Philadelphia, PA 19106   Phone: (215) 238-7800
First Published: 1983. Frequency: Quarterly. ISSN: 0733-8651.

★3217★   CARDIOVASCULAR CLINICS
F.A. Davis Co.
1915 Arch St.
Philadelphia, PA 19103   Phone: (215) 568-2270
First Published: 1969. Frequency: 3/yr. ISSN: 0069-0384.

★3218★   CHEMICAL IMMUNOLOGY
S. Karger Publishers, Inc.
26 W. Avon Rd.
PO Box 529
Farmington, CT 06085   Phone: (203) 675-7834
First Published: 1939. Frequency: Irregular.

★3219★   CLINICAL REVIEWS IN ALLERGY
Humana Press, Inc.
PO Box 2148
Clifton, NJ 07015   Phone: (201) 773-4389
First Published: 1983. Frequency: Quarterly. ISSN: 0731-8235.

★3220★   CLINICS IN CHEST MEDICINE
W.B. Saunders Co.
Curtis Center
Independence Sq., W.
Philadelphia, PA 19106   Phone: (215) 238-7800
First Published: 1980. Frequency: Quarterly. ISSN: 0272-5231.

★3221★   CLINICS IN GERIATRIC MEDICINE
W.B. Saunders Co.
Curtis Center
Independence Sq., W.
Philadelphia, PA 19106   Phone: (215) 238-7800
First Published: 1985. Frequency: Quarterly. ISSN: 0749-0690.

★3222★ CLINICS IN LABORATORY MEDICINE
W.B. Saunders Co.
Curtis Center
Independence Sq., W.
Philadelphia, PA 19106   Phone: (215) 238-7800
First Published: 1981. **Frequency:** Quarterly. **ISSN:** 0272-2712.

★3223★ CLINICS IN PERINATOLOGY
W.B. Saunders Co.
Curtis Center
Independence Sq., W.
Philadelphia, PA 19106   Phone: (215) 238-7800
First Published: 1974. **Frequency:** Quarterly. **ISSN:** 0095-5108.

★3224★ CLINICS IN PLASTIC SURGERY
W.B. Saunders Co.
Curtis Center
Independence Sq., W.
Philadelphia, PA 19106   Phone: (215) 238-7800
First Published: 1974. **Frequency:** Quarterly. **ISSN:** 0094-1298.

★3225★ CLINICS IN PODIATRIC MEDICINE AND SURGERY
W.B. Saunders Co.
Curtis Center
Independence Sq., W.
Philadelphia, PA 19106   Phone: (215) 238-7800
First Published: 1984. **Frequency:** Quarterly. **ISSN:** 0891-8422.

★3226★ CLINICS IN SPORTS MEDICINE
W.B. Saunders Co.
Curtis Center
Independence Sq., W.
Philadelphia, PA 19106   Phone: (215) 238-7800
First Published: 1982. **Frequency:** Quarterly. **ISSN:** 0278-5919.

★3227★ CONTEMPORARY ENDOCRINOLOGY
Plenum Publishing Corp.
233 Spring St.
New York, NY 10013   Phone: (212) 620-8000
First Published: 1977. **Frequency:** Annual.

★3228★ CONTEMPORARY GERIATRIC MEDICINE
Plenum Publishing Corp.
233 Spring St.
New York, NY 10013   Phone: (212) 620-8000
First Published: 1983. **Frequency:** Irregular.

★3229★ CONTEMPORARY HEMATOLOGY/ONCOLOGY
Plenum Publishing Corp.
233 Spring St.
New York, NY 10013   Phone: (212) 620-8000
First Published: 1977. **Frequency:** Irregular. **ISSN:** 0197-3649.

★3230★ CONTEMPORARY METABOLISM
Plenum Publishing Corp.
233 Spring St.
New York, NY 10013   Phone: (212) 620-8000
First Published: 1976. **Frequency:** Irregular.

★3231★ CONTEMPORARY NEPHROLOGY
Plenum Publishing Corp.
233 Spring St.
New York, NY 10013   Phone: (212) 620-8000
First Published: 1981. **Frequency:** Biennial.

★3232★ CONTEMPORARY NEUROSURGERY
Williams & Wilkins
428 E. Preston St.
Baltimore, MD 21202   Phone: (301) 528-4000
Frequency: Biweekly. **ISSN:** 0163-2108.

★3233★ CONTEMPORARY PSYCHIATRY
Plenum Publishing Corp.
233 Spring St.
Philadelphia, PA 10013   Phone: (212) 620-8000
First Published: 1982. **Frequency:** Quarterly. **ISSN:** 0277-8041.

★3234★ CONTEMPORARY PSYCHOLOGY: A JOURNAL OF REVIEWS
American Psychological Association
1200 17th St., NW
Washington, DC 20036   Phone: (202) 955-7600
Frequency: Monthly.

★3235★ CONTEMPORARY REVIEWS IN OBSTETRICS AND GYNAECOLOGY
Butterworth-Heinemann
80 Montvale Ave.
Stoneham, MA 02180   Phone: (617) 438-8464
Frequency: Quarterly. **ISSN:** 0953-9182.

★3236★ CONTEMPORARY TOPICS IN IMMUNOBIOLOGY
Plenum Publishing Corp.
233 Spring St.
New York, NY 10013   Phone: (212) 620-8000
First Published: 1972. **Frequency:** Irregular. **ISSN:** 0093-4054.

★3237★ CONTEMPORARY TOPICS IN MOLECULAR IMMUNOLOGY
Plenum Publishing Corp.
233 Spring St.
New York, NY 10013   Phone: (212) 620-8000
First Published: 1972. **Frequency:** Irregular. **ISSN:** 0090-8800.

★3238★ CONTRIBUTIONS TO GYNECOLOGY AND OBSTETRICS
S. Karger Publishers, Inc.
26 W. Avon Rd.
PO Box 529
Farmington, CT 06085   Phone: (203) 675-7834
First Published: 1950. **Frequency:** Irregular. **ISSN:** 0304-4246.

★3239★ CONTRIBUTIONS TO HUMAN DEVELOPMENT
S. Karger Publishers, Inc.
26 W. Avon Rd.
PO Box 529
Farmington, CT 06085   Phone: (203) 675-7834
First Published: 1962. **Frequency:** Irregular. **ISSN:** 0301-4193.

★3240★ CONTRIBUTIONS IN MEDICAL STUDIES
Greenwood Press
88 Post Rd., W.
PO Box 5007
Westport, CT 06881-9990   Phone: (203) 226-3571
First Published: 1978. **Frequency:** Irregular. **ISSN:** 0886-8220.

★3241★ CONTRIBUTIONS TO MICROBIOLOGY AND IMMUNOLOGY
S. Karger Publishers, Inc.
26 W. Avon Rd.
PO Box 529
Farmington, CT 06085   Phone: (203) 675-7834
First Published: 1973. **Frequency:** Irregular. **ISSN:** 0301-3081.

★3242★ CONTRIBUTIONS TO NEPHROLOGY
S. Karger Publishers, Inc.
26 W. Avon Rd.
PO Box 529
Farmington, CT 06085   Phone: (203) 675-7834
First Published: 1975. **Frequency:** Irregular. **ISSN:** 0302-5144.

★3243★ CRITICAL CARE CLINICS
W.B. Saunders Co.
Curtis Center
Independence Sq., W.
Philadelphia, PA 19106   Phone: (215) 238-7800
First Published: 1985. **Frequency:** Quarterly. **ISSN:** 0749-0704.

★3244★ CRITICAL REVIEWS IN BIOCHEMISTRY
CRC Press, Inc.
2000 Corporate Blvd., NW
Boca Raton, FL 33431   Phone: (407) 994-0555
First Published: 1971. **Frequency:** Bimonthly. **ISSN:** 0045-6411.

★3245★ CRITICAL REVIEWS IN BIOCOMPATIBILITY
CRC Press, Inc.
2000 Corporate Blvd., NW
Boca Raton, FL 33431   Phone: (407) 994-0555
First Published: 1984. Frequency: Quarterly. ISSN: 0748-5204.

★3246★ CRITICAL REVIEWS IN BIOMEDICAL ENGINEERING
CRC Press, Inc.
2000 Corporate Blvd., NW
Boca Raton, FL 33431   Phone: (407) 994-0555
First Published: 1974. Frequency: Bimonthly. ISSN: 0278-940X.

★3247★ CRITICAL REVIEWS IN BIOTECHNOLOGY
CRC Press, Inc.
2000 Corporate Blvd., NW
Boca Raton, FL 33431   Phone: (407) 994-0555
First Published: 1983. Frequency: Quarterly. ISSN: 0738-8551.

★3248★ CRITICAL REVIEWS IN CLINICAL LABORATORY
SCIENCES
CRC Press, Inc.
2000 Corporate Blvd., NW
Boca Raton, FL 33431   Phone: (407) 994-0555
First Published: 1970. Frequency: Bimonthly. ISSN: 0590-8191.

★3249★ CRITICAL REVIEWS IN DIAGNOSTIC IMAGING
CRC Press, Inc.
2000 Corporate Blvd., NW
Boca Raton, FL 33431   Phone: (407) 994-0555
First Published: 1970. Frequency: Quarterly. ISSN: 0147-6750.

★3250★ CRITICAL REVIEWS IN ENVIRONMENTAL
CONTROL
CRC Press, Inc.
2000 Corporate Blvd., NW
Boca Raton, FL 33431   Phone: (407) 994-0555
First Published: 1970. Frequency: Quarterly.

★3251★ CRITICAL REVIEWS IN FOOD SCIENCE AND
NUTRITION
CRC Press, Inc.
2000 Corporate Blvd., NW
Boca Raton, FL 33431   Phone: (407) 994-0555
First Published: 1970. Frequency: Quarterly. ISSN: 0099-0248.

★3252★ CRITICAL REVIEWS IN IMMUNOLOGY
CRC Press, Inc.
2000 Corporate Blvd., NW
Boca Raton, FL 33431   Phone: (407) 994-0555
First Published: 1980. Frequency: Quarterly. ISSN: 0197-3355.

★3253★ CRITICAL REVIEWS IN MICROBIOLOGY
CRC Press, Inc.
2000 Corporate Blvd., NW
Boca Raton, FL 33431   Phone: (407) 994-0555
First Published: 1971. Frequency: Bimonthly. ISSN: 0045-6454.

★3254★ CRITICAL REVIEWS IN NEUROBIOLOGY
CRC Press, Inc.
2000 Corporate Blvd., NW
Boca Raton, FL 33431   Phone: (407) 994-0555
Frequency: 4/yr.

★3255★ CRITICAL REVIEWS IN NEUROSURGERY
Springer-Verlag New York, Inc.
175 5th Ave.
New York, NY 10010   Phone: (212) 460-1500
First Published: 1991. Frequency: Monthly. ISSN: 0939-0146.

★3256★ CRITICAL REVIEWS IN ONCOGENESIS
CRC Press, Inc.
2000 Corporate Blvd., NW
Boca Raton, FL 33431   Phone: (407) 994-0555
First Published: 1989. Frequency: Quarterly. ISSN: 0893-9675.

★3257★ CRITICAL REVIEWS IN ONCOLOGY/HEMATOLOGY
CRC Press, Inc.
2000 Corporate Blvd., NW
Boca Raton, FL 33431   Phone: (407) 994-0555
First Published: 1983. Frequency: Quarterly. ISSN: 0737-9587.

★3258★ CRITICAL REVIEWS IN ORAL BIOLOGY AND
MEDICINE
CRC Press, Inc.
2000 Corporate Blvd., NW
Boca Raton, FL 33431   Phone: (407) 994-0555
First Published: 1989. Frequency: Quarterly. ISSN: 1045-4411.

★3259★ CRITICAL REVIEWS IN PHYSICAL AND
REHABILITATION MEDICINE
CRC Press, Inc.
2000 Corporate Blvd., NW
Boca Raton, FL 33431   Phone: (407) 994-0555
First Published: 1989. Frequency: Quarterly. ISSN: 0896-2960.

★3260★ CRITICAL REVIEWS IN THERAPEUTIC DRUG
CARRIER SYSTEMS
CRC Press, Inc.
2000 Corporate Blvd., NW
Boca Raton, FL 33431   Phone: (407) 884-0555
First Published: 1984. Frequency: Quarterly. ISSN: 0743-4863.

★3261★ CRITICAL REVIEWS IN TOXICOLOGY
CRC Press, Inc.
2000 Corporate Blvd., NW
Boca Raton, FL 33431   Phone: (407) 994-0555
First Published: 1971. Frequency: Bimonthly. ISSN: 0045-6446.

★3262★ CURRENT ANAESTHESIA AND CRITICAL CARE
Churchill Livingstone, Inc.
1560 Broadway
New York, NY 10036   Phone: (212) 819-5400
First Published: 1989. Frequency: Quarterly. ISSN: 0953-7112.

★3263★ CURRENT CANCER THERAPEUTICS
Current Science
20 N. 3rd St.
Philadelphia, PA 19106   Phone: (215) 514-2266
First Published: 1992.

★3264★ CURRENT CARDIOVASCULAR DRUGS
Current Science
20 N. 3rd St.
Philadelphia, PA 19106   Phone: (215) 514-2266
First Published: 1992.

★3265★ CURRENT CONCEPTS IN NUTRITION
John Wiley & Sons, Inc.
605 3rd Ave.
New York, NY 10158   Phone: (212) 850-6000
First Published: 1972. Frequency: Irregular. ISSN: 0090-0443.

★3266★ CURRENT DIRECTIONS IN PSYCHOLOGICAL
SCIENCE
Cambridge University Press
40 W. 20th St.
New York, NY 10011   Phone: (212) 924-3900
First Published: 1991. Frequency: Bimonthly. ISSN: 0963-7214.

★3267★ CURRENT GASTROENTEROLOGY
Mosby-Year Book, Inc.
11830 Westline Industrial Dr.
St. Louis, MO 63146   Phone: (314) 872-8370
First Published: 1980. Frequency: Annual. ISSN: 0198-8085.

★3268★ CURRENT HEPATOLOGY
Mosby-Year Book, Inc.
11830 Westline Industrial Dr.
St. Louis, MO 63146   Phone: (314) 872-8370
First Published: 1980. Frequency: Annual. ISSN: 0798-8085.

★3269★   CURRENT IMAGING
Churchill Livingstone, Inc.
1560 Broadway
New York, NY 10036   Phone: (212) 819-5400
First Published: 1988. **Frequency:** Quarterly. **ISSN:** 0952-0619.

★3270★   CURRENT NEPHROLOGY
Mosby-Year Book, Inc.
11830 Westline Industrial Dr.
St. Louis, MO 63146   Phone: (314) 872-8370
First Published: 1977. **Frequency:** Annual. **ISSN:** 0148-4265.

★3271★   CURRENT NEUROLOGY
Mosby-Year Book, Inc.
11830 Westline Industrial Dr.
St. Louis, MO 63146   Phone: (314) 872-8370
First Published: 1980. **Frequency:** Annual. **ISSN:** 0161-780X.

★3272★   CURRENT NEURO-OPHTHALMOLOGY
Mosby-Year Book, Inc.
11830 Westline Industrial Dr.
St. Louis, MO 63146   Phone: (314) 872-8370
First Published: 1987. **Frequency:** Biennial. **ISSN:** 0893-0147.

★3273★   CURRENT OBSTETRICS AND GYNAECOLOGY
Churchill Livingstone, Inc.
1560 Broadway
New York, NY 10036   Phone: (212) 819-5400
First Published: 1991. **Frequency:** Quarterly. **ISSN:** 0957-5847.

★3274★   CURRENT OPINION IN ANAESTHESIOLOGY
Current Science
20 N. 3rd St.
Philadelphia, PA 19106   Phone: (215) 514-2266
Frequency: Bimonthly. **ISSN:** 0952-7907.

★3275★   CURRENT OPINION IN CARDIOLOGY
Current Science
20 N. 3rd St.
Philadelphia, PA 19106   Phone: (215) 514-2266
Frequency: Bimonthly. **ISSN:** 0268-4705.

★3276★   CURRENT OPINION IN DENTISTRY
Current Science
20 N. 3rd St.
Philadelphia, PA 19106   Phone: (215) 514-2266
Frequency: Quarterly. **ISSN:** 1046-0764.

★3277★   CURRENT OPINION IN GASTROENTEROLOGY
Current Science
20 N. 3rd St.
Philadelphia, PA 19106   Phone: (215) 514-2266
Frequency: Bimonthly. **ISSN:** 0267-1379.

★3278★   CURRENT OPINION IN INFECTIOUS DISEASES
Current Science
20 N. 3rd St.
Philadelphia, PA 19106   Phone: (215) 514-2266
Frequency: Bimonthly. **ISSN:** 0951-7375.

★3279★   CURRENT OPINION IN LIPIDOLOGY
Current Science
20 N. 3rd St.
Philadelphia, PA 19106   Phone: (215) 514-2266
Frequency: Bimonthly. **ISSN:** 0957-9672.

**★3280★   CURRENT OPINION IN NEPHROLOGY AND
   HYPERTENSION**
Current Science
20 N. 3rd St.
Philadelphia, PA 19106   Phone: (215) 514-2266
First Published: 1992.

**★3281★   CURRENT OPINION IN NEUROLOGY AND
   NEUROSURGERY**
Current Science
20 N. 3rd St.
Philadelphia, PA 19106   Phone: (215) 514-2266
Frequency: Bimonthly. **ISSN:** 0951-7383.

**★3282★   CURRENT OPINION IN OBSTETRICS AND
   GYNECOLOGY**
Current Science
20 N. 3rd St.
Philadelphia, PA 19106   Phone: (215) 514-2266
Frequency: Bimonthly. **ISSN:** 1040-872X.

★3283★   CURRENT OPINION IN ONCOLOGY
Current Science
20 N. 3rd St.
Philadelphia, PA 19106   Phone: (215) 514-2266
Frequency: Bimonthly. **ISSN:** 1040-8746.

★3284★   CURRENT OPINION IN OPHTHALMOLOGY
Current Science
20 N. 3rd St.
Philadelphia, PA 19106   Phone: (215) 514-2266
Frequency: Bimonthly. **ISSN:** 1040-8738.

★3285★   CURRENT OPINION IN ORTHOPAEDICS
Current Science
20 N. 3rd St.
Philadelphia, PA 19106   Phone: (215) 514-2266
Frequency: Bimonthly. **ISSN:** 1041-9918.

★3286★   CURRENT OPINION IN PEDIATRICS
Current Science
20 N. 3rd St.
Philadelphia, PA 19106   Phone: (215) 514-2266
Frequency: Bimonthly. **ISSN:** 1040-8703.

★3287★   CURRENT OPINION IN PSYCHIATRY
Current Science
20 N. 3rd St.
Philadelphia, PA 19106   Phone: (215) 514-2266
Frequency: Bimonthly. **ISSN:** 0951-7367.

★3288★   CURRENT OPINION IN RADIOLOGY
Current Science
20 N. 3rd St.
Philadelphia, PA 19106   Phone: (215) 514-2266
Frequency: Bimonthly. **ISSN:** 1040-869X.

★3289★   CURRENT OPINION IN RHEUMATOLOGY
Current Science
20 N. 3rd St.
Philadelphia, PA 19106   Phone: (215) 514-2266
Frequency: Bimonthly. **ISSN:** 1040-8711.

★3290★   CURRENT OPINION IN UROLOGY
Current Science
20 N. 3rd St.
Philadelphia, PA 19106   Phone: (215) 514-2266
Frequency: Bimonthly. **ISSN:** 0963-0643.

★3291★   CURRENT ORTHOPAEDICS
Churchill Livingstone, Inc.
1560 Broadway
New York, NY 10036   Phone: (212) 819-5400
First Published: 1986. **Frequency:** Quarterly. **ISSN:** 0268-0890.

★3292★   CURRENT PEDIATRICS
Churchill Livingstone, Inc.
1560 Broadway
New York, NY 10036   Phone: (212) 819-5400
First Published: 1991. **Frequency:** Quarterly. **ISSN:** 0957-5839.

★3293★ CURRENT PRACTICE IN SURGERY
Churchill Livingstone, Inc.
1560 Broadway
New York, NY 10036   Phone: (212) 819-5400
Frequency: Quarterly. ISSN: 0952-0627.

★3294★ CURRENT PROBLEMS IN CANCER
Mosby-Year Book, Inc.
11830 Westline Industrial Dr.
St. Louis, MO 63146   Phone: (314) 872-8370
First Published: 1976. Frequency: Bimonthly. ISSN: 0147-0272.

★3295★ CURRENT PROBLEMS IN CARDIOLOGY
Mosby-Year Book, Inc.
11830 Westline Industrial Dr.
St. Louis, MO 63146   Phone: (314) 872-8370
First Published: 1976. Frequency: Monthly. ISSN: 0146-2806.

★3296★ CURRENT PROBLEMS IN DERMATOLOGY
S. Karger Publishers, Inc.
26 W. Avon Rd.
PO Box 529
Farmington, CT 06085   Phone: (203) 675-7834
First Published: 1959. Frequency: Irregular. ISSN: 0070-2064.

★3297★ CURRENT PROBLEMS IN DIAGNOSTIC RADIOLOGY
Mosby-Year Book, Inc.
11830 Westline Industrial Dr.
St. Louis, MO 63146   Phone: (314) 872-8370
First Published: 1972. Frequency: Bimonthly. ISSN: 0363-0188.

★3298★ CURRENT PROBLEMS IN OBSTETRICS AND
GYNECOLOGY AND FERTILITY
Mosby-Year Book, Inc.
11830 Westline Industrial Dr.
St. Louis, MO 63146   Phone: (314) 872-8370
First Published: 1977. Frequency: Monthly. ISSN: 8756-0410.

★3299★ CURRENT PROBLEMS IN PEDIATRICS
Mosby-Year Book, Inc.
11830 Westline Industrial Dr.
St. Louis, MO 63146   Phone: (314) 872-8370
First Published: 1970. Frequency: Monthly. ISSN: 0045-9380.

★3300★ CURRENT PROBLEMS IN SURGERY
Mosby-Year Book, Inc.
11830 Westline Industrial Dr.
St. Louis, MO 63146   Phone: (314) 872-8370
First Published: 1964. Frequency: Monthly. ISSN: 0011-3840.

★3301★ CURRENT PROBLEMS IN UROLOGY
Mosby-Year Book, Inc.
11830 Westline Industrial Dr.
St. Louis, MO 63146   Phone: (314) 872-8370
First Published: 1991. Frequency: Bimonthly.

★3302★ CURRENT PULMONOLOGY
Mosby-Year Book, Inc.
11830 Westline Industrial Dr.
St. Louis, MO 63146   Phone: (314) 872-8370
First Published: 1977. Frequency: Annual. ISSN: 0798-8085.

★3303★ CURRENT STUDIES IN HEMATOLOGY AND BLOOD
TRANSFUSION
S. Karger Publishers, Inc.
26 W. Avon Rd.
Farmington, CT 06085   Phone: (203) 675-7834
ISSN: 0258-0330.

★3304★ CURRENT SURGERY
J.B. Lippincott Co.
E. Washington Sq.
Philadelphia, PA 19105   Phone: (215) 238-4200
First Published: 1933. Frequency: Bimonthly. ISSN: 0149-7944.

★3305★ CURRENT TOPICS IN BIOENERGETICS
Academic Press, Inc.
1250 6th Ave.
San Diego, CA 92101   Phone: (619) 231-0926
First Published: 1966. Frequency: Irregular. ISSN: 0070-2129.

★3306★ CURRENT TOPICS IN CELLULAR REGULATION
Academic Press, Inc.
1250 6th Ave.
San Diego, CA 92101   Phone: (619) 231-0926
First Published: 1969. Frequency: Irregular. ISSN: 0070-2137.

★3307★ CURRENT TOPICS IN DEVELOPMENTAL BIOLOGY
Academic Press, Inc.
1250 6th Ave.
San Diego, CA 92101   Phone: (619) 231-0926
First Published: 1966. Frequency: Irregular. ISSN: 0070-2153.

★3308★ CURRENT TOPICS IN EXPERIMENTAL
ENDOCRINOLOGY
Academic Press, Inc.
1250 6th Ave.
San Diego, CA 92101   Phone: (619) 231-0926
First Published: 1972. Frequency: Irregular. ISSN: 0091-7397.

★3309★ CURRENT TOPICS IN EYE RESEARCH
Academic Press, Inc.
1250 6th Ave.
San Diego, CA 92101   Phone: (619) 231-0926
First Published: 1979. Frequency: Irregular. ISSN: 0190-2970.

★3310★ CURRENT TOPICS IN MEMBRANES AND
TRANSPORT
Academic Press, Inc.
1250 6th Ave.
San Diego, CA 92101   Phone: (619) 231-0926
First Published: 1970. Frequency: Irregular. ISSN: 0070-2161.

★3311★ CURRENT TOPICS IN MICROBIOLOGY AND
IMMUNOLOGY
Springer-Verlag New York, Inc.
175 5th Ave.
New York, NY 10010   Phone: (212) 460-1500
First Published: 1914. Frequency: Irregular. ISSN: 0070-217X.

★3312★ CURRENT TOPICS IN NUTRITION AND DISEASE
John Wiley & Sons, Inc.
605 3rd Ave.
New York, NY 10158   Phone: (212) 850-6000
First Published: 1977. Frequency: Irregular. ISSN: 0191-2453.

★3313★ CURRENT TOPICS IN PATHOLOGY
Springer-Verlag New York, Inc.
175 5th Ave.
New York, NY 10010   Phone: (212) 460-1500
First Published: 1976. Frequency: Irregular. ISSN: 0070-2188.

★3314★ DENTAL CLINICS OF NORTH AMERICA
W.B. Saunders Co.
Curtis Center
Independence Sq., W.
Philadelphia, PA 19106   Phone: (215) 238-8405
First Published: 1956. Frequency: Quarterly. ISSN: 0011-8532.

★3315★ DERMATOLOGIC CLINICS
W.B. Saunders Co.
Curtis Center
Independence Sq., W.
Philadelphia, PA 19106   Phone: (215) 238-7800
First Published: 1983. Frequency: Quarterly. ISSN: 0733-8635.

★3316★ DEVELOPMENTS IN IMMUNOLOGY
Elsevier Science Publishing Co., Inc.
655 Avenue of the Americas
New York, NY 10010   Phone: (212) 989-5800
First Published: 1978. Frequency: Irregular.

★3317★ DEVELOPMENTS IN OPHTHALMOLOGY
S. Karger Publishers, Inc.
26 W. Avon Rd.
PO Box 529
Farmington, CT 06085   Phone: (203) 675-7834
First Published: 1980. **Frequency:** Irregular. **ISSN:** 0250-3751.

★3318★ DIABETES/METABOLISM REVIEWS
John Wiley & Sons, Inc.
605 3rd Ave.
New York, NY 10158   Phone: (212) 850-6000
First Published: 1985. **Frequency:** 8/yr. **ISSN:** 0742-4221.

★3319★ DIGEST OF GERIATRICS
W.B. Saunders Co.
Curtis Center
Independence Sq., W.
Philadelphia, PA 19106   Phone: (215) 238-7800
Frequency: Monthly.

★3320★ DM/DISEASE-A-MONTH
Mosby-Year Book, Inc.
11830 Westline Industrial Dr.
St. Louis, MO 63146   Phone: (314) 872-8370
First Published: 1954. **Frequency:** Monthly. **ISSN:** 0011-5029.

★3321★ DRUG METABOLISM REVIEWS
Marcel Dekker, Inc.
270 Madison Ave.
New York, NY 10016   Phone: (212) 696-9000
First Published: 1972. **Frequency:** Bimonthly. **ISSN:** 0360-2532.

**★3322★ EMERGENCY MEDICINE CLINICS OF NORTH
       AMERICA**
W.B. Saunders Co.
Curtis Center
Independence Sq., W.
Philadelphia, PA 19106   Phone: (215) 238-8405
First Published: 1983. **Frequency:** Quarterly. **ISSN:** 0733-8627.

★3323★ ENDOCRINE REVIEWS
Williams & Wilkins
428 E. Preston St.
Baltimore, MD 21202   Phone: (301) 528-4223
First Published: 1980. **Frequency:** Quarterly. **ISSN:** 0163-769X.

**★3324★ ENDOCRINOLOGY AND METABOLISM CLINICS OF
       NORTH AMERICA**
W.B. Saunders Co.
Curtis Center
Independence Sq., W.
Philadelphia, PA 19106   Phone: (215) 238-7800
First Published: 1972. **Frequency:** Quarterly. **ISSN:** 0889-8529.

★3325★ EPIDEMIOLOGIC REVIEWS
School of Hygiene and Public Health
Johns Hopkins University
624 N. Broadway, Rm. 225
Baltimore, MD 21205   Phone: (301) 955-3441
First Published: 1979. **Frequency:** Annual. **ISSN:** 0193-936X.

★3326★ EXERCISE AND SPORT SCIENCES REVIEWS
Macmillan Publishing Co.
866 3rd Ave.
New York, NY 10022
First Published: 1973. **Frequency:** Annual. **ISSN:** 0091-6331.

★3327★ FETAL MEDICINE REVIEW
Cambridge University Press
40 W. 20th St.
New York, NY 10011   Phone: (212) 924-3900
Frequency: Semiannual. **ISSN:** 0953-8267.

★3328★ FRONTIERS IN DIABETES
S. Karger Publishers, Inc.
26 W. Avon Rd.
PO Box 529
Farmington, CT 06085   Phone: (203) 675-7834
First Published: 1981. **Frequency:** Annual. **ISSN:** 0251-5342.

★3329★ FRONTIERS OF GASTROINTESTINAL RESEARCH
S. Karger Publishers, Inc.
26 W. Avon Rd.
PO Box 529
Farmington, CT 06085   Phone: (203) 675-7834
First Published: 1960. **Frequency:** Irregular.

★3330★ FRONTIERS OF HORMONE RESEARCH
S. Karger Publishers, Inc.
26 W. Avon Rd.
PO Box 529
Farmington, CT 06085   Phone: (203) 675-7834
First Published: 1972. **Frequency:** Irregular. **ISSN:** 0301-3073.

★3331★ FRONTIERS OF MATRIX BIOLOGY
S. Karger Publishers, Inc.
26 W. Avon Rd.
PO Box 529
Farmington, CT 06085   Phone: (203) 675-7834
First Published: 1973. **Frequency:** Irregular. **ISSN:** 0301-0155.

★3332★ FRONTIERS OF ORAL PHYSIOLOGY
S. Karger Publishers, Inc.
26 W. Avon Rd.
PO Box 529
Farmington, CT 06085   Phone: (203) 675-7834
First Published: 1974. **Frequency:** Irregular. **ISSN:** 0301-536X.

**★3333★ FRONTIERS OF RADIATION THERAPY AND
       ONCOLOGY**
S. Karger Publishers, Inc.
26 W. Avon Rd.
PO Box 529
Farmington, CT 06085   Phone: (203) 675-7834
First Published: 1967. **Frequency:** Irregular. **ISSN:** 0071-9676.

★3334★ HAND CLINICS
W.B. Saunders Co.
Curtis Center
Independence Sq., W.
Philadelphia, PA 19106   Phone: (215) 238-7800
First Published: 1985. **Frequency:** Quarterly. **ISSN:** 0749-0712.

★3335★ HEALTH LIBRARIES REVIEW
Blackwell Scientific Publications
3 Cambridge Center, Ste. 208
Cambridge, MA 02142
Frequency: Quarterly. **ISSN:** 0265-6647.

**★3336★ HEMATOLOGY/ONCOLOGY CLINICS OF NORTH
       AMERICA**
W.B. Saunders Co.
Curtis Center
Independence Sq., W.
Philadelphia, PA 19106   Phone: (215) 238-7800
First Published: 1972. **Frequency:** Quarterly. **ISSN:** 0889-8588.

★3337★ IMMUNOLOGICAL INVESTIGATIONS
Marcel Dekker, Inc.
270 Madison Ave.
New York, NY 10016   Phone: (212) 696-9000
First Published: 1972. **Frequency:** 7/yr. **ISSN:** 0882-0139.

★3338★ IMMUNOLOGICAL REVIEWS
Blackwell Scientific Publications, Inc.
3 Cambridge Center, Ste. 208
Cambridge, MA 02142   Phone: (617) 225-0401
First Published: 1969. **Frequency:** Bimonthly. **ISSN:** 0105-2896.

★3339★ IMMUNOLOGY AND ALLERGY CLINICS OF NORTH
AMERICA
W.B. Saunders Co.
Curtis Center
Independence Sq., W.
Philadelphia, PA 19106   Phone: (215) 238-8405
First Published: 1981. Frequency: 3/yr. ISSN: 0889-8561.

★3340★ INTERNATIONAL NURSING REVIEW
International Council of Nurses
Imprimeries Reunies Lausanne S.A.
3 Place Jean-Marteau
CH-1201 Geneva, Switzerland
First Published: 1926. Frequency: Bimonthly. ISSN: 0020-8132.

★3341★ INTERNATIONAL REVIEW OF CYTOLOGY
Academic Press, Inc.
1250 6th Ave.
San Diego, CA 92101   Phone: (619) 231-0926
First Published: 1952. Frequency: Irregular. ISSN: 0074-7696.

★3342★ INTERNATIONAL REVIEW OF EXPERIMENTAL
PATHOLOGY
Academic Press, Inc.
1250 6th Ave.
San Diego, CA 92101   Phone: (619) 231-0926
First Published: 1962. Frequency: Irregular. ISSN: 0074-7718.

★3343★ INTERNATIONAL REVIEW OF NEUROBIOLOGY
Academic Press, Inc.
1250 6th Ave.
San Diego, CA 92101   Phone: (619) 231-0926
First Published: 1959. Frequency: Irregular. ISSN: 0074-7742.

★3344★ INTERNATIONAL REVIEW OF RESEARCH IN
MENTAL RETARDATION
Academic Press, Inc.
1250 6th Ave.
San Diego, CA 92101   Phone: (619) 231-0926
First Published: 1966. Frequency: Irregular. ISSN: 0074-7750.

★3345★ ISSUES IN BIOMEDICINE
S. Karger Publishers, Inc.
26 W. Avon Rd.
PO Box 529
Farmington, CT 06085   Phone: (203) 675-7834
First Published: 1967. Frequency: Irregular.

★3346★ JOURNAL OF TOXICOLOGY—TOXIN REVIEWS
Marcel Dekker, Inc.
270 Madison Ave.
New York, NY 10016   Phone: (212) 696-9000
First Published: 1982. Frequency: 3/yr. ISSN: 0731-3837.

★3347★ LEGAL MEDICINE
Praeger Publishers
1 Madison Ave.
New York, NY 10010   Phone: (212) 685-5300
First Published: 1969. Frequency: Annual. ISSN: 0197-9981.

★3348★ MEDICAL CARE REVIEW
Health Administration Press
1021 E. Huron
Ann Arbor, MI 48104-9990   Phone: (313) 943-0544
First Published: 1944. Frequency: Quarterly. ISSN: 0025-7087.

★3349★ MEDICAL CLINICS OF NORTH AMERICA
W.B. Saunders Co.
Curtis Center
Independence Sq., W.
Philadelphia, PA 19106   Phone: (215) 238-7800
First Published: 1916. Frequency: Bimonthly. ISSN: 0025-7125.

★3350★ METHODS AND ACHIEVEMENTS IN
EXPERIMENTAL PATHOLOGY
S. Karger Publishers, Inc.
26 W. Avon Rd.
PO Box 529
Farmington, CT 06085   Phone: (203) 675-7834
First Published: 1965. Frequency: Irregular. ISSN: 0076-681X.

★3351★ NEUROLOGIC CLINICS
W.B. Saunders Co.
Curtis Center
Independence Sq., W.
Philadelphia, PA 19106   Phone: (215) 238-7800
First Published: 1983. Frequency: Quarterly. ISSN: 0733-8619.

★3352★ NEUROSCIENCE AND BIOBEHAVIORAL REVIEWS
Pergamon Press, Inc.
Maxwell House, Fairview Park
Elmsford, NY 10523   Phone: (914) 592-7700
First Published: 1977. Frequency: Quarterly. ISSN: 0149-7634.

★3353★ NEW HORIZONS IN THERAPEUTICS
Plenum Publishing Corp.
233 Spring St.
New York, NY 10013   Phone: (212) 620-8000
First Published: 1984. Frequency: Annual.

★3354★ NUCLEAR MEDICINE ANNUAL
Raven Press
1185 Avenue of the Americas
New York, NY 10036   Phone: (212) 930-9500
First Published: 1980. Frequency: Annual. ISSN: 0272-0108.

★3355★ NURSING CLINICS OF NORTH AMERICA
W.B. Saunders Co.
Curtis Center
Independence Sq., W.
Philadelphia, PA 19106   Phone: (215) 238-7800
First Published: 1966. Frequency: Quarterly. ISSN: 0029-6465.

★3356★ OBSTETRICAL AND GYNECOLOGICAL SURVEY
Williams & Wilkins
428 E. Preston St.
Baltimore, MD 21202   Phone: (301) 528-4223
First Published: 1946. Frequency: Monthly. ISSN: 0029-7828.

★3357★ OBSTETRICS AND GYNECOLOGY CLINICS OF
NORTH AMERICA
W.B. Saunders Co.
Curtis Center
Independence Sq., W.
Philadelphia, PA 19106   Phone: (215) 238-7800
First Published: 1974. Frequency: Quarterly. ISSN: 0889-8545.

★3358★ OPTOMETRY: CURRENT LITERATURE IN
PERPECTIVE
Mosby-Year Book, Inc.
11830 Westline Industrial Dr.
St. Louis, MO 63146   Phone: (314) 872-8370
First Published: 1991. Frequency: Quarterly.

★3359★ ORTHOPAEDIC REVIEW
Core Medical Journals
3131 Princeton Pike
Lawrenceville, NJ 08648   Phone: (609) 896-9450
First Published: 1972. Frequency: Monthly. ISSN: 0094-6591.

★3360★ ORTHOPEDIC CLINICS OF NORTH AMERICA
W.B. Saunders Co.
Curtis Center
Independence Sq., W.
Philadelphia, PA 19106   Phone: (215) 238-7800
First Published: 1970. Frequency: Quarterly. ISSN: 0030-5898.

★3361★ OTOLARYNGOLOGIC CLINICS OF NORTH AMERICA
W.B. Saunders Co.
Curtis Center
Independence Sq., W.
Philadelphia, PA 19106   Phone: (215) 238-7800
First Published: 1968. **Frequency:** Quarterly. ISSN: 0030-6665.

★3362★ PAIN AND HEADACHE
S. Karger Publishers, Inc.
26 W. Avon Rd.
PO Box 529
Farmington, CT 06085   Phone: (203) 675-7834
First Published: 1967. **Frequency:** Irregular. ISSN: 0255-3910.

★3363★ PATHOBIOLOGY ANNUAL
Raven Press
1185 Avenue of the Americas
New York, NY 10036   Phone: (212) 930-9500
First Published: 1972. **Frequency:** Annual. ISSN: 0362-3025.

★3364★ PATHOLOGY ANNUAL
Appleton & Lange
25 Van Zant St.
East Norwalk, CT 06855   Phone: (203) 838-4400
First Published: 1966. **Frequency:** Semiannual. ISSN: 0079-0184.

★3365★ PEDIATRIC CLINICS OF NORTH AMERICA
W.B. Saunders Co.
Curtis Center
Independence Sq., W.
Philadelphia, PA 19106   Phone: (215) 238-7800
First Published: 1954. **Frequency:** Bimonthly. ISSN: 0031-3955.

★3366★ PERSPECTIVES IN PEDIATRIC PATHOLOGY
S. Karger Publishers, Inc.
26 W. Avon Rd.
Farmington, CT 06085   Phone: (203) 675-7834
ISSN: 0091-2921.

★3367★ PHARMACOLOGICAL REVIEWS
Williams & Wilkins
428 E. Preston St.
Baltimore, MD 21202   Phone: (301) 528-4223
First Published: 1951. **Frequency:** Quarterly. ISSN: 0031-6997.

★3368★ PHYSIOLOGICAL REVIEWS
American Physiological Society
9650 Rockville Pike
Bethesda, MD 20814   Phone: (301) 530-7070
First Published: 1921. **Frequency:** Quarterly. ISSN: 0031-9333.

★3369★ POSTGRADUATE RADIOLOGY
Mosby-Year Book, Inc.
11830 Westline Industrial Dr.
St. Louis, MO 63146   Phone: (314) 872-8370
First Published: 1981. **Frequency:** Quarterly.

★3370★ PRIMARY CARE: CLINICS IN OFFICE PRACTICE
W.B. Saunders Co.
Curtis Center
Independence Sq., W.
Philadelphia, PA 19106   Phone: (215) 238-7800
First Published: 1974. **Frequency:** Quarterly. ISSN: 0095-4543.

★3371★ PROGRESS IN ANESTHESIOLOGY
Raven Press
1185 Avenue of the Americas
New York, NY 10036   Phone: (212) 930-9500
First Published: 1975. **Frequency:** Irregular. ISSN: 0099-1546.

★3372★ PROGRESS IN BEHAVIOR MODIFICATION
Academic Press, Inc.
1250 6th Ave.
San Diego, CA 92101   Phone: (619) 231-0926
First Published: 1975. **Frequency:** Annual. ISSN: 0099-037X.

★3373★ PROGRESS IN BIOCHEMICAL PHARMACOLOGY
S. Karger Publishers, Inc.
26 W. Avon Rd.
PO Box 529
Farmington, CT 06085   Phone: (203) 675-7834
First Published: 1965. **Frequency:** Irregular. ISSN: 0079-6085.

★3374★ PROGRESS IN BIOPHYSICS AND MOLECULAR BIOLOGY
Pergamon Press, Inc.
Maxwell House, Fairview Park
Elmsford, NY 10523   Phone: (914) 592-7700
First Published: 1950. **Frequency:** Quarterly. ISSN: 0079-6107.

★3375★ PROGRESS IN CANCER RESEARCH AND THERAPY
Raven Press
1185 Avenue of the Americas
New York, NY 10036   Phone: (212) 930-9500
First Published: 1976. **Frequency:** Irregular. ISSN: 0145-3726.

★3376★ PROGRESS IN CARDIOLOGY
Lea & Febiger
600 S. Washington Sq.
Philadelphia, PA 19106   Phone: (800) 444-1785
First Published: 1972. **Frequency:** Semiannual. ISSN: 0097-109X.

★3377★ PROGRESS IN CHEMICAL FIBRINOLYSIS AND THROMBOLYSIS
Raven Press
1185 Avenue of the Americas
New York, NY 10036   Phone: (212) 930-9500
First Published: 1975. **Frequency:** Irregular. ISSN: 0361-0233.

★3378★ PROGRESS IN CLINICAL AND BIOLOGICAL RESEARCH
John Wiley & Sons, Inc.
605 3rd Ave.
New York, NY 10158   Phone: (212) 850-6000
First Published: 1975. **Frequency:** Irregular. ISSN: 0361-7742.

★3379★ PROGRESS IN DRUG RESEARCH
Birkhaeuser Verlag
PO Box 133
CH4010 Basel, Switzerland
First Published: 1959. **Frequency:** Irregular. ISSN: 0071-786X.

★3380★ PROGRESS IN EXPERIMENTAL TUMOR RESEARCH
S. Karger Publishers, Inc.
26 W. Avon Rd.
PO Box 529
Farmington, CT 06085   Phone: (203) 675-7834
First Published: 1960. **Frequency:** Irregular. ISSN: 0079-6263.

★3381★ PROGRESS IN FOOD AND NUTRITION SCIENCE
Pergamon Press, Inc.
Maxwell House, Fairview Park
Elmsford, NY 10523   Phone: (914) 592-7700
First Published: 1975. **Frequency:** Quarterly. ISSN: 0306-0632.

★3382★ PROGRESS IN HEMATOLOGY
W. B. Saunders Co.
Curtis Center
Independence Sq., W.
Philadelphia, PA 19106   Phone: (215) 238-7800
First Published: 1956. **Frequency:** Irregular. ISSN: 0079-6301.

★3383★ PROGRESS IN HEMOSTASIS AND THROMBOSIS
W. B. Saunders Co.
Curtis Center
Independence Sq., W.
Philadelphia, PA 19106   Phone: (215) 238-7800
First Published: 1972. **Frequency:** Irregular. ISSN: 0362-6350.

★3384★ PROGRESS IN HISTOCHEMISTRY AND
CYTOCHEMISTRY
Gustav Fischer New York, Inc.
220 E. 23rd St., Ste. 909
New York, NY 10010
First Published: 1970. Frequency: Irregular. ISSN: 0079-6336.

★3385★ PROGRESS IN MEDICAL VIROLOGY
S. Karger Publishers, Inc.
26 W. Avon Rd.
PO Box 529
Farmington, CT 06085   Phone: (203) 675-7834
First Published: 1958. Frequency: Irregular. ISSN: 0079-645X.

★3386★ PROGRESS IN MOLECULAR AND SUBCELLULAR
BIOLOGY
Springer-Verlag New York, Inc.
175 5th Ave.
New York, NY 10010   Phone: (212) 460-1500
First Published: 1969. Frequency: Irregular. ISSN: 0079-6484.

★3387★ PROGRESS IN NEUROBIOLOGY
Pergamon Press, Inc.
Maxwell House, Fairview Park
Elmsford, NY 10523   Phone: (914) 592-7700
First Published: 1973. Frequency: Monthly. ISSN: 0301-0082.

★3388★ PROGRESS IN NEUROPATHOLOGY
Raven Press
1185 Avenue of the Americas
New York, NY 10036   Phone: (212) 930-9500
First Published: 1971. Frequency: Irregular.

★3389★ PROGRESS IN NEURO-PSYCHOPHARMACOLOGY
AND BIOLOGICAL PSYCHIATRY
Pergamon Press, Inc.
Maxwell House, Fairview Park
Elmsford, NY 10523   Phone: (914) 592-7700
First Published: 1977. Frequency: Bimonthly. ISSN: 0278-5846.

★3390★ PROGRESS IN NUCLEIC ACID RESEARCH AND
MOLECULAR BIOLOGY
Academic Press, Inc.
1250 6th Ave.
San Diego, CA 92101   Phone: (619) 231-0926
First Published: 1963. Frequency: Irregular. ISSN: 0079-6603.

★3391★ PROGRESS IN PSYCHOBIOLOGY AND
PHYSIOLOGICAL PSYCHOLOGY
Academic Press, Inc.
1250 6th Ave.
San Diego, CA 92101   Phone: (619) 231-0926
First Published: 1967. Frequency: Irregular.

★3392★ PROGRESS IN REPRODUCTIVE BIOLOGY AND
MEDICINE
S. Karger Publishers, Inc.
26 W. Avon Rd.
PO Box 529
Farmington, CT 06085   Phone: (203) 675-7834
First Published: 1976. Frequency: Irregular. ISSN: 0254-105X.

★3393★ PROGRESS IN RESPIRATION RESEARCH
S. Karger Publishers, Inc.
26 W. Avon Rd.
PO Box 529
Farmington, CT 06085   Phone: (203) 675-7834
First Published: 1963. Frequency: Irregular. ISSN: 0079-6751.

★3394★ PROGRESS IN RETINAL RESEARCH
Pergamon Press, Inc.
Maxwell House, Fairview Park
Elmsford, NY 10523   Phone: (914) 592-7700
First Published: 1982. Frequency: Annual. ISSN: 0278-4327.

★3395★ PROGRESS IN SENSORY PHYSIOLOGY
Springer-Verlag New York, Inc.
175 5th Ave.
New York, NY 10010   Phone: (212) 460-1500
First Published: 1981. Frequency: Irregular. ISSN: 0721-9156.

★3396★ PROGRESS IN SURGERY
S. Karger Publishers, Inc.
26 W. Avon Rd.
PO Box 529
Farmington, CT 06085   Phone: (203) 675-7834
First Published: 1961. Frequency: Irregular. ISSN: 0079-6824.

★3397★ PROGRESS IN VETERINARY MICROBIOLOGY AND
IMMUNOLOGY
S. Karger Publishers, Inc.
26 W. Avon Rd.
PO Box 529
Farmington, CT 06085   Phone: (203) 675-7834
First Published: 1985. Frequency: Irregular.

★3398★ PSYCHIATRIC ANNALS
Slack, Inc.
6900 Grove Rd.
Thorofare, NJ 08086   Phone: (609) 848-1000
First Published: 1971. Frequency: Monthly. ISSN: 0048-5713.

★3399★ PSYCHIATRIC CLINICS OF NORTH AMERICA
W.B. Saunders Co.
Curtis Center
Independence Sq., W.
Philadelphia, PA 19106   Phone: (215) 238-7800
First Published: 1978. Frequency: Quarterly. ISSN: 0193-953X.

★3400★ PSYCHOANALYTIC STUDY OF THE CHILD
Yale University Press
92A Yale Sta.
New Haven, CT 06520   Phone: (203) 432-0940
First Published: 1945. Frequency: Annual. ISSN: 0079-7308.

★3401★ PSYCHOLOGICAL REVIEW
American Psychological Association
1200 17th St., NW
Washington, DC 20036   Phone: (202) 955-7600
Frequency: Quarterly.

★3402★ QDT
Quintenssence Publishing Co., Inc.
870 Oak Creek Dr.
Lombard, IL 60148   Phone: (708) 620-4443
First Published: 1976. Frequency: Annual.

★3403★ RADIOLOGIC CLINICS OF NORTH AMERICA
W.B. Saunders Co.
Curtis Center
Independence Sq., W.
Philadelphia, PA 19106   Phone: (215) 238-7800
First Published: 1963. Frequency: Bimonthly. ISSN: 0033-8389.

★3404★ RECENT ADVANCES IN NUCLEAR MEDICINE
W. B. Saunders Co.
Curtis Center
Independence Sq., W.
Philadelphia, PA 19106   Phone: (215) 238-7800
First Published: 1965. Frequency: Irregular. ISSN: 0163-6170.

★3405★ RECENT ADVANCES IN RADIOLOGY AND MEDICAL
IMAGING
Churchill Livingstone, Inc.
1560 Broadway
New York, NY 10036   Phone: (212) 819-5400
First Published: 1979. Frequency: Irregular. ISSN: 0143-6961.

★3406★   **RECENT DEVELOPMENTS IN ALCOHOLISM**
Plenum Publishing Corp.
233 Spring St.
New York, NY 10013   Phone: (212) 620-8000
First Published: 1984. **Frequency:** Irregular. **ISSN:** 0738-422X.

★3407★   **RECENT RESULTS IN CANCER RESEARCH**
Springer-Verlag New York, Inc.
175 5th Ave.
New York, NY 10010   Phone: (212) 460-1500
First Published: 1965. **Frequency:** Irregular. **ISSN:** 0080-0015.

★3408★   **REPRODUCTIVE MEDICINE REVIEW**
Cambridge University Press
40 W. 20th St.
New York, NY 10011   Phone: (212) 924-3900
Frequency: Semiannual. **ISSN:** 0962-2799.

★3409★   **REVIEW OF BEHAVIOR THERAPY: THEORY AND PRACTICE**
Guilford Press
72 Spring St., 4th Fl.
New York, NY 10012   Phone: (212) 431-9800
First Published: 1973. **Frequency:** Biennial.

★3410★   **REVIEW OF MEDICAL AND VETERINARY MYCOLOGY**
C.A.B. International
845 N. Park Ave.
Tucson, AZ 85719   Phone: (800) 528-4841
First Published: 1943. **Frequency:** Quarterly. **ISSN:** 0034-6624.

★3411★   **REVIEWS IN BIOCHEMICAL TOXICOLOGY**
Elsevier Science Publishing Co., Inc.
655 Avenue of the Americas
New York, NY 10010   Phone: (212) 989-5800
First Published: 1979. **Frequency:** Annual. **ISSN:** 0163-7673.

★3412★   **REVIEWS IN CLINICAL AND BASIC PHARMACOLOGY**
Freund Publishing House, Ltd.
Chesham House, Ste. 500
150 Regent St.
London W1R 5FA, England
First Published: 1980. **Frequency:** Quarterly. **ISSN:** 0334-1534.

★3413★   **REVIEWS IN CLINICAL GERONTOLOGY**
Cambridge University Press
40 W. 20th St.
New York, NY 10011   Phone: (212) 924-3900
First Published: 1992. **Frequency:** Quarterly. **ISSN:** 0959-2598.

★3414★   **REVIEWS OF INFECTIOUS DISEASES**
University of Chicago Press
5801 Ellis Ave.
Chicago, IL 60637   Phone: (312) 702-7700
First Published: 1979. **Frequency:** Bimonthly. **ISSN:** 0162-0886.

★3415★   **REVIEWS OF MAGNETIC RESONANCE IN MEDICINE**
Pergamon Press, Inc.
Maxwell House, Fairview Park
Elmsford, NY 10523   Phone: (914) 592-7700
First Published: 1986. **Frequency:** 2/yr. **ISSN:** 0883-8291.

★3416★   **REVIEWS IN MEDICAL MICROBIOLOGY**
Churchill Livingstone, Inc.
1560 Broadway
New York, NY 10036   Phone: (212) 819-5400
First Published: Quarterly. **ISSN:** 0954-139X.

★3417★   **REVIEWS OF PHYSIOLOGY, BIOCHEMISTRY AND PHARMACOLOGY**
Springer-Verlag New York, Inc.
175 5th Ave.
New York, NY 10010   Phone: (212) 460-1500
First Published: 1983. **Frequency:** Irregular. **ISSN:** 0303-4240.

★3418★   **RHEUMATIC DISEASE CLINICS OF NORTH AMERICA**
W.B. Saunders Co.
Curtis Center
Independence Sq., W.
Philadelphia, PA 19106   Phone: (215) 238-7800
First Published: 1975. **Frequency:** 3/yr. **ISSN:** 0889-857X.

★3419★   **RHEUMATOLOGY**
S. Karger Publishers, Inc.
26 W. Avon Rd.
PO Box 529
Farmington, CT 06085   Phone: (203) 675-7834
First Published: 1966. **Frequency:** Irregular. **ISSN:** 0080-2727.

★3420★   **RHEUMATOLOGY REVIEW**
Churchill Livingstone, Inc.
1560 Broadway
New York, NY 10036   Phone: (212) 819-5400
First Published: 1991. **Frequency:** Quarterly. **ISSN:** 0958-2584.

★3421★   **SELECTED READINGS IN PLASTIC SURGERY**
University of Texas Health Science Center
Plastic Surgery Division
3600 Gaston Ave., Ste. 852
Dallas, TX 75246   Phone: (214) 824-0154
First Published: 1980. **Frequency:** 20/yr. **ISSN:** 0739-5523.

★3422★   **SEMINARS IN ARTHRITIS AND RHEUMATISM**
W. B. Saunders Co.
Curtis Center
Independence Sq., W.
Philadelphia, PA 19106   Phone: (215) 238-7800
First Published: 1971. **Frequency:** Quarterly. **ISSN:** 0049-0172.

★3423★   **SEMINARS IN AVIAN AND EXOTIC PET MEDICINE**
W.B. Saunders Co.
Curtis Center
Independence Sq., W.
Philadelphia, PA 19106   Phone: (215) 238-7800
First Published: 1992. **Frequency:** Quarterly.

★3424★   **SEMINARS IN DERMATOLOGY**
W. B. Saunders Co.
Curtis Center
Independence Sq., W.
Philadelphia, PA 19106   Phone: (215) 238-7800
First Published: 1982. **Frequency:** Quarterly. **ISSN:** 0278-145X.

★3425★   **SEMINARS IN DIAGNOSTIC PATHOLOGY**
W. B. Saunders Co.
Curtis Center
Independence Sq., W.
Philadelphia, PA 19106   Phone: (215) 238-7800
First Published: 1984. **Frequency:** Quarterly. **ISSN:** 0740-2570.

★3426★   **SEMINARS IN GASTROINTESTINAL DISEASE**
W.B. Saunders Co.
Curtis Center
Independence Sq., W.
Philadelphia, PA 19106   Phone: (215) 238-7800
Frequency: Quarterly.

★3427★   **SEMINARS IN HEMATOLOGY**
W. B. Saunders Co.
Curtis Center
Independence Sq., W.
Philadelphia, PA 19106   Phone: (215) 238-7800
First Published: 1964. **Frequency:** Quarterly. **ISSN:** 0037-1963.

★3428★　SEMINARS IN LIVER DISEASES
Thieme Medical Publishers, Inc.
381 Park Ave., S., Ste. 1501
New York, NY 10016　　　　　　　Phone: (212) 683-5088
First Published: 1981. Frequency: Quarterly. ISSN: 0272-8087.

★3429★　SEMINARS IN NEPHROLOGY
W. B. Saunders Co.
Curtis Center
Independence Sq., W.
Philadelphia, PA 19106　　　　　Phone: (215) 238-7800
First Published: 1981. Frequency: Quarterly. ISSN: 0270-9295.

★3430★　SEMINARS IN NUCLEAR MEDICINE
W. B. Saunders Co.
Curtis Center
Independence Sq., W.
Philadelphia, PA 19106　　　　　Phone: (215) 238-7800
First Published: 1981. Frequency: Quarterly. ISSN: 0001-2998.

★3431★　SEMINARS IN ONCOLOGY
W. B. Saunders Co.
Curtis Center
Independence Sq., W.
Philadelphia, PA 19106　　　　　Phone: (215) 238-7800
First Published: 1974. Frequency: Quarterly. ISSN: 0093-7754.

★3432★　SEMINARS IN ONCOLOGY NURSING
W. B. Saunders Co.
Curtis Center
Independence Sq., W.
Philadelphia, PA 19106　　　　　Phone: (215) 238-7800
First Published: 1985. Frequency: Quarterly. ISSN: 0749-2081.

★3433★　SEMINARS IN OPHTHALMOLOGY
W. B. Saunders Co.
Curtis Center
Independence Sq., W.
Philadelphia, PA 19106　　　　　Phone: (215) 238-7800
First Published: 1986. Frequency: Quarterly. ISSN: 0882-0538.

★3434★　SEMINARS IN ORTHOPAEDICS
W. B. Saunders Co.
Curtis Center
Independence Sq., W.
Philadelphia, PA 19106　　　　　Phone: (215) 238-7800
First Published: 1986. Frequency: Quarterly. ISSN: 0882-052X.

★3435★　SEMINARS IN PEDIATRIC SURGERY
W.B. Saunders Co.
Curtis Center
Independence Sq., W.
Philadelphia, PA 19106　　　　　Phone: (215) 238-7800
Frequency: Quarterly.

★3436★　SEMINARS IN PERINATOLOGY
W. B. Saunders Co.
Curtis Center
Independence Sq., W.
Philadelphia, PA 19106　　　　　Phone: (215) 238-7800
First Published: 1977. Frequency: Quarterly. ISSN: 0146-0005.

★3437★　SEMINARS IN PERIOPERATIVE NURSING
W.B. Saunders Co.
Curtis Center
Independence Sq., W.
Philadelphia, PA 19106　　　　　Phone: (215) 238-7800
Frequency: Quarterly.

★3438★　SEMINARS IN RADIATION ONCOLOGY
W.B. Saunders Co.
Curtis Center
Independence Sq., W.
Philadelphia, PA 19106　　　　　Phone: (215) 238-7800
Frequency: Quarterly.

★3439★　SEMINARS IN RESPIRATORY INFECTIONS
W. B. Saunders Co.
Curtis Center
Independence Sq., W.
Philadelphia, PA 19106　　　　　Phone: (215) 238-7800
First Published: 1986. Frequency: Quarterly. ISSN: 0882-0546.

★3440★　SEMINARS IN ROENTGENOLOGY
W. B. Saunders Co.
Curtis Center
Independence Sq., W.
Philadelphia, PA 19106　　　　　Phone: (215) 238-7800
First Published: 1966. Frequency: Quarterly. ISSN: 0037-198X.

★3441★　SEMINARS IN SURGICAL ONCOLOGY
John Wiley & Sons, Inc.
605 3rd Ave.
New York, NY 10158　　　　　　Phone: (212) 850-6000
Frequency: Quarterly. ISSN: 8756-0437.

★3442★　SEMINARS IN THROMBOSIS AND HEMOSTASIS
Thieme Medical Publishers, Inc.
381 Park Ave., S., 4th Fl.
New York, NY 10016　　　　　　Phone: (212) 683-5088
Frequency: Quarterly. ISSN: 0094-6176.

★3443★　SEMINARS IN ULTRASOUND, CT, AND MR
W. B. Saunders Co.
Curtis Center
Independence Sq., W.
Philadelphia, PA 19106　　　　　Phone: (215) 238-7800
First Published: 1980. Frequency: Quarterly. ISSN: 0194-1720.

★3444★　SEMINARS IN UROLOGY
W. B. Saunders Co.
Curtis Center
Independence Sq., W.
Philadelphia, PA 19106　　　　　Phone: (215) 238-7800
First Published: 1983. Frequency: Quarterly. ISSN: 0730-9147.

★3445★　SEMINARS IN VETERINARY MEDICINE AND
　　　　SURGERY: SMALL ANIMAL
W. B. Saunders Co.
Curtis Center
Independence Sq., W.
Philadelphia, PA 19106　　　　　Phone: (215) 238-7800
First Published: 1986. Frequency: Quarterly. ISSN: 0882-0511.

★3446★　STATISTICAL METHODS IN MEDICAL RESEARCH
Cambridge University Press
40 W. 20th St.
New York, NY 10011　　　　　　Phone: (212) 924-3900
First Published: 1991. Frequency: Triannual. ISSN: 0962-2802.

★3447★　SURGERY ANNUAL
Appleton & Lange
25 Van Zant St.
East Norwalk, CT 06855　　　　　Phone: (203) 838-4400
First Published: 1969. Frequency: Annual. ISSN: 0081-9638.

★3448★　SURGICAL CLINICS
W.B. Saunders Co.
Curtis Center
Independence Sq., W.
Philadelphia, PA 19106　　　　　Phone: (215) 238-7800
First Published: 1912. Frequency: Bimonthly. ISSN: 0039-6109.

★3449★　SURVEY OF ANESTHESIOLOGY
Williams & Wilkins
428 E. Preston St.
Baltimore, MD 21202　　　　　　Phone: (301) 528-4223
First Published: 1957. Frequency: Bimonthly. ISSN: 0039-6206.

★3450★ SURVEY OF OPHTHALMOLOGY
Survey of Ophthalmology, Inc.
Seven Kent St., Ste. 4
Brookline, MA 02146   Phone: (617) 566-2138
First Published: 1956. **Frequency:** Bimonthly. **ISSN:** 0039-6257.

★3451★ TRANSFUSION MEDICINE REVIEWS
W. B. Saunders Co.
Curtis Center
Independence Sq., W.
Philadelphia, PA 19106   Phone: (215) 238-7800
First Published: 1987. **Frequency:** 3/yr. **ISSN:** 0887-7963.

★3452★ UROLOGIC CLINICS
W.B. Saunders Co.
Curtis Center
Independence Sq., W.
Philadelphia, PA 19106   Phone: (215) 238-8405
First Published: 1974. **Frequency:** Quarterly. **ISSN:** 0094-0143.

★3453★ VASCULAR MEDICINE REVIEW
Cambridge University Press
40 W. 20th St.
New York, NY 10011   Phone: (212) 924-3900
Frequency: Semiannual. **ISSN:** 0954-2582.

★3454★ VETERINARY CLINICS: SMALL ANIMAL PRACTICE
W.B. Saunders Co.
Curtis Center
Independence Sq., W.
Philadelphia, PA 19106   Phone: (215) 238-7800
First Published: 1971. **Frequency:** Bimonthly. **ISSN:** 0195-5616.

★3455★ VITAMINS AND HORMONES
Academic Press, Inc.
1250 6th Ave.
San Diego, CA 92101   Phone: (619) 231-0926
First Published: 1943. **Frequency:** Irregular. **ISSN:** 0083-6729.

★3456★ WORLD REVIEW OF NUTRITION AND DIETETICS
S. Karger Publishers, Inc.
26 W. Avon Rd.
PO Box 529
Farmington, CT 06085   Phone: (203) 675-7834
First Published: 1964. **Frequency:** Irregular. **ISSN:** 0084-2230.

★3457★ YEAR BOOK OF ANESTHESIA
Mosby-Year Book, Inc.
11830 Westline Industrial Dr.
St. Louis, MO 63146   Phone: (314) 872-8370
First Published: 1961. **Frequency:** Annual. **ISSN:** 0084-3652.

★3458★ YEAR BOOK OF CARDIOLOGY
Mosby-Year Book, Inc.
11830 Westline Industrial Dr.
St. Louis, MO 63146   Phone: (314) 872-8370
First Published: 1968. **Frequency:** Annual. **ISSN:** 0145-4145.

★3459★ YEAR BOOK OF CRITICAL CARE MEDICINE
Mosby-Year Book, Inc.
11830 Westline Industrial Dr.
St. Louis, MO 63146   Phone: (314) 872-8370
First Published: 1983. **Frequency:** Annual. **ISSN:** 0734-3299.

★3460★ YEAR BOOK OF DENTISTRY
Mosby-Year Book, Inc.
11830 Westline Industrial Dr.
St. Louis, MO 63146   Phone: (314) 872-8370
First Published: 1936. **Frequency:** Annual. **ISSN:** 0084-3717.

★3461★ YEAR BOOK OF DERMATOLOGY
Mosby-Year Book, Inc.
11830 Westline Industrial Dr.
St. Louis, MO 63146   Phone: (314) 872-8370
First Published: 1933. **Frequency:** Annual. **ISSN:** 0093-3619.

★3462★ YEAR BOOK OF DIAGNOSTIC RADIOLOGY
Mosby-Year Book, Inc.
11830 Westline Industrial Dr.
St. Louis, MO 63146   Phone: (314) 872-8370
First Published: 1932. **Frequency:** Annual. **ISSN:** 0098-1672.

★3463★ YEAR BOOK OF DIGESTIVE DISEASES
Mosby-Year Book, Inc.
11830 Westline Industrial Dr.
St. Louis, MO 63146   Phone: (314) 872-8370
First Published: 1984. **Frequency:** Annual.

★3464★ YEAR BOOK OF DRUG THERAPY
Mosby-Year Book, Inc.
11830 Westline Industrial Dr.
St. Louis, MO 63146   Phone: (314) 872-8370
First Published: 1933. **Frequency:** Annual. **ISSN:** 0084-3733.

★3465★ YEAR BOOK OF EMERGENCY MEDICINE
Mosby-Year Book, Inc.
11830 Westline Industrial Dr.
St. Louis, MO 63146   Phone: (314) 872-8370
First Published: 1981. **Frequency:** Annual. **ISSN:** 0271-7964.

★3466★ YEAR BOOK OF ENDOCRINOLOGY
Mosby-Year Book, Inc.
11830 Westline Industrial Dr.
St. Louis, MO 63146   Phone: (314) 872-8370
First Published: 1950. **Frequency:** Annual. **ISSN:** 0084-3741.

★3467★ YEAR BOOK OF FAMILY PRACTICE
Mosby-Year Book, Inc.
11830 Westline Industrial Dr.
St. Louis, MO 63146   Phone: (314) 872-8370
First Published: 1977. **Frequency:** Annual. **ISSN:** 0147-1996.

★3468★ YEAR BOOK OF GERIATRICS AND GERONTOLOGY
Mosby-Year Book, Inc.
11830 Westline Industrial Dr.
St. Louis, MO 63146   Phone: (314) 872-8370
Frequency: Annual.

★3469★ YEAR BOOK OF HAND SURGERY
Mosby-Year Book, Inc.
11830 Westline Industrial Dr.
St. Louis, MO 63146   Phone: (314) 872-8370
Frequency: Annual.

★3470★ YEAR BOOK OF HEMATOLOGY
Mosby-Year Book, Inc.
11830 Westline Industrial Dr.
St. Louis, MO 63146   Phone: (314) 872-8370
First Published: 1986. **Frequency:** Annual.

★3471★ YEAR BOOK OF INFECTIOUS DISEASES
Mosby-Year Book, Inc.
11830 Westline Industrial Dr.
St. Louis, MO 63146   Phone: (314) 872-8370
Frequency: Annual.

★3472★ YEAR BOOK OF INFERTILITY
Mosby-Year Book, Inc.
11830 Westline Industrial Dr.
St. Louis, MO 63146   Phone: (314) 872-8370
Frequency: Annual.

★3473★ YEAR BOOK OF MEDICINE
Mosby-Year Book, Inc.
11830 Westline Industrial Dr.
St. Louis, MO 63146   Phone: (314) 872-8370
First Published: 1933. **Frequency:** Annual. **ISSN:** 0084-3873.

★3474★   YEAR BOOK OF NEONATAL AND PERINATAL
MEDICINE
Mosby-Year Book, Inc.
11830 Westline Industrial Dr.
St. Louis, MO 63146   Phone: (314) 872-8370
Frequency: Annual.

★3475★   YEAR BOOK OF NEUROLOGY AND
NEUROSURGERY
Mosby-Year Book, Inc.
11830 Westline Industrial Dr.
St. Louis, MO 63146   Phone: (314) 872-8370
First Published: 1902. Frequency: Annual.

★3476★   YEAR BOOK OF NUCLEAR MEDICINE
Mosby-Year Book, Inc.
11830 Westline Industrial Dr.
St. Louis, MO 63146   Phone: (314) 872-8370
First Published: 1966. Frequency: Annual. ISSN: 0084-3903.

★3477★   YEAR BOOK OF OBSTETRICS AND GYNECOLOGY
Mosby-Year Book, Inc.
11830 Westline Industrial Dr.
St. Louis, MO 63146   Phone: (314) 872-8370
First Published: 1933. Frequency: Annual. ISSN: 0084-3911.

★3478★   YEAR BOOK OF OCCUPATIONAL AND
ENVIRONMENTAL MEDICINE
Mosby-Year Book, Inc.
11830 Westline Industrial Dr.
St. Louis, MO 63146   Phone: (314) 872-8370
First Published: 1990. Frequency: Annual.

★3479★   YEAR BOOK OF ONCOLOGY
Mosby-Year Book, Inc.
11830 Westline Industrial Dr.
St. Louis, MO 63146   Phone: (314) 872-8370
First Published: 1957. Frequency: Annual. ISSN: 0084-3679.

★3480★   YEAR BOOK OF OPHTHALMOLOGY
Mosby-Year Book, Inc.
11830 Westline Industrial Dr.
St. Louis, MO 63146   Phone: (314) 872-8370
First Published: 1901. Frequency: Annual. ISSN: 0084-392X.

★3481★   YEAR BOOK OF ORTHOPEDICS
Mosby-Year Book, Inc.
11830 Westline Industrial Dr.
St. Louis, MO 63146   Phone: (314) 872-8370
First Published: 1940. Frequency: Annual. ISSN: 0276-1092.

★3482★   YEAR BOOK OF OTOLARYNGOLOGY-HEAD AND
NECK SURGERY
Mosby-Year Book, Inc.
11830 Westline Industrial Dr.
St. Louis, MO 63146   Phone: (314) 872-8370
First Published: 1900. Frequency: Annual. ISSN: 0146-7247.

★3483★   YEAR BOOK OF PATHOLOGY AND CLINICAL
PATHOLOGY
Mosby-Year Book, Inc.
11830 Westline Industrial Dr.
St. Louis, MO 63146   Phone: (314) 872-8370
First Published: 1940. Frequency: Annual. ISSN: 0084-3946.

★3484★   YEAR BOOK OF PEDIATRICS
Mosby-Year Book, Inc.
11830 Westline Industrial Dr.
St. Louis, MO 63146   Phone: (314) 872-8370
First Published: 1933. Frequency: Annual. ISSN: 0084-3954.

★3485★   YEAR BOOK OF PLASTIC AND RECONSTRUCTIVE
SURGERY
Mosby-Year Book, Inc.
11830 Westline Industrial Dr.
St. Louis, MO 63146   Phone: (314) 872-8370
First Published: 1970. Frequency: Annual. ISSN: 0084-3962.

★3486★   YEAR BOOK OF PODIATRIC MEDICINE AND
SURGERY
Mosby-Year Book, Inc.
11830 Westline Industrial Dr.
St. Louis, MO 63146   Phone: (314) 872-8370
Frequency: Annual.

★3487★   YEAR BOOK OF PSYCHIATRY AND APPLIED
MENTAL HEALTH
Mosby-Year Book, Inc.
11830 Westline Industrial Dr.
St. Louis, MO 63146   Phone: (314) 872-8370
First Published: 1970. Frequency: Annual. ISSN: 0084-3970.

★3488★   YEAR BOOK OF PULMONARY DISEASE
Mosby-Year Book, Inc.
11830 Westline Industrial Dr.
St. Louis, MO 63146   Phone: (314) 872-8370
First Published: 1986. Frequency: Annual.

★3489★   YEAR BOOK OF REHABILITATION
Mosby-Year Book, Inc.
11830 Westline Industrial Dr.
St. Louis, MO 63146   Phone: (314) 872-8370
First Published: 1986. Frequency: Annual.

★3490★   YEAR BOOK OF SPEECH, LANGUAGE AND
HEARING
Mosby-Year Book, Inc.
11830 Westline Industrial Dr.
St. Louis, MO 63146   Phone: (314) 872-8370
First Published: 1990. Frequency: Annual.

★3491★   YEAR BOOK OF SPORTS MEDICINE
Mosby-Year Book, Inc.
11830 Westline Industrial Dr.
St. Louis, MO 63146   Phone: (314) 872-8370
First Published: 1979. Frequency: Annual. ISSN: 0162-0908.

★3492★   YEAR BOOK OF SURGERY
Mosby-Year Book, Inc.
11830 Westline Industrial Dr.
St. Louis, MO 63146   Phone: (314) 872-8370
First Published: 1971. Frequency: Annual. ISSN: 0090-3671.

★3493★   YEAR BOOK OF UROLOGY
Mosby-Year Book, Inc.
11830 Westline Industrial Dr.
St. Louis, MO 63146   Phone: (314) 872-8370
First Published: 1933. Frequency: Annual. ISSN: 0084-4071.

★3494★   YEAR BOOK OF VASCULAR SURGERY
Mosby-Year Book, Inc.
11830 Westline Industrial Dr.
St. Louis, MO 63146   Phone: (314) 872-8370
First Published: 1986. Frequency: Annual.

(4) Abstracting and Indexing Services

Entries listed below are arranged alphabetically by publication titles. For further information, see the User's Guide located at the front of this directory.

★3495★ ABORTION BIBLIOGRAPHY
Whitson Publishing Co.
PO Box 958
Troy, NY 12181　　　　　　　Phone: (518) 283-4363
First Published: 1970. **Frequency:** Annual. **ISSN:** 0092-9522.

★3496★ ABRIDGED INDEX MEDICUS
U.S. National Library of Medicine
8600 Rockville Pike
Bethesda, MD 20894　　　　　　Phone: (202) 783-3238
First Published: 1970. **Frequency:** Monthly. **ISSN:** 0001-3331.

**★3497★ ABSTRACT NEWSLETTER: BIOMEDICAL
TECHNOLOGY AND HUMAN FACTORS ENGINEERING**
U.S. National Technical Information Service
5285 Port Royal Rd.
Springfield, VA 22161　　　　　Phone: (703) 487-4630
Frequency: Weekly. **ISSN:** 0163-1497.

★3498★ ABSTRACT NEWSLETTER: HEALTH CARE
U.S. National Technical Information Service
5285 Port Royal Rd.
Springfield, VA 22161　　　　　Phone: (703) 487-4630
Frequency: Weekly.

★3499★ ABSTRACT NEWSLETTER: MEDICINE AND BIOLOGY
U.S. National Technical Information Service
5285 Port Royal Rd.
Springfield, VA 22161　　　　　Phone: (703) 487-4630
Frequency: Weekly. **ISSN:** 0364-6432.

**★3500★ ABSTRACTS OF BULGARIAN SCIENTIFIC MEDICAL
LITERATURE**
Center for Scientific Information in Medicine and Public Health
8 Ul. Bialo More
1527 Sofia, Bulgaria
First Published: 1970. **Frequency:** Quarterly. **ISSN:** 0001-3536.

★3501★ ABSTRACTS: CELLULAR PATHOLOGY
Charnlind, Ltd.
PO Box 29
Woking, Surrey GU21 1AE, England
First Published: 1979. **Frequency:** Quarterly. **ISSN:** 0268-4993.

★3502★ ABSTRACTS OF ENTOMOLOGY
BIOSIS
2100 Arch St.
Philadelphia, PA 19103　　　　Phone: (215) 587-4800
First Published: 1970. **Frequency:** Monthly. **ISSN:** 0001-3579.

**★3503★ ABSTRACTS ON HYGIENE AND COMMUNICABLE
DISEASES**
Bureau of Hygiene and Tropical Diseases
Keppel St.
London WC1E 7HT, England
First Published: 1926. **Frequency:** Monthly. **ISSN:** 0260-5511.

★3504★ ABSTRACTS OF MYCOLOGY
BIOSIS
2100 Arch St.
Philadelphia, PA 19103　　　　Phone: (215) 587-4800
First Published: 1967. **Frequency:** Monthly. **ISSN:** 0001-3617.

**★3505★ ADDICTION RESEARCH FOUNDATION
BIBLIOGRAPHIC SERIES**
Addiction Research Foundation of Ontario
33 Russell St.
Toronto, ON, Canada M5S 2S1　　Phone: (416) 595-6123
First Published: 1967. **Frequency:** Irregular. **ISSN:** 0065-1885.

**★3506★ AEROSPACE MEDICINE AND BIOLOGY: A
CONTINUING BIBLIOGRAPHY**
Scientific & Technical Information Facility
U.S. National Aeronautics and Space Administration
Box 8757
Washington Intl. Airport, MD 21240　　Phone: (202) 453-8545
First Published: 1964. **Frequency:** Monthly. **ISSN:** 0001-9410.

★3507★ AIDS LITERATURE AND NEWS REVIEW
University Publishing Group
107 E. Church St.
Frederick, MD 21701　　　　　Phone: (800) 654-8188
First Published: 1987. **Frequency:** Monthly. **ISSN:** 0893-1526.

★3508★ AIDS RESEARCH TODAY
BIOSIS
2100 Arch St.
Philadelphia, PA 19103　　　　Phone: (215) 587-4800
First Published: 1987. **Frequency:** Monthly. **ISSN:** 0895-3201.

**★3509★ AIDS SCAN: CURRENT LITERATURE IN
PERSPECTIVE**
Mosby-Year Book, Inc.
11830 Westline Industrial Dr.
St. Louis, MO 63146　　　　　Phone: (314) 872-8370
First Published: 1989. **Frequency:** Quarterly. **ISSN:** 1040-6778.

★3510★ ANIMAL DISEASE OCCURRENCE
C.A.B. International
845 N. Park Ave.
Tucson, AZ 85719   Phone: (800) 528-4841
First Published: 1980. **Frequency:** Semiannual. **ISSN:** 0144-3879.

★3511★ APPLIED HEALTH PHYSICS ABSTRACTS AND NOTES
Nuclear Technology Publishing
Box 7
Ashford, Kent TN25 4NW, England
First Published: 1975. **Frequency:** Quarterly. **ISSN:** 0305-7615.

★3512★ ATIN: AIDS TARGETED INFORMATION NEWSLETTER
Williams & Wilkins
428 E. Preston St.
Baltimore, MD 21202   Phone: (301) 528-4223
First Published: 1987. **Frequency:** Monthly. **ISSN:** 0892-0125.

★3513★ BEHAVIORAL MEDICINE ABSTRACTS
Society of Behavioral Medicine
PO Box 8530, University Sta.
Knoxville, TN 37996   Phone: (615) 974-5164
First Published: 1980. **Frequency:** Quarterly. **ISSN:** 0197-7717.

★3514★ BIBLIOGRAPHIC GUIDE TO PSYCHOLOGY
G.K. Hall & Co.
70 Lincoln St.
Boston, MA 02111   Phone: (617) 423-3990
Frequency: Annual. **ISSN:** 0360-277X.

★3515★ BIBLIOGRAPHIES AND INDEXES IN GERONTOLOGY
Greenwood Press
88 Post Rd., W.
PO Box 5007
Westport, CT 06881-9990   Phone: (203) 226-3571
First Published: 1985. **Frequency:** Irregular. **ISSN:** 0743-7560.

★3516★ BIBLIOGRAPHIES AND INDEXES IN PSYCHOLOGY
Greenwood Press
88 Post Rd., W.
PO Box 5007
Westport, CT 06881-9990   Phone: (203) 226-3571
First Published: 1984. **Frequency:** Irregular. **ISSN:** 0742-681X.

★3517★ BIBLIOGRAPHY OF BIOETHICS
Kennedy Institute for Ethics
National Reference Center for Bioethics Literature
Georgetown University
Washington, DC 20057   Phone: (202) 687-6771
First Published: 1975. **Frequency:** Annual. **ISSN:** 0363-0161.

★3518★ BIBLIOGRAPHY OF DEVELOPMENTAL MEDICINE AND CHILD NEUROLOGY
J.B. Lippincott Co.
E. Washington Sq.
Philadelphia, PA 19105   Phone: (215) 238-4200
First Published: 1963. **Frequency:** Annual. **ISSN:** 0067-7183.

★3519★ BIBLIOGRAPHY OF THE HISTORY OF MEDICINE
U.S. National Library of Medicine
8600 Rockville Pike
Bethesda, MD 20894   Phone: (202) 783-3238
First Published: 1965. **Frequency:** Annual. **ISSN:** 0067-7280.

★3520★ BIBLIOGRAPHY OF REPRODUCTION
Reproduction Research Information Service Ltd.
141 Newmarket Rd.
Cambridge CB5 8HA, England
First Published: 1963. **Frequency:** Monthly. **ISSN:** 0006-1565.

★3521★ BIBLIOGRAPHY ON SMOKING AND HEALTH
Office on Smoking and Health
U.S. Public Health Service
Park Bldg., Rm. 116
5600 Fishers Ln.
Rockville, MD 20857   Phone: (301) 443-1575
First Published: 1967. **Frequency:** Annual. **ISSN:** 0067-7361.

★3522★ BIBLIOGRAPHY OF SURGERY OF THE HAND
American Society for Surgery of the Hand
3025 S. Parker Rd., Ste. 65
Aurora, CO 80014   Phone: (303) 755-4588
First Published: 1967. **Frequency:** Annual. **ISSN:** 0067-7264.

★3523★ BIO-CONTROL NEWS AND INFORMATION
C.A.B. International
845 N. Park Ave.
Tucson, AZ 85719   Phone: (800) 528-4841
First Published: 1980. **Frequency:** Quarterly. **ISSN:** 0143-1404.

★3524★ BIOLOGICAL ABSTRACTS
BIOSIS
2100 Arch St.
Philadelphia, PA 19103   Phone: (215) 587-4800
First Published: 1927. **Frequency:** Biweekly. **ISSN:** 0006-3169.

★3525★ BIOLOGICAL ABSTRACTS/RRM
BIOSIS
2100 Arch St.
Philadelphia, PA 19103   Phone: (215) 587-4800
First Published: 1965. **Frequency:** Biweekly. **ISSN:** 0192-6985.

★3526★ BIOLOGICAL AND AGRICULTURAL INDEX
H.W. Wilson Co.
950 University Ave.
Bronx, NY 10452   Phone: (212) 588-8400
First Published: 1964. **Frequency:** Monthly. **ISSN:** 0006-3177.

★3527★ BIOLOGY DIGEST
Plexus Publishing, Inc.
143 Old Marlton Pike
Medford, NJ 08055   Phone: (609) 654-6500
First Published: 1974. **Frequency:** Monthly. **ISSN:** 0095-2958.

★3528★ BIOMETRIKA
University College London
Gower St.
London WC1E 6BT, England
First Published: 1901. **Frequency:** Quarterly. **ISSN:** 0006-3444.

★3529★ BIORESEARCH TODAY: BIOENGINEERING AND INSTRUMENTATION
BIOSIS
2100 Arch St.
Philadelphia, PA 19103   Phone: (215) 587-4800
First Published: 1972. **Frequency:** Monthly. **ISSN:** 0149-0990.

★3530★ BIORESEARCH TODAY: CANCER A— CARCINOGENESIS
BIOSIS
2100 Arch St.
Philadelphia, PA 19103   Phone: (215) 587-4800
First Published: 1972. **Frequency:** Monthly. **ISSN:** 0149-1016.

★3531★ BIORESEARCH TODAY: CANCER B—ANTICANCER AGENTS
BIOSIS
2100 Arch St.
Philadelphia, PA 19103   Phone: (215) 587-4800
First Published: 1972. **Frequency:** Monthly. **ISSN:** 0149-1024.

★3532★ BIORESEARCH TODAY: CANCER C—IMMUNOLOGY
BIOSIS
2100 Arch St.
Philadelphia, PA 19103   Phone: (215) 587-4800
First Published: 1972. **Frequency:** Monthly. **ISSN:** 0149-1032.

★3533★ BIORESEARCH TODAY: FOOD MICROBIOLOGY
BIOSIS
2100 Arch St.
Philadelphia, PA 19103   Phone: (215) 587-4800
First Published: 1972. Frequency: Monthly. ISSN: 0149-0974.

★3534★ BIORESEARCH TODAY: HUMAN AND ANIMAL
AGING
BIOSIS
2100 Arch St.
Philadelphia, PA 19103   Phone: (215) 587-4800
First Published: 1972. Frequency: Monthly. ISSN: 0149-0966.

★3535★ BIORESEARCH TODAY: HUMAN AND ANIMAL
PARASITOLOGY
BIOSIS
2100 Arch St.
Philadelphia, PA 19103   Phone: (215) 587-4800
First Published: 1972. Frequency: Monthly. ISSN: 0149-094X.

★3536★ BIORESEARCH TODAY: INDUSTRIAL HEALTH AND
TOXICOLOGY
BIOSIS
2100 Arch St.
Philadelphia, PA 19103   Phone: (215) 587-4800
First Published: 1972. Frequency: Monthly. ISSN: 0149-0923.

★3537★ BIOTECHNOLOGY RESEARCH ABSTRACTS
Cambridge Scientific Abstracts
7200 Wisconsin Ave., 6th Fl.
Bethesda, MD 20814   Phone: (301) 961-6750
Frequency: Bimonthly. ISSN: 0733-5709.

★3538★ BPA QUARTERLY
Black Psychiatrists of America
c/o Dr. Thelissa Harris
664 Prospect Ave.
Hartford, CT 06105   Phone: (203) 236-2320
First Published: 1969. Frequency: Quarterly.

★3539★ BREASTFEEDING ABSTRACTS
La Leche League International
9616 Minneapolis Ave.
PO Box 1209
Franklin Park, IL 60131   Phone: (708) 455-7730
First Published: 1981. Frequency: Quarterly.

★3540★ CA SELECTS: ALLERGY AND ANTIALLERGY
Chemical Abstract Service
2540 Olentangy River Rd.
Box 3012
Columbus, OH 43210   Phone: (614) 447-3600
First Published: 1981. Frequency: Biweekly. ISSN: 0276-3095.

★3541★ CA SELECTS: ALZHEIMER'S DISEASE AND
RELATED MEMORY DYSFUNCTIONS
Chemical Abstracts Service
2540 Olentangy River Rd.
Box 3012
Columbus, OH 43210   Phone: (614) 447-3600
First Published: 1986. Frequency: Biweekly.

★3542★ CA SELECTS: ANIMAL LONGEVITY AND AGING
Chemical Abstracts Service
2540 Olentangy River Rd.
Box 3012
Columbus, OH 43210   Phone: (614) 447-3600
First Published: 1979. Frequency: Biweekly. ISSN: 0162-7694.

★3543★ CA SELECTS: ANTIARRHYTHMIC
Chemical Abstracts Service
2540 Olentangy River Rd.
Box 3012
Columbus, OH 43210   Phone: (614) 447-3600
First Published: 1988. Frequency: Biweekly.

★3544★ CA SELECTS: ANTICONVULSANTS AND
ANTIEPILEPTICS
Chemical Abstracts Service
2540 Olentangy River Rd.
Box 3012
Columbus, OH 43210   Phone: (614) 477-3600
First Published: 1986. Frequency: Biweekly.

★3545★ CA SELECTS: ANTIFUNGAL AND ANTIMYCOTIC
AGENTS
Chemical Abstracts Service
2540 Olentangy River Rd.
Box 3012
Columbus, OH 43210   Phone: (614) 477-3600
First Published: 1988. Frequency: Biweekly.

★3546★ CA SELECTS: ANTI-INFLAMMATORY AGENTS AND
ARTHRITIS
Chemical Abstracts Service
2540 Olentangy River Rd.
Box 3012
Columbus, OH 43210   Phone: (614) 447-3600
First Published: 1978. Frequency: Biweekly. ISSN: 0148-2394.

★3547★ CA SELECTS: ANTITUMOR AGENTS
Chemical Abstracts Service
2540 Olentangy River Rd.
Box 3012
Columbus, OH 43210   Phone: (614) 447-3600
First Published: 1978. Frequency: Biweekly. ISSN: 0148-2386.

★3548★ CA SELECTS: ATHEROSCLEROSIS AND HEART
DISEASE
Chemical Abstracts Service
2540 Olentangy River Rd.
Box 3012
Columbus, OH 43210   Phone: (614) 447-3600
First Published: 1978. Frequency: Biweekly. ISSN: 0148-2378.

★3549★ CA SELECTS: BIOGENIC AMINES AND THE
NERVOUS SYSTEM
Chemical Abstracts Service
2540 Olentangy River Rd.
Box 3012
Columbus, OH 43210   Phone: (614) 447-3600
First Published: 1979. Frequency: Biweekly. ISSN: 0162-7716.

★3550★ CA SELECTS: BIOLOGICAL INFORMATION
TRANSFER
Chemical Abstracts Service
2540 Olentangy River Rd.
Box 3012
Columbus, OH 43210   Phone: (614) 447-3600
First Published: 1979. Frequency: Biweekly. ISSN: 0162-7724.

★3551★ CA SELECTS: BLOOD COAGULATION
Chemical Abstracts Service
2540 Olentangy River Rd.
Box 3012
Columbus, OH 43210   Phone: (614) 447-3600
First Published: 1979. Frequency: Biweekly. ISSN: 0162-7732.

★3552★ CA SELECTS: CARCINOGENS, MUTAGENS, AND
TERATOGENS
Chemical Abstracts Service
2540 Olentangy River Rd.
Box 3012
Columbus, OH 43210   Phone: (614) 447-3600
First Published: 1978. Frequency: Biweekly. ISSN: 0148-2408.

★3553★ CA SELECTS: CHEMICAL HAZARDS, HEALTH AND
SAFETY
Chemical Abstracts Service
2540 Olentangy River Rd.
Box 3012
Columbus, OH 43210   Phone: (614) 447-3600
First Published: 1977. Frequency: Biweekly. ISSN: 0190-9398.

★3554★　CA SELECTS: DRUG AND COSMETIC TOXICITY
Chemical Abstracts Service
2540 Olentangy River Rd.
Box 3012
Columbus, OH 43210　　　　Phone: (614) 447-3600
First Published: 1979. **Frequency:** Biweekly. **ISSN:** 0162-7775.

★3555★　CA SELECTS: DRUG INTERACTIONS
Chemical Abstracts Service
2540 Olentangy River Rd.
Columbus, OH 43210　　　　Phone: (614) 447-3600
First Published: 1987. **Frequency:** Biweekly.

★3556★　CA SELECTS: FOOD TOXICITY
Chemical Abstracts Service
2540 Olentangy River Rd.
Box 3012
Columbus, OH 43210　　　　Phone: (614) 447-3600
First Published: 1979. **Frequency:** Biweekly. **ISSN:** 0162-7813.

★3557★　CA SELECTS: IMMUNOCHEMICAL METHODS
Chemical Abstracts Service
2540 Olentangy River Rd.
Box 3012
Columbus, OH 43210　　　　Phone: (614) 447-3600
First Published: 1981. **Frequency:** Biweekly. **ISSN:** 0276-3168.

★3558★　CA SELECTS: INDOOR AIR POLLUTION
Chemical Abstracts Service
2540 Olentangy River Rd.
Box 3012
Columbus, OH 43210　　　　Phone: (614) 447-3600
First Published: 1988. **Frequency:** Biweekly.

★3559★　CA SELECTS: LEUKOTRIENES
Chemical Abstracts Service
2540 Olentangy River Rd.
Box 3012
Columbus, OH 43210　　　　Phone: (614) 447-3600
First Published: 1985. **Frequency:** Biweekly.

★3560★　CA SELECTS: MONOCLONAL ANTIBODIES
Chemical Abstracts Service
2540 Olentangy River Rd.
Box 3012
Columbus, OH 43210　　　　Phone: (614) 447-3600
First Published: 1985. **Frequency:** Biweekly.

★3561★　CA SELECTS: NITROGEN FIXATION
Chemical Abstracts Service
2540 Olentangy River Rd.
Columbus, OH 43210　　　　Phone: (614) 447-3600
Frequency: Biweekly.

★3562★　CA SELECTS: NUTRITIONAL ASPECTS OF CANCER
Chemical Abstracts Service
2540 Olentangy River Rd.
Box 3012
Columbus, OH 43210　　　　Phone: (614) 447-3600
First Published: 1985. **Frequency:** Biweekly.

★3563★　CA SELECTS: OCCUPATIONAL EXPOSURE AND HAZARDS
Chemical Abstracts Service
2540 Olentangy River Rd.
Box 3012
Columbus, OH 43210　　　　Phone: (614) 447-3600
First Published: 1988. **Frequency:** Biweekly.

★3564★　CA SELECTS: OSTEOPOROSIS AND RELATED BONE LOSS
Chemical Abstracts Service
2540 Olentangy River Rd.
Box 3012
Columbus, OH 43210　　　　Phone: (614) 447-3600
First Published: 1989. **Frequency:** Biweekly.

★3565★　CA SELECTS: PHOTOBIOCHEMISTRY
Chemical Abstracts Service
2540 Olentangy River Rd.
Box 3012
Columbus, OH 43210　　　　Phone: (614) 447-3600
First Published: 1978. **Frequency:** Biweekly. **ISSN:** 0148-2335.

★3566★　CA SELECTS: PSYCHOBIOCHEMISTRY
Chemical Abstracts Service
2540 Olentangy River Rd.
Box 3012
Columbus, OH 43210　　　　Phone: (614) 447-3600
First Published: 1976. **Frequency:** Biweekly. **ISSN:** 0362-9848.

★3567★　CA SELECTS: STEROIDS
Chemical Abstracts Service
2540 Olentangy River Rd.
Box 3012
Columbus, OH 43210　　　　Phone: (614) 447-3600
First Published: 1978. **Frequency:** Biweekly. **ISSN:** 0160-9173.

★3568★　CA SELECTS: ULCER INHIBITORS
Chemical Abstracts Service
2540 Olentangy River Rd.
Box 3012
Columbus, OH 43210　　　　Phone: (614) 447-3600
First Published: 1986. **Frequency:** Biweekly.

★3569★　CA SELECTS: VIRUCIDES AND VIRYSTATS
Chemical Abstracts Service
2540 Olentangy River Rd.
Box 3012
Columbus, OH 43210　　　　Phone: (614) 447-3600
First Published: 1986. **Frequency:** Biweekly.

★3570★　CALCIFIED TISSUE ABSTRACTS
Cambridge Scientific Abstracts
7200 Wisconsin Ave., 6th Fl.
Bethesda, MD 20814　　　　Phone: (301) 961-6700
First Published: 1969. **Frequency:** Quarterly. **ISSN:** 0008-0586.

★3571★　CAMBRIDGE SCIENTIFIC BIOCHEMISTRY ABSTRACTS, PART 1: BIOLOGICAL MEMBRANES
Cambridge Scientific Abstracts
7200 Wisconsin Ave., 6th Fl.
Bethesda, MD 20814　　　　Phone: (301) 961-6700
First Published: 1973. **Frequency:** Monthly. **ISSN:** 0143-330X.

★3572★　CAMBRIDGE SCIENTIFIC BIOCHEMISTRY ABSTRACTS, PART 2: NUCLEIC ACIDS
Cambridge Scientific Abstracts
7200 Wisconsin Ave., 6th Fl.
Bethesda, MD 20814　　　　Phone: (301) 961-6700
First Published: 1971. **Frequency:** Monthly. **ISSN:** 0143-3318.

★3573★　CAMBRIDGE SCIENTIFIC BIOCHEMISTRY ABSTRACTS, PART 3: AMINO ACIDS, PEPTIDES AND PROTEINS
Cambridge Scientific Abstracts
7200 Wisconsin Ave., 6th Fl.
Bethesda, MD 20814　　　　Phone: (301) 961-6700
First Published: 1972. **Frequency:** Monthly. **ISSN:** 0143-3326.

★3574★　CENTRAL PATENTS INDEX
Derwent, Inc.
1313 Dolley Madison Blvd., Ste. 303
McLean, VA 22101
First Published: 1970. **Frequency:** Weekly.

★3575★ CHEMICAL ABSTRACTS
Chemical Abstracts Service
2540 Olentangy River Rd.
Box 3012
Columbus, OH 43210   Phone: (614) 447-3600
First Published: 1907. Frequency: Weekly. ISSN: 0009-2258.

★3576★ CHEMICAL ABSTRACTS—BIOCHEMISTRY SECTIONS
Chemical Abstracts Service
2540 Olentangy River Rd.
Box 3012
Columbus, OH 43210   Phone: (614) 447-3600
First Published: 1963. Frequency: Biweekly. ISSN: 0009-2304.

★3577★ CHEMICAL TITLES
Chemical Abstracts Service
2450 Olentangy River Rd.
Box 3012
Columbus, OH 43210   Phone: (614) 447-3600
First Published: 1961. Frequency: Biweekly. ISSN: 0009-2711.

★3578★ CHEMORECEPTION ABSTRACTS
Cambridge Scientific Abstracts
7200 Wisconsin Ave., 6th Fl.
Bethesda, MD 20814   Phone: (301) 961-6700
First Published: 1973. Frequency: Quarterly. ISSN: 0300-1261.

★3579★ CHICAGO PSYCHOANALYTIC LITERATURE INDEX
Chicago Institute for Psychoanalysis
180 N. Michigan Ave.
Chicago, IL 60601   Phone: (312) 726-6300
First Published: 1958. Frequency: Quarterly. ISSN: 0009-3661.

★3580★ CHILD DEVELOPMENT ABSTRACTS AND
   BIBLIOGRAPHY
Society for Research in Child Development
University of Chicago Press
5720 Woodlawn Ave.
Chicago, IL 60637   Phone: (312) 702-7470
First Published: 1927. Frequency: 3/yr. ISSN: 0009-3939.

★3581★ CLIN-ALERT
Learned Information, Inc.
143 Old Marlton Pike
Medford, NJ 08055   Phone: (609) 654-6266
First Published: 1962. Frequency: 26/yr. ISSN: 0069-4770.

★3582★ CLINICAL RESEARCH
American Federation for Clinical Research
6900 Grove Rd.
Thorofare, NJ 08086   Phone: (609) 848-1000
First Published: 1953. Frequency: 4/yr. ISSN: 0009-9279.

★3583★ COMBINED CUMULATIVE INDEX TO PEDIATRICS
Numarc Book Corp.
60 Alcona Ave.
Buffalo, NY 14226   Phone: (716) 834-1390
First Published: 1979. Frequency: Annual. ISSN: 0190-4981.

★3584★ CONFERENCE PAPERS INDEX
Cambridge Scientific Abstracts
7200 Wisconsin Ave., 6th Fl.
Bethesda, MD 20814   Phone: (301) 961-6700
First Published: 1973. Frequency: Monthly. ISSN: 0162-704X.

★3585★ CONSUMER HEALTH AND NUTRITION INDEX
Oryx Press
4041 N. Central at Indian School Rd.
Phoenix, AZ 85102   Phone: (602) 265-6250
First Published: 1985. Frequency: Quarterly. ISSN: 0883-1963.

★3586★ CORE JOURNALS IN CLINICAL NEUROLOGY
Elsevier Science Publishing Co., Inc.
655 Avenue of the Americas
New York, NY 10010   Phone: (212) 989-5800
First Published: 1978. Frequency: 11/yr. ISSN: 0165-1056.

★3587★ CORE JOURNALS IN OBSTETRICS/GYNECOLOGY
Elsevier Science Publishing Co., Inc.
655 Avenue of the Americas
New York, NY 10010   Phone: (212) 989-5800
First Published: 1977. Frequency: 11/yr. ISSN: 0376-5059.

★3588★ CORE JOURNALS IN OPHTHALMOLOGY
Elsevier Science Publishing Co., Inc.
655 Avenue of the Americas
New York, NY 10010   Phone: (212) 989-5800
First Published: 1978. Frequency: 11/yr. ISSN: 0165-1005.

★3589★ CORE JOURNALS IN PEDIATRICS
Elsevier Science Publishing Co., Inc.
655 Avenue of the Americas
New York, NY 10010   Phone: (212) 989-5800
First Published: 1977. Frequency: Monthly. ISSN: 0376-5040.

★3590★ CUMULATED INDEX MEDICUS
U.S. National Library of Medicine
8600 Rockville Pike
Bethesda, MD 20894   Phone: (202) 783-3238
Frequency: Annual. ISSN: 0090-1423.

★3591★ CUMULATED INDEX TO NURSING AND ALLIED
   HEALTH LITERATURE
CINHAL Information Systems
Box 871
Glendale, CA 91209   Phone: (818) 409-8005
First Published: 1961. Frequency: Bimonthly. ISSN: 0146-5554.

★3592★ CURRENT AWARENESS IN BIOLOGICAL SCIENCES
Pergamon Press, Inc.
Maxwell House, Fairview Park
Elmsford, NY 10523   Phone: (914) 592-7700
First Published: 1954. Frequency: 144/yr. ISSN: 0733-4443.

★3593★ CURRENT BIBLIOGRAPHY OF PLASTIC AND
   RECONSTRUCTIVE SURGERY
Plastic Surgery Education Foundation
c/o American Society of Plastic Surgeons
444 E. Algonquin Rd.
Arlington Heights, IL 60005   Phone: (301) 252-4022
First Published: 1973. Frequency: Bimonthly. ISSN: 0149-5348.

★3594★ CURRENT BIOTECHNOLOGY ABSTRACTS
Thomas Graham House
Science Park, Milton Rd.
Cambridge CB4 4WF, England
First Published: 1983. Frequency: Monthly. ISSN: 0264-3391.

★3595★ CURRENT CITATION ON STRABISMUS, AMBLYOPIA
   AND OTHER DISEASES OF OCULAR MOTILITY
Wills Eye Hospital
9th and Walnut Sts.
Philadelphia, PA 19107   Phone: (215) 928-3003
First Published: 1970. Frequency: Quarterly. ISSN: 0090-1164.

★3596★ CURRENT CONTENTS/AGRICULTURE, BIOLOGY
   AND ENVIRONMENTAL SCIENCES
Institute for Scientific Information
3501 Market St.
Philadelphia, PA 19104   Phone: (215) 386-0100
First Published: 1973. Frequency: Weekly. ISSN: 0090-0508.

★3597★ CURRENT CONTENTS/CLINICAL MEDICINE
Institute for Scientific Information
3501 Market St.
Philadelphia, PA 19104   Phone: (215) 386-0100
First Published: 1973. Frequency: Weekly. ISSN: 0091-1704.

★3598★ CURRENT CONTENTS/LIFE SCIENCES
Institute for Scientific Information
3501 Market St.
Philadelphia, PA 19104   Phone: (215) 386-0100
First Published: 1958. Frequency: Weekly. ISSN: 0011-3409.

★3599★ CURRENT CONTENTS/SOCIAL AND BEHAVIORAL SCIENCES
Institute for Scientific Information
3501 Market St.
Philadelphia, PA 19104   Phone: (215) 386-0100
First Published: 1969. **Frequency:** Weekly. **ISSN:** 0092-6361.

★3600★ CURRENT LITERATURE ON AGING
National Council on the Aging
600 Maryland Ave., SW, W. Wing 100
Washington, DC 20024   Phone: (202) 479-1200
First Published: 1957. **Frequency:** Quarterly. **ISSN:** 0011-3662.

★3601★ CURRENT LITERATURE IN FAMILY PLANNING
Katharine Dexter McCormick Library
Planned Parenthood Federation of America, Inc.
810 7th Ave.
New York, NY 10019   Phone: (212) 603-4637
First Published: 1972. **Frequency:** Monthly. **ISSN:** 0092-6000.

★3602★ CURRENT LITERATURE IN NEPHROLOGY, HYPERTENSION, AND TRANSPLANTATION
Current Literature Publications, Inc.
1513 E St.
Bellingham, WA 98225   Phone: (206) 671-6664
First Published: 1982. **Frequency:** Monthly. **ISSN:** 0743-8036.

★3603★ CURRENT WORK IN THE HISTORY OF MEDICINE
Professional & Scientific Publications
Tavistock Sq.
London WCIH 9JR, England
First Published: 1954. **Frequency:** Quarterly. **ISSN:** 0011-3999.

★3604★ DENTAL ABSTRACTS
American Dental Association
211 E. Chicago Ave.
Chicago, IL 60611   Phone: (312) 440-2500
First Published: 1956. **Frequency:** Monthly. **ISSN:** 0011-8486.

★3605★ DIGEST OF NEUROLOGY AND PSYCHIATRY
Institute of Living
400 Washington St.
Hartford, CT 06106   Phone: (203) 241-6824
First Published: 1932. **Frequency:** Monthly. **ISSN:** 0012-2769.

★3606★ DRUG ABUSE BIBLIOGRAPHY
Whitston Publishing Co., Inc
PO Box 958
Troy, NY 12181   Phone: (518) 283-4363
First Published: 1970. **Frequency:** Annual. **ISSN:** 0093-2515.

★3607★ DRUGS IN PROSPECT
Paul de Haen International, Inc.
2750 S. Shoshone St.
Englewood, CO 80110   Phone: (800) 438-0296
First Published: 1965. **Frequency:** Bimonthly.

★3608★ DRUGS IN RESEARCH
Paul de Haen International, Inc.
2750 S. Shoshone St.
Englewood, CO 80110   Phone: (800) 438-0296
First Published: 1965. **Frequency:** Bimonthly.

★3609★ DRUGS IN USE
Paul de Haen International, Inc.
2750 S. Shoshone St.
Englewood, CO 80110   Phone: (800) 438-0296
First Published: 1965. **Frequency:** Bimonthly.

★3610★ ELECTRON MICROSCOPY ABSTRACTS
PRM Science & Technology Agency, Ltd.
261A Finchley Rd.
Hampstead, London NW3 6LU, England
First Published: 1973. **Frequency:** Quarterly. **ISSN:** 0306-9869.

★3611★ ENDOCRINOLOGY ABSTRACTS
Cambridge Scientific Abstracts
7200 Wisconsin Ave., 6th Fl.
Bethesda, MD 20814   Phone: (301) 961-6700
Frequency: Monthly. **ISSN:** 0749-8020.

★3612★ ENTOMOLOGY ABSTRACTS
Cambridge Scientific Abstracts
7200 Wisconsin Ave., 6th Fl.
Bethesda, MD 20814   Phone: (301) 961-6700
First Published: 1969. **Frequency:** Monthly. **ISSN:** 0013-8924.

★3613★ ENVIRONMENTAL POLLUTION AND CONTROL: AN ABSTRACT NEWSLETTER
U.S. National Technical Information Service
5285 Port Royal Rd.
Springfield, VA 22161   Phone: (703) 487-4650
Frequency: Weekly. **ISSN:** 0364-4936.

★3614★ EXCEPTIONAL CHILD EDUCATION RESOURCES
Council for Exceptional Children
1920 Association Dr.
Reston, VA 22091   Phone: (703) 620-3660
First Published: 1969. **Frequency:** Quarterly. **ISSN:** 0160-4309.

★3615★ EXCERPTA MEDICA: ADVERSE REACTIONS TITLES
Elsevier Science Publishing Co., Inc.
655 Avenue of the Americas
New York, NY 10010   Phone: (212) 989-5800
First Published: 1966. **Frequency:** Monthly. **ISSN:** 0001-8848.

★3616★ EXCERPTA MEDICA: ANATOMY, ANTHROPOLOGY, EMBRYOLOGY AND HISTOLOGY
Elsevier Science Publishing Co., Inc.
655 Avenue of the Americas
New York, NY 10010   Phone: (212) 989-5800
First Published: 1947. **Frequency:** 10/yr. **ISSN:** 0014-4053.

★3617★ EXCERPTA MEDICA: ANESTHESIOLOGY
Elsevier Science Publishing Co., Inc.
655 Avenue of the Americas
New York, NY 10010   Phone: (212) 989-5800
First Published: 1966. **Frequency:** 10/yr. **ISSN:** 0014-4282.

★3618★ EXCERPTA MEDICA: ARTHRITIS AND RHEUMATISM
Elsevier Science Publishing Co., Inc.
655 Avenue of the Americas
New York, NY 10010   Phone: (212) 989-5800
First Published: 1965. **Frequency:** 8/yr. **ISSN:** 0014-4355.

★3619★ EXCERPTA MEDICA: BIOPHYSICS, BIOENGINEERING AND MEDICAL INSTRUMENTATION
Elsevier Science Publishing Co., Inc.
655 Avenue of the Americas
New York, NY 10010   Phone: (212) 989-5800
First Published: 1967. **Frequency:** 10/yr. **ISSN:** 0014-4312.

★3620★ EXCERPTA MEDICA: CANCER
Elsevier Science Publishing Co., Inc.
655 Avenue of the Americas
New York, NY 10010   Phone: (212) 989-5800
First Published: 1953. **Frequency:** 32/yr. **ISSN:** 0014-4207.

★3621★ EXCERPTA MEDICA: CARDIOVASCULAR DISEASE AND CARDIOVASCULAR SURGERY
Elsevier Science Publishing Co., Inc.
655 Avenue of the Americas
New York, NY 10010   Phone: (212) 989-5800
First Published: 1957. **Frequency:** 24/yr. **ISSN:** 0014-4223.

★3622★ EXCERPTA MEDICA: CHEST DISEASES, THORACIC
SURGERY AND TUBERCULOSIS
Elsevier Science Publishing Co., Inc.
655 Avenue of the Americas
New York, NY 10010   Phone: (212) 989-5800
First Published: 1948. Frequency: 20/yr. ISSN: 0014-4193.

★3623★ EXCERPTA MEDICA: CLINICAL BIOCHEMISTRY
Elsevier Science Publishing Co., Inc.
655 Avenue of the Americas
New York, NY 10010   Phone: (212) 989-5800
First Published: 1948. Frequency: 32/yr. ISSN: 0300-5372.

★3624★ EXCERPTA MEDICA: DERMATOLOGY AND
VENEREOLOGY
Elsevier Science Publishing Co., Inc.
655 Avenue of the Americas
New York, NY 10010   Phone: (212) 989-5800
First Published: 1947. Frequency: 16/yr. ISSN: 0014-4177.

★3625★ EXCERPTA MEDICA: DEVELOPMENTAL BIOLOGY
AND TERATOLOGY
Elsevier Science Publishing Co., Inc.
655 Avenue of the Americas
New York, NY 10010   Phone: (212) 989-5800
First Published: 1961. Frequency: 8/yr. ISSN: 0014-4258.

★3626★ EXCERPTA MEDICA: DRUG DEPENDENCE,
ALCOHOL ABUSE AND ALCOHOLISM
Elsevier Science Publishing Co., Inc.
655 Avenue of the Americas
New York, NY 10010   Phone: (212) 989-5800
First Published: 1973. Frequency: 6/yr. ISSN: 0304-4041.

★3627★ EXCERPTA MEDICA: DRUG LITERATURE INDEX
Elsevier Science Publishing Co., Inc.
655 Avenue of the Americas
New York, NY 10010   Phone: (212) 989-5800
First Published: 1969. Frequency: 24/yr. ISSN: 0376-5091.

★3628★ EXCERPTA MEDICA: ENDOCRINOLOGY
Elsevier Science Publishing Co., Inc.
655 Avenue of the Americas
New York, NY 10010   Phone: (212) 989-5800
First Published: 1947. Frequency: 24/yr. ISSN: 0014-407X.

★3629★ EXCERPTA MEDICA: ENVIRONMENTAL HEALTH
AND POLLUTION CONTROL
Elsevier Science Publishing Co., Inc.
655 Avenue of the Americas
New York, NY 10010   Phone: (212) 989-5800
First Published: 1971. Frequency: 10/yr. ISSN: 0300-5194.

★3630★ EXCERPTA MEDICA: EPILEPSY ABSTRACTS
Elsevier Science Publishing Co., Inc.
655 Avenue of the Americas
New York, NY 10010   Phone: (212) 989-5800
First Published: 1971. Frequency: 6/yr. ISSN: 0303-8459.

★3631★ EXCERPTA MEDICA: FORENSIC SCIENCE
ABSTRACTS
Elsevier Science Publishing Co., Inc.
655 Avenue of the Americas
New York, NY 10010   Phone: (212) 989-5800
First Published: 1975. Frequency: 6/yr. ISSN: 0031-0743.

★3632★ EXCERPTA MEDICA: GASTROENTEROLOGY
Elsevier Science Publishing Co., Inc.
655 Avenue of the Americas
New York, NY 10010   Phone: (212) 989-5800
First Published: 1971. Frequency: 20/yr. ISSN: 0031-3580.

★3633★ EXCERPTA MEDICA: GENERAL PATHOLOGY AND
PATHOLOGICAL ANATOMY
Elsevier Science Publishing Co., Inc.
655 Avenue of the Americas
New York, NY 10010   Phone: (212) 989-5800
First Published: 1948. Frequency: 24/yr. ISSN: 0014-4096.

★3634★ EXCERPTA MEDICA: GERONTOLOGY AND
GERIATRICS
Elsevier Science Publishing Co., Inc.
655 Avenue of the Americas
New York, NY 10010   Phone: (212) 989-5800
First Published: 1958. Frequency: 8/yr. ISSN: 0014-424X.

★3635★ EXCERPTA MEDICA: HEALTH POLICY, ECONOMICS
AND MANAGEMENT
Elsevier Science Publishing Co., Inc.
655 Avenue of the Americas
New York, NY 10010   Phone: (212) 989-5800
First Published: 1971. Frequency: 10/yr. ISSN: 0300-5321.

★3636★ EXCERPTA MEDICA: HEMATOLOGY
Elsevier Science Publishing Co., Inc.
655 Avenue of the Americas
New York, NY 10010   Phone: (212) 989-5800
First Published: 1967. Frequency: 24/yr. ISSN: 0014-4290.

★3637★ EXCERPTA MEDICA: HUMAN GENETICS
Elsevier Science Publishing Co., Inc.
655 Avenue of the Americas
New York, NY 10010   Phone: (212) 989-5800
First Published: 1963. Frequency: 24/yr. ISSN: 0014-4266.

★3638★ EXCERPTA MEDICA: IMMUNOLOGY, SEROLOGY
AND TRANSPLANTATION
Elsevier Science Publishing Co., Inc.
655 Avenue of the Americas
New York, NY 10010   Phone: (212) 989-5800
First Published: 1967. Frequency: 32/yr. ISSN: 0014-4304.

★3639★ EXCERPTA MEDICA: INTERNAL MEDICINE
Elsevier Science Publishing Co., Inc.
655 Avenue of the Americas
New York, NY 10010   Phone: (212) 989-5800
First Published: 1947. Frequency: 24/yr. ISSN: 0014-410X.

★3640★ EXCERPTA MEDICA: MICROBIOLOGY
BACTERIOLOGY, MYCOLOGY AND PARASITOLOGY
Elsevier Science Publishing Co., Inc.
655 Avenue of the Americas
New York, NY 10010   Phone: (212) 989-5800
First Published: 1948. Frequency: 24/yr. ISSN: 0167-4285.

★3641★ EXCERPTA MEDICA: NEUROLOGY AND
NEUROSURGERY
Elsevier Science Publishing Co., Inc.
655 Avenue of the Americas
New York, NY 10010   Phone: (212) 989-5800
First Published: 1948. Frequency: 32/yr. ISSN: 0014-4126.

★3642★ EXCERPTA MEDICA: NUCLEAR MEDICINE
Elsevier Science Publishing Co., Inc.
655 Avenue of the Americas
New York, NY 10010   Phone: (212) 989-5800
First Published: 1964. Frequency: 20/yr. ISSN: 0014-4274.

★3643★ EXCERPTA MEDICA: OBSTETRICS AND
GYNECOLOGY
Elsevier Science Publishing Co., Inc.
655 Avenue of the Americas
New York, NY 10010   Phone: (212) 989-5800
First Published: 1948. Frequency: 20/yr. ISSN: 0014-4142.

★3644★ EXCERPTA MEDICA: OCCUPATIONAL HEALTH AND INDUSTRIAL MEDICINE
Elsevier Science Publishing Co., Inc.
655 Avenue of the Americas
New York, NY 10010   Phone: (212) 989-5800
First Published: 1971. **Frequency:** 16/yr. **ISSN:** 0014-4398.

★3645★ EXCERPTA MEDICA: OPHTHALMOLOGY
Elsevier Science Publishing Co., Inc.
655 Avenue of the Americas
New York, NY 10010   Phone: (212) 989-5800
First Published: 1947. **Frequency:** 10/yr. **ISSN:** 0014-4169.

★3646★ EXCERPTA MEDICA: ORTHOPEDIC SURGERY
Elsevier Science Publishing Co., Inc.
655 Avenue of the Americas
New York, NY 10010   Phone: (212) 989-5800
First Published: 1956. **Frequency:** 10/yr. **ISSN:** 0014-4371.

★3647★ EXCERPTA MEDICA: OTORHINOLARYNGOLOGY
Elsevier Science Publishing Co., Inc.
655 Avenue of the Americas
New York, NY 10010   Phone: (212) 989-5800
First Published: 1948. **Frequency:** 10/yr. **ISSN:** 0014-4150.

★3648★ EXCERPTA MEDICA: PEDIATRICS AND PEDIATRIC SURGERY
Elsevier Science Publishing Co., Inc.
655 Avenue of the Americas
New York, NY 10010   Phone: (212) 989-5800
First Published: 1947. **Frequency:** 24/yr.

★3649★ EXCERPTA MEDICA: PHARMACOLOGY
Elsevier Science Publishing Co., Inc.
655 Avenue of the Americas
New York, NY 10010   Phone: (212) 989-5800
First Published: 1948. **Frequency:** 16/yr. **ISSN:** 0167-9643.

★3650★ EXCERPTA MEDICA: PHYSIOLOGY
Elsevier Science Publishing Co., Inc.
655 Avenue of the Americas
New York, NY 10010   Phone: (212) 989-5800
First Published: 1948. **Frequency:** 24/yr. **ISSN:** 0014-4061.

★3651★ EXCERPTA MEDICA: PLASTIC SURGERY
Elsevier Science Publishing Co., Inc.
655 Avenue of the Americas
New York, NY 10010   Phone: (212) 989-5800
First Published: 1970. **Frequency:** 6/yr. **ISSN:** 0014-438X.

★3652★ EXCERPTA MEDICA: PSYCHIATRY
Elsevier Science Publishing Co., Inc.
655 Avenue of the Americas
New York, NY 10010   Phone: (212) 989-5800
First Published: 1948. **Frequency:** 20/yr. **ISSN:** 0014-4363.

★3653★ EXCERPTA MEDICA: PUBLIC HEALTH, SOCIAL MEDICINE AND EPIDEMIOLOGY
Elsevier Science Publishing Co., Inc.
655 Avenue of the Americas
New York, NY 10010   Phone: (212) 989-5800
First Published: 1955. **Frequency:** 24/yr. **ISSN:** 0014-4215.

★3654★ EXCERPTA MEDICA: RADIOLOGY
Elsevier Science Publishing Co., Inc.
655 Avenue of the Americas
New York, NY 10010   Phone: (212) 989-5800
First Published: 1947. **Frequency:** 24/yr. **ISSN:** 0014-4185.

★3655★ EXCERPTA MEDICA: REHABILITATION AND PHYSICAL MEDICINE
Elsevier Science Publishing Co., Inc.
655 Avenue of the Americas
New York, NY 10010   Phone: (212) 989-5800
First Published: 1958. **Frequency:** 8/yr. **ISSN:** 0014-4231.

★3656★ EXCERPTA MEDICA: SURGERY
Elsevier Science Publishing Co., Inc.
655 Avenue of the Americas
New York, NY 10010   Phone: (212) 989-5800
First Published: 1947. **Frequency:** 20/yr. **ISSN:** 0014-4134.

★3657★ EXCERPTA MEDICA: UROLOGY AND NEPHROLOGY
Elsevier Science Publishing Co., Inc.
655 Avenue of the Americas
New York, NY 10010   Phone: (212) 989-5800
First Published: 1967. **Frequency:** 20/yr. **ISSN:** 0014-4320.

★3658★ EXCERPTA MEDICA: VIROLOGY
Elsevier Science Publishing Co., Inc.
655 Avenue of the Americas
New York, NY 10010   Phone: (212) 989-5800
First Published: 1971. **Frequency:** 10/yr. **ISSN:** 0304-4084.

★3659★ FAMLI (FAMILY MEDICINE LITERATURE INDEX)
College of Family Physicians of Canada
4000 Leslie St.
Willowdale, ON, Canada M2K 2R9
First Published: 1980. **Frequency:** Annual. **ISSN:** 0227-2393.

★3660★ FIVE-YEAR CUMULATIVE INDEX TO THE JOURNAL OF ALLERGY AND CLINICAL IMMUNOLOGY
Mosby-Year Book, Inc.
11830 Westline Industrial Dr.
St. Louis, MO 63146   Phone: (314) 872-8370

★3661★ FIVE-YEAR CUMULATIVE INDEX TO OTOLARYNGOLOGY—HEAD AND NECK SURGERY
Mosby-Year Book, Inc.
11830 Westline Industrial Dr.
St. Louis, MO 63146   Phone: (314) 872-8370

★3662★ FOODS ADLIBRA
Foods Adlibra Publications
9000 Plymouth Ave., N.
Minneapolis, MN 55427   Phone: (612) 540-2720
First Published: 1974. **Frequency:** Semimonthly. **ISSN:** 0146-9304.

★3663★ GENERAL SCIENCE INDEX
H.W. Wilson Co.
950 University Ave.
Bronx, NY 10452   Phone: (212) 588-8400
Frequency: Monthly. **ISSN:** 0162-1963.

★3664★ GENETICS ABSTRACTS
Cambridge Scientific Abstracts
7200 Wisconsin Ave., 6th Fl.
Bethesda, MD 20814   Phone: (301) 961-6700
First Published: 1968. **Frequency:** Monthly. **ISSN:** 0016-674X.

★3665★ GERMAN JOURNAL OF PSYCHOLOGY
Hogrefe & Huber Publishers, Inc.
12-14 Bruce Park Ave.
Toronto, ON, Canada M4P 2S3   Phone: (416) 482-6339
First Published: 1977. **Frequency:** Quarterly. **ISSN:** 0705-5870.

★3666★ GERONTOLOGICAL ABSTRACTS
University Information Services, Inc.
University of Michigan
5212 School of Dentistry
Ann Arbor, MI 48109-1078   Phone: (313) 764-1555
First Published: 1978. **Frequency:** Bimonthly.

★3667★ GOVERNMENT REPORTS ANNOUNCEMENTS AND INDEX
U.S. National Technical Information Service
5285 Port Royal Rd.
Springfield, VA 22161   Phone: (703) 487-4650
Frequency: Biweekly. **ISSN:** 0097-9007.

★3668★ HEALTH BUILDINGS LIBRARY BULLETIN
Great Britain Dept. of Health and Social Security
Alexander Fleming House
Elephant and Castle
London SE1 6BY, England
First Published: 1971. Frequency: Monthly.

★3669★ HEALTH DEVICES ALERTS
Emergency Care Research Institute
5200 Butler Pike
Plymouth Meeting, PA 19462   Phone: (215) 825-6000
First Published: 1976. Frequency: Weekly. ISSN: 0163-0458.

★3670★ HEALTH EDUCATION INDEX
B. Edsall & Co., Ltd.
124 Belgrave Rd.
London SW1V 2BL, England
First Published: 1967. Frequency: 2/yr. ISSN: 0140-3273.

★3671★ HEALTH, PHYSICAL EDUCATION AND RECREATION
    MICROFORM PUBLICATIONS BULLETIN
Microform Publications
College of Human Development and Performance
University of Oregon
1479 Moss St.
Eugene, OR 97403   Phone: (503) 686-4117
First Published: 1949. Frequency: Semiannual. ISSN: 0090-5119.

★3672★ HEALTH PHYSICS RESEARCH ABSTRACTS
International Atomic Energy Agency
Wagramerstrasse 5
PO Box 100
A-1400 Vienna, Austria
First Published: 1967. Frequency: Irregular. ISSN: 0085-1450.

★3673★ HEALTH AND SAFETY SCIENCE ABSTRACTS
Cambridge Scientific Abstracts
7200 Wisconsin Ave., 6th Fl.
Bethesda, MD 20814   Phone: (301) 961-6700
First Published: 1973. Frequency: Quarterly. ISSN: 0892-9351.

★3674★ HEALTH SCIENCES SERIALS
U.S. National Library of Medicine
8600 Rockville Pike
Bethesda, MD 20894   Phone: (202) 783-3238
First Published: 1979. Frequency: Quarterly. ISSN: 0162-0843.

★3675★ HEALTH SERVICE ABSTRACTS
Great Britain Dept. of Health and Social Security
Library, Rm. A 109
Alexander Fleming House
Elephant and Castle
London SE1 6BY, England
First Published: 1974. Frequency: Monthly.

★3676★ HEALTHCARE TRENDS REPORT
Health Trends
PO Box 151026
Chevy Chase, MD 20815-9944   Phone: (301) 652-8937
First Published: 1987. Frequency: Monthly. ISSN: 0894-7961.

★3677★ HELMINTHOLOGICAL ABSTRACTS: SERIES A,
    ANIMAL AND HUMAN HELMINTHOLOGY
C.A.B. International
845 N. Park Ave.
Tucson, AZ 85719   Phone: (800) 528-4841
First Published: 1932. Frequency: Monthly. ISSN: 0300-8339.

★3678★ HOSPITAL LITERATURE INDEX
American Hospital Association
840 N. Lake Shore Dr.
Chicago, IL 60611   Phone: (312) 280-6000
First Published: 1945. Frequency: Quarterly. ISSN: 0018-5736.

★3679★ ICRDB CANCERGRAM: ANTITUMOR AND
    ANTIVIRAL AGENTS—EXPERIMENTAL THERAPEUTICS,
    TOXICOLOGY, PHARMACOLOGY
U.S. National Cancer Institute
International Cancer Research Data Bank
International Cancer Information Center, Bldg. 82
National Institutes of Health
Bethesda, MD 20892   Phone: (301) 496-7403
First Published: 1977. Frequency: Monthly.

★3680★ ICRDB CANCERGRAM: ANTITUMOR AND
    ANTIVIRAL AGENTS—MECHANISM OF ACTION
U.S. National Cancer Institute
International Cancer Research Data Bank
International Cancer Information Center, Bldg. 82
National Institutes of Health
Bethesda, MD 20892   Phone: (301) 496-7403
First Published: 1977. Frequency: Monthly.

★3681★ ICRDB CANCERGRAM: BREAST CANCER—
    DIAGNOSIS, TREATMENT, PRECLINICAL BIOLOGY
U.S. National Cancer Institute
International Cancer Research Data Bank
International Cancer Information Center, Bldg. 82
National Institutes of Health
Bethesda, MD 20892   Phone: (301) 496-7403
First Published: 1977. Frequency: Monthly.

★3682★ ICRDB CANCERGRAM: CANCER DETECTION AND
    MANAGEMENT—BIOLOGICAL MARKERS
U.S. National Cancer Institute
International Cancer Research Data Bank
International Cancer Information Center, Bldg. 82
National Institutes of Health
Bethesda, MD 20892   Phone: (301) 496-7403
First Published: 1977. Frequency: Monthly.

★3683★ ICRDB CANCERGRAM: CANCER DETECTION AND
    MANAGEMENT—DIAGNOSTIC RADIOLOGY
U.S. National Cancer Institute
International Cancer Research Data Bank
International Cancer Information Center, Bldg. 82
National Institutes of Health
Bethesda, MD 20892   Phone: (301) 496-7403
First Published: 1977. Frequency: Monthly.

★3684★ ICRDB CANCERGRAM: CANCER DETECTION AND
    MANAGEMENT—NUCLEAR MEDICINE
U.S. National Cancer Institute
International Cancer Research Data Bank
International Cancer Information Center, Bldg. 82
National Institutes of Health
Bethesda, MD 20892   Phone: (301) 496-7403
Frequency: Monthly.

★3685★ ICRDB CANCERGRAM: CLINICAL TREATMENT OF
    CANCER—RADIATION THERAPY
U.S. National Cancer Institute
International Cancer Research Data Bank
International Cancer Information Center, Bldg. 82
National Institutes of Health
Bethesda, MD 20892   Phone: (301) 496-7403
First Published: 1977. Frequency: Monthly.

★3686★ ICRDB CANCERGRAM: COLO-RECTAL CANCERS—
    DIAGNOSIS, TREATMENT
U.S. National Cancer Institute
International Cancer Research Data Bank
International Cancer Information Center, Bldg. 82
National Institutes of Health
Bethesda, MD 20892   Phone: (301) 496-7403
First Published: 1977. Frequency: Monthly.

★3687★   ICRDB CANCERGRAM: CNS MALIGNANCIES—
   DIAGNOSIS, TREATMENT
U.S. National Cancer Institute
International Cancer Research Data Bank
International Cancer Information Center, Bldg. 82
National Institutes of Health
Bethesda, MD 20892   Phone: (301) 496-7403
First Published: 1977. Frequency: Monthly.

★3688★   ICRDB CANCERGRAM: ENDOCRINE TUMORS—
   DIAGNOSIS, TREATMENT, PATHOPHYSIOLOGY
U.S. National Cancer Institute
International Cancer Research Data Bank
International Cancer Information Center, Bldg. 82
National Institutes of Health
Bethesda, MD 20892   Phone: (301) 496-7403
First Published: 1977. Frequency: Monthly.

★3689★   ICRDB CANCERGRAM: GENITO-URINARY
   CANCERS—DIAGNOSIS, TREATMENT
U.S. National Cancer Institute
International Cancer Research Data Bank
International Cancer Information Center, Bldg. 82
National Institutes of Health
Bethesda, MD 20892   Phone: (301) 496-7403
First Published: 1977. Frequency: Monthly.

★3690★   ICRDB CANCERGRAM: GYNECOLOGICAL TUMORS—
   DIAGNOSIS, TREATMENT
U.S. National Cancer Institute
International Cancer Research Data Bank
International Cancer Information Center, Bldg. 82
National Institutes of Health
Bethesda, MD 20892   Phone: (301) 496-7403
First Published: 1977. Frequency: Monthly.

★3691★   ICRDB CANCERGRAM: LEUKEMIA AND MULTIPLE
   MYELOMA—DIAGNOSIS AND TREATMENT
U.S. National Cancer Institute
International Cancer Research Data Bank
International Cancer Information Center, Bldg. 82
National Institutes of Health
Bethesda, MD 20892   Phone: (301) 496-7403
First Published: 1977. Frequency: Monthly.

★3692★   ICRDB CANCERGRAM: LUNG CANCER—DIAGNOSIS,
   TREATMENT
U.S. National Cancer Institute
International Cancer Research Data Bank
International Cancer Information Center, Bldg. 82
National Institutes of Health
Bethesda, MD 20892   Phone: (301) 496-7403
First Published: 1977. Frequency: Monthly.

★3693★   ICRDB CANCERGRAM: LYMPHOMAS—DIAGNOSIS,
   TREATMENT
U.S. National Cancer Institute
International Cancer Research Data Bank
International Cancer Information Center, Bldg. 82
National Institutes of Health
Bethesda, MD 20892   Phone: (301) 496-7403
First Published: 1977. Frequency: Monthly.

★3694★   ICRDB CANCERGRAM: MELANOMA AND OTHER
   SKIN CANCERS—DIAGNOSIS, TREATMENT
U.S. National Cancer Institute
International Cancer Research Data Bank
International Cancer Information Center, Bldg. 82
National Institutes of Health
Bethesda, MD 20982   Phone: (301) 496-7403
First Published: 1977. Frequency: Monthly.

★3695★   ICRDB CANCERGRAM: NEOPLASIA OF THE HEAD
   AND NECK—DIAGNOSIS, TREATMENT
U.S. National Cancer Institute
International Cancer Research Data Bank
International Cancer Information Center, Bldg. 82
National Institutes of Health
Bethesda, MD 20892   Phone: (301) 496-7403
First Published: 1977. Frequency: Monthly.

★3696★   ICRDB CANCERGRAM: PEDIATRIC ONCOLOGY
U.S. National Cancer Institute
International Cancer Research Data Bank
International Cancer Information Center, Bldg. 82
National Institutes of Health
Bethesda, MD 20892   Phone: (301) 496-7403
First Published: 1977. Frequency: Monthly.

★3697★   ICRDB CANCERGRAM: REHABILITATION AND
   SUPPORTIVE CARE
U.S. National Cancer Institute
International Cancer Research Data Bank
International Cancer Information Center, Bldg. 82
National Institutes of Health
Bethesda, MD 20892   Phone: (301) 496-7403
First Published: 1977. Frequency: Monthly.

★3698★   ICRDB CANCERGRAM: SARCOMAS AND RELATED
   TUMORS—DIAGNOSIS, TREATMENT
U.S. National Cancer Institute
International Cancer Research Data Bank
International Cancer Information Center, Bldg. 82
National Institutes of Health
Bethesda, MD 20892   Phone: (301) 496-7403
First Published: 1977. Frequency: Monthly.

★3699★   ICRDB CANCERGRAM: UPPER GASTROINTESTINAL
   TUMORS—DIAGNOSIS, TREATMENT
U.S. National Cancer Institute
International Cancer Research Data Bank
International Cancer Information Center, Bldg. 82
National Institutes of Health
Bethesda, MD 20892   Phone: (301) 496-7403
First Published: 1977. Frequency: Monthly.

★3700★   IMMUNOLOGY ABSTRACTS
Cambridge Scientific Abstracts
7200 Wisconsin Ave., 6th Fl.
Bethesda, MD 20814   Phone: (301) 961-6700
First Published: 1976. Frequency: Monthly. ISSN: 0307-112X.

★3701★   INDEX TO DENTAL LITERATURE
American Dental Association
Bureau of Library Services
211 E. Chicago Ave.
Chicago, IL 60611   Phone: (312) 440-2500
First Published: 1921. Frequency: Quarterly. ISSN: 0019-3992.

★3702★   INDEX TO HEALTH INFORMATION
Congressional Information Service, Inc.
4520 East-West Hwy., Ste 800-DM
Bethesda, MD 20814-3389   Phone: (301) 654-1550
First Published: 1988. Frequency: Quarterly.

★3703★   INDEX TO INDIAN MEDICAL PERIODICALS
Controller of Publications
Civil Lines
Delhi 110054, India
First Published: 1959. Frequency: Quarterly. ISSN: 0019-4042.

★3704★   INDEX MEDICUS
U.S. National Library of Medicine
8600 Rockville Pike
Bethesda, MD 20894   Phone: (202) 783-3238
First Published: 1960. Frequency: Monthly. ISSN: 0019-3879.

★3705★ INDEX OF NLM SERIAL TITLES
U.S. National Library of Medicine
8600 Rockville Pike
Bethesda, MD 20894 Phone: (202) 783-3238
First Published: 1972. Frequency: Annual. ISSN: 0162-6639.

★3706★ INDEX TO PERIODICAL LITERATURE ON AGING
Lorraine Publications
2162 Chene
Detroit, MI 48207 Phone: (313) 834-4570
First Published: 1982. Frequency: Biennial. ISSN: 0882-3405.

★3707★ INDEX OF PSYCHOANALYTIC WRITINGS
International Universities Press, Inc.
59 Boston Post Rd.
PO Box 1524
Madison, CT 06443-1524 Phone: (203) 245-4000
First Published: 1966. Frequency: Irregular. ISSN: 0073-5884.

★3708★ INDEX TO SCIENTIFIC REVIEWS
Institute for Scientific Information
3501 Market St.
Philadelphia, PA 19104 Phone: (215) 386-0100
First Published: 1974. Frequency: Semiannual.

★3709★ INDEX TO SCIENTIFIC AND TECHNICAL
PROCEEDINGS
Institute for Scientific Information
3501 Market St.
Philadelphia, PA 19104 Phone: (215) 386-0100
First Published: 1978. Frequency: Monthly. ISSN: 0149-8088.

★3710★ INDEX VETERINARIUS
C.A.B. International
845 N. Park Ave.
Tucson, AZ 85719 Phone: (800) 528-4841
First Published: 1933. Frequency: Monthly. ISSN: 0019-4123.

★3711★ INDIAN PSYCHOLOGICAL ABSTRACTS
Indian Council of Social Science Research
35 Ferozshah Rd.
New Delhi 110001, India
First Published: 1972. Frequency: Quarterly. ISSN: 0250-9679.

★3712★ INDUSTRIAL HYGIENE DIGEST
Industrial Health Foundation, Inc.
34 Penn Circle, W.
Pittsburgh, PA 15206 Phone: (412) 363-6600
First Published: 1937. Frequency: Monthly. ISSN: 0019-8382.

★3713★ INFORMATIONSDIENST
KRANKENHAUSWESEN/HEALTH CARE INFORMATION
SERVICE
Institut fuer Krankenhausbau
Technische Universitaet Berlin
Strasse des 17, Juni 135
1000 Berlin 12, Germany
First Published: 1969. Frequency: Bimonthly. ISSN: 0341-0595.

★3714★ INPHARMA
ADIS Press, Ltd.
Private Bag, Mairingi Bay
Auckland 10, New Zealand
First Published: 1975. Frequency: Weekly. ISSN: 0156-2703.

★3715★ INTERNATIONAL BIBLIOGRAPHY ON BURNS
National Institute for Burn Medicine
909 E. Ann St.
Ann Arbor, MI 48104 Phone: (313) 769-9000
First Published: 1969. Frequency: Annual. ISSN: 0090-0575.

★3716★ INTERNATIONAL NURSING INDEX
American Journal of Nursing Co.
555 W. 57th St.
New York, NY 10019 Phone: (212) 582-8820
First Published: 1966. Frequency: Quarterly. ISSN: 0020-8124.

★3717★ INTERNATIONAL PHARMACEUTICAL ABSTRACTS
American Society of Hospital Pharmacists
4630 Montgomery Ave.
Bethesda, MD 20814 Phone: (301) 657-3000
First Published: 1964. Frequency: Semimonthly. ISSN: 0020-8264.

★3718★ KEY NEUROLOGY AND NEUROSURGERY
Mosby-Year Book, Inc.
11830 Westline Industrial Dr.
St. Louis, MO 63146 Phone: (314) 872-8370
First Published: 1986. Frequency: Quarterly. ISSN: 0886-8018.

★3719★ KEY OBSTETRICS AND GYNECOLOGY
Mosby-Year Book, Inc.
11830 Westline Industrial Dr.
St. Louis, MO 63146 Phone: (314) 872-8370
Frequency: Quarterly. ISSN: 0896-4467.

★3720★ KEY OPHTHALMOLOGY
Mosby-Year Book, Inc.
11830 Westline Industrial Dr.
St. Louis, MO 63146 Phone: (314) 872-8370
Frequency: Quarterly. ISSN: 0886-8026.

★3721★ KOREAN MEDICAL ABSTRACTS
Institute for Economics and Technology
PO Box 250
206-9 Cheongryangri-Dong
Dongdaimun-Ku, Republic of Korea
First Published: 1971. Frequency: Quarterly. ISSN: 0047-360X.

★3722★ LABORATORY HAZARDS BULLETIN
Royal Society of Chemistry
Burlington House
Piccadilly
London W1V 0BN, England
First Published: 1981. Frequency: Monthly. ISSN: 0261-2917.

★3723★ LABORATORY MEDICINE ABSTRACT AND
COMMENT
Churchill Livingstone, Inc.
1560 Broadway
New York, NY 10036 Phone: (212) 819-5400
First Published: 1991. Frequency: 10/yr. ISSN: 1050-9658.

★3724★ LATEST LITERATURE IN FAMILY PLANNING
Family Planning Information Service
27-35 Mortimer St.
London W1N 7RJ, England
First Published: 1974. Frequency: Bimonthly. ISSN: 0308-8774.

★3725★ LINGUISTICS AND LANGUAGE BEHAVIOR
ABSTRACTS
Sociological Abstracts, Inc.
PO Box 22206
San Diego, CA 92122 Phone: (619) 565-6603
Frequency: Quarterly.

★3726★ LIST BIO-MED: BIOMEDICAL SERIALS IN
SCANDINAVIAN LIBRARIES
Karolinska Institutets Bibliotek och Informationscentral
Box 60201
S-104 01 Stockholm, Sweden
First Published: 1965. Frequency: Irregular. ISSN: 0075-9813.

★3727★ LIST OF JOURNALS INDEXED IN INDEX MEDICUS
U.S. National Library of Medicine
8600 Rockville Pike
Bethesda, MD 20894 Phone: (202) 783-3238
First Published: 1960. Frequency: Annual. ISSN: 0093-3821.

★3728★ MEDICAL ABSTRACTS NEWSLETTER
Communi-T Publications
PO Box 2170
Teaneck, NJ 07666 Phone: (201) 836-5030
First Published: 1981. Frequency: Monthly. ISSN: 0730-7810.

★3729★   MEDICAL ELECTRONICS AND COMMUNICATIONS ABSTRACTS
Parjon Information Services
Hayward Heath
PO Box 144
Sussex RH16 2YX, England
First Published: 1966. **Frequency:** Quarterly. **ISSN:** 0025-7222.

★3730★   MEDICAL AND HEALTH CARE BOOKS AND SERIALS IN PRINT
R.R. Bowker Co.
121 Chanlon Rd.
New Providence, NJ 07974   Phone: (908) 464-6800
First Published: 1972. **Frequency:** Annual. **ISSN:** 0000-085X.

★3731★   MEDICAL INFORMATION SYSTEMS: ALLERGY
References & Index Services, Inc.
3951 N. Meridian, Ste. 100
Indianapolis, IN 46208   Phone: (317) 923-1575
First Published: 1966. **Frequency:** Monthly.

★3732★   MEDOC: INDEX TO U.S. GOVERNMENT PUBLICATIONS IN THE MEDICAL AND HEALTH SCIENCES
Spencer S. Eccles Health Sciences Library
University of Utah
Bldg. 589
Salt Lake City, UT 84112   Phone: (801) 581-5268
First Published: 1975. **Frequency:** Quarterly. **ISSN:** 0097-9732.

★3733★   MICROBIOLOGY ABSTRACTS, SECTION A: INDUSTRIAL AND APPLIED MICROBIOLOGY
Cambridge Scientific Abstracts
7200 Wisconsin Ave., 6th Fl.
Bethesda, MD 20814   Phone: (301) 961-6700
First Published: 1965. **Frequency:** Monthly. **ISSN:** 0300-838X.

★3734★   MICROBIOLOGY ABSTRACTS, SECTION B: BACTERIOLOGY
Cambridge Scientific Abstracts
7200 Wisconsin Ave., 6th Fl.
Bethesda, MD 20814   Phone: (301) 961-6700
First Published: 1966. **Frequency:** Monthly. **ISSN:** 0300-8398.

★3735★   MICROBIOLOGY ABSTRACTS, SECTION C: ALGOLOGY, MYCOLOGY AND PROTOZOOLOGY
Cambridge Scientific Abstracts
7200 Wisconsin Ave., 6th Fl.
Bethesda, MD 20814   Phone: (301) 961-6700
First Published: 1972. **Frequency:** Monthly. **ISSN:** 0301-2328.

★3736★   MIMS
Monthly Index of Medical Specialties, Ltd.
Box 2059
Pretoria 0001, Republic of South Africa
First Published: 1960. **Frequency:** Monthly. **ISSN:** 0027-0431.

★3737★   NATIONAL LIBRARY OF MEDICINE AUDIOVISUALS CATALOG
U.S. National Library of Medicine
8600 Rockville Pike
Bethesda, MD 20894   Phone: (202) 783-3238
First Published: 1978. **Frequency:** Quarterly. **ISSN:** 0149-9939.

★3738★   NEUROSCIENCES ABSTRACTS
Cambridge Scientific Abstracts
7200 Wisconsin Ave., 6th Fl.
Bethesda, MD 20814   Phone: (301) 961-6700
First Published: 1983. **Frequency:** Monthly. **ISSN:** 0141-7711.

★3739★   NEW LITERATURE ON OLD AGE
Centre for Policy on Ageing
25/31 Ironmonger Row
London EC1V 3QP, England
First Published: 1977. **Frequency:** Bimonthly. **ISSN:** 0140-2447.

★3740★   NURSING ABSTRACTS
Nursing Abstracts Co., Inc.
PO Box 295
Forest Hills, NY 11375
First Published: 1979. **Frequency:** Bimonthly. **ISSN:** 0195-3354.

★3741★   NURSING RESEARCH ABSTRACTS
Great Britain Department of Health and Social Security
Alexander Fleming House
Elephant & Castle
London SE1 6BY, England
First Published: 1978. **Frequency:** Quarterly. **ISSN:** 0141-3899.

★3742★   NUTRITION ABSTRACTS AND REVIEWS: SERIES A, HUMAN AND EXPERIMENTAL
C.A.B. International
845 N. Park Ave.
Tucson, AZ 85719   Phone: (800) 528-4841
First Published: 1977. **Frequency:** Monthly. **ISSN:** 0309-1295.

★3743★   ONCOLOGY OVERVIEW
National Cancer Institute
00, Bldg. 82, Rm. ADV
Bethesda, MA 20892
Frequency: Annual.

★3744★   OPHTHALMIC LITERATURE
Institute of Ophthalmology
Judd St.
London WC1H 9QS, England
First Published: 1947. **Frequency:** Quarterly. **ISSN:** 0030-3720.

★3745★   ORTHOPAEDIC TRANSACTIONS
Journal of Bone and Joint Surgery, Inc.
10 Shattuck St.
Boston, MA 02115   Phone: (617) 734-2835
First Published: 1977. **Frequency:** 3/yr. **ISSN:** 0162-9379.

★3746★   PHARMACEUTICAL NEWS INDEX
UMI Data Courier, Inc.
620 S. 3rd St.
Louisville, KY 40202   Phone: (800) 626-2823
First Published: 1975. **Frequency:** Weekly. **ISSN:** 0362-4439.

★3747★   PHARMINDEX
Skyline Publishers, Inc.
PO Box 1029, University Sta.
Portland, OR 97207   Phone: (503) 228-6568
First Published: 1958. **Frequency:** Monthly. **ISSN:** 0031-7152.

★3748★   PHYSICAL EDUCATION INDEX
Ben Oak Publishing Co.
PO Box 474
Cape Girardeau, MO 63701   Phone: (314) 334-8789
First Published: 1978. **Frequency:** Quarterly. **ISSN:** 0191-9202.

★3749★   PHYSICAL FITNESS/SPORTS MEDICINE
President's Council on Physical Fitness and Sports
450 5th St., NW, Ste. 7130
Washington, DC 20001   Phone: (202) 272-3421
First Published: 1978. **Frequency:** Quarterly. **ISSN:** 0163-2582.

★3750★   PLEXUS: ANNUAL MEDICAL SPECIALTY UPDATES
References & Index Services, Inc.
3951 N. Meridian, Ste. 100
Indianapolis, IN 46208   Phone: (317) 923-1575
First Published: 1966. **Frequency:** Monthly.

★3751★   POLLUTION ABSTRACTS
Cambridge Scientific Abstracts
7200 Wisconsin Ave., 6th Fl.
Bethesda, MD 20814   Phone: (301) 961-6700
First Published: 1970. **Frequency:** Bimonthly. **ISSN:** 0032-3624.

★3752★ POPULATION INDEX
Office of Population Research
Princeton University
21 Prospect Ave.
Princeton, NJ 08544-2091   Phone: (609) 258-4873
First Published: 1935. **Frequency:** Quarterly. **ISSN:** 0032-4701.

★3753★ PROTOZOOLOGICAL ABSTRACTS
C.A.B. International
845 N. Park Ave.
Tucson, AZ 85719   Phone: (800) 528-4841
First Published: 1977. **Frequency:** Monthly. **ISSN:** 0309-1287.

★3754★ PSYCHIATRIC ABSTRACT AND COMMENT
Churchill Livingstone, Inc.
1560 Broadway
New York, NY 10036   Phone: (212) 819-5400
First Published: 1991. **Frequency:** 10/yr. **ISSN:** 1042-041X.

★3755★ PSYCHOLOGICAL ABSTRACTS
American Psychological Association
1200 17th St., NW
Washington, DC 20036   Phone: (202) 955-7600
First Published: 1927. **Frequency:** Monthly. **ISSN:** 0033-2887.

★3756★ PSYCSCAN: APPLIED PSYCHOLOGY
American Psychological Association
1200 17th St., NW
Washington, DC 20036   Phone: (202) 955-7600
Frequency: Quarterly. **ISSN:** 0271-7506.

★3757★ PSYCSCAN: CLINICAL PSYCHOLOGY
American Psychological Association
1200 17th St., NW
Washington, DC 20036   Phone: (202) 955-7600
Frequency: Quarterly. **ISSN:** 0197-1484.

★3758★ PSYCSCAN: DEVELOPMENTAL PSYCHOLOGY
American Psychological Association
1200 17th St., NW
Washington, DC 20036   Phone: (202) 955-7600
Frequency: Quarterly. **ISSN:** 0197-1492.

★3759★ PSYCSCAN: LEARNING AND COMMUNICATION DISORDERS AND MENTAL RETARDATION
American Psychological Association
1200 17th St., NW
Washington, DC 20036   Phone: (202) 955-7600
Frequency: Quarterly.

★3760★ PSYCSCAN NEUROPSYCHOLOGY
American Psychological Association
1200 17th St. NW
Washington, DC 20036   Phone: (202) 955-7600
Frequency: Quarterly.

★3761★ PSYCSCAN: PSYCHOANALYSIS
American Psychological Association
1200 17th St., NW
Washington, DC 20036   Phone: (202) 955-7600
Frequency: Quarterly.

★3762★ REACTIONS
ADIS Press, Ltd.
Private Bag, Mairingi Bay
Auckland 10, New Zealand
First Published: 1979. **Frequency:** Semimonthly. **ISSN:** 0157-7271.

★3763★ REVIEW OF MEDICAL AND VETERINARY ENTOMOLOGY
C.A.B. International
845 N. Park Ave.
Tucson, AZ 85719   Phone: (800) 528-4841
First Published: 1913. **Frequency:** Monthly.

★3764★ SAFETY AND HEALTH AT WORK
International Occupational Safety and Health Information Centre (CIS)
International Labour Office
CH-1211 Geneva 22, Switzerland
First Published: 1974. **Frequency:** Bimonthly. **ISSN:** 1010-7053.

★3765★ SCIENCE CITATION INDEX
Institute for Scientific Information
3501 Market St.
Philadelphia, PA 19104   Phone: (215) 386-0100
First Published: 1961. **Frequency:** Bimonthly. **ISSN:** 0036-827X.

★3766★ SELECTED ABSTRACTS ON OCCUPATIONAL DISEASES
Great Britain Dept. of Health and Social Security
Alexander Fleming House
Elephant and Castle
London SE1 6BY, England
First Published: 1982. **Frequency:** Quarterly.

★3767★ SEXUALLY TRANSMITTED DISEASES ABSTRACTS AND BIBLIOGRAPHY
U.S. Centers for Disease Control
1600 Clifton Rd., NE
Atlanta, GA 30333
First Published: 1978. **Frequency:** Annual. **ISSN:** 0195-7708.

★3768★ SMOKING AND HEALTH BULLETIN
Office on Smoking and Health
U.S. Public Health Service
Park Bldg., Rm. 116
5600 Fishers Ln.
Rockville, MD 20857   Phone: (301) 443-1575
First Published: 1967. **Frequency:** Semimonthly. **ISSN:** 0081-0363.

★3769★ SOCIAL SCIENCES INDEX
H.W. Wilson Co.
950 University Ave.
Bronx, NY 10452   Phone: (212) 588-8400
First Published: 1965. **Frequency:** Quarterly. **ISSN:** 0094-4920.

★3770★ SOCIAL WORK RESEARCH AND ABSTRACTS
National Association of Social Workers
7981 Eastern Ave.
Silver Spring, MD 20910   Phone: (301) 565-0333
First Published: 1965. **Frequency:** Quarterly. **ISSN:** 0148-0847.

★3771★ SUBSTANCE ABUSE INDEX AND ABSTRACTS
Scientific DataLink
270 Lafayette St., Suite 704
New York, NY 10012   Phone: (212) 334-1922
First Published: 1989. **Frequency:** 3/yr.

★3772★ TOXICOLOGY ABSTRACTS
Cambridge Scientific Abstracts
7200 Wisconsin Ave., 6th Fl.
Bethesda, MD 20814   Phone: (301) 961-6700
First Published: 1978. **Frequency:** Monthly. **ISSN:** 0140-5365.

★3773★ TROPICAL DISEASES BULLETIN
Bureau of Hygiene and Tropical Diseases
Keppel St.
London WC1E 7HT, England
First Published: 1912. **Frequency:** Monthly. **ISSN:** 0041-3240.

★3774★ U.S. NATIONAL LIBRARY OF MEDICINE CURRENT CATALOG
U.S. National Library of Medicine
8600 Rockville Pike
Bethesda, MD 20894   Phone: (202) 783-3238
First Published: 1966. **Frequency:** Quarterly. **ISSN:** 0027-9641.

★3775★ VETERINARY BULLETIN
C.A.B. International
845 N. Park Ave.
Tucson, AZ 85719   Phone: (800) 528-4841
First Published: 1931. **Frequency:** Monthly. **ISSN:** 0042-4854.

★3776★ VIROLOGY AND AIDS ABSTRACTS
Cambridge Scientific Abstracts
7200 Wisconsin Ave., 6th Fl.
Bethesda, MD 20814   Phone: (301) 961-6700
First Published: 1967. **Frequency:** Monthly. **ISSN:** 0042-6830.

(5) Directories

Entries in this chapter are listed alphabetically by publication titles. Consult the User's Guide located at the front of this directory for additional information.

★3777★ **AA GUIDE FOR THE DISABLED TRAVELLER**
Automobile Association
Information Research Unit
Fanum House
Basingstoke, Hampshire RG21 2EA, England
Covers: Over 400 hotels, guesthouses, and inns in the United Kingdom and Ireland which provide accommodations suitable for persons in wheelchairs; lists of accessible hotel restaurants, highway service areas, heritage properties, firms which repair wheelchairs, Department of Health and Social Security Application Centres, picnic sites, associations for the handicapped, highway service areas, hotels on selected routes in Europe, and other information. **Entries Include:** All listings include name and address; most also include phone. For hotel and hotel restaurants—Services, facilities, and ratings. **Pages (approx.):** 140. **Frequency:** Annual, April. **Available in the U.S. from:** Salem House Publishers (formerly Merimack Publishers Circle), 462 Boston, Topsfield, MA 01983 (617-887-8191).

★3778★ **ABMS COMPENDIUM OF CERTIFIED MEDICAL SPECIALISTS**
American Board of Medical Specialties
1 Rotary Center, Ste. 805
Evanston, IL 60201   Phone: (708) 491-9091
Covers: Over 400,000 doctors and medical specialists certified in the United States by 23 medical specialty boards. **Entries Include:** Name, office address, phone, year and place of birth, school from which M.D. degree obtained, year of M.D. degree, places of residency and internship, fellowships, type of practice, principal academic and hospital staff appointments, memberships in professional associations, certifications. **Pages (approx.):** 11,000 (in seven volumes). **Frequency:** Biennial, even years, with supplement in odd years.

★3779★ **ABMS—DIRECTORY OF CERTIFIED ALLERGISTS/IMMUNOLOGISTS**
American Board of Medical Specialties
1 Rotary Center, Ste. 805
Evanston, IL 60201   Phone: (708) 491-9091
Covers: 3,100 certified allergists and immunologists. **Entries Include:** Name, address, phone, educational data, professional association membership. **Pages (approx.):** 110. **Frequency:** Biennial, odd years.

★3780★ **ABMS—DIRECTORY OF CERTIFIED ANESTHESIOLOGISTS**
American Board of Medical Specialties
1 Rotary Center, Ste. 805
Evanston, IL 60201   Phone: (708) 491-9091
Covers: 17,500 certified anesthesiologists. **Entries Include:** Name, address, phone, certification data, professional association membership. **Pages (approx.):** 370. **Frequency:** Biennial, odd years.

★3781★ **ABMS—DIRECTORY OF CERTIFIED COLON AND RECTAL SURGEONS**
American Board of Medical Specialties
1 Rotary Center, Ste. 805
Evanston, IL 60201   Phone: (708) 491-9091
Covers: 850 certified colon and rectal surgeons. **Entries Include:** Name, address, phone, certification data, professional association membership. **Pages (approx.):** 40. **Frequency:** Biennial, even years.

★3782★ **ABMS—DIRECTORY OF CERTIFIED DERMATOLOGISTS**
American Board of Medical Specialties
1 Rotary Center, Ste. 805
Evanston, IL 60201   Phone: (708) 491-9091
Covers: About 7,000 certified dermatologists. **Entries Include:** Name, address, phone, education, professional association membership. **Pages (approx.):** 110. **Frequency:** Biennial, even years.

★3783★ **ABMS—DIRECTORY OF CERTIFIED EMERGENCY PHYSICIANS**
American Board of Medical Specialties
1 Rotary Center, Ste. 805
Evanston, IL 60201   Phone: (708) 491-9091
Covers: About 9,000 certified physicians specializing in emergency diagnosis and treatment. **Entries Include:** Name, address, phone, education, professional association membership. **Pages (approx.):** 110. **Frequency:** Biennial, even years.

★3784★ **ABMS—DIRECTORY OF CERTIFIED FAMILY PHYSICIANS**
American Board of Medical Specialties
1 Rotary Center, Ste. 805
Evanston, IL 60201   Phone: (708) 491-9091
Covers: About 36,700 certified family physicians. **Entries Include:** Name, address, phone, education, professional association membership. **Pages (approx.):** 725. **Frequency:** Biennial, odd years.

★3785★ **ABMS—DIRECTORY OF CERTIFIED INTERNISTS**
American Board of Medical Specialties
1 Rotary Center, Ste. 805
Evanston, IL 60201   Phone: (708) 491-9091
Covers: About 96,000 certified physicians specializing in internal medicine. **Entries Include:** Name, address, phone, education, professional association membership. **Pages (approx.):** 2,035. **Frequency:** Biennial, even years.

★3786★ **ABMS—DIRECTORY OF CERTIFIED NEUROLOGICAL SURGEONS**
American Board of Medical Specialties
1 Rotary Center, Ste. 805
Evanston, IL 60201   Phone: (708) 491-9091
Covers: About 3,180 certified surgeons specializing in nervous system disorders. **Entries Include:** Name, address, phone, education, professional

association membership. **Pages (approx.):** 110. **Frequency:** Biennial, even years.

★3787★ ABMS—DIRECTORY OF CERTIFIED NEUROLOGISTS
American Board of Medical Specialties
1 Rotary Center, Ste. 805
Evanston, IL 60201   Phone: (708) 491-9091
Covers: About 6,500 certified neurologists. **Entries Include:** Name, address, phone, educational data, professional association membership. **Pages (approx.):** 175. **Frequency:** Biennial, even years.

★3788★ ABMS—DIRECTORY OF CERTIFIED NUCLEAR MEDICINE SPECIALISTS
American Board of Medical Specialties
1 Rotary Center, Ste. 805
Evanston, IL 60201   Phone: (708) 491-9091
Covers: About 3,600 certified physicians specializing in the radioactive diagnosis and treatment of disease. **Entries Include:** Name, address, phone, education, professional association membership. **Pages (approx.):** 110. **Frequency:** Biennial, even years.

★3789★ ABMS—DIRECTORY OF CERTIFIED OBSTETRICIANS AND GYNECOLOGISTS
American Board of Medical Specialties
1 Rotary Center, Ste. 805
Evanston, IL 60201   Phone: (708) 491-9091
Covers: About 25,000 certified gynecologists and obstetricians. **Entries Include:** Name, address, phone, education data, professional association membership. **Pages (approx.):** 560. **Frequency:** Biennial, odd years.

★3790★ ABMS—DIRECTORY OF CERTIFIED OPHTHALMOLOGISTS
American Board of Medical Specialties
1 Rotary Center, Ste. 805
Evanston, IL 60201   Phone: (708) 491-9091
Covers: About 14,300 certified medical doctors specializing in treating diseases of the eye. **Entries Include:** Name, address, phone, education, professional association membership. **Pages (approx.):** 325. **Frequency:** Biennial, even years.

★3791★ ABMS—DIRECTORY OF CERTIFIED ORTHOPAEDIC SURGEONS
American Board of Medical Specialties
1 Rotary Center, Ste. 805
Evanston, IL 60201   Phone: (708) 491-9091
Covers: About 15,500 certified physicians who correct skeletal deformities through surgery. **Entries Include:** Name, address, phone, education, professional association membership. **Pages (approx.):** 400. **Frequency:** Biennial, odd years.

★3792★ ABMS—DIRECTORY OF CERTIFIED OTOLARYNGOLOGISTS
American Board of Medical Specialties
1 Rotary Center, Ste. 805
Evanston, IL 60201   Phone: (708) 491-9091
Covers: About 8,500 certified ear, nose, and throat specialists. **Entries Include:** Name, address, phone, education data, professional association membership. **Pages (approx.):** 220. **Frequency:** Biennial, odd years.

★3793★ ABMS—DIRECTORY OF CERTIFIED PATHOLOGISTS
American Board of Medical Specialties
1 Rotary Center, Ste. 805
Evanston, IL 60201   Phone: (708) 491-9091
Covers: About 16,500 certified pathologists. **Entries Include:** Name, address, phone, educational background, professional association membership. **Pages (approx.):** 415. **Frequency:** Biennial, odd years.

★3794★ ABMS—DIRECTORY OF CERTIFIED PEDIATRICIANS
American Board of Medical Specialties
1 Rotary Center, Ste. 805
Evanston, IL 60201   Phone: (708) 491-9091
Covers: About 40,000 certified pediatricians. **Entries Include:** Name, address, phone, education, professional association membership. **Pages (approx.):** 880. **Frequency:** Biennial, even years.

★3795★ ABMS—DIRECTORY OF CERTIFIED PHYSICAL MEDICINE AND REHABILITATION SPECIALISTS
American Board of Medical Specialties
1 Rotary Center, Ste. 805
Evanston, IL 60201   Phone: (708) 491-9091
Covers: 2,900 certified physical therapists and other physical medicine specialists. **Entries Include:** Name, address, phone, education, professional association membership. **Pages (approx.):** 85. **Frequency:** Biennial, odd years.

★3796★ ABMS—DIRECTORY OF CERTIFIED PLASTIC SURGEONS
American Board of Medical Specialties
1 Rotary Center, Ste. 805
Evanston, IL 60201   Phone: (708) 491-9091
Covers: 3,400 certified plastic surgeons. **Entries Include:** Name, address, phone, education, professional association membership. **Pages (approx.):** 110. **Frequency:** Biennial, even years.

★3797★ ABMS—DIRECTORY OF CERTIFIED PREVENTIVE MEDICINE PHYSICIANS
American Board of Medical Specialties
1 Rotary Center, Ste. 805
Evanston, IL 60201   Phone: (708) 491-9091
Covers: Nearly 3,800 certified preventive medicine physicians. **Entries Include:** Name, address, phone, credentials, professional association membership. **Pages (approx.):** 100. **Frequency:** Biennial, odd years.

★3798★ ABMS—DIRECTORY OF CERTIFIED PSYCHIATRISTS
American Board of Medical Specialties
1 Rotary Center, Ste. 805
Evanston, IL 60201   Phone: (708) 491-9091
Covers: 23,000 certified psychiatrists. **Entries Include:** Name, address, phone, education data, professional association membership. **Pages (approx.):** 600. **Frequency:** Biennial, even years.

★3799★ ABMS—DIRECTORY OF CERTIFIED RADIOLOGISTS
American Board of Medical Specialties
1 Rotary Center, Ste. 805
Evanston, IL 60201   Phone: (708) 491-9091
Covers: 26,000 certified radiologists. **Entries Include:** Name, address, phone, education, professional association membership. **Pages (approx.):** 600. **Frequency:** Biennial, odd years.

★3800★ ABMS—DIRECTORY OF CERTIFIED SURGEONS
American Board of Medical Specialties
1 Rotary Center, Ste. 805
Evanston, IL 60201   Phone: (708) 491-9091
Covers: 30,500 certified surgeons. **Entries Include:** Name, address, phone, credentials, education, professional association membership. **Pages (approx.):** 810. **Frequency:** Biennial, odd years.

★3801★ ABMS—DIRECTORY OF CERTIFIED THORACIC SURGEONS
American Board of Medical Specialties
1 Rotary Center, Ste. 805
Evanston, IL 60201   Phone: (708) 491-9091
Covers: 4,800 certified thoracic surgeons. **Entries Include:** Name, address, phone, credentials, professional association membership. **Pages (approx.):** 150. **Frequency:** Biennial, even years.

★3802★ ABMS—DIRECTORY OF CERTIFIED UROLOGISTS
American Board of Medical Specialties
1 Rotary Center, Ste. 805
Evanston, IL 60201   Phone: (708) 491-9091
Covers: About 6,500 certified physicians specializing in diseases of the urinary tract. **Entries Include:** Name, address, phone, educational data, professional association membership. **Pages (approx.):** 210. **Frequency:** Biennial, even years.

★3803★ ABORTION ALTERNATIVE ORGANIZATIONS DIRECTORY
American Business Directories, Inc.
American Business Information, Inc.
5711 S. 86th Circle
Omaha, NE 68127   Phone: (402) 593-4600
Number of Listings: 1,131. **Entries Include:** Name, address, phone, size of

advertisement, name of owner or manager, number of employees, year first in "Yellow Pages." **Frequency:** Annual.

★3804★ ACADEMY OF AMBULATORY FOOT SURGERY— MEMBERSHIP DIRECTORY
Academy of Ambulatory Foot Surgery
Box 2730
Tuscaloosa, AL 35403   Phone: (205) 758-3678
Covers: 1,500 podiatrists who perform surgery in their offices. **Entries Include:** Name, address, and phone. **Pages (approx.):** 35. **Frequency:** Annual, August.

★3805★ ACADEMY OF BEHAVIORAL MEDICINE RESEARCH—MEMBERSHIP DIRECTORY
Department of Medical Psychology
Uniformed Services University of the Health Sciences
Academy of Behavioral Medicine Research (ABMR)
4301 Jones Bridge Rd.
Bethesda, MD 20889-4799   Phone: (301) 295-3270
Covers: Approximately 375 member doctors and researchers in the field of behavioral medicine. **Entries Include:** Name, address, phone, degree held, research involvement. **Pages (approx.):** 22. **Frequency:** Annual, December.

★3806★ ACADEMY OF DENTISTRY FOR THE HANDICAPPED—REFERRAL/MEMBERSHIP ROSTER
Academy of Dentistry for the Handicapped
211 E. Chicago Ave., 16th Fl.
Chicago, IL 60611   Phone: (312) 440-2660
Covers: 500 dentists, dental hygienists, and other professionals specializing in treatment of handicapped persons; international coverage. **Entries Include:** Name, primary address, phone. **Pages (approx.):** 50. **Frequency:** Annual, July.

★3807★ ACADEMY OF DISPENSING AUDIOLOGISTS— MEMBERSHIP DIRECTORY
Academy of Dispensing Audiologists
3008 Millwood Ave.
Columbia, SC 29205   Phone: (803) 252-5646
Covers: Nearly 250 member audiologists. **Entries Include:** Name, address, phone. **Frequency:** Annual.

★3808★ ACADEMY FOR HEALTH SERVICES MARKETING— MEMBERSHIP DIRECTORY AND SERVICES GUIDE
Academy for Health Services Marketing
250 S. Wacker Dr., Ste. 200
Chicago, IL 60606   Phone: (312) 648-0536
Covers: About 3,300 member marketing professionals and suppliers of services in the health care field. **Entries Include:** Name, address, phone. **Pages (approx.):** 125. **Frequency:** Annual, fall.

★3809★ ACCENT ON LIVING—BUYER'S GUIDE
Accent Special Publications
Cheever Publishing, Inc.
PO Box 700
Bloomington, IL 61702   Phone: (309) 378-2961
Covers: Over 400 manufacturers and distributors of products for disabled persons, ranging from wheelchairs to bowling ball pushers and talking calculators. **Entries Include:** Company name, address. **Pages (approx.):** 150. **Frequency:** Biennial, December of odd years.

★3810★ ACCESS AMERICA: AN ATLAS AND GUIDE TO THE NATIONAL PARKS FOR VISITORS WITH DISABILITIES
Northern Cartographic
Box 133
Burlington, VT 05402   Phone: (802) 860-2886
Covers: About 40 national parks with facilities for visitors with mobility impairments, hearing, visual, or developmental disabilities. **Entries Include:** Name and location of park; description of park attractions and facilities; access evaluations based on national and federal standards. **Pages (approx.):** 465. **Frequency:** Irregular; latest edition 1988; next edition expected 1992. **Also Includes:** 300 full color maps and photographs.

★3811★ ACCESS TO ART: A MUSEUM DIRECTORY FOR BLIND AND VISUALLY IMPAIRED PEOPLE
American Foundation for the Blind
15 W. 16th St.
New York, NY 10011   Phone: (212) 620-2143
Covers: Over 300 museums, galleries, and exhibits in the U.S. with special

access facilities for blind or visually impaired students, including tactile exhibits, Braille and large print labeling, cassette tours, workshops, and specially trained guides. Printed in large print. **Entries Include:** Museum name, address, phone; description of necessary arrangements, facilities, permanent collections, and special exhibits. **Pages (approx.):** 144. **Frequency:** Published 1989.

★3812★ ACCESS GUIDE TO EFFECTIVE LABORATORY EQUIPMENT AND SUPPLY DEALERS
Market Pace Associates
c/o Theta Corp.
Theta Bldg.
Middlefield, CT 06455   Phone: (203) 349-1054
Covers: Over 5,000 distributors of laboratory, X-ray, and monitoring equipment, medical disposables, surgical instruments, computers, and spirometers; coverage includes Canada. **Entries Include:** Company name, address, phone, name and title of contact, number of years in business, geographical area served, annual sales volume, type of ownership, parent organization, number of branches, size of sales and service departments, major line of products, principal type of client, companies whose products are carried. **Frequency:** Irregular; latest edition 1986; update 1988.

★3813★ ACCESS TO THE SCIENCE AND ENGINEERING LABORATORY AND CLASSROOM
Higher Education and Adult Training for People with Handicaps
American Council on Education
1 Dupont Circle NW, Ste. 800
Washington, DC 20036   Phone: (202) 939-9320
Publication Includes: List of about 60 manufacturers and suppliers of products to aid the visually impaired, mobility impaired, hearing impaired, and learning disabled student; list of publishers of material about handicapped students in the science classroom. **Entries Include:** For producers and suppliers—Name, address, phone, product or service provided. For publishers—Name, address, phone, publications. **Frequency:** Published 1986.

★3814★ ACCESS TRAVEL: AIRPORTS
Airport Operators Council International
1220 19th St. NW, Ste. 200
Washington, DC 20036   Phone: (202) 293-8500
Covers: About 400 airports in 42 countries; dot chart tabulation. **Entries Include:** Airport name, location, indication of presence or absence of about 60 facilities and services of special importance to persons in wheelchairs and to blind, deaf, and aged persons. **Pages (approx.):** 40. **Frequency:** Irregular; previous edition February 1986; latest edition May 1991. **Send Orders to:** Access America, Washington, DC 20202.

★3815★ ACCESSIBILITY BOOK: BUILDING CODE SUMMARY AND PRODUCTS DIRECTORY
jqp, inc.
PO Box 28093
Crystal, MN 55428   Phone: (612) 553-1246
Covers: Over 200 national manufacturers and suppliers of products that are accessible to or enhance access to facilities for the handicapped. **Entries Include:** Company name and address, illustrations and approximate prices of access equipment. **Pages (approx.):** 170. **Frequency:** Latest edition January 1990. **Also Includes:** Information on federal and state building codes related to handicap access.

★3816★ ACCREDITED ADVANCED DENTAL EDUCATIONAL PROGRAMS
Commission on Dental Accreditation
American Dental Association
211 E. Chicago Ave.
Chicago, IL 60611   Phone: (312) 440-2690
Covers: About 700 dental education programs accredited for postdoctoral work, dentistry specialties, general practice residency, and advanced general dentistry; coverage includes Canada. **Entries Include:** Institution name, address, years of past and next accreditation reviews. **Pages (approx.):** 20. **Frequency:** Semiannual, January and June.

★3817★ ACCREDITED EDUCATIONAL PROGRAMS IN HEALTH RECORD ADMINISTRATION AND HEALTH RECORD TECHNOLOGY
American Health Information Management Association
919 N. Michigan Ave., Ste. 1400
Chicago, IL 60611   Phone: (312) 787-2672
Covers: Over 50 schools that offer accredited baccalaureate programs or post-baccalaureate certificates in health record administration; approxi-

mately 120 associate degree programs in health record technology. **Entries Include:** College or university name, location, name of school or department, name of program director, prerequisites, length of program, whether a degree is awarded, month that classes begin. **Pages (approx.):** 10. **Frequency:** Four to six per year.

★3818★ **ACCREDITED EDUCATIONAL PROGRAMS IN MEDICAL RECORD TECHNOLOGY**
American Medical Record Association
919 N. Michigan Ave., Ste. 1400
Chicago, IL 60611   Phone: (312) 787-2672
Covers: About 100 accredited associate degree programs in medical record technology. **Entries Include:** School name, location; prerequisites, length of program, month classes begin; name of program director. **Pages (approx.):** 5. **Frequency:** Semiannual, March and September.

★3819★ **ACCREDITED PROFESSIONAL PROGRAMS OF COLLEGES AND SCHOOLS OF PHARMACY**
American Council on Pharmaceutical Education
311 W. Superior St., Ste. 512
Chicago, IL 60610   Phone: (312) 664-3575
Covers: Accredited pharmacy colleges with professional degree programs in the United States and Puerto Rico. **Entries Include:** College name, address, phone, dean's name, date of most recent and of next accreditation evaluation. **Pages (approx.):** 20. **Frequency:** Annual, July.

★3820★ **ACR DIRECTORY OF FELLOWSHIP PROGRAMS**
American College of Radiology (ACR)
1891 Preston White Dr.
Reston, VA 22091   Phone: (703) 648-8900
Frequency: Latest edition 1990.

★3821★ **ACUPUNCTURE DIRECTORY**
American Business Directories, Inc.
American Business Information, Inc.
5711 S. 86th Circle
Omaha, NE 68127   Phone: (402) 593-4600
Covers: Approximately 3,161 acupuncturists who advertise their services. **Entries Include:** Name, address, phone (including area code), size of advertisement, year first in "Yellow Pages," name of owner or manager, number of employees. **Frequency:** Annual.

★3822★ **ADDRESS LIST, REGIONAL AND SUBREGIONAL LIBRARIES FOR THE BLIND PHYSICALLY HANDICAPPED**
National Library Service for the Blind and Physically Handicapped
Library of Congress
1291 Taylor St., NW
Washington, DC 20542   Phone: (202) 707-5100
Covers: Over 148 state and local libraries that serve blind and physically handicapped persons as part of the Library of Congress cooperating network. **Entries Include:** Name, address, contact name, phone. **Pages (approx.):** 25. **Frequency:** Semiannual, winter and summer.

★3823★ **ADMISSION REQUIREMENTS OF U.S. AND CANADIAN DENTAL SCHOOLS**
American Association of Dental Schools
1625 Massachusetts Ave. NW
Washington, DC 20036   Phone: (202) 667-9433
Covers: Nearly 70 schools. **Entries Include:** School name, dean, address, program, admission requirements, calendar, expenses, characteristics of entering class, financial aid. **Pages (approx.):** 200. **Frequency:** Annual, summer.

★3824★ **ADRESSBUCH DER DEUTSCHEN TIERARZTESCHAFT**
Schlutersche Verlagsanstalt
Georgswall 4
W-3000 Hannover 1, Germany
Covers: Veterinarians and those otherwise involved with veterinary medicine in Germany. **Entries Include:** Name, address, function. **Pages (approx.):** 670. **Frequency:** Triennial; latest edition 1989; new edition expected 1992.

★3825★ **ADRESSBUCH DER KASSENARZTE IN NORDWURTTEMBERG**
Thebal-Verlag
Bussenstrasse 56
W-7000 Stuttgart 1, Germany
Covers: Approximately 4,300 doctors, clinics, and sanatoriums in the

northeast region of the German state of Baden-Wurttemberg. **Entries Include:** For doctors—Name, address, phone, hours available. For institutions—Name, address, phone, name of director. **Pages (approx.):** 700. **Frequency:** Biennial, fall of even years.

★3826★ **ADRESSBUCH DER KASSENARZTE IN SUDWURTTEMBERG**
Thebal-Verlag
Bussenstrasse 56
W-7000 Stuttgart 1, Germany
Covers: Approximately 2,400 doctors, clinics, and sanatoriums in the southeast region of the West German state of Baden-Wurttemberg. **Entries Include:** For doctors—Name, address, phone, hours available. For institutions—Name, address, phone, name of director. **Pages (approx.):** 300. **Frequency:** Biennial, fall of odd years.

★3827★ **ADVERTISERS AND THEIR AGENCIES**
Engel Communications, Inc.
820 Bear Tavern Rd., Ste. 302
West Trenton, NJ 08628   Phone: (609) 530-0044
Covers: Manufacturers and suppliers of pharmaceuticals and health care products, including pharmaceutical companies, medical device and diagnostic manufacturers, hospitals, and HMOs. **Entries Include:** Company name, address, phone, key personnel, products, agency assignments, names of product managers and account executives. **Pages (approx.):** 450. **Frequency:** Annual, spring.

★3828★ **AFB DIRECTORY OF SERVICES FOR BLIND AND VISUALLY IMPAIRED PERSONS IN THE UNITED STATES**
American Foundation for the Blind
15 W. 16th St.
New York, NY 10011   Phone: (212) 620-2000
Covers: About 1,500 government and national voluntary agencies and other organizations, and school for blind and visually impaired persons; all were established through local, state, or federal legislation. **Entries Include:** Agency or organization name, address, phone, name and title of contact, services offered, accreditation, memberships. **Pages (approx.):** 475. **Frequency:** Irregular; previous edition 1984; latest edition September 1988; quarterly updates.

★3829★ **AFFORDABLE SPAS AND FITNESS RESORTS: THE INSIDER'S GUIDE TO HEALTH-ORIENTED VACATIONS AND WEEKENDS**
Ventana Press
PO Box 2468
Chapel Hill, NC 27515-2408   Phone: (919) 942-0220
Covers: More than 80 health spas and fitness resorts in the United States. **Entries Include:** Resort name, address, phone, cost; description of services, including menus, lodging facilities, and activities offered. **Pages (approx.):** 220. **Frequency:** Irregular; latest edition February 1988.

★3830★ **AGING MYTHS: REVERSIBLE CAUSES OF MIND AND MEMORY LOSS**
McGraw-Hill, Inc.
1221 Avenue of the Americas
New York, NY 10020   Phone: (212) 512-2000
Publication Includes: List of organizations that are concerned with the problems of mental dysfunction in the elderly.

★3831★ **AGRICULTURAL AND VETERINARY SCIENCES INTERNATIONAL WHO'S WHO**
Longman Group UK Ltd.
Westgate House
The High
Harlow, Essex CM20 1YR, England
Covers: Over 7,500 directors and senior staff of research establishments, academic establishments, and international advisory bodies in all areas of agricultural research, including agricultural engineering, animal production, botany, fisheries, aquaculture, food science, forestry and forest products, horticulture, plant production, soil science, veterinary science, and zoology; international coverage of over 100 countries. **Entries Include:** Name, address, phone, qualifications, biographical data, subjects of major interest, memberships, publications, scientific and research interest, positions held during past 10 years. **Pages (approx.):** 1,240. **Frequency:** Triennial; latest edition February 1990. **Available in the U.S. from:** Gale Research Inc., 835 Penobscot Bldg., Detroit, MI 48226.

★3832★ AHA DIRECTORY OF HEALTH CARE
PROFESSIONALS
American Hospital Association (AHA)
840 N. Lake Shore Dr.
Chicago, IL 60611   Phone: (312) 280-6000
Covers: Over 140,000 hospital professionals and 3,000 health care system
professionals. Entries Include: Hospital or system headquarters name,
mailing address, street address (if different), phone, fax, bed size range;
name, title, and phone of key personnel. Pages (approx.): 2,380. Frequency:
Annual, May. Send Orders to: AHA Services, Inc., PO Box 92683, Chicago,
IL 60675-2683.

★3833★ AHA GUIDE TO THE HEALTH CARE FIELD
Data Services Business Group
American Hospital Association (AHA)
840 N. Lake Shore Dr.
Chicago, IL 60611   Phone: (312) 280-6000
Covers: Hospitals, multi-health care systems, freestanding ambulatory
surgery centers, psychiatric facilities, long-term care facilities, substance
abuse programs, hospices, Health Maintenance Organizations (HMOs),
and other health-related organizations. Entries Include: For hospitals—
Facility name, address, phone, administrator's name, number of beds,
facilities and services, number of employees, expenses, other statistics. For
other organizations—Name, address, phone, name and title of contact.
Pages (approx.): 945. Frequency: Annual, July.

★3834★ AIDS: FACTS AND ISSUES
Rutgers University Press
109 Church St.
New Brunswick, NJ 08903   Phone: (201) 932-7762
Publication Includes: List of resources for information on Acquired
Immune Deficiency Syndrome (AIDS). Frequency: Published late 1986.

★3835★ AIDS FUNDING: A GUIDE TO GIVING BY
FOUNDATIONS AND CHARITABLE ORGANIZATIONS
The Foundation Center
79 5th Ave.
New York, NY 10003   Phone: (212) 620-4230
Covers: Approximately 55 public and 435 private foundations, and 50
direct corporate giving programs that provide funding for AIDS/HIV
programs and services. Entries Include: Organization name, address, phone
number, name and title of contact, purpose and activities, grants awarded,
financial data, types of support, limitations, publications, application
information, names and titles of key personnel, number of staff, employer
identification number, and recent grants paid (where available). Pages
(approx.): 300. Frequency: Biennial, spring of odd years.

★3836★ AIDS/HIV RECORD DIRECTORY OF KEY AIDS
PROGRAM OFFICIALS IN FEDERAL, STATE, COUNTY, AND
CITY GOVERNMENTS
Bio-Data Publishers
PO Box 66020
Washington, DC 20035   Phone: (202) 393-2437
Pages (approx.): 205. Frequency: Biennial, even years.

★3837★ AIDS INFORMATION RESOURCES DIRECTORY
American Foundation for AIDS Research
5900 Wilshire Blvd., 2nd Fl.
E. Satellite
Los Angeles, CA 90036-5032   Phone: (213) 857-5900
Covers: Organizations providing educational materials and products, such
as brochures, posters, and audiovisual materials, designed to fight the
spread of AIDS (Acquired Immunodeficiency Syndrome). Entries Include:
Organization name, address, material or product, reviewer's comments.
Pages (approx.): 195. Frequency: Quarterly.

★3838★ AIDS INFORMATION SOURCEBOOK
Oryx Press
4041 N. Central, No. 700
Phoenix, AZ 85012   Phone: (602) 265-2651
Covers: Organizations providing information about Acquired Immune
Deficiency Syndrome (AIDS); coverage includes Canada. Entries Include:
Organization or facility name, address, phone, names and titles of key
personnel, organizational affiliations, type of organization or facility,
financial information, list of publications, description of activities and
services, and statement of purpose. Pages (approx.): 225. Frequency:
Annual, June. Also Includes: Chronology of the AIDS epidemic; bibliography of recent publications.

★3839★ AIDS: PUBLIC POLICY DIMENSIONS
United Hospital Fund of New York
55 5th Ave.
New York, NY 10003   Phone: (212) 645-2500
Publication Includes: List of about 150 national and local organizations
offering AIDS (Acquired Immune Deficiency Syndrome) programs and
related services. Entries Include: Organization name, address, phone.
Frequency: Published 1987.

★3840★ AJAO DIRECTORY OF PEDIATRIC RHEUMATOLOGY
SERVICES
American Juvenile Arthritis Organization
1314 Spring St. NW
Atlanta, GA 30309   Phone: (404) 872-7100
Covers: More than 100 pediatric rheumatology centers and related services
in the United States, Canada, and Puerto Rico. Entries Include: Organiza-
tion name, address, phone.

★3841★ ALCOHOL, DRUG ABUSE, MENTAL HEALTH,
RESEARCH GRANT AWARDS
U.S. Alcohol, Drug Abuse, and Mental Health Administration
5600 Fishers Ln., Rm. 13-103
Rockville, MD 20857   Phone: (301) 443-1596
Covers: Recipients of alcohol, drug abuse, and mental health research
grants. Entries Include: Institution name, location; name of investigator,
project title, grant number, amount awarded for fiscal year covered. Pages
(approx.): 187. Frequency: Annual, July.

★3842★ ALCOHOLISM INFORMATION AND TREATMENT
DIRECTORY
American Business Directories, Inc.
American Business Information, Inc.
5711 S. 86th Circle
Omaha, NE 68127   Phone: (402) 593-4600
Number of Listings: 13,397. Entries Include: Name, address, phone
(including area code), size of advertisement, year first in "Yellow Pages,"
name of owner or manager, number of employees. Frequency: Annual.

★3843★ ALLERGY PRODUCTS DIRECTORY
Allergy Publications, Inc.
PO Box 640
Menlo Park, CA 94026   Phone: (415) 322-1663
Covers: Approximately 1,780 U.S., Canadian, and British manufacturers
and suppliers of products and services to aid allergy sufferers. Entries
Include: Company name, address, phone, brand name, description of
product or service. Pages (approx.): 130. Frequency: Irregular; latest edition
1987; new edition expected 1991.

★3844★ ALLIED HEALTH EDUCATION DIRECTORY
American Medical Association
515 N. State St.
Chicago, IL 60610   Phone: (312) 464-5000
Covers: 2,800 health career educational programs in about 28 allied health
occupations for which the AMA Committee on Allied Health Education
and Accreditation (CAHEA) accredits programs. Entries Include: Name
and address of hospital or institution sponsoring program, phone, length of
program, date classes begin, prerequisites, class size, tuition rate,
award/degree granted, names of program director and educational coordinator, degree or certificate awarded, clinical affiliates. Pages (approx.):
350. Frequency: Annual, April. Also Includes: Descriptions of the occupations and of the process by which programs become accredited; allied
health education and accreditation glossary, and a large compilation of
education statistics.

★3845★ ALTENHEIM ADRESSBUCH
Curt R. Vincentz Verlag
Schiffgraben 41-43
W-3000 Hannover 1, Germany
Covers: About 8,000 nursing homes, geriatric clinics and psychology
institutions, welfare organizations, affiliated government agencies, and
schools specializing in care for the aged in western Germany. Entries
Include: Institution name, address, phone, telex, names and titles of key
personnel, number of rooms, date of establishment, proximity to public
transportation, description of facilities and amenities. Pages (approx.):
500. Frequency: Annual, November/December.

★3846★   ALZHEIMER'S DISEASE: A GUIDE FOR FAMILIES
Addison-Wesley Publishing Co. Inc.
1 Jacob Way
Rte. 128
Reading, MA 01867   Phone: (617) 944-3700
Publication Includes: List of about 60 chapters of the Alzheimer's Disease and Related Disorders Association. **Entries Include:** Chapter name, address, phone, name of contact person. **Frequency:** Published 1983.

★3847★   ALZHEIMER'S DISEASE TREATMENT FACILITIES AND HOME HEALTH CARE PROGRAMS
Oryx Press
4041 N. Central, No. 700
Phoenix, AZ 85012   Phone: (602) 265-2651
Pages (approx.): 275. **Frequency:** Published October 1989.

★3848★   AMBULANCE SERVICE DIRECTORY
American Business Directories, Inc.
American Business Information, Inc.
5711 S. 86th Circle
Omaha, NE 68127   Phone: (402) 593-4600
Number of Listings: 6,501. **Entries Include:** Name, address, phone (including area code), size of advertisement, year first in "Yellow Pages," name of owner or manager, number of employees. **Frequency:** Annual.

★3849★   AMBULATORY MATERNAL HEALTH CARE AND FAMILY PLANNING SERVICES
Professional Education Department
March of Dimes Birth Defects Foundation
1275 Mamaroneck Ave.
White Plains, NY 10605   Phone: (914) 428-7100
Publication Includes: List of professional organizations concerned with family planning and newborn care. **Entries Include:** Name of organization, address.

★3850★   AMBULATORY PEDIATRIC ASSOCIATION— MEMBERSHIP DIRECTORY
Ambulatory Pediatric Association
Degnon Associates
6728 Old McLean Village
McLean, VA 22101   Phone: (703) 556-9222
Covers: About 1,300 medical personnel, social workers, and others interested in the care of children in ambulatory care facilities. **Entries Include:** Name, office address and phone, fax, electronic mail, highest degree held, special interest group memberships. **Pages (approx.):** 70. **Frequency:** Biennial, fall of odd years.

★3851★   AMERICAN ACADEMY OF ALLERGY AND IMMUNOLOGY—MEMBERSHIP DIRECTORYIT2
American Academy of Allergy & Immunology
611 E. Wells St.
Milwaukee, WI 53202   Phone: (414) 272-6071
Covers: Over 4,000 physicians specializing in allergies and allergic diseases; also institutions offering residencies and fellowships for allergy training. **Entries Include:** For physicians—Name, office address and phone, year of birth, educational data. For institutions—Name, address, number of residencies, name of program director, programs. **Pages (approx.):** 350. **Frequency:** Biennial, even years.

★3852★   AMERICAN ACADEMY OF CHILD AND ADOLESCENT PSYCHIATRY—MEMBERSHIP DIRECTORY
American Academy of Child and Adolescent Psychiatry
3615 Wisconsin Ave., NW
Washington, DC 20016   Phone: (202) 966-7300
Covers: 4,450 members. **Entries Include:** Name, home or office address, phone, type of membership. **Pages (approx.):** 120. **Frequency:** Biennial, even years.

★3853★   AMERICAN ACADEMY OF FORENSIC PSYCHOLOGY—DIRECTORY OF DIPLOMATES
American Board of Forensic Psychology
Park Plaza
128 N. Craig St.
Pittsburgh, PA 15213   Phone: (412) 681-3000
Covers: Approximately 130 forensic psychologists. **Entries Include:** Personal name, home and office addresses and phone numbers, biographical data, services. **Pages (approx.):** 70. **Frequency:** Biennial, fall of even years.

★3854★   AMERICAN ACADEMY OF IMPLANT DENTISTRY— DIRECTORY
American Academy of Implant Dentistry
6900 Grove Rd.
Thorofare, NJ 08086   Phone: (609) 848-7027
Covers: 440 dentists and others engaged in the study of buried metals in the jaw and dental procedures involving implantation. **Entries Include:** Name, address, phone. **Pages (approx.):** 50. **Frequency:** Annual, December.

★3855★   AMERICAN ACADEMY OF NATURAL FAMILY PLANNING—DIRECTORY
American Academy of Natural Family Planning
615 S. New Ballas Rd.
St. Louis, MO 63141   Phone: (314) 569-6495
Covers: About 250 natural family planning instructors, practitioners, supervisors, educators, and medical consultants. **Entries Include:** Name, address, phone, credentials. **Pages (approx.):** 20. **Frequency:** Annual.

★3856★   AMERICAN ACADEMY OF NEUROLOGICAL AND ORTHOPAEDIC SURGERY—DIRECTORY
American Academy of Neurological & Orthopaedic Surgery
2320 Rancho Dr., Ste. 108
Las Vegas, NV 89102   Phone: (702) 385-6886
Covers: About 2,500 neurological and orthopedic surgeons and professionals in allied specialties. **Entries Include:** Name, address, phone, specialty. **Frequency:** Biennial.

★3857★   AMERICAN ACADEMY OF ORTHOTISTS AND PROSTHETISTS—DIRECTORY
American Academy of Orthotists and Prosthetists
717 Pendleton St.
Alexandria, VA 22314   Phone: (703) 836-7118
Covers: 1,700 certified orthotists and prosthetists concerned with the design, fabrication, and fitting of orthopedic braces, artificial limbs, and other major body parts, and with cosmetic replacement of minor parts. **Entries Include:** Name, home address, highest degree held. **Pages (approx.):** 110. **Frequency:** Annual, spring.

★3858★   AMERICAN ACADEMY OF PEDIATRIC DENTISTRY— MEMBERSHIP ROSTER
American Academy of Pediatric Dentistry
211 E. Chicago Ave., Ste. 1036
Chicago, IL 60611   Phone: (312) 337-2169
Covers: 3,100 pediatric dentists in practice, teaching, and research. **Entries Include:** Name, address, phone. **Pages (approx.):** 80. **Frequency:** Annual, August.

★3859★   AMERICAN ACADEMY OF PEDIATRICS— FELLOWSHIP LIST
American Academy of Pediatrics
141 Northwest Point Blvd.
Elk Grove Village, IL 60007   Phone: (708) 981-7638
Covers: Member pediatricians worldwide. **Entries Include:** Name, address, phone, year of graduation from medical school. **Pages (approx.):** 450. **Frequency:** Annual, December.

★3860★   AMERICAN ACADEMY OF PSYCHIATRISTS IN ALCOHOLISM AND ADDICTION—MEMBERSHIP DIRECTORY
American Academy of Psychiatrists in Alcoholism & Addictions
Box 376
Greenbelt, MD 20768   Phone: (301) 220-0951
Covers: About 900 member psychiatrists, and psychiatric-medical residents concerned with alcohol and drug abuse. **Entries Include:** Name, address, phone. **Pages (approx.):** 70. **Frequency:** Annual, May.

★3861★   AMERICAN ACADEMY OF PSYCHOANALYSIS— MEMBERSHIP ROSTER
American Academy of Psychoanalysis
30 E. 40th St., Ste. 206
New York, NY 10016   Phone: (212) 679-4105
Covers: About 800 physicians practicing psychoanalysis. **Entries Include:** Name, office address and phone; home address and phone (if supplied). **Pages (approx.):** 70. **Frequency:** Approximately triennial; latest edition 1989. **Also Includes:** List of Academy officers, committee chairpersons, and past presidents.

★3862★ AMERICAN ACADEMY OF SOMNOLOGY—MEMBERSHIP DIRECTORY
American Academy of Somnology
Box 29124
Las Vegas, NV 89126   Phone: (702) 594-5746
Covers: About 75 physicians, dentists, nurses, psychologists, technicians, and students and sponsoring organizations, including associations, institutions, and corporations, with a special interest in sleep. **Entries Include:** For individuals—Name, degrees, address, phone, specialty, affiliations. For others—Name, address, phone, products (if applicable). **Pages (approx.):** 25. **Frequency:** Annual, June.

★3863★ AMERICAN ANNALS OF THE DEAF—REFERENCE ISSUE
Convention of American Instructors of the Deaf
Gallaudet College
KDESPAS-6
800 Florida Ave., NE
Washington, DC 20002   Phone: (202) 651-5340
Publication Includes: Educational programs and services, supportive and rehabilitation programs and services, and research and information programs and services focusing on the deaf and aurally handicapped. **Entries Include:** Generally, name of sponsoring organization, address, and description of programs offered. School listings include staff and enrollment data. **Frequency:** Annual, summer.

★3864★ AMERICAN ASSOCIATION OF BLOOD BANKS—MEMBERSHIP DIRECTORY
American Association of Blood Banks
1117 N. 19th St., Ste. 600
Arlington, VA 22209   Phone: (703) 528-8200
Covers: Institutional and individual members. **Entries Include:** Name, address, phone. **Pages (approx.):** 260. **Frequency:** Biennial, odd years.

★3865★ AMERICAN ASSOCIATION OF CHILDREN'S RESIDENTIAL CENTERS—DIRECTORY OF ORGANIZATIONAL MEMBERS
American Association of Children's Residential Centers
440 1st St., NW, Ste. 310
Washington, DC 20001   Phone: (202) 638-1604
Covers: About 85 residential treatment centers for emotionally disturbed children. **Entries Include:** Facility name, address, phone; name and title of chief executive officer; name of admissions contact; accreditation and licensing; year established; geographic area covered; capacity; age range and sex of patients accepted; average annual admissions; usual length of stay, categories not accepted; rates; comments on treatment, orientation, etc. **Pages (approx.):** 85. **Frequency:** Annual, July.

★3866★ AMERICAN ASSOCIATION OF COLLEGES OF PHARMACY—ROSTER OF TEACHING PERSONNEL IN COLLEGES AND SCHOOLS OF PHARMACY
American Association of Colleges of Pharmacy
1426 Prince St.
Alexandria, VA 22314   Phone: (703) 739-2330
Covers: Faculty members teaching in schools of pharmacy in the United States and Puerto Rico; similar information is given for schools in Canada, the Philippines, and Malaysia. **Entries Include:** Name, title, rank, institution name, address, phone, area of instruction. **Pages (approx.):** 145. **Frequency:** Annual, September.

★3867★ AMERICAN ASSOCIATION FOR CORRECTIONAL PSYCHOLOGY—DIRECTORY
American Association for Correctional Psychology
Counseling Program
University of West Virginia
College of Graduate Studies
Institute, WV 25112   Phone: (304) 766-1929
Covers: 400 mental health professionals engaged in correctional and rehabilitative work in prisons, reformatories, juvenile institutions, probation and parole agencies, and in other aspects of criminal justice. **Entries Include:** Name, affiliation, address, phone. **Pages (approx.):** 30. **Frequency:** Continuously updated.

★3868★ AMERICAN ASSOCIATION OF DENTAL SCHOOLS—DIRECTORY OF INSTITUTIONAL MEMBERS
American Association of Dental Schools
1625 Massachusetts Ave. NW
Washington, DC 20036   Phone: (202) 667-9433
Covers: Over 170 member dental schools, dental education programs, and dental service programs offered by hospitals and other institutions not affiliated with dental schools. **Entries Include:** Name, address, name and title of chief administrator, phone numbers of institution and administrator. **Pages (approx.):** 80. **Frequency:** Annual, June.

★3869★ AMERICAN ASSOCIATION OF DIABETES EDUCATORS—ROSTER OF MEMBERSHIP
American Association of Diabetes Educators (AADE)
500 N. Michigan Ave., No. 1400
Chicago, IL 60611   Phone: (312) 661-1700
Covers: About 6,000 AADE members. **Entries Include:** For individual members—Name, address, title, phone, credentials, type of membership, chapter affiliation. For institutional members—Name, address, names and titles of representatives. **Pages (approx.):** 150. **Frequency:** Annual, January.

★3870★ AMERICAN ASSOCIATION FOR FUNCTIONAL ORTHODONTICS—MEMBERS' DIRECTORY
American Association for Functional Orthodontics
106 S. Kent St.
Winchester, VA 22601   Phone: (703) 662-2200
Covers: More than 2,000 member orthodontists, pedodontists, and general dentists who have an interest in functional appliance treatment for orthodontic malocclusions and temporomandibular joint (TMJ) syndrome; international membership. **Entries Include:** Dentist's name and address. **Pages (approx.):** 190. **Frequency:** Annual, June.

★3871★ AMERICAN ASSOCIATION OF HEALTHCARE CONSULTANTS—DIRECTORY OF MEMBER CONSULTANTS AND AFFILIATED FIRMS
American Association of Healthcare Consultants
11208 Waples Mill Rd., Ste. 109
Fairfax, VA 22030   Phone: (703) 691-2242
Covers: About 230 individuals and 70 firms with over 90 practice locations that offer consulting services related to facilities planning, strategy, marketing, finance, organization management, operations and information systems, and human resource management. **Entries Include:** Name, address, phone, services offered, geographic area served; company listings include contact, individual listings include company affiliation, membership status. **Pages (approx.):** 30. **Frequency:** Annual, January, with mid-year update. **Also Includes:** Educational programs offered by the association.

★3872★ AMERICAN ASSOCIATION FOR THE HISTORY OF MEDICINE—MEMBERSHIP DIRECTORY
American Association for the History of Medicine
c/o J. Worth Estes, M.D.
Boston University School of Medicine
80 E. Concord St.
Boston, MA 02118-2394   Phone: (617) 638-4328
Covers: 1,400 members. **Entries Include:** Name, address. **Pages (approx.):** 85. **Frequency:** Biennial.

★3873★ AMERICAN ASSOCIATION OF HOMES FOR THE AGING—DIRECTORY OF MEMBERS
American Association of Homes for the Aging
901 E St. NW, Ste. 500
Washington, DC 20004-2037   Phone: (202) 783-2242
Covers: Over 3,500 nonprofit member homes and health facilities; over 800 business firm suppliers, individuals, and other associate members. **Entries Include:** Name of home, address, phone, names of administrative staff, sponsorship, levels of care, services. **Pages (approx.):** 300. **Frequency:** Annual, January.

★3874★ AMERICAN ASSOCIATION FOR LABORATORY ANIMAL SCIENCE—MEMBERSHIP DIRECTORY
American Association for Laboratory Animal Science
70 Timber Creek Dr., Ste. 5
Cordova, TN 38018   Phone: (901) 754-8620
Covers: 4,500 persons and institutions professionally concerned with the production, use, care, and study of laboratory animals. **Entries Include:** Name, address, phone, degree. **Pages (approx.):** 150. **Frequency:** Annual, June.

★3875★ AMERICAN ASSOCIATION FOR MEDICAL SYSTEMS AND INFORMATICS—COMMUNICATION NETWORK

★3876★ AMERICAN ASSOCIATION FOR MUSIC THERAPY—MEMBERSHIP DIRECTORY
American Association for Music Therapy
PO Box 80012
King of Prussia, PA 19484-0012   Phone: (215) 265-4006
Covers: Approximately 530 music therapists and 130 students. **Entries Include:** Name, address, phone. **Pages (approx.):** 48. **Frequency:** Annual.

★3877★ AMERICAN ASSOCIATION OF NEUROPATHOLOGISTS—ROSTER
American Association of Neuropathologists
c/o Reid R. Heffner, Jr., M.D.
State University of New York
Buffalo, NY 14214   Phone: (716) 898-3510
Covers: 670 members. **Entries Include:** Name, address, phone. **Pages (approx.):** 50. **Frequency:** Annual, March.

★3878★ AMERICAN ASSOCIATION OF ORAL AND MAXILLOFACIAL SURGEONS—MEMBERSHIP DIRECTORY
American Association of Oral & Maxillofacial Surgeons
9700 W. Bryn Mawr
Rosemont, IL 60618   Phone: (708) 678-6200
Covers: Over 6,100 dental specialists in the diagnosis, surgical and adjunctive treatment of diseases, injuries, and defects of the oral and maxillofacial region. **Entries Include:** Name, office address and phone, hospital affiliation. **Pages (approx.):** 310. **Frequency:** Annual, January.

★3879★ AMERICAN ASSOCIATION OF PUBLIC HEALTH PHYSICIANS—MEMBERSHIP ROSTER
American Association of Public Health Physicians
Department of Family Medicine and Practice
University of Wisconsin Medical School
777 S. Mills St.
Madison, WI 53715   Phone: (405) 271-4476
Covers: 200 physicians. **Entries Include:** Name, address, professional affiliation. **Pages (approx.):** 10. **Frequency:** Annual.

★3880★ AMERICAN BOARD OF EXAMINERS IN PSYCHODRAMA, SOCIOMETRY, AND GROUP PSYCHOTHERAPY—DIRECTORY
American Board of Examiners in Psychodrama, Sociometry, and Group Psychotherapy
Box 15572
Washington, DC 20003   Phone: (202) 965-4115
Covers: More than 300 certified psychodramatists providing services, training, and consultation in psychodrama, sociometry, and group psychotherapy. **Entries Include:** Name, address, phone, credentials. **Pages (approx.):** 20. **Frequency:** Annual, August.

★3881★ AMERICAN BOARD OF ORTHODONTICS—DIRECTORY OF DIPLOMATES
American Board of Orthodontics
225 S. Meramec Ave.
St. Louis, MO 63105   Phone: (314) 727-5039
Publication Includes: List of diplomates of the board (specialists in prevention or correction of irregularities in position of teeth). **Entries Include:** Name, address, phone. **Frequency:** Annual, July.

★3882★ AMERICAN BOARD OF ORTHOPAEDIC SURGERY—DIRECTORY OF DIPLOMATES
American Board of Orthopaedic Surgery
737 N. Michigan Ave., Ste. 1150
Chicago, IL 60611   Phone: (312) 664-9444
Covers: About 15,950 orthopedic surgeons certified by the board. **Entries Include:** Name, address. **Pages (approx.):** 600. **Frequency:** Annual, spring.

★3883★ AMERICAN BOARD OF PROFESSIONAL PSYCHOLOGY—DIRECTORY OF DIPLOMATES
American Board of Professional Psychology
2100 E. Broadway, Ste. 313
Columbia, MO 65201   Phone: (314) 875-1267
Covers: 3,200 psychologists who have passed the board's examination. **Entries Include:** Name, office address, highest degree held, date of certification. **Pages (approx.):** 300. **Frequency:** Irregular; previous edition 1988; latest edition January 1991.

★3884★ AMERICAN BRONCHO-ESOPHAGOLOGICAL ASSOCIATION—TRANSACTIONS
American Broncho-Esophagological Association
c/o Stanley M. Shapshay, M.D.
Lahey Clinic
41 Mall Rd.
Burlington, MA 01805-0001   Phone: (617) 273-8854
Publication Includes: List of 300 member otolaryngologists, chest specialists, thoracic surgeons, and gastroenterologists engaged in the practice of broncho-esophagology. **Entries Include:** Name, affiliation, address, phone. **Frequency:** Annual, May.

★3885★ AMERICAN BURN ASSOCIATION—MEMBERSHIP DIRECTORY
American Burn Association
c/o Dr. Andrew M. Munster, Secretary
Baltimore Regional Burn Center
4940 Eastern Ave.
Baltimore, MD 21224
Covers: 3,150 physicians, occupational and physical therapists, nurses, social workers, dietitians, biomedical engineers, emergency medical technicians, and others with special competence or interest in care of patients suffering from burns. **Entries Include:** Name, address, title. **Pages (approx.):** 125. **Frequency:** Irregular; latest edition January 1990; new edition expected fall 1990.

★3886★ AMERICAN CANCER SOCIETY CANCER BOOK
Doubleday & Co., Inc.
666 5th Ave.
New York, NY 10103   Phone: (212) 765-6500
Publication Includes: List of about 135 cancer organizations, centers, information and support services and programs. **Entries Include:** Organization name, address, phone; some include description of program or service. **Frequency:** Published September 1986.

★3887★ AMERICAN CHIROPRACTIC ASSOCIATION—MEMBERSHIP DIRECTORY
American Chiropractic Association
1701 Clarendon Blvd.
Arlington, VA 22209   Phone: (703) 276-8800
Covers: 16,000 chiropractors. **Entries Include:** Name, affiliation, address, phone. **Pages (approx.):** 400. **Frequency:** Annual, January.

★3888★ AMERICAN CLEFT PALATE-CRANIOFACIAL ASSOCIATION MEMBERSHIP AND TEAM DIRECTORY
American Cleft Palate-Craniofacial Association
1218 Grandview Ave.
Pittsburgh, PA 15211   Phone: (412) 481-1376
Covers: 2,500 physicians, dentists, speech pathologists, audiologists, psychologists, and others actively concerned with care of individuals with cleft palates and related deformities; international coverage. **Entries Include:** For individuals—Name, address, phone; educational and professional data; affiliations. For teams—Institution name, address, phone, name of director. **Pages (approx.):** 250. **Frequency:** Annual, fall.

★3889★ AMERICAN COLLEGE OF CHEST PHYSICIANS—MEMBERSHIP DIRECTORY
American College of Chest Physicians
3300 Dundee Rd.
Northbrook, IL 60062-2303   Phone: (708) 498-1400
Covers: 14,000 physicians and surgeons specializing in diseases of the heart and lungs. **Entries Include:** Name, personal and career data, address, certifications, specialty. **Pages (approx.):** 1,050. **Frequency:** Annual, winter.

★3890★ AMERICAN COLLEGE OF HEALTHCARE EXECUTIVES—DIRECTORY
American College of Healthcare Executives
840 N. Lake Shore Dr.
Chicago, IL 60611   Phone: (312) 943-0544
Covers: 16,000 member executives, worldwide. **Entries Include:** Name, title, health service-related affiliation, office and home addresses, memberships; personal, education, and career data; some listings include phone numbers. **Pages (approx.):** 1,200. **Frequency:** Biennial, February of even years. **Send Orders to:** American College of Healthcare Executives, 1951 Cornell Avenue, Melrose Park, IL 60160.

★3891★ AMERICAN COLLEGE OF INTERNATIONAL
PHYSICIANS—MEMBERSHIP DIRECTORY
American College of International Physicians
5530 Wisconsin Ave. NW, Ste. 1149
Washington, DC 20815   Phone: (301) 986-8741
Covers: 2,000 physicians and surgeons interested in promoting national
efforts in international health, education, research, training, and welfare.
Entries Include: Name, address, phone. **Frequency:** Latest edition 1985;
suspended indefinitely .

★3892★ AMERICAN COLLEGE OF OBSTETRICIANS AND
GYNECOLOGISTS—DIRECTORY OF FELLOWS WITH BY-
LAWS, COUNCILS, COMMISSIONS, COMMITTEES & TASK
FORCES
American College of Obstetricians & Gynecologists
409 12th St. SW
Washington, DC 20024   Phone: (202) 638-5577
Pages (approx.): 400. **Frequency:** Latest edition 1990; new edition expected
1992.

★3893★ AMERICAN COLLEGE OF OCCUPATIONAL
MEDICINE—MEMBERSHIP DIRECTORY
American College of Occupational Medicine
55 W. Seegers Rd.
Arlington Heights, IL 60005   Phone: (708) 228-6850
Covers: 5,200 medical directors and plant physicians specializing in
occupational medicine and surgery; coverage includes Canada and other
foreign countries. **Entries Include:** Name, title, affiliation, address, phone,
degree; codes for membership class, medical specialty certifications, and
type of practice. **Pages (approx.):** 400. **Frequency:** Annual, July.

★3894★ AMERICAN COLLEGE OF PHYSICIAN
EXECUTIVES—MEMBERSHIP DIRECTORY
American College of Physician Executives
4890 W. Kennedy Blvd., Ste. 200
Tampa, FL 33609   Phone: (813) 287-2000
Covers: About 5,800 physicians who are managers of group practices,
health maintenance organizations, and hospitals, or who are also directors
of medical areas in universities, private industry, the military, or other
government agencies. **Entries Include:** Name, title, organization, address,
phone, description of organization. **Pages (approx.):** 550. **Frequency:**
Annual, January.

★3895★ AMERICAN COLLEGE OF VETERINARY
PATHOLOGISTS—MEMBERSHIP DIRECTORY
American College of Veterinary Pathologists
c/o Gary L. Cockerell, Secretary-Treasurer
Department of Pathology
College of Veterinary Medicine and Biomedical Science
Fort Collins, CO 80523   Phone: (303) 491-0599
Covers: About 970 veterinary and veterinary clinical pathologists. **Entries
Include:** Name, office address, phone. **Pages (approx.):** 30. **Frequency:**
Annual, January. **Send Orders to:** Coley Lyons, Executive Secretary,
ACVP, 875 Kings Hwy., Ste. 200, West Deptford, NJ 08096 (609-848-
7784).

★3896★ AMERICAN DANCE THERAPY ASSOCIATION—
MEMBERSHIP DIRECTORY
American Dance Therapy Association
2000 Century Plaza, Ste. 108
Columbia, MD 21044   Phone: (301) 997-4040
Number of Listings: 1,100. **Entries Include:** Name, address; career informa-
tion is given in alternate volumes in odd years. **Pages (approx.):** 50.
Frequency: Annual, February.

★3897★ AMERICAN DENTAL ASSOCIATION—ANNUAL
REPORT ON DENTAL EDUCATION
Educational Measurements Division
Council on Dental Education
American Dental Association
211 E. Chicago Ave.
Chicago, IL 60611   Phone: (312) 440-2642
Covers: Dental schools in the United States and Canada; graduates. **Entries
Include:** For schools—Name, address, phone, names and titles of key
personnel, admission requirements, financial assistance available, type of
work performed by students. **Pages (approx.):** 30. **Frequency:** Annual.

★3898★ AMERICAN DENTAL ASSOCIATION—REPORT ON
ADVANCED DENTAL EDUCATION
Educational Measurements Division
Council on Dental Education
American Dental Association
211 E. Chicago Ave.
Chicago, IL 60611   Phone: (312) 440-2690
Covers: Nearly 60 dental schools and more than 300 other schools that
have advanced dental education programs. **Entries Include:** Institution
name, address, programs, program directors, whether program directors
are board certified and full-time, enrollment, graduates, fees and tuition
for each program, application deadline, program starting dates. **Pages
(approx.):** 70. **Frequency:** Latest edition 1988.

★3899★ AMERICAN DENTAL DIRECTORY
American Dental Association
211 E. Chicago Ave.
Chicago, IL 60611   Phone: (312) 440-2500
Covers: Over 180,000 dentists. Also includes list of active and historic
dental schools, dental organizations, dental consultants, and state dental
examining boards. **Entries Include:** Name, address, year of birth, educational data, specialty, membership status. **Pages (approx.):** 1,400. **Frequency:** Annual, January.

★3900★ AMERICAN DRUG INDEX
J. B. Lippincott Co.
PO Box 1580
Hagerstown, MD 21740   Phone: (301) 714-2300
Publication Includes: List of manufacturers of prescription drugs, patent
medicines, and other drug store items. **Entries Include:** Company name,
address. **Frequency:** Annual, February. **Also Includes:** Listings for over
20,000 prescription and over-the-counter drug items, toiletries, etc., giving
information on manufacturer, forms and strengths, packaging, trade
names, etc.; for drugs, correlates generic and brand names.

★3901★ AMERICAN DRUGGIST BLUE BOOK
Hearst Corp.
60 E. 42nd St.
New York, NY 10165   Phone: (212) 297-9680
Publication Includes: List of manufacturers of prescription and over-the-
counter drugs, sold in retail drug stores. **Entries Include:** Company name,
address, phone. **Frequency:** Annual, August. **Also Includes:** Alphabetical list
of products with price and package information; manufacturers' catalogs.

★3902★ AMERICAN ELECTROLOGY ASSOCIATION—ROSTER
American Electrology Association
106 Oak Ridge Rd.
Trumbull, CT 06611   Phone: (203) 374-6667
Covers: About 2,000 electrologists (persons engaged in the permanent
removal of body hair by electrolysis or thermolysis); international cover-
age. **Entries Include:** Name, address, phone, board certification, modality.
Pages (approx.): 130. **Frequency:** Annual, January; addendum, June.

★3903★ AMERICAN FITNESS ASSOCIATION—FITNESS
DIRECTORY
American Fitness Association
820 N. Hillside Dr.
Long Beach, CA 90815-4715   Phone: (213) 596-6036
Entries Include: Name, address, phone, products or services, geographical
area covered, sports and fitness interests. **Pages (approx.):** 50. **Frequency:**
Annual, summer.

★3904★ AMERICAN GROUP PRACTICE ASSOCIATION—
DIRECTORY
American Group Practice Association
1422 Duke St.
Alexandria, VA 22314   Phone: (703) 838-0033
Covers: About 300 private group medical practices and their professional
staffs, totalling about 23,000 physicians. **Entries Include:** Group member
name, address, phone, names of administrator and other executives, names
of physician listed by medical specialties. **Pages (approx.):** 700. **Frequency:**
Annual, January.

**★3905★ AMERICAN GROUP PSYCHOTHERAPY
ASSOCIATION—MEMBERSHIP DIRECTORY**
American Group Psychotherapy Association
25 E. 21st St., 6th Fl.
New York, NY 10010   Phone: (212) 477-2677
Covers: 3,500 physicians, psychologists, clinical social workers, psychiatric nurses, and other mental health professionals interested in treatment of emotional problems by group methods. **Entries Include:** Name, office or home address, highest degree held, office or home phone number. **Pages (approx.):** 160. **Frequency:** Reported as biennial; previous edition 1987; latest edition summer 1990.

**★3906★ AMERICAN HOLISTIC MEDICAL ASSOCIATION—
DIRECTORY OF MEMBERS**
American Holistic Medical Association
4101 Lake Boone Trail, Ste. 201
Raleigh, NC 27607   Phone: (919) 787-5146
Covers: 550 doctors of medicine and other health practitioners who practice or are interested in holistic medicine. **Entries Include:** Name, address, specialty. **Pages (approx.):** 80. **Frequency:** Annual, June.

**★3907★ AMERICAN INDUSTRIAL HYGIENE ASSOCIATION—
DIRECTORY**
American Industrial Hygiene Association
475 Wolf Ledges Pkwy.
Akron, OH 44311   Phone: (216) 762-7294
Covers: Approximately 8,900 members concerned with the study and control of environmental factors affecting people at work. **Entries Include:** Name, address, phone, affiliation. **Pages (approx.):** 220. **Frequency:** Annual, September.

**★3908★ AMERICAN INSTITUTE OF ULTRASOUND IN
MEDICINE—MEMBERSHIP ROSTER**
American Institute of Ultrasound in Medicine
11200 Rockville Pk., Ste. 205
Rockville, MD 20854-3139   Phone: (301) 881-AIUM
Covers: About 9,000 physicians, engineers, scientists, sonographers, and others interested in the use of ultrasonic radiation clinically and in research. **Entries Include:** Name, address, phone, specialty. **Pages (approx.):** 334. **Frequency:** Biennial, fall of odd years.

**★3909★ AMERICAN JOURNAL OF NURSING—DIRECTORY
OF NURSING ORGANIZATIONS ISSUE**
American Journal of Nursing Co.
555 W. 57th St.
New York, NY 10019   Phone: (212) 582-8820
Publication Includes: Directory of nursing organizations and agencies. **Entries Include:** Name, address, names of officers or nursing representative. **Frequency:** Annual, April.

**★3910★ AMERICAN MEDICAL CARE AND REVIEW
ASSOCIATION FOUNDATION—PPO DIRECTORY**
American Medical Care and Review Association Foundation
1227 25th St. NW, Ste. 710
Washington, DC 20037-1156
Covers: Preferred provider organizations. **Frequency:** Latest edition December 1988.

★3911★ AMERICAN MEDICAL DIRECTORY
American Medical Association
515 N. State St.
Chicago, IL 60610   Phone: (312) 464-5000
Covers: In four volume set, more than 633,000 physicians in the United States and United States physicians in foreign countries. **Entries Include:** Name, address, year licensed, medical school, type of practice, primary and secondary specialties, and board certifications. **Pages (approx.):** 5,500. **Frequency:** Biennial, September of even years.

**★3912★ AMERICAN MEDICAL PUBLISHING ASSOCIATION—
DIRECTORY**
American Medical Publishing Association
PO Box 944
Crystal Lake, IL 60014   Phone: (815) 459-3712
Covers: Approximately 50 member companies and individuals. **Entries Include:** Name, address, phone, fax, telex, name and title of contact, names and titles of key personnel. **Pages (approx.):** 60. **Frequency:** Biennial, January of even years.

**★3913★ AMERICAN MEDICAL WRITERS' ASSOCIATION—
AMWA FREELANCE DIRECTORY**
American Medical Writers Association (AMWA)
9650 Rockville Pike
Bethesda, MD 20814   Phone: (301) 493-0003
Covers: Over 250 members of the association who are primarily freelance writers and editors on biomedical subjects; includes consultants, photographers, translators, educators, audiovisual specialists, lecturers, reporters, indexers, researchers, and reviewers. **Entries Include:** Name, address, phone, specialties, types of media with which familiar, subjects, publications in which work has appeared. **Pages (approx.):** 70. **Frequency:** Biennial, June.

**★3914★ AMERICAN MEDICAL WRITERS' ASSOCIATION—
MEMBERSHIP DIRECTORY**
American Medical Writers Association
9650 Rockville Pike
Bethesda, MD 20814   Phone: (301) 493-0003
Covers: 3,400 medical writers, editors, publishers, audiovisual specialists, and others concerned with communication in medicine and allied sciences. **Entries Include:** Name, address. **Pages (approx.):** 100. **Frequency:** Annual, May. **Also Includes:** List of the association chapters.

**★3915★ AMERICAN ORTHODONTIC SOCIETY—TECHNIQUE
REFERRAL DIRECTORY**
American Orthodontic Society
9550 Forest Ln., No. 215
Dallas, TX 75243   Phone: (214) 343-0805
Covers: About 2,100 general dentists and pedodontists who practice orthodontics; international coverage. **Entries Include:** Name, address, whether a member, orthodontic technique, type of pratice, specialty. **Pages (approx.):** 270. **Frequency:** Biennial, summer of even years.

**★3916★ AMERICAN OSTEOPATHIC ASSOCIATION—
YEARBOOK AND DIRECTORY OF OSTEOPATHIC
PHYSICIANS**
American Osteopathic Association
142 E. Ontario St.
Chicago, IL 60611   Phone: (312) 280-5800
Covers: Member and nonmember osteopathic physicians; also includes student members, associate members, osteopathic colleges, student aid and training programs, hospitals. **Entries Include:** Name, office or home address, specialty, type of practice, age, date and institution granting degree; code indicates whether member. **Pages (approx.):** 685. **Frequency:** Annual, January.

**★3917★ AMERICAN OSTEOPATHIC HOSPITAL
ASSOCIATION—DIRECTORY**
American Osteopathic Hospital Association
1454 Duke St.
Alexandria, VA 22314   Phone: (703) 684-7700
Covers: About 200 osteopathic hospitals. Includes list of individual and institutional members; also lists osteopathic colleges and state osteopathic hospital associations. **Entries Include:** For hospitals—Name of hospital, name of chief executive officer, address, phone, number of beds and other hospital data, including multi-hospital systems. Similar data given for other lists. **Pages (approx.):** 60. **Frequency:** Annual, January.

**★3918★ AMERICAN PSYCHIATRIC ASSOCIATION—
BIOGRAPHICAL DIRECTORY**
American Psychiatric Association
1400 K St. NW, Ste. 1101
Washington, DC 20005   Phone: (202) 682-6262
Covers: 35,000 member psychiatrists. **Entries Include:** Name, address, phone, secondary address and phone, type of membership, current work status, birth date, gender, professional titles and memberships, education, medical education, graduate degrees held, training, certification, current hospital affiliations, offices currently and/or previously held in professional organizations, special interests, customary services, foreign languages used in practice, number of books or articles authored, bibliographic citation of books or articles published. **Pages (approx.):** 1,900. **Frequency:** Irregular; previous edition 1983; latest edition 1989.

**★3919★ AMERICAN PSYCHOANALYTIC ASSOCIATION—
ROSTER**
American Psychoanalytic Association
309 E. 49th St.
New York, NY 10017   Phone: (212) 752-0450
Covers: Over 3,000 APA members. **Entries Include:** Name, address, phone.

Pages (approx.): 120. **Frequency:** Biennial, fall of even years. **Also Includes:** Lists of accredited training institutions and affiliated societies.

★3920★ **AMERICAN PSYCHOLOGICAL ASSOCIATION— DIRECTORY**
American Psychological Association
1200 17th St. NW
Arlington, VA 22201   Phone: (202) 955-7600
Covers: Over 70,000 members in the United States, Canada, and abroad. **Entries Include:** Name, office or home address, office and/or home phone, date of birth, major field, areas of specialization, highest degree (year, field, and institution), present position(s) and immediate past positions, state licensure/certification as a psychologist, and membership and divisional affiliations. **Pages (approx.):** 1,800 (in two volumes). **Frequency:** Quadrennial; latest edition July 1989; new edition expected July 1993. **Send Orders to:** American Psychological Association, Box 2710, Hyattsville, MD 20784.

★3921★ **AMERICAN PSYCHOLOGICAL ASSOCIATION— MEMBERSHIP REGISTER**
American Psychological Association
1200 17th St. NW
Washington, DC 20036   Phone: (202) 955-7600
Covers: Over 70,000 members in the United States, Canada, and abroad; also includes membership rosters of American Board of Professional Psychology and American Board of Psychological Hypnosis. **Entries Include:** Name, office or home address, phone, membership and divisional affiliations. **Pages (approx.):** 750. **Frequency:** Reported as annual, April, in years when APA "Directory" (see separate entry) is not published ("Directory" is quadrennial from 1981). **Send Orders to:** American Psychological Association, Box 2710, Hyattsville, MD 20784.

★3922★ **AMERICAN SLEEP DISORDERS ASSOCIATION ROSTER OF MEMBER CENTERS AND LABORATORIES**
American Sleep Disorders Association
1610 14th St. NW, Ste. 300
Rochester, MN 55901   Phone: (507) 287-6006
Covers: About 145 member sleep disorders centers, some associated with hospitals, directed by a medical doctor, and allowing on-site inspection by association officials; also lists about 25 accredited laboratories for sleep-related breathing disorders. **Entries Include:** For centers—Name unit and of hospital (if unit is hospital-based), address, phone, name of medical contact. For laboratories—Name of organization and parent hospital or center, address, phone, name of physician contact. **Pages (approx.):** 48. **Frequency:** Approximately semi-annually; latest edition September 1991.

★3923★ **AMERICAN SOCIETY FOR ADOLESCENT PSYCHIATRY—MEMBERSHIP DIRECTORY**
American Society for Adolescent Psychiatry
4330 East West Hwy., No. 1117
Bethesda, MD 20814   Phone: (301) 718-6502
Covers: 1,500 members. **Entries Include:** Name, office address and phone, home address and phone (when given). **Pages (approx.):** 200. **Frequency:** Biennial, fall of even years.

★3924★ **AMERICAN SOCIETY OF BARIATRIC PHYSICIANS— DIRECTORY**
American Society of Bariatric Physicians
5600 S. Quebec, Ste. 160-D
Englewood, CO 80111   Phone: (303) 779-4833
Number of Listings: 850. **Entries Include:** Name, address, phone. **Pages (approx.):** 50. **Frequency:** Annual, August.

★3925★ **AMERICAN SOCIETY OF CATARACT AND REFRACTIVE SURGERY AND AMERICAN SOCIETY OF OPHTHALMIC ADMINISTRATORS—MEMBERSHIP ROSTER**
American Society of Cataract and Refractive Surgery
3702 Pender Dr., Ste. 250
Fairfax, VA 22030   Phone: (703) 591-2220
Covers: About 4,500 ophthamologists and ophthalmic administrators who are interested in or perform cataract surgery, anterior segment surgery, and intraocular lens implantation. **Entries Include:** Name, address, phone. **Pages (approx.):** 200. **Frequency:** Biennial, even years; supplement, odd years.

★3926★ **AMERICAN SOCIETY FOR CLINICAL EVOKED POTENTIALS—MEMBERSHIP DIRECTORY**
American Society for Clinical Evoked Potentials
14 Soundview Ave., No. 51
White Plains, NY 10606
Covers: Over 400 physicians engaged in the study of the nervous system's transmissions. Members are in physical medicine and rehabilitation, neurology, neurosurgery, ophthalmology, and anesthesiology. **Entries Include:** Name, address. **Frequency:** Updated as needed.

★3927★ **AMERICAN SOCIETY OF CLINICAL HYPNOSIS— MEMBERSHIP DIRECTORY**
American Society of Clinical Hypnosis
2200 E. Devon, Ste. 291
Des Plaines, IL 60018   Phone: (708) 297-3317
Covers: About 3,500 physicians, dentists, and psychologists who use hypnosis. **Entries Include:** Name, office address, highest degree held, specialty. **Pages (approx.):** 165. **Frequency:** Biennial, odd years.

★3928★ **AMERICAN SOCIETY FOR COLPOSCOPY AND CERVICAL PATHOLOGY—MEMBERSHIP LIST**
American Society for Colposcopy and Cervical Pathology
c/o Slack, Inc.
6900 Grove Rd.
Thorofare, NJ 08086   Phone: (609) 848-1000
Description: Mailing labels. Covers more than 2,000 obstetricians, gynecologists, and others concerned with treatment of diseases of the female lower genital tract. **Entries Include:** Name, title, address. **Pages (approx.):** 100. **Frequency:** Biennial, odd years.

★3929★ **AMERICAN SOCIETY FOR HEALTH CARE MARKETING AND PUBLIC RELATIONS—MEMBERSHIP DIRECTORY**
American Society for Health Care Marketing and Public Relations
840 N. Lake Shore Dr.
Chicago, IL 60611   Phone: (312) 280-6359
Covers: 3,100 members. **Entries Include:** Hospital name, name and title of contact, address, phone. **Pages (approx.):** 115. **Frequency:** Annual, February.

★3930★ **AMERICAN SOCIETY FOR HOSPITAL MATERIALS MANAGEMENT—ROSTER**
American Society for Hospital Materials Management
840 N. Lake Shore Dr.
Chicago, IL 60611   Phone: (312) 280-6155
Covers: 1,945 members. **Entries Include:** Member name, address, hospital affiliation, and phone. **Pages (approx.):** 160. **Frequency:** Annual, fall.

★3931★ **AMERICAN SOCIETY FOR NEUROLOGICAL INVESTIGATION—DIRECTORY**
American Society for Neurological Investigation
c/o Dr. Marc R. Nuwer
81 Winthorp St.
Augusta, ME 04330
Covers: About 200 physicians who are pursuing academic careers in neurology and fellowships in neurology available at institutions in the United States and Canada. **Entries Include:** For junior faculty, fellows, and residents—Name, address, residency, interests, whether recipient of a fellowship. For fellowships—Institution name, address, contact, content of fellowship. **Pages (approx.):** 75. **Frequency:** Irregular; previous edition September 1985; latest edition winter 1987.

★3932★ **AMERICAN SOCIETY OF OUTPATIENT SURGEONS— MEMBERSHIP DIRECTORY**
American Society of Outpatient Surgeons
3960 Park Blvd., Ste. E
San Diego, CA 92103   Phone: (619) 692-9918
Covers: Approximately 400 board certified physicians performing outpatient surgery. **Entries Include:** Physician name, address, phone. **Pages (approx.):** 60. **Frequency:** Annual, May.

★3933★   AMERICAN SOCIETY OF PEDIATRIC HEMATOLOGY/ONCOLOGY—DIRECTORY OF MEMBERS
American Society of Pediatric Hematology/Oncology
c/o Carl Pochedly, M.D.
King/Drew Medical Center
12021 S. Wilmington Ave.
Los Angeles, CA 90059   Phone: (213) 603-4641
Covers: About 850 physicians and others concerned with the understanding and management of cancer and of disorders of the blood in children. **Entries Include:** Name, address, phone, institution and department or division where practicing. **Pages (approx.):** 44. **Frequency:** Annual, August.

★3934★   AMERICAN SOCIETY OF PSYCHOANALYTIC PHYSICIANS—MEMBERSHIP DIRECTORY
American Society of Psychoanalytic Physicians
4804 Jasmine Dr.
Rockville, MD 20853   Phone: (301) 929-1623
Covers: About 350 member physicians, psychiatrists, psychoanalysts; international coverage. **Entries Include:** Name, address, phone. **Pages (approx.):** 45. **Frequency:** Annual, May.

★3935★   AMERICAN SOCIETY OF VETERINARY OPHTHALMOLOGY—DIRECTORY
American Society of Veterinary Ophthalmology
1528 Shalamar
Stillwater, OK 74074   Phone: (405) 377-2134
Covers: 230 member veterinarians interested in animal ophthalmology. **Entries Include:** Name, address, office and home phone numbers, and year of graduation. **Pages (approx.):** 30. **Frequency:** Annual, December.

★3936★   AMERICAN SPEECH-LANGUAGE-HEARING ASSOCIATION—MEMBERSHIP DIRECTORY
American Speech-Language-Hearing Association
10801 Rockville Pike
Rockville, MD 20852   Phone: (301) 897-5700
Covers: About 60,000 speech/language pathologists and audiologists; also lists accredited educational programs in this field. **Entries Include:** For members—Name, address, phone, and type of certification (coded). For educational programs—Name and address of institution. **Pages (approx.):** 990. **Frequency:** Irregular; new edition expected 1992. **Also Includes:** List of relevant state associations.

★3937★   AMERICAN VETERINARY MEDICAL ASSOCIATION—DIRECTORY
American Veterinary Medical Association
930 N. Meacham Rd.
Schaumburg, IL 60196   Phone: (708) 605-8070
Covers: 48,600 veterinarians; not limited to AVMA members. **Entries Include:** Name, spouse's name, address, and codes for practice activity, type of employer, institution granting degree, and year received. **Pages (approx.):** 700. **Frequency:** Annual, December. **Also Includes:** Extensive list of veterinary medical and related associations, veterinary schools, related government agencies.

★3938★   ANIMAL HOSPITALS DIRECTORY
American Business Directories, Inc.
American Business Information, Inc.
5711 S. 86th Circle
Omaha, NE 68127   Phone: (402) 593-4600
Number of Listings: 12,135. **Entries Include:** Name, address, phone (including area code), size of advertisement, year first in "Yellow Pages," name of owner or manager, number of employees. **Frequency:** Annual.

★3939★   ANIMAL ORGANIZATIONS AND SERVICES DIRECTORY
Animal Stories
3004 Maple Ave.
Manhattan Beach, CA 90266
Covers: Over 500 U.S. and Canadian organizations involved in animal protection and welfare; also lists veterinary and medical organizations such as clinics, pet insurance companies, zoological societies, pet transporting and other services, pet fancier clubs, consultants, and publishers of magazines and newsletters concerned with animals. **Entries Include:** Name of organization, address, phone, branch offices, year established, key personnel, membership information, objectives, description of materials available by mail. **Pages (approx.):** 250. **Frequency:** Biennial, fall of odd years.

★3940★   ANNALS OF HUMAN BIOLOGY—SOCIETY FOR THE STUDY OF HUMAN BIOLOGY MEMBERSHIP LIST ISSUE
Society for the Study of Human Biology
London School of Hygiene and Tropical Medicine
Keppel St.
London WC1E 7HT, England
Publication Includes: List of about 500 scientists worldwide whose special field is human biology. **Entries Include:** Name, affiliation, address. **Frequency:** Annual, January.

★3941★   ANNUAIRE CNRS: SCIENCES DE LA VIE
Centre National de la Recherche Scientifique
15, quai Anatole France
F-75700 Paris, France
Covers: Over 410 current research projects in biology, pharmacology, and medicine which are sponsored by the National Center for Scientific Research (CNRS) in France. **Entries Include:** Name of research center, address, phone, telex, staff, research in progress, technical developments, technical equipment, keywords describing research. **Pages (approx.):** 930. **Frequency:** Irregular; latest edition December 1984. **Send Orders to:** Librairie des Editions du CNRS, 295, rue Saint Jacques, F-75005 Paris, France.

★3942★   APA GUIDE TO RESEARCH SUPPORT
American Psychological Association (APA)
1200 17th St. NW
Washington, DC 20036   Phone: (202) 955-7600
Covers: Over 180 federal programs and 55 private organizations providing support for research in psychological, cognitive, and behavioral sciences. **Entries Include:** Program name, address, names and phone numbers of contacts, types of research supported, funding mechanisms, application procedures. **Pages (approx.):** 275. **Frequency:** Irregular; latest edition August 1987; suspended indefinitely. **Send Orders to:** American Psychological Association, Box 2710, Hyattsville, MD 20784 (703-247-7705).

★3943★   APNEA AND NEONATAL MONITORING
Theta Corp.
Theta Bldg.
Middlefield, CT 06455   Phone: (203) 349-1054
Publication Includes: List of companies that manufacture home and hospital apnea and neonatal monitoring equipment. **Entries Include:** Company name, address, phone, key personnel, background information, description of products, annual sales, research and development efforts, distribution systems, five year projection. **Frequency:** Irregular; previous edition November 1987; latest edition September 1990.

★3944★   APOTHEKEN TELEFONREGISTER
Osterreichische Apothekerverlagsgesellschaft m.b.H.
Spitalgasse 31
A-1090 Vienna, Austria
Covers: Pharmacies and pharmacists in Austria. **Pages (approx.):** 125. **Frequency:** Annual, spring.

★3945★   APPROVED PROVIDERS OF CONTINUING PHARMACEUTICAL EDUCATION
American Council on Pharmaceutical Education
311 W. Superior St., Ste. 512
Chicago, IL 60610   Phone: (312) 664-3575
Covers: About 280 universities, colleges, associations, publishers, and corporations that provide continuing pharmaceutical education seminars, workshops, publications, audiovisual materials, and correspondence courses. **Entries Include:** Organization name, type of organization, address, phone, name and title of contact. **Pages (approx.):** 35. **Frequency:** Annual, July.

★3946★   ARIS FUNDING REPORTS
Academic Research Information System (ARIS)
2940 16th St., Ste. 314
San Francisco, CA 94103   Phone: (415) 558-8133
Covers: Grant and fellowship programs of private organizations and federal government agencies. Published in three editions: "T Creative Arts and Humanities Report," "T Social and Natural Sciences Report," and "T Biomedical Sciences Report" (formerly "T Medical Sciences Report"). Each issue of each edition includes 125-200 listings. **Entries Include:** Name of funding source, address, phone, contact name, program information with particular attention to procedures and deadlines. **Pages (approx.):** 45 per issue. **Frequency:** Every six weeks; social and natural sciences and biomedical sciences reports are supplemented.

★3947★ ARTIFICIAL BREASTS DIRECTORY
American Business Directories, Inc.
American Business Information, Inc.
5711 S. 86th Circle
Omaha, NE 68127   Phone: (402) 593-4600
Number of Listings: 1,019. **Entries Include:** Name, address, phone, size of advertisement, name of owner or manager, number of employees, year first in "Yellow Pages." **Frequency:** Annual.

★3948★ ARTIFICIAL LIMBS DIRECTORY
American Business Directories, Inc.
American Business Information, Inc.
5711 S. 86th Circle
Omaha, NE 68127   Phone: (402) 593-4600
Number of Listings: 1,793. **Entries Include:** Name, address, phone, size of advertisement, name of owner or manager, number of employees, year first in "Yellow Pages." **Frequency:** Annual.

★3949★ ASK YOUR DOCTOR, ASK YOURSELF
Schiffer Publishing Ltd.
1469 Morstein Rd.
West Chester, PA 19380   Phone: (215) 696-1001
Publication Includes: List of about 40 health care organizations involved in medical self-care. **Entries Include:** Organization name and address. **Frequency:** Published April 1986.

★3950★ ASSISTIVE TECHNOLOGY SOURCEBOOK
RESNA
1101 Connecticut Ave., NW, Ste. 700
Washington, DC 20036   Phone: (202) 857-1199
Publication Includes: List of suppliers of equipment for the handicapped, as well as publishers of material pertinent to independent living for the handicapped. **Frequency:** Irregular; previous edition 1984; latest edition March 1990.

★3951★ ASSOCIACAO PORTUGUESA DA INDUSTRIA FARMACEUTICA—LISTA DE ASSOCIADOS
Associacao Portuguesa da Industria Farmaceutica
Avenida Duque de Avila, 95-2
P-1000 Lisbon, Portugal
Covers: Member associations of pharmaceutical manufacturers and importers in Portugal. **Entries Include:** Member name, address, phone, telex. **Pages (approx.):** 10. **Frequency:** Monthly.

★3952★ ASSOCIATE DEGREE EDUCATION FOR NURSING
National League for Nursing
350 Hudson St.
New York, NY 10014   Phone: (212) 989-9393
Covers: About 415 two-year associate degree nursing programs accredited by the National League for Nursing. **Entries Include:** Institution name, address, length of program, residential facilities, fees, advanced placement programs, part-time evening programs, linkage with BS-RN program, estimated costs, number of graduates, number of enrollments. **Pages (approx.):** 160. **Frequency:** Annual.

★3953★ ASSOCIATION FOR ADVANCEMENT OF BEHAVIOR THERAPY—MEMBERSHIP DIRECTORY
Association for Advancement of Behavior Therapy
15 W. 36th St.
New York, NY 10018   Phone: (212) 279-7970
Covers: Over 4,000 psychologists, psychiatrists, and others interested in behavior therapy. **Entries Include:** Name, office or home address, phone, certifications or licenses, degree specialty, population served, and personal data. **Pages (approx.):** 160. **Frequency:** Biennial, spring of even years.

★3954★ ASSOCIATION FOR THE ADVANCEMENT OF BEHAVIOR THERAPY, NEUROPSYCHOLOGY SPECIAL INTEREST GROUP—DIRECTORY
Behavioral Neuropsychology Special Interest Group
Association for the Advancement of Behavior Therapy
Chestnut Ridge Hospital
930 Chestnut Ridge Rd.
Morgantown, WV 26505   Phone: (304) 293-2411
Covers: 250 member neuropsychologists involved with behavior therapy. **Entries Include:** Name, address. **Pages (approx.):** 5. **Frequency:** Annual, June.

★3955★ ASSOCIATION FOR THE ADVANCEMENT OF MEDICAL INSTRUMENTATION—MEMBERSHIP DIRECTORY
Association for the Advancement of Medical Instrumentation
3330 Washington Blvd., Ste. 400
Arlington, VA 22201-4598   Phone: (703) 525-4890
Covers: 5,000 physicians, clinical engineers, biomedical engineers and technicians, and medical equipment manufacturers. **Entries Include:** Name, title, affiliation, office address, phone, code for occupational specialization. **Pages (approx.):** 150. **Frequency:** Biennial, January of even years.

★3956★ ASSOCIATION OF AMERICAN MEDICAL COLLEGES—CURRICULUM DIRECTORY
Association of American Medical Colleges
2450 N St. NW
Washington, DC 20037-1126   Phone: (202) 828-0400
Covers: Accredited medical schools in the U.S., Puerto Rico, and Canada. **Entries Include:** School name, address, contact person, academic programs offered, required and elective courses, length of program, type of instruction, conditions for learning, grading evaluation, and instructional innovations. **Pages (approx.):** 335. **Frequency:** Annual, October.

★3957★ ASSOCIATION OF AMERICAN MEDICAL COLLEGES—DIRECTORY OF AMERICAN MEDICAL EDUCATION
Association of American Medical Colleges
2450 N St. NW
Washington, DC 20037-1126   Phone: (202) 828-0400
Covers: Accredited medical schools; coverage includes U.S., Puerto Rico, and Canada. **Entries Include:** Name of school, address, phone, fax, history, whether public or private, enrollment, names of clinical facilities; names and titles of university officials, medical school administrative staff, and department, division, or section chairpersons and a brief historical statement. Officers and members of various AAMC organizations are listed, including member medical academic societies and teaching hospitals. **Pages (approx.):** 490. **Frequency:** Annual, September.

★3958★ ASSOCIATION OF AMERICAN MEDICAL COLLEGES GROUP ON PUBLIC AFFAIRS—MEMBERSHIP DIRECTORY
Association of American Medical Colleges
2450 N St. NW
Washington, DC 20037-1126   Phone: (202) 828-0400
Covers: 126 medical schools and over 400 teaching hospitals and their key personnel in public relations, alumni, and development areas. **Entries Include:** School or hospital name, address, phone, name and title of contact. **Pages (approx.):** 100. **Frequency:** Annual, March.

★3959★ ASSOCIATION OF BRITISH HEALTH-CARE INDUSTRIES DIRECTORY
Directory Profiles Ltd.
148 Upper Richmond Rd. W.
London SW14 8DP, England
Covers: Over 200 member manufacturers and suppliers of health care equipment, supplies, and services in Great Britain. **Entries Include:** Company name, address, phone, telex, fax, name of contact, product or service, trade name. **Pages (approx.):** 85. **Frequency:** Annual, April.

★3960★ ASSOCIATION OF THE BRITISH PHARMACEUTICAL INDUSTRY—DATA SHEET COMPENDIUM
Datapharm Publications Ltd.
12 Whitehall
London SW1A 2DY, England
Covers: Manufacturers of pharmaceutical products. **Entries Include:** Company name, address, phone, description of products. **Pages (approx.):** 1,660. **Frequency:** Every 15 months.

★3961★ ASSOCIATION OF THE BRITISH PHARMACEUTICAL INDUSTRY—DIRECTORY OF MEMBERS
Association of the British Pharmaceutical Industry
12 Whitehall
London SW1A 2DY, England
Covers: Manufacturers of pharmaceutical products. **Entries Include:** Company name, address, phone. **Pages (approx.):** 39. **Frequency:** Annual.

★3962★ ASSOCIATION OF THE BRITISH PHARMACEUTICAL INDUSTRY—VETERINARY DATA SHEET COMPENDIUM
Datapharm Publications Ltd.
12 Whitehall
London SW1A 2DY, England
Covers: Manufacturers of veterinary pharmaceutical products. **Entries Include:** Company name, address, phone, description of products. **Pages (approx.):** 600. **Frequency:** Every 15 months.

★3963★ ASSOCIATION OF FEDERAL SAFETY AND HEALTH PROFESSIONALS—DIRECTORY
Association of Federal Safety and Health Professionals
7549 Wilhelm Dr.
Lanham, MD 20706-3737   Phone: (202) 523-8045
Covers: 400 safety and health specialists employed by the federal government. **Entries Include:** Name, home address, business address and phone, title. **Pages (approx.):** 40. **Frequency:** Annual, winter.

★3964★ ASSOCIATION OF HALFWAY HOUSE ALCOHOLISM PROGRAMS OF NORTH AMERICA—MEMBERSHIP DIRECTORY
Association of Halfway House Alcoholism Programs of North America
786 E. 7th St.
St. Paul, MN 55106   Phone: (612) 771-0933
Covers: About 600 alcoholism programs. **Entries Include:** For organizations—Name, address, phone, director's name, number of beds, target population and substance abused. For individuals—Name, address. **Pages (approx.):** 40. **Frequency:** Biennial, odd years.

★3965★ ASSOCIATION OF HEALTH FACILITY SURVEY AGENCIES—DIRECTORY
Association of Health Facility Survey Agencies
Division of Licensing and Regulation
Office of Inspector General, Cabinet for Human Resources
275 E. Main St., No. 4E
Frankfort, KY 40621   Phone: (502) 564-2800
Covers: State government officials primarily responsible for administering health facilities licensure and certification programs. **Entries Include:** Name, address, phone, title, and department. **Pages (approx.):** 12. **Frequency:** Annual.

★3966★ ASSOCIATION OF MEDICAL ILLUSTRATORS— MEMBERSHIP DIRECTORY
The Association of Medical Illustrators
1819 Peachtree St. NE, Ste. 560
Atlanta, GA 30309   Phone: (404) 350-7900
Covers: About 835 medical illustrators and allied health professionals; schools with accredited medical illustration programs. **Entries Include:** For members—Name, business address and phone, home phone (when given), fax, freelance availability. For programs—Program name, department name, school name, address, phone, degree offered, length of curriculum. **Pages (approx.):** 78. **Frequency:** Annual.

★3967★ ASSOCIATION OF MEDICAL REHABILITATION ADMINISTRATORS—MEMBERSHIP DIRECTORY
Association of Medical Rehabilitation Administrators
PO Box 1964
Parkersburg, WV 26102-2964   Phone: (508) 877-0517
Number of Listings: 250. **Entries Include:** Member name, home address, business address, phone, type of membership, year joined association. **Pages (approx.):** 75. **Frequency:** Annual, March.

★3968★ ASSOCIATION OF MEDICAL RESEARCH CHARITIES—HANDBOOK
Association of Medical Research Charities
Tavisrock House, S.
Tavisrock Sq.
London WC1H 9LG, England
Covers: Nearly 60 member and affiliated charities. **Entries Include:** Charity name, address, phone, telex, name and title of contact, financial data, research interest, description of activities and projects. **Pages (approx.):** 60. **Frequency:** Annual, October.

★3969★ ASSOCIATION OF OTOLARYNGOLOGY ADMINISTRATORS—RESOURCE NOTEBOOK
Association of Otolaryngology Administrators
PO Box 3150
Iowa City, IA 52244   Phone: (319) 356-2371
Publication Includes: List of managers of private and academic group medical practices specializing in head and neck surgery (often referred to as "ear, nose, throat"). **Entries Include:** Name, address, phone, name of contact, product or service, number of staff. **Frequency:** Annual, January.

★3970★ ASSOCIATION OF PHYSICIAN'S ASSISTANTS IN CARDIOVASCULAR SURGERY—MEMBERSHIP DIRECTORY
Association of Physician's Assistants in Cardiovascular Surgery
2000 Tate Springs Rd.
Lynchburg, VA 24501   Phone: (804) 847-8745
Covers: About 800 physician's assistants who work with cardiovascular surgeons. **Entries Include:** Name, address, phone. **Pages (approx.):** 10. **Frequency:** Annual.

★3971★ ASSOCIATION OF SURGEONS OF GREAT BRITAIN AND IRELAND—HANDBOOK
Association of Surgeons of Great Britain & Ireland
35/43 Lincoln's Inn Fields
London WC2A 3PN, England
Covers: Fellow members of the Association. **Entries Include:** Fellow name, address. **Pages (approx.):** 95. **Frequency:** Annual, September. **Also Includes:** List of rules.

★3972★ ASTHMA RESOURCES DIRECTORY
Allergy Publications Inc.
PO Box 640
Menlo Park, CA 94026   Phone: (415) 322-1663
Covers: Approximately 700 organizations, companies, and publishers that provide more than 2,500 services, programs, products, camps, books, self-help groups, and references for asthma sufferers. **Entries Include:** Company name, address, phone, description of services. **Pages (approx.):** 320. **Frequency:** Published August 1990.

★3973★ AUDIOLOGISTS DIRECTORY
American Business Directories, Inc.
American Business Information, Inc.
5711 S. 86th Circle
Omaha, NE 68127   Phone: (402) 593-4600
Number of Listings: 2,906. **Entries Include:** Name, address, phone (including area code), size of advertisement, year first in "Yellow Pages," name of owner or manager, number of employees. **Frequency:** Annual.

★3974★ AUDIO-VISUAL RESOURCES RELATED TO FAMILY INTERACTION WITH A HANDICAPPED MEMBER: AN ANNOTATED BIBLIOGRAPHY
Department of Child and Family Development
University of Minnesota at Duluth
Montague Hall, Rm. 120
Duluth, MN 55812   Phone: (218) 726-7233
Covers: Nearly 80 films, videotapes, and other audiovisual aids for use with the handicapped. **Entries Include:** Title, description, length, format, intended audience, whether for sale or for rent, price, supplier name; supplier's address and phone given in a separate list. **Pages (approx.):** 18. **Frequency:** Published 1985.

★3975★ AUTISM SOCIETY OF CANADA—DIRECTORY OF SERVICES AND RESOURCES
Autism Society Canada
45 Shepphard
Toronto, ON, Canada M2N 5W9   Phone: (416) 512-6475
Frequency: Latest edition 1984.

★3976★ AUTOMATED BLOOD GAS ANALYZERS AND NONINVASIVE BLOOD GAS MONITORS
Theta Corp.
Theta Bldg.
Middlefield, CT 06455   Phone: (203) 349-1054
Publication Includes: List of about 10 manufacturers that produce blood-gas analyzers and transcutaneous blood gas monitors and oximeters. **Entries Include:** Company name, address, phone, key personnel, background information, description of products, annual sales, research and development efforts, distribution efforts, five year projection. **Frequency:** Irregular; previous edition February 1983; latest edition October 1986.

★3977★ BABIES WITH DOWN'S SYNDROME: A NEW PARENTS' GUIDE
Woodbine House
5615 Fishers Ln.
Rockville, MD 20852　　　Phone: (301) 468-8800
Publication Includes: List of organizations and facilities providing information and services for parents with infants who have Down's syndrome. **Entries Include:** Company name, address, phone; name and title of contact. **Frequency:** Published 1986.

★3978★ BACCALAUREATE EDUCATION IN NURSING: KEY TO A PROFESSIONAL CAREER IN NURSING
National League for Nursing
350 Hudson St.
New York, NY 10014　　　Phone: (212) 989-9393
Covers: About 600 NLN-accredited four-year nursing schools and accredited nursing programs in colleges and universities. **Entries Include:** Name of institution, address, contact, entrance requirements, length of program, policy on acceptance of two-year college graduates, living accommodations, study arrangements, tuition and fees, number of graduates, number of enrollments. **Pages (approx.):** 100. **Frequency:** Previously annual; latest edition August 1989; new edition expected 1991.

★3979★ BARRON'S GUIDE TO FINANCING A MEDICAL SCHOOL EDUCATION
Barron's Educational Series, Inc.
250 Wireless Blvd.
Hauppauge, NY 11788　　　Phone: (516) 434-3311
Covers: Financial aid programs for medical students offered by federal agencies, state agencies, and individual medical schools. **Entries Include:** Granting institution name, address, phone, program name, eligibility requirements, application process, other regulations, sources of further information. **Pages (approx.):** 393. **Frequency:** Published 1990. **Also Includes:** Bibliography; information on medical education incentives in the military; discussion of financial aid eligibility and process.

★3980★ BARRON'S GUIDE TO MEDICAL AND DENTAL SCHOOLS
Barron's Educational Series, Inc.
250 Wireless Blvd.
Hauppauge, NY 11788　　　Phone: (800) 645-3476
Covers: About 220 medical, osteopathic, and dental schools. **Entries Include:** School name, address, admission requirements, housing, grading and promotion policies, facilities, description of curriculum. **Pages (approx.):** 340. **Frequency:** Biennial, odd years.

★3981★ BATTERED WOMEN'S DIRECTORY
Terry Mehlman
Box E-94
Earlham College
Richmond, IN 47374
Covers: Over 2,000 shelters, hotlines, YWCA's, hospitals, mental health services, legal service agencies, and other organizations and agencies which offer services to abused wives in the United States and abroad; includes listings of many educational resources on the problem. **Entries Include:** Name, address, phone; additional information as available. **Pages (approx.):** 285. **Frequency:** Irregular; previous edition August 1985; latest edition spring 1989.

★3982★ BEHAVIOR THERAPY AUDIO-VISUAL DIRECTORY
Association for Advancement of Behavior Therapy
15 W. 36th St.
New York, NY 10018
Pages (approx.): 65. **Frequency:** Latest edition 1987.

★3983★ THE BEST HOSPITALS IN AMERICA
Henry Holt & Co.
115 W. 18th St.
New York, NY 10011　　　Phone: (212) 633-0605
Covers: Over 150 hospitals. **Entries Include:** Hospital name, requirements for admission, description of services, costs, number of beds, length of average patient stay, emergency room statistics, names of specialists. **Frequency:** Latest edition 1987.

★3984★ BILLIAN'S HOSPITAL BLUE BOOK
Billian Publishing Co.
2100 Powers Ferry Rd., Ste. 300
Atlanta, GA 30339　　　Phone: (404) 955-5656
Covers: More than 7,100 hospitals; some listings also appear in a separate southern edition of this publication. **Entries Include:** Name of hospital, accreditation, mailing address, phone, number of beds, type of facility (nonprofit, general, state, etc.); list of administrative personnel and chiefs of medical services, with titles. **Pages (approx.):** National edition, 1,100; southern edition, 600. **Frequency:** Annual, spring.

★3985★ BIOFEEDBACK EQUIPMENT
Theta Corp.
Theta Bldg.
Middlefield, CT 06455　　　Phone: (203) 349-1054
Publication Includes: List of companies that produce biofeedback devices such as electromyography (EMG), thermal deviation, or galvanic skin responses (GSR). **Entries Include:** Company name, address, phone, key personnel, background information, description of products, annual sales, research and development efforts, distribution systems, five year projection. **Frequency:** Irregular; previous edition February 1983; latest edition March 1988.

★3986★ BIOFEEDBACK THERAPISTS DIRECTORY
American Business Directories, Inc.
American Business Information, Inc.
5711 S. 86th Circle
Omaha, NE 68127　　　Phone: (402) 593-4600
Number of Listings: 1,177. **Entries Include:** Name, address, phone, size of advertisement, name of owner or manager, number of employees, year first in "Yellow Pages." **Frequency:** Annual.

★3987★ BIOLOGICAL PHOTOGRAPHIC ASSOCIATION— MEMBERSHIP DIRECTORY
Biological Photographic Association
115 Stoneridge Dr.
Chapel Hill, NC 27514　　　Phone: (919) 967-8247
Covers: 1,200 photographers, technicians, doctors, scientists, educators, and others concerned with photography in the health sciences and related fields. **Entries Include:** Name, address. **Pages (approx.):** 60. **Frequency:** Annual.

★3988★ BIOMEDICAL INDEX TO PHS SUPPORTED RESEARCH
U.S. National Institutes of Health
5333 Westbard Ave., Rm. 148
Bethesda, MD 20892　　　Phone: (301) 496-7543
Covers: Over 55,000 research grants and contracts supported by the United States Public Health Service. **Entries Include:** Project title, project number, name and address of principal investigator. **Pages (approx.):** 2,450 (in two volumes). **Frequency:** Annual, July.

★3989★ BIOMEDICAL PRODUCTS—CELL BIOLOGY BUYER'S GUIDE ISSUE
Gordon Publications, Inc.
301 Gibralter, Box 650
Morris Plains, NJ 07950-6050　　　Phone: (201) 292-5100
Publication Includes: Over 100 manufacturers of chemicals, products, and equipment for use in cell biology laboratory procedures. **Entries Include:** Company name, address, products. **Frequency:** Annual, June.

★3990★ BIOMEDICAL PRODUCTS MAGAZINE—ANTIBODY AND ANTISERA BUYER'S GUIDE ISSUE
Gordon Publications, Inc.
301 Gibraltor Dr.
Morris Plains, NJ 07950　　　Phone: (201) 292-5100
Publication Includes: Listing of early 100 manufacturers of antibodies, antiseras, and other related products. **Entries Include:** Company name, address, products. **Frequency:** Annual, January.

★3991★ BIOMEDICAL RESEARCH TECHNOLOGY RESOURCES—A RESEARCH RESOURCES DIRECTORY
National Center for Research Resources
U.S. National Institutes of Health
9000 Rockville Pike
Bethesda, MD 20892　　　Phone: (301) 496-5665
Covers: Over 60 Division of Research Resources grantee facilities (specialized computer systems, nuclear magnetic resonance spectrometers, electric

spin resonancy spectrometers, etc.) that can be used by biomedical investigators. **Entries Include:** Facility name, address, phone, names of principal investigators, name of contact person, and details on the installation. **Pages (approx.):** 115. **Frequency:** Latest edition 1990. **Send Orders to:** Research Resources Information Center, 1601 Research Boulevard, Rockville, MD (301-984-2870).

★3992★   **BIOPHYSICAL SOCIETY—DIRECTORY**
Biophysical Society
c/o Emily M. Gray
9650 Rockville Pike, Rm. 2503/5
Bethesda, MD 20814   Phone: (301) 530-7114
Covers: 4,000 scientists, including biophysicists, physical biochemists, and physical and biological scientists, interested in the application of physical laws and techniques to the analysis of biological or living phenomena. **Entries Include:** Name, title, affiliation, address. **Pages (approx.):** 125. **Frequency:** Annual.

★3993★   **BLOOD PRESSURE EQUIPMENT MARKETS: UNITED STATES, WESTERN EUROPE, AND JAPAN**
Theta Corp.
Theta Bldg.
Middlefield, CT 06455   Phone: (203) 349-1054
Publication Includes: List of about 20 manufacturers of blood pressure equipment. **Entries Include:** Company name, address, phone, key personnel, background information, description of products, annual sales, research and development efforts, distribution systems, five year projection. **Frequency:** Irregular; previous edition April 1985; latest edition January 1990.

★3994★   **BLUE BOOK DIGEST OF HMOS**
National Association of Employers on Health Care Action
240 Crandon Blvd., Ste. 110
PO Box 220
Key Biscayne, FL 33149   Phone: (305) 361-2810
Covers: Over 575 health maintenance organizations in the United States. **Entries Include:** Organization name, address, phone, names of key officials, type, date of initial operation, date federally qualified, profit or nonprofit, enrollment, employer groups, open-ended HMO and provider employment data reports. **Pages (approx.):** 135. **Frequency:** Annual, summer.

★3995★   **BLUE BOOK DIGEST OF PPOS UTILIZATION REVIEW**
National Association of Employers on Health Care Action
240 Crandon Blvd., Ste. 110
PO Box 220
Key Biscayne, FL 33149   Phone: (305) 361-2810
Covers: About 668 medical, dental, podiatry, physical therapy, and mental health preferred provider organizations (PPOs); 128 utilization review firms. **Entries Include:** Organization name, address, phone, names of key personnel; whether profit or nonprofit, independent or chain; operational date, type of sponsor, number of hospitals and physicians, service area, subscribers, member groups, utilization review, professional and retainer staff. **Pages (approx.):** 155. **Frequency:** Annual, summer.

★3996★   **BLUE BOOK OF OPTOMETRISTS**
Butterworth-Heinemann
80 Montvale Ave.
Stoneham, MA 02180   Phone: (617) 438-8464
Covers: Nearly 30,000 optometrists, optical supply houses, manufacturers and import firms, associations, national and state examining board members, colleges and programs concerned with optometry and para-optometry; coverage includes Canada. **Entries Include:** For optometrists—Name, office address, phone; personal, education, and career data; specialty. **Pages (approx.):** 465. **Frequency:** Biennial, late fall of odd years.

★3997★   **BONE GROWTH STIMULATORS**
Theta Corp.
Theta Bldg.
Middlefield, CT 06455   Phone: (203) 349-1054
Publication Includes: List of manufacturers of products for bone growth stimulators. **Entries Include:** Company name, address, phone, key personnel, background information, description of products, annual sales, research and development efforts, distribution systems, five year projection. **Pages (approx.):** 59. **Frequency:** Irregular; previous edition February 1984; latest edition May 1987.

★3998★   **BRITAIN'S PHARMACEUTICAL INDUSTRY**
Jordan & Sons Ltd.
21 St. Thomas St.
Bristol BS1 6JS, England
Covers: Manufacturers and suppliers of pharmaceutical products in the United Kingdom. **Entries Include:** Company name, address, phone, names and titles of key personnel, financial data for previous three years, corporate ownership and shareholder data. **Pages (approx.):** 100. **Frequency:** Irregular, latest edition 1989. **Also Includes:** Industry market profiles.

★3999★   **BRITISH ACUPUNCTURE ASSOCIATION AND REGISTER—YEAR BOOK AND REGISTER**
British Acupuncture Association
34 Alderney St.
London SW1V 4EU, England
Entries Include: Name, address, and phone. **Pages (approx.):** 35. **Frequency:** Reported as every four years, latest edition 1982; no recent edition.

★4000★   **BRITISH ASSOCIATION FOR COUNSELLING— COUNSELLING AND PSYCHOTHERAPY RESOURCES DIRECTORY**
British Association for Counselling
37a Sheep St.
Rugby, Warwickshire CV21 3BX, England
Covers: National and local organizations and individuals specializing in counseling in Great Britain. **Entries Include:** Center or personal name, address, phone, specialty field, branch office names and addresses. **Pages (approx.):** 620. **Frequency:** Annual, July.

★4001★   **BRITISH ASSOCIATION OF UROLOGICAL SURGEONS—HANDBOOK**
British Association of Urological Surgeons
c/o The Royal College of Surgeons
35/43 Lincoln's Inn Fields
London WC2A 3PN, England
Covers: Approximately 1,100 member urological surgeons and association officers. **Entries Include:** Name, address, phone. **Pages (approx.):** 72. **Frequency:** Biennial, even years. **Also Includes:** Rules and history of the association.

★4002★   **BRITISH OSTEOPATHIC ASSOCIATION—DIRECTORY**
British Osteopathic Association
8-10 Boston Pl.
London NW1 6QH, England
Covers: Approximately 100 member certified osteopaths practicing in the United Kingdom. **Entries Include:** Name, address, phone, certification. **Pages (approx.):** 35. **Frequency:** Annual, February.

★4003★   **BRITISH PSYCHOLOGICAL SOCIETY—LIST OF MEMBERS OF THE DIVISION OF OCCUPATIONAL PSYCHOLOGY OFFERING CONSULTANCY SERVICES**
Occupational Psychology Division
British Psychological Society
St. Andrews House
48 Princess Rd., E.
Leicester LE1 7DR, England
Covers: About 200 member psychologists offering consulting services. **Entries Include:** Member name, address, phone. **Pages (approx.):** 200. **Frequency:** Irregular; previous edition 1986, latest edition 1990.

★4004★   **BURN CARE SERVICES IN NORTH AMERICA**
American Burn Association
c/o Dr. Andrew M. Munster, Secretary
Baltimore Regional Burn Center
4940 Eastern Ave.
Baltimore, MD 21224
Covers: About 200 burn care facilities; approximately 25 skin banks. **Entries Include:** Facility name, address, phone; name and phone of contact, number of beds available. **Pages (approx.):** 25. **Frequency:** Annual, early in year.

★4005★   **BUSINESS INSURANCE—DIRECTORY OF HMOS AND PPOS ISSUE**
Crain Communications, Inc.
740 N. Rush St.
Chicago, IL 60611   Phone: (312) 649-5279
Publication Includes: List of more than 1,000 health maintenance and preferred provider organizations nationwide. **Entries Include:** Organiza-

tion name, address, phone, dates of inception and federal qualification, sponsorship, names and titles of contact and other key personnel, number of employees, geographical area served, financial data, description of products and services provided. **Frequency:** Annual, December. **Send Orders to:** Business Insurance, 965 N. Jefferson, Detroit, MI 48207 (313-446-6000).

★4006★ **BUYERS GUIDE FOR THE HEALTH CARE INDUSTRY**
American Hospital Publishing, Inc.
211 E. Chicago Ave., Ste. 700
Chicago, IL 60611   Phone: (312) 440-6800
Covers: 1,200 manufacturers and suppliers of equipment, products, and services to the health care industry. **Entries Include:** Company name, address, products. **Pages (approx.):** 80. **Frequency:** Annual, December.

★4007★ **CALENDAR OF CONGRESSES OF MEDICAL SCIENCES**
Council for International Organizations of Medical Sciences
c/o World Health Organization
20 Avenue Appia
CH-1211 Geneva 27, Switzerland
Covers: International and regional congresses of the international biomedical community. **Entries Include:** Congress title, date, and location; name of sponsoring organization; name, title, and address of contact. **Pages (approx.):** 65. **Frequency:** Annual, January.

★4008★ **CALENDAR OF THE PHARMACEUTICAL SOCIETY OF IRELAND**
Pharmaceutical Society of Ireland
37 Northumberland Rd.
Dublin 4, Ireland
Covers: More than 2,800 member pharmaceutical chemists, pharmacists, registered druggists, and pharmaceutical assistants in Ireland. **Entries Include:** Member name, address. **Pages (approx.):** 170. **Frequency:** Annual, March.

★4009★ **CAMPUS GANG RAPE: PARTY GAMES?**
Project on the Status and Education of Women
Association of American Colleges
1818 R St. NW
Washington, DC 20009   Phone: (202) 387-1300
Publication Includes: List of about 10 publishers and organizations concerned with gang rape on college campuses. **Frequency:** Published November 1985.

★4010★ **CANADIAN HOSPITAL DIRECTORY**
Canadian Hospital Association
17 York St., Ste. 100
Ottawa, ON, Canada K1N 9J6   Phone: (613) 238-8005
Covers: About 1,250 hospitals, health centers, and nursing stations; 700 health associations and other professional related associations; manufacturers and suppliers of hospital equipment and supplies. **Entries Include:** For hospitals—Hospital name, address, phone, fax, whether public or private; accreditation, year established, number of beds, number of employees, budget, other statistical data; names and titles of key personnel. For others—Name of organization or firm, address, phone; description of product, services, or activities. **Pages (approx.):** 365. **Frequency:** Annual, September.

★4011★ **CANADIAN HOSPITAL MARKET DIRECTORY**
SMG Marketing Group, Inc.
1342 N. LaSalle Dr.
Chicago, IL 60610   Phone: (312) 642-3026
Covers: Approximately 1,500 hospitals in Canada. **Entries Include:** Hospital name, address, phone, number of beds, yearly admissions. **Pages (approx.):** 150. **Frequency:** Annual, July.

★4012★ **CANADIAN LOCATIONS OF JOURNALS INDEXED FOR MEDLINE**
Canada Institute for Scientific and Technical Information
National Research Council Canada
Montreal Rd.
Ottawa, ON, Canada K1A 0S2   Phone: (613) 993-3854
Publication Includes: List of Canadian libraries holding health science publications as indexed in MEDLINE. **Entries Include:** Library name and address. **Frequency:** Annual.

★4013★ **CANADIAN MEDICAL DIRECTORY**
Southam Business Communications Inc.
1450 Don Mills Rd.
Don Mills, ON, Canada M3B 2X7   Phone: (416) 445-6641
Covers: Over 45,000 physicians who replied to questionnaires mailed by the publisher. Lists of medical schools, universities, government health agencies, and medical societies for Canada are also given. **Entries Include:** For physicians—Name, address, year and school of medical degree, professional memberships, hospital affiliations, address, phone. For others—Name, address, phone. **Pages (approx.):** 910. **Frequency:** Annual, June.

★4014★ **CANCER FACTS AND FIGURES**
American Cancer Society
1599 Clifton Rd, NE
Atlanta, GA 30329   Phone: (404) 320-3333
Publication Includes: List of cancer treatment centers and 57 American Cancer Society division offices. **Entries Include:** Center name, phone. **Frequency:** Annual, February.

★4015★ **CANCER SOURCEBOOK**
Omnigraphics
Penobscot Bldg.
Detroit, MI 48226   Phone: (313) 961-1340
Publication Includes: List of support groups and services available for cancer victims and their families. **Frequency:** Latest editon 1990.

★4016★ **CAREER PLANNING AND PLACEMENT STRATEGIES FOR POSTSECONDARY STUDENTS WITH DISABILITIES**
Higher Education and Adult Training of People with Handicaps
1 Dupont Circle, NW, Ste. 800
Washington, DC 20036   Phone: (202) 939-9320
Covers: About 30 educational institutions and organizations offering career placement programs for handicapped postsecondary students. **Entries Include:** Institution name, address, phone, name and title of contact, program name, description of program. **Pages (approx.):** 10. **Frequency:** Published 1990. **Also Includes:** Annotated bibliography on job placement for handicapped students.

★4017★ **CAREERS THAT COUNT**
American Hospital Association
840 N. Lake Shore Dr.
Chicago, IL 60611   Phone: (312) 280-6117
Publication Includes: List of about 50 professional organizations in health care fields serving hospitals, including hospital administration, medical records administration, therapy, nursing, biomedical engineering, etc. **Entries Include:** Name and address. **Frequency:** Irregular; previous edition 1985; latest edition 1987.

★4018★ **CARING FOR ALZHEIMER'S PATIENTS: A GUIDE FOR FAMILY AND HEALTH CARE PROVIDERS**
Plenum Publishing Corp.
233 Spring St.
New York, NY 10013   Phone: (212) 620-8460
Publication Includes: List of about 5 organizations that provide information and resources concerning Alzheimer's disease support groups, hospitals, and other caregiving organizations. **Entries Include:** Organization name, address, phone, fax, description of services and activities. **Frequency:** Published August 1989.

★4019★ **CARING FOR THE MENTALLY IMPAIRED ELDERLY: A FAMILY GUIDE**
Henry Holt & Company
115 W. 18th St.
New York, NY 10011   Phone: (212) 886-9200
Publication Includes: In appendixes—list of resources to aid mentally impaired elderly, including publications, institutions, and other sources of information. **Frequency:** Published 1989.

★4020★ **CARING FOR THE SICK**
Facts on File, Inc.
460 Park Ave. S.
New York, NY 10016   Phone: (212) 683-2244
Publication Includes: List of about 10 health care organizations that provide assistance or information in the field of home health care. **Entries Include:** Company or organization name and address. **Frequency:** Published 1985.

★4021★ CARING FOR YOUR OWN DEAD
Upper Access Publishers
1 Upper Access Rd.
Hinesburg, VT 05461   Phone: (802) 482-2988
Publication Includes: List of crematories that work directly with families, medical schools that accept body donations, and state agencies in charge of regulating care for the dead. **Entries Include:** Agency, organization, or institution name, address, phone, description of service, geographic territory served. **Frequency:** First edition 1987.

★4022★ CASE MANAGEMENT RESOURCE GUIDE
Center for Consumer Healthcare Information
4000 Birch St., Ste. 112
Newport Beach, CA 92660-2211   Phone: (714) 752-2335
Covers: In four regional volumes, lists about 65,000 health care facilities and support services, including homecare, rehabilitation, psychiatric, and addiction treatment programs; hospices, adult day care, and burn and cancer centers. **Entries Include:** Facility name, address, phone, names and titles of key personnel; number of employees, geographic area covered, type of service or program provided, branch office or parent organization and phone number, and credentials. **Pages (approx.):** 2,800. **Frequency:** Annual, February. **Send Orders to:** Center for Consumer Healthcare Information, PO Box 16067, Irvine, CA 92713 .

★4023★ CATALOG OF CELL LINES
National Institutes of General Medical Sciences
U.S. National Institutes of Health
9000 Rockville Pike
Bethesda, MD 20892   Phone: (301) 496-4000
Publication Includes: List of 610 physicians and other scientists interested in human genetics who have submitted cultures of genetically normal and abnormal human cell cultures to the repository. **Entries Include:** Name, address. **Frequency:** Annual, October. **Send Orders to:** Human Genetic Mutant Cell Repository, Coriell Institute for Medical Research, Copewood & Davis Sts., Camden, NJ 08103 (609-966-7377);.

★4024★ CATHETERS
Theta Corp.
Theta Bldg.
Middlefield, CT 06455   Phone: (203) 349-1054
Publication Includes: List of about 30 manufacturers and distributors of medical catheter devices. **Entries Include:** Company name, address, phone, key personnel, background information, description of products, annual sales, research and development efforts, distribution systems, five year projection. **Frequency:** Irregular; latest edition September 1988; updated November 1990.

**★4025★ CHEMIST AND DRUGGIST DIRECTORY AND
    TABLET AND CAPSULE IDENTIFICATION GUIDE**
Benn Business Information Services Ltd.
PO Box 20
Sovereign Way
Tonbridge, Kent TN9 1RQ, England
Covers: 6,500 manufacturers, distributors, and wholesalers of pharmaceuticals, medical products, cosmetics, toiletries, and pharmacy equipment. **Entries Include:** Company name, address, phone, fax, trade and brand names, products and services. **Pages (approx.):** 380. **Frequency:** Annual, November. **Also Includes:** List of hospital pharmacists and a capsule and tablet identification guide, with data on drug interactions. **Available in the U.S. from:** Nichols Publishing Co., 155 W. 72nd St., New York, NY 10023 (212-580-8079).

**★4026★ CHILD ABUSE AND NEGLECT AND FAMILY
    VIOLENCE AUDIOVISUAL CATALOG**
Clearinghouse on Family Violence Information
Box 1182
Washington, DC 20013   Phone: (703) 821-2086
Covers: Distributors of over 550 films, videotapes, filmstrips with tapes, slides with tapes, and audiovisual packages about child abuse and neglect and family violence. **Entries Include:** Title, name of producer, distributor name and address; description of materials, including length, format, and price. **Pages (approx.):** 250. **Frequency:** Irregular; latest edition February 1990; new edition expected March 1991.

**★4027★ CHILD ABUSE AND NEGLECT: AN INFORMATION
    AND REFERENCE GUIDE**
Garland Publishing Inc.
136 Madison Ave.
New York, NY 10016   Phone: (212) 686-7942
Publication Includes: Listings of child abuse and neglect prevention agencies and programs; and national reporting, training, treatment, and prevention sources.

**★4028★ CHILDREN AND ADOLESCENTS WITH MENTAL
    ILLNESS: A PARENTS GUIDE**
Woodbine House
5615 Fishers Ln.
Rockville, MD 20852   Phone: (301) 468-8800
Publication Includes: List of organizations and facilities providing information and services for families with mentally ill children. **Entries Include:** Company or institution name, address, phone, contact person (if appropriate). **Frequency:** Published 1988. **Also Includes:** Appendix on medications; bibliographies.

★4029★ CHILDREN WITH EPILEPSY: A PARENTS' GUIDE
Woodbine House
5615 Fishers Ln.
Rockville, MD 20852   Phone: (301) 468-8800
Publication Includes: List of organizations and facilities providing information and services for families with epilectic children. **Frequency:** Published 1988. **Also Includes:** Bibliography, resource guide, references, glossary, and cassettes list.

**★4030★ CHINESE AMERICAN MEDICAL SOCIETY—
    MEMBERSHIP DIRECTORY**
Chinese American Medical Society
630 W. 168th St.
New York, NY 10032   Phone: (212) 305-3569
Covers: 550 physicians of Chinese origin now residing in the United States and Canada. **Entries Include:** Name, address, phone, specialty, affiliation. **Pages (approx.):** 90. **Frequency:** Biennial, December of even years.

★4031★ CHIROPODISTS REGISTER
Chiropodists Board
184 Kennington Park Rd.
London SE11 4BU, England
Covers: Chiropodists registered to practice within the United Kingdom National Health Service and overseas. **Entries Include:** Name, address, qualifications, office name and location, geographic territory covered. **Pages (approx.):** 200. **Frequency:** Annual, September.

**★4032★ THE CHIROPRACTIC COLLEGE ADMISSIONS AND
    CURRICULUM DIRECTORY**
K M Enterprises
3407 Cabrillo Blvd.
Los Angeles, CA 90066   Phone: (213) 398-9135
Covers: Over 20 chiropractic colleges, state and national licensing boards, national associations. international coverage. **Entries Include:** College name, address, phone, names and titles of key personnel, history, financial data, admissions requirements, curriculum, typical questions, clinical opportunities, postgraduate and residency programs. **Pages (approx.):** 250. **Frequency:** Biennial, January of even years. **Send Orders to:** K M Enterprises, PO Box 25978, Los Angeles, CA 90025.

★4033★ CHIROPRACTORS DIRECTORY
American Business Directories, Inc.
American Business Information, Inc.
5711 S. 86th Circle
Omaha, NE 68127   Phone: (402) 593-4600
Number of Listings: 53,660. **Entries Include:** Name, address, phone (including area code), size of advertisement, year first in "Yellow Pages," name of owner or manager, number of employees. **Frequency:** Annual.

**★4034★ CHOICES: REALISTIC ALTERNATIVES IN CANCER
    TREATMENT**
Avon Books
1350 Avenue of the Americas
New York, NY 10019   Phone: (212) 261-6895
Publication Includes: Chapter titled "Where to Get Help," which lists American Cancer Society offices, National Cancer Institute research study groups and cancer treatment centers, and other organizations and associations of assistance to cancer patients and their families in the United

States, Canada, and Europe. **Entries Include:** Organization name, name of contact (for research programs), address, phone. Research and treatment programs may also include some indication of the emphasis. **Frequency:** Irregular; previous edition 1980; latest edition 1987.

★4035★ **CLINICAL CHEMISTRY ANALYZERS**
Theta Corp.
Theta Bldg.
Middlefield, CT 06455   Phone: (203) 349-1054
Publication Includes: List of manufacturers of clinical chemistry analysis instruments. **Entries Include:** Company name, address, phone, key personnel, background information, description of products, annual sales, research and development efforts, distribution systems, five year projection. **Frequency:** Irregular; latest edition January 1990.

★4036★ **CLINICAL PHARMACOLOGY: A GUIDE TO TRAINING PROGRAMS**
Peterson's Guides, Inc.
PO Box 2123
Princeton, NJ 08543-2123   Phone: (609) 243-9111
Covers: About 50 colleges and universities that offer postdoctoral training programs in clinical pharmacology. **Entries Include:** Institution name, address, department name, name of program director, program requirements, clinical and research facilities, financial support, application procedures, faculty, faculty research areas and publications. **Pages (approx.):** 180. **Frequency:** Irregular; latest edition 1988.

★4037★ **CLINICAL PROGRAMS FOR MENTALLY RETARDED CHILDREN**
National Center for Education in Maternal and Child Health
38th & R Sts., NW
Washington, DC 20057   Phone: (202) 625-8400
Covers: About 280 outpatient medical facilities providing comprehensive evaluation, treatment, or follow-up services primarily to children suspected of or diagnosed with mental retardation; also includes list of state maternal and child health and crippled children's services directors. **Entries Include:** For facilities—Name, address, phone, name of director, geographic area served, ages accepted. For directors—Name, department, address, phone. **Pages (approx.):** 35. **Frequency:** Irregular; previous edition July 1984; latest edition November 1985. **Send Orders to:** National Maternal and Child Health Clearinghouse, 38th & R Sts., NW, Washington, D.C. 20057.

★4038★ **CLINICS DIRECTORY**
American Business Directories, Inc.
American Business Information, Inc.
5711 S. 86th Circle
Omaha, NE 68127   Phone: (402) 593-4600
Number of Listings: 37,362. **Entries Include:** Clinic name, address, phone (including area code), size of advertisement, year first in "Yellow Pages," name of owner or manager, number of employees. **Frequency:** Annual.

★4039★ **CLINLAB PRODUCTS COMPANY DIRECTORY**
RSF International Group, Inc.
Box 368
Mount Kisco, NY 10549   Phone: (914) 241-6360
Covers: More than 450 manufacturers of equipment and supplies for clinical laboratories. **Entries Include:** Company name, parent company, address, phone, fax, telex, ownership, names and titles of key personnel, financial information, distributors in the United States and Europe, total number of employees and number of employees in sales, service, and research and development; products. **Pages (approx.):** 450. **Frequency:** Biennial, even years.

★4040★ **CODEX GALENICA**
Galenica AG
Box 2653
CH-3001 Bern, Switzerland
Publication Includes: List of manufacturers of drugs, serums, immune globulines, and vaccines available in Switzerland. **Frequency:** Triennial; latest edition 1989. **Available in the U.S. from:** Drug Intelligence and Clinical Pharmacy, Harvey Whitney Books, Box 42435, Cincinnati, OH 45242 (513-793-3555).

★4041★ **COLLEGE AND CAREER PROGRAMS FOR DEAF STUDENTS**
Gallaudet Research Institute
800 Florida Ave., NE
Washington, DC 20002   Phone: (202) 651-5575
Covers: About 155 postsecondary institutions offering special services for deaf students. **Entries Include:** Institution name, address, phone, program coordinators and information officers, enrollment, tuition and fees, accreditations, date established, admission requirements, special services available, preparatory programs, major areas of study. **Pages (approx.):** 150. **Frequency:** Irregular; previous edition 1988; latest edition 1991.

★4042★ **COLLEGE OF OPTOMETRISTS IN VISION DEVELOPMENT—FELLOW MEMBER ROSTER**
College of Optometrists in Vision Development
Box 285
Chula Vista, CA 91912   Phone: (619) 425-6191
Covers: About 980 members. **Entries Include:** Name, address, phone. **Pages (approx.):** 95. **Frequency:** Annual, January.

★4043★ **COLLEGE OF OSTEOPATHIC HEALTHCARE EXECUTIVES—DIRECTORY**
College of Osteopathic Healthcare Executives
1454 Duke St.
Alexandria, VA 22314   Phone: (703) 684-7700
Covers: 200 fellows, members, and nominees. **Entries Include:** Name, address, hospital affiliation. **Pages (approx.):** 55. **Frequency:** Annual, May.

★4044★ **COLLEGE OF SPEECH THERAPISTS—DIRECTORY**
The College of Speech Therapists
Harold Poster House
6 Lechmere Rd.
London NW2 5BU, England
Covers: 4,400 member speech therapists primarily in the United Kingdom. **Entries Include:** Name, address, phone, whether full or part time, languages (other than English) used in treatment, and employing authority. **Pages (approx.):** 140. **Frequency:** Triennial, latest edition 1990.

★4045★ **COLLEGES OFFERING PROGRAMS FOR STUDENTS WITH A LEARNING DISABILITY**
Continuing Education Department
Simsbury Public School District
754 Hopmeadow St.
Simsbury, CT 06070   Phone: (203) 658-0009
Covers: Over 60 colleges that offer programs for learning disabled students. **Entries Include:** Institution name, address, phone, program title, cost, name and title of contact, number of employees, admission criteria, orientation requirements, description of services. **Pages (approx.):** 135. **Frequency:** Published 1988.

★4046★ **COLLEGES OF VETERINARY MEDICINE ACCREDITED OR APPROVED BY AMERICAN VETERINARY MEDICAL ASSOCIATION**
American Veterinary Medical Association
930 N. Meacham Rd.
Schaumburg, IL 60196   Phone: (708) 605-8070
Number of Listings: About 32; coverage includes Canada and Europe. **Entries Include:** Institution name, address; name of dean, accreditation status, year of latest review. **Pages (approx.):** 5. **Frequency:** Semiannual; latest edition August 1990.

★4047★ **COMMON GROUND: RESOURCES FOR PERSONAL TRANSFORMATION**
Common Ground
305 San Anselmo Ave.
San Anselmo, CA 94960   Phone: (415) 459-4900
Covers: Music schools; art instructors; educational programs; conferences and festivals; natural and health food restaurants and suppliers; medicine and dentistry professionals who emphasize preventive health care; holistic health practitioners; individuals engaged in the psychic arts, psychology, and psychic healing; retreat sites, camps, hot springs, and inns; publications, book publishers, and other sources of materials; gyms, dance studios, yoga instructors, and instructors in the martial arts; palmists and astrologists. All listings are paid. Coverage is primarily of northern California. **Entries Include:** Generally, name, address, phone, name of contact, description of services, program, or merchandise. **Pages (approx.):** 152. **Frequency:** Quarterly. **Also Includes:** Articles of relating to personal growth and transformation.

★4048★ COMMONWEALTH ASSOCIATION OF MENTAL HANDICAP AND DEVELOPMENTAL DISABILITIES— DIRECTORY
Commonwealth Association of Mental Handicap and Developmental Disabilities
Beehives
90 Hay Ln.
Kingsbury NW9 0LG, England
Covers: 400 individuals and professionals in fields dealing with mental handicaps and developmental disability working to prevent mental retardation, especially in developing countries. **Entries Include:** Personal name, address, names and titles of key personnel. **Pages (approx.):** 80 per volume. **Frequency:** Annual, January.

★4049★ COMMONWEALTH NURSES FEDERATION— DIRECTORY
Commonwealth Nurses Federation
c/o Royal Commonwealth Society
18 Northumberland Ave.
London WC2N 5BJ, England
Covers: Approximately 55 national nurses associations in Commonwealth countries and correspondents in 9 countries, associated states, and dependencies. **Pages (approx.):** 20. **Frequency:** Semiannual, March and November. **Also Includes:** Reports of workshops, seminars, meetings, and conferences; list of books and visual aids.

★4050★ COMPLETE DIRECTORY OF PEOPLE WITH DISABILITIES
Gale Research Inc.
835 Penobscot Bldg.
Detroit, MI 48226   Phone: (313) 961-2242
Covers: 6,000 products, services, organizations and facilities available for the disabled, including assistive devices, publications, camps, educational programs, housing, recreation, rehabilitation services, associations, travel and transportation services, and conference shows. **Entries Include:** Name, address, phone, description of product, service, facility, or program. **Pages (approx.):** 700. **Frequency:** Biennial, November of odd years.

★4051★ COMPREHENSIVE CLINICAL GENETIC SERVICES CENTERS: A NATIONAL DIRECTORY
National Center for Education in Maternal and Child Health
38th and R Sts., NW
Washington, DC 20057   Phone: (202) 625-8400
Number of Listings: 215. **Entries Include:** Center name, address, phone, names and titles of key personnel, geographical area served, services provided. **Pages (approx.):** 110. **Frequency:** Irregular; latest edition 1985. **Also Includes:** Lists of state genetic service coordinators, state newborn screening directors, and state maternal, child health, crippled children agencies.

★4052★ COMPUTER USE IN PSYCHOLOGY: A DIRECTORY OF SOFTWARE
American Psychological Association
1200 17th St. NW
Washington, DC 20036   Phone: (202) 955-7600
Frequency: Latest edition November 1988.

★4053★ COMPUTERS IN HEALTHCARE—MARKET DIRECTORY ISSUE
Cardiff Publishing Co., Inc.
6300 S. Syracuse Way, Ste. 650
Englewood, CO 80111   Phone: (303) 220-0600
Publication Includes: Directory of 750 suppliers, consultants, and associations of computer software and hardware with specific application to the health care field. **Entries Include:** Company name, address, phone, fax, name and title of contact, geographical territory covered; description of products, including hardware system requirements, training programs available, and applications. **Frequency:** Annual, August.

★4054★ COMPUTERTALK FOR THE PHARMACIST—BUYERS GUIDE ISSUE
ComputerTalk Associates, Inc.
482 Norristown Rd., Ste. 112
Blue Bell, PA 19422   Phone: (215) 825-7686
Publication Includes: List of 40 retail pharmacy data processing system suppliers. All listings are paid. **Entries Include:** Company name, address, phone; number of installations, entry-level system configuration and price, software available, expandability, additional costs, length and cost of training period, largest system installed, map showing states where systems

are marketed, supplier's statement. **Frequency:** Annual, March. **Also Includes:** Table summarizing contents of listings.

★4055★ CONGRESS AND HEALTH: AN INTRODUCTION TO THE LEGISLATIVE PROCESS AND ITS KEY PARTICIPANTS
National Health Council
350 5th Ave., Ste. 1118
New York, NY 10118   Phone: (212) 268-8900
Publication Includes: List of key legislators in the United States Senate and House of Representatives concerned with health, and members of Senate and House committees and subcommittees on health, and their staffs. **Entries Include:** Name, address, phone; legislators' listings include photograph. **Frequency:** Biennial, July of odd years.

★4056★ CONSUMER HEALTH INFORMATION SOURCE BOOK
R. R. Bowker Co.
121 Chanlon Rd.
New Providence, NJ 07974   Phone: (908) 464-6800
Publication Includes: Names of publishers of over 700 reference books, pamphlets, and other materials on health education for lay persons. **Entries Include:** Publisher name, address. **Frequency:** Irregular; previous edition 1981; latest edition June 1984.

★4057★ CONSUMERS' GUIDE TO HOSPITALS
Consumers Checkbook
806 15th St. NW, Ste. 925
Washington, DC 20005   Phone: (202) 347-9612
Covers: Almost 6,000 acute-care hospitals. **Entries Include:** Hospital name, address, description of services, advanced teaching programs for doctors, university affiliation, death rate statistics. **Pages (approx.):** 200. **Frequency:** Published 1988, now out of print; new edition possible 1991.

★4058★ CONTACT LENS MANUFACTURERS ASSOCIATION— DIRECTORY OF MEMBERS
Contact Lens Manufacturers Association
421 King St., Ste. 224
Alexandria, VA 22314   Phone: (703) 739-0122
Number of Listings: 140. **Entries Include:** Company name, address, phone, name and title of contact. **Pages (approx.):** 30. **Frequency:** Annual, March.

★4059★ CONTACT LENSES-RETAIL DIRECTORY
American Business Directories, Inc.
American Business Information, Inc.
5711 S. 86th Circle
Omaha, NE 68127   Phone: (402) 593-4600
Number of Listings: 14,704. **Entries Include:** Name, address, phone (including area code), size of advertisement, year first in "Yellow Pages," name of owner or manager, number of employees. **Frequency:** Annual.

★4060★ CONTEMPORARY DIALYSIS AND NEPHROLOGY— BUYER'S GUIDE AND DIRECTORY ISSUE
Contemporary Dialysis, Inc.
20335 Ventura Blvd., Ste. 400
Woodland Hills, CA 91364   Phone: (818) 704-5555
Publication Includes: List of more than 400 manufacturers and suppliers of dialysis, nephrology, and transplantation products and services for renal care and a directory of renal care associations. **Entries Include:** For companies—Name of firm, address, phone, names and titles of key personnel, customer service and telex numbers, and coded product classification. For associations—Name of organization, address, phone, chief officers. **Frequency:** Annual, January. **Also Includes:** List of renal hospital units which are approved transplant centers, with statistics on recent year's kidney transplants performed.

★4061★ CONTEMPORARY LONG-TERM CARE—PRODUCT DIRECTORY AND BUYERS' GUIDE ISSUE
Bill Communications, Inc.
633 3rd Ave.
New York, NY 10017   Phone: (212) 984-2235
Publication Includes: Lists of over 900 manufacturers and suppliers of furnishings, products, equipment, and services for long-term patient care in nursing homes and retirement communities. **Entries Include:** Company name, address, phone, fax. **Frequency:** Annual, November.

★4062★ CORE COLLECTION IN NURSING AND THE ALLIED HEALTH SCIENCES: BOOKS, JOURNALS, MEDIA
Oryx Press
4041 N. Central, No. 700
Phoenix, AZ 85012-3397   Phone: (602) 265-2651
Publication Includes: Lists of publishers, distributors, and producers of print and non-print materials dealing with nursing and the allied health sciences. **Entries Include:** Publisher, distributor, or producer name, address, phone. **Frequency:** Latest edition 1990.

★4063★ COUNCIL FOR HEALTH AND HUMAN SERVICE MINISTRIES—DIRECTORY OF SERVICES
Council for Health and Human Service Ministries
760 Prospect Ave.
Cleveland, OH 44115   Phone: (216) 736-2250
Covers: About 250 social welfare agencies, retirement homes, children's residential homes, hospitals, and other health and human service facilities affiliated with the United Church of Christ. **Entries Include:** Agency name, type of institution and summary of services offered, certifications and memberships, name of chief administrator, mailing address, phone, and conference assignment. **Pages (approx.):** 90. **Frequency:** Irregular; latest edition 1989; new edition expected 1992.

★4064★ COUNCIL FOR INTERNATIONAL ORGANIZATIONS OF MEDICAL SCIENCES—ORGANIZATION, ACTIVITIES, MEMBERS
Council for International Organizations of Medical Sciences
c/o World Health Organization
20 avenue Appia
CH-1211 Geneva 27, Switzerland
Covers: Approximately 95 international and national organizations and associate members involved in the medical sciences. **Entries Include:** Organization name, address, names and titles of key personnel. **Pages (approx.):** 75. **Frequency:** Irregular; latest edition 1989.

★4065★ COUNSELLING AND PSYCHOTHERAPY RESOURCES DIRECTORY
British Association for Counselling
37a Sheep St.
Rugby, Warwickshire CV21 3BX, England
Covers: Approximately 2,500 national organizations, local independent agencies, counselors, and therapists offering counseling and psychotherapy services in the United Kingdom. **Entries Include:** Organization or individual name, address, phone. **Pages (approx.):** 500. **Frequency:** Annual, June.

★4066★ THE COURAGE TO HEAL: A GUIDE FOR WOMEN SURVIVORS OF CHILD SEXUAL ABUSE
HarperCollins
10 E. 53rd St.
New York, NY 10022   Phone: (212) 207-7000
Publication Includes: List of organizations and support groups that provide assistance to women who were sexually abused as children; also includes publications dealing with child sexual abuse. **Entries Include:** Organization name, address, phone, geographical area served, description of services. **Frequency:** Irregular; most recent reprint, February 1990.

★4067★ CPA WORLD DIRECTORY OF OLD AGE
Longman Group UK Ltd.
Westgate House
The High
Harlow, Essex CM20 1YR, England
Publication Includes: List of old age advocacy groups and related organizations worldwide. **Entries Include:** Organization name, address, phone, leadership, membership, history, policies, budget, and international affiliations. **Frequency:** Latest edition 1989. **Available in the U.S. from:** St. James Press, 233 E. Ontario St., Ste. 600, Chicago, IL 60611 (312-787-5800).

★4068★ CRCD INFORMATION DIRECTORY: REHABILITATION TREATMENT CENTRES FOR PHYSICALLY DISABLED PERSONS IN CANADA
Canadian Rehabilitation Council for the Disabled
45 Sheppard Ave. E., Ste. 801
Toronto, ON, Canada M2N 5W9   Phone: (416) 250-7490
Covers: 70 Centers. **Entries Include:** Center name, address, phone, names and titles of key executives or contacts, services provided, specialized programs and facilities, average caseload per day, restrictions concerning clients served, organizational structure, source of funding. **Pages (approx.):** 120. **Frequency:** latest edition 1984; suspended indefinitely.

★4069★ CRITICAL CARE CHOICES
Springhouse Corp.
1111 Bethlehem Pike
Springhouse, PA 19477   Phone: (215) 646-8700
Covers: Non-profit and investor-owned hospitals and departments of the United States government that hire critical care nurses. Does not report specific positions available. **Entries Include:** Unit name, location, areas of nursing specialization, educational requirements for nurses, licensing, facilities, benefits. **Pages (approx.):** 145. **Frequency:** Annual, May.

★4070★ CURRENT ISSUES: CHILD ABUSE
Omnigraphics, Inc.
Penobscot Bldg.
645 Griswold, 24th Fl.
Detroit, MI 48226   Phone: (313) 961-1340
Publication Includes: Lists of contacts to whom suspected child abuse should be reported, resource materials on child abuse, and related organizations. **Entries Include:** Agency, distributor, or organization name, address, phone. **Frequency:** Published 1990.

★4071★ CURRENT MEDICAL AND HEALTH-RELATED PERIODICALS PUBLISHED IN THE WESTERN PACIFIC REGION OF THE WORLD HEALTH ORGANIZATION—A DIRECTORY
Regional Office for the Western Pacific
World Health Organization
Box 2932
Manila 1099, Philippines
Number of Listings: Over 1,200. **Entries Include:** Title, name of publisher or sponsoring organization, address, frequency of publication, date of first issue, and outside publications that index the periodical. **Pages (approx.):** 285. **Frequency:** Irregular; latest edition 1983.

★4072★ DATA RESOURCES IN GERONTOLOGY: A DIRECTORY OF SELECTED INFORMATION VENDORS, DATABASES, AND ARCHIVES
Gerontological Society of America
1275 K St., NW, Ste. 350
Washington, DC 20005-4006   Phone: (202) 842-1275
Covers: Approximately 50 vendors of database access/information sources, bibliographic or reference databases, and data archives related to aging; regional census offices; state agencies, universities, libraries, and regional and local governments that provide census information. **Entries Include:** For vendors—Company name, address, phone, description of products and services. For regional census offices—Name, address, phone, geographical area served. For others—Name, address, phone, name and title of contact, geographical area served. **Pages (approx.):** 35. **Frequency:** Published August 1989.

★4073★ DENTAL CLINICS DIRECTORY
American Business Directories, Inc.
American Business Information, Inc.
5711 S. 86th Circle
Omaha, NE 68127   Phone: (402) 593-4600
Number of Listings: 18,607. **Entries Include:** Name, address, phone, size of advertisement, name of owner or manager, number of employees, year first in "Yellow Pages." **Frequency:** Annual.

★4074★ DENTAL EQUIPMENT AND SUPPLIES WHOLESALERS/MANUFACTURERS DIRECTORY
American Business Directories, Inc.
American Business Information, Inc.
5711 S. 86th Circle
Omaha, NE 68127   Phone: (402) 593-4600
Number of Listings: 2,172. **Entries Include:** Name, address, phone, size of advertisement, name of owner or manager, number of employees, year first in "Yellow Pages." **Frequency:** Annual.

★4075★ DENTAL LABORATORIES DIRECTORY
American Business Directories, Inc.
American Business Information, Inc.
5711 S. 86th Circle
Omaha, NE 68127   Phone: (402) 593-4600
Number of Listings: 11,659. **Entries Include:** Name, address, phone (including area code), size of advertisement, year first in "Yellow Pages," name of owner or manager, number of employees. **Frequency:** Annual.

★4076★ DENTAL SCHOOLS OF THE WORLD
Office of International Affairs
American Dental Association
211 E. Chicago Ave.
Chicago, IL 60611   Phone: (312) 440-2726
Covers: 155 institutions affiliated with dentistry worldwide. **Entries Include:** Institution name, address. **Pages (approx.):** 25. **Frequency:** Irregular; latest edition January 1984; new edition expected 1990.

★4077★ DENTAL SUPPLIES
Theta Corp.
Theta Bldg.
Middlefield, CT 06455   Phone: (203) 349-1054
Publication Includes: List of about 20 dental supplies companies. **Entries Include:** Company name, address, phone, key personnel, background information, sales, market shares, distribution, product development, marketing strategy, corporate outlook. **Frequency:** Irregular; previous edition November 1987; latest edition February 1990.

★4078★ DENTAL TECHNICIAN YEARBOOK AND DIRECTORY
A. E. Morgan Publications Ltd.
Stanley House
9 West St.
Epsom, Surrey KT18 7RL, England
Covers: About 25 dental associations, over 1,660 laboratories, and 200 manufacturers and suppliers of dental products and equipment in the United Kingdom. **Entries Include:** For associations—Name; name, title, and address of contact; background, description of membership, founding date. For manufacturers and suppliers—Company name, address, phone, telex, subsidiary and branch names and locations. For laboratories—Name, address, phone. **Pages (approx.):** 164. **Frequency:** Annual, January. **Also Includes:** List of dental conferences and seminars, with dates and locations.

★4079★ DENTISTRY JOURNALS AND SERIALS: AN ANALYTICAL GUIDE
Greenwood Publishing Group, Inc.
88 Post Rd. W.
PO Box 5007
Westport, CT 06881   Phone: (203) 226-3571
Publication Includes: Lists of publishers of English-language serials and journals, database suppliers, and publishers of microforms and reprints. **Entries Include:** Publisher or supplier name, address. **Frequency:** Published 1985.

★4080★ DENTISTS DIRECTORY
American Business Directories, Inc.
American Business Information, Inc.
5711 S. 86th Circle
Omaha, NE 68127   Phone: (402) 593-4600
Number of Listings: 163,104. **Entries Include:** Name, address, phone (including area code), size of advertisement, code indicating specialty, year first in "Yellow Pages," name of owner or manager, number of employees. **Frequency:** Annual.

★4081★ DENTISTS REGISTER
General Dental Council
37 Wimpole St.
London W1M 8DQ, England
Covers: Registered dentists in the United Kingdom. **Entries Include:** Name, address, date of registration, qualifications. **Pages (approx.):** 480. **Frequency:** Annual, June.

★4082★ DIAGNOSTIC IMAGING CENTERS DIRECTORY
SMG Marketing Group, Inc.
1342 N. LaSalle Dr.
Chicago, IL 60610   Phone: (312) 642-3026
Covers: About 1,200 hospital-based, freestanding, and mobile diagnostic imaging centers in the United States. **Entries Include:** Center or hospital name, address, phone, type of unit, equipment utilized. **Pages (approx.):** 200. **Frequency:** Annual, August.

★4083★ DIAL 800 FOR HEALTH
People's Medical Society
462 Walnut St.
Allentown, PA 18102   Phone: (215) 770-1670
Covers: Health related organizations providing toll-free numbers. **Entries Include:** Organization name, location, toll-free phone number, geographi-

cal area served, description of service. **Pages (approx.):** 70. **Frequency:** Published 1987.

★4084★ DIALYSIS AND TRANSPLANTATION—BUYER'S GUIDE/REFERENCE ISSUE
Dialysis & Transplantation, Inc.
7628 Densmore Ave.
Van Nuys, CA 91406   Phone: (818) 782-7328
Publication Includes: List of suppliers of products, equipment, and services used in dialysis treatments and kidney transplants; "The List of Transient Dialysis Centers"; directory of renal transplant centers; organ procurement facilities; and dialysis and transplant organizations. **Entries Include:** For suppliers of products, equipment, and services—Company name, address, phone, name and title of contact, brief description of products or services. **Frequency:** Annual, July.

★4085★ DICTIONNAIRE DES MEDICAMENTS VETERINAIRES
Editions du Point Veterinaire
25 rue Bourgelat
F-94700 Maisons-Alfort, France
Publication Includes: List of laboratories, manufacturers, and distributors of veterinary medicines. **Entries Include:** Name of company, address, phone, telex, product, trade name, logo. **Frequency:** Biennial.

★4086★ DICTIONNAIRE VIDAL
Office de Vulgarisation Pharmaceutique
11, rue Quentin-Bauchart
F-75384 Paris Cedex 08, France
Publication Includes: List of manufacturers of drugs, pharmaceuticals, personal hygiene products, medical and surgical equipment, and disinfectants; international coverage. **Entries Include:** Laboratory name, address, phone, products. **Frequency:** Annual, April; quarterly supplements. **Also Includes:** Description of drug interactions; list of drugs prohibited by the International Olympic Committee for the 1984 Olympic games.

★4087★ DIETITIANS REGISTER
Dietitians Board
184 Kennington Park Rd.
London SE11 4BU, England
Covers: Dietitians in the United Kingdom and overseas. **Entries Include:** Personal name, address, qualifications, and courses. **Pages (approx.):** 60. **Frequency:** Annual, July.

★4088★ DIFFERENT DRUMMER: HOMOSEXUALITY IN AMERICA
Julian A. Messner
Silver Burdett Press
190 Sylvan Ave.
Englewood Cliffs, NJ 07632   Phone: (201) 461-4969
Publication Includes: List of resource centers that provide information on Acquired Immune Deficiency Syndrome (AIDS). **Pages (approx.):** 115. **Frequency:** Published April 1986. **Also Includes:** Bibliography. **Send Orders to:** Simon and Schuster, 20 Old Tappan Rd., Old Tappan, NJ 07675.

★4089★ DIRECTORIO PROFESIONAL HISPANO
Blanca Balbi
PO Box 408
Flushing, NY 11352   Phone: (718) 762-1432
Covers: About 3,500 Hispanic doctors, optometrists, dentists, lawyers, architects, and accountants, with offices in the eastern United States. **Entries Include:** Name, address, phone. **Pages (approx.):** 100. **Frequency:** Annual, July.

★4090★ DIRECTORY OF ADULT DAY CARE IN AMERICA
National Institute on Adult Daycare
National Council on the Aging, Inc.
600 Maryland Ave., SW, West Wing 100
Washington, DC 20024   Phone: (202) 479-1200
Covers: Nearly 850 adult day care centers in the United States; 40 state adult day care associations. **Entries Include:** For centers—Name, address, phone, name and title of contact, description of services and facilities, number of employees. For associations—Name, address, phone, name and title of contact. **Pages (approx.):** 150. **Frequency:** Irregular; previous edition 1987; latest edition summer 1990.

★4091★ DIRECTORY OF ADVENTURE ALTERNATIVES IN CORRECTIONS, MENTAL HEALTH AND SPECIAL POPULATIONS
Association for Experiential Education
PO Box 249-CU
Boulder, CO 80309   Phone: (303) 492-1547
Covers: About 115 organizations and agencies providing programs that link traditional therapeutic strategies with alternative practices to treat children and adults who have corrections, substance abuse, or mental health problems, or are physically or mentally handicapped. Entries Include: Organization name, address, phone, name of director, description of program, and coded indication of target population location, sex, and age. Pages (approx.): 60. Frequency: Irregular; previous edition 1985; latest edition 1988.

★4092★ DIRECTORY OF AGENCIES AND ORGANIZATIONS SERVING DEAF-BLIND INDIVIDUALS
Helen Keller National Center
111 Middle Neck Rd.
Sands Point, NY 11050   Phone: (516) 944-8900
Covers: Approximately 440 public and private agencies that provide programs and services for deaf-blind persons. Entries Include: Agency name, address, phone, names and titles of key personnel, geographical area served, financial data, requirements for eligibility, description of services. Pages (approx.): 200. Frequency: Published 1987; annual updates.

★4093★ DIRECTORY OF ALCOHOL AND DRUG TREATMENT RESOURCES IN ONTARIO
Addiction Research Foundation
33 Russell St.
Toronto, ON, Canada M5S 2S1   Phone: (416) 595-6000
Frequency: Irregular; previous edition 1985; latest edition spring 1991.

★4094★ DIRECTORY OF AMERICAN BAPTIST RETIREMENT HOMES, HOSPITALS, NURSING HOMES, CHILDREN'S HOMES AND SPECIAL SERVICES
American Baptist Homes and Hospitals Association
Box 851
Valley Forge, PA 19482   Phone: (215) 768-2382
Covers: About 90 member American Baptist related retirement, nursing, and children's homes and hospitals. Entries Include: Institution name, address, phone, facilities available. Frequency: Annual.

★4095★ DIRECTORY OF ANIMAL DISEASE DIAGNOSTIC LABORATORIES
National Veterinary Services Laboratories
Animal and Plant Health Inspection Service
U.S. Department of Agriculture
PO Box 844
Ames, IA 50010   Phone: (515) 239-8571
Number of Listings: 200. Entries Include: Laboratory name, address, description of services. Pages (approx.): 235. Frequency: Biennial, January of odd years.

★4096★ DIRECTORY—AVIATION MEDICAL EXAMINERS
Office of Aviation Medicine
Federal Aviation Administration
Aeronautical Center
Box 25082
Oklahoma City, OK 73125   Phone: (405) 680-4881
Covers: Physicians who are authorized to perform physical examinations and issue airman medical certificates for the Administrator of the Federal Aviation Administration. Available as a "consolidated" directory covering all of the United States, or in 10 regional directories covering Alaska, Northwest Mountain, Western Pacific, Great Lakes, Central, Southwest, New England, Eastern, and Southern areas, and International. Also includes military installations where FAA exams may be administered for military personnel. Entries Include: For physicians—Name, address, phone, class of exams authorized to conduct, year authorized to administer exams, whether an accident investigator. For military installations— Name, address. Pages (approx.): Consolidated directory, 370; regional directories, 70 each. Frequency: Annual, late in year.

★4097★ DIRECTORY OF AWARDS, BHPR SUPPORT, FISCAL YEAR 1989
U.S. Bureau of Health Professions
Rockville, MD 20857   Phone: (301) 443-6936
Covers: Several hundred institutions having education programs in conventional and osteopathic medicine, dentistry, optometry, pharmacy,

podiatry, veterinary medicine, nursing, allied health professions, and public health, which are funded through awards of the Bureau of Health Professions. Entries Include: Institution name, grant number, name of contact, program title, number of awards, total amount awarded. Pages (approx.): 270. Frequency: Annual; covers previous fiscal year. Send Orders to: National Technical Information Service, Springfield, VA 22161.

★4098★ DIRECTORY OF BILINGUAL SPEECH-LANGUAGE PATHOLOGISTS AND AUDIOLOGISTS
American Speech-Language-Hearing Association
10801 Rockville Pike
Rockville, MD 20852   Phone: (301) 897-5700
Covers: More than 900 members who have speaking proficiency in English and at least one other language. Entries Include: Personal name, address, phone, area of certification (i.e. speech-language pathology, audiology, or both). Pages (approx.): 65. Frequency: Biennial, even years.

★4099★ DIRECTORY OF BIOMEDICAL AND HEALTH CARE GRANTS
Oryx Press
4041 N. Central, No. 700
Phoenix, AZ 85012   Phone: (602) 265-2651
Covers: More than 2,000 federal, state, and private grant programs in health and related fields. Entries Include: Program name, sponsor name and address, description, requirements, amount of grant, application deadline, renewal information; federal programs include Catalog of Federal Domestic Assistance program number. Pages (approx.): 700. Frequency: Approximately annual; latest edition 1990.

★4100★ DIRECTORY OF BLUE CROSS AND BLUE SHIELD PLANS
Blue Cross and Blue Shield Association
676 St. Clair
Chicago, IL 60611   Phone: (312) 440-6000
Covers: About 100 providers of Blue Cross and Blue Shield plans. Entries Include: NAP and name of chief executive. Pages (approx.): 25. Frequency: Semiannual, January and June.

★4101★ DIRECTORY OF CANADIAN ORGANIZATIONS INVOLVED IN FOOD AND NUTRITION
Ryerson Polytechnical Institute
350 Victoria St., L-284
Toronto, ON, Canada M5B 2K3
Frequency: Latest edition 1982.

★4102★ DIRECTORY OF CERTIFIED HEALTH CARE ENGINEERING PROFESSIONALS
International Certification Commission for Instrumentation Clinical Engineering and Biomedical Technology
c/o Association for Advancement of Medical
3330 Washington Blvd., Ste. 400
Arlington, VA 22201   Phone: (703) 525-4890
Covers: Nearly 3,000 clinical engineers, and engineering technicians and technologists in health care fields. Entries Include: Name, address, phone, certification number, level of certification. Pages (approx.): 80. Frequency: Irregular; latest edition September 1985; new edition possible 1988. Also Includes: Necrology and list of certified professionals whose addresses are not known.

★4103★ DIRECTORY OF CERTIFIED HEALTHCARE SAFETY PROFESSIONALS
International Healthcare Safety Professional Certification Board
8009 Carita Ct.
Bethesda, MD 20817   Phone: (301) 984-8969
Covers: About 300 persons "working in a medical activity (or similar functions) who are charged with responsibility for hazard control activities." Entries Include: Name, address (often with affiliation), phone, title. Pages (approx.): 20. Frequency: Irregular; previous edition spring 1987; latest edition fall 1989.

★4104★ DIRECTORY OF CERTIFIED OPHTHALMIC MEDICAL PERSONNEL
Joint Commission on Allied Health Personnel in Ophthalmology
2025 Woodlane Dr.
St. Paul, MN 55125-2995   Phone: (612) 731-2944
Covers: About 7,000 certified ophthalmic medical personnel trained to assist ophthalmologists in various medical procedures involving eye care. Entries Include: Name, address, code indicating level of certification, codes

indicating whether a member of the Association of Technical Personnel in Ophthalmology or American Association of Certified Orthoptists. **Pages (approx.):** 105. **Frequency:** Annual, May.

★4105★   DIRECTORY OF CHILD LIFE PROGRAMS IN NORTH AMERICA
Association for the Care of Children's Health
7910 Woodmont Ave., Ste. 300
Bethesda, MD 20814   Phone: (301) 654-6549
Covers: Approximately 350 pediatric health programs. **Entries Include:** Department name, name and address of hospital, department phone, name of contact, average number of patients, pediatric age range, staff number and training level, program times, number of activity centers, source of funding, administrative structure, student internship availability, initial year of program. **Pages (approx.):** 90. **Frequency:** Triennial; new edition expected 1993.

★4106★   DIRECTORY OF COLLEGE FACILITIES AND SERVICES FOR PEOPLE WITH DISABILITIES
Oryx Press
4041 N. Central, No. 700
Phoenix, AZ 85012   Phone: (602) 265-2651
Covers: Approximately 1,600 universities and colleges with facilities for disabled students. **Entries Include:** Institution name, address, phone, name and title of contact; institution type, degrees offered, enrollment; campus facilities (including those that are handicapped accessible); services provided for specific disability groups. **Pages (approx.):** 361. **Frequency:** Irregular; previous edition 1986; latest edition 1991. **Also Includes:** Bibliography; list of 66 national associations and centers concerned with disabilities; list of 15 clearing houses and databases (with address and phone); list of nearly 150 grant programs for higher education institutions with disabled student programs, including program description, restrictions, requirements, amount of grant, dates for application, sponsor.

★4107★   DIRECTORY OF COMMUNITY BLOOD CENTERS
American Association of Blood Banks
1117 N. 19th St., Ste. 600
Arlington, VA 22209   Phone: (703) 528-8200
Covers: About 130 community blood centers throughout the states and in Puerto Rico; institutional members of the Council of Community Blood Centers, the American R ed Cross Blood Services, and the American Association of Blood Banks. **Entries Include:** For community blood centers—Name, main address, phone; subcenter addresses and phone numbers; number of employees (including part-time), names and titles of key staff members; budget; counties, hospitals, and population served; rates of blood draw and outdate; number of blood products produced by type. For association members—Institution name, address, phone. **Pages (approx.):** 145. **Frequency:** Biennial, summer of odd years.

★4108★   DIRECTORY OF CREDENTIALS IN COUNSELING AND PSYCHOTHERAPY
G. K. Hall & Co.
70 Lincoln St.
Boston, MA 02111   Phone: (617) 423-3990
Covers: About 60 organizations issuing certification in various aspects of counseling and psychotherapy. **Entries Include:** Organization name, address, phone, titles conferred, certification requirements, training available. **Pages (approx.):** 300. **Frequency:** First edition November 1989.

★4109★   DIRECTORY OF CROSS-CULTURAL RESEARCH AND RESEARCHERS
International Association for Cross-Cultural Psychology
Wake Forest University
PO Box 7778, Reynolds Sta.
Psychology Department
Winston-Salem, NC 27109   Phone: (919) 759-5424
Covers: Researchers in psychology, anthropology, and psychiatry with an interest in the development of comparative dimensions in behavioral sciences. **Entries Include:** Name, address, phone, telex, fax, areas of interest. **Pages (approx.):** 30. **Frequency:** Irregular, latest edition 1988.

★4110★   DIRECTORY OF DENTAL EDUCATORS
American Association of Dental Schools
1625 Massachusetts Ave. NW
Washington, DC 20036   Phone: (202) 667-9433
Covers: About 15,000 full- and part-time faculty members at 60 United States and 10 Canadian dental schools. **Entries Include:** Name, academic rank, primary discipline, degrees, whether full- or part-time; title is shown

for administrative personnel. **Pages (approx.):** 230. **Frequency:** Biennial, spring of even years.

★4111★   DIRECTORY OF DEPARTMENTS OF ANATOMY OF THE UNITED STATES AND CANADA
American Association of Anatomists
1430 Tulane Ave.
New Orleans, LA 70112   Phone: (504) 584-2727
Covers: About 2,800 anatomy department faculty members in about 190 colleges of medicine, dentistry, osteopathic, and veterinary medicine in the United States and Canada. **Entries Include:** Name, office address and phone, academic rank, highest degree held and granting institution, teaching and research interests. **Pages (approx.):** 195. **Frequency:** Irregular; latest edition 1987; new edition expected 1991.

★4112★   DIRECTORY OF DIETETIC PROGRAMS
American Dietetic Association
216 W. Jackson Blvd., Ste. 800
Chicago, IL 60606-6995   Phone: (312) 899-0040
Covers: About 600 approved or accredited dietetic education programs. **Entries Include:** Institution name, department name, address, phone, name and title of contact, program concentration. **Pages (approx.):** 55. **Frequency:** Annual, August.

★4113★   DIRECTORY OF DIGESTIVE DISEASES ORGANIZATIONS
National Digestive Diseases Information Clearinghouse
Box NDDIC
9000 Rockville Pike
Bethesda, MD 20892   Phone: (301) 468-6344
Covers: Lay and voluntary, and professional digestive disease and digestive disease-related organizations. **Entries Include:** Organization name, address, phone, purpose, publications, and other materials provided. **Pages (approx.):** 7 (in two volumes). **Frequency:** Approximately biennial; latest edition April 1991.

★4114★   DIRECTORY FOR DISABLED PEOPLE: A HANDBOOK OF INFORMATION AND OPPORTUNITIES FOR DISABLED AND HANDICAPPED PEOPLE
Woodhead-Faulkner Ltd.
Fitzwilliam House
32 Trumpington St.
Cambridge CB2 1QY, England
Covers: Firms and other organizations in the United Kingdom providing services to or concerned with handicapped and disabled persons. **Entries Include:** Organization name, address, phone, services or activities. **Pages (approx.):** 370. **Frequency:** Irregular; latest edition February 1988. **Available in the U.S. from:** Longwood, 51 Washington St., Dover, NH 03820.

★4115★   DIRECTORY OF EDUCATIONAL SOFTWARE FOR NURSING
National League of Nursing
350 Hudson St.
New York, NY 10014   Phone: (212) 989-9393
Covers: Suppliers of over 400 instructional IBM and Apple compatible software packages in the area of health care. **Entries Include:** Program title, supplier name, address, phone, description of program, style of instruction, hardware compatibility, price; ratings on quality, interest, accessibility, and micro attributes. **Pages (approx.):** 745. **Frequency:** Biennial.

★4116★   DIRECTORY OF EPISCOPAL FACILITIES FOR THE ELDERLY
Episcopal Society for Ministry on Aging
323 Wyandotte St.
Bethlehem, PA 18015   Phone: (215) 868-5400
Covers: About 100 hospitals, nursing homes, retirement homes, and other facilities for the aging sponsored by the Episcopal Church. **Entries Include:** Name of facility, address, phone, name of administrator; number of beds or units, type of care provided. **Pages (approx.):** 85. **Frequency:** Latest edition September 1985.

★4117★   DIRECTORY OF ETHNIC MINORITY PROFESSIONALS IN PSYCHOLOGY
American Psychological Association
Office of Ethnic Minority Affairs
1200 17th St. NW
Washington, DC 20036   Phone: (202) 955-7763
Covers: Over 2,000 ethnic minority psychologists nationwide and in Puerto

Rico. **Entries Include:** Company name, address, phone. **Pages (approx.):** 264. **Frequency:** Latest edition January 1991; new edition expected 1992.

★4118★ DIRECTORY OF THE EUROPEAN ASSOCIATION FOR CANCER RESEARCH
European Association for Cancer Research
Cancer Research Campaign Laboratories
University of Nottingham
Nottingham NG7 2RD, England
Covers: About 1,400 members active in cancer research and holding academic degrees. **Entries Include:** Member name, address, phone, fax, areas of interest. **Pages (approx.):** 100. **Frequency:** Latest edition 1991.

★4119★ DIRECTORY FOR EXCEPTIONAL CHILDREN
Porter Sargent Publishers, Inc.
11 Beacon St., Ste. 1400
Boston, MA 02108   Phone: (617) 523-1670
Covers: Over 3,000 public and private schools, clinics, and treatment centers for children and young adults with emotional, developmental, and organic disabilities; includes lists of governmental and private agencies, associations, etc. **Entries Include:** Name of facility, address, names of key personnel, primary and secondary handicaps accepted, enrollment; list of faculty with specialties, fees, financial assistance available, therapies conducted, treatment emphases, educational activities. **Pages (approx.):** 1,400. **Frequency:** Approximately biennial; latest edition January 1990.

★4120★ DIRECTORY OF FACILITIES OBLIGATED TO PROVIDE UNCOMPENSATED SERVICES
Bureau of Health Resources Development
Health Resources and Services Administration
U.S. Public Health Service
5600 Fishers Ln., Rm. 11-03
Rockville, MD 20857   Phone: (301) 443-5656
Covers: About 2,750 hospitals and other health care facilities that are obligated to provide some uncompensated services to patients as payment for loans disbursed through the Public Health Service under the Hospital Survey and Construction Act of 1946, as amended. **Entries Include:** Facility name, city, county, facility ID number, type of facility, type of control, year obligation expires. **Pages (approx.):** 125. **Frequency:** Annual, January.

★4121★ DIRECTORY OF FACILITIES AND SERVICES FOR THE LEARNING DISABLED
Academic Therapy Publications
20 Commercial Blvd.
Novato, CA 94949   Phone: (415) 883-3314
Covers: About 500 facilities which help children and adults with diagnosed learning disabilities; publishers and producers of books and other materials; organizations and agencies; educational journals; special education technology clearing houses. **Entries Include:** For facilities—Name, address, phone, name of director, number of staff, and coded information describing type of facility (educational, summer camp, etc.), age ranges accepted, whether coed, day-length of program, fee information, and related professional services provided. For other listings—Name, address, phone. **Pages (approx.):** 185. **Frequency:** Biennial, spring of odd years.

★4122★ DIRECTORY OF FAMILY PLANNING GRANTEES, DELEGATES, AND CLINICS
Family Life Information Exchange
PO Box 37299
Washington, DC 20013-7299   Phone: (301) 585-6636
Covers: About 4,500 family planning clinics and recipients of grants funded by Title X of the Public Health Service Act through the Department of Health and Human Services. **Entries Include:** Name, address. **Pages (approx.):** 170. **Frequency:** Irregular; previous edition 1989; latest edition 1991-1992.

★4123★ DIRECTORY OF FAMILY PRACTICE RESIDENCY PROGRAMS
American Academy of Family Physicians
1740 W. 92nd St.
Kansas City, MO 64114   Phone: (816) 333-9700
Covers: Over 380 accredited residency programs in family practice. **Entries Include:** Name of program; name and phone of director; name of primary care hospital and its size; number of residents, remuneration and benefits, faculty to resident ratio, level of responsibility for residents. **Pages (approx.):** 775. **Frequency:** Annual, February.

★4124★ DIRECTORY OF GRADUATE MEDICAL EDUCATION PROGRAMS
American Medical Association
515 N. State St.
Chicago, IL 60610   Phone: (312) 464-5000
Covers: About 6,500 residency and fellowship programs accredited by the Accreditation Council for Graduate Medical Education. **Entries Include:** Program name, name and address of director, specialty, requirements, length of program, names of teaching hospitals. **Pages (approx.):** 760. **Frequency:** Annual, March.

★4125★ DIRECTORY OF HEALTH CARE COALITIONS IN THE UNITED STATES
Office of Health Coalitions and Private Sector Initiatives
American Hospital Association (AHA)
840 N. Lake Shore Dr.
Chicago, IL 60611   Phone: (312) 280-6124
Covers: Over 175 health care coalitions, including business coalitions on health, purchasing alliances, health action councils, and others with unified interests in health care. **Entries Include:** Organization name, address, phone, name and title of contact, organizational status, year established, geographic area served, groups and organizations involved in the coalition, materials produced, annual cash budget, dues, and activities and issues being addressed. **Pages (approx.):** 400. **Frequency:** Annual, January; supplements in spring and fall.

★4126★ DIRECTORY OF HEALTH CARE GROUP PURCHASING ORGANIZATIONS
McKnight Medical Communications, Inc.
1419 Lake Cook Rd.
Deerfield, IL 60015   Phone: (708) 945-0345
Covers: About 275 hospital and nursing home materials purchasing groups. **Entries Include:** Name and location of buying group, total number of beds in each group, approximate dollar expenditures, executives' and purchasing directors' names, number and names of institutions represented. **Pages (approx.):** 400. **Frequency:** Annual, spring.

★4127★ DIRECTORY OF HEALTH CARE HUMAN RESOURCE CONSULTANTS
American Society for Healthcare Human Resources Administration
c/o American Hospital Association
840 N. Lake Shore Dr.
Chicago, IL 60611   Phone: (312) 280-6000
Covers: More than 60 human resource consultants and suppliers of related services to the health care industry; international coverage. **Entries Include:** Company name, address, phone, names and titles of key personnel, branch office or subsidiary names and addresses, geographical area served, and description of services. **Pages (approx.):** 35. **Frequency:** Annual, spring.

★4128★ DIRECTORY OF HEALTH CENTRES
Longman Group UK Ltd.
Longman House
Burnt Mill
Harlow, Essex CM20 2JE, England
Covers: Over 1,300 health centers in the United Kingdom, including dental and community nursing care institutions. **Entries Include:** Institution name, address, phone, names and titles of key personnel, services and facilities available. **Pages (approx.):** 500.

★4129★ DIRECTORY OF HEALTH AND WELFARE MINISTRIES
General Board of Global Ministries
United Methodist Church
475 Riverside Dr., Rm. 350
New York, NY 10115   Phone: (212) 870-3871
Covers: 70 hospitals, 65 child care agencies, and 180 long-term care agencies related to the United Methodist Church. **Entries Include:** Institution name, address, phone, name of executive, list of services. **Pages (approx.):** 45. **Frequency:** Irregular; previous edition 1984; latest edition 1987. **Send Orders to:** The Service Center, General Board of Global Ministries, United Methodist Church, 7820 Reading Rd., Cincinnati, OH 45237.

★4130★ DIRECTORY OF HOLISTIC MEDICINE AND ALTERNATIVE HEALTH CARE SERVICES IN THE U.S.
Health Plus Publishers
PO Box 1027
Sherwood, OR 97140   Phone: (503) 625-0589
Covers: Nearly 1,100 health professionals, such as osteopaths, other

225

physicians, nurses, chiropractors, dentists, nutrition consultants, and clinics and health centers involved in holistic medicine; associations, foundations, and schools and institutes that have courses in holistic medicine. **Entries Include:** For practitioners—Name, address, phone, services provided, hospital affiliation; some entries also include memberships and school from which degree obtained. For associations and schools—Name, address. **Pages (approx.):** 265. **Frequency:** Irregular; latest edition 1986.

**★4131★   DIRECTORY OF HOMEMAKER-HOME HEALTH
     AIDE SERVICES—ACCREDITED/APPROVED**
National HomeCaring Council, Division
Foundation for Hospice and Homecare
519 C St., NE
Washington, DC 20002   Phone: (202) 547-6586
Covers: Local programs supplying homemaker-home health aid services which are accredited/approved by the Council. **Entries Include:** Agency name, address, phone. **Pages (approx.):** 10. **Frequency:** Semiannual, April and September.

★4132★   DIRECTORY OF HORMONAL CONTRACEPTIVES
International Planned Parenthood Federation
Regent's College
Inner Circle
Regent's Park
London NW1 4NS, England
Publication Includes: List of approximately 10 major manufacturers of hormonal contraceptives worldwide. **Entries Include:** Company name, address, brand names, hormonal composition, availability. **Frequency:** Irregular; previous edition 1981; latest edition 1988.

**★4133★   DIRECTORY OF HOSPITAL INFORMATION SYSTEM
     PRODUCTS**
Richard Sneider
29 Crafts St., Ste. 380
Newton, MA 02160   Phone: (617) 965-7075
Covers: Over 150 hardware and software suppliers for hospital information systems. **Entries Include:** Company name, address, phone, product line, number of previous installations, annual sales. **Frequency:** Irregular; latest edition 1986.

★4134★   DIRECTORY OF HOSPITAL PERSONNEL
Medical Device Register
5 Paragon Dr.
Montvale, NJ 07645-1725
Covers: 110,000 executives at 7,000 U.S. hospitals. **Entries Include:** Name of hospital, address, phone, number of beds, type and JACHO status of hospital, names and titles of key department heads and staff. **Pages (approx.):** 1,100. **Frequency:** Annual, latest edition December 1990.

**★4135★   DIRECTORY OF HOSPITAL PSYCHOSOCIAL
     POLICIES AND PROGRAMS**
Association for the Care of Children's Health
7910 Woodmont Ave., Ste. 300
Bethesda, MD 20814   Phone: (301) 654-6549
Covers: Psychosocial profiles of approximately 300 hospitals in the U.S. and Canada. **Entries Include:** Hospital name, address, phone, contact information, and description of institution's policies and programs involving psychological and social concerns. **Pages (approx.):** 128. **Frequency:** Latest edition 1988. **Also Includes:** Comparisons between survey data compiled in 1981 and 1988, and a list of hospitals offering "innovative" policies or services.

★4136★   DIRECTORY OF HOSPITALS
SMG Marketing Group Inc.
1342 N. LaSalle Dr.
Chicago, IL 60610   Phone: (312) 642-3026
Covers: Over 7,600 hospitals in the United States. **Entries Include:** Hospital name, address, phone, geographic service area, description of services. **Pages (approx.):** 500. **Frequency:** Annual, January.

★4137★   DIRECTORY OF HOSPITALS
Longman Group UK Ltd.
Westgate House, 6th Fl.
The High
Harlow, Essex CM20 1YR, England
Covers: Approximately 2,440 National Health Service hospitals in England, Wales, Scotland, and Northern Ireland; nearly 225 independent

hospitals throughout the United Kingdom. **Entries Include:** Hospital name, address, phone; type of facility, number of beds; specialties, name of specialties consultants. **Pages (approx.):** 310. **Frequency:** Annual, spring.

**★4138★   DIRECTORY OF HOTLINES AND CRISIS
     INTERVENTION CENTERS**
Covenant House
c/o Patricia Connors
346 W. 17th St.
New York, NY 10011   Phone: (212) 727-4000
Covers: About 2,150 crisis intervention and hotline programs. **Entries Include:** Name of program, address, phone, referral houses, ages served, brief service description. **Pages (approx.):** 230. **Frequency:** Irregular; previous edition 1986; latest edition 1989.

★4139★   DIRECTORY OF HYPERBARIC CHAMBERS
Undersea and Hyperbaric Medical Society
9650 Rockville Pike
Bethesda, MD 20814   Phone: (301) 571-1818
Covers: About 250 high pressure chambers for medical and other testing and research; coverage includes Canada. **Entries Include:** Institution or company name, address, phone; type of chamber, usage, availability. **Pages (approx.):** 26 (loose-leaf). **Frequency:** Irregular; latest edition July 1990; annual updates.

**★4140★   DIRECTORY OF INDEPENDENT HOSPITALS AND
     HEALTH SERVICES**
Longman Group UK Ltd.
Westgate House, 6th Fl.
The High
Harlow, Essex CM20 1YR, England
Covers: More than 10,000 independent hospitals, screening clinics, nursing and rest homes, private pathology laboratories, and major U.K. group owners in the United Kingdom. **Entries Include:** Name of institution, address, phone, contact name, number of beds, facilities available. **Pages (approx.):** 775. **Frequency:** Annual, December. **Also Includes:** Geographical list of private-room accommodations in National Health Service hospitals.

★4141★   DIRECTORY OF INFORMATION RESOURCES
National Arthritis and Musculoskeletal and Skin Diseases Information
   Clearinghouse
Box AMS
Bethesda, MD 20892   Phone: (301) 468-3235
Covers: About 130 organizations, clearinghouses, government agencies, international organizations, and databases with information regarding arthritis and musculoskeletal and skin diseases. **Entries Include:** Organization name, address, phone, description of purpose or activities, publications. **Pages (approx.):** 55. **Frequency:** Latest edition 1986.

**★4142★   DIRECTORY OF INFORMATION RESOURCES ON
     VICTIMIZATION OF WOMEN**
Response
4136 Leland St.
Chevy Chase, MD 20815   Phone: (301) 951-0039
Covers: Special libraries, clearinghouses, and online database offering resource information on women and children as victims of abuse. **Send Orders to:** Response, Box 2462, Ada, OK 74820.

**★4143★   DIRECTORY OF THE INTERNATIONAL FEDERATION
     OF ASSOCIATIONS OF ANATOMISTS**
International Federation of Associations of Anatomists
Institut fur Anatomie
Medizinizche Universitat zu Lubeck
Ratzeburger Alles 160
D-2400 Lubeck 1, Germany
Covers: 56 member associations. **Entries Include:** Organization name, address, phone, number of members, names and titles of officers, funding, publications. **Pages (approx.):** 140. **Frequency:** Irregular; latest edition 1990; new edition expected 1993. **Also Includes:** History and constitution of the federation.

**★4144★   DIRECTORY OF THE INTERNATIONAL FEDERATION
     OF SPORTS MEDICINE**
International Federation of Sports Medicine
Rua Felipe Becker 95
91330 Porto Alegre, Brazil
Covers: About 80 national branches worldwide. **Entries Include:** Executive

committee and commissions, history, by-laws, position statements. **Pages (approx.):** 115.

★4145★ DIRECTORY OF INTERNATIONAL FELLOWSHIPS AND GRANTS IN THE HEALTH SCIENCES
Fogarty International Center
U.S. National Institutes of Health
Bldg. 31, Rm. B2C39
Bethesda, MD 20892   Phone: (301) 496-1653
Covers: More than 180 agencies, foundations and organizations that provide fellowships and grants in biomedical and behavioral sciences for research abroad. **Entries Include:** Name of program sponsor, address, phone, name of grant, particular focus and purpose of program, financial provisions, duration of support, number of fellowships available, application dates; name and address of foundations abroad. **Pages (approx.):** 70. **Frequency:** Biennial, October of odd years.

★4146★ DIRECTORY OF INVESTOR-OWNED HOSPITALS, RESIDENTIAL TREATMENT FACILITIES AND CENTERS, HOSPITAL MANAGEMENT COMPANIES
Federation of American Health Systems
1405 N. Pierce, Ste. 311
Little Rock, AR 72207   Phone: (501) 661-9555
Covers: Approximately 1,500 investor-owned hospitals and over 80 hospital management companies in the United States and Puerto Rico. **Entries Include:** For hospitals—Name, address, phone, name of administrator, number of beds, code for name of parent company (if applicable). For management companies—Company name, address, phone, officers' names; names of hospitals owned, addresses, phone numbers, names of chief administrators, regional offices and subsidiaries. **Pages (approx.):** 300. **Frequency:** Annual, November.

★4147★ DIRECTORY OF LONG-TERM CARE CENTRES IN CANADA
Canadian Hospital Association
17 York St., Ste. 100
Ottawa, ON, Canada K1N 9J6   Phone: (613) 238-8005
Covers: More than 3,000 long-term care facilities; long-term care facilities in general and special hospitals; manufacturers and suppliers of equipment and supplies; health care organizations and education programs. **Entries Include:** Facility name, address, phone, type of facility, number of beds, names and titles of key personnel. **Pages (approx.):** 230. **Frequency:** Annual, September.

★4148★ DIRECTORY OF MEDICAL COMPUTER SYSTEMS
ComputerTalk Associates, Inc.
482 Norristown Rd., Ste. 112
Blue Bell, PA 19422   Phone: (215) 825-7686
Covers: About 100 medical office data processing system suppliers. All listings are paid. **Entries Include:** Company name, location, hardware used, software capabilities, price, expandability, number of installations. **Pages (approx.):** 70. **Frequency:** Three times per year; January, May, and September.

★4149★ DIRECTORY OF MEDICAL AND HEALTH CARE LIBRARIES IN THE UNITED KINGDOM AND REPUBLIC OF IRELAND
Library Association Publishing Ltd.
7 Ridgmount St.
London WC1E 7AE, England
Covers: About 950 libraries. **Entries Include:** Institution name, address, phone, names and titles of key personnel, number of staff, type of library, hours, permitted users, stocking and lending policies, holdings, special collections, classification system used, computer data retrieval facilities and fee (if any), network affiliations. **Pages (approx.):** 285. **Frequency:** Irregular; previous edition 1986; latest edition May 1990. **Also Includes:** Geographical listing of names and addresses of the 13 members of British National Health Services Librarians Group.

★4150★ DIRECTORY OF MEDICAL PRODUCTS DISTRIBUTORS AND MANUFACTURER'S REPRESENTATIVES
McKnight Medical Communications, Inc.
1419 Lake Cook Rd.
Deerfield, IL 60015   Phone: (708) 945-0345
Covers: Over 5,000 distributors of medical products, with over 2,000 wholesale/retail supply locations; 400 medical product manufacturers' representatives. **Entries Include:** Company name, address, branches, phone, name of principal executives, type of distributor (i.e., hospital

supply, rental, etc.), number of salesmen, financial data (keyed), area served, association affiliations. **Pages (approx.):** 400. **Frequency:** Annual, spring.

★4151★ DIRECTORY OF MEDICAL SCHOOLS WORLDWIDE
U.S. Directory Service, Publishers
655 NW 128th St.
PO Box 68-1700
Miami, FL 33168   Phone: (305) 769-1700
Covers: Nearly 1,200 medical schools in 100 countries. **Entries Include:** School name, address, phone, admissions requirements, curriculum, language, statistical data. **Frequency:** Irregular; latest edition 1987.

★4152★ DIRECTORY OF MEDICAL SPECIALISTS
Marquis Who's Who/Macmillan Directory Division
Macmillan, Inc.
3002 Glenview Rd.
Wilmette, IL 60091   Phone: (800) 621-9669
Covers: More than 350,000 board-certified specialists in over 20 areas of medical practice from allergy to urology. **Entries Include:** Name, office address, phone, date and place of birth, education, career data, date certified, type of practice, professional memberships, selected writings, awards, achievements. **Pages (approx.):** 5,806 (in three volumes). **Frequency:** Biennial, October of odd years. **Also Includes:** List of state licensing information resoures; overview of each medical specialty.

★4153★ DIRECTORY OF MOSQUITO CONTROL AGENCIES
American Mosquito Control Association
PO Box 5416
Lake Charles, LA 70606   Phone: (318) 474-2723
Covers: About 740 mosquito control agencies in the United States and Canada, of which about 150 control other disease carriers as well. **Entries Include:** Company name, address, phone, geographic area covered, methods used. **Pages (approx.):** 40. **Frequency:** Irregular; previous edition 1981; latest edition 1990.

★4154★ DIRECTORY OF NARCOTIC TREATMENT PROGRAMS
U.S. Food and Drug Administration
Rockville, MD 20857   Phone: (301) 443-3414
Covers: About 800 outpatient mental health centers, drug treatment centers, and methadone clinics; and inpatient detoxification centers and hospitals. **Entries Include:** For outpatient centers—Name, address, name and title of sponsor, phone, mailing address. For hospitals—Name, unit name if different, address, phone. **Pages (approx.):** 50. **Frequency:** Latest edition November 1984; suspended indefinitely.

★4155★ DIRECTORY OF THE NATIONAL BLOOD EXCHANGE
American Association of Blood Banks
1117 N. 19th St., Ste. 600
Arlington, VA 22209   Phone: (703) 528-8200
Covers: About 2,400 Blood Replacement Exchange and Cooperative Participants of the NBE; also hospitals and other transfusion facilities that share reciprocity through blood banks in the Blood Replacement Exchange and for which donor replacements can be drawn. **Entries Include:** Hospital or facility name, address, phone, description of services. **Pages (approx.):** 300. **Frequency:** First edition 1988; new edition expected 1991.

★4156★ DIRECTORY OF NATIONAL INFORMATION SOURCES ON HANDICAPPING CONDITIONS AND RELATED SERVICES
Office of Special Education and Rehabilitative Services
U.S. National Institute of Disability and Rehabilitation Research
Washington, DC 20202   Phone: (202) 732-1202
Covers: Approximately 400 major national organizations that disseminate information on disabilities and services for disabled persons. **Entries Include:** Organization name, address, phone, handicapping conditions served, type of user served, organization description, information services offered. **Pages (approx.):** 350. **Frequency:** Irregular; previous edition 1982; latest edition July 1986; new edition expected 1991. **Send Orders to:** Government Printing Office, Washington, DC 20402.

★4157★   DIRECTORY OF NON-MEDICAL RESEARCH RELATING TO HANDICAPPED PEOPLE
Handicapped Persons Research Unit
Newcastle upon Tyne Polytechnic
1 Coach Ln.
Newcastle upon Tyne NE7 7TW, England
Covers: Agencies and organizations in the United Kingdom sponsoring about 450 non-medical research projects for the physically and mentally handicapped in areas such as communications, health and social services, training, and rehabilitation. **Entries Include:** Organization name, address, phone, names and titles of key personnel, description of project, financial data, start and completion date for each study and relevant articles and publications. **Pages (approx.):** 410. **Frequency:** Annual, January.

★4158★   DIRECTORY OF NORTH, CENTRAL AND SOUTH AMERICAN MEDICAL SCHOOLS
Pan American Federation of Associations of Medical Schools
Apartado 60.411
Caracas 1060-A, Venezuela
Covers: Nearly 355 international institutions, national and regional associations, medical schools, and individuals in about 20 countries, including approximately 130 in the United States, that work to meet the medical service needs of Pan American countries. **Entries Include:** For institutions, associations, and medical schools—Organization name, address, names and titles of key personnel, geographic territory covered. For individual members—Personal name, address, geographic territory covered. **Pages (approx.):** 305. **Frequency:** Irregular; latest edition November 1986; new edition expected 1990.

★4159★   DIRECTORY OF NURSE-MIDWIFERY PRACTICES
American College of Nurse-Midwives
1522 K St. NW, Ste. 1000
Washington, DC 20005   Phone: (202) 289-0171
Covers: About 600 nurse and midwifery practices. **Entries Include:** Name of practice, address, phone, name of contact, site of birth. **Pages (approx.):** 99. **Frequency:** Annual, spring.

★4160★   DIRECTORY OF NURSES WITH DOCTORAL DEGREES
American Nurses' Association
2420 Pershing Rd.
Kansas City, MO 64108   Phone: (816) 436-8917
Covers: More than 3,500 nurses who have earned doctoral degrees. **Entries Include:** Name, office or home address, phone, educational and career data, areas of research and/or specialization. **Pages (approx.):** 130. **Frequency:** Irregular; latest edition 1984.

★4161★   DIRECTORY OF NURSING HOMES
Oryx Press
4041 N. Central, No. 700
Phoenix, AZ 85012   Phone: (602) 265-2651
Covers: 16,140 state-licensed long-term care facilities. **Entries Include:** Name of facility, address, phone, licensure status, number of beds; many listings also include name of administrator and health services supervisor; number of nursing, dietary, and auxiliary staff members; availability of social, recreational, and religious programs; and medicaid/medicare certification status. **Pages (approx.):** 1,460. **Frequency:** Reported as triennial; latest edition July 1990; new edition expected July 1991.

★4162★   DIRECTORY OF NURSING PRECEPTORSHIPS IN THE UNITED STATES
Fetters Infomanagement Co.
PO Box 386
Port Aransas, TX 78373   Phone: (512) 749-6634
Covers: Approximately 1,000 hospitals offering training programs, internships, and externships for graduate nurses or experienced nurses returning to the field after an absence. **Entries Include:** Institution name, address, phone, names and titles of key personnel, geographical area served, requirements for eligibility, description of programs. **Pages (approx.):** 600. **Frequency:** Biennial, fall of even years.

★4163★   DIRECTORY OF ON-GOING RESEARCH IN CANCER EPIDEMIOLOGY
International Agency for Research on Cancer
150, cours Albert Thomas
F-69372 Lyons Cedex 08, France
Covers: About 1,300 ongoing cancer epidemiology research projects in 80 countries and about 50 projects in mutation epidemiology; also includes lists of population-based cancer registries and biological materials banks.

Entries Include: Name and address of principal investigator; name of collaborator(s); description of project; keywords; term of project; cancer registry involved. **Pages (approx.):** 800. **Frequency:** Annual, January. **Available in the U.S. from:** Oxford University Press New York, Inc., 200 Madison Ave., New York, NY 10016.

★4164★   DIRECTORY OF ONLINE HEALTHCARE DATABASES
Medical Data Exchange
445 S. San Antonio Rd.
Los Altos, CA 94022   Phone: (415) 941-3600
Covers: About 245 producers of online databases concerned with the health care industry. **Entries Include:** Producer name, host name, cost per hour of use, size of file, dates of coverage, description of content. **Pages (approx.):** 78. **Frequency:** Annual, February.

★4165★   DIRECTORY OF ORGANIZATIONS INTERESTED IN PEOPLE WITH DISABILITIES
People to People Committee for the Handicapped
1020 Ashton Rd.
Ashton, MD 20861   Phone: (301) 774-7446
Covers: Approximately 100 organizations that provide assistance or support for persons with disabilities; state employment security agencies and vocational rehabilitation agencies; about 40 additional organizations concerned with the problems of the handicapped. **Entries Include:** For organizations—Name, address, phone, names and titles of key officers, description and purpose of organization, principal programs and services, titles of publications. For agencies—Agency name, address, phone. For additional organizations—Name and address. **Pages (approx.):** 70. **Frequency:** Every four years.

★4166★   DIRECTORY OF ORGANIZATIONS SERVING PEOPLE WITH DISABILITIES
Commission on Accreditation of Rehabilitation Facilities
101 N. Wilmot Rd., Ste. 500
Tucson, AZ 85711   Phone: (602) 748-1212
Covers: About 2,900 organizations offering more than 8,000 hospital-based, outpatient medical rehabilitation, spinal cord injury, and chronic pain management programs; brain injury, work hardening, infant and early childhood development programs; vocational evaluation, work adjustment, occupational skill training, and job placement; work services, personal and social adjustment services, supported employment, and industry-based programs; residential services; respite and psychosocial programs; and alcoholism and drug abuse treatment programs that have been accredited by the Commission. **Entries Include:** Organization name, address, phone, name and title of chief executive, accredited programs offered. **Pages (approx.):** 175. **Frequency:** Annual, January.

★4167★   DIRECTORY OF OSTEOPATHIC POSTDOCTORAL EDUCATION OPPORTUNITIES
American Osteopathic Hospital Association
5301 Wisconsin Ave. NW, Ste. 630
Washington, DC 20015   Phone: (202) 686-1700
Covers: Over 100 postdoctoral education programs approved by the American Osteopathic Association. **Entries Include:** Name and address of hospital, names of administrator and director of medical education, operating statistics, description of internship program, residencies offered. **Pages (approx.):** 78. **Frequency:** Annual, October.

★4168★   DIRECTORY OF PAIN TREATMENT CENTERS IN THE U.S. AND CANADA
Oryx Press
4041 N. Central, No. 700
Phoenix, AZ 85012   Phone: (602) 265-2651
Covers: Approximately 500 facilities specializing in pain treatment. **Entries Include:** Facility name, address, phone, names and titles of key personnel, description of facilities and programs. **Pages (approx.):** 225. **Frequency:** Latest edition April 1989.

★4169★   DIRECTORY OF PARTICIPATING PHYSICIANS AND MEDICAL INSTITUTIONS ABROAD
Foundation for the Support of International Medical Training
International Association for Medical Assistance to Travellers
417 Center St.
Lewiston, NY 14092   Phone: (716) 754-4883
Covers: 450 association centers in 120 countries, and English-speaking physicians affiliated with the association worldwide. **Entries Include:** Name of center, phone, names of contacts. **Pages (approx.):** 70. **Frequency:** Annual.

★4170★ DIRECTORY OF PATHOLOGY TRAINING PROGRAMS
Intersociety Committee on Pathology Information
4733 Bethesda Ave., Ste. 700
Bethesda, MD 20814   Phone: (301) 656-2944
Covers: Over 200 institutions offering pathologist training programs; coverage includes Canada; all listings are paid. **Entries Include:** Name and address of institution, programs offered, stipends, types and numbers of appointments, facilities, type of specialization, names of staff. **Pages (approx.):** 600. **Frequency:** Annual, June. **Also Includes:** Information on communities and fellowship programs.

★4171★ DIRECTORY OF PERSONNEL RESPONSIBLE FOR RADIOLOGICAL HEALTH PROGRAMS
Conference of Radiation Control Program Directors
205 Capital Ave.
Frankfort, KY 40601-2832   Phone: (502) 227-4543
Covers: About 350 individuals who conduct radiological health program activities in federal, state, and local government agencies; members of the conference. **Entries Include:** For directors—Name and title, name of agency, address, phone; office hours listed with state heading. For members—Name, address, phone, affiliation, department, and title. **Pages (approx.):** 75. **Frequency:** Annual, January.

★4172★ DIRECTORY OF THE PHARMACEUTICAL INDUSTRY IN JAPAN
Survey Japan
6 Kojimachi Bldg., Ste. 61
4-5 Kojimachi
Chiyoda-ku
Toyko 102, Japan
Covers: Over 110 pharmaceutical firms, industry-related organizations, and 1,200 pharmaceutical companies and wholesalers in Japan. **Entries Include:** Company name, address, phone, fax, telex, financial data, number of employees, names and titles of key personnel, product/service, products under development, domestic and international company connections. **Pages (approx.):** 400. **Also Includes:** Japanese pharmaceutical regulations.

★4173★ DIRECTORY OF PHYSICIANS AND SUPPLIERS THAT ACCEPT MEDICARE
U.S. Health Care Financing Administration
200 Independence Ave. SW
Washington, DC 20201   Phone: (202) 245-6113
Covers: Physicians and medical products suppliers who serve Medicare patients; separate editions for geographic areas served by Medicare's 38 carriers. **Entries Include:** Physician or company name, address, phone. **Frequency:** Reported as annual; latest edition January 1990. Annual, April.

★4174★ DIRECTORY OF PLANNING AND DESIGN PROFESSIONALS FOR HEALTH FACILITIES
American Hospital Association
840 N. Lake Shore Dr.
Chicago, IL 60611   Phone: (312) 280-5223
Covers: Architectural firms with experience or special interest in health care facilities. **Entries Include:** Firm name, address, phone, number of personnel with health-care specialty, description of activities, subsidiary offices. **Pages (approx.):** 70. **Frequency:** Annual, January.

★4175★ DIRECTORY OF PREFERRED PROVIDER ORGANIZATIONS
American Managed Care and Review Association
1227 25th St., NW, Ste. 610
Washington, DC 20037   Phone: (202) 728-0506
Covers: About 815 operating and planned preferred provider health care groups physicians and/or hospitals offering health care with fees and other terms negotiated with third-party payers; approximately 760 health maintenance organizations (HMOs). **Entries Include:** For physicians and hospitals—Organization name, address, type of sponsorship, name of contact, whether operating or planned, operational date, geographical area covered; number of hospitals, physicians, PPO eligibles. For HMOs—Name, address, phone, national HMO, affiliation number of hospitals and physicians participating, types of benefits offered, types of membership offered. **Pages (approx.):** 460. **Frequency:** Annual, spring.

★4176★ DIRECTORY OF PRIMARY CARE NURSE PRACTITIONER/SPECIALIST PROGRAM FOR REGISTERED NURSES AND NURSE MIDWIFERY PROGRAMS FOR REGISTERED NURSES
Division of Nursing
U.S. Health Resources and Services Administration
Rockville, MD 20857   Phone: (301) 443-6333
Covers: About 135 certificate, bachelor's, and master's programs for nurse practitioners. **Entries Include:** Institution name, address, phone, specialties offered. **Pages (approx.):** 17. **Frequency:** Irregular; previous edition October 1984; latest edition July 1989.

★4177★ DIRECTORY OF PRIVATE MEDICAL COMPANIES
Biomedical Business International
1524 Brookhollow Dr.
Santa Ana, CA 92705   Phone: (714) 755-5757
Covers: Approximately 300 private companies involved in the healthcare industry that have been in operation less than ten years. **Entries Include:** Company name, address, phone, fax, telex, names and titles of key personnel, number of employees, financial data, description of products or services, and agreements or financing being sought. **Pages (approx.):** 150. **Frequency:** Annual, September.

★4178★ DIRECTORY OF PROFESSIONAL ELECTROLOGISTS
Gordon Blackwell
Box 26
Eastchester, NY 10709   Phone: (914) 793-6633
Covers: 600 permanent hair removal services; international coverage. **Entries Include:** Name, office address and phone, modalities used (short wave, galvanic, blended current). **Pages (approx.):** 30. **Frequency:** Annual, spring.

★4179★ DIRECTORY OF PSYCHIATRY RESIDENCY TRAINING PROGRAMS
American Psychiatric Association
1400 K St. NW, Ste. 1101
Washington, DC 20005   Phone: (202) 682-6262
Covers: About 225 general and child psychiatric residency training programs; coverage includes Canada. An appendix also lists members of the American Association of Directors of Medical Student Education in Psychiatry. **Entries Include:** Name of sponsoring hospital or other facility, address; name, title, and phone of contact; other key personnel; type of program; university affiliations; facilities used with number of psychiatric beds, total admissions per year, number of outpatient visits per year, and length of assignment; other residencies used for required rotations; number of full-time faculty by degree; remuneration and fringe benefits; average patient load and night-call frequency; other continuing and postgraduate education opportunities offered; theoretical orientation; and other details. For association members—Name, affiliation, address. **Pages (approx.):** 615. **Frequency:** Biennial, spring of even years.

★4180★ DIRECTORY OF PSYCHOLOGY STAFFING AND SERVICES
Psychology Services
Veterans Administration Medical Center
1900 E. Main St.
116B VAMC
Danville, IL 61832   Phone: (217) 442-8000
Covers: About 155 staffing, research, and training programs in psychology for Department of Veterans Affairs medical facilities; includes universities cooperating in VA programs. **Entries Include:** Program title, sponsor's name, address, phone, name of program director, staffing and credential requirements, description of program. **Pages (approx.):** 335. **Frequency:** Biennial, spring of odd years.

★4181★ DIRECTORY OF REGISTERED DIETITIANS
American Dietetic Association
216 W. Jackson Blvd., Ste. 800
Chicago, IL 60606-6995   Phone: (312) 899-0040
Covers: Approximately 660 registered dietitians in the fifty states, the District of Columbia, and Canada. **Entries Include:** Personal name, address, phone. **Pages (approx.):** 55.

★4182★ DIRECTORY OF RESIDENTIAL ACCOMMODATION FOR THE MENTALLY HANDICAPPED IN ENGLAND, WALES AND NORTHERN IRELAND
Royal Society for Mentally Handicapped Children and Adults
Mencap National Centre
123 Golden Lane
London EC1Y 0RT, England
Covers: Group homes, hotels, and other residential facilities for the mentally handicapped in Great Britain, Wales, and Northern Ireland. **Entries Include:** Facility name, address, phone, telex, type of accommodations, special cases treated, special features. **Pages (approx.):** 155. **Frequency:** Latest edition 1982; suspended indefinitely.

★4183★ DIRECTORY OF RESIDENTIAL CENTERS FOR ADULTS WITH DEVELOPMENTAL DISABILITIES
Oryx Press
4041 N. Central, No. 700
Phoenix, AZ 85012   Phone: (602) 265-2651
Pages (approx.): 410. **Frequency:** Latest edition December 1988.

★4184★ DIRECTORY OF RESIDENTIAL FACILITIES FOR EMOTIONALLY HANDICAPPED CHILDREN AND YOUTH
Oryx Press
4041 N. Central, No. 700
Phoenix, AZ 85012   Phone: (602) 265-2651
Covers: More than 300 public and private facilities. **Entries Include:** Facility name, address, phone, name of admissions contact, specialty, ages and sexes of children accepted, costs, financial aid or other sources of funding, services. **Pages (approx.):** 305. **Frequency:** Irregular; previous edition 1985; latest edition December 1988.

★4185★ DIRECTORY OF RESIDENTIAL FACILITIES IN SCOTLAND
Scottish Council for Voluntary Organisations
18-19 Claremont Crescent
Edinburgh EH7 4QD, Scotland
Covers: Private and public residential facilities catering to people with special needs. **Entries Include:** Facility name, address, phone, description of services offered, age range served. **Pages (approx.):** 220. **Frequency:** Annual.

★4186★ DIRECTORY OF RESOURCES FOR ADULTS WITH DISABILITIES
U.S. Office of Vocational and Adult Education
400 Maryland Ave. SW
Washington, DC 20202   Phone: (202) 708-5750
Covers: Over 95 federal and non-federal agencies and programs, associations, clearinghouses, foundations, and other resources for educators working with disabled adults. **Entries Include:** Resource name, address, phone, program description, resources available. **Pages (approx.):** 125. **Frequency:** Irregular; latest edition 1985.

★4187★ DIRECTORY OF RESOURCES OF BIOMEDICAL AND ZOOLOGICAL SPECIMENS
Registry of Comparative Pathology
Armed Forces Institute of Pathology
Washington, DC 20306   Phone: (202) 576-2452
Covers: About 100 collections of biomedical and zoological specimens; international coverage. **Entries Include:** Type of collection; description of collection, including number of specimens, species, use of collection in research; restrictions on accessibility of collection; name and title of contact, organization name, address, phone. **Pages (approx.):** 50. **Frequency:** Irregular; previous edition 1981; latest edition 1990.

★4188★ DIRECTORY OF SCHOOL PSYCHOLOGY GRADUATE PROGRAMS
National Association of School Psychologists
8455 Colesville Rd., Ste. 1000
Silver Spring, MD 20910   Phone: (301) 608-0500
Covers: Approximately 225 school psychology graduate programs. **Entries Include:** Institution name, address; degrees offered; admission requirements; ratio of graduates to enrollment; description of program; names and specialties of faculty. **Pages (approx.):** 240. **Frequency:** Irregular; previous edition 1984; latest edition 1989. **Also Includes:** Survey of programs characteristics and comparative information for 1977, 1984, and 1989.

★4189★ DIRECTORY OF SELECTED EARLY CHILDHOOD PROGRAMS
Handicapped Children's Early Education Program
U.S. Office of Special Education Programs
400 Maryland Ave. SW, MES
Washington, DC 20202   Phone: (202) 732-1166
Covers: Over 250 projects in educational research, personnel preparation, and handicapped children's services sponsored by government agencies, universities, and other organizations and funded under the Handicapped Children's Early Education Program and the National Institute for Disability and Rehabilitation Research; other divisions of the Office of Special Education Programs. **Entries Include:** Project name, address, phone, fax, SpecialNet number, director's name, name of sponsoring agency, years funded, grant number, project characteristics such as target population, statement of project objective, and additional services provided. **Pages (approx.):** 300. **Frequency:** Annual, March.

★4190★ DIRECTORY OF SERVICES FOR ELDERLY PEOPLE
Longman Group UK Ltd.
Westgate House, 6th Fl.
The High
Harlow, Essex CM2 1YR, England
Covers: Organizations, government agencies, academic and research institutions, and publications in the United Kingdom offering services or information regarding care of the elderly. **Entries Include:** Company name, address, phone, telex, names and titles of key personnel, number of employees, geographical area served, branch office or subsidiary names and addresses, descriptions of information or services available. **Pages (approx.):** 272. **Frequency:** Annual, August.

★4191★ DIRECTORY OF SERVICES FOR VISUALLY HANDICAPPED SOUTH AFRICANS
South African National Council for the Blind
PO Box 11149
Brooklyn
Pretoria 0011, Republic of South Africa
Covers: National, state, and local agencies and organizations such as hostels, libraries, publishers, self-help groups, and optometrists serving visually impaired South Africans. **Entries Include:** For national, state, and local agencies—Agency name, address, date established, geographical areas and populations served, objectives, and services provided. For organizations—Name, address, phone, description of services, conditions of eligibility; libraries and publications also include description of materials available and circulation information; schools include admission requirements, languages of instruction, and curriculum specifications. **Pages (approx.):** 329. **Frequency:** Irregular; previous edition 1985; latest edition 1990; new edition expected 1992. **Also Includes:** Explanation of the Blindness System in South Africa; South African definition of legal blindness, procedures for registering as such.

★4192★ DIRECTORY OF STATE AND AREA AGENCIES ON AGING
National Association of Area Agencies on Aging
1112 16th St. NW, Ste. 100
Washington, DC 20036   Phone: (202) 296-8130
Covers: State and area offices on aging; Native American aging organizations; federal aging offices. **Entries Include:** Name, address, phone, name of director. **Pages (approx.):** 156. **Frequency:** Published 1989. **Also Includes:** Maps showing planning and service areas for each agency.

★4193★ DIRECTORY OF STATE AND TERRITORIAL ALCOHOLISM PROGRAM DIRECTORS
National Clearinghouse for Alcohol and Drug Information
PO Box 2345
Rockville, MD 20852   Phone: (301) 468-2600
Covers: State and territorial alcoholism program directors. **Entries Include:** Agency name, address, phone, director. **Pages (approx.):** 5. **Frequency:** Latest edition 1985.

★4194★ DIRECTORY OF STD CLINICS
Technical Information Services
Center for Prevention Services
Centers for Disease Control
Atlanta, GA 30333   Phone: (404) 639-1819
Covers: Clinics providing treatment of sexually transmitted diseases. **Entries Include:** Facility name, address, phone, hours of operation, appointment and cost information, list of illnesses diagnosed and/or treated.

★4195★ DIRECTORY OF STUDENT PLACEMENTS IN HEALTH CARE SETTINGS IN NORTH AMERICA
Association for the Care of Children's Health
7910 Woodmont Ave., Ste. 300
Bethesda, MD 20814   Phone: (301) 654-6549
Covers: Nearly 150 internships, fellowships, and other practical teaching experiences in hospitals for students of "child life activity." **Entries Include:** Facility name, address, phone, name of individual in charge of the practicum; number of hours and number of weeks for practicum; beginning dates, if specified; number of students accepted each term; total number of students accepted for year; colleges from which students are generally referred; areas of study from which students generally come; fees; stipend and other benefits; prerequisites; whether application is to be made to college or hospital; level of student generally accepted; practicum experiences available; form of evaluation. **Pages (approx.):** 20. **Frequency:** Irregular; latest edition 1985.

★4196★ DIRECTORY OF SUDDEN INFANT DEATH SYNDROME PROGRAMS AND RESOURCES
National Sudden Infant Death Syndrome Clearinghouse
8201 Greensboro Dr., Ste. 600
McLean, VA 22102   Phone: (703) 821-8955
Covers: About 110 federal, state, and private agencies and organizations that provide information and counseling on sudden infant death syndrome and related problems. **Entries Include:** Company or organization name, address, phone, name and title of contact. **Pages (approx.):** 20. **Frequency:** Latest edition spring 1988; new edition possible, date not set.

★4197★ DIRECTORY OF SUICIDE PREVENTION/CRISIS INTERVENTION AGENCIES IN THE UNITED STATES
American Association of Suicidology
2459 S. Ash
Denver, CO 80222   Phone: (303) 692-0985
Covers: About 600 suicide prevention and crisis intervention centers. **Entries Include:** Center name, sponsoring organization name (if different), address, phone, emergency phone number, hours of service. **Pages (approx.):** 60. **Frequency:** Annual, October.

★4198★ DIRECTORY OF SURVIVORS OF SUICIDE SUPPORT GROUPS
American Association of Suicidology
2459 S. Ash
Denver, CO 80222   Phone: (303) 692-0985
Covers: 220 support groups in the U.S. and Canada for family, friends, and other survivors of people who commit suicide. **Entries Include:** Name, address, phone. **Pages (approx.):** 28. **Frequency:** Annual, fall.

★4199★ DIRECTORY OF TEACHING HOSPITALS
SMG Marketing Group, Inc.
1342 N. LaSalle Dr.
Chicago, IL 60610   Phone: (312) 642-3026
Covers: Hospitals in the United States with teaching facilities for residents. **Entries Include:** Hospital name, address, phone, geographical area served, description of services and teaching facilities. **Pages (approx.):** 250. **Frequency:** Annual, January.

★4200★ DIRECTORY OF TEEN CHALLENGE CENTERS
National Teen Challenge
1525 N. Campbell Ave.
Springfield, MO 65803   Phone: (417) 862-6969
Covers: About 100 evangelical Christian rehabilitation centers for teenagers and young adults. **Entries Include:** Center name, address, phone, name and title of contact. **Pages (approx.):** 15. **Frequency:** Semiannual, January and June.

★4201★ DIRECTORY OF TRAINING PROGRAMS IN INTERNAL MEDICINE: RESIDENCY AND SUBSPECIALTY FELLOWSHIPS
National Study of Internal Medicine Manpower
Center for Health Administration Studies
University of Chicago
969 E. 60th St.
Chicago, IL 60637   Phone: (312) 702-7753
Covers: About 440 training programs accredited by the Accreditation Council for Graduate Medical Education and about 1,700 fellowships in internal medicine and 15 subspecialties. **Entries Include:** Name of institution, center, or medical department, address, contact name, category or subspecialty in which residency or fellowship is offered, number of residents and fellows trained annually, size of institution, type of owner-

ship, number of filled positions. **Pages (approx.):** 200. **Frequency:** Annual, March. **Also Includes:** Tables and discussion of training in internal medicine.

★4202★ DIRECTORY OF U.S.-BASED AGENCIES INVOLVED IN INTERNATIONAL HEALTH ASSISTANCE
National Council for International Health
1701 K St. NW, Ste. 600
Washington, DC 20006   Phone: (202) 833-5900
Covers: Over 400 private voluntary organizations, universities, civic groups, professional associations, and other groups which have health, nutrition, and population/family planning programs in developing countries. **Entries Include:** Organization name, address, services provided, territory covered. **Pages (approx.):** 200. **Frequency:** Irregular; previous edition June 1980; latest edition 1988; new edition expected 1991.

★4203★ DIRECTORY OF UNITED STATES HOMEOPATHIC PRACTITIONERS
National Center for Homeopathy
1500 Massachusetts Ave., N.W., Ste. 42
Washington, DC 20005   Phone: (202) 223-6182
Covers: About 400 doctors of medicine and osteopathy, dentists, chiropractors, acupuncturists, and veterinarians who include homeopathy in their practices. **Entries Include:** Name, address, degree, medical specialty (if any). **Pages (approx.):** 100. **Frequency:** Approximately biennial; latest edition February 1990.

★4204★ DIRECTORY OF U.S. NURSING HOMES AND NURSING HOME CHAINS
McKnight Medical Communications Company
1419 Lake Cook Rd., Ste. 110
Deerfield, IL 60015   Phone: (708) 945-0345
Covers: More than 17,500 nursing homes and about 100 nursing home chains. **Entries Include:** Facility name, address, phone, name and title of contact, number of beds. **Pages (approx.):** 600. **Frequency:** Annual, December.

★4205★ DIRECTORY OF WOMEN'S HEALTH CARE CENTERS
Oryx Press
4041 N. Central, No. 700
Phoenix, AZ 85012   Phone: (602) 265-2651
Covers: More than 200 women's health care facilities and organizations. **Entries Include:** Facility or organization name, address, phone, names and titles of key personnel, type of facility, year established, parent company or organization affiliation, description of facilities, services, programs, and publications. **Pages (approx.):** 160. **Frequency:** Latest edition July 1989.

★4206★ DISTRIBUTOR PROFILES
Medical Device Register
655 Washington Blvd., Ste. 706
Stamford, CT 06901   Phone: (203) 348-6319
Covers: More than 21,000 medical products distributors and manufacturers' representatives; international coverage. **Entries Include:** Company name, address, phone, names and titles of key personnel, number of employees, medical products sales volume (in dollars), geographical area served, distribution specialities, companies represented. **Pages (approx.):** 2,000 (in two volumes). **Frequency:** Annual, November.

★4207★ DR. GREENBERGER'S WHAT EVERY MAN SHOULD KNOW ABOUT HIS PROSTATE
Walker & Co.
Walker Publishing Co., Inc.
720 5th Ave.
New York, NY 10019   Phone: (212) 265-3632
Publication Includes: List of prostate cancer support organizations. **Pages (approx.):** 180. **Frequency:** Latest edition 1988.

★4208★ DORLAND'S MEDICAL DIRECTORY: EASTERN PENNSYLVANIA AND SOUTHERN NEW JERSEY
Legal Communications Ltd.
1617 John F. Kennedy Blvd., Ste. 1245
Philadelphia, PA 19103   Phone: (215) 563-2700
Covers: Over 11,000 practicing medical and osteopathic physicians, hospitals and their staffs, and local health and human resource organizations in Eastern Pennsylvania and Southern New Jersey. **Entries Include:** For physicians—Name, office and home addresses and phone numbers, medical school attended and year graduated, medical specialties, certifications, hospital affiliations. For hospitals—Name, address, names and

specialties of staff members. **Pages (approx.):** 750. **Frequency:** Annual, November.

★4209★ **DRUG ABUSE AND ADDICTION INFO/TREATMENT DIRECTORY**
American Business Directories, Inc.
American Business Information, Inc.
5711 S. 86th Circle
Omaha, NE 68127   Phone: (402) 593-4600
Number of Listings: 8,471. **Entries Include:** Name, address, phone (including area code), size of advertisement, year first in "Yellow Pages," name of owner or manager, number of employees. **Frequency:** Annual.

★4210★ **DRUG, ALCOHOL, AND OTHER ADDICTIONS: A DIRECTORY OF TREATMENT CENTERS AND PREVENTION PROGRAMS NATIONWIDE**
Oryx Press
4041 N. Central, No. 700
Phoenix, AZ 85012   Phone: (602) 265-2651
Covers: Nearly 18,000 federal, state, and local addiction treatment programs including public and private centers. **Entries Include:** Center or program name, address, phone, name and title of contact, addictions treated, treatments used, description of services available, number of clients for the year, specialty groups, ownership, funding statistics. **Pages (approx.):** 785. **Frequency:** First edition 1989; new edition expected March 1991.

★4211★ **DRUG DELIVERY SYSTEMS**
Theta Corp.
Theta Bldg.
Middlefield, CT 06455   Phone: (203) 349-1054
Publication Includes: List of companies that produce or are developing drug delivery systems. **Entries Include:** Company name, address, phone, key personnel, background information, description of products, annual sales, research and development efforts, distribution efforts, five year projection. **Frequency:** Irregular; previous edition November 1988; latest edition December 1990.

★4212★ **DRUG TOPICS RED BOOK**
Medical Economics Data Co.
Medical Economics Co.
5 Paragon Dr.
Montvale, NJ 07645   Phone: (201) 358-7200
Publication Includes: Manufacturers of prescription drugs, patent medicines, and other drug store items. **Entries Include:** Company name, address, trade and brand names, wholesale prices. **Frequency:** Annual, March; monthly updates. **Also Includes:** Company catalogs; sections titled "Emergency Information," "Organizations," "Practice Aids," "Pharmacy Quick Facts," "Merchandising Information," "Product Identification Illustration," "Home Health Care Information," "Pharmacy Computer Suppliers."

★4213★ **DRUGS AVAILABLE ABROAD**
Gale Research Inc.
835 Penobscot Bldg.
Detroit, MI 48226-4094   Phone: (313) 961-2242
Covers: 1,000 therapeutic drugs approved and in use abroad, but not generally available in the U.S.; coverage includes Western Europe, Central America, Mexico, the Caribbean, Australia, Canada, Scandinavia, and South Africa. **Entries Include:** Generic drug name, countries where available and release dates, synonyms for generic drug name, brand names and manufacturers, drug action (purpose), indications/usage, form (tablet, suppository, liquid), dosage, precautions and warnings, contraindications, drug interactions, adverse effects, U.S. status, equivalent U.S. treatments. **Pages (approx.):** 410. **Frequency:** First edition October 1990.

★4214★ **DRUGS MADE IN AUSTRIA**
Fachverband der Chemischen Industrie Osterreichs
Wiedner Hauptstrasse 63
A-1045 Vienna, Austria
Covers: Austrian companies producing and exporting industrial pharmaceuticals. **Entries Include:** Company name, address, phone, telex. **Pages (approx.):** 120. **Frequency:** Irregular; previous edition 1983; new edition expected 1991.

★4215★ **DUN'S GUIDE TO HEALTHCARE COMPANIES**
Dun's Marketing Services
Dun & Bradstreet Corp.
3 Sylvan Way
Parsippany, NJ 07054-3896   Phone: (201) 605-6000
Covers: Approximately 15,000 manufacturers and suppliers of health care products.

★4216★ **THE DYSLEXIA INSTITUTE—SPECIAL NEEDS, SPECIAL PROVISION**
The Dyslexia Institute
133 Gresham Rd.
Staines TW18 2AJ, England
Publication Includes: List of approximately 20 branches of the Dyslexia Institute in the United Kingdom. **Entries Include:** Address, phone, additional outreach locations, services offered. **Frequency:** Annual.

★4217★ **EARTH STAR/WHOLE LIFE NEW ENGLAND—HOLISTIC HEALTH**
Earth Star Press Inc.
PO Box 110
Temple, NH 03084   Phone: (603) 878-4090
Publication Includes: About 500 preventive and holistic health practitioners and schools. **Entries Include:** Name, address, phone, specialties; practitioner listings include qualifications. **Frequency:** Bimonthly.

★4218★ **EDTA—EUROPEAN RENAL ASSOCIATION—DIRECTORY OF MEMBERS**
EDTA - European Renal Association
Department of Nephrology
Hospital Puerta Hierro
E-28035 Madrid, Spain
Covers: 1,645 scientific workers in nephrology. **Frequency:** Irregular.

★4219★ **EDUCATION ASSISTANCE FOR AMERICAN INDIANS AND ALASKA NATIVES**
Master of Public Health Program for American Indians
School of Public Health
University of California
Warren Hall, Rm. 140
Berkeley, CA 94720   Phone: (415) 642-3228
Publication Includes: Sources of information regarding health careers, training for health careers, and financial aid available to American Indians and Alaska natives from the Bureau of Indian Affairs, institutions, tribal councils, and other sources. **Entries Include:** Name of organization or publisher, address, name of contact, phone, service programs offered. **Frequency:** Biennial, June of even years.

★4220★ **EDUCATION FOR EMPLOYMENT: A GUIDE TO POSTSECONDARY VOCATIONAL EDUCATION FOR STUDENTS WITH DISABILITIES**
Higher Education and Adult Training for People with Handicaps Resource Center
American Council on Education
1 Dupont Circle NW, Ste. 800
Washington, DC 20036   Phone: (202) 939-9320
Publication Includes: Lists of over 25 resources and books available to assist disabled students and their educators. **Entries Include:** Name of resource or book, source, address, phone, description. **Frequency:** Published August 1986.

★4221★ **EDUCATION-FOR-HEALTH: THE SELECTIVE GUIDE**
National Center for Health Education
30 E. 29th St.
New York, NY 10016   Phone: (212) 689-1886
Publication Includes: List of distributors of films, videotapes, and audiocassettes on topics of mental health and family life education. **Entries Include:** Name, address, and phone; title, synopsis, and descriptive evaluation of film or tape, name of producer, running time, whether in black and white or color, type of audience, sale or rental price. **Frequency:** Irregular; latest edition 1985. **Also Includes:** List of related publications and plays.

★4222★ **EDUCATION FOR NURSING: THE DIPLOMA WAY**
National League for Nursing
350 Hudson St.
New York, NY 10014   Phone: (212) 989-9393
Covers: Accredited diploma programs in nursing for high school graduates;

most take three years and are hospital based. **Entries Include:** Name of institution and program, address, contact, educational requirements, length of program, policy on advanced placement and transfers, living accommodations, possibility of outside courses, estimated costs of tuition, fees, room and board, number of graduates, number of enrollments. **Pages (approx.):** 50. **Frequency:** Annual.

★4223★ **EDUCATIONAL OPPORTUNITIES IN COMPARATIVE PATHOLOGY, UNITED STATES AND FOREIGN COUNTRIES**
Registry of Comparative Pathology
Armed Forces Institute of Pathology
Washington, DC 20306   Phone: (202) 576-2452
Covers: About 90 institutions offering programs in comparative pathology. **Entries Include:** School name, address, name of director; description of program, including residencies or preceptorships offered, degree offered, specializations possible, and extramural affiliations. **Pages (approx.):** 41. **Frequency:** Biennial, even years.

★4224★ **EDUCATIONAL PROGRAMS IN OCCUPATIONAL THERAPY PROGRAMS**
American Occupational Therapy Association, Inc.
1383 Piccard Dr.
PO Box 1725
Rockville, MD 20849-1725   Phone: (301) 948-9626
Covers: Over 80 accredited and developing programs in occupational therapy and over 80 accredited and developing occupational therapy assistant programs. **Entries Include:** Institution name, address, level of program. **Pages (approx.):** 10. **Frequency:** Annual.

★4225★ **EDUCATORS GUIDE TO FREE HEALTH, PHYSICAL EDUCATION AND RECREATION MATERIALS**
Educators Progress Service, Inc.
214 Center St.
Randolph, WI 53956   Phone: (414) 326-3126
Covers: Sources for about 2,060 films, filmstrips/audiotapes, videotapes, scripts, phonograph records, and printed materials useful in study of health, physical education, and recreation. Materials are provided by industrial, governmental, and other sponsors for free use by teachers and other educators. **Entries Include:** Title, brief description, length or running time, whether sound or scripts are available for silent tapes and films, whether color or black and white, source. **Pages (approx.):** 490. **Frequency:** Annual, September.

★4226★ **ELDER NEGLECT AND ABUSE: AN ANNOTATED BIBLIOGRAPHY**
Greenwood Publishing Group, Inc.
88 Post Rd. W.
PO Box 5007
Westport, CT 06881   Phone: (203) 226-3571
Publication Includes: List of national and state mental health offices, medicaid agencies, and national protective agencies for the elderly. **Entries Include:** Agency or office name, address, phone. **Frequency:** Irregular; previous edition August 1985; latest edition 1987.

★4227★ **ELECTROLYSIS DIRECTORY**
American Business Directories, Inc.
American Business Information, Inc.
5711 S. 86th Circle
Omaha, NE 68127   Phone: (402) 593-4600
Number of Listings: 6,507. **Entries Include:** Name, address, phone (including area code), size of advertisement, year first in "Yellow Pages," name of owner or manager, number of employees. **Frequency:** Annual.

★4228★ **EMERGENCY MEDICAL SERVICES—BUYERS GUIDE ISSUE**
Creative Age Publications
7628 Densmore Ave.
Van Nuys, CA 91406   Phone: (818) 782-7328
Publication Includes: Lists of about 1,000 manufacturers, suppliers, and distributors of equipment and other products used in emergency medical services; coverage includes Canada. Also covers 45 emergency medical service associations, state agencies, and meetings, workshops, and other conferences of interest. **Entries Include:** For companies—Company name, address, phone, name of principal executive, product/service. For associations—Name, address, phone, name of director, number of members, description of membership, publications, meeting time. **Frequency:** Annual, December. **Also Includes:** List of toll-free phone numbers.

★4229★ **EMERGENCY MEDICAL AND SURGICAL SERVICE DIRECTORY**
American Business Directories, Inc.
American Business Information, Inc.
5711 S. 86th Circle
Omaha, NE 68127   Phone: (402) 593-4600
Number of Listings: 1,106. **Entries Include:** Name, address, phone, size of advertisement, name of owner or manager, number of employees, year first in "Yellow Pages." **Frequency:** Annual.

★4230★ **EMERGENCY MEDICINE MAGAZINE—LIST OF POISON CONTROL CENTERS**
Health Care Group
Cahners Publishing Co.
249 W. 17th St.
New York, NY 10011   Phone: (212) 645-0067
Covers: About 250 poison control centers across the United States that are officially recognized as such by their respective state departments of health. **Entries Include:** Name of center, address, phone. **Pages (approx.):** 10. **Frequency:** Annual.

★4231★ **THE ENCYCLOPEDIA OF CHILD ABUSE**
Facts on File, Inc.
460 Park Ave. S.
New York, NY 10016   Phone: (212) 683-2244
Publication Includes: Listings of child abuse prevention organizations. **Entries Include:** Organization name, address, phone. **Frequency:** Published 1989.

★4232★ **ENCYCLOPEDIA OF DRUG ABUSE**   ·
Facts on File, Inc.
460 Park Ave. S.
New York, NY 10016   Phone: (212) 683-2244
Publication Includes: Directories of government agencies and private organizations concerned with medical, legal, biological, and social facets of drug abuse. **Frequency:** Irregular; previous edition 1984; latest edition April 1991.

★4233★ **ENCYCLOPEDIA OF HEALTH INFORMATION SOURCES**
Gale Research Inc.
835 Penobscot Bldg.
Detroit, MI 48226-4094   Phone: (313) 961-2242
Covers: Over 13,000 sources of information of interest to health care personnel, such as publications, health organizations, research centers, and databases. **Entries Include:** For publications—Title, editor or author, publisher name, address, frequency or date of publication. For organizations, institutes, or agencies—Name, address. For databases—Title, producer, addresses, distributor, frequency of revision. **Pages (approx.):** 490. **Frequency:** Irregular; first edition 1987; new edition possible 1992.

★4234★ **ENCYCLOPEDIA OF MEDICAL ORGANIZATIONS AND AGENCIES**
Gale Research Inc.
835 Penobscot Bldg.
Detroit, MI 48226-4094   Phone: (313) 961-2242
Covers: Over 12,200 state, national, and international medical associations, foundations, research institutes, federal and state agencies, and medical and allied health schools. **Entries Include:** Organization name, address, phone; many listings include names and titles of key personnel, descriptive annotations. **Pages (approx.):** 1,210. **Frequency:** Biennial, November of odd years.

★4235★ **END-STAGE RENAL DISEASE SOURCEBOOK**
Techne Research
1100 Massachusetts Ave.
Arlington, MA 02174   Phone: (617) 646-6297
Covers: Over 100 manufacturers, service companies, and distributors of products and equipment for treatment of end-stage renal disease; over 1,000 United States treatment centers and 2,000 foreign treatment centers (ESRD); related federal, state, and local government agencies; over 125 professional associations, foundations, and nonprofit groups; investigators who have received grants or contracts for research in this area; publishers of about 90 periodicals that have published articles on this topic. **Entries Include:** All listings include organization or investigator name, address, and phone. In addition, for manufacturers—Names of key personnel; name, address, and phone of ESRD division; products and services; some listings include financial information, corporate officers, and principal sales and distribution offices and manufacturing plants. For treatment

centers—Most listings include types of services offered, number of patient stations, name of director. For government agencies and associations—Names of key personnel. For investigators—Name of granting agency, title of project, institutional affiliation, amount of grant. For periodical publishers—Name of editor. **Pages (approx.):** 400. **Frequency:** Approximately quadrennial; latest edition October 1984; new edition expected 1988. **Also Includes:** Bibliography; statistical data.

★4236★ EQUIPMENT FOR DISABLED PEOPLE
Disability Information Trust
Mary Marlborough Lodge
Nuffield Orthopaedic Centre
Headington, Oxfordshire OX3 7LD, England
Covers: Equipment and self-help devices for the disabled and elderly in the United Kingdom, with information on manufacturers and suppliers. **Entries Include:** Company name, address, phone, product or service, and comments. **Pages (approx.):** 250. **Frequency:** Irregular; previous edition August 1991; latest edition November 1991.

★4237★ EQUIPMENT FOR VISUALLY DISABLED PEOPLE—AN INTERNATIONAL GUIDE
Technical Research Section
Royal National Institute for the Blind
224 Great Portland St.
London W1N 6AA, England
Covers: Over 200 manufacturers of products for the visually handicapped. **Entries Include:** Company name, address, descriptions and prices of products. **Frequency:** Annual.

★4238★ ESSENTIAL GUIDE TO GENERIC DRUGS
HarperCollins
10 E. 53rd St.
New York, NY 10022   Phone: (212) 207-7000
Covers: Manufacturers of generic drugs approved by the Food and Drug Administration. **Entries Include:** Drug, brand name, manufacturers' names, dosage form, use, precautions, side effects, percentage of possible savings by using generic product, drug patent expiration dates. **Pages (approx.):** 350. **Frequency:** Latest edition March 1986.

★4239★ EUROPEAN ACADEMY OF FACIAL SURGERY—MEMBERSHIP/BY-LAWS BOOK
European Academy of Facial Surgery
c/o T. R. Bull
107 Harley St.
London W1, England
Publication Includes: List of approximately 350 consultant surgeons qualified as specialists in ear, nose, and throat treatment, plastic and allied surgical specialities. **Also Includes:** Regulations and by-laws.

★4240★ EUROPEAN ASSOCIATION OF NEUROSURGICAL SOCIETIES—ANNUAL DIRECTORY
European Association of Neurosurgical Societies
c/o Department of Neurological Society
University Hospital
De Pintelaan 185
B-9000 Ghent, Belgium
Covers: Member associations. **Frequency:** Annual.

★4241★ EUROPEAN CHIROPRACTORS' UNION DIRECTORY
European Chiropractors' Union
Ahlgade 3
4300 Holbaek, Denmark
Covers: About 1,400 chiropractors in Europe. **Entries Include:** Name, address, phone. **Pages (approx.):** 50. **Frequency:** Annual, May/June.

★4242★ EUROPEAN CONSUMER HEALTHCARE MARKETING DIRECTORY
Euromonitor Publications Ltd.
87-88 Turnmill St.
London EC1M 5QU, England
Covers: Approximately 500 European consumer health care producers; producers and publishers of marketing information sources. **Entries Include:** For consumer health care producers—Company name, address, phone, fax, summary of company activities, financial data, products and brands, number of employees, subsidiary and branch names and locations, names and titles of key personnel. For publishers and producers—Name, address, phone, fax, purchase information, description of coverage, language, circulation, frequency, name and title of contact. **Pages (ap-

prox.):** 400. **Frequency:** Published 1991. **Also Includes:** Market overview and statistics. **Available in the U.S. from:** Find/SVP, 625 Avenue of the Americas, New York, NY 10011 (212-645-4500).

★4243★ EUROPEAN PHARMACEUTICAL MARKETING RESEARCH ASSOCIATION—LIST OF AGENCIES
European Pharmaceutical Marketing Research Association
c/o Mr. D. S. Mitchell
9 Paterson Dr.
Woodhouse Eaves, Leicestershire LE12 8RL, England
Frequency: Annual.

★4244★ EUROPEAN PROPRIETARY ASSOCIATION—GENERAL INFORMATION DIRECTORY
European Proprietary Association
18, rue Jean Giraudoux
F-75116 Paris, France
Covers: 15 European national proprietary medicines associations. **Frequency:** Irregular.

★4245★ EUROPEAN SOCIETY FOR NEUROCHEMISTRY—MEMBERSHIP DIRECTORY
European Society for Neurochemistry
Institute of Neurobiology
University of Goteborg
PO Box 33 031
S-400 33 Goteborg, Sweden
Covers: Approximately 800 researchers in neurochemistry, neurology, molecular neurobiology, molecular neuropharmacology, and psychiatry, including about 30 researchers from the United States. **Entries Include:** Personal name, address, phone, fax, when available. **Pages (approx.):** 100. **Frequency:** Irregular; latest edition 1990.

★4246★ EUROPEAN SOCIETY OF NEURORADIOLOGY—DIRECTORY
European Society of Neuroradiology
c/o Centre Hospitalier L. Pasteur
F-68021 Colmar, France
Covers: Over 600 members. **Frequency:** Irregular.

★4247★ EUROPEAN SOCIETY OF REGIONAL ANAESTHESIA—YEARBOOK
European Society of Regional Anaesthesia
Kempenlaan 12
B-2300 Turnhout, Belgium
Publication Includes: List of medical doctors specializing in anesthesiology. **Frequency:** Annual.

★4248★ EUROPEAN STUDY GROUP ON LYSOSOMAL DISEASES—REGISTER OF LABORATORIES
European Study Group on Lysosomal Diseases
Department of Biochemistry
Kings College
Campden Hill Rd.
London W8 7AH, England
Covers: Approximately 90 laboratories conducting research on lysosomal storage diseases. **Frequency:** Biennial.

★4249★ EXERCISE AND PHYSICAL FITNESS PROGRAMS DIRECTORY
American Business Directories, Inc.
American Business Information, Inc.
5711 S. 86th Circle
Omaha, NE 68127   Phone: (402) 593-4600
Number of Listings: 10,985. **Entries Include:** Name, address, phone (including area code), size of advertisement, year first in "Yellow Pages," name of owner or manager, number of employees. **Frequency:** Annual.

★4250★ EXERSAFETY ASSOCIATION—MEMBER DIRECTORY
Exersafety Association
PO Box 394166
Solon, OH 44139   Phone: (216) 687-1718
Covers: Over 3,000 fitness instructors, health clubs and spas, YMCA's, community recreation departments, aerobics studios, universities, hospital wellness programs, and others concerned with educational aspects of exercise; international coverage. **Entries Include:** Member name, membership status, location (city, state, country). **Pages (approx.):** 10. **Frequency:** Biennial, January of odd years.

★4251★ EXPERTNET
ExpertNet, Ltd.
225 W. Ohio St., Ste. 325
Chicago, IL 60610   Phone: (312) 527-0470
Covers: More than 1,000 medical malpractice and personal injury experts that serve as consultants and trial witnesses.

★4252★ FACULTY DIRECTORY OF THE SCHOOLS AND COLLEGES OF OPTOMETRY
Association of Schools and Colleges of Optometry
6110 Executive Blvd., Ste. 514
Rockville, MD 20852   Phone: (301) 231-5944
Covers: Optometric schools and colleges. **Entries Include:** Institution name, address, names and titles of key personnel, teaching and research disciplines offered. **Pages (approx.):** 80. **Frequency:** Biennial.

★4253★ FACULTY OF OPHTHALMOLOGISTS—ANNUAL REPORT
Faculty of Ophthalmologists
Bramber Court
2 Bramber Rd.
London W14 9PQ, England
Publication Includes: List of members. **Entries Include:** Member name, address. **Frequency:** Annual, May.

★4254★ FAMILY PLANNING INFORMATION CENTERS DIRECTORY
American Business Directories, Inc.
American Business Information, Inc.
5711 S. 86th Circle
Omaha, NE 68127   Phone: (402) 593-4600
Number of Listings: 3,958. **Entries Include:** Name, address, phone (including area code), size of advertisement, year first in "Yellow Pages," name of owner or manager, number of employees. **Frequency:** Annual.

★4255★ FEDERAL HOSPITAL PHONE BOOK
U.S. Directory Service
655 NW 128th St.
PO Box 68-1700
Miami, FL 33168   Phone: (305) 769-1700
Covers: Nearly 1,000 U.S. military, Veterans Administration, and Public Health Service hospitals in the United States and abroad; miscellaneous random listings for state correctional institution medical facilities. **Entries Include:** Facility name, address, phone. **Pages (approx.):** 85. **Frequency:** Irregular; previous edition 1983; latest edition 1988.

★4256★ FEDERALLY QUALIFIED REPORT
Office of Prepaid Health Care
U.S. Health Care Financing Administration
200 Independence Ave. SW, Rm. 423H
Washington, DC 20201   Phone: (202) 245-0197
Covers: About 600 Health Maintenance Organizations (HMO's) currently or previously qualified by the federal government. **Entries Include:** HMO name, address, phone, plan code number, contact name, whether for- or non-profit, date qualified, date qualification revoked (if applicable), amount of loan commitment, date of end of fiscal year, name of assigned compliance officer. **Pages (approx.):** 75. **Frequency:** Monthly.

★4257★ FERTILITY AWARENESS AND NATURAL FAMILY PLANNING RESOURCE DIRECTORY
Fertility Awareness Services
828 NW 33rd.
PO Box 986
Corvallis, OR 97339   Phone: (503) 753-8530
Pages (approx.): 200. **Frequency:** Latest edition May 1988; new edition expected 1991.

★4258★ FETAL MONITORING
Theta Co.
Theta Bldg.
Middlefield, CT 06455   Phone: (203) 349-1054
Publication Includes: List of about 10 companies that market or produce electronic fetal monitors (EFM). **Entries Include:** Company name, address, phone, key personnel, background information, description of products, annual sales, research and development efforts, distribution systems, five year projection. **Frequency:** Irregular; previous edition January 1985; latest edition September 1987.

★4259★ FINANCIAL AID FOR THE DISABLED AND THEIR FAMILIES
Reference Service Press
1100 Industrial Rd., Ste. 9
San Carlos, CA 94070   Phone: (415) 594-0743
Covers: Foundations, corporations, government agencies, professional associations, and other organizations that offer 900 scholarships, fellowships, grants, loans, and awards to disabled persons or their family members. **Entries Include:** Program name, sponsor name, address, phone, description of program including purpose, financial data, and eligibility requirements. **Pages (approx.):** 307. **Frequency:** Biennial, January even years. **Also Includes:** List of sources of financial aid and information about financial aid for the disabled.

★4260★ FIRE CHIEF—EMS/RESCUE BUYERS' GUIDE ISSUE
Communication Channels, Inc.
6255 Barfield Rd.
Atlanta, GA 30328   Phone: (404) 256-9800
Publication Includes: List of 650 suppliers of equipment for emergency medical and rescue service. **Entries Include:** Company name, address, phone, fax, telex, products. **Frequency:** Annual, November. **Send Orders to:** Communication Channels, Inc., 307 N. Michigan Ave., Chicago, IL 60601 (312-726-7277).

★4261★ FIRST AID SUPPLIES RETAIL DIRECTORY
American Business Directories, Inc.
American Business Information, Inc.
5711 S. 86th Circle
Omaha, NE 68127   Phone: (402) 593-4600
Number of Listings: 1,860. **Entries Include:** Name, address, phone, size of advertisement, name of owner or manager, number of employees, year first in "Yellow Pages." **Frequency:** Annual.

★4262★ THE FIRST WHOLE REHAB CATALOG: A COMPREHENSIVE GUIDE TO PRODUCTS AND SERVICES FOR THE PHYSICALLY DISADVANTAGED
Betterway Publications, Inc.
PO Box 219
Crozet, VA 22932   Phone: (804) 823-5661
Covers: Manufacturers of products that help physically handicapped people to live independently. **Entries Include:** Manufacturer name, address, phone and fax numbers, product descriptions. **Pages (approx.):** 240. **Frequency:** Latest edition 1990. **Also Includes:** Appendix listing support groups, independent-living centers, magazines and newsletters, accessible travel, state protection and advocacy agencies, and legal resources.

★4263★ FOCUS ON FAMILIES: A REFERENCE HANDBOOK
ABC-CLIO
PO Box 1911
Santa Barbara, CA 93116-1911   Phone: (805) 968-1911
Publication Includes: List of agencies, organizations, and hotlines that service the public for a variety of social concerns including child abuse, incest, drug abuse, poverty, step-families, communication problems, alcoholism, runaways, and single-parent families. **Frequency:** Published 1989. **Also Includes:** Annotated bibliography of fiction, non-fiction, and audio-visual materials.

★4264★ FREESTANDING AMBULATORY CENTER DIRECTORY
SMG Marketing Group, Inc.
1342 N. LaSalle Dr.
Chicago, IL 60610   Phone: (312) 642-3026
Covers: Over 2,800 emergency centers. **Entries Include:** Center name, address, phone, corporate affiliation. **Pages (approx.):** 300. **Frequency:** Annual, November. **Also Includes:** General information about the freestanding ambulatory center industry; alphabetical list of corporate chains owning and managing the covered emergency centers.

★4265★ FREESTANDING OUTPATIENT SURGERY CENTER DIRECTORY
SMG Marketing Group, Inc.
1342 N. LaSalle Dr.
Chicago, IL 60610   Phone: (312) 642-3026
Covers: More than 1,200 ambulatory surgical centers. **Entries Include:** Facility name, address, phone, ownership; number of operating suites, number of surgeries performed each year and types of surgery performed. **Pages (approx.):** 300. **Frequency:** Annual, August.

★4266★ FUND-RAISING RESEARCH: FRI PROSPECT-RESEARCH RESOURCE DIRECTORY
Fund-Raising Institute
12300 Twin Brook Parkway, Ste. 450
Rockville, MD 20852   Phone: (800) 888-8238
Covers: In Volume 2—Over 500 publishers and suppliers of databases and other sources that provide information on potential donors of philanthropic gifts and government grants to philanthropic causes; associations, corporations, foundations, government agencies, individuals, and other sources of philanthropic income. **Entries Include:** For publications—Publisher name, address, and phone; title, type of resource, year first available, date of latest edition or frequency, price, number of pages, and description of contents. For databases—Supplier name, address, phone, description of services provided. **Pages (approx.):** 360. **Frequency:** Triennial; latest edition spring 1986.

★4267★ GENERAL CLINICAL RESEARCH CENTERS
National Center for Research Resources
U.S. National Institutes of Health
Bethesda, MD 20892   Phone: (301) 496-5545
Covers: About 80 research centers located in academic medical centers nationwide, funded by the National Center for Research Resources, National Institutes of Health for controlled studies of human disorders. **Entries Include:** Institution name; name, title, address, and phone of program director; name and title of associate director; name, title, address, and phone of principal investigator; address of facility; description of on-site resources; description of major areas of investigation. Some listings have less detailed information. **Pages (approx.):** 120. **Frequency:** Irregular; previous edition 1988; latest edition 1991. **Send Orders to:** Research Resources Information Center, 1601 Research Blvd., Rockville, MD 20850.

★4268★ GLOBAL GUIDE TO MEDICAL INFORMATION
Elsevier Science Publishing Co., Inc.
655 Avenue of the Americas
New York, NY 10010   Phone: (212) 989-5800
Covers: International and regional health organizations; national government departments concerned with health and medicine, medical associations, and publishers of medical journals, serials, and books. **Pages (approx.):** 810. **Frequency:** Irregular; latest edition 1988.

★4269★ GRADUATE EDUCATION IN NURSING
National League for Nursing
350 Hudson St.
New York, NY 10014   Phone: (212) 582-1022
Covers: About 150 colleges and universities offering National League for Nursing accredited Master's degree programs; about 35 universities that offer doctoral degree programs administered by the schools' nursing education divisions. **Entries Include:** Institution name, address, type of control, name of nursing education administrator, areas of study available, degree offered. **Pages (approx.):** 40. **Frequency:** Annual.

★4270★ GRADUATE STUDY IN PSYCHOLOGY AND ASSOCIATED FIELDS
American Psychological Association
1200 17th St. NW
Washington, DC 20036   Phone: (202) 955-7600
Covers: Over 600 programs in the United States and Canada offering graduate education in psychology and associated fields. **Entries Include:** Institution name, address, name of department offering degree, department phone, year program established, chairperson, size of faculty, APA accreditation, academic year system, programs and degrees offered, application procedure, admission requirements, student statistics for the previous year, degree requirements, tuition, financial aid available, and comments on special programs, goals, etc. **Pages (approx.):** 660. **Frequency:** Annual, April. **Send Orders to:** American Psychological Association, Box 2710, Hyattsville, MD 20784.

★4271★ GRADUATE TRAINING IN BEHAVIOR THERAPY AND EXPERIMENTAL CLINICAL PSYCHOLOGY
Association for Advancement of Behavior Therapy
15 W. 36th St.
New York, NY 10018   Phone: (212) 279-7970
Covers: 400 programs throughout the U.S. and Canada offering masters and doctorate level training in the area of behavior psychology. **Entries Include:** Company name, address, phone, names and titles of key personnel, number of employees, requirements for membership, product/service. **Pages (approx.):** 200. **Frequency:** Biennial, September of odd years.

★4272★ GRANTS FOR HOSPITALS AND MEDICAL CARE
The Foundation Center
79 5th Ave.
New York, NY 10003   Phone: (212) 620-4230
Covers: 460 foundations which, in the year prior to that of publication, gave grants to hospitals and medical centers. **Frequency:** Annual. **Also Includes:** Statistics on health care funding.

★4273★ GROUP HEALTH ASSOCIATION OF AMERICA—NATIONAL DIRECTORY OF HMOS
Group Health Association of America
1129 20th St. NW, Ste. 600
Washington, DC 20036   Phone: (202) 778-3245
Covers: About 750 health maintenance organizations (prepaid health organizations that provide members with their medical and hospital care for a set fee), state regulatory agencies, and state associations. **Entries Include:** For HMOs—Name, address, phone, names of key personnel, model type, affiliation, owner/management, whether for-profit or nonprofit, benefit options. For others—Agency or association name, address, phone, name of contact. **Pages (approx.):** 150. **Frequency:** Annual, June.

★4274★ GROUPEMENT DES ALLERGOLOGISTES ET IMMUNOLOGISTES DE LANGUES LATINES—ANNUAIRE
Groupement des Allergologistes et Immunologistes de Langues Latines
c/o CAIC
Rua Sampaioe Pina, 16-4
P-1000 Lisbon, Portugal
Covers: 250 member allergists and immunologists who speak French, Spanish, Portuguese, Italian, or Romanian. **Entries Include:** Personal name, address, phone, medical specialty. **Pages (approx.):** 20. **Frequency:** Triennial.

★4275★ GUIDA MONACI—ANNUARIO SANITARIO
Guida Monaci SpA
Via Crispi 10
I-00187 Rome, Italy
Covers: Hospitals, clinics, public health services, etc. in Italy. **Entries Include:** Hospital or clinic name, address, phone, telex, names and titles of key personnel, description of services. **Pages (approx.):** 1,350 in two volumes. **Frequency:** Annual, May.

★4276★ GUIDE TO BIOMEDICAL STANDARDS
Quest Publishing Co.
1351 Titan Way
Brea, CA 92621   Phone: (714) 738-6400
Publication Includes: List of over 60 organizations that issue standards for medical devices, equipment, and medical care facilities; worldwide coverage. **Entries Include:** Organization name, address, phone, brief description of organization, list of standards. **Frequency:** Annual, October.

★4277★ GUIDE TO COMPASSIONATE CARING OF THE AGING
Thomas Nelson Publishers
PO Box 141000
Nashville, TN 37214-1000   Phone: (615) 889-9000
Publication Includes: Sources of information, publications, assistance, and funding for care of the aging. Also includes federal agencies that provide funding for adult day care services (the Department of Health and Human Services, Labor, Education, Transportation, Treasury, Housing and Urban Development, and ACTION); regional offices of the Administration of Aging, HUD, and religious and interfaith programs for the aging. **Entries Include:** Agency, program, or publication name and address. **Frequency:** Published August 1985.

★4278★ GUIDE TO GIFTS AND BEQUESTS: A DIRECTORY OF PHILANTHROPICALLY SUPPORTED INSTITUTIONS
The Institutions Press, Inc.
142 Lexington Ave.
New York, NY 10016   Phone: (212) 532-0367
Description: Publishes paid listings for hospitals, colleges, social service agencies, museums, and other institutions and organizations that wish to bring their activities to the notice of lawyers, accountants, trust officers and prospective donors; separate editions for Illinois, California, New York, and Florida, with 150-300 listings per edition. **Entries Include:** Organization name, address, phone, tax exempt status, financial data, financial needs, donor opportunities, activities, programs, names and titles of chief officers and directors. **Pages (approx.):** 160-240. **Frequency:** Triennial; California, latest edition 1991; Illinois, latest edition 1990; New York and Florida, latest edition 1991.

★4279★ GUIDE TO GRADUATE EDUCATION IN SPEECH-LANGUAGE PATHOLOGY AND AUDIOLOGY
American Speech-Language-Hearing Association
10801 Rockville Pike
Rockville, MD 20852   Phone: (301) 897-5700
Covers: More than 240 colleges and universities offering graduate training in speech-language pathology and audiology. **Entries Include:** Institution name, location, size, faculty, student characteristics, admission requirements, tuition, degrees granted, program description, costs, availability of financial aid. **Pages (approx.):** 210. **Frequency:** Irregular; previous edition 1988; latest edition 1991.

★4280★ GUIDE TO HEALTH-ORIENTED PERIODICALS
Sprouting Publications
Box 62
Ashland, OR 97520   Phone: (503) 488-2326
Covers: Over 250 newsletters, magazines, journals, and newspapers. **Entries Include:** Title, publisher name, address, phone, description of content, frequency, number of pages, type of paper used, amount of advertising carried, subscription and sample issue prices, name of editor, size, year established, ISSN, affiliations. **Pages (approx.):** 110. **Frequency:** Annual. **Also Includes:** List of periodicals that recently ceased publication.

★4281★ GUIDE TO MANUSCRIPT COLLECTIONS IN THE HISTORY OF PSYCHOLOGY AND PSYCHIATRY AND RELATED AREAS
Kraus International Publications
Kraus Organization Ltd.
Rte. 100
Millwood, NY 10546   Phone: (914) 762-2200
Covers: About 500 libraries and other organizations with manuscript collections in the history of psychology and similar subjects. **Entries Include:** Library, university, or organization name; address, phone, name and title of contact; description of collection, including subject scope, time period, form of material, individuals and institutions cited, correspondents; finding aids, and accessibility of collection. **Pages (approx.):** 220. **Frequency:** Published May 1982.

★4282★ GUIDE TO THE NATION'S HOSPICES
National Hospice Organization
1901 N. Moore St., Ste. 901
Arlington, VA 22209   Phone: (703) 243-5900
Covers: About 1,500 hospices, palliative care centers, and other programs serving terminally ill persons. **Entries Include:** Name of hospice program, institution name, address, and phone, name and title of principal executive, service area, scope of services. **Pages (approx.):** 205. **Frequency:** Annual, July.

★4283★ GUIDE TO POSTGRADUATE DEGREES, DIPLOMAS AND COURSES IN MEDICINE
IntelliGene
Woodlands
Ford, Midlothian EH37 5RE, Scotland
Covers: Colleges and universities offering medical degrees, diplomas, and specialized training in the United Kingdom. **Entries Include:** College name, address, phone, degree requirements. **Pages (approx.):** 76. **Frequency:** Annual, February.

★4284★ GUIDE TO PROFESSIONAL SERVICES IN SPEECH-LANGUAGE PATHOLOGY AND AUDIOLOGY
American Speech-Language-Hearing Association
10801 Rockville Pike
Rockville, MD 20852   Phone: (301) 897-5700
Covers: Accredited and nonaccredited clinical speech and hearing programs in the United States and Canada; personnel of government agencies; and ASHA members in full-time private practice. **Entries Include:** For accredited clinics—Clinic name, address, phone, director, size and certification of staff, type of clinic, referrals, and services offered. For members—Name, address, phone, specialty, and certification status. For nonaccredited clinics—Name, address, phone, specialty, director, referrals, languages, size and certification of staff. **Pages (approx.):** 240. **Frequency:** Irregular; latest edition April 1987; new edition expected, date not set.

★4285★ GUIDE TO PROGRAMS IN NURSING IN FOUR YEAR COLLEGES AND UNIVERSITIES
American Council on Education
1 Dupont Circle NW, Ste. 535
Washington, DC 20036   Phone: (202) 939-9300
Covers: About 590 educational institutions offering baccalaureate, masters, and/or doctoral programs in nursing. **Entries Include:** Institution name, address, phone, name of contact; description of programs, faculty, number of students, library facilities, affiliated health-care facilities, enrollment data, degree(s) offered, fees. **Pages (approx.):** 470. **Frequency:** Published 1987.

★4286★ GUIDE ROSENWALD
Guide Rosenwald Annuaire du Corps Medical Francais
10, rue Vineuse
F-75116 Paris, France
Covers: About 140,000 physicians, hospitals, medical laboratories, clinics, and other medical and health-related facilities, including health spas; medical equipment manufacturers and suppliers. **Entries Include:** All listings include name, address, phone; doctor listings include date of graduation and medical specialty; supplier listings include products. **Pages (approx.):** 5,000 (3 volumes). **Frequency:** Annual, December. **Available in the U.S. from:** I. C. Publications, 380 Lexington Ave., Suite 1121, New York, NY 10168.

★4287★ GUIDE TO SELECTED NATIONAL GENETIC VOLUNTARY ORGANIZATIONS
National Center for Education in Maternal and Child Health
38th & R Sts., NW
Washington, DC 20057   Phone: (202) 625-8410
Covers: About 150 mutual support groups focused on genetic and congenital conditions, such as Alzheimer's disease, arthritis, autism, cerebral palsy, cystic fibrosis, Down's syndrome, epilepsy, hemophilia, Huntington's disease, hydrocephalus, leukemia, lupus, multiple sclerosis, Parkinson's disease, scoliosis, spina bifida, and others. **Entries Include:** Organization name, address, phone, director name, contact, chapters, purpose, publications, audiovisuals, newsletters. **Pages (approx.):** 225. **Frequency:** Approximately biennial; latest edition 1989.

★4288★ GUIDE TO U.K. ORGANIZATIONS FOR VISUALLY DISABLED PEOPLE
Technical Research Section
Royal National Institute for the Blind
224 Great Portland St.
London WIN 6AA, England
Covers: Organizations in the United Kingdom serving the visually disabled person. **Entries Include:** Organization name, address, phone, name of director, description of activities, publications. **Pages (approx.):** 200. **Frequency:** Latest edition December 1990.

★4289★ GUILD OF PRESCRIPTION OPTICIANS OF AMERICA—GUILD REFERENCE DIRECTORY
Guild of Prescription Opticians of America, Division
Opticians Association of America
10341 Democracy Ln.
PO Box 10110
Fairfax, VA 22030   Phone: (703) 691-8355
Covers: 250 member firms with a total of 300 retail locations. **Entries Include:** Company name, address, name of manager, services. **Pages (approx.):** 40. **Frequency:** Annual, January.

★4290★ HANDBOOK OF CERTIFICATION AND LICENSURE REQUIREMENTS FOR SCHOOL PSYCHOLOGISTS
National Association of School Psychologists
8455 Colesville Rd., Ste. 1000
Silver Spring, MD 20910   Phone: (301) 608-0500
Covers: State departments of education and state licensing/examining boards for school psychology. **Entries Include:** Agency name, address, phone, fees, requirements, contacts. **Pages (approx.):** 230. **Frequency:** approximately biennial, latest edition 1987. **Also Includes:** Introductory chapter providing overview of certification and licensure processes, experience requirements, and credential levels; glossary.

★4291★ HANDBOOK—A DIRECTORY OF HEALTH CARE MEETINGS AND CONVENTIONS
Healthcare Convention & Exhibitors Association
5775 Peachtree Dunwoody Rd., Ste. 500G
Atlanta, GA 30342   Phone: (404) 252-3663
Covers: More than 1,600 health care meetings, most of which have an

exhibit program. **Entries Include:** Name of association/meeting, name, address, phone of contact, meeting and exhibit dates for current year, number of members, number of exhibit booths, average cost and net square feet of booth space, attendance at previous meeting, date and site for next meeting, attendee & exhibitor profiles. **Pages (approx.):** 390. **Frequency:** Semiannual, June and December.

★4292★ **HANDBOOK OF MEDICAL EDUCATION**
Association of Indian Universities
16 Kotla Marg
New Delhi 110002, India
Covers: About 200 medical programs in India, covering western, homeopathic, ayurvedic, and unani systems; includes dentistry, nursing, and pharmacy. **Entries Include:** Name, location, application deadline; scholarships, fellowships, and other programs; boarding and other facilities; admission requirements and procedures; tuition and other fees. **Pages (approx.):** 270. **Frequency:** Annual.

★4293★ **HANDICAPPED DRIVER'S MOBILITY GUIDE**
American Automobile Association
1000 AAA Dr.
Heathrow, FL 32746-5063   Phone: (407) 444-7000
Covers: Approximately 1,000 manufacturers of driving aids, driving schools, publishers, government agencies, universities, and other organizations and companies offering services and products to the handicapped driver; about 15 VA-approved hand control and lift manufacturers, and augmented driving systems. **Entries Include:** Organization, publisher, or manufacturer name, address, phone, code for products or services. **Pages (approx.):** 130. **Frequency:** Biennial. **Also Includes:** Summary of types of driving aids recommended by Veterans Administration for various handicaps. **Send Orders to:** Local AAA Club office.

★4294★ **HANDICAPPED FUNDING DIRECTORY**
Research Grant Guides
PO Box 1214
Loxahatchee, FL 33470   Phone: (407) 795-6129
Covers: More than 1,200 foundations, associations, and government agencies that grant funds to nonprofit organizations for projects related to handicapped persons. **Entries Include:** Name of granting organization, address, contact name, information concerning type and size of grants, application details. **Pages (approx.):** 225. **Frequency:** Biennial, April of even years.

★4295★ **HAVING YOUR BABY BY DONOR INSEMINATION: A COMPLETE RESOURCE GUIDEIT2**
Houghton Mifflin Company
2 Park St.
Boston, MA 02108   Phone: (617) 725-5000
Publication Includes: List of organizations and facilities providing information about donor insemination. **Frequency:** Published November 1987. **Also Includes:** Bibliography.

★4296★ **HAYES CHAIN DRUG STORE GUIDE**
Edward N. Hayes, Publisher
4229 Birch St.
Newport Beach, CA 92660   Phone: (714) 756-9063
Covers: About 20,000 chain drug stores in the United States; a chain drug store comprises six or more stores. **Entries Include:** Store headquarters name, address, phone; names, addresses, and phone numbers of franchises. **Pages (approx.):** 950. **Frequency:** Annual, September.

★4297★ **HAYES DIRECTORY OF DENTAL SUPPLY HOUSES**
Edward N. Hayes, Publisher
4229 Birch St.
Newport Beach, CA 92660   Phone: (714) 756-9063
Number of Listings: About 655. **Entries Include:** Company name, address, phone, financial strength and credit rating. **Pages (approx.):** 40. **Frequency:** Annual, September.

★4298★ **HAYES DIRECTORY OF MEDICAL SUPPLY HOUSES**
Edward N. Hayes, Publisher
4229 Birch St.
Newport Beach, CA 92660   Phone: (714) 756-9063
Covers: Over 4,635 firms. **Entries Include:** Company name, address, phone, financial strength, credit rating. **Pages (approx.):** 213. **Frequency:** Annual, September.

★4299★ **HAYES DRUGGIST DIRECTORY**
Edward N. Hayes, Publisher
4229 Birch St.
Newport Beach, CA 92660   Phone: (714) 756-9063
Covers: About 53,000 retail and about 700 wholesale drug companies. **Entries Include:** Company name, address, phone, address, financial strength, and credit rating. **Pages (approx.):** 1,170. **Frequency:** Annual, March.

★4300★ **HAYES INDEPENDENT DRUGGIST GUIDE**
Edward N. Hayes, Publisher
4229 Birch St.
Newport Beach, CA 92660   Phone: (714) 756-9063
Covers: Approximately 31,000 independent U.S. drug stores (those with 5 or fewer affiliate stores). **Entries Include:** Store name, address, phone. **Pages (approx.):** 850. **Frequency:** Annual, September.

★4301★ **HEALTH AGENCIES DIRECTORY**
American Business Directories, Inc.
American Business Information, Inc.
5711 S. 86th Circle
Omaha, NE 68127   Phone: (402) 593-4600
Number of Listings: 1,441. **Entries Include:** Name, address, phone, size of advertisement, name of owner or manager, number of employees, year first in "Yellow Pages." **Frequency:** Annual.

★4302★ **HEALTH CARE MATERIAL MANAGEMENT SOCIETY—MEMBERSHIP DIRECTORY**
Health Care Material Management Society
13223 Black Mountain Rd., No. 1-432
San Diego, CA 92129   Phone: (619) 538-0863
Covers: More than 1,000 member material management and purchasing directors in health care and hospital fields. **Entries Include:** Name, title, company, address, phone. **Frequency:** Annual, spring. **Also Includes:** Sources of information and services in the industry.

★4303★ **THE HEALTH CARE STRATEGIST: THE EXECUTIVE'S DIRECTORY OF MEDICAL TRANSACTIONS**
Windhover Information, Inc.
PO Box 360
South Norwalk, CT 06856   Phone: (203) 838-4401
Covers: Companies involved in approximately 2,000 health care industry acquisitions, alliances, and financing ventures. **Entries Include:** Company name, address, phone, names and titles of key personnel, financial data, description of transaction, terms, valuations. **Pages (approx.):** 700. **Frequency:** Annual, April.

★4304★ **HEALTH CARE SYSTEMS—DIRECTORY ISSUE**
Gralla Publications
1515 Broadway, Ste. 3201
New York, NY 10036   Phone: (212) 869-1300
Publication Includes: List of 2,500 manufacturers of equipment, supplies, and services for hospitals and nursing homes. **Entries Include:** Company name, address, phone, products or services. **Frequency:** Annual, January.

★4305★ **HEALTH CLUBS DIRECTORY**
American Business Directories, Inc.
American Business Information, Inc.
5711 S. 86th Circle
Omaha, NE 68127   Phone: (402) 593-4600
Number of Listings: 12,623. **Entries Include:** Name, address, phone (including area code). **Frequency:** Annual, January.

★4306★ **HEALTH DEVICES SOURCEBOOK**
Emergency Care Research Institute
5200 Butler Pike
Plymouth Meeting, PA 19462   Phone: (215) 825-6000
Covers: Over 5,000 manufacturers of patient care equipment, medical and surgical instruments, implants, clinical laboratory equipment and supplies, medical and hospital disposable supplies, and testing instruments; also lists companies that service, recondition, lease, or buy and sell used equipment; coverage includes Canada. **Entries Include:** Company name, address, phone, toll-free phone, telex, TWX, names of key executive and contact, product categories handled, trade names, methods of distribution, typical pricing. **Pages (approx.):** 2,000. **Frequency:** Annual, December.

★4307★ THE HEALTH DIRECTORY
National Council for Voluntary Organizations
Bedford Sq. Press
26 Bedford Sq.
London WC1B 3HU, England
Covers: 1,000 organizations who service patients interested in self-help and their families. **Entries Include:** Organization name, address, phone, description of services. **Pages (approx.):** 120. **Frequency:** Irregular; latest edition 1990.

★4308★ HEALTH EDUCATION—ASSOCIATION FOR THE ADVANCEMENT OF HEALTH EDUCATION DIRECTORY OF INSTITUTIONS ISSUE
Association for the Advancement of Health Education
1900 Association Dr.
Reston, VA 22091   Phone: (703) 476-3437
Publication Includes: Directory of about 300 institutions offering undergraduate and/or graduate programs in school, community, and/or public health education. **Entries Include:** Institution name, address, program offered; most listings include contact name and phone. **Frequency:** Biennial, summer of even years.

★4309★ HEALTH AND FITNESS PROGRAM CONSULTANTS DIRECTORY
American Business Directories, Inc.
American Business Information, Inc.
5711 S. 86th Circle
Omaha, NE 68127   Phone: (402) 593-4600
Number of Listings: 3,226. **Entries Include:** Name, address, phone (including area code), size of advertisement, year first in "Yellow Pages," name of owner or manager, number of employees. **Frequency:** Annual.

★4310★ HEALTH FUNDS GRANTS RESOURCES YEARBOOK
Health Resources Publishing
Brinley Professional Plaza
3100 Hwy. 138
Wall Township, NJ 07719-1442   Phone: (908) 681-1133
Covers: Foundations, government agencies, and corporations which award grants in areas of health care. **Entries Include:** Name, address, funding priorities, description of grants and programs. **Pages (approx.):** 210. **Frequency:** Approximately annual; latest edition April 1990; new edition expected 1992. **Also Includes:** Bibliography of information sources for healthcare grant seekers.

★4311★ HEALTH GRANTS AND CONTRACTS WEEKLY
Capitol Publications, Inc.
1101 King St., Ste. 444
Alexandria, VA 22314   Phone: (703) 683-4100
Covers: All newly available health-related federal contracts and grants. **Entries Include:** Description of project, funding information, deadlines, eligibility; contact name, address, phone. **Pages (approx.):** 8. **Frequency:** Weekly.

★4312★ HEALTH AND HUMAN SERVICES TELEPHONE DIRECTORY
U.S. Department of Health and Human Services
200 Independence Ave. SW
Washington, DC 20201   Phone: (202) 245-1605
Covers: Health, Education, and Welfare Department offices and key personnel in the metropolitan Washington area, and selected offices elsewhere. **Entries Include:** Office, institute, or other unit name, address, names of principal personnel with titles, room numbers, and phone numbers. **Pages (approx.):** 250. **Frequency:** Irregular; previous edition 1987; latest edition 1990.

★4313★ HEALTH, ILLNESS, AND DISABILITY: A GUIDE TO BOOKS FOR CHILDREN AND YOUNG ADULTS
R. R. Bowker
121 Chanlon Rd.
New Providence, NJ 07974   Phone: (908) 464-6800
Publication Includes: List of publishers of books designed for preschoolers through young adults on hospitalization, medical treatment, and physical and mental handicaps. **Entries Include:** Company name, address. **Frequency:** Irregular; latest edition 1983.

★4314★ HEALTH INDUSTRY BUYERS GUIDE
SN Publications, Inc.
103 N. 2nd St.
West Dundee, IL 60118   Phone: (708) 426-6100
Covers: 3,000 manufacturers of hospital and physician's supplies and equipment, including medical laboratory, oxygen therapy, and X-ray supplies, home health care products, and orthopedic appliances. **Entries Include:** Manufacturer name, address, phone. **Pages (approx.):** 650. **Frequency:** Annual, November.

★4315★ HEALTH INDUSTRY MANUFACTURERS ASSOCIATION—DIRECTORY
Health Industry Manufacturers Association
1030 15th St., NW, Ste. 1100
Washington, DC 20005   Phone: (202) 452-8240
Covers: About 300 member manufacturers of medical devices and diagnostic products. **Entries Include:** Company name, address, phone, name of official representative or correspondent; product or service provided. **Pages (approx.):** 100. **Frequency:** Annual, October.

★4316★ HEALTH INDUSTRY REPRESENTATIVES ASSOCIATION—MEMBERSHIP DIRECTORY
Health Industry Representatives Association
5818 Reeds Rd.
Mission, KS 66202   Phone: (913) 262-4512
Covers: Over 140 manufacturers' representatives in the health care industry, and manufacturers of health care products. **Entries Include:** Firm name, name of representative to the association, address, phone, date of membership in the association, representative firm listings include geographic area covered; related firm listings include products. **Pages (approx.):** 50. **Frequency:** Annual, winter.

★4317★ HEALTH INFORMATION HANDBOOK
Gower Publishing Company Ltd.
Gower House
Croft Rd.
Aldershot, Hants GU11 3HR, England
Publication Includes: List of organizations, publishers, and voluntary and self-help groups that provide health information services in the United Kingdom. **Frequency:** Latest edition 1986.

★4318★ HEALTH INFORMATION RESOURCES IN THE FEDERAL GOVERNMENT
ODPHP National Health Information Center
Office of Disease Prevention and Health Promotion
U.S. Public Health Service
330 C St. SW, Rm. 2132
Washington, DC 20201   Phone: (301) 565-4167
Covers: Over 120 federal and federally sponsored offices and programs providing health information and assistance. **Entries Include:** Organization name, address, phone, name of administrator, description of services, intended users, restrictions on use, fees, publications, online databases (if any). **Pages (approx.):** 68. **Frequency:** Irregular; previous edition 1987; latest edition 1990. **Send Orders to:** ONHIC, PO Box 1133, Washington, DC 20013-1133.

★4319★ HEALTH MAINTENANCE ORGANIZATIONS DIRECTORY
American Business Directories, Inc.
American Business Information, Inc.
5711 S. 86th Circle
Omaha, NE 68127   Phone: (402) 593-4600
Number of Listings: 2,113. **Entries Include:** Name, address, phone, size of advertisement, name of owner or manager, number of employees, year first in "Yellow Pages." **Frequency:** Annual.

★4320★ HEALTH MARKETING BUYERS GUIDE
CPS Communications, Inc.
7200 W. Camino Real, Ste. 215
Boca Raton, FL 33433   Phone: (407) 368-9301
Covers: Over 1,200 journals specializing in the health care industry. **Entries Include:** Company or publisher name, address, phone, fax, name of contact, key personnel, price rates, circulation, advertising rates, editorial directions. **Pages (approx.):** 1,200. **Frequency:** Semiannual, June and December. **Also Includes:** Section on alternative media and circulation by physician specialty for major health-care journals.

★4321★ HEALTH AND MEDICAL CARE DIRECTORY
Yellow Pages of America, Inc.
719 Main St.
Niagara Falls, NY 14301   Phone: (800) 387-4209
Covers: More than 70,000 physical and mental health care facilities and practitioners, medical equipment manufacturers, and suppliers of medicines throughout the United States; nearly 400 U.S. medical libraries; medical services, including 350 overseas hospitals and physicians, members of the Association for Medical Assistance to Travellers; state chapters of national medical organizations; and about 360 poison control centers. **Entries Include:** Facility, association, company, library, or personal name, address, phone. **Pages (approx.):** 675. **Frequency:** Annual. **Also Includes:** Lists of toll-free phone numbers for medical information, brief descriptions of common prescription and nonprescription medications.

★4322★ HEALTH ORGANIZATIONS OF THE UNITED STATES, CANADA, AND THE WORLD
Gale Research Inc.
835 Penobscot Building
Detroit, MI 48226   Phone: (313) 961-2242
Covers: About 1,600 professional groups, voluntary associations, foundations, and other organizations concerned with health, medicine, and related fields; includes national and international organizations. **Entries Include:** Organization name, address, phone, date founded, name of principal executive, and description of activities, publications, etc. **Pages (approx.):** 410. **Frequency:** Irregular; latest edition 1981.

★4323★ HEALTH RESOURCE BUILDER: FREE AND INEXPENSIVE MATERIALS FOR LIBRARIES AND TEACHERS
McFarland & Co., Inc.
Box 611
Jefferson, NC 28640   Phone: (919) 246-4460
Covers: Associations, government departments, foundations, and institutions involved in health care fields. **Entries Include:** Organization name, address, phone, types of publications or other materials issued. **Pages (approx.):** 263. **Frequency:** Latest edition 1988. **Also Includes:** Health care hotlines, National Health Observances calendar, state and regional offices of public agencies.

★4324★ HEALTH RESOURCES DIRECTORY
Health Research Institute
1600 S. Main Plaza, No. 170
Walnut Creek, CA 94596   Phone: (415) 676-2320
Covers: More than 10,000 organizations providing medical and health care programs and cost containment services to employers, government agencies, and labor unions. Organizations include hospitals, health maintenance organizations, preferred provider organizations, health and wellness counselors, and communications services. **Entries Include:** Organization name, address, phone, name of contact, description of service provided, including locations of programs and scope of services. **Pages (approx.):** 600. **Frequency:** Reported as annual; suspended indefinitely. **Send Orders to:** Health Publishing Co., 2837 Willow Pass Rd., Concord, CA 94596.

★4325★ HEALTH AND SAFETY DIRECTORY
Croner Publications Ltd.
Croner House
London Rd.
Kingston upon Thames, Surrey KT2 6SR, England
Covers: National and local government agencies, trade unions, pressure groups, trade organizations, and other groups involved in occupational health and safety, primarily in the United Kingdom. **Entries Include:** Organization or agency name, address, phone, telex, fax, name and title of contact, names and titles of key personnel, description of activities, committees, publications. **Pages (approx.):** 1,200. **Frequency:** Annual, June. **Also Includes:** Diary of events, bibliography, acronyms and abbreviations section, and name-changes sections.

★4326★ HEALTH AND SAFETY MARKET GUIDE
Aydee Marketing Ltd.
Nithsdale House
159 Cambridge St.
Aylesbury, Buckinghamshire HP20 1BQ, England
Covers: Approximately 870 organizations and associations concerned with occupational health and safety, security, fire protection, and safe materials handling in the United Kingdom. **Entries Include:** Company name, address, phone, telex, name and title of contact. **Pages (approx.):** 210. **Frequency:** Annual, March.

★4327★ HEALTH SCIENCES INFORMATION IN CANADA: ASSOCIATIONS
Canada Institute for Scientific and Technical Information
National Research Council of Canada
Montreal Rd., Bldg. M-58
Ottawa, ON, Canada K1A 0R6   Phone: (613) 993-9101
Covers: Canadian organizations whose objectives focus on the physical and emotional well-being of Canadians. **Entries Include:** Organization name, address, phone, telex, name and title of contact, number of members, date of establishment, statement of objectives, names of affiliated associations, publications. **Pages (approx.):** 340. **Frequency:** Irregular; latest edition 1984.

★4328★ HEALTH SCIENCES INFORMATION IN CANADA: LIBRARIES
Canada Institute for Scientific and Technical Information
National Research Council of Canada
Montreal Rd., Bldg. M-58
Ottawa, ON, Canada K1A 0S2   Phone: (613) 993-9101
Covers: Over 500 health science libraries in Canada. **Entries Include:** Institution name, address, phone, telex, number of employees, geographical area served, size and subject speciality of collection, languages of service, subject and classification system. **Pages (approx.):** 200. **Frequency:** Irregular, latest edition 1986.

★4329★ HEALTH SERVICE BUYER'S GUIDE
Benns Business Information Services Ltd.
PO Box 20
Sovereign Way
Towbridge, Kent TN9 1RQ, England
Covers: About 3,000 suppliers of health care products, equipment, and services in the United Kingdom. **Pages (approx.):** 300. **Frequency:** Annual, October.

★4330★ HEALTH SERVICE DIRECTORY
American Business Directories, Inc.
American Business Information, Inc.
5711 S. 86th Circle
Omaha, NE 68127   Phone: (402) 593-4600
Number of Listings: 3,160. **Entries Include:** Name, address, phone (including area code), size of advertisement, year first in "Yellow Pages," name of owner or manager, number of employees. **Frequency:** Annual.

★4331★ HEALTH SERVICES ADMINISTRATION EDUCATION
Association of University Programs in Health Administration
1911 N. Fort Myer Dr., Ste. 503
Arlington, VA 22209   Phone: (703) 524-5500
Covers: Undergraduate, graduate, and nontraditional member programs in health services administration; coverage includes Canada. **Entries Include:** Program name, address, department name, name of director, phone; program history and description; curriculum description; admission procedures and requirements; financial assistance available; placement services; enrollment and student characteristics; fees. **Pages (approx.):** 360. **Frequency:** Biennial, odd years.

★4332★ HEALTH SERVICES MANAGEMENT EDUCATION DEVELOPMENT AND RESEARCH DIRECTORY
European Healthcare Management Association
Vergemount Hall
Clonskeagh
Dublin 6, Ireland
Covers: Over 100 organizations offering educational programs in health services management in Europe. **Entries Include:** Organization name, address, phone. **Pages (approx.):** 250. **Frequency:** Biennial, even years.

★4333★ HEALTH SPAS AROUND THE WORLD
Globe Pequot Press
138 W. Main St.
Chester, CT 06412   Phone: (203) 526-9571
Covers: About 130 traditional and modern health resorts in 22 European countries. **Entries Include:** Resort address, price ranges, descriptions, and "practical" details. **Pages (approx.):** 170.

★4334★ HEALTHCARE AND BIOTECHNOLOGY COMPANIES
IN SCOTLAND
Scottish Development Agency
120 Bothwell St.
Glasgow G2 7JP, Scotland
Covers: About 250 companies involved in health care and biotechnology
industry in Scotland. Entries Include: Company name, address, phone,
telex, name and title of contact, number of employees, geographical area
covered, description of services. Pages (approx.): 50. Frequency: Annual,
winter. Available in the U.S. from: Scottish Development Agency, 1
Landmark Sq., Ste. 810, Stamford, CT 06901.

★4335★ HEALTHCARE FINANCIAL MANAGEMENT
ASSOCIATION—MEMBERSHIP LABELS
Healthcare Financial Management Association
2 Westbrook Corporate Center, Ste. 700
Westchester, IL 60154   Phone: (312) 531-9600
Description: Mailing labels. Covers more than 28,000 member financial
management executives, accountants and financial consultants involved in
the health care field. Entries Include: Individual name, address, job title,
and company name. Frequency: Updated as needed.

★4336★ HEALTHCARE FOODSERVICE WHO'S WHO
Information Central, Inc.
Box 3900
Prescott, AZ 86302   Phone: (602) 778-1513
Covers: 4,500 hospitals, nursing homes, retirement facilities, homes for the
aged, and other health care institutions; all institutions listed have at least
180 beds. Also included are multi-unit operators, purchasing groups, and
food management companies. Listings are in two volumes: volume I, short-
term hospitals; volume II, long-term institutions. Entries Include: Facility
name, type of institution, address, phone, food service director, number of
beds, annual food purchases, number of meals served per day, types of
food service offered, name of food management company, and/or cooperative buying organization. Pages (approx.): 250. Frequency: Triennial; latest
edition December 1990.

★4337★ HEALTHCARE STANDARDS DIRECTORY
ECRI
5200 Butler Pike
Plymouth Meeting, PA 19462   Phone: (215) 825-6000
Covers: Approximately 13,000 healthcare standards and guidelines issued
by federal and state governments, professional societies, medical societies,
and accreditation agencies; coverage includes Canada. Entries Include: In
"Organizations and Their Standards" section—Organization name, address, phone, standards or guidelines, year of issue, non-member price,
catalog number, authorizing committee, bibliographic information. In
"Names and Addresses" section—Organization or agency name, address,
phone. Pages (approx.): 1,400. Frequency: Annual; regular updates in
"Healthcare Standards Update" newsletter. Also Includes: Separate "Laws,
Legislation, and Regulation" sections tracing citations to specific state and
federal legislation.

★4338★ HEALTHCARE STANDARDS DIRECTORY AND
INFORMATION SERVICE
ECRI
5200 Butler Pike
Plymouth Meeting, PA 19462
Publication Includes: List of organizations and state and federal agencies
that have issued health care guidelines, laws, and standards. Entries
Include: Organization or agency name, address, phone. Frequency: Annual,
December.

★4339★ HEALTHIEST DINING IN AMERICA: A GUIDE TO
WHOLESOME MEALS WHEN TRAVELING
Tensleep Publications
Melius & Peterson Publishing, Inc.
526 Citizens Building
Aberdeen, SD 57401   Phone: (605) 226-0488
Covers: About 400 restaurants, cafeterias, airline services, and university
food programs offering meals that adhere to specific dietary guidelines.
Entries Include: Restaurant name, address, phone, name of owner or
manager, number of locations, credit cards accepted, hours of operation,
specialties, price range, description of services, menu samplings, handicapped accessibility. Pages (approx.): 240. Frequency: Published 1986.

★4340★ HEALTHY MOTHERS, HEALTHY BABIES—
DIRECTORY OF EDUCATIONAL MATERIALS
Healthy Mothers, Healthy Babies Coalition
409 12th St., SW, Rm. 309
Washington, DC 20023   Phone: (202) 863-2458
Covers: Approximately 70 member organizations providing educational
services and materials (primarily literature) concerning prenatal and infant
care; approximately 15 additional nonmember organizations offering
similar services or products. Entries Include: Organization name and
address; brief statement outlining objectives and projects; list of materials
or services provided. Pages (approx.): 170. Frequency: Irregular; latest
edition 1985; new edition possible 1990.

★4341★ HEARING AIDS RETAILERS DIRECTORY
American Business Directories, Inc.
American Business Information, Inc.
5711 S. 86th Circle
Omaha, NE 68127   Phone: (402) 593-4600
Number of Listings: 9,345. Entries Include: Name, address, phone (includ-
ing area code), size of advertisement, year first in "Yellow Pages," name of
owner or manager, number of employees. Frequency: Annual.

★4342★ HEARING INSTRUMENTS—INTERNATIONAL
DIRECTORY OF HEARING HEALTH CARE PRODUCTS
ISSUE
Edgell Communications, Inc.
1 E. 1st St.
Duluth, MN 55802   Phone: (218) 723-9200
Publication Includes: List of over 900 manufacturers and distributors of
hearing aids, ear molds, audiometric test equipment, audiometers, and
noise control products, worldwide. Entries Include: Company name,
address, phone, names of executives. Frequency: Annual, May.

★4343★ HEARING JOURNAL—HEARING HEALTH INDUSTRY
WORLD DIRECTORY ISSUE
The Laux Co.
63 Great Rd.
Maynard, MA 01754   Phone: (508) 897-5552
Covers: Manufacturers and suppliers of hearing aids, ear molds, audiometers, testing equipment, calibrators, and accessory items; hearing aid repair
laboratories; services; related publishers, trade associations, organizations;
international coverage. Entries Include: Company name, address, phone,
names and titles of executives, whether manufacturer or distributor, trade
and brand names, list of products or services provided. Frequency: Annual,
December.

★4344★ HEART VALVES AND SOFT TISSUE IMPLANT
MARKETS
Theta Corp.
Theta Bldg.
Middlefield, CT 06455   Phone: (203) 349-1054
Publication Includes: List of corporations involved in the heart valve
market. Entries Include: Company name, address, phone, key personnel,
background information, description of products, annual sales, research
and development efforts, distribution systems, five year projection.
Frequency: Irregular; latest edition April 1989.

★4345★ HEMATOLOGY INSTRUMENTATION FOR THE
CLINICAL LAB
Theta Corp.
Theta Bldg.
Middlefield, CT 06455   Phone: (203) 349-1054
Publication Includes: List of about 10 manufacturers of hematology and
coagulation instruments. Entries Include: Company name, address, phone,
key personnel, background information, description of products, annual
sales, research and development efforts, distribution systems, five year
projection. Frequency: Irregular; latest edition September 1989.

★4346★ HERITAGE OF AVIATION MEDICINE: AN
ANNOTATED DIRECTORY OF EARLY ARTIFACTS
Aerospace Medical Association
320 S. Henry St.
Alexandria, VA 22314   Phone: (703) 739-2240
Covers: About 75 private collections, museums, and other collections of
over 500 aviation medicine artifacts. Entries Include: Collection or
museum name, address, name of contact, description of collection
including specific objects held. Pages (approx.): 125. Frequency: Published
1979; no new edition expected.

★4347★ HIGH GROWTH IMMUNODIAGNOSTICS
Theta Corp.
Theta Bldg.
Middlefield, CT 06455 Phone: (203) 349-1054
Publication Includes: List of companies involved in the immunodiagnostic testing market. **Entries Include:** Company name, address, phone, key personnel, background information, description of products, annual sales, research and development efforts, distribution systems, five year projection. **Frequency:** Irregular; previous edition April 1984; latest edition March 1988.

★4348★ HMO/PPO DIRECTORY
Medical Device Register
5 Paragon Dr.
Montvale, NJ 07645-1725
Covers: 600 health maintenance organizations (HMOs) and 400 preferred provider organizations (PPOs). **Entries Include:** Name of organization, address, phone, number of members, names of officers, employer references, geographical area served, parent company, average fees and copayments, financial data, and cost control procedures. **Pages (approx.):** 300. **Frequency:** Annual.

★4349★ HOLIDAYS IN THE BRITISH ISLES: A GUIDE FOR DISABLED PEOPLE
Royal Association for Disability & Rehabilitation
25 Mortimer St.
London W1N 8AB, England
Covers: About 2,000 hotels, motels, and other overnight accommodations for the disabled traveler in the United Kingdom. **Entries Include:** Facility name, address, phone, telex, name and title of contact, room measurements and specifications, special adaptations, rates. **Pages (approx.):** 600. **Frequency:** Annual, January.

★4350★ HOLIDAYS AND TRAVEL ABROAD: A GUIDE FOR DISABLED PEOPLE
Royal Association for Disability and Rehabilitation
25 Mortimer St.
London W1N 8AB, England
Covers: Approximately 500 international hotel chains, single hotels, transportation services and national advisory organizations worldwide (outside the United Kingdom) which cater to disabled travelers. **Entries Include:** Company name, address, phone, description of facilities and services. **Pages (approx.):** 230. **Frequency:** Irregular; latest edition July 1991.

★4351★ THE HOLISTIC NETWORK DIRECTORY
The Holistic Network
172 Archway Rd.
London N6 5BB, England
Covers: 7,500 health clinics, practitioners, associations, training organizations, and suppliers in the United Kingdom and Ireland dealing with holistic health car e, psychic healing, and spirituality. **Entries Include:** Company name, address, phone, type of service provided. **Pages (approx.):** 240. **Frequency:** Biennial, May of odd years.

★4352★ HOLISTIC PRACTITIONERS DIRECTORY
American Business Directories, Inc.
American Business Information, Inc.
5711 S. 86th Circle
Omaha, NE 68127 Phone: (402) 593-4600
Number of Listings: 1,243. **Entries Include:** Name, address, phone, size of advertisement, name of owner or manager, number of employees, year first in "Yellow Pages." **Frequency:** Annual.

★4353★ HOLISTIC RESOURCES DIRECTORY
Holistic Resources
c/o Quality Books, Inc.
918 Sherwood Dr.
Lake Bluff, IL 60044 Phone: (708) 295-2010
Covers: Publishers, organizations, retailers, and practitioners of holistic products and services. **Entries Include:** Company, organization, or personal name, address, phone, product or service. **Pages (approx.):** 265. **Frequency:** Published 1988.

★4354★ HOME CARE MARKET ATLAS
SMG Marketing Group, Inc.
1342 N. LaSalle
Chicago, IL 60610 Phone: (312) 642-3026
Covers: About 7,500 home health care agencies and medical equipment suppliers. **Entries Include:** Agency or company name, address, phone, number of employees, products or services. **Pages (approx.):** 300. **Frequency:** Annual, July; suspended indefinitely.

★4355★ HOME HEALTH AGENCY CHAIN DIRECTORY
SMG Marketing Group, Inc.
1342 N. LaSalle
Chicago, IL 60610 Phone: (312) 642-3026
Covers: Over 250 corporate home health agency chains which own 2 or more facilities. **Entries Include:** Company name, location, subsidiary and branch names and locations, type of agency, number of employees, types of services offered. **Pages (approx.):** 300. **Frequency:** Annual, December.

★4356★ HOME HEALTH CARE: A COMPLETE GUIDE FOR PATIENTS AND THEIR FAMILIES
W. W. Norton & Co., Inc.
500 5th Ave.
New York, NY 10110 Phone: (212) 354-5500
Publication Includes: List of adult day care centers. **Frequency:** Published 1986.

★4357★ HOME HEALTH SERVICE DIRECTORY
American Business Directories, Inc.
American Business Information, Inc.
5711 S. 86th Circle
Omaha, NE 68127 Phone: (402) 593-4600
Number of Listings: 10,974. **Entries Include:** Name, address, phone (including area code), size of advertisement, year first in "Yellow Pages," name of owner or manager, number of employees. **Frequency:** Annual.

★4358★ HOME HEALTHCARE AGENCY DIRECTORY
SMG Marketing Group, Inc.
1342 N. LaSalle Dr.
Chicago, IL 60610 Phone: (312) 642-3026
Covers: Approximately 8,500 agencies providing health care to patients at home. **Entries Include:** Agency name, address, phone, type of agency, number of employees, types of services offered. **Pages (approx.):** 350. **Frequency:** Annual, December.

★4359★ HOME/SELF HEALTH CARE
Techne Research
1100 Massachusetts Ave.
Arlington, MA 02174 Phone: (617) 646-6297
Covers: Over 600 manufacturers, service providers, and national distributors; over 7,000 home health care agencies, including home health service associations, public health nursing services, and visiting nurse associations, related federal, state, and local government agencies; over 200 professional associations, foundations, and nonprofit groups concerned with home health care, and publishers of about 60 related periodicals. **Entries Include:** All listings include organization name, address, and phone. In addition, for manufacturers—Names of key personnel, names of divisions involved with home and self health care, products and services; some listings include financial information, corporate officers, and principal offices. For home health care agencies—Services, name of chief executive officer, type of ownership (proprietary, corporate not-for-profit, hospital, county, etc.). For government agencies—Key personnel. For associations—Key personnel, annual meeting or convention dates. For periodical publishers—Name of editor. **Pages (approx.):** 700. **Frequency:** Annual, November.

★4360★ HOMECARE PRODUCT DIRECTORY AND BUYERS' GUIDE
Miramar Publishing Co.
6133 Bristol Pkwy.
PO Box 3640
Culver City, CA 90231-3640 Phone: (213) 337-9717
Publication Includes: List of about 750 manufacturers and distributors of home health care and rehabilitation products. **Entries Include:** Company name, address, phone, names and titles of key personnel, trade names, product or service provided; also by product category. **Frequency:** Annual, July.

★4361★ HOMECARE PRODUCT REFERENCE
Medical Economic Data
5 Paragon Dr.
Montvale, NJ 07645-1742   Phone: (201) 358-7500
Covers: Over 3,000 suppliers of 26,000 products in the home health care industry; coverage includes Canada. **Entries Include:** Company name, address, phone, fax and telex numbers, names and titles of key personnel, contacts, number of employees, company ownership, sales volume, financial data, products. **Pages (approx.):** 700. **Frequency:** Annual, summer.

★4362★ HOMES—RESIDENTIAL CARE FACILITY DIRECTORY
American Business Directories, Inc.
American Business Information, Inc.
5711 S. 86th Circle
Omaha, NE 68127   Phone: (402) 593-4600
Number of Listings: 2,345. **Entries Include:** Name, address, phone (including area code), size of advertisement, year first in "Yellow Pages," name of owner or manager, number of employees. **Frequency:** Annual.

★4363★ HOSPICE ALTERNATIVE: A NEW CONTEXT FOR DEATH AND DYING
Basic Books, Inc.
10 E. 53rd St.
New York, NY 10022   Phone: (212) 207-7057
Publication Includes: Appendix of hospice referral centers. **Entries Include:** Name, address. **Frequency:** Published August 1986.

★4364★ HOSPICES DIRECTORY
American Business Directories, Inc.
American Business Information, Inc.
5711 S. 86th Circle
Omaha, NE 68127   Phone: (402) 593-4600
Number of Listings: 1,019. **Entries Include:** Name, address, phone, size of advertisement, name of owner or manager, number of employees, year first in "Yellow Pages." **Frequency:** Annual.

★4365★ HOSPITAL CONSULTANTS DIRECTORY
American Business Directories, Inc.
American Business Information, Inc.
5711 S. 86th Circle
Omaha, NE 68127   Phone: (402) 593-4600
Number of Listings: 1,070. **Entries Include:** Name, address, phone, size of advertisement, name of owner or manager, number of employees, year first in "Yellow Pages." **Frequency:** Annual.

★4366★ HOSPITAL EQUIPMENT AND SUPPLIES DIRECTORY
American Business Directories, Inc.
American Business Information, Inc.
5711 S. 86th Circle
Omaha, NE 68127   Phone: (402) 593-4600
Number of Listings: 17,048. **Entries Include:** Name, address, phone (including area code), size of advertisement, year first in "Yellow Pages," name of owner or manager, number of employees. **Frequency:** Annual.

★4367★ HOSPITAL MARKET ATLAS
SMG Marketing Group, Inc.
1342 N. LaSalle Dr.
Chicago, IL 60610   Phone: (312) 642-3026
Covers: Over 8,200 hospitals, clinical laboratories, hospital systems, group purchasing organizations, health maintenance organizations, outpatient surgery centers, and diagnostic imaging centers. **Entries Include:** Hospital or organization name, address, phone, county code, management, type of hospital service, number of beds, admissions, surgical operations, and emergency room visits. **Pages (approx.):** 450. **Frequency:** Annual. **Also Includes:** Maps of states and cities with hospital locations keyed.

★4368★ HOSPITAL PHONE BOOK
U.S. Directory Service
655 NW 128th St.
Miami, FL 33168   Phone: (305) 769-1700
Covers: About 7,975 hospitals, including military and other federal facilities. **Entries Include:** Institution name, address, phone. **Pages (approx.):** 220. **Frequency:** Irregular; previous edition 1988; latest edition 1991/92.

★4369★ HOSPITAL PHONE BOOK/CANADA
U.S. Directory Service
655 NW 128th St.
Miami, FL 33168   Phone: (305) 769-1700
Covers: Nearly 1,200 hospitals in Canada. **Entries Include:** Hospital name, address, phone, number of beds. **Frequency:** Latest edition 1986.

★4370★ HOSPITAL SOFTWARE SOURCEBOOK
Aspen Publishers, Inc.
200 Orchard Ridge Dr.
Gaithersburg, MD 20878   Phone: (301) 417-7500
Publication Includes: List of over 2,000 computer software packages or systems that can be used by hospitals and are available from approximately 500 manufacturers or suppliers. **Entries Include:** Company name, address, phone, name of contact, toll-free phone, fax, description of software package or system, price of program, compatability considerations. **Pages (approx.):** 1,200. **Frequency:** Annual, December. **Send Orders to:** Aspen Publishers, Inc., 7201 McKinney Circle, Frederick, Maryland 21701 (301-698-7100).

★4371★ HOSPITALIZATION PLANS DIRECTORY
American Business Directories, Inc.
American Business Information, Inc.
5711 S. 86th Circle
Omaha, NE 68127   Phone: (402) 593-4600
Number of Listings: 10,284. **Entries Include:** Name, address, phone (including area code), size of advertisement, year first in "Yellow Pages," name of owner or manager, number of employees. **Frequency:** Annual.

★4372★ HOSPITALS DIRECTORY
American Business Directories, Inc.
American Business Information, Inc.
5711 S. 86th Circle
Omaha, NE 68127   Phone: (402) 593-4600
Number of Listings: 10,978. **Entries Include:** Name, address, phone (including area code), size of advertisement, year first in "Yellow Pages," name of owner or manager, number of employees. **Frequency:** Annual.

★4373★ HOSPITALS AND HEALTH SERVICES YEARBOOK AND DIRECTORY OF HOSPITAL SUPPLIERS
Institute of Health Services Management
75 Portland Pl.
London W1N 4AN, England
Covers: National Health Service and independent hospitals; health authorities; private medical insurance plans; postgraduate training hospitals; government departments, councils, etc., concerned with health services; manufacturers and suppliers of hospital equipment. **Entries Include:** For health service authorities—Name, address, phone, principal officials, services or responsibilities. For hospitals—Name, address, phone, number of beds, facilities; health center listings have less detail. For suppliers—Company name, address, phone. **Pages (approx.):** 1,000. **Frequency:** Annual, spring.

★4374★ HOSPITALS WITH RESIDENCY PROGRAMS
SMG Marketing Group, Inc.
1342 N. LaSalle Dr.
Chicago, IL 60610   Phone: (312) 642-3026
Covers: U.S. hospitals with residency programs. **Entries Include:** Hospital name, address, phone, total residency openings, breakdown of openings by hospital unit; annual number of admissions, emergency room patients, and births. **Pages (approx.):** 300. **Frequency:** Quarterly.

★4375★ HOW TO FIND INFORMATION ABOUT AIDS
The Haworth Press, Inc.
10 Alice St.
Binghamton, NY 13904   Phone: (607) 722-5857
Covers: Approximately 600 organizations; counseling, educational, and referral services; treatment facilities; local and state health departments; federal and private sources of research and grant funding; hotlines. **Entries Include:** Organization, agency, or hotline name, address, phone, brief description. **Pages (approx.):** 130. **Frequency:** Irregular; previous edition 1988; latest edition winter 1991.

★4376★ HUMAN FACTORS SOCIETY—DIRECTORY
Human Factors Society
Box 1369
Santa Monica, CA 90406   Phone: (213) 394-1811
Covers: 5,200 psychologists, engineers, physiologists, and other scientists in

related fields who are concerned with the use of human factors in the development of systems and devices of all kinds. **Entries Include:** Name, affiliation, address, degrees, specialties. **Pages (approx.):** 336. **Frequency:** Annual, April.

★4377★   HYPNOTISTS DIRECTORY
American Business Directories, Inc.
American Business Information, Inc.
5711 S. 86th Circle
Omaha, NE 68127   Phone: (402) 593-4600
Number of Listings: 3,851. **Entries Include:** Name, address, phone (including area code), size of advertisement, year first in "Yellow Pages," name of owner or manager, number of employees. **Frequency:** Annual.

**★4378★   THE ILLUSTRATED DIRECTORY OF HANDICAP
      PRODUCTS**
Trio Publications Inc.
3600 W. Timber Ct.
Lawrence, KS 66049-2149   Phone: (913) 749-1453
Covers: Approximately 1,000 products for the handicapped, such as wheelchairs, lifts, elevators, ramps, and dressing and eating aids. **Entries Include:** Manufacturer name, address, phone; product description and photo. **Pages (approx.):** 250. **Frequency:** Annual.

**★4379★   THE IMPOSSIBLE CHILD—IN SCHOOL, AT HOME:
      A GUIDE FOR CARING TEACHERS AND PARENTS**
Practical Allergy Research Foundation
Box 60
Buffalo, NY 14223-0060   Phone: (716) 875-5578
Publication Includes: List of about 20 companies that provide allergy supplies, air purifiers, heater, cotton clothes, mattresses, bedding, less allergenic vitamins and medicines, and other products for people with food, inhalant, or chemical sensitivities; nearly 60 publishers of books that contain information about allergies, environmental and chemical irritants, and children's behavioral and learning problems. **Entries Include:** For companies—Name, address, phone, products. For publishers—Name, address, name of author, book title, year published, price. **Frequency:** Irregular; previous edition October 1986; latest edition 1989.

★4380★   IMPOTENCE: HOW TO OVERCOME IT
HealthProInk & Thirty Three Publishing
Spelman Productions, Inc.
582 Wind Cliff
Spring Lake, MI 49456   Phone: (616) 847-2843
Publication Includes: List of approximately 150 support groups and institutions and manufacturers of penile implants. **Entries Include:** Organizations or company name, address, phone, name and title of contact, product or service. **Frequency:** Approximately biennial, summer of odd years. **Send Orders to:** HealthProInk & Thirty Three Publishing, Box 3333, Farmington Hills, MI 48333.

**★4381★   IN TOUCH: HANDBOOK FOR BLIND AND
      PARTIALLY SIGHTED PEOPLE**
Broadcasting Support Services
252 Western Ave.
London W3 6XJ, England
Covers: Manufacturers and suppliers of products, services, and equipment to the visually handicapped in Great Britain. **Entries Include:** Company name, address, phone, product or service. **Pages (approx.):** 400. **Frequency:** Annual, May.

**★4382★   INDEPENDENT MEDICAL DISTRIBUTORS
      ASSOCIATION—MEMBERSHIP DIRECTORY**
Independent Medical Distributors Association
5818 Reeds Rd.
Shawnee Mission, KS 66202   Phone: (913) 262-4510
Covers: Member distributors of specialized high technology medical products. **Entries Include:** Name, address, product or service provided. **Pages (approx.):** 40. **Frequency:** Annual, March.

**★4383★   INDEX MEDICUS FOR WHO EASTERN
      MEDITERRANEAN REGION (IMEMR)**
Eastern Mediterranean Regional Office
World Health Organization
Box 1517
Alexandria, Egypt
Publication Includes: List of approximately 100 medical periodicals issued in the Eastern Mediterranean region. **Entries Include:** Title, publisher

name, address, and frequency. **Pages (approx.):** 1,000. **Frequency:** Annual, March.

★4384★   INDEX OF VETERINARY SPECIALITIES
A. E. Morgan Publications Ltd.
Stanley House
9 West St.
Epsom, Surrey KT18 7RL, England
Publication Includes: List of about 20 manufacturers of veterinary products in the United Kingdom; all listing are paid. **Entries Include:** Company name, address, phone, product or service. **Frequency:** Bimonthly.

★4385★   INFACT MEDICAL SCHOOL INFORMATION SYSTEM
Dataflow Systems Inc.
7758 Wisconsin Ave.
Bethesda, MD 20814   Phone: (301) 654-9133
Description: Microfiche. Not a directory, but a compilation of about 240 microfiche containing the complete catalogs of over 140 North American medical schools; coverage includes Canada. **Pages (approx.):** 17,000 (frames/pages). **Frequency:** Updated 3 times per year on microfiche.

★4386★   INFERTILITY: MEDICAL AND SOCIAL CHOICES
Office of Technology Assessment
600 Pennsylvania Ave., SE
Washington, DC 20510   Phone: (202) 224-3827
Publication Includes: List of approximately 170 facilities that perform in vitro fertilization (IVF) and gamete intrafallopian transfer (GIFT) surgery; approximately 20 surrogate mothering matching services. **Entries Include:** For IVF/GIFT facilities—Company or institution name, address, phone. For surrogate mothering matching services—Company name, address. **Frequency:** Published May 1988.

★4387★   INFORMATION FOR HANDICAPPED TRAVELERS
Reference Section
National Library Service for the Blind and Physically Handicapped
Library of Congress
Washington, DC 20542   Phone: (202) 707-9286
Covers: About 55 travel agencies, travel information centers, and transportation services for disabled travelers. **Entries Include:** Company name, address, phone, description of services. **Pages (approx.):** 10. **Frequency:** Irregular; latest edition July 1987. **Also Includes:** Selected listing of print and special format books on the topic.

**★4388★   THE INSIDER'S GUIDE TO MEDICAL AND DENTAL
      SCHOOLS**
Arco Publishing, Inc.
Simon & Schuster, Inc.
15 Columbus Circle, 16th Fl.
New York, NY 10023   Phone: (212) 373-8931
Covers: 120 medical and dental schools. **Entries Include:** School name, address, faculty/student ratio, enrollment data, graduate studies offered, financial data, student services. **Pages (approx.):** 340. **Frequency:** Latest edition fall 1988. **Send Orders to:** Arco Publishing, Inc., Ordering Department, 200 Old Tappan Road, Old Tappan, NJ 07675 (201-767-5937).

★4389★   INSURANCE—HEALTH AND ACCIDENT DIRECTORY
American Business Directories, Inc.
American Business Information, Inc.
5711 S. 86th Circle
Omaha, NE 68127   Phone: (402) 593-4600
Number of Listings: 2,110. **Entries Include:** Name, address, phone, size of advertisement, name of owner or manager, number of employees, year first in "Yellow Pages." **Frequency:** Annual.

★4390★   INTERACTIVE HEALTHCARE DIRECTORY
Stewart Publishing, Inc.
6471 Merritt Court
Alexandria, VA 22312   Phone: (703) 354-8155
Covers: Sponsors and producers of over 400 videodisc and CD-ROM projects developed for the health science field. **Entries Include:** Project name, sponsor name, address, and phone; producer name, address, and phone; description of project, including purpose, subject, intended audience, hardware system, authoring language, and availability. **Pages (approx.):** 206. **Frequency:** Annual, spring.

★4391★ INTERNATIONAL ACADEMY OF NUTRITION AND PREVENTIVE MEDICINE—MEMBERSHIP DIRECTORY
International Academy of Nutrition and Preventive Medicine
PO Box 18433
Asheville, NC 28814 Phone: (704) 258-3243
Covers: 500 persons having doctoral degrees in one of the health care professions (medicine, osteopathy, dentistry, etc.). Entries Include: Name, office address, highest degree held, areas of occupational specialization. Pages (approx.): 50. Frequency: Reported as annual; latest edition 1988.

★4392★ INTERNATIONAL ASSOCIATION FOR ANALYTICAL PSYCHOLOGY—LIST OF MEMBERS
International Association for Analytical Psychology
Postfach 115
CH-8042 Zurich, Switzerland
Covers: 1,500 Jungian analysts who are members of one or more of about 25 professional Jungian groups worldwide. Entries Include: Name, address, phone, membership classification. Pages (approx.): 240. Frequency: Triennial, autumn; latest edition December 1989; annual supplements.

★4393★ INTERNATIONAL ASSOCIATION OF ASTHMOLOGY—MEMBERSHIP DIRECTORY
International Association of Asthmology
c/o Prof. P. Godard
Clinique L'Aiguelongue
Ave. Major Flandre
F-34059 Montpellier Cedex, France
Covers: 1,300 doctors and other individuals interested in asthmology. Entries Include: Member name, address, phone. Pages (approx.): 50. Frequency: Triennial.

★4394★ INTERNATIONAL ASSOCIATION OF DENTO-MAXILLO-FACIAL RADIOLOGY NEWSLETTER—DIRECTORY ISSUE
International Association of Dento-Maxillo-Facial Radiology
Department of Dental Diagnostic Science
UTHSCSA
7703 Floyd Curl Dr.
San Antonio, TX 78284
Covers: 500 dento-maxillo-facial radiologists and others professionally interested in radiology and allied diagnostic procedures. Frequency: Triennial.

★4395★ INTERNATIONAL ASSOCIATION OF LARYNGECTOMEES—DIRECTORY OF INSTRUCTORS OF ALARYNGEAL SPEECH
International Association of Laryngectomees
c/o American Cancer Society
1599 Clifton Rd., NE
Atlanta, GA 30329 Phone: (404) 320-3333
Covers: About 600 instructors of speech to laryngectomees. Entries Include: Name, affiliation, address, phone. Pages (approx.): 35. Frequency: Irregular; previous edition March 1987; latest edition spring 1991; updated in quarterly issues of "IAL News."

★4396★ INTERNATIONAL ASSOCIATION OF LOGOPEDICS AND PHONIATRICS—LIST OF INDIVIDUAL MEMBERS, LIST OF AFFILIATED SOCIETIES
International Association of Logopedics and Phoniatrics
c/o Dr. A. Muller
6, avenue de la Gare
CH-1003 Lausanne, Switzerland
Covers: 600 phoniaters (voice disorder specialists), logopedists (speech-language defect therapists), and audiologists (hearing specialists) and 50 affiliated societies in nearly 35 countries. Entries Include: For IALP members—Name, address. For affiliated societies—Organization name, address, name and title of contact. Pages (approx.): 40. Frequency: Annual, January.

★4397★ INTERNATIONAL ASSOCIATION OF ORAL PATHOLOGISTS—MEMBERSHIP LIST
International Association of Oral Pathologists
c/o Dr. William H. Binnie
3302 Gaston Ave.
Dallas, TX 75246 Phone: (214) 828-8110
Covers: 325 dentists who have had postgraduate instruction in oral pathology. Entries Include: Personal name, address. Pages (approx.): 25. Frequency: Annual.

★4398★ INTERNATIONAL ASSOCIATION FOR ORTHODONTICS—MEMBERSHIP DIRECTORY
International Association for Orthodontics
211 E. Chicago Ave., Ste. 915
Chicago, IL 60611 Phone: (312) 642-2602
Covers: 1,700 general and children's dentists specializing in prevention or correction of facial and jaw irregularities. Entries Include: Name, office address and phone, orthodontic techniques practiced. Pages (approx.): 100. Frequency: Annual, June.

★4399★ INTERNATIONAL ASSOCIATION FOR THE STUDY OF PAIN—DIRECTORY OF MEMBERS
International Association for the Study of Pain
909 NE 43rd St., Rm. 306
Seattle, WA 98105 Phone: (206) 547-6409
Covers: Over 4,500 scientists, physicians, and other health professionals interested in pain research and therapy. Entries Include: Name, title, address, code for type of membership, medical or scientific specialty; some listings include phone. Pages (approx.): 184. Frequency: Annual, July.

★4400★ INTERNATIONAL BRAIN RESEARCH ORGANIZATION—DIRECTORY OF MEMBERS
International Brain Research Organization
51, boulevard de Montmorency
F-75016 Paris, France
Covers: 24,000 scientists working in neuroscience. Entries Include: Name, address, phone, fax. Frequency: Irregular; previous edition 1988; latest edition 1991.

★4401★ INTERNATIONAL CHILDBIRTH EDUCATION ASSOCIATION—ICEA MEMBERSHIP DIRECTORY
International Childbirth Education Association (ICEA)
Box 20048
Minneapolis, MN 55420 Phone: (612) 854-8660
Covers: Cesarean educators, childbirth educators, counselors, family physicians, homebirth specialists, nurses, nurse midwives, obstetricians and gynecologists, parent educators, pediatricians, and physical therapists and other individuals and associations involved in family-centered maternity care; international coverage. Entries Include: Personal or organization name, address, names and titles of key personnel, services. Pages (approx.): 160. Frequency: Annual, February.

★4402★ INTERNATIONAL COLLEGE OF SURGEONS—MEMBERSHIP DIRECTORY
International College of Surgeons
1516 N. Lake Shore Dr.
Chicago, IL 60610 Phone: (312) 642-3555
Covers: About 14,000 surgeons; international coverage. Entries Include: Personal name, address, specialization. Pages (approx.): 235. Frequency: Irregular; previous edition 1985; latest edition 1990.

★4403★ INTERNATIONAL COUNCIL OF PSYCHOLOGISTS—YEARBOOK
International Council of Psychologists
4805 Regent St.
Madison, WI 53705 Phone: (608) 238-5373
Covers: About 1,800 psychologists and related mental health professionals. Entries Include: Name, office and home address, career data, languages spoken and written, highest degree, fields of interest. Pages (approx.): 100. Frequency: Biennial, November of even years.

★4404★ INTERNATIONAL COUNCIL OF SPORT SCIENCE AND PHYSICAL EDUCATION—CALENDAR OF EVENTS
International Council of Sport Science and Physical Education
c/o University of Jyvaskyla
Dept. of Biology of Physical Activity
Seminaarinkatu 15
SF-40100 Jyvaskyla, Finland
Covers: Congresses, conferences, symposia, and meetings in the field of sport science and physical education. Entries Include: Organization name, address, phone, fax, telex, name and title of contact; title, date, and location of scheduled event. Pages (approx.): 20. Frequency: Semiannual, October and March.

★4405★ INTERNATIONAL COURSES IN OCCUPATIONAL HEALTH AND SAFETY
Nordic Institute for Advanced Training in Occupational Health
Topeliuksenkatu 41 a A
SF-00250 Helsinki, Finland
Covers: Training programs in occupational health. **Frequency:** Annual, July.

★4406★ INTERNATIONAL DIABETES FEDERATION DIRECTORY: A GUIDE TO THE ACTIVITIES OF IDF MEMBER ASSOCIATIONS
International Diabetes Federation (IDF)
40, rue Washington
B-1050 Brussels, Belgium
Frequency: Irregular; previous edition November 1988; latest edition June 1991.

★4407★ INTERNATIONAL DIRECTORY OF ADULT-ORIENTED ASSISTIVE DEVICE SOURCES
Lifeboat Press
Box 11782
Marina Del Rey, CA 90295   Phone: (213) 305-1600
Covers: Suppliers of implements and tools enabling adults with impaired functions or disabilities to perform daily living activities. **Entries Include:** Company name, address, phone, contact name, products or services, illustrations. **Pages (approx.):** 350. **Frequency:** Biennial, May of even years.

★4408★ INTERNATIONAL DIRECTORY OF AGENCIES FOR THE VISUALLY DISABLED
Technical Research Section
Royal National Institute for the Blind
224 Great Portland St.
London W1N 6AA, England
Covers: Organizations serving the handicapped in 142 countries. **Entries Include:** Organization name, English translation of name, address, phone, contact name, description of activities. **Pages (approx.):** 160. **Frequency:** Latest edition 1991.

★4409★ INTERNATIONAL DIRECTORY OF BIONIC AND PROSTHETIC ASSISTIVE DEVICE SOURCES
Lifeboat Press
Box 11782
Marina Del Rey, CA 90295   Phone: (213) 305-1600
Covers: Suppliers of bionic and prosthetic equipment. **Entries Include:** Company name, address, phone, contact name, products or services, illustrations. **Pages (approx.):** 350. **Frequency:** Biennial, June of even years.

★4410★ INTERNATIONAL DIRECTORY OF CHILD-ORIENTED ASSISTIVE DEVICE SOURCES
Lifeboat Press
Box 11782
Marina Del Rey, CA 90295   Phone: (213) 305-1600
Covers: Suppliers of implements and tools enabling children with impaired functions or disabilities to perform daily living activities. **Entries Include:** Company or organization name, address, phone, contact name, products or services, illustrations. **Pages (approx.):** 350. **Frequency:** Biennial, April of even years.

★4411★ INTERNATIONAL DIRECTORY OF CONSCIOUS BREATHING TEACHERS
Conscious Breathers Association
Box 234
Sierraville, CA 96126   Phone: (916) 994-3737
Covers: Approximately 500 teachers of breathing techniques for stress reduction, emotional release, and spiritual development. **Entries Include:** Teacher name, address, phone, and description of training. **Pages (approx.):** 100. **Frequency:** Semiannual, January and July; latest edition January 1991.

★4412★ INTERNATIONAL DIRECTORY OF GENETIC SERVICES
March of Dimes Birth Defects Foundation
1275 Mamaroneck Ave.
White Plains, NY 10605   Phone: (914) 428-7100
Covers: About 90 medical genetic units engaged in research or counseling. **Entries Include:** Name of unit director, unit name, address, phone, code for services offered or special capabilities. **Pages (approx.):** 60. **Frequency:** Irregular; previous edition July 1986; latest edition April 1990.

★4413★ INTERNATIONAL DIRECTORY OF JOB-ORIENTED ASSISTIVE DEVICE SOURCES
Lifeboat Press
Box 11782
Marina del Rey, CA 90292   Phone: (213) 305-1600
Covers: About 250 sources of implements and tools enabling workers with handicaps to do their jobs. **Entries Include:** Source name, address, phone, contact; disability and resulting problem, description of device, occupation involved. **Pages (approx.):** 350. **Frequency:** Irregular; previous edition 1983; latest edition March 1987.

★4414★ INTERNATIONAL DIRECTORY OF LIBRARIES AND PRODUCTION FACILITIES FOR THE BLIND
International Federation of Library Associations and Institutions
Box 95312
NL-2509 CH The Hague, Netherlands
Covers: About 710 organizations, institutes, libraries, and government agencies that produce braille materials or recordings (talking books) for the blind, or that maintain collections of such materials; 28 languages covered. **Entries Include:** Company or institution name, address, phone, key personnel. **Pages (approx.):** 115. **Frequency:** Irregular; latest edition 1984. **Available in the U.S. from:** National Library Service for the Blind and Physically Handicapped, Library of Congress, Washington, DC 20542.

★4415★ INTERNATIONAL DIRECTORY OF MENTAL RETARDATION RESOURCES
Office of Human Development Services
U.S. Department of Health and Human Services
Washington, DC 20201
Publication Includes: Voluntary organizations, government agencies, United Nations agencies, and others concerned with mental retardation; international coverage. **Entries Include:** Organization name, address, phone, founding date, name and title of contact, description.

★4416★ INTERNATIONAL DIRECTORY OF PEDIATRIC PATHOLOGISTS
Hemisphere Publishing Corp.
79 Madison Ave., Ste. 110
New York, NY 10016

★4417★ INTERNATIONAL DIRECTORY OF PERIODICALS RELATED TO DEAFNESS
Gallaudet University Library
800 Florida Ave., NE
Washington, DC 20002   Phone: (202) 651-5220
Covers: More than 500 periodical titles related to deafness; international coverage. **Entries Include:** Publication title, editor name, publisher name and address, date of initial publication, frequency, price (including subscription information), languages used, affiliations, description of subject matter. **Pages (approx.):** 125. **Frequency:** Irregular; latest edition 1985; new edition expected 1991.

★4418★ INTERNATIONAL DIRECTORY OF PSYCHOLOGISTS
International Union of Psychological Science
Psychologisches Institut
Von-Melle-Park 11
W-2000 Hamburg 13, Germany
Covers: Psychologists acting as members of about 50 national psychological societies and committees. **Entries Include:** Name, business address, fax, specialization. **Pages (approx.):** 1,200. **Frequency:** Every 5-6 years. **Available in the U.S. from:** Elsevier Science Publishing Co., Inc., 52 Vanderbilt Ave., New York, NY 10017 (212-370-5520).

★4419★ INTERNATIONAL DIRECTORY OF RECREATION-ORIENTED ASSISTIVE DEVICE SOURCES
Lifeboat Press
Box 11782
Marina del Rey, CA 90295   Phone: (213) 305-1600
Covers: Approximately 240 suppliers of sport and recreation assistive equipment for the disabled. **Entries Include:** Company name, address, phone, name and title of contact, product or service, photo of device. **Pages (approx.):** 260. **Frequency:** Biennial, July of even years.

★4420★ INTERNATIONAL DIRECTORY OF RESEARCH AND RESEARCHERS IN COMPARATIVE GERONTOLOGY
Publications Division
International Federation on Aging
601 E St. NW
Washington, DC 20049   Phone: (202) 434-2430
Covers: Over 150 research projects in comparative gerontology conducted since 1980; international coverage. **Entries Include:** Project title; sponsoring institution, organization, or individual name, address, phone; biographical data for researchers, description of study. **Pages (approx.):** 195. **Frequency:** Irregular; previous edition 1987; latest edition 1990.

★4421★ INTERNATIONAL EYECARE—REFERENCE FOR CONTACT LENS PRACTICE ISSUE
Professional Press Group
Fairchild Publications, Inc.
7 E. 12th St.
New York, NY 10003   Phone: (212) 741-6640
Publication Includes: List of about 300 companies providing products and services to the contact lens industry. **Entries Include:** Company name, address, local and toll-free phone; letter code indicating products or services provided. **Frequency:** Annual, July.

★4422★ INTERNATIONAL FEDERATION OF CATHOLIC PHARMACISTS—LISTING-FIPC
International Federation of Catholic Pharmacists
Bergstrasse 59
B-4700 Eupen, Belgium
Covers: National associations of Catholic pharmacists. **Frequency:** Biennial.

★4423★ INTERNATIONAL FEDERATION OF CLINICAL CHEMISTRY—HANDBOOK
International Federation of Clinical Chemistry
Centre du Medicament
Universite de Nancy 1
30, rue l'Ionnois
F-54000 Nancy, France
Covers: 52 national societies of clinical chemistry. **Entries Include:** IFCC member name, address. **Pages (approx.):** 74. **Frequency:** Triennial; latest edition 1991. **Also Includes:** Information about clinical chemistry and chemists; federation statutes and rules.

★4424★ INTERNATIONAL FEDERATION FOR FAMILY HEALTH—MEMBERSHIP ROSTER
International Federation for Family Health
Jalan Makmur 24
Bandung, Indonesia
Covers: About 20 national fertility research programs engaged in the evaluation of family planning projects designed to improve the quality of life in the Third World. **Frequency:** Irregular.

★4425★ INTERNATIONAL FEDERATION FOR MEDICAL AND BIOLOGICAL ENGINEERING—MEMBERSHIP DIRECTORY
International Federation for Medical and Biological Engineering
c/o National Research Council of Canada
Bldg. M-50, Rm. 305
Ottawa, ON, Canada K1A 0R8   Phone: (613) 993-1686
Covers: Over 33 member national engineering and physical science organizations; international coverage. **Entries Include:** Organization name, address, phone, fax, telex, name and title of contact. **Pages (approx.):** 20. **Frequency:** Every 18 months. **Also Includes:** List of administrative councils and federation committees, giving name, address, phone.

★4426★ INTERNATIONAL FEDERATION OF PHARMACEUTICAL MANUFACTURERS ASSOCIATIONS—STRUCTURE AND ACTIVITIES
International Federation of Pharmaceutical Manufacturers Associations
67, rue de Saint-Jean
CH-1201 Geneva, Switzerland
Publication Includes: List of over 50 member national pharmaceutical manufacturers' organizations. **Entries Include:** Association name, address, phone, telex, cable address, telefax. **Frequency:** Biennial, odd years.

★4427★ INTERNATIONAL FILARIASIS ASSOCIATION—MEMBERSHIP LIST
International Filariasis Association
c/o Dr. Ralph Muller
Commonwealth Institute of Parasitology
395 A Hatfield Rd.
St. Albans, Hertfordshire AL4 OXU, England
Covers: 200 persons interested in the study and control of filariasis, diseases caused by nematode worms, affecting chiefly the lymph glands and connective tissues.

★4428★ INTERNATIONAL GROUP OF SCIENTIFIC, TECHNICAL AND MEDICAL PUBLISHERS—STM INFORMATION BOOKLET
International Group of Scientific, Technical and Medical Publishers
462 Keizersgracht
NL-1016 GE Amsterdam, Netherlands
Covers: About 115 member publishing companies in 20 countries specializing in the fields of science, technology, medicine, and the social and behavioral sciences. **Entries Include:** Company name, address, phone, names of key personnel. **Pages (approx.):** 80. **Frequency:** Annual, spring. **Also Includes:** Bylaws and membership rules, permissions guidelines.

★4429★ INTERNATIONAL GUIDE TO LOCATING AUDIO-VISUAL MATERIALS IN THE HEALTH SCIENCES
Ashgate Publishing Co.
Old Post Rd.
Brookfield, VT 05036   Phone: (802) 276-3162
Covers: Directories, catalogs, periodicals and databases that list sources of medical audiovisual aids. **Entries Include:** Description of the medical/audio-visual aid and publisher/manufacturer address. **Pages (approx.):** 55. **Frequency:** Irregular; latest edition 1986.

★4430★ INTERNATIONAL HEALTH ELECTIVES FOR MEDICAL STUDENTS
American Medical Student Association
1890 Preston White Dr.
Reston, VA 22091   Phone: (703) 620-6600
Covers: More than about 200 foreign and United States institutions and organizations that offer learning experiences outside the United States to American medical students. **Entries Include:** Institution or organization name, funding agency name, countries in which active, duration of program, number of students permitted in program, time of year program is offered, fees, financial aid available, nature of duties and other details, name and address of contact, evaluative comments from students who have participated in some of the electives. **Pages (approx.):** 88. **Frequency:** Irregular; previous edition 1986; latest edition 1990; new edition expected 1992.

★4431★ INTERNATIONAL INTRA-OCULAR IMPLANT CLUB—MEMBERSHIP LIST
International Intra-Ocular Implant Club
38 Mt. Ash Rd.
Sydenham
London SE26, England
Covers: 150 members. **Frequency:** Annual.

★4432★ INTERNATIONAL LEPROSY ASSOCIATION—DIRECTORY
International Leprosy Association
c/o Dr. R. H. Thangaraj
No. 5 Amrita Shergill Marg
New Delhi 110003, India
Frequency: Annual.

★4433★ INTERNATIONAL PEDIATRIC ASSOCIATION—MEMBERSHIP LIST
International Pediatric Association
Chateau de Longchamp
Bois de Boulogne
F-75016 Paris, France
Covers: Approximately 110 national pediatric societies and associations that belong to the International Pediatric Association.

**★4434★   INTERNATIONAL PSYCHOANALYTICAL
        ASSOCIATION—ROSTER**
International Psychoanalytical Association
Broomhills
Woodside Ln.
London N12 8UD, England
Covers: About 6,800 members of the regional association, component
societies, and study groups of the association; also lists affiliate societies
and approved training institutes of the American Psychoanalytic Associa-
tion. **Entries Include:** Member name, address. **Pages (approx.):** 160.
Frequency: Annual, January.

**★4435★   INTERNATIONAL SOCIETY FOR COMPARATIVE
        PSYCHOLOGY—DIRECTORY**
International Society for Comparative Psychology
c/o Ethel Tobach
University Center
33 W. 42nd St., Rm. 615
New York, NY 10036-8099   Phone: (212) 769-5487
Covers: About 200 psychologists, biologists, anthropologists, and educators
concerned with comparative psychology. **Frequency:** Annual.

**★4436★   INTERNATIONAL SOCIETY FOR DEVELOPMENTAL
        NEUROSCIENCE—MEMBERSHIP DIRECTORY**
International Society for Developmental Neuroscience
c/o Bernard Haber, Secretary General ISDN
University of Texas Medical Branch
Marine Biomedical Institute
Galveston, TX 77550   Phone: (409) 761-2108
Covers: 800 members. **Entries Include:** Institution or personal name,
address, phone, fax, area of specialty. **Pages (approx.):** 110. **Frequency:**
Irregular; latest edition 1986; new edition expected 1991.

**★4437★   INTERNATIONAL SOCIETY OF HEMATOLOGY—
        CONSTITUTION, RULES AND BY-LAWS, AND LIST OF
        MEMBERS**
International Society of Hematology
Haematology Laboratory Department
Hospital Clinic i Provincial
Villavroel 170
E-08036 Barcelona, Spain
Covers: About 3,000 physicians and scientists who have spent more than 5
years in the research or practice of hematology. **Entries Include:** Member
name, address, phone. **Pages (approx.):** 140. **Frequency:** Biennial, odd
years. **Also Includes:** Constitution, rules, and bylaws of the society.

**★4438★   INTERNATIONAL SOCIETY FOR HUMAN AND
        ANIMAL MYCOLOGY—MEMBERSHIP LIST**
International Society for Human and Animal Mycology
Laboratory for Mycology
Institute of Tropical Medicine
Nationalestraat 155
B-2000 Antwerp, Belgium
Covers: 850 physicians, veterinarians, pathologists, microbiologists, and
others interested in human and animal mycology. **Pages (approx.):** 130.
Frequency: Biennial, odd years.

**★4439★   INTERNATIONAL SOCIETY OF HYPERTENSION—
        MEMBERSHIP DIRECTORY**
International Society of Hypertension
Departments of Pharmacotheraphy and Cardiology
Academic Medical Centre and Academic Hospital
University of Amsterdam, Meiberg dreef 15
NL-1105 AZ Amsterdam, Netherlands
Covers: 900 researchers and corporate members with an interest in the field
of hypertension. **Pages (approx.):** 120. **Frequency:** Biennial.

**★4440★   INTERNATIONAL SOCIETY FOR
        NEUROCHEMISTRY—MEMBERSHIP DIRECTORY**
International Society for Neurochemistry
Division for Toxicology
Norwegian Defence Research Establishment
Box 25
2007 Kjeller, Norway
Covers: About 1,500 scientists interested in promoting research in neuro-
chemistry. **Entries Include:** Name, affiliation, address, phone. **Pages
(approx.):** 140. **Frequency:** Biennial, even years.

**★4441★   INTERNATIONAL SOCIETY OF
        NEUROPATHOLOGY—MEMBERSHIP DIRECTORY**
International Society of Neuropathology
Department of Pathology
Richardson Laboratory
Queen's University
Kingston, ON, Canada K7L 3N6   Phone: (613) 545-2818
Covers: Approximately 2,000 members of national societies of neuropa-
thology, including over 700 members from the United States. **Entries
Include:** Personal name, address. **Pages (approx.):** 150. **Frequency:** Irregu-
lar; previous edition 1985, latest edition 1990.

**★4442★   INTERNATIONAL SOCIETY OF PODIATRIC LASER
        SURGERY—MEMBERSHIP BOOKLET**
International College of Podiatric Laser Surgery
2945 Snake Hill Rd.
Doylestown, PA 18901-1750   Phone: (215) 794-5180
Covers: About 300 member podiatrists who utilize lasers in surgeries;
coverage includes Canada and Puerto Rico. **Entries Include:** Individual
name, address, phone, type of CO_2 laser utilized, membership status.
Pages (approx.): 60. **Frequency:** Latest edition 1992.

**★4443★   INTERNATIONAL SOCIETY FOR PROSTHETICS AND
        ORTHOTICS—DIRECTORY OF OFFICERS AND MEMBERS**
International Society for Prosthetics and Orthotics
Borgervaenget 5
DK-2100 Copenhagen, Denmark
Covers: 1,800 medical and paramedical professionals, in 65 countries,
interested in prosthetics, orthotics, and other fields of rehabilitation
engineering. **Pages (approx.):** 110. **Frequency:** Irregular; latest edition 1989,
new edition expected 1992.

**★4444★   INTERNATIONAL SOCIETY FOR RESEARCH ON
        CIVILIZATION DISEASES AND ENVIRONMENT—
        MEMBERSHIP LIST**
International Society for Research on Civilization Diseases and
Environment
29 Sq. Larousse
B-1060 Brussels, Belgium
Covers: Approximately 600 researchers interested in the adverse effects of
industrialization on humans and the environment. **Frequency:** Annual, fall.

**★4445★   INTERNATIONAL SOCIETY OF UROLOGY—
        MEMBERSHIP LIST**
International Society of Urology
3. Place dela Republique
F-59000 Lille, France
Covers: 2,500 surgeons and other specialists in 65 national groups in the
field of urology. **Frequency:** Irregular.

**★4446★   INTERNATIONAL STRABISMOLOGICAL
        ASSOCIATION—MEMBERSHIP DIRECTORY**
International Strabismological Association
c/o Texas Children's Hospital
Dr. Gunther Von Noorden
6621 Fannin
Houston, TX 77030   Phone: (713) 798-1470
Covers: Ophthalmologists specializing in strabismus (eye movement disor-
ders).

**★4447★   INTERNATIONAL TELEPHONE DIRECTORY OF TDD
        USERS**
Telecommunications for the Deaf, Inc.
8719 Colesville Rd., Ste. 300
Silver Spring, MD 20910-3919   Phone: (301) 589-3786
Covers: About 26,000 organizations, services, and deaf persons who use the
hearing device called TDD on their telephones. **Entries Include:** Name,
address, TDD and voice phone number. **Pages (approx.):** 275. **Frequency:**
Annual, January.

**★4448★   INTERNATIONAL UNION OF NUTRITIONAL
        SCIENCES—DIRECTORY**
International Union of Nutritional Sciences
c/o Department of Human Nutrition
Agricultural University
2, PO Box 8129
NL-6400 EV Wageningen, Netherlands
Covers: Approximately 65 national nutritional societies and about 500

individual members. **Entries Include:** Organization or personal name, address, name and title of contact. **Pages (approx.):** 95. **Frequency:** Biennial; latest edition 1991. **Also Includes:** List of officers and committees; statutes and rules of procedure.

★4449★ **INTERNATIONAL VEGETARIAN HANDBOOK**
Vegetarian Society
Parkdale
Dunham Rd.
Altrincham, Cheshire WA14 4QG, England
Covers: Resources for vegetarian food throughout the world, including restaurants and hotels; includes vegetarian publications. **Entries Include:** Name, address; listings may also include phone, hours, and capacity. **Pages (approx.):** 350. **Frequency:** Biennial; latest edition December 1986.

★4450★ **INTERNATIONAL VEGETARIAN UNION—YEARBOOK**
International Vegetarian Union
10 Kings Dr.
Marple
Stockport, Cheshire SK6 6NQ, England
Covers: Societies whose members are vegetarians; vegetarian accommodation, restaurants, and health food stores worldwide. **Frequency:** Annual.

★4451★ **INTERNSHIP PROGRAMS IN PROFESSIONAL PSYCHOLOGY, INCLUDING POST-DOCTORAL TRAINING PROGRAMS**
Association of Psychology Postdoctoral and Internship Centers
733 15th St. NW, Ste. 717
Washington, DC 20005   Phone: (202) 347-0022
Covers: Institutions offering internship programs in professional psychology. **Entries Include:** Institution name, name and address of contact, description of program including percentage of time spent in supervision and in seminar attendance, theoretical orientation, number of interns, stipend, admission requirements. **Pages (approx.):** 600. **Frequency:** Annual, September.

★4452★ **INVENTORY OF MEDICAL AND HEALTH RELATED RESEARCH INSTITUTIONS IN COMMONWEALTH COUNTRIES OF EAST, CENTRAL, AND SOUTHERN AFRICA**
Commonwealth Regional Health Secretariat
Box 1009
Arusha, United Republic of Tanzania
Covers: Schools, colleges, universities, and research institutions involved in health care research. **Pages (approx.):** 182. **Frequency:** Irregular; latest edition 1990.

★4453★ **INVENTORY OF U.S. HEALTH CARE DATA BASES, 1976-1987**
Office of Data Analysis and Management
U.S. Bureau of Health Professions
5600 Fishers Ln.
Rockville, MD 20857   Phone: (301) 443-6936
Covers: About 350 health care databases sponsored by government or private agencies, associations, and universities, that are available to researchers. Databases listed contain data obtained since 1976. **Entries Include:** Database title, sponsoring organization, address, phone, purpose, subject headings, source of data, size of sample population, frequency of sampling, time period, availability, cost, related publications. **Pages (approx.):** 175. **Frequency:** Irregular; previous edition May 1984; latest edition May 1988.

★4454★ **ITALIAN DIRECTORY OF DRUGS AND MANUFACTURERS**
Organizzazione Editoriale Medico Farmaceutica SpA
Via Edolo 42
I-20125 Milan, Italy
Publication Includes: List of about 2,200 Italian pharmaceutical manufacturers. **Entries Include:** Company name, address. **Frequency:** Annual, March. **Available in the U.S. from:** Drug Intelligence and Clinical Pharmacy, Box 42435, Cincinnati, OH 45242 (513-793-3555).

★4455★ **I.V. INSTRUMENTATION**
Theta Corp.
Theta Bldg.
Middlefield, CT 06455   Phone: (203) 349-1054
Publication Includes: List of companies that produce or market intravenous therapy equipment. **Entries Include:** Company name, address, phone, key personnel, background information, description of products, annual sales, research and development efforts, distribution systems, five year projection. **Frequency:** Irregular; previous edition April 1984; latest edition November 1986.

★4456★ **JAPAN DIAGNOSTIC REAGENTS COMPANY DIRECTORY**
RSF International Group, Inc.
Box 368
Mount Kisco, NY 10549   Phone: (914) 241-6360
Covers: About 110 Japanese diagnostic reagent companies whose products and equipment are used in the medical field and for other biotechnology applications. **Entries Include:** Company name, address, phone, fax, names and titles of key personnel, owner, number of employees, capital, date established, total sales volume and breakdown for diagnostic reagents, number and location of sales offices, factory/distributor locations, products, corporate affiliations. **Pages (approx.):** 100. **Frequency:** Biennial, odd years. **Also Includes:** Data on Japanese general health care; "major" health care-related meetings in Japan; list of "important" Japanese medical publications.

★4457★ **JAPANESE HEALTHCARE INDUSTRY**
Japan Publications, Inc.
Shin-Nichibo Bldg.
1-2-1 Sarugaku-Cho
Chiyoda-Ku
Tokyo 101, Japan
Covers: Over 810 public, private, and foreign capital companies in the Japanese health care industry. **Entries Include:** Company name, address, phone, subsidiary and branch names and locations, products, and sales data. **Pages (approx.):** 550. **Frequency:** Annual. **Available in the U.S. from:** International Publications Service, Taylor & Francis, Inc., 1900 Frost Rd., Ste. 101, Bristol, PA 19007-1598 (215-238-0939).

★4458★ **JAPANESE MEDICAL RESEARCHERS DIRECTORY**
Igaku-Shoin Ltd.
5-24-3 Hongo
Bunkyo-ku
Tokyo 113-91, Japan
Covers: About 170 colleges and research institutes in Japan specializing in the medical and dental sciences. **Entries Include:** Institution name, address, name of contact. **Pages (approx.):** 780. **Frequency:** Annual, November.

★4459★ **JOURNAL OF THE AMERICAN MEDICAL ASSOCIATION—PHYSICIAN SERVICE OPPORTUNITIES OVERSEAS ISSUE**
American Medical Association
515 N. State St.
Chicago, IL 60610   Phone: (312) 464-5000
Publication Includes: List of more than 170 organizations that provide assignments overseas for physicians from the United States. **Entries Include:** Organization name, address, phone, contact person, countries served, medical specialties sought, length of assignment, stipend or salary (if provided), whether facilities or equipment, housing, and transportation are provided, and additional requirements. **Frequency:** Triennial; latest edition June 1990.

★4460★ **JOURNAL OF BEHAVIOR THERAPY AND EXPERIMENTAL PSYCHIATRY—DIRECTORY ISSUE**
Behavior Therapy and Research Society
Department of Psychology
Pepperdine University
400 Corporate Pointe
Culver City, CA 90230   Phone: (213) 568-5753
Publication Includes: List of about 250 clinical and clinical research fellows with training and experience in behavior therapy. **Entries Include:** Name, office address, phone, highest degree held. **Frequency:** Annual, December.

★4461★ **JOURNAL OF DENTAL EDUCATION—DIRECTORY OF ASSOCIATION OFFICERS**
American Association of Dental Schools (AADS)
1625 Massachusetts Ave. NW
Washington, DC 20036   Phone: (202) 667-9433
Publication Includes: List of AADS executive officers, council members, and section officers. **Entries Include:** For executive and section officers—Personal name, address, phone. For council members—Personal name, location, phone. **Frequency:** Annual, July.

★4462★ JOURNAL OF HISTOCHEMISTRY AND CYTOCHEMISTRY—HISTOCHEMICAL SOCIETY DIRECTORY ISSUE
Histochemical Society
c/o Susan Crowley
Slack, Inc.
6900 Grove Rd.
Thorofare, NJ 08086   Phone: (609) 848-1000
Publication Includes: Listing of 550 physicians and scientists interested in histochemistry (study of the chemical substances in body or cells). **Entries Include:** Name, affiliation, address, phone and fax numbers. **Frequency:** Biennial, even years.

★4463★ JOURNAL OF NURSING ADMINISTRATION—DIRECTORY OF CONSULTANTS NURSING ADMINISTRATION ISSUE
J. B. Lippincott Co.
E. Washington Sq.
Philadelphia, PA 19105   Phone: (215) 238-4273
Publication Includes: About 500 consultants (primarily registered nurses) and firms employing registered nurses, who specialize in nursing administration, training, patient ser vices, etc. Criteria for inclusion are registered nurse license (for most specialties), Master's degree or equivalent level of experience, and charging of fees for consultation. **Entries Include:** Consultant or firm name, address, phone, areas of occupational specialization, agency setting, geographical area of consultation, years of consulting experience or year consulting first offered; firm listings include number of consultants. Some listings include basic fee, services. **Pages (approx.):** 65. **Frequency:** Semiannual, February and August.

★4464★ JOURNAL OF PROSTHETIC DENTISTRY—INDEX ISSUE
Mosby-Year Book, Inc.
11830 Westline Industrial Dr.
St. Louis, MO 63146   Phone: (314) 872-8370
Publication Includes: List of prosthetics and implant dentistry associations and their officers. **Entries Include:** Association name; names and addresses of president, president-elect, vice president, secretary-treasurer, and other officials, dates and location of next meeting. **Frequency:** Semiannual, January and July.

★4465★ JOURNALS IN PSYCHOLOGY: A RESOURCE LISTING FOR AUTHORS
American Psychological Association
1200 17th St. NW
Washington, DC 20036   Phone: (202) 955-7600
Covers: Over 200 U.S. periodicals in the behavioral and social sciences to which papers may be submitted for publication. **Entries Include:** Title, editor name and address, editorial policy, circulation, index terms, publisher, submission requirements. **Pages (approx.):** 145. **Frequency:** Latest edition 1990. **Send Orders to:** American Psychological Association, PO Box 2710, Hyattsville, MD 20784-0710 (703-247-7705).

★4466★ JUNGIAN PSYCHOLOGY RESOURCE GUIDE
Inner Growth Books
Box 520
Chiloquin, OR 97624   Phone: (503) 783-3126
Covers: National and local professional groups, sponsors of conferences and training programs, publishers of books and periodicals, mail order book suppliers, libraries and archives, and other organizations that utilize or provide information about the teachings of psychologist and psychiatrist Dr. Carl Jung. **Entries Include:** Organization name, address, phone, description of services or publications. **Pages (approx.):** 150. **Frequency:** Irregular; latest edition 1987.

★4467★ THE K & W GUIDE—COLLEGES FOR THE LEARNING DISABLED STUDENT
Kravets, Wax and Associates
PO Box 187
Deerfield, IL 60015-0187
Covers: 160 colleges and universities with specialized services and facilities for learning-disabled students. **Entries Include:** Institution name, address, phone, name of coordinator of learning-disabled programs, number of learning-disabled students, description of facilities and services. **Pages (approx.):** 370. **Frequency:** Published 1990.

★4468★ KEITHWOOD DIRECTORY OF MEDICAL/HOME HEALTH CARE SUPPLY DEALERS
Keithwood Publishing Co.
Box 2693
Upper Darby, PA 19082   Phone: (215) 352-7550
Covers: More than 6,500 medical supply dealers. **Entries Include:** Company name, address (including branches, divisions, etc.), phone, fax, product and services. **Pages (approx.):** 400. **Frequency:** Annual.

★4469★ KEYGUIDE TO INFORMATION SOURCES IN PARAMEDICAL SCIENCES
Mansell Publishing
Cassell PLC
Villiers House
41-47 Strand
London WC2N 5JE, United Kingdom
Publication Includes: International directory of paramedical science organizations. **Available in the U.S. from:** Publishers Distribution Center, PO Box C831, Rutherford, NJ 07070.

★4470★ KEYGUIDE TO INFORMATION SOURCES IN PHARMACY
Mansell Publishing
Casselle PLC
Villiers House
41-47 Strand
London WC2N 5JE, England
Publication Includes: International directory of pharmaceutical organizations. **Available in the U.S. from:** Publishers Distribution Center, PO Box C831, Rutherford, NJ 07070.

★4471★ KIDNEY DIALYSIS AND SUPPLIES
Theta Corp.
Theta Bldg.
Middlefield, CT 06455   Phone: (203) 349-1054
Publication Includes: Manufacturers of kidney dialysis equipment. **Entries Include:** Company name, address, phone, key personnel, background information, description of products, annual sales, research and development efforts, distribution systems, five year projection. **Frequency:** Irregular; latest edition October 1988.

★4472★ KOREAN MEDICAL ASSOCIATION OF AMERICA—MEMBERSHIP DIRECTORY
Korean Medical Association of America
c/o Dr. Chan-Sung Ko
1801 Mahantongo St.
Pottsville, PA 17901   Phone: (717) 622-6463
Covers: About 4,000 member medical doctors of Korean descent and others interested in Korean medicine. **Frequency:** Latest edition 1982.

★4473★ KYM INTERNATIONAL DIRECTORY OF PHARMACEUTICAL COMPANIES
KYM Consultancy Ltd.
Prospect House
20 High St.
Westerham, Kent TN16 1RG, England
Covers: Over 15,000 pharmaceutical companies in over 100 countries. **Entries Include:** Subsidiary company name, address, phone, fax, telex, corporate ownership, major therapy interests. **Pages (approx.):** 1,300. **Frequency:** Annual.

★4474★ KYM INTERNATIONAL DIRECTORY OF PHARMACEUTICAL PERSONNEL
KYM Consultancy Ltd.
Prospect House
20 High St.
Westerham, Kent TN16 1RG, England
Covers: Over 22,000 executives and other key personnel employed by over 4,000 pharmaceutical companies in over 80 countries. **Entries Include:** Company name, address, phone, telex, fax, employee name, job title, department, job specialty. **Pages (approx.):** 800 (loose-leaf). **Frequency:** Quarterly.

★4475★ KYM INTERNATIONAL DIRECTORY OF
PHARMACEUTICAL PRODUCTS
KYM Consultancy Ltd.
Prospect House
20 High St.
Westerham, Kent TN16 1RG, England
Covers: Marketers of over 34,000 pharmaceutical drugs in approximately
70 countries. Entries Include: Brand name, marketing company, country
location, therapy area code. Pages (approx.): 800 (loose-leaf). Frequency:
Annual.

★4476★ LABORADRESSBUCH
Verlag Neuer Merkur GmbH
Ingolstadter Strasse 63 A
W-8000 Munich 46, Germany
Covers: More than 5,000 dental laboratories and dental technicians in
Germany; about 50 schools for dental technology; related organizations.
Entries Include: For laboratories, technicians, and schools—Name, ad-
dress, phone. For organizations—Name, address, phone; name, address,
phone of chairman; contact name. Pages (approx.): 280. Frequency:
Biennial, fall of odd years.

★4477★ LABORATORIES MEDICAL DIRECTORIES
DIRECTORY
American Business Directories, Inc.
American Business Information, Inc.
5711 S. 86th Circle
Omaha, NE 68127   Phone: (402) 593-4600
Number of Listings: 6,821. Entries Include: Name, address, phone (includ-
ing area code), size of advertisement, year first in "Yellow Pages," name of
owner or manager, number of employees. Frequency: Annual.

★4478★ THE LARYNGOSCOPE—DIRECTORY OF
OTOLARYNGOLOGIC SOCIETIES ISSUE
Triological Foundation, Inc.
10 S. Broadway, Ste. 1401
St. Louis, MO 63102   Phone: (314) 621-6550
Publication Includes: List of more than 50 international otolaryngologic
societies. Entries Include: Organization name, address, phone, names and
titles of key personnel. Frequency: Monthly.

★4479★ LATIN AMERICAN ASSOCIATION OF
PHARMACEUTICAL INDUSTRIES—DIRECTORY OF
MEMBERS
Latin American Association of Pharmaceutical Industries
Esmeralda 130, Piso 5
1035 Buenos Aires, Argentina
Frequency: Annual, June.

★4480★ LEARNING DISABILITIES ASSOCIATION OF
CANADA—LDAC DIRECTORY OF RESOURCES
Learning Disabilities Association of Canada
323 Chapel St., Ste. 200
Ottawa, ON, Canada K1N 7Z2   Phone: (613) 238-5721
Covers: Publishers of audiovisual material, books, periodicals, and journals; technology, schools, resource centers, camps, organizations, postsecondary education programs, and other agencies concerned with people
with learning disabilities. Entries Include: Company or organization name,
address, phone, name and title of contact, names and titles of key
personnel, geographical area covered, eligibility requirements, description
of services. Pages (approx.): 150. Frequency: Biennial, odd years.

★4481★ LEARNING DISABILITIES: NATIONAL
INFORMATION AND ADVOCACY ORGANIZATIONS
National Library Service for the Blind and Physically Handicapped
Library of Congress
1291 Taylor St. NW
Washington, DC 20542   Phone: (202) 707-5000
Covers: Approximately 20 national information and advocacy organizations for learning-disabled youths and adults, their families, and professionals who serve them; approximately 55 publishers and distributors of
books, periodicals, magazines, and other literature for the learning-disabled and those who serve them; and over 100 state-level agencies that
administer public programs providing special education and rehabilitation
for learning disabled persons. Entries Include: For national organizations—Name, address, phone, description. For publishers and distributors—Name, address, title, year published, number of pages, price. For
state agencies—Name, address, phone. Pages (approx.): 21. Frequency:
Published March 1990.

★4482★ LEONARD CHESHIRE FOUNDATION
INTERNATIONAL—DIRECTORY
Leonard Cheshire Foundation International
26-29 Maunsel St.
London SW1P 2QN, England
Covers: Over 180 residential care facilities, day care centers, and rehabilita-
tion centers for the handicapped in 48 countries. Entries Include: Facility
name, address, phone, year founded, description. Pages (approx.): 60.
Frequency: Irregular; latest edition 1989; new edition possible 1991.

★4483★ LETTERS TO JUDY: WHAT YOUR KIDS WISH THEY
COULD TELL YOU
Putnam Publishing Group
G. P. Putnam's Sons
390 Murray Hill Parkway
East Rutherford, NJ 07073   Phone: (800) 631-8571
Publication Includes: List of agencies concerned with children's welfare and
development. Frequency: Published 1986.

★4484★ LIBRARY RESOURCES FOR THE BLIND AND
PHYSICALLY HANDICAPPED
National Library Service for the Blind and Physically Handicapped
Library of Congress
1291 Taylor St., NW
Washington, DC 20542   Phone: (202) 707-9274
Covers: More than 55 regional and 91 subregional libraries, and 6 machine-
lending agencies in the United States, Puerto Rico, the U.S. Virgin Islands,
and Guam that provide a free library service of braille and recorded books
and magazines to visually and physically handicapped persons; other
agencies distributing braille materials and talking book machines are also
indicated. Entries Include: Name of library, address, phone, fax, TWX
number (if any), in-WATS number, TDD number (for the deaf), name of
librarian, name of contact for machines (if any), hours of operation, list of
book collections (includes disc, cassette, braille, large type), list of special
collections (films, foreign language cassettes), list of special services. Pages
(approx.): 75. Frequency: Annual, July. Also Includes: Library readership
and circulation appendix.

★4485★ LICENSURE REQUIREMENTS FOR NURSING HOME
ADMINISTRATORS: ROSTER OF STATE LICENSURE
BOARDS
National Association of Boards of Examiners of Nursing Home
Administrators
808 17th St., NW, Ste. 200
Washington, DC 20006   Phone: (202) 223-9750
Covers: More than 50 state nursing home administrator licensing boards,
and about 500 board members. Entries Include: For boards—Name,
address, phone, names of key officials, licensing requirements. For board
members—Name, address, phone, title. Pages (approx.): 95. Frequency:
Annual.

★4486★ LIST OF APPROVED HOSPITALS AND HOUSE
OFFICER POSTS IN THE UNITED KINGDOM
General Medical Council
44 Hallam St.
London W1N 6AE, England
Covers: Training posts in the United Kingdom for doctors at pre-registra-
tion house officer level. Entries Include: Hospital name, location, type of
post available. Pages (approx.): 70. Frequency: Biennial, January of odd
years.

★4487★ LIST OF CANADIAN HOSPITALS
Canadian Centre for Health Information
Statistics Canada
R. H. Coats Bldg., 18th Fl.
Tunney's Pasture
Ottawa, ON, Canada K1A OT6   Phone: (613) 951-1650
Covers: About 1,200 hospitals in Canada. Entries Include: Facility name,
location; whether public, private, or federal; type of hospital, registered
owner or type of owner, number of beds and cribs, number of bassinets.
Pages (approx.): 45. Frequency: Annual.

★4488★ LIST OF SCHOOLS FOR CHILDREN WITH AUTISM
National Autistic Society
276 Willesden Ln.
London NW2 5RB, England
Covers: Member and local society schools for children with autism in
England and Wales. Entries Include: School name, address, phone, number

of students, age range. **Pages (approx.):** 15. **Frequency:** Irregular; latest edition July 1989.

★4489★   LIVING WITH DYING: A LOVING GUIDE FOR FAMILY AND FRIENDS
McGraw-Hill, Inc.
11 W. 19th St.
New York, NY 10011   Phone: (212) 512-2000
Publication Includes: Directory of organizations that can assist individuals caring for a dying person. **Frequency:** Published April 1985.

★4490★   LIVING WITH ENDOMETRIOSIS: HOW TO COPE WITH THE PHYSICAL AND EMOTIONAL CHALLENGES
Addison-Wesley Publishing Co., Inc.
1 Jacob Way
Rte. 128
Reading, MA 01867   Phone: (617) 944-3700
Publication Includes: Lists of about 20 pain management centers and 10 other organizations that provide resource information on endometriosis, a common gynecological disorder. **Entries Include:** Organization name, address, phone. **Frequency:** Published June 1987. **Also Includes:** Glossary of terms and lists of related publications.

★4491★   LIVING WITH LOW VISION: A RESOURCE GUIDE FOR PEOPLE WITH SIGHT LOSS
Resources for Rehabilitation
33 Bedford St., Ste. 19A
Lexington, MA 02173   Phone: (617) 862-6455
Covers: Resources and services for people with vision loss, including national organizations, publications, distributors of large print publications, reading services, technological aids, and organizations and publications for groups such as the elderly, adolescents, veterans, and those with hearing loss as well. **Pages (approx.):** 151. **Frequency:** Published 1990.

★4492★   LOCAL AIDS SERVICES: THE NATIONAL DIRECTORY
U.S. Conference of Mayors
1620 I St., NW
Washington, DC 20006   Phone: (202) 293-7330
Covers: Nearly 2,500 organizations that provide AIDS-related services and information, including counseling, financial and legal services, health care, local health departments, community-based organizations, housing assistance, state AIDS coordinators, social security regional AIDS coordinators, NIAID (National Institute of Allergy and Infectious Diseases) AIDS Treatment and Evaluation Units, AIDS information hotlines. **Entries Include:** Organization, agency, or facility name, address, phone; description of services. **Pages (approx.):** 160. **Frequency:** Annually; previous edition 1988; latest edition 1990. **Also Includes:** List of state and local AIDS-related directories.

★4493★   LOCAL HEALTH DEPARTMENT DIRECTORY
United States Conference of Local Health Officers
c/o Steve Horn, Publications
1620 I St., NW
Washington, DC 20006   Phone: (202) 293-7330
Covers: Over 2,000 local health departments. **Entries Include:** Facility name, address, phone, name of director/health officer, classification of local health department (i.e., city, city-county, district). **Pages (approx.):** 100. **Frequency:** Irregular.

★4494★   LONDON HEALTH ACTION NETWORK
National Community Health Resource
57 Chalton St.
London NW1 1HU, England
Covers: Community health councils and community based health initiatives in London. **Entries Include:** Organization name, address, phone, name and title of contact. **Pages (approx.):** 50. **Frequency:** Irregular; latest edition 1986.

★4495★   LOSS OF SELF: A FAMILY RESOURCE FOR THE CARE OF ALZHEIMER'S DISEASE AND RELATED DISORDERS
W. W. Norton & Co., Inc.
500 5th Ave.
New York, NY 10110   Phone: (212) 354-5500
Publication Includes: List of organizations that provide help to victims of Alzheimer's disease and their families. **Entries Include:** Name, address. **Frequency:** Published February 1986.

★4496★   LOVEJOY'S COLLEGE GUIDE FOR THE LEARNING DISABLED
Monarch Press
Simon & Schuster, Inc.
15 Columbus Circle, 16th Fl.
New York, NY 10023   Phone: (212) 373-8500
Covers: Over 270 colleges or universities offering special services and programs for the learning disabled. **Entries Include:** Institution name, address, phone, contact person, enrollment, tuition, cost of room and board, mean SAT scores, degrees offered, admission criteria, special services and programs, description of academic requirement, list of schools or colleges, facilities. **Pages (approx.):** 120. **Frequency:** Published 1988.

★4497★   LYNDA MADARAS TALKS TO TEENS ABOUT AIDS— AN ESSENTIAL GUIDE FOR PARENTS, TEACHERS, AND YOUNG PEOPLE
Newmarket Press
18 E. 48th St.
New York, NY 10017   Phone: (212) 832-3575
Publication Includes: List of five organizations that provide printed or audiovisual materials on AIDS; 76 AIDS hotlines around the U.S. **Entries Include:** Organization name, address, phone, geographical area served.

★4498★   MADE IN EUROPE—MEDICAL EQUIPMENT AND SUPPLY GUIDE
Made in Europe Marketing Organization GmbH
Hahnstrasse 70
Postfach 710601
W-6000 Frankfurt 71, Germany
Covers: Several hundred manufacturers of hospital and medical equipment, supplies, and furnishings for diagnosis, therapy, surgery, orthopedics, rehabilitation, and laboratories; all listings are paid. **Entries Include:** Company name, address, phone, and telex, in ad format; information such as product lines, ordering information payment terms, sales literature, and trade fair participation is given in some ads. **Pages (approx.):** 450. **Frequency:** Annual, May.

★4499★   MAGAZINES IN SPECIAL MEDIA
National Library Service for the Blind and Physically Handicapped
Library of Congress
1291 Taylor St., NW
Washington, DC 20542   Phone: (202) 287-9286
Publication Includes: List of over 90 public and private organizations that publish magazines in braille, on cassette, on disc, in large type or moon type for the blind and physically handicapped. **Entries Include:** Name of publisher, address, price. **Frequency:** Biennial, even years; new edition expected 1991.

★4500★   MAGNETIC RESONANCE IMAGING MARKETS
Theta Corp.
Theta Bldg.
Middlefield, CT 06455   Phone: (203) 349-1054
Publication Includes: List of about 20 manufacturers of magnetic resonance imaging (MRI) equipment. **Entries Include:** Company name, address, phone, key personnel, background information, description of products, annual sales, research and development efforts, distribution systems, five year projection. **Frequency:** Irregular; latest edition September 1988.

★4501★   MARHGN DIRECTORY: GENETIC SERVICES IN THE MID-ATLANTIC REGION
Mid-Atlantic Regional Human Genetics Network
Department of Pediatrics/Genetics
University of Virginia School of Medicine
Box 386
Charlottesville, VA 22908   Phone: (804) 924-9477
Covers: About 100 medical genetics facilities in Delaware, District of Columbia, Maryland, New Jersey, Pennsylvania, Virginia, and West Virginia. **Entries Include:** Name, address, phone, name of contact, services. **Pages (approx.):** 70. **Frequency:** Biennial, August of odd years.

★4502★   MARRIAGE AND FAMILY COUNSELORS DIRECTORY
American Business Directories, Inc.
American Business Information, Inc.
5711 S. 86th Circle
Omaha, NE 68127   Phone: (402) 593-4600
Number of Listings: 51,056. **Entries Include:** Name, address, phone (including area code), size of advertisement, year first in "Yellow Pages," name of owner or manager, number of employees. **Frequency:** Annual.

★4503★ MARTINDALE: THE EXTRA PHARMACOPOEIA
Pharmaceutical Press
Pharmaceutical Society of Great Britain
1 Lambeth High St.
London SE1 7JN, England
Publication Includes: List of over 4,600 pharmaceutical manufacturers, the majority outside Great Britain. **Entries Include:** Company name, address. **Frequency:** Irregular; previous edition December 1982; latest edition January 1989. **Available in the U.S. from:** Rittenhouse Book Distributors, Inc., 511 Feheley Dr., King of Prussia, PA 19406.

★4504★ MASSAGE THERAPISTS DIRECTORY
American Business Directories, Inc.
American Business Information, Inc.
5711 S. 86th Circle
Omaha, NE 68127   Phone: (402) 593-4600
Number of Listings: 1,859. **Entries Include:** Name, address, phone, size of advertisement, name of owner or manager, number of employees, year first in "Yellow Pages." **Frequency:** Annual.

★4505★ MATERIALS AND STRATEGIES FOR THE EDUCATION OF TRAINABLE MENTALLY RETARDED LEARNERS
Garland Publishing, Inc.
136 Madison Ave.
New York, NY 10016   Phone: (212) 686-7492
Publication Includes: List of agencies providing services to retarded individuals and their families, doctors, and teachers; list of publishers of materials useful in educating retarded students, including handbooks, measurement tools, professional periodicals, pamphlets of professional and parent groups, kits, computer software, and recipe books. **Entries Include:** For agencies—Name, address, phone. For publishers—Name, address. **Frequency:** Published 1990.

★4506★ MATERNAL AND CHILD HEALTH RESEARCH PROGRAM: I. ACTIVE PROJECTS
National Maternal and Child Health Clearinghouse
38th & R Sts. NW
Washington, DC 20057

★4507★ MCKNIGHT'S LONG-TERM CARE NEWS—BUYER'S GUIDE ISSUE
McKnight Medical Communications
1419 Lake Cook Rd., Ste. 110
Deerfield, IL 60015   Phone: (708) 945-0345
Publication Includes: List of suppliers of products and services for nursing homes. **Entries Include:** Company name, address, phone, fax, name and title of contact. **Frequency:** Annual, May.

★4508★ MED TECH DIRECTORY
Med Tech Services, Inc.
D. H. Blair & Co.
44 Wall St.
New York, NY 10005   Phone: (212) 495-4507
Covers: Over 1000 international and domestic publicly owned health-care companies, including suppliers of services, disposable and other products, medical devices, equipment, pharmaceuticals, and biotechnology research. **Entries Include:** Company name, address, phone, names and titles of officers with percentage of ownership (if data was furnished), activity in medical field; number of employees, four-year review of net sales, net profits, revenues, earnings per share, and stock price range; exchange on which traded, stock exchange symbol, balance sheet summaries, and other financial data. **Pages (approx.):** 400. **Frequency:** Annual.

★4509★ MEDICAL DEVICE AND DIAGNOSTIC INDUSTRY—ANNUAL BUYERS GUIDE TO MEDICAL PACKAGING ISSUE
Canon Communications, Inc.
3340 Ocean Park Blvd., Ste. 1000
Santa Monica, CA 90405   Phone: (213) 392-5509
Publication Includes: List of about 240 packagers of medical devices and suppliers of packaging equipment, materials, and services. **Entries Include:** Company name, location, phone, products and services provided, toll-free number, fax. **Frequency:** Annual, August.

★4510★ MEDICAL DEVICE AND DIAGNOSTIC INDUSTRY—ANNUAL BUYERS GUIDE TO MEDICAL PLASTICS ISSUE
Canon Communications, Inc.
3340 Ocean Park Blvd., Ste. 1000
Santa Monica, CA 90405   Phone: (213) 392-5509
Publication Includes: List of approximately 300 suppliers of medical device equipment, products, and services. **Entries Include:** Company name, location, phone, toll-free number, fax, products and services. **Frequency:** Annual, April.

★4511★ MEDICAL DEVICE REGISTER
Medical Device Register, Inc.
5 Paragon Dr.
Montvale, NJ 07645-1725   Phone: (203) 348-6319
Covers: More than 11,000 manufacturers of medical devices and clinical laboratory products; also includes 20,000 medical product distributors. Published in three volumes; volumes 1 & 2 cover the United States and Canada; volume 3 lists 6,000 manufacturers and 4,000 distributors operating outside the United States and Canada. **Entries Include:** For manufacturers—Company name, address, phone, fax, telex, names and titles of key personnel, ownership, medical product sales volume, number of employees, method of distribution, medical product subsidiaries; public company listings include annual revenues and net income. For distributors—Company name, address, phone. **Pages (approx.):** 2,700 (volumes 1 & 2), 880 (volume 3). **Frequency:** Annual, December; interedition update.

★4512★ MEDICAL DIRECTORY
Industry and Public Management Division
Longman Group UK Ltd.
Westgate House, 6th Fl.
The High
Harlow, Essex CM20 1YR, England
Covers: About 2,440 hospitals and 115,000 physicians registered with the General Medical Council in the United Kingdom and Republic of Ireland; also includes medical schools, universities, medical offices of government agencies, and research institutions. **Entries Include:** For physicians—Name, address, career and medical education data, professional association membership, publications. For hospitals—Name, address, phone, number of beds, names of heads of each medical specialty. **Pages (approx.):** 5,000 (in two volumes). **Frequency:** Annual, summer. **Available in the U.S. from:** St. James Press, 233 E. Ontario St., Ste. 600, Chicago, IL 60611.

★4513★ MEDICAL ELECTRONICS—MEDICAL EQUIPMENT BUYERS GUIDE ISSUES
Measurements & Data Corp.
2994 W. Liberty Ave.
Pittsburgh, PA 15216   Phone: (412) 343-9666
Publication Includes: Manufacturers of biomedical instruments. **Entries Include:** Manufacturer name, address, phone, name of contact. **Frequency:** Bimonthly.

★4514★ MEDICAL GROUP MANAGEMENT ASSOCIATION—DIRECTORY
Medical Group Management Association
104 Inverness Terrace, E.
Englewood, CO 80112-5306   Phone: (303) 753-1111
Covers: More than 10,500 individual members and 4,700 member groups representing over 95,000 physicians. **Entries Include:** Group or clinic name, address, phone, size, services provided, types of specialties, statistical data; name, title, and biographical data of administrator(s). **Pages (approx.):** 750. **Frequency:** Annual, December.

★4515★ MEDICAL GROUPS DIRECTORY
American Business Directories, Inc.
American Business Information, Inc.
5711 S. 86th Circle
Omaha, NE 68127   Phone: (402) 593-4600
Number of Listings: 1,667. **Entries Include:** Name, address, phone, size of advertisement, name of owner or manager, number of employees, year first in "Yellow Pages." **Frequency:** Annual.

★4516★ MEDICAL AND HEALTH CARE BOOKS AND SERIALS IN PRINT
R. R. Bowker Co.
121 Chanlon Rd.
New Providence, NJ 07974   Phone: (908) 464-6800
Publication Includes: List of 2,500 publishers and distributors of books, micropublishers of serials, and abstracting and indexing services concerned with health sciences and health care, including medicine, dentistry,

psychiatry, nursing, etc. **Entries Include:** Name, address, phone, ISBN prefix, ordering address, imprints. **Frequency:** Annual, March.

★4517★   MEDICAL AND HEALTH INFORMATION DIRECTORY
Gale Research Inc.
835 Penobscot Bldg.
Detroit, MI 48226-4094   Phone: (313) 961-2242
Covers: In volume 1, medical and health oriented associations, organizations, institutions, and government agencies, including health maintenance organizations (HMOs), preferred provider organizations (PPOs), insurance companies, pharmaceutical companies, research centers, and medical and allied health schools. In volume 2, medical book publishers; medical periodicals, review serials, etc.; audiovisual producers and services, medical libraries and information centers, and computer-readable databases. In volume 3, clinics, treatment centers, care programs, and counseling/diagnostic services for 31 subject areas. **Entries Include:** Institution, service, or firm name, address, phone; many include names of key personnel and, when pertinent, descriptive annotation. **Pages (approx.):** Volume 1, 1,330; volume 2, 700; volume 3, 860. **Frequency:** Each volume published separately on a biennial basis; volume 1, latest edition 1992; volume 2, latest edition 1992; volume 3, latest edition 1992.

★4518★   MEDICAL AND HEALTHCARE MARKETPLACE GUIDE
IDD, Inc.
MLR Publishing Co.
229 S. 18th St.
Philadelphia, PA 19103   Phone: (215) 790-7000
Covers: Over 5,500 American firms, including over 300 subsidiaries of foreign firms operating in the United States, which offer medical products and services; covers over 4,200 separate operating units. **Entries Include:** Company name, address, phone, fax, toll-free phone (if any), names and titles of key personnel, description of company, products or services, financial information, and number of employees. **Pages (approx.):** 2,000. **Frequency:** Annual, July. **Send Orders to:** 2 World Trade Center, 18th Fl., New York, NY 10048 (212-227-1200).

★4519★   MEDICAL ILLUSTRATION SOURCEBOOK
The Association of Medical Illustrators
1819 Peachtree St. NE, Ste. 560
Atlanta, GA 30309   Phone: (404) 350-7900
Covers: Over 130 member illustrators available for freelance work; listings are paid. **Entries Include:** Name, address, phone, affiliation, specialties, education, awards, professional memberships, names of clients, samples of work. **Pages (approx.):** 162. **Frequency:** Biennial, spring of odd years.

★4520★   MEDICAL INFORMATION SOURCES: A REFERRAL DIRECTORY
American Medical Association
515 N. State St.
Chicago, IL 60610   Phone: (312) 464-4818
Publication Includes: List of medical organizations that provide information to the public on all aspects of medical education and science. **Entries Include:** Company name, address, phone, branch offices and addresses. **Pages (approx.):** 135. **Frequency:** Semiannual. **Send Orders to:** AMA Library, PO Box 10623, Chicago, IL 60610-0623.

★4521★   MEDICAL LABORATORY DIRECTORY
U.S. Directory Service, Publishers
655 N. 128th St.
PO Box 68-1700
Miami, FL 33168   Phone: (305) 769-1700
Covers: 4,000 medicare-approves and state licensed medical laboratories. **Entries Include:** Center name, address, type of services provided. **Frequency:** Irregular; latest edition 1987.

★4522★   MEDICAL LABORATORY OBSERVER—CLINICAL LABORATORY REFERENCE ISSUE
Medical Economics Publishing
Medical Economics Co.
5 Paragon Dr.
Montvale, NJ 07645   Phone: (201) 358-7200
Publication Includes: List of about 170 manufacturers of diagnostic reagents, tests, systems, instruments, supplies, and services used in clinical laboratories; listings are paid. **Entries Include:** Company name, address, phone, products or services provided. **Frequency:** Annual, July.

★4523★   MEDICAL LABORATORY SCIENTIFIC OFFICER'S REGISTER
Medical Laboratory Technicians Board
184 Kennington Park Rd.
London SE11 4BU, England
Covers: Individuals registered to practice with the UK National Health Services. **Entries Include:** Name, address, biographical data, qualifications, courses. **Pages (approx.):** 350. **Frequency:** Annual, January.

★4524★   MEDICAL LASER—BUYERS GUIDE
PennWell Publishing Co.
1 Technology Park Dr.
Westford, MA 01886   Phone: (508) 692-0700
Covers: Approximately 100 manufacturers and suppliers of medical lasers worldwide. **Entries Include:** Company name, address, phone, telex, names and titles of key personnel, descriptions of products and services. **Pages (approx.):** 100. **Frequency:** Annual, January.

★4525★   MEDICAL LIBRARY ASSOCIATION—DIRECTORY
Medical Library Association
6 N. Michigan Ave., No. 300
Chicago, IL 60602   Phone: (312) 419-9094
Covers: 5,000 member individuals and institutions; includes list of vendors. **Entries Include:** For individuals—Name, address, phone, fax. For institutions—Name, address, phone, fax, names of representatives. For vendors—Name, address, phone, fax, product description. **Pages (approx.):** 175. **Frequency:** Annual, September.

★4526★   MEDICAL MARKETING AND MEDIA—HEALTHCARE AGENCY PROFILES ISSUE
CPS Communications, Inc.
7200 W. Camino Real, Ste. 215
Boca Raton, FL 33433   Phone: (407) 368-9301
Publication Includes: List of about 130 health care advertising agencies. **Entries Include:** Company name, address, phone, key personnel, financial revenue, percentages of regional markets, market breakdown, current accounts, new accounts and accounts lost, number of employees, year established, special services, divisions. **Pages (approx.):** 135. **Frequency:** Annual, December.

★4527★   MEDICAL MEETING/ASSOCIATION REGISTER
Medical Device Register, Inc.
5 Paragon Dr.
Montvale, NJ 07645-1725
Covers: Over 3,000 medical meetings and sponsoring associations; international coverage. **Pages (approx.):** 600. **Frequency:** Latest edition 1989; suspended indefinitely.

★4528★   MEDICAL MEETINGS—DIRECTORY OF MEDICAL ASSOCIATIONS AND MEETINGS ISSUE
The Laux Co., Inc.
63 Great Rd.
Maynard, MA 01754   Phone: (508) 897-5552
Publication Includes: List of about 2,000 meetings of medical, osteopathic, dental, nursing, hospital and nursing home, podiatry, optometry, veterinary, chiropractic, and allied health associations and societies. **Entries Include:** Name of organization, address, phone, names of executive director and/or meeting planner; number of members, number on staff, annual budget; annual meeting date, site, number attending, whether exhibits are included. **Frequency:** Annual, November.

★4529★   MEDICAL MEETINGS—FACILITIES GUIDE ISSUE
The Laux Co., Inc.
63 Great Rd.
Maynard, MA 01754   Phone: (508) 897-5552
Publication Includes: About 1,000 hotels and conference centers that can accommodate medical conferences; local convention bureaus; coverage is primarily the United States and Canada. **Entries Include:** For convention bureaus—Name, address, phone; name of director; medical schools and hospitals in area. For others—Facility name, address, phone, name of contact; number of guest rooms, information on meeting rooms and exhibit space, major recreation facilities, type of facility (convention center, city hotel, resort hotel, etc.). **Frequency:** Annual, May.

★4530★ MEDICAL OFFICERS OF SCHOOLS ASSOCIATION—RULES AND LIST OF MEMBERS
Medical Officers of Schools Association
11 Chandos St.
Cavendish Sq.
London W1M 0EB, England
Frequency: Irregular; previous edition 1984; latest edition January 1991.

★4531★ MEDICAL PLASTICS DIRECTORY AND BUYERS GUIDE
Healthcare Division
Society of the Plastics Industry
1275 K St., NW, Ste. 400
Washington, DC 20005   Phone: (202) 371-5230
Covers: More than 500 Healthcare Division member manufacturers and distributors of medical products; consultants to the medical industry. **Entries Include:** Member name, address, phone, name of contact, product or service provided. **Pages (approx.):** 80. **Frequency:** Irregular; previous edition 1986; latest edition July 1989.

★4532★ MEDICAL REGISTER
General Medical Council
44 Hallam St.
London W1N 6AE, England
Covers: Medical practitioners who hold full or provisional registration in the Principal List of the Register kept by the General Medical Council. Three supplements include information regarding recent additions to the list (Group A), changes of addresses (Group B), and names removed from the list (Group C). **Entries Include:** Name, address, initial registration date, registered qualifications, registration number, sex. **Pages (approx.):** 4,600 (in 3 volumes). **Frequency:** Annual, April; biweekly supplements. **Also Includes:** General information about registration.

★4533★ MEDICAL REMARKETER—ANNUAL BUYER'S GUIDE ISSUE
Ledgewood Publications
5 Colony Rd.
Canton, CT 06019   Phone: (203) 693-9055
Publication Includes: List of approximately 100 manufacturers and suppliers of equipment for the medical and health care industry. **Entries Include:** Company name, address, phone, fax, names and titles of key personnel, name and title of contact, product/service, brief company profile. **Frequency:** Annual, February.

★4534★ MEDICAL RESEARCH CENTRES
Longman Group UK Ltd.
Westgate House
The High
Harlow, Essex CM20 1YR, England
Covers: Over 10,525 hospitals, universities, companies, research centers, and other organizations, involved in research in medicine, dentistry, pharmacy, biochemistry, and related subjects; international coverage. **Entries Include:** Name of center in native language and in English, acronym, address, phone, fax, telex, affiliation or parent body, products, names of director and senior staff member for each laboratory, annual research & development expenditure, number of graduate research staff, research interests, major clients, publications. **Frequency:** Biennial, summer of even years. **Available in the U.S. from:** Gale Research Inc., 835 Penobscot Bldg., Detroit, MI 48226.

★4535★ MEDICAL RESEARCH FUNDING BULLETIN
Science Support Center
Box 7507
New York, NY 10150   Phone: (212) 371-3398
Description: Each bulletin describes about 15-35 federal contracts available for research in health and science fields, and 10-40 grants from both federal and private organizations (including scholarships, fellowships, and research grants), with deadines in the coming two months. **Entries Include:** For contracts—Agency, acronym, project title, request for proposal number and due date, description of project, name and address of agency contact. For grants—Agency or organization name, acronym, department, description of grant, deadline for application; name, address, and phone of contact. **Pages (approx.):** 10-35. **Frequency:** Published on the 10th, 20th, and 30th of each month.

★4536★ MEDICAL SCHOOL ADMISSION REQUIREMENTS—UNITED STATES AND CANADA
Association of American Medical Colleges
2450 N St. NW
Washington, DC 20037-1126   Phone: (202) 828-0400
Covers: Accredited medical schools; in the U.S., Canada, and Puerto Rico. **Entries Include:** School name, address, name and title of contact, admission requirements, application procedures, premedical planning, financial aid programs, fees, selection factors, curriculum features, first year current expenses, premedical planning, MCAT and AMCAS information, applicant statistics. **Pages (approx.):** 423. **Frequency:** Annual, April.

★4537★ MEDICAL AND SCIENCE NEWS MEDIA
Larriston Communications
Box 20229
New York, NY 10025   Phone: (212) 864-0150
Covers: Over 300 daily newspapers of 50,000 or more circulation; radio and television networks, about 40 market areas, and local programs that focus on scientific or medical topics; general magazines, medical and science magazines; wire services, newspaper groups, and news bureaus; syndicated columnists, and over 200 independent writers in this field. **Entries Include:** For newspapers—Name of paper, address, phone, name of managing editor and city editor, name of contact person, news services. For radio and television stations—Name, address, and phone; name of news director or science editor, audience figures, network affiliation. For programs—Program name, address, phone, name of host, station affiliation. Magazines have similar information and may include frequency of publication. Listings for independent writers are coded according to subject area preferred and indicate credits and availability for freelance assignment. **Pages (approx.):** 180. **Frequency:** Annual, mid-year update.

★4538★ MEDICAL SCIENCES INTERNATIONAL WHO'S WHO
Longman Group UK Ltd.
Westgate House
The High
Harlow, Essex CM20 1YR, England
Covers: Over 8,000 research workers in medicine, dentistry and pharmacy in 90 countries. **Entries Include:** Name, address, phone, qualifications, biographical data, present and past positions, memberships, research interests, publications. **Pages (approx.):** 1,340. **Frequency:** Triennial; latest edition February 1990. **Available in the U.S. from:** Gale Research Inc., 835 Penobscot Bldg., Detroit, MI 48226.

★4539★ MEDICAL AND SURGICAL SERVICE ORGANIZATIONS DIRECTORY
American Business Directories, Inc.
American Business Information, Inc.
5711 S. 86th Circle
Omaha, NE 68127   Phone: (402) 593-4600
Number of Listings: 1,359. **Entries Include:** Name, address, phone, size of advertisement, name of owner or manager, number of employees, year first in "Yellow Pages." **Frequency:** Annual.

★4540★ MEDICAL TECHNOLOGY ASSESSMENT DIRECTORY
National Academy Press
2101 Constitution Ave., NW
Washington, DC 20418   Phone: (202) 334-3180
Covers: Approximately 70 institutions worldwide conducting programs for the assessment of current medical technology; 75 information resources, including online database producers, publishers, and abstracting services; and 75 United States organizations involved in the field of medical technology. **Entries Include:** For programs—Institution name, address, phone, name and title of contact; description of program, including purpose, types of technology assessed, intended users, size of budget, and preferred topics; bibliography of reports with dates completed or expected completion dates. For information resources—Title and/or producer or publisher name, subject, description of contents, sources utilized, access information (in dot chart format); producer/publisher address and phone given in index. For other organizations—Name, address, phone, name and title of contact, description of membership and activities. **Pages (approx.):** 700. **Frequency:** Published spring 1988. **Also Includes:** Subject index to assessment reports, technology thesaurus.

★4541★ MEDICAL UTILIZATION REVIEW DIRECTORY
Faulkner & Gray's Healthcare Information Center
1133 15th St. NW, Ste. 450
Washington, DC 20005   Phone: (202) 828-1022
Covers: Approximately 500 medical utilization review companies providing review for insurance companies, employers, health maintenance

organizations, group medical practices, and consumers. **Entries Include:** Company name, address, phone, names and titles of key personnel, number of employees, geographical area served, financial data, subsidiary and branch names and locations, services provided. **Pages (approx.):** 400. **Frequency:** Annual, September; first edition 1990.

★4542★   **THE MEDICARE HANDBOOK**
Superintendent of Documents
U.S. Government Printing Office
Dept. 33
Washington, DC 20402   Phone: (202) 783-3238
Publication Includes: Lists of medicare carriers in individual states. **Pages (approx.):** 44. **Frequency:** Latest edition 1989.

★4543★   **MEDPARD DIRECTORY**
U.S. Health Care Financing Administration
6325 Security Blvd.
Baltimore, MD 21207   Phone: (301) 966-6962
Covers: Physicians and other medical service suppliers who have signed an agreement to accept fixed, standard fees on Medicare claims in cooperation with a cost control program established by Congress. Available only in state editions purchased from local or state health and human services offices.

★4544★   **MEETING THE NEEDS OF EMPLOYEES WITH DISABILITIES**
Resources for Rehabilitation
33 Bedford St., Ste. 19A
Lexington, MA 02173   Phone: (617) 862-6455
Publication Includes: List of organizations that assist those involved in the employment of people with disabilities. **Entries Include:** Organization name, address, phone, geographical area served, requirements for membership, admission, or eligibility, description. **Frequency:** Biennial, summer of even years.

★4545★   **MEETINGS INMED**
Scientific Meetings Publications
Box 81662
San Diego, CA 92138   Phone: (619) 270-2910
Covers: Medical, dental, and health science conferences scheduled for the forthcoming 12 months; international coverage. **Entries Include:** Conference name, address. **Pages (approx.):** 80. **Frequency:** Quarterly; February, May, August, and November.

★4546★   **MENTAL HEALTH DIRECTORY**
U.S. National Institute of Mental Health
5600 Fishers Ln., Rm. 15C-05
Rockville, MD 20857   Phone: (301) 443-4513
Covers: Hospitals, treatment centers, outpatient clinics, day/night facilities, residential treatment centers for emotionally disturbed children, residential supportive programs such as halfway houses, and mental health centers offering mental health assistance; not included are substance abuse programs, Veteran's Administration programs, nursing homes, programs for the developmentally disabled, and organizations in which fees are retained by individual members. **Entries Include:** Name, address, phone. **Pages (approx.):** 468. **Frequency:** Irregular; previous edition 1985; latest edition 1990. **Also Includes:** Lists of state mental health agencies.

★4547★   **MENTAL HEALTH SERVICES DIRECTORY**
American Business Directories, Inc.
American Business Information, Inc.
5711 S. 86th Circle
Omaha, NE 68127   Phone: (402) 593-4600
Number of Listings: 12,868. **Entries Include:** Name, address, phone (including area code), size of advertisement, year first in "Yellow Pages," name of owner or manager, number of employees. **Frequency:** Annual.

★4548★   **MENTAL HEALTH SYSTEMS SOFTWARE DIRECTORY**
American Association for Medical Systems and Informatics
1101 Connecticut Ave. NW, Ste. 700
Washington, DC 20036   Phone: (202) 857-1189
Covers: Approximately 60 producers of software with mental health program applications. **Entries Include:** Company name, address, phone, description of software. **Pages (approx.):** 70. **Frequency:** Irregular; latest edition 1985.

★4549★   **MENTAL RETARDATION AND DEVELOPMENTALLY DISABLED SERVICES DIRECTORY**
American Business Directories, Inc.
American Business Information, Inc.
5711 S. 86th Circle
Omaha, NE 68127   Phone: (402) 593-4600
Number of Listings: 1,134. **Entries Include:** Name, address, phone, size of advertisement, name of owner or manager, number of employees, year first in "Yellow Pages." **Frequency:** Annual.

★4550★   **MIDDLE EAST COMMITTEE FOR THE WELFARE OF THE BLIND—DIRECTORY**
Middle East Committee for the Welfare of the Blind
c/o Regional Bureau for the Blind
Box 3465
Riyadh 11471, Saudi Arabia
Covers: Representatives of Middle Eastern countries who work to assist the blind, especially with respect to education and vocational training.

★4551★   **MIGRANT HEALTH SERVICES DIRECTORY**
Midwest Migrant Health Information Office
National Migrant Worker Council
6131 W. Outer Dr., 4th Fl.
Detroit, MI 48235   Phone: (313) 927-7545
Covers: About 60 federally funded migrant health clinics in Michigan, Ohio, Indiana, Illinois, Iowa, Wisconsin, and Minnesota. **Entries Include:** Clinic name, address, phone, contact name, hours of operation, description of services provided, eight month calendar. **Pages (approx.):** 30. **Frequency:** Annual, March. **Also Includes:** Maps of each state, with location of clinics, major highways, and cities noted; pictograms of services.

★4552★   **MINORITY BIOMEDICAL SUPPORT PROGRAM: A RESEARCH RESOURCES DIRECTORY**
Division of Research Resources
U.S. National Institutes of Health
Bethesda, MD 20892   Phone: (301) 984-2876
Covers: Institutions granting research awards to minority faculty and students engaged in biomedical research. **Entries Include:** Institution name, name of program director, address, phone, names of individual project investigators, number of student participants, projects, equipment available. **Pages (approx.):** 90. **Frequency:** Latest edition January 1988; suspended indefinitely. **Send Orders to:** Research Resources Information Center, 1601 Research Blvd., Rockville, MD 20850.

★4553★   **MINORITY HEALTH RESOURCES DIRECTORY**
ANROW Publishing
5515 Security Ln., Ste. 510
Rockville, MD 20852
Covers: 360 federal government programs and agencies, organizations, and foundations offering health services and products to minority group members. **Entries Include:** Name, address, phone, description, activities for minorities, publications and other communications, meetings and conferences. **Pages (approx.):** 355. **Frequency:** Published 1991.

★4554★   **MINORITY STUDENT OPPORTUNITIES IN UNITED STATES MEDICAL SCHOOLS**
Association of American Medical Colleges
1 Dupont Circle NW, Ste. 200
Washington, DC 20036   Phone: (202) 828-0400
Covers: Programs for minority group students at nearly 130 medical schools. **Entries Include:** Name of school, name of parent institution, if applicable, address, phone, name of contact; descriptions of recruitment, admissions, financial aid, and academic assistance programs for the minority student; statistical table on minority admissions and enrollment. **Pages (approx.):** 325. **Frequency:** Biennial, August of even years. **Also Includes:** List of schools offering summer programs.

★4555★   **MONOCLONAL ANTIBODIES**
Theta Corp.
Theta Bldg.
Middlefield, CT 06455   Phone: (203) 349-1054
Publication Includes: List of nearly 95 manufacturers of monoclonal antibodies (MCAs). **Entries Include:** Company name, address, phone, key personnel, background information, description of products, annual sales, research and development efforts, distribution systems, five year projection. **Pages (approx.):** 110. **Frequency:** Irregular; previous edition November 1987; latest edition December 1989.

★4556★ MONTREAL WOMEN'S DIRECTORY
Les Editions Communiqu'Elles
3585 St. Urbain
Montreal, PQ, Canada H2X 2N6   Phone: (514) 844-1761
Covers: Resource centers, civic organizations, health services, day care centers, legal services, and other groups for women in Montreal, Quebec, Canada. Pages (approx.): 240. Frequency: Biennial, odd years.

★4557★ MOTORING AND MOBILITY FOR DISABLED PEOPLE
Royal Association for Disability & Rehabilitation
25 Mortimer St.
London W1N 8AB, England
Publication Includes: Companies and organizations that provide special vehicular services for handicapped automobile drivers. Entries Include: Company or organization name, address, phone, services. Frequency: Irregular; latest edition 1985.

★4558★ MULTI-HOSPITAL SYSTEMS AND GROUP PURCHASING ORGANIZATIONS DIRECTORY
SMG Marketing Group, Inc.
1342 N. LaSalle
Chicago, IL 60610   Phone: (312) 642-3026
Covers: Over 420 multi-hospital systems and group purchasing organizations. Entries Include: Company name, address, phone, hospital name, address, phone, type of hospital service, licensed number of beds, number of staffed beds, annual admission data, annual surgical information, status of hospital, activity in recent quarter as well as date and length of management contract with the hospital. Pages (approx.): 600. Frequency: Quarterly.

★4559★ MUSIC THERAPY CLINICAL TRAINING FACILITIES DIRECTORY
National Association for Music Therapy
8455 Colesville Rd., Ste. 930
Silver Spring, MD 20910   Phone: (301) 589-3300
Covers: About 160 clinical training sites in the United States. Entries Include: Facility name, address, phone, name of clinical training director, code indicating type of population served. Pages (approx.): 10. Frequency: Annual, March.

★4560★ NAN DIRECTORY OF AIDS EDUCATION AND SERVICE ORGANIZATIONS
National AIDS Network
2033 M St., NW, No. 800
Washington, DC 20036   Phone: (202) 293-2437
Covers: About 700 groups providing services to people with Acquired Immune Deficiency Syndrome or involved in AIDS education. Entries Include: Organization name, address, phone, geographical area covered, client service and education programs offered, minority community programs offered, and hotline information. Pages (approx.): 120. Frequency: Annual.

★4561★ NAPSAC DIRECTORY OF ALTERNATIVE BIRTH SERVICES AND CONSUMER GUIDE
National Association of Parents & Professionals for Safe Alternatives in Childbirth
Rt. 1, Box 646
Marble Hill, MO 63764   Phone: (314) 238-2010
Covers: 2,000 birth centers, midwifery schools, midwives, doctors attending to home births, childbirth educators, and others in the field of alternative childbirth; international coverage. Entries Include: Name, address, phone, medically related degree, and services offered. Pages (approx.): 150. Frequency: Annual, spring. Also Includes: List of state and regional associations and referral services belonging to NAPSAC.

★4562★ NARCOTICS AND DRUG ABUSE: A-Z
Croner Publications, Inc.
34 Jericho Turnpike
Jericho, NY 11753   Phone: (516) 333-9085
Covers: Agencies, organizations, facilities, companies and persons actively opposed to the use and/or abuse of narcotics and drugs. In three volumes: Volume 1, Connecticut, New Jersey, New York; volume 2, Alaska, Arizona, California, Colorado, Hawaii, Iowa, Montana, New Mexico, Nevada, Oregon, Vermont, Washington, and Wyoming; volume 3, all others. Entries Include: For agencies, commissions, and facilities—Name, address, name of administrator, description of services. For companies—Name, location, products or activities. Frequency: Annual; quarterly

updates. Also Includes: Descriptions of drugs, with glossary of slang terms used in English and Spanish to refer to specific drugs; bibliography.

★4563★ NARIC DIRECTORY OF LIBRARIANS AND INFORMATION SPECIALISTS IN DISABILITY AND REHABILITATION
National Rehabilitation Information Center (NARIC)
8455 Colesville Rd., Ste. 935
Silver Spring, MD 20910-3319   Phone: (301) 588-9284
Covers: Approximately 445 librarians and information specialists in the U.S. who work with disability and rehabilitation information. Entries Include: Individual's name, address, phone, biographical data, areas of special interest and expertise. Pages (approx.): 60. Frequency: Irregular; latest edition January 1990.

★4564★ NARIC GUIDE TO DISABILITY AND REHABILITATION PERIODICALS
National Rehabilitation Information Center
8455 Colesville Rd., Ste. 935
Silver Spring, MD 20910   Phone: (301) 588-9284
Covers: Over 400 local, national, and international rehabilitation journals and newsletters. Entries Include: Periodical title, name and address of publisher, frequency, volumes held by NARIC, description, subjects covered, subscription rates, audience. Pages (approx.): 200. Frequency: Irregular; previous edition 1989, latest edition 1991.

★4565★ NATIONAL ABORTION FEDERATION—MEMBERSHIP DIRECTORY
National Abortion Federation
1436 U St. NW, Ste. 103
Washington, DC 20009   Phone: (202) 667-5881
Covers: 310 member abortion clinics, hospitals, professional corporations (medical practices), and research organizations. Entries Include: Facility name, address, phone, name of representative to the federation, names and titles of key personnel, services offered, fees, code for type of facility. Pages (approx.): 110. Frequency: Annual, January.

★4566★ NATIONAL ACCREDITATION COUNCIL FOR AGENCIES SERVING THE BLIND AND VISUALLY HANDICAPPED—LIST OF MEMBER ORGANIZATIONS
National Accreditation Council for Agencies Serving the Blind and Visually Handicapped
232 Madison Ave., Ste. 907
New York, NY 10016   Phone: (212) 779-8080
Covers: About 100 accredited agencies and schools for service to the blind. Entries Include: Organization name, date first accredited, date of next re-evaluation, city and state. Pages (approx.): 10. Frequency: Semiannual, June and December; reprinted in council's annual report.

★4567★ NATIONAL ALLIANCE FOR THE MENTALLY ILL—ANNOTATED READING LIST
National Alliance for the Mentally Ill
2101 Wilson Blvd., Ste. 302
Arlington, VA 22201   Phone: (703) 524-7600
Covers: Distributors of books, periodicals, and videotapes dealing with mental illnesses and treatments. Entries Include: Publisher or producer name, address; title of publication, author, price, description of content. Pages (approx.): 45. Frequency: Irregular; previous edition 1986; latest edition March 1989.

★4568★ NATIONAL ASSOCIATION OF CHAIN DRUG STORES—MEMBERSHIP DIRECTORY
National Association of Chain Drug Stores
413 Lee St.
Alexandria, VA 22314   Phone: (703) 549-3001
Covers: About 170 chain drug retailers and their 21,000 individual pharmacies; 800 supplier companies; state boards of pharmacy, pharmaceutical and retail associations, colleges of pharmacy; drug trade associations. Entries Include: For chain drug retailers—Firm name, headquarters address and phone, number of retail outlets and pharmacies operated, names and titles of key personnel, buying hours, warehouse address. For suppliers—Firm name, address, phone, product/service provided, names and titles of key personnel. For individual drug stores—Name, address; parent company not identified if not included in store name. For other listings—Company or other name, address, phone, name of chief executive. Pages (approx.): 240. Frequency: Annual, December.

★4569★ NATIONAL ASSOCIATION OF DEVELOPMENTAL DISABILITIES COUNCILS—MEMBERSHIP LIST
National Association of Developmental Disabilities Councils
1234 Massachusetts Ave., NW, Ste. 103
Washington, DC 20005   Phone: (202) 347-1234
Covers: About 55 state and territorial councils on developmental disabilities. **Entries Include:** Names, addresses, and phone numbers of each council's executive director, chairperson, and council delegate. **Pages (approx.):** 10. **Frequency:** Annual, March.

★4570★ NATIONAL ASSOCIATION FOR MUSIC THERAPY—MEMBERSHIP DIRECTORY
National Association for Music Therapy
8455 Colesville Rd., Ste. 930
Silver Spring, MD 20910   Phone: (301) 589-3300
Covers: 3,000 members. **Entries Include:** Name, home address, phone, type of membership. **Pages (approx.):** 70. **Frequency:** Annual, spring.

★4571★ NATIONAL ASSOCIATION OF PRIVATE PSYCHIATRIC HOSPITALS—MEMBERSHIP ROSTER
National Association of Private Psychiatric Hospitals
1319 F St., NW, Ste. 1000
Washington, DC 20004   Phone: (202) 393-6700
Covers: Over 300 psychiatric hospitals. **Entries Include:** Hospital name, address, phone and fax numbers, bed size, CEO, medical director, and administrator. **Pages (approx.):** 48. **Frequency:** Annual.

★4572★ NATIONAL ASSOCIATION OF PRIVATE RESIDENTIAL RESOURCES—DIRECTORYOF MEMBERS
National Association of Private Residential Resources
4200 Evergreen Ln., Ste. 315
Annandale, VA 22003   Phone: (703) 642-6614
Covers: 625 agencies serving people with mental retardation. **Entries Include:** Name of organization, address, phone, name of administrator; description of persons served including number, sex, age, level of disability, and special conditions served; licensing and certification. **Pages (approx.):** 115. **Frequency:** Approximately biennial; latest edition February 1990.

★4573★ NATIONAL ASSOCIATION OF PRIVATE SCHOOLS FOR EXCEPTIONAL CHILDREN—MEMBERSHIP DIRECTORY
National Association of Private Schools for Exceptional Children
1522 K St., NW, Ste. 1032
Washington, DC 20005   Phone: (202) 408-3338
Number of Listings: About 200. **Entries Include:** Name, address, facilities, type of child and ages accepted, services. **Pages (approx.):** 400. **Frequency:** Biennial; lastest edition 1989-90. **Also Includes:** List of affiliated state associations.

★4574★ NATIONAL ASSOCIATION OF SUBSTANCE ABUSE TRAINERS AND EDUCATORS—DIRECTORY
National Association of Substance Abuse Trainers and Educators
Thomas P. Lief, Ph.D.
1521 Hillary St.
New Orleans, LA 70118
Covers: About 70 universities offering educational programs in the treatment of substance abuse. **Entries Include:** Name of college or university, location, contact name, courses and degree programs offered. **Pages (approx.):** 40. **Frequency:** Annual, summer.

★4575★ NATIONAL BLACK HEALTH LEADERSHIP DIRECTORY
NRW Associates
1315 Hamlin St. NE
Washington, DC 20017   Phone: (202) 635-4804
Covers: Approximately 420 Black health professionals serving in leadership roles in private and public sector organizations, including the Department of Health and Human Services, public health departments, hospitals and hospital systems, associations, agencies, educational institutions, health maintenance organizations, long-term health care administration, community and family care centers, health policy, planning, and research. **Entries Include:** Name, address, phone, name and title of contact. **Pages (approx.):** 212. **Frequency:** Annual, September.

★4576★ NATIONAL COMMISSION FOR ELECTROLOGIST CERTIFICATION—DIRECTORY OF CERTIFIED CLINICAL ELECTROLOGISTS
National Commission for Electrologist Certification
Box 52
Killeen, TX 76540   Phone: (817) 526-6515
Covers: About 1,000 certified electrologists; coverage includes Canada, Europe, and Japan. **Entries Include:** Name, address, phone. **Pages (approx.):** 50. **Frequency:** Annual, January.

★4577★ NATIONAL CONTINUING CARE DIRECTORY
Scott, Foresman and Co.
1900 E. Lake Ave.
Glenview, IL 60025   Phone: (708) 729-3000
Covers: More than 365 retirement communities in 39 states, which provide board, lodging, and health services. **Entries Include:** Community name, address, phone, special features and services, costs, other information. **Pages (approx.):** 460. **Frequency:** Irregular; previous edition spring 1984; latest edition March 1988.

★4578★ NATIONAL CUED SPEECH ASSOCIATION—MEMBERSHIP DIRECTORY
National Cued Speech Association
Box 31345
Raleigh, NC 27622   Phone: (919) 828-1218
Covers: About 500 hearing-impaired individuals, friends, family, associates, and professionals who use Cued Speech, a system which clarifies lipreading by adding hand signals to the natural mouth movements of speech to provide a means of accurately identifying all speech sounds. **Entries Include:** Individual or organization name, address, phone. **Pages (approx.):** 10. **Frequency:** Annual, spring.

★4579★ NATIONAL DIRECTORY OF ADULT DAY CARE CENTERS
Health Resources Publishing
Brinley Professional Plaza
3100 Highway 138
Wall Township, NJ 07719-1442   Phone: (908) 681-1133
Covers: Over 1,000 centers and programs providing adult day care. **Entries Include:** Center or program name, address, phone, director or coordinator name; separate section details programs, providing sponsor information, geographic area served, client profiles, fees, number of clients and staff, services, and sources of funding. **Frequency:** Irregular; previous edition October 1986; latest edition summer 1991. **Also Includes:** Bibliography of resources.

★4580★ NATIONAL DIRECTORY OF CERTIFIED COUNSELORS
National Board for Certified Counselors
5999 Stevenson Ave., Ste. 402
Alexandria, VA 22304   Phone: (703) 461-6222
Covers: 20,000 certified counselors, career counselors, and clinical mental health counselors. **Entries Include:** Personal name, address, phone. **Pages (approx.):** 300. **Frequency:** Irregular; previous edition spring 1988; latest edition spring 1991.

★4581★ NATIONAL DIRECTORY OF CHILD ABUSE PROSECUTORS
National Center for Prosecution of Child Abuse
1033 N. Fairfax St., Ste. 200
Alexandria, VA 22314   Phone: (703) 739-0321
Covers: Over 800 prosecutors and district attorneys specializing in child abuse cases. **Entries Include:** District attorney name, assistant district attorney name, address, phone, jurisdiction size. **Pages (approx.):** 170. **Frequency:** Reported as annual; previous edition March 1988; latest edition December 1989.

★4582★ NATIONAL DIRECTORY OF CHILDREN AND YOUTH SERVICES
Marion L. Peterson, Publisher
Box 1837
Longmont, CO 80502   Phone: (303) 776-7539
Covers: Child, youth, and family-oriented social services, health and mental health services, and juvenile court and youth advocacy services in state and private agencies, major cities, and 3,100 counties; also covers runaway youth centers, child abuse projects, congressional committees, clearinghouses, and national organizations concerned with child health and welfare; buyers' guide to specialized services and products. **Entries Include:** Agency listings include agency name, address, phone, names of

principal executives and staff, description of services. **Pages (approx.):** 725. **Frequency:** Biennial, July of odd years. **Also Includes:** Listings of child abuse hotlines and instructions for their use.

★4583★ **NATIONAL DIRECTORY OF CHIROPRACTIC**
One Directory Of Chiropractic
PO Box 10056
Olathe, KS 66061-1358
Covers: Chiropractors; chiropractic colleges, state boards of examiners, and associations. **Entries Include:** For chiropractors—Name, address, phone, school attended, year graduated, specialties. **Pages (approx.):** 464. **Frequency:** Latest edition 1991. **Also Includes:** Listing of each state's licensing requirements and reciprocity policies; professional statistics.

★4584★ **NATIONAL DIRECTORY OF DRUG ABUSE AND ALCOHOLISM TREATMENT AND PREVENTION PROGRAMS**
U.S. National Institute on Drug Abuse
5600 Fishers Ln.
Rockwall II, Ste. 620
Rockville, MD 20857   Phone: (301) 443-6637
Covers: 9,000 federal, state, local, and privately funded agencies administering or providing drug abuse and alcoholism treatment and prevention services. **Entries Include:** Name of agency, address, phone; whether the agency's purpose is treatment or prevention of drug, alcohol, or drug/alcohol abuse. **Pages (approx.):** 400. **Frequency:** Reported as annual; latest edition 1989.

★4585★ **NATIONAL DIRECTORY OF EDUCATIONAL PROGRAMS IN GERONTOLOGY AND GERIATRICS**
Association for Gerontology in Higher Education
1001 Connecticut Ave. NW, Ste. 410
Washington, DC 20036-5504   Phone: (202) 429-9277
Covers: Degree and certificate programs and course offerings in the field of gerontology available at nearly 300 institutions of higher education. **Entries Include:** Institution name, name and title of contact, address, phone, fax, overview of campus gerontology instruction/activity, description of gerontology programs(s), other educational, research, and community activities, and financial aid available for students. **Pages (approx.):** 650. **Frequency:** Every 2-3 years; new edition expected 1993.

★4586★ **NATIONAL DIRECTORY OF FACILITIES AND SERVICES FOR LESBIAN AND GAY ALCOHOLICS**
National Association of Lesbian and Gay Alcoholism Professionals
204 W. 20th St.
New York, NY 10011   Phone: (212) 713-5074
Covers: Over 300 treatment facilities, private counselors, etc.; facilities and services are not necessarily limited to homosexuals. **Entries Include:** Facility name, address, phone, name of contact, services provided, fees; eligibility requirements (if any), percentages of staff and clientele openly gay or lesbian. **Pages (approx.):** 95. **Frequency:** Irregular; latest edition 1987.

★4587★ **NATIONAL DIRECTORY OF FOUR YEAR...TWO YEAR COLLEGES AND POST HIGH SCHOOL TRAINING PROGRAMS FOR YOUNG PEOPLE...LEARNING DISABILITIES**
Partners in Publishing Co.
1419 W. 1st St.
Tulsa, OK 74127   Phone: (918) 584-5906
Covers: About 200 postsecondary institutions offering programs for learning disabled students. **Entries Include:** School name, address, and name of contact; description of program including type of program, admission policies, courses offered and curriculum modifications; enrollment; percentage of learning disabled students completing the program; remedial clinic available. **Pages (approx.):** 115. **Frequency:** Irregular; previous edition December 1989; new edition expected 1991. **Send Orders to:** PIP Box 50347 Tulsa, OK 74150 (918-584-5906).

★4588★ **NATIONAL DIRECTORY OF HEAD INJURY REHABILITATION SERVICES**
National Head Injury Foundation
1140 Connecticut Ave. NW, Ste. 613
Washington, DC 20036-4001   Phone: (202) 296-6443
Covers: More than 500 facilities offering specialized treatment for head injuries. **Entries Include:** Facility name, address, phone, name of contact; type of rehabilitation program, accreditations. **Frequency:** Annual, March.

★4589★ **NATIONAL DIRECTORY OF MEDICAL PSYCHOTHERAPISTS**
American Board of Medical Psychotherapists
300 25th Ave. N, Ste. 11
Nashville, TN 37203   Phone: (615) 327-2984
Covers: About 2,600 psychiatrists, psychologists, psychiatric nurses, counselors, and social workers. **Entries Include:** Name, address, phone, credentials. **Pages (approx.):** 180. **Frequency:** Annual, April.

★4590★ **NATIONAL DIRECTORY OF ORGANIZATIONS SERVING PARENTS OF CHILDREN AND YOUTH WITH EMOTIONAL AND BEHAVIORAL DISORDERS**
Research and Training Center on Family Support and Children's Mental Health
Regional Research Institute
Portland State University
PO Box 751
Portland, OR 97207-0751   Phone: (503) 725-4040
Covers: Approximately 345 organizations that provide assistance to parents of children with serious emotional disabilities. **Entries Include:** Organization name, address, phone, names and titles of contact and key personnel, geographical area of service, services. **Pages (approx.):** 315. **Frequency:** Irregular; previous edition September 1986; latest edition September 1988.

★4591★ **NATIONAL DIRECTORY OF PHYSICIAN ASSISTANT PROGRAMS**
Association of Physician Assistant Programs
950 N. Washington St.
Alexandria, VA 22314   Phone: (703) 836-2272
Covers: Over 50 programs that educate physician assistants. **Entries Include:** Program name, institution name, address, phone; description of program, including curriculum, selection criteria, degrees or certificates offered. **Pages (approx.):** 105. **Frequency:** Biennial, spring/summer of even years.

★4592★ **NATIONAL DIRECTORY OF REHABILITATION FACILITIES OFFERING VOCATIONAL EVALUATION AND ADJUSTMENT TRAINING TO HEARING IMPAIRED PERSONS**
Rehabilitation Research and Training Center on Deafness and Hearing Impairment
University of Arkansas
4601 W. Markham
Little Rock, AR 72205   Phone: (501) 686-9691
Covers: Institutions and programs that offer vocational evaluation and assistance in adjustment to deaf and hearing impaired people. **Pages (approx.):** 215. **Frequency:** Latest edition 1984.

★4593★ **NATIONAL DIRECTORY OF REHABILITATION, SHORT TERM CARE AND CONVALESCENCE**
Independent Healthcare Association
22 Little Russell St.
London WC1, England
Covers: Panel-approved short term care facilities such as nursing homes, convalescent homes, and other active rehabilitation institutions for the disabled in the United Kingdom. **Entries Include:** Facility name, address, phone, names of titles of key personnel, fees, amenities, type of care given, number of patients, review by the Panel. **Pages (approx.):** 175. **Frequency:** Annual, January.

★4594★ **NATIONAL DIRECTORY OF RETIREMENT FACILITIES**
Oryx Press
4041 N. Central, No. 700
Phoenix, AZ 85012   Phone: (602) 265-2651
Covers: Over 12,250 retirement facilities in the United States and Puerto Rico. **Entries Include:** Facility name, address, phone, name of contact, types of services available, capacity. **Pages (approx.):** 1,075. **Frequency:** Irregular; latest edition January 1991; new edition expected January 1992.

★4595★ **NATIONAL DIRECTORY OF RUNAWAY PROGRAMS**
American Youth Work Center
1751 N St. NW, Ste. 302
Washington, DC 20036   Phone: (202) 785-0764
Covers: Over 300 programs serving runaway youth. **Entries Include:** Sponsoring agency, address, name and phone of contact, facilities and services offered, funding sources, number of staff, number of runaways

served, success rate and other statistics. **Pages (approx.):** 130. **Frequency:** Irregular; previous edition 1983; latest edition January 1988.

★4596★ NATIONAL DIRECTORY: TRAINING AND EMPLOYMENT PROGRAMS FOR AMERICANS WITH DISABILITIES
Administration on Developmental Disabilities
Office of Human Development Services
U.S. Department of Health and Human Services
200 Independence Ave. SW, Rm. 3290
Washington, DC 20201   Phone: (202) 245-2890
Covers: About 650 job training programs and referral services in the private sector for disabled people; state agencies such as vocational rehabilitation agencies, governor's committees on employment of the handicapped, and developmental disability planning councils. **Entries Include:** Program name, sponsoring organization name and address, description, including training areas and levels, placement, and disabilities served. **Pages (approx.):** 460. **Frequency:** Latest edition September 1985.

★4597★ NATIONAL DRUG CODE DIRECTORY
U.S. Food and Drug Administration
5600 Fishers Ln. (HFN-315)
Rockville, MD 20857   Phone: (301) 443-6597
Publication Includes: List of manufacturers of commercially marketed human prescription drugs. **Entries Include:** Drug company name, address, labeler code, product name, description of product, National Drug Code (NDC) number. **Frequency:** Irregular; latest edition 1986, with supplement 1987.

★4598★ NATIONAL GUIDE TO FUNDING IN AGING
Foundation Center
79 5th Ave.
New York, NY 10003   Phone: (212) 620-4230
Covers: Nearly 600 foundations, federal and state government agencies, and private organizations that offer public and private sources of funding for programs about aging. **Entries Include:** For federal government agencies—Agency name, address, phone; regional office name, address, phone; description of program, types of assistance awarded, eligibility requirements, description of past programs funded by the agency, application procedure. For state government agencies—Agency name, address, phone. For private organizations—Organization name, address, phone, description of funding program, types of financial assistance available, description of publications. For foundations—Foundation name, address, phone, names of key personnel, description of program, assets, amount of money awarded, deadline date for application, description of publications. **Pages (approx.):** 280. **Frequency:** Irregular; previous edition 1986; latest edition January 1990. **Also Includes:** Over 1,100 recently awarded foundation grants.

★4599★ NATIONAL HEAD INJURY FOUNDATION NEWSLETTER—NHIF STATE ASSOCIATIONS SECTION
National Head Injury Foundation, Inc. (NHIF)
1140 Connecticut Ave. NW, Ste. 812
Washington, DC 20036-4001   Phone: (202) 296-6443
Covers: About 55 state associations and support groups involved in research and treatment of head injuries. **Entries Include:** Group or association name, address, phone. **Pages (approx.):** 1. **Frequency:** Quarterly.

★4600★ NATIONAL HEALTH COUNCIL—LISTING OF MEMBER ORGANIZATIONS
National Health Council
350 5th Ave., Ste. 1118
New York, NY 10118   Phone: (212) 268-8900
Covers: Approximately 100 national voluntary, professional, nonprofit, business, and federal government agencies with active interests in national health planning. **Entries Include:** Agency name, address of national headquarters, chief executive. **Pages (approx.):** 10. **Frequency:** Irregular; latest edition September 1989.

★4601★ NATIONAL HEALTH DIRECTORY
Aspen Publishers, Inc.
200 Orchard Ridge Dr.
Gaithersburg, MD 20878   Phone: (301) 417-7500
Covers: About 11,500 public health-care officials at policy-making levels. Covers federal and state agencies, including personnel of state health planning agencies and health systems agencies, and county and city health officials. **Entries Include:** Agency name, address; names, titles, addresses,

and phone numbers of key personnel. **Pages (approx.):** 740. **Frequency:** Annual, May.

★4602★ NATIONAL HEARING AID SOCIETY—DIRECTORY OF MEMBERS
National Hearing Aid Society
20361 Middlebelt Rd.
Livonia, MI 48152   Phone: (313) 478-2610
Covers: 2,500 hearing instrument specialists and provisional members. **Entries Include:** Name, address, phone. **Pages (approx.):** 50. **Frequency:** Annual, April. **Also Includes:** Manufacturers and suppliers of hearing aids.

★4603★ NATIONAL HEARING CONSERVATION ASSOCIATION—MEMBERSHIP DIRECTORY
National Hearing Conservation Association
900 Des Moines, Ste. 200
Des Moines, IA 50309   Phone: (515) 266-2189
Covers: About 450 members, including professional service organizations concerned with hearing protection; manufacturers and suppliers of products used for occupational noise reduction or monitoring; audiologists, industrial hygienists, nurses, safety engineers, and other individuals and organizations involved in hearing conservation programs. **Entries Include:** For organizations—Name, address, phone, contact name, branch offices addresses and phone numbers, years in business, description of services, equipment utilized, consulting issues. For manufacturers and suppliers—Name, address, phone, contact name, description of services, products available, years in business. For individuals—Name, address, phone, title, company name. **Pages (approx.):** 110. **Frequency:** Annual, March. **Also Includes:** Occupational Hearing Conservationist Training Guidelines and NHCA bylaws.

★4604★ NATIONAL HOME CARE AND HOSPICE DIRECTORY
National Association of Home Care
519 C St. NE
Washington, DC 20002   Phone: (202) 547-7424
Covers: Approximately 14,000 home care providers in the U.S. **Entries Include:** Agency name, address, phone, director's name, product/service provided. **Pages (approx.):** 500. **Frequency:** Annual, January.

★4605★ NATIONAL INSTITUTE OF DENTAL RESEARCH PROGRAMS
National Institute of Dental Research
U.S. National Institutes of Health
9000 Rockville Pike, Rm. B4BNO8
Bethesda, MD 20892   Phone: (301) 496-7220
Covers: About 170 organizations sponsoring dental research and training projects funded by the National Institute of Dental Research during the previous fiscal year. **Entries Include:** Name, city and state of performing organization, name and institution of principal investigator, grant award amount. **Pages (approx.):** 190. **Frequency:** Annual, March. **Also Includes:** Charts showing breakdowns of awards by type and other details, many ranked by amount of award.

★4606★ NATIONAL INSTITUTE FOR THE PSYCHOTHERAPIES—MEMBERSHIP DIRECTORY
National Institute for the Psychotherapies
330 W. 58th St., Ste. 200
New York, NY 10019   Phone: (212) 582-1566
Covers: Psychotherapists, psychologists, psychoanalysts, counselors, and other mental health professionals certified by the organization. **Frequency:** Annual.

★4607★ NATIONAL INSTITUTES OF HEALTH—R&D CONTRACTS, AND GRANTS FOR TRAINING, CONSTRUCTION, AND MEDICAL LIBRARIES
Division of Research Grants
National Institutes of Health
Westwood Bldg., Rm. 449
Bethesda, MD 20892   Phone: (301) 496-7441
Covers: R&D contracts, training grants, construction grants, and medical library grants made by the National Institutes of Health from funds for the fiscal year covered. **Entries Include:** Organization name, zip code, name of program director or responsible official; area of training, purpose of grant, or project title; grant number and amount; total number of grants and total amount awarded that institution. **Pages (approx.):** 450. **Frequency:** Annual.

★4608★ NATIONAL INSTITUTES OF HEALTH—RESEARCH GRANTS
U.S. National Institutes of Health
5333 Westbard Ave.
Bethesda, MD 20892   Phone: (301) 496-7441
Covers: New grants and awards by the National Institutes of Health made during the past year. Entries Include: Company or institution name, name of principal investigator, location. Pages (approx.): 560. Frequency: Annual.

★4609★ NATIONAL HEARING CONSERVATION ASSOCIATION—PROFESSIONAL SERVICE ORGANIZATION DIRECTORY
National Hearing Conservation Association
900 Des Moines St., No. 200
Des Moines, IA 50309   Phone: (515) 266-2189
Covers: Approximately 45 companies in the United States and Canada that provide services related to protection of hearing. Entries Include: Company name, address, phone, fax, telex, names and titles of key personnel, geographical area served, subsidiary and branch names and locations, description of service. Pages (approx.): 40. Frequency: Annual, spring.

★4610★ NATIONAL AND INTERNATIONAL DENTAL ORGANIZATIONS OF THE WORLD
Office of International Affairs
American Dental Association
211 E. Chicago Ave.
Chicago, IL 60611   Phone: (312) 440-2726
Number of Listings: 156. Entries Include: Association name, address. Pages (approx.): 22. Frequency: Irregular.

★4611★ NATIONAL LIBRARY OF MEDICINE AUDIOVISUALS CATALOG
U.S. National Library of Medicine
8600 Rockville Pike
Bethesda, MD 20894   Phone: (301) 496-5497
Publication Includes: List of about 900 distributors and other sources for audiovisual materials and computer software described. Entries Include: Source or distributor name, address, phone. Frequency: Quarterly; fourth issue cumulative.

★4612★ NATIONAL REGISTER
American Association of Sex Educators, Counselors, and Therapists
435 N. Michigan Ave., Ste. 1717
Chicago, IL 60611   Phone: (312) 644-0828
Covers: About 1,400 sex educators, 1,300 sex therapists, and 200 sex counselors. Entries Include: Name, address, highest degree. Pages (approx.): 145. Frequency: Irregular; previous edition 1984; latest edition 1987; new edition possible 1990. Also Includes: Details of certification requirements and procedures.

★4613★ NATIONAL REGISTER OF HEALTH SERVICE PROVIDERS IN PSYCHOLOGY
Council for the National Register of Health Service Providers in Psychology
1730 Rhode Island Ave., NW, Ste. 1200
Washington, DC 20036   Phone: (202) 833-2377
Covers: About 16,000 psychologists who are licensed or certified, have had at least 2 years of supervised experience, and practice independently. Entries Include: Name, degree, address, phone, where licensed/certified, theoretical orientations, health services and specialized health services offered, age group of patients served, foreign language and sign language fluency. Pages (approx.): 665. Frequency: Biennial; two supplements between editions.

★4614★ NATIONAL REGISTRY OF PSYCHOANALYSTS
National Association for the Advancement of Psychoanalysis and the American Boards for Accreditation & Certification
80 8th Ave., Ste. 1501
New York, NY 10011   Phone: (212) 741-0515
Covers: Over 1,500 certified psychoanalysts, psychoanalytic psychotherapists and associates at approved training institutions; coverage includes Canada, Mexico, and Europe. Entries Include: Name, preferred address and phone, name of institution granting certificate, year granted, certification number, educational and career data. Pages (approx.): 160. Frequency: Annual. Also Includes: Criteria for certification, code of ethics, training curriculum, research and academic affiliates, and supporters of psychoanalysis.

★4615★ NATIONAL RESOURCE DIRECTORY
National Spinal Cord Injury Association
600 W. Cummings Park, Ste. 2000
Woburn, MA 01801   Phone: (617) 935-2722
Covers: Agencies, aids, services, and opportunities for persons with spinal cord injury or disease. Entries Include: Name of agency or organization, location; some entries provide toll-free phone numbers. Pages (approx.): 150. Frequency: Published 1985; suspended indefinitely. Also Includes: Bibliographies appropriate to the separate topics; glossary.

★4616★ NATIONAL SURVEY OF TREATMENT PROGRAMS FOR PKU AND SELECTED OTHER INHERITED METABOLIC DISEASES
U.S. Office of Maternal and Child Health
5600 Fishers Ln.
Rockville, MD 20857
Covers: About 115 clinical centers with programs for phenylketonuria (PKU) and similar metabolic disorders in infants, children, and mothers; about 50 state directors of newborn screening. Entries Include: For centers—Name, address, phone; names, titles, and phone numbers of key personnel. For directors—Name, title, department name, address, phone. Pages (approx.): 65. Send Orders to: National Center for Education in Maternal and Child Health Clearinghouse, 38th & R Sts., NW, Washington, DC 20057 (202-625-8400).

★4617★ NATIONAL TREATMENT DIRECTORY
International Publishing Group
4959 Commerce Pkwy.
Cleveland, OH 44128   Phone: (216) 464-1210
Covers: 3,000 drug and alcohol treatment programs and facilities, addiction counselors, and physicians. Entries Include: Institution name, address, phone, addictions treated, type of facility, size. Pages (approx.): 150. Frequency: Annual, January.

★4618★ NATIONAL WELLNESS ASSOCIATION—DIRECTORY
National Wellness Association
South Hall
1319 Fremont St.
Stevens Point, WI 54481-3899   Phone: (715) 346-2172
Covers: More than 1,700 health and wellness promotion professionals in corporations, hospitals, colleges, government agencies, universities, community organizations, schools (K-12), and consulting firms. Entries Include: Member name, address, and phone. Pages (approx.): 108. Frequency: Annual.

★4619★ NATIONAL WHEELCHAIR BASKETBALL ASSOCIATION—DIRECTORY
National Wheelchair Basketball Association
Seaton Building, No. 100
University of Kentucky
Lexington, KY 40506-0219   Phone: (606) 257-1623
Covers: Approximately 315 officers, team representatives, and game officials for each conference in the National Wheelchair Basketball Association. Entries Include: Name, address, and team name. Entries for team representatives include phone. Pages (approx.): 20. Frequency: Annual, December.

★4620★ NATIONAL WHOLESALE DRUGGISTS' ASSOCIATION—MEMBERSHIP AND EXECUTIVE DIRECTORY
National Wholesale Druggists' Association
Box 238
Alexandria, VA 22313   Phone: (703) 684-6400
Covers: Wholesalers, manufacturers, national drug-trade associations, and colleges of pharmacy. Entries Include: For industry—Company name, address, phone, fax, names of principal executives. For colleges—Institution name, address. Pages (approx.): 130. Frequency: Annual, January.

★4621★ NATIONAL WOMEN'S DIRECTORY OF ALCOHOL AND DRUG ABUSE TREATMENT AND PREVENTION PROGRAMS
Human Services Institute, Inc.
4301 32nd St. S.W., No. C8
Bradenton, FL 34205-2743   Phone: (813) 746-7088
Pages (approx.): 80. Frequency: Latest edition March 1988; no new edition planned.

★4622★   NATIONWIDE HOSPITAL INSURANCE BILLING DIRECTORY
Francis B. Kelly & Associates
123 Veteran Ave.
Los Angeles, CA 90024   Phone: (213) 472-6570
Covers: Payment offices for more than 800 health insurance companies, Blue Cross and Blue Shield, Champus, Medicaid, Medicare, and federal employee plans. **Entries Include:** Company name, address, phone, name and title of contact, addresses and phone numbers of branch offices, affiliated hospitals and physicians. **Pages (approx.):** 280. **Frequency:** Annual. **Also Includes:** Sample forms.

★4623★   NCOA DIRECTORY OF SENIOR CENTERS
Oryx Press
4041 N. Central, No. 700
Phoenix, AZ 85012   Phone: (602) 265-2651
Covers: In six regional volumes, more than 10,000 centers that offer a variety of services to senior citizens, such as counseling, employment, transportation, education, and recreation. **Entries Include:** Facility name, address, name and title of contact, organizational structure, year established, geographic area served, hours of operation, number of staff, membership, average daily attendance, eligibility requirements, fees, location, special facilities, description of services. **Pages (approx.):** 420. **Frequency:** Published 1988. **Also Includes:** List of officers and state delegates of the National Institute of Senior Centers.

★4624★   NEPHROLOGY RESOURCE DIRECTORY
Virgil Smirnow Associates
8501 Burdette Rd.
PO Box 34425
Bethesda, MD 20827   Phone: (301) 469-7933
Covers: Approximately 7,200 U.S. nephrologists and other doctors who treat kidney disorders; transplant surgeons; organ procurement agencies; companies involved in nephrology-related supplies, services, or equipment; End Stage Renal Disease (ESRD) facilities; state kidney programs; related organizations; publishers of related materials; Canadian kidney doctors, facilities and organizations, foreign ESRD facilities providing visitor dialysis. **Entries Include:** For nephrologists and physicians—Name, office address, phone, medical school attended, year graduated, hospital affiliation, teaching title, specialities, board certifications, years in specialities. For others—Name, address, phone, fax. **Pages (approx.):** 800. **Frequency:** Irregular; latest edition January 1991.

★4625★   NEUROSCIENCE TRAINING PROGRAMS IN NORTH AMERICA
Society for Neuroscience
11 Dupont Circle NW Ste. 500
Washington, DC 20036   Phone: (202) 462-6688
Covers: About 300 institutions in North America offering undergraduate, graduate, and postdoctoral neuroscience training. **Entries Include:** Institution name, department or program name, level of training, degrees offered, current enrollment, financial aids, assistance for minorities; names, addresses, and phone numbers of program contacts, program description. **Pages (approx.):** 320. **Frequency:** Triennial, latest edition September 1990.

★4626★   NIH GUIDE FOR GRANTS AND CONTRACTS
National Institutes of Health
9000 Rockville Pike, Rm. B4BNO8
Bethesda, MD 20892   Phone: (301) 496-1787
Covers: Research grants and contracts currently offered in the fields of anatomy, biomedical engineering, health care, diseases, etc.; and the awarding agency for each. **Entries Include:** Description of grant or contract; bibliographic references for further information on topic; agency name, address, phone; and name and title of contact. **Pages (approx.):** 15. **Frequency:** Weekly.

★4627★   NONGOVERNMENTAL ORGANIZATIONS IN INTERNATIONAL POPULATION AND FAMILY PLANNING
Population Crisis Committee
1120 19th St., NW, Ste. 550
Washington, DC 20036   Phone: (202) 659-1833
Covers: About 100 organizations concerned with population issues and family planning; international coverage. **Entries Include:** Organization name, address, phone, names of director and president or chairpersons, description of activities and concerns. **Pages (approx.):** 20. **Frequency:** Latest December edition 1988; suspended indefinitely.

★4628★   NON-ISOTOPIC IMMUNOASSAY
Theta Corp.
Theta Bldg.
Middlefield, CT 06455   Phone: (203) 349-1054
Publication Includes: List of about 10 companies manufacturing products for non-isotopic immunoassay. **Entries Include:** Company name, address, phone, key personnel, background information, description of products, annual sales, research and development efforts, distribution systems, five year projection. **Frequency:** Irregular; latest edition November 1988.

★4629★   NORTH AMERICAN DIRECTORY OF PROGRAMS FOR RUNAWAYS, HOMELESS YOUTH AND MISSING CHILDREN
American Youth Work Center
1751 N St. NW, Ste. 302
Washington, DC 20036   Phone: (202) 785-0764
Covers: Over 500 organizations offering programs or providing resources for youth workers and other professionals concerned with either runaway or homeless teenagers or missing children. **Entries Include:** Organization name, address, phone, telex, name and title of contact, names and titles of key personnel, geographical area served, financial data, description of services. **Pages (approx.):** 200. **Frequency:** Reported as biennial; latest edition summer 1988; new edition expected summer 1991.

★4630★   NORTH AMERICAN SOCIETY OF PACING AND ELECTROPHYSIOLOGY—MEMBERSHIP DIRECTORY
North American Society of Pacing and Electrophysiology
377 Elliot St.
Newton Upper Falls, MA 02164   Phone: (617) 244-7300
Covers: Over 1,100 member physicians, nurses, technicians, biomedical engineers, and other professionals concerned with cardiac pacing and cardiac electrophysiology. **Entries Include:** Name, address, phone. **Pages (approx.):** 76. **Frequency:** Annual, fall.

★4631★   NURSES CALL SYSTEMS
Theta Corp.
Theta Bldg.
Middlefield, CT 06455   Phone: (203) 349-1054
Publication Includes: List of manufacturers of nurses' call systems. **Entries Include:** Company name, address, phone, key personnel, background information, description of products, annual sales, research and development efforts, distribution systems, five year projection. **Frequency:** Irregular; latest edition May 1985.

★4632★   NURSES AND NURSES' REGISTRIES DIRECTORY
American Business Directories, Inc.
American Business Information, Inc.
5711 S. 86th Circle
Omaha, NE 68127   Phone: (402) 593-4600
Number of Listings: 12,340. **Entries Include:** Name, address, phone (including area code), size of advertisement, year first in "Yellow Pages," name of owner or manager, number of employees. **Frequency:** Annual.

★4633★   NURSING CAREER DIRECTORY
Springhouse Corp.
1111 Bethlehem Pike
PO Box 908
Springhouse, PA 19477-0908   Phone: (215) 646-8700
Covers: Nonprofit and investor-owned hospitals and departments of the United States government which hire nurses. Does not report specific positions available. **Entries Include:** Unit name, location, areas of nursing specialization, educational requirements for nurses, licensing, facilities, benefits, etc. **Pages (approx.):** 500. **Frequency:** Annual, January.

★4634★   NURSING HOME CHAIN DIRECTORY
SMG Marketing Group, Inc.
1342 N. LaSalle Dr.
Chicago, IL 60610   Phone: (312) 642-3026
Covers: Over 265 for-profit and nonprofit corporate owners of nursing homes, each of which owns two or more facilities. **Entries Include:** Corporation name, address, phone, name of director; facilities owned, each including nursing home name, address, phone, number of beds, total number of residents. **Pages (approx.):** 500. **Frequency:** Annual, October.

★4635★ NURSING HOME MARKET DIRECTORY
SMG Marketing Group, Inc.
1342 N. LaSalle Dr.
Chicago, IL 60610   Phone: (312) 642-3026
Covers: More than 15,600 nursing homes in the United States. **Entries Include:** Nursing home name, address, phone, number of skilled and unskilled beds, total number of residents. **Pages (approx.):** 500. **Frequency:** Annual, October.

★4636★ NURSING HOMES DIRECTORY
American Business Directories, Inc.
American Business Information, Inc.
5711 S. 86th Circle
Omaha, NE 68127   Phone: (402) 593-4600
Number of Listings: 17,917. **Entries Include:** Name, address, phone (including area code), size of advertisement, year first in "Yellow Pages," name of owner or manager, number of employees. **Frequency:** Annual.

★4637★ NURSINGWORLD JOURNAL NURSING JOB GUIDE
Prime National Publishing Corp.
470 Boston Post Rd.
Weston, MA 02193   Phone: (617) 899-2702
Covers: Over 7,000 hospitals and medical centers, infirmaries, government hospitals, and other hospitals in the United States; in tabular format, provides information about each facility that would be of interest to nurses considering employment there, but does not list specific openings. **Entries Include:** Hospital name, address, phone, name of nurse recruiter; number of beds, number of admissions, number of patient days, type of control, whether a teaching institution; nurses salary range; nursing specialties utilized; list of fringe benefits; whether relocation assistance is given; educational opportunities; special programs. **Pages (approx.):** 700. **Frequency:** Annual, January.

★4638★ NUTRIENT DATA BANK DIRECTORY
Department of Human Nutrition, Foods, and Food Systems
  Management
College of Home Economics
University of Missouri
217 Gwynn Hall
Columbia, MO 65211   Phone: (314) 882-4288
Covers: Producers of more than 100 software packages for the analysis of nutrient content and information. **Entries Include:** Software title, producer name and address, system requirements, hardware compatibility, programming language used; specific proteins, fats, carbohydrates, vitamins, and minerals available in each program. **Frequency:** Latest edition 1988.

★4639★ THE NUTRITION FUNDING REPORT
Nutrition Legislation Services
PO Box 75035
Washington, DC 20013
Covers: Approximately 30 foundations, government agencies, associations, and other sources of grants, contracts, scholarships, fellowships, publications, and other information products and services of interest to food, nutrition, and health care professionals in the U.S. and Canada. **Entries Include:** Source name, address, phone, name and title of contact, description. **Pages (approx.):** 8. **Frequency:** Monthly.

★4640★ NUTRITIONISTS DIRECTORY
American Business Directories, Inc.
American Business Information, Inc.
5711 S. 86th Circle
Omaha, NE 68127   Phone: (402) 593-4600
Number of Listings: 2,599. **Entries Include:** Name, address, phone (including area code), size of advertisement, year first in "Yellow Pages," name of owner or manager, number of employees. **Frequency:** Annual.

★4641★ OCCUPATIONAL HEALTH AND SAFETY PURCHASING SOURCEBOOK
Stevens Publishing Corp.
225 N. New Rd.
Waco, TX 76710   Phone: (817) 776-9000
Covers: Over 2,700 manufacturers and distributors of products, equipment, and services in the field of industrial medicine and health care; consultants in the field. **Entries Include:** Company name, address, phone, toll-free phone, name of contact, names and titles of key personnel, list of products or services, trade and brand names. **Pages (approx.):** 200. **Frequency:** Annual, August.

★4642★ OCCUPATIONAL THERAPISTS DIRECTORY
American Business Directories, Inc.
American Business Information, Inc.
5711 S. 86th Circle
Omaha, NE 68127   Phone: (402) 593-4600
Number of Listings: 1,249. **Entries Include:** Name, address, phone, size of advertisement, name of owner or manager, number of employees, year first in "Yellow Pages." **Frequency:** Annual.

★4643★ OCCUPATIONAL THERAPISTS REGISTER
Occupational Therapists Board
184 Kennington Park Rd.
London SE11 4BU, England
Covers: About 15,000 registered occupational therapists, worldwide. **Entries Include:** Name, address, qualifications, courses. **Pages (approx.):** 210. **Frequency:** Annual, December. **Also Includes:** Requirements for registration.

★4644★ OLD AGE: A REGISTER OF SOCIAL RESEARCH
Centre for Policy on Ageing
25-31 Ironmonger Row
London EC1V 3QP, England
Covers: Organizations sponsoring British research in progress on social aspects of aging, including health, psychology, sociology, and services to older people. **Entries Include:** Project title, organization name, address, name of principal investigator, phone, aims of research, methodology, name(s) of investigator or type of staff, dates of study, publications, name of source of funding (if separate). **Pages (approx.):** 280. **Frequency:** Irregular; previous edition 1986; latest edition April 1991. **Send Orders to:** Bailey Distribution Ltd., Book Distribution Centre, Learoyd Rd., Mountfield Rd. Industrial Estate, New Romney, Kent TN28 8XU, England (679 66668).

★4645★ THE 100 BEST TREATMENT CENTERS FOR ALCOHOLISM AND DRUG ABUSE
Avon Books
1350 Avenue of the Americas
New York, NY 10019   Phone: (212) 261-6895
Covers: 100 substance abuse treatment centers; therapists, family counseling organizations, and support groups. **Entries Include:** For treatment centers—Name, address, phone, number of employees, requirements for admission, description of program, financial data. For others—Personal or organization name, address, phone. **Pages (approx.):** 455. **Frequency:** Published 1988.

★4646★ 120 CAREERS IN THE HEALTHCARE FIELD
U.S. Directory Service
655 NW 128th St.
PO Box 68-1700
Miami, FL 33168   Phone: (305) 769-1700
Publication Includes: Nearly 5,500 accredited training programs for over 120 health care professions. **Entries Include:** Program name, address. **Pages (approx.):** 500. **Frequency:** Irregular, latest edition 1989.

★4647★ ONLINE MEDICAL DATABASES
Aslib
Information House
20-24 Old St.
London EC1V 9AP, England
Covers: Over 100 online medical and biomedical databases worldwide, plus hosts, producers, and suppliers. **Entries Include:** For databases—Name and acronym of database, content, producer and host names, costs, user aids available. For hosts, producers, and suppliers—Company name, address, phone. **Pages (approx.):** 100. **Frequency:** Biennial, even years.

★4648★ OPHTHALMIC INSTRUMENTS AND INTRAOCULAR LENSES
Theta Corp.
Theta Bldg.
Middlefield, CT 06455   Phone: (203) 349-1054
Publication Includes: List of about 30 manufacturers of ophthalmic equipment. **Entries Include:** Company name, address, phone, key personnel, background information, description of products, annual sales, research and development efforts, distribution systems, five year projection. **Frequency:** Irregular; previous edition March 1989; latest edition February 1991.

★4649★ OPHTHALMIC PHOTOGRAPHERS' SOCIETY—DIRECTORY
Ophthalmic Photographers' Society, Inc.
c/o Mark Maio, President
Erie County Medical Center
462 Grider St.
Buffalo, NY 14215   Phone: (716) 898-3940
Covers: Over 1,200 member ophthalmic photographers. **Entries Include:** Name, address, phone. **Frequency:** Annual.

★4650★ OPPORTUNITIES IN CHIROPRACTIC HEALTH CARE CAREERS
VGM Career Books
National Textbook Co.
4255 W. Touhy Ave.
Lincolnwood, IL 60646   Phone: (708) 679-5500
Publication Includes: List of chiropractic associations and state boards. **Entries Include:** Association or organization name, address. **Pages (approx.):** 160. **Frequency:** Irregular; latest edition 1988.

★4651★ OPPORTUNITIES IN NUTRITION CAREERS
VGM Career Books
National Textbook Co.
4255 W. Touhy Ave.
Lincolnwood, IL 60646   Phone: (708) 679-5500
Publication Includes: List of colleges and universities offering graduate programs and internships in nutrition. **Frequency:** Published 1986.

★4652★ OPPORTUNITIES IN VETERINARY MEDICINE
VGM Career Books
National Textbook Co.
4255 W. Touhy Ave.
Lincolnwood, IL 60646   Phone: (708) 679-5500
Publication Includes: List of colleges of veterinary medicine; coverage includes Canada. **Frequency:** Latest edition 1987.

★4653★ OPPORTUNITY PLACEMENT REGISTER
Physicians Career Resource
American Medical Association
515 N. State St.
Chicago, IL 60610   Phone: (312) 464-4712
Covers: Employment or practice opportunities for physicians. Also has lists of practices for sale, state medical societies, executive and professional recruiting firms, hospital or clinic management companies, medical schools, national medical specialty societies, health maintenance organizations, etc. **Entries Include:** Medical specialty, location and type of practice, beginning financial arrangements, income range, size of community, physician population, date available. For entries in other lists—Name, address, phone. **Pages (approx.):** 14. **Frequency:** Monthly.

★4654★ OPTICAL GOODS RETAILERS DIRECTORY
American Business Directories, Inc.
American Business Information, Inc.
5711 S. 86th Circle
Omaha, NE 68127   Phone: (402) 593-4600
Number of Listings: 11,442. **Entries Include:** Name, address, phone (including area code), size of advertisement, year first in "Yellow Pages," name of owner or manager, number of employees. **Frequency:** Annual.

★4655★ OPTICAL GOODS-WHOLESALE AND MANUFACTURERS DIRECTORY
American Business Directories, Inc.
American Business Information, Inc.
5711 S. 86th Circle
Omaha, NE 68127   Phone: (402) 593-4600
Number of Listings: 2,622. **Entries Include:** Name, address, phone (including area code), size of advertisement, year first in "Yellow Pages," name of owner or manager, number of employees. **Frequency:** Annual.

★4656★ OPTICIANS DIRECTORY
American Business Directories, Inc.
American Business Information, Inc.
5711 S. 86th Circle
Omaha, NE 68127   Phone: (402) 593-4600
Number of Listings: 16,152. **Entries Include:** Company name, address, phone (including area code), size of advertisement, year first in "Yellow Pages," name of owner or manager, number of employees. **Frequency:** Annual.

★4657★ OPTICIANS REGISTER
General Optical Council
41 Harley St.
London W1N 2DJ, England
Covers: 11,000 registered opticians and optician companies in the United Kingdom. **Entries Include:** Name, address, professional qualifications. **Pages (approx.):** 385. **Frequency:** Annual, March.

★4658★ OPTOMETRISTS DIRECTORY
American Business Directories, Inc.
American Business Information, Inc.
5711 S. 86th Circle
Omaha, NE 68127   Phone: (402) 593-4600
Number of Listings: 35,721. **Entries Include:** Name, address, phone (including area code), size of advertisement, year first in "Yellow Pages," name of owner or manager, number of employees. **Frequency:** Annual.

★4659★ OPTOMETRY: A CAREER WITH VISION
American Optometric Association
243 N. Lindbergh Blvd.
St. Louis, MO 63141   Phone: (314) 991-4100
Covers: About 20 optometry schools. **Entries Include:** School name, address, phone; name of contact; admission requirements; statistical profile of students in program. **Pages (approx.):** 20. **Frequency:** Annual, January. **Also Includes:** List of sources of additional information on optometry.

★4660★ OPTOMETRY AND VISION SCIENCE—GEOGRAPHICAL DIRECTORY, AMERICAN ACADEMY OF OPTOMETRY ISSUE
American Academy of Optometry
5530 Wisconsin Ave. NW, Ste. 1149
Washington, DC 20015   Phone: (301) 652-0905
Publication Includes: List of 3,400 members; international coverage. **Entries Include:** Name, title, affiliation; office address, phone. **Frequency:** Biennial, odd years.

★4661★ O.R. PRODUCT DIRECTORY
Association of Operating Room Nurses
10170 E. Mississippi Ave.
Denver, CO 80231   Phone: (303) 369-9560
Covers: Approximately 2,500 manufacturers and distributors of products of use particularly to operating room nurses. **Entries Include:** Company name, address, phone, telex, subsidiary and branch names and locations, description of products provided. **Pages (approx.):** 1,100. **Frequency:** Annual, October.

★4662★ ORGANIC ACIDEMIA ASSOCIATION—MEMBERSHIP ROSTER
Organic Acidemia Association
522 Lander St.
Reno, NV 89509   Phone: (702) 322-5542
Covers: About 300 parents and relatives of children with metabolic disorders leading to enzyme deficiencies and dietitians, geneticists, and researchers concerned with the treatment of such disorders; international coverage. **Entries Include:** Name, address, phone. **Frequency:** Annual.

★4663★ ORTHODONTIC DIRECTORY OF THE WORLD
Orthodontic Directory of the World
4525 Harding Rd., No. 110
Nashville, TN 37205   Phone: (615) 383-5152
Covers: 9,000 main and branch orthodontic offices in the United States and Canada and 6,000 orthodontists overseas. **Entries Include:** Name, affiliation, address, phone, year graduated from dental school, school of graduate orthodontic training and year completed, whether exclusive or nonexclusive practice, techniques used. **Pages (approx.):** 550. **Frequency:** Biennial, April of even years.

★4664★ ORTHOPEDIC APPLIANCES-RETAIL DIRECTORY
American Business Directories, Inc.
American Business Information, Inc.
5711 S. 86th Circle
Omaha, NE 68127   Phone: (402) 593-4600
Number of Listings: 3,192. **Entries Include:** Name, address, phone (including area code), size of advertisement, year first in "Yellow Pages," name of owner or manager, number of employees. **Frequency:** Annual.

★4665★ ORTHOPEDIC IMPLANTS
Theta Corp.
Theta Bldg.
Middlefield, CT 06455   Phone: (203) 349-1054
Publication Includes: List of manufacturers of orthopedic implant products. **Entries Include:** Company name, address, phone, background information, description of products, annual sales, research and development efforts, distribution systems, five year projection. **Frequency:** Irregular; latest edition April 1988.

★4666★ ORTHOPTISTS REGISTER
Orthoptists Board
184 Kennington Park Rd.
London SE11 4BU, England
Covers: Optical specialists belonging to the Orthoptists Board in the United Kingdom. **Entries Include:** Member name, address, qualifications, courses. **Pages (approx.):** 45. **Frequency:** Annual, September. **Also Includes:** List of training courses approved by the board.

★4667★ OUTPATIENT HEALTH CARE: MEDICAL SPECIALTY CLINICS
Techne Research
1100 Massachusetts Ave.
Arlington, MA 02174   Phone: (617) 646-6297
Covers: About 100 companies that own or manage medical specialty clinics; over 1,700 clinics that provide services in cardiac rehabilitation, diagnosis, substance abuse treatment, diabetes management, pain management, treatment of obesity and other eating disorders, and industrial medicine; government agencies, professional associations, and publishers of periodicals. **Entries Include:** For companies—Name, address, phone, names of key personnel, divisions and subsidiaries, clinic locations, financial information. For clinics—Name, address, phone, name of key executive, service and ownership codes. For government agencies—Name, address, phone, contact name, state licensing requirements. For associations—Name, address, phone, contact name, publications, description of activities. For publishers—Name, periodical name, address, phone. **Pages (approx.):** 400. **Frequency:** Irregular; latest edition 1986; new edition expected fall 1988.

★4668★ OUTPATIENT HEALTH CARE: SURGICAL AND URGENT CARE CENTERS
Techne Research
1100 Massachusetts Ave.
Arlington, MA 02174   Phone: (617) 646-6297
Covers: Over 400 surgical and 1,350 urgent care centers; companies providing such services or owning centers; related federal and state government agencies; and professional associations in the field. **Entries Include:** For centers—Name, address, phone, name of director. For companies—Name, address, phone, key personnel, clinic locations, financial information (when available). For government agencies—Name, address, phone, names of key personnel. For associations—Name, address, phone. **Pages (approx.):** 200. **Frequency:** Triennial; new edition expected 1988. **Also Includes:** Bibliography; statistical data.

★4669★ OVERCOMING AGORAPHOBIA: CONQUERING FEAR OF THE OUTSIDE WORLD
Penguin USA
PO Box 999
Bergenfield, NJ 07621   Phone: (201) 366-2000
Publication Includes: List of treatment programs for those suffering from agoraphobia. **Entries Include:** Organization name, address, phone, name and title of contact, description of services provided. **Frequency:** Published spring 1987.

★4670★ OXYGEN THERAPY EQUIPMENT DIRECTORY
American Business Directories, Inc.
American Business Information, Inc.
5711 S. 86th Circle
Omaha, NE 68127   Phone: (402) 593-4600
Number of Listings: 1,635. **Entries Include:** Name, address, phone, size of advertisement, name of owner or manager, number of employees, year first in "Yellow Pages." **Frequency:** Annual.

★4671★ OXYGEN-WHOLESALE DIRECTORY
American Business Directories, Inc.
American Business Information, Inc.
5711 S. 86th Circle
Omaha, NE 68127   Phone: (402) 593-4600
Number of Listings: 6,508. **Entries Include:** Name, address, phone (including area code), size of advertisement, year first in "Yellow Pages," name of owner or manager, number of employees. **Frequency:** Annual.

★4672★ PACIFIC RESEARCH CENTRES: A DIRECTORY OF ORGANIZATIONS IN SCIENCE, TECHNOLOGY, AGRICULTURE, AND MEDICINE
Longman Group UK Ltd.
Westgate House
The High
Harlow, Essex CM20 1YR, England
Covers: Nearly 3,000 government, state, and private company laboratories, government and university research departments, industrial research centers, and hospital research laboratories in Australia, Brunei, China, Fiji, Hong Kong, Indonesia, Japan, Korea, Malaysia, New Caledonia, New Zealand, Papua New Guinea, Philippines, Samoa, Singapore, Solomon Islands, Taiwan, Thailand, Vanuatu, Vietnam, and some Pacific Islands. **Entries Include:** Name of organization, name of parent company, English translation and acronym (where applicable), address, phone, fax, telex, names of key personnel, number of graduate research staff, description of product or service, summary of current projects, annual expenditure (in local monetary units) for research and development, status (whether unit of government, university, industrial company, or an independent), name, description of publications. **Pages (approx.):** 530. **Frequency:** Biennial, January of even years. **Available in the U.S. from:** Gale Research Inc., 835 Penobscot Bldg., Detroit, MI 48226.

★4673★ PASSPORT—GUIDE FOR TRAVELLING HEMOPHILIACS
World Federation of Hemophilia
4616 St. Catherine St., W.
Montreal, PQ, Canada H3Z 1S3   Phone: (514) 933-7944
Covers: Treatment centers for hemophilia in nearly 60 countries. **Entries Include:** Facility name, location, name of doctor/director, outpatient and inpatient fees, blood products available, services, size of facility. **Pages (approx.):** 188. **Frequency:** Irregular; previous edition May 1983; latest edition August 1990.

★4674★ PC PHYSICIAN GUIDE
PC Physician Guide
3300 Mitchell Ln., Ste. 390
Boulder, CO 80301   Phone: (303) 443-8085
Description: Diskette. Covers books, magazines, online services, professional organizations, and other resources supporting the use of computers in medicine.

★4675★ PEDIATRIC ORTHOPAEDIC SOCIETY OF NORTH AMERICA—MEMBERSHIP DIRECTORY
Pediatric Orthopaedic Society of North America
222 S. Prospect Ave.
Park Ridge, IL 60068   Phone: (708) 698-1628
Covers: About 500 member orthopedic surgeons for children. **Frequency:** Annual.

★4676★ PERINATOLOGY/NEONATOLOGY—BUYERS GUIDE ISSUE
Macmillan Healthcare Information
30 Vreeland Rd.
Florham Park, NJ 07932   Phone: (201) 822-1622
Publication Includes: About 300 manufacturers and exclusive distributors of products and services to professionals and practices in perinatology and neonatology (including obstetricians, gynecologists, nurses, pediatricians, and others). **Entries Include:** Firm name, address, phone, TWX and telex numbers, names of key personnel, foreign subsidiaries. **Frequency:** Reported as annual; out of print.

★4677★ PETERSON'S GUIDE TO COLLEGES WITH PROGRAMS FOR LEARNING-DISABLED STUDENTS
Peterson's Guides, Inc.
PO Box 2123
Princeton, NJ 08543-2123   Phone: (609) 243-9111
Covers: Over 900 two- and four-year United States colleges and universities with services and programs for students with such learning disabilities as aphasia, dyslexia, and minimal brain dysfunction; list of resource organizations. **Entries Include:** Institution name, location, special services offered (note takers, diagnostic testing, special orientation, etc.); description of school, admission procedures, tutoring and advising offered, testing, housing, staff information. **Pages (approx.):** 400. **Frequency:** Irregular; new edition expected fall 1991.

★4678★ PETERSON'S GUIDE TO GRADUATE PROGRAMS IN BUSINESS, EDUCATION, HEALTH, AND LAW
Peterson's Guides, Inc.
PO Box 2123
Princeton, NJ 08543-2123   Phone: (609) 243-9111
Covers: Colleges and universities in the United States and Canada that offer more than 12,000 accredited graduate programs in business, education, health, and law. **Entries Include:** School name, address, phone, name and title of contact, admission requirements, description of school and programs. **Pages (approx.):** 1,600. **Frequency:** Annual, December.

★4679★ PHARMACEUTICAL ACTIVITIES INDEX—DIRECTORY
Pharmaco Medical Documentation Inc.
Box 429
Chatham, NJ 07928   Phone: (201) 822-9200
Publication Includes: Section with manufacturers of medicinal drugs and research chemicals; international coverage. **Entries Include:** Company name, address, phone, mnemonic company code. **Frequency:** Irregular; new edition expected January 1992.

★4680★ PHARMACEUTICAL MARKETERS DIRECTORY
CPS Communications, Inc.
7200 W. Camino Real, Ste. 215
Boca Raton, FL 33433   Phone: (407) 368-9301
Covers: About 7,000 marketing personnel of pharmaceutical, medical equipment, and biotechnology companies; advertising agencies with clients in the medical field; health care publications; and medical industry suppliers. **Entries Include:** Company name, address, list of marketing personnel by department or section (with titles, and phone and fax numbers). **Pages (approx.):** 700. **Frequency:** Annual, April. **Also Includes:** List of publishers' representatives and a list of industry suppliers.

★4681★ PHARMACEUTICAL PRODUCTS-WHOLESALERS AND MANUFACTURERS DIRECTORY
American Business Directories, Inc.
American Business Information, Inc.
5711 S. 86th Circle
Omaha, NE 68127   Phone: (402) 593-4600
Number of Listings: 2,656. **Entries Include:** Name, address, phone (including area code), size of advertisement, year first in "Yellow Pages," name of owner or manager, number of employees. **Frequency:** Annual.

★4682★ PHARMACEUTICAL TECHNOLOGY—BUYERS' GUIDE ISSUE
Aster Publishing Corp.
PO Box 10460
Eugene, OR 97440   Phone: (503) 343-1200
Publication Includes: List of 750 manufacturers and suppliers in the pharmaceutical industry, including suppliers of chemical raw materials and ingredients, equipment and manufacturing supplies, packaging materials, lab instrumentation, clean room equipment. **Entries Include:** Company name, address, phone. **Frequency:** Annual, July.

★4683★ PHARMACISTS IN OPHTHALMIC INSTITUTIONS—DIRECTORY
Pharmacists in Ophthalmic Institutions
c/o Wills Eye Hospital
9th & Walnut Sts.
Philadelphia, PA 19107   Phone: (215) 928-3334
Covers: About 25 member pharmacists in the U.S. and Great Britain who are either directors or chief pharmacists of institutions dealing primarily with ophthalmology or otolaryngology (ear, nose, throat). **Entries Include:** Hospital name, name of pharmacist, address, phone, fax, specialty, phone mail numbers. **Pages (approx.):** 2. **Frequency:** Annual.

★4684★ PHARMACY SCHOOL ADMISSION REQUIREMENTS
American Association of Colleges of Pharmacy
1426 Prince St.
Alexandria, VA 22314   Phone: (703) 739-2330
Covers: 74 colleges and schools with pharmacy programs accredited by the American Council on Pharmaceutical Education. **Entries Include:** School name, address, admission requirements, tuition, contact name, timetables for application and admission for one-year period in advance. Descriptions of student life and housing, facilities, curriculum, and advanced placement are provided. **Pages (approx.):** 175. **Frequency:** Annual, September.

★4685★ PHI DELTA EPSILON NEWS AND SCIENTIFIC JOURNAL—DIRECTORY ISSUE
Phi Delta Epsilon Medical Fraternity
1140 Broadway, Ste. 807
New York, NY 10001   Phone: (212) 889-3386
Covers: National, regional, district, chapter, and club officers; chapters, committee, and other members of the Phi Delta Epsilon medical fraternity. **Entries Include:** For chapters—Name, address, names of members. For officers and committee members—Name, title, address. For others—Name, address, chapter, year of graduation. **Pages (approx.):** 30. **Frequency:** Quarterly.

★4686★ PHYSICAL EDUCATION GOLD BOOK: DIRECTORY OF PHYSICAL EDUCATION IN HIGHER EDUCATION
Human Kinetics Publishers, Inc.
Box 5076
Champaign, IL 61825-5076   Phone: (217) 351-5076
Covers: Approximately 600 college and university physical education departments; about 6,000 faculty members in physical education. **Entries Include:** Institution name; address of physical education department; degrees offered by department; names, interest areas, and phone numbers of professional staff. **Pages (approx.):** 140. **Frequency:** Irregular; previous edition 1982; latest edition May 1987.

★4687★ PHYSICAL THERAPISTS DIRECTORY
American Business Directories, Inc.
American Business Information, Inc.
5711 S. 86th Circle
Omaha, NE 68127   Phone: (402) 593-4600
Number of Listings: 16,643. **Entries Include:** Name, address, phone (including area code), size of advertisement, year first in "Yellow Pages," name of owner or manager, number of employees. **Frequency:** Annual.

★4688★ PHYSICIAN INSURERS ASSOCIATION OF AMERICA—MEMBERSHIP DIRECTORY
Physician Insurers Association of America
65 S. Main St., Bldg. D
Pennington, NJ 08534-2827   Phone: (609) 737-7193
Covers: Over 40 state medical societies and their affiliated cooperative insurance companies. **Entries Include:** For medical societies—Name, address, phone, name and title of president or chief executive officer. For insurance companies—Name, address, mailing address, phone, names and titles of officers, date established, members, licensing information, insurance coverage and rates, assets, surplus, premium range. **Pages (approx.):** 70. **Frequency:** Annual, May.

★4689★ PHYSICIAN OFFICE: CLINICAL CHEMISTRY INSTRUMENTATION
Theta Corp.
Theta Bldg.
Middlefield, CT 06455   Phone: (203) 349-1054
Publication Includes: List of about 25 suppliers of laboratory equipment for physician's and clinical offices. **Entries Include:** Company name, address, phone, key personnel, background information, description of products, annual sales, research and development efforts, distribution systems, five year projection. **Frequency:** Irregular; latest edition September 1985.

★4690★ PHYSICIAN OFFICE DISTRIBUTION
Theta Corp.
Theta Bldg.
Middlefield, CT 06455   Phone: (203) 349-1054
Publication Includes: List of distributors of physician's office equipment. **Entries Include:** Company name, address, phone, key personnel, background information, description of products, annual sales, research and development efforts, distribution systems, five year projection. **Frequency:** Irregular; latest edition November 1988.

★4691★ PHYSICIAN OFFICE PRODUCTS
Theta Corp.
Theta Bldg.
Middlefield, CT 06455   Phone: (203) 349-1054
Publication Includes: List of suppliers of products for physician's offices. **Entries Include:** Company name, address, phone, key personnel, background information, description of products, annual sales, research and development efforts, distribution systems, five year projection. **Frequency:** Irregular; latest edition November 1988.

★4692★ PHYSICIANS' CLINICS DIRECTORY
American Business Directories, Inc.
American Business Information, Inc.
5711 S. 86th Circle
Omaha, NE 68127   Phone: (402) 593-4600
Number of Listings: 70,994. **Entries Include:** Name, address, phone, size of advertisement, name of owner or manager, number of employees, year first in "Yellow Pages." **Frequency:** Annual.

★4693★ PHYSICIANS' DESK REFERENCE
Medical Economics Data
5 Paragon Dr.
Montvale, NJ 07645   Phone: (201) 358-7200
Publication Includes: List of several hundred manufacturers of more than 2,000 commonly prescribed drug products; distributed primarily to physicians, though it is available to laypersons. **Entries Include:** Manufacturer name, address, phone; address and phone of branch office or distribution center; reference to the product information and product identification sections (see "Other Information" below). **Frequency:** Annual, January. **Also Includes:** List of poison control centers. **Send Orders to:** Physicians' Desk Reference, Box 10689, Des Moines, IA 50336.

★4694★ PHYSICIANS' DESK REFERENCE FOR OPHTHALMOLOGY
Medical Economics Data
Medical Economics Co.
5 Paragon Dr.
Montvale, NJ 07645   Phone: (201) 358-7200
Publication Includes: List of manufacturers of eyecare equipment and drug products; distributed primarily to ophthalmologists, though it is available to laypersons. **Entries Include:** Manufacturer name, address, phone, subsidiary and branch names and locations, product information and identification. **Frequency:** Annual, December.

★4695★ PHYSICIANS AND SURGEONS DIRECTORY
American Business Directories, Inc.
American Business Information, Inc.
5711 S. 86th Circle
Omaha, NE 68127   Phone: (402) 593-4600
Number of Listings: 420,249. **Entries Include:** Name, address, phone, size of advertisement, year first in "Yellow Pages," name of owner or manager, number of employees. **Frequency:** Annual.

★4696★ PHYSICIANS AND SURGEONS EQUIPMENT AND SUPPLIES DIRECTORY
American Business Directories, Inc.
American Business Information, Inc.
5711 S. 86th Circle
Omaha, NE 68127   Phone: (402) 593-4600
Number of Listings: 6,749. **Entries Include:** Name, address, phone (including area code), size of advertisement, year first in "Yellow Pages," name of owner or manager, number of employees. **Frequency:** Annual.

★4697★ PHYSICIANS AND SURGEONS INFORMATION BUREAUS DIRECTORY
American Business Directories, Inc.
American Business Information, Inc.
5711 S. 86th Circle
Omaha, NE 68127   Phone: (402) 593-4600
Number of Listings: 2,374. **Entries Include:** Name, address, phone (including area code), size of advertisement, year first in "Yellow Pages," name of owner or manager, number of employees. **Frequency:** Annual.

★4698★ PHYSIOTHERAPISTS REGISTER
Physiotherapists Board
184 Kennington Park Rd.
London SE11 4BU, England
Covers: Practicing physical therapists and institutions offering training courses; international coverage. **Entries Include:** Personal or institution name, address, qualifications or courses offered. **Pages (approx.):** 480. **Frequency:** Annual, June.

★4699★ PIERRE FAUCHARD ACADEMY—MEMBERSHIP DIRECTORY
Pierre Fauchard Academy
c/o Dr. Richard Kozal
8021 W. 79th St.
Justice, IL 60458   Phone: (708) 594-5884
Covers: 5,000 dentists "of high standards and leadership" who are nominated to the Academy by present members; international coverage. **Entries Include:** Name, address. **Pages (approx.):** 35. **Frequency:** Irregular; latest edition 1985.

★4700★ PLANNED PARENTHOOD AFFILIATES, CHAPTER & STATE PUBLIC AFFAIRS OFFICES DIRECTORY
Planned Parenthood Federation of America
810 7th Ave.
New York, NY 10019   Phone: (212) 603-4736
Number of Listings: 250. **Entries Include:** Affiliate or chapter name, address, phone, code for whether medical, educational, provisional member, or public affairs office. **Pages (approx.):** 30. **Frequency:** Annual, September.

★4701★ PODIATRISTS DIRECTORY
American Business Directories, Inc.
American Business Information, Inc.
5711 S. 86th Circle
Omaha, NE 68127   Phone: (402) 593-4600
Number of Listings: 20,161. **Entries Include:** Name, address, phone (including area code), size of advertisement, year first in "Yellow Pages," name of owner or manager, number of employees. **Frequency:** Annual.

★4702★ PODIATRY MANAGEMENT—BUYER'S GUIDE ISSUE
Kane Communications, Inc.
7000 Terminal Sq.
Upper Darby, PA 19082   Phone: (215) 734-2420
Publication Includes: List of manufacturers and suppliers of equipment, products, or services to podiatrists. **Entries Include:** Company name, address, phone, name of contact, products or services. **Frequency:** Annual, February.

★4703★ PORTABLE DEFIBRILLATORS
Theta Corp.
Theta Bldg.
Middlefield, CT 06455   Phone: (203) 349-1054
Publication Includes: List of about 15 companies involved in the portable defibrillator equipment industry. **Entries Include:** Company name, address, phone, key personnel, background information, description of products, annual sales, research and development efforts, distribution systems, five year projection. **Frequency:** Irregular; latest edition April 1989.

★4704★ PORTS DESIGNATED IN APPLICATION OF THE INTERNATIONAL HEALTH REGULATIONS
Division of Epidemiological Surveillance and Health Situation and Trend Assessment
World Health Organization
20, avenue Appia
CH-1211 Geneva 27, Switzerland
Covers: Ports worldwide designated to issue deratting certificates and/or deratting exemption certificates under the International Health Regulations. **Entries Include:** Name of port, official designation. **Pages (approx.):** 35. **Frequency:** Irregular; latest edition January 1984. **Available in the U.S. from:** World Health Organizations Publications Centre, 49 Sheridan Avenue, Albany, NY 10017.

★4705★ POST POLIO DIRECTORY
International Polio Network
5100 Oakland Ave., No. 206
St. Louis, MO 63110   Phone: (314) 534-0475
Covers: Doctors, clinics, and support groups for polio survivors; international coverage. **Entries Include:** Name, address, phone. **Pages (approx.):** 27. **Frequency:** Annual, February; quarterly supplements.

★4706★ POST-TRAUMATIC STRESS DISORDER, RAPE TRAUMA, DELAYED STRESS AND RELATED CONDITIONS: A BIBLIOGRAPHY
McFarland & Co., Inc.
Box 611
Jefferson, NC 28640   Phone: (919) 246-4460
Publication Includes: List of 1,895 outreach programs for war veterans seeking counseling for a variety of battle-related mental disorders: post-traumatic stress disorder (PTSD), delayed stress, war neurosis, shell-shock, combat fatigue, acute combat reaction, combat-related stress, gross stress reaction, combat exhaustion, battle-induced mental disorder, and battle shock. **Entries Include:** Institution, address, phone, type of service provided. **Frequency:** Published 1986.

★4707★ PRACTICAL NURSING CAREER
National League for Nursing
350 Hudson St.
New York, NY 10014   Phone: (212) 989-9393
Covers: League-accredited programs in practical nursing; most are one-year programs. **Entries Include:** Name of program, address, name of contact person, requirements, whether evening courses are offered, administrative control and source of financing, approximate cost to applicant, living accommodations, number of graduates, number of enrollments. **Pages (approx.):** 50. **Frequency:** Annual, summer.

★4708★ PREVENTION EDUCATION: A GUIDE TO RESEARCH
Garland Publishing, Inc.
136 Madison Ave.
New York, NY 10016   Phone: (212) 686-7492
Publication Includes: Appendixes listing organizations and periodicals providing information on substance abuse. **Frequency:** Published 1990.

★4709★ PRIVATE PRACTICE SECTION OF THE AMERICAN PHYSICAL THERAPY ASSOCIATION—MEMBERSHIP DIRECTORY
Private Practice Section
American Physical Therapy Association
1101 17th St. NW, Ste. 1000
Washington, DC 20036   Phone: (202) 457-1114
Covers: About 4,700 member physical therapists in private practice. **Entries Include:** Firm name, home address, business address and phone, fax, names and titles of key personnel, specialty, type of practice, congressional district. **Pages (approx.):** 200. **Frequency:** Biennial, April of even years.

★4710★ PRODUCT DEVELOPMENT DIRECTORY
Medical Device Register, Inc.
5 Paragon Dr.
Montvale, NJ 07645-1725
Covers: Approximately 5,100 manufacturers of medical products who filed for FDA product approval. **Entries Include:** Manufacturer name, product name, application date, approval date, 510 (k) number, FDA device code. **Pages (approx.):** 800. **Frequency:** Irregular previous edition 1986; latest edition 1991.

★4711★ PRODUCT S.O.S. (SITUATION OCCURRENCE SERVICE)
Medical Device Register, Inc.
5 Paragon Dr.
Montvale, NJ 07645-1725   Phone: (203) 348-6319
Publication Includes: List of manufacturers of medical devices with FDA problem reports. **Entries Include:** Company name, address, phone, products, description of problem. **Frequency:** Annual, November.

★4712★ PROFESSIONAL BUSINESS MANAGEMENT CONSULTANTS
Practice Management Information Center
621 Plainfield Rd., Ste. 308
Willowbrook, IL 60521   Phone: (708) 850-7100
Covers: Nearly 400 professional business consulting firms to physicians and dentists. **Entries Include:** Firm name, address, phone, name and title of contact. **Pages (approx.):** 15. **Frequency:** Annual, November.

★4713★ PROFILES OF ORGANIZATIONS CONTRACTING WITH HOSPITALS
California Association of Hospitals and Health Systems
PO Box 1100
Sacramento, CA 95812   Phone: (916) 443-7401
Covers: About 70 PPOs and 54 HMOs that possess active contracts with hospitals; utilization review firms in California. **Entries Include:** For HMOs and PPOs—Company name, address, phone, name and title of key personnel, organization type, regulatory agency, sponsor, source of capital, controlling interest, tax status, number of employees, geographical area served, hospital services, coverage incentives, management services, professional liability coverage, claims payment policy, risk, requirement for membership, hospital and physician pricing, member fee, marketing, patient sources, enrollment, number of contracted physicians, and utilization services. **Pages (approx.):** 140. **Frequency:** Annual, December; 1989 edition omitted.

★4714★ PROGRAMS TO STRENGTHEN FAMILIES: A RESOURCE GUIDE
Family Resource Coalition
200 S. Michigan, Ste. 1520
Chicago, IL 60604   Phone: (312) 341-0900
Covers: Descriptions of 72 organizations offering programs providing a variety of service models for working with families of varied economic and ethnic backgrounds in different geographic (urban, rural, etc.) settings; includes parent education, prevention of child abuse and neglect, day care, neighborhood-based self-help and information support programs, and others. **Entries Include:** Organization name, address, phone, program name, description, goals, history, community served, services, participants, staff, evaluation (by program or independent evaluator), source of funding, materials available. **Pages (approx.):** 140. **Frequency:** Irregular; previous edition 1983 (out of print); latest edition May 1988.

★4715★ PROOFS—BUYERS' GUIDE AND MANUFACTURERS' DIRECTORY ISSUE
Dental Economics Division
PennWell Publishing Co.
Box 3408
Tulsa, OK 74101   Phone: (918) 835-3161
Publication Includes: List of over 390 manufacturers of dental products and equipment; coverage includes Canada. **Entries Include:** Company name, address, phone, names of key personnel, distribution method, coded product list. **Frequency:** Annual, January.

★4716★ PROOFS—CALENDAR OF DENTAL MEETINGS
Pennwell Publishing Co.
Box 3408
Tulsa, OK 74101   Phone: (918) 835-3161
Frequency: Annual, October.

★4717★ PROOFS—DIRECTORY OF DENTAL DEALERS
Dental Economics Division
PennWell Publishing Co.
Box 3408
Tulsa, OK 74101   Phone: (918) 835-3161
Publication Includes: List of over 750 companies which are retail outlets for dental supplies, equipment, and services in the U.S., Canada, Puerto Rico, and overseas. **Entries Include:** Company name, address, phone, names of principal executives, number of outside sales representatives (if applicable). **Frequency:** Annual, July/August.

★4718★ PROVIDER—LTC BUYERS' GUIDE ISSUE
American Health Care Association
1201 L St., NW
Washington, DC 20005   Phone: (202) 898-2838
Publication Includes: List of several hundred manufacturers and suppliers of products and services to the nursing home and long term care industries. **Entries Include:** Company name, address, phone, products or services. **Frequency:** Annual, August.

★4719★ PSYCHIATRIC HOSPITAL DIRECTORY
National Association of Private Psychiatric Hospitals
1319 F St., NW, Ste. 1000
Washington, DC 20004   Phone: (202) 393-6700
Covers: 350 hospitals. **Entries Include:** Name of hospital, address, name of administrator, description of treatment program(s), accreditation, number of beds, room rates. **Pages (approx.):** 200. **Frequency:** Biennial, July of odd years.

★4720★ PSYCHOIMMUNITY AND THE HEALING PROCESS: A HOLISTIC APPROACH TO IMMUNITY AND AIDS
Celestial Arts
PO Box 7327
Berkeley, CA 94707   Phone: (415) 524-1801
Publication Includes: List of about 60 holistic health practitioners and organizations and centers that provide information about the treatment of immune dysfunction and Acquired Immune Deficiency Syndrome (AIDS). **Entries Include:** Organization, center or individual name, address, phone, background information, description of services. **Frequency:** Approximately annual, February.

★4721★ PSYCHOLOGISTS DIRECTORY
American Business Directories, Inc.
American Business Information, Inc.
5711 S. 86th Circle
Omaha, NE 68127   Phone: (402) 593-4600
Number of Listings: 37,473. **Entries Include:** Name, address, phone (including area code), size of advertisement, year first in "Yellow Pages," name of owner or manager, number of employees. **Frequency:** Annual.

★4722★ PSYCHOTHERAPISTS DIRECTORY
American Business Directories, Inc.
American Business Information, Inc.
5711 S. 86th Circle
Omaha, NE 68127   Phone: (402) 593-4600
Number of Listings: 6,512. **Entries Include:** Name, address, phone (including area code), size of advertisement, year first in "Yellow Pages," name of owner or manager, number of employees. **Frequency:** Annual.

★4723★ PSYCHWARE SOURCEBOOK
Pro-Ed, Inc.
8700 Shoal Creek Blvd.
Austin, TX 78758   Phone: (512) 451-3246
Covers: Over 450 computer-based products that have applications for assessing or modifying human behavior; also covers the suppliers of these products. **Entries Include:** Supplier name, product name, address, product applications, product category, description, type and cost of services provided, sample printout of product. **Pages (approx.):** 615. **Frequency:** Previous edition June 1987; latest edition 1988.

★4724★ PUBLIC COMPANY PROFILES
Medical Device Register, Inc.
655 Washington Blvd.
Stamford, CT 06901   Phone: (203) 348-6319
Covers: Over 500 publicly owned companies that manufacture or supply medical or health care equipment. **Entries Include:** Company name, address, phone, names of key personnel, number of employees, subsidiaries, products provided, sales volume, income statement. **Pages (approx.):** 150. **Frequency:** Irregular; latest edition July 1987.

★4725★ PUBLIC HEALTH
Swiss Office for the Development of Trade
4, avenue de l'Avant
CH-1001 Lausanne, Switzerland
Covers: Swiss manufacturers and distributors of public health products and services.

★4726★ PUBLIC HEALTH LABORATORY SERVICE—PHLS DIRECTORY
Public Health Laboratory Service Board
61 Colindale Ave.
London NW9 5DF, England
Covers: Laboratories and units of the Public Health Service in England and Wales. **Entries Include:** Name, address, phone, names and titles of key personnel. **Pages (approx.):** 80. **Frequency:** Annual. **Also Includes:** List of committees with members' names.

★4727★ PULMONARY SPIROMETRY
Theta Corp.
Theta Bldg.
Middlefield, CT 06455   Phone: (203) 349-1054
Publication Includes: List of manufacturers of pulmonary spirometry equipment. **Entries Include:** Company name, address, phone, key personnel, background information, description of products, annual sales, research and development efforts, distribution systems, five year projection. **Frequency:** Irregular; previous edition February 1983; latest edition November 1985.

★4728★ P.U.S.H.—A STEP AHEAD: SERVICES FOR DISABLED IN SOUTHWESTERN ONTARIO
Persons United for Self Help
PO Box 24026
301 Oxford St., W.
London, ON, Canada N6H 5C4   Phone: (519) 673-4010
Covers: About 800 organizations and agencies offering services available to disabled persons in southwestern Ontario. **Entries Include:** Organization or agency name, address, phone, name and title of contact, geographical area served, description of services. **Pages (approx.):** 300. **Frequency:** Annual, March.

★4729★ RADIATION RESEARCH SOCIETY—DIRECTORY AND CONSTITUTION
Radiation Research Society
1891 Preston White Dr.
Reston, VA 22091   Phone: (703) 648-3780
Covers: 1,900 biologists, physicists, chemists, and physicians contributing to knowledge of radiation and its effects. **Entries Include:** Name, affiliation, address, phone, year joined, membership classification, highest degree. **Pages (approx.):** 70. **Frequency:** Annual, spring.

★4730★ RADIOGRAPHERS REGISTER
Radiographers Board
184 Kennington Park Rd.
London SE11 4BU, England
Covers: Registered radiographers; international coverage. **Entries Include:** Radiographer name, address, qualifications. **Pages (approx.):** 320. **Frequency:** Annual, April. **Also Includes:** List of approved training courses.

★4731★ RARE DISEASES: A RESOURCE DIRECTORY
Office of Orphan Products Development
U.S. Food and Drug Administration
5600 Fishers Ln.
Rockville, MD 20857   Phone: (301) 443-4903
Covers: Over 140 associations and other organizations and 30 federal government agencies that provide information or other services on rare diseases. **Entries Include:** For associations and organizations—Name, address, phone, type of organization, disease focus, services offered, publications, affiliated medical or advisory boards. For agencies—Name, address, phone, publications. **Pages (approx.):** 225. **Frequency:** Published March 1986. **Send Orders to:** National Technical Information Service, Springfield, VA 22161.

★4732★ REACHING OUT: A DIRECTORY OF NATIONAL ORGANIZATIONS RELATED TO MATERNAL AND CHILD HEALTH
National Center for Education in Maternal and Child Health
38th & R Sts., NW
Washington, DC 20057   Phone: (202) 625-8400
Covers: Over 500 national and international voluntary organizations for health professionals, educators, and the public; mutual support groups; self-help clearinghouses; and selected federal Maternal and Child Health Information Centers. **Entries Include:** Name, address, phone, name of contact; code indicates whether a newsletter is published. **Pages (approx.):** 130. **Frequency:** Approximately biennial; previous edition December 1987; latest edition March 1989; new edition expected 1991.

★4733★ A READER'S GUIDE FOR PARENTS OF CHILDREN WITH MENTAL, PHYSICAL, OR EMOTIONAL DISABILITIES
Woodbine House
5615 Fishers Ln.
Rockville, MD 20852   Phone: (301) 468-8800
Covers: 660 books, nearly 380 agencies and associations, and over 100 periodicals and directories providing information about cleft palate, learning disabilities, autism, epilepsy, visual or hearing impairment, mental retardation, mental illness, and speech and language disabilities. **Entries Include:** For publications—Title, publisher name and address, annotation. For associations and agencies—Name, address, disability concern. **Pages (approx.):** 248. **Frequency:** Irregular; latest edition 1990.

★4734★ RECOVERING FROM RAPE
Henry Holt & Co.
4375 West 1980 South
Salt Lake City, UT 84104   Phone: (801) 972-2221
Publication Includes: List of rape crisis centers in the United States. **Frequency:** Irregular; previous edition April 1986; latest edition July 1989.

★4735★ RECOVERY, INCORPORATED—DIRECTORY OF GROUP MEETING INFORMATION
Recovery, Inc.
802 N. Dearborn St.
Chicago, IL 60610   Phone: (312) 337-5661
Covers: Approximately 1,000 weekly group meetings providing a professionally developed method of self-help aftercare to help prevent relapses in former mental patients and relieve chronic nervous conditions. **Entries Include:** Group meeting location, time and date. **Pages (approx.):** 50. **Frequency:** Annual, January.

★4736★ THE RECOVERY RESOURCE BOOK
Simon & Schuster, Inc.
Simon & Schuster Bldg.
1230 Avenue of the Americas
New York, NY 10020   Phone: (212) 698-7000
Publication Includes: Lists of self-help clearinghouses, U.S. state and Canadian province addiction agencies, state departments of rehabilitation, and publishers of books concerned with overcoming addictions. **Frequency:** Latest edition 1990.

★4737★ RED BOOK OF OPHTHALMOLOGY
Butterworth-Heinemann
80 Montvale Ave.
Stoneham, MA 02180   Phone: (617) 438-8464
Covers: 16,000 ophthalmologists; optical supply houses, manufacturers, and importers; hospitals with ophthalmology residencies; eye banks; international, national, state, and local organizations; coverage includes Canada. **Entries Include:** For ophthalmologists—Name, office address and phone, special interests; personal, educational, and career data. **Pages (approx.):** 300. **Frequency:** Biennial, January of even years.

★4738★ RED NOTEBOOK
Friends of Libraries for Deaf Action
Box 50045
Washington, DC 20091-9998   Phone: (202) 727-1186
Covers: Sources of information, services, library and other resources concerning the culture, language, arts, technology, and history of the deaf. **Pages (approx.):** 100 (loose-leaf). **Frequency:** Base edition published 1980; annual updates.

★4739★ REFERENCE BOOK OF REGISTERED NURSING HOMES
Registered Nursing Home Association
Calthorpe House
Hagley Rd.
Edgbaston
Birmingham B16 8QY, England
Covers: About 4,500 registered nursing homes, clinics, and hospitals in the United Kingdom. **Entries Include:** Name, address, phone. **Pages (approx.):** 195. **Frequency:** Annual, January.

★4740★ REGISTER OF DENTISTS
Dental Council
57 Merrion Sq.
Dublin 2, Ireland
Covers: About 1,250 registered dentists in Ireland. **Entries Include:** Name, address, date of registration, qualifications. **Pages (approx.):** 140. **Frequency:** Every 5 years; latest edition 1987; new edition expected 1992.

★4741★ REGISTER OF OSTEOPATHS—DIRECTORY OF MEMBERS
BPCC Whitefriars Ltd.
56 London St.
Tunbridge Wells, Kent, England
Covers: About 1,000 registered osteopaths in the United Kingdom and overseas. **Entries Include:** Name, address, phone, school of training, graduation date. **Pages (approx.):** 160. **Frequency:** Annual, October.

★4742★ REHAB: A COMPREHENSIVE GUIDE TO THE BEST DRUG-ALCOHOL TREATMENT CENTERS IN THE U.S.
HarperCollins
10 E. 53rd St.
New York, NY 10022   Phone: (212) 207-7000
Covers: Over 140 drug and alcohol treatment centers; centers exclusively for women are listed in an appendix. **Entries Include:** Center name, costs, admission policy, insurance accepted, staff qualifications, description of

programs, resources, and facilities. **Pages (approx.):** 320. **Frequency:** Latest edition December 1988.

★4743★ REHABILITATION RESOURCE MANUAL: VISION
Resources for Rehabilitation
33 Bedford St., Ste. 19A
Lexington, MA 02173   Phone: (617) 862-6455
Publication Includes: List of information sources in North America for people who are visually impaired or blind. **Entries Include:** Company or organization name, address, phone, description. **Frequency:** Biennial, summer of even years. **Also Includes:** Chapters discussing issues relevant to those helping vision-impaired people, such as informing someone of permanent vision loss and starting support groups.

★4744★ REHABILITATION SERVICES DIRECTORY
American Business Directories, Inc.
American Business Information, Inc.
5711 S. 86th Circle
Omaha, NE 68127   Phone: (402) 593-4600
Number of Listings: 9,586. **Entries Include:** Name, address, phone (including area code), size of advertisement, year first in "Yellow Pages," name of owner or manager, number of employees. **Frequency:** Annual.

★4745★ REPORT ON DENTAL AUXILIARY EDUCATION
Educational Measurements Division
Council on Dental Education
American Dental Association
211 E. Chicago Ave.
Chicago, IL 60611   Phone: (312) 440-2642
Covers: About 550 institutions conducting dental assisting, dental hygiene, and dental laboratory technology programs. **Entries Include:** Institution name, address, name of program director. **Pages (approx.):** 45. **Frequency:** Annual. **Also Includes:** Tables giving admission data and costs, and enrollment and graduate statistics in geographical and by-program arrangements.

★4746★ REPRESENTANTFORENINGEN FOR UTLANDSKA FARMACEVTISKA INDUSTRIE—RUFI MEDLEMSFORTECKNING OCH STADGAR
Representantforeningen for Utlandska Farmacevtiska Industrier
Kungsgatan 32
S-111 83 Stockholm, Sweden
Covers: About 55 member Swedish pharmaceutical firms acting as representatives for foreign firms worldwide. **Entries Include:** Representative company name, address, phone, telex, telefax; names, titles, addresses, and phone numbers of key personnel; names and addresses of represented firms. **Pages (approx.):** 35. **Frequency:** Annual, September. **Also Includes:** Constitution and committees of the organization.

★4747★ RESEARCH BOOKLET: A DIRECTORY OF PROJECTS AND PEOPLE INVOLVED IN PSYCHOSOCIALLY-ORIENTED CHILD HEALTH RESEARCH
Association for the Care of Children's Health
7910 Woodmont Ave., Ste. 300
Bethesda, MD 20814   Phone: (301) 654-6549
Pages (approx.): 50. **Frequency:** Latest edition 1988.

★4748★ RESEARCH AND HUMAN NEEDS
United Nations Educational, Scientific, and Cultural Organization
7, place de Fontenoy
F-75700 Paris, France
Covers: About 840 organizations with activities or interests in the area of appropriate technology; about 500 publishers of related periodicals and publications; worldwide coverage. **Entries Include:** For organizations—Name, address. For publishers—Name, title, address, frequency, price, description of content. **Pages (approx.):** 185. **Frequency:** First edition 1979; latest edition 1981.

★4749★ RESEARCH IN PROGRESS
Pan American Health Organization
525 23rd St., NW
Washington, DC 20037   Phone: (202) 861-3200
Covers: About 125 research projects sponsored by the organization on infectious diseases and in fields of public health, biomedicine, socioepidemiology, and operational research in member nations of the Pan American Health Organization. **Entries Include:** Name of project, institution name, names of key researchers, address, phone, source of funding. **Pages**

(approx.): 320. **Frequency:** Annual, June; suspended indefinitely. **Also Includes:** Statistical tables.

★4750★ RESEARCH SOCIETY ON ALCOHOLISM— DIRECTORY
Research Society on Alcoholism
4314 Medical Pkwy., No. 300
Austin, TX 78756-3332   Phone: (512) 454-0022
Covers: About 700 member researchers concerned with alcoholism and other related problems. **Entries Include:** Name, address, phone, fax. **Pages (approx.):** 65. **Frequency:** Annual, January.

★4751★ RESEARCH FOR VISUALLY DISABLED PEOPLE: AN INTERNATIONAL GUIDE
Technical Research Section
Royal National Institute for the Blind
224 Great Portland St.
London W1N 6AA, England
Covers: Over 600 non-medical research agencies serving visually disabled people worldwide. **Entries Include:** Agency name, address, phone, name of contact, description of projects and services. **Pages (approx.):** 100. **Frequency:** Approximately annual; previous edition December 1989; latest edition April 1990.

★4752★ THE RESOURCE BOOK: DIRECTORY OF ORGANIZATIONS, ASSOCIATIONS, SELF HELP GROUPS, AND HOTLINES FOR MENTAL HEALTH AND HUMAN SERVICES...
The Haworth Press, Inc.
10 Alice St.
Binghamton, NY 13904   Phone: (607) 722-5857
Description: Complete title, "The Resource Book: Directory of Organizations, Associations, Self Help Groups, and Hotlines for Mental Health and Human Services Professionals and Their Clients"; includes agencies, hotlines, and organizations providing information and services to children, youth, minorities, the handicapped, senior citizens, families, the mentally retarded, the homeless, women, and others with special social or emotional needs. **Entries Include:** Agency, hotline, or organization name, address, phone, brief description. **Pages (approx.):** 165. **Frequency:** Published 1987.

★4753★ RESOURCE DIRECTORY
Association for Humanistic Psychology
325 9th St.
San Francisco, CA 94103   Phone: (415) 453-3333
Covers: 800 psychologists, clergy, social workers, educators, psychiatrists, and others in detail. 5,500 members are covered in name-and-address entries. **Entries Include:** Name, affiliation, address, phone, credentials and certifications. **Pages (approx.):** 125. **Frequency:** Latest edition 1984; suspended indefinitely.

★4754★ RESOURCE DIRECTORY
Closing the Gap
Box 68
Henderson, MN 54044   Phone: (612) 248-3294
Covers: About 300 suppliers of computer hardware and software designed for use by physically and/or emotionally handicapped persons. **Entries Include:** Company or organization name, address, phone, description of products. **Pages (approx.):** 175. **Frequency:** Annual, February/March.

★4755★ RESOURCE DIRECTORY FOR OLDER PEOPLE
U.S. National Institute on Aging
Federal Bldg., Rm. 6C12
7550 Wisconsin Ave.
Bethesda, MD 20892   Phone: (301) 496-1752
Covers: About 200 national self-care and self-help groups, professional organizations, government agencies, and other organizations with related programs for the elderly, their families, and health care professionals. **Entries Include:** Organization name, address, phone, number of members, purpose, description of programs, titles of periodicals with frequency and circulation, other publications. **Pages (approx.):** 225. **Frequency:** Irregular; previous edition fall 1989; latest edition spring 1991.

★4756★ RESOURCE LIST FOR INFORMATIONAL MATERIALS ON SEXUALLY TRANSMITTED DISEASES
Technical Information Services
Center for Prevention Services
Centers for Disease Control
Atlanta, GA 30333   Phone: (404) 639-1819
Publication Includes: List of organizations that provide information on sexually transmitted diseases. **Pages (approx.):** 30. **Frequency:** Published March 1987.

★4757★ RESOURCES FOR COMPARATIVE BIOMEDICAL RESEARCH
National Center for Research Resources
National Institutes of Health
Westwood Bldg., Rm. 857
Bethesda, MD 20892   Phone: (301) 496-5545
Covers: Regional primate research centers, primate breeding and research projects, animal diagnostic laboratories, information projects, animal reference centers, special animal colonies and model studies centers, and institutional training awards supported by the Comparative Medicine Program, Division of Research Resources, NIH. **Entries Include:** Resource name, address, phone, names of principal investigators, name of contact person, principal areas of research, and details on the resource. **Pages (approx.):** 75. **Send Orders to:** Research Resources Information Center, 1601 Research Blvd., Rockville, MD 20850 (301-984-2870).

★4758★ RESOURCES FOR ELDERS WITH DISABILITIES
Resources for Rehabilitation
33 Bedford St., No. 19A
Lexington, MA 02173   Phone: (617) 862-6455
Covers: Services, products, and publications that enable people with hearing loss, vision loss, diabetes, stroke, arthritis, and osteoporosis to function independently. **Entries Include:** Name, address, phone, requirements for membership, admission, or eligibility, description of product/service. **Pages (approx.):** 168. **Frequency:** Biennial, winter of even years. **Also Includes:** Brief information about laws affecting older people with disabilities and about travel; information about aspects and effects of given disability.

★4759★ RESOURCES FOR HEALTH, FITNESS AND LEARNING
David I. Weiss Publishing
PO Box 1705
Brookline, MA 02146   Phone: (617) 277-7547
Covers: About 800 holistic health practitioners in Massachusetts, Rhode Island, and adjacent areas including physicians, acupuncturists, chiropractors, dentists, psychotherapists, massage therapists, teachers of workshops and seminars relating to yoga, personal growth, wellness, healing, and exercise. **Entries Include:** Name, address, phone, and description of services. **Pages (approx.):** 220. **Frequency:** Irregular; latest edition April 1990.

★4760★ RESOURCES FOR PEOPLE WITH DISABILITIES AND CHRONIC CONDITIONS
Resources for Rehabilitation
33 Bedford St., Ste. 19A
Lexington, MA 02173   Phone: (617) 862-6455
Description: Lists rehabilitation services and laws affecting people with disabilities, within chapters on hearing and speech disorders, visual impairment, spinal cord injury, epilepsy, multiple sclerosis and lower back pain. **Entries Include:** Company name, address, phone, requirements for membership, admission, or eligibility, description of services provided. **Pages (approx.):** 215. **Frequency:** Biennial, summer, odd years.

★4761★ REVIEW OF THE PUBLIC HEALTH SERVICE'S RESPONSE TO AIDS
Office of Technology Assessment
United States Congress
600 Pennsylvania Ave., SE
Washington, DC 20510
Publication Includes: Lists of projects and grants sponsored or funded by the National Institutes of Health for research into Acquired Immune Deficiency Syndroms (AIDS). **Entries Include:** Institute or organization name, location, research subject, date established. **Frequency:** Published February 1985. **Send Orders to:** Government Printing Office, Washington, DC 20402.

★4762★ ROADS TO RECOVERY: A NATIONAL DIRECTORY OF RESIDENTIAL ALCOHOLISM TREATMENT CENTERS
Macmillan Publishing Co.
866 3rd Ave.
New York, NY 10022   Phone: (212) 702-4296
Covers: Over 500 alcoholism treatment centers. **Entries Include:** Facility name, address, names and titles of key personnel, admission requirements, size of facility, accreditation, description of program, whether insurance-approved. **Pages (approx.):** 350. **Frequency:** Irregular; latest edition 1986.

★4763★ ROLF INSTITUTE INTERNATIONAL DIRECTORY
Rolf Institute
Box 1868
Boulder, CO 80306   Phone: (303) 449-5903
Covers: About 600 practitioners and teachers of the Rolfing technique of physical manipulation of the human body, including Rolfing and Rolfing Movement Integration; worldwide coverage. **Entries Include:** Name, address, phone. **Pages (approx.):** 50. **Frequency:** Semiannual, June and January.

★4764★ ROLLS OF DENTAL AUXILIARIES
General Dental Council
37 Wimpole St.
London W1M 8DQ, England
Covers: Over 2,650 registered dental hygienists and therapists in the United Kingdom. **Entries Include:** Name, address, date of registration, qualifications. **Pages (approx.):** 60. **Frequency:** Annual, June.

★4765★ ROTE LISTE
Editio Cantor Verlag
4 Bandelstockweg 20
W-7960 Aulendorf, Germany
Publication Includes: List of over 410 drug manufacturing firms in Germany. **Entries Include:** Firm name, address, phone, telex, cable address, emergency phone, products. **Frequency:** Annual. **Available in the U.S. from:** I.P.S. Division, Taylor & Francis, Inc., 242 Cherry St., Philadelphia, PA 19106.

★4766★ ROYAL COLLEGE OF OBSTETRICIANS AND GYNAECOLOGISTS—REGISTER OF FELLOWS AND MEMBERS
Royal College of Obstetricians & Gynaecologists
27 Sussex Pl.
Regent's Park
London NW1 4RG, England
Covers: About 7,950 member obstetricians and gynaecologists. **Entries Include:** Member name, address, biographical data, geographical area covered. **Pages (approx.):** 250. **Frequency:** Biennial, odd years; latest edition June 1991.

★4767★ ROYAL COLLEGE OF PATHOLOGISTS—HANDBOOK
Royal College of Pathologists
2 Carlton House Terrace
London SW1Y 5AF, England
Publication Includes: List of member pathologists. **Frequency:** Annual.

★4768★ ROYAL COLLEGE OF RADIOLOGISTS—MEMBERS HANDBOOK
Royal College of Radiologists
38 Portland Pl.
London WIN 3DG, England
Covers: 3,650 member diagnostic radiologists, radiotherapists, oncologists, nuclear medicine specialists, interventional radiologists, and ultrasound specialists. **Frequency:** Biennial.

★4769★ ROYAL NATIONAL INSTITUTE FOR THE DEAF—INFORMATION DIRECTORY
Royal National Institute for the Deaf
105 Gower St.
London WC1E 6AH, England
Covers: National and local deaf institutions and associations, social workers, and schools, homes, hostels, and other services and resources for deaf people in the United Kingdom. **Entries Include:** Contact name, address, phone; description. **Pages (approx.):** 370. **Frequency:** Annual.

★4770★ ROYAL SOCIETY OF TROPICAL MEDICINE AND HYGIENE—YEAR BOOK
Royal Society of Tropical Medicine and Hygiene
Manson House
26 Portland Place
London W1N 4EY, England
Covers: About 3,000 members. **Entries Include:** Member name, address, date of election, appointment. **Pages (approx.):** 120. **Frequency:** Annual, September.

★4771★ RX HOME CARE—BUYERS GUIDE ISSUE
Bill Communications Inc.
PO Box 3599
Akron, OH 44309   Phone: (216) 867-4401
Publication Includes: Listings of more than 11,300 manufacturers and exclusive distributors of home health care products and services worldwide. **Entries Include:** Company name, address, phone, telex, TWX, names of contact or key personnel. **Frequency:** Annual, October.

★4772★ SAFE, STRONG, AND STREETWISE
Joy Street Books
Little, Brown & Co.
34 Beacon St.
Boston, MA 02108   Phone: (617) 227-0730
Publication Includes: List of 40 organizations concerned with crisis and informative counseling and prevention of sexual assault, particularly involving teenagers. **Entries Include:** Organization name, address, phone. **Pages (approx.):** 180. **Frequency:** Published March 1987.

★4773★ SAFETY AND HEALTH—INDUSTRIAL HYGIENE BUYERS' GUIDE ISSUE
National Safety Council
444 N. Michigan Ave.
Chicago, IL 60611   Phone: (312) 527-4800
Publication Includes: List of manufacturers and suppliers of industrial hygiene products and services. **Entries Include:** Name of company, address, phone, contacts. **Frequency:** Annual, May.

★4774★ SAFETY AND HEALTH—SAFETY EQUIPMENT BUYERS' GUIDE ISSUE
National Safety Council
444 N. Michigan Ave.
Chicago, IL 60611   Phone: (312) 527-4800
Publication Includes: Directory of manufacturers and distributors of occupational health and safety products and services. **Entries Include:** Company or institution name, address, phone; some listings include addresses and phone numbers of branch offices or local distributors. **Frequency:** Annual, March.

★4775★ SCALP TREATMENT DIRECTORY
American Business Directories, Inc.
American Business Information, Inc.
5711 S. 86th Circle
Omaha, NE 68127   Phone: (402) 593-4600
Number of Listings: 2,552. **Entries Include:** Name, address, phone (including area code), size of advertisement, year first in "Yellow Pages," name of owner or manager, number of employees. **Frequency:** Annual.

★4776★ SCHIZOPHRENIA: STRAIGHT TALK FOR FAMILY AND FRIENDS
William Morrow & Co., Inc.
1350 Avenue of the Americas
New York, NY 10019   Phone: (212) 261-6500
Publication Includes: List of more than 150 local chapters of the National Alliance for the Mentally Ill. **Entries Include:** Chapter name, address, phone, names of key personnel. **Frequency:** Published February 1986. **Also Includes:** Bibliography. **Send Orders to:** Warner Books, 666 5th Ave., New York, NY 10103.

★4777★ SCHOLARSHIPS AND LOANS FOR NURSING EDUCATION
National League for Nursing
350 Hudson St.
New York, NY 10014   Phone: (212) 989-9393
Covers: Over 70 organizations offering fellowships, traineeships, grants, scholarships, and loans for nursing education. **Entries Include:** Organization name, address, name of scholarship, fellowship or other program, eligibility restrictions, application deadline. **Pages (approx.):** 80. **Frequen-**

cy: Annual, August. **Also Includes:** Bibliography; appendix of State Boards of Nursing; tips on obtaining aid; explanation of the licensing process.

★4778★ **SCIENTIFIC DIRECTORY AND ANNUAL BIBLIOGRAPHY**
U.S. National Institutes of Health
Bldg. 31, Rm. 2B03
Bethesda, MD 20892   Phone: (301) 496-4143
Covers: Professional staff and publications of 13 National Institutes of Health, two Divisions of Research, three National Centers, the National Library of Medicine, the Fogarty International Center for Advanced Study in the Health Sciences, and the Magnuson Clinical Center, two components of the Alcohol, Drug House, and Mental Health Administration, and one center of the Food and Drug Administration. **Entries Include:** Institution name, names and titles of key personnel, publications; divisions and subdivisions and their staff and publications. **Pages (approx.):** 490. **Frequency:** Annual, December.

★4779★ **SCIENTIFIC AND TECHNICAL SOCIETIES OF CANADA**
Canada Institute for Scientific and Technical Information
National Research Council of Canada
Ottawa, ON, Canada K1A 0S2   Phone: (613) 993-8242
Covers: 540 national, provincial, and regional associations in Canada devoted to a scientific, technical or medical discipline. **Entries Include:** Association name, address, phone, names and titles of contact and other key personnel, geographical area covered, brief history, statement of objectives, requirements for membership, number of members, schedule of regular meetings, description of projects and services, description of library, and list of publications, including name and address of editors. **Pages (approx.):** 230. **Frequency:** Formerly biennial; latest edition 1988.

★4780★ **SCRIP DIRECTORY OF WORLDWIDE PHARMACEUTICAL COMPANIES**
PJB Publications Ltd.
18-20 Hill Rise
Richmond, Surrey TW10 6UA, England
Covers: About 14,000 firms in the pharmaceutical industry and their subsidiaries, representatives, and agents; and nearly 220 related associations, 200 regulatory agencies, and 100 institutions. Published in 4 volumes; The European edition, American and Caribbean Section (including North and South America), the Australasian and Asian edition, and Rest of the World edition. **Entries Include:** Name, address, phone, telex, fax. **Pages (approx.):** 1,000. **Frequency:** Irregular; European edition published July 1989; American and Caribbean Section published October 1990; Australasian and Asian edition published April 1989; Rest of the World edition published May 1990. **Available in the U.S. from:** Pharmabooks Ltd., 1775 Broadway, Ste. 511, New York, NY 10019.

★4781★ **SEIBT DIRECTORY OF MEDICAL APPLIANCES**
Seibt Verlag GmbH
Leopoldstrasse 208
W-8000 Munich 40, Germany
Covers: About 8,000 European suppliers and manufacturers of medical instruments, devices, and equipment, including laboratory equipment, X-ray equipment, orthopedic appliances, furnishings, disposable paper and plastic items, audiovisual instructional materials, publications, and equipment and supplies for veterinary medicine and dentistry. **Entries Include:** Company name, address, phone, telex, cable address, products, line of business (manufacturer, distributor, service, importer, or exporter). **Pages (approx.):** 400. **Frequency:** Annual, December.

★4782★ **SEIBT PHARMA-TECHNIK**
Seibt Verlag GmbH
Leopoldstrasse 208
W-8000 Munich 40, Germany
Covers: 6,000 suppliers of chemicals, laboratory equipment, equipment for packaging, storing, and conditioning pharmaceutical products, and other materials and equipment used by the pharmaceutical industry. **Entries Include:** Company name, address, phone; some listings also show telex, cable address. **Pages (approx.):** 300. **Frequency:** Annual, December.

★4783★ **SELECTED STATE LEGISLATION: A GUIDE FOR EFFECTIVE STATE LAWS TO PROTECT CHILDREN**
National Center for Missing and Exploited Children
2101 Wilson Blvd., Ste. 550
Arlington, VA 22201   Phone: (703) 235-3900
Publication Includes: List of agencies and organizations working to end child abuse and parental kidnapping. **Entries Include:** Agency or organiza-

tion name, address, phone; names of key personnel. **Frequency:** Published 1989.

★4784★ **SELF-HELP SOURCEBOOK**
American Self-Help Clearinghouse
St. Clares-Riverside Medical Center
Pocono Rd.
Denville, NJ 07834   Phone: (201) 625-9565
Covers: Over 600 national and selected self-help groups for addictions, disabilities, illnesses, parenting, and other stress-causing problems. **Entries Include:** Group name, address, phone, purpose, number of chapters, name and title of contact. **Pages (approx.):** 160. **Frequency:** Biennial, summer of even years. **Also Includes:** General suggestions for starting a self-help group; list of national toll-free helplines.

★4785★ **THE SENIOR CITIZEN'S HANDBOOK: A NUTS AND BOLTS APPROACH TO MORE COMFORTABLE LIVING**
Price/Stern/Sloan, Inc.
360 N. La Cienega Blvd.
Los Angeles, CA 90048   Phone: (213) 657-6100
Publication Includes: List of organizations that provide information on issues relevant to senior citizens. **Entries Include:** Organization name, address. **Frequency:** Published April 1989.

★4786★ **SENIOR CITIZENS SERVICE ORGANIZATIONS DIRECTORY**
American Business Directories, Inc.
American Business Information, Inc.
5711 S. 86th Circle
Omaha, NE 68127   Phone: (402) 593-4600
Number of Listings: 7,157. **Entries Include:** Name, address, phone (including area code), size of advertisement, year first in "Yellow Pages," name of owner or manager, number of employees. **Frequency:** Annual.

★4787★ **SERIALS ON AGING: AN ANALYTICAL GUIDE**
Greenwood Publishing Group, Inc.
88 Post Rd. W.
PO Box 5007
Westport, CT 06881   Phone: (203) 226-3571
Publication Includes: Lists of publishers of English-language serials and journals and database suppliers and publishers of microforms and reprints. **Entries Include:** Publisher or supplier name, address. **Frequency:** Published 1986.

★4788★ **THE SEX DIRECTORY**
Woodhead-Faulkner Ltd.
Fitzwilliam House
32 Trumpington St.
Cambridge CB2 1Q4, England
Covers: Sex counseling services, family planning clinics, abortion facilities, and facilities for treatment of sexually transmitted diseases. **Entries Include:** Name, address, phone, services. **Pages (approx.):** 275. **Frequency:** First edition November 1987. **Available in the U.S. from:** Longwood, 51 Washington Street, Dover, NH 03820 (603-569-4576).

★4789★ **SEXUAL ABUSE PREVENTION EDUCATION: AN ANNOTATED BIBLIOGRAPHY**
Network Publications
Box 1830
Santa Cruz, CA 95601   Phone: (408) 438-4060
Publication Includes: List of almost 50 organizations and consultants of help in establishing child sexual abuse prevention programs, and publishers or distributors of films, filmstrips, and videocassettes used in teaching prevention techniques or coping strategies. **Entries Include:** Organization or publisher name, title of program or other material, address, phone. **Frequency:** Irregular; latest edition 1986.

★4790★ **SEXUALITY EDUCATION: A RESOURCE BOOK**
Garland Publishing, Inc.
136 Madison Ave.
New York, NY 10016   Phone: (212) 686-7492
Publication Includes: List of suppliers of audiovisual materials for use in sexuality education. **Entries Include:** Company name, address, phone. **Pages (approx.):** 470. **Frequency:** Published 1989. **Also Includes:** Annotated bibliographies listing books, periodicals, curricula, audiovisuals, and other resources for educators and parents to use in sexuality education.

★4791★ SHOES—ORTHOPEDIC RETAIL DIRECTORY
American Business Directories, Inc.
American Business Information, Inc.
5711 S. 86th Circle
Omaha, NE 68127   Phone: (402) 593-4600
Number of Listings: 1,783. **Entries Include:** Name, address, phone, size of advertisement, name of owner or manager, number of employees, year first in "Yellow Pages." **Frequency:** Annual.

★4792★ SICKNESS AND WELLNESS PUBLICATIONS
John Gordon Burke Publisher, Inc.
PO Box 1492
Evanston, IL 60204   Phone: (708) 866-8625
Covers: About 500 newsletters and publications on health-related issues for the layperson. **Entries Include:** Publication title, year first published, if known; sponsoring organization and address and phone; editor, subscription address, frequency, cost, ISSN when available, number of pages, size, special features, annotation by publication editor along with a description of the publication. **Pages (approx.):** 320. **Frequency:** Annual.

★4793★ SIGN LANGUAGE OF THE DEAF IN ISRAEL
World Organization of Jewish Deaf
c/o Association of the Deaf in Israel
Box 9001
61090 Tel Aviv, Israel
Frequency: Irregular.

★4794★ SJOGREN'S SYNDROME: THE SNEAKY "ARTHRITIS"
Pixel Press
319 Ridge Rd.
Jupiter, FL 33477   Phone: (407) 744-8775
Publication Includes: List of about 10 national support groups for sufferers of Sjogren's Syndrome, a rare disease affecting the autoimmune system. **Entries Include:** Organization name, address, phone. **Frequency:** Irregular; latest edition September 1988. **Send Orders to:** Pixel Press, Box 3151, Tequesta, FL 33469.

★4795★ SKIN TREATMENTS DIRECTORY
American Business Directories, Inc.
American Business Information, Inc.
5711 S. 86th Circle
Omaha, NE 68127   Phone: (402) 593-4600
Number of Listings: 7,670. **Entries Include:** Name, address, phone (including area code), size of advertisement, year first in "Yellow Pages," name of owner or manager, number of employees. **Frequency:** Annual.

★4796★ SMART DRUGS AND NUTRIENTS: HOW TO IMPROVE YOUR MEMORY AND INCREASE OUR INTELLIGENCE USING THE LATEST DISCOVERIES IN NEUROSCIENCE
B & J Publications
PO Box 483
Santa Cruz, CA 95061   Phone: (408) 429-1596
Publication Includes: Directory of suppliers of drugs and nutrients that are purported to enhance cognition; international coverage. **Entries Include:** Company and address. **Frequency:** Published July 1991.

★4797★ SMG UNITED STATES NURSING HOME DIRECTORY
SMG Marketing Group, Inc.
1342 N. LaSalle
Chicago, IL 60610   Phone: (312) 642-3026
Covers: Over 15,000 nursing homes with 50 beds or more. **Entries Include:** Nursing home name, address, phone, numbers of skilled nursing care beds, unskilled nursing care beds, and residents. **Pages (approx.):** 320. **Frequency:** Annual, October.

★4798★ SMOKERS INFORMATION AND TREATMENT CENTERS DIRECTORY
American Business Directories, Inc.
American Business Information, Inc.
5711 S. 86th Circle
Omaha, NE 68127   Phone: (402) 593-4600
Number of Listings: 1,412. **Entries Include:** Name, address, phone, size of advertisement, name of owner or manager, year first in "Yellow Pages." **Frequency:** Annual.

★4799★ SOCIETY OF CHIROPODISTS—DIRECTORY OF MEMBERS
Society of Chiropodists
53 Welbeck St.
London W1M 7HE, England
Covers: Approximately 5,500 chiropodists in the U.K. **Entries Include:** Member name, address, phone. **Pages (approx.):** 150. **Frequency:** Every 2-3 years; latest edition 1990.

★4800★ SOCIETY FOR CLINICAL AND EXPERIMENTAL HYPNOSIS—DIRECTORY
Society for Clinical and Experimental Hypnosis
128-A Kings Park Dr.
Liverpool, NY 13090   Phone: (315) 652-7299
Covers: 1,200 United States and Canadian physicians, psychologists (licensed or certified), and dentists who use hypnosis in their practices. **Entries Include:** Name, office and home addresses, highest degree held, areas of occupational specialization, whether diplomate of American Board of Clinical Hypnosis and/or specialty boards of the American Medical Association, American Dental Association, and American Psychological Association. **Pages (approx.):** 140. **Frequency:** Irregular; previous edition April 1988; latest edition February 1989.

★4801★ SOCIETY FOR EPIDEMIOLOGIC RESEARCH— MEMBERSHIP DIRECTORY
Society for Epidemiologic Research
c/o American Journal of Epidemiology
2007 E. Monument St.
Baltimore, MD 21205   Phone: (919) 966-2110
Covers: 2,600 epidemiologists, psychologists, sociologists, biostatisticians, and others interested in epidemiologic research. **Entries Include:** Name, address, phone. **Pages (approx.):** 100. **Frequency:** Irregular; previous edition 1983; latest edition 1988.

★4802★ SOCIETY OF MEDICAL-DENTAL MANAGEMENT CONSULTANTS—MEMBERSHIP DIRECTORY
Society of Medical-Dental Management Consultants
6215 Larson
Kansas City, MO 64133   Phone: (816) 353-8488
Covers: About 115 consultants in business and financial aspects of the management of medical and dental practices. **Entries Include:** Name, name and address of company or affiliation, phone, geographic area served. **Pages (approx.):** 50. **Frequency:** Annual, June.

★4803★ SOCIETY FOR NEUROSCIENCE MEMBERSHIP DIRECTORY
Society for Neuroscience
11 Dupont Circle, NW, Ste. 500
Washington, DC 20036   Phone: (202) 462-6688
Covers: 15,300 scientists who have done research relating to the brain and central nervous system. **Entries Include:** Name, degree, department, affiliated organization name, address, phone, fax, and electronic mail address. **Pages (approx.):** 222. **Frequency:** Biennial, March of even years. **Also Includes:** Lists of chapters, emeritus members, committee members, sustaining associates, and members of Congress.

★4804★ SOCIETY FOR PERSONALITY ASSESSMENT— DIRECTORY
Lawrence Erlbaum Associates, Inc.
365 Broadway
Hillsdale, NJ 07642   Phone: (201) 666-4110
Publication Includes: List of 2,000 psychologists, physicians, and other professional assessment specialists. **Entries Include:** Name, address, date of affiliation. **Frequency:** Annual.

★4805★ SOCIETY FOR RESEARCH IN CHILD DEVELOPMENT—DIRECTORY
Society for Research in Child Development
c/o University of Chicago Press
5720 Woodlawn Ave.
Chicago, IL 60637   Phone: (312) 702-7470
Covers: 4,600 anthropologists, educators, nurses, pediatricians, psychiatrists, psychologists, sociologists, statisticians. **Entries Include:** Name, affiliation, address, phone, highest degree. **Pages (approx.):** 300. **Frequency:** Irregular; previous edition December 1987; latest edition 1990.

★4806★ SOCIETY FOR THE SCIENTIFIC STUDY OF SEX—DIRECTORY OF MEMBERS
Society for the Scientific Study of Sex
c/o Howard J. Ruppel, M.A.
Box 208
Mount Vernon, IA 52314   Phone: (319) 895-8407
Covers: Member therapists, educators, physicians, scientists, nurses, psychologists, and social workers who share an interest and competency in the scientific pursuit of knowledge concerning sexuality. **Entries Include:** Name, address, phone, professional affiliation. **Frequency:** Annual, May.

★4807★ SOCIETY OF TEACHERS OF FAMILY MEDICINE—MEMBERSHIP DIRECTORY
Society of Teachers of Family Medicine
8880 Ward Pkwy.
Kansas City, MO 64114   Phone: (816) 333-9700
Covers: About 3,000 physicians and other individuals involved in teaching or promotion of family medicine; international coverage. **Entries Include:** Name, office address and phone, highest degree held. **Pages (approx.):** 250. **Frequency:** Biennial, January of even years.

★4808★ SOCIETY FOR TRAUMATIC STRESS STUDIES—MEMBERSHIP LIST
Society for Traumatic Stress Studies
435 N. Michigan Ave., Ste. 1717
Chicago, IL 60611-4067   Phone: (312) 644-0828
Description: Mailing labels. Covers more than 3,000 psychologists, social workers, clergy, and lawyers who are concerned with the treatment of individuals suffering from traumatic disorders as a result of rape, robbery, domestic or criminal violence, natural disasters, technological disasters, war, or intense mental or emotional stress; international coverage. **Entries Include:** Name, address, phone. **Pages (approx.):** 50. **Frequency:** Continuous updating.

★4809★ SOURCE BOOK
The Healthcare Forum
830 Market St.
San Francisco, CA 94102   Phone: (415) 421-8810
Covers: About 7,500 hospitals and multi-hospital systems, and manufacturers and suppliers to hospitals nationwide. **Entries Include:** For hospitals—Name, address, and phone; name of administrator or chief executive officer, names and titles of department heads, number of beds. **Pages (approx.):** 400. **Frequency:** Annual.

★4810★ SOURCEBOOK FOR INNOVATIVE DRUG DELIVERY
Canon Communications, Inc.
3340 Ocean Park Blvd., Ste. 1000
Santa Monica, CA 90405   Phone: (213) 392-5509
Covers: Approximately 300 suppliers of drug delivery products and services. **Entries Include:** Company name, address, phone, names and titles of key personnel, branch office or subsidiary names and addresses, products and services. **Pages (approx.):** 155. **Frequency:** Published 1987.

★4811★ SOUTHERN CALIFORNIA SENIOR LIFE DIRECTORY
Senior Media, Inc.
6022 W. Pico Blvd., No. 7
Los Angeles, CA 90035   Phone: (213) 933-9228
Pages (approx.): 128. **Frequency:** Annual, November.

★4812★ SPA BOOK: A GUIDE TO THE TOP 101 HEALTH RESORTS IN AMERICA
G. P. Putnam's Sons
200 Madison Ave.
New York, NY 10016   Phone: (212) 951-8400
Covers: Approximately 100 health spa resort facilities in the United States. **Entries Include:** Facility name, address, phone, name and title of contact, number of employees, geographical area served, description of facility, programs and services provided, and general statement of philosophy. **Pages (approx.):** 300. **Frequency:** Published 1988. **Also Includes:** General information about health spas and fitness resorts. **Send Orders to:** Putnam/Berkeley Warehouse, 1 Grosset Dr., Kirkwood, NY 13795 (607-775-17 40).

★4813★ SPECIAL OLYMPICS—LIST OF INTERNATIONAL SPECIAL OLYMPICS PROGRAMS
Special Olympics International
1350 New York Ave., NW, Ste. 500
Washington, DC 20005   Phone: (202) 628-3630
Covers: About 125 directors of Special Olympics programs promoting sports training and competition for the mentally retarded; limited international coverage. **Entries Include:** Director name, address, phone, location of program. **Pages (approx.):** 10. **Frequency:** Quarterly.

★4814★ SPECIAL RECREATION COMPENDIUM OF 1,500 RESOURCES FOR PEOPLE WITH DISABILITIES
Special Recreation Digest
362 Koser Ave.
Iowa City, IA 52246-3038   Phone: (319) 337-7578
Covers: Over 1,500 associations, national and state government agencies, companies, colleges and universities, and other contacts for 40 recreation activities for the disabled, including amusement and theme parks, toll-free phone services, suppliers of adapted equipment and special products, rehabilitation therapies, recreation vehicles, sports organizations, travel agencies, and wildlife resource agencies; worldwide coverage. **Entries Include:** Organization name, address, phone, names of key personnel, number of members, number of affiliates, description of programs and services, publications, committees, and meetings. **Pages (approx.):** 500 (loose-leaf). **Frequency:** Irregular; latest edition 1988; new edition expected 1992.

★4815★ SPECIALIZED PROGRAMS FOR MEDICAL LABORATORY TECHNICIANS AND MEDICAL ASSISTANTS AND INSTITUTIONS OF ALLIED HEALTH
Accrediting Bureau of Health Education Schools/Programs
29089 U.S. 20 W.
Elkhart, IN 46514   Phone: (219) 293-0124
Covers: Nearly 165 institutions offering programs accredited by the Accrediting Bureau of Health Education Schools; includes programs of preparation for medical laboratory technician, medical assistant, and allied health education careers. **Entries Include:** Institution name, address, phone, name and title of director, programs accredited, year of initial accreditation, year of next accreditation review. **Pages (approx.):** 35. **Frequency:** Annual, March. **Also Includes:** Profiles of the commissioners of the Accrediting Bureau of Health Education Schools/Programs.

★4816★ SPECTROSCOPY
Theta Corp.
Theta Bldg.
Middlefield, CT 06455   Phone: (203) 349-1054
Publication Includes: List of suppliers of spectroscopy instruments. **Entries Include:** Company name, address, phone, key personnel, background information, description of products, annual sales, research and development efforts, distribution systems, five year projection. **Frequency:** Irregular; latest edition October 1985.

★4817★ SPEECH PATHOLOGISTS DIRECTORY
American Business Directories, Inc.
American Business Information, Inc.
5711 S. 86th Circle
Omaha, NE 68127   Phone: (402) 593-4600
Number of Listings: 3,605. **Entries Include:** Name, address, phone (including area code), size of advertisement, year first in "Yellow Pages," name of owner or manager, number of employees. **Frequency:** Annual.

★4818★ SPINAL NETWORK: THE TOTAL RESOURCE FOR THE WHEELCHAIR COMMUNITY
Spinal Associates
1911 11th St., No. 307
PO Box 4162
Boulder, CO 80306   Phone: (303) 449-5412
Publication Includes: List of nearly 100 national resource organizations for those disabled by spinal cord injuries; list of vocational rehabilitation agencies, governors' committees, independent living centers, Model System Centers (hospitals that promote a "total care" model for spinal cord injuries), and other local organizations and companies serving the wheelchair community. **Entries Include:** Organization or institution name, address, phone; national organizations also include descriptions of services and activities. **Frequency:** First edition 1988; latest edition 1989.

★4819★   SPORTS AND LEISURE: AN ACCESS GUIDE FOR DISABLED SPECTATORS
Royal Association for Disability & Rehabilitation
25 Mortimer St.
London W1N 8AB, England
Covers: Sports facilities in England and Wales that accommodate such sports as car racing, cricket, football, horse racing, horse show jumping, rugby, and tennis and offer special facilities for the handicapped. **Entries Include:** Facility name, address, phone.

★4820★   STARTING EARLY: A GUIDE TO FEDERAL RESOURCES IN MATERNAL AND CHILD HEALTH
National Center for Education in Maternal and Child Health
38th & R Sts. NW
Washington, DC 20057   Phone: (202) 625-8410
Covers: Federal government agencies and federally supported organizations offering over 500 print and non-print resources (posters, audiovisual materials, software) on prenatal, infant, and adolescent health; state and regional maternal and child health contacts; regional genetics services networks. **Entries Include:** Agency name, address, phone; description of publication, including title, length, order number, price. **Pages (approx.):** 170. **Frequency:** Irregular; latest edition November 1988.

★4821★   STATE-APPROVED SCHOOLS OF NURSING: L.P.N./L.V.N.
National League for Nursing
350 Hudson St.
New York, NY 10014   Phone: (212) 989-9393
Covers: Licensed practical nurse and licensed vocational nurse programs in about 1,320 schools. **Entries Include:** Name of school, address, types of programs, admission policies, type of administrative control, sources of financial support, length of program, information on state board approval and National League for Nursing accreditation. **Pages (approx.):** 80. **Frequency:** Annual, fall.

★4822★   STATE-APPROVED SCHOOLS OF NURSING: R.N.
National League for Nursing
350 Hudson St.
New York, NY 10014   Phone: (212) 989-9393
Covers: Associate degree, baccalaureate degree, and diploma programs offered in over 1,475 schools, leading to licensure as a registered nurse. **Entries Include:** Name of school, address, names of deans and directors of programs, type of administrative control, sources of financial support, and information on National League for Nursing accreditation status. **Pages (approx.):** 100. **Frequency:** Annual, August. **Also Includes:** Summary tables of new programs and programs recently closed.

★4823★   STATE PLANNING COUNCIL ON DEVELOPMENTAL DISABILITIES—LIST OF MEMBER EXECUTIVE DIRECTORS
National Association of Developmental Disabilities
1234 Massachusetts Ave. NW, Ste. 103
Washington, DC 20005   Phone: (202) 347-1234
Covers: The executive in each state government responsible for planning programs for the mentally handicapped. **Entries Include:** Name, title, agency name, address, phone. **Pages (approx.):** 10. **Frequency:** Annual, March.

★4824★   STATE VOCATIONAL REHABILITATION AGENCIES
U.S. Office of Special Education and Rehabilitative Services
330 C St. SW
Washington, DC 20202   Phone: (202) 732-1370
Covers: State government agencies responsible for vocational rehabilitation activities, including those for the blind. **Entries Include:** Agency name, address, phone, name and title of director, federal Rehabilitation Services Administration region number. **Pages (approx.):** 10. **Frequency:** Three times a year; April, August, and December.

★4825★   STROKE: FROM CRISIS TO VICTORY
Franklin Watts
387 Park Ave. South
New York, NY 10016   Phone: (212) 686-7070
Publication Includes: Stroke clubs and other organizations providing assistance for stroke victims. **Frequency:** Published 1985.

★4826★   STUDENT NATIONAL DENTAL ASSOCIATION— DIRECTORY
Student National Dental Association
c/o Dr. Robert Knight
Howard University School of Dentistry
600 W St., NW
Washington, DC 20059   Phone: (202) 806-0301
Covers: About 1,000 minority dental students. **Entries Include:** Name, address, phone, minority classification. **Pages (approx.):** 50. **Frequency:** Annual.

★4827★   STUDENTS WHO ARE DEAF AND HARD OF HEARING IN POSTSECONDARY EDUCATION
Higher Education and Adult Training for People with Handicaps Resource Center
1 Dupont Circle NW, Ste. 800
Washington, DC 20036   Phone: (202) 939-9320
Publication Includes: List of nearly 50 organizations involved with the physical, social, and educational well-being of college students who are deaf or hard of hearing. **Entries Include:** Organization name, address, phone, service provided. **Frequency:** Biennial, even years. **Also Includes:** Annotated bibliography of publications about students who are deaf or hard of hearing and their educational concerns.

★4828★   SUBSTANCE ABUSE AND KIDS: A DIRECTORY OF EDUCATION, INFORMATION, PREVENTION, AND EARLY INTERVENTION PROGRAMS
Oryx Press
4041 N. Central, No. 700
Phoenix, AZ 85012   Phone: (602) 265-2651
Pages (approx.): 490. **Frequency:** Published November 1989.

★4829★   SUBSTANCE ABUSE RESIDENTIAL TREATMENT CENTERS FOR TEENS
Oryx Press
4041 N. Central Ave., No. 700
Phoenix, AZ 85012   Phone: (602) 265-2651
Covers: Over 1,000 drug and alcohol abuse residential treatment centers for patients aged nine to nineteen. **Entries Include:** Organization name, address, phone, "hotline" number, name and title of contact, licensure, means of facility evaluation, addictions and disorders treated, treatment methods, program setting, additional client services, staff, specialty groups served, ownership, admission requirements, fees, and funding sources. **Pages (approx.):** 304. **Frequency:** Published 1990.

★4830★   SURVEY OF PHARMACEUTICAL ENTERPRISES IN CHINA
Xinhua News Agency
57 Xidajie Xuanwumen Wai
Beijing 668521-787, People's Republic of China
Description: Pharmaceutical companies in China. **Entries Include:** Company name, address, description, including product information and management. **Pages (approx.):** 670. **Frequency:** Latest edition 1989.

★4831★   SURVIVING CANCER: A PRACTICAL GUIDE FOR THOSE FIGHTING TO WIN
Acropolis Books Ltd.
13950 Park Center Rd.
Herndon, VA 22071   Phone: (703) 709-0006
Publication Includes: List of sources of support and information for cancer patients such as books, pamphlets, tapes, counseling services, alternative practitioners, etc. **Entries Include:** Organization or publisher name, address, product or service. **Pages (approx.):** 176. **Frequency:** Published May 1987.

★4832★   SVERIGES LEGITIMERADE OPTIKERS RIKSFORBUND—MATRIKEL
Sveriges Legitimerade Optikers Riksforbund
Arstaangsvagen 1 C
S-117 43 Stockholm, Sweden
Covers: Member licensed opticians in Sweden. **Entries Include:** Personal name, address. **Pages (approx.):** 190. **Frequency:** Irregular; latest edition 1986.

★4833★ TANGLED TONGUE: LIVING WITH A STUTTER
University of Toronto Press
St. George Campus
Toronto, ON, Canada M5S 1A6   Phone: (416) 978-2239
Publication Includes: List of approximately 180 centers for speech therapy and programs of research concerned with stuttering. **Pages (approx.):** 260. **Frequency:** Published 1985.

★4834★ T.A.P.P. SOURCES: A NATIONAL DIRECTORY OF TEENAGE PREGNANCY PREVENTION
Women's Action Alliance
370 Lexington Ave.
New York, NY 10017   Phone: (212) 532-8330
Covers: About 600 teenage pregnancy prevention programs. **Entries Include:** Program name, address, phone, names and titles of key personnel, number of employees, geographical area served, financial data, description of services. **Pages (approx.):** 560. **Frequency:** Published 1989.

★4835★ 3RD OPINION: INTERNATIONAL DIRECTORY TO COMPLEMENTARY THERAPY CENTERS FOR TREATMENT/PREVENTION OF CANCER AND OTHER DEGENERATIVE DISEASES
Avery Publishing Group, Inc.
120 Old Broadway
Garden City Park, NY 11040   Phone: (516) 741-2155
Covers: Over 300 alternative treatment cancer centers, educational centers, support groups, and information services; international coverage. **Entries Include:** Center name, address, phone, driving directions, names and titles of key personnel, geographical area served background financial data, description of philosophical approaches and methods of treatment. **Pages (approx.):** 290. **Frequency:** Reported as biennial; latest edition January 1992. **Also Includes:** List of related publications.

★4836★ 330/329-FUNDED COMMUNITY AND MIGRANT HEALTH CENTERS DIRECTORY
National ClearingHouse for Primary Care Information
8201 Greensboro Dr., Ste. 600
McLean, VA 22102   Phone: (703) 821-8955
Covers: About 1,500 community and migrant health centers in the United States and its territories funded under Sections 330 and 329 of the Public Health Services Act; also includes (in an index) state and regional primary care associations. **Entries Include:** Center name, address, phone, name and title of chief administrator, medical director, head of governing board, source of funding (if not 330), Congressional District, and service area. **Pages (approx.):** 150. **Frequency:** Annual, April. **Also Includes:** List of Department of Health and Human Services regional offices.

★4837★ TISSUE CULTURE ASSOCIATION—MEMBERSHIP ROSTER
Tissue Culture Association
8815 Centre Park Dr., Ste. 210
Columbia, MD 21045   Phone: (301) 992-0946
Covers: 2,300 international tissue culture researchers. **Entries Include:** Name, address, phone, affiliation, and type of membership. **Pages (approx.):** 80. **Frequency:** Biennial, March of odd years.

★4838★ TOTAL NUTRITION FOR BREAST-FEEDING MOTHERS
Little, Brown & Co., Inc.
34 Beacon St.
Boston, MA 02108-1493   Phone: (617) 227-0730
Publication Includes: List of about 25 resources for nursing mothers, such as organizations, books, and magazines. **Entries Include:** Organization name, address, phone. **Frequency:** Published July 1986.

★4839★ TOXSERV: A DIRECTORY OF ANALYTICAL SERVICES FOR TOXICOLOGY IN WESTERN CANADA
Toxicology Research Centre
University of Saskatchewan
Saskatoon, SK, Canada S7N 0W0   Phone: (306) 966-7441
Covers: Nearly 50 laboratories and persons supplying toxicological and analytical services (including analyses of drugs, metals, mycotoxins, and mutagenicity testing) to western Canada; and 50 members of the Toxicology Group of the University of Saskatchewan who have indicated willingness to provide expert advice in emergency situations, primarily in Saskatchewan. (About one-third of the listings are duplicated between sections.). **Entries Include:** For suppliers of analytical services—Name, affiliation, address, phone. For Toxicology Group members—Name, title and specialty, affiliation, location (if other than the university), phone.

Pages (approx.): 25. **Frequency:** Irregular; latest edition December 1983. **Also Includes:** Emergency phone numbers for poison control centers, environmental spills, major accidents, and disasters.

★4840★ TRADITIONAL ACUPUNCTURE SOCIETY—REGISTER OF MEMBERS
Traditional Acupuncture Society
1 The Ridgeway
Stratford-upon-Avon, Warwickshire CV37 9JL, England
Covers: About 500 members. **Frequency:** Semiannual.

★4841★ TRAINING IN COUNSELING AND PSYCHOTHERAPY—A DIRECTORY
British Association for Counseling
37a Sheep St.
Rugby, Warwickshire CV21 3BX, England
Covers: 380 institutions in the United Kingdom offering training in counseling and psychotherapy. **Entries Include:** Name, address, phone, length of training, entry requirements, description of courses. **Pages (approx.):** 140. **Frequency:** Annual, November.

★4842★ TRAVEL FOR THE DISABLED
Twin Peaks Press
Box 129
Vancouver, WA 98666   Phone: (206) 694-2462
Covers: Publishers of about 500 access guides; travel agencies and resources for the disabled; international coverage. **Entries Include:** Company or organization name, address, phone, name and title of contact, services provided, geographical area served. **Pages (approx.):** 190. **Frequency:** Irregular; previous edition October 1985; latest edition July 1990; new edition expected 1991.

★4843★ TUMOR MARKERS IN THE CLINICAL LABORATORY
Theta Corp.
Theta Bldg.
Middlefield, CT 06455   Phone: (203) 349-1054
Publication Includes: List of companies that produce or market tumor markers including CEA, Ca-119, Ca-125, LASA, HCG, a-fetoprotein, and B-protein used in clinical laboratories. **Entries Include:** Company name, address, phone, key personnel, background information, description of projects, annual sales, research and development efforts, distribution systems, five year projection. **Frequency:** Irregular; previous edition July 1985; latest edition January 1986.

★4844★ 200 WAYS TO PUT YOUR TALENT TO WORK IN THE HEALTH FIELD
National Health Council, Inc.
350 5th Ave., Ste. 118
New York, NY 10118   Phone: (212) 268-8900
Covers: Professional associations, government agencies, institutions, and other organizations offering information or assistance concerning health career education. **Entries Include:** Organization name, address, whether financial aid is offered. **Pages (approx.):** 30. **Frequency:** Irregular; previous edition December 1985; latest edition September 1990.

★4845★ UICC INTERNATIONAL DIRECTORY OF CANCER INSTITUTES AND ORGANIZATIONS
International Union against Cancer
3, rue du Conseil-General
CH-1205 Geneva, Switzerland
Covers: About 800 major institutions with specialized competence in the field of cancer research and/or treatment; international coverage. **Entries Include:** Institution name, address, phone, telex; affiliations; names of directors and department heads; number of personnel; annual cancer patient statistics; description of research and treatment activities; availability of postgraduate training opportunities. **Pages (approx.):** 300. **Frequency:** Biennial, August of even years.

★4846★ UNDERSTANDING ARTHRITIS: WHAT IT IS, HOW IT'S TREATED, HOW TO COPE WITH IT
Charles Scribner's Sons
866 3rd Ave.
New York, NY 10022   Phone: (212) 702-7830
Publication Includes: List of organizations and agencies that provide information or assistance to arthritis patients and their families. **Frequency:** Published 1985.

★4847★ UNIFORMED SERVICES MEDICAL/DENTAL FACILITIES IN THE U.S.A.
American Forces Information Service
U.S. Department of Defense
601 N. Fairfax St.
Alexandria, VA 22314
Covers: Hospitals, medical clinics, and dental facilities for members of the armed forces and their dependents. **Entries Include:** Facility name, address; hospital listings include phone. **Pages (approx.):** 25. **Frequency:** Irregular; latest edition 1989.

★4848★ UNITED STATES OF AMERICA-PHYSICIANS AND SURGEONS ASSOCIATION—MEMBERSHIP DIRECTORY AND CONCORDANCE
United States of America-Physicians and Surgeons Association
Box 9010
Scottsdale, AZ 85252   Phone: (702) 644-1923
Covers: About 9,300 practitioners of all branches of medicine, including osteopathy, naturopathy, allopathy, acupuncture, hypnosis, and drugless medical practice. **Entries Include:** Member name, address, phone, area of specialty. **Frequency:** Semiannual.

★4849★ UNITED STATES AND CANADIAN PROGRAMS FOR GRADUATE TRAINING IN PHARMACOLOGY
American Society for Pharmacology and Experimental Therapeutics
9650 Rockville Pike
Bethesda, MD 20814   Phone: (301) 530-7060
Covers: More than 200 institutions; limited Canadian coverage. **Entries Include:** Institution name, department name, address, name of department chairperson, phone, pharmacological specialties offered, highest degree offered. **Pages (approx.):** 15. **Frequency:** Triennial; latest edition January 1991.

★4850★ U.S. HOSPITALS IN COUNTY ORDER
SMG Marketing Group, Inc.
1342 N. LaSalle Dr.
Chicago, IL 60610   Phone: (312) 642-3026
Covers: Over 7,600 hospitals in the United States. **Entries Include:** Hospital name, address, phone, number of beds, emergency room visits, number of staff. **Pages (approx.):** 300. **Frequency:** Quarterly.

★4851★ U.S. MEDICAL DIRECTORY
U.S. Directory Service, Publishers
655 NW 128th St.
PO Box 68-1700
Miami, FL 33168   Phone: (305) 769-1700
Covers: Medical doctors, hospitals, nursing facilities, medical research laboratories, poison control centers, medical schools and libraries, and other medical services, organizations, facilities, and institutes. **Pages (approx.):** 1,000. **Frequency:** Latest edition 1989.

★4852★ U.S. MEDICINE—DIRECTORY OF MAJOR FEDERAL MEDICAL TREATMENT FACILITIES ISSUE
U.S. Medicine, Inc.
2033 M St., NW
Washington, DC 20036   Phone: (202) 463-6000
Covers: Approximately 1,100 federal government medical treatment facilities and administrative headquarters in the United States and abroad. **Entries Include:** Facility or center name, address, commercial and government phone numbers, chiefs of staff, administrators. **Pages (approx.):** 48. **Frequency:** Annual, June.

★4853★ U.S. SCHOOLS OF PUBLIC HEALTH AND GRADUATE PUBLIC HEALTH PROGRAMS ACCREDITED BY THE COUNCIL ON EDUCATION FOR PUBLIC HEALTH
Council on Education for Public Health
1015 15th St., NW
Washington, DC 20005   Phone: (202) 789-1050
Covers: About 40 graduate schools of public health, community health education programs, and community health and preventive medicine programs in the United States. **Entries Include:** Institution name, address, name of dean or director, date of next accreditation review. **Frequency:** Annual, January.

★4854★ U.S. STROKE CLUB LISTING
National Stroke Association
300 E. Hampden Ave., Ste. 240
Englewood, CO 80110-2622   Phone: (303) 762-9922
Covers: About 750 state stroke clubs and support groups that assist stroke survivors and their families. **Entries Include:** Organization name, address, phone, coordinator name, sponsor name. **Frequency:** Irregular.

★4855★ UNLISTED DRUGS INDEX-GUIDE
Pharmaco-Medical Documentation, Inc.
Box 429
Chatham, NJ 07928   Phone: (201) 822-9200
Covers: Medicinal drugs and pharmaceutical research chemicals originally not listed in "Drug Compendia," and their manufacturers; international coverage. **Entries Include:** Company name, address. **Pages (approx.):** 720. **Frequency:** Irregular; Previous edition May 1987; latest edition April 1990; new edition expected January 1992.

★4856★ UROLOGICAL SUPPLIES AND IMPLANTS
Theta Corp.
Theta Bldg.
Middlefield, CT 06455   Phone: (203) 349-1054
Publication Includes: List of manufacturers of urological supplies. **Entries Include:** Company name, address, phone, key personnel, background information, description of products, annual sales, research and development efforts, distribution systems, five year projection. **Frequency:** Irregular; latest edition November 1985.

★4857★ VEGETARIAN HEALTH DIRECTORY
21st Century Publications
401 N. Fourth St.
Fairfield, IA 52556   Phone: (515) 472-5105
Covers: Over 1,200 New Age centers, publishers, periodicals, bookstores, and products; health resorts; traditional and non-traditional physicians interested in holistic approaches; natural healing centers; communes; spiritual centers and courses; and extensive listings of vegetarian, fruitarian, and other natural food resources. **Entries Include:** Organization or personal name, address, description of product, service, or interest. **Pages (approx.):** 65. **Frequency:** Irregular; previous edition 1981; latest edition January 1988; suspended indefinitely.

★4858★ VEGETARIAN VOICE—LOCAL VEGETARIAN ORGANIZATIONS SECTION
North American Vegetarian Society
Box 72
Dogleville, NY 13329   Phone: (518) 568-7970
Publication Includes: List of about 100 affiliated vegetarian societies and information centers. **Entries Include:** Organization name, address; some listings include name of contact. **Frequency:** Quarterly.

★4859★ VERZEICHNIS DER KRANKENHAUSER IN DER BUNDESREPUBLIK DEUTSCHLAND
Verlag W. Kohlhammer GmbH
2 Metzler-Poeschel Verlag
Kernerstrasse
W-7000 Stuttgart 1, Germany
Covers: Hospitals, sanatoriums, and maternity hospitals in the Federal Republic of Germany. **Entries Include:** Institution name, address, financial institution, specialty, departments, number of beds, affiliated school of medicine (where applicable). **Pages (approx.):** 250. **Frequency:** Irregular; latest edition 1982;.

★4860★ VETERINARIAN CLINICS DIRECTORY
American Business Directories, Inc.
American Business Information, Inc.
5711 S. 86th Circle
Omaha, NE 68127   Phone: (402) 593-4600
Number of Listings: 18,078. **Entries Include:** Name, address, phone, size of advertisement, name of owner or manager, number of employees, year first in "Yellow Pages." **Frequency:** Annual.

★4861★ VETERINARIANS DIRECTORY
American Business Directories, Inc.
American Business Information, Inc.
5711 S. 86th Circle
Omaha, NE 68127   Phone: (402) 593-4600
Number of Listings: 45,369. **Entries Include:** Name, address, phone

(including area code), size of advertisement, year first in "Yellow Pages," name of owner or manager, number of employees. **Frequency:** Annual.

★4862★ **VETERINARIANS EQUIPMENT AND SUPPLIES DIRECTORY**
American Business Directories, Inc.
American Business Information, Inc.
5711 S. 86th Circle
Omaha, NE 68127   Phone: (402) 593-4600
Number of Listings: 2,133. **Entries Include:** Name, address, phone (including area code), year first in "Yellow Pages," name of owner or manager, number of employees. **Frequency:** Annual.

★4863★ **VETERINARY AND HUMAN TOXICOLOGY— DIRECTORY ISSUES**
Comparative Toxicology Laboratories
Kansas State University
Manhattan, KS 66506-5606   Phone: (913) 532-5679
Publication Includes: Lists of about 2,500 toxicologists, physicians, veterinarians, clinicians, nurses; poison control centers, emergency rooms and their directors; and hospitals and similar institutions. Directory issues are published for the following organizations: American Academy of Veterinary and Comparative Toxicology (formerly American College of Veterinary Toxicologists), American Board of Veterinary Toxicologists, American Association of Poison Control Centers, American Academy of Clinical Toxicology, American Board of Medical Toxicology, and American Board of Toxicology. **Entries Include:** For institutions—Name, address, phone. For individuals—Name, address, phone, affiliation, highest degree earned. **Frequency:** Annual.

★4864★ **VETERINARY REGISTER OF IRELAND**
Veterinary Council
53 Lansdowne Rd.
Ballsbridge
Dublin 4, Ireland
Covers: About 1,765 registered veterinarians in Ireland. **Entries Include:** Name, address, phone. **Pages (approx.):** 194. **Frequency:** Annual, March. **Also Includes:** List of qualifications necessary for becoming registered as a veterinarian in Ireland.

★4865★ **VOLUNTEERS WHO PRODUCE BOOKS: BRAILLE, TAPE, LARGE TYPE**
National Library Service for the Blind and Physically Handicapped
Library of Congress
1291 Taylor St., NW
Washington, DC 20542   Phone: (202) 707-5100
Covers: Volunteer organizations and individuals who produce books for visually and physically handicapped persons. Includes proofreaders and special education specialists. **Entries Include:** For organizations—Name, address, and phone; chairperson's name, address, phone; type of media, specialty. For individuals—Name, address, and phone. **Pages (approx.):** 90. **Frequency:** Biennial, odd years.

★4866★ **WEIGHT CONTROL SERVICES DIRECTORY**
American Business Directories, Inc.
American Business Information, Inc.
5711 S. 86th Circle
Omaha, NE 68127   Phone: (402) 593-4600
Number of Listings: 14,591. **Entries Include:** Name, address, phone (including area code), size of advertisement, year first in "Yellow Pages," name of owner or manager, number of employees. **Frequency:** Annual.

★4867★ **WEST AFRICAN COLLEGE OF SURGEONS— MEMBERS LIST**
West African College of Surgeons
West African Health Community Bldg.
6 Taylor Dr., Edmund Cresent
P.M.B. 1067
Yaba, Lagos, Nigeria
Covers: 1,020 anesthetists, dental surgeons, obstetricians, gynecologists, ophthalmologists, otorhinolaryngologists, radiologists, surgeons, and surgical subspecialists. **Frequency:** Biennial.

★4868★ **WHEEL CHAIRS DIRECTORY**
American Business Directories, Inc.
American Business Information, Inc.
5711 S. 86th Circle
Omaha, NE 68127   Phone: (402) 593-4600
Number of Listings: 5,231. **Entries Include:** Name, address, phone (including area code), size of advertisement, year first in "Yellow Pages," name of owner or manager, number of employees. **Frequency:** Annual.

★4869★ **WHEEL CHAIRS RENTING DIRECTORY**
American Business Directories, Inc.
American Business Information, Inc.
5711 S. 86th Circle
Omaha, NE 68127   Phone: (402) 593-4600
Number of Listings: 1,120. **Entries Include:** Name, address, phone, size of advertisement, name of owner or manager, number of employees, year first in "Yellow Pages." **Frequency:** Annual.

★4870★ **WHEN SOMEONE YOU KNOW HAS AIDS: A PRACTICAL GUIDE**
Crown Publishers, Inc.
201 E. 50th St.
New York, NY 10022   Phone: (212) 572-6142
Publication Includes: List of organizations dealing with AIDS (Acquired Immune Deficiency Syndrome) related issues. **Entries Include:** Organization name, address, phone, geographical area served. **Frequency:** Published May 1987.

★4871★ **WHERE CAN MOM LIVE? A FAMILY GUIDE TO LIVING ARRANGEMENTS FOR ELDERLY PARENTS**
D. C. Heath & Co.
Lexington Books
125 Spring St.
Lexington, MA 02173   Phone: (617) 860-1580
Publication Includes: List of state government and private agencies that deal with the elderly and housing for the elderly. **Entries Include:** Agency name, address, phone. **Frequency:** Published October 1987.

★4872★ **WHO USES DRUGS?**
Chelsea House Publishers
Main Line Book Co.
95 Madison Ave.
New York, NY 10016   Phone: (212) 683-4400
Publication Includes: List of state agencies offering information and services relevant to drug use and abuse. **Frequency:** Published 1988.

★4873★ **WHO'S WHO IN AMERICAN NURSING**
Society of Nursing Professionals
3004 Glenview Rd.
Wilmette, IL 60091   Phone: (708) 441-2387
Covers: Approximately 30,000 nursing professionals, including educators, administrators, deans of nursing, directors of nursing, nurse practitioners, clinical supervisors, and others. **Entries Include:** Name, address, personal history, area of specialization, professional experience, education, professional organization membership, research interests, honors, publications, experience in public speaking. **Pages (approx.):** 1,000 (in two volumes). **Frequency:** Biennial, July of odd years.

★4874★ **WHO'S WHO IN AMERICAN PHARMACY**
American Pharmaceutical Association
2215 Constitution Ave. NW
Washington, DC 20037   Phone: (202) 429-7586
Covers: National organizations, state associations, colleges and state boards of pharmacy, and publications concerned with pharmacy and related subjects. **Entries Include:** Association name, address, phone. **Pages (approx.):** 60. **Frequency:** Annual, December.

★4875★ **WHO'S WHO IN THE BIOBEHAVIORAL SCIENCES**
Research Institute of Psychophysiology
525 Boynton Canyon Rd.
Sedona, AZ 86336   Phone: (602) 282-2900
Covers: Approximately 1,400 professionals in the biobehavioral sciences, including such disciplines as behavioral medicine, psychophysiology, biopsychiatry, health psychology, and holistic medicine. **Entries Include:** Name, address, credentials, current activities, association membership, awards or honors. **Pages (approx.):** 320. **Frequency:** Triennial; latest edition 1987.

★4876★   WHO'S WHO IN THE DENTAL LABORATORY INDUSTRY
National Association of Dental Laboratories
3801 Mt. Vernon Ave.
Alexandria, VA 22305   Phone: (703) 683-5263
Covers: About 3,300 dental laboratories; 12,000 certified dental technicians, manufacturers, and schools of dental technology. **Entries Include:** Company name, address, phone, name of owner, certification status, product or service. **Pages (approx.):** 200. **Frequency:** Annual, September.

★4877★   WHO'S WHO IN GERONTOLOGY: GSA MEMBERSHIP DIRECTORY
Gerontological Society of America (GSA)
1275 K St., NW, Ste. 350
Washington, DC 20005   Phone: (202) 842-1275
Number of Listings: 5,050. **Entries Include:** Personal name, address, phone. **Pages (approx.):** 150. **Frequency:** Published 1986.

★4878★   WOMEN'S AUXILIARY OF THE INTERNATIONAL CHIROPRACTORS ASSOCIATION—MEMBERSHIP ROSTER
Women's Auxiliary of the International Chiropractors Association
1925 Apple Ave.
Muskegon, MI 49442   Phone: (616) 777-2622
Covers: About 500 women who are chiropractic assistants, chiropractors, or related to members of the ICA. **Frequency:** Biennial.

★4879★   WORLD ASSOCIATION FOR THE ADVANCEMENT OF VETERINARY PARASITOLOGY—STATUTES/LIST OF MEMBERS
World Association for the Advancement of Veterinary Parasitology
SmithKline Beecham Animal Health
Applebrook Center
1600 Paoli Dr.
West Chester, PA 19380   Phone: (215) 251-7416
Covers: Approximately 385 veterinarians and other scientists in 55 countries interested in veterinary parasitology. **Frequency:** Biennial.

★4880★   WORLD ASSOCIATION OF SOCIETIES OF PATHOLOGY-ANATOMIC AND CLINICA L—DIRECTORY
World Association of Societies of Pathology-Anatomic and Clinical
Department of Clinical Pathology
Jichi Medical School
Minamikawachi-Machi
Tochigi-Ken 329-04, Japan
Covers: 45 national societies of anatomic and clinical pathology. **Entries Include:** Organization name, address, names and titles of key personnel, geographical. **Pages (approx.):** 70. **Frequency:** Biennial, spring of odd years.

★4881★   WORLD DIRECTORY OF BIOLOGICAL AND MEDICAL SCIENCES LIBRARIES
K. G. Saur, Inc.
R. R. Bowker Co.
121 Chanlon Rd.
New Providence, NJ 07974   Phone: (201) 665-2874
Pages (approx.): 215. **Frequency:** Latest edition March 1988.

★4882★   WORLD DIRECTORY OF GAY/LESBIAN GROUPS OF ALCOHOLICS ANONYMOUS
International Advisory Council for Homosexual Men and Women in Alcoholics Anonymous
Box 90
Washington, DC 20044   Phone: (202) 293-4022
Number of Listings: About 450. **Entries Include:** Group name, address, meeting information; some listings include name and phone of contact. **Pages (approx.):** 40. **Frequency:** Biennial, even years.

★4883★   WORLD DIRECTORY OF MEDICAL SCHOOLS
Division of Development of Human Resources for Health
World Health Organization
Avenue Appia
CH-1211 Geneva 27, Switzerland
Covers: Undergraduate medical teaching institutions in about 130 countries and territories. **Entries Include:** Name of institution, address, year in which instruction began, admission requirements, duration of program, language of instruction, degree awarded, number of students and graduates (separate figures are given for men and women, nationals and foreigners) number of teaching staff, license to practice. **Pages (approx.):** 310. **Frequency:** Irregular; latest edition 1988 (1983-84 data); new edition

possible 1994. **Available in the U.S. from:** WHO Publications Center USA, 49 Sheridan Ave., Albany, NY 12210 (518-436-9686).

★4884★   WORLD DIRECTORY OF SCHOOLS OF PUBLIC HEALTH
Division of Development of Human Resources for Health
World Health Organization
Avenue Appia
CH-1211 Geneva 27, Switzerland
Covers: About 215 educational institutions worldwide that have public health postgraduate degree or diploma programs. **Entries Include:** Name, address, year course established, number of teaching staff, number of students in all courses, number of students in public health course. **Pages (approx.):** 190. **Frequency:** Irregular; latest edition 1985; new edition possible 1993. **Available in the U.S. from:** WHO Publications Center USA, 49 Sheridan Ave., Albany, NY 12210.

★4885★   WORLD FEDERATION OF ASSOCIATIONS OF CLINICAL TOXICOLOGY CENTERS AND POISON CONTROL CENTERS—MEMBERSHIP LIST
World Federation of Associations of Clinical Toxicology Centers and
    Poison Control Centers
c/o CIRC
150, cours Albert-Thomas
F-69372 Lyon, France
Covers: National and international organizations dealing with toxicology; associations of poison control centers; and national poison control centers. **Pages (approx.):** 40. **Frequency:** Irregular.

★4886★   WORLD FEDERATION OF NEUROSURGICAL SOCIETIES—WORLD DIRECTORY
World Federation of Neurosurgical Societies
c/o Dr. Sean Mullen
Medical Center, Neurosurgery
5841 S. Maryland Ave.
Chicago, IL 60637

★4887★   WORLD FEDERATION OF SOCIETIES OF ANAESTHESIOLOGISTS—DIRECTORY OF MEMBER SOCIETIES
World Federation of Societies of Anaesthesiologists
Pantai Medical Center
8 Jalan Bukit Panti
Kuala Lumpur, Malaysia
Covers: Approximately 80 societies of anesthesiologists. **Frequency:** Annual.

★4888★   WORLD LIST OF FAMILY PLANNING ADDRESSES
International Planned Parenthood Federation
Regent's College
Inner Circle
Regent's Park
London NW1 4NS, England
Covers: National family planning associations in nearly 150 countries. **Entries Include:** Organization name, address, phone, cable address, whether member of the IPPF or of the Caribbean Family Planning Affiliation. **Pages (approx.):** 30. **Frequency:** Annual, July; latest edition 1991.

★4889★   A WORLD OF OPTIONS FOR THE 1990S: A GUIDE TO INTERNATIONAL EDUCATIONAL EXCHANGE, COMMUNITY SERVICE...FOR PERSONS WITH DISABILITIES
Mobility International USA
PO Box 3551
Eugene, OR 97403   Phone: (503) 343-1284
Covers: About 200 educational programs, workcamps, transportation and travel advisory services for persons with disabilities. **Entries Include:** Name, address, phone, geographical area served, financial data, eligibility requirements, descriptions of projects and services. **Pages (approx.):** 338. **Frequency:** Irregular; latest edition 1990. **Also Includes:** Personal accounts written by past participants, describing international educational and travel experiences.

★4890★ WORLD ORGANIZATION OF GASTROENTEROLOGY—NEWSLETTER
World Organization of Gastroenterology
2nd Department of Medicine
Technical University
Ismaningerstr. 22
W-8000 Munich, Germany
Publication Includes: List of the medical doctors and professors who are presidents and secretaries of the organization's more than 70 national member societies. **Entries Include:** Association name, name and address of president, name and address of secretary. **Frequency:** Irregular; latest edition 1990; new edition expected 1991.

★4891★ WORLD PHARMACEUTICALS DIRECTORY
Pharmaco-Medical Documentation Inc.
PO Box 429
Chatham, NJ 07928   Phone: (201) 822-9200
Covers: Companies that manufacture medicinal drugs and pharmaceutical research chemicals, originally not listed in "Known Drug Compendia", international coverage. **Entries Include:** Company name, address, phone, mnemonic company code name, type of drug or chemical produced, ingredients. **Pages (approx.):** 600. **Frequency:** Biennial, January of even years.

★4892★ WORLD VETERINARY ASSOCIATION—LIST OF MEMBERS
World Veterinary Association
Calle Isabel la Catolica, Numero 12
E-28018 Madrid, Spain
Covers: Approximately 20 international, 75 national, and 5 commercial organizations. **Entries Include:** Name, address, voting rights. **Pages (approx.):** 20. **Frequency:** Annual, April.

★4893★ WORLD VETERINARY DIRECTORY
World Veterinary Association
Principe de Vergara 276, 60E
E-28016 Madrid, Spain
Covers: Veterinary schools and faculties worldwide; distributors of approximately 3,000 audiovisual aids; veterinary associations, journals, and research institute s. **Entries Include:** For schools and faculties—Name, address, phone, fax, telex, year founded, type of center, clinical resources, experimental farms, length of study, number of faculty, number of students (male and female), admission criteria, post-graduate studies available. For distributors—Title, year of production; distributor name, address, phone, fax; language, duration. For associations and research institutes—Name, address, phone. For journals—Title; publisher name, address, phone. **Pages (approx.):** 430. **Frequency:** First edition 1991; new edition expected 1995. **Also Includes:** General information on each country, such as population, number of veterinarians, etc.

★4894★ WORLDWIDE AIDS DIRECTORY
Technology Management Group
25 Science Park
New Haven, CT 06511   Phone: (203) 786-5445
Covers: Nearly 800 manufacturers, 700 research institutions, and 540 other AIDS-related organizations; international coverage. **Entries Include:** Company or institution name, address, phone, names and titles of key personnel; products or services provided, collaborating organizations, current research projects and product development, conferences held, etc. **Pages (approx.):** 545. **Frequency:** Published October 1987.

★4895★ X-RAY APPARATUS AND SUPPLIES DIRECTORY
American Business Directories, Inc.
American Business Information, Inc.
5711 S. 86th Circle
Omaha, NE 68127   Phone: (402) 593-4600
Number of Listings: 1,913. **Entries Include:** Name, address, phone, size of advertisement, name of owner or manager, number of employees, year first in "Yellow Pages." **Frequency:** Annual.

★4896★ X-RAY FILMS
Theta Corp.
Theta Bldg.
Middlefield, CT 06455   Phone: (203) 349-1054
Publication Includes: List of about 20 manufacturers of X-ray films and supplies. **Entries Include:** Company name, address, phone, key personnel, background information, description of products, marketing strategy, annual sales, research and development efforts, distribution systems, five year projection. **Frequency:** Irregular; previous edition February 1988; latest edition April 1990.

★4897★ X-RAY LABORATORIES MEDICAL DIRECTORY
American Business Directories, Inc.
American Business Information, Inc.
5711 S. 86th Circle
Omaha, NE 68127   Phone: (402) 593-4600
Number of Listings: 1,796. **Entries Include:** Name, address, phone, size of advertisement, name of owner or manager, number of employees, year first in "Yellow Pages." **Frequency:** Annual.

★4898★ YEARBOOK OF THE ROYAL SOCIETY
The Royal Society
6 Carlton House Terrace
London SW1Y 5AG, England
Covers: 1,100 fellows of the society in fields of science, engineering, and medicine. **Entries Include:** Name, address, phone, telex. **Pages (approx.):** 390. **Frequency:** Annual, February. **Also Includes:** Description of services and activities of the society.

★4899★ YELLOW FEVER VACCINATING CENTRES FOR INTERNATIONAL TRAVEL
Division of Epidemiological Surveillance and Health Situation and Trend Assessment
World Health Organization
20, avenue Appia
CH-1211 Geneva 27, Switzerland
Covers: Designated yellow fever vaccinating centers worldwide. **Entries Include:** Name of vaccination center, location. **Pages (approx.):** 70. **Frequency:** Irregular; previous edition January 1985; latest edition January 1991. **Available in the U.S. from:** World Health Organization Publications Centre, 49 Sheridan Avenue, Albany, NY 10017.

★4900★ YOUTH IN TRANSITION: A DESCRIPTION OF SELECTED PROGRAMS SERVING ADOLESCENTS WITH EMOTIONAL DISABILITIES
Portland State University
Mental Health
Regional Research Institute for Human Services
PO Box 751
Portland, OR 97207-0751   Phone: (503) 725-4040
Covers: Residential treatment, hospital and school-based, case management, and multi-service agencies for young people with emotional disabilities. **Entries Include:** Program name, address, phone, funding, philosophy, staffing, programs components, services. **Pages (approx.):** 163.

(6) Publishers

The following are listed alphabetically by publisher names. For additional information, see the User's Guide located at the front of this directory.

★4901★ **A GRANITE PUBLISHERS**
80 Granada Dr.
Kenner, LA 70065   Phone: (504) 443-5765
Description: Publishes a nonfiction paperback in the consumer health or personal finance fields for educated adults interested in in consumer health or entrepreneurship.

★4902★ **AACC PRESS**
2029 K St. NW, 7th Fl.
Washington, DC 20006
Description: "A nonprofit national organization of chemists, physicians, and other scientists who specialize in clinical chemistry." Publishes on clinical chemistry and related health sciences.

★4903★ **ABBE PUBLISHERS ASSOCIATION OF WASHINGTON, DC**
4111 Gallows Rd.
Annandale, VA 22003-1862   Phone: (703) 750-0255
Description: Publishes on all subjects particularly scientific, medical, and scholarly books.

★4904★ **ABILITY WORKSHOP PRESS**
24861 Alicia Pkwy., No. 292
Laguna Hills, CA 92653   Phone: (714) 661-5779
Description: Publishes fiction and nonfiction books on self-help, psychology, philosophy, and learning disabilities.

★4905★ **ABLEX PUBLISHING CORPORATION**
355 Chestnut St.
Norwood, NJ 07648   Phone: (201) 767-8450
Description: Publishes textbooks, research journals, edited volumes, and monographs on computers and social sciences, including psychology.

★4906★ **ABLIN PRESS**
c/o Ablin Press Distributors
3332 Hadfield Greene
Sarasota, FL 34235   Phone: (813) 377-4512
Description: Publishes art therapy books.

★4907★ **ABRAHAMSON PUBLISHING COMPANY**
10164 Norell Ave.
Stillwater, MN 55082   Phone: (612) 439-2680
Description: Publishes health and fitness books.

★4908★ **ACADEMIC GUILD PUBLISHERS**
PO Box 397
Cambridge, MA 02238   Phone: (617) 491-1354
Description: Publishes on medicine, nutrition, developmental disability, and mental retardation for reference use, professionals, and for parents.

★4909★ **ACADEMIC PRESS, INC.**
1250 6th Ave.
San Diego, CA 92101   Phone: (619) 699-6412
Description: Publishes scientific and technical materials, including textbooks in the medical sciences.

★4910★ **ACADEMIC THERAPY PUBLICATIONS**
20 Commercial Blvd.
Novato, CA 94949-6191   Phone: (415) 883-3314
Description: Publishes tests, remedial curriculum materials, and professional/parent resourse books to identify and remediate learning disabilities. **Subject Specialties:** Learning disabilities, remedial reading, ESL, adult education.

★4911★ **A.C.A.T. PRESS**
1275 4th St.
Santa Rosa, CA 95404   Phone: (707) 576-7564
Description: Publishes materials for adult children of alcoholics.

★4912★ **ACCELERATED DEVELOPMENT, INC.**
3400 Kilgore
Muncie, IN 47304   Phone: (317) 284-7511
Description: Publishes psychology materials for psychologists, professional counselors, and clients. Offers textbooks and audio tapes.

★4913★ **ACCORD PRESS**
PO Box 9432
San Jose, CA 95157   Phone: (408) 446-2423
Description: Publishes on psychology and self-help.

★4914★ **ACHIEVEMENT PRESS**
1501 Fort Mackenzie Rd.
PO Box 608
Sheridan, WY 82801
Description: Publishes consumer-oriented publications on health-related topics. **Subject Specialties:** Health, Wyoming, breastfeeding, childbirth.

★4915★ **ACORN PUBLISHING**
PO Box 7067
Syracuse, NY 13261   Phone: (315) 689-7072
Description: Publishes on fitness and recreation.

★4916★ ACTIVITY FACTORY
2227 Rock Island Ct.
Snellville, GA 30278   Phone: (404) 979-5727
Description: Publishes books on recreation ideas for nursing home activity programs.

★4917★ ACU PRESS
1533 Shattuck Ave.
Berkeley, CA 94709   Phone: (415) 845-1069
Description: Publishes self-help and how-to books and cassettes on stress management, fitness, first aid, beauty, diet, and health.

★4918★ ACUPINCH OUTREACH CENTER
2989 McCully Dr. NE
Atlanta, GA 30345   Phone: (404) 939-1678
Subject Specialties: Health, self-help, how-to, sports, the elderly.

★4919★ ADAPTIVE LIVING
PO Box 60857
Rochester, NY 14606   Phone: (716) 458-5455
Description: Publishes on dwarfism and other disabilities.

★4920★ ADDICTION REVIEW
Box 396
Mendham, NJ 07945   Phone: (201) 543-5775
Description: Publishes a children's book on drug and alcohol abuse.

★4921★ ADDISON-WESLEY LONGMAN
Rte. 128
Reading, MA 01867   Phone: (617) 944-3700
Description: Publishes books on medicine, as well as other subjects.

★4922★ ADRENAL METABOLIC RESEARCH SOCIETY OF THE HYPOGLYCEMIA FOUNDATION
153 Pawling Ave.
Troy, NY 12180   Phone: (518) 272-7154
Description: Publishes information on hypoglycemia.

★4923★ AEROBICS AND FITNESS ASSOCIATION OF AMERICA
15250 Ventura Blvd., No. 310
Sherman Oaks, CA 91403   Phone: (818) 905-0040
Description: Publishes on aerobic exercise for fitness professionals and enthusiasts, sports enthusiasts, and aerobic exercise instructors. **Subject Specialties:** Fitness industry news, health, travel, fashion.

★4924★ AERO-MEDICAL CONSULTANTS
10912 Hamlin Blvd.
Largo, FL 34644   Phone: (813) 596-2551
Subject Specialties: Aviation, medical.

★4925★ AEROSPACE MEDICAL ASSOCIATION
320 S. Henry St.
Alexandria, VA 22314-3524   Phone: (703) 739-2240
Subject Specialties: Aerospace medicine.

★4926★ AESCULAPIUS PUBLISHING COMPANY
700 18th St. S., Ste. 511
Birmingham, AL 35233-1800   Phone: (205) 933-6888
Description: Publishes on ophthalmology.

★4927★ AFCOM PUBLISHING
24147 Eastvale
Rolling Hills Estate, CA 90274   Phone: (213) 335-1534
Description: Self-publisher of fiction, nonfiction, how to, and business books. **Subject Specialties:** Health, how-to, children's books, business books on total management.

★4928★ AFTERWORDS PUBLISHING
5124 Grove St.
Minneapolis, MN 55436   Phone: (612) 929-6448
Description: Publishes on suicide and suicide grief.

★4929★ AGATHON PRESS
111 8th Ave.
New York, NY 10011   Phone: (212) 741-3087
Description: Publishes scholarly books for academics in the fields of political science, higher education, early childhood education, and childhood sexual development.

★4930★ AIGA PUBLICATIONS
PO Box 148
Laie, HI 96762   Phone: (808) 293-5277
Description: Publishes public health information in many languages on Hansen's disease. **Subject Specialties:** Medical/health, computers, contract bridge, anthropology.

★4931★ AIR-PLUS ENTERPRISES
PO Box 190
Garrisonville, VA 22463
Description: An information agency dealing with women's health and sexuality. In addition to publishing, does some research of medical literature, provides information for students' term papers, etc. **Subject Specialties:** Legal abortion, women's health and sexuality.

★4932★ ALAMITOS HEALTH PUBLICATIONS
3801 Katella Ave., Ste. 230
Los Alamitos, CA 90720   Phone: (213) 598-9428
Subject Specialties: Health.

★4933★ ALAN GUTTMACHER INSTITUTE
111 5th Ave.
New York, NY 10003   Phone: (212) 254-5656
Description: Publishes research and policy analysis in the field of reproductive health. **Subject Specialties:** Family planning, population, abortion, sex education, prenatal and maternity care, adolescent sexuality, women's rights, law, and policy.

★4934★ ALCOHOLICS ANONYMOUS WORLD SERVICES, INC.
468 Park Ave. S.
New York, NY 10016   Phone: (212) 686-1100
Description: Presents the recovery program of Alcoholics Anonymous.

★4935★ ALDINE DE GRUYTER
200 Saw Mill River Rd.
Hawthorne, NY 10532   Phone: (914) 747-0110
Description: Publishes books and journals in the behavioral and social sciences. **Subject Specialties:** Sociology, social work, anthropology, political science, communications, psychology.

★4936★ ALEF BET COMMUNICATIONS
14809 Bremer Rd.
New Haven, IN 46774   Phone: (219) 749-0182
Description: Publishes materials on medicine and religion.

★4937★ ALEXA PRESS, INC.
PO Box 523
East Hampton, NY 11937   Phone: (516) 324-0405
Subject Specialties: Psychoanalysis, psychohistory.

★4938★ ALEXANDER GRAHAM BELL ASSOCIATION FOR THE DEAF
3417 Volta Pl. NW
Washington, DC 20007   Phone: (202) 337-5220
Description: Publishes special education books, journals, monographs, and audio-visual materials mainly for hearing impaired people.

★4939★ ALFRED ADLER INSTITUTE OF CHICAGO
618 S. Michigan Ave., 6th Fl.
Chicago, IL 60605-1901   Phone: (312) 294-7100
Description: Publishes materials on Adlerian psychology for professionals and laymen.

★4940★ ALIN FOUNDATION PRESS
1 Alin Plaza
2107 Dwight at Shattuck
Berkeley, CA 94704   Phone: (415) 644-3366
Description: Publishes scientific and biomedical information, as well as information on topics of broad social and economic concern.

★4941★   ALINDA PRESS
PO Box 553
Eureka, CA 95502   Phone: (707) 442-6856
Subject Specialties: Deaf education, sign language, public enlightenment about deafness.

★4942★   ALLERGY PUBLICATIONS INC.
1259 El Camino Real, Ste. 254
Menlo Park, CA 94025   Phone: (415) 322-1663
Description: Publishes allergy information for allergy sufferers and the professionals who work with them. Also offers recipe books, educational booklets, and directories. **Subject Specialties:** Allergy, asthma.

★4943★   ALLIANCE PRESS
3911 5th Ave., Ste. 202
San Diego, CA 92103   Phone: (619) 296-1116
Description: Self-publishes a book on aging and mental health.

★4944★   ALM PUBLISHERS, INC.
12230 N. 103rd Pl.
Scottsdale, AZ 85260   Phone: (800) 367-3981
Description: Publishes books on health and the prevention and treatment of diseases.

★4945★   ALORAY, INC.
215 Greenwich Ave.
Goshen, NY 10924   Phone: (914) 294-9143
Description: Publishes occupational health safety and industrial hygiene books for college students and professionals.

★4946★   AMBERLY PUBLICATIONS
PO Box 4153
Chapel Hill, NC 27515   Phone: (919) 968-3963
Description: Publishes on human interest topics and social issues such as adoption and drug and alcohol abuse.

★4947★   AMBLESIDE PUBLISHERS, INC.
2122 E. Concorda Dr.
Tempe, AZ 85282   Phone: (602) 967-3457

★4948★   AMERICAN ACADEMY OF ALLERGY AND IMMUNOLOGY
611 E. Wells St., 4th Fl.
Milwaukee, WI 53202   Phone: (414) 272-6071
Description: A nonprofit association founded for the advancement of the knowledge and practice of allergy and immunology, by discussion at meetings, by fostering the education of students and the public, by encouraging union and cooperation among those engaged in the field, and by promoting and stimulating research and study in allergy and immunology.

★4949★   AMERICAN ACADEMY OF ORTHOPAEDIC SURGEONS
222 S. Prospect Ave.
Park Ridge, IL 60068   Phone: (708) 823-7186
Description: Publishes medical and educational books for orthopedists, emergency medical services personnel, and athletic trainers.

★4950★   AMERICAN ACADEMY OF PEDIATRICS
141 Northwest Point Blvd.
Elk Grove Village, IL 60007   Phone: (800) 433-9016
Description: Offers professional education for pediatricians and other health professionals with reference manuals on topics such as infectious diseases, nutrition, and perinatal care. Offers a newsletter and brochures.

★4951★   AMERICAN ALLERGY ASSOCIATION
PO Box 7273
Menlo Park, CA 94026   Phone: (415) 322-1663
Description: Publishes materials on allergies and asthma.

★4952★   AMERICAN ALLIANCE FOR HEALTH, PHYSICAL EDUCATION, RECREATION & DANCE
1900 Association Dr.
Reston, VA 22091   Phone: (703) 476-3400
Description: Publishes professional literature on teaching physical education, recreation, and dance.

★4953★   AMERICAN ASSOCIATION OF AVIAN PATHOLOGISTS
c/o R. J. Eckroade
New Bolton Center
382 W. Street Rd.
Kennett Square, PA 19348   Phone: (215) 444-5800
Description: Assists teachers, researchers, and scientists in avian pathology and avian diseases. **Subject Specialties:** Avian pathology, avian diseases.

★4954★   AMERICAN ASSOCIATION OF BLOOD BANKS
1117 N. 19th St., Ste. 600
Arlington, VA 22209   Phone: (703) 528-8200
Description: Publishes monographs of technical scientific and administrative workshops. **Subject Specialties:** Blood banking, immunohematology, hematology.

★4955★   AMERICAN ASSOCIATION OF CHILDREN'S RESIDENTIAL CENTERS
440 1st St. NW, Ste. 310
Washington, DC 20001   Phone: (202) 638-1604
Description: Publishes proceedings from meetings and a directory of members.

★4956★   AMERICAN ASSOCIATION FOR CLINICAL CHEMISTRY
2029 K St. NW, 7th Fl.
Washington, DC 20006   Phone: (202) 857-0717
Description: "A nonprofit national organization of chemists, physicians, and other scientists who specialize in clinical chemistry." Publishes on clinical chemistry and related health sciences.

★4957★   AMERICAN ASSOCIATION OF COLLEGES OF PHARMACY
4720 Montgomery Ln.
Ste. 602
Bethesda, MD 20814   Phone: (301) 654-9060
Subject Specialties: Pharmacy education.

★4958★   AMERICAN ASSOCIATION FOR COUNSELING AND DEVELOPMENT
5999 Stevenson Ave.
Alexandria, VA 22304   Phone: (703) 823-9800
Description: Publishes books, journals, films, and videotapes for use by counselors, educators, administrators, students, other counseling and human development specialists. In addition, AACD produces some material for use by the general public.

★4959★   AMERICAN ASSOCIATION OF CRITICAL-CARE NURSES
101 Columbia
Aliso Viejo, CA 92656   Phone: (714) 362-2000
Description: Offers educational and research publications and computer-assisted instruction for critical-care nurses.

★4960★   AMERICAN ASSOCIATION OF DENTAL SCHOOLS
1625 Massachusetts Ave. NW
Washington, DC 20036   Phone: (202) 667-9433
Description: Designed to inform readers of new and pertinent information in the dental education field.

★4961★   AMERICAN ASSOCIATION OF DIABETES EDUCATORS
500 N. Michigan Ave., Ste. 1400
Chicago, IL 60611   Phone: (312) 661-1700
Description: Publishes original literature from all disciplines involved in diabetes patient education.

★4962★   AMERICAN ASSOCIATION OF HOMES FOR THE AGING
1129 20th St. NW, Ste. 400
Washington, DC 20036-3489   Phone: (202) 296-5960
Description: Publishes paperback books about homes for the aging. **Subject Specialties:** Retirement homes, nursing homes, volunteers.

★4963★ AMERICAN ASSOCIATION ON MENTAL RETARDATION
1719 Kalorama Rd. NW
Washington, DC 20009   Phone: (202) 387-1968
Description: Disseminates basic and applied research, program advances, and public policyguidelines among professionals in a variety of disciplines and interested lay advocates. **Subject Specialties:** Mental retardation: psychology, education, medicine, administration, etc.

★4964★ AMERICAN ASSOCIATION OF SEX EDUCATORS, COUNSELORS, AND THERAPISTS
435 N. Michigan Ave., Ste. 1717
Chicago, IL 60611   Phone: (312) 644-0828
Description: A nonprofit, professional association promoting standards of education, training, research, ethics, and patient care in the diverse aspects of human sexuality. Publishes a journal, a newsletter, monographs, and related materials.

★4965★ AMERICAN BOARD OF EXAMINERS IN CLINICAL SOCIAL WORK
8484 Georgia Ave., Ste. 800
Silver Spring, MD 20910-5604   Phone: (301) 587-8783
Description: Publishes a directory of advanced clinical social workers.

★4966★ AMERICAN BOARD OF MEDICAL SPECIALTIES
1 Rotary Center, Ste. 805
Evanston, IL 60201-4889   Phone: (708) 491-9091
Description: Publishes biographical directories biennially for each of twenty-four medical specialty areas. Also publishes case bound books on topics relevant to the evaluations of physicians and the validity of testing methods. Also offers mailing labels of physicians.

★4967★ AMERICAN BOARD OF ORTHODONTICS
225 S. Meramec
St. Louis, MO 63105   Phone: (317) 727-5039
Description: Publishes a directory of orthodontists.

★4968★ AMERICAN CITIZENS CONCERNED FOR LIFE, INC./ACCL COMMUNICATIONS CENTER
PO Box 179
Excelsior, MN 55331   Phone: (612) 474-0885
Description: A national nonprofit organization engaged in educational, research, and service activities "to promote respect for all human life in contemporary society." Also publishes a counseling manual and booklets.

★4969★ AMERICAN COLLEGE OF APOTHECARIES
205 Daingerfield Rd.
Alexandria, VA 22314   Phone: (703) 684-8603
Description: Disseminates research data and developments in professional practice for practicing pharmacists, pharmacy students, the pharmaceutical industry, and the public.

★4970★ AMERICAN COLLEGE OF CHEST PHYSICIANS
3300 Dundee Rd.
Northbrook, IL 60062-2303   Phone: (708) 698-2200
Description: Sponsors postgraduate courses, meetings, cassettes, periodicals, and books for physicians.

★4971★ AMERICAN COLLEGE HEALTH ASSOCIATION
1300 Piccard Dr., Ste. 200
Rockville, MD 20850   Phone: (301) 963-1100
Description: Publishes a variety of education materials and literature to promote wellness in the higher education community.

★4972★ AMERICAN COLLEGE OF NURSE-MIDWIVES
1522 K St. NW, Ste. 1000
Washington, DC 20005   Phone: (202) 347-5445
Description: Publishes articles and information of interest to certified nurses-midwives, women of child-bearing age, and health care.

★4973★ AMERICAN COLLEGE OF OSTEOPATHIC SURGEONS
123 N. Henry St.
Alexandria, VA 22314   Phone: (703) 684-0416
Description: Publishes a monthly newsletter and an annual directory.

★4974★ AMERICAN COLLEGE OF PHYSICIAN EXECUTIVES
4890 W. Kennedy Blvd., Ste. 200
Tampa, FL 33609   Phone: (813) 287-2000
Description: Publishes current information on health care management as it pertains to physicians managing health care organizations.

★4975★ AMERICAN COLLEGE OF SPORTS MEDICINE
PO Box 1440
Indianapolis, IN 46206-1440   Phone: (215) 922-1330
Description: Publishes monographs and other major publications.

★4976★ AMERICAN CONFERENCE OF GOVERNMENTAL INDUSTRIAL HYGIENISTS
6500 Glenway Ave., Bldg. D-7
Cincinnati, OH 45211   Phone: (513) 661-7881
Description: Devoted to the development of administrative and technical aspects of worker health protection. Publishes material in this field. **Subject Specialties:** Industrial hygiene.

★4977★ AMERICAN COUNCIL ON ALCOHOLISM
5024 Campbell Blvd., Ste. H
Baltimore, MD 21236   Phone: (301) 529-9206
Description: Promotes public education on alcoholism and alcohol abuse by distributing pamphlets and other literature.

★4978★ AMERICAN COUNCIL FOR DRUG EDUCATION
204 Monroe St.
Rockville, MD 20850   Phone: (301) 294-0600
Description: A nonprofit organization dedicated to educating the American public about problems associated with illicit drug use. Produces educational materials which include monographs, brochures, newsletters and films.

★4979★ AMERICAN DANCE THERAPY ASSOCIATION
2000 Century Plaza, Ste. 108
Columbia, MD 21044   Phone: (301) 997-4040
Description: A professional organization to promote education and competency in the field. Publishes a newsletter, journal, monographs, bibliographies, and conference proceedings.

★4980★ AMERICAN DEAFNESS AND REHABILITATION ASSOCIATION
PO Box 251554
Little Rock, AR 72225   Phone: (501) 663-7074
Description: Promotes the development and expansion of professional rehabilitation services for the adult deaf, provides a forum and a common meeting ground to bring about a better understanding of deaf people. **Subject Specialties:** Deafness, handicapped, mental health, social work, rehabilitation.

★4981★ AMERICAN DENTAL ASSOCIATION
211 E. Chicago Ave.
Chicago, IL 60611   Phone: (312) 440-2500
Description: Publishes professional books, journals, and aids. Also dental health education materials for the public, school curriculum guides, posters, models, kits, and pamphlets.

★4982★ AMERICAN DIETETIC ASSOCIATION
216 W. Jackson Blvd.
Chicago, IL 60606-6995   Phone: (312) 899-0040
Description: Publishes refereed reports of original research and other papers covering the broad aspects of dietetics, including nutrition and diet therapy, community nutrition, education and training, and administration.

★4983★ AMERICAN FOUNDATION FOR THE BLIND
15 W. 16th St.
New York, NY 10011   Phone: (212) 620-2000
Description: Publishes professional, research, and public education materials about blindness and visual impairment. **Subject Specialties:** Blindness, visual impairment, training, education, technology.

★4984★ AMERICAN GROUP PRACTICE ASSOCIATION
1422 Duke St.
Alexandria, VA 22314   Phone: (703) 838-0033
Description: Serves the needs and interests of physicians engaged in group practice.

★4985★ AMERICAN GROUP PSYCHOTHERAPY ASSOCIATION
25 E. 21st St., 6th Fl.
New York, NY 10010   Phone: (212) 477-2677
Subject Specialties: Group psychotherapy.

★4986★ AMERICAN HEALTH AND NUTRITION
262 Larkspur Plaza Dr.
Larkspur, CA 94939-1404
Description: Publishes books on physical and mental health and nutrition.

★4987★ AMERICAN HOSPITAL ASSOCIATION
840 N. Lake Shore Dr.
Chicago, IL 60611   Phone: (800) AHA-2626
Description: Publishes books on hospitals and health care.

★4988★ AMERICAN HOSPITAL PUBLISHING, INC.
211 E. Chicago Ave.
Chicago, IL 60611   Phone: (312) 440-6800
Description: Publishes administration books, reference books, and manuals on health care.

★4989★ AMERICAN INSTITUTE OF THE HISTORY OF PHARMACY
University of Wisconsin
School of Pharmacy
425 N. Charter St.
Madison, WI 53706   Phone: (608) 262-5378
Description: Publishes the quarterly *Pharmacy in History* and other booklets on the history of pharmaceuticals and the history of the field of pharmacy. Offers notecards, slides, and calendars. **Subject Specialties:** History of pharmacy and pharmaceuticals.

★4990★ AMERICAN INSTITUTE FOR PSYCHOLOGICAL RESEARCH
PO Box 27040
Albuquerque, NM 87125-7040   Phone: (505) 296-2320
Subject Specialties: Psychology.

★4991★ AMERICAN INSTITUTE OF ULTRASOUND IN MEDICINE
11200 Rockville Pike, Ste. 205
Rockville, MD 20852-3139   Phone: (301) 656-6117
Description: Publishes journals and texts "to advance the art and science of ultrasound in medicine and research."

★4992★ AMERICAN MEDIA
PO Box 4646
Westlake Village, CA 91359   Phone: (805) 496-1649
Description: Publishes nonfiction in areas such as health, nutrition, politics, creation. Reaches market through direct mail.

★4993★ AMERICAN MEDICAL ASSOCIATION
515 N. State St.
Chicago, IL 60610   Phone: (312) 464-5000
Description: Publishes books on medicine with a wide variety of medical topics, including medical law, insurance, children's issues, statistics, and medical practice.

★4994★ AMERICAN NATURAL HYGIENE SOCIETY
PO Box 30630
Tampa, FL 33630   Phone: (813) 855-6607
Subject Specialties: Natural living, health.

★4995★ AMERICAN NURSES' ASSOCIATION
2420 Pershing Rd.
Kansas City, MO 64108   Phone: (816) 474-5720
Description: The professional organization for registered nurses in the United States. Address orders to: Publications Distribution Center, PO Box 90660, Washington, DC 20090-0660. **Subject Specialties:** Nursing education, practice, research, statistics, economic and general welfare of nurses.

★4996★ AMERICAN OCCUPATIONAL THERAPY ASSOCIATION
1383 Piccard Dr.
PO Box 1725
Rockville, MD 20850-4375   Phone: (301) 948-9626
Description: Publishes materials on improving the quality of occupational therapy services.

★4997★ AMERICAN OSTEOPATHIC HOSPITAL ASSOCIATION
1454 Duke St.
Alexandria, VA 22314   Phone: (703) 684-7700
Description: Publishes various manuals, periodicals, and guidelines on management of osteopathic hospitals.

★4998★ AMERICAN PHARMACEUTICAL ASSOCIATION
2215 Constitution Ave. NW
Washington, DC 20037   Phone: (202) 628-4410
Description: The national professional society of pharmacists; publishes books on a broad range of pharmacy and drug-related, scientific and non-scientific topics.

★4999★ AMERICAN PHYSICAL THERAPY ASSOCIATION
1111 N. Fairfax St.
Alexandria, VA 22314   Phone: (703) 684-2782
Description: Publishes reference guides, monographs, brochures, and periodicals for physical therapy professionals on education, practice, research, and administration.

★5000★ AMERICAN PRINTING HOUSE FOR THE BLIND
PO Box 6085
Louisville, KY 40206   Phone: (505) 895-2405
Description: Publishes literature in all media (braille, large type, recorded) for the blind. Manufactures educational aids for special use by visually impaired students, such as K-12 textbooks, preschool and vocational materials, and talking educational software.

★5001★ AMERICAN PSYCHIATRIC PRESS, INC.
1400 K St. NW
Washington, DC 20005   Phone: (202) 682-6262
Description: A nonprofit company that publishes educational materials for psychiatrists.

★5002★ AMERICAN PSYCHOLOGICAL ASSOCIATION
1200 17th St. NW
Washington, DC 20036   Phone: (202) 955-7600
Description: Established to advance psychology as a science and profession. Produces material for professionals, students, and the public including books, scientific journals, microform publications, videos, and computer databases.

★5003★ AMERICAN PUBLIC HEALTH ASSOCIATION
1015 15th St. NW
Washington, DC 20005   Phone: (202) 789-5600
Description: Publishes on the public health and health care fields in the areas of laboratory science, epidemiology, and clinical investigation of use to researchers and practitioners.

★5004★ AMERICAN RUNNING AND FITNESS ASSOCIATION
9310 Old Georgetown Rd.
Bethesda, MD 20814   Phone: (301) 897-0197
Description: A non-profit educational association of athletes and sports medicine professionals. Publishes materials dealing with health and fitness, especially running.

★5005★ AMERICAN SCHOOL HEALTH ASSOCIATION
PO Box 708
Kent, OH 44240   Phone: (216) 678-1601
Description: Publishes on learning disabilities, tobacco and alcohol education, and school athletics.

★5006★ AMERICAN SOCIETY FOR ADOLESCENT PSYCHIATRY
4330 East-West Hwy., Ste. 1117
Bethesda, MD 20814   Phone: (301) 718-6502
Description: Offers an annual volume of papers, most of which were given at meetings. **Subject Specialties:** Mental health.

★5007★   AMERICAN SOCIETY OF ANIMAL SCIENCE
309 W. Clark St.
Champaign, IL 61820   Phone: (217) 356-3182
Description: Publishes papers presented at symposiums. **Subject Specialties:** Veterinary science.

★5008★   AMERICAN SOCIETY FOR HOSPITAL MATERIALS MANAGEMENT
840 N. Lake Shore Dr.
Chicago, IL 60611   Phone: (312) 280-6155
Description: Publishes handbooks and guideline reports that were developed to address current issues and new techniques, or to be used in the daily work setting of the hospital material or purchasing manager as a reference source.

★5009★   AMERICAN SOCIETY OF HOSPITAL PHARMACISTS
4630 Montgomery Ave.
Bethesda, MD 20814   Phone: (301) 657-3000
Description: Publishes books, journals, software, and videotapes on rational drug therapy in hospitals and other health care facilities.

★5010★   AMERICAN SOCIETY OF SAFETY ENGINEERS
1800 E. Oakton St.
Des Plaines, IL 60018-2187   Phone: (708) 692-4121
Description: Publishes the magazine *Professional Safety,* books, and course materials. Also provides technical material to practicing safety professionals. **Subject Specialties:** Safety engineering, safety management, fire protection, industrial hygiene, occupational health.

★5011★   AMERICAN SPEECH-LANGUAGE-HEARING ASSOCIATION
10801 Rockville Pike
Rockville, MD 20852   Phone: (301) 897-5700
Description: Publishes on speech and hearing.

★5012★   AMERICAN STUDENT DENTAL ASSOCIATION
211 E. Chicago Ave., Ste. 840
Chicago, IL 60611   Phone: (312) 440-2795
Description: Publishes guides to post-doctoral dental programs. Also offers three membership publications and reprints of national board exams. **Subject Specialties:** Dentistry for dental students and recent graduates.

★5013★   AMERICAN VETERINARY PUBLICATIONS, INC.
5782 Thornwood Dr.
Goleta, CA 93117-3896   Phone: (805) 967-5988
Description: Publishes text and reference books for the veterinary profession.

★5014★   AMERICAN YOUTH WORK CENTER
1751 N St. NW, Ste. 302
Washington, DC 20036   Phone: (202) 785-0764
Description: Assists youth programs and youth workers, conferences, and exchange programs. **Subject Specialties:** Youth, youth services, delinquency prevention, alcohol and drug abuse, runaways.

★5015★   AMY'S
PO Box 1718
Fort Myers, FL 33902   Phone: (313) 732-2118
Description: Self-publisher of book about nutrition to get rid of aches and pains.

★5016★   A/N ENTERPRISES, INC.
1129 20th St. NW, Ste. 400
Washington, DC 20036   Phone: (202) 296-5960
Description: A national nonprofit organization that represents nonprofit homes, housing, and health-related services and facilities for the elderly. Produces books, newsletters, and consumer brochures.

★5017★   ANALYTIC PRESS
365 Broadway
Hillsdale, NJ 07642   Phone: (201) 358-9477
Description: Publishes psychoanalytic books for mental health professionals. **Subject Specialties:** Psychoanalysis, Freud studies, science of man, applied analysis, women's studies.

★5018★   AND/OR PRESS, INC.
PO Box 2246
Berkeley, CA 94702   Phone: (415) 548-2124
Subject Specialties: Health, controlled substances.

★5019★   ANN WIGMORE FOUNDATION
196 Commonwealth Ave.
Boston, MA 02116-2503   Phone: (617) 267-9424
Description: A nonprofit organization and learning center implementing the principles of living food, wheatgrass chlorophyll, and care of the body for the restoration and maintenance of health.

★5020★   ANNUAL REVIEWS, INC.
4139 El Camino Way
Palo Alto, CA 94306   Phone: (415) 493-4400
Description: A nonprofit science publisher established to promote, by its publications and various activities, the advancement of the sciences. Publishes books and microforms. **Subject Specialties:** Life sciences, physical sciences, medical sciences, social sciences, naturalsciences, computer science.

★5021★   ANTHROPOSOPHIC PRESS INC.
RR 4, Box 94-A-1
Hudson, NY 12534   Phone: (518) 851-2054
Description: Publishes the works of Rudolf Steiner and other anthroposophic books. **Subject Specialties:** Agriculture, medicine, health, nutrition, education, spiritual science.

★5022★   ANTLER PUBLISHING COMPANY
3033 E. 3rd St.
Tucson, AZ 85716   Phone: (602) 881-0492
Description: Publishes medical, self-help, and how-to books for general markets and specialized markets such as libraries, schools and universities, community relations programs, police departments, and service organizations.

★5023★   APHRA BEHN PRESS
8080 W. Slope Dr. SW
Portland, OR 97225   Phone: (503) 646-0471
Description: Publishes biomedical texts and on the history and philosophy of modern science and technology.

★5024★   APLIC-INTERNATIONAL
c/o Population Council Library
1 Dag Hammarskjold Plaza
New York, NY 10017
Description: Publishes on the field of population and family planning for libraries and information centers.

★5025★   APPLE PRESS
5536 SE Harlow
Milwaukie, OR 97222   Phone: (503) 659-2475
Description: Publishes on food and health. Reaches market through commission representatives, direct mail, trade sales, Pacific Pipeline, and Royal Publications.

★5026★   APPLETON DAVIES, INC.
32 S. Raymond Ave., Ste. 4
Pasadena, CA 91105-1935   Phone: (818) 792-3046
Description: Publishes books and journals on medicine and surgery for professionals.

★5027★   APPLETON & LANGE
25 Van Zant St.
East Norwalk, CT 06855   Phone: (203) 838-4400
Description: Publishes medical and nursing periodicals and reference materials.

★5028★   APPLIED THERAPEUTICS, INC.
PO Box 5077
Vancouver, WA 98668-5077   Phone: (206) 253-7123
Description: Publishes textbooks for pharmacy students, physicians, nurses and other allied health professionals.

★5029★   APPRENTICE ACADEMICS
PO Box 788
Claremore, OK 74018-0788   Phone: (918) 342-1335
Description: Publishes on midwifery and childbirth education.

★5030★   AQUARIAN RESEARCH FOUNDATION
5620 Morton St.
Philadelphia, PA 19144   Phone: (215) 849-3237
Subject Specialties: Natural birth control, alternative lifestyles, peace research.

★5031★   ARIES RISING PRESS
PO Box 29532
Los Angeles, CA 90029-0532   Phone: (818) 504-6569
Description: Self-publishes medical books for the layperson.

★5032★   ARIS BOOKS
1621 5th St.
Berkeley, CA 94710   Phone: (415) 527-5171
Description: General trade publisher of hardcover and paperback books and periodicals. **Subject Specialties:** Cookbooks, travel, nutrition, gardening.

★5033★   ARLIN J. BROWN INFORMATION CENTER, INC.
PO Box 251
Fort Belvoir, VA 22060   Phone: (703) 752-9511
Description: Publishes information on non-toxic and natural therapies for cancer and other diseases.

★5034★   ARS PUBLISHING COMPANY
6 W. Main St., Ste. I & P
Stockton, CA 95202   Phone: (209) 465-8243
Subject Specialties: Pro-life, health, social issues.

★5035★   ART THERAPY PUBLICATIONS
Craftsbury Common, VT 05827   Phone: (802) 586-2255
Subject Specialties: Art therapy.

★5036★   ARTEMIS PRESS, INC.
PO Box 4295
Boulder, CO 80306   Phone: (303) 939-0202
Description: Publishes books and software programs on ecological and holistic healing methods using medicinal plants and foods.

★5037★   ARTS & IMAGES
10485 Dupont Rd. S.
Bloomington, MN 55431   Phone: (612) 888-7712
Description: Publishes resource manuals and how-to books on health and social service issues.

★5038★   ARVILLA PRESS
H.C.R. Box 314
Van Buren, AR 72956   Phone: (501) 474-6101
Subject Specialties: Nutrition.

★5039★   ASCP PRESS
2100 W. Harrison St.
Chicago, IL 60612   Phone: (312) 738-4866
Description: Publishes on medical topics for medical professionals, laboratorians, and students. Offers books, slides, plate atlases, audio-visual seminars, professional educational videotapes, and microcomputer software.

★5040★   ASHWINS PUBLICATIONS
PO Box 1686
Ojai, CA 93024   Phone: (805) 646-6622
Description: Publishes books on holistic health.

★5041★   ASKON PUBLISHING COMPANY
1998 Industrial Blvd., No. C
Abilene, TX 79602-7842   Phone: (915) 672-3640
Description: Publishes a book about breast diseases, breast cancer, and cosmetic breast surgery.

★5042★   ASLAN PUBLISHING
PO Box 887
Boulder Creek, CA 95006-0887   Phone: (408) 338-7504
Description: Publishes books aimed to expand consciousness through "the correlation between the physical and spiritual worlds." **Subject Specialties:** Holistic health, new consciousness, parenting.

★5043★   ASPEN PUBLISHERS, INC.
200 Orchard Ridge Dr.
Gaithersburg, MD 20878   Phone: (301) 417-7500
Description: Publishes health care, nursing, medical, law, and special educational materials.

★5044★   ASSOCIATES IN THANATOLOGY
115 Blue Rock Rd.
South Yarmouth, MA 02664   Phone: (508) 394-6520
Description: Publishes on innovative ways of caring for the terminally ill.

★5045★   ASSOCIATION FOR THE ADVANCEMENT OF HEALTH EDUCATION
1900 Association Dr.
Reston, VA 22091   Phone: (703) 476-3437
Description: Has published books, filmstrips, films, microcomputer software, pamphlets, and brochures. Aims to assist in professional preparation programs and assistance of classroom teachers and health educators. Offers resource guides on specific health education topics.

★5046★   ASSOCIATION FOR THE ADVANCEMENT OF MEDICAL INSTRUMENTATION
3330 Washington Blvd., Ste. 400
Arlington, VA 22201   Phone: (703) 525-4890
Description: Promotes improved patient care through the application and management of medical instrumentation and technology. Offers a journal, a newsletter, and technical documents intended for medical equipment manufacturers and health care professionals.

★5047★   ASSOCIATION FOR THE CARE OF CHILDREN'S HEALTH
3615 Wisconsin Ave. NW
Washington, DC 20016   Phone: (202) 244-1801
Description: A multidisciplinary association to meet the psychosocial needs of children and families in health care settings. Publishes guidelines, bibliographies, books for health professionals, parents, and children.

★5048★   ASSOCIATION FOR GERONTOLOGY IN HIGHER EDUCATION
600 Maryland Ave. SW
W. Wing, Ste. 204
Washington, DC 20024   Phone: (202) 484-7505
Description: Nonprofit association committed to gerontology education, training, and research. Publishes a national directory, a series of brief bibliographies, research reports, and occasional proceedings.

★5049★   ASSOCIATION OF HALFWAY HOUSE ALCOHOLISM PROGRAMS OF NORTH AMERICA
786 E. 7th St.
St. Paul, MN 55106   Phone: (612) 771-0933
Description: Publishes to facilitate opening and managing halfway houses.

★5050★   ASSOCIATION FOR HUMANISTIC PSYCHOLOGY
1772 Vallejo St., No. 3
San Francisco, CA 94123   Phone: (415) 346-7929
Description: A worldwide network for the development of the human sciences which works toward fulfillment of people as individuals and as members of society. **Subject Specialties:** Humanistic psychology, holistic health, education, organizational development.

★5051★   ASSOCIATION OF MEDICAL REHABILITATION ADMINISTRATORS
PO Box 1964
Parkersburg, WV 26102   Phone: (304) 485-5842
Description: Publishes an annual membership directory and a standards manual. **Subject Specialties:** Rehabilitation administration and management.

★5052★   **ASSOCIATION OF OFFICIAL ANALYTICAL CHEMISTS**
2200 Wilson Blvd., Ste. 400
Arlington, VA 22201-3301   Phone: (703) 522-3032
Description: A professional organization of scientists devoted to developing, testing, and publishing methods for the analysis of foods, drugs, pesticides, fertilizers, feeds, cosmetics, hazardous substances, and other materials related to agriculture and public health and welfare.

★5053★   **ASSOCIATION FOR RETARDED CITIZENS OF THE U.S.**
500 E. Border St., Ste. 300
PO Box 1047
Arlington, TX 76004   Phone: (817) 261-6003
Description: Publishes on mental retardation for parents, employers, and people with mental retardation. Offers newsletters and brochures.

★5054★   **ASSOCIATION OF UNIVERSITY PROGRAMS IN HEALTH ADMINISTRATION**
1191 N. Fort Myer Dr., Ste. 503
Arlington, VA 22209   Phone: (703) 524-5500
Description: The publications reach academics, practitioners, and students in the health care administration field in the effort to improve health services through education for health management. Offers brochures, a quarterly journal, a field directory, a newsletter, books on various related topics, and a catalog of publications in the field.

★5055★   **ASTER PUBLISHING CORPORATION**
320 N. A St.
Springfield, OR 97477   Phone: (503) 726-1200
Description: Publishes technical manuals for research scientists and manufacturers in the pharmaceutical and analytical instrumentation industries.

★5056★   **ATCOM, INC.**
2315 Broadway, Rm. 300
New York, NY 10024   Phone: (212) 873-5900
Description: Publishes newsletters, journals, and books for the business community and behavioral/helping professions.

★5057★   **ATLANTIS PUBLISHING COMPANY**
3325 Hollywood Blvd., Ste. 404
Hollywood, FL 33021-6926   Phone: (305) 962-8301
Description: Publishes educational texts on spelling, arithmetic, beginning language development, computers, and cancer.

★5058★   **AUBURN HOUSE PUBLISHING COMPANY**
14 Dedham St.
Dover, MA 02030   Phone: (617) 785-2220
Description: Publishes professional and scholarly books on human needs, business, labor relations, and health to "link theory to practice."

★5059★   **AURA PUBLISHING COMPANY**
20 Sunnyside Ave., A150
Mill Valley, CA 94941   Phone: (415) 383-7813
Description: Provides practical, inspiring information about epilepsy for doctors, health workers, family and friends of those with epilepsy, and to everyone who wants to understand this problem.

★5060★   **AURICLE PRESS**
18917 Lomita Ave.
Sonoma, CA 95476   Phone: (707) 996-2323
Description: Publishes books concerning health and well-being, based upon a synthesis of Eastern and Western methodologies of the martial arts and healing arts.

★5061★   **AURORA PRESS**
205 3rd Ave., Apt. 2A
New York, NY 10003   Phone: (212) 673-1831
Subject Specialties: Alternative healthcare, astrology, yoga.

★5062★   **AURORA PUBLISHING COMPANY**
310 1/2 N. Main
PO Box 1729
Garden City, KS 67846   Phone: (316) 275-7488
Description: Publishes books on medical terminology for the layman. Topics include personal health and cancer.

★5063★   **AUTHORS COOPERATIVE, INC.**
PO Box 53
Boston, MA 02199   Phone: (617) 267-9809
Description: Publishes on behavioral science.

★5064★   **AVERY PUBLISHING GROUP**
120 Old Broadway
Garden City Park, NY 11040   Phone: (516) 741-2155
Description: Publishes college texts, reference books, and trade titles specializing in childbirth, child care, natural cooking, health, and military books.

★5065★   **AXELROD PUBLISHING OF TAMPA BAY**
1304 De Soto Ave., No. 308
Tampa, FL 33606   Phone: (813) 251-5269
Subject Specialties: Food, health, biography, regional, photographic essays, humor.

★5066★   **AZURE ZEPHYR PUBLICATIONS**
9395 Harritt Ln., No. 125
Lakeside, CA 92040   Phone: (619) 561-0690
Description: Publishes on alcoholism.

★5067★   **B.C. DECKER, INC.**
320 Walnut St., Ste. 400
Philadelphia, PA 19106   Phone: (215) 625-0001
Description: Publishes on health science for students and practitioners.

★5068★   **B & J PUBLICATIONS**
PO Box 483
Santa Cruz, CA 95061   Phone: (408) 429-1596
Description: Publishes popular science and medical books.

★5069★   **BACKWOODS BOOKS**
McClellan Ln.
PO Box 9
Gibbon Glade, PA 15440   Phone: (412) 329-4581
Description: Publishes health and poetry booklets.

★5070★   **BADER & ASSOCIATES, INC.**
5640 Nicholson Ln., Ste. 226
Rockville, MD 20852-2952   Phone: (301) 468-1610
Description: Specializes in publications for healthcare leaders and hospital governing board members on quality of care and quality and resource management.

★5071★   **BAGGEBODA PRESS**
RR 1, Box 2315
Unity, ME 04988-9716   Phone: (207) 437-2746
Description: Publishes a pictorial symbol system for non-speech communication. Also includes instructions for creating new picsyms and suggestions for personalizing picsyms for individual children's needs. **Subject Specialties:** Augmentative education, speech, handicapped children.

★5072★   **BALBOA PUBLISHING**
11 Library Pl.
San Anselmo, CA 94960   Phone: (415) 453-8886
Subject Specialties: Nutrition, exercise, self-esteem, weight management for adolescents and children.

★5073★   **BARRETT BOOK COMPANY**
1123 High Ridge Rd.
Stamford, CT 06905   Phone: (203) 322-8270
Subject Specialties: Occupational medicine.

★5074★ **BASIC BOOKS, INC.**
10 E. 53rd St.
New York, NY 10022 Phone: (212) 207-7057
Description: Publishes general nonfiction titles and college textbooks.
Subject Specialties: Behavioral sciences, social sciences, economics, political science, science, professional books.

★5075★ **BASK INDUSTRIES**
3240 Vail View Dr.
Daytona Beach, FL 32124 Phone: (904) 760-0989
Description: Publishes medical books.

★5076★ **BAYWOOD PUBLISHING COMPANY, INC.**
26 Austin Ave.
Amityville, NY 11701 Phone: (516) 691-1270
Subject Specialties: Anthropology, archaeology, education, psychology, psychiatry, health, labor relations, sociology, mathematics, computers, thanatology, environment.

★5077★ **BEACON HOUSE INC.**
Welsh Rd. & Butler Pike
Ambler, PA 19002 Phone: (215) 643-7800
Description: Specializes in group psychotherapy and psychodrama works for students and professionals in all fields of therapy.

★5078★ **BEEKMAN PUBLISHERS, INC.**
Rte. 212
PO Box 888
Woodstock, NY 12498 Phone: (914) 679-2300
Description: Publishes and distributes books on health, business, history and medicine.

★5079★ **BEHAVIORAL MEDICINE PRESS**
2101 Devonshire
Ann Arbor, MI 48104
Description: Publishes on behavioral problems.

★5080★ **BEHAVIORAL PUBLISHING COMPANY**
710 Old Mill Rd.
San Marino, CA 91108 Phone: (818) 798-5491
Subject Specialties: Psychology, human behavior, human sexuality.

★5081★ **BEHAVIORAL SCIENCE RESEARCH PRESS**
2695 Villa Creek Dr., Ste. 100
Dallas, TX 75234 Phone: (214) 243-8543

★5082★ **BEING BOOKS INC.**
19834 Gresham St.
Northridge, CA 91324 Phone: (818) 341-0283
Description: Publishes books for mental health professionals.

★5083★ **BELLERAPHON PRESS**
18829 Farmington Rd.
Livonia, MI 48152 Phone: (313) 478-7860
Description: Publishes a book for rheumatologists who are new to private practice or who would like to make strategic and economic changes in their present practice. **Subject Specialties:** Rheumatology.

★5084★ **BENCHMARK PRESS, INC.**
701 Congressional Blvd., No. 340
Carmel, IN 46032
Description: Publishes college texts and reference books and videos on health, physical education, and sports medicine.

★5085★ **BENJAMIN-CUMMINGS PUBLISHING COMPANY**
390 Bridge Pkwy.
Redwood City, CA 94065 Phone: (415) 594-4400
Subject Specialties: Mathematics, science, computers, health, nursing.

★5086★ **BERKELEY PLANNING ASSOCIATES**
440 Grand Ave., Ste. 500
Oakland, CA 94610-5085 Phone: (415) 465-7885
Description: Private research and planning firm specializing in program and policy planning and evaluations, and in contract research in the fields of social and health services, urban and regional development, child care, energy, housing, and transportation. Reports and documents available in microform from NTIS, and Educational Resources Information Center.

★5087★ **BERKELEY SCIENTIFIC PUBLICATIONS**
5401 E. Dakota Ave., No. 1
Denver, CO 80222 Phone: (303) 355-2675
Description: Provides review material to help medical technologists pass board examinations. **Subject Specialties:** Clinical laboratory, medical technology.

★5088★ **BETA BOOKS**
PO Box 404954
Brooklyn, NY 11240-4954 Phone: (718) 499-3822
Description: Publishes books about biomedicine and art. Reaches market through direct mail, reviews, and wholesalers. **Subject Specialties:** AIDS, art photography.

★5089★ **BETTERWAY PUBLICATION, INC.**
Box 219
Crozet, VA 22932 Phone: (804) 823-5661
Description: Publishes resource guides and handbooks on home building and remodeling, small business and finance, theather crafts, and parenting and family health.

★5090★ **BETZ PUBLISHING COMPANY, INC.**
PO Box 34631
Bethesda, MD 20827 Phone: (301) 340-0030
Description: Serve pre-med, college, and el-hi students and their advisors through publication of books and materials for advancement in education through self-directed study, focusing on premedical preparation materials.

★5091★ **BEYOND WORDS PUBLISHING INC.**
Rte. 3, Box 492B
Hillsboro, OR 97123 Phone: (503) 647-5109
Description: Publishes nature, self-help, health, and children's books. Offers calendars, planners, and art prints.

★5092★ **BGC PUBLISHING COMPANY**
9550 Collegeview Rd.
Minneapolis, MN 55437-2160 Phone: (612) 830-1043
Description: Publishes on Alzheimer's disease. Offers audio tapes for the blind.

★5093★ **BIBULOPHILE PRESS**
24 Old Mt. Tom Rd.
PO Box 757
Bantam, CT 06750-0750 Phone: (203) 567-5543
Description: Publishes information on alcoholism/addiction.

★5094★ **BIG A & COMPANY**
2303 26 1/2 Ave. SW
Fargo, ND 58103 Phone: (701) 298-0272
Description: Publishes on children's bereavement.

★5095★ **BIOBEHAVIORAL PUBLISHERS AND DISTRIBUTORS, INC.**
9725 Louedd Ave.
Houston, TX 77070 Phone: (713) 890-8575
Description: Publishes on stress management psychology, relaxation, and vocational guidance.

★5096★ **BIO-COMMUNICATIONS PRESS**
3100 N. Hillside
Wichita, KS 67219 Phone: (316) 682-3100
Description: Publishes on health. **Subject Specialties:** Vitamins, nutrition, self-help.

★5097★ **BIO-DATA PUBLISHERS**
PO Box 66020
Washington, DC 20035 Phone: (202) 393-2437
Description: Publishes health/lifestyle information, currently concentrating on the AIDS/HIV epidemic.

★5098★ BIOFEEDBACK AND ADVANCED THERAPY INSTITUTE, INC.
5979 W. 3rd St., Ste. 205
Los Angeles, CA 90036   Phone: (213) 938-0478
Description: Publishes on biofeedback, electromyometry, referred pain, treatment modalities.

★5099★ BIOFEEDBACK PRESS
3428 Sacramento St.
San Francisco, CA 94118   Phone: (415) 921-5455
Description: Provides educational resources (books, tapes, sound/slide programs) in behavioral medicine, stress management, and biofeedback for health care professionals, general public, and students.

★5100★ BIOFEEDBACK RESEARCH INSTITUTE
6399 Wilshire Blvd., Ste. 1010
Los Angeles, CA 90048   Phone: (213) 933-9451
Description: Publishes research done by workers within the institute.
Subject Specialties: Biofeedback in clinical practice and neuromuscular re-education.

★5101★ BIOHISTORICAL PRESS
8215 Belden Blvd.
Cottage Grove, MN 55016   Phone: (612) 459-2379
Description: Publishes on history, biology, and medicine.

★5102★ BIOKINESIOLOGY INSTITUTE
5432 Hwy. 227
Trail, OR 97541   Phone: (503) 878-2080
Description: An educational and research organization promoting a better understanding of how the mind and body function, as well as better health, using many health-building methodologies. Publishes books and issues anatomy flash cards, acupuncture flash cards, and an emotional chart.
Subject Specialties: Wholistic health, biokinesiology.

★5103★ BIOMEDICAL PUBLICATIONS
PO Box 8209
Foster City, CA 94404   Phone: (415) 573-6224
Description: Publishes textbooks on the graduate school level and reference and technical manuals intended for the scientific specialist. **Subject Specialties:** Clinical laboratory manuals, clinical forensic and environmental toxicology, medical texts.

★5104★ BION PUBLISHING
1113 Golden W.
Ojai, CA 93023   Phone: (805) 646-3096
Description: Publishes books on health and nutrition.

★5105★ BIO-PROBE, INC.
4401 Real Ct.
Orlando, FL 32808   Phone: (407) 299-4149
Description: Provides scientific information on the use of toxic metals in dentistry.

★5106★ BIOTECHNICAL VETERINARY CONSULTANTS
32050 Lynx Hollow Rd.
Cresswell, OR 97426   Phone: (619) 756-1344
Description: Publishes veterinary textbooks, especially dog books.

★5107★ BISHOP OF BOOKS
46 Eureka Ave.
Wheeling, WV 26003   Phone: (304) 242-2937
Description: Publishes books on alcoholism. Offers calendars and databases.

★5108★ BITTERSWEET
32 Ocean Ave.
Bay Shore, NY 11706   Phone: (516) 665-5382
Description: Publishes on the adult children of alcoholics.

★5109★ BJO'S ENTERPRISES
837 Archie St.
Eugene, OR 97402   Phone: (503) 688-5400
Description: Publishes children's books on disability awareness issues.

★5110★ BLACKWELL SCIENTIFIC PUBLICATIONS, INC.
3 Cambridge Center, Ste. 208
Cambridge, MA 02142   Phone: (617) 225-0401
Description: Publishes books and journals on medicine, veterinary medicine, earth sciences, life science, and the environment.

★5111★ BLUE DOLPHIN PUBLISHING, INC.
PO Box 1908
Nevada City, CA 95959   Phone: (916) 265-6925
Description: Publishes books on health, psychology, cross-cultural comparative spiritual traditions, science, and humor.

★5112★ BLUE POPPY ENTERPRISES/PRESS
1775 Linden Ave.
Boulder, CO 80304   Phone: (303) 442-0796
Description: Publishes information on Oriental medicine in the West. Audience is largely practitioners and students of acupuncture and other types of Oriental medicine (Japanese, Korean, Tibetan, Auyervedic).

★5113★ BOATHOUSE PRESS
3600 Conshohocken Ave., Ste. 1501A
Philadelphia, PA 19131   Phone: (215) 473-4054
Description: Publishes on health and fitness.

★5114★ BONNIE PRUDDEN PRESS
Prospect Hill Rd.
PO Box 625
Stockbridge, MA 01262   Phone: (413) 298-3066
Description: Publishes Bonnie Prudden's books to promote physical fitness for all ages.

★5115★ BOOKMAKERS GUILD, INC.
9655 W. Colfax Ave.
Lakewood, CO 80215   Phone: (202) 785-4061
Description: Dedicated to publishing materials for and about children, especially child welfare and abuse and neglect. Also publishes on natural sciences, history and literature, and family management.

★5116★ BOSC-BOOKS ON SPECIAL CHILDREN
PO Box 305
Congers, NY 10920   Phone: (914) 638-1236
Description: Publishes a directory for parents and professionals of learning disabled people. Offers catalogs. Distributes products for many different publishers who specialize in books for people with handicaps.

★5117★ BOSTON CHINESE MEDICINE
8 Whittier Pl., No. 19-D
Boston, MA 02114   Phone: (617) 720-4448
Description: Publishes a book on Chinese herbal medicines explaining how to use them in pill form.

★5118★ BOSTON UNIVERSITY
PIKE INSTITUTE FOR THE HANDICAPPED
765 Commonwealth Ave.
Boston, MA 02215   Phone: (617) 353-2904
Description: A component of Boston University School of Law that publishes on the advancement of disability law through research, advocacy, public service, and the training of law students. **Subject Specialties:** Rights of people with physical and mental disabilities.

★5119★ BOSTON WOMEN'S HEALTH BOOK COLLECTIVE, INC.
240 A Elm St.
Somerville, MA 02144   Phone: (617) 924-0271
Description: Compiles, publishes, and disseminates information on wide range of health and women's issues.

★5120★ BOXWOOD PRESS
183 Ocean View Blvd.
Pacific Grove, CA 93950   Phone: (408) 375-0430
Subject Specialties: Natural history, invertebrates, ecology, psychiatry.

★5121★ **BOWLING GREEN PRESS, INC.**
1435 Rosewood Dr.
Bowling Green, OH 43402   Phone: (419) 352-0493
Description: Specializes in publications dealing with deafness and American sign language.

★5122★ **BRAILLE, INC.**
205 Worcester Ct., Ste. C-3
Falmouth, MA 02540   Phone: (508) 540-0800
Description: Publishes braille versions of various literary and mathematical materials. Subjects include computers, engineering, science, foreign languages, and graphics.

★5123★ **BRAILLE INSTITUTE PRESS**
741 N. Vermont Ave.
Los Angeles, CA 90029   Phone: (213) 663-1111
Description: Publishes braille books and magazines.

★5124★ **BRANDON HOUSE, INC.**
PO Box 240
Bronx, NY 10471
Description: Seeks to advance the mental imagery field. **Subject Specialties:** Psychology, psychiatry, literature.

★5125★ **BREAKTHRU PUBLISHING**
3605 Piedmont
Oakland, CA 94611   Phone: (415) 530-1256
Description: Publishes on weight control, dieting, and hair care.

★5126★ **BRIAN'S HOUSE, INC.**
1300 S. Concord Rd.
West Chester, PA 19382   Phone: (215) 363-1205
Subject Specialties: Handicapped, social service.

★5127★ **BRIDGEVIEW BOOKS**
1065 Central Blvd.
Hayward, CA 94542   Phone: (415) 889-6355
Subject Specialties: Self-help, health, fitness, nutrition.

★5128★ **BRIGGS CORPORATION**
PO Box 1698
Des Moines, IA 50306-1698   Phone: (515) 274-9221
Description: Publishes on health care related subjects.

★5129★ **BROOKE-RICHARDS PRESS**
9420 Reseda Blvd., Ste. 511
Northridge, CA 91343   Phone: (818) 893-4405
Description: Publishes books on social studies for people with reading disabilities.

★5130★ **BROOKLINE BOOKS**
PO Box 1046
Cambridge, MA 02238-1046   Phone: (617) 868-0360
Subject Specialties: General education, special education, computers in schools, developmental disabilities, clinical and child psychology, psychotherapy, special needs of handicapped children.

★5131★ **BRUNNER/MAZEL, INC.**
19 Union Sq. W.
New York, NY 10003   Phone: (212) 924-3344
Description: Publishes professional books. **Subject Specialties:** Psychoanalysis, psychiatry, psychology, neurology, social work, special education, child development, marriage, family therapy.

★5132★ **BRUNO PRESS**
2627 General Pershing St.
New Orleans, LA 70115   Phone: (504) 899-2367
Description: Publishes for mental health professionals and patients.

★5133★ **BUBBA PRESS**
2100 Cactus Ct., No. 2
Walnut Creek, CA 94595
Description: Publishes to educate the public on epilepsy.

★5134★ **BUDLONG PRESS COMPANY**
5915 N. Northwest Hwy.
Chicago, IL 60631   Phone: (312) 763-7720
Description: Publishes health and medical books directed to doctors to be used as patient education aids.

★5135★ **BULL PUBLISHING COMPANY**
110 Gilbert Ave.
Menlo Park, CA 94025   Phone: (415) 322-2855
Description: Publishes books on health, nutrition, fitness, and cancer care written by professionals for both professionals and the general public.

★5136★ **BUREAU OF ECONOMIC AND BEHAVIORAL RESEARCH**
211 E. Chicago Ave.
Chicago, IL 60611   Phone: (312) 440-2500
Description: Conducts economic research and publishes reports to assist policy-makers of the dental profession. **Subject Specialties:** Statistics of a dental practice, the number of dentists.

★5137★ **BURNELL COMPANY/PUBLISHERS, INC.**
PO Box 304
821 N. 2nd St.
Mankato, MN 56002   Phone: (507) 625-4302
Description: Publishes on education in radiologic technology and emergency medical services.

★5138★ **BURNS ARCHIVE**
140 E. 38th St.
New York, NY 10016   Phone: (212) 889-1938
Description: Publishes books and journals on medical photography from 1839 to 1920.

★5139★ **BUTTERFLY PRESS**
PO Box 19571
Houston, TX 77224   Phone: (713) 464-7570
Subject Specialties: Cookbooks, diet and weight loss, exercise, self-help.

★5140★ **BUTTERWORTH-HEINEMANN**
80 Montvale Ave.
Stoneham, MA 02180   Phone: (617) 438-8464
Description: Publishers of books and journals in medicine, engineering, security, and architecture. **Subject Specialties:** Science, medicine, technology, photography, cinematography, broadcasting, optometry.

★5141★ **C. ANTONIO PROVOST**
4474 Sunburst Dr.
Oceanside, CA 92056-3540   Phone: (619) 758-8754
Description: Publishes nonfiction literature mainly on health, philosophy, sociology, and education. Aims to "inform the general public of the nature of social problems and provide viable solutions to them."

★5142★ **C. G. JUNG FOUNDATION FOR ANALYTICAL PSYCHOLOGY**
28 E. 39th St.
New York, NY 10016   Phone: (212) 697-6430
Description: A nonprofit educational foundation whose purpose is to disseminate the work and thought of C. G. Jung, to develop understanding of the range and applicability of analytical psychology, and to foster the preparation and training of new Jungian analysts.

★5143★ **C. G. JUNG INSTITUTE OF LOS ANGELES**
10349 W. Pico Blvd.
Los Angeles, CA 90064   Phone: (213) 556-1193
Description: Nonprofit corporation whose primary purpose is to train therapists to become Jungian analysts. Publishes *Psychological Perspectives* as well as books on psychology.

★5144★ **C. HENRY KEMPE NATIONAL CENTER FOR THE PREVENTION AND TREATMENT OF CHILD ABUSE**
University of Colorado
Health Science Center
1205 Oneida St.
Denver, CO 80220   Phone: (303) 321-3963
Description: Publishes a variety of books related to the prevention and treatment of child abuse.

★5145★   C. OLSON & COMPANY
PO Box 5100
Santa Cruz, CA 95063-5100   Phone: (408) 458-3365
Description: Publishes on popular health, the environment, and philosophy.

★5146★   CAB INTERNATIONAL—NORTH AMERICA
845 N. Park Ave.
Tucson, AZ 85719   Phone: (602) 621-7897
Description: Publishes books and other information services on medicine, nutrition, and animal sciences.

★5147★   CABALLERO PRESS
1936 Caballero Way
Las Vegas, NV 89109   Phone: (702) 735-3406
Subject Specialties: Weight control, self-help.

★5148★   CALIFORNIA COLLEGE FOR HEALTH SCIENCES
CALIFORNIA COLLEGE PUBLISHING
222 W. 24th St.
National City, CA 92050   Phone: (619) 477-4800
Description: Publishes allied health care education information.

★5149★   CALIFORNIA PSYCHOLOGICAL PUBLISHERS
1223 Wilshire Blvd.
Santa Monica, CA 90403   Phone: (213) 451-3118
Description: Publishes self-help books on psychology and stress management for workers and professionals.

★5150★   CAMBRIDGE UNIVERSITY PRESS
20 W. 20th St.
New York, NY 10011   Phone: (212) 924-3900
Description: Publishes scholarly and reference books, including medical books, Bibles, and textbooks. **Subject Specialties:** Humanities, social sciences, mathmatics, sciences, and medicine.

★5151★   CAMELBACK RECORDS
7306 E. Rancho Vista Dr.
Scottsdale, AZ 85251-1333   Phone: (602) 945-1101
Description: Publishes health, exercise, and fitness oriented books, articles, cassettes, and video tapes.

★5152★   CANCER CONTROL SOCIETY/CANCER BOOK HOUSE
2043 N. Berendo St.
Los Angeles, CA 90027   Phone: (213) 663-7801
Description: Publishes and distributes books on such cancer therapies as Laetrile, and on the importance of nutrition in the prevention and control of cancer and other diseases.

★5153★   CAPITOL PUBLICATIONS, INC.
1101 King St., Ste. 444
Alexandria, VA 22314   Phone: (703) 683-4100
Description: Publishes newsletters, special reports and information services. **Subject Specialties:** Special education.

★5154★   CARE COMMUNICATIONS, INC.
101 E. Ontario, 6th Fl.
Chicago, IL 60611   Phone: (312) 943-0463
Description: Provides consultation, training, and publications to health care facilities on such subjects as quality assurance, risk management, medical record systems, documentation, and utilization management.

★5155★   CARLINSHAR & ASSOCIATES APPLIED RESEARCH
519 E. Briarcliff
Bolingbrook, IL 60439   Phone: (312) 739-7720
Subject Specialties: Minority issues, mental health, community, corrections.

★5156★   CARLOS V. PESTANA
PO Box 790617
San Antonio, TX 78279-0617
Description: Self-publishes books for medical school applicants.

★5157★   CAROLANDO PRESS
6545 W. North Ave.
Oak Park, IL 60302   Phone: (708) 383-6480
Description: Provides podiatric surgeons and students with up-to-date surgical techniques in foot surgery.

★5158★   CAROLINA PRESS
PO Box 24906
Winston-Salem, NC 27114   Phone: (919) 768-9180
Description: Publishes health and self-help materials.

★5159★   CASSANDRA PRESS, INC.
PO Box 868
San Rafael, CA 94915   Phone: (415) 382-8507
Description: Publishes metaphysical, astrology, and holistic health books.

★5160★   CASTALIA PUBLISHING COMPANY
PO Box 1587
Eugene, OR 97440   Phone: (503) 343-4433
Description: Disseminates research-based books and videos for parents, educators, guidance counselors, family therapists, and mental health professionals. The focus is on social learning and cognitive-behavioral approaches to adult and adolescent depression.

★5161★   CATALYST
PO Box 20572
Sarasota, FL 34276-3572   Phone: (813) 349-1613
Description: Self-publishes a book dealing with cancer.

★5162★   CATHOLIC HEALTH ASSOCIATION OF THE UNITED STATES
4455 Woodson Rd.
St. Louis, MO 63134-3797   Phone: (314) 427-2500
Description: Publishes books, pamphlets, manuals, journals, and newspapers on health care ethics and management. **Subject Specialties:** Bioethics, management, governance, allied health, health ministry.

★5163★   CECOM PUBLISHING
PO Box 3059
Homer, AK 99603-3059   Phone: (907) 235-6378
Description: Publishes on health.

★5164★   CEDAR CREEK PUBLISHERS
2310 Sawmill Rd.
Fort Wayne, IN 46825   Phone: (219) 637-3856
Description: Publishes books on special diet problems, e.g. hyperactivity, low-sugar, milk-free.

★5165★   CENTER FOR APPLICATIONS OF PSYCHOLOGICAL TYPE
2720 NW 6th St.
Gainesville, FL 32609   Phone: (904) 375-0160
Description: A nonprofit publisher and distributor of informational, research, and training materials about the Myers-Briggs Type Indicator (MBTI) and psychological types for educators, counselors, researchers, other professionals, and the general public.

★5166★   CENTER FOR BIO-GERONTOLOGY
PO Box 11097
Pensacola, FL 32524   Phone: (904) 484-0595
Description: Publishes books related to biological aging, aging retardation, and life extension.

★5167★   CENTER FOR CONSUMER HEALTHCARE INFORMATION
4000 Birch St., No. 112
Newport Beach, CA 92660   Phone: (714) 752-2335
Description: Publishes on health care providers and managed care organizations.

★5168★   CENTER FOR CORPORATE HEALTH PROMOTION
1850 Centennial Park Dr., Ste. 520
Reston, VA 22091   Phone: (703) 391-2400
Description: Publishes books on health and medical self-care.

★5169★ CENTER FOR EMPIRICAL MEDICINE
4221 45th St. NW
Washington, DC 20016   Phone: (202) 364-0898
Description: Publishes books on homeopathic medicine, medical history, vaccination, AIDS , and syphilis.

★5170★ CENTER FOR GESTALT DEVELOPMENT
PO Box 990
Highland, NY 12528
Description: Publishes books on gestalt therapy.

★5171★ CENTER FOR MODERN PSYCHOANALYTIC STUDIES PUBLICATIONS DIVISION
16 W. 10th St.
New York, NY 10011   Phone: (212) 260-7052
Description: Publishes a journal, *Modern Psychoanalysis* and other materials in the field of psychoanalytic literature.

★5172★ CENTER PRESS
2045 Francisco St.
Berkeley, CA 94709   Phone: (415) 526-8373
Description: Publishes books, monographs, and a journal to explore "a somatic understanding of human experience." **Subject Specialties:** Psychology, holistic health, philosophy.

★5173★ CENTER FOR PUBLIC REPRESENTATION
121 S. Pinckney St.
Madison, WI 53703   Phone: (608) 251-4008
Description: Publishes materials relevant to the elderly and health care providers.

★5174★ CENTER FOR RESEARCH IN AMBULATORY HEALTH CARE ADMINISTRATION
104 Inverness Ter. E.
Englewood, CO 80112-5306   Phone: (303) 753-1111
Description: Promotes improved administration of ambulatory health care in general and group practice in particular by developing innovative publications, demonstration programs, and educational, research, and data services.

★5175★ CENTER FOR SCIENCE IN THE PUBLIC INTEREST
1875 Connecticut Ave. NW, No. 300
Washington, DC 20009   Phone: (202) 332-9110
Description: Publishes reports in the fields of nutrition and health.

★5176★ CENTER FOR THE STUDY OF MULTIPLE BIRTH
333 E. Superior St., Ste. 464
Chicago, IL 60611   Phone: (312) 266-9093
Description: Stimulates and fosters medical and social research in the area of multiple birth and provides help to mothers with the special problems they and their offspring will encounter.

★5177★ CENTER FOR THANATOLOGY RESEARCH AND EDUCATION
391 Atlantic Ave.
Brooklyn, NY 11217-1701   Phone: (718) 858-3026
Description: Objective is to distribute and promote all publications on aging, dying, and death and release relevant titles in these subjects.

★5178★ CENTRE FOR TRADITIONAL ACUPUNCTURE
American City Bldg., Ste. 108
Columbia, MD 21044   Phone: (301) 997-3770
Description: Publishes acupuncture books for schools, practitioners, and bookstores. Offers acupuncture charts.

★5179★ CENTURY PUBLISHER
210 Partridge
Holts Summit, MO 65043   Phone: (314) 896-4968
Description: Self-publisher; also distributes for the National Association of the Deaf. **Subject Specialties:** Sign language.

★5180★ CGM, INC.
107-12th St.
Racine, WI 53403   Phone: (414) 633-0100
Description: Publishes health materials for professionals and the general public.

★5181★ CHAMPION PRESS
Centinela Hospital
555 E. Hardy St.
Inglewood, CA 90301   Phone: (213) 673-4660
Description: Publishes fitness guides based on research conducted at the hospital by physicians, physical therapists, and technicians. Titles are geared toward professional and amateur athletes, including baseball players, golfers, and little leaguers.

★5182★ CHANEY ALLEN ENTERPRISES
PO Box 13011
San Diego, CA 92113   Phone: (619) 427-8763
Description: Publishes on alcohol and drug addiction.

★5183★ CHANNING L. BETE COMPANY, INC.
200 State Rd.
South Deerfield, MA 01373   Phone: (413) 665-7611
Description: Publishes informational booklets in a scriptographic format—brief blocks oftext and simple graphics. Offers calendars, coloring books, activity books, videos, and list rentals. **Subject Specialties:** Health, energy, military life, customer service, religion, substance abuse, safety, career planning.

★5184★ CHARLES C. THOMAS, PUBLISHER
2600 S. 1st St.
Springfield, IL 62794-9265   Phone: (217) 789-8980
Description: Publishes trade and textbooks in the biomedical sciences, behavioral sciences, special education, criminal justice, and speech-language-hearing topics. Produces on-demand photocopy editions of out-of-print titles.

★5185★ CHARLES E. WEBER
Box 60
Aransas Pass, TX 78336   Phone: (512) 758-5219
Description: Publishes on physiology and nutrition.

★5186★ CHARLES PRESS PUBLISHERS, INC.
PO Box 15715
Philadelphia, PA 19103   Phone: (215) 735-3665
Description: Publishes monographs in the fields of medicine, psychology, nursing, and thanatology.

★5187★ CHAS. FRANKLIN PRESS
PO Box 524
Lynnwood, WA 98046   Phone: (206) 774-6979
Subject Specialties: Childbirth, women's issues, child safety.

★5188★ CHATSWORTH PRESS
9135 Alabama Ave., Ste. B
Chatsworth, CA 91311   Phone: (818) 341-3156
Description: Publishes erotica and books on human sexuality intended for the professional as well as the layman.

★5189★ CHC PUBLISHING
105 Locust Ave.
Larkspur, CA 94939   Phone: (415) 924-6106
Description: Publishes on colon health.

★5190★ CHEEVER PUBLISHING, INC.
PO Box 700
Bloomington, IL 61702   Phone: (309) 378-2961
Description: Provides information for handicapped individuals and professionals working with the disabled.

★5191★ CHEM-ORBITAL
PO Box 134
Park Forest, IL 60466   Phone: (708) 748-0440
Description: Publishes a book on nutrition and a book on lymphomas.

★5192★ CHINESE CULTURE BOOKS COMPANY
1601 Clay St.
Oakland, CA 94612   Phone: (510) 763-3866
Description: Publishes on Chinese culture and traditional Chinese medicine.

★5193★ CHIRON PUBLICATIONS
400 Linden Ave.
Wilmette, IL 60091   Phone: (312) 256-7551
Description: Publishes clinical literature in the field of analytical psychology, to make the field of Jungian psychology a clinically vital approach to psychological treatment. **Subject Specialties:** Psychology, religion, literature.

★5194★ CHOICE (CONCERN FOR HEALTH OPTIONS: INFORMATION CARE AND EDUCATION)
1233 Locust St., 3rd. Fl.
Philadelphia, PA 19107   Phone: (215) 985-3355
Description: A consumer education and advocacy organization concerned with reproductive health care, AIDS, sexuality education, maternity care, and child care. It is a nonprofit agency which produces educational books, pamphlets, brochures, and flyers for teens, working parents, women, and anyone interested in AIDS and reproductive health.

★5195★ CHURCHILL LIVINGSTONE, INC.
1560 Broadway
New York, NY 10036   Phone: (212) 819-5400
Description: Produces a line of medical books and journals.

★5196★ CIN PUBLICATIONS
PO Box 11277
San Francisco, CA 94101   Phone: (415) 861-5018
Description: Offers films, videotapes, and audio cassettes as well as books. **Subject Specialties:** General health, longevity, rejuvenation, gas economy.

★5197★ CITY SPIRIT PUBLICATIONS
590 Pacific St.
Brooklyn, NY 11217   Phone: (718) 857-1545
Description: Publishes directories on alternative health care and environmentally "safe" products.

★5198★ CLARKE PUBLISHING
191 University Blvd., Ste. 249
Denver, CO 80206   Phone: (303) 333-2254
Description: Publishes books on health education.

★5199★ CLEVELAND CLINIC FOUNDATION
9500 Euclid Ave., M17
Cleveland, OH 44195-5146   Phone: (216) 444-6453
Description: Publishes on health care for consumers and professionals. Offers nutrition education booklets, cookbooks, newsletters, and video cassettes.

★5200★ CLINICAL HEARING CONSULTANTS
8100 E. Indian School Rd.
Scottsdale, AZ 85251   Phone: (602) 941-1200
Description: Publishes on hearing health care.

★5201★ CLINICAL PHARMACOLOGY CONSULTANTS
PO Box 772
Goodlettsville, TN 37072-0772   Phone: (615) 859-1348
Description: Publishes medical pharmacology, private research, and patient drug information.

★5202★ CLINICAL PSYCHOLOGY PUBLISHING COMPANY, INC.
4 Conant Sq.
Brandon, VT 05733   Phone: (802) 247-6871
Description: Publishes psychological and educational journals, monographs, books, and tests. **Subject Specialties:** School psychology, clinical psychology, special education.

★5203★ CLINTWORTH PUBLICATIONS
2018 Griffith Park Blvd.
Los Angeles, CA 90039   Phone: (213) 661-3469
Description: Publishes an annual resource for use by medical librarians. **Subject Specialties:** Medical bibliographic database searching.

★5204★ CLOVERNOOK PRINTING HOUSE FOR THE BLIND
7000 Hamilton Ave.
Cincinnati, OH 45231   Phone: (513) 522-3860
Description: Publishes fiction and nonfiction in Braille.

★5205★ CMD RESEARCH
Syracuse University
Dept. of Psychology
Syracuse, NY 13244   Phone: (315) 446-7012
Description: Publishes research on sexuality.

★5206★ COLD SPRING HARBOR LABORATORY PRESS
PO Box 100
Cold Spring Harbor, NY 11724   Phone: (516) 367-8423
Description: Publishes books and videotapes in biological science, molecular and cell biology, genetics, immunology, virology, microbiology, neurobiology, cancer research, and biological risk assessment.

★5207★ COLLEGE-HILL PRESS
34 Beacon St.
Boston, MA 02108   Phone: (617) 227-0730
Description: Specializes in speech-language pathology, publishing special education books and software, clinical books, and college-level textbooks.

★5208★ COLOR CODED CHARTING AND FILING SYSTEMS
7759 California Ave.
Riverside, CA 92504   Phone: (714) 688-0800
Description: Color Coded Systems is a dental bookkeeping supply company which also publishes the texts of Dr. Robert Peshek. **Subject Specialties:** Oral health, nutrition.

★5209★ COMMISSION ON THE MENTALLY DISABLED
1800 M St. NW
Washington, DC 20036   Phone: (202) 331-2240
Description: Sponsors research and public information regarding the laws that affect mentally and physically disabled persons. **Subject Specialties:** Disability law.

★5210★ COMMITTEE FOR ABORTION RIGHTS AND AGAINST STERILIZATION ABUSE
17 Murray Street, 5th Fl.
New York, NY 10007   Phone: (212) 964-1350
Description: Publishes to educate about and promote reproductive freedom for all women.

★5211★ COMMITTEE FOR NUCLEAR RESPONSIBILITY
PO Box 11207
San Francisco, CA 94101   Phone: (415) 776-8299
Description: Aims to "clarify the first principles of public health science and human rights on which consistent rules about pollution and contamination, hazardous jobs, hazardous consumer products, and diagnostic X-rays can be soundly based within a free market." **Subject Specialties:** Radiation injury, nuclear power, public health principles, individual human rights.

★5212★ COMMON KNOWLEDGE PRESS
451 Mesa Rd.
PO Box 316
Bolinas, CA 94924   Phone: (415) 868-0970
Description: Commonweal, an affiliated nonprofit corporation, conducts service and research activities concerning environmental factors affecting health and innovative approaches to health promotion for the elderly and chronically ill. Offers integral cancer therapy and alternative cancer therapy information services. Common Knowledge Press publishes works resulting from research.

★5213★ COMMUNICATION STUDIES
6145 Anita St.
Dallas, TX 75214-2612   Phone: (214) 823-1981
Description: Self-publisher of books and cassettes on self-help, staff training, and classes. **Subject Specialties:** Psychiatry, emotions, psychology.

★5214★ COMMUNITY INTERVENTION, INC.
529 7th St., Ste. 570
Minneapolis, MN 55415   Phone: (612) 332-6537
Description: Publishes on drug abuse, adolescence.

★5215★ COMMUNITY RECOVERY PRESS
PO Box 20979
Milwaukee, WI 53220   Phone: (414) 321-9455
Description: Publishes alcohol and drug abuse materials for educators.

★5216★ COMMUNITY SERVICE SOCIETY
Office of Information
105 E. 22nd St.
New York, NY 10010   Phone: (212) 254-8900
Description: Conducts policy research on conditions in New York City on behalf of the poor. Conditions include health, education, housing, child care, and community development.

★5217★ COMPCARE PUBLISHERS
2415 Annapolis Ln.
Minneapolis, MN 55441   Phone: (612) 559-4800
Description: Publishes and distributes books and pamphlets on personal well-being. **Subject Specialties:** Alcohol and drug abuse, health, relationships, parenting, weight loss.

★5218★ COMPREHENSIVE HEALTH EDUCATION FOUNDATION
22323 Pacific Hwy. S.
Seattle, WA 98198   Phone: (206) 824-2907
Description: A nonprofit organization promoting health education in the home, school, and community. Publishes a drug abuse prevention curriculum and health-oriented programs for school children. Offers books, videos, audiotapes, posters, banners, games, and *CHEF* newsletter. **Subject Specialties:** Drug and alcohol education, AIDS prevention, sex education, self-esteem.

★5219★ CONCERN FOR DYING
250 W. 57th St., Rm. 831
New York, NY 10107   Phone: (212) 246-6962
Description: A nonprofit educational organization that educates the public and health professionals about legal, ethical, and psychological issues in treatment refusal. Distributes information about living wills. **Subject Specialties:** Medical, legal, ethical, and personal aspects of refusal of life-sustaining treatment.

★5220★ CONCERNED UNITED BIRTHPARENTS, INC.
2000 Walker St.
Des Moines, IA 50317   Phone: (515) 263-9558
Subject Specialties: Adoption, birthparenthood, teen pregnancy.

★5221★ CONSCIOUS LIVING FOUNDATION
PO Box 9
Drain, OR 97435   Phone: (503) 836-2358
Description: Researches and teaches healthier ways to manage stress.

★5222★ CONSULTING PSYCHOLOGISTS PRESS, INC.
577 College Ave.
Palo Alto, CA 94306   Phone: (415) 857-1444
Description: Publishes psychological tests, books, and software for psychologists, career counselors, training and development professionals, and educators.

★5223★ CONSUMER INFORMATION PUBLICATIONS, INC.
2245 Curlew Rd.
Palm Harbor, FL 34683   Phone: (813) 784-7795
Description: A nonprofit company promoting alternative medical therapy and prevention of disease. Reaches market through direct mail and wholesalers.

★5224★ CONSUMING PASSIONS
PO Box 802
Georgetown, CT 06829   Phone: (203) 544-9663
Description: Publishes on eating disorders affecting women and men.

★5225★ CONTEMPORARY BOOKS, INC.
180 N. Michigan Ae.
Chicago, IL 60601   Phone: (312) 782-9181
Subject Specialties: Health, martial arts, cooking, sports, business, childcare, biography, GED preparation.

★5226★ CONTINENTAL ASSOCIATION OF FUNERAL AND MEMORIAL SOCIETIES
33 University Sq., Ste. 333
Madison, WI 53715
Description: Publishes materials to aid consumers in pre-arranging funerals that are dignified, simple, and low cost.

★5227★ CONTINUING PROFESSIONAL EDUCATION CENTER, INC.
PO Box 305
Skillman, NJ 08558-0305   Phone: (609) 924-4500
Description: Publishes home-study continuing medical education materials for physicians and nurses. **Subject Specialties:** Medicine.

★5228★ COPESTHETIC PUBLISHERS
2032 Belmont Rd. NW, No. 612
Washington, DC 20009   Phone: (202) 667-0470
Description: Publisher of consumer, environmental, health, and education advocacy materials for citizen and educator networks, particularly global organizations and developing countries.

★5229★ COSMOENERGETICS PUBLICATIONS
PO Box 86353
San Diego, CA 92138   Phone: (619) 295-1664
Description: Publishes on the use of touch and language in healing. **Subject Specialties:** Healing, symbolism, psychology, language, metaphysics.

★5230★ COTTAGE BOOKS
731 Treat Ave.
San Francisco, CA 94110   Phone: (415) 536-4514
Description: Publishes how-to books for families and caregivers looking after Alzheimers patients and books of Celtic interest.

★5231★ COUGAR PASS PUBLISHING COMPANY
PO Box 463060
Escondido, CA 92046-3060   Phone: (619) 738-0682
Description: Publishes access information for disabled persons.

★5232★ COUNCIL FOR EXCEPTIONAL CHILDREN
1920 Association Dr.
Reston, VA 22091   Phone: (703) 620-3660
Description: Publishes to provide professional literature and resources to special educators including teachers, administrators, and teacher educators.

★5233★ COUNCIL ON SOCIAL WORK EDUCATION
1600 Duke St.
Alexandria, VA 22314   Phone: (202) 667-2300
Description: Accrediting body for social work education authorized by the U.S. Office of Education, the Department of Health, Education, and Welfare, and the Council on Postsecondary Accreditation. Exists to enhance the efforts of social work education at all levels.

★5234★ COUNSELING AND CONSULTING SERVICES PUBLICATIONS
c/o Joseph Gill
4020 Moorpark Avenue, Ste. 206
San Jose, CA 95117   Phone: (408) 246-1128
Description: Publishes self-help and preventive mental health books that are essentially geared towards the general public and serve as a supplemental aid to mental health professionals.

★5235★ COUNSELING RESOURCE CENTER, INC.
5 Spruce St.
Winchester, MA 01890   Phone: (617) 729-8044
Description: Publishes on personal growth, psychological health, and religious orientation.

★5236★ COUNSELOR PUBLICATIONS
PO Box 515
Marlborough, CT 06447   Phone: (203) 295-9185
Description: Publishes on substance abuse counselor training.

★5237★ COUPLE TO COUPLE LEAGUE
3621 Glenmore Ave.
Cincinnati, OH 45211   Phone: (513) 661-7612
Subject Specialties: Natural family planning, birth control, teen sexuality.

★5238★   COVER PUBLISHING COMPANY
PO Box 1092
Tampa, FL 33601   Phone: (813) 237-0266

★5239★   COX PUBLICATIONS
PO Box 20316
Billings, MT 59104-0316   Phone: (406) 256-8822
Description: Cox Publications grew out of the activities of Meridith B. Cox Associates in 1977. Publishes newsletters and books for health care professionals. **Subject Specialties:** Risk management and medical-legal.

★5240★   C.P.S., INC.
PO Box 83
Larchmont, NY 10538   Phone: (914) 833-1633
Description: Publishes psychological test materials for practitioners in psychotherapy. **Subject Specialties:** Psychological testing, psychotherapy.

★5241★   CRAB COVE BOOKS
PO Box 214
Alameda, CA 94501   Phone: (415) 945-0854
Description: Publishes health/nutrition books for adults and a book on household hints.

★5242★   CRANBROOK PUBLISHING COMPANY
2302 Windmere
Flint, MI 48503   Phone: (313) 338-6403
Description: Publishes science and technology books and journals, including many in the medical field. **Subject Specialties:** Counseling, death, and divorce help for children.

★5243★   CRC PRESS, INC.
2000 Corporate Blvd. NW
Boca Raton, FL 33431   Phone: (407) 994-0555
Description: Publishes science and technology books and journals, including many in the medical field.

★5244★   CRCS PUBLICATIONS
PO Box 1460
Sebastopol, CA 95472   Phone: (707) 829-0735
Description: Publishes on astrology, self-help, and holistic health.

★5245★   CREATIVE ASSISTANCE PRESS
7101 Coachwhip Hollow
Austin, TX 78750   Phone: (512) 345-2404
Description: Publishes books on drug addiction.

★5246★   CREATIVE WALKING, INC.
PO Box 50296
Clayton, MO 63105   Phone: (314) 721-3600
Description: Publishes on health and fitness with special emphasis on school and corporate walking programs.

★5247★   CREATIVITY UNLIMITED PRESS
30819 Casilina
Rancho Palos Verdes, CA 90274   Phone: (213) 541-4844
Description: Publishes poetry, short stories, and a series of cassette tapes promoting personal growth through self-hypnosis. **Subject Specialties:** Psychology, self-help, occult, poetry, hypnosis.

★5248★   CRITTENDEN-NORTH CONCEPTS
30131 Town Center Dr., No. 35
Laguna Niguel, CA 92677-2034   Phone: (714) 495-8550
Description: Publishes medical self-help materials.

★5249★   CROMLECH BOOKS, INC.
175 Nobska Rd.
Woods Hole, MA 02543   Phone: (508) 540-1185
Description: Publishes on AIDS.

★5250★   CRONER PUBLICATION, INC.
34 Jericho Tpke.
Jericho, NY 11753   Phone: (516) 333-9085
Subject Specialties: Schools, drug abuse, international trade.

★5251★   CROSS RIVER PRESS
PO Box 473
Cross River, NY 10518   Phone: (914) 763-8050
Description: Publishes books on travel and medicine.

★5252★   CTB INTERNATIONAL PUBLISHING, INC.
PO Box 218
Maplewood, NJ 07040   Phone: (201) 763-6855
Description: Publishes on biotechnology and pharmacology.

★5253★   CTM ASSOCIATES
1 Randell Pl., Rte. 2
Denison, TX 75020   Phone: (903) 465-0882
Description: Publishes self-help books on stress reduction. **Subject Specialties:** 21st century human cybernetic science.

★5254★   CURRENT CLINICAL STRATEGIES PUBLISHING
4200 Park Newport, Ste. 214
Newport Beach, CA 92660   Phone: (714) 721-0710
Description: Publishes on medical topics for physicians, nurses, and medical students.

★5255★   CYBELE SOCIETY
1603 W. 9th Ave.
Spokane, WA 99204-3406   Phone: (509) 838-2332
Subject Specialties: Family-centered maternity care.

★5256★   DALLAS SANDT COMPANY
3104 E. Camelback Rd., Ste. 301
Phoenix, AZ 85016   Phone: (602) 279-1166
Description: Publishes "books about good nutrition which are easy to use and to understand." Also offers a nutrition learning game, *Play for Your Life.*

★5257★   DAYSTAR PUBLISHING COMPANY
PO Box 707
Angwin, CA 94508   Phone: (707) 965-2085
Subject Specialties: Holistic health, vegetarianism, travel.

★5258★   DAYTON PRESS
3235 Dayton Ave.
Lorain, OH 44055   Phone: (216) 246-1397
Description: Publishes books in the area of the health sciences and folklore.

★5259★   D'CARLIN PUBLISHING
PO Box 534
Carlsbad, CA 92008   Phone: (619) 720-9468
Subject Specialties: Health.

★5260★   DCI PUBLISHING
13911 Ridgedale Dr.
Minnetonka, MN 55343   Phone: (612) 541-0239
Description: Publishes health, wellness, and nutrition books written for the general reader interested in health issues and for the health professional for use with patients.

★5261★   DE-FEET PRESS
2401 W. 15th St.
Panama City, FL 32401   Phone: (904) 763-3333
Subject Specialties: Foot care, health, history.

★5262★   DELMAR PUBLISHERS, INC.
PO Box 15015
2 Computer Dr., W.
Albany, NY 12212   Phone: (518) 459-1150
Description: Publishes vocational, technical, and professional reference books. **Subject Specialties:** Vocational trades, nursing & allied health, early childhood education, technology education.

★5263★   DENALI PUBLISHING
134 Old Washington
Hanover, MA 02339   Phone: (617) 826-4465
Description: Publishes health and materials science textbooks.

★5264★ DENTAL FOLKLORE BOOKS OF K.C.
8221 NW 39th St.
Bethany, OK 73008   Phone: (405) 495-2578
Description: Publishes on dental history and folklore and the collection of dental antiques. Also offers prints, postcards, posters, and calendars.

★5265★ DENTAL HEALTH CENTER
2440 W. 3rd St.
Los Angeles, CA 90057   Phone: (213) 383-3833
Subject Specialties: Dentistry, health.

★5266★ DENTAL INFO
2509 N. Campbell, No. 9
Tucson, AZ 85719
Description: Publishes self-help, holistic, and naturalistic health information with a focus on herbs, dentistry, nutrition, and stress.

★5267★ DEVIN-ADAIR PUBLISHERS, INC.
6 N. Water St.
Greenwich, CT 06830   Phone: (203) 531-7755
Description: Publishes materials on health, conservative politics, gardening and ecology, cooking, travel, and glossy photographic books.

★5268★ DIETARY RESEARCH
5201 16th Avenue, NE
Seattle, WA 98105   Phone: (206) 524-2176
Description: Prepares and updates innovative dietary cookbooks for general public or medical teaching.

★5269★ DILLMAN PUBLISHING
2009 Bechtel Rd.
Indianapolis, IN 46260   Phone: (317) 872-8987
Description: Publishes manuals for pre-hospital care personnel.

★5270★ DIMI PRESS
3820 Oak Hollow Ln. SE
Salem, OR 97302   Phone: (503) 364-7698
Description: Publishes books and cassettes, emphasizing psychological self-help and relaxation techniques.

★5271★ D.I.N. PUBLICATIONS
PO Box 27568
Tempe, AZ 85285-7568   Phone: (602) 491-0393
Description: A nonprofit, national drug, alcohol, and health education project. Publishes a quarterly newsletter, pamphlets, booklets, and posters on substances, behavior, and health.

★5272★ DISPATCH PUBLICATIONS
1263 Canyon Side Ave.
San Ramon, CA 94583   Phone: (415) 946-4555
Description: Provides publications for public safety dispatchers including police, fire, and emergency medical services.

★5273★ DMI ASSOCIATES
615 Clark Ave.
Owosso, MI 48867
Description: Publishes books on coping and defense mechanisms for mental health professionals. Subject Specialties: Defense mechanisms.

★5274★ DNR PRESS
5652 Lake Murray Blvd.
La Mesa, CA 92041   Phone: (714) 465-3393
Subject Specialties: Dentistry for the consumer.

★5275★ DON QUIXOTE PUBLISHING COMPANY, INC.
PO Box 9442
Amarillo, TX 79105   Phone: (806) 352-5271
Description: Publishes self-help medical, environmental, and clinical ecology materials.

★5276★ DOWN THERE PRESS
PO Box 2086
Burlingame, CA 94011-2086   Phone: (415) 342-2536
Description: Publishes exclusively sexual self-help books for adults and children.

★5277★ DRAY PUBLICATIONS, INC.
Rte. 5
Deerfield, MA 01342   Phone: (413) 773-5491
Description: Produces employee and public information booklets and visual aids on workplace and home safety.

★5278★ DRELWOOD PUBLICATIONS
PO Box 10605
Portland, OR 97210   Phone: (503) 223-9106
Description: Publishes books written by Elizabeth and Elton Baker. Subject Specialties: Nutrition.

★5279★ DRUG INTELLIGENCE PUBLICATIONS, INC.
4720 Montgomery Ln.
Ste. 807
Bethesda, MD 20814   Phone: (301) 654-8736
Description: Publishes drug information geared for health professionals.

★5280★ DRUGREF, INC.
32 Loockerman Sq., Ste. L-100
Dover, DE 19901   Phone: (415) 365-0656
Description: Publishes medical reference texts.

★5281★ DUKE UNIVERSITY
CENTER FOR THE STUDY OF AGING AND HUMAN DEVELOPMENT
Medical Center
Box 3003
Durham, NC 27710   Phone: (919) 684-2248
Description: A research and training facility within Duke University Medical Center. Publishes periodic reports and books based on research on the physical and psychological effects of aging conducted at the Center.

★5282★ DUO ASSOCIATES
10211 SW Barbur Blvd., Ste. 109-A
Portland, OR 97219
Description: Publishes a guide and reference manual to Medicare to help health care providers and people on Medicare get the most for their Medicare dollars; also simplifies the Medicare process and tells people how to get all the benefits they are entitled to.

★5283★ E & L PRESS
PO Box 1967
Chicago, IL 60690   Phone: (312) 883-1734
Description: Publishes on philosophy and health.

★5284★ EAGLE WING BOOKS, INC.
PO Box 9972
Memphis, TN 38109   Phone: (901) 377-4593
Description: Publishes materials on substance abuse, mental health, and sex offender treatment.

★5285★ EARTH RITES PRESS
c/o Sherry Mestel
398 8th St.
Brooklyn, NY 11215   Phone: (718) 768-8148
Description: Publishes on alternative methods of healing and creation of personal rituals with a focus on earth awareness and ecology. Subject Specialties: Health, occult, ecology.

★5286★ EAST WEST HEALTH BOOKS
17 Station St.
Brookline, MA 02147   Phone: (617) 232-1000
Description: Publishes on health and nutrition from the Orient to the Occident. Subject Specialties: Natural health and living.

★5287★ EASTLAND PRESS
119 1st Ave. S., Ste. 400
Seattle, WA 98104   Phone: (206) 587-6013
Description: Publishes medical books, with emphasis on osteopathy, manual medicine, and Oriental medicine.

★5288★ EBS PRESS
1011 Boren Ave.
PO Box 179
Seattle, WA 98104　　　Phone: (206) 763-2381
Description: Publishes books on nutrition and occult writings.

★5289★ ECLECTIC PRESS
205 Pigeon St.
Waynesville, NC 28786　　　Phone: (704) 456-6736
Description: Publishes books on holistic health.

★5290★ ECRI
5200 Butler Pike
Plymouth Meeting, PA 19462　　　Phone: (215) 825-6000
Description: Health care technology consultants. Publishes two annual directories, journals, and newsletters.

★5291★ EDEN MEDICAL RESEARCH INC.
PO Box 51
St. Albans, VT 05478　　　Phone: (514) 931-3910
Subject Specialties: Scholarly, medical, scientific, and general nonfiction.

★5292★ EDGEHILL PUBLICATIONS
200 Harrison Ave.
Newport, RI 02840　　　Phone: (401) 849-5700
Description: Publishes books and monographs on alcoholism, drugs, and gambling addictions.

★5293★ EDITORIAL CONCEPTS, INC.
11980 SW 46th St.
Miami, FL 33175　　　Phone: (305) 661-6588
Description: Publishes dictionaries, encyclopedias, and children's books.
Subject Specialties: Food, health, nutrition, parapsychology.

★5294★ EDITORIAL CONSULTANTS, INC.
1738 Union St.
San Francisco, CA 94123　　　Phone: (415) 474-5010
Subject Specialties: Health care, history.

★5295★ EDITS PUBLISHERS
PO Box 7234
San Diego, CA 92107　　　Phone: (619) 488-1666
Description: Publishes psychological and educational books and testing materials and a career awareness program.

★5296★ EDUCATIONAL MEDIA CORPORATION
PO Box 21311
Minneapolis, MN 55421　　　Phone: (612) 781-0088
Description: Publishes books, films, and software for counselors and psychologists. **Subject Specialties:** Counseling.

★5297★ EDWARD N. HAYES, PUBLISHER
4229 Birch St.
Newport Beach, CA 92660　　　Phone: (714) 756-9063
Description: Publishes specialized directories on the financial strength and credit ratings of retail pharmacies, medical supply houses, and dental supply houses in U.S.

★5298★ E.G.L. ENTERPRISES, INC.
5438 Fernwood Ave.
Los Angeles, CA 90027　　　Phone: (213) 465-7121
Description: Publishes works on behaviorial sciences dealing with human sexuality and related educational programs. **Subject Specialties:** Body taboo neurosis, self-esteem, life enhancement, new living alternatives, nudism, naturism.

★5299★ EHG INTERMEDIC, INC.
777 3rd Ave.
New York, NY 10017
Description: Publishes a directory of physicians in over 200 foreign cities that Americans may call if a doctor is suddenly needed.

★5300★ ELBERN PUBLICATIONS
PO Box 09497
Columbus, OH 43209　　　Phone: (614) 235-2643
Description: Publishes vocational/career assessment materials for the physically and mentally handicapped.

★5301★ ELFIN COVE PRESS
PO Box 924
Redmond, WA 98052　　　Phone: (206) 868-4547
Description: Publishes a book on nutrition and a story on Minnesota in the early 1900's.

★5302★ ELLIOTT E. CARTER
PO Box 2487
Christiansburg, VA 24068　　　Phone: (703) 382-1874
Description: Publishes on job search techniques for recovering alcoholics, drug addicts, and ex-offenders.

★5303★ ELM PRESS
3555 5th Ave.
San Diego, CA 92103　　　Phone: (619) 298-7135
Description: Publishes a book for health care professionals.

★5304★ ELSEVIER SCIENCE PUBLISHING COMPANY, INC.
655 Avenue of the Americas
New York, NY 10010　　　Phone: (212) 989-5800
Description: Publishes books on the sciences, including medicine.

★5305★ EMERGENCY RESPONSE INSTITUTE, INC.
4537 Foxhall Dr. NE
Olympia, WA 98506　　　Phone: (206) 491-7785
Subject Specialties: Emergency management, emergency preparedness, disaster planning, search and rescue, emergency response.

★5306★ EMERGENCY TRAINING
150 N. Miller Rd., Bldg. No. 200
Akron, OH 44313　　　Phone: (216) 864-0878
Description: Publishes textbooks and audio-visual training materials for emergency medical personnel (pre-hospital), including the general public, industrial personnel, office personnel, and trained professionals.

★5307★ ENERGY PUBLICATIONS, INC.
RD 1
Morrisville, NY 13408　　　Phone: (315) 684-9284
Description: Publishes on breakthroughs in health and energy.

★5308★ ENSMINGER PUBLISHING COMPANY/PEGUS PRESS
648 W. Sierra Ave.
Clovis, CA 93612　　　Phone: (209) 299-2263
Description: Aim to promote better livestock production and human nutrition around the world.

★5309★ ENVIRONMENTAL PRESS
1201 Dusky Thrush
Austin, TX 78746　　　Phone: (512) 327-5479
Subject Specialties: Health.

★5310★ EPIDEMIOLOGY RESOURCES INC.
PO Box 339
Chestnut Hill, MA 02167　　　Phone: (617) 734-9100
Description: Publishes educational materials in epidemiology.

★5311★ EPILEPSY FOUNDATION OF AMERICA
4351 Garden City Dr.
Landover, MD 20785　　　Phone: (301) 459-3700
Description: Publishes a monthly newsletter, public service announcement materials, public health and professional education materials, teaching guidelines, bibliographies, audiovisual materials, catalogs on epilepsy, and epilepsy program guidelines.

★5312★ ESHA RESEARCH, INC.
1193 Royvonne SE, Ste. 23
Salem, OR 97302　　　Phone: (503) 585-6242
Description: Publishes a reference on nutrition and offers nutrition analysis software for IBM, Apple II, and Macintosh personal computers.

★5313★ ESKUALDUN PUBLISHERS, LTD.
PO Box 50266
Phoenix, AZ 85076-0266   Phone: (602) 893-2394
Subject Specialties: Self-help, inspirational, sharing, health, cancer, alcoholism.

★5314★ ESSENTIAL MEDICAL INFORMATION SYSTEMS, INC.
PO Box 1607
Durant, OK 74702-1607   Phone: (800) 225-0694
Description: Publishes medical texts and handbooks for physicians and clinicians.

★5315★ ETERNA PRESS
PO Box 157941
Chicago, IL 60615
Description: Publishes books relative to child and family services, special education, health, mental health, and social work. Subject Specialties: Medicine, social services, special education, continental philosophy.

★5316★ EUGENE V. WHITE
1 W. Main St.
Berryville, VA 22611-0286   Phone: (703) 955-2280
Subject Specialties: Pharmacy office practice.

★5317★ EVALUATION RESEARCH ASSOCIATES
RR 1, Box 203 G
Mullica Hill, NJ 08062   Phone: (609) 863-6077
Description: Publishes a directory of hotlines and crisis intervention centers.

★5318★ EXCEPTIONAL PARENT PRESS
1170 Commomwealth Ave.
Boston, MA 02134   Phone: (617) 730-5800
Description: Publishes books helpful to parents of children with disabilities.

★5319★ EXER FUN PUBLISHERS
3089C Clairemont Dr., Ste. 130
San Diego, CA 92117   Phone: (619) 268-0684
Description: Publishes fitness books with accompanying audio cassettes for home or class use by children, teachers, parents, and people with limited mobility.

★5320★ EXPRESSION COMPANY
PO Box 153
Londonderry, NH 03053   Phone: (603) 432-5232
Subject Specialties: Speech and reading problems.

★5321★ EYE CARE CONCEPTS, INC.
6552 Neosho St.
St. Louis, MO 63109-2642   Phone: (314) 832-3236
Description: Publishes educational and informational books and forms on eye and vision care subjects.

★5322★ F. A. DAVIS COMPANY
1915 Arch St.
Philadelphia, PA 19103   Phone: (215) 568-2270
Description: Publishes textbooks on medicine, nursing, and allied health.

★5323★ F. E. PEACOCK PUBLISHERS, INC.
PO Box 397
Itasca, IL 60143-0397   Phone: (708) 350-0777
Description: Publishes college level textbooks on education, social science, and behavioral science. Accepts unsolicited manuscripts.

★5324★ F. FERGESON PUBLICATIONS
160 John Dr.
Mount Zion, IL 62549   Phone: (217) 864-5620
Description: Specializes in medical communications with an emphasis on the "wellness" movement. Future publications will be on preventive medicine. Subject Specialties: Medicine, music.

★5325★ FACT PUBLISHING
PO Box 26B42
Los Angeles, CA 90026   Phone: (213) 665-5140
Subject Specialties: Public health, religion.

★5326★ FALKYNOR BOOKS
4950 SW 70th Ave.
Davie, FL 33314   Phone: (305) 791-1562
Description: Publishes on alternative health and healing techniques.

★5327★ FAMILY HEALTH INTERNATIONAL
RTP Branch
PO Box 13950
Durham, NC 27709   Phone: (919) 544-7261
Description: Conducts, analyzes, and disseminates research on contraceptive methods, family planning services, maternity care, and primary health care. Research reported in journals and in an occasional monograph series.

★5328★ FAMILY HEALTH MEDIA
1811 N. Jay
Aberdeen, SD 57401   Phone: (605) 229-5990
Subject Specialties: Sexuality, medicine, mental health.

★5329★ FAMILY PROCESS, INC.
841 Broadway, Ste. 504
New York, NY 10003   Phone: (212) 505-6517
Description: A multi-disciplinary organization that publishes clinical research, training, and theoretical contributions in the broad area of family therapy.

★5330★ FAMILY PUBLICATIONS
PO Box 490398
Maitland, FL 32794-0398   Phone: (407) 539-1411
Description: Publishes on childbirth education and consumer health education.

★5331★ FAMILY PUBLISHING COMPANY
PO Box 462
Bodega Bay, CA 94923   Phone: (707) 875-3373
Subject Specialties: Fiction, cattle management, local history, poetry, drug abuse, comedy, child care.

★5332★ FC & A
103 Clover Green
Peachtree City, GA 30269   Phone: (404) 487-6307
Description: Publishes on health and nutrition.

★5333★ F.D.M. DISTRIBUTOR
7807 Hohman Ave.
Munster, IN 46321   Phone: (219) 836-8107
Description: Self-publishes materials on exercise and care of the aging body (after fifty).

★5334★ FEDERATION OF AMERICAN HEALTH SYSTEMS
1405 N. Pierce, Ste. 311
Little Rock, AR 72207   Phone: (501) 661-9555
Description: Publishes a bimonthly magazine, Health Systems Review, an annual report, a directory, and a biweekly newsletter Hotline. Subject Specialties: Health legislation, regulatory matters.

★5335★ FELIX MORROW, PUBLISHER
13 Welwyn Rd.
Great Neck, NY 11021   Phone: (516) 482-1044
Description: Publishes books on the psychophysical disciplines.

★5336★ FERTILITY AWARENESS SERVICES
828 NW 33rd.
PO Box 986
Corvallis, OR 97339   Phone: (503) 753-8530
Description: Publishes on fertility.

★5337★ F.I. COMMUNICATIONS
PO Box 3121
Stanford, CA 94309   Phone: (415) 851-0254
Subject Specialties: Psychology, cross-cultural personality and values, self and clinical health care, philosophy.

★5338★ FIREPLACE BOOKS
5705 SE Belmont
Portland, OR 97215   Phone: (503) 236-5335
Description: Publishes on women alcoholics.

★5339★ FIRST PUBLICATIONS, INC.
PO Box 5072
Evanston, IL 60204   Phone: (312) 869-7210
Description: Publishes practical information for people who care for those with mental disabilities.

★5340★ FITNESS ALTERNATIVES PRESS
28551 Moss Rock Rd.
Golden, CO 80401   Phone: (303) 674-7476
Subject Specialties: Physical fitness, time management.

★5341★ FITNESS FIRST
3 Haskins Rd.
Hanover, NH 03755   Phone: (603) 643-4059
Description: Publishes an illustrated book and cassette tape for women's at-home exercising. **Subject Specialties:** Physical fitness, health.

★5342★ FITNESS PUBLICATIONS
1991 Country Pl.
Ojai, CA 93023   Phone: (805) 646-0350
Description: Publishes cookbooks devoted to fitness, health, and weight loss.

★5343★ FITNESS PUBLICATIONS
521 Old Corvallis Rd.
Hamilton, MT 59840   Phone: (406) 363-6970
Description: Publishes on health and general well-being for individuals, schools, hospitals, insurance companies, and corporate fitness programs.

★5344★ FOCUS PRACTICE MANAGEMENT PUBLISHERS
Century Center, Ste. 3585
1750 Kalakaua Ave.
Honolulu, HI 96826   Phone: (808) 599-2790
Description: Publishes practice management literature for acupuncturists and other health care professionals.

★5345★ FOLIO ASSOCIATES, INC.
111 Perkins St.
Boston, MA 02130   Phone: (617) 522-5200
Description: Publishes annual medical directories of Massachusetts, Rhode Island, and Connecticut.

★5346★ FOOD AND NUTRITION PRESS, INC.
6527 Main St.
PO Box 374
Trumbull, CT 06611   Phone: (203) 261-8587
Description: Publishes books for reference and college and secondary textbook use on food and nutrition.

★5347★ FORDHAM UNIVERSITY HISPANIC RESEARCH CENTER
Fordham Rd., Thebaud Hall
Bronx, NY 10458   Phone: (212) 579-2678
Description: Disseminates the findings of the center's work on issues affecting the mental health of the Hispanic population in the northeast region of the U.S. **Subject Specialties:** Mental health.

★5348★ FORMUR INTERNATIONAL
4200 Laclede Ave.
St. Louis, MO 63108   Phone: (314) 289-9200
Description: Publishes on homeopathy and biochemistry.

★5349★ FOUNDATION FOR BLOOD IRRADIATION
1315 Apple Ave.
Silver Spring, MD 20910   Phone: (301) 587-8686
Description: Researches and promotes ultraviolet blood irradiation therapy in treatment of blood diseases and other degenerative diseases. Publishes reports and documents.

★5350★ FOUNDATION OF HUMAN UNDERSTANDING
8780 Venice Blvd.
PO Box 34036
Los Angeles, CA 90034   Phone: (213) 559-3711
Description: Publishes works on metaphysics and psychology, as well as self-help books. Alternate address is: PO Box 811, 111 Evelyn St. NW, Grants Pass, OR 97526.

★5351★ FOUNDATION FOR SCIENCE AND THE HANDICAPPED
1141 Iroquois Dr., No. 114
Naperville, IL 60563   Phone: (708) 357-7908
Description: Publishes a book to promote career options for talented people with physical handicaps. **Subject Specialties:** Education, counseling, special education, career guidance.

★5352★ FRANCIS CLARK WOOD INSTITUTE FOR THE HISTORY OF MEDICINE
19 S. 22nd St.
Philadelphia, PA 19103   Phone: (215) 563-3737
Description: Publishes on current and historical issues in medicine.

★5353★ FRASER PRODUCTS COMPANY
10730 Wheatland Ave.
Sunland, CA 91040   Phone: (818) 767-3334
Description: Publishes self-help books for individuals to reach his/her maximum potential. **Subject Specialties:** Health, nutrition, cookbooks, self-improvement, sports, exercise.

★5354★ FREESTONE PUBLISHING COLLECTIVE
PO Box 398
Monroe, UT 84754   Phone: (801) 527-3738
Description: Publishes self-help books that emphasize power, confidence, and healing. **Subject Specialties:** Health, sexuality, yoga, family planning.

★5355★ FUTURA PUBLISHING COMPANY, INC.
2 Bedford Ridge Rd.
PO Box 330
Mount Kisco, NY 10549   Phone: (914) 666-3505
Description: Medical publisher of single topic monographs.

★5356★ G & G PUBLISHING
615 Brandenburg Way
Roswell, GA 30075   Phone: (404) 992-8654
Subject Specialties: Nutrition, weight reduction, dieting.

★5357★ GABRIEL PRESS
4018 N. 40th St.
Phoenix, AZ 85018   Phone: (602) 955-0551
Description: Publishes books to "illustrate the healing potential of the body-mind-spirit relationship." **Subject Specialties:** Holistic health.

★5358★ GAINING GROUND
PO Box 9184
Portland, OR 97207   Phone: (503) 232-1871
Description: Self-publisher of an exercise book. **Subject Specialties:** Exercise, health.

★5359★ GALE RESEARCH INC.
835 Penobscot Bldg.
Detroit, MI 48226-4094   Phone: (313) 961-2242
Description: Publishes reference books for libraries and businesses. **Subject Specialties:** Directories, indexex, biographical references, literary criticism, author biographies, dictionaries, bibliographies.

★5360★ GALLAUDET UNIVERSITY
GALLAUDET RESEARCH INSTITUTE
800 Florida Ave. NE
Washington, DC 20002   Phone: (202) 651-5400
Description: Conducts multidisciplinary research on topics concerning deafness and deaf people, including studies in education, demographics, psychology, sociology, linguistics, cultural anthropology, mental health, and rehabilitation engineering. Offers *Research at Gallaudet*, a triannual newsletter and *A Tradition of Discovery*, an annual report.

★5361★ GALLAUDET UNIVERSITY
GALLAUDET UNIVERSITY PRESS
800 Florida Ave. NE
Washington, DC 20002   Phone: (202) 651-5488
Description: Publishes books for and about hearing impaired people.

★5362★ GARDNER PRESS, INC.
19 Union Sq. W.
New York, NY 10003   Phone: (212) 924-8293
Description: Publishes reference and textbooks on social sciences, behavioral sciences, biographies; also publishes trade books and nonfiction.

★5363★ GAZETTE INTERNATIONAL NETWORKING
INSTITUTE
4502 Maryland Ave.
St. Louis, MO 63108   Phone: (314) 361-0475
Description: An organization dedicated to empowering polio survivors and other persons with disabilities by supplying accurate information and a network of knowledgeable, caring people. **Subject Specialties:** Late effects of polio, home mechanical ventilation, experiences of persons with disabilities.

★5364★ GEMINI PUBLICATIONS
177-31 Edgerton Rd.
Jamaica Estates, NY 11432   Phone: (718) 380-1787
Subject Specialties: Natural health, self-development, nutrition.

★5365★ GENERAL MEDICAL PUBLISHERS
318 Lincoln Blvd., No. 117
Venice, CA 90291   Phone: (213) 392-4911
Description: Publishes books on clinical nursing.

★5366★ GENTLE WORLD, INC.
PO Box U
Paia, Maui, HI 96779   Phone: (808) 572-1560
Description: Publishes educational and philosophical materials on pure vegetarian nutrition for the health oriented community.

★5367★ GEORGE OHSAWA MACROBIOTIC FOUNDATION
1511 Robinson St.
Oroville, CA 95965   Phone: (916) 533-7702
Subject Specialties: Macrobiotics, nutrition, health, Eastern philosophy.

★5368★ GEORGE WASHINGTON UNIVERSITY
INTERGOVERNMENTAL HEALTH POLICY PROJECT
2011 Eye St. NW, Ste. 200
Washington, DC 20006   Phone: (202) 872-1445
Description: Publishes information on health policy, particularly state legislation and trends. Also provides technical assistance, research service, a state legislative clearinghouse, and legislative summaries.

★5369★ GEORGETOWN UNIVERSITY
KENNEDY INSTITUTE OF ETHICS
Washington, DC 20057   Phone: (202) 687-3885
Description: Publishes on ethical and public policy issues in health care and biomedical research, including such topics as professional patient relationship, resource allocation, contraception and abortion, reproductive technologies, genetic intervention, mental health therapies, human experimentation, organ transplantation, death and dying, and the use of animals in research.

★5370★ GE-PS CANCER MEMORIAL
519 Austin St.
Park Ridge, IL 60068   Phone: (312) 381-2815
Subject Specialties: Cancer treatment, religion, cancer prevention and detection, congressional investigation.

★5371★ GERIATRIC EDUCATIONAL CONSULTANTS
43 Middleton Ln.
Willingboro, NJ 08046   Phone: (609) 877-5972
Description: Publishes books on aging.

★5372★ GERI-REHAB, INC.
170 Hibbler Rd.
Lebanon, NJ 08833   Phone: (201) 735-8918
Description: Publishes materials on occupational therapy and rehabilitation.

★5373★ GERONTOLOGICAL SOCIETY OF AMERICA
1275 K St. NW, Ste. 350
Washington, DC 20005   Phone: (202) 842-1275
Description: Publishes on aging.

★5374★ GETWELL STAYWELL, AMERICA!
4390 Bidwell Dr.
Fremont, CA 94538   Phone: (408) 637-1919
Description: Aim is "to launch a health revolution in America whereby the suffering class of America can learn the truth about how to get well and stay well, without doctors, drugs, and surgery."

★5375★ GILGAL PUBLICATIONS
PO Box 3386
Sunriver, OR 97707   Phone: (503) 593-8639
Description: Publishes books on coping with stress and resolving grief. **Subject Specialties:** Bereavement, stress, inspiration, faith.

★5376★ GLEN ABBEY BOOKS
PO Box 31329
Seattle, WA 98103   Phone: (206) 548-9360
Description: Publishes books for people in 12 step recovery programs. **Subject Specialties:** Recovery from alcoholism, drug addiction.

★5377★ GLUTEN INTOLERANCE GROUP OF NORTH
AMERICA
PO Box 23053
Seattle, WA 98102-0353   Phone: (206) 325-6980
Description: "Offers assistance to persons with Celiac Sprue, their families, and health professionals." Publishes on diet and nutrition. Also publishes *GIG Newsletter* quarterly and fact sheets.

★5378★ GOEHRINGER & SONS ASSOCIATES
PO Box 9626
Pittsburgh, PA 15226   Phone: (412) 531-9549
Subject Specialties: Drug abuse, law enforcement, alcohol abuse.

★5379★ GOLDEN QUILL PUBLISHERS, INC.
PO Box 1278
Colton, CA 92324   Phone: (714) 783-0119
Subject Specialties: Holistic health, preventive medicine, New Age.

★5380★ GOOD THINGS INC.
610 W. Main St.
Greenfield, IN 46140   Phone: (317) 326-4608
Description: Publishes on nutrition and health.

★5381★ GORDON & BREACH, SCIENCE PUBLISHERS, INC.
270 8th Ave.
New York, NY 10011   Phone: (212) 206-8900
Description: Publishes college textbooks, magazines, books, and journals. **Subject Specialties:** Technology, science, business, medicine, behavioral science, research, reference.

★5382★ GORDON HANDWERK PUBLISHERS
PO Box 685
Madison, NJ 07940   Phone: (201) 377-8232
Description: Publishes psychology books for university courses and libraries.

★5383★ GORSUCH SCARISBRICK PUBLISHERS
8233 Via Paseo del Norte, Ste. F-400
Scottsdale, AZ 85258   Phone: (602) 991-7881
Description: A college-level educational publisher. Accepts unsolicited

manuscripts. Reaches market through direct mail and telephone sales.
Subject Specialties: Speech communication, health, physical education, recreation, real estate, career planning.

★5384★   **GOWER MEDICAL PUBLISHING LTD.**
101 5th Ave.
New York, NY 10003   Phone: (212) 929-6290
Description: Publishes full-color text-atlases in all areas of medicine.

★5385★   **GRACEWAY PUBLISHING COMPANY**
PO Box 159, Sta. C.
Flushing, NY 11367   Phone: (718) 463-3914
Description: Publishes medicine and economics titles geared for academia and business professionals.

★5386★   **GRAIN AND SALT SOCIETY**
14351 Wyclif
PO Box GDD
Magalia, CA 95954   Phone: (916) 873-0294
Description: Publishes on alternative nutrition, health, and food preparation.

★5387★   **GREAT OCEAN PUBLISHERS**
1823 N. Lincoln St.
Arlington, VA 22207   Phone: (703) 525-0909
Description: Publishes trade books on education, music, health, and fine arts.

★5388★   **GREENSWARD PRESS**
1600 Larkin, No. 104
San Francisco, CA 94109   Phone: (415) 928-4142
Description: Publishes alternative and mainstream health publications for physicians, dentists, general public, and health practitioners.

★5389★   **GREENWOOD PUBLISHING GROUP, INC.**
88 Post Rd. W.
PO Box 5007
Westport, CT 06881   Phone: (203) 226-3571
Description: Publishes nonfiction books, reference books, and hardcover monographs, scholarly books, and journals. **Subject Coverage:** Business, social sciences, humanities, business law, medicine.

★5390★   **GRINNEN-BARRETT PUBLISHING COMPANY**
36 Winchester St., No. 8
PO Box 779
Brookline, MA 02146   Phone: (617) 232-1993
Description: Publishes on pregnancy and nutrition. Offers posters and dieting materials.

★5391★   **GT INTERNATIONAL**
PO Box 1550
Pomona, CA 91769   Phone: (714) 623-1738
Description: Publishes trade books and limited editions on yoga, meditation, and nutrition.

★5392★   **GUILD FOR THE BLIND**
180 N. Michigan, No. 1720
Chicago, IL 60601   Phone: (312) 236-8569
Description: Publications foster independent living for the blind and visually impaired. Offers books on audio cassette. Also offers books with directions specially designed to accomodate the needs of the blind and visually impaired.

★5393★   **GUILFORD PUBLICATIONS, INC.**
72 Spring St.
New York, NY 10012   Phone: (212) 431-9800
Description: Publishes books, cassettes, educational programs, and journals in psychology, psychiatry, sociology, communication, family studies, criminology, geography, and molecular biology for clinical and academic readers.

★5394★   **GURZE BOOKS**
PO Box 2238
Carlsbad, CA 92008   Phone: (619) 434-7533
Description: Publishes on bulimia, an eating disorder of binge eating and vomiting.

★5395★   **H. & B. HESS COMPANY**
548 Majorca Ct.
Satellite Beach, FL 32937   Phone: (305) 773-2867
Description: Publishes textbooks for supervisors and faculty in nursing and the health professions.

★5396★   **H.W. WILSON COMPANY**
950 University Ave.
Bronx, NY 10452   Phone: (212) 588-8400
Description: Publishes reference tools for libraries and book trade, including works in the sciences.

★5397★   **HAIGHT-ASHBURY PUBLICATIONS**
409 Clayton St., 2nd Fl.
San Francisco, CA 94117   Phone: (415) 565-1904
Description: Publishes medical and scientific information on psychoactive substances (both licit and illicit) for professional health and mental health care providers as well as the interested lay reader. **Subject Specialties:** Drugs (including alcohol, tobacco, medicines).

★5398★   **HALLELUJAH ACRES PUBLISHING**
Mt.ain Valley Rd.
Eidson, TN 37731   Phone: (615) 272-7800
Description: Publishes on health and nutrition for the Christian community.

★5399★   **HAMILTON PUBLICATIONS**
PO Box 3222
Boulder, CO 80307-3222   Phone: (303) 499-3183
Description: Publishes materials for educators of students with special educational needs.

★5400★   **HAND-D-CAP PUBLISHING**
1027 E. Palmaritas Dr.
Phoenix, AZ 85020   Phone: (602) 944-6560
Description: Publishes a book on gardening for the handicapped.

★5401★   **HANLEY & BELFUS, INC.**
210 S. 13th St.
Philadelphia, PA 19107   Phone: (215) 546-4995
Description: Publishes professional books and periodicals in human medicine.

★5402★   **HAPPY HEALTH PUBLISHERS**
13048 Del Monte Dr., No. 42-D
Seal Beach, CA 90740   Phone: (213) 431-0069
Description: Publishes information on sex, nutrition, and health.

★5403★   **HAPPY HISTORY, INC.**
PO Box 2160
Boca Raton, FL 33432   Phone: (305) 483-8093
Subject Specialties: American history, women's history, the handicapped.

★5404★   **HARBOR PRESS**
6712 38th Ave. NW
PO Box 1656
Gig Harbor, WA 98335   Phone: (206) 851-5190
Description: Publishes health and metaphysical books.

★5405★   **HARBOR PUBLISHING COMPANY**
80 N. Moore St., Ste. 4J
New York, NY 10013   Phone: (212) 349-1818
Description: Publishes interdisciplinary material in the social sciences and artifical intelligence. **Subject Specialties:** Psychology, sociology, anthropology.

★5406★   **HARCOURT BRACE JOVANOVICH, INC.**
6277 Sea Harbor Dr.
Orlando, FL 32887   Phone: (407) 345-2000
Description: Publishes elementary and secondary school and college textbooks, general fiction and nonfiction children's books, and scientific and medical books and journals.

★5407★ HARPERCOLLINS INC.
10 E. 53rd St.
New York, NY 10022   Phone: (212) 207-7000
Description: Publishes general fiction and nonfiction. Also publishes audio tapes, medical and nursing textbooks, and college textbooks.

★5408★ HARVARD UNIVERSITY
HARVARD UNIVERSITY PRESS
79 Garden St.
Cambridge, MA 02138   Phone: (617) 495-2600
Description: Publishes general scholarly titles, scientific titles, and titles on medicine.

★5409★ HARVEY WHITNEY BOOKS COMPANY
PO Box 42696
Cincinnati, OH 45242   Phone: (513) 793-3555
Description: Provides publications on drug therapy for physicians, pharmacists, and other health care professionals.

★5410★ HARWAL PUBLISHING COMPANY
605 W. State St.
PO Box 96
Media, PA 19063   Phone: (215) 565-0746
Description: Publishes review books and other titles for medical and veterinary practitioners; co-publishes the National Medical Series for Independent Study with John Wiley Medical.

★5411★ HASTINGS CENTER
255 Elm Rd.
Briarcliff, NY 10510   Phone: (914) 762-8500
Description: Publishes texts and reports on ethical questions in medicine, law, and other professions.

★5412★ HAWKES PUBLISHING, INC.
5947 S. 350 W.
PO Box 65735
Salt Lake City, UT 84107   Phone: (801) 266-5555
Subject Specialties: Self-help, food storage, cooking, health, inspirational.

★5413★ HAWORTH PRESS, INC.
10 Alice St.
Binghamton, NY 13904   Phone: (607) 722-5857
Description: Publishes books and 100 biannual or quarterly journals on the social and behavioral sciences for professionals. **Subject Specialties:** Gerontology, chemical dependency, social work, marketing, pharmaceutical sciences, agriculture, nutrition.

★5414★ HAYES PUBLISHING COMPANY, INC.
6304 Hamilton Ave.
Cincinnati, OH 45224   Phone: (513) 681-7559
Subject Specialties: Sex education, pro-life publication on abortion.

★5415★ HAYMARKET DOYMA, INC.
53 Park Pl.
New York, NY 10007   Phone: (212) 766-4300
Description: Publishes medical books and journals.

★5416★ HAZELDEN EDUCATIONAL MATERIALS
PO Box 176
Center City, MN 55012   Phone: (612) 257-4010
Description: Publishes books and produces audiovisual material on alcoholism, drug abuse, eating disorders, and other addictions. Provides information to dependent people, their families, and professionals about all aspects of addictions and compulsive behaviors. **Subject Specialties:** Alcoholism, drug dependency, eating disorders, self-help, employee assistance, AIDS, codependency.

★5417★ HEALTH ACTION PRESS
PO Box 270
Springfield, MA 01138   Phone: (413) 782-2115
Description: Publishes educational literature on the subject of freedom of choice in personal health and of compulsory water fluoridation.

★5418★ HEALTH ADMINISTRATION PRESS
1021 E. Huron
Ann Arbor, MI 48104-9990   Phone: (313) 764-1380
Description: Publishes books on health services management. **Subject Specialties:** Health services management, health policy, medical-legal issues.

★5419★ HEALTH ALERT PRESS
PO Box 2060
Cambridge, MA 02238   Phone: (617) 497-4190
Description: Publishes an illustrated, easy to read book for the layperson on AIDS. **Subject Specialties:** Health, education.

★5420★ HEALTH CARE COMMUNICATIONS, INC.
1 Bridge Plaza N.
Fort Lee, NJ 07024-7502   Phone: (201) 947-5545
Description: Publishes medical books on cardiology, psychology, and out patient therapy.

★5421★ HEALTH CHALLENGE PRESS
c/o Guy Fasciana
7721 E. 39th St.
Tucson, AZ 85730   Phone: (602) 991-9824
Description: A publishing company that addresses the dental health needs of concerned dental consumers. **Subject Specialties:** Health, medicine, dentistry.

★5422★ HEALTH COMMUNICATIONS, INC.
3201 SW 15th St.
Deerfield Beach, FL 33442   Phone: (305) 360-0909
Description: Distributes information and educational resources for the professional, para-profesional, and lay person in the drug and alcohol abuse field.

★5423★ HEALTH EDUCATION PUBLISHING CORPORATION
PO Box 2388
Eugene, OR 97402   Phone: (503) 998-6003
Description: Publishes on chiropractic.

★5424★ HEALTH EDUCATOR PUBLICATIONS, INC.
1580 Kirkland Rd.
Old Town, ME 04468   Phone: (207) 827-3633
Description: Publishes health related books.

★5425★ HEALTH FACTS PUBLISHING
3521 Broadway
Kansas City, MO 64111   Phone: (816) 753-8850
Description: Publishes on health education.

★5426★ HEALTH INDUSTRY REPRESENTATIVES
ASSOCIATION
5818 Reeds Rd.
Mission, KS 66202   Phone: (913) 262-4513
Description: Publishes a directory covering 170 manufacturers' representatives in the health care industry and manufacturers of health care products.

★5427★ HEALTH PLUS PUBLISHERS
PO Box 1027
Sherwood, OR 97140   Phone: (503) 625-0589
Description: Publishes to promote the art and study of holistic health and to advance public understanding of the individual's responsibility for his/her own health and well-being. **Subject Specialties:** Health, food, nutrition, fitness, holistic/biological medicine.

★5428★ HEALTH POLICY ADVISORY CENTER
17 Murray St.
New York, NY 10007   Phone: (212) 267-8890
Description: Publishes on health policy as it affects all Americans, toward the goal of quality, affordable, appropriate health care for all.

★5429★ HEALTH PRESS
PO Box 367
Santa Fe, NM 87501   Phone: (505) 982-9373
Description: Publishes health related books on food, nutrition, aging, cancer, pregnancy, and travel health.

★5430★   HEALTH PSYCHOLOGY PUBLICATIONS
710 11th Ave., Ste. 106
Greeley, CO 80631   Phone: (303) 353-6552
Description: Publishes on health, sports, and child psychology.

★5431★   HEALTH PUBLISHING COMPANY
3700 California St.
PO Box 3805
San Francisco, CA 94119   Phone: (415) 750-6165
Description: Publishes psychological and educational test materials, remedial activities, and health care books.

★5432★   HEALTH RESEARCH
PO Box 19420
Las Vegas, NV 89132   Phone: (702) 733-8476
Description: Publishes alternative health care materials for health care professionals. **Subject Specialties:** Preventive medicine, dentistry, psychology, New Age.

★5433★   HEALTH RESEARCH ASSOCIATES
PO Box 5280
Santa Cruz, CA 95063
Description: Publishes books on health and fitness.

★5434★   HEALTH AND SAFETY PUBLICATIONS
2265 Westwood Blvd., No. 563
Los Angeles, CA 90064   Phone: (213) 837-7003
Description: Publishes health education materials for industry. Offers self-improvement calendars, cards, flyers, and statement stuffers.

★5435★   HEALTH SCIENCE
7340 Hollister Ave.
PO Box 7
Santa Barbara, CA 93102   Phone: (805) 968-1028
Subject Specialties: Health, nutrition, exercise, triathlon training.

★5436★   HEALTHCARE FINANCIAL MANAGEMENT ASSOCIATION
2 Westbrook Corporate Center, Ste. 700
Westchester, IL 60154   Phone: (708) 531-9600
Description: Publishes books aimed toward the healthcare financial manager.

★5437★   HEALTHCARE PRESS
PO Box 4488
Rollingbay, WA 98061   Phone: (206) 842-5243
Description: Publishes a book on Alzheimer's disease.

★5438★   HEALTHCARE SAFETY PROFESSIONAL CERTIFICATION BOARD
8009 Carita Ct.
Bethesda, MD 20817   Phone: (301) 984-8969
Description: A nonprofit corporation dedicated to upgrading professional practice.

★5439★   HEALTHFUL CHEF, INC.
9 Shady Ln.
Danville, IL 61832   Phone: (217) 446-1060
Description: Publishes a health-related cookbook.

★5440★   HEALTHMERE PRESS, INC.
PO Box 986
Evanston, IL 60204   Phone: (312) 251-5950
Description: Publishes on fitness, health, and nutrition.

★5441★   HEALTHRIGHT PUBLISHING
92 Golden Hinde Blvd.
San Rafael, CA 94903-3817   Phone: (415) 776-0969
Description: Publishes on health and rejuvenation.

★5442★   HEALTHWISE, INC.
PO Box 1989
Boise, ID 83701-1989   Phone: (208) 345-1161
Description: Produces self-help health education programs and materials for individuals, organizations, and government agencies.

★5443★   HEALTHY CHANGES
47 Bedard St.
Derry, NH 03038-4214
Description: Publishers of nutritional literature, cookbooks for allergy, diabetics, and natural whole grain cooking.

★5444★   HEALTHY LIVING INSTITUTE
402 S. 14th St.
Hettinger, ND 58639   Phone: (701) 567-2646
Description: Publishes on the health effects of obesity.

★5445★   HEARST BOOKS
105 Madison Ave.
New York, NY 10016   Phone: (212) 889-3050
Description: Publishes fiction, nonfiction and marine titles.

★5446★   HEINZ PRESS
2629 Riverview Dr.
Eau Claire, WI 54703   Phone: (715) 835-4147
Description: Publishes "selected material pertinent to clinical practice of psychology."

★5447★   HELLINGER ENTERPRISES
1728 Laurel Canyon Blvd., No. F
West Hollywood, CA 90046   Phone: (213) 874-7607
Subject Specialties: Whole health, exercise, poetry, art, photography.

★5448★   HEMISPHERE PUBLISHING CORPORATION
1900 Frost Rd., Ste. 101
Bristol, PA 19007   Phone: (215) 785-5800
Description: Publishes professional, reference, and advanced-level textbooks on engineering, social sciences, life sciences, and environmental sciences.

★5449★   HEMLOCK SOCIETY
PO Box 11830
Eugene, OR 97440   Phone: (503) 342-5748
Description: Publishes books on voluntary euthanasia. Aims to "educate the public on the option of voluntary euthanasia for the terminally ill". **Subject Specialties:** Euthanasia, right to die, medical ethics.

★5450★   HENDERSON PRESS
5 Bee S. Main
Henderson, KY 42420   Phone: (502) 826-2586
Description: Self-publishes a book on the author's career as a surgeon.

★5451★   HERITAGE COMMUNICATIONS
12055 Cooperwood Ln.
Cincinnati, OH 45242   Phone: (513) 771-2230
Description: Publishes books on dentistry and dental fear.

★5452★   HERITAGE PUBLICATIONS
PO Box 71
Virginia Beach, VA 23458   Phone: (804) 428-0400
Description: Publishes books on the Edgar Cayce reading about natural health remedies.

★5453★   HESPERIAN FOUNDATION
PO Box 1692
Palo Alto, CA 94302   Phone: (415) 325-9017
Description: A nonprofit organization publishing books, papers, and a slide series on health care and health education for the rural poor. **Subject Specialties:** Primary health care, community based rehabilitation, health and social justice.

★5454★   HEURISTICUS PUBLISHING COMPANY
401 Tolbert St.
Brea, CA 92621   Phone: (714) 996-1270
Description: Self-publishes a reference work on human sexuality.

★5455★   HILARY HOUSE PUBLISHERS, INC.
980 N. Federal Hwy., Ste. 206
Boca Raton, FL 33432-2704   Phone: (407) 393-5656
Description: Publishes reference books, directories, health and fitness books, and how-to books.

★5456★ HILL PUBLICATIONS, INC.
235 Fox Tail Dr., No. 235-A
West Palm Beach, FL 33415-6194   Phone: (407) 968-7722
Description: Publishes books on health and nutrition, public speaking, and humor. **Subject Specialties:** Nutrition, cancer, public speaking, divorce humor.

★5457★ HIMALAYAN PUBLISHERS
RR 1, Box 400
Honesdale, PA 18431   Phone: (717) 253-5551
Description: Publishes materials on holistic health, preventive medicine, yoga, meditation, diet and nutrition, philosophy, psychology, and self-development.

★5458★ HINSDALE PRESS
PO Box 591481
San Francisco, CA 94159   Phone: (415) 752-8748
Description: Publishes books presenting new and possibly controversial ideas related to nutritional medicine and social concerns. Books are intended to serve both general readers and professionals, the latter through appendices and/or reference notes. **Subject Specialties:** Nutritional medicine, social concerns, yachting.

★5459★ HIPPOCRATES HEALTH INSTITUTE
1443 Palmdale Ct.
West Palm Beach, FL 33411   Phone: (407) 471-8876
Description: Promotes the vital health and well-being of mankind through proper nourishment, proper breathing and exercise, and proper mental attitude. **Subject Specialties:** Indoor gardening, colon health, sprouting, child care, pet care.

★5460★ HOFSTRA UNIVERSITY
INSTITUTE FOR ADVANCED RESEARCH IN ASIAN SCIENCE
  AND MEDICINE
Hempstead, NY 11550   Phone: (212) 270-1629
Description: Offers *The American Journal of Clinical Medicine.* Publishes a periodical and monographs.

★5461★ HOGREFE & HUBER PUBLISHERS
PO Box 51
Lewiston, NY 14092   Phone: (716) 282-1610
Description: Publishes books and journals in the fields of psychology, psychiatry, neuroscience, and medicine. Also has a Canadian office: 12 Bruce Park Ave., Toronto, ON, Canada M4P 2S3.

★5462★ HOHM PRESS
219 W. Gurley St.
Prescott, AZ 86301   Phone: (602) 778-9189
Subject Specialties: Philosophy, religion, health.

★5463★ HOLISTIC EXCHANGE
PO Box 1621
Muncie, IN 47308   Phone: (317) 741-7850
Description: Publishes books and catalogs on holistic health, women, and black studies.

★5464★ HOSPITAL COMPENSATION SERVICE
115 Watchung Dr.
PO Box 321
Hawthorne, NJ 07507   Phone: (201) 427-2221
Description: Publishes reports on hospital and nursing home employee compensations.

★5465★ HOSPITAL RESEARCH AND EDUCATIONAL TRUST
840 N. Lake Shore Dr.
Chicago, IL 60611   Phone: (312) 280-6000
Description: Conducts research and administration projects related to critical issues affecting health care, finance, and delivery. This work results in development of projects to help hospital executives increase the efficiency and effectiveness of their institutions. Offers publications, slide packages, *Executive Subscription Series on Economic Trends Affecting Health Care Industry,* and educational programs.

★5466★ HOUGHTON MIFFLIN COMPANY
1 Beacon St.
Boston, MA 02108   Phone: (617) 725-5000
Description: Publishes general literature, fiction, biographies, autobiographies, history, poetry, children's books, reference books, and elementary, secondary school, and college textbooks, including a medical reference titled "The Medical Health and Science Wordbook".

★5467★ HP BOOKS
360 N. La Cienga Blvd.
Los Angeles, CA 90048-1925   Phone: (213) 657-6100
Subject Specialties: Leisure, hobbies, automotive, cooking, photography, home improvement, computers, gardening, family health, arts and crafts, sports, fitness, medicine, business, finance.

★5468★ HUMAN ECOLOGY BALANCING SCIENCES, INC.
PO Box 737
Mahopac, NY 10541   Phone: (914) 751-3105
Description: Publishes on human ecology, human energy, New Age practices, nutrition, and diet. Offers audio cassettes, a newsletter, wall charts, and diet cards. **Subject Specialties:** New Age, nutrition, health, self-help, learning disorders.

★5469★ HUMAN ENERGY PRESS
1020 Foster City Blvd., No. 205
Foster City, CA 94404   Phone: (415) 349-0718
Description: Publishes on natural healing, AIDS, and metaphysics.

★5470★ HUMAN KINETICS PUBLISHERS, INC.
1607 N. Market St.
PO Box 5076
Champaign, IL 61825-5076   Phone: (217) 351-5076
Description: Publishes on physical education, sport and exercise sciences, sports medicine, and physical fitness. Also publishes sports books for coaches and players.

★5471★ HUMAN POLICY PRESS
PO Box 127, University Sta.
Syracuse, NY 13210   Phone: (315) 443-2761
Description: A vehicle for the distribution of books, slide shows, pamphlets, and posters on advocacy and attitude change toward people with disabilities.

★5472★ HUMAN SCIENCES PRESS
233 Spring St.
New York, NY 10013   Phone: (212) 620-8000
Description: Publishes on social, medical, and behavioral sciences.

★5473★ HUMAN SERVICES INSTITUTE, INC.
4301 32nd St. W., Ste. C-8
Bradenton, FL 34205   Phone: (813) 746-7088
Description: Publishes and distributes books on alcoholism, drug abuse, domestic violence, and self-help psychology.

★5474★ HUMANA PRESS, INC.
PO Box 2148
Clifton, NJ 07015   Phone: (201) 773-4389
Description: Publishes scientific and biomedical books and journals for professional audiences; also publishes a trade line for general audiences.

★5475★ HUNTER HOUSE, INC., PUBLISHERS
PO Box 847
Claremont, CA 91711-0847   Phone: (714) 624-2277
Description: Publishes titles on women's health, psychology, and family health.

★5476★ IDEAL WORLD PUBLISHING COMPANY
PO Box 252
Langhorne, PA 19047   Phone: (407) 254-6003
Subject Specialties: Health, nutrition, electric vehicles.

★5477★ IGAKU-SHOIN MEDICAL PUBLISHERS, INC.
1 Madison Ave.
New York, NY 10010   Phone: (212) 779-0123
Description: Publishes medical books and atlases for clinicians, students, and other medical professionals.

★5478★   IMAGE AWARENESS CORPORATION
1271 High St.
Auburn, CA 95603   Phone: (916) 823-7092
Subject Specialties: Nutrition.

★5479★   IMAGES UNLIMITED
124 N. Grand Ave.
PO Box 305
Maryville, MO 64468   Phone: (816) 582-4279
Description: Publishes on nutrition, cooking, and health.

★5480★   IMAGINART PRESS
307 Arizona St.
Bisbee, AZ 85603   Phone: (800) 828-1376
Description: Publishes books on speech-impairment.

★5481★   IMPACT PUBLISHERS, INC.
9774 Phillips Rd.
Lafayette, CO 80026-9756   Phone: (805) 543-5911
Description: Publishes books on human development. Subject Specialties:
Popular psychology, self-help, personal growth, relationships, families,
communities.

★5482★   IMPULSE PUBLISHING
PO Box 3321
Danbury, CT 06813-3321   Phone: (203) 790-8430
Description: Publishes books on natural and holistic health care.

★5483★   INDIANA UNIVERSITY
INSTITUTE FOR THE STUDY OF DEVELOPMENTAL
   DISABILITIES
2853 E. 10th St.
Bloomington, IN 47405   Phone: (812) 855-6508
Description: Provides curriculum guides, position papers, training materi-
als, and other resource materials in the area of developmental disabilities.

★5484★   INDUSTRIAL HEALTH FOUNDATION
34 Penn Circle W.
Pittsburgh, PA 15206   Phone: (412) 363-6600
Description: Publishes proceedings of technical meetings. Subject Specialties: Occupational health, industrial hygiene, toxicology.

★5485★   INFANT HEARING RESOURCE
3930 SW Macadam Ave.
Portland, OR 97201   Phone: (503) 494-4206
Description: Publishes a guide to help educators structure programs for
habilitating infants and helping parents during the critical early years.
Subject Specialties: Guides for educators of children with hearing disabilities.

★5486★   INFINITY IMPRESSIONS, LTD.
88 E. Main St., Ste. 500
Mendham, NJ 07945   Phone: (201) 543-9211
Description: Publishes nutrition and curriculum information for educators.

★5487★   INFORMATION, PROTECTION, AND ADVOCACY
   CENTER FOR HANDICAPPED INDIVIDUALS, INC.
300 Eye St. NE, Ste. 202
Washington, DC 20002   Phone: (202) 547-8081
Description: Publishes directories of resources and services for the handi-
capped.

★5488★   INGHAM PUBLISHING, INC.
5650 1st Ave.
PO Box 12642
St. Petersburg, FL 33733-2642   Phone: (813) 343-4811
Description: Publishes books in the health field dealing with foot reflexolo-
gy. Books are published in seven different languages.

★5489★   INNER GROWTH BOOKS
PO Box 520
Chiloquin, OR 97624   Phone: (503) 783-3126
Description: Publishes on simple living, Jungian psychology, metaphysics,
and Christian mysticism.

★5490★   INNER TRADITIONS INTERNATIONAL LTD.
1 Park St.
Rochester, VT 05767   Phone: (802) 767-3174
Description: Publishes on esoteric philosophy and health. Subject Specialties: Metaphysics, philosophy, art, alternative health.

★5491★   INNER VISION PUBLISHING COMPANY
PO Box 1117, Seapines Sta.
Virginia Beach, VA 23451   Phone: (804) 671-1777
Subject Specialties: Psychology, self-help, inspiration, consciousness.

★5492★   INQUIRY PRESS
1880 N. Eastman
Midland, MI 48640   Phone: (517) 631-0009
Description: Publishes for Wysong Corporation on health, medical, and
nutrition topics. Subject Specialties: Nutrition, healthy lifestyles, pet
nutrition.

★5493★   INSIGHT PRESS
535 Cordova Rd., Ste. 228
Santa Fe, NM 87501   Phone: (505) 471-7511
Description: Publishes educational and training books. Subject Specialties:
Health.

★5494★   INSIGHT PRESS
4001 Manchaca Rd.
Austin, TX 78704   Phone: (512) 440-0888
Description: Publishes books on alternative health care and medicines.

★5495★   INSTITUTE FOR THE ADVANCEMENT OF HEALTH
16 E. 53rd St.
New York, NY 10022   Phone: (212) 832-8282
Description: Publishes annotated bibliographies on mind-body-health
research. The bibliographies "systematically assemble research abstracts
on treating major medical disorders with psychological and behavioral
techniques."

★5496★   INSTITUTE FOR CLINICAL SCIENCE, INC.
1833 Delancey Pl.
Philadelphia, PA 19103   Phone: (215) 829-7507
Description: Publishes a bimonthly journal, Annals of Clinical and Laboratory Science and a yearly manual on clinical pathology and chemistry in
conjunction with scientific presentations at meetings of the Association of
Clinical Scientists. Additional books are published by the director.
Alternate phone number is (215) 829-7068. Subject Specialties: Clinical
pathology, clinical chemistry, laboratory medicine.

★5497★   INSTITUTE OF MIND AND BEHAVIOR
PO Box 522, Village Sta.
New York, NY 10014   Phone: (212) 595-4853
Description: Publishes a philosophical psychology journal, The Journal of
Mind and Behavior. Also publishes as books special issues pertaining to
mind/body interactionism in the social sciences, medicine, and social
philosophy. Subject Specialties: Psychology, psychiatry, medicine, psychol-
ogy of literature, philosophy of science.

★5498★   INSTITUTE FOR PERSONALITY AND ABILITY
   TESTING, INC.
PO Box 188
Champaign, IL 61820
Description: Publishes psychological tests and related books and materials.
Also sells computer reports to professional audiences. Subject Specialties:
Psychology, behavioral medicine.

★5499★   THE INSTITUTE FOR PHOBIC AWARENESS
PO Box 1180
Palm Springs, CA 92263   Phone: (619) 322-2673
Description: Offers resources for persons afflicted with phobias and panic
related disorders. Also offers posters.

★5500★   INSTITUTE PRESS
2210 Wilshire Blvd., Ste. 171
Santa Monica, CA 90403   Phone: (213) 828-6541
Description: Publishes professional books in various fields. Subject Specialties: Mental health, creativity in the arts, restaurant management.

★5501★ INSTITUTE FOR PSYCHOANALYSIS, CHICAGO
180 N. Michigan Ave.
Chicago, IL 60601 Phone: (312) 726-6300
Description: Offers a series of professional studies. **Subject Specialties:** Psychoanalysis, psychosomatic medicine, psychiatry, psychology.

★5502★ INSTITUTE FOR PSYCHOHISTORY
PO Box 401
New York, NY 10024 Phone: (212) 873-5900
Description: Provides an outlet for the emerging discipline of psychohistory and psychoanalytic anthropology. Publishes books and journals.

★5503★ INSTITUTE FOR RATIONAL-EMOTIVE THERAPY
45 E. 65th St.
New York, NY 10021 Phone: (212) 535-0822
Description: Publishes monographs, journals, audio and video tapes, software, and posters. **Subject Specialties:** Psychology, self-help.

★5504★ INSTITUTE FOR SCIENTIFIC INFORMATION
University City Science Centers
3501 Market St.
Philadelphia, PA 19104 Phone: (215) 386-0100
Description: Publishes scientific books, including some dealing with medicine.

★5505★ INSTITUTE OF SOCIAL SCIENCES AND ARTS, INC.
817 Lizabeth St.
Johnson City, TN 37604 Phone: (615) 282-9023
Description: A small academic publishing group composed of academicians in social science and arts disciplines. Specializes in short run projects for academic classroom adoptions. **Subject Specialties:** Psychology, criminal justice, religion, history.

★5506★ INSTITUTE FOR THE STUDY OF HUMAN ISSUES
1530 Locust St., Ste. 80
Philadelphia, PA 19102 Phone: (215) 732-9729
Description: Conducts research in the social and behavioral sciences and the humanities. Publishes books, monographs, translations, reprints, and essays.

★5507★ INSTITUTE FOR SUBSTANCE ABUSE RESEARCH
2501 27th Ave., Ste. F-6
Vero Beach, FL 32960 Phone: (305) 569-3121
Description: Publishes to educate the public on the dangers of drug abuse and misusing prescription drugs. Offers two games, *Yeah, But* and *Addictionary,* as well as a Drug Abuse Recognition Slideguide and a Substance Abuse Wall Calendar.

★5508★ INTERNATIONAL ACADEMY OF CHEST
PHYSICIANS AND SURGEONS
3300 Dundee Rd.
Northbrook, IL 60062-2303 Phone: (708) 498-1400
Description: Not-for-profit medical society devoted to the continuing education of medical professionals involved with the chest specialties. Publishes a scientific journal, a quarterly bulletin, newsletters, and scientific and medical monographs.

★5509★ INTERNATIONAL ACADEMY OF NUTRITION AND
PREVENTIVE MEDICINE
PO Box 18433
Asheville, NC 28814-0433 Phone: (704) 258-3243
Description: Publishes scientific reports, reviews, case studies, editorials, etc. on stressing the human applications of nutritional knowledge.

★5510★ INTERNATIONAL ASSOCIATION OF CANCER
VICTORS AND FRIENDS
7740 W. Manchester Ave.
Ste. 110
Playa del Rey, CA 90293 Phone: (213) 822-5032
Description: Publishes information concerning non-toxic cancer therapies.

★5511★ INTERNATIONAL ASSOCIATION FOR MEDICAL
ASSISTANCE TO TRAVELERS
417 Center St.
Lewiston, NY 14092 Phone: (716) 754-4883
Description: Gathers and disseminates health and sanitary information world-wide, information on health hazards, sanitation, tropical diseases, information on prevention of the above and information on qualified medical care overseas.

★5512★ INTERNATIONAL ASSOCIATION OF
TRICHOLOGISTS
37320 22nd St.
Kalamazoo, MI 49009 Phone: (616) 372-3224
Description: Publishes books and newsletters on hair and scalp diseases.

★5513★ INTERNATIONAL BIO-MEDICAL INFORMATION
SERVICE, INC.
c/o Amy D'Orazio
229 S. 18th St.
Philadelphia, PA 19103 Phone: (215) 790-7000
Description: Publishes a guide to the medical and health care industry.

★5514★ INTERNATIONAL CENTER FOR ARTIFICIAL
ORGANS AND TRANSPLANTATION
8937 Euclid Ave.
Cleveland, OH 44106 Phone: (216) 229-1800
Subject Specialties: Artificial organs.

★5515★ INTERNATIONAL CHILDBIRTH EDUCATION
ASSOCIATION, INC.
PO Box 20048
Minneapolis, MN 55420 Phone: (612) 854-8660
Description: Publishes for health care professionals and consumers who work with the childbearing family. Also offers four periodicals per year, a review book catalog, and teaching aids for childbirth educators.

★5516★ INTERNATIONAL COMMISSION FOR THE
PREVENTION OF ALCOHOLISM AND DRUG DEPENDENCY
12501 Old Columbia Pike
Silver Spring, MD 20904 Phone: (301) 680-6719
Description: Promotes the scientific study of intoxicants and their effects on the social, economic, political, and religious life of the countries of the commission. Publishes periodicals, reports, and books.

★5517★ INTERNATIONAL FEDERATION ON AGING
PUBLICATIONS DIVISION
601 E. St. NW
Bldg. A, 10th Fl.
Washington, DC 20049 Phone: (202) 434-2429
Description: Publishes a semi-annual journal and other information on developments in aging around the world, with an emphasis on programs and policies for the elderly.

★5518★ INTERNATIONAL FOUNDATION FOR BIOSOCIAL
DEVELOPMENT AND HUMAN HEALTH, INC.
1 Madison Ave., 7th Fl.
New York, NY 10010-3603 Phone: (212) 935-8900
Subject Specialties: Health communications, biopsychosocial health, biologos, creative health.

★5519★ INTERNATIONAL HEALTH COUNCIL
PO Box 151
Fairbanks, AK 99707
Description: Provides data on cancer that does not appear in medical journals. **Subject Specialties:** Health, religion.

★5520★ INTERNATIONAL HEALTH ECONOMICS AND
MANAGEMENT INSTITUTE
Southern Illinois University
Box 1101
Edwardsville, IL 62026-1101 Phone: (618) 692-2291
Description: Publishes the selected papers presented at each annual conference of the Institute. **Subject Specialties:** Health care.

★5521★ INTERNATIONAL HEALTH PUBLICATIONS, INC.
PO Box 17535
San Diego, CA 92117 Phone: (619) 692-1439
Description: Produces books and audio tapes on clinical hypnosis. **Subject Specialties:** Psychology.

★5522★ INTERNATIONAL INSTITUTE FOR BIOENERGETIC ANALYSIS
144 E. 36th St. 1A
New York, NY 10016   Phone: (212) 532-7742
Description: Offers workshops and conferences in bioenergetic therapy.

★5523★ INTERNATIONAL INSTITUTE OF PREVENTIVE PSYCHIATRY
11445 Dona Dolores Pl.
Studio City, CA 91604   Phone: (213) 650-6276
Subject Specialties: Mental health and related fields.

★5524★ INTERNATIONAL LIFE SCIENCES INSTITUTE NUTRITION FOUNDATION
1126 16th St. NW, Ste. 300
Washington, DC 20036   Phone: (202) 659-0074
Description: Publishes food safety and nutrition materials for use by professionals. **Subject Specialties:** Nutrition, toxicology, food safety, risk assessment.

★5525★ INTERNATIONAL SCHOOL PSYCHOLOGY
92 S. Dawson Ave.
Columbus, OH 43209   Phone: (614) 863-6687
Description: Publishes works of interest to school psychologists. Address for orders: c/o Gretchen Catterall, 6258 Braiden Court, Columbus, OH 43213.

★5526★ INTERNATIONAL SOCIETY ON METABOLIC EYE DISEASE
1200 5th Ave.
New York, NY 10029   Phone: (212) 427-1246
Description: Publishes a journal, proceedings of symposia, and books with information on metabolic diseases affecting the eye or diagnosed via an ophthalmological involvement or examination.

★5527★ INTERNATIONAL UNIVERSITIES PRESS, INC.
59 Boston Post Rd.
Madison, CT 06443-1524   Phone: (203) 245-4000
Description: Publishes books and journals in psychiatry, psychology, psychoanalysis, and medical and social sciences.

★5528★ INTERPHARM PRESS
1358 Busch Pkwy.
Buffalo Grove, IL 60089-4505   Phone: (708) 459-8480
Description: Publishes books and booklets for the pharmaceutical, medical device, and health care industries. Makes available various national and international documents in the field and distributes simular material for other publishers. **Subject Specialties:** Applications, legislation, and regulations pertinent to drug and medical device industries.

★5529★ INTERPRETIVE LABORATORY DATA
2902 S. Memorial
Greenville, NC 27834   Phone: (919) 756-6113
Description: Publishes material on medical subjects.

★5530★ INTERSOCIETY COMMITTEE ON PATHOLOGY INFORMATION, INC.
4733 Bethesda Ave.
Ste. 700
Bethesda, MD 20814   Phone: (301) 656-2944
Description: Publishes a directory of training programs in the U.S. and Canada in anatomic and clinical pathology for medical residents; includes fellowships and post graduate opportunities in certifiable subspecialties. Offers a brochure, *Pathology as a Career in Medicine*. **Subject Specialties:** Medicine (pathology).

★5531★ INTERSTUDY
5715 Christmas Lake Rd.
PO Box 458
Excelsior, MN 55331-0458   Phone: (612) 474-1176
Description: A private nonprofit health care research and policy studies firm publishing in the areas of managed care (HMOs, PPOs), competition in health care, and evaluation of quality/patient outcomes. Publications include a biannual census of the HMO industry and two periodicals, *The Interstudy Competitive Edge,* and *The Interstudy Quality Edge.*

★5532★ IRL PRESS
PO Box Q
McLean, VA 22101-0850   Phone: (703) 442-0048
Description: Publishes books, journals, videos, and software in the biological and medical sciences.

★5533★ ISHIYAKU EUROAMERICA, INC.
716 Hanley Industrial Ct.
St. Louis, MO 63144   Phone: (314) 644-4322
Description: Publishes medical, dental, and nursing books.

★5534★ ISLE OF GUAM INTERNATIONAL PUBLISHING AND DISTRIBUTING COMPANY
PO Box 21119
Guam Main Facility, GU 96921   Phone: (808) 963-6317
Description: Publishes on psychology for parents, teachers, and mental health professionals.

★5535★ J.B. LIPPINCOTT COMPANY
227 E. Washington Sq.
Philadelphia, PA 19106   Phone: (215) 238-4200
Description: Publishes books on medicine, dentistry, nursing, and veterinary medicine.

★5536★ J.G. FERGUSON PUBLISHING COMPANY
200 W. Monroe
Chicago, IL 60606   Phone: (312) 580-5480
Description: Publishes reference works for home and office use sold through subscription sales. Also used in elementary, junior, and senior high schools and colleges and universities.

★5537★ J & J PUBLISHING
PO Box 8549
Middletown, OH 45042
Description: A small press publishing for the health, food, and children's markets.

★5538★ JAI PRESS, INC.
55 Old Post Rd. No. 2
PO Box 1678
Greenwich, CT 06830   Phone: (203) 661-0792
Description: Publishes reference works for research and professionals in business, economics, finance, management, library science, sociology, psychology, political science, chemistry, and life sciences.

★5539★ JALSCO, INC.
PO Box 30226
Cincinnati, OH 45230   Phone: (513) 791-7001
Description: Publishes educational material on occupational and public health.

★5540★ JANES PUBLISHING
25671 Fleck Rd.
Veneta, OR 97487   Phone: (503) 935-7654
Description: Publishes on alternative communities and midwifery.

★5541★ JASON ARONSON, INC.
230 Livingston St.
Northvale, NJ 07647   Phone: (201) 767-4093
Description: Publishes professional books in psychiatry, psychoanalysis, behavioral sciences, and Judaica.

★5542★ JB PRESS
PO Box 4843, Duke Sta.
Durham, NC 27706   Phone: (919) 644-0736
Description: Publishes self-help, health, and wellness books and tapes.

★5543★ JBBA PUBLISHING, INC.
225 N. Richmond St., Ste. 102
Appelton, WI 54914   Phone: (414) 731-5222
Description: Publishes on weight training, bodybuilding, and general health and fitness.

★5544★ JBK PUBLISHING, INC.
1863 SW Montgomery Dr.
Portland, OR 97201   Phone: (503) 248-0717
Description: Publishes medical dental books and medical histories.

★5545★ J.C. PRINTING COMPANY
1847 Washington Rd.
East Point, GA 30344   Phone: (404) 265-2030
Subject Specialties: Law, taxation, health.

★5546★ JEN HOUSE PUBLISHING COMPANY
119 Cherry Valley Rd.
Reisterstown, MD 21136   Phone: (301) 526-3805
Description: Publishes textbooks and bibliographic reference titles on medicine, dentistry and allied fields.

★5547★ JESMAN PUBLISHING COMPANY
87 West St.
Danbury, CT 06810   Phone: (203) 792-5831
Description: Produces medical publications for both professionals and non-professionals.

★5548★ JEWISH BRAILLE INSTITUTE OF AMERICA, INC.
110 E. 30th St.
New York, NY 10016   Phone: (212) 889-2525
Description: Prepares large print books and transcriptions to braille.

★5549★ JIGSAW PUBLISHING HOUSE
PO Box 702558
Tulsa, OK 74136   Phone: (913) 492-5112
Description: Publishes self-help books on arthritis.

★5550★ JOANNE FRIEDMAN
66 N. Mitchell Ave.
Livingston, NJ 07039   Phone: (201) 994-6644
Description: Publishes on nutrition during pregnancy and infancy.

★5551★ JOHMAX BOOKS, INC.
48 Pine Brook Dr.
PO Box 625
Larchmont, NY 10538   Phone: (914) 834-0822
Subject Specialties: Health, education, food.

★5552★ JOHN CURLEY & ASSOCIATES, INC.
PO Box 37
South Yarmouth, MA 02664   Phone: (508) 394-1282
Description: Publishes books in large print for visually handicapped and elderly people. **Subject Specialties:** Current fiction, biographies, popular authors.

★5553★ JOHN K. CHAR INC.
850 Kam Hwy.
Pearl City, HI 96782   Phone: (808) 456-1022
Description: Publishes on holistic dentistry and nutrition.

★5554★ JOHN MILTON SOCIETY FOR THE BLIND
475 Riverside Dr., Ste. 455
New York, NY 10115   Phone: (212) 870-3335
Description: Publishes free materials for the blind and visually impaired. Publications are in large print, braille, and on records. **Subject Specialties:** Religion, family, denominational news, inspirational, stories, poems, how-to, theme topics on social issues.

★5555★ JOHN TRACY CLINIC
806 W. Adams Blvd.
Los Angeles, CA 90007   Phone: (213) 748-5481
Description: Publishes material designed to aid parents and teachers of deaf and deaf-blind pre-school children.

★5556★ JOHN WILEY & SONS, INC.
605 3rd Ave.
New York, NY 10158   Phone: (212) 850-6088

★5557★ JOHNS HOPKINS UNIVERSITY
JOHNS HOPKINS UNIVERSITY PRESS
701 W. 40th St., Ste. 275
Baltimore, MD 21211   Phone: (301) 338-6900
Description: Publishes in such subject areas as literary studies, classics, history, economics, political sciences, the history of science and medicine, environmental studies, and the Chesapeake Bay region.

★5558★ JOHNSON INSTITUTE
7151 Metro Blvd.
Minneapolis, MN 55439-2122   Phone: (612) 944-0511
Description: Publications are written for chemically dependent people, their families, and the professionals who serve them. They contain state-of-the-art information based on the latest research findings that teach how to prevent, intervene with, and provide treatment for alcohol/drug dependence and co-dependence. **Subject Specialties:** Chemical dependence.

★5559★ JOINT COMMISSION ON ACCREDITATION OF
HEALTHCARE ORGANIZATIONS
1 Renaissance Blvd.
Oakbrook Terrace, IL 60181   Phone: (708) 916-5600
Description: Publishes accreditation standards manuals for hospitals, long term care facilities, ambulatory health care facilities, hospice, psychiatric facilities, and mental health services.

★5560★ JONES AND BARTLETT PUBLISHERS, INC.
20 Park Plaza
Boston, MA 02116   Phone: (617) 482-5243
Description: Publishes on biology, biochemistry, genetics, chemistry, astronomy, mathematics, computer science, and marine science.

★5561★ JONES MEDICAL PUBLICATIONS
355 Los Cerros Dr.
Greenbrae, CA 94904   Phone: (415) 461-3749
Description: Publishes medical texts and reference books.

★5562★ JOSSEY-BASS, INC., PUBLISHERS
350 Sansome St.
San Francisco, CA 94104   Phone: (415) 433-1740
Subject Specialties: Education, business, health, public administration, social and behavioral science, nonprofit sector.

★5563★ JOURNEY PRESS
PO Box 9036
Berkeley, CA 94709   Phone: (415) 540-5500
Description: Self-publisher. **Subject Specialties:** Jungian psychology, dreamwork.

★5564★ JOYCE MEDIA, INC.
2654 Diamond St.
Rosamond, CA 93560   Phone: (805) 269-1169
Description: Publishes for and about deaf people. Offers videotapes, cards, games, and weekly newspapers.

★5565★ JUDY M. STRUM
c/o Anatomy Dept.
University of Maryland
655 W. Baltimore St.
Baltimore, MD 21201   Phone: (301) 328-3532
Description: Publishes an atlas of electron micrographs which includes a self-study guide text for medical students in histology courses and graduate students interested in electron microscopy and cell biology.

★5566★ JUDY'S SPLASH AEROBICS
1738 Briarwood Dr.
Lansing, MI 48917   Phone: (517) 321-2669
Description: Publishes a water exercise book. Audience includes instructors and persons wanting to exercise in their backyard pool. Offers laminated poster of water exercises.

★5567★ JUNIUS-VAUGHN PRESS
PO Box 85
Fairview, NJ 07022   Phone: (201) 868-7725
Subject Specialties: Sociology, medical history, bibliography.

★5568★ JUVENESCENT RESEARCH CORPORATION
807 Riverside Dr.
New York, NY 10032   Phone: (212) 795-3749
Subject Specialties: Physiology.

★5569★ JYM ENTERPRISES
PO Box 73
Batavia, OH 45103
Subject Specialties: Sports and fitness.

**★5570★ KANSAS STATE UNIVERSITY
COMPARATIVE TOXICOLOGY LABORATORIES**
Veterinary Clinical Science Bldg.
Manhattan, KS 66506-5606   Phone: (913) 532-4334
Description: Publishes scientific material in toxicology for professionals
and health scientists dealing with humans, animals, and the environment.
Subject Specialties: Toxicology, chemically-induced disease and health
effects.

★5571★ KEATS PUBLISHING, INC.
27 Pine St.
New Canaan, CT 06840   Phone: (203) 966-8721
Subject Specialties: Nonfiction, health, medicine, sports and fitness,
regional, nutrition.

★5572★ KEITHWOOD PUBLISHING COMPANY
PO Box 2693
Upper Darby, PA 19082   Phone: (215) 352-7550

★5573★ KEMPLER INSTITUTE
PO Box 1692
Costa Mesa, CA 92628   Phone: (714) 472-4155
Subject Specialties: Psychiatry, family life.

★5574★ KEYSTONE PRESS
PO Box 6163
Bradenton, FL 34281   Phone: (813) 753-5179
Description: Publishes a series of pocket-sized editions of the U.S. Federal
regulations covering the pharmaceutical, medical device, and diagnostic
industries, available in English and Spanish.

★5575★ KINETOMATIC
Rte. 1, Box 63C
Templeton, CA 93465   Phone: (805) 238-7750
Description: Publishes on subjects in life science and biomedical science.

**★5576★ KING COUNTY SEXUAL ASSAULT RESOURCE
CENTER**
PO Box 300
Renton, WA 98057   Phone: (206) 226-5062
Description: Publishes on child sexual abuse education and prevention.

★5577★ KISSLINGER PUBLICATIONS
541 Sturgeon Eddy Rd.
Wausau, WI 54401   Phone: (715) 848-2232
Description: Publishes a cookbook for a gluten-free diet. Also provides
information on Celiac disease and diet therapy.

★5578★ KLUWER ACADEMIC PUBLISHERS
101 Philip Dr.
Assinippi Park
Norwell, MA 02061   Phone: (617) 871-6600
Description: Publishes on the humanities, social, natural, and life sciences,
technology, medicine, and law.

★5579★ KM ASSOCIATES
4711 Overbrook Rd.
Bethesda, MD 20816   Phone: (301) 652-4536
Description: Produces, publishes, and markets educational materials on
natural family planning and related topics.

★5580★ KM ENTERPRISES
PO Box 25978
Los Angeles, CA 90025   Phone: (213) 398-9135
Description: Publishes health career directories, financial aid directories,
informative newsletters, educational handbooks, and other media. Intended audience is the prospective health care student, career advisor, and
current health careers student.

★5581★ KRIEGER PUBLISHING COMPANY, INC.
PO Box 9542
Melbourne, FL 32902   Phone: (407) 724-9542
Description: Publishes in the scientific-technical field. **Subject Specialties:**
Business science and economics, technology and engineering, chemistry,
physical and natural sciences, medical sciences, history, religion.

★5582★ LA LECHE LEAGUE INTERNATIONAL
9616 Minneapolis Ave.
PO Box 1209
Franklin Park, IL 60131-8209   Phone: (708) 455-7730
Description: Publishes and distributes information about breastfeeding,
including books, periodicals, and calendars. **Subject Specialties:** Breastfeeding, child care, nutrition, family life.

★5583★ LACTATION ASSOCIATES PUBLISHING COMPANY
1818 Stonecrest Ct.
PO Box 7092
Lakeland, FL 33813   Phone: (813) 644-7714
Description: Self-publishes on breast-feeding.

★5584★ LAKE PRESS
PO Box 7934, Avondale Sta.
Paducah, KY 42002   Phone: (502) 575-2200
Description: Publishes women's health books.

★5585★ LANCASTER CLEFT PALATE CLINIC
223 N. Lime St.
Lancaster, PA 17603   Phone: (717) 394-3793
Description: A nonprofit organization to provide total coordinated care of
children and adults with oral and facial handicaps. Conducts research and
publishes results in books, periodicals, annual report, newsletter, and
educational brochures.

★5586★ LANG ENT PUBLISHING
PO Box 6846
Jefferson City, MO 65101   Phone: (314) 893-5545
Description: Publishes self-care books related to ear, nose, and throat
medicine.

★5587★ LASENDA PUBLISHERS
1590 Via Chaparral
Fallbrook, CA 92028   Phone: (619) 723-1407
Description: Publishes books on medicine and on private flying.

★5588★ LAUNCH PRESS
PO Box 31491
Walnut Creek, CA 94598   Phone: (415) 943-7603
Description: Publishes psychology books for professionals in the mental
health field.

★5589★ LAWRENCE ERLBAUM ASSOCIATES, INC.
365 Broadway
Hillsdale, NJ 07642   Phone: (201) 666-4110
Description: Publishes textbooks. **Subject Specialties:** Communications,
computer science, social sciences, medicine, and psychology.

★5590★ LAWTON-TEAGUE PUBLICATIONS
PO Box 12353
Oakland, CA 94604   Phone: (415) 839-8145
Subject Specialties: Natural healing (nutritional, herbal, massage, naturo-
pathic), mental birth control.

★5591★ LEA & FEBIGER
200 Chester Field Pkwy.
Malvern, PA 19355   Phone: (215) 251-2230
Subject Specialties: Medicine, dentistry, veterinary science, physical education, pharmacy, life sciences.

★5592★ **LEARNING PUBLICATIONS, INC.**
Box 1338
3008 Ave. C
Holmes Beach, FL 34218-1326   Phone: (813) 778-6651
Description: Publishes materials in social science for educators and human service workers.

★5593★ **LEARTA MOULTON**
PO Box 482
509 East 2100 North
Provo, UT 84604   Phone: (801) 377-2239
Description: Publishes full-color medicinal, edible, and poisonous plant identification books and cards. Also produces a wheat-gluten cookbook and films.

★5594★ **LEISURE PRESS**
PO Box 5076
Champaign, IL 61825-5076   Phone: (217) 351-5076
Subject Specialties: Sports, fitness, physical education.

★5595★ **LEONARD ROY FRANK**
2300 Webster St.
San Francisco, CA 94115   Phone: (415) 922-3029
Description: Publishes anti-psychiatry books.

★5596★ **LEXINGTON BOOKS**
c/o Publicity Dept.
125 Spring St.
Lexington, MA 02173   Phone: (617) 862-6650
Subject Specialties: Science, behavioral science, social science, economics, business, international relations, political science.

★5597★ **LIAISON PRESS**
602 W. 231st St.
Bronx, NY 10463
Description: Publishes psychoanalytic works.

★5598★ **LIBRA PRESS**
4328 N. Lincoln Ave.
Chicago, IL 60618   Phone: (312) 478-2410
Description: Publishes on health, numerology, and the occult.

★5599★ **LIFE ENERGY MEDIA**
14755 Ventura Blvd., Ste. 1908
Sherman Oaks, CA 91403   Phone: (213) 874-7100
Description: Publishes on psychology, health, organizational development, and mysticism.

★5600★ **LIFE PUBLISHING**
36 Bates Ave.
Wenthrop, MA 02152   Phone: (617) 539-0771
Description: Publishes on health and fitness, self-improvement, and organizational methods. **Subject Specialties:** Education, health and fitness, business, self-improvement.

★5601★ **LIFE SCIENCES PRESS**
PO Box 1174
Tacoma, WA 98401   Phone: (206) 922-0442
Description: Publishes scientific books ranging from medicine to political science analysis for the layman and professional. **Subject Specialties:** Nutritional science, organic chemistry, environmental toxicology, medicine, political science.

★5602★ **LIFEBOAT PRESS**
PO Box 11782
Marina del Rey, CA 90295   Phone: (213) 305-1600
Description: Publishes books and audio-visual materials for the handicapped and professionals that work with them.

★5603★ **LIFE'S RESOURCES, INC.**
114 E. Main St.
Addison, MI 49220   Phone: (517) 547-7494
Description: Publishes books on the environment and how it affects health and welfare.

★5604★ **LIFETIME BOOKS, INC.**
2131 Hollywood Blvd., Ste. 204
Hollywood, FL 33020   Phone: (305) 925-5242
Subject Specialties: Self-help, spiritual, health, business.

★5605★ **LIFEWORK PRESS**
700 S. Sparks St.
State College, PA 16801   Phone: (814) 237-1980
Description: Publishes resources for adapting to chronic illnesses, and physical handicaps.

★5606★ **LIGHTHOUSE PUBLISHING**
1420 Windsor Dr.
Gladstone, OR 97027-2651   Phone: (503) 650-8840
Subject Specialties: Addiction, philosophy, psychology, sociology, religion.

★5607★ **LINSTOK PRESS**
9306 Mintwood St.
Silver Spring, MD 20901-3599   Phone: (301) 585-1939
Subject Specialties: Linguistics, anthropology, communication, sign language.

★5608★ **LITTLE, BROWN & COMPANY, INC.**
34 Beacon St.
Boston, MA 02108   Phone: (617) 227-0730
Description: Publishes general fiction, nonfiction, children's books, art, professional, and photography books. Offers large-print editions, calendars, and posters. **Subject Specialties:** Biographies, history, drama, art, photography, travel, law, medicine, health, cookbooks, mysteries, reference, science, sports, poetry, inspirational, education.

★5609★ **LIVINGQUEST**
Box 3306
Boulder, CO 80307   Phone: (303) 444-1319
Description: Publishes on addiction, eating disorders, and personal and planetary transformation.

★5610★ **LOTUS PRESS**
PO Box 6265
Santa Fe, NM 87502   Phone: (505) 982-5534
Description: Publishes books on ayurvedic medicine, the science of self healing.

★5611★ **LOTUS PRESS**
PO Box 800
Lotus, CA 95651   Phone: (916) 621-4374
Description: Publishes self-help recovery materials that offer an alternative to traditional "12 Step" programs like Alcoholics Anonymous.

★5612★ **LOVEGLO & COMFORT PUBLICATIONS**
PO Box 88
Tempe, AZ 85280-0088   Phone: (602) 894-2997
Subject Specialties: Nutrition, health, self-help, environment.

★5613★ **LOWELL HOUSE**
1875 Century Park E., No. 220
Los Angeles, CA 90067   Phone: (213) 203-8407
Subject Specialties: Women's issues, health, parenting.

★5614★ **LUC DE SCHEPPER**
2901 Wilshire Blvd., Ste. 435
Santa Monica, CA 90403   Phone: (213) 828-4480
Description: Publishes two books on acupuncture.

★5615★ **LUTHERAN BRAILLE WORKERS, INC.**
LARGE PRINT DIVISION
PO Box 5000
Yucaipa, CA 92399   Phone: (415) 221-7500
Description: Provides Christian religious braille for the blind and large print for the visually impaired with dimming eyesight. Offers the entire bible in braile, as well as large print copies of the New Testament.

★5616★ LYNN PUBLICATIONS
PO Box 2323
Iowa City, IA 52244   Phone: (319) 337-9890
Description: Publishes materials for people who have lost someone to
suicide and for the professionals who treat them.

★5617★ LYONS VISUALIZATION SERIES
19065 St. Croy Rd.
Red Bluff, CA 96080   Phone: (916) 527-7386
Description: Supplies material on visual training to the optometric
profession, other professions, and interested individuals.

★5618★ M. C. WINCHESTER
PO Box 817
Hermosa Beach, CA 90254
Subject Specialties: Health.

★5619★ M. M. DONAHUE-GANDY
6228 Westbrook Dr.
Citrus Heights, CA 95621   Phone: (916) 722-5611
Description: Provides program and guidance to aquatics teachers of
individuals with disabilities/handicaps.

★5620★ M & S PRESS, INC.
45 Colpitts Rd.
PO Box 311
Weston, MA 02193   Phone: (617) 891-5650
Description: Publishes new editions of books important in American
intellectual history, chiefly rare materials first published in the nineteenth
century, with new materials prepared by scholars, including biographical
and bibliographical information. **Subject Specialties:** Political reform,
philosophy, psychology, economics, science information, medicine, literature.

★5621★ MAC PUBLISHING
5005 E. 39th Ave.
Denver, CO 80207   Phone: (303) 331-0148
Description: Produces books, films, and games on substance and physical
abuse.

★5622★ MACK PUBLISHING COMPANY
20th and Northampton Sts.
Easton, PA 18042   Phone: (215) 258-9111
Description: Publishes and distributes pharmaceutical books.

★5623★ MACKINAC PUBLISHING
PO Box 215
Mackinac Island, MI 49757   Phone: (313) 542-4194
Description: Publishes books on travel and health care.

★5624★ M.A.D. HOUSE
PO Box 1716
Sanford, FL 32771   Phone: (305) 323-5159
Subject Specialties: Drugs.

★5625★ MAGIC LANTERN PUBLICATIONS
200 Midlike Dr., Ste. C
Knoxville, TN 37918   Phone: (615) 688-1303
Description: Publishes psychological and therapy help books on sexually
abused children.

★5626★ MAGNOLIA STREET PUBLISHERS
1250 W. Victoria
Chicago, IL 60660   Phone: (312) 561-2121
Description: Publishes psychology and art books.

★5627★ MAITLAND ENTERPRISES
8118 N. 28th Ave.
Phoenix, AZ 85051   Phone: (602) 995-4365
Description: Publishes a book on training young athletes to use weights
safely.

★5628★ MALLICOTE PUBLICATIONS
152 Boower Rd.
Bristol, TN 37620-2602   Phone: (615) 968-1100
Description: Publishes patient education information for physicians,
hospitals, and clinics nationwide.

★5629★ MANAGEMENT LEARNING LABORATORIES
302 W. Hill St.
Champaign, IL 61824   Phone: (217) 359-5940
Description: Provides books, monographs, and tapes for managers and
administrators in general and for parks, recreation, and leisure personnel
in particular. Also develops titles in health and wellness areas, including
sports health and corporate health strategies.

★5630★ MANDALA SOCIETY
PO Box 1233
Del Mar, CA 92014   Phone: (619) 481-7751
Description: Publishes on holistic health.

★5631★ MANKIND RESEARCH UNLIMITED, INC.
1315 Apple Ave.
Silver Spring, MD 20910   Phone: (301) 587-8686
Description: Research and development organization on future-oriented
technology and its impact on health, education, and energy resources.
Publishes monographs, books, bibliographies, and technical reports.

**★5632★ MANPOWER DEMONSTRATION RESEARCH
CORPORATION**
3 Park Ave.
New York, NY 10016   Phone: (212) 532-3200
Description: Purpose is to test alternative approaches to the solution of
social problems in the U.S. **Subject Specialties:** Work welfare, teen
pregnancy, supported work for mentally retarded.

★5633★ MARATHON CONSULTING AND PRESS
PO Box 09189
Columbus, OH 43209-0189   Phone: (614) 235-5509
Description: Publishes mainly psychological tests for practice and research.

★5634★ MARCEL DEKKER, INC.
270 Madison Ave.
New York, NY 10016   Phone: (212) 696-9000
Description: Publishes research books, reference books, professional books,
textbooks, encyclopedias, and journals.

★5635★ MARIAN KURTZ GEORGE
215 W. 12th St., No. 1
Maryville, MO 64468   Phone: (816) 582-4462
Subject Specialties: Nursing.

★5636★ MARK BOOKS
382 Hollyberry Ln.
Boulder, CO 80303
Description: Publishes on personal and group development, self-improvement, health, and fitness.

★5637★ MARY ANN LIEBERT
1651 3rd Ave.
New York, NY 10128   Phone: (212) 289-2300
Description: Publishes books on medicine. **Subject Coverage:** Nursing.

★5638★ MASS PRESS
1129 New Hampshire Ave. NW, No. 610
Washington, DC 20037   Phone: (202) 659-9580
Description: Publishes psychology and political science titles.

**★5639★ MASSACHUSETTS INSTITUTE OF TECHNOLOGY
MIT PRESS**
55 Hayward St.
Cambridge, MA 02142   Phone: (617) 253-5646
Description: Publishes scholarly books. **Subject Specialties:** Architecture,
computer science, cognitive science, economics, philosophy, linguistics,
neuroscience, technology studies.

★5640★ MASTERWORKS PUBLISHING, INC.
PO Box 1677
Norman, OK 73070   Phone: (405) 799-6306
Description: Publishes juvenile books on nutrition.

★5641★ MATERNITY CENTER ASSOCIATION
48 E. 92nd St.
New York, NY 10128   Phone: (212) 369-7300
Description: A national nonprofit health agency dedicated to the improvement of maternal and child health. Publishes booklets, a newsletter, pamphlets, teaching charts, books, and slide sets.

★5642★ MATRIX PUBLISHING
405 N. Wabash Ave., No. 3908
Chicago, IL 60611   Phone: (312) 822-0935
Description: Publications are designed to educate and assist physicians.

★5643★ MCBOOKS PRESS
908 Steammill Rd.
Ithaca, NY 14850-9423   Phone: (607) 272-2114
Description: Publishes books of interest to local residents. Also publishes on vegetarian nutrition. Subject Specialties: Nutrition, poetry, photography, local interest, parenting.

★5644★ MCDOWELL PUBLISHING COMPANY
PO Box 980005
Houston, TX 77098   Phone: (713) 933-4617
Description: Publishes health-related materials for the general public and textbooks on diagnosis and treatment for chiropractic doctors.

★5645★ MCKNIGHT MEDICAL COMMUNICATIONS INC.
1419 Lake Cook Rd.
Deerfield, IL 60015   Phone: (312) 945-0345
Description: Publishes several magazines and directories in the health care field.

★5646★ MCS PUBLICATIONS
PO Box 486
Murray, KY 42071   Phone: (502) 753-7750
Description: Publishes books on medical finance and health insurance consumerism.

★5647★ MCSA
10223 NE 58th St.
Kirkland, WA 98033   Phone: (206) 828-4263
Description: Publishes conference and research works. Subject Specialties: Medical research, service, educational.

★5648★ M.D. PUBLISHING COMPANY
675 Water St.
Excelsior, MN 55331   Phone: (612) 474-4167
Description: Publishes a book on a health care system that promotes warm, personal health care relationships.

★5649★ MEADOWBROOK PRESS, INC.
18318 Minnetonka Blvd.
Deephaven, MN 55391   Phone: (612) 473-5400
Description: Publishes books on pregnancy, newborn and child care, the environment, travel, and cooking.

★5650★ MED SALES PRO PUBLICATIONS
1713 E.Broadway, Ste. 273
Tempe, AZ 85282
Description: Publishes a book for college students, nurses, and sales representatives. Subject Specialties: Medical sales.

★5651★ MEDI COMP PRESS
1168 Sterling Ave.
Berkeley, CA 94708   Phone: (415) 841-1260
Description: Presently publishes information on cannabis. Planning to also publish biographical works in medical history. Subject Specialties: Cannabis, medical history.

★5652★ MEDIAHEALTH PUBLICATIONS
PO Box 541
St. Helena, CA 94574   Phone: (707) 963-1493
Description: Publishes health-related materials by professionals for patients or health conscious adults. Disseminates useful medical and psychological information through books, audio, and video channels.

★5653★ MEDIC PUBLISHING COMPANY
PO Box 89
Redmond, WA 98073   Phone: (206) 881-2883
Subject Specialties: Patient education.

★5654★ MEDICAL ECONOMICS DATA
655 Washington Blvd.
Stamford, CT 06901   Phone: (203) 348-6319
Description: Directory publishing house dealing with the healthcare industry.

★5655★ MEDICAL EDUCATION CONSULTANTS
PO Box 67159
Los Angeles, CA 90067   Phone: (213) 475-5141
Subject Specialties: Medical, nursing, pharmacy, psychology.

★5656★ MEDICAL HISTORY PUBLISHING ASSOCIATES
1 Claremont Ct.
Arlington, MA 02174   Phone: (617) 646-6762
Description: Publishes titles related to the history of medicine.

★5657★ MEDICAL LETTER INC.
56 Harrison St.
New Rochelle, NY 10801   Phone: (914) 235-0500
Description: Publishes books on evaluating drugs as well as a biweekly bulletin, The Medical Letter.

★5658★ MEDICAL LIBRARY ASSOCIATION
6 N. Michigan Ave., Ste. 300
Chicago, IL 60602   Phone: (312) 419- 4094
Description: Fosters medical and allied scientific libraries, promotes the educational and professional growth of health sciences librarians, and exchanges medical literature among its members.

★5659★ MEDICAL MANAGEMENT ANALYSIS INTERNATIONAL, INC.
133 Rollins Ave., Ste. 3
Rockville, MD 20850   Phone: (301) 468-1610
Description: Offers a full range of services designed to help healthcare organizations meet the challenge of managing quality risk and resource use.

★5660★ MEDICAL MANOR BOOKS
3501 Newberry Rd.
Philadelphia, PA 19154   Phone: (215) 637-9255
Description: Publishes health, fitness, and nutrition books and a medical newsletter.

★5661★ MEDICAL MEDIA CORPORATION
7405 Mt. Vista Rd.
Kingsville, MD 21087
Description: Publishes catalogs for booksellers and buyers in the medical field.

★5662★ MEDICAL MEDIA PUBLISHERS
947 Valleyview Rd.
Pittsburgh, PA 15243-1062 Phone: (412) 681-9385
Description: Formed by medical consultants to publish a single purpose directory. Subject Specialties: Medical audio-visual tapes.

★5663★ MEDICAL PHYSICS PUBLISHING CORPORATION
1300 University Ave., Rm. 27B
Madison, WI 53706   Phone: (608) 262-4021
Description: A nonprofit organization which publishes on medical physics.

★5664★   MEDICAL PRODUCTIONS, INC.
5308 Elm, Bldg. C
Houston, TX 77081   Phone: (713) 666-4269
Description: Publishes guides to Houston's medical community and social services. Also specializes in medical marketing, brochures, and promotional materials for area doctors, hospitals, and medical companies. Offers data on labels and lists.

★5665★   MEDICAL PRODUCTS MARKETING SERVICES
3633 W. Lake Ave., No. 415
Glenview, IL 60025
Description: Market research and sales support organization providing services to the medical equipment manufacturing industry. Publishes annual surveys of installed equipment and purchasing patterns at United States hospitals and other healthcare facilities. Reports and documents copyrighted and available in printed and electronic form from organization.

★5666★   MEDICINE IN THE PUBLIC INTEREST, INC.
1 State St., Ste. 400
Boston, MA 02109   Phone: (617) 227-3654
Description: Publishes on current issues relating to medicine, science, and society in the U.S. for the development of standards and programs designed to meet public health and welfare needs.

★5667★   MEDI-PUBLISHING GROUP
2809 Bird Ave., No. 133
Coconut Grove, FL 33133   Phone: (305) 854-0087
Subject Specialties: Office planning and practice management of physician's medical practice.

★5668★   MEDMASTER, INC.
17500 NE 9th Ave.
North Miami Beach, FL 33162   Phone: (305) 653-3480
Description: Publishes medical books and brief overviews of clinically relevant material for medical students and other health professionals.

★5669★   MEGABOOKS, INC.
4300 NW 23rd Ave., Ste. 192
PO Box 1702
Gainesville, FL 32606-9990   Phone: (904) 371-6342
Description: Publishes textbooks and study cards for health professionals.

★5670★   MELIUS AND PETERSON PUBLISHING, INC.
PO Box 925
Aberdeen, SD 57401   Phone: (605) 226-0488
Description: Publishes on nutrition, self-help, cookbooks, and general outdoor recreation.

★5671★   MENDOCINO FOUNDATION FOR HEALTH EDUCATION
PO Box 1377
Mendocino, CA 95460   Phone: (707) 964-0425
Description: Specializes in health publications and books for aspiring pre-medical students.

★5672★   MENTAL HEALTH MATERIALS CENTER, INC.
PO Box 304
Bronxville, NY 10708   Phone: (914) 337-6596
Description: Provides consultation services to national agencies with major concerns in the field of health, mental health, and family life education. Develops publishing properties in the above fields.

★5673★   META PUBLICATIONS, INC.
PO Box 565
Cupertino, CA 95015   Phone: (415) 965-0954
Description: Publishes psychology books.

★5674★   MEYERBOOKS, PUBLISHER
235 W. Main St.
PO Box 427
Glenwood, IL 60425   Phone: (708) 757-4950
Description: Publishes books on herbs, herbal recipes, folk medicine, Americana, cooking, and conjuring.

★5675★   MHM PUBLISHING
6105 Tilden Ln., Rm. 10-D
Rockville, MD 20852   Phone: (301) 881-7337
Description: Publishes nutrition and diet guides.

★5676★   MICHAEL KESEND PUBLISHING LTD.
1025 5th Ave.
New York, NY 10028   Phone: (212) 249-5150
Description: Publishes books on nature, animals, travel, sports, history, and health.

★5677★   MICHELLE PUBLISHING COMPANY
2317 Silas Deane Hwy.
Rocky Hill, CT 06067   Phone: (203) 721-8800
Description: Publishes on health care.

★5678★   MICKEY A. CHRISTIASON
11066 Gonsalves Pl.
Cerritos, CA 90701   Phone: (215) 724-2107
Description: Publishes a resource book for the handicapped, their families, and professionals.

★5679★   MIDEWIWIN PRESS
797 Goodrich Ave.
St. Paul, MN 55105   Phone: (612) 224-7039
Description: Publishes medical history for physicians, historians, and lay people interested in medicine.

★5680★   MIDWEST ALLIANCE IN NURSING
2511 E. 46th St., Ste.E-3
Indianapolis, IN 46205   Phone: (317) 541-3600
Description: Publishes proceedings from semiannual program conferences; focuses on issues in nursing or health care. Publishes *MAIN*, a triannual journal. Offers a bimonthly newsletter and a directory of nursing consultants.

★5681★   MIDWEST HEALTH CENTER FOR WOMEN
825 S. 8th St., No. 902
Minneapolis, MN 55404   Phone: (612) 332-2311
Description: Publishes books for and about women. Also produces newsletters, brochures, and family planning information.

★5682★   MILLS PUBLISHING COMPANY
PO Box 6158, King Sta.
Santa Ana, CA 92706   Phone: (714) 541-5750
Description: Publishes books on Spanish for health professionals who work with Spanish-speaking patients and for adults wishing to learn Spanish for everyday situations. **Subject Specialties:** Autobiography, philosophy, learning Spanish, medical Spanish.

★5683★   MILLS & SANDERSON, PUBLISHERS
41 North Rd., Ste. 201
Bedford, MA 01730   Phone: (617) 861-0992
Description: Publishes nonfiction books for adults on lifestyle improvement. **Subject Specialties:** Independent travel, health and fitness, parenting.

★5684★   MINDBODY PRESS
3339 Kipling St.
Palo Alto, CA 94306   Phone: (415) 493-6628
Description: Publishes on holistic ideas and applications in medicine and philosophy.

★5685★   MKW PUBLISHING COMPANY
RFD 1, Box 134
Benton, MO 63736   Phone: (314) 545-3918
Description: Publishes a story directed at seven to eleven-year-old children on the effects of drug use.

★5686★   MND PUBLISHING, INC.
7163 Old Harding Rd.
Nashville, TN 37221   Phone: (615) 646-9879
Description: Publishes on natural family planning for family planning agencies, book trade, health food markets, and libraries.

★5687★ **MODERN PUBLISHING**
155 E. 55th St.
New York, NY 10022   Phone: (212) 826-0850
Subject Specialties: Nonfiction, reference, cookbooks, humor, health, nutrition, children's books.

★5688★ **MODERN SIGNS PRESS, INC.**
PO Box 1181
Los Alamitos, CA 90720   Phone: (213) 596-8548
Description: Publishes on sign language. Offers greeting cards, posters, video cassettes, software, a newsletter, and flash cards.

★5689★ **MOLLICA PRESS, LTD.**
313 Highridge Dr.
Syracuse, NY 13215   Phone: (315) 476-5002
Subject Specialties: Health.

★5690★ **MORRIS PUBLISHING COMPANY**
3 Blue Ridge Rd.
Plymouth Meeting, PA 19462   Phone: (215) 828-4865
Description: Publications on health and wellbeing. **Subject Specialties:** Health, nutrition, sex, exercise.

★5691★ **MOSAIC**
3923 Partridge Ln.
Baton Rouge, LA 70809   Phone: (504) 925-1604
Description: Self-publisher of diet and other self-help books.

★5692★ **MOSBY-YEAR BOOK, INC.**
11830 Westline Industrial Dr.
St. Louis, MO 63146   Phone: (314) 872-8370
Description: Publishes college textbooks, reference books, and professional journals on health related topics. Also offers software and standardized tests for health sciences.

★5693★ **MOSCATO CARDS**
2735 Lytelle Pl.
Los Angeles, CA 90065   Phone: (818) 502-0122
Description: Publishes alternative health care, self-help, and metaphysical titles. Offers greeting cards and audio cassettes.

★5694★ **MOSES PUBLICATIONS**
2001 Rocky Dells Dr.
Prescott, AZ 86303   Phone: (602) 778-7804
Description: Publishes on critical thinking and drug use.

★5695★ **MOTAMED MEDICAL PUBLISHER, INC.**
7141 N. Kedzie Ave., Ste. 1504
Chicago, IL 60645   Phone: (312) 761-6667
Description: Publishes medical books.

★5696★ **MOTHERING MAGAZINE**
PO Box 1690
Santa Fe, NM 87504   Phone: (505) 984-8116
Description: Publishes *Mothering Magazine,* an alternative parenting magazine. Also publishes books and booklets pertaining to pregnancy, birth, and parenting.

★5697★ **MOUNTAIN HOME PUBLISHING**
PO Box 829
Ingram, TX 78025   Phone: (512) 367-4492
Description: Publishes a variety of health books and cassette tapes on a number of health topics-cholesterol, hypoglycemia, vision improvement, thyroid, weight loss, adrenal problems, etc.

★5698★ **MOUNTAIN SPRING PRESS LTD.**
24 W. 760 Geneva Rd.
Carol Stream, IL 60188   Phone: (312) 653-2244
Description: Publishes books on chiropractic principles and special interest magazines.

★5699★ **MOUNTAINTOP CONSCIOUSNESS PUBLISHING**
5333 Agnes Ave., No. 1
North Hollywood, CA 91607   Phone: (702) 829-7179
Description: Publishes self-help, psychology, philosophy, and religious and spiritual materials.

★5700★ **MULTI-FIT PUBLICATIONS**
8033 Sunset Blvd., Ste. 726
Los Angeles, CA 90046   Phone: (818) 957-1895
Description: Publishes fitness books.

★5701★ **MURIEL C. CLAUSEN COMPANY**
780 W. Grand Ave.
Oakland, CA 94612   Phone: (415) 836-1131
Subject Specialties: Vitamins, nutrition, exercise.

★5702★ **NAPSAC INTERNATIONAL**
PO Box 646
Marble Hill, MO 63764   Phone: (314) 238-2010
Subject Specialties: Childbirth, maternity care, obstetrics, pediatrics, early infant rearing, home birth.

★5703★ **NARCOTICS EDUCATION, INC.**
12501 Old Columbia Pike
Silver Spring, MD 20904-1608   Phone: (301) 680-6740
Description: Publishes and distributes books, pamphlets, visual aids, and audio-visual materials on drug abuse prevention.

★5704★ **NATIONAL ACADEMY PRESS**
2101 Constitution Ave. NW
PO Box 285
Washington, DC 20055   Phone: (202) 334-3313
Subject Specialties: Health, science, technology.

★5705★ **NATIONAL ACCREDITATION COUNCIL FOR AGENCIES SERVING THE BLIND AND VISUALLY HANDICAPPED**
232 Madison Ave., Ste. 907
New York, NY 10016   Phone: (212) 496-5880
Description: Publishes standards for management and human services used in accreditation of agencies and schools for the blind and visually handicapped.

★5706★ **NATIONAL ASSOCIATION FOR THE ADVANCEMENT OF PSYCHOANALYSIS**
80 8th Ave., Ste. 1501
New York, NY 10011   Phone: (212) 741-0515
Description: Publishes *National Registry of Psychoanalysts* yearly and a newspaper, *NAAP News* quarterly. **Subject Specialties:** Psychiatry.

★5707★ **NATIONAL ASSOCIATION OF BLIND TEACHERS**
1010 Vermont Ave., Ste. 1100
Washington, DC 20005   Phone: (202) 393-3666
Description: Publishes resource material for blind teachers.

★5708★ **NATIONAL ASSOCIATION OF BOARDS OF PHARMACY**
1300 Higgins, Ste. 103
Park Ridge, IL 60601   Phone: (312) 698-6227
Description: Publishes material of the NABP as well as more general pharmaceutical topics.

★5709★ **NATIONAL ASSOCIATION OF THE DEAF**
814 Thayer Ave.
Silver Spring, MD 20910   Phone: (301) 587-1788
Description: Publishes textbooks on American Sign Language and other systems of manual communication.

★5710★ **NATIONAL ASSOCIATION OF DENTAL LABORATORIES**
3801 Mt. Vernon Ave.
Alexandria, VA 22305   Phone: (703) 683-5263
Description: Publishes texts and newsletters informing members of latest trends in dental laboratories.

★5711★ NATIONAL ASSOCIATION OF DEVELOPMENTAL DISABILITIES COUNCILS
1234 Massachusetts Ave. NW, Ste. 103
Washington, DC 20005   Phone: (202) 347-1234
Description: A nonprofit organization to improve the lives of persons with developmental disabilities by promoting cooperation among agencies in the field and educating the public about the needs and rights of those so handicapped.

★5712★ NATIONAL ASSOCIATION OF LESBIAN AND GAY ALCOHOLISM PROFESSIONALS
1208 E. State Blvd.
Fort Wayne, IN 46805   Phone: (219) 483-8280
Description: Publishes books, brochures, and monographs concerning alcoholism and substance abuse in the lesbian and gay communities.
Subject Specialties: Alcoholism, chemical addiction, lesbian and gay issues.

★5713★ NATIONAL ASSOCIATION OF PARENTS AND PROFESSIONALS FOR SAFE ALTERNATIVES IN CHILDBIRTH
Rte. 1, Box 646
Marble Hill, MO 63764
Description: Publishes information on childbirth, nutrition, and family life.

★5714★ NATIONAL ASSOCIATION OF SCHOOL PSYCHOLOGISTS
8455 Colesville Rd., No. 1000
Silver Spring, MD 20910-3319   Phone: (301) 608-0500
Description: Publishes on topics dealing with helping the school psychology practice, research, and training.

★5715★ NATIONAL BRAILLE ASSOCIATION
1290 University Ave.
Rochester, NY 14607   Phone: (716) 473-0900
Description: Publishes manuals and other material outlining guidelines for transcription procedures, format, and uniform standards for the production and distribution of reading material for the visually impaired.

★5716★ NATIONAL BRAILLE PRESS, INC.
88 St. Stephen St.
Boston, MA 02115   Phone: (617) 266-6160
Description: Publishes books for children and adults in print and braille and booklets on cooking and handicrafts. Provides a braille book club for children. Offers a newsletter, *National Braille Press Release,* a guide for blind job seekers, *Take Charge,* and a blind programmer's guide for programming in the C language. Also offers a calendar in print and in braille.

★5717★ NATIONAL CANCER CARE FOUNDATION
1180 Avenue of the Americas
New York, NY 10036   Phone: (212) 221-3300
Description: Publishes results of its own social research studies and the proceedings of various symposia on catastrophic illness in families.

★5718★ NATIONAL CITIZENS' COALITION FOR NURSING HOME REFORM
1224 M St. NW, Ste. 301
Washington, DC 20005-5183   Phone: (202) 393-2018

★5719★ NATIONAL COMMISSION ON CORRECTIONAL HEALTH CARE
2105 N. Southport, Ste. 200
Chicago, IL 60614   Phone: (312) 528-0818
Description: Publishes and distributes various materials on improving health care in correctional institutions.

★5720★ NATIONAL COMMITTEE FOR CLINICAL LABORATORY STANDARDS
771 E. Lancaster Ave.
Villanova, PA 19085   Phone: (215) 525-2435
Description: Publishes guidelines and standards for clinical laboratories and manufacturers of clinical laboratory products. Also publishes *Update,* a newsletter and conference proceedings.

★5721★ NATIONAL COUNCIL FOR INTERNATIONAL HEALTH
1701 K St. NW, Ste. 600
Washington, DC 20006   Phone: (202) 833-5900
Description: Publishes on international health issues.

★5722★ NATIONAL DOWN SYNDROME CONGRESS
1800 Dempster St.
Park Ridge, IL 60068-1146   Phone: (708) 823-7550
Description: Publishes journals, pamphlets, and other material to disseminate accurate information concerning Down syndrome. Distributes information from other publishers.

★5723★ NATIONAL EASTER SEAL SOCIETY
70 E. Lake St.
Chicago, IL 60601   Phone: (312) 726-6200
Description: A national, voluntary health agency which provides practical and technical information relating to persons with disabilities and their families.

★5724★ NATIONAL ENVIRONMENTAL HEALTH ASSOCIATION
720 S. Colorado Blvd.
Ste. 970, South Tower
Denver, CO 80222   Phone: (303) 756-9090
Description: Publishes educational materials and on-the-job assistance material for personnel in environmental health and protection employed by local, state, and federal governments, institutions, industry, and post-secondary education.

★5725★ NATIONAL HEALTH COUNCIL
350 5th Ave., Ste. 1118
New York, NY 10118   Phone: (212) 268-8900
Description: Publishes as a service to members and general public interested in current issues in the health field.

★5726★ NATIONAL HEALTH PUBLISHING
428 E. Preston St.
Baltimore, MD 21202   Phone: (301) 528-4100
Description: Publishes health care manuals for professionals.

★5727★ NATIONAL HEARING AID SOCIETY
20361 Middlebelt Rd.
Livonia, MI 48152   Phone: (313) 478-2610
Description: Publishes materials for professional hearing instrument specialists and other members of the hearing health care team.

★5728★ NATIONAL HOSPICE ORGANIZATION
1901 N. Moore St., Ste. 901
Arlington, VA 22209   Phone: (703) 243-5900
Description: Publications are designed to meet the educational, informational, legislative, and developmental needs of hospice programs, professionals and volunteers. **Subject Specialties:** Death, grief, funeral planning.

★5729★ NATIONAL INSTITUTE FOR BURN MEDICINE
909 E. Ann St.
Ann Arbor, MI 48104   Phone: (313) 769-9000
Description: Publishes and distributes information regarding care of burn victims and their families. Materials include slides, films, posters, and teaching packages.

★5730★ NATIONAL LEAGUE FOR NURSING
350 Hudson St.
New York, NY 10014   Phone: (212) 989-9393
Description: Disseminates information directly related to important developments in nursing and health care for the improvement of nursing and nursing education; publishes management guides, issues and trends monographs, evaluation tools, and reference materials. **Subject Specialties:** Nursing, health care, education.

★5731★ NATIONAL MALE NURSE ASSOCIATION
2309 State St.
Saginaw, MI 48602   Phone: (517) 799-8208
Subject Specialties: Professional nursing.

★5732★ NATIONAL MARFAN FOUNDATION
382 Main St.
Port Washington, NY 11050   Phone: (516) 883-8712
Description: Publishes materials about the Marfan Syndrome for the layperson and the medical fields.

★5733★ NATIONAL MEDICAL SEMINARS, INC.
735 Sunrise Ave., No. 100
Roseville, CA 95661-4568   Phone: (916) 784-6200
Description: Publishes quality books for the general public and medical continuing education courses for health professionals.

★5734★ NATIONAL NURSING REVIEW, INC.
342 State St., No. 6
Los Altos, CA 94022   Phone: (415) 941-5784
Description: Publishes materials to assist student nurses in preparing for the National Council Licensure Examinations for RN's and PN's.

★5735★ NATIONAL ORGANIZATION ON DISABILITY
910 16th St. NW, Ste. 600
Washington, DC 20037   Phone: (202) 293-5960
Description: Publishes to foster public understanding and acceptance of disabled persons.

★5736★ NATIONAL PARENTS' RESOURCE INSTITUTE FOR DRUG EDUCATION
The Hurt Bldg., Ste. 210
50 Hurt Plaza
Atlanta, GA 30303   Phone: (404) 577-4500
Description: A nonprofit organization with the purpose of diminishing drug and alcohol use among youth by educating the public through the development and maintenance of an international information network. Publishes pamphlets, books, and audio-visuals for parents, students, researchers, educators, and others.

★5737★ NATIONAL PUBLISHERS OF THE BLACK HILLS, INC.
Rte. 59, Brook Hill Dr.
West Nyack, NY 10994
Description: Publishes texts geared for vocational and technical schools. Topics include travel and tourism careers, medical careers, and computer careers.

★5738★ NATIONAL REHABILITATION INFORMATION CENTER
8455 Colesville Rd., Ste. 935
Silver Spring, MD 20910-3319   Phone: (301) 588-9284
Description: Compiles and publishes information on rehabilitation of persons with disabilities. Publishes reports, directories, a newsletter, *NARIC Quarterly,* resource guides, and mailing list labels. **Subject Specialties:** Physical disabilities, mental retardation, rehabilitation.

★5739★ NATIONAL SAFETY COUNCIL
444 N. Michigan Ave.
Chicago, IL 60611   Phone: (312) 527-4800
Description: Publishes current information designed to help identify problems and develop methods and procedures that will eliminate or decrease the seriousness of accident problems. **Subject Specialties:** Occupational, traffic, school, farm, labor, youth, motor transportation and public (governmental) employee safety.

★5740★ NATIONAL SOCIETY TO PREVENT BLINDNESS
500 E. Remington Rd.
Schaumburg, IL 60173   Phone: (708) 843-2020
Description: Provides programs and services designed for the prevention of blindness. Also publishes pamphlets, teaching materials, and curriculum aids. **Subject Specialties:** Eye health, eye safety.

★5741★ NATIONAL TAY-SACHS AND ALLIED DISEASES
2001 Beacon St.
Ste. 304
Brookline, MA 02146   Phone: (617) 964-5508
Description: A nonprofit organization committed to the eradication of Tay-Sachs and the allied diseases. Programs include public education, carrier screening, family services, lab quality control, research, and financial services. Offers video cassettes, newsletters, posters, and a lending library.

★5742★ NATIONAL TUBEROUS SCLEROSIS ASSOCIATION
8000 Corporate Dr., Ste. 120
Landover, MD 20785-2239   Phone: (301) 459-9888
Description: Provides information on problems associated with tuberous sclerosis through a telephone referral service, support group data, a quarterly newsletter, and other publications.

★5743★ NATIONAL VETERINARY SERVICES LABORATORIES
PO Box 844
Ames, IA 50010   Phone: (515) 239-8266
Subject Specialties: Veterinary medicine.

★5744★ NATIONAL WELLNESS INSTITUTE
South Hall
1319 Fremont
Stevens Point, WI 54481   Phone: (715) 346-2172
Description: Publishes for health-care professionals, doctors, and dieticians.

★5745★ NATIONAL WHEELCHAIR BASKETBALL ASSOCIATION
110 Seaton Bldg.
University of Kentucky
Lexington, KY 40506   Phone: (606) 257-1623
Description: Publishes information on wheelchair basketball.

★5746★ NATURAL PRESS
PO Box 730
Manitowoc, WI 54221-0730   Phone: (414) 758-2500
Subject Specialties: Nutrition.

★5747★ NATUREGRAPH PUBLISHERS, INC.
3543 Indian Creek Rd.
PO Box 1075
Happy Camp, CA 96039   Phone: (916) 493-5353
Description: Publishes on natural history, gardening, health, and Native American studies.

★5748★ NATURO-VET SERVICES
857 El Pintado Rd.
Danville, CA 94526   Phone: (415) 837-7759
Description: Publishes to give the consumer information and option of holistic healing for their animals. **Subject Specialties:** Veterinary science.

★5749★ NETWORK PUBLICATIONS
PO Box 1830
Santa Cruz, CA 95061-1830   Phone: (408) 438-4060
Description: Nonprofit publisher of family life, health, and sex education books, videos curricula, research reports, and pamphlets.

★5750★ NEUROPSYCHOLOGY PRESS
2920 S. 4th Ave.
Tucson, AZ 85713-4819   Phone: (602) 795-3717
Description: Publishes neuropsychological and head injury books and diskettes.

★5751★ NEUROTICS ANONYMOUS INTERNATIONAL LIAISON, INC.
11140 Bainbridge Dr.
Little Rock, AR 72212   Phone: (501) 221-2809
Description: Publishes books and pamphlets describing recovery program for the mentally and emotionally ill to aid them in "getting well and staying well."

★5752★ NEW HARBINGER PUBLICATIONS INC.
5674 Shattuck Ave.
Oakland, CA 94609   Phone: (415) 652-0215
Description: Publishes psychology and self-help books and cassette tapes.

★5753★ NEW HORIZON PRESS
PO Box 669
Far Hills, NJ 07931   Phone: (201) 221-1858
Description: Publishes books in the fields of social science, human interest, and psychology.

★5754★ NEW LIFESTYLE BOOKS
Rte. 1, Box 441
Seale, AL 36875-9127   Phone: (205) 855-4708
Description: Publishes books to promote vegetarianism, a low-stress lifestyle, and non-drug healing therapies.

★5755★ NEW NATIVITY PRESS
PO Box 6223
Leawood, KS 66206   Phone: (913) 341-8369
Description: Publishes on childbirth.

★5756★ NEW NURSE, PUBLISHER
PO Box 803
Plattsburgh, NY 12901
Subject Specialties: Nursing, nursing education, public relations, personnel relations, nutrition.

★5757★ NEW OPTIONS PUBLISHING
360 S. Monroe St., Ste. 310
Denver, CO 80209   Phone: (303) 830-7718
Description: Assists self-publishers on psychology and personal development.

★5758★ NEW VIEW PUBLICATIONS
510 Yorktown Dr.
Chapel Hill, NC 27516   Phone: (919) 968-6337
Description: Publishes self-help and psychology books.

★5759★ NEW WIN PUBLISHING INC.
PO Box 5159
Clinton, NJ 08809   Phone: (201) 735-9701
Description: Publishes dictionaries, books on health and business, and books for sportsmen.

★5760★ NEW WORLD LIBRARY
58 Paul Dr.
San Rafael, CA 94903   Phone: (415) 472-2100
Description: Publishes books on ecology, careers, and psychology.

★5761★ NEWCASTLE PUBLISHING COMPANY, INC.
13419 Saticcy St.
North Hollywood, CA 91605   Phone: (213) 873-3191
Subject Specialties: Child rearing, education, health, how-to, nutrition, psychology, occult.

★5762★ NEWMARK PUBLISHING COMPANY
729 Ellington Rd.
South Windsor, CT 06074   Phone: (203) 282-7265
Description: Publishes fiction, nonfiction, and health books.

★5763★ NEWMARKET PRESS
18 E. 48th St.
New York, NY 10017   Phone: (212) 832-3575
Description: General trade publisher specializing in nonfiction. **Subject Specialties:** Parenting, child care, psychology, health, nutrition, inspiration, history, biography, film study, music, performing arts, communications, business.

★5764★ NOMIS PUBLICATIONS, INC.
PO Box 5122
Poland, OH 44514   Phone: (216) 788-9608
Description: Publishes a funeral home directory.

★5765★ NORMAN GELLER
PO Box 3217
Auburn, ME 04210   Phone: (207) 783-2400
Description: Publishes books for children dealing with aging, death and dying, mourning, and cremation.

★5766★ NORMAN PUBLISHING
720 Market St.
San Francisco, CA 94102   Phone: (415) 781-6402
Description: Publishes on the history of science and medicine.

★5767★ NORMED VERLAG, INC.
291 Audubon Rd.
Englewood, NJ 07631   Phone: (201) 569-5386
Description: Publishes on medicine and science.

★5768★ NORTH ATLANTIC BOOKS
2800 Woolsey St.
Berkeley, CA 94705   Phone: (415) 652-5309
Description: Publishes materials on a wide range of subjects from health and medicine to baseball.

★5769★ NORTHERN PUBLISHING
2399 School Lake Rd.
PO Box 136
Maple City, MI 49664   Phone: (616) 334-3360
Description: Publishes on Alzheimer's disease.

★5770★ NORTHWEST LEARNING ASSOCIATES, INC.
5728 N. Via Umbrosa
Tucson, AZ 85715   Phone: (602) 299-8435
Description: Publishes on dietary habits and smoking cessation.

★5771★ NOURISHING THOUGHTS ENTERPRISES
PO Box 1402
Hudson, OH 44236   Phone: (216) 686-2662
Subject Specialties: Nutritional facts for children.

★5772★ NOVEMBER MOON
PO Box 6265
Santa Fe, NM 87502   Phone: (505) 982-5534
Description: Publishes books on health, ethnic studies, and the environment.

★5773★ NPP BOOKS
PO Box 1491
Ann Arbor, MI 48106-1491   Phone: (313) 971-7363
Description: Publishes scientific books. **Subject Specialties:** Nervous system, drugs, pharmacology.

★5774★ NUCLEUS PUBLICATIONS
Rte. 2, Box 49
Willow Springs, MO 65793   Phone: (417) 469-4310
Description: Publishes books on health, spirituality, and social transformation. Offers catalogs and a newsletter.

★5775★ NUMARC BOOK CORPORATION
60 Alcona Ave.
Buffalo, NY 14226   Phone: (716) 834-1390
Subject Specialties: Health sciences.

★5776★ NURSING MANAGEMENT SYSTEM
c/o G.S. Foundation
1310 Southern Ave. SE
Washington, DC 20032   Phone: (703) 284-7706
Description: Publishes practical guides to various healthcare management needs describing systems which are currently working successfully.

★5777★ NURSING RESEARCH ASSOCIATES
3752 Cummings St.
Eau Claire, WI 54701   Phone: (715) 832-0034
Description: Provides nursing schools with personality tests and empathy inventories which allow nursing school faculty members to increase their understanding of themselves and their students.

★5778★ NUTRI-BOOKS CORPORATION
PO Box 5793
Denver, CO 80217   Phone: (303) 778-8383
Description: Publishes books on health.

★5779★ NUTRITION COUNSELING/EDUCATION SERVICES
14135 Murlen Rd.
Olathe, KS 66062   Phone: (913) 782-8230
Description: Publishes materials on client health education, especially dieting.

★5780★ NUTRITION EDUCATION ASSOCIATION PUBLISHING COMPANY
3647 Glen Haven
Houston, TX 77025   Phone: (713) 665-2946
Description: Publishes information for the general public on the importance of nutrition to good health.

★5781★ NUTRITION EDUCATION CENTER
9500 Nall Ave., Ste. 304
Overland Park, KS 66207   Phone: (913) 383-3464
Description: Provides diet instruction material for lay-person education.

★5782★ NUTRITION LEGISLATION SERVICES
PO Box 75035
Washington, DC 20013   Phone: (202) 488-8879
Description: Publishes on nutrition regulation, nutrition legislation, and nutrition funding.

★5783★ NUTRITION FOR OPTIMAL HEALTH ASSOCIATION
PO Box 380
Winnetka, IL 60093   Phone: (708) 835-5030
Description: Publishes a nutritional cookbook.

★5784★ NUTRITIONAL DEVELOPMENT, INC.
PO Box 3130
Holiday, FL 33590-0130   Phone: (813) 848-5498
Subject Specialties: Health.

★5785★ NUTRITIONAL RESEARCH CONSULTANTS
PO Box 801333
Dallas, TX 75380   Phone: (913) 469-8878
Description: Publishes medical nutritional information.

★5786★ ODN PRODUCTIONS
8 E. 12th St., 7th Fl.
New York, NY 10003   Phone: (212) 366-0303
Description: Publishes video cassettes, books, discussion guides, and films on a variety of health issues.

★5787★ OK PUBLISHING
8151 Mary Ellen Ave.
North Hollywood, CA 91605   Phone: (818) 901-8445
Subject Specialties: Sign language.

★5788★ OMNI LEARNING INSTITUTE
2508 5th Ave., No. 110
Seattle, WA 98121   Phone: (704) 452-1866
Description: Publishes on medical research and consciousness development.

★5789★ OMNICOMM PUBLICATIONS
7233 Alliance Ct.
San Diego, CA 92119   Phone: (619) 465-7960
Description: Publishes health information booklets. **Subject Specialties:** Sexuality, nutrition, fitness, family life.

★5790★ ONE-EIGHT INC., PUBLISHER
4th Ave. and Boyachiel Way
Forks, WA 98331   Phone: (206) 374-6500
Description: Publishes home chiropractic handbooks.

★5791★ ONESS PRESS
PO Box 1064
Kurtistown, HI 96760   Phone: (707) 462-9957
Description: Publishes on holistic health and family life.

★5792★ OPEN COURT PUBLISHING COMPANY
315 5th St.
Peru, IL 61354   Phone: (815) 223-2520
Description: General Books Division publishes works in philosophy, psychology, religion, and public policy.

★5793★ ORGANICA PRESS
4419 N. Manhattan Ave.
Tampa, FL 33614   Phone: (813) 876-4879
Description: Publishes books on the arts and alternative health.

★5794★ ORYX PRESS
4041 N. Central at Indian School Rd., Ste. 700
Phoenix, AZ 85012-3397   Phone: (602) 265-2651
Description: Publishes directories, periodicals, textbooks, general reference books, and library and information science materials.

★5795★ OSTEOGENESIS IMPERFECTA FOUNDATION
PO Box 24776
Tampa, FL 33623-4776   Phone: (813) 855-7077
Description: Publishes information concerning osteogenesis imperfecta. Offers a quarterly newsletter, pamphlets, and articles.

★5796★ OUTCOMES UNLIMITED PRESS, INC.
1015 Gayley Ave., Ste. 1165
Los Angeles, CA 90024   Phone: (213) 208-2952
Description: Publishes self-help books on psychology.

★5797★ OVULATION METHOD TEACHERS ASSOCIATION
PO Box 10-1780
Anchorage, AK 99510   Phone: (907) 344-8606
Subject Specialties: Ovulation.

★5798★ OXFORD UNIVERSITY PRESS, INC.
200 Madison Ave.
New York, NY 10016   Phone: (212) 679-7300
Description: Publishes scholarly, reference, and professional books and journals. **Subject Specialties:** History, science, medicine, social sciences, humanitites, music.

★5799★ P. GAINES COMPANY
333 S. Taylor Ave.
PO Box 2253
Oak Park, IL 60303   Phone: (708) 524-1073
Description: Publishes midwest guidebooks, business publications, and other regional interest publications. Also publishes nonfictional titles of special topical interest.

★5800★ PAL PRESS
PO Box 487
199 San Francisco Blvd.
San Anselmo, CA 94960   Phone: (415) 453-8547
Description: Publishes health books by the owner as well as books on other subjects. **Subject Specialties:** Religion, health, history.

★5801★ PALAMORA PUBLISHING COMPANY
PO Box 370
Burton, OH 44021   Phone: (216) 834-1695
Description: Publishes books and booklets dealing with psychology and self-help.

★5802★ PALM PUBLICATIONS
2654 Gough St., No. 102
San Francisco, CA 94123   Phone: (415) 928-3369
Description: Publishes "a metaphysical explanation of the AIDS crisis."

★5803★ PANAEROBICS PRESS
PO Box 81867
Pittsburgh, PA 15217-1131
Description: Publishes on exercise and fitness.

★5804★ PANDA PRESS
4111 Watkins Trail
Annandale, VA 22003   Phone: (703) 256-2461
Description: Publishes books on alcohol and drug abuse.

★5805★ PANJANDRUM BOOKS
5428 Hermitage Ave.
North Hollywood, CA 91607   Phone: (818) 985-7259
Description: Publishes paperbacks on health, diet, cooking, music and drama, and literature.

★5806★ PARADON PUBLISHING COMPANY
2920 Dean Pkwy., No. 209
Minneapolis, MN 55416   Phone: (612) 929-3949
Description: Publishes trade paperbacks for the health care and humor markets, books on small business management and books for gifted children, their parents, and teachers.

★5807★ PARAMOUNT PUBLISHING, INC.
800 Roosevelt Rd.
Glen Ellyn, IL 60137   Phone: (312) 790-2483
Description: Trade book publisher of cookbooks, dictionaries, and medical subjects.

★5808★ PARENT EDUCATION PROGRAMS PRESS
3007 22nd St.
Lubbock, TX 79410   Phone: (806) 799-6021
Description: Publishes teaching materials for Lamaze childbirth preparation class use.

★5809★ PARENTERAL DRUG ASSOCIATION
1617 JFK Blvd., Ste. 640
Philadelphia, PA 19103   Phone: (215) 564-6466
Description: Collects and disseminates information on parenteral products, sterile products, and related processes in the form of bulletins, monographs, and reports.

★5810★ PARKINSON'S DISEASE FOUNDATION
650 W. 168th St.
New York, NY 10032   Phone: (212) 923-4700
Description: Established to seek the cause and cure of Parkinson's and related disorders through research.

★5811★ PARKINSON'S EDUCATIONAL PROGRAM-USA
3900 Birch St., Ste. 105
Newport Beach, CA 92660   Phone: (714) 250-2975
Description: Publishes to provide information about Parkinson's disease.

★5812★ PARTHENON GROUP, INC.
120 Mill Rd.
Park Ridge, NJ 07656   Phone: (201) 391-6796
Description: Publishes science, technical, and medical materials.

★5813★ PASSAGES, INC.
PO Box 1565
Fayetteville, AR 72702
Description: Disseminates information about psychiatric problems.

★5814★ PATHWAY BOOKS
700 Parkview Ter.
Golden Valley, MN 55416   Phone: (612) 377-1521
Subject Specialties: Self-help, health, time-management, psychology, fiction.

★5815★ PAUL H. BROOKES PUBLISHING COMPANY, INC.
PO Box 10624
Baltimore, MD 21285-0624   Phone: (301) 337-9580
Description: Publishes scholarly books in the human services, including special education, rehabilitation, therapeutic services, early childhood intervention, speech, hearing, and language.

★5816★ PAUL M. D'AMICO, D.O.
Main St.
Livingston Manor, NY 12758   Phone: (914) 439-4990
Subject Specialties: Behavior, addiction, medicine.

★5817★ PAUL PAREY SCIENTIFIC PUBLISHERS
PO Box 1815
New York, NY 10156-0610   Phone: (212) 679-0782
Description: Publishes books and journals on agriculture, veterinary medicine, and horticulture, as well as on biology, plant protection, forestry, ecology, behavior research and ethology. **Subject Specialties:** Biology, veterinary medicine, horticulture, ariculture.

★5818★ PEDIATRIC PROJECTS, INC.
PO Box 571555
Tarzana, CA 91357   Phone: (818) 705-3660
Description: Publishes a monograph series, children's books, and two newsletters. **Subject Specialties:** Health psychology for children, teens, parents, and professionals.

★5819★ PEDIPRESS, INC.
125 Red Gate Ln.
Amherst, MA 01002   Phone: (413) 549-7798
Description: Publishes books on child health care which are geared to parents.

★5820★ PENINSULA CENTER FOR THE BLIND
4151 Middlefield Rd., Ste. 101
Palo Alto, CA 94303   Phone: (415) 858-0202
Description: Published one book for families of people who are losing their sight.

★5821★ PENNANT BOOKS
3463 State St., Ste. 238
Santa Barbara, CA 93105   Phone: (805) 683-1079
Description: Publishes on health, nutrition, business, and investment.

★5822★ PENNWELL BOOKS
PO Box 1260
Tulsa, OK 74101   Phone: (918) 835-3161
Description: Publishes technical information for petroleum industry professionals, pratice management books for dentistry, computers, lasers, telecommunications, and other professsional information for high-tech industries.

★5823★ PENNYPRESS, INC.
1100 23rd Ave. E.
Seattle, WA 98112   Phone: (206) 325-1419
Description: Publishes pamphlets and books exploring controversial issues and new areas of concern in maternity care. **Subject Specialties:** Childbirth, parenting.

★5824★ PERFORMANCE RESOURCE PRESS, INC.
1863 Technology Dr., Ste. 200
Troy, MI 48083   Phone: (313) 588-7733
Description: Publishes on alcohol and drugs in schools and the workplace.

★5825★ PERGAMON PRESS, INC.
Maxwell House, Fairview Park
Elmsford, NY 10523   Phone: (914) 592-7700
Description: Publishes STM journals and upper level graduate/undergraduate textbooks, handbooks, proceedings volumes, and major reference works, including those in the field of medicine.

★5826★ PERINATAL LOSS
2116 NE 18th Ave.
Portland, OR 97212   Phone: (503) 284-7426
Description: Publishes on how to deal with the death of a baby.

★5827★ PERINATOLOGY PRESS
507 Cayuga Heights Rd.
Ithaca, NY 14850   Phone: (607) 257-3278
Description: Produces state-of-the-art research and writings in medical and scientific areas. Offers a poster.

★5828★ PHARMACEUTICAL MANUFACTURERS ASSOCIATION
1100 15th St. NW
Washington, DC 20005   Phone: (202) 763-2000
Description: Publishes numerous pamphlets and some books related to the industry. Also distributes publications prepared by member companies.

★5829★ PHILLIPS-NEUMAN COMPANY
1606 Noyes Dr.
Silver Spring, MD 20910-2224
Subject Specialties: Health, education.

★5830★ PHOENIX INTERNATIONAL
PO Box 1569
Pompano Beach, FL 33060   Phone: (305) 481-9883
Description: Publishes books on all subjects. **Subject Specialties:** How-to, self-help, cookbooks, fiction, poetry, health.

★5831★ PHYSICIANS AND SCIENTISTS PUBLISHING COMPANY
PO Box 435
Glenview, IL 60025   Phone: (708) 724-3303
Description: Publishes medical and research books. Not for the public.

★5832★ P.I. INDUSTRIES PUBLISHING COMPANY
300 S. Loomis Ave.
Fort Collins, CO 80521   Phone: (303) 224-9381
Description: Publishes a medical self-care manual. **Subject Specialties:** Health, nutrition, how-to, survival.

★5833★ PIA PRESS
19 Prospect St.
Summit, NJ 07901   Phone: (201) 277-9191
Description: Publishes self-help books on mental health for families and professionals. Offers posters.

★5834★ PINK INC.! PUBLISHING
PO Box 866
Atlantic Beach, FL 32233-0866   Phone: (904) 731-7120
Description: Publishes on pregnancy, birth, and parenting.

★5835★ PIXEL PRESS
PO Box 3151
Tequesta, FL 33469   Phone: (407) 744-8775
Description: Publishes general trade and graphic arts books on health, the arts, and history.

★5836★ PIZZAZZ PRESS, INC.
5114 Chicago
Omaha, NE 68132   Phone: (402) 466-5311
Subject Specialties: Fitness for women.

★5837★ PJD PUBLICATIONS LTD.
PO Box 966
Westbury, NY 11590   Phone: (516) 626-0650
Description: Publishes scholarly, medicinal, scientific, and philosophical titles.

★5838★ PLANNED PARENTHOOD FEDERATION OF AMERICA
Marketing Dept.
810 7th Ave.
New York, NY 10019   Phone: (212) 541-7800
Description: Publishes information on reproductive health, sexuality, and family planning.

★5839★ PLENUM PUBLISHING CORPORATION
233 Spring St.
New York, NY 10013   Phone: (212) 620-8000
Description: Publishes college textbooks in science, mathematics, computers, and medicine.

★5840★ PLYMOUTH PRESS/PLYMOUTH BOOKS
PO Box 2044
Miami, FL 33140   Phone: (305) 673-0771
Subject Specialties: Health, medicine, sex, nutrition, languages, weight loss, exercise.

★5841★ PMA PUBLISHING CORPORATION
3176 Pullman St., Ste. 104
Costa Mesa, CA 92626   Phone: (714) 545-1162
Description: Offers books, journals, and videos aimed primarily at the medical field.

★5842★ POCKET POWER
PO Box 898
Poway, CA 92064   Phone: (619) 485-1860
Description: Publishes a series of pocket-size books designed to help get the most from professional encounters.

★5843★ POPULAR MEDICINE PRESS
PO Box 1212
San Carlos, CA 94070   Phone: (415) 594-1855
Description: Publishes books on health topics based on assessment of scientific literature. **Subject Specialties:** Nutrition, science, health.

★5844★ POPULATION COUNCIL
1 Dag Hammarskjold Plaza
New York, NY 10017   Phone: (212) 644-1300
Description: An international, nonprofit organization; undertakes social science and biomedical research, advises and assists governments and international agencies, and is a leading source of information on population issues. **Subject Specialties:** Population, development, economics, women's and children's health, and family planning programs.

★5845★ A POSITIVE APPROACH, INC.
1600 Malone St., Municipal Airport
Millville, NJ 08332   Phone: (609) 327-4040
Description: Publishes a cookbook, quarterly magazine, and a "barrier-free design" book for the disabled. **Subject Specialties:** Education, computers, driving, art, photography, barrier-free design, religion.

★5846★ POTENTIALS DEVELOPMENT FOR HEALTH AND AGING SERVICES, INC.
775 Main St., Ste. 604
Buffalo, NY 14203   Phone: (716) 842-2658
Subject Specialties: Aging.

★5847★ PRACTICAL ALLERGY RESEARCH FOUNDATION
PO Box 60
Buffalo, NY 14223   Phone: (716) 875-5578
Description: Publishes books, videotapes, and audio tapes on behavior and learning problems related to unsuspected and unrecognized allergy.

★5848★ PRACTICE DYNAMICS
2290 S. 1st St.
Lake City, FL 32055   Phone: (904) 752-6673
Description: Publishes on private healthcare management. Toll-free telephone number: (800) 552-4060.

★5849★ PRADER-WILLI SYNDROME ASSOCIATION
6490 Excelsior Blvd., E-102
St. Louis Park, MN 55426   Phone: (612) 926-1947
Description: Publishes to educate parents and medical professionals on the problems associated with the Prader-Willi syndrome.

★5850★ PRAIRIE LARK PRESS
PO Box 699
Springfield, IL 62705
Description: Publishes books to help parents, children, and professionals in the area of grief counseling.

★5851★ PRECEPT PRESS
160 E. Illinois St.
Chicago, IL 60611   Phone: (312) 467-0424
Description: Publishes medical books for professionals within that field.

★5852★ PRENTICE HALL
Rte. 9W
Englewood Cliffs, NJ 07632   Phone: (201) 592-2000
Description: Publishes college textbooks and professional books, including some in the medical field.

★5853★ PRESIDENT'S COMMITTEE ON EMPLOYMENT OF PEOPLE WITH DISABILITIES
1111 20th St. NW, Rm. 600
Washington, DC 20036   Phone: (202) 653-5044
Description: Publishes "to create an atmosphere which will increase employment opportunities for individuals with disabilities."

★5854★ PRESS WEST
1855-304 McKelvey Hill Dr.
Maryland Heights, MO 63043
Description: Publishes self-help books in the areas of health, medical science, physical science and psychology.

★5855★ PRESTIGE PRESS
PO Box 2608
Falls Church, VA 22042-0608   Phone: (703) 573-8521
Description: Publishes a book on the personal experience of a victim of Alzheimer's disease and her caregiver spouse.

★5856★ PRICE-POTTENGER NUTRITION FOUNDATION
PO Box 2614
La Mesa, CA 92044-0702   Phone: (619) 582-4168
Description: Supports ongoing research, development, evaluation, and dissemination of nutritional information and materials.

★5857★ PRICKLY PAIR PUBLISHING AND CONSULTING COMPANY
9628 W. Oregon Pl.
Denver, CO 80232   Phone: (303) 986-3505
Description: Publishes education books on AIDS.

★5858★ P.R.I.D.E. FOUNDATION
71 Plaza Ct.
Groton, CT 06340   Phone: (203) 445-1448
Description: Purpose is to "promote real independence for the disabled and elderly through solutions to clothing, home management, and grooming special needs."

★5859★ PRIDE PUBLISHING LTD.
900 Larkspur Landing Circle, No. 105
Larkspur, CA 94939   Phone: (415) 461-5200
Description: Publishes practice management training manuals and reference books for the dentist and dental staff members.

★5860★ PRIME NATIONAL PUBLISHING CORPORATION
470 Boston Post Rd.
Weston, MA 02193   Phone: (617) 899-2702
Subject Specialties: Nursing.

★5861★ PRINCIPIA PRESS
5743 Kimbark Ave.
Chicago, IL 60637
Description: Publishes on philosophy, psychology, and education.

★5862★ PRISM PRESS
c/o Avery Publishing Group Inc.
120 Old Broadway
Garden City Park, NY 11040-5015   Phone: (516) 741-2155
Description: Publishes an extensive general trade list that penetrates into the health, cooking, New Age, and metaphysics markets, and has strengthened concentration in the self-sufficiency field. Also publishes a number of do-it-yourself titles.

★5863★ PRITCHETT & HULL ASSOCIATES, INC.
3440 Oakcliff Rd. NE, Ste. 110
Atlanta, GA 30340   Phone: (404) 451-0602
Description: Publishes and distributes patient education materials. Also produces slides and offers medication cards.

★5864★ PRO-ED, INC.
8700 Shoal Creek Blvd.
Austin, TX 78758   Phone: (512) 451-3246
Description: Publishes tests, books, journals, and other materials on special education, remedial education, and psychology.

★5865★ PROFESSIONAL ASSOCIATES NETWORK PRESS
PO Box 902
Fayetteville, AR 72702   Phone: (501) 751-1412
Description: Publishes reference material for professionals who work with handicapped people. Also deal with private school and residential placement for handicapped adolescents and adults.

★5866★ PROFESSIONAL BOOKS
PO Box 3246
Jackson, TN 38301   Phone: (901) 423-5400
Description: Publishes books and booklets about food, chemical, and yeast allergies, and related illnesses in children and adults. Also publishes material on child guidance, hyperactivity, learning disabilities, clinical ecology, preventive medicine, and nutrition. Directed toward physicians and the general public.

★5867★ PROFESSIONAL EXAMINATION REVIEW SYSTEM
1020 Kidder Rd.
Carencro, LA 70520   Phone: (318) 896-4780
Description: Publishes study materials for persons taking the Nursing Home Administrator Licensure Examination.

★5868★ PROFESSIONAL PRESS
PO Box 50343
Santa Barbara, CA 93150   Phone: (805) 565-1351
Description: Publishes guides on finding a psychotherapist, harmful psychotherapists, and designing a new future for those in midlife crisis.

★5869★ PROFESSIONAL RESOURCE EXCHANGE, INC.
PO Box 15560
Sarasota, FL 34277-1560   Phone: (813) 366-7913
Description: Produces "publications and continuing education programs for practicing mental health clinicians."

★5870★ PROFICIENCY EXAMINATION REVIEW
818 Olive St., Ste. 918
St. Louis, MO 63101   Phone: (314) 241-1445
Subject Specialties: Clinical laboratory technology.

★5871★ PROJECT RELEASE
PO Box 396, FDR Sta.
New York, NY 10022   Phone: (212) 447-6804
Description: Purpose is to "educate consumers of psychiatric mental health services of the dangers involved in routine treatment."

★5872★ PROMETHEUS NEMESIS BOOK COMPANY
PO Box 2748
Del Mar, CA 92014   Phone: (619) 632-1575
Description: Publishes materials on personality and behavior for psychology professionals and laymen. Also offers tests, reprints, and software.
Subject Specialties: Psychology, psychiatry, sociology.

★5873★ PRYTANEUM PRESS
1015 Bryan
Amarillo, TX 79102   Phone: (806) 372-7888
Subject Specialties: Psychology, philosophy, anthropology.

★5874★ PSYCH/GRAPHIC PUBLISHERS
13626 Orchard Gate Dr.
Poway, CA 92064   Phone: (619) 486-3404
Subject Specialties: Psychology, anthropology.

★5875★ PSYCHEGENICS PRESS
PO Box 332
Gaithersburg, MD 20884   Phone: (301) 948-1122
Description: Conducts research, tests, practices, and teaches ways to enhance human capabilities and human experience.

★5876★ PSYCHOANALYTIC QUARTERLY, INC.
175 5th Ave., Rm. 210
New York, NY 10010   Phone: (212) 982-9358
Subject Specialties: Psychoanalysis and related topics.

★5877★ PSYCHOHISTORY PRESS
PO Box 401
New York, NY 10024   Phone: (212) 873-5900
Description: Publishes works on psychohistory.

★5878★ PSYCHOLOGICAL ASSESSMENT RESOURCES, INC.
16204 N. Florida Ave.
Lutz, FL 33556
Description: Publishes psychological, career interest, and educational tests,

software and related assessment materials, and books of interest to psychologists, educators, counselors, and other mental health professionals.

★5879★ **PSYCHOLOGICAL DIMENSIONS, INC.**
301 E. 87th St., Ste. 21A
New York, NY 10128   Phone: (212) 289-5158
Description: Publishes materials on the architecture of the brain, neurotransmitters, psychotropic drugs, and medical genetics. Offers psychological publications in genetics, perception, the psychology of women, and social psychology.

★5880★ **PSYCHOLOGY AND CONSULTING ASSOCIATES PRESS**
9834 Genesee Ave., No. 321
La Jolla, CA 92037   Phone: (619) 455-7535
Description: Publishes psychology, self-help, and religious books. **Subject Specialties:** Psychology, self-help, religion.

★5881★ **PSYCHOLOGY SOCIETY**
100 Beekman St.
New York, NY 10038-1810   Phone: (212) 285-1872
Description: Organization of clinical psychologists that produces reports and documents on the use of psychology in dealing with and treating human problems such as crime, domestic/marital relations, drug use, youth culture, and aggression.

★5882★ **PSYTEC, INC.**
PO Box 564
De Kalb, IL 60115   Phone: (815) 758-1415
Description: Provides books and testing materials that benefit psychologists, social workers, and family court mediators in dealing with family violence and divorce.

★5883★ **PUBLIC AFFAIRS COMMITTEE**
381 Park Ave. South
New York, NY 10016   Phone: (212) 683-4331
Description: Nonprofit organization publishing educational material on health and mental health, family life, child development, alcohol and drug abuse, and social and economic issues.

★5884★ **PUBLIC CITIZEN HEALTH RESEARCH GROUP**
2000 P St. NW
Washington, DC 20036   Phone: (202) 872-0320
Description: "Nonprofit public interest consumer advocacy organization which works on drug safety, medical device safety, and occupational health and safety."

★5885★ **PUBLIC INFORMATION PRESS, INC.**
PO Box 402611
Miami Beach, FL 33140   Phone: (305) 538-5308
Subject Specialties: Reproductive health care.

★5886★ **PUBLIC RESPONSIBILITY IN MEDICINE AND RESEARCH**
132 Boylston St., 4th Fl.
Boston, MA 02116   Phone: (617) 423-4112
Description: "Founded to provide a multi-disciplinary forum for developing practical approaches to bioethical problems, including the protection of both human and animal subjects in biomedical and behavioral research."

★5887★ **PUBLIC SAFETY PRESS**
1320 Trancas St., Ste. 211
Napa, CA 94558   Phone: (707) 963-2559
Description: Publishes self-help books and training manuals. **Subject Specialties:** Women's survival, self defense, school emergency action plans.

★5888★ **PUBLICATIONS INTERNATIONAL, LTD.**
7373 N. Cicero
Lincolnwood, IL 60646   Phone: (312) 676-3470
Description: Publishes books by *Consumer Magazine* on health, automobiles, medicine, fitness, collectibles, entertainment, and consumer information. Offers calendars, videos, and exercise tapes.

★5889★ **PUBLISHERS CONSULTANTS**
PO Box 1908
Fort Collins, CO 80522   Phone: (303) 482-2286
Description: Publishes on political science and psychology.

★5890★ **PUBLISHERS MARK**
PO Box 6939
Incline Village, NV 89450   Phone: (702) 831-5139
Description: Publishes materials on death education for adults and children.

★5891★ **PUBLITEC EDITIONS**
271 Lower Cliff Dr., Ste. A
PO Box 4342
Laguna Beach, CA 92652   Phone: (714) 497-6100
Description: Publishes on hang gliding, health, and fitness.

★5892★ **PURCELL PRODUCTIONS, INC.**
484 W. 43rd St., 23M
New York, NY 10036   Phone: (212) 279-0795
Description: Publishes coloring books on substance abuse, alcoholism, family life, and sex education.

★5893★ **PURITAN PUBLISHING COMPANY**
749 N. 3rd St.
Coeur d'Alene, ID 83814-3016   Phone: (408) 296-6951
Description: Publishes a diet book.

★5894★ **PWJ PUBLISHING**
PO Box 238
Tehama, CA 96090   Phone: (916) 384-1341
Description: Self-publisher of texts for psychologists and graphologists.

★5895★ **QUAIL VALLEY PUBLICATIONS**
19234 Vanowen St.
Reseda, CA 91335   Phone: (818) 705-1157
Description: Publishes medical and health materials in English and in Spanish. **Subject Specialties:** Health, nutrition, travel, pregnancy, childcare.

★5896★ **QUALITY MEDICAL PUBLISHING INC.**
2086 Craigshire Dr.
St. Louis, MO 63146   Phone: (314) 878-7808
Description: Publishes medical books for medical field professionals.

★5897★ **QUEST PUBLISHING COMPANY**
1351 Titan Way
Brea, CA 92621   Phone: (714) 738-6400
Description: Specializes in publications in the field of medical device technology.

★5898★ **QUINTESSENCE PUBLISHING COMPANY, INC.**
870 Oak Creek Dr.
Lombard, IL 60148-6405   Phone: (708) 620-4443
Description: Publishes professional and scholarly books, journals, and video cassettes. **Subject Specialties:** Medicine, medical history, health, nutrition, dentistry.

★5899★ **QUOTIDIAN, INC.**
1325 Cherry Valley Rd.
Stroudsburg, PA 18360   Phone: (717) 424-5505
Description: Publishes alcoholism, addiction, and personal growth books.

★5900★ **RAE PUBLICATIONS**
PO Box 731
Brush Prairie, WA 98606   Phone: (206) 687-3767
Description: Publishes cookbooks for people afflicted with allergies.

★5901★ **RALPH R. HOVNANIAN**
2128 Prospect Ave.
Evanston, IL 60201   Phone: (312) 869-4346
Description: Publishes on overlooked cures of disease, especially cancer.

★5902★   RAMA PUBLISHING COMPANY
PO Box 793
Carthage, MO 64836   Phone: (417) 358-1093
Description: Publishes on health from a Christian standpoint, to promote the upkeep of a healthy body, mind, and spirit.

★5903★   RAMSCO PUBLISHING COMPANY
414 Main St.
PO Box N
Laurel, MD 20707   Phone: (301) 953-3699
Description: Provides information for allied health professionals.

★5904★   RAVEN PRESS
1185 Avenue of the Americas
New York, NY 10036   Phone: (212) 930-9500
Description: Publishes books and journals on the medical and life sciences.

★5905★   READER'S DIGEST GENERAL BOOKS
260 Madison Ave.
New York, NY 10016   Phone: (212) 953-0030
Description: Publishes reference books on a wide variety of subjects.
Subject Specialties: Crafts and hobbies, home repair, cooking, travel, history, geography, gardening, money management, language, medicine, Bible.

★5906★   RED FLAG GREEN FLAG RESOURCES
PO Box 2984
Fargo, ND 58108
Description: A nonprofit agency serving victims of sexual abuse, sexual assault, and domestic violence through educational materials for children and young adults. Also holds training seminars. Provides materials in coloring book form, storybook form, workbooks, manuals, videotapes, and filmstrips.

★5907★   RED LYON PUBLICATIONS
c/o Midwifery Today
PO Box 2672
Eugene, OR 97402   Phone: (503) 753-5019
Subject Specialties: Midwifery, birthing, women's health, biography, self development.

★5908★   REGENT PRESS
6020-A Adeline
Oakland, CA 94608   Phone: (415) 547-7602
Description: Publishes academic books on psychology and general trade publishing.

★5909★   REGISTRY OF INTERPRETERS FOR THE DEAF, INC.
8719 Colesville Rd., No. 310
Silver Spring, MD 20910-3919   Phone: (301) 279-0555
Description: Publishes texts used in the teaching, education, and professional development of interpretation for the hearing impaired. **Subject Specialties:** Cross cultural communication and mediation, interpreting for the hearing impaired.

★5910★   RESEARCH GRANT GUIDES
PO Box 1214
Loxahatchee, FL 33470
Description: Publishes directory of handicapped funding for nonprofit organizations.

★5911★   RESEARCH PRESS
2612 N. Mattis Ave.
Champaign, IL 61821   Phone: (217) 352-3273
Subject Specialties: Psychology, education.

★5912★   RESOURCE DIRECTORY
1038 N. Tustin, Ste. 241
Orange, CA 92667   Phone: (714) 997-1191
Description: Provides resources for professionals who help people.

★5913★   RESOURCES FOR CHILDREN IN HOSPITALS
PO Box 10
Belmont, MA 02178   Phone: (617) 648-8033
Description: Assists young children in becoming familiar with the hospital environment and hospital experiences.

★5914★   RESOURCES FOR REHABILITATION
33 Bedford St., No. 19A
Lexington, MA 02173   Phone: (617) 862-6455
Description: Publishes books designed to help people with disabilities function independently. Offers desk references for professionals and large print publications for people with disabilities.

★5915★   RIPPED ENTERPRISES
528 Chama NE
Albuquerque, NM 87108   Phone: (505) 266-5858
Description: Self-publishes on bodybuilding.

★5916★   RISING SUN CHRISTIANITY PUBLISHERS
196 Commonwealth Ave.
Boston, MA 02116   Phone: (617) 267-9525
Description: Publishes on natural health care, living foods, indoor gardening, childcare, pet care, survival, and spirituality.

★5917★   ROBERT BRIGGS ASSOCIATES
400 2nd St., Ste. 108
Lake Oswego, OR 97034   Phone: (503) 635-0435
Description: Publishes on health, philosophy, science, and psychology.

★5918★   ROCIN PRESS
8 E. 62nd St.
New York, NY 10021   Phone: (212) 355-0109
Description: Publishes to educate the public in skin care and self-improvement through surgical means.

★5919★   ROCKEFELLER UNIVERSITY
ROCKEFELLER UNIVERSITY PRESS
222 E. 70th St.
New York, NY 10021   Phone: (212) 570-8572
Description: Publishes scientific journals and books.

★5920★   RODALE PRESS, INC.
33 E. Minor St.
Emmaus, PA 18098   Phone: (215) 967-5171
Description: Publishes books on gardening, health, fitness, and the environment.

★5921★   ROMAINE PIERSON PUBLISHERS, INC.
80 Shore Rd.
PO Box 911
Port Washington, NY 11050   Phone: (516) 883-6350
Description: Publishes on the medical profession.

★5922★   RONALD S. BIVIANO, M.D., INC.
451 Scarborough Rd.
Valparaiso, IN 46383-8008
Subject Specialties: Medical education.

★5923★   ROS BERNARD PUBLICATIONS
17 Minell Pl.
Teaneck, NJ 07666   Phone: (919) 596-0859
Subject Specialties: Health education.

★5924★   ROSECOTT PUBLISHING
PO Box 9876
Riviera Beach, FL 33404   Phone: (305) 842-7170
Description: Focuses on women's health issues and lifestyles.

★5925★   ROUTLEDGE, CHAPMAN & HALL, INC.
29 W. 35th St.
New York, NY 10001-2291   Phone: (212) 244-3336
Subject Specialties: History, geography, business, engineering, science, theatre, dance, sociology, anthropology, education, film, philosophy, literature, women's studies.

★5926★   ROYAL COURT REPORTS, PUBLISHERS
3720 NE 28th Terrace
Ocala, FL 32670   Phone: (601) 324-3578
Description: Health, communications and self-help booklets designed to provide the layman with information on specific subjects.

★5927★ RUBEN PUBLISHING
PO Box 414
Avon, CT 06001   Phone: (203) 673-0740
Description: Publishes works on yoga and exercise for the elderly.

★5928★ RUDI PUBLISHING
1901 Broadway, Ste. 321
Iowa City, IA 52240   Phone: (319) 337-5057
Description: Publishes health-related and history books.

★5929★ RUTGERS UNIVERSITY
CENTER OF ALCOHOL STUDIES PUBLICATIONS DIVISION
PO Box 969
Piscataway, NJ 08855-0969   Phone: (908) 932-2190
Description: Publishes scientific and non-technical books, pamphlets, and reprints on all aspects of alcohol and its use. Subject Specialties: All aspects of alcohol and alcohol-related problems.

★5930★ S. KARGER PUBLISHERS, INC.
26 W. Avon Rd.
PO Box 529
Farmington, CT 06085   Phone: (203) 675-7834
Description: Publishes research and clinical books in the field of medicine and its related disciplines.

★5931★ SAFER SOCIETY PRESS
RR 1, Box 24-B
Orwell, VT 05760   Phone: (802) 897-7541
Description: A nonprofit religious organization publishing books and other materials on nonrepressive alternatives for sex-crime victims and offenders, including strategies for prevention.

★5932★ SAFETY NOW COMPANY INC.
PO Box 567
Jenkintown, PA 19046   Phone: (215) 884-0210
Description: Publishes child safety books and materials.

★5933★ SAGE PUBLICATIONS, INC.
2111 W. Hillcrest Dr.
Newbury Park, CA 91320   Phone: (805) 499-0721
Description: Publishes on social and behavioral sciences.

★5934★ ST. DENIS PRESS
PO Box 442
Northfield, MN 55057   Phone: (507) 529-1172
Description: Publishes on health and fitness and humor.

★5935★ SANDPIPER PRESS
PO Box 286
Brookings, OR 97415   Phone: (503) 469-5588
Description: Produces low-cost, large-type books for the vision-impaired. Offers audio tapes, bookmarks, notecards, and greeting cards. Subject Specialties: Religion, short stories, poetry, cookbook, classics, handicapped.

★5936★ SANDRIDGE PUBLISHING
15348 Sandridge Rd.
Bowling Green, OH 43402   Phone: (419) 352-1055
Description: Publishes nurtition/health books for adults and children.

★5937★ SANUK, INC.
836 Lookout Mountain Rd.
Golden, CO 80401   Phone: (303) 526-1992
Description: Publishes educational books, fiction and nonfiction on helicopter medevac, trauma care, and emergency medicine systems.

★5938★ SAUK RIVER PRESS
812 Bay St., Ste. 3
PO Box 2475
San Francisco, CA 94126   Phone: (415) 771-8253
Description: Publishes on the use of vitamins and minerals for women and senior citizens.

★5939★ SCHOLIUM INTERNATIONAL, INC.
99 Seaview Blvd.
Port Washington, NY 11050   Phone: (516) 484-3290
Description: Publishes and distributes books on science, technology, and medicine.

★5940★ SCIENCE AND BEHAVIOR BOOKS
PO Box 60519
Palo Alto, CA 94306   Phone: (415) 965-0954
Description: Publishes psychology and self-help titles. Subject Specialties: Psychotherapy, family therapy, marriage counseling, drug and alcohol addiction.

★5941★ SCIENCE SAFETY SPECIALISTS
318 N. Russel St.
Mount Prospect, IL 60056   Phone: (708) 259-2938
Description: Publishes on science safety.

★5942★ SCIENTIFIC AND MEDICAL PUBLICATIONS OF FRANCE
100 E. 42nd St., Ste. 1002
New York, NY 10017   Phone: (212) 983-6278
Description: Publishes medical and scientific books.

★5943★ SCINTA, INC.
2421 Homestead Dr.
Silver Spring, MD 20902   Phone: (301) 593-9478
Description: Publishes educational and reference material on radiation for health physicists, radiation technicians, doctors, and nurses.

★5944★ SCOLIOSIS ASSOCIATION
PO Box 51353
Raleigh, NC 27609   Phone: (919) 846-2639
Description: Publishes information on scoliosis and other spinal disorders.

★5945★ SCOTTLAND EDUCATIONAL SPECIALTIES, INC.
PO Box 14483
Oklahoma City, OK 73113   Phone: (405) 348-3864
Description: Publishes on medical and allied health education.

★5946★ SEACOAST INFORMATION SERVICES, INC.
4446 S. County Trail
Charlestown, RI 02813   Phone: (401) 364-6419
Description: Publishes on the visual stress that computers can cause.

★5947★ SELF HELP FOR HARD OF HEARING PEOPLE
7800 Wisconsin Ave.
Bethesda, MD 20814   Phone: (301) 657-2248
Description: A nonprofit, non-sectarian educational organization devoted to the welfare and interests of persons with a hearing loss, their families and friends, and the hearing health professionals. Publications deal with various aspects of hearing loss: speechreading, coping strategies, assertiveness training, stress reduction, and personal interest stories.

★5948★ SELF-HELP MANUAL
5481 Kingley Ave., Apt. A
Mountclaire, CA 91763   Phone: (714) 626-8600
Description: Publishes self-help manual providing sexual information to disabled men.

★5949★ SELF-PROGRAMMED CONTROL PRESS
PO Box 49939
Los Angeles, CA 90049   Phone: (213) 301-3317
Description: Publishes on self-actualization, self-hypnosis, bio-feedback, holistic medicine, and education.

★5950★ SENAY PUBLISHING, INC.
PO Box 397
Chesterland, OH 44026   Phone: (216) 256-8519
Subject Specialties: General reference, health, nutrition.

★5951★ SENIOR LIFE DIRECTORY
6022 W. Pico Blvd., No. 7
Los Angeles, CA 90035   Phone: (213) 933-9228
Description: Publishes a directory of special services, help lines, medical care, legal and financial information, etc., for seniors.

★5952★ SERALA PRESS
PO Box 3876
Oakland, CA 94609   Phone: (415) 933-7777
Description: Publishes an anthology of stories about Alzheimer's disease.

★5953★ SERRELL & SIMONS, PUBLISHERS
PO Box 64
Winnebago, WI 54985   Phone: (414) 231-1939
Subject Specialties: Psychology, also suitable for young adults (high school students).

★5954★ SEX INFORMATION AND EDUCATION COUNCIL OF THE U.S.
130 W. 42nd St., Ste. 2500
New York, NY 10036   Phone: (212) 819-9770
Description: Nonprofit information and education organization which acts as a clearinghouse and resource center on all aspects of human sexuality. Publishes *SIECUS Report*, pamphlets, booklets, training manuals, reprints, and specialized bibliographies.

★5955★ SHAMBHALA PUBLICATIONS, INC.
Horticultural Hall
300 Massachusetts Ave.
Boston, MA 02115   Phone: (617) 424-0030
Description: Publishes on art, literature, philosophy, science, Asian studies, psychology, children's literature, and comparative religion.

★5956★ SHARED LEARNING INC.
975 Walnut, Ste. 104
Cary, NC 27511   Phone: (919) 467-4602
Description: Publishes substance abuse prevention materials for schools.

★5957★ SHERRY SIEGEL
28 W. Chestnut
Chicago, IL 60610
Description: Publishes how-to/health books.

★5958★ SHOTWELL & CARR, INC.
3003 LBJ Fwy., Ste. 100
Dallas, TX 75234   Phone: (214) 243-1634
Description: Publishes veterinary drug references, with quarterly update service.

★5959★ SIERRA PUBLISHING COMPANY
133 Bright Ave.
PO Box 213
Jackson, CA 95642   Phone: (209) 223-3760
Description: Publishes professional and scholarly books. **Subject Specialties:** Health, religion, history, philosophy.

★5960★ SIGO PRESS
25 New Chardon St., No. 8748
Boston, MA 02114   Phone: (508) 281-4722
Description: Publishes books by auxillary writers of psychology of C. G. Jung and on health, death and dying, and human growth and development. **Subject Specialties:** Psychology, women's studies, death and dying, health, New Age, religion.

★5961★ SIMMONS & HALL PUBLISHING
4419 Praire Willow Ct.
Concord, CA 94521-4440   Phone: (415) 686-9041
Description: Publishes books in medicine and psychology.

★5962★ SIMON J. CARMEL
25 Branchbrook Dr.
Henrietta, NY 14467
Description: Self-publisher. **Subject Specialties:** Sign language, linguistics, deaf culture, deafness, education for the deaf.

★5963★ SINAUER ASSOCIATES, INC.
N. Main St.
Sunderland, MA 01375-0407   Phone: (413) 665-3722
Description: Publishes college textbooks and reference works on biological and behavioral sciences.

★5964★ SKIDMORE-ROTH PUBLISHING
207 Cincinnati Ave.
El Paso, TX 79902   Phone: (800) 825-3150
Description: Publishes books on medicine, nursing, allied health, consumer health, and New Age. Offers calendars and card sets.

★5965★ SKILLBOOK COMPANY
1111 Bethlehem Pike
Spring House, PA 19477   Phone: (215) 646-8700
Description: Publishes professional books for nurses.

★5966★ SLACK, INC.
6900 Grove Rd.
Thorofare, NJ 08086-9447   Phone: (609) 848-1000
Description: Publishes medical reference books and textbooks in medical and health services specialties. **Subject Specialties:** Medicine, health professions.

★5967★ SMOOTH STONE PRESS, INC.
PO Box 19875
St. Louis, MO 63144   Phone: (314) 968-2596
Description: Publishes on women's health.

★5968★ SMT GUILD, INC.
PO Box 313
Indianapolis, IN 46206   Phone: (317) 784-3483
Description: Nonprofit corporation that publishes alcoholic rehabilitation material by Father Ralph S. Pfau, who was founder of the National Catholic Council on Alcoholism.

★5969★ SOCIETY OF CRITICAL CARE MEDICINE
251 E. Imperial Hwy., No. 480
Fullerton, CA 92635   Phone: (714) 449-8700
Description: Publishes materials for critical care practitioners.

★5970★ SOCIETY OF NUCLEAR MEDICINE
136 Madison Ave.
New York, NY 10016-6784   Phone: (212) 889-0717
Description: A multidisciplinary organization of physicians, physicists, chemists, radiopharmacists, technologists, and others interested in the diagnostic, therapeutic, and investigational use of radionuclides. **Subject Specialties:** Nuclear medicine, nuclear medicine technology, nuclear magnetic resonance.

★5971★ SOCIETY OF NURSING PROFESSIONALS
3004 Glenview Rd.
Wilmette, IL 60091   Phone: (708) 441-2387
Description: Publishes a biographical reference directory of the nursing profession.

★5972★ SOCIETY FOR NUTRITION EDUCATION
2001 Killebrew Dr., Ste. 340
Minneapolis, MN 55425-1882   Phone: (612) 854-0035
Description: "Disseminates scientifically sound information on food and nutrition."

★5973★ SOCIETY FOR OCCUPATIONAL AND ENVIRONMENTAL HEALTH
6728 Old McLean Village Dr.
McLean, VA 22101   Phone: (202) 737-5045
Description: A nonprofit organization that publishes the proceedings of its conferences.

★5974★ SOCIETY OF TEACHERS OF FAMILY MEDICINE
PO Box 8729
Kansas City, MO 64114   Phone: (816) 333-9700
Description: Publishes for family medicine educators within medical schools, community hospitals, and university teaching hospitals. Offers curriculum guides, predoctoral education handbooks, and practice management and patient education monographs.

★5975★ SOFTWIND PUBLISHING
15948 Caminito Aire Puro
San Diego, CA 92128   Phone: (619) 673-9999
Description: Publishes materials on health, weight loss, and nutrition.

★5976★ SOUND FEELINGS PUBLISHING
24266 Walnut St., Ste. 49
Newhall, CA 91321   Phone: (805) 254-4938
Description: Book and tape publishing, specializing in music, education, and health-related fields.

★5977★ SP MEDICAL AND SCIENTIFIC BOOKS
200 Park Ave. S.
New York, NY 10003-1503   Phone: (212) 658-0888
Description: Publishes medical, psychiatric, and biomedical research books and journals.

★5978★ SPA FINDERS TRAVEL ARRANGEMENTS LTD.
91 5th Ave., 3rd Fl.
New York, NY 10003   Phone: (212) 924-6800
Description: Publishes catalogs on spas, fitness and health resorts, and New Age retreats.

★5979★ SPECIAL CHILD PUBLICATIONS
PO Box 33548
Seattle, WA 98133   Phone: (206) 522-2036
Description: Publishes professional books, programs, and tests in the fields of special education and psychology.

★5980★ SPECIAL LEARNING CORPORATION
42 Boston Post Rd.
Guilford, CT 06437   Phone: (203) 453-8579
Description: Publishers university and college textbooks and reference books in education and learning disabilities.

★5981★ SPECIAL RECREATION, INC.
362 Koser Ave.
Iowa City, IA 52246   Phone: (319) 337-7578
Description: National nonprofit organization dedicated to serving the recreation needs, rights, and aspirations of people with disabilities. Reports and documents available in print and microform from ERIC and in printed form from the National Rehabilitation Information Center.

★5982★ SPECTRA PUBLISHING COMPANY, INC.
PO Box 1403
Dillon, CO 80435   Phone: (303) 468-6439
Description: Publishes law books for law students and attorneys. Also publishes a medical book on the fragile X syndrome.

★5983★ SPEECH BIN, INC.
1766 20th Ave.
Vero Beach, FL 32960   Phone: (407) 770-0007
Description: Publishes books and materials for use by special educators, speech-language pathologists, and audiologists.

★5984★ SPEECH FOUNDATION OF AMERICA
PO Box 11749
Memphis, TN 38111   Phone: (202) 363-3199
Description: Established to supply information about the prevention and treatment of stuttering.

★5985★ SPELMAN PUBLISHERS, INC.
26941 Pebblestone
Southfield, MI 48034   Phone: (313) 355-3686
Description: Publishes in the areas of biography/history, health, and automobiles.

★5986★ SPICE WEST PUBLISHING COMPANY
PO Box 2044
Pocatello, ID 83201   Phone: (208) 233-0962
Description: Publishes a guide to medicinal plants.

★5987★ SPINAL NETWORK
PO Box 4162
Boulder, CO 80306   Phone: (303) 449-5412
Description: Publishes consumer resource guides and news journals for spinal cord injured persons and related professionals. Subject Specialties: Medicine, sports, travel, sexuality, civil rights, regeneration.

★5988★ SPRING
c/o David V. Forrest, M.D.
155 W. 68th
New York, NY 10023   Phone: (212) 873-7750
Subject Specialties: Psychiatry, language.

★5989★ SPRING PUBLICATIONS, INC.
PO Box 222069
Dallas, TX 75222   Phone: (214) 943-4094
Description: Publishes on Jungian and archetypal psychology, mythology, fairy tales, literary studies, and related topics.

★5990★ SPRINGER PUBLISHING COMPANY
536 Broadway
New York, NY 10012   Phone: (212) 431-4370
Description: Publishers of scholarly books and journals in fields of psychology, social work, medicine/public health, gerontology and geriatrics, nursing, and rehabilitation.

★5991★ SPRINGER-VERLAG NEW YORK, INC.
175 5th Ave., 19th Fl.
New York, NY 10010   Phone: (212) 460-1500
Description: Publishes reference and non-trade scientific and medical books.

★5992★ SPRINGHOUSE CORPORATION
1111 Bethlehem Pike
Spring House, PA 19477   Phone: (215) 646-8700
Description: Publishes text and reference books for doctors and nurses relating to the nursing field.

★5993★ STADION PUBLISHING COMPANY
PO Box 447
Island Pond, VT 05846   Phone: (802) 723-6175
Description: Publishes sports and fitness manuals, bringing East European sports know-how to Western athletes and coaches.

★5994★ STAR PUBLISHING
1000 Jousting
Austin, TX 78746   Phone: (512) 327-8310
Description: Publishes information on birth, parenting, the family, metaphysics, and spiritual life.

★5995★ STAR VALLEY PUBLICATIONS
PO Box 421
Noti, OR 97461   Phone: (503) 935-3032
Description: Publishes consumer medical guides.

★5996★ STARBRIGHT BOOKS
1611 E. Dow Rd.
Freeland, WA 98249   Phone: (206) 321-6138
Subject Specialties: Nutrition, preventive medicine, holistic health.

★5997★ STATE MUTUAL BOOK AND PERIODICAL SERVICE LTD.
521 5th Ave., 17th Fl.
New York, NY 10175   Phone: (212) 682-5844
Description: Publishes and distributes academic titles on history, autobiography, management, and medicine.

★5998★ STATFORD PUBLISHING
1259 El Camino Real, Ste. 1500
Menlo Park, CA 94025   Phone: (415) 854-9355
Description: Publishes books on nutrition.

★5999★   STATION HILL PRESS
Station Hill Rd.
Barrytown, NY 12507   Phone: (914) 758-5840
Description: Publishes on literature, art, and health. **Subject Specialties:**
Poetry, fiction, Blake criticism, translations, health, mind and body.

★6000★   STEP AHEAD PRESS
6509 Brecksville Rd.
PO Box 31360
Cleveland, OH 44131   Phone: (216) 526-6727
Description: Publishes on health, self-improvement, and adult nonfiction.

★6001★   STEREO PUBLICATIONS
57 Montague St.
Brooklyn, NY 11201   Phone: (718) 852-0258
Description: Publishes a study of the anatomy of the arteries and veins of
the brain using View-Master custom stereo picture reels.

★6002★   STERLING PUBLISHING COMPANY, INC.
387 Park Ave. S.
New York, NY 10016-8810   Phone: (212) 532-7160
Subject Specialties: Business, health, cookbooks, woodworking, history,
military, knitting, body building, sports, gardening, hobbies, New Age,
medical reference.

★6003★   STOELTING COMPANY
620 Wheat Ln.
Wood Dale, IL 60191-1109   Phone: (708) 860-9700
Description: Publishes psychological tests, special education materials, and
employee screening materials with related software.

★6004★   STOKESVILLE PUBLISHING COMPANY
PO Box 14401
Atlanta, GA 30324   Phone: (404) 658-3075
Description: Publishes and distributes volumes primarily of interest to
physical and occupational therapists.

★6005★   STOP AIDS PROJECT, INC.
40 Plympton St.
Boston, MA 02118   Phone: (617) 542-5679
Description: Publishes on understanding, coping, and helping the victims
of the AIDS virus.

★6006★   STRESSPRESS
PO Box 474
Putney, VT 05346
Description: Publishers of stress and human development materials.
Subject Specialties: Psychology.

★6007★   STRETCHING INC.
PO Box 767
Palmer Lake, CO 80133   Phone: (719) 481-3928
Description: Self-publisher of book on fitness and exercise. Also produces
stretching charts, pads, cards, software program, and videos.

★6008★   SUN EAGLE PUBLISHING
17038 Chatsworth St.
PO Box 33545
Granada Hills, CA 91394-8545   Phone: (818) 360-2224
Description: Publishes self-help books and videos. **Subject Specialties:**
Health, yoga, martial arts.

★6009★   SUNBELT MEDICAL PUBLISHERS
PO Box 13512
Tallahassee, FL 32317   Phone: (904) 386-8918
Description: Publishes medical textbooks, workbooks, and manuals for
nurses, midlevel practitioners, and physicians in training.

★6010★   SUNSHINE PRESS
PO Box 8147
Longmont, CO 80501   Phone: (303) 772-3556
Description: Publishes nonfictional works of current interest in health,
lifestyle, psychology, and small business operations.

★6011★   SUPER G PUBLISHING COMPANY
302 Willow Oaks Blvd.
Hampton, VA 23669   Phone: (804) 851-2261
Description: Publishes books on health.

★6012★   SUPPORT SOURCE
420 Rutgers Ave.
Swarthmore, PA 19081-2417   Phone: (215) 544-3605
Description: Publications help families deal with the complex emotional
and practical problems of caring for a frail older person and help
individuals face their own aging with courage.

★6013★   SURREY BOOKS
230 E. Ohio St., Ste. 120
Chicago, IL 60611   Phone: (312) 751-7330
Description: Publishes health and diet cookbooks, and several job search
titles.

★6014★   SUTTON MOVEMENT WRITING PRESS
PO Box 517
La Jolla, CA 92038-0517   Phone: (619) 456-0098
Description: Devoted to spread the use of Sutton Movement Writing,
Dance Writing, and Sign Writing for the sign languages used by deaf
communities worldwide.

★6015★   SVERGE-HAUS PUBLISHERS
11 Indian Spring Rd.
Milton, MA 02186   Phone: (617) 773-2709
Description: Publishes books mostly pertaining to medicine and linguistics.
Subject Specialties: Poetry, novels, philosophy, pre-history, etymologic
linguistics.

★6016★   SWEET CH'I PRESS
662 Union St.
Brooklyn, NY 11215   Phone: (718) 857-0449
Description: Publishes works on traditional Chinese health sciences, mostly
translations from Chinese. **Subject Specialties:** Herbology, Chinese health
sciences.

★6017★   SYMPOSIA FOUNDATION
PO Box 611857
1175 NE 129th Street, Ste. 509
Miami, FL 33161   Phone: (305) 891-0658
Description: Nonprofit organization dedicated to public health care.
Publishes proceedings and books of interest to the medical, paramedical,
and scientific professions.

★6018★   SYNAPSE PUBLICATIONS, INC.
3093 Shelly Dr.
Library, PA 15129-8860   Phone: (412) 765-3140
Description: International medical writing and communication firm providing research, writing, editing, graphics, and publication and distribution
for the health industry.

★6019★   SYNERGETICS HEALTH PUBLICATIONS
2090 Versailles Rd.
Frankfort, KY 40601-9255   Phone: (502) 695-5665
Description: Publishes self-help books on exercise, fitness, and health.

★6020★   SYSTEMS PLANNING ASSOCIATION, INC.
Publications Division
PO Box 1447
Keene, NH 03431   Phone: (603) 357-4005
Description: Promotes the distribution and publication of materials for
social service agencies, gerontological practitioners, and others interested
in the aging process and service.

★6021★   TAOIST PUBLISHERS
c/o EDT, Inc.
917 Woodcrest
Royal Oak, MI 48067   Phone: (313) 545-6624
Description: Publishes books on natural health, fitness, spiritual development, and yoga "to aid individuals in realizing their highest potentials in
mind, body, and spirit."

★6022★ TAPESTRY PRESS
371 N. 900 E.
Springville, UT 84663   Phone: (801) 489-9432
Description: Publishes on health and personal improvement.

★6023★ TARANTULA PRESS
PO Box 17211
Tucson, AZ 85731   Phone: (602) 296-5332
Description: Publishes books in sports and health areas.

★6024★ TASH: THE ASSOCIATION FOR PERSONS WITH SEVERE HANDICAPS
7010 Roosevelt Way NE
Seattle, WA 98115   Phone: (206) 523-8446
Description: TASH publishes a quarterly journal and a monthly newsletter. Videos, books, monographs, and reprints from back issues of the journal and bibliographies are available on subjects such as supported employment, non-aversive behavior management techniques, and working with families.

★6025★ TATERHILL PRESS
PO Box 5100
Santa Cruz, CA 95063   Phone: (408) 458-3365
Description: Publishes on health issues.

★6026★ TECHKITS, INC.
PO Box 105
Demarest, NJ 07627   Phone: (201) 768-7334
Subject Specialties: Nutrition.

★6027★ TECHNOMIC PUBLISHING COMPANY, INC.
851 Holland Ave.
PO Box 3535
Lancaster, PA 17604-3535   Phone: (717) 291-5609
Subject Specialties: Science, engineering, education, energy, health, environmental science and technology, software.

★6028★ T.E.D. ASSOCIATES
42 Lowell Rd.
Brookline, MA 02146   Phone: (617) 277-8446
Subject Specialties: Psychology, psychological testing.

★6029★ TEN STAR PRESS
2417 W. 78th St.
Inglewood, CA 90305   Phone: (213) 758-2123
Description: Publishes books on history, politics, social issues, health, and yoga.

★6030★ TEST CORPORATION OF AMERICA
4050 Pennsylvania, Ste. 310
Kansas City, MO 64111   Phone: (816) 756-1490
Description: Publishes professional reference books in psychology, education, and business.

★6031★ TETRAHEDRON INC.
10 B Drumlin Rd.
PO Box 402
Rockport, MA 01966   Phone: (508) 546-6586
Description: Publishes on the principles and practices of holistic health. **Subject Specialties:** Self-help, health, psychology.

★6032★ THEOSOPHICAL BOOK ASSOCIATION FOR THE BLIND
54 Krotona Hill
Ojai, CA 93023   Phone: (805) 646-2121
Description: Publishes a quarterly braille magazine, braille books, and "talking book" cassette tapes of theosophical interest for the blind and visually impaired.

★6033★ THEOSOPHICAL PUBLISHING HOUSE
306 W. Geneva Rd.
PO Box 270
Wheaton, IL 60189-0270   Phone: (708) 665-0130
Description: Publishes on healing, health, diet, occultism, mysticism, philosophy, transpersonal psychology, theosophy, reincarnation, religion, yoga, and meditation.

★6034★ THERAPEUTIC MEDIA INC.
PO Box 21056
Santa Barbara, CA 93121   Phone: (805) 736-6792
Description: A company designed to disseminate information about therapeutic approaches in pediatrics and, more specifically, treatments for children with neuromuscular disorders.

★6035★ THETA CORPORATION
Theta Bldg.
Middlefield, CT 06455   Phone: (203) 349-1054
Description: Publishes technological and market research reports for worldwide manufacturers of medical equipment, pharmaceuticals, and biotechnology.

★6036★ THIEME MEDICAL PUBLISHERS, INC.
381 Park Ave. S.
New York, NY 10016   Phone: (212) 683-5088
Description: Publishes books and journals on clinical medicine.

★6037★ THINKING PUBLICATIONS
1731 Westgate Rd.
PO Box 163
Eau Claire, WI 54702-0163   Phone: (715) 832-2488
Description: Publishes materials addressing oral communication and thinking skills for special educators, particularly speech-language pathologists and learning disabilities specialists.

★6038★ THIRD LINE PRESS, INC.
4751 Viviana Dr., Ste. 101
Tarzana, CA 91356   Phone: (818) 996-0076
Description: Publishes on medicine and nutrition.

★6039★ THIRD PARTY PUBLISHING COMPANY
PO Box 13306, Montclair Sta.
Oakland, CA 94661-0306   Phone: (415) 339-2323
Description: Publishes books for students and practitioners of the applied behavioral sciences, with emphasis on organizations, communities, and social systems. Office address: 6933 Armour Dr. **Subject Specialties:** Health education, medical care, organizations development.

★6040★ THOMAS-HENNING PUBLISHING
PO Box 121176
Arlington, TX 76012   Phone: (817) 265-8297
Description: Publishes on health related travel.

★6041★ THOMPSON & COMPANY, INC.
4600 Longfellow Ave.
Minneapolis, MN 55407-3638   Phone: (612) 331-3963
Description: Publishes nonfiction books on healthcare and business. Offers college textbooks.

★6042★ THREE WISHES PRESS
PO Box 81033
Pittsburgh, PA 15217   Phone: (412) 521-1057
Description: Publishes a series of books for psychologists, social workers, and nurses.

★6043★ THROUGH THICK AND THIN
6216 Hills Dr.
Birmingham, MI 48010   Phone: (313) 642-4252
Description: Provides research and food information concerning health and natural eating.

★6044★ TIDE BOOK PUBLISHING COMPANY
PO Box 101
York Harbor, ME 03911-0101   Phone: (207) 363-4534
Description: Publishes on social science, health, aging, women, and the arts.

★6045★ TIRESIAS PRESS, INC.
116 Pinehurst Ave.
New York, NY 10033   Phone: (212) 568-9570
Description: Publishes books in the health field and on adoption. **Subject Specialties:** Nursing, aging, occupational therapy, adoption.

★6046★ TISSA, INC.
Rte. 8, Box 90
Culpeper, VA 22701   Phone: (703) 547-2149
Description: Researches and publishes cures of mental conditions leading to psychopathy.

★6047★ T.J. PUBLISHER, INC.
817 Silver Spring Ave., Ste. 206
Silver Spring, MD 20910   Phone: (301) 585-4440
Description: Publishes books primarily on American sign language and deafness, including books by deaf authors.

★6048★ TOM FEDERLIN
47 Cardinal Ct.
Saratoga Springs, NY 12866   Phone: (518) 587-3704
Description: Publishes books on sign language.

★6049★ TOPPING INTERNATIONAL INSTITUTE
2622 Birchwood Ave., No. 7
Bellingham, WA 98225   Phone: (206) 647-2703
Description: Publishes to increase the focus on holistic health through education.

★6050★ TRADITIONAL ACUPUNCTURE INSTITUTE, INC.
American City Bldg., Ste. 100
Columbia, MD 21044   Phone: (301) 596-6006
Description: Publishes books on traditional acupuncture and Oriental medicine.

★6051★ TRANQUILITY PRESS
200 Leslie Dr., Box 516
Hallandale, FL 33009   Phone: (305) 454-8082
Description: Publishes information for parents before and after the birth of their child. **Subject Specialties:** Health-stress management.

★6052★ TRAVEL MEDICINE, INC.
351 Pleasant St., Ste. 312
Northampton, MA 01060   Phone: (413) 584-0381
Description: Publishes an annual guide for traveler's seeking health information.

★6053★ TREE OF LIFE PUBLICATIONS
PO Box 126
Joshua Tree, CA 92252-0126   Phone: (619) 366-2478
Description: Publishes books on natural health and holistic healing.

★6054★ TRIAD PUBLISHING COMPANY, INC.
1110 NW 8th Ave.
Gainesville, FL 32601   Phone: (904) 373-5800
Description: Publishes on health, medicine, and healthful cooking.

★6055★ TRI-MED PRESS
47 Portland Pl.
Montclair, NJ 07042-2821   Phone: (201) 746-9132
Description: Publishes medical books for the layman and professional.

★6056★ TRINGA PRESS
PO Box 8181
Saint Paul, MN 55108-0181   Phone: (603) 647-9776
Description: Publishes a glossary of healthcare industry terms for use by hospital trustees, administrators, and laypersons.

★6057★ TUCKER PUBLICATIONS, INC.
PO Box 580
Lisle, IL 60532   Phone: (708) 969-3809
Description: Publishes on health care issues concerning Black Americans.

★6058★ TURNING POINT PUBLICATIONS
1122 M St.
Eureka, CA 95501-2442   Phone: (707) 445-2290
Description: Publishes natural healthcare books dealing with vegetarian (macrobiotic) cooking and traditional natural healing techniques.

★6059★ TWENTY-FIRST CENTURY PUBLICATIONS
PO Box 702
401 N. 4th St.
Fairfield, IA 52556   Phone: (515) 472-5105
Description: Educates public to self-sufficency in matters of health and diet. **Subject Specialties:** Sprouting, wheatgrass therapy, holistic health, raw foods.

★6060★ TWIN PEAKS PRESS
PO Box 129
Vancouver, WA 98666   Phone: (205) 694-2462
Description: Publishes several titles for the disabled.

★6061★ UNITED HOSPITAL FUND OF NEW YORK
55 5th Ave., 16th Fl.
New York, NY 10003   Phone: (212) 645-2500
Description: Publishes on the provision and financing of health care in New York City and the nation. Offers two newsletters and one quarterley summary of hospital statistics.

★6062★ UNITED PRESS, INC.
PO Box 4064
Sarasota, FL 33578
Subject Specialties: Health, diet, fasting.

★6063★ UNITED SCLERODERMA FOUNDATION
PO Box 350
Watsonville, CA 95077-0350   Phone: (408) 728-2202
Description: A patient-oriented foundation responding to inquiries about scleroderma. Furnishes literature to patients, health professionals, or any interested party.

★6064★ U.S. ASSOCIATION FOR BLIND ATHLETES
33 N. Institute
Brown Hall, Ste. 015
Colorado Springs, CO 80903   Phone: (719) 630-0422
Description: Publishes rules of sanctioned sports for visually impaired persons.

★6065★ U.S. DIRECTORY SERVICE, PUBLISHERS
655 NW 128th St.
PO Box 68-1700
Miami, FL 33168   Phone: (305) 769-1700
Description: Publishes medical directories.

★6066★ U.S. LIBRARY OF CONGRESS
NATIONAL LIBRARY SERVICE FOR THE BLIND AND PHYSICALLY HANDICAPPED
1291 Taylor St., NW
Washington, DC 20542   Phone: (202) 707-5100
Description: Talking and braille books and magazines are distributed through 159 regional and subregional libraries to blind and physically handicapped residents of the U.S. and its territories.

★6067★ U.S. NATIONAL INSTITUTES OF HEALTH
NATIONAL CENTER FOR RESEARCH RESOURCES
9000 Rockville Pike
Bethesda, MD 20892   Phone: (301) 496-5545
Description: Produces materials for health professionals and the general public on scientific and medical research.

★6068★ U.S. NATIONAL LIBRARY OF MEDICINE
8600 Rockville Pike
Bethesda, MD 20894   Phone: (301) 496-6221
Description: Serves as the nation's chief medical information source.

★6069★ U.S. PHARMACOPEIAL CONVENTION INC.
12601 Twinbrook Pkwy.
Rockville, MD 20852   Phone: (301) 881-0666
Description: Publishes information for health care providers on drugs they prescribe or dispense. Offers books on patient counseling.

★6070★ UNIVERSITY PUBLISHING GROUP
107 E. Church St.
Frederick, MD 21701   Phone: (301) 694-8531
Description: Publishes on law, medicine, and public policy.

★6071★ UNIVERSITY OF TEXAS, AUSTIN
HOGG FOUNDATION FOR MENTAL HEALTH
PO Box 7998
Austin, TX 78713   Phone: (512) 471-5041
Description: Publishes materials on mental health. Offers audio cassettes of radio interviews, proceedings of seminars, and quarterly newsletters.

★6072★ UNIVERSITY OF WISCONSIN, STOUT
MATERIALS DEVELOPMENT CENTER
Menomonie, WI 54751   Phone: (715) 232-1342
Description: Publishes books designed to provide how-to information in topic areas of interest to professionals in the field of rehabilitation.

★6073★ UPLIFT BOOKS
PO Box 5233
Carmel, CA 93921   Phone: (408) 646-9246
Description: Publishes a book on hypoglycemia-how it feels and what to do.
Subject Specialties: Health, nutrition.

★6074★ URBAN & SCHWARZENBERG, INC.
428 E. Preston St.
Baltimore, MD 21202   Phone: (301) 528-4000
Description: Publishes textbooks and reference books in medicine and bioscience. **Subject Specialties:** Anatomy, cell biology, neurology, orthopaedics, pain medicine, pediatrics, radiology, sports medicine, surgery, obstetrics and gynocology, family practice.

★6075★ VALET PUBLISHING COMPANY
220 Main St.
Clayton, GA 30525   Phone: (800) 227-6269
Description: Publishes books on alternative medicine and violence control.

★6076★ VALLEY PRESS
1907 Vinton St.
Lafayette, IN 47904   Phone: (317) 742-2347
Description: Publishes books on nursing. Offers calendars.

★6077★ VALLEY PUBLISHING
333 Michigan Dr.
Lower Burrell, PA 15068   Phone: (412) 337-0635
Description: Publishes medical information for the lay public.

★6078★ VAN NOSTRAND REINHOLD COMPANY, INC.
115 5th Ave.
New York, NY 10003   Phone: (212) 254-3232
Description: Publishes reference books, periodicals, and software including some that relate to medicine.

★6079★ VCH PUBLISHERS, INC.
220 E. 23rd St., Ste. 909
New York, NY 10010-4606   Phone: (212) 683-8333
Description: Publishes professional and reference works in the sciences, chemistry engineering, law, medicine, and psychology.

★6080★ VEGETUS PUBLICATIONS
171 Madison Ave.
New York, NY 10016   Phone: (212) 679-3590
Description: Publishes books and periodicals about medicine, nutrition, and psychology.

★6081★ VENTNOR PUBLISHERS
PO Box G
Ventnor, NJ 08406-0078
Subject Specialties: Near and Middle East texts, medicine, medical history.

★6082★ VETERINARY MEDICINE PUBLISHING COMPANY
9073 Lenexa Dr.
Lenexa, KS 66215   Phone: (913) 492-4300
Description: Publishes clinical and practice-management books for veterinarians, a monthly clinical magazine, a monthly practice-management magazine, and a newsletter.

★6083★ VETERINARY PRACTICE PUBLISHING COMPANY
PO Box 4457
Santa Barbara, CA 93140   Phone: (805) 965-1028
Description: Publishes materials for use by veterinarians and students.

★6084★ VETERINARY TEXTBOOKS
36 Woodcrest Ave.
Ithaca, NY 14850   Phone: (607) 272-1860
Subject Specialties: Veterinary anatomy.

★6085★ VICKTOR, INC.
10467 White Granite Dr., Ste. 300
Oakton, VA 22124   Phone: (703) 218-8400
Description: Purpose is to "educate employees and dependents nationwide about leading healthy lifestyles and using the medical care system appropriately."

★6086★ VINCENTE BOOKS, INC.
PO Box 7388
Berkeley, CA 94707-0388   Phone: (415) 524-7343
Description: Publishes books explaining science in lay language.

★6087★ VISION FOUNDATION, INC.
818 Mt. Auburn St.
Watertown, MA 02172   Phone: (617) 926-4232
Description: Publishes on vision and sight loss.

★6088★ VITAL BODY MARKETING COMPANY, INC.
PO Box 1067
Manhasset, NY 11030   Phone: (516) 759-5200
Subject Specialties: Publishes relaxation and self-help audio cassettes.

★6089★ VOICE FOUNDATION
40 W. 57th St.
New York, NY 10019   Phone: (212) 688-1897
Description: A nonprofit organization promoting prevention and treatment of voice disorders. Publishes monographs, proceedings of annual symposia, and audiovisual cassettes.

★6090★ VOLCANO PRESS, INC.
PO Box 270
Volcano, CA 95689   Phone: (209) 296-4515
Subject Specialties: Women's health, domestic violence, art, children's books.

★6091★ VORTEX COMMUNICATIONS, INC.
PO Box 1008
Topanga, CA 90290   Phone: (213) 455-7221
Description: Publishes health resource guides that "awaken and enliven the human spirit."

★6092★ W. B. PATTERSON
3080 Alaneo Pl.
Wailuku, HI 96793   Phone: (808) 244-5437
Description: Self-publisher of a medical monograph, *Fetal Adrenal Hyperplasia: Its Relationship to Late Toxemia.*

★6093★ W. B. SAUNDERS COMPANY
Curtis Center
Independence Sq. W.
Philadelphia, PA 19106   Phone: (215) 238-7800
Description: Publishes on medicine, nursing, veterinary medicine, dentistry, and allied health.

★6094★ W. D. HOARD & SONS COMPANY
28 Milwaukee Ave. W.
Fort Atkinson, WI 53538   Phone: (414) 563-5551
Description: Publishes an international dairy magazine and a newspaper as well as dairy and agricultural titles aimed at farmers and students of dairy and veterinary science.

★6095★ WALLCUR INC.
3287 F St., Ste. G
San Diego, CA 92102   Phone: (619) 233-9628
Description: Publishes texts for nursing education at the junior college and university level.

★6096★ WARFIELD COMMUNICATIONS, INC.
PO Box 553
Winsted, CT 06098-0553
Subject Specialties: Medical equipment, operations, service, financing.

★6097★ WARREN BOOK PUBLISHING COMPANY
7515 Yacht St.
Warren, MI 48090   Phone: (313) 756-7886
Description: Self-publisher of a book on alcoholism.

★6098★ WARREN H. GREEN, INC.
8356 Olive Blvd.
St. Louis, MO 63132   Phone: (314) 991-1335
Description: Publishes books on medicine and classic philosophy.

★6099★ WASHINGTON BUSINESS INFORMATION, INC.
1117 N. 19th St., No. 200
Arlington, VA 22209-1798   Phone: (703) 247-3400
Description: Publishes books on product safety, food and drug issues, devices and diagnostics issues, and plastics.

**★6100★ WASHINGTON UNIVERSITY
CENTRAL INSTITUTE FOR THE DEAF**
818 S. Euclid Ave.
St. Louis, MO 63110
Description: Publishes on the evaluation and instruction of hearing impaired children. Produces test kits.

★6101★ WATSON PUBLISHING INTERNATIONAL
PO Box 493
Canton, MA 02021   Phone: (617) 828-8450
Description: Publishes college textbooks and scholarly books on science and medicine.

★6102★ WEEHAWKEN BOOK COMPANY
4221 45th St. NW
Washington, DC 20016   Phone: (202) 362-3185
Description: Publishes on the history of medical thought.

★6103★ WELLBEING BOOKS
PO Box 396
Newtonville, MA 02160   Phone: (617) 332-7845
Description: Publishes books and audio cassettes on health and technology.

★6104★ WELLNESS, INC.
PO Box 33063
Granada Hills, CA 91344   Phone: (818) 891-2084
Description: Founded as a preventive health service, to teach prevention of disease and healthy lifestyles. Publishes respiratory therapy learning aids for certification exams and a preventive health guide.

★6105★ WELLNESS PUBLICATIONS
PO Box 2397
Holland, MI 49422-2398   Phone: (616) 396-5477
Description: Publishes health and wellness information.

★6106★ WEST BEND HIGH SCHOOLS
1305 E. Decorah Rd.
West Bend, WI 53095   Phone: (414) 338-5563
Description: Publishes a handbook to help other school districts and agencies set up pregnancy prevention programs in their communities.

★6107★ WEST PINE PUBLISHING COMPANY
912 W. Pine St.
Hattiesburg, MS 39401   Phone: (601) 582-1978
Description: Publishes a self-help book on women's health.

★6108★ WHALEHALL, INC.
277 West End Avenue, No. 15A
New York, NY 10023   Phone: (212) 787-5897
Description: Publishes on acupuncture.

★6109★ WHITE DOVE PUBLISHING COMPANY
10711 Winmer Rd.
Independence, MO 64052
Description: Publishes to educate the uninformed about the efficacy of chiropractic medicine. Also publishes a book on fat reduction.

★6110★ WHITMORE PUBLISHING COMPANY
35 Cricket Ter.
Ardmore, PA 19003   Phone: (215) 896-6116
Subject Specialties: Nutrition, education, community life, philosophy, self-improvement, family and career planning.

★6111★ WHOLE PERSON ASSOCIATES INC.
PO Box 3151
Duluth, MN 55803   Phone: (218) 728-4077
Description: Designs workshops and publishes innovative training materials. **Subject Specialties:** Stress management, burnout prevention, wellness promotion, communication skills.

★6112★ WILDWOOD RESOURCES, INC.
9085 E. Mineral Circle, Ste. 300
Englewood, CO 80112   Phone: (303) 790-7580
Description: Publishes and distributes educational books and materials for parents, family day care homes, day care centers, and preschools. **Subject Specialties:** Nutrition, child care.

★6113★ WILEY-LISS
605 3rd Ave.
New York, NY 10158   Phone: (212) 850-8800
Description: Publishes scientific and medical books.

★6114★ WILLETT PUBLISHING COMPANY
710 Bluff St.
Glencoe, IL 60022   Phone: (708) 835-0900
Description: Publishes mental health books for patients, universities, and Recovery, Inc. (a community mental health organization.).

★6115★ WILLIAM AND ALLEN
PO Box 6147
Olympia, WA 98502   Phone: (206) 866-7417
Subject Specialties: Travel, health.

★6116★ WILLIAM M. MERCER, INC.
Louisville Galleria
2600 Meidinger Tower
Louisville, KY 40202   Phone: (502) 561-4555
Description: Publishes booklets and newsletters. **Subject Specialties:** Social Security, Medicare.

★6117★ WILLIAMS & WILKINS
428 E. Preston St.
Baltimore, MD 21202   Phone: (301) 528-4000
Subject Specialties: Medicine, pharmacy, nursing, podiatry, veterinary medicine, allied health, science, chiropractic medicine.

★6118★ WILLOW PUBLISHING INC.
PO Box 6636 - AH
San Antonio, TX 78209   Phone: (512) 822-5263
Description: Publishes books by Herbert M. Shelton on nutrition and health.

★6119★ WILLYSHE PUBLISHING COMPANY, INC.
112 Mountain Rd.
Linthicum Heights, MD 21090   Phone: (301) 789-0241
Subject Specialties: Devotional, folklore, history, Germanic research, archaeology, physical fitness for handicapped children.

★6120★ WILSON, BROWN & COMPANY
23200 Chagrin Blvd., No. 160
Cleveland, OH 44122-5403   Phone: (216) 464-1820
Description: Publishes health care books and manuals.

★6121★ WINTERGREEN PRESS
3630 Eileen St.
Maple Plain, MN 55359   Phone: (612) 476-1303
Description: Publishes books for families on infant death. Also offers cards and videos.

★6122★ WOMEN FOR SOBRIETY, INC.
PO Box 618
109 W. Broad St.
Quakertown, PA 18951   Phone: (215) 536-8026
Description: Publishes material for women alcoholics in recovery. Offers books, booklets, cassettes, video tapes, and posters.

★6123★ WOODBRIDGE PRESS
815 De La Vina St.
Santa Barbara, CA 93101   Phone: (805) 237-6053
Description: Publishes on nutrition and health, foods, and gardening. Also publishes general how-to books. Offers greeting cards.

★6124★ WOODLAND BOOKS
PO Box 1422
Provo, UT 84603   Phone: (801) 785-8100
Description: Publishes health and nutrition books.

★6125★ WOODLAND PUBLISHING COMPANY, INC.
Box 85
Wayzata, MN 55391   Phone: (612) 473-2725
Subject Specialties: Religion, health.

★6126★ WOODMERE PRESS
PO Box 20190
Park West Finance Sta.
New York, NY 10025   Phone: (212) 678-7839
Description: Publishes books on drug prevention, particularly the health hazards of marijuana, alcohol, drugs, and driving while impaired.

★6127★ WORDSCOPE ASSOCIATES
8040 Floral Ave., Ste. 304
Skokie, IL 60077   Phone: (312) 677-0506
Description: Publishes health education materials for laymen. **Subject Specialties:** Diabetes control, high blood pressure, headaches, arthritis, menopause, phobias.

★6128★ WORLD CLASS ENTERPRISES, INC.
3209 Jacqueline Dr.
Albany, GA 31705   Phone: (912) 436-7434
Description: Promotes and publishes materials on physical and mental excellence. **Subject Specialties:** Health, fitness, performance enhancement.

★6129★ WORLD HEALTH ORGANIZATION
49 Sheridan Ave.
Albany, NY 12210   Phone: (518) 436-9686
Description: Publishes non-serial publications, directories, and serials concerned with international health matters.

★6130★ WORLD SERVICE OFFICE OF NARCOTICS ANONYMOUS, INC.
PO Box 9999
Van Nuys, CA 91409   Phone: (818) 780-3951
Description: A nonprofit organization which handles publication and distribution of literature and other items for worldwide Fellowship of Narcotics Anonymous. Materials available in several foreign languages.
Subject Specialties: Recovery from drug addiction.

★6131★ WOSS PUBLISHING COMPANY
6821 SR 366
Huntsville, OH 43324   Phone: (513) 686-3183
Description: Publishes conservative, fundamental religious materials and self-help materials, especially in the field of health.

★6132★ WRITE AGE
c/o McCormick & Schilling
N82 W15855 Valley View Dr.
Menomonee Falls, WI 53051   Phone: (414) 251-3615
Description: Publishes writing therapy books primarily for teachers of gerontology/writing, physically impaired people, and activity directors.

★6133★ WWIC INTERNATIONAL PUBLISHING COMPANY
PO Box 2615
Littleton, CO 80161   Phone: (303) 798-5128
Description: Publishes a biographical reference source on doctors of chiropractic both past and present.

★6134★ YALE UNIVERSITY YALE UNIVERSITY PRESS
92A Yale Sta.
New Haven, CT 06520   Phone: (203) 432-0960
Description: Publishes reference works on medicine.

★6135★ YOGA TOOLS, INC.
PO Box 3286
New Haven, CT 06515   Phone: (203) 387-2028
Description: Publishes on yoga and health.

★6136★ ZAHRA PUBLICATIONS
PO Box 730
Blanco, TX 78606   Phone: (512) 833-5334
Description: Publishes on religion and health sciences.

★6137★ ZEITLIN & VER BRUGGE, BOOKSELLERS
815 N. La Cienega Blvd.
Los Angeles, CA 90069   Phone: (213) 655-7581
Description: Publishes annual rare book catalogs on science, medicine, art, and California.

★6138★ ZILPHA MAIN
2701 Wilshire Blvd., No. 809
Los Angeles, CA 90057
Description: Self-publisher on travel, health, and marriage.

(7) Audiovisual Producers and Services

Chapter 7 is arranged alphabetically by organization names. Consult the User's Guide located at the front of this directory for additional information.

★6139★ AA WORLD SERVICES, INC.
PO Box 459, Grand Central Sta.
New York, NY 10163   Phone: (212) 686-1100
Description: Materials available for alcoholism education include films, slides, and videocassettes.

★6140★ ABC DISTRIBUTION COMPANY
CAPITAL CITIES/ABC VIDEO ENTERPRISES
825 7th Ave.
New York, NY 10019   Phone: (212) 887-1731
Description: Videocassettes are available, for purchase only, on a wide variety of topics, including health and safety, family and community issues, and energy and the environment. ABC also licenses programs for educational distribution.

★6141★ ACTRONICS, INC.
810 River Ave.
Pittsburgh, PA 15212   Phone: (412) 231-6200
Description: Distributes the American Heart Association's CPR and Advanced Cardiac Life Support multimedia courseware. The interactive videodisc medium trains and certifies individuals in Basic and Advanced Cardiac Life support. Toll-free number: (800) 851-3780.

★6142★ THE ACUPUNCTURE EDUCATION CENTER
DIALECTIC PUBLISHING, INC.
3805 NE 167th St.
North Miami Beach, FL 33160-3540   Phone: (305) 945-5359
Description: Videos available for purchase about the types, techniques, and concepts of acupuncture.

★6143★ ADDICTION EDUCATION SERVICES, INC.
PO Box 30380
Indianapolis, IN 46230   Phone: (317) 547-8273
Description: Produces audio and video tapes about chemical dependency. Accepts unsolicited manuscripts. Distributes for Gateway Productions, Johnson Institute, Herald House, and Reallife Productions. Reaches market through direct mail, telephone and trade sales, Human Services Institute, WRS Group, NIMCO, and CompCare Publications.

★6144★ ADDICTION RESEARCH FOUNDATION OF ONTARIO
33 Russell St.
Toronto, ON, Canada M5S 2S1   Phone: (416) 595-6059
Description: Offers films, videocassettes, and audiocassettes, for professionals and general audiences, on alcohol and other drugs.

★6145★ AGENCY FOR INSTRUCTIONAL TECHNOLOGY (AIT)
Box A
Bloomington, IN 47402   Phone: (812) 339-2203
Description: AIT videotapes are primarily directed to K-12 classrooms and focus on core curricular disciplines, including a number of topics in the areas of mental health, physical health, and safety. Videos are available for rental or purchase. Toll-free number: (800) 457-4509.

★6146★ AIDS IMPACT
PO Box 9443
Seattle, WA 98109   Phone: (206) 284-3865
Description: Produces and distributes educational audiocassette programs on HIV and AIDS for health professionals. Toll-free number: (800) 763-AIDS.

★6147★ AIDSFILMS
50 W. 34th St., Ste. 6B6
New York, NY 10001   Phone: (212) 629-6288
Description: Non-profit organization that produces and distributes AIDS educational films free of charge to community-based organizations.

★6148★ AIMS MEDIA
9710 DeSoto Ave.
Chatsworth, CA 91311-4409   Phone: (818) 773-4300
Description: Offers 16mm films and videos on health care for patient education, continuing education, and general audiences. Toll-free number: (800) 367-2467.

★6149★ ALBANY MEDICAL COLLEGE
AUDIOVISUAL SERVICES
Administration Bldg., Rm. 203
47 New Scotland Ave.
Albany, NY 12208   Phone: (518) 445-5487
Description: Video production services available, either on-site or in the studio; video editing and duplicating also available.

★6150★ ALBERTA EDUCATIONAL COMMUNICATIONS
CORPORATION
ACCESS NETWORK
16930 114th Ave.
Edmonton, AB, Canada T5M 3S2   Phone: (403) 451-7272
Description: Produces and distributes educational videotapes for general and professional audiences. Topics include child development, human growth and development, and medicine and health.

★6151★ ALEXANDER GRAHAM BELL ASSOCIATION FOR
THE DEAF
3417 Volta Pl., NW
Washington, DC 20007   Phone: (202) 337-5220
Description: Audiovisual programs for sale to aid families and teachers in understanding and educating hearing impaired children and adults, including oral options in education.

★6152★ ALFRED HIGGINS PRODUCTIONS, INC.
6350 Laurel Canyon Blvd., Ste. 305
North Hollywood, CA 91606-3223   Phone: (818) 762-3300
Description: Films and videocassettes produced and distributed for public education with a primary focus on AIDS, sexually transmitted diseases, and sex education.

★6153★ ALLERGAN, INC.
Corporate and Professional Communications
2525 Dupont Dr.
PO Box 19534
Irvine, CA 92713-9534   Phone: (714) 752-4500
Description: Educational materials are distributed free of charge in the fields of optometry and ophthalmology.

★6154★ ALPHA OMEGA ALPHA HONOR MEDICAL SOCIETY
525 Middlefield Rd., Ste. 130
Menlo Park, CA 94025   Phone: (415) 329-0291
Description: Sponsors a videotape series, "Leaders in American Medicine".

★6155★ THE ALTSCHUL GROUP, INC.
1560 Sherman Ave.
Evanston, IL 60201   Phone: (708) 328-6700
Description: Comprised of Visions Video, Inc., Lawren Productions, Inc., Medical Electronic Educational Services, Inc., Perennial Education, Inc., Professional Research, Inc., Spectrum Films, Inc., and Teaching Films, Inc.. Altschul distributes educational and training programs on a wide variety of medical and health topics for professional and general audiences. Programs are available in 1/2 and 3/4 inch vidoecassette formats for preview, purchase, or rental. Toll-free number: (800) 421-2363.

★6156★ AMBROSE VIDEO PUBLISHING, INC.
1290 6th Ave., No. 2245
New York, NY 10104-0101   Phone: (212) 696-4545
Description: Distributes films and videotapes for general audiences, including a variety of subjects relating to health and medicine.

★6157★ AMERICAN ACADEMY OF CHILD AND ADOLESCENT PSYCHIATRY
3615 Wisconsin Ave., NW
Washington, DC 20016   Phone: (202) 966-7300
Description: Offers a series of videotapes on various topics in child and adolescent psychiatry; available for sale to Academy members, medical and mental health professionals, and the general public.

★6158★ AMERICAN ACADEMY OF DERMATOLOGY
930 N. Meacham
PO Box 4014
Schaumburg, IL 60173-4014   Phone: (708) 330-0230
Description: Produces dermatological slides, audiocassettes, and videocassettes for health professionals and public education.

★6159★ AMERICAN ACADEMY OF FACIAL PLASTIC AND RECONSTRUCTIVE SURGERY
1110 Vermont Ave., NW, Ste. 220
Washington, DC 20005   Phone: (202) 842-4500
Description: Develops and distributes videotapes and publications for rental and sale on various topics relating to facial plastic and reconstructive surgery.

★6160★ AMERICAN ACADEMY OF FAMILY PHYSICIANS
8880 Ward Pkwy.
Kansas City, MO 64114   Phone: (816) 333-9700
Description: Reviews and accredits audiovisuals for continuing medical education; also produces and distributes programs relating to family practice.

★6161★ AMERICAN ACADEMY OF HUSBAND-COACHED CHILDBIRTH
Box 5224
Sherman Oaks, CA 91413-5224   Phone: (818) 788-6662
Description: Offers videos on the Bradley method of husband-coached childbirth; available for purchase only. Toll-free number: (800) 42-BIRTH.

★6162★ AMERICAN ACADEMY OF OPHTHALMOLOGY
655 Beach St.
PO Box 7424
San Francisco, CA 94120-7424   Phone: (415) 561-8500
Description: Offers slide/script programs for use by ophthalmologists in presentations and lectures to groups of physicians and allied health care providers and videotapes for continuing education in ophthalmology.

★6163★ AMERICAN ACADEMY OF ORTHOPAEDIC SURGEONS
222 S. Prospect Ave.
Park Ridge, IL 60068   Phone: (708) 823-7186
Description: Produces professional and patient education programs in several formats. Distribution sources are listed in the Academy's catalog.

★6164★ AMERICAN ACADEMY OF OTOLARYNGOLOGY— HEAD AND NECK SURGERY FOUNDATION
1 Prince St.
Alexandria, VA 22314   Phone: (703) 836-4444
Description: Through the Academy's Continuing Education with Television programs, residents and practitioners can purchase videotapes containing presentations on new ideas, clinical information, and surgical techniques in otolaryngology-head and neck surgery. A slide lecture series for use in presentations to medical students, civic organizations, and non-otolaryngologists in general is also available for sale. The Academy also offers patient education videos, a quarterly patient newsletter, and a patient education leaflet series of over thirty titles.

★6165★ AMERICAN ASSOCIATION OF BLOOD BANKS
1117 N. 19th St., Ste. 600
Arlington, VA 22209   Phone: (703) 528-8200
Description: Produces slides, audio- and videotapes on topics in transfusion medicine.

★6166★ AMERICAN ASSOCIATION FOR COUNSELING AND DEVELOPMENT
5999 Stevenson Ave.
Alexandria, VA 22304   Phone: (703) 823-9800
Description: Offers videotapes and films on a broad range of topics in counseling and human development.

★6167★ AMERICAN ASSOCIATION OF ORAL AND MAXILLOFACIAL SURGEONS
9700 W. Bryn Mawr
Rosemont, IL 60018   Phone: (708) 678-6200
Description: Audiocassettes and videocassettes are available for sale.

★6168★ AMERICAN ASSOCIATION OF ORTHODONTISTS
401 N. Lindbergh Blvd.
St. Louis, MO 63141   Phone: (314) 993-1700
Description: Continuing education programs are available for rental in videotape format.

★6169★ AMERICAN ASSOCIATION FOR RESPIRATORY CARE
11030 Ables Ln.
Dallas, TX 75229   Phone: (214) 243-2272
Description: Provides a videotape series covering a wide range of subjects for those in the respiratory care field. Available on 3/4 inch, Beta, or VHS; for sale only.

★6170★ AMERICAN BAR ASSOCIATION DIVISION FOR PROFESSIONAL EDUCATION
750 N. Lake Shore Dr.
Chicago, IL 60611   Phone: (312) 988-6191
Description: Offers an ABA VideoLaw Seminar series on medical malpractice litigation designed for attorneys, risk managers, and health professionals; available for rent or purchase in 3/4 inch U-matic and 1/2 inch VHS and Beta formats. Toll-free number: (800) 621-8986.

★6171★ AMERICAN CANCER SOCIETY
1599 Clifton Rd., NE
Atlanta, GA 30329   Phone: (404) 320-3333
Description: Professional education films are available for free short term loans or leases to medical, nursing and dental educators. State chapters distribute the cancer programs.

★6172★ AMERICAN CHEMICAL SOCIETY
1155 16th St., NW
Washington, DC 20036   Phone: (202) 872-4600
Description: Professional development courses for scientists available for sale on either audiocassette or videocassette format. Topics include laboratory techniques, industrial marketing and management, and biochemistry, medicine, and polymer science.

★6173★ AMERICAN COLLEGE OF ALLERGY AND
IMMUNOLOGY
800 E. Northwest Hwy., Ste. 1080
Palatine, IL 60067   Phone: (708) 359-2800
Description: Records proceedings of the College's scientific meetings and postgraduate courses for distribution on audiocassettes.

★6174★ AMERICAN COLLEGE OF CARDIOLOGY
Heart House
9111 Old Georgetown Rd.
Bethesda, MD 20814-1699   Phone: (301) 897-5400
Description: Offers, for sale, a 12-tape videocassette series covering echocardiography and a monthly audiocassette subscription program covering cardiology.

★6175★ AMERICAN COLLEGE OF CHEST PHYSICIANS
3300 Dundee Rd.
Northbrook, IL 60062-2303   Phone: (708) 498-1400
Description: Professional education audiovisuals in cardiology and pulmonary medicine are available for purchase.

★6176★ AMERICAN COLLEGE OF HEALTHCARE
EXECUTIVES
840 N. Lake Shore Dr., Ste. 1103-W
Chicago, IL 60611   Phone: (312) 943-0544
Description: Distributes videocassettes on issues in healthcare management.

★6177★ AMERICAN COLLEGE OF OBSTETRICIANS AND
GYNECOLOGISTS
409 12th St., SW
Washington, DC 20024   Phone: (202) 638-5577
Description: Offers professional education videocassettes, audiocassettes, and slide/tape programs for purchase. Home exercise programs are available for patient education on video and audiocassette, or record album.

★6178★ AMERICAN COLLEGE OF PHYSICIANS
Independence Mall, W.
6th St. at Race
Philadelphia, PA 19106   Phone: (215) 351-2400
Description: Offers videotapes and slide shows on radiology for public and professional audiences.

★6179★ AMERICAN COLLEGE OF RADIOLOGY
1891 Preston White Dr.
Reston, VA 22091   Phone: (703) 648-8900
Description: Film productions in radiology are available from the American Medical Association Film Library, c/o Association Films, LaGrange, IL.

★6180★ AMERICAN COLLEGE OF SURGEONS
55 Erie St.
Chicago, IL 60611   Phone: (312) 664-4050
Description: Produces surgical motion pictures and audiocassettes.

★6181★ AMERICAN CYANAMID COMPANY
DAVIS AND GECK FILM LIBRARY
1 Casper St.
Danbury, CT 06810   Phone: (203) 796-9539
Description: Surgical motion pictures available for rental include the collections of Davis and Geck, American College of Surgeons, American College of Obstetricians and Gynecologists, and Association of Operating Room Nurses.

★6182★ AMERICAN DENTAL ASSOCIATION
DIVISION OF COMMUNICATIONS
211 E. Chicago Ave.
Chicago, IL 60611   Phone: (312) 440-2805
Description: Produces films, videocassettes, and slides for professionals and the general public; available for sale or rental. For purchase call (312) 440-2808.

★6183★ AMERICAN DIABETES ASSOCIATION
1970 Chain Bridge Rd.
McLean, VA 22109-0592   Phone: (703) 549-1500
Description: Offers informational videos and slides about diabetes for health care professionals, patients and the public. Toll-free number: (800) ADA-DISC, ext. 363.

★6184★ AMERICAN DIETETIC ASSOCIATION
216 W. Jackson Blvd., Ste. 800
Chicago, IL 60606   Phone: (312) 899-0040
Description: Produces audiocassettes for dieticians to earn continuing education credit; available to members and nonmembers.

★6185★ AMERICAN EDWARDS LABORATORIES
17221 Red Hill
Irvine, CA 92714   Phone: (714) 250-2500
Description: Distributes films, videotapes, and slide educational programs relating to hemodynamic monitoring.

★6186★ AMERICAN HEART ASSOCIATION
7272 Greenville Ave.
Dallas, TX 75231-4596   Phone: (214) 706-1486
Description: Produces films and videotapes for professional and public education relating to cardiovascular disease. Requests by groups, clubs, and individuals not affiliated with the American Heart Association should be made through local AHA's.

★6187★ AMERICAN HOSPITAL ASSOCIATION
840 N. Lake Shore Dr.
Chicago, IL 60611   Phone: (312) 280-6000
Description: Educational videocassettes and audiotapes are available for sale. Topics include administration, planning, and financing of health care facilities, as well as delivery of health care services. Toll-free number: (800) 242-2626.

★6188★ AMERICAN HUMANIST ASSOCIATION
7 Harwood Dr.
PO Box 146
Amherst, NY 14226   Phone: (716) 839-5080
Description: Produces and distributes videocassettes on ethics and morals in today's society, including the ethics of medicine and psychiatry. Available for rental or sale. Preview tapes available on request.

★6189★ AMERICAN INSTITUTE OF BIOLOGICAL SCIENCES
730 11th St., NW
Washington, DC 20001-4521   Phone: (202) 628-1500
Description: Offers Biotech series of self-instructional slide/tape and filmstrip productions on animal handling and allied health skills, such as specimen and culture preparation.

★6190★ AMERICAN INSTITUTE OF ULTRASOUND IN
MEDICINE
11200 Rockville Pike, No. 205
Rockville, MD 20852-3139   Phone: (301) 881-AIUM
Description: Videotape programs in diagnostic ultrasound are available for lease or purchase.

★6191★ AMERICAN JOURNAL OF NURSING COMPANY
EDUCATIONAL SERVICES DIVISION
555 W. 57th St.
New York, NY 10019   Phone: (212) 582-8820
Description: Nursing education videotapes, films, slide/tape programs, computer-related media, and interactive videos are available for rental or sale. Toll-free number: (800) 223-2282.

★6192★ AMERICAN LUNG ASSOCIATION
1740 Broadway
New York, NY 10019   Phone: (212) 315-8000
Description: Distributes audio and videotapes, films, leaflets, and slide programs which provide physicians, educators, patients, and students with reviews of current concepts in pulmonary medicine.

★6193★ AMERICAN MEDIA, INC.
1454 30th St.
West Des Moines, IA 50265-1390   Phone: (515) 224-0919
Description: Produces and distributes training films and videos for the health care field. Available for preview, rental, or lease/purchase in 16mm, videocassette, or B eta. Toll-free number: (800) 262-2557.

★6194★ AMERICAN OCCUPATIONAL THERAPY ASSOCIATION
PO Box 1725
Rockville, MD 20849-1725   Phone: (301) 948-9626
Description: Distributes, for rental or sale, 16mm films and videocassettes for occupational therapists.

★6195★ AMERICAN OPTOMETRIC ASSOCIATION
243 N. Lindbergh Blvd.
St. Louis, MO 63141   Phone: (314) 991-4100
Description: Produces films, videotapes, and slide shows on vision and eye care for public and professional audiences. Available for loan or purchase.

★6196★ AMERICAN PHYSICAL THERAPY ASSOCIATION
1111 N. Fairfax St.
Alexandria, VA 22314   Phone: (703) 684-2782
Description: Offers, for sale or rental, films, slide/tapes, and videotapes on topics relating to physical therapy.

★6197★ AMERICAN PODIATRIC MEDICAL ASSOCIATION AUDIOVISUAL SECTION
9312 Old Georgetown Rd.
Bethesda, MD 20814   Phone: (301) 571-9200
Description: Distributes films, filmstrips, slides, and tape recordings for professional education.

★6198★ AMERICAN PSYCHIATRIC ASSOCIATION HOSPITAL AND COMMUNITY PSYCHIATRY SERVICE
1400 K St., NW
Washington, DC 20005   Phone: (202) 682-6173
Description: Films and videotapes are available for rental to psychiatric and mental health professionals. Materials are suitable for professional education, development, and community education.

★6199★ AMERICAN PSYCHOLOGICAL ASSOCIATION CONTINUING EDUCATION PROGRAM
750 1st St., NE
Washington, DC 20002-4242   Phone: (202) 336-5500
Description: Offers recordings of lectures and symposia given by leading psychologists at the annual convention of the American Psychological Association. Covers a broad range of subjects.

★6200★ AMERICAN RED CROSS FRANK STANTON PRODUCTION CENTER
5816 Seminary Rd.
Falls Church, VA 22041   Phone: (703) 379-8160
Description: Produces films, videocassettes, filmstrips, and slide/tape programs. Topics for general and professional audiences include various aspects of Red Cross blo od services, youth services, nursing and health services, disaster services, safety services, and services to the armed forces and veterans.

★6201★ AMERICAN SOCIETY OF CLINICAL PATHOLOGISTS
2100 W. Harrison
Chicago, IL 60612   Phone: (312) 738-1336
Description: Produces and distributes slides, videos and audiocassettes in pathology. Materials are designed for continuing education and approved for credit by the AMA.

★6202★ AMERICAN SOCIETY FOR CONTEMPORARY OPHTHALMOLOGY
233 E. Erie St.
Chicago, IL 60611   Phone: (312) 951-1400
Description: Distributes videocassettes to physicians; programs meet AMA credit standards.

★6203★ AMERICAN SOCIETY OF DENTISTRY FOR CHILDREN
211 E. Chicago Ave., Ste. 1430
Chicago, IL 60611   Phone: (312) 943-1244
Description: Produces, for purchase, slide/tape programs on prenatal and early infant tooth development and care, nursing caries syndrome, and the responsibility of the dental office to recognize and report child abuse.

★6204★ AMERICAN SOCIETY OF HOSPITAL PHARMACISTS
4630 Montgomery Ave.
Bethesda, MD 20814   Phone: (301) 657-3000
Description: Videotape programs available from the Society are designed for pharmacists, hospital personnel, and patient education.

★6205★ AMERICAN SOCIETY FOR MICROBIOLOGY
1325 Massachusetts Ave., NW
Washington, DC 20005   Phone: (202) 737-3600
Description: Produces professional and student education audiocassettes on microbiology, and career information in microbiology.

★6206★ AMERICAN SOCIETY OF PLASTIC AND RECONSTRUCTIVE SURGEONS PLASTIC SURGERY EDUCATIONAL FOUNDATION
444 E. Algonquin Rd.
Arlington Heights, IL 60005   Phone: (708) 228-9900
Description: Produces videotape programs and sound slides on plastic surgery education for members.

★6207★ AMERICAN SOCIETY OF POST ANESTHESIA NURSES
11512 Allecingie Pkwy.
Richmond, VA 23235   Phone: (804) 379-5516
Description: Offers audio and videocassettes on various health and medical topics relati ng to post anesthesia nursing. For sale in 3/4 inch, VHS, or Beta to members or non-members of the Society.

★6208★ AMERICAN SOCIETY OF RADIOLOGIC TECHNOLOGISTS EDUCATIONAL FOUNDATION
15000 Central Ave., SE
Albuquerque, NM 87123   Phone: (505) 298-4500
Description: Produces and distributes videotapes, radiographs, and audio-cassettes for education in radiology.

★6209★ AMERICAN SOCIETY FOR SURGERY OF THE HAND VIDEOTAPE LIBRARY
3025 S. Parker Rd., Ste. 65
Aurora, CO 80014-2911   Phone: (303) 755-4588
Description: Continuing medical education videotapes are available for purchase from Medical Audio Video Transcripts, Inc., 4465 Washington St., Denver, CO 80216, (303) 292-2739. Toll-free number (800) 373-2952.

★6210★ AMS DISTRIBUTORS, INC.
PO Box 457
Roswell, GA 30077   Phone: (800) 424-3464
Description: Offers video training programs about on-the-job safety; available for preview and purchase.

★6211★ APM-STERNGOLD
23 Frank Mossberg Dr.
PO Box 839A
Attleboro, MA 02703   Phone: (508) 226-5660
Description: Offers, for rental or sale, a variety of slides and videotapes relating to dentistry. Toll-free number: (800) 243-9942.

★6212★ APOGEE COMMUNICATIONS GROUP
159 Alpine Way
Boulder, CO 80304   Phone: (303) 443-8473
Description: Produces and sells videotapes on osteoporosis, breast self-examination, and mammography.

★6213★ APPALSHOP FILMS
306 Madison St.
Whitesburg, KY 41858   Phone: (606) 633-0108
Description: Produces and distributes educational films and videos on the history, culture, and social issues of Appalachia and rural America, including topics relating to health care. Available for rental or sale.

★6214★ APPLE TREE PRODUCTIONS
5200 N. Sawyer Ave.
Boise, ID 83714-1491   Phone: (208) 322-6155
Description: Production and post-production facilities provide professional firms with a complete range of video services, including marketing and training tapes, corporate communications, film to tape transfers, and tape duplication. Clients include those in the medical field. Toll-free number: (800) 321-6155.

★6215★ APPLETON DAVIES, INC.
32 S. Raymond Ave., Ste. 4
Pasadena, CA 91105-1935   Phone: (818) 792-3046
Description: Provides instructional videos for professionals in the medical field about cardiovascular and abdominal procedures.

★6216★ APPLETON & LANGE
25 Van Zant St.
PO Box 5630
Norwalk, CT 06855   Phone: (203) 838-4400
Description: Distributes media programs on a wide range of health topics. Formats include filmstrips, audiocassettes, videocassettes, and slides. Preview kits are available. Toll-free number: (800) 423-1359.

★6217★ ARC AUDIO-VIDEO INC.
250 W. 57th St., Ste. 1527
New York, NY 10107   Phone: (212) 956-6235
Description: Produces and distributes audiocassettes featuring various topics relating to holistic health and spiritual healing; available for purchase.

★6218★ ARTHRITIS FOUNDATION
1314 Spring St., NW
Atlanta, GA 30309   Phone: (404) 872-7100
Description: Produces slide programs for health professionals on rheumatism and arthritis.

★6219★ ARTHUR MOKIN PRODUCTIONS, INC.
PO Box 1866
Santa Rosa, CA 95402   Phone: (707) 542-4868
Description: Produces and distributes films and videotapes on a wide variety of subjects, including psychology and aging. Available for rental or purchase.

★6220★ ASSOCIATION OF AMERICAN MEDICAL COLLEGES
2450 N St., NW
Washington, DC 20037-1129   Phone: (202) 828-0416
Description: Videos for high school and college students about attending medical school, topics also include applying to medical school and preparing for the MCAT.

★6221★ ASSOCIATION FOR THE CARE OF CHILDREN'S
    HEALTH
7910 Woodmont Ave., Ste. 300
Bethesda, MD 20814-3015   Phone: (301) 654-6549
Description: Produces and distributes videotapes focusing on children with special health needs; designed for use by families and medical professionals. Topics include Pediatric AIDS and caring for children with disabilities. Tapes are available for preview and purchase.

★6222★ ASSOCIATION OF OPERATING ROOM NURSES
10170 E. Mississippi Ave.
Denver, CO 80231   Phone: (303) 755-6300
Description: Sponsors the production of motion pictures for nursing education.

★6223★ THE ASSOCIATION FOR PERSONS WITH SEVERE
    HANDICAPS
11201 Greenwood Ave., N.
Seattle, WA 98133   Phone: (206) 361-8870
Description: Produces video and audio cassettes pertaining to individuals with severe cognitive disabilities.

★6224★ ASTRA PHARMACEUTICAL PRODUCTS, INC.
50 Otis St.
Westboro, MA 01581   Phone: (508) 366-1100
Description: Medical and dental motion pictures are loaned at no charge to professional organizations and educational institutions. Recent titles available for VCR; specify 3/4 inch or 1/2 inch. For direct order call: (212) 921-0966.

★6225★ AUDIO-DIGEST FOUNDATION
1577 E. Chevy Chase Dr.
Glendale, CA 91206   Phone: (213) 245-8505
Description: Produces audiocassettes and videocassettes for continuing medical education in the following specialty areas: anesthesiology, emergency medicine, family practice, internal medicine, obstetrics and gynecology, ophthalmology, otolaryngology, pediatrics, psychiatry, surgery, orthopaedics, urology, and gastroenterology. Printed subject indexes are published annually.

★6226★ AUDIO-LEARNING, INC.
15 Terrace Rd.
Norristown, PA 19401   Phone: (215) 279-1422
Description: Offers audiocassettes and videocassettes for the continuing education of health professionals in the areas of neurophysiology and orthopedic medicine.

★6227★ AUDIOVISUAL MEDICAL MARKETING, INC.
235 Park Ave., S.
New York, NY 10003   Phone: (212) 460-9300
Description: Distributes slide/tape programs for continuing medical education. Toll-free number: (800) 221-3995.

★6228★ AVC CORPORATION
PO Box 1060
Petaluma, CA 94953   Phone: (415) 883-7701
Description: Videocassette packages for use in nursing education are available for preview, purchase, and rental. Free catalog available. Toll-free number for all states except Alaska, Hawaii, and California: (800) 227-2020.

★6229★ AVEKTA PRODUCTIONS, INC.
164 Madison Ave.
New York, NY 10016   Phone: (212) 686-4550
Description: Motion picture design and marketing firm. Products include video press releases that have been designed for pharmaceutical companies and other clients in the medical field.

★6230★ AYERST LABORATORIES
AUDIOVISUAL SERVICES
145 King of Prussia Rd.
Radnor, PA 19087   Phone: (215) 341-2041
Description: Continuing education film and video programs for health professionals are produced for free loan. Most medical specialty areas are included in the program topics.

★6231★ BANDERA ENTERPRISES, INC.
PO Box 1107
Studio City, CA 91604   Phone: (818) 985-5050
Description: Child care programs for pediatricians and general audiences are available for rental and purchase on videotape or 16mm film.

★6232★ BANJO VIDEO AND FILM PRODUCTIONS
1188 St. Andrews Rd.
Columbia, SC 29210
Description: Produces commercial, medical, forensic, and scientific educational films, filmstrips, slides, and art. Also offers slide duplication services and maintains an extensive stock of medical and scientific transparencies, prints, and motion pictures.

★6233★ BARR FILMS
12801 Schabarum
PO Box 7878
Irwindale, CA 91706-7808   Phone: (818) 338-7878
Description: Distributes educational and motivational films for general audiences. Includes a variety of topics, such as chemical dependency, mental health, safety, sexuality, physical and emotional abuse, maternal and child health, and staff training. Toll-free number: (800) 234-7878.

★6234★ BAUSCH & LOMB
SOFLENS DIVISION
Optics Center
1400 N. Goodman St.
PO Box 450
Rochester, NY 14617-0450   Phone: (716) 338-6000
Description: Loans, free of charge, films and slide shows for use as speaker's aids by eye care professionals.

★6235★ BAXTER HEALTHCARE CORPORATION
RENAL DIVISION
1425 Lake Cook Rd.
Deerfield, IL 60015   Phone: (708) 940-6385
Description: Provides a wide selection of educational materials on the various aspects of peritoneal and hemodialysis.

★6236★ BAYLOR COLLEGE OF MEDICINE
LEARNING RESOURCES CENTER
1 Baylor Plaza, Rm. M202
Houston, TX 77030   Phone: (713) 798-4746
Description: Motion pictures produced by the College are available for rental. Topics include surgery and the cardiovascular system.

★6237★ BENCHMARK FILMS, INC.
145 Scarborough Rd.
Briarcliff Manor, NY 10510   Phone: (914) 762-3838
Description: Sells and rents films and videocassettes for schools, colleges, and public libraries. Subjects include biology, mental health, dying, and nutrition.

★6238★ BENHAVEN
85 Willow St.
New Haven, CT 06511   Phone: (203) 782-1307
Description: Offers a training videotape series designed to assist professionals working in the field of autism and neurological impairment. Entire series or individual tapes are available for rental or purchase.

★6239★ BETHESDA LUTHERAN HOME
700 Hoffmann Dr.
Watertown, WI 53094   Phone: (414) 261-3050
Description: Distributes films, videos, and audiocassettes to help people understand mental retardation and issues of concern to retarded persons. Available for rental or sale. Toll-free number: (800) 369-4636.

★6240★ BILLY BUDD FILMS, INC.
235 E. 57th St.
New York, NY 10022   Phone: (212) 755-3968
Description: Offers, for rental or sale, a variety of films and videos in many fields of healthcare and medicine. Material is suitable for groups, organizations, hospitals, corporations, schools, and individuals.

★6241★ BIOFEEDBACK REVIEW SEMINARS
PO Box 38474
Los Angeles, CA 90038   Phone: (213) 851-2065
Description: Audiocassettes that serve as a review for medical professionals preparing for the national certification examination offered by the Biofeedback Certification Institute of America.

★6242★ BNA COMMUNICATIONS, INC.
9439 Key West Ave.
Rockville, MD 20850-3396   Phone: (301) 948-0540
Description: Produces and distributes training videos for professionals in management and labor relations. Topics include drug testing, emergency procedures, accident prevention, and safety in the workplace. Available for purchase. Toll-free number: (800) 233-6067.

★6243★ BOSTON FAMILY INSTITUTE
580 Dedham St.
Newton, MA 02159-2943   Phone: (617) 244-1589
Description: Distributes videotapes for mental health training programs and family therapy.

★6244★ BOSTON UNIVERSITY
SARGENT COLLEGE OF ALLIED HEALTH PROFESSIONS
CENTER FOR PSYCHIATRIC REHABILITATION
730 Commonwealth Ave.
Boston, MA 02215   Phone: (617) 353-3550
Description: Produces and distributes a variety of video and audio cassettes related to the field of psychology and psychiatry; available for preview and purchase.

★6245★ BOSTON UNIVERSITY
SARGENT COLLEGE OF ALLIED HEALTH PROFESSIONS
GEORGE K. MAKECHNIE INSTRUCTIONAL RESOURCE
  CENTER
635 Commonwealth Ave.
Boston, MA 02215   Phone: (617) 353-7474
Description: Offers videos that discuss the rehabilitation and therapy used with a number of health disorders or diseases; available for rental or purchase.

★6246★ BRIGHAM YOUNG UNIVERSITY
AUDIOVISUAL SERVICES
101 FB
Provo, UT 84602   Phone: (801) 378-3456
Description: Videotapes for physicians, nurses, and laboratory technicians are produced and are available for rental.

★6247★ BRITANNICA FILMS
Britannica Centre
310 S. Michigan Ave.
Chicago, IL 60604   Phone: (312) 347-7400
Description: Offers 1/2 and 3/4 inch videotapes on a variety of health education topics; available for purchase. Toll-free number: (800) 554-9862.

★6248★ BRUNNER/MAZEL, INC.
19 Union Sq., W.
New York, NY 10003   Phone: (800) 825-3089
Description: Videotapes focusing on marital therapy, spouse abuse and stress management are available for purchase.

★6249★ BUREAU OF BUSINESS PRACTICE
24 Rope Ferry Rd.
Waterford, CT 06386   Phone: (800) 243-0876
Description: Film and videotape training programs covering a wide variety of subjects, including safety and health, substance abuse, and medical emergencies are available for rental or sale.

★6250★ BURROUGHS WELLCOME COMPANY
3030 Cornwallis Rd.
Research Triangle Park, NC 27709   Phone: (919) 248-4904
Description: Depending on availability, loans, slide/tape programs and videocassettes for continuing medical, pharmacy, and nursing education free of charge.

★6251★ CALIFORNIA BIOMEDICAL RESEARCH
  ASSOCIATION
48 Shattuck Sq.
Box 114
Berkeley, CA 94704   Phone: (415) 644-0829
Description: Produces and distributes a videotape featuring the use of animals in biomedical research. Available for purchase.

★6252★ CALLY CURTIS COMPANY
1111 N. Las Palmas Ave.
Hollywood, CA 90038   Phone: (213) 467-1101
Description: Produces and distributes videotapes covering AIDS, drugs, and other safety and health issues in the workplace. Available for preview, purchase or rental. Toll-free number: (800) 522-2559.

★6253★ CAMBRIDGE CAREER PRODUCTS
Dept. CC6
PO Box 2153
Charleston, WV 25328-2153   Phone: (304) 744-9323
Description: Educational and motivational videocassettes and filmstrips, on a variety of subjects, including teen suicide, sex education, substance abuse, AIDS, and nutrition are available for purchase. Designed for a high school audience. Toll-free number: (800) 468-4227.

★6254★ CAMBRIDGE DOCUMENTARY FILMS, INC.
PO Box 385
Cambridge, MA 02139   Phone: (617) 354-3677
Description: Distributes films and videocassettes on a variety of social issues, including those relating to medicine, health, and reproductive health.

★6255★ CAMBRIDGE HOME ECONOMICS
PO Box 2153, Dept. HE4
Charleston, WV 25328-2153   Phone: (304) 744-9323
Description: Offers educational videocassettes and filmstrips for purchase. Topics include: drug and alcohol education, sex education, pregnancy, newborn and child care, health education, first aid, and nutrition. Toll-free number: (800) 468-4227.

★6256★ CAMBRIDGE PHYSICAL EDUCATION AND HEALTH
90 MacCorkle Ave., SW
So. Charleston, WV 25303   Phone: (304) 744-9323
Description: Distributes videocassettes and filmstrips on a variety of sports-related topics, including injury care and prevention, nutrition, first aid, substance abuse education, sex education, exercise, and physical fitness. Available for purchase. Toll-free number: (800) 468-4227.

★6257★ CAMPUS FILM AND VIDEO DISTRIBUTORS CORPORATION
24 Depot Sq.
Tuckahoe, NY 10707   Phone: (914) 961-1900
Description: Films on mental health, rehabilitation, patient education, and professional health care are available for rental or purchase. Formats include videotape, 16mm, super 8mm films, and 8mm video equipment.

★6258★ CANADIAN REHABILITATION COUNCIL FOR THE DISABLED
45 Sheppard Ave., E., Ste. 801
Willowdale, ON, Canada M2N 5W9   Phone: (416) 250-7490
Description: Produces videos covering various aspects of physical disabilities.

★6259★ CARE VIDEO PRODUCTIONS
1650 Crossings Pkwy.
Westlake, OH 44145   Phone: (216) 835-5872
Description: Services include production, duplication, and distribution of medical education programs.

★6260★ CAREER AIDS
941 Hickory Ln.
Mansfield, OH 44905   Phone: (419) 589-1700
Description: Audiocassettes, 35mm filmstrips, computer software, and videocassettes focusing on patient care and allied health training are available for sale and preview.

★6261★ CAREER PUBLISHING, INC.
910 N. Main St.
PO Box 5486
Orange, CA 92613   Phone: (714) 771-5155
Description: Distributes a cassette/transcript program to assist in the development of listening skills of those who transcribe dictation from physicians and paraprofessionals who speak with foreign accents.

★6262★ CARLE MEDIA
611 W. Park
Urbana, IL 61801   Phone: (217) 384-4838
Description: Produces and distributes films and videos covering many areas of healthcare, including treatment, legal, ethical, and psychosocial aspects. Available, for rental or purchase, to professionals and the general public.

★6263★ CARLOCKE/LANGDEN, INC.
4122 Main St.
Dallas, TX 75226   Phone: (214) 826-9380
Description: Videos for health care professionals on the topic of patient and care giver relations; available for preview and purchase.

★6264★ CAROLINA BIOLOGICAL SUPPLY COMPANY
2700 York Rd.
Burlington, NC 27215   Phone: (919) 584-0381
Description: Distributes anatomical models and skeletons.

★6265★ CAROUSEL FILM AND VIDEO
260 5th Ave.
New York, NY 10001   Phone: (212) 683-1660
Description: Offers films and videos on a wide variety of subjects, including health and medicine, the handicapped, aging, mental health, nursing, and psychology. Materials are available for preview with purchase consideration, or rental from various libraries.

★6266★ CASE WESTERN RESERVE UNIVERSITY SCHOOL OF MEDICINE INSTRUCTION AND RESEARCH INFORMATION SERVICES
10900 Euclid Ave.
Cleveland, OH 44106   Phone: (216) 368-2000
Description: Produces films and videocassettes for medical and nursing education in obstetrics and pediatrics.

★6267★ CATHOLIC HEALTH ASSOCIATION OF THE UNITED STATES
4455 Woodson Rd.
St. Louis, MO 63134   Phone: (314) 427-2500
Description: Produces and distributes, for rental or sale, videos on topics relating to health care and Catholic health care issues.

★6268★ CAVALCADE PRODUCTIONS, INC.
7360 Potter Valley Rd.
Ukiah, CA 95482   Phone: (707) 743-1168
Description: Provides a full range of production services to a variety of clients and offers, for sale, a videotape on back care and professional training videos on ritual child abuse and multiple personality disorders.

★6269★ CENTER FOR INTERDISCIPLINARY STUDIES
1115 Grant St.
Denver, CO 80203   Phone: (303) 837-1700
Description: Offers videotape educational program which presents an interdisciplinary model for understanding various substance abuse issues from the perspectives of medicine, psychiatry, biochemistry, psychology, society, and law enforcement. Available for purchase.

★6270★ CENTER FOR MARITAL AND SEXUAL STUDIES
5251 E. Los Altos Plaza
Long Beach, CA 90815   Phone: (310) 597-4425
Description: Distributes audiovisual materials to health professionals for use in treatm ent of sexual dysfunction. Orders may be placed through Focus International (see separate entry).

★6271★ CENTRAL HOSPITAL SERVICES, INC.
1226 Huron Rd., Playhouse Sq.
Cleveland, OH 44115   Phone: (216) 696-6900
Description: Offers a videotape-conveyed education service, the Health Education Television Network (HETN), to hospitals and other health care organizations. HETN consists of two parts, including the Staff Education Videotape Library and the Patient Education Videotape Package. The Staff Education Videotape Library contains over 1500 video programs of interest to physicians, nurses, therapists, technicians, dieticians, and most other members of the hospital staff. The individual programs deal with surgery, drug therapy, safety, nutrition, management, and numerous other medically-relevant subjects. The Patient Education Videotape Package is composed of ten hours of updated video program material dealing with

general health concerns, such as diabetes. These patient programs are transmitted to patient rooms within the hospital via closed-circuit television. Each part of the service involves an annual subscription fee based on the hospital's bed size and other factors.

★6272★ CENTRE COMMUNICATIONS
1800 30th St., No. 207
Boulder, CO 80301   Phone: (303) 444-1166
Description: Produces and distributes 16mm films and videos on a variety of subjects, including health and medicine.

★6273★ CENTRE FILMS, INC.
1103 N. El Centro Ave.
Hollywood, CA 90038   Phone: (213) 466-5123
Description: Distributes films and videocassettes on prepared childbirth and offers videotape production services.

★6274★ CENTRON PRODUCTIONS
708 9th St.
PO Box 687
Lawrence, KS 66044   Phone: (913) 843-0400
Description: Producers of custom videos for a variety of clients, including the health care field.

★6275★ CHANNEL ONE VIDEO TAPE, INC.
3341 NW 82nd Ave.
Miami, FL 33122   Phone: (305) 592-1764
Description: Producer of videos for television commercials and programs, sporting events, and education programs, including medical training tapes for doctors and informational programs for health professionals and patients.

★6276★ CHILDREN'S NATIONAL MEDICAL CENTER
DESIGN CENTRAL
111 Michigan Ave., NW
Washington, DC 20010   Phone: (202) 745-5065
Description: Distributes slides, films and videocassettes relating to the needs of hospitalized children and their families; available for rental or purchase.

★6277★ CHURCHILL MEDIA
12210 Nebraska Ave.
Los Angeles, CA 90025-3600   Phone: (310) 207-6600
Description: Produces and distributes general audience and staff development films, videos and laser videodiscs on topics including substance abuse, patient education, parenting, childbirth, first aid, nutrition, mental health education, death and dying, AIDS, eating disorders, cancer, and CPR.

★6278★ CINCINNATI CENTER FOR DEVELOPMENTAL
DISORDERS
MEDIA DEVELOPMENT
3300 Elland Ave.
Cincinnati, OH 45229   Phone: (513) 559-4688
Description: Videocassettes relating to the developmentally disabled are available for purchase or rental.

★6279★ THE CINEMA GUILD
1697 Broadway
New York, NY 10019   Phone: (212) 246-5522
Description: Producer and distributor of films and videos covering a wide range of subjects, including health, substance abuse, nutrition, and mental health. Material available for rental or sale.

★6280★ CINEMA MEDICA, INC.
6652 N. Western Ave.
Chicago, IL 60645   Phone: (312) 973-2297
Description: 16mm films and videocassettes on childbirth are available for rental and sale. Programs are for professional and patient audiences.

★6281★ CNS PRODUCTIONS
130 3rd St.
PO Box 96
Ashland, OR 97520-1962   Phone: (503) 488-2805
Description: Creates, produces, and distributes films, video, and audio programs for health care professionals and pharmaceutical representatives

on drugs of abuse for training, and also for the treatment and prevention of drug abuse.

★6282★ CODE RED PRODUCTIONS, LTD.
PO Box 317
Bright's Grove, ON, Canada N0N 1C0   Phone: (519) 339-0157
Description: Offers the Complete CPR Overhead Transparency Teaching Aid Kit for purchase. Available in the U.S. from: Code Red Corporation, PO Box 34102, Louisville, KY 40232; (502) 368-3071.

★6283★ COLORADO STATE UNIVERSITY
COLLEGE OF VETERINARY MEDICINE AND BIOMEDICAL
  SCIENCES
W102 Anatomy Bldg.
Ft. Collins, CO 80523   Phone: (303) 491-7053
Description: Videotapes and slide/sound programs in the field of veterinary science are available for rental or sale.

★6284★ COMPONENTS CORPORATION
6 Kinsey Pl.
Denville, NJ 07834   Phone: (201) 627-0290
Description: Distributes intraocular lens implantation videocassettes for rental or purchase.

★6285★ CONCEPT MEDIA
PO Box 19542
Irvine, CA 92713   Phone: (714) 660-0727
Description: Nursing education productions focus on all aspects of professional care. Programs are on videocassette. Previews available to selected institutions. Toll-free number: (800) 233-7078.

★6286★ CORNELL UNIVERSITY
AUDIO VISUAL RESOURCE CENTER
8 Research Park
Ithaca, NY 14850   Phone: (607) 255-2091
Description: Produces and distributes, for rental or sale, films, slides, videotapes, and audiotapes on a variety of health and medical subjects, including nutrition, public health, child abuse, and toxicology.

★6287★ CORONET/MTI FILM VIDEO
108 Wilmot Rd.
Deerfield, IL 60015   Phone: (708) 940-1260
Description: Distributors of general audience films, videotapes, and Disney Educational Productions; available for long-term lease and preview. Topics include health, safety, physical fitness, biological and life sciences, and family living. Toll-free number: (800) 621-2131.

★6288★ COUNCIL FOR EXCEPTIONAL CHILDREN
1920 Association Dr.
Reston, VA 22091   Phone: (703) 620-3660
Description: Offers filmstrip and audiocassette programs for the training of those who serve the educational needs of exceptional children.

★6289★ CREATIVE LEARNING ENVIRONMENTS
507 Park Blvd.
Austin, TX 78751   Phone: (512) 454-4489
Description: Produces and distributes, for rental or sale, documentary films and videos on the life and works of mentally and physically handicapped artists.

★6290★ CREATIVE PRODUCTIONS, INC.
200 Main St.
Orange, NJ 07050   Phone: (201) 676-4422
Description: Offers various audio-visual services to health care professionals and pharmaceutical organizations.

★6291★ CREIGHTON UNIVERSITY
BIO-INFORMATION CENTER
LEARNING RESOURCE CENTER
719 N. 24th St.
Omaha, NE 68178   Phone: (402) 280-5130
Description: Loans audiovisuals for health professionals. Formats include audiocassettes, films, slides, and videocassettes.

★6292★   CRM FILMS
2215 Faraday
Carlsbad, CA 92008   Phone: (800) 421-0833
Description: Training films and videocassettes are distributed for sale and rental. Topics include stress management, AIDS in the workplace, and mental health.

★6293★   CRYSTAL PRODUCTIONS
PO Box 2159
Glenview, IL 60025   Phone: (708) 657-8144
Description: Offers videotapes and 16mm films for hospital and rehabilitation center use in such areas as patient education, family service, community awareness, nurses' training, hospital staff training, and physical therapy. Subjects include spinal cord injury, rehabilitation, oncology, alcohol and drug abuse, and sight and hearing impairment. Toll-free number: (800) 255-8629.

★6294★   CYSTIC FIBROSIS FOUNDATION
6931 Arlington Rd.
Bethesda, MD 20814   Phone: (301) 951-4422
Description: Films and slides on cystic fibrosis may be borrowed without charge.

★6295★   DANA FARBER CANCER INSTITUTE
SOCIAL WORK ONCOLOGY GROUP
44 Binney St.
Boston, MA 02115   Phone: (617) 732-3301
Description: Offers, for rental or purchase, a videotape which addresses the subject of death and dying.

★6296★   DANA PRODUCTIONS
6249 Babcock Ave.
North Hollywood, CA 91606   Phone: (213) 877-9246
Description: 16mm films and videos for community health services on drug and alcohol prevention and rehabilitation are available for rental and purchase.

★6297★   DARTMOUTH-HITCHCOCK MEDICAL CENTER
CONNECTIVE TISSUE DISEASE SECTION
1 Medical Center Dr.
Lebanon, NH 03756   Phone: (603) 650-7700
Description: Produces and distributes professional and patient education slide/tape programs on arthritis. Available for purchase or rental.

★6298★   DARTMOUTH-HITCHCOCK MEDICAL CENTER
DEPARTMENT OF VISUAL COMMUNICATIONS
Medical Center Dr.
Lebanon, NH 03756   Phone: (603) 650-7041
Description: Medical Center audiovisual productions include a video program currently viewed on PBS nationally. Each show deals with a specific medical topic and stresses illness prevention.

★6299★   DARTNELL
4660 Ravenswood Ave.
Chicago, IL 60640   Phone: (312) 561-4000
Description: Offers, for rental or sale, training films for business and industry, as well as films for the healthcare profession. Toll-free number: (800) 621-5463.

★6300★   DAVID J. WITHERSTY, M.D. & ASSOCIATES
1303 Riddle Ave.
Morgantown, WV 26505   Phone: (304) 599-6968
Description: Video titled "The Patient-Physician Partnership: A Literature Review," designed for practicing physicians is available for purchase.

★6301★   DAVIDSON FILMS
231 E St.
Davis, CA 95616   Phone: (916) 753-9604
Description: Topics of films for rental and sale include infant development, psychotherapy, Down's syndrome, and learning disabilities.

★6302★   DAYTON LAB
3235 Dayton Ave.
Lorain, OH 44055   Phone: (216) 246-1397
Description: Produces slides and slide/tapes in the basic and clinical sciences.

★6303★   DCM SYSTEMS, INC.
INSTRUCTIONAL SYSTEMS DIVISION
80 Wilson Way
Westwood, MA 02090   Phone: (800) 348-0025
Description: Markets unique audiovisual teaching systems for introductory human anatomy, medical terminology, and dental terminology.

★6304★   DE NONNO PIX, INC.
7119 Shore Rd.
Brooklyn, NY 11209   Phone: (718) 745-3937
Description: Produces and distributes 16mm films and videocassettes for general audiences. Subjects include blindness and the architectural/attitudinal barriers that handicapped people face. Available for sale or rental.

★6305★   DELPHI PRODUCTIONS, LTD.
3159 6th St.
Boulder, CO 80304   Phone: (303) 443-2100
Description: Offers a complete video production service for a wide range of clients, including those in the medical field.

★6306★   DEMOSTHENES PRODUCTIONS
39572 Stevenson Pl., Ste. 225
Fremont, CA 95438   Phone: (415) 792-2077
Description: Produces and sells a videotape titled "Growing Through Time" that is aimed at learning to assess psychological, biological, and social problems in young people.

★6307★   DENTSPLY INTERNATIONAL, INC.
550 W. College Ave.
York, PA 17404   Phone: (717) 845-7511
Description: Motion pictures and slides for professional dental education are distributed for sale and rental.

★6308★   DERMATOPATHOLOGY FOUNDATION
PO Box 377
Canton, MA 02021   Phone: (617) 821-0648
Description: 35mm slide sets on gross and microscopic skin pathology and clinical dermatology are produced and distributed. The Foundation sponsors courses and seminars in the field of skin pathology.

★6309★   D4 FILM STUDIOS, INC.
PO Box 187
Needham, MA 02192   Phone: (617) 235-1119
Description: Produces 16mm films and provides complete post-production services. Has done numerous film productions in the medical field.

★6310★   DIALYRN
REGIONAL KIDNEY DISEASE PROGRAM
900 S. 8th St., Ste. 904
Minneapolis, MN 55404   Phone: (612) 347-5949
Description: Produces the Dialyrn education system, a training program for staff and patients that outlines renal disease and the principles of dialysis.

★6311★   DIDIK TV PRODUCTIONS
Box 7460
Rego Park, NY 11374   Phone: (718) 843-6839
Description: Company specializes in high technology imaging systems and production, including 3D. Services directed to the medical field, among others.

★6312★   DIRECT CINEMA LIMITED
PO Box 10003
Santa Monica, CA 90410   Phone: (800) 525-0000
Description: Distributes films and videotapes for rental or sale. Some topics include AIDS, Alzheimer's disease, the history of nursing, and mental institutions, and fitness, eating disorders, and aging.

★6313★   DOCUMENTARIES FOR LEARNING
74 Fenwood Rd.
Boston, MA 02115   Phone: (617) 566-6793
Description: Produces films and videotapes for health care professional in-service training and education. Topics include various medical, psychological, and social issues.

★6314★   DYNAMEDIA, INC.
2 Fulham Ct.
Silver Springs, MD 20902   Phone: (800) 468-4680
Description: Produces and distributes videos demonstrating echocardiography and color flow imaging in vascular and radiology applications.

**★6315★   EAST CENTRAL AIDS EDUCATION AND TRAINING
CENTER**
Department of Family Medicine
1314 Kinnear Rd., Area 300
Columbus, OH 43212-1194   Phone: (614) 292-1400
Description: Offers educational videos on various aspects of AIDS and the HIV virus.

★6316★   ECC MEDIA PLUS
150 Bergen St., Rm B105
Newark, NJ 07103   Phone: (201) 456-5343
Description: Complete audio/visual production facility for medical illustration, graphics, photography, video and writing.

★6317★   EDITORIAL ENTERPRISES CORPORATION
PO Box 1267
Gainesville, FL 32602   Phone: (904) 375-0821
Description: Offers educational slides covering a variety of medical issues, including developmental pathology, perinatal neuropathology, and pediatric lung disease. Available for purchase.

★6318★   EDUCATIONAL COMMUNICATIONS, INC.
761 5th Ave.
King of Prussia, PA 19406   Phone: (215) 337-1011
Description: Offers a full range of customized production services to the pharmaceutical and health care industries; a wide variety of formats is available.

★6319★   EDUCATIONAL GRAPHIC AIDS
2695 E. Long Lane
Littleton, CO 80121   Phone: (303) 796-0088
Description: Distributes slides, filmstrips, and videotapes for patient education in the areas of childbirth, parenting, family planning, and pregnancy. Toll-free number: (800) 227-0731.

★6320★   EDUCATIONAL IMAGES
PO Box 3456, West Side Sta.
Elmira, NY 14905   Phone: (607) 732-1090
Description: Produces and distributes educational videocassettes, slide sets, and filmstrips in the area of science, including medical and health topics. Toll-free number: (800) 527-4264.

**★6321★   EDUCATIONAL MATERIALS FOR HEALTH
PROFESSIONALS, INC.**
607 Watervliet Ave.
Dayton, OH 45420   Phone: (513) 254-0990
Description: Offers self-instructional units that include a paper pack, slides, and videos for continuing education of individuals in the health professions.

★6322★   EDUCATIONAL PRODUCTIONS
17412 SW Beaverton Hillsdale Hwy., Ste. 210
Portland, OR 97225   Phone: (503) 688-3950
Description: Offers, for rental or sale, videotapes covering various health topics of interest to professionals and the general public, including a training series for kidney patients and their families, and special needs children.

★6323★   EDUCATIONAL REVIEWS, INC.
6801 Cahaba Valley Rd.
Birmingham, AL 35242   Phone: (205) 991-5188
Description: Subscription service of audiocassette programs in 25 medical, dental, and allied health specialties. Tapes review articles selected from current specialty and clinical journals.

★6324★   EDWARD FEIL PRODUCTIONS
4614 Prospect Ave.
Cleveland, OH 44103   Phone: (216) 881-0040
Description: Gerontology, Alzheimer's disease, and laboratory safety films are available for rental and sale.

★6325★   EFFECTIVE COMMUNICATION ARTS, INC.
221 W. 57th St.
New York, NY 10019   Phone: (212) 333-5656
Description: Full-service producer of films, videotapes, and interactive videodiscs for many industries, businesses, and the medical field.

★6326★   EMERGENCY FILM GROUP
225 Water St.
Plymouth, MA 02360   Phone: (800) 842-0999
Description: Produces emergency response programs specializing in hazmat training videos; available for preview and purchase.

★6327★   EMERGENCY TRAINING
Miller Landing Bldg. 200
150 N. Miller Rd.
Akron, OH 44333   Phone: (216) 836-0600
Description: Offers emergency training teaching programs and lectures on videocassette for those in the emergency medical service field.

**★6328★   EMORY UNIVERSITY
SCHOOL OF MEDICINE
HEALTH SCIENCES CENTER LIBRARY**
1462 Clifton Rd.
Atlanta, GA 30322   Phone: (404) 727-5817
Description: Serves as rental and sale distributor for medical videotape programs produced by the Emory Medical Television Network.

★6329★   ENVISION CORPORATION
270 Congress St.
Boston, MA 02210   Phone: (617) 482-3444
Description: A full-service production company creating videos, slides, and films for varied industries and businesses, including many medical institutions.

★6330★   EPILEPSY FOUNDATION OF AMERICA
4351 Garden City Dr., Ste. 406
Landover, MD 20785   Phone: (301) 577-0100
Description: Sponsors a loan service of epilepsy films for general and professional audiences. Offers films, videos, audiocassettes, and slides on epilepsy for purchase.

★6331★   ERIC MILLER COMPANY
PO Box 443
Narberth, PA 19072   Phone: (215) 667-3360
Description: Offers, for sale, several video programs for the health care industry, including a custom-produced hospital orientation video and community cable television show.

★6332★   ETHICON, INC.
Rte. 22
Somerville, NJ 08876   Phone: (201) 218-0707
Description: Sponsors medical education films.

**★6333★   EXECUTIVE COMMUNICATIONS, INC.
AMERICAN REHABILITATION EDUCATIONAL NETWORK**
3120 William Pitt Way
Pittsburgh, PA 15238   Phone: (412) 826-3608
Description: Produces and distributes corporate videotapes concerned with allied health education. Available for purchase. Toll-free number: (800) 331-5190.

★6334★   EXTENDED-CARE VIDEO LIBRARY
PO Box 255394
Sacramento, CA 95865   Phone: (916) 722-3456
Description: Produces and distributes video-taped training programs for nurse assistants in long-term care facilities. Toll-free number: (800) 423-6124.

★6335★   F.A. DAVIS COMPANY
1915 Arch St.
Philadelphia, PA 19103   Phone: (215) 568-2270
Description: Slide/tape sets relating to emergency medicine, medical assisting/medical secretary, and medical technology are available for purchase. Toll-free number: (800) 523-4049.

★6336★ **FAIRVIEW AUDIO-VISUALS**
17909 Groveland Ave.
Cleveland, OH 44111   Phone: (216) 476-7054
Description: Nursing education, risk management, and personnel educa-
tion programs are produced. Programs in 1/2 inch VHS and 3/4 inch U-
MATIC videocassette formats are available for rental or purchase.

★6337★ **FAMILY COMMUNICATIONS, INC.**
4802 5th Ave.
Pittsburgh, PA 15213   Phone: (412) 687-2990
Description: Produces and distributes a variety of materials covering
subjects of concern to children and families, including videocassettes
which provide basic information and reassurance about hospital experiences.

★6338★ **FANLIGHT PRODUCTIONS**
47 Halifax St.
Boston, MA 02130   Phone: (617) 524-0980
Description: Offers films and videos, for rental or sale, on a variety of
health, education, work, and family-life issues, including AIDS, death and
dying, mental illness, nursing ethics, birth control, infertility, abortion,
spinal cord injuries, and eating disorders.

★6339★ **FEELING FINE PROGRAMS**
3575 Cahuenga Blvd., W., Ste. 440
Los Angeles, CA 90068   Phone: (213) 851-1027
Description: Distributes physical fitness and exercise programs on VHS
and Beta videocassettes for purchase.

★6340★ **FEMINIST MAJORITY FOUNDATION**
1600 Wilson Blvd., No. 704
Arlington, VA 22209   Phone: (703) 522-2214
Description: Media center offers videos on national abortion rights;
available to activists, educators, and researchers.

★6341★ **FILM IDEAS, INC.**
3575 Commercial Ave.
Northbrook, IL 60062   Phone: (708) 480-5760
Description: Distributes educational films and videos on such topics as
substance abuse, sexually transmitted diseases, steroid use, AIDS, life
saving techniques, and physical disabilities. Programs are available for
rental and/or sale. Toll free number: (800) 475-3456.

★6342★ **FILMAKERS LIBRARY, INC.**
124 E. 40th St., Ste. 901
New York, NY 10016   Phone: (212) 808-4980
Description: Distributes 16mm films and videos for public education
purposes. Topics include mental health, rehabilitation, child development,
and aging.

★6343★ **FILMFAIR COMMUNICATIONS**
10621 Magnolia Blvd.
North Hollywood, CA 91601   Phone: (818) 985-0244
Description: First aid and general health programs are distributed on
16mm film and videocassette. Toll free numbers: (800) 423-2461.

★6344★ **FILMS INC.**
5547 N. Ravenswood Ave.
Chicago, IL 60640   Phone: (312) 878-2600
Description: Distributor of 16mm films and videocassettes in a variety of
areas, including health and medicine. Toll-free number: (800) 323-4222.

★6345★ **FILMS FOR THE HUMANITIES AND SCIENCES, INC.**
PO Box 2053
Princeton, NJ 08543   Phone: (609) 452-1128
Description: Offers films and videos on a wide range of medical and health
topics, including the physical and biological sciences, guidance, counseling,
handicaps, sex education, and substance abuse; available for rental or sale.
Toll-free number: (800) 257-5126.

★6346★ **FIRE PREVENTION THROUGH FILMS, INC.**
PO Box 11
Newton Highlands, MA 02161   Phone: (617) 965-4444
Description: Fire prevention and safety training audiovisuals for health
care facility p ersonnel, emergency medical technicians, and those working
with chemicals in laboratories; may be rented or purchased.

★6347★ **FIRST RUN/ICARUS FILMS**
153 Waverly Pl., 6th Fl.
New York, NY 10014   Phone: (212) 727-1711
Description: Distributes films and videos from around the world covering a
wide range of subjects, including medicine and health, and psychology.
Available for rental or sale.

★6348★ **FISHER SCIENTIFIC COMPANY
ADVERTISING DEPARTMENT**
711 Forbes Ave.
Pittsburgh, PA 15219   Phone: (412) 562-8300
Description: Markets models and slides.

★6349★ **FLORIDA STATE UNIVERSITY
INSTRUCTIONAL SUPPORT CENTER
FILM/VIDEO LIBRARY**
056 Johnston Bldg.
Tallahassee, FL 32306   Phone: (904) 644-2820
Description: Motion picture and video rental service includes subjects in
mental health, general health education, nursing, physiology, psychology,
psychiatry, sociology, chemistry, biology, injury prevention, handicapped,
health safety, and nutrition.

★6350★ **FMS PRODUCTIONS, INC.**
PO Box 5016
Carp, CA 93014   Phone: (805) 564-2488
Description: Distributes, for rental and purchase, films for public audi-
ences on alcohol and drug treatment and education. Toll-free number:
(800) 421-4609.

★6351★ **FOCUS INTERNATIONAL, INC.**
14 Oregon Dr.
Huntington Station, NY 11746-2627   Phone: (516) 549-5320
Description: Produces and distributes videos and 16mm films on medical
education, human sexuality, and behavioral psychology topics. Toll-free
number: (800) 843-0305.

★6352★ **THE FORTUNE GROUP**
1 Concourse Pkwy., Ste. 155
Atlanta, GA 30328   Phone: (404) 395-2808
Description: Distributes a videotape training program on alcoholism and
drug addiction.

★6353★ **FOTO-COMM CORPORATION**
2000 York Rd., No. 112
Oak Brook, IL 60521-8820   Phone: (708) 575-2900
Description: Company specializes in developing educational audiovisual
materials from lectures presented at meetings. Services are provided
exclusively to associations.

★6354★ **FOUNDATION FOR BIOMEDICAL RESEARCH**
818 Connecticut Ave., NW, Ste. 303
Washington, DC 20006   Phone: (202) 457-0654
Description: Produces and distributes videotapes concerning the use of
animals in biomedical research.

★6355★ **FULD INSTITUTE FOR TECHNOLOGY IN NURSING
EDUCATION**
28 Station St.
Athens, OH 45701   Phone: (614) 592-2511
Description: Distributes a series of videos on the life and work of notable
nurse theorists.

★6356★ **GALLAUDET UNIVERSITY LIBRARY
GALLAUDET MEDIA DISTRIBUTION**
800 Florida Ave., NE
Washington, DC 20002   Phone: (202) 651-5579
Description: Distributes deafness-related programs on videocassette, film,
or slide; available for loan or purchase.

★6357★ **GARY WHITEAKER CORPORATION**
PO Box 307
Belleville, IL 62222   Phone: (618) 233-0005
Description: Produces and distributes drug and alcohol education videos
for patients, families, and public education programs. Toll-free number:
(800) 851-5406.

★6358★ GAUMARD SCIENTIFIC COMPANY, INC.
7030 SW 46th St.
Miami, FL 33155   Phone: (305) 666-8548
Description: Manufactures anatomical and clinical teaching models for medical and nursing educators and students, including SIMA brand CPR mannequins, hospital training mannequins, clinical simulators, patient training arms, OB/GYN, family planning and sex education models and simulators, and a complete line of anatomical artwork models.

★6359★ GEIGY PHARMACEUTICALS
556 Morris Ave.
Summit, NJ 07901   Phone: (908) 277-5000
Description: Produces medical teaching films which are distributed for free loan.

**★6360★ GILLETTE CHILDREN'S HOSPITAL
MEDICAL MEDIA SERVICES**
200 E. University Ave.
St. Paul, MN 55101   Phone: (612) 229-3947
Description: Produces and distributes medical education video programs for pediatric and orthopaedic health professionals. Offers medical illustration, photography, and videographic production services.

★6361★ GILLIS W. LONG HANSEN'S DISEASE CENTER
5445 Point Clair Rd.
Carville, LA 70721   Phone: (504) 642-4737
Description: Distributes instructional materials (35mm slide series, videocassettes, television programs, and printed materials), on Hansen's disease, to other medical and educational institutions for teaching purposes. The audiovisuals are loaned free of charge.

★6362★ GLENCOE PUBLISHING COMPANY
15319 Chatsworth St.
PO Box 9609
Mission Hills, CA 91346-9609   Phone: (818) 898-1391
Description: Audiovisual products include a health media kit consisting of filmstrips and audiocassettes on topics relevant to high school health curriculums. Toll-free number: (800) 423-9534.

★6363★ GOLDEN PRODUCTIONS
249 Sunset Dr.
Encinitas, CA 92024
Description: Offers a series of videotape programs developed for classroom or self-instructional training of health and mental health professionals. Individual programs or entire series available for purchase only.

**★6364★ GOOD SAMARITAN HOSPITAL AND MEDICAL
CENTER
VISION WORKS, INC.**
1015 NW 22nd Ave.
Portland, OR 97210   Phone: (503) 229-8038
Description: Offers videotape programs on a variety of medical topics, including neurological disorders, epilepsy, stroke, family violence, aging, multiple sclerosis, and sleep problems. Available for rental or purchase.

★6365★ GOWER MEDICAL PUBLISHING LTD.
101 5th Ave.
New York, NY 10003   Phone: (212) 929-6290
Description: Offers slide collections based on the company's color-illustrated medical texts and atlases; a wide variety of topics that includes dermatology, neurology, obstetrics, pathology, and pediatrics.

★6366★ GPN
PO Box 80669
Lincoln, NE 68501   Phone: (402) 472-2007
Description: Distributes videotaped instructional courses and programs, plus videodiscs and specialized slides, to educational institutions and public broadcasting stations. Topics include alcoholism, child abuse, crisis intervention, and sexuality and aging. Toll-free number: (800) 228-4630.

★6367★ GRANDVIEW HOSPITAL AND MEDICAL CENTER
405 Grand Ave.
Dayton, OH 45405   Phone: (513) 226-3956
Description: Produces and distributes patient education and staff education videotapes for the health care markets. Toll-free number: (800) 426-3812.

★6368★ GRAPHIC FILMS CORPORATION
3341 Cahuenga Blvd., W.
Los Angeles, CA 90068   Phone: (213) 851-4100
Description: Distributes medical films on the embryology and pathology of the intestinal tract, and on the molecular activity that creates and sustains life.

★6369★ GRASSLAND MEDIA
535 Science Dr., Ste. A
Madison, WI 53711   Phone: (608) 238-7575
Description: Offers complete video production services to business, industry, and the medical field.

★6370★ GREAT ATLANTIC RADIO CONSPIRACY
2743 Maryland Ave.
Baltimore, MD 21218   Phone: (410) 243-6987
Description: Produces and distributes audiotapes and cassettes which examine current events in many areas, including the medical industry. For sale to individuals and institutions.

★6371★ GROUP FIVE COMMUNICATIONS
500 Commercial St., Ste. 302
Manchester, NH 03101   Phone: (603) 627-2599
Description: Specializes in the custom design and development of films, videos, and slide productions for a variety of industries, including healthcare and medicine. Toll-free number: (800) 553-2599.

★6372★ GROVE PRESS FILM DIVISION
841 Broadway, 4th Fl.
New York, NY 10003   Phone: (212) 614-7850
Description: Offers, for rental or sale, films and videos on a wide variety of subjects, including medicine, health, and psychology.

★6373★ GUIDANCE ASSOCIATES
PO Box 1000
Mt. Kisco, NY 10549   Phone: (914) 666-4100
Description: Educational videos available for purchase or preview on topics that include AIDS, genetics, reproduction, anatomy, and human biology, health and nutrition, and psychology. Toll-free number: (800) 431-1242.

★6374★ GUILFORD PUBLICATIONS, INC.
72 Spring St.
New York, NY 10012   Phone: (212) 431-9800
Description: Produces educational materials, including video- and audiocassette programs for psychologists and psychiatrists in the behavioral sciences. Topics include behavior therapy; hypnosis; family and marital therapy; school and child psychology; neuropsychology; and clinical, cognitive, and experimental psychology. Toll-free number: (800) 365-7006.

★6375★ GURZE BOOKS
Box 2238
Carlsbad, CA 92008   Phone: (619) 434-7533
Description: Offers videotapes on topics such as anorexia nervosa, bulimia, compulsive eating, sexual abuse, and related topics. Available for purchase.

★6376★ H.E. BEERNINK RELEASING
20 El Camino Real
Berkeley, CA 94705   Phone: (510) 845-0344
Description: Films or videotapes relating to Lamaze and Cesarean births are available for preview and purchase.

★6377★ HANDEL FILM CORPORATION
8730 Sunset Blvd.
West Hollywood, CA 90069   Phone: (310) 657-8990
Description: 16mm films and/or videocassettes include programs on medical applications of atomic energy; also included are films on general health and safety.

**★6378★ HARPER & ROW
CUSTOMER SERVICE**
PO Box 1580
Hagerstown, MD 21741   Phone: (301) 714-2300
Description: Distributes audiovisual materials for purchase and preview. Rental programs may be obtained from the Film Rental office in New York.

★6379★ HARPER & ROW MEDIA
FILM RENTALS
10 E. 53rd St.
New York, NY 10022   Phone: (212) 207-7000
Description: Slides, films and audiocassettes for nursing and allied health sciences, and on speech disorders, are available for rental. AV purchases may be made from the Hagerstown, MD, office.

★6380★ HARRIS-TUCHMAN PRODUCTIONS, INC.
4293 Sarah St.
Burbank, CA 91505   Phone: (818) 841-4100
Description: Nursing and patient education filmstrips are distributed and are available for purchase.

★6381★ HARTLEY FILM FOUNDATION, INC.
Cat Rock Rd.
Cos Cob, CT 06807   Phone: (203) 869-1818
Description: Films and videotapes on stress reduction, biofeedback, therapeutic touch, holistic health, and meditation are available for rental or purchase.

★6382★ HARVEST FILMS/HARVEST AV, INC.
98 Riverside Dr.
New York, NY 10024   Phone: (212) 873-6900
Description: Produces and distributes, for rental or sale, 16mm films and videotapes on industrial safety and health.

★6383★ HARWYN MEDICAL PHOTOGRAPHERS
17291 NE 19th Ave.
North Miami Beach, FL 33162   Phone: (305) 947-0618
Description: 35mm color photomicrographs are distributed for hematology, histology, pathology, parasitology and tropical medicine, obstetrics and gynecology, and tumor microscopy.

★6384★ HAYES PRODUCTIONS, INC.
PO Box 780875
San Antonio, TX 78278   Phone: (512) 493-3551
Description: Film, video, and animation production company offers a wide variety of products and services to advertising, architectural, educational, legal, and medical clients.

★6385★ HAYES PUBLISHING COMPANY, INC.
6304 Hamilton Ave.
Cincinnati, OH 45224   Phone: (513) 681-7559
Description: Company offers slide/tape sets and videotapes dealing with human life and abortion issues.

★6386★ HAZELDEN EDUCATIONAL MATERIALS
Pleasant Valley Rd.
PO Box 176
Center City, MN 55012   Phone: (612) 257-4010
Description: Distributes films, video and audiocassettes for use in alcohol consulting services. Toll-free number: (800) 328-9000.

★6387★ HEALING ARTS HOME VIDEO
321 Hampton Dr., No. 203
Venice, CA 90291   Phone: (310) 399-3700
Description: Offers health and fitness video- and audiocassettes for purchase. Topics in clude massage, yoga, and back pain. Toll-free number: (800) 722-7347.

★6388★ HEALTH COMMUNICATIONS PRODUCTIONS, INC.
255 E. Brown St., Ste. 310
Birmingham, MI 48009   Phone: (313) 540-6006
Description: Produces patient information videotapes to explain and promote medical practices and procedures. Also offers videos on HIV testing and baldness.

★6389★ HEALTH EDCO
PO Box 21207
Waco, TX 76702   Phone: (817) 776-6461
Description: Produces models, charts, slides, audiocassettes, games, displays, and specimens for use in medical and patient education. Toll-free number: (800) 299-3366.

★6390★ HEALTH EDUCATION AIDS
PO Box 3311
Kansas City, KS 66103   Phone: (816) 753-7812
Description: Distributes programs for pre-clinical and nursing education; available for preview. Formats include audiocassettes, filmstrips, and videotapes.

★6391★ HEALTH AND EDUCATION MULTIMEDIA, INC.
501 E. 79th St., No. 18D
New York, NY 10021-0774   Phone: (212) 288-2297
Description: Distributes videotape programs on human development and psychiatry for professional education.

★6392★ HEALTH AND EDUCATION RESOURCES
4733 Bethesda Ave.
Bethesda, MD 20814   Phone: (301) 656-3178
Description: Distributes audiovisual materials on medical laboratory techniques; available for sale.

★6393★ HEALTH SCIENCES COMMUNICATIONS
ASSOCIATION
6105 Lindell Blvd.
St. Louis, MO 63112   Phone: (314) 725-4722
Description: Association members design, develop, and distribute health-related teaching materials in human and veterinary medicine.

★6394★ HEALTH SCIENCES CONSORTIUM
201 Silver Cedar Ct.
Chapel Hill, NC 27514   Phone: (919) 942-8731
Description: Publisher and marketer of instructional materials for medical, nursing, and allied health education. Formats include videotape, slide/tape, CAI, and videodisc.

★6395★ HEALTHTAPES, INC.
13320 Northend Ave.
Oak Park, MI 48237-3213   Phone: (313) 548-3222
Description: Produces and distributes 1/2 inch, 3/4 inch and Beta home exercise videocassettes for women who have had breast surgery, persons with Parkinson's disease, and people over fifty; available for purchase.

★6396★ HEART TALK/TAMPA TRACINGS
PO Box 4809
Indian Rocks Beach, FL 34685   Phone: (813) 596-2047
Description: Cardiology slides and audiocassettes for physicians, nurses, and medical students are sold.

★6397★ HIGH/SCOPE EDUCATIONAL RESEARCH
FOUNDATION
600 N. River St.
Ypsilanti, MI 48198-2898   Phone: (313) 485-2000
Description: Public education programs on child development are available for rental and sale in book, videotape, and cassette formats.

★6398★ HOECHST-CELANESE PHARMACEUTICALS
Rte. 202-206, N.
PO Box 2500
Somerville, NJ 08876-1258   Phone: (908) 231-2000
Description: Films produced for medical groups and hospital personnel are available for free loan.

★6399★ HOSPITAL HOME HEALTH CARE AGENCY
2601 Airport Dr., Ste. 110
Torrance, CA 90505   Phone: (310) 530-3800
Description: Distributes films and videotapes relating to hospice/home health care.

★6400★ HOUSE EAR INSTITUTE
VISUAL COMMUNICATIONS
2100 W. 3rd St.
Los Angeles, CA 90057   Phone: (213) 483-4431
Description: Institute produces and distributes educational slides and videotapes for physicians, audiologists, patients, and the lay public. Direct orders to the Finance department.

★6401★ HRM VIDEO
175 Tompkins Ave.
Pleasantville, NY 10570-9973   Phone: (800) 431-2050
Description: Produces and distributes videos on drug education and health and fitness for a pre-teen and teenage audience.

★6402★ HUBBARD SPECTRUM
PO Box 760
Chippewa Falls, WI 54729-1468   Phone: (715) 723-4427
Description: Offers, for sale, a series of videocassettes on the systems of the human body. Free preview tape available. Toll-free number: (800) 323-8368.

★6403★ HUMAN RELATIONS MEDIA
175 Tompkins Ave.
Pleasantville, NY 10570   Phone: (914) 769-7496
Description: Distributes filmstrips, filmstrips-on-video, and videocassettes on medicine, mental health, family life, sex education, AIDS, and substance abuse topics. Programs are available for free preview and purchase. Toll-free number: (800) 431-2050.

★6404★ HUXLEY INSTITUTE
900 N. Federal Hwy., No. 160
Boca Raton, FL 33432-2753   Phone: (407) 393-6167
Description: Offers, for sale, tapes on orthomolecular medicine and psychiatry.

★6405★ HYMAN W. FISHER, INC.
121 E. Northfield Rd.
Livingston, NJ 07039   Phone: (201) 994-9480
Description: Consultants to healthcare-related industries. Offers a wide range of audiovisual support services, including film and video programs, slide programs, speakers' and instructors' kits, audiocassette kits, and exhibit components.

★6406★ ICI AMERICUS, INC.
PO Box 751
Wilmington, DE 19897   Phone: (302) 886-3000
Description: Produces professional education programs on 16mm film, slides, and 3/4 inch videocassette. Loaned free of charge.

★6407★ IEA PRODUCTIONS, INC.
520 E. 77th St.
New York, NY 10021   Phone: (212) 988-9244
Description: Professional education videotapes on family and group therapy are distributed for rental and purchase.

★6408★ IFEX FILMS
201 W. 52nd St.
New York, NY 10019   Phone: (212) 582-4318
Description: Distributes 16mm educational films, including medical and health-related titles on such subjects as mental retardation, drug addiction, leukemia, cancer, and aging.

★6409★ IGAKU-SHOIN MEDICAL PUBLISHERS, INC.
1 Madison Ave.
New York, NY 10010   Phone: (212) 779-0123
Description: Produces and distributes videotapes covering a variety of topics in the medical field. Videotapes are available for purchase in VHS or Beta format. Toll-free number: (800) 765-0800.

★6410★ IMAGE ASSOCIATES
352 Conejo Rd.
PO Box 40106
Santa Barbara, CA 93140   Phone: (805) 962-6009
Description: Offers 16mm films and videotapes for sale on a variety of medical, health, psychology, and safety topics.

★6411★ IMS CREATIVE COMMUNICATIONS
MEDICAL VIDEO LIBRARY
University of Toronto
One King's College Circle
Toronto, ON, Canada M5S 1A8   Phone: (416) 978-6302
Description: Professional, paraprofessional, and patient education materials are produced and distributed for sale and rental. Formats include films and videocassettes.

★6412★ INDIANA UNIVERSITY
CENTER FOR MEDIA AND TEACHING RESOURCES
Bloomington, IN 47405-5901   Phone: (812) 855-8087
Description: Programs on 16mm film and videotape are available for rental and sale. Many topics in medicine and health are included.

★6413★ INDIANA UNIVERSITY
SCHOOL OF MEDICINE
DEPARTMENT OF OBSTETRICS AND GYNECOLOGY
1001 Walnut St., MF104
Indianapolis, IN 46202-5196   Phone: (317) 274-7129
Description: Professional education programs in obstetrics and gynecology are distributed for purchase in 16mm film and video formats.

★6414★ INDIANA UNIVERSITY
SCHOOL OF MEDICINE
MEDICAL EDUCATIONAL RESOURCES PROGRAM
1226 W. Michigan St., BR156
Indianapolis, IN 46202-5178   Phone: (317) 274-4083
Description: Video, film, slide/tape, audio, and computer assisted learning programs are produced on medical and health subjects for physician, medical student, and patient education/information. Also offered to health care facilities in Indiana are closed circuit television networks, the Medical Television Network of Indiana and the Patient Television Network, and a videotape mailing network, the Medical Mailing Network of Indiana. Also distributes educational videocassettes for the nursing and health care fields produced by the Indiana University School of Nursing.

★6415★ INFOMEDIX
12800 Garden Grove Blvd., Ste. F
Garden Grove, CA 92643   Phone: (714) 530-3454
Description: A full-service production company specializing in videotaping, audio taping, and high speed tape duplicating services serving a variety of clients, including those in the medical field.

★6416★ INSTA-TAPE, INC.
810 S. Myrtle Ave.
PO Box 1729
Monrovia, CA 91017-5729   Phone: (213) 303-2531
Description: Produces audio recordings of medical conferences, symposiums, and workshops; available for purchase.

★6417★ INSTITUTE FOR RATIONAL/EMOTIVE THERAPY
45 E. 65th St.
New York, NY 10021   Phone: (212) 535-0822
Description: Audio and video cassettes on cognitive therapy for professionals, and self-help tapes for the general public, are available for purchase.

★6418★ INSTITUTE FOR REHABILITATION AND RESEARCH
1333 Moursund Ave.
Houston, TX 77030-3405   Phone: (713) 797-5945
Description: Offers videotapes, audiotapes and slide/sound programs for health care and rehabilitation professionals, as well as for disabled consumers and patient/family education; available for purchase.

★6419★ INTERACTIVE HEALTHCARE CONSORTIUM
Stewart Publishing, Inc.
6471 Merritt Ct.
Alexandria, VA 22312   Phone: (703) 354-8155
Description: Produces and distributes videotapes and videodiscs for the health sciences. Available for purchase.

★6420★ INTERCOLLEGIATE CENTER FOR NURSING EDUCATION
LEARNING RESOURCES UNIT
W. 2917 Ft. George Wright Dr.
Spokane, WA 99204-5277   Phone: (509) 325-6141
Description: Produces videos on a wide range of subjects relating to the practice of nursing.

★6421★ INTERNATIONAL CENTER FOR SPORTS NUTRITION
502 S. 44th St., Ste. 3012
Omaha, NE 68105-1065   Phone: (402) 559-5505
Description: Offers for purchase a video titled "Eating Disorders and Athletic Performance."

★6422★ INTERNATIONAL DIABETES CENTER
5000 W. 39th St.
Minneapolis, MN 55416   Phone: (612) 927-3393
Description: Center markets patient education videos on diabetes and nutrition topics.

★6423★ INTERNATIONAL FILM BUREAU INC.
332 S. Michigan Ave.
Chicago, IL 60604-4382   Phone: (312) 427-4545
Description: Distributes educational films, videocassettes, audiocassettes, filmstrips, and slides to schools and universities, cultural and public institutions, business and industry. Topics include human physiology and occupational safety. Available for preview, purchase or rental. Toll-free number: (800) 432-2241.

★6424★ INTERNATIONAL FILM EXCHANGE, LTD.
201 W. 52nd St.
New York, NY 10019   Phone: (212) 582-4318
Description: Distributes a film dealing with mental retardation.

★6425★ INTERNATIONAL TELECOMMUNICATION SERVICES
PO Box 1290
State College, PA 16804-1290   Phone: (814) 234-4011
Description: Offers video-training programs in all video formats for support personnel in medical and health care facilities.

★6426★ INTERNATIONAL TELE-FILM ENTERPRISES, LTD.
47 Densley Ave.
Toronto, ON, Canada M6M 5A8   Phone: (416) 241-4483
Description: Distributes films and videos, for general and professional audiences, on topics which include health and safety.

★6427★ IPO ASSOCIATES LIMITED
PO Box 339
Flourtown, PA 19031   Phone: (215) 836-2383
Description: Produces and distributes videotape and audiocassette programs on legal aspects of nursing practice.

★6428★ IRL PRESS AT OXFORD UNIVERSITY PRESS
200 Madison Ave.
New York, NY 10016   Phone: (212) 679-7300
Description: Offers three video series, Techniques in Genetic Engineering, Immunology in Focus, and Physiology Classics, for teaching and individual study. Available for sale only.

★6429★ IRVINGTON PUBLISHERS, INC.
195 McGregor St.
Manchester, NH 03102   Phone: (603) 669-5933
Description: Produces and distributes videotapes on hypnosis.

★6430★ IVANHOE COMMUNICATIONS, INC.
401 S. Rosalind Ave.
PO Box 865
Orlando, FL 32801   Phone: (407) 423-8045
Description: Specializes in television programming and in the development and production of broadcast quality video for medical facilities nationwide.

★6431★ J.B. LIPPINCOTT COMPANY
E. Washington Sq.
Philadelphia, PA 19105   Phone: (215) 238-4200
Description: Distributes videocassettes in medical and clinical sciences, nursing skills, patient care, and allied health fields. Materials are available for 10-day free examination. Toll-free number: (800) 523-2945.

★6432★ J.J. KELLER & ASSOCIATES, INC.
3003 W. Breezewood Ln.
PO Box 368
Neenah, WI 54957-0368   Phone: (414) 722-2848
Description: Produces and distributes a video dealing with healthcare in the workplace; available for purchase. Toll-free number: (800) 558-5011.

★6433★ J.M. NEY COMPANY
Ney Industrial Park
Bloomfield, CT 06002   Phone: (203) 242-2281
Description: Produces and distributes slide presentations in anatomy and dentistry.

★6434★ JACOBY/STORM PRODUCTIONS, INC.
22 Crescent Rd.
Westport, CT 06880   Phone: (203) 227-2220
Description: A full-service audiovisual company producing educational, training, and mot ivational materials for schools and businesses on a wide variety of subjects, including health and medical topics.

★6435★ JEFFREY NORTON PUBLISHERS, INC.
AUDIO-FORUM
96 Broad St., Dept. R
Guilford, CT 06437   Phone: (203) 453-9794
Description: Publishes audio- and videocassettes for professional education in the areas of psychology and psychiatry and a language course, Medical Spanish: A Conversational Approach. Also distributes Medically Speaking: English for the Medical Profession, an audiocassette program produced by the BBC; and videocassettes on child abuse and treatment. Toll free number: (800) 243-1234.

★6436★ JIM STOKES COMMUNICATIONS
453 S. Cedar Lake Rd.
Minneapolis, MN 55405   Phone: (612) 377-6251
Description: Writer, director, and producer of films, videos, audiotapes, and slide/tapes in the medical and healthcare fields.

★6437★ JOHN WILEY & SONS, INC.
605 3rd Ave.
New York, NY 10158   Phone: (212) 850-8800
Description: Offers video tutorials for purchase on the subject of coronary angioplasty and cell motility and the cytoskeleton.

★6438★ JOHNS HOPKINS UNIVERSITY
SCHOOL OF MEDICINE
MEDICAL VIDEO PRODUCTION
720 Rutland Ave.
Baltimore, MD 21205   Phone: (410) 955-3562
Description: Offers films and videocassettes for medical professionals; available for rental and sale. Produces film, video, tape and slide/tape programs, and video teleconferencing.

★6439★ JOHNSON INSTITUTE
7205 Ohms Ln.
Edina, MN 55439-2159   Phone: (612) 831-1630
Description: Films, videocassettes, and audiotapes on alcoholism and drug abuse are available for purchase.

★6440★ JOSEPH P. KENNEDY, JR. FOUNDATION
1350 New York Ave. NW, Ste. 500
Washington, DC 20005-4709   Phone: (202) 393-1250
Description: Produces films which focus on medical ethics issues. Topics include the right to die, the right to live, and the right to give treatment to those unable to give consent. Films are distributed by Bono Films and Video Services; 3200 Lee Hwy.; Arlington, VA 22207; (703) 243-0800.

★6441★ JOSLIN DIABETES CENTER
1 Joslin Pl.
Boston, MA 02215   Phone: (617) 732-2429
Description: Provides informative videos for people with diabetes; available for purchase.

★6442★ KENT STATE UNIVERSITY
AUDIOVISUAL SERVICES
PO Box 5190
Kent, OH 44242   Phone: (216) 672-3456
Description: A rental source for 16mm films and videocassettes on all subjects, including a complete range of medical- and health-related topics. Toll-free number: (800) 338-5718.

★6443★   KILGORE INTERNATIONAL, INC.
36 W. Pearl St.
Coldwater, MI 49036   Phone: (517) 279-9123
Description: Models and skeletons for use in anatomical science education are distributed. Toll-free number: (800) 892-9999.

★6444★   KINETIC
255 Delaware Ave., Ste. 340
Buffalo, NY 14202   Phone: (716) 856-7631
Description: Specializes in audiovisuals on social issues, with particular emphasis on hospital staff development, substance abuse, child abuse and neglect, and aging. Films and videotapes available for rent or purchase.

★6445★   LAERDAL MEDICAL CORPORATION
1 Labriola Ct.
PO Box 190
Armonk, NY 10504   Phone: (914) 273-9404
Description: Markets resuscitation training aids and emergency medical equipment. Toll-free number: (800) 431-1055.

★6446★   LANDMARK FILMS INC.
3450 Slade Run Dr.
Falls Church, VA 22042   Phone: (703) 241-2030
Description: Produces and distributes videotapes and 16 mm films covering a variety of subjects, including substance abuse and sexual diseases. Available for preview, purchase or rental. Toll-free number: (800) 342-4336.

★6447★   LEARNER MANAGED DESIGNS, INC.
2201-K W. 25th St.
Lawrence, KS 66044   Phone: (913) 842-9088
Description: Produces and distributes video training resources on such topics as home and school care for children with special health needs, genetic applications for counseling families, birth crisis intervention, controlling blood-borne diseases, and caring for young children with disabilities and chronic conditions. Available for rent or purchase.

★6448★   LEARNING CORPORATION OF AMERICA
108 Wilmot Rd.
Deerfield, IL 60015   Phone: (708) 940-1260
Description: Distributes 16 mm films and videotapes covering a variety of subjects, including teenage sexuality/sex education, death and dying, and interacting with the aging. Available for purchase. Toll-free number: (800) 621-2131.

**★6449★   LEARNING DISABILITIES ASSOCIATION OF
    AMERICA**
4156 Library Rd.
Pittsburgh, PA 15234   Phone: (412) 341-1515
Description: Videos available for rent on the subject of learning disabled individuals.

★6450★   LEARNING RESOURCES AND COMMUNICATIONS
Television-Radion-Print-AV
Box 100016 U.F. Health Science Center
Gainesville, FL 32610-0016   Phone: (904) 392-4143
Description: Offers a wide range of educational media, graphics, photography, and television production services to health science center faculty and others.

★6451★   LEXCOM PRODUCTIONS
2720 Sunset Blvd.
West Columbia, SC 29169   Phone: (803) 739-4711
Description: Company specializes in the creation of videotape training programs for the health care industry. Maintains a library of programs and offers writing, editing, production, and post-production services.

★6452★   LIFE SCIENCE ASSOCIATES
One Fenimore Rd.
Bayport, NY 11705   Phone: (516) 472-2111
Description: Distributes educational cassette/slide programs in the field of neuroscience and psychology for pre-med and medical schools.

★6453★   LIFECIRCLE
2378 Cornell Dr.
Costa Mesa, CA 92626   Phone: (714) 546-1427
Description: Educational videos and slide/tape sets that provide parents and their families with information on all aspects of pregnancy, labor, birth, and the infant's first year; available for rent and purchase.

★6454★   LIFECYCLE PRODUCTIONS
PO Box 183
Newton, MA 02165   Phone: (617) 964-0047
Description: Develops, produces, and distributes informational and instructional videotapes for healthcare professionals and patients. Videos are designed to help people cope with life changes and stress associated with birth, growth, illness, and death. Programs are available for sale.

★6455★   THE LIVING SERIES
121 W. 27th St., Ste. 902
New York, NY 10001   Phone: (212) 675-7722
Description: Offers videotape series of 3 videos, which discusses the emotional issues o f living with a chronic illness; areas include diabetes, arthritis, and heart disease. Available in 1/2 and 3/4 inch formats for purchase, rental or preview.

★6456★   LONG ISLAND FILM STUDIOS
2895 Whitby Dr.
Atlanta, GA 30340   Phone: (404) 939-4030
Description: Distributes educational, children's, and health education films.

★6457★   LONG ISLAND PRODUCTIONS
6787 Snowdon Ave.
El Cerrito, CA 94530   Phone: (510) 232-5215
Description: Produces and distributes videotapes on first aid, laboratory safety, radiation safety, psychosocial care, and patient education for hospital employees. Available for preview and purchase.

**★6458★   LOS AMIGOS RESEARCH AND EDUCATION
    INSTITUTE, INC. OF THE RANCHO LOS AMIGOS MEDICAL
    CENTER**
12841 Dahlia St.
PO Box 500, Los Amigos Sta.
Downey, CA 90242   Phone: (310) 940-8111
Description: Physical medicine and rehabilitation programs are available for rental and purchase. Formats include videocassettes, audiocassettes, and slide/tapes.

★6459★   LUCERNE MEDIA
37 Ground Pine Rd.
Morris Plains, NJ 07950   Phone: (201) 538-1401
Description: Distributes a wide variety of educational videocassettes. Topics include alcohol education, seat belt safety, and viruses; also offers a series on the human body and the safe child program which teaches personal safety skills to young children. Toll-free number: (800) 341-2293.

**★6460★   LUPUS FOUNDATION OF AMERICA
BAY AREA CHAPTER**
2635 N. 1st St., Ste. 206
San Jose, CA 95134   Phone: (408) 954-8600
Description: Offers a two-part program, to health professionals and lay persons, on the diagnosis, treatment, and management of lupus. Available for rental or sale in 35mm sound/slide, video, or videocassette formats. In California call toll free: (800) 523-3363.

★6461★   MAINE HUMANITIES COUNCIL
PO Box 7202
Portland, ME 04112   Phone: (207) 773-5051
Description: Distributes a videotape on AIDS and its effects on human values. Available for purchase.

★6462★   MANISSES COMMUNICATIONS GROUP, INC.
205 Governor St.
Providence, RI 02906-0757   Phone: (401) 831-6020
Description: Videotapes of teleconferences given by professionals on alcoholism and substance abuse; the psychological impact of divorce on children; and suicide, pregnancy, and AIDS as they affect teenagers.

★6463★ MARCH OF DIMES BIRTH DEFECTS FOUNDATION
1275 Mamaroneck Ave.
White Plains, NY 10605   Phone: (914) 428-7100
Description: Public and professional education materials on birth defects, genetics, and pregnancy are produced on 1/2 and 3/4 inch videocassettes, 16mm film, and radio cassettes.

★6464★ THE MARIONS SUPPORT SYSTEM
INTEGRATIVE HEALTH CENTRE
14 Ellis Potter Ct., Ste. 2A
Madison, WI 53705   Phone: (608) 277-1979
Description: Offers a six week audiocassette self-help, support group program with accompanying manual and handbook for individuals dealing with life-threatening/chronic illnesses, for their families, and for health care professionals. Available for sale.

★6465★ MARSH MEDIA
PO Box 8082
Shawnee Mission, KS 66208   Phone: (816) 523-1059
Description: Develops health guidance and medical educational programs for schools. Available as filmstrips or videos; for sale only. Toll-free number: (800) 821-3303.

★6466★ MARSHFIELD CLINIC
OFFICE OF MEDICAL EDUCATION
1000 N. Oak Ave.
Marshfield, WI 54449   Phone: (715) 387-5127
Description: Offers videotape, slide/lecture, demonstration and/or discussion group formats in many areas of health and medicine. Programs are directed to physicians, nurses, and allied health personnel for supplemental education; CME credit available. Also offers documentary programs for patient education. Available for rental or sale. Toll-free number: (800) 782-8581.

★6467★ MARTHA STUART COMMUNICATIONS, INC.
147 W. 22nd St., No. 6S
New York, NY 10011   Phone: (212) 255-2718
Description: Produces and distributes programs on health issues for general audiences; formats include videocassettes and motion pictures.

★6468★ MARYLAND PUBLIC TELEVISION
11767 Owings Mills Blvd.
Owings Mills, MD 21117   Phone: (410) 356-5600
Description: Produces video programs on alcoholism and pediatrics.

★6469★ MASSACHUSETTS GENERAL HOSPITAL
TELEVISION DEPARTMENT
Fruit St.
Boston, MA 02114   Phone: (617) 726-5055
Description: Distributes video television programs on a variety of medical subjects for health care professionals.

★6470★ MCGILL UNIVERSITY
INSTRUCTIONAL COMMUNICATIONS CENTER
550 Sherbrooke St., W., Ste. 400
Montreal, PQ, Canada H3A 1B9   Phone: (514) 398-7200
Description: Produces videocassettes on a variety of medical and health related topics, including examination of the musculoskeletal system and speech teaching to the hearing impaired. Available for purchase, rental, or preview in VHS format.

★6471★ MEDCOM/TRAINEX
PO Box 3225
Garden Grove, CA 92642   Phone: (714) 891-1443
Description: Produces audiovisual educational materials for health professionals, patients, and consumers. Preview and sale of videos. Toll-free number: (800) 877-1443.

★6472★ MEDFILMS, INC.
6841 N. Cassim Pl.
Tucson, AZ 85704   Phone: (602) 575-8900
Description: Offers educational videotapes on a variety of topics for the training of nurses and other hospital employees, including videotape programs to help hospitals comply with the training requirements of OSHA's Bloodborne Pathogens Standard and the FDA's Safe Medical Devices Act.

★6473★ MEDIA DESIGN ASSOCIATES, INC.
PO Box 3189
Boulder, CO 80307-3189   Phone: (303) 443-2800
Description: Produces and distributes videocassettes on a variety of health issues, such as alcohol and drug abuse, AIDS, smoking, and nutrition. Company has also produced a number of interactive videodiscs. Programs are available for purchase.

★6474★ MEDIA GUILD
11722 Sorrento Valley Rd., Ste. E
San Diego, CA 92121   Phone: (619) 755-9191
Description: Distributes general audience programs on such topics as mental health, AIDS, drugs and alcohol, prenatal care and childbirth, and depression; available for rental and purchase.

★6475★ MEDIA RESOURCES, INC.
2614 Fort Vancouver Way
Vancouver, WA 98661-3997   Phone: (206) 693-3344
Description: Offers videos for preview or purchase on emergency services training, and business safety and health management. Toll-free number: (800) 666-0106.

★6476★ MEDICAL EDUCATION PROGRAMS, LTD.
372 Danbury Rd.
Wilton, CT 06897   Phone: (203) 834-1811
Description: Creates and produces marketing communications programs for medical and health care companies. Programs which include film, video, and audio materials, are aimed at informing physician audiences of appropriate role of client products.

★6477★ MEDICAL GROUP MANAGEMENT ASSOCIATION
104 Inverness Terrace E.
Englewood, CO 80112-5306   Phone: (303) 799-1111
Description: Slide/tape programs, videocassettes, and audiocassettes for medical group administrators and physicians on health care and medical group office management are available for rental or purchase.

★6478★ MEDICAL ILLUSTRATIONS COMPANY
800 Cox's Lane
PO Box 944
Cutchogue, NY 11935   Phone: (516) 222-1717
Description: Company produces medical graphics in any medium, including print, television, film, and display.

★6479★ MEDICAL INFORMATION SERVICES, INC.
1995 Broadway
New York, NY 10023   Phone: (212) 580-3466
Description: Produces and distributes educational audiocassettes and videotapes covering a variety of topics in the medical field.

★6480★ MEDICAL INFORMATION SYSTEMS, INC.
2 Seaview Blvd.
Port Washington, NY 11050   Phone: (516) 621-7200
Description: Publishes and distributes continuing education programs in the areas of obstetrics-gynecology, pediatrics, psychiatry, and dentistry. Sponsored by the American College of Obstetricians and Gynecologists, the American Academy of Pediatrics, the American College of Psychiatrists, and the Academy of General Dentistry.

★6481★ MEDICAL MEDIA SYSTEMS
2421 W. Pratt Blvd.
Chicago, IL 60645   Phone: (312) 764-1144
Description: Facility produces medical education video and audio programs for schools of medicine and nursing, medical licensure agencies, and other allied health care organizations. Available for sale. Scriptwriting, narrating, and producers' services available.

★6482★ MEDICAL UNIVERSITY OF SOUTH CAROLINA
DIVISION OF TELEVISION SERVICES
HEALTH COMMUNICATIONS NETWORK
171 Ashley Ave.
Charleston, SC 29425   Phone: (803) 792-4435
Description: Professional health education materials are produced for broadcast to network members on closed circuit television. Programs are available for sale or rental.

★6483★   MEDICAL VIDEO PRODUCTIONS
450 N. New Ballas Rd., Ste. 205
St. Louis, MO 63141   Phone: (314) 991-5510
Description: Produces and distributes medical videotapes for physicians.
Topics include OB/GYN, ophthalmology, orthopaedics, and cardiology.
The tapes are available to physicians by subscription for 1, 2 or 3 years.
Toll-free number: (800) 822-3100.

★6484★   MEDI-LEGAL INSTITUTE
15301 Ventura Blvd., Ste. 300
Sherman Oaks, CA 91403   Phone: (818) 995-7189
Description: Produces and distributes audio- and videocassette programs
designed for legal, health, and insurance professionals. Topics include
health related issues, such as injury, disability, malpractice, and litigation
from a medical and legal perspective. Available for purchase.

★6485★   MED-SCENE
217 S. Payne St.
Alexandria, VA 22314   Phone: (703) 548-7039
Description: Produces and distributes audiotapes, videotapes, and films
that cover medical meetings, conferences, and special events. Also distributes over 400 videotapes with continuing medical education credit for
physicians, nurses, and technicians.

★6486★   MELEAR MULTI-MEDIA, INC.
1344 Johnson Ferry Rd., Ste. 14
Marietta, GA 30067   Phone: (404) 971-5665
Description: Provides media production services for regional, national, and
international communications campaigns related to public health, behavioral science, and substance abuse prevention.

**★6487★   MERCK SHARP AND DOHME HEALTH
INFORMATION SERVICES**
Sumney Town Pke.
West Point, PA 19486   Phone: (215) 661-7484
Description: A video service on key health topics, for general audiences, is
available on a preview-for-purchase basis.

★6488★   MERRELL DOW AUDIOVISUAL LIBRARY
c/o NKY Distribution Center, Inc.
7172 New Buffington Rd.
Florence, KY 41042   Phone: (606) 525-2138
Description: Pharmacy, surgical and clinical medicine, psychiatry, and a
series on medicine and the law are among the 16mm films and videotapes
available on a free loan basis to health professionals.

**★6489★   MICHIGAN DEPARTMENT OF MENTAL HEALTH
CENTER FOR FORENSIC PSYCHIATRY**
PO Box 2060
Ann Arbor, MI 48106   Phone: (313) 429-2531
Description: Lends forensic science psychiatry and psychology materials
designed for health professionals. Programs are on videocassettes and
audiocassettes.

**★6490★   MICHIGAN STATE UNIVERSITY
INSTRUCTIONAL MEDIA CENTER**
Marketing Division
PO Box 710
East Lansing, MI 48826   Phone: (517) 353-9229
Description: Audiovisuals in medicine, nursing, mental health, and veteri-
nary medicine are produced on slide/tape, videotape, and 16mm film.
Film rentals are available through the Scheduling Office (Phone: 517-353-
3960).

**★6491★   MICRO X-RAY RECORDER
MEDICAL FILM SLIDE DIVISION**
120 W. Illinois, 2nd Fl., W.
Chicago, IL 60610   Phone: (312) 527-5111
Description: Provides 35mm slides and slide/tape materials for medical
education.

**★6492★   MILES INC.
DIAGNOSTICS DIVISION**
PO Box 70
Elkhart, IN 46515   Phone: (219) 264-8111
Description: Collection of 16mm films is available for free loan.

★6493★   MILNER-FENWICK, INC.
2125 Greenspring Dr.
Timonium, MD 21093   Phone: (301) 252-1700
Description: Produces and distributes video programs for patient and
professional education. Toll-free number: (800) 432-8433.

**★6494★   MILWAUKEE REGIONAL MEDICAL INSTRUCTIONAL
TELEVISION STATION, INC.**
5000 W. National Ave.
Milwaukee, WI 53295   Phone: (414) 384-2000
Description: Operates a closed circuit educational TV network for hospitals
in the Milwaukee region. Programs are designed for both the health
professional and the non-professional hospital staff. Videocassettes are
also available to member hospitals.

★6495★   MOBILTAPE COMPANY, INC.
25061 W. Avenue Stanford, Ste. 70
Valencia, CA 91355   Phone: (805) 295-0504
Description: Provides an audiocassette taping and distribution service for
conventions of health science organizations.

★6496★   MODERN TALKING PICTURE SERVICE, INC.
5000 Park St., N.
St. Petersburg, FL 33709   Phone: (813) 541-5763
Description: Distributes free loan films and videocassettes for public
education. Also available for purchase are a selection of videos and
videodiscs. Topics include health and hygiene. Toll-free number: (800)
243-MTPS.

★6497★   MOSBY-YEAR BOOK, INC.
11830 Westline Industrial Dr.
St. Louis, MO 63146   Phone: (314) 872-8370
Description: Distributes audiocassettes, videotapes, laser discs, and slides
on a variety of health topics that include the human anatomy and nurse
training.

★6498★   MOTIVATIONAL MEDIA, INC.
12001 Ventura Pl., Ste. 202
Studio City, CA 91604   Phone: (818) 508-6553
Description: Produces and distributes videotapes dealing with substance
abuse and recovery/treatment programs for patients and clients. Available
for preview and purchase. Toll-free number: (800) 331-8454.

★6499★   MRI EDUCATION FOUNDATION, INC.
400 Oak St., Ste. 227
Cincinnati, OH 45219   Phone: (513) 281-3400
Description: Produces and distributes Magnetic Resonance Imaging (MRI)
videos and slides; includes orthopedic, spine, neuro, body, and general
MRI.

★6500★   MULTI-FOCUS, INC.
1525 Franklin St.
San Francisco, CA 94109   Phone: (415) 673-5100
Description: Distributes films, videotapes, filmstrips, and slides on human
sexuality to clinics, classrooms, community centers, and medical facilities.
Available for rental or sale.

**★6501★   NAACOG: THE ORGANIZATION FOR OBSTETRIC,
GYNECOLOGIC, AND NEONATAL NURSES**
409 12th St., SW
Washington, DC 20024   Phone: (202) 638-0026
Description: Distributes audiovisual programs that meet the continuing
education standards of NAACOG and the American Nursing Association.

★6502★   NATIONAL ASSOCIATION OF THE DEAF
814 Thayer Ave.
Silver Spring, MD 20910   Phone: (301) 587-1788
Description: Films on sign language and deafness can be purchased.

★6503★   NATIONAL DOWN SYNDROME SOCIETY
666 Broadway
New York, NY 10012   Phone: (212) 460-9330
Description: NDSS has produced a videotape which explores parents'
feelings about raising a child with Down's Syndrome; available on a ten-
day loan basis. Toll-free number: (800) 221-4602.

★6504★ NATIONAL FILM BOARD OF CANADA
U.S. Distribution Representative
1251 Avenue of the Americas, 16th Fl.
New York, NY 10020   Phone: (212) 586-5131
Description: Health care topics are covered in films produced for general distribution.

★6505★ NATIONAL FIRE PROTECTION ASSOCIATION
Batterymarch Park
Quincy, MA 02269   Phone: (617) 770-3000
Description: Safety programs include films designed for hospital personnel.

★6506★ NATIONAL GEOGRAPHIC SOCIETY
EDUCATIONAL SERVICES
PO Box 98019
Washington, DC 20090   Phone: (800) 368-2728
Description: Offers, for sale, science, health, and social studies teaching aids in a variety of formats, including learning kits and sound filmstrips on such topics as tooth and dental hygiene, foods and nutrition, and the human body.

★6507★ NATIONAL INSTITUTE FOR BURN MEDICINE
909 E. Ann St.
Ann Arbor, MI 48104   Phone: (313) 769-9000
Description: Produces teaching packages and slides on burn prevention and the care, treatment, and rehabilitation of burn victims.

★6508★ NATIONAL LEAGUE FOR NURSING
350 Hudson St.
New York, NY 10014   Phone: (212) 989-9393
Description: Distributes a wide variety of health and medical videos that relate to the nursing profession; available for purchase. Toll-free number: (800) 669-1656.

★6509★ NATIONAL NEUROFIBROMATOSIS FOUNDATION
141 5th Ave., Ste. 7-S
New York, NY 10010   Phone: (212) 460-8980
Description: VHS videotapes on neurofibromatosis are available for purchase.

★6510★ NATIONAL SAFETY COUNCIL
1121 Spring Lake Dr.
Itasca, IL 60143-3201   Phone: (708) 285-1121
Description: 16mm films, video, and slides for purchase and rental (excluding slides), cover all aspects of safety and health.

★6511★ NATIONAL SAFETY COUNCIL
GREATER LOS ANGELES CHAPTER
FILM LIBRARY
3450 Wilshire Blvd., Ste. 700
Los Angeles, CA 90010-8215   Phone: (213) 385-6461
Description: Films and videotapes are available for rent and purchase. Topics include health, health care training, and employee safety and training. Some titles are available in Spanish.

★6512★ NATIONAL SOCIETY TO PREVENT BLINDNESS
500 E. Remington Rd.
Schaumburg, IL 60173-4557   Phone: (708) 843-2020
Description: Offers 16mm films, 1/2 and 3/4 inch videos, slides, and audiocassettes on a variety of topics including cataracts, glaucoma, and home/industry/sports eye safety for professional and general audiences of all ages. Available for rental, purchase, or preview. Toll-free number: (800) 331-2020.

★6513★ NCES: NUTRITION COUNSELING AND EDUCATION SERVICES
PO Box 3018
Olathe, KS 66062-8018   Phone: (913) 782-8230
Description: Offers a variety of videos on nutrition and other health matters, including fitness, high blood pressure, and breast-feeding; available for purchase. Toll-free number: (800) 445-5653.

★6514★ NEBRASKA LIBRARY COMMISSION
1420 P St.
Lincoln, NE 68508   Phone: (402) 471-2045
Description: Rents films on a wide range of subjects, including psychology, and health and safety.

★6515★ NEMIROFF PRODUCTIONS, INC.
152 Cold Spring Rd.
Syosset, NY 11791   Phone: (212) 832-7600
Description: Produces films, videotape programs, and audiovisual presentations for a wide variety of clients, including the U.S. Surgical Corp., American Cancer Society, and National Society to Prevent Blindness. Programs range from those intended for public education to others for professional education.

★6516★ NETCHE VIDEOTAPE LIBRARY
PO Box 83111
Lincoln, NE 68501   Phone: (402) 472-3611
Description: Produces and distributes 1/2 and 3/4 inch videocassette educational programs in health-related areas of genetics, nursing, psychology, sociology, safety, physiology, human development, and community health.

★6517★ NETWORK FOR CONTINUING MEDICAL
EDUCATION
1 Harmon Plaza, 7th Fl.
Secaucus, NJ 07094   Phone: (201) 867-3550
Description: A videocassette subscription service, accredited by the Accreditation Council for Continuing Medical Education, that offers continuing medical education credits for physicians.

★6518★ NEW DAY FILM CO-OP, INC.
121 W. 27th St., Ste. 902
New York, NY 10001   Phone: (212) 645-8210
Description: Cooperative of independent film and video producers who distribute films and tapes about contemporary social issues. Subjects covered include health and the environment; young adult issues; birth, parenting, and the family; sexuality; aging; and special needs.

★6519★ NEW DIMENSION MEDIA, INC.
85803 Lorane Hwy.
Eugene, OR 97405   Phone: (503) 484-7125
Description: Distributes 16mm film and videocassette programs that are available for purchase or rental on a variety of health topics including AIDS education, drug education, and teen sexuality.

★6520★ NEW DIMENSIONS FOUNDATION
PO Box 410510
San Francisco, CA 94141   Phone: (415) 563-8899
Description: Audiocassettes on community health care, psychology, and psychiatry are produced and distributed.

★6521★ NEW ENGLAND SLIDE SERVICE, LTD.
76 Olcott Dr.
White River Junction, VT 05001-0685   Phone: (802) 295-7300
Description: Offers a complete slide production service, such as computer generated presentation slides from Macintosh and IBM/DOS programs and slides from X-rays, to a variety of clients, including hospitals, extended care facilities, and physicians.

★6522★ THE NEW FILM COMPANY, INC.
7 Mystic St., Ste. 315
Arlington, MA 02174   Phone: (617) 641-2580
Description: Offers, for rental or sale, films and videos on the subject of aging.

★6523★ NEW YORK STATE EDUCATION DEPARTMENT
BUREAU OF TECHNOLOGY APPLICATIONS
Cultural Education Center, Rm. C-7, Concourse Level
Albany, NY 12230   Phone: (518) 474-1265
Description: Bureau duplicates and distributes videotaped programs in a wide range of subject areas. Health-related topics include alcohol and drug abuse, mental illness, nutrition, and handicapping conditions. Programs are geared to audiences of all ages.

★6524★ NEW YORK STATE PSYCHIATRIC INSTITUTE
722 W. 168th St.
New York, NY 10032   Phone: (212) 960-2200
Description: Programs for mental health professionals are produced and distributed for purchase on videocassettes.

★6525★ NEW YORK UNIVERSITY
COLLEGE OF DENTISTRY
DAVID B. KRISER DENTAL CENTER
345 E. 24th St.
New York, NY 10010   Phone: (212) 998-9800
Description: Produces instructional television programs, slide and audio tape programs, and other audiovisual materials. Offers design and consulting services.

★6526★ NEW YORK UNIVERSITY
FILM LIBRARY
35 W. 4th St., Rm. 777
New York, NY 10003   Phone: (212) 998-1212
Description: 16mm film topics include child development and mental health; available for rental.

★6527★ NORTH CAROLINA STATE UNIVERSITY
SCHOOL OF VETERINARY MEDICINE
BIOMEDICAL COMMUNICATIONS
4700 Hillsborough St.
Raleigh, NC 27606   Phone: (919) 829-4212
Description: Produces and distributes videotapes, videodiscs, and slide/tape programs covering many areas of veterinary medicine. Topics include dentistry, laboratory, orthopedics, and surgical. Available for purchase.

★6528★ NORWICH EATON PHARMACEUTICALS, INC.
AUDIOVISUAL LIBRARY
350 N. Pennsylvania
Wilkes-Barre, PA 18773   Phone: (800) 637-4123
Description: Offers educational films, videotapes, and slide programs in the fields of urology, nutrition, obstetrics and gynecology, bones, anesthesiology, and patient education.

★6529★ NOVELA HEALTH EDUCATION
934 E. Main St.
Stamford, CT 06902   Phone: (203) 967-8900
Description: Produces and distributes educational videotapes on vital health subjects, including AIDS, geriatrics, drug abuse and prenatal care. Novela's emphasis is on cross-cultural health education with programs offered in both English and Spanish. Tapes are available for rental or purchase. Toll-free number: (800) 677-4799.

★6530★ NUCLEAR ASSOCIATES
100 Voice Rd.
Carle Place, NY 11514   Phone: (516) 741-6360
Description: Nuclear medicine and radiologic technology audiovisuals approved for AMA continuing education credit are produced and available for sale. Formats include slide/tape and filmstrips.

★6531★ NURSING MANAGEMENT VIDEOS
103 N. 2nd St., Ste. 200
West Dundee, IL 60118   Phone: (708) 426-6100
Description: Distributes films and videotapes for staff development, continuing education, and nursing education.

★6532★ NUS TRAINING CORPORATION
910 Clopper Rd.
PO Box 6032
Gaithersburg, MD 20877-0962   Phone: (301) 258-2500
Description: Produces and distributes work safety videos; available for preview and purchase.

★6533★ OAK WOODS MEDIA, INC.
PO Box 19127
Kalamazoo, MI 49019-0127   Phone: (616) 375-5621
Description: Produces multiple sets of slides and audiocassettes for clients in the medi cal field.

★6534★ OHIO STATE UNIVERSITY
COLLEGE OF MEDICINE
BIOMEDICAL COMMUNICATIONS
School of Allied Medical Professions Bldg.
1583 Perry St.
Columbus, OH 43210   Phone: (614) 292-3323
Description: Produces medical and allied health education programs which are available for rental and purchase. Formats include slide/tape, audio and videotape.

★6535★ OHIO STATE UNIVERSITY
COLLEGE OF MEDICINE
CONTINUING MEDICAL EDUCATION
320 W. 10th Ave.
Columbus, OH 43210   Phone: (614) 292-4985
Description: Sponsors satellite television network for physician education. Also distributes slide/tape packages and sponsors a slide/tape network for physician education; programs are accredited by the AMA.

★6536★ OHIO STATE UNIVERSITY
NISONGER CENTER
1581 Dodd Dr.
Columbus, OH 43210   Phone: (614) 292-8365
Description: Produces and distributes, for preview and purchase, videotapes and slide/tape programs relating to mental retardation and developmental disability.

★6537★ OKLAHOMA STATE UNIVERSITY
AUDIOVISUAL CENTER
Stillwater, OK 74078   Phone: (405) 744-7212
Description: Educational films and videotapes are available for rent to schools, individuals, and organizations throughout the U.S. Topics include many in the medical and health care fields.

★6538★ OKLAHOMA STATE UNIVERSITY
COLLEGE OF VETERINARY MEDICINE
LEARNING RESOURCES CENTER
102 Veterinary Medical Bldg.
Stillwater, OK 74078   Phone: (405) 744-6729
Description: Slide/tape programs and videocassettes on topics relating to veterinary medicine are available for rental or purchase.

★6539★ ORGANON, INC.
375 Mt. Pleasant Ave.
West Orange, NJ 07052   Phone: (201) 325-4500
Description: Distributes medical and pharmaceutical films at no charge.

★6540★ ORTHO PHARMACEUTICAL CORPORATION
EDUCATIONAL PROGRAMS DEPARTMENT
Rte. 202 S.
PO Box 300
Raritan, NJ 08869   Phone: (908) 218-6443
Description: Professional education films are distributed on a free-loan basis.

★6541★ ORTHOPAEDIC AUDIO-SYNOPSIS FOUNDATION
PO Box H
South Pasadena, CA 91031   Phone: (213) 682-1760
Description: Distributes a monthly audiocassette accredited by the AMA for continuing medical education in orthopaedic surgery.

★6542★ PACIFICA RADIO ARCHIVE
3729 Cahuenga Blvd., W.
North Hollywood, CA 91604-3584   Phone: (818) 506-1077
Description: Audiotapes and cassettes in medicine, health care, and psychology are distributed to professional and general audiences.

★6543★ PADRE KINO VIDEOLIBRERIA
Tucson Medical Park
5230 E. Farness, No. 106
Tucson, AZ 85712   Phone: (800) 922-8638
Description: Produces and distributes videos on chemical dependency in Spanish.

★6544★ PAIN RESOURCE CENTER, INC.
PO Box 2836
Durham, NC 27705   Phone: (919) 286-9180
Description: Produces and distributes educational and testing materials on the subject of pain; applicable to all medical specialties.

★6545★ PARENTING PICTURES
121 NW Crystal St.
Crystal River, FL 32629   Phone: (904) 795-2156
Description: Educational films on child care for parental audiences can be rented or purchased.

★6546★ PATHFINDER INTERNATIONAL
COMMODITIES DEPARTMENT
9 Galen St., Ste. 217
Watertown, MA 02172   Phone: (617) 924-7200
Description: Offers 3 training films relating to family planning and free for distribution in developing countries.

★6547★ PBS VIDEO
1320 Braddock Pl.
Alexandria, VA 22314   Phone: (703) 739-5380
Description: Distributes videocassette programs on a wide range of subjects, including health and medicine. Available for rental or sale. Toll-free number: (800) 424-7963.

★6548★ PENNSYLVANIA COLLEGE OF PODIATRIC
MEDICINE
8th at Race St.
Philadelphia, PA 19107   Phone: (215) 629-0300
Description: Distributes audiocassette recordings of seminars conducted at the institution.

★6549★ PENNSYLVANIA MEDICAL SOCIETY
777 E. Park Dr.
PO Box 8820
Harrisburg, PA 17105-8820   Phone: (717) 558-7750
Description: Distributes practice management programs for the medical profession; also provides an audio and videocassette duplication service for physicians.

★6550★ PENNSYLVANIA STATE UNIVERSITY
AUDIO-VISUAL SERVICES
Special Services Bldg.
1127 Fox Hill Rd.
University Park, PA 16803-1824   Phone: (814) 865-6314
Description: Videos produced for health care professionals and educators includes topics on the hospitalization of children, special education, emotional disturbances of children, delinquency, drug abuse and pregnancy, and counseling and psychiatry. Toll-free number: (800) 826-0132.

★6551★ PENNSYLVANIA STATE UNIVERSITY
MILTON S. HERSHEY MEDICAL CENTER
SLEEP RESEARCH AND TREATMENT CENTER
PO Box 850
Hershey, PA 17033   Phone: (717) 531-8520
Description: Offers, for rental or sale, a Center-produced film for physicians on advances in sleep research and their clinical applications.

★6552★ PEP-USA
3900 Birch, Ste. 105
Newport Beach, CA 92660   Phone: (714) 250-2975
Description: Audiotapes relating to Parkinson's disease are available for loan, rental, or purchase.

★6553★ PHILADELPHIA CHILD GUIDANCE CENTER
34th and Civic Center Blvd.
Philadelphia, PA 19104   Phone: (215) 243-2600
Description: Family therapy materials are distributed to mental health facilities for professional use. Programs are on videotape.

★6554★ PHOENIX FILMS, INC.
468 Park Ave., S.
New York, NY 10016   Phone: (212) 684-5910
Description: Films and videos for sale and rental include topics of child development, mental health, gerontology, teen pregnancy, and sexually transmitted diseases.

★6555★ PLANNED PARENTHOOD FEDERATION OF
AMERICA
810 7th Ave.
New York, NY 10019   Phone: (800) 669-0156
Description: Distributes films for physicians and health professionals on family planning and reproductive health topics.

★6556★ POINT OF VIEW PRODUCTIONS
2477 Folsom St.
San Francisco, CA 94110   Phone: (415) 821-0435
Description: Produces and distributes videotapes, for rental or sale, on water birth and on holistic health, wellness and preventive health care.

★6557★ POLYMORPH FILMS
118 South St.
Boston, MA 02111   Phone: (617) 542-2004
Description: Educational programs for the public and professionals on maternal and child care are distributed on 16mm film and videotape. Toll-free number (800) 370- 3456.

★6558★ POSTGRADUATE INSTITUTE FOR MEDICINE
11031 S. Pike's Peak Dr.
PO Box 158
Parker, CO 80134   Phone: (303) 841-5102
Description: Develops and distributes accredited video and slide/cassette continuing medical education programs for physicians. Topics include clinical electrocardiography; fluids, electrolyte, and acid-base disorders; pulmonary function and disease; and diabetes mellitus. Also develops custom medical education programs for pharmaceutical companies which include slide presentation kits, audiocassettes, videos, seminars, and monographs.

★6559★ PRIMARY EYECARE, INC.
1200 Godfrey Ave.
Philadelphia, PA 19141   Phone: (215) 276-6259
Description: Offers, for sale, audio- and videocassette programs for the optometric profession.

★6560★ PROSPECT MEDIA
73 College Rd., W.
Princeton, NJ 08540   Phone: (609) 921-2631
Description: Develops, produces and distributes 16mm films and video-tapes on a variety of subjects, including many for the healthcare field. Topics include a 3-part series about living with chronic illness: diabetes, arthritis, and heart disease.

★6561★ PSYCHOLOGICAL AND EDUCATIONAL FILMS
3334 E. Coast Hwy., No. 252
Corona Del Mar, CA 92625   Phone: (714) 494-5079
Description: Distributes films and videos on a variety of psychology subjects; available for purchase or rent.

★6562★ PURDUE UNIVERSITY
SCHOOL OF VETERINARY MEDICINE
MEDICAL ILLUSTRATION AND COMMUNICATIONS
Lynn Hall, Rm. 33
West Lafayette, IN 47907-1245   Phone: (317) 494-1153
Description: Produces videotape programs for use in veterinary medical education.

★6563★ PURDUE UNIVERSITY
SELF-DIRECTED LEARNING PROGRAMS
Continuing Education
1586 Stewart Center
West Lafayette, IN 47907-1586   Phone: (317) 494-2748
Description: Educational videotapes are offered to health care professionals for purchase. Topic areas include veterinary medicine, speech-language pathology and audiology, nursing, mainstreaming handicapped, and substance abuse. Toll-free number: (800) 359-2968.

★6564★   PYRAMID FILM AND VIDEO
PO Box 1048
Santa Monica, CA 90406-1048   Phone: (800) 421-2304
Description: Distributes film and videos for educating public audiences on health isssues. Media formats include video and 16mm film; available for purchase or rental.

★6565★   QUALITY MEDICAL PUBLISHING, INC.
2086 Craigshire Dr.
St. Louis, MO 63146   Phone: (314) 878-7808
Description: Videotape programs covering plastic surgery, laparoscopic surgery and neurological surgery are available for purchase. Toll-free number: (800) 423-6865.

★6566★   QUEEN'S TELEVISION
McArthur Hall, Queen's University
Kingston, ON, Canada K7L 3N6   Phone: (613) 545-2817
Description: Produces and distributes post-secondary teaching and learning materials for the health sciences division of Queen's University. In addition to in-house production of videotapes to complement University causes, QTV contracts with various agencies and private medical practitioners for programming.

★6567★   RADIOLOGICAL SOCIETY OF NORTH AMERICA
EDUCATIONAL MATERIALS DIVISION
PO Box 5316
Oak Brook, IL 60522-5316   Phone: (708) 575-2900
Description: Offers continuing education courses to physicians on video and slide/tape format. Most medical discipline areas are included in the AMA accredited programs.

★6568★   RANCHO LOS AMIGOS MEDICAL CENTER
LOS AMIGOS RESEARCH AND EDUCATION INSTITUTE, INC.
7601 E. Imperial Hwy.
PO Box 3500, Los Amigos Sta.
Downey, CA 90242   Phone: (213) 940-7165
Description: Produces and distributes videotapes for medical professionals and patients. Topics include brain injury, spinal cord injury and rehabilitation programs. Programs are available for preview and purchase or rental.

★6569★   REELIZATIONS
PO Box 555
Woodstock, NY 12498   Phone: (914) 679-8363
Description: Produces and distributes videotape programs on the treatment of, and recovery from, addictions of all kinds.

★6570★   REGIONAL CANCER FOUNDATION
2107 Van Ness Ave., Ste. 408
San Francisco, CA 94109   Phone: (415) 755-9956
Description: Offers, for sale or free loan, audio and videotapes on many subjects relating to cancer and the cancer patient. Tapes are available for children as well as adults.

★6571★   REHABILITATION INSTITUTE OF CHICAGO
EDUCATION AND TRAINING CENTER
345 E. Superior St.
Chicago, IL 60611   Phone: (312) 908-6184
Description: Videotape programs for physical therapy education are distributed for rental and purchase.

★6572★   RESEARCH PRESS
2612 N. Mattis Ave.
PO Box 9177
Champaign, IL 61826   Phone: (217) 352-3273
Description: Offers films, videocassettes, and audiocassettes, for rental or sale, on a variety of behavioral and social issues.

★6573★   RHODE ISLAND EDUCATION AND TRAINING
SYSTEMS, INC.
PO Box 959
East Greenwich, RI 02818
Description: Distributes a videocassette educational program which discusses Class II Type A, B1, B2, and B3 biological safety cabinets. Intended for pharmacists, nurses, industrial hygienists, laboratory technicians, physicians, and other health care personnel.

★6574★   RIDGEVIEW INSTITUTE
3995 S. Cobb Dr.
Smyrna, GA 30080   Phone: (404) 434-4567
Description: Distributes a videotape dealing with multiple personality disorder. Available for rental or purchase. Toll-free number: (800) 345-9775.

★6575★   RMC MEDICAL
5301 Tacony St.
Box 208
Philadelphia, PA 19137-2309   Phone: (215) 537-0672
Description: Produces and distributes a medical training video covering hazardous material accidents.

★6576★   RMI MEDIA PRODUCTIONS, INC.
2807 W. 47th St.
Shawnee Mission, KS 66205   Phone: (800) 821-5480
Description: Distributes videotape training materials for the health occupations field, including topics on health issues, nutrition, stress management, and management training.

★6577★   THE ROEHER INSTITUTE
York University
Kinsmen Bldg.
4700 Keele St.
North York, ON, Canada M3J IP3   Phone: (416) 661-5701
Description: Offers videos and films for the public, professionals, and community groups about individuals with an intellectual impairment; available for rent or purchase.

★6578★   ROSS LABORATORIES
625 Cleveland Ave.
Columbus, OH 43215   Phone: (614) 227-3333
Description: Produces motion pictures and slide/tape programs on pediatrics and nutrition.

★6579★   SACRED HEART MEDICAL CENTER
W. 101 8th Ave.
TAF-C9
Spokane, WA 99220   Phone: (509) 455-3131
Description: Produces videotapes on a wide variety of medical subjects for patient and staff education. Available for rental or sale.

★6580★   SAI COMMUNICATIONS
SCHORR ASSOCIATES, INC.
125 S. 9th St., Ste. 400
Philadelphia, PA 19107   Phone: (215) 923-6466
Description: Produces customized computer generated slide programs designed for business, sales, and training in large corporations, manufacturers, and hospitals.

★6581★   ST. ELIZABETH HOSPITAL
AUDIOVISUAL SERVICES
2209 Genesee St.
Utica, NY 13501   Phone: (315) 798-8199
Description: Produces in-service training tapes and slide presentations for hospital personnel and medical seminars. Topics include: pre-operative, post-operative, and public relations programs.

★6582★   ST. LOUIS UNIVERSITY MEDICAL CENTER
EDUCATIONAL MEDIA DEPARTMENT
3525 Caroline
St. Louis, MO 63104   Phone: (314) 577-8604
Description: Offers videocassettes on the subjects of death and dying, and medical communication skills, and other biomedical topics.

★6583★   ST. LUKE'S HOSPITAL MEDICAL CENTER
EDUCATION DEPARTMENT
1800 E. Van Buren
Phoenix, AZ 85006   Phone: (602) 251-8100
Description: Produces and distributes, for preview and purchase, slide/tape patient education programs.

★6584★ SALENGER FILMS
1635 12th St.
Santa Monica, CA 90404   Phone: (310) 450-1300
Description: Offers films and videos on common safety and health problems in the work environment; available for preview, purchase, or rent.

★6585★ SAN ANTONIO STATE HOSPITAL
6711 S. New Braunfel
San Antonio, TX 78223   Phone: (512) 532-8811
Description: Offers slide/sound programs for adult education, vocational, and mental health personnel training; available for sale.

★6586★ SAN JOSE STATE UNIVERSITY
DEPARTMENT OF OCCUPATIONAL THERAPY
1 Washington Sq.
San Jose, CA 95192-0059   Phone: (408) 924-3070
Description: Videotapes dealing with occupational therapy education are available for purchase.

★6587★ SAVANT
801 E. Chapman Ave.
PO Box 3670
Fullerton, CA 92634   Phone: (714) 870-7880
Description: Produces and distributes videotapes and slide/tape training programs concerning chemical laboratory instrumentation and safety in the workplace for laboratory employees, as well as other health care workers. Toll-free number: (800) 472-8268.

★6588★ SCHERING CORPORATION
PROFESSIONAL SERVICES DEPARTMENT
Galloping Hill Rd., Bldg. 5
Kenilworth, NJ 07033   Phone: (908) 298-4915
Description: Produces films and slide/tape programs for medical, nursing and pharmacy education.

★6589★ SCIENCE SOFTWARE SYSTEMS, INC.
3576 Woodcliff Rd.
Sherman Oaks, CA 91403   Phone: (818) 501-7855
Description: Distributes 35mm slide sets for allied health sciences and 16mm motion pictures for physician education.

★6590★ SCIENCE-THRU-MEDIA, INC.
303 5th Ave., Ste. 803
New York, NY 10016   Phone: (212) 684-5366
Description: Produces and distributes a variety of medical education audiocassettes and accompanying materials. Available for sale.

★6591★ SCRIPPS MEMORIAL HOSPITAL
CANCER CENTER
PO Box 28
La Jolla, CA 92038-0028   Phone: (619) 457-6756
Description: Provides, for rental or sale, oncology nursing educational materials in videotape and audiocassette formats. Also sells cancer prevention and early detection videotapes.

★6592★ SHIELD PRODUCTIONS/STREETERVILLE STUDIOS, INC.
161 E. Grand Ave.
Chicago, IL 60611   Phone: (312) 644-1666
Description: Provides audio production services to a variety of clients, including those in the medical field.

★6593★ SHIRLEY A. SELBY
336 Country Club Dr.
San Francisco, CA 94132   Phone: (415) 661-3807
Description: Offers videotape training packages for hospital volunteer programs.

★6594★ SIMULAIDS, INC.
12 Dixon Ave.
Woodstock, NY 12498   Phone: (914) 679-2475
Description: Produces first aid and emergency medical training aids, models, and simulators. Toll-free number: (800) 431-4310; in NY, (800) 626-6676.

★6595★ SINGER-SHARRETTE PRODUCTIONS
52370 DeQuindre
Shelby Township, MI 48316   Phone: (313) 731-5199
Description: Producers and distributors of educational films/videotapes relating to traditional healing.

★6596★ SMITHKLINE BEECHAM PHARMACEUTICALS
HEALTH MEDIA CENTER
c/o West Glen
1430 Broadway
New York, NY 10018   Phone: (212) 764-8815
Description: Maintains a free-loan library of medical programs in the areas of surgery, gastroenterology, rheumatology, cardiology, psychiatry, and patient education. Formats include films and videotapes. Toll-free number: (800) 223-2342.

★6597★ SOCIETY FOR FRENCH AMERICAN CULTURAL
SERVICES AND EDUCATIONAL AID
972 5th Ave.
New York, NY 10021   Phone: (212) 439-1439
Description: Medical and psychology films are rented for short-term loans. Programs are from the Ministry of Foreign Affairs in Paris and are in English.

★6598★ SOCIETY FOR NUTRITION EDUCATION
2001 Killbrew Dr., No. 340
Minneapolis, MN 55425-1882   Phone: (612) 854-0035
Description: Distributes 16mm films, videotapes, and audiocassettes for sale, on nutrition for children, pregnant women, and older adults.

★6599★ SOCIETY FOR VISUAL EDUCATION, INC.
1345 Diversey Pkwy., Dept. DJ
Chicago, IL 60614-1299   Phone: (312) 525-1500
Description: Offers educational videos, filmstrips, laserdiscs, and microcomputer software on a wide variety of subjects, including health and safety. Appropriate for elementary school children through high school age. Available for sale. Toll-free number: (800) 829-1900.

★6600★ SOUTHERN ILLINOIS UNIVERSITY
SCHOOL OF MEDICINE
BIOMEDICAL COMMUNICATIONS CENTER FOR
EDUCATIONAL TELEVISION
PO Box 19230
Springfield, IL 62794-9230   Phone: (217) 782-7420
Description: Produces training and instructional videos for hospital, health care, and safety related organizations. Programs, stock footage, and graphics available for purchase. Complete post-production facilities including 1-inch mastering, avid offlin, Betacam SP and Dubner Graphics are available to qualified medical producers for grant or contract work.

★6601★ SOUTHERN MEDICAL ASSOCIATION
35 Lakeshore Dr.
PO Box 190088
Birmingham, AL 35219   Phone: (800) 423-4992
Description: Association's multi-media resources include audiocassette educational programs for physicians (available for sale only), videocassette programs for professional and patient education (rental or sale), and a comprehensive audiotape library for physician continuing medical education (available via subscription to the telephone service).

★6602★ SPRINGER-VERLAG NEW YORK, INC.
175 5th Ave., 19th Fl.
New York, NY 10010   Phone: (212) 460-1573
Description: Slides and videotapes on a wide variety of medical subjects are available for sale to professionals and medical institutions.

★6603★ SPRINGHOUSE PUBLISHING COMPANY
1111 Bethlehem Pike
Springhouse, PA 19477   Phone: (215) 646-4670
Description: Produces and distributes videotapes and audiocassettes on various aspects of nursing and health care; available for purchase. Toll-free number: (800) 331-3170 (except 215 area code).

★6604★ STACY KEACH PRODUCTIONS
3969 Longridge Ave.
Sherman Oaks, CA 91423   Phone: (818) 905-9601
Description: Offers, for sale, an audiocassette on exercise for senior

citizens. Also offers videos and 8 and 16mm films on topics including fear of heart surgery and on the rehabilitation process for those who have had heart surgery or heart attacks.

★6605★ STANFIELD HOUSE
PO Box 3208, Dept. H
Santa Monica, CA 90403   Phone: (213) 820-4568
Description: Offers educational films, videos, filmstrips, and audiocassettes on a variety of subjects, including health, mental health, the disabled, sexuality, and nutrition. Available for rental or sale.

★6606★ STANFORD UNIVERSITY
SCHOOL OF MEDICINE
STANFORD GERIATRIC EDUCATION CENTER
703 Welch Rd., Ste. H1
Stanford, CA 94305   Phone: (415) 723-7063
Description: Produces and distributes an instructional video on geriatric assessment. Available for purchase.

★6607★ STANFORD UNIVERSITY
SCHOOL OF MEDICINE
VISUAL ART SERVICES
MSOB, Rm. 100
Stanford, CA 94305   Phone: (415) 723-6813
Description: Videotape productions focusing on cancer victims are distributed for rental and purchase.

★6608★ STANTON FILMS
2417 Artesia Blvd.
Redondo Beach, CA 90278   Phone: (213) 542-6573
Description: Produces educational films and videos on a variety of subjects, including health. Available for rental and sale.

★6609★ STARWEST PRODUCTIONS
1391 N. Speer Blvd., Ste. 490
Denver, CO 80204   Phone: (303) 623-0636
Description: A full-service production company serving a variety of clients, including those in the medical field.

★6610★ STATE UNIVERSITY OF NEW YORK AT BUFFALO
EDUCATIONAL TECHNOLOGY SERVICES
MEDIA LIBRARY
24 Capen Hall
Buffalo, NY 14260   Phone: (716) 636-2802
Description: Rental service includes films, slides, and videotape recordings on child care, nursing, nutrition, and general health education.

★6611★ STATE UNIVERSITY OF NEW YORK HEALTH
SCIENCE CENTER AT SYRACUSE
EDUCATIONAL COMMUNICATIONS
c/o Edward Elsner
766 Irving Ave., Rm. 1257 WH
Syracuse, NY 13210   Phone: (315) 464-4860
Description: Produces and distributes, for rental or sale, videocassettes covering topics from basic health sciences to complex clinical procedures.

★6612★ STUART PHARMACEUTICALS
New Murphy and Concord Pike
Wilmington, DE 19897   Phone: (302) 886-3000
Description: Produces professional education programs on 16mm film, slides, and 3/4 inch videocassette; loaned free of charge.

★6613★ THE SUN GROUP
1133 Broadway
New York, NY 10010   Phone: (212) 255-1000
Description: A full-service audio production company specializing in recording and production of audio tracks for the medical and pharmaceutical industries.

★6614★ SUNBURST COMMUNICATIONS
39 Washington Ave.
Pleasantville, NY 10570   Phone: (914) 769-5030
Description: Distributes videotapes and 35mm filmstrips for schools, colleges, and health agencies in areas including health studies, drug education, sex education, nutrition, and first aid. Toll-free number: (800) 431-1934.

★6615★ SUTHERLAND LEARNING ASSOCIATES, INC.
8700 Reseda Blvd., Ste. 108
Northridge, CA 91324   Phone: (818) 701-1344
Description: Produces and distributes films, videocassettes, and print materials on aspects of cardiology, nursing quality assurance, and child care for health professionals.

★6616★ SYRACUSE UNIVERSITY
FILM RENTAL CENTER
1455 E. Colvin St.
Syracuse, NY 13244   Phone: (315) 443-2452
Description: Offers educational films specializing in hospital in-patient and nursing skills, staff development, and administrative skills; available for rent. Toll-free number: (800) 223-2409; in NY, (800) 345-6797.

★6617★ T.J. PUBLISHERS
817 Silver Spring Ave., Ste. 206
Silver Spring, MD 20910   Phone: (301) 585-4440
Description: Distributes sign language- and deafness-related programs on videocassette; available for sale. Toll-free number (voice and TDD): (800) 999-1168.

★6618★ TANE, INC.
11005 Garland Rd.
Dallas, TX 75218   Phone: (214) 328-7255
Description: Distributes filmstrip programs for drug education.

★6619★ TEACH 'EM, INC.
160 E. Illinois St.
Chicago, IL 60611   Phone: (312) 467-0424
Description: Provides on-location audiocassette recording, producing, and duplication services at professional meetings. The company's clients include many in the medical field. Toll-free number: (800) 225-3775.

★6620★ TEACHING AIDS, INC.
PO Box 1798
Costa Mesa, CA 92628   Phone: (714) 548-9321
Description: Videotapes relating to health care, drug and alcohol problems, nutrition, and eating disorders are available for purchase.

★6621★ TELEDYNE HANAU
80 Sonwil Dr.
Buffalo, NY 14225   Phone: (716) 684-0110
Description: Slides for professional dental education may be rented or purchased.

★6622★ TELESOURCE, INC.
525 E. 14th St., Ste. 10B
New York, NY 10009   Phone: (212) 353-3939
Description: Offers concept development, full production services, and videocassette marketing and distribution for instructional, medical, business and sales training, made-for-home video, corporate, government, and non-profit foundation communications.

★6623★ TELSTAR, INC.
10 10th Ave. N.
Hopkins, MN 55343-7504   Phone: (612) 938-5611
Description: Produces and distributes videocassettes for basic science courses in nursing education, specializing in listening skills for health care workers.

★6624★ TEMPLE UNIVERSITY
HEALTH SCIENCES CENTER
DEPARTMENT OF MEDICAL COMMUNICATIONS
3400 N. Broad St.
Philadelphia, PA 19140   Phone: (215) 221-7912
Description: Publishes listing of materials collected by the School of Medicine. Designated videocassette productions in medical education can be purchased.

★6625★ TEXAS A&M UNIVERSITY
COLLEGE OF VETERINARY MEDICINE
MEDIA RESOURCES
College Station, TX 77843   Phone: (409) 845-1780
Description: Offers production services, including videotape, color

slide/sound programs, original medical art, and computer-generated graphics and art.

★6626★ TEXAS HEART INSTITUTE
BIO-COMMUNICATIONS LABORATORY
PO Box 20345
Houston, TX 77225   Phone: (713) 791-4287
Description: Produces and distributes videotaped cardiovascular educational programs.

★6627★ TEXAS HEART INSTITUTE
PUBLICATIONS AND COMMUNICATIONS DEPARTMENT
PO Box 20345
Houston, TX 77225-0345   Phone: (713) 522-7060
Description: Produces and distributes videocassettes for cardiovascular educational purposes. Programs are available for purchase in VHS or Beta format.

★6628★ THE THERAPLAY INSTITUTE
180 N. Michigan Ave., Ste. 1928
Chicago, IL 60601   Phone: (312) 332-1260
Description: Distributes videotapes that demonstrate the application of interactional therapy to a variety of child and adult developmental/behavioral situations, both normal and abnormal. Programs are available for rental or sale.

★6629★ 3M COMPANY
MEDICAL, SURGICAL AND MEDICAL DEVICE DIVISION
3M Center, Bldg. 225-55-01
St. Paul, MN 55144   Phone: (800) 228-3957
Description: Films and videocassettes available on free loan include demonstrations of medical and surgical procedures.

★6630★ TISSUE CULTURE ASSOCIATION
AUDIOVISUAL LIBRARY
8815 Centre Park Dr., No. 210
Columbia, MD 21045-0000   Phone: (410) 992-0946
Description: Association maintains a large collection of films and videocassettes on cell culture and cell culture techniques; available for rental.

★6631★ TOTAL VIDEO COMPANY
432 N. Canal St., Unit 12
South San Francisco, CA 94080   Phone: (415) 583-8236
Description: Offers a full range of production and post-production video services to a variety of clients, including the healthcare industry.

★6632★ TRANSTAR PRODUCTIONS, INC.
9520 E. Jewell Ave., Ste. C
Denver, CO 80231   Phone: (303) 695-4207
Description: A full-service video, film, and multi-image production company serving a wide variety of clients, including those in the medical field.

★6633★ TRICEPTS PRODUCTIONS
22-D Hollywood Ave.
Ho-Ho-Kus, NJ 07423   Phone: (201) 652-1989
Description: Produces and distributes educational videotapes dealing with gerontology. Available for preview, purchase or rental.

★6634★ TRI-COUNTY DENTAL HEALTH COUNCIL
29350 Southfield Rd., No. 35
Southfield, MI 48076-2020
Description: Provides dental health slide/tape series on oral healthcare for geriatric and handicapped persons for health professionals; may be rented or purchased.

★6635★ TUTORIALS OF CYTOLOGY
1640 E. 50th St., Ste. 20-B
Chicago, IL 60615-3161   Phone: (312) 947-0098
Description: Produces slide sets in cytopathology and diagnostic cytology for professional and student audiences.

★6636★ UNIFOUR PRODUCTIONS, INC.
1020 3rd Ave. Dr. NW
Hickory, NC 28601-4855   Phone: (704) 324-1314
Description: Offers custom creative and producer video services. Experienced in patient information, hospital promotion, and training programs.

★6637★ UNITED CEREBRAL PALSY ASSOCIATIONS
7 Penn Plaza, No. 804
New York, NY 10001   Phone: (212) 481-6300
Description: Audiovisual resources for professional and general education relating to cerebral palsy are distributed for loan, rental and purchase.

★6638★ UNITED HOSPITAL
NURSING EDUCATION AND RESEARCH DEPARTMENT
333 N. Smith Ave.
St. Paul, MN 55102   Phone: (612) 220-8224
Description: Slide/tape and videotape educational programs in critical care and special care nursing are available for purchase.

★6639★ UNITED LEARNING
6633 W. Howard St.
PO Box 718
Niles, IL 60648   Phone: (708) 647-0600
Description: Offers educational films and videos on a variety of subjects, including many in the medical and health fields; available for purchase. Toll-free number: (800) 424-0362.

★6640★ UNITED TRAINING MEDIA
6633 W. Howard St.
Niles, IL 60648   Phone: (312) 647-0600
Description: Distributes training videos on a variety of management/supervision, staff development, and sales/marketing issues, including substance abuse and AIDS in the workplace. Also offers several videos designed exclusively for the health care industry. Available for purchase or rental. Toll-free number: (800) 759-0364.

★6641★ U.S. ARMED FORCES INSTITUTE OF PATHOLOGY
MEDIA CENTER
Bldg. 54, Rm. G124
Washington, DC 20306-6000   Phone: (202) 576-2979
Description: Medical nursing and allied health films can be rented at no cost from area headquarters. Most specialty areas in medicine are included in the coverage.

★6642★ U.S. NATIONAL AUDIOVISUAL CENTER
8700 Edgeworth Dr.
Capitol Heights, MD 20743-3701   Phone: (301) 763-1896
Description: Center serves as a central clearinghouse for all federally produced audiovisuals. Materials (films, videocassettes, audiocassettes, slides, and multimedia kits) covering a wide range of subjects, including medicine, dentistry, and allied health sciences, are available to the public for rental or sale.

★6643★ U.S. NATIONAL LIBRARY OF MEDICINE
8600 Rockville Pike
Bethesda, MD 20894   Phone: (301) 496-6095
Description: NLM acquires and makes available for distribution audiovisual instructional materials in a variety of formats, including videocassettes, audiocassettes, 16mm films, filmstrips and slides, X-rays, computer software, and videodiscs. Most audiovisuals are in core biomedical subjects, are in English, and are available for loan to any library in the U.S. Loans are not made directly to individuals. The Library also develops prototype interactive audiovisual communication programs for the health educational community (formerly the functions of the now defunct U.S. National Medical Audiovisual Center), and maintains the Learning Center for Interactive Technology, which makes a variety of audiovisual and computer-based interactive instructional programs available for demonstration. In addition, NLM indexes and catalogs audiovisuals for the AVLINE data base of MEDLARS. This computer system prints the National Library of Medicine Audiovisuals Catalog which contains bibliographic and content information.

★6644★ U.S. DEPARTMENT OF VETERANS AFFAIRS
CENTRAL OFFICE FILM LIBRARY
810 Vermont Ave.
Washington, DC 20420   Phone: (202) 233-4000
Description: Motion picture films, filmstrips, slides, audiocassettes, and videocassettes are available on free-loan from the library. Subject areas include dentistry, health, medicine, nursing, rehabilitation, and safety. Films are for use in support of medical and scientific research programs and studies, and for orientation, training, and information.

★6645★   **UNIVERSAL HEALTH ASSOCIATES**
PO Box 65465
Washington, DC 20035-5465   Phone: (202) 429-9506
Description: Distributes educational videos on a variety of subjects, including diabetes, maternal-child health, nutrition, and stroke rehabilitation and recovery. Also offers professional education videos. Tapes are available for preview and purchase. Toll-free number: (800) 229-1UHA.

★6646★   **UNIVERSITY OF ALABAMA AT BIRMINGHAM**
SCHOOL OF DENTISTRY
University Sta.
Dental Television, Rm. 631
Birmingham, AL 35294   Phone: (205) 934-4562
Description: Produces and distributes programs on videocassette and 16mm film for dental education; available for purchase and preview. Also has a dental television studio.

★6647★   **UNIVERSITY OF ALABAMA AT BIRMINGHAM**
SPAIN REHABILITATION CENTER
TRAINING DEPARTMENT
1717 6th Ave., S., Ste. 506
Birmingham, AL 35233   Phone: (205) 934-3283
Description: Produces and distributes professional and patient education videotapes and slide/tape programs concerned with preventing and treating secondary complications associated with spinal cord injury.

★6648★   **UNIVERSITY OF ALBERTA**
HEALTH SCIENCES MEDIA SERVICES AND DEVELOPMENT
Rm. 0J1 W.C. Mackenzie Health Sciences Centre
Edmonton, AB, Canada T6G 2B7   Phone: (403) 432-6560
Description: Produces and distributes videocassettes and slide/tape programs for use in medical education.

★6649★   **UNIVERSITY OF ARIZONA**
ARIZONA HEALTH SCIENCES CENTER
Division of Biomedical Communications
Tucson, AZ 85724   Phone: (602) 626-7343
Description: Instructional media productions designed for professional, patient, and hospital personnel are distributed on videotapes and slide/tapes.

★6650★   **UNIVERSITY OF BRITISH COLUMBIA**
HEALTHMEDIA CENTRE
Biomedical Communications
2194 Health Sciences Mall, Rm. B32
Vancouver, BC, Canada V6T 1W5   Phone: (604) 228-3467
Description: Produces and distributes programs on many health related subjects addressed to both lay and professional audiences. Programs may be previewed or purchased.

★6651★   **UNIVERSITY OF CALGARY**
DEPARTMENT OF COMMUNICATIONS MEDIA
MacKimmie Library Block
2500 University Dr., NW
Calgary, AB, Canada T2N 1N4   Phone: (403) 220-3709
Description: Produces and distributes videos on community health, health professions, occupational health, safety and training, and programs for sports, recreation, and fitness; available for preview, rental, and purchase.

★6652★   **UNIVERSITY OF CALIFORNIA**
CENTER FOR MEDIA AND INDEPENDENT LEARNING
2176 Shattuck Ave.
Berkeley, CA 94704   Phone: (510) 642-0460
Description: Distributes videocassettes and 16mm films on a wide variety of medical and health topics; available for purchase or rental.

★6653★   **UNIVERSITY OF CALIFORNIA—DAVIS**
SCHOOL OF VETERINARY MEDICINE
OFFICE OF THE DEAN
Davis, CA 95616   Phone: (916) 752-6521
Description: Produces and distributes videotapes and slide/tape programs for students and practitioners of veterinary medicine. Available for purchase or rental.

★6654★   **UNIVERSITY OF CALIFORNIA—LOS ANGELES**
INSTRUCTIONAL MEDIA LIBRARY
Powell Library-46
Los Angeles, CA 90024   Phone: (213) 825-0755
Description: Films and video productions include topics in medical ethics, psychology, and animal behavior.

★6655★   **UNIVERSITY OF CALIFORNIA—LOS ANGELES**
NEUROPSYCHIATRIC INSTITUTE
BEHAVIORAL SCIENCES MEDIA LABORATORY
760 Westwood Plaza, Rm. 37-451
Los Angeles, CA 90024   Phone: (213) 825-0448
Description: Produces and distributes, for rental or sale, educational and documentary films and videotapes in the fields of mental health and the behavioral sciences.

★6656★   **UNIVERSITY OF CALIFORNIA—SAN DIEGO**
SCHOOL OF MEDICINE
OFFICE OF LEARNING RESOURCES-TV 0615
9500 Gilman Dr.
La Jolla, CA 92093-0615   Phone: (619) 534-4134
Description: Videotape productions for medical education may be rented or purchased.

★6657★   **UNIVERSITY OF CALIFORNIA—SAN FRANCISCO**
DEPARTMENT OF RADIOLOGY
521 Parnassus Ave., Rm. C324
San Francisco, CA 94143   Phone: (415) 476-5731
Description: Postgraduate medicine courses in radiology are produced and are available for rent or sale on VHS; AMA accredited.

★6658★   **UNIVERSITY OF CALIFORNIA—SAN FRANCISCO**
EDUCATIONAL TELEVISION
1855 Folsam, CED, Rm. 646
San Francisco, CA 94143-0876   Phone: (415) 476-1958
Description: Produces and distributes videotapes for postgraduate medical education. Subject areas include pediatrics, obstetrics and gynecology, psychiatry, and medicine.

★6659★   **UNIVERSITY OF COLORADO—BOULDER**
ACADEMIC MEDIA SERVICES
Campus Box 379
Boulder, CO 80309-0379   Phone: (303) 492-8282
Description: Film rental service includes health education programs for professional and student audiences.

★6660★   **UNIVERSITY HOSPITALS OF CLEVELAND**
MEDICINE TODAY
2074 Adelbert Rd.
Cleveland, OH 44106   Phone: (216) 844-5050
Description: Offers 3 weekly medical education broadcasts; Medicine Today, Surgery Today, and Pediatril Grand Rounds.

★6661★   **UNIVERSITY OF ILLINOIS**
FILM CENTER
1325 S. Oak St.
Champaign, IL 61820   Phone: (217) 333-1360
Description: Offers films, videos, laserdiscs, and laserstacks in a variety of subject areas, including mental health, nursing, and medical topics. Available for purchase or rental. Toll-free number: (800) 367-3456.

★6662★   **UNIVERSITY OF ILLINOIS AT CHICAGO**
OFFICE OF MEDIA SERVICES
PO Box 6998
Chicago, IL 60680   Phone: (312) 996-7912
Description: Offers a full range of illustration, design, photography, and television production services to internal and external organizations.

★6663★   **UNIVERSITY OF KANSAS MEDICAL CENTER**
EDUCATIONAL RESOURCE CENTER
3901 Rainbow Blvd.
Kansas City, KS 66160-7182   Phone: (913) 588-7343
Description: Professional and patient education programs are available for rental and purchase. Formats include 35mm slide kits, 3/4 inch U-matic and 1/2 inch videocassettes, and 16mm films.

★6664★ UNIVERSITY OF LOUISVILLE
UNIVERSITY MEDIA SERVICES
BIOMEDICAL COMMUNICATIONS CENTER
230 Health Services Instructional Bldg.
Louisville, KY 40292   Phone: (502) 588-6464
Description: Offers biomedical and instructional television, photography services, computer graphics, medical illustration, film and slide processing, audiovisual services, and videoconferencing services.

★6665★ UNIVERSITY OF MARYLAND
DENTAL SCHOOL
DEPARTMENT OF EDUCATIONAL AND INSTRUCTIONAL
   RESOURCES
DIVISION OF DENTAL INFORMATICS
666 W. Baltimore St.
Baltimore, MD 21201-1586   Phone: (301) 328-3388
Description: Produces and distributes slide/tape and videotape programs for use in dental education.

★6666★ UNIVERSITY OF MARYLAND
SCHOOL OF MEDICINE
DEPARTMENT OF PHYSICAL THERAPY
VIDEO PRESS
100 Penn St., 1st Fl.
Baltimore, MD 21201   Phone: (410) 328-5497
Description: Produces and distributes video instructional materials and humanistic documentaries on health-related issues appropriate for the disciplines of medicine, nursing, social work, psychology, psychiatry, physical therapy, occupational therapy, and gerontology. Also offers video production services.

★6667★ UNIVERSITY OF MICHIGAN
FILM AND VIDEO LIBRARY
919 S. University Ave.
Ann Arbor, MI 48109-1185   Phone: (313) 764-5360
Description: A videotape and film rental service is available to educational institutions and community groups; topics include basic sciences and health care.

★6668★ UNIVERSITY OF MICHIGAN
MEDIA LIBRARY
1327 Jones Dr., Ste. 104
Ann Arbor, MI 48109-0518   Phone: (313) 763-2074
Description: Produces and distributes videos, slides, and instructional resources on a wide variety of medical topics, including AIDS, child abuse, dermatology, genetics, geriatrics, nutrition, obstetrics, pharmacology, psychiatry, and radiology; available for rent or purchase.

★6669★ UNIVERSITY OF MICHIGAN
SCHOOL OF DENTISTRY
EDUCATIONAL RESOURCES
Ann Arbor, MI 48109   Phone: (313) 763-0205
Description: Produces and distributes instructional material for professional and patient education in dentistry and dental hygiene.

★6670★ UNIVERSITY OF MINNESOTA
DEPARTMENT OF INDEPENDENT STUDY
45 Wesbrook Hall
77 Pleasant St., SE
Minneapolis, MN 55455   Phone: (612) 624-4393
Description: Independent study courses available on audio- and videocassette, television, and radio are offered in a wide range of areas, including health topics.

★6671★ UNIVERSITY OF MINNESOTA
MEDIA DISTRIBUTION
Box 734 Mayo Bldg.
420 Delaware St., S.E.
Minneapolis, MN 55455   Phone: (612) 624-7906
Description: Distributes instructional materials produced at the University, including video and audiotapes. Program topics include various health-related subjects.

★6672★ UNIVERSITY OF MISSOURI—COLUMBIA
SCHOOL OF MEDICINE
EDUCATIONAL RESOURCES GROUP
MA119 Medical Science Bldg.
Columbia, MO 65212   Phone: (314) 882-6172
Description: Slide/tape and videocassette programs for medical education and several allied health fields are produced and distributed for sale.

★6673★ UNIVERSITY OF MISSOURI—KANSAS CITY
SCHOOL OF DENTISTRY
BIOMEDICAL COMMUNICATIONS
650 E. 25th St., Rm. 260M
Kansas City, MO 64108-2795   Phone: (816) 235-2070
Description: Distributes slides and videocassettes which have been produced for dental and dental hygiene education.

★6674★ UNIVERSITY OF MISSOURI—KANSAS CITY
SCHOOL OF MEDICINE
OFFICE OF EDUCATIONAL RESOURCES
2411 Holmes St.
Kansas City, MO 64108   Phone: (816) 235-1830
Description: Produces and distributes films, videocassettes, audiocassettes, and slides on a broad range of medical specialties.

★6675★ UNIVERSITY OF NEBRASKA
MEDICAL CENTER
BIOMEDICAL COMMUNICATIONS DEPARTMENT
600 S. 42nd St.
Omaha, NE 68198-5170   Phone: (402) 559-7100
Description: Produces and distributes videocassettes, printed materials, and slide/tape packages for professional and public health sciences education; special focus on problems of the developmentally disabled.

★6676★ UNIVERSITY OF NEBRASKA MEDICAL CENTER
MEYER REHABILITATION INSTITUTE
MEDIA RESOURCE CENTER
600 S. 42nd St.
Omaha, NE 68198-5450   Phone: (402) 559-7467
Description: Produces and distributes videotapes and slide/tape programs dealing with children's developmental disabilities and other chronic handicapping conditions. Designed for use by parents, students and medical professionals. Available for rental or purchase.

★6677★ UNIVERSITY OF NEW MEXICO
SCHOOL OF MEDICINE
BIOMEDICAL COMMUNICATIONS
Albuquerque, NM 87131   Phone: (505) 277-3633
Description: Produces and distributes, for purchase only, videotapes for medical and allied health professionals.

★6678★ UNIVERSITY OF NORTH DAKOTA
MEDICAL CENTER REHABILITATION HOSPITAL AND
   CLINICS
1300 S. Columbia Rd.
Grand Forks, ND 58201   Phone: (701) 780-2311
Description: Videotape and slide/tape programs relating to rehabilitation of the physically handicapped are available for rental or purchase.

★6679★ UNIVERSITY OF OKLAHOMA
HEALTH SCIENCES CENTER
DEPARTMENT OF TELEVISION SERVICES
PO Box 26901
Oklahoma City, OK 73190   Phone: (405) 271-2318
Description: Videotape programs for medical education are available for purchase.

★6680★ UNIVERSITY OF THE PACIFIC
SCHOOL OF DENTISTRY
COMMUNICATION SERVICES
2155 Webster St., Rm. 103
San Francisco, CA 94115   Phone: (415) 929-6584
Description: Offers photos and slides, primarily aimed at education of dental undergraduates. Services include photography; graphic design; and computer slide design, production, and slide duping.

★6681★ UNIVERSITY OF PITTSBURGH
CREATIVE SERVICES
230 McKee Pl., Ste. 102
Pittsburgh, PA 15213   Phone: (412) 624-5050
Description: Provides a variety of audiovisual services to six schools of the health sciences at the University, affiliated hospitals, and not-for-profit health-related agencies. These services include photography, slide/tape programs, producing audio and videotapes, and graphic design.

★6682★ UNIVERSITY OF PITTSBURGH
WESTERN PSYCHIATRIC INSTITUTE AND CLINIC LIBRARY
BENEDUM AUDIOVISUAL CENTER
3811 O'Hara St.
Pittsburgh, PA 15213   Phone: (412) 624-1920
Description: Loans videocassettes on a wide range of mental health-related issu es. Media collection is designed for mental health professionals and students in the healthcare professions. Secondary groups of intended users are the regional mental health agencies, hospitals, schools, and other institutions.

★6683★ UNIVERSITY OF SOUTH ALABAMA
SOUTH ALABAMA MEDICAL SCIENCE FOUNDATION
CSAB, Rm. 104
Mobile, AL 36688   Phone: (205) 460-6041
Description: Produces and distributes a biosafety training video for professionals working with human biohazardous material. Available for purchase.

★6684★ UNIVERSITY OF SOUTHERN CALIFORNIA
SCHOOL OF MEDICINE
BIOMEDICAL COMMUNICATIONS
1975 Zonal Ave., KAM 205A
Los Angeles, CA 90033   Phone: (213) 342-1502
Description: Produces health care-related audiovisual materials and offers illustration, photography, and production services to the health care community.

★6685★ UNIVERSITY OF TEXAS
M.D. ANDERSON CANCER CENTER
DEPARTMENT OF BIOMEDICAL COMMUNICATIONS
1515 Holcombe, MDA-TV, 126
Houston, TX 77030   Phone: (713) 792-7287
Description: Videocassettes, slide/tape programs, and 16mm films on oncology and cancer-related topics are distributed to health professionals and patients. All are available for rental and sale.

★6686★ UNIVERSITY OF TEXAS HEALTH SCIENCE CENTER
AT SAN ANTONIO
DEPARTMENT OF CELLULAR AND STRUCTURAL BIOLOGY
7703 Floyd Curl Dr.
San Antonio, TX 78284-7762   Phone: (512) 567-3900
Description: Videotaped displays of human anatomy prosections are distributed for sale.

★6687★ UNIVERSITY OF TEXAS SOUTHWESTERN MEDICAL
CENTER AT DALLAS
BIOMEDICAL COMMUNICATIONS DEPARTMENT
Medical Television Center, Rm. E1-500
5323 Harry Hines Blvd.
Dallas, TX 75235   Phone: (214) 688-3692
Description: A full service video unit is available.

★6688★ UNIVERSITY OF TORONTO
MEDIA CENTRE
121 St. George St.
Toronto, ON, Canada M5S 1A1   Phone: (416) 978-6049
Description: Produces and distributes, for rental and sale, videotapes, films, and slide/tape programs on a variety of subjects, including health sciences, medicine, nursing, and pharmacy.

★6689★ UNIVERSITY OF VERMONT
OFFICE OF HEALTH PROMOTION RESEARCH
235 Rowell Bldg.
Burlington, VT 05405   Phone: (802) 656-4187
Description: Offers, for rental or sale, several educational videocassettes dealing with lung disease.

★6690★ UNIVERSITY OF VIRGINIA
MEDICAL CENTER
MEDICAL TELEVISION SERVICES
Box 418
Charlottesville, VA 22908   Phone: (804) 924-9100
Description: Provides a full range of production, equipment repair, and maintenance services.

★6691★ UNIVERSITY OF WASHINGTON
CHILD DEVELOPMENT AND MENTAL RETARDATION
CENTER
CDMRC MEDIA
Seattle, WA 98195   Phone: (206) 543-4011
Description: Videotapes and slide/tape presentations relating to child development and mental retardation are available for rental or purchase.

★6692★ UNIVERSITY OF WASHINGTON
HEALTH SCIENCES CENTER FOR EDUCATIONAL
RESOURCES
T281 Health Science Bldg., SB-56
Seattle, WA 98195   Phone: (206) 685-1186
Description: Produces and distributes slide/tape programs for medical and allied health education. Topics include laboratory animal medicine and science, nursing, hematology, and professional and continuing education.

★6693★ UNIVERSITY OF WASHINGTON
INSTRUCTIONAL MEDIA SERVICES
35 D Kane Hall, DG-10
Seattle, WA 98195   Phone: (206) 543-9909
Description: Offers rental 16mm films and videocassettes on a wide range of subjects, including many topics relating to health and medicine.

★6694★ UNIVERSITY OF WASHINGTON PRESS
4045 Brooklyn Ave., NE
Seattle, WA 98105   Phone: (206) 543-4050
Description: Produces and distributes films, slides, videotapes, and audiotapes in medicine, allied health, and nursing as part of the Life Sciences series. Programs are available for rent.

★6695★ UNIVERSITY OF WISCONSIN—MADISON
BUREAU OF AUDIOVISUAL INSTRUCTION
1327 University Ave.
PO Box 2093
Madison, WI 53715-2499   Phone: (608) 262-1644
Description: Film and video rental service includes medical, allied health, and mental health topics.

★6696★ UNIVERSITY OF WISCONSIN—MADISON
CENTER FOR HEALTH SCIENCES
OFFICE OF EDUCATIONAL RESOURCES
1300 University Ave., Rm. 4285 MSC
Madison, WI 53706   Phone: (608) 263-4713
Description: Health education programs on videotape and slide tape include basic science and clinical science topics. Programs are available for preview and purchase.

★6697★ UNIVERSITY OF WISCONSIN—MADISON
SCHOOL OF NURSING
CONTINUING EDUCATION IN NURSING
600 Highland Ave.
Madison, WI 53792   Phone: (608) 262-0566
Description: Distributes, for sale, self-instructional audiocassettes for nursing education.

★6698★ UNIVERSITY OF WYOMING
AUDIO VISUAL SERVICE
PO Box 3273, University Sta.
Laramie, WY 82071   Phone: (307) 766-3184
Description: Rental film service includes programs for use in medical, nursing, and allied health education.

★6699★ UPJOHN COMPANY
7000 Portage Rd.
Kalamazoo, MI 49001   Phone: (616) 323-4000
Description: Films for medical and allied health professionals are available for purchase or loan; also a small collection of patient education films.

★6700★ VANGUARD PRODUCTIONS
7064 Huntley Rd.
Columbus, OH 43229   Phone: (614) 436-4610
Description: Produces video programs for a variety of clients, including those in the medical field.

★6701★ VICTORIA HOSPITAL CORPORATION
DEPARTMENT OF VISUAL SERVICES
375 South St.
London, ON, Canada N6A 4G5   Phone: (519) 667-6502
Description: Produces customized VHS videos and computer generated slides on various medical topics.

★6702★ VIDA HEALTH COMMUNICATIONS
6 Bigleow St.
Cambridge, MA 02139   Phone: (617) 864-4334
Description: Produces and sells videos for patients and professionals on the subjects of parenting, peri-natal substance abuse, childbirth, and AIDS.

★6703★ VIDEO FARM
156 Drakes Ln.
Box 12, The Farm
Summertown, TN 38483-2519   Phone: (615) 964-3574
Description: Offers, for rental or sale, instructional videotapes and films of childbirth techniques.

★6704★ VIDEO TRAINING RESOURCE, INC.
7900 W. 78th St., Ste. 250
Edina, MN 55439   Phone: (612) 829-1555
Description: Distributes and produces complete video training courses for patient care technical assignments in the pre-hospital areas. Also available are programs on chemical hazards and training the trainer.

★6705★ VIDEOLEARNING SYSTEMS, INC.
354 W. Lancaster Ave., Ste. 105
Haverford, PA 19041   Phone: (215) 896-6600
Description: Distributes videotapes in the areas of patient relations, supervisory training, and fire prevention/safety in healthcare facilities; stress management; substance abuse; and AIDS in the workplace. Available for preview, rental, lease, or purchase. Toll free number: (800) 622-3610.

★6706★ VIDEOMED
5109 Ridge Rd.
Minneapolis, MN 55436   Phone: (612) 938-6994
Description: Offers videotape and laserdisc patient education systems to health and medical professionals on eye, infertility, and gynecological problems. Also offers custom production of educational, sales training, product introduction, and interactive multi-media projects related to the health field. Toll-free number: (800) 332-0633.

★6707★ VIDEOSURGERY LTD.
c/o Dr. Robert A. Chase
Stanford University
Dept. of Surgery
Stanford, CA 94305   Phone: (415) 725-6618
Description: Produces and distributes videocassettes covering a wide range of surgeries.

★6708★ VIRGINIA COMMONWEALTH UNIVERSITY
MEDICAL COLLEGE OF VIRGINIA
VIRGINIA HOSPITAL TELEVISION NETWORK
Office of Medical Education
Box 48
Richmond, VA 23298   Phone: (804) 786-0494
Description: Produces videotapes of videoconferences on health care topics. Available for sale.

★6709★ VIRGINIA COMMONWEALTH UNIVERSITY
UNIVERSITY LIBRARY SERVICES
MEDIA PRODUCTION SERVICES
P.O. Box 62, MCV Station
Richmond, VA 23298-0062   Phone: (804) 786-9590
Description: Produces medical, allied health, and patient education materials for Virginia Commonwealth University and other state agencies.

★6710★ VISTAR VIDEO
4567 E. 9th Ave.
Denver, CO 80220   Phone: (303) 320-2121
Description: Offers, for rental or sale, videotape programs for patient and hospital staff education.

★6711★ VISUAL INFORMATION SYSTEMS INC.
1 Harmon Plaza
Secaucus, NJ 07094   Phone: (201) 867-7600
Description: Produces and distributes videotapes and audiocassettes covering the medical field.

★6712★ VISUCOM PRODUCTIONS, INC.
PO Box 5472
Redwood City, CA 94063   Phone: (415) 364-5566
Description: Produces and distributes videotapes specializing in health and safety training programs. Available for preview, purchase or rental. Toll-free number: (800) 222-4002.

★6713★ VOICE TAPES, INC.
PO Box 5772
Bellingham, WA 98227   Phone: (206) 647-3737
Description: Produces and distributes educational videotapes and audio-cassettes covering speech-language pathology, audiology, and related fields. All video programs come with an instructional manual for preview, purchase or rental.

★6714★ W.B. SAUNDERS COMPANY
Curtis Center
Independence Sq., W.
Philadelphia, PA 19106   Phone: (215) 238-7800
Description: Anatomy, dentistry, audiology, and medical specialties are among the topics of slides and filmstrips produced and distributed for professionals.

★6715★ WAKE FOREST UNIVERSITY
BOWMAN GRAY SCHOOL OF MEDICINE
Medical Center Blvd.
Winston-Salem, NC 27157-1069   Phone: (919) 748-4691
Description: Distributes slide/tape programs on radiographic anatomy for medical students.

★6716★ WALTER J. KLEIN COMPANY, LTD.
6311 Carmel Rd.
PO Box 2087
Charlotte, NC 28247-2087   Phone: (704) 542-1403
Description: Produces and distributes films and videotapes for general audiences, from children to adults, on a variety of topics, including food and nutrition, and health. Films are offered for 24 hour free-loan or for purchase.

★6717★ WALTER REED ARMY MEDICAL CENTER
WRAMC-TV
Rm. 1063, Bldg. 54
Washington, DC 20306-6000   Phone: (202) 576-2878
Description: Videotape productions designed for the professional WRAMC staff. Some titles are available for public non-profit exhibition and medical education purposes. Programs are available for duplication onto 3/4 inch videocassette or 1/2 inch VHS; requesting institute provides blank tape stock and return postage.

★6718★ WARD'S NATURAL SCIENCE ESTABLISHMENT, INC.
5100 W. Henrietta Rd.
PO Box 92912
Rochester, NY 14692   Phone: (716) 359-2502
Description: Distributes slides and transparencies on human biological systems; also manufactures models, skeletons, and prepared microscope slides for histology and parasitology.

★6719★ WASHINGTON STATE UNIVERSITY
INSTRUCTIONAL MEDIA SERVICES
Pullman, WA 99164-5602   Phone: (509) 335-5618
Description: Loans educational films on a wide range of topics, including medicine and health.

★6720★   WASHINGTON UNIVERSITY
GEORGE W. BROWN SCHOOL OF SOCIAL WORK
LEARNING RESOURCES VIDEO CENTER
Campus Box 1196
St. Louis, MO 63130   Phone: (314) 889-6612
Description: Produces and distributes 1/2 and 3/4 inch videotapes on a variety of medical topics including health care, diabetes, sudden infant death syndrome, heart attack, mental health, and child development; also offers a training package for child abuse workers. Available for rental or purchase.

★6721★   WAYNE STATE UNIVERSITY
COLLEGE OF NURSING
DENT PROJECT
5557 Cass Ave.
Detroit, MI 48202   Phone: (313) 577-4082
Description: Instructional audiovisual materials for use in nursing education are issued on videotape and 16mm film formats. Sale, rental, and preview terms are available.

★6722★   WAYNE STATE UNIVERSITY
MEDIA LIBRARY
5265 Cass
Detroit, MI 48202   Phone: (313) 577-1980
Description: Instructional audiovisual materials in basic medical science, physical diagnosis, and pediatrics and nursing can be rented. Types of media include film, slides, video- and audiotapes.

★6723★   WELLBEING BOOKS
PO Box 396
Newtonville, MA 02146   Phone: (617) 232-8585
Description: Offers audiocassettes on health and technology.

★6724★   WEST GLEN FILMS
1430 Broadway
New York, NY 10018   Phone: (212) 921-0966
Description: Films, slides, and videocassettes are available for free loan, rental, and purchase. Topics include health, medicine, and nutrition.

★6725★   WESTERN MICHIGAN UNIVERSITY
MEDIA SERVICES
1450 Dunbar Hall
Kalamazoo, MI 49008-5001   Phone: (616) 387-5000
Description: Produces and distributes video programs for allied health care professionals; topics include communication disorders of infants and adults, geriatrics and physicians assistants programs, health promotion and disease prevention, reproductive health and sexuality, and multidisciplinary diagnostic clinical programs devoted to evaluation of multi-handicapped children and adults.

★6726★   WEXLER FILM PRODUCTIONS
801 N. Seward St.
Los Angeles, CA 90038   Phone: (213) 462-6671
Description: Producer of films and videos for health professionals and patient education.

★6727★   WHALLEY & ASSOCIATES
2005 Palo Verde Ave., Ste. 210
Long Beach, CA 90815   Phone: (213) 799-1477
Description: Distributes films and videocassettes on a variety of subjects, including alcohol and drug abuse, handicaps, aging, and health.

★6728★   WINTHROP-BREON LABORATORIES
90 Park Ave.
New York, NY 10016   Phone: (212) 907-2000
Description: Educational films for physicians and nursing personnel are available for preview and purchase.

★6729★   WNET/THIRTEEN
356 W. 58th St.
New York, NY 10019   Phone: (212) 560-2000
Description: Produces a variety of television shows for PBS, some of which are available on videocassette; topics include comprehensive explorations of the brain and the mind.

★6730★   WOMEN MAKE MOVIES, INC.
225 Lafayette St., No. 211
New York, NY 10012   Phone: (212) 925-0606
Description: Organization is devoted to the distribution of media by and about women. Films and videotapes on a wide range of subjects, including a number of health-related topics, are available for rental or sale.

★6731★   WOODY CLARK PRODUCTIONS, INC.
1024 Warfield Ave.
Oakland, CA 94103   Phone: (510) 451-1668
Description: Health-related films and videos include a Norman Cousins series on health, heart attack, and cancer, as well as a documentary on his positive attitude philosophy. Also offers a film on the issue of age discrimination in the workplace.

★6732★   WRS MOTION PICTURE AND VIDEO LABORATORY
1000 Napor Blvd.
Pittsburgh, PA 15205   Phone: (412) 937-7700
Description: A complete motion picture and video laboratory offering processing, duplication, tape-to-film, film-to-tape, distribution and fulfillment, and captioning services to a variety of clients, including those in medical and health-related fields. Toll-free number: (800) 345-6977.

★6733★   YALE UNIVERSITY
SCHOOL OF MEDICINE
Communications Media 1-E96
333 Cedar St.
New Haven, CT 06510   Phone: (203) 785-2647
Description: Produces and distributes films and videotapes for health science education.

(8) Computer-Readable Databases

Entries listed below are arranged alphabetically by database names. See the User's Guide located at the front of this directory for additional information.

★6734★   A.M. BEST LIFE/HEALTH INSURANCE COMPANIES
A.M. Best Co.
Best DataBase Services
Ambest Rd.
Oldwick, NJ 08858   Phone: (908) 439-2200
General Description: Provides financial information for more than 1400 life and health insurance companies. Includes expenses, operating and financial ratios, balance sheet flow of funds, business by line and state, income and operating statements, marketing results, investment results, and loss reserve development. **Language of Database:** English. **Subject Coverage:** The financial aspects of operating life and health insurance companies.

★6735★   ABDA-PHARMA
Bundesvereinigung Deutscher Apothekerverbande
Postfach 970108
D-6000 Frankfurt am Main 97, Germany
General Description: Covers drug preparations marketed in Germany. Provides information on manufacturer, dosage form, and qualitative composition for drugs marketed in other European countries, the United States, and Japan. **Language of Database:** German. **Subject Coverage:** Pharmaceutical drugs, drug ingredients, and manufacturers.

★6736★   ABLEDATA
Newington Children's Hospital
Adaptive Equipment Center
181 E. Cedar St.
Newington, CT 06111   Phone: (203) 667-5405
General Description: Contains descriptions of more than 17,000 commercially available products made available by 2200 manufacturers for rehabilitation and independent living. **Language of Database:** English. **Subject Coverage:** Rehabilitation aids and equipment for personal care, home management, mobility, communication, and vocational, educational, and therapeutic needs.

★6737★   ACCENT ON INFORMATION (AOI)
Accent on Living
Gillum Rd. and High Dr.
PO Box 700
Bloomington, IL 61702   Phone: (309) 378-2961
General Description: Provides abstracts of documents in more than 400 subject areas of interest to the handicapped, including persons with disabilities, their relatives, and rehabilitation professionals. **Language of Database:** English. **Subject Coverage:** All subjects pertaining to the physically handicapped, including eating, feeding, bathing, clothing, toilet, mobility problems and aids, architectural barriers, homemaking, communications, recreation, travel, education, and sexual adjustment.

★6738★   ADONIS
PO Box 839
NL-1000 Amsterdam, Netherlands
General Description: Contains the complete text of all issues of 437 biomedical journal titles published worldwide. **Subject Coverage:** Biomedical sciences, including biology, chemistry, medicine, pharmacology, physics, veterinary medicine, and general science.

★6739★   ADVANCED MEDICAL INFORMATION SERVICES
AMS Corp.
2-6-2 Marunouchi, Chiyoda-ku
Tokyo 100, Japan
General Description: Provides medical and health-related news, literature references, and other information and electronic services for physicians, hospital administrators, and public health officials in Japan. Includes press releases from public agencies, infectious disease surveillance alerts, adverse drug reaction reports, health care products recalls, and other items of interest to health care workers. Offers information on approximately 160,000 therapeutic drugs. **Language of Database:** Japanese. **Subject Coverage:** Japanese health and medical industry.

★6740★   AFTERCARE INSTRUCTIONS
Micromedex, Inc.
600 Grant St.
Denver, CO 80203-3527   Phone: (303) 831-1400
General Description: Provides instructions for health care professionals to distribute to patients regarding the care of illnesses and injuries after discharge from the hospital or clinic. Includes brief information on 30 generic drugs specific to the emergency department or clinic setting. Enables the user to print 620 different aftercare documents in 22 subject categories, and more than 340 drug information leaflets for patients from an optional United States Pharmacopeia Dispensing Information (USP-DI) component. **Language of Database:** English; Spanish. **Subject Coverage:** Patient instructions for the aftercare of injuries and illnesses, including information on drugs.

★6741★   AGE BASE
The Brookdale Foundation Group
126 E. 56th St.
New York, NY 10022   Phone: (212) 308-7355
General Description: Contains information on direct service programs for the elderly. **Language of Database:** English. **Subject Coverage:** Service programs for the elderly, including programs for the home-bound elderly, health promotion programs for seniors, and senior citizen classes.

★6742★   AGELINE
American Association of Retired Persons (AARP)
National Gerontology Resource Center
601 E St., NW
Washington, DC 20049   Phone: (202) 434-6231
General Description: Provides citations and abstracts of journal articles, books, and reports concerning the sociological, psychological, economic, and political aspects of aging. **Also Known as:** AARP Database. **Language of Database:** English. **Subject Coverage:** Middle age and aging, including

aging and the future, demographics, economics, financial planning and pensions, retirement and retirement planning, family caregiving, health care services and costs, housing, intergenerational relationships, longterm care and nursing homes, mental and physical health assessment, nutrition and exercise, psychology of aging, public policy and legislation, services for older adults, social and family relationships, Social Security, Medicare and Medicaid, and theories of aging.

★6743★ **AGENCIES: AN INTERNATIONAL GUIDE FOR VISUALLY DISABLED PEOPLE**
Royal National Institute for the Blind
Technical Development Department
224 Great Portland St.
London W1N 6AA, England
General Description: Provides descriptions and contact information for national agencies providing services for visually disabled people worldwide. **Language of Database:** English. **Subject Coverage:** National agencies worldwide serving the blind and visually impaired.

★6744★ **AGRICOLA**
U.S. National Agricultural Library
10301 Baltimore Blvd.
Beltsville, MD 20705   Phone: (301) 344-3813
General Description: Contains complete bibliographic and cataloging information for all monographs and serials received at the National Agricultural Library and indexing records for articles from agricultural literature. **Also Known as:** Agricultural Online Access. **Language of Database:** English. **Subject Coverage:** All aspects of agricultural sciences, including agricultural economics, rural sociology, agricultural engineering, agricultural products, animal husbandry, animal welfare, energy in agriculture, botany, entomology, food and human nutrition, forestry, pesticides, plant and animal sciences, soils and fertilizers, veterinary medicine, chemistry, and environmental pollution.

★6745★ **AHA ANNUAL SURVEY OF HOSPITALS**
American Hospital Association (AHA)
Hospital Data Center
840 N. Lake Shore Dr.
Chicago, IL 60611   Phone: (312) 280-6000
General Description: Profiles the facilities and services of more than 7000 U.S. hospitals. **Language of Database:** English. **Subject Coverage:** Hospital facilities and services, utilization, hospital expenses, and staffing.

★6746★ **AIDS CLINICAL CARE**
Massachusetts Medical Society
Medical Publishing Group
1440 Main St.
Waltham, MA 02254   Phone: (617) 893-3800
General Description: Provides information on the clinical aspects of Acquired Immune Deficiency Syndrome (AIDS). **Language of Database:** English. **Subject Coverage:** Acquired Immune Deficiency Syndrome.

★6747★ **AIDS DAILY SUMMARY**
BT North America, Inc.
2560 N. 1st St.
PO Box 49019
San Jose, CA 95161-9019   Phone: (408) 922-0250
General Description: Covers developments in Acquired Immune Deficiency Syndrome (AIDS) research, treatment, and policy. Provides references and summaries to relevant material appearing in journals, magazines, and other sources. **Language of Database:** English. **Subject Coverage:** Acquired Immune Deficiency Syndrome, including public policy, population, and research; human resources; precedent-setting legislation and litigation; education, prevention, and treatment; and confidentiality and discrimination.

★6748★ **AIDS DATABASE**
Bureau of Hygiene and Tropical Diseases
Keppel St.
London WC1E 7HT, England
General Description: Provides citations and abstracts of published materials covering all aspects of Acquired Immune Deficiency Syndrome (AIDS), the HTLV-I and -II viruses, and human immunodeficiency viruses (HIV). **Language of Database:** English. **Subject Coverage:** All aspects of AIDS and other related immunodeficiency viruses, including transmission, epidemiology, immunology, pathology, etiology, research, clinical aspects, serology, treatment, control, public health policy and education, and behavioral aspects.

★6749★ **AIDS INFORMATION AND EDUCATION WORLDWIDE**
CD Resources, Inc.
118 W. 74th St., Ste. 2A
New York, NY 10023   Phone: (212) 580-2263
General Description: Contains the complete text of more than 300 publications, articles, technical reports, and case studies covering all aspects of Acquired Immune Deficiency Syndrome (AIDS). Includes abstracts and bibliographic citations for each document. **Language of Database:** English. **Subject Coverage:** Acquired Immune Deficiency Syndrome, including medical aspects, biology and epidemiology, consumer health, treatment and care in and out of institutions, geography, attitudinal and behavioral change, legislation, control, and prevention.

★6750★ **AIDS KNOWLEDGE BASE**
Massachusetts Medical Society
Medical Publishing Group
1440 Main St.
Waltham, MA 02254   Phone: (617) 893-4610
General Description: Provides information and guidelines on the treatment of Acquired Immune Deficiency Syndrome (AIDS) as established by physicians at San Francisco General Hospital. Covers new developments and practices in all areas of the diagnosis and treatment of AIDS. **Also Known as:** AIDS Knowledge Base from San Francisco General Hospital. **Language of Database:** English. **Subject Coverage:** Acquired Immune Deficiency Syndrome, including new developments and practices in the areas of epidemiology, pathogenesis, diagnosis, prevention and treatment strategies, and societal and psychological implications.

★6751★ **AIDS NEWSLETTER**
Bureau of Hygiene and Tropical Diseases
Keppel St.
London WC1E 7HT, England
General Description: Reports news and developments concerning all aspects of Acquired Immune Deficiency Syndrome (AIDS), the HTVL-I and -II viruses, and human immunodeficiency viruses (HIV). Contains synopses of important news stories from the United Kingdom and elsewhere, commentaries on the latest social, occupational, and scientific developments, and notices of relevant publications and meetings. **Language of Database:** English. **Subject Coverage:** All aspects of AIDS and other related immunodeficiency viruses, including medical, social, statistical, and other scientific trends.

★6752★ **AIDS POLICY AND LAW**
The Bureau of National Affairs, Inc. (BNA)
BNA ONLINE
1231 25th St., NW
Washington, DC 20037   Phone: (202) 452-4132
General Description: Focuses on the practical and legal issues of Acquired Immune Deficiency Syndrome (AIDS) through coverage of the latest developments at the federal, state, and local levels. Discusses what employers are doing, insurance company problems, how testing is being used, pending legislation, and active and potential court cases. **Language of Database:** English. **Subject Coverage:** AIDS and its impact on employment, insurance, schools, housing, medical care, and other areas.

★6753★ **AIDS SCHOOL HEALTH EDUCATION DATABASE**
U.S. Centers for Disease Control
Center for Chronic Disease Prevention and Health Promotion
1600 Clifton Rd., Bldg. 1/SSB-249/MS-A34
Atlanta, GA 30333   Phone: (404) 639-3492
General Description: Contains bibliographic descriptions of published materials dealing with promoting education and awareness among students on the subject of Acquired Immune Deficiency Syndrome (AIDS). **Language of Database:** English. **Subject Coverage:** Educational materials covering Acquired Immune Deficiency Syndrome (AIDS).

★6754★ **AIDSCAN**
Ryerson Polytechnical Institute Library
350 Victoria St.
Toronto, ON, Canada M5B 2K3   Phone: (416) 979-5083
General Description: Contains citations and abstracts of materials held in the Ryerson Polytechnical Institute Library relating to concerns of health care workers and psychosocial aspects of caring for Acquired Immune Deficiency Syndrome (AIDS) patients. **Language of Database:** English. **Subject Coverage:** Psychosocial aspects involving the care of AIDS patients.

★6755★ AIDSDRUGS
U.S. National AIDS Information Clearinghouse
AIDS Clinical Trials Information Service (ACTIS)
PO Box 6421
Rockville, MD 20850
General Description: Provides current information on the safety and efficacy of drugs and vaccines being tested as treatment against AIDS (Acquired Immune Deficiency Syndrome) and related diseases. Maintained as part of the ACTIS internal database. Serves as a companion file to AIDSTRIALS (described in a separate entry). **Language of Database:** English. **Subject Coverage:** Experimental drugs and vaccines for treatment of Acquired Immune Deficiency Syndrome.

★6756★ AIDSLINE
U.S. National Library of Medicine
MEDLARS Management Section
8600 Rockville Pike
Bethesda, MD 20894   Phone: (301) 496-6193
General Description: Provides references to the world's medical journal literature dealing with AIDS (Acquired Immune Deficiency Syndrome), focusing on the biomedical, epidemiologic, and social and behavioral aspects of the disease. **Language of Database:** English. **Subject Coverage:** Acquired Immune Deficiency Syndrome, including research and clinical aspects, epidemiology, social and behavioral issues, and health policy.

★6757★ AIDSTRIALS
U.S. National AIDS Information Clearinghouse
AIDS Clinical Trials Information Service (ACTIS)
PO Box 6421
Rockville, MD 20850
General Description: Provides current information on clinical trials of drugs and vaccines as treatment against AIDS (Acquired Immune Deficiency Syndrome) and related diseases. Describes the general criteria for participating in the trials. Maintained as part of the ACTIS internal database. Serves as a companion file to AIDSDRUGS (described in a separate entry). **Language of Database:** English. **Subject Coverage:** Clinical trials of drugs and vaccines for treatment of Acquired Immune Deficiency Syndrome.

★6758★ ALCOHOL AND ALCOHOL PROBLEMS SCIENCE
  DATABASE
U.S. National Institute on Alcohol Abuse and Alcoholism
Office of Scientific Affairs
5600 Fishers Ln.
Rm. 16C-14
Rockville, MD 20857   Phone: (202) 443-3860
General Description: Provides citations and abstracts of international published and unpublished clinical and scientific literature dealing with alcohol and alcoholism. **Language of Database:** English. **Subject Coverage:** Alcoholism research, including psychology, psychiatry, physiology, biochemistry, epidemiology, sociology, animal studies, treatment, prevention, education, accidents and safety, legislation, employment, labor and industry, and public policy.

★6759★ ALCOHOL AND DRUGS IN THE WORKPLACE:
  COSTS, CONTROLS, AND CONTROVERSIES
The Bureau of National Affairs, Inc. (BNA)
BNA ONLINE
1231 25th St., NW
Washington, DC 20037   Phone: (202) 452-4132
General Description: Addresses the growing concern and controversy about drugs and alcohol in the workplace and what employers, unions, legislators, regulators, and consultants are doing about it. **Language of Database:** English. **Subject Coverage:** Alcohol and drug use in the workplace, including financial and human costs involved; identification of users; abuse control strategies; plans for combatting abuse; case studies; and laws, regulations, and legal principles.

★6760★ ALCOHOL INFORMATION FOR CLINICIANS AND
  EDUCATORS DATABASE
Dartmouth Medical School
Project CORK Institute
Hanover, NH 03756   Phone: (603) 646-7540
General Description: Contains citations and abstracts of published literature covering all aspects of alcohol use and abuse. Includes clinically relevant information from literature in the biological and social sciences. **Language of Database:** English. **Subject Coverage:** All aspects of alcohol use and abuse, including information about other drugs as related to alcohol.

★6761★ ALCOHOL USE/ABUSE
University of Minnesota - College of Pharmacy
Drug Information Services
3-160 Health Sciences Unit F
308 Harvard St., SE
Minneapolis, MN 55455   Phone: (612) 624-6492
General Description: Provides citations and abstracts of journal articles, books, and other materials covering alcoholism and chemical dependency, and related topics. **Language of Database:** English. **Subject Coverage:** Evaluation of treatment for alcoholism/chemical dependency; the chemically-dependent female; alcoholism among the elderly and adolescents; family therapy, counselor and clergy training, and industry programs.

★6762★ ALCONARC
Centralforbundet for Alkohol- och Narkotikaupplysning
PO Box 27302
S-102 54 Stockholm, Sweden
General Description: Contains complete bibliographic descriptions and holdings information for books, technical reports, conference proceedings, and theses acquired by the CAN Library. **Language of Database:** English; Swedish; Norwegian; Danish. **Subject Coverage:** Alcohol and drug dependence and related topics.

★6763★ ALCONLINE
Centralforbundet for Alkohol- och Narkotikaupplysning
PO Box 27302
S-102 54 Stockholm, Sweden
General Description: Provides citations and abstracts of literature and research projects covering drug abuse and alcoholism and their effects on transportation and traffic safety. Comprises selections from the DALCTRAF and NORDRUG databases, each of which is described in a separate entry. **Language of Database:** English. **Subject Coverage:** Alcohol and drug dependence and related topics.

★6764★ ALLIED AND ALTERNATIVE MEDICINE
British Library
Medical Information Service
Boston Spa
Wetherby, W. Yorks LS23 7BQ, England
General Description: Contains citations and abstracts of biomedical journal literature and relevant articles published in other journals, newspapers, or books. **Language of Database:** English. **Subject Coverage:** Allied and alternative medicine, including acupuncture, homeopathy, hypnosis, chiropractic, osteopathy, psychotherapy, diet therapy, herbalism, holistic treatment, traditional Chinese medicine, occupational therapy, physiotherapy, rehabilitation, ayurdevic medicine, reflexology, iridology, moxibustion, meditation, yoga, healing research, and the Alexander technique.

★6765★ ALZHEIMER'S DISEASE DATABASE (AZ)
U.S. National Institute on Aging
Alzheimer's Disease Education and Referral Center
PO Box 8250
Silver Spring, MD 20907-8250   Phone: (301) 495-3311
General Description: Contains references to books, journal articles, and other published literature dealing with Alzheimer's disease. **Language of Database:** English. **Subject Coverage:** Alzheimer's disease, including clinical aspects, research projects, and resources.

★6766★ AMERICAN FAMILY PHYSICIAN
American Academy of Family Physicians
8880 Ward Pkwy.
Kansas City, MO 64114
General Description: Contains the complete text of articles in American Family Physician, a monthly journal for doctors practicing family medicine. Includes all images, tables, and figures from the original articles. **Language of Database:** English. **Subject Coverage:** Family medicine, including diagnostic and therapeutic techniques and developments in medicine.

★6767★ AMERICAN MEDICAL DIRECTORY
American Medical Association (AMA)
515 N. State St.
Chicago, IL 60610   Phone: (312) 645-5000
General Description: Provides professional and personal information for physicians practicing medicine in the United States. Covers both AMA members and nonmembers. **Language of Database:** English. **Subject Coverage:** Physicians, including non-federal physicians, physicians in military service, physicians practicing in government agencies, physicians

in the U.S. Public Health Service, and U.S. physicians temporarily residing outside the United States.

★6768★   AMERICAN PRINTING HOUSE FOR THE BLIND CENTRAL AUTOMATED RESOURCE LIST (APH-CARL)
American Printing House for the Blind
1839 Frankfort Ave.
PO Box 6085
Louisville, KY 40206-0085   Phone: (502) 895-2405
General Description: Provides information on materials for educating blind and visually impaired students. Covers more than 20,000 books available from volunteer and commercial producers. Enables the user to place federal orders for materials online. **Language of Database:** English. **Subject Coverage:** Educational materials for blind and visually impaired students, including braille, large type, and recorded books.

★6769★   THE AMERICAN PSYCHO/INFO EXCHANGE (AMPIE)
PO Box 20533
New York, NY 10025   Phone: (212) 864-5838
General Description: Contains information regarding mental health issues, current literature and text reviews, and online questionnaires for ongoing research. Provides facilities for electronic mail and special-interest bulletin boards as well as copies of public domain software programs. **Language of Database:** English. **Subject Coverage:** Mental health, including aging, alcoholism, child and adolescent disorders, clergy, drug addiction, eating disorders, forensic science, measurement, neuropsychology, psychopathology, psychopharmacology, psychotherapy, sexuality, teaching, and thanatology.

★6770★   AMERICAN RHEUMATISM ASSOCIATION MEDICAL INFORMATION SYSTEM (ARAMIS)
701 Welch Rd., Ste. 3301
Palo Alto, CA 94304   Phone: (415) 723-7814
General Description: Contains clinical and investigative data on different types of rheumatic diseases. Data are based on 24,000 patients, 150,000 patient visits, and 75,000 years of patient follow-up; up to 490 variables are maintained for each patient. **Language of Database:** English. **Subject Coverage:** Rheumatic diseases, with emphasis on systemic lupus erythematosus, rheumatoid arthritis, osteoarthritis, and connective tissue diseases.

★6771★   AMIA MEDICAL FORUM
American Medical Informatics Association (AMIA)
4915 St. Elmo Ave., Ste. 302
Bethesda, MD 20814   Phone: (301) 657-1291
General Description: Provides a forum for the exchange of news and information of interest to the medical community. Features real-time conferences. **Language of Database:** English. **Subject Coverage:** Medicine, including paramedics, mental health, physical therapy, surgery, neurology, drugs, codes and standards, nursing, anesthesiology, and pediatrics.

★6772★   APPLIED SOCIAL SCIENCES INDEX AND ABSTRACTS (ASSIA)
Bowker-Saur Ltd.
60 Grosvenor St.
London W1X 9DA, England
General Description: Provides news and information on social services and sociological issues, with particular emphasis on the applied aspects of the social sciences. **Language of Database:** English. **Subject Coverage:** Social sciences and services, including child development, industrial relations, social welfare, criminology, politics, child abuse, pollution, geriatrics, immigration, housing, child psychiatry, probation and prison services, nervous disorders, effects of European regulations, unemployment, social effects of television, dyslexia, public administration, illegal drugs, Acquired Immune Deficiency Syndrome (AIDS), National Health Service, retirement pensions, riots, race relations, manpower, inner city problems, rural depredation, and ethnic problems.

★6773★   AREA RESOURCE FILE (ARF)
U.S. Public Health Service
Health Resources and Services Administration
Parklawn Bldg., Rm. 8-43
5600 Fishers Ln.
Rockville, MD 20857   Phone: (301) 443-6936
General Description: Provides information on the county-by-county distribution of the health workforce and other health resources in the United States. Contains current and some historical data for health professions and data on personnel shortages; health facilities, hospitals, and nursing homes information; health training data on schools, enrollments, and graduates; population characteristics; economic data by income; utilization data, including hospital utilization levels; expenditure data, including hospital expenditures; and environment information, including land area and large animal population. **Language of Database:** English. **Subject Coverage:** Health resources in the United States, including demographics, manpower, facilities, training, utilization, expenditures, and environment.

★6774★   ARTHRITIS AND MUSCULOSKELETAL AND SKIN DISEASES DATABASE (AMS)
U.S. National Arthritis and Musculoskeletal and Skin Diseases Information Clearinghouse
Box AMS
9000 Rockville Pike
Bethesda, MD 20892   Phone: (301) 495-4484
General Description: Contains references and abstracts of print and audiovisual educational materials concerning arthritis and related rheumatic, musculoskeletal, and skin diseases. **Language of Database:** English. **Subject Coverage:** Arthritis and related rheumatic, musculoskeletal, and skin diseases.

★6775★   ARZTE ZEITUNG DATENBANK
Arzte Zeitung Verlagsgesellschaft mbH
Am Forsthaus Gravenbruch 5
D-6078 Neu-Isenburg 2, Germany
General Description: Contains the complete text of the Arzte-Zeitung, a daily newspaper covering the general field of medicine and health-related sciences. **Language of Database:** German. **Subject Coverage:** Medicine and health-related sciences, including current medical and clinical research, therapy, health-related social issues, office management, as well as health-related industries and individuals connected with the medical profession.

★6776★   ATOMIC VETERANS STATUS INFORMATION SYSTEM
National Association of Atomic Veterans
PO Box 4424
Salem, MA 01970   Phone: (508) 744-9396
General Description: Contains information on more than 50,000 veterans of U.S. nuclear weapons testing and Nagasaki/Hiroshima occupation forces, some of whom now have cancers and other diseases presumed to be radiation-related under Public Law 100-321. **Language of Database:** English. **Subject Coverage:** U.S. veterans exposed to ionizing radiation.

★6777★   AVLINE
U.S. National Library of Medicine
MEDLARS Management Section
8600 Rockville Pike
Bethesda, MD 20894   Phone: (301) 496-6193
General Description: Provides citations to audiovisual material in clinical medicine as cataloged by the MEDLARS. Covers motion pictures, videocassettes, and slide/cassette and filmstrip/cassette programs. **Also Known as:** Audiovisuals Online. **Language of Database:** English. **Subject Coverage:** Audiovisual material in clinical medicine, ranging from anatomy to zoology.

★6778★   BANQUE D'INFORMATIONS AUTOMATISEE SUR LES MEDICAMENTS (BIAM)
15, rue Rieux
F-92100 Boulogne, France
General Description: Provides detailed descriptions of drugs used in therapy in France. Comprises two complementary data files covering 8000 pharmaceutical products and the 2600 active ingredients used to produce them. **Language of Database:** French. **Subject Coverage:** Pharmaceutical products used in drug therapy in France.

★6779★   BANQUE D'INFORMATIONS SUR LES RECHERCHES (BIR)
France Institut National de la Sante et de la Recherche Medicale
Bureau d'Evaluation Scientifique
101, rue de Tolbiac
F-75654 Paris Cedex 13, France
General Description: Provides descriptions of ongoing biomedical research projects conducted or sponsored by Institut National de la Sante et de la Recherche Medicale. **Language of Database:** French. **Subject Coverage:** Biomedical research, especially in the areas of genetic engineering, biotechnology, immunology, pharmacology, nutrition, reproduction, clinical investigations, mental health, and public health.

★6780★ BAU LITDOK
Deutsche Bundesanstalt fur Arbeitsschutz
Informations- und Dokumentationszentrum fur Arbeitsschutz
Vogelpothsweg 50-52
Postfach 17 02 02
D-4600 Dortmund 1, Germany
General Description: Provides citations and abstracts of literature covering occupational safety and health and related labor topics. **Also Known as:** Labour Safety. **Language of Database:** German. **Subject Coverage:** Occupational safety and health, including accident prevention, ergonomics, humanization of work, industrial medicine, and security technology.

★6781★ BIBLIOMED
U.S. National Library of Medicine
MEDLARS Management Section
8600 Rockville Pike
Bethesda, MD 20894   Phone: (301) 496-6193
General Description: Contains citations and abstracts to biomedical literature published worldwide. A subset of the MEDLINE database (described in a separate entry). **Language of Database:** English. **Subject Coverage:** Biomedicine.

★6782★ BIBLIOMED CARDIOLOGY SERIES
U.S. National Library of Medicine
MEDLARS Management Section
8600 Rockville Pike
Bethesda, MD 20894   Phone: (301) 496-6193
General Description: Contains citations and abstracts of worldwide literature on cardiology and cardiovascular diseases. A subset of the MEDLINE database (described in a separate entry). **Language of Database:** English. **Subject Coverage:** Cardiology and cardiovascular diseases.

★6783★ BIOBUSINESS
BIOSIS
2100 Arch St.
Philadelphia, PA 19103-1399   Phone: (215) 587-4800
General Description: Provides references and abstracts of current and retrospective published literature dealing with the business applications and economic implications of biological and biomedical research in the areas of agriculture, biotechnology, food and beverages, and pharmaceuticals. **Language of Database:** English. **Subject Coverage:** Business and economic aspects of the following life sciences areas: agriculture, animal production, biomass conversion, biotechnology, cosmetics, crop production, diet and nutrition, energy, environment, fermentation, food technology, forestry, genetic engineering, health care, industrial microbiology, medical diagnostics, medical instrumentation, occupational health, pesticides, pharmaceuticals, protein production, toxicology, veterinary science, and waste treatment.

★6784★ BIOCOMMERCE ABSTRACTS AND DIRECTORY
BioCommerce Data Ltd.
Prudential Bldgs.
95 High St.
Slough, Berks. SL1 1DH, England
General Description: Provides abstracts of commercial biotechnology news from trade journals, periodicals, and newspapers for use in business planning, science policy review, and investment analysis. Includes directory information for approximately 1800 worldwide organizations involved in biotechnology, including companies, academic groups, and financial bodies. **Language of Database:** English. **Subject Coverage:** Commercial aspects of biochemistry, genetics, immunology, microbiology, and molecular biology and their applications in such areas as agriculture, brewing, chemicals, energy, foods, health care, and waste treatment; worldwide organizations involved in biotechnology.

★6785★ BIOETHICSLINE
Georgetown University
Kennedy Institute of Ethics
Center for Bioethics
Washington, DC 20057   Phone: (202) 687-3885
General Description: Indexes and abstracts the world's English-language literature related to the ethical and public policy aspects of medicine, health care, and biomedical and behavioral research. **Language of Database:** English. **Subject Coverage:** Bioethics, including patient's rights, allocation of health care resources, human experimentation, animal experimentation, euthanasia and allowing to die, abortion, contraception, mental health therapies, genetic intervention, reproductive technologies, organ transplantation, and medical worker-patient relationship.

★6786★ BIOEXPRESS
BIOSIS
2100 Arch St.
Philadelphia, PA 19103-1399   Phone: (215) 587-4800
General Description: Contains citations to articles appearing in life science periodicals. **Language of Database:** English. **Subject Coverage:** Life sciences.

★6787★ BIOLOGICAL ABSTRACTS (BA)
BIOSIS
2100 Arch St.
Philadelphia, PA 19103-1399   Phone: (215) 587-4800
General Description: Provides references and abstracts of international biological and biomedical journal articles and other literature dealing with research in the life sciences. **Language of Database:** English. **Subject Coverage:** Life sciences dealing with animals (including humans), plants and microorganisms, including aerospace and underwater biological effects, agronomy, allergy, anatomy and histology, animal production, bacteriology, behavioral biology, biochemistry, biophysics, blood and body fluids, botany (general and systematic), cardiovascular system, chemotherapy, Circadian rhythm and other life cycles, cytology and cytochemistry, dental and oral biology, developmental biology, digestive system, disinfection and sterilization, ecology, economic botany, economic entomology, endocrine system, enzymes, evolution, food and industrial microbiology, food technology, forestry and forest products, general biology, genetics and cytogenetics, gerontology, horticulture, immunology, integumentary system, invertebra (comparative and experimental), laboratory animals, mathematical biology and statistical methods, medical and clinical microbiology, metabolism, methods and materials, microbiological apparatus, morphology and anatomy of plants, morphology and cytology of bacteria, muscle, neoplasms and neoplastic agents, nervous system, nutrition, paleobiology, paleobotany, paleozoology, palynology, parasitology, pathology, pediatrics, pest control, pharmacognosy and pharmaceutical botany, pharmacology, physical anthropology (ethnobiology), physiology and biochemistry of bacteria, physiology (general), phytopathology, plant physiology (biochemistry and biophysics), poultry production, psychiatry, public health, radiation biology, reproductive system, sense organs, skeletal system, social biology, soil microbiology, soil science, temperature (measurements, effects, and regulation), tissue culture, toxicology, urinary system and external secretions, veterinary science, and virology (general).

★6788★ BIOLOGICAL AND AGRICULTURAL INDEX
H.W. Wilson Co.
950 University Ave.
Bronx, NY 10452   Phone: (212) 588-8400
General Description: Provides citations to English-language periodical literature in the life sciences. **Language of Database:** English. **Subject Coverage:** Life sciences, including agriculture; agricultural chemicals, economics, engineering, and research; animal husbandry; biochemistry; biology; botany; cytology; ecology; entomology; environmental science; food science; forestry; genetics; horticulture; marine biology and limnology; microbiology; nutrition; physiology; plant pathology; soil science; veterinary medicine; and zoology.

★6789★ BIOLOGY DIGEST
Plexus Publishing Inc.
143 Old Marlton Pike
Medford, NJ 08055   Phone: (609) 654-6500
General Description: Contains citations and abstracts of worldwide life science literature. Covers research papers and articles published in scientific and medical journals, newspapers, and popular news magazines. **Language of Database:** English. **Subject Coverage:** Life sciences, including botany, ecology, medicine, nutrition, psychology, and zoology.

★6790★ BIOREP
Royal Netherlands Academy of Arts and Sciences
Joan Muyskenweg 25
PO Box 41950
NL-1009 DD Amsterdam, Netherlands
General Description: Provides descriptions of biotechnological research projects currently in progress in European Economic Community (EEC) countries. **Subject Coverage:** Biotechnology research.

★6791★ BIOSIS PREVIEWS
BIOSIS
2100 Arch St.
Philadelphia, PA 19103-1399   Phone: (215) 587-4800
General Description: Provides citations to international biological and biomedical journal articles and other literature dealing with research in the

life sciences. **Language of Database:** English. **Subject Coverage:** Life sciences dealing with animals (including humans), plants and microorganisms, including aerospace and underwater biological effects, agronomy, allergy, anatomy and histology, animal production, bacteriology, behavioral biology, biochemistry, biophysics, blood and body fluids, botany (general and systematic), cardiovascular system, chemotherapy, Circadian rhythm and other life cycles, cytology and cytochemistry, dental and oral biology, developmental biology, digestive system, disinfection and sterilization, ecology, economic botany, economic entomology, endocrine system, enzymes, evolution, food and industrial microbiology, food technology, forestry and forest products, general biology, genetics and cytogenetics, gerontology, horticulture, immunology, integumentary system, invertebra (comparative and experimental), laboratory animals, mathematical biology and statistical methods, medical and clinical microbiology, metabolism, methods and materials, microbiological apparatus, morphology and anatomy of plants, morphology and cytology of bacteria, muscle, neoplasms and neoplastic agents, nervous system, nutrition, paleobiology, paleobotany, paleozoology, palynology, parasitology, pathology, pediatrics, pest control, pharmacognosy and pharmaceutical botany, pharmacology, physical anthropology (ethnobiology), physiology and biochemistry of bacteria, physiology (general), phytopathology, plant physiology (biochemistry and biophysics), poultry production, psychiatry, public health, radiation biology, reproductive system, sense organs, skeletal system, social biology, soil microbiology, soil science, temperature (measurements, effects, and regulation), tissue culture, toxicology, urinary system and external secretions, veterinary science, and virology (general).

★6792★   BIOTECHNOLOGY ABSTRACTS
Derwent Publications Ltd.
Rochdale House
128 Theobalds Rd.
London WC1X 8RP, England
General Description: Provides citations and abstracts of international journal articles and patent literature dealing with all aspects of biotechnology. **Language of Database:** English. **Subject Coverage:** Biotechnology, including genetic engineering, biochemical engineering, fermentation, tissue culture, plant cell culture and breeding, biological control, downstream processing, and waste disposal.

★6793★   BIOTECHNOLOGY NEWSWATCH
McGraw-Hill, Inc.
1221 Avenue of the Americas
New York, NY 10020-1095   Phone: (212) 512-2000
General Description: Reports scientific, financial, commercial, and governmental developments in the field of biotechnology. Includes information on international patent disclosures, current literature, meetings, symposia, and courses. Features news of research, book reviews, and a calendar of events. **Language of Database:** English. **Subject Coverage:** Biotechnology, including genetic engineering, hybridoma technology, applied plant genetics, enzymology, and biomass conversion.

★6794★   BIOTECHNOLOGY RESEARCH ABSTRACTS
Cambridge Scientific Abstracts
7200 Wisconsin Ave.
Bethesda, MD 20814   Phone: (301) 961-6750
General Description: Contains citations and abstracts of international periodical and other literature covering biotechnology research ranging from basic genetic engineering to state-of-the-art applications in medical, chemical, pharmaceutical, and agricultural fields. **Language of Database:** English. **Subject Coverage:** Biotechnology research. Specific topics covered include genetic engineering, including gene manipulation, transfer, and expression; immobilization; cell culture, including algae and higher plants and animals; products of biotechnology, including interferons, vaccines, antibiotics, antitumor agents, food, amino acids, and other substances; biotechnological applications in medicine, agriculture, waste treatment, energy, chemicals, minerals, environment, and pollution; fermentation and process engineering; and hybridoma technology.

★6795★   BIRTH DEFECTS INFORMATION SYSTEM (BDIS)
Center for Birth Defects Information Services, Inc.
Dover Medical Building
Box 1776
Dover, MA 02030   Phone: (617) 785-2525
General Description: Provides clinical, diagnosis, prognosis, and related data on birth defects. Divided into two subsystems: • The Information Retrieval Facility contains t he complete text of articles that summarize the clinical features, history, complications, treatment, and prognosis of 1800 birth defects. • Micro BDIS cons ists of two files: 1) The Diagnostic Assist Facility—provides interactive decision support for differential diagnosis. Accepts case descriptions and provides a list of the best matches from a

knowledge base of more than 1000 conditions. 2) The Unknowns Registry Facility—stores clinical, demographic, and epidemiologic information on birth defect cases which do not correspond to established syndromes. The file is regularly analyzed for matches in the reported cases. **Language of Database:** English. **Subject Coverage:** Birth defects and human genetics.

★6796★   BLOOD RESOURCE DATABASE
U.S. National Heart, Lung, and Blood Institute Information Center
4733 Bethesda Ave., Ste. 530
Bethesda, MD 20814   Phone: (301) 951-3260
General Description: Contains references to published materials concerning the supply and safety of blood and blood components. **Language of Database:** English. **Subject Coverage:** Blood donation, transfusion medicine, transfusion alternatives.

★6797★   BMA PRESS CUTTINGS DATABASE (BMAP)
British Medical Association (BMA)
Tavistock Sq.
London WC1H 9JP, England
General Description: Contains brief summaries of articles and information in the media concerning key medical topics. **Language of Database:** English. **Subject Coverage:** Medical news and related ethical and sociological issues.

★6798★   BNA OCCUPATIONAL SAFETY AND HEALTH DAILY
The Bureau of National Affairs, Inc. (BNA)
BNA ONLINE
1231 25th St., NW
Washington, DC 20037   Phone: (202) 452-4132
General Description: Covers legislative, regulatory, and judicial developments involving worker safety and health at both the federal and state levels. **Language of Database:** English. **Subject Coverage:** Worker safety and health, including federal and state standards, regulations and policies, state and federal programs, enforcement efforts, research, and labor relations.

★6799★   BULLETIN ON THE RHEUMATIC DISEASES
Arthritis Foundation
1314 Spring St., NW
Atlanta, GA 30309   Phone: (404) 872-7100
General Description: Provides concise discussions on aspects of current developments in research and management of rheumatic diseases by experts in the field. **Language of Database:** English. **Subject Coverage:** Research and management of rheumatic diseases.

★6800★   CA FILE
Chemical Abstracts Service
2540 Olentangy River Rd.
PO Box 3012
Columbus, OH 43210-0012   Phone: (614) 447-3600
General Description: Contains bibliographic data and Chemical Abstracts (CA) index entries for documents cited in CA since 1967. Includes complete CA abstract text for documents abstracted since 1970. Covers more than 1,200,000 patent records. **Language of Database:** English. **Subject Coverage:** All areas of chemistry and chemical engineering, including applied chemistry and chemical engineering; biochemistry; macromolecular chemistry; organic chemistry; and physical, inorganic, and analytical chemistry.

★6801★   CA INDEX GUIDE
Chemical Abstracts Service
2540 Olentangy River Rd.
PO Box 3012
Columbus, OH 43210-0012   Phone: (614) 447-3600
General Description: Provides cross-references from commonly used subject terms and substance names to the controlled Chemical Abstracts index terminology and CAS Registry numbers where applicable. Also contains information on CA indexing policies. **Language of Database:** English. **Subject Coverage:** Equivalent chemical substance names covering terms in all areas of chemistry and chemical engineering, including applied chemistry and chemical engineering; biochemistry; macromolecular chemistry; organic chemistry; and physical, inorganic, and analytical chemistry.

★6802★   CA REGISTRY FILE
Chemical Abstracts Service
2540 Olentangy River Rd.
PO Box 3012
Columbus, OH 43210-0012   Phone: (614) 447-3600
General Description: Contains name and formula information for more

than 10.5 million substances identified by Chemical Abstracts Service. Covers 16,000,000 substance names. Includes Markush structure diagrams for patent information. Enables the user to access the ten most recent citations from CA File (described in a separate entry) on the substance identified in the search, or cross over into CA or CAOLD (described in separate entries) to retrieve more information on the substance. **Language of Database:** English. **Subject Coverage:** Substance information and identification, including organic compounds, coordination compounds, polymers, alloys, mixtures, and minerals.

★6803★   CA SEARCH
Chemical Abstracts Service
2540 Olentangy River Rd.
PO Box 3012
Columbus, OH 43210-0012   Phone: (614) 447-3600
General Description: Contains bibliographic data and Chemical Abstracts index entries for documents cited in CA since 1967. Includes CA General Subject headings from a controlled vocabulary and CAS Registry Numbers. **Language of Database:** English. **Subject Coverage:** All areas of chemistry and chemical engineering, including applied chemistry and chemical engineering; biochemistry; macromolecular chemistry; organic chemistry; and physical, inorganic, and analytical chemistry.

★6804★   CAB ABSTRACTS
C.A.B. International
Wallingford, Oxon. OX10 8DE, England
General Description: Provides citations and abstracts of worldwide journal articles and other literature covering agriculture and the related areas of applied biology, sociology, and economics. Comprises approximately 50 subfiles, each covering a specialized area of agricultural research. (For a complete list of the CAB Abstracts subfiles described in this directory, consult the Producer's section under C.A.B. International.). **Language of Database:** English. **Subject Coverage:** Agricultural science, including animal sciences, dairy science and technology, agricultural economics, engineering, forestry, human nutrition, rural development and regional planning, veterinary medicine, taxonomy, and horticulture, as well as the related areas of applied biology, sociology, and economics.

★6805★   CALCIFIED TISSUE ABSTRACTS
Cambridge Scientific Abstracts
7200 Wisconsin Ave.
Bethesda, MD 20814   Phone: (301) 961-6750
General Description: Contains citations and abstracts of international periodical and other literature covering all aspects of calcium and related mineral metabolism. **Language of Database:** English. **Subject Coverage:** All aspects of calcium and related mineral metabolism. Specific topics covered include intestinal absorption of calcium, phosphorus, and magnesium; factors controlling bone composition and kidney functions; ectopic calcification; bone diseases such as osteoporosis, osteomalacia, rickets, Paget's Disease, parathyroid disorders and bone fractures; effects of pregnancy, menopause, aging, and immobilization on bone structure and calcium metabolism; and enzymes.

★6806★   CAMBRIDGE SCIENTIFIC BIOCHEMISTRY
ABSTRACTS, PART 1: BIOLOGICAL MEMBRANES
Cambridge Scientific Abstracts
7200 Wisconsin Ave.
Bethesda, MD 20814   Phone: (301) 961-6750
General Description: Contains citations and abstracts of international periodical and other literature covering cell membranes in a wide variety of biological systems, with emphasis on the structure and function of cell membranes. **Language of Database:** English. **Subject Coverage:** Cell membranes in all types of biological systems. Specific topics covered include membrane components, physical properties, receptors, model and reconstituted systems, methodology, ultrastructures, transport and related phenomena (subcellular components, single cells, and tissues), regulation of membrane function, clinical aspects, cell interactions, cell membranes and immune response, membrane turnover, membrane-bound enzymes, and bioenergetics.

★6807★   CAMBRIDGE SCIENTIFIC BIOCHEMISTRY
ABSTRACTS, PART 2: NUCLEIC ACIDS
Cambridge Scientific Abstracts
7200 Wisconsin Ave.
Bethesda, MD 20814   Phone: (301) 961-6750
General Description: Contains citations and abstracts of international periodical and other literature covering all aspects of nucleic acids. **Language of Database:** English. **Subject Coverage:** Nucleic acids, including purines, pyrimidines, and analogs; nucleosides and analogs; nucleotides,

nucleoside di- and tri-phosphates, and analogs; oligonucleotides, polynucleotides, and analogs; transfer RNA; protein biosynthesis; RNA, including structure, physical properties, biosynthesis, virus and phage infections, effect of hormones, biological properties, role as messenger, and chemical reactions; DNA, including chemical reactions and properties, the effects of radiation, structure and sequence, biosynthesis, virus and phage infections, DNA repair, effect of antibiotics and other agents, gene regulation, transduction, transfection, conjugation, transformation, transposition, micro-injection, cloning, mutagenesis, host systems, and expression of cloned genes; enzymes, including RNases, DNases, polymerases, phosphorylases, phosphatases, and DNA unwinding enzymes; immunological aspects; and protein-nucleic acid association.

★6808★   CAMBRIDGE SCIENTIFIC BIOCHEMISTRY
ABSTRACTS, PART 3: AMINO-ACIDS, PEPTIDES AND
PROTEINS
Cambridge Scientific Abstracts
7200 Wisconsin Ave.
Bethesda, MD 20814   Phone: (301) 961-6750
General Description: Contains citations and abstracts of international periodical and other literature covering all aspects of amino acids, peptides, and proteins. **Language of Database:** English. **Subject Coverage:** Amino acids; purification and preliminary characterization of peptides and proteins; primary structure of peptides and proteins; chemical modification of proteins; conformation and solution studies; x-ray, electron microscope, and neutron diffraction studies; theoretical aspects of protein structure; peptide synthesis; enzyme assay; mechanisms of enzyme action; immobilized enzymes; peptide and protein hormones and related substances; insect and reptile toxins and related substances; peptides with structural features not found in proteins; and evolutionary aspects.

★6809★   CANADIAN DIRECTORY OF COMPLETED MASTER'S
THESES IN NURSING (CAMN)
University of Alberta
Faculty of Nursing
Clinical Sciences Bldg., 5th Fl.
Edmonton, AB, Canada T6G 2G3   Phone: (403) 432-6250
General Description: Provides descriptions of all completed master's theses submitted for nursing degrees in Canada. **Also Known as:** Le Repertoire des Theses de Maitrise Completees en Nursing. **Language of Database:** English; French. **Subject Coverage:** Canadian master's theses in, or related to nursing.

★6810★   CANADIAN STUDIES/ETUDES CANADIENNES
Canadian Centre for Occupational Health and Safety
250 Main St. E.
Hamilton, ON, Canada L8N 1H6   Phone: (416) 572-2981
General Description: Provides descriptions of current or recently completed studies on occupational health and safety conducted by Canadians, or about the Canadian workplace. Provides information on the field of study, performing organization, and funding body. **Language of Database:** English; French. **Subject Coverage:** Canadian occupational health and safety studies.

★6811★   CANADIAN UNION CATALOGUE OF LIBRARY
MATERIALS FOR THE HANDICAPPED (CANUC:H)
National Library of Canada
Public Services Branch
Union Catalogue Division
395 Wellington St.
Ottawa, ON, Canada K1A 0N4   Phone: (613) 996-7507
General Description: Contains full bibliographic descriptions of monograph and serial titles which are in special media format (braille, large print, and talking books) for visually-impaired persons. **Language of Database:** English. **Subject Coverage:** Special imprints for the visually impaired.

★6812★   CANCER-CD
SilverPlatter Information, Inc.
River Ridge Office Park
100 River Ridge Rd.
Norwood, MA 02062   Phone: (617) 769-2599
General Description: Contains citations and abstracts of the world's published literature dealing with all aspects of cancer, including clinical, drug, and pharmaceutical aspects. Corresponds to the following three products: • EMCANCER (Excerpta Medica, Section 16: Cancer) (described in a separate entry). • The Year Book of Cancer. • CANCERLIT (described in a separate entry). **Also Known as:** Ca-CD. **Language of Database:**

English. **Subject Coverage:** Cancer and related topics, including drug, clinical, and pharmaceutical information.

★6813★ CANCER ON DISC
J.B. Lippincott Co.
East Washington Sq.
Philadelphia, PA 19105   Phone: (215) 238-4206
General Description: Contains the complete text of each of the preceding year's issues of Cancer, the semimonthly journal of the American Cancer Society. Includes all articles, tables, color and black & white images, and references cited. **Language of Database:** English. **Subject Coverage:** Cancer, including the diagnostic and clinical aspects of the disease.

★6814★ CANCER FORUM
CompuServe Information Service
5000 Arlington Centre Blvd.
PO Box 20212
Columbus, OH 43220   Phone: (614) 457-8600
General Description: Provides a forum for cancer-stricken patients and their family and friends to exchange information and offer mutual support. Includes standard and supplemental methods of cancer treatment, research, and cancer in children. **Language of Database:** English. **Subject Coverage:** Individuals diagnosed with cancer.

★6815★ CANCER LITERATURE (CANCERLIT)
U.S. National Cancer Institute
International Cancer Information Center
Bldg. 82, Rm. 102
Bethesda, MD 20892   Phone: (301) 496-7403
General Description: Contains citations and abstracts of published cancer research results appearing in U.S. and foreign periodicals and other literature. Maintained as part of CANCERLINE. **Also Known as:** Cancer Literature Information Online. **Language of Database:** English. **Subject Coverage:** All aspects of cancer, including the etiology, prevention, diagnosis, treatment, and biology.

★6816★ CANTECH DATABASE
Hutchison Research
King West Centre
2 Pardee Ave., Ste. 202
Toronto, ON, Canada M6K 3H5   Phone: (416) 539-9220
General Description: Provides descriptions of advanced technology companies, products, and services in Canada. Includes a coding and classification system designed for the identification of advanced technology products and services. **Language of Database:** English. **Subject Coverage:** Advanced technology products and services, including computer hardware and software, telecommunications, photonics, artificial intelligence, advanced materials, biotechnology, aerospace, advanced manufacturing systems, medical technology, and measurement and control systems.

★6817★ CAOLD
Chemical Abstracts Service
2540 Olentangy River Rd.
PO Box 3012
Columbus, OH 43210-0012   Phone: (614) 447-3600
General Description: Contains bibliographic data and Chemical Abstracts index entries for documents prior to 1967 that are covered in the printed Chemical Abstracts. Currently under development. **Language of Database:** English. **Subject Coverage:** All areas of chemistry and chemical engineering, including applied chemistry and chemical engineering; biochemistry; macromolecular chemistry; organic chemistry; and physical, inorganic, and analytical chemistry.

★6818★ CAPREVIEWS
Chemical Abstracts Service
2540 Olentangy River Rd.
PO Box 3012
Columbus, OH 43210-0012   Phone: (614) 447-3600
General Description: Provides bibliographic citations (before abstracts and indexing have been added) for documents which are to be added within six to eight weeks to the printed Chemical Abstracts (CA) or the CA File database (described in a separate entry). Includes information on the content of 1700 recent patents each week from all areas of chemistry and chemical engineering. Documents are deleted from the file as they are added to the Chemical Abstracts and CA File. **Language of Database:** English. **Subject Coverage:** All areas of chemistry and chemical engineering, including applied chemistry and chemical engineering; biochemistry; macromolecular chemistry; organic chemistry; and physical, inorganic, and analytical chemistry.

★6819★ CARCINOGENICITY INFORMATION DATABASE OF ENVIRONMENTAL SUBSTANCES (CIDES)
Technical Database Services, Inc.
10 Columbus Circle
New York, NY 10019   Phone: (212) 245-0044
General Description: Provides experimental data on the carcinogenicity and mutagenicity of approximately 1000 substances of environmental or health concern. Includes both positive and negative results of human and animal exposure, and features the Carcinogenicity Ratio (CR), a pair of values providing an objective measure of the likelihood of carcinogenicity in substances and the weight of evidence indicating the extent of testing upon which the likelihood is based. **Language of Database:** English. **Subject Coverage:** Carcinogenicity and mutagenicity of environmental substances.

★6820★ THE CARCINOGENICITY PREDICTOR (CPBS)
Technical Database Services, Inc.
10 Columbus Circle
New York, NY 10019   Phone: (212) 245-0044
General Description: Provides analyses of actual or hypothetical results from testing for mutagenicity and genetic activity of potential carcinogens. By inputting results from 32 short term assays, the user can retrieve a calculation of the probability that a compound is a carcinogen or noncarcinogen. Graphic analyses show progression as test results are added to the battery. **Language of Database:** English. **Subject Coverage:** Carcinogenicity and mutagenicity prediction.

★6821★ CASE LAW/JURISPRUDENCE
Canadian Centre for Occupational Health and Safety
250 Main St. E.
Hamilton, ON, Canada L8N 1H6   Phone: (416) 572-2981
General Description: Provides summaries of cases and decisions relating to occupational health and safety from jurisdictions across Canada. Includes such information as jurisdiction, forum, year, and summary. **Language of Database:** English; French. **Subject Coverage:** Canadian occupational health and safety case law.

★6822★ CASREACT
Chemical Abstracts Service
2540 Olentangy River Rd.
PO Box 3012
Columbus, OH 43210-0012   Phone: (614) 447-3600
General Description: Provides information on approximately 800,000 reactions of organic substances, including organometallics and biomolecules selected from papers reported in more than 100 journals. Includes reaction participants listed in CA File (described in a separate entry) and not listed, multi-step reactions, percent yields for some reactions, and safety and reaction condition information when provided. Also provides bibliographic information on the source and CAS Registry Numbers for the substances involved. **Language of Database:** English. **Subject Coverage:** Chemical catalysts, products, reactants, reagents, and solvents, covering general organic chemistry; physical organic chemistry; aliphatic compounds; alicyclic compounds; benzene, its derivatives, and condensed benzenoid compounds; biomolecules and their synthetic analogs; heterocyclic compounds; organometallic and organomelloidal compounds; terpenes and terpenoids; alkaloids; steroids; carbohydrates; and amino acids, peptides, and proteins.

★6823★ CATLINE
U.S. National Library of Medicine
MEDLARS Management Section
8600 Rockville Pike
Bethesda, MD 20894   Phone: (301) 496-6193
General Description: Provides full bibliographic descriptions of books and serials cataloged at the National Library of Medicine. **Also Known as:** Catalog Online. **Language of Database:** English. **Subject Coverage:** Books and serials in the biomedical sciences.

★6824★ CD-GENE
Hitachi America, Ltd.
2000 Sierra Point Pkwy.
Brisbane, CA 94005-1819   Phone: (415) 589-8300
General Description: Covers genetic sequencing data. Comprises the following four DNA and amino acid sequence data bases: • GenBank. • EMBL Data Library. • NBRF-PIR Protein Sequence Database. • SWISS-PROT. **Language of Database:** English. **Subject Coverage:** Genetic sequencing data covering DNA, nucleic acids, amino acids, and proteins.

★6825★ CDC AIDS WEEKLY
CDC AIDS WEEKLY/NCI CANCER WEEKLY
206 Rogers St., NE, Ste. 104
PO Box 5528
Atlanta, GA 30307-0528　　　　　Phone: (404) 377-8895
General Description: Provides comprehensive coverage of world news and developments relating to AIDS (Acquired Immune Deficiency Syndrome), with emphasis on research and clinical findings. **Language of Database:** English. **Subject Coverage:** AIDS research.

★6826★ CHEMICAL EXPOSURE
Science Applications International Corp.
800 Oak Ridge Tpke.
PO Box 2501
Oak Ridge, TN 37831　　　　　Phone: (615) 482-9031
General Description: Contains references and abstracts of published literature relating to some 1820 chemicals which are not natural constituents identified in human and animal biological media. **Language of Database:** English. **Subject Coverage:** Chemicals identified in the tissues and body fluids of humans and feral and food animals, including tissue levels, health effects, and toxicological and pathological aspects.

★6827★ CHEMICAL JOURNALS OF THE AMERICAN
　　　CHEMICAL SOCIETY (CJACS)
American Chemical Society
1155 16th St., NW
Washington, DC 20036　　　　　Phone: (202) 872-8065
General Description: Contains the complete text of 18 primary American Chemical Society (ACS) journals. **Language of Database:** English. **Subject Coverage:** Chemistry, biochemistry, chemical engineering, and related topics.

★6828★ CHEMICAL TITLES (CT)
Chemical Abstracts Service
2540 Olentangy River Rd.
PO Box 3012
Columbus, OH 43210-0012　　　　　Phone: (614) 447-3600
General Description: Provides titles of important research articles appearing in 800 leading scientific journals published worldwide. **Language of Database:** English. **Subject Coverage:** All areas of chemistry and chemical engineering, including applied chemistry and chemical engineering; biochemistry; macromolecular chemistry; organic chemistry; and physical, inorganic, and analytical chemistry.

★6829★ CHEMLINE
U.S. National Library of Medicine
Toxicology Information Program
8600 Rockville Pike
Bethesda, MD 20894　　　　　Phone: (301) 496-1131
General Description: Contains various nomenclature and structural fragments for a collection of chemical compounds. Covers primarily chemicals that are identified by CAS Registry Numbers in the TOXLINE, TOXLINE65, TOXLIT, TOXLIT65, RTECS, MEDLINE, HSDB, CCRIS, and CANCERLIT databases, as well as the EPA Toxic Substances Control Act Inventory of Chemical Substances. **Also Known as:** Chemical Dictionary Online. **Language of Database:** English. **Subject Coverage:** Chemical substances.

★6830★ CHEMORECEPTION ABSTRACTS
Cambridge Scientific Abstracts
7200 Wisconsin Ave.
Bethesda, MD 20814　　　　　Phone: (301) 961-6750
General Description: Contains citations and abstracts of international periodical and other literature covering the sciences of taste, smell, and related phenomena. **Language of Database:** English. **Subject Coverage:** The sciences of taste, smell, and related phenomena, including internal chemoreception, chemotaxis, and associated forms of sensitivity such as psychophysics, animal behavior studies, odor pollution, flavor and aroma studies of food, and perfumery. Specific topics covered include peripheral and central sensory mechanisms; human physiology and pathology; neuroanatomy, histology, and histochemistry; animal behavior and chemical communication, including pheromones; chemistry of odorous materials; molecular structure and odor qualities; chemistry of sapid materials; molecular structure and taste qualities; odor control; apparatus and methodology; and new products and marketing.

★6831★ CHEMTOX DATABASE
Resource Consultants, Inc.
The CHEMTOX System
7121 CrossRoads Blvd.
PO Box 1848
Brentwood, TN 37024-1848　　　　　Phone: (615) 373-5040
General Description: Covers chemicals regulated by government agencies. Provides information on more than 6100 chemical substances that are hazardous and that are common to the environment and the workplace due to their economic importance. **Language of Database:** English. **Subject Coverage:** Hazardous materials regulated by government agencies, including such aspects as toxicology, industrial hygiene, occupational medicine and safety, environmental sciences and engineering, emergency response, and hazardous materials transport.

★6832★ CHICANO DATABASE ON CD-ROM
University of California, Berkeley
Chicano Studies Library
3404 Dwinelle Hall
Berkeley, CA 94720　　　　　Phone: (415) 642-3859
General Description: Provides citations to periodical articles, books, and other published literature dealing with the Chicano (Mexican-American) experience. Includes the Latinos and AIDS Database compiled by the Chicano Research Center at the University ofCalifornia, Los Angeles. **Language of Database:** English. **Subject Coverage:** All topics pertaining to the Chicano (Mexican-American) experience.

★6833★ CHILD ABUSE AND NEGLECT
U.S. National Center on Child Abuse and Neglect
Clearinghouse on Child Abuse and Neglect Information
PO Box 1182
Washington, DC 20013　　　　　Phone: (703) 821-2086
General Description: Covers publications, programs, research projects, and laws concerning child abuse and neglect. Comprises the following five files: Annotated citations to published literature and court decisions; descriptions of service programs; descriptions of ongoing research projects; excerpts of current state laws; and descriptions of audiovisual materials. **Language of Database:** English. **Subject Coverage:** Child abuse and neglect.

★6834★ CHINESE PHARMACEUTICAL LITERATURE
　　　DATABASE (CPLDB)
State Pharmaceutical Administration of China
Scientific and Technical Information Research Institute
A-38 Bei Lishi Lu
Beijing 100810, People's Republic of China
General Description: Provides references and abstracts of Chinese pharmaceutical and medical literature. Includes coverage of Western pharmaceutical literature. **Language of Database:** Chinese. **Subject Coverage:** Chinese and Western pharmaceuticals, including traditional Chinese medicines, philosophy of Western and traditional Chinese practices, pharmacognosy and materia medica, pharmaceutical chemistry, pharmaceutical technology, toxicology, pharmacodynamics, pharmacokinetics, drug analysis, clinical trial and drug evaluation, adverse drug reactions and interaction, manufacturing management and quality control, processing machinery and plant design, and new products.

★6835★ CHOLESTEROL, HIGH BLOOD PRESSURE, AND
　　　SMOKING EDUCATION DATABASE
U.S. National Heart, Lung, and Blood Institute Information Center
4733 Bethesda Ave., Ste. 530
Bethesda, MD 20814　　　　　Phone: (301) 951-3260
General Description: Contains references and abstracts of published materials concerning disease prevention and health promotion aspects of blood resources, cholesterol, high blood pressure, asthma, and smoking. **Language of Database:** English. **Subject Coverage:** Blood research, cholesterol, high blood pressure, and smoking, with emphasis on educational and disease prevention/health promotion aspects.

★6836★ CIS ABSTRACTS
International Labour Office
Centre International d'Informations de Securite et de Sante au
　　　Travail
CH-1211 Geneva 22, Switzerland
General Description: Provides references and abstracts to journal articles, books, and other literature covering topics in occupational safety and health. **Also Known as:** CISILO. **Language of Database:** English; French. **Subject Coverage:** Occupational health and safety, including occupational medicine and physiology; industrial toxicology; environmental hygiene; accident and disease prevention; safety engineering; loss control; condi-

tions of work; health effects of dust, noise, and vibration exposures; ergonomics and work organization; occupational psychology; labor administration; workers compensation; training and education; and legislation and standards.

★6837★   CISTI MONOGRAPHS
Canada Institute for Scientific and Technical Information
Montreal Rd.
Ottawa, ON, Canada K1A 0S2   Phone: (613) 993-1600
General Description: Provides bibliographic descriptions of monographs, technical reports, and conference proceedings held by CISTI and covering topics in the fields of science, technology, and medicine. **Language of Database:** English. **Subject Coverage:** Science, technology, engineering, medicine, and health sciences.

★6838★   CISTI SERIALS
Canada Institute for Scientific and Technical Information
Montreal Rd.
Ottawa, ON, Canada K1A 0S2   Phone: (613) 993-1600
General Description: Contains cataloging information for periodicals, annuals, journals, monographic series, and conference proceedings held by CISTI and its branches. **Language of Database:** English. **Subject Coverage:** Serials in all areas of science, technology, and medicine; selected materials in other disciplines relating to activities of National Research Council Canada.

★6839★   CLINICAL PROTOCOLS (CLINPROT)
U.S. National Cancer Institute
International Cancer Information Center
Bldg. 82, Rm. 102
Bethesda, MD 20892   Phone: (301) 496-7403
General Description: Provides summaries of clinical cancer therapy protocols for use by researchers and clinical investigators. Maintained as part of CANCERLINE. **Language of Database:** English. **Subject Coverage:** Clinical cancer treatment protocols.

★6840★   COLLEAGUE MAIL
BRS Information Technologies
BRS/COLLEAGUE
8000 Westpark Dr.
McLean, VA 22102   Phone: (703) 442-0900
General Description: Provides physicians and health care professionals with the facilities to exchange ideas and information through a series of bulletin boards on various medical and health care topics. Also offers private bulletin board facilities for medical organizations. **Language of Database:** English. **Subject Coverage:** Medical and health care topics, including AIDS/HIV, critical care, dermatology, immunology, medical ethics, neurology, and oncology.

★6841★   COMBINED HEALTH INFORMATION DATABASE (CHID)
U.S. National Institutes of Health
PO Box NDIC
Bethesda, MD 20892   Phone: (301) 496-2162
General Description: Provides references and abstracts of published materials as well as descriptions of information resources dealing with patient and professional education in a number of specific health care specialties. Emphasis is on materials unavailable through libraries, online databases, or other traditional sources. Comprises the following 13 files: • AIDS Education Materials. • AIDS School Heal h Education. • Alzheimer's Disease. • Arthritis and Musculoskeletal and Skin Diseases. • Blood Resource. • Cholesterol, High Blood Pressure, and Smoking Education. • Diabetes. • Digestive Diseases. • Disease Prev ention/Health Promotion. • Health Education and Promotion. • Kidney and Urologic Diseases. • National Eye Health Education Program. • VA Patient Education. **Language of Database:** English. **Subject Coverage:** Health resources, patient and professional education materials, patient education programs and curricula, evaluation materials, and specific disease information, with emphasis on AIDS (Acquired Immune Deficiency Syndrome), Alzheimer's, arthritis, blood, diabetes, digestive diseases, cardiovascular diseases, eye health, and kidney and urologic diseases.

★6842★   COMMUNITY HEALTHCARE CLINICS
FIRSTMARK
34 Juniper Ln.
Newton Center, MA 02159   Phone: (617) 965-7989
General Description: Provides listings for U.S. government-funded (Title 330) community health centers and clinics. **Language of Database:** English. **Subject Coverage:** Community health centers and clinics.

★6843★   COMPACT LIBRARY: AIDS
Maxwell Electronic Publishing
124 Mount Auburn St.
Cambridge, MA 02138   Phone: (617) 661-2955
General Description: Provides a comprehensive collection of the latest medical information on all aspects of Acquired Immune Deficiency Syndrome (AIDS). **Language of Database:** English. **Subject Coverage:** Acquired Immune Deficiency Syndrome, including transmission, treatment, prevention, and education.

★6844★   COMPACT LIBRARY: VIRAL HEPATITIS
Maxwell Electronic Publishing
124 Mount Auburn St.
Cambridge, MA 02138   Phone: (617) 661-2955
General Description: Provides a comprehensive collection of the latest medical information on hepatitis research. **Language of Database:** English. **Subject Coverage:** Viral hepatitis, including research activities, clinical aspects, and public health considerations.

★6845★   COMPREHENSIVE CORE MEDICAL LIBRARY (CCML)
BRS Information Technologies
8000 Westpark Dr.
McLean, VA 22102   Phone: (703) 442-0900
General Description: Provides the complete text of current editions of selected medical reference works and textbooks, plus current and retrospective issues of more than 80 English-language medical journals published worldwide. **Language of Database:** English. **Subject Coverage:** Emergency, internal, and critical care medicine.

★6846★   COMPUTER RETRIEVAL OF INFORMATION ON SCIENTIFIC PROJECTS (CRISP)
U.S. National Institutes of Health
Division of Research Grants
Research Documentation Section
5333 Westbard Ave., Rm. 148
Bethesda, MD 20892   Phone: (301) 496-7543
General Description: Provides descriptions and indexing of biomedical research projects supported by U.S. Public Health Service grants, cooperative agreements, and career award and research contracts, as well as intramural projects conducted by the National Institutes of Health; the Alcohol, Drug Abuse, and Mental Health Administration; the Centers for Disease Control; the Food and Drug Administration; and others. **Language of Database:** English. **Subject Coverage:** Research in biomedical and allied health fields.

★6847★   COMPUTERIZED AIDS INFORMATION NETWORK (CAIN)
Los Angeles Gay and Lesbian Community Services Center
1213 N. Highland Ave.
Los Angeles, CA 90038   Phone: (213) 464-7400
General Description: Provides information on the medical and social aspects of AIDS (Acquired Immune Deficiency Syndrome). Contains articles, transcripts, reports, and records dealing with HIV/AIDS and related topics. Provides a forum enabling the user to interact with other users in an exchange of questions and answers, experiences, concerns, suggestions, and solutions. **Language of Database:** English. **Subject Coverage:** Acquired Immune Deficiency Syndrome (AIDS).

★6848★   COMPUTERIZED CLINICAL INFORMATION SYSTEM (CCIS)
Micromedex, Inc.
600 Grant St.
Denver, CO 80203-3527   Phone: (303) 831-1400
General Description: Provides current information on toxicology, drug therapy, and acute care of interest to health care professionals. Comprises the following ten files: Aftercare Instructions; Drugdex System; Emerginde System; Identidex System; Martindale Online; Poisindex System; Dosing and Therapeutic Tools; TOMES (Toxicology, Occupational Medicine & Environmental Series); REPRORISK; Drug Interactions from MEDIS-PAN. **Language of Database:** English. **Subject Coverage:** Toxicology, drug therapy, and acute care.

★6849★   CONFERENCE PAPERS INDEX (CPI)
Cambridge Scientific Abstracts
7200 Wisconsin Ave.
Bethesda, MD 20814   Phone: (301) 961-6750
General Description: Contains citations to current research findings and papers presented at scientific and technical conferences worldwide. **Language of Database:** English. **Subject Coverage:** Conference papers in science

and technology, including aerospace science and engineering, civil and mechanical engineering, chemistry and chemical engineering, electronic and general engineering and technology, materials science and engineering, nuclear and power engineering, animal and plant science, biology, physics, astronomy, geosciences, mathematics and computer science, biochemistry, clinical and experimental medicine, and pharmacology.

★6850★ CONSUMER DRUG INFORMATION (CDIF)
American Society of Hospital Pharmacists
4630 Montgomery Ave.
Bethesda, MD 20814   Phone: (301) 657-3000
General Description: Contains descriptions of the most commonly prescribed drugs in the United States. Covers more than 260 drugs, representing more than 14,000 brand names and 95 percent of the prescriptions written in the United States. Language of Database: English. Subject Coverage: Commonly prescribed drugs in the United States.

★6851★ CRITICAL CARE MEDICINE ON DISC
Williams & Wilkins
428 E. Preston St.
Baltimore, MD 21202   Phone: (301) 528-4000
General Description: Contains the complete text of all articles, tables, and images appearing in Critical Care Medicine, the monthly journal of the Society of Critical Care Med icine. Language of Database: English. Subject Coverage: Critical care medicine.

★6852★ CSA LIFE SCIENCES COLLECTION
Cambridge Scientific Abstracts
7200 Wisconsin Ave.
Bethesda, MD 20814   Phone: (301) 961-6750
General Description: Contains citations and abstracts of international periodical and other research literature covering all fields of the life sciences, including biology, medicine, biochemistry, and selected areas of agriculture, and veterinary science. Language of Database: English. Subject Coverage: Life sciences, including animal behavior, biochemistry (biological membranes, nucleic acids, and amino acids, peptides, and proteins), biotechology, calcified tissue, chemoreception, ecology, endocrinology, entomology, genetics, immunology, marine biotechnology, microbiology (industrial and applied microbiology, bacteriology, and algology, mycology, and protozoology), neurosciences (including endocrinology), oncology, toxicology, and virology and AIDS.

★6853★ CSA NEUROSCIENCES ABSTRACTS
Cambridge Scientific Abstracts
7200 Wisconsin Ave.
Bethesda, MD 20814   Phone: (301) 961-6750
General Description: Contains citations and abstracts of international periodical and other literature covering neurology, endocrinology, and the related fields of metabolism and reproduction. Language of Database: English. Subject Coverage: The sciences of neurology and endocrinology. Specific topics covered include methods and apparatus; neuroanatomy, histology and cytology; growth and development; aging, degeneration and repair; neurophysiology; neurochemistry; neuroendocrinology; neuropharmacology; neurotoxicology; immunology; genetics; experimental pathology; neural correlates of behavior; sleep; clinical endocrinology; hypothalamic releasing hormones and factors; growth hormone, thyroid-stimulation hormone, and other human hormones; prostaglandins; reproductive biology; and pheromones.

★6854★ CURRENT AWARENESS IN BIOLOGICAL SCIENCES (CABS)
Pergamon Press Plc
Headington Hill Hall
Oxford OX3 0BW, England
General Description: Provides references to the world's journal and other published literature dealing with the biological sciences and related areas. Language of Database: English. Subject Coverage: Biological sciences and related areas, including biochemistry, cell and developmental biology, ecological and environmental sciences, endocrinology, genetics and molecular biology, immunology, microbiology, neuroscience, pharmacology and toxicology, physiology, plant science, and clinical chemistry.

★6855★ CURRENT BIOTECHNOLOGY ABSTRACTS (CBA)
Royal Society of Chemistry
Information Services
Thomas Graham House
Science Park
Cambridge CB4 4WF, England
General Description: Provides citations and abstracts of international

journal and other literature covering the scientific, technical, and techno-commercial aspects of biotechnology. Language of Database: English. Subject Coverage: Biotechnology, including microbiology, genetics, medicine, biochemistry, immunology, pharmaceutics, fermentation, and other topics.

★6856★ CURRENT CONTENTS SEARCH
Institute for Scientific Information
3501 Market St.
Philadelphia, PA 19104   Phone: (215) 386-0100
General Description: Indexes the tables of contents pages from the latest issues of more than 6500 leading scientific journals. Searchable in its entirety or limited to one of the seven Current Contents editions that comprise the file. Also Known as: CC Search. Language of Database: English. Subject Coverage: Life sciences, including biochemistry, cytology, experimental medicine, genetics, hematology, immunology, molecular biology, neuroscience, pathology, pharmaceutical chemistry, radiology and nuclear medicine, toxicology, and virology; clinical medicine, including allergy, critical care medicine, epidemiology, geriatrics and gerontology, nuclear medicine, oncology, radiology, surgery, and tropical medicine; agriculture, biology, and environmental sciences, including veterinary medicine and pathology; and social and behavioral sciences, includinghuman development, public health,and substance abuse. n studies, and women's studies.

★6857★ CURRENT PATENTS EVALUATION
Current Patents Ltd.
34-42 Cleveland St.
London W1P 5FB, England
General Description: Provides evaluations and merit ratings of current therapeutic patents registered worldwide covering cardiovascular, central nervous system (CNS), and antimicrobial. Coverage is expected to be extended to cover anticancer therapy, hormones, anti-inflammatory, anti-allergics, gastrointestinal therapy, and metabolic diseases. Language of Database: English. Subject Coverage: Patents covering cardiovascular, central nervous system, and antimicrobial therapies.

★6858★ DALCTRAF
DALCTRAF HB
PO Box 5815
S-102 48 Stockholm, Sweden
General Description: Contains references to worldwide literature dealing with the incidence and effects of alcohol and drugs on transportation. Language of Database: English. Subject Coverage: Alcohol and drug use in relation to transportation and traffic safety.

★6859★ DATA ARCHIVE ON ADOLESCENT PREGNANCY AND PREGNANCY PREVENTION (DAAPP)
Sociometrics Corp.
170 State St., No. 260
Los Altos, CA 94022   Phone: (415) 949-3282
General Description: Covers studies dealing with adolescent family life, sexuality, contraception, pregnancy, childbearing, parenting, and family planning. Language of Database: English. Subject Coverage: Adolescent sexuality, health, marriage, employment, and education; general information on family planning, infant health, and attitudes toward sexual issues; information on social demographics.

★6860★ DATABASE OF ANTIVIRAL AND IMMUNOMODULATORY THERAPIES FOR AIDS (DAITA)
CDC AIDS WEEKLY/NCI CANCER WEEKLY
206 Rogers St., NE, Ste. 104
PO Box 5528
Atlanta, GA 30307-0528   Phone: (404) 377-8895
General Description: Covers current published and unpublished research findings on every drug or therapy that has been presented as a potential treatment for AIDS (Acquired Immune Deficiency Syndrome). Language of Database: English. Subject Coverage: AIDS-related pharmaceutical and therapeutic products, including antivirals, immune modulators, and treatments for opportunistic infections.

★6861★ DATABASE AND DIRECTORY OF AIDS-SPECIFIC PERIODICALS AND DATABASES
CDC AIDS WEEKLY/NCI CANCER WEEKLY
206 Rogers St., NE, Ste. 104
PO Box 5528
Atlanta, GA 30307-0528   Phone: (404) 377-8895
General Description: Provides coverage of information resources dealing with AIDS (Acquired Immune Deficiency Syndrome). Comprises the

following four files: AIDS-Specific Periodicals; AIDS Databases; AIDS Information/Support Services; and AIDS Meetin gs. **Language of Database:** English. **Subject Coverage:** AIDS information resources.

★6862★ DATABASE AND DIRECTORY OF CANCER-SPECIFIC PERIODICALS AND DATABASES
CDC AIDS WEEKLY/NCI CANCER WEEKLY
206 Rogers St., NE, Ste. 104
PO Box 5528
Atlanta, GA 30307-0528   Phone: (404) 377-8895
General Description: Provides coverage of information resources dealing with any form of cancer. Comprises the following four files: Cancer-Specific Periodicals; Cancer Databases; Cancer Information/Support Services; Cancer Meetings. **Language of Database:** English. **Subject Coverage:** Cancer-related information resources.

★6863★ DBS-MDI
Toyo Information Systems Co., Ltd.
Shinbashi-Sanwa-Toyo Bldg.
1-11-7, Shinbashi, Minato-ku
Tokyo 105, Japan
General Description: Contains personal medical records. Covers medical history, present medical status, and present treatment and prescriptions. **Language of Database:** Japanese. **Subject Coverage:** Japanese medical records.

★6864★ DE HAEN DRUG DATA
Paul De Haen International, Inc.
2750 S. Shoshone St.
Englewood, CO 80110   Phone: (303) 781-6683
General Description: Provides specific information on pharmaceuticals, including information on drug synthesis, research and development, preclinical and clinical testing, adverse reactions and interactions, and marketing statistics. **Language of Database:** English. **Subject Coverage:** New and existing drugs, including drug synthesis, chemical structure, therapeutic classification, pharmacology, toxicology, and marketing.

★6865★ DECHEMA BIOTECHNOLOGY EQUIPMENT SUPPLIERS (BIOQUIP)
DECHEMA
Theodor-Heuss-Allee 25
D-6000 Frankfurt am Main 97, Germany
General Description: Provides information on 400 companies that manufacture or supply some 1000 products in the field of biotechnology. **Language of Database:** German; English; French. **Subject Coverage:** Manufacturers and suppliers of plants, apparatus, equipment, and machinery for biotechnology, including pumps, compressors, valves, and seals; packaging and storage technology; control and instrumentation engineering; laboratory equipment and apparatus; analysis equipment and chemicals; and safety engineering.

★6866★ DERMAL ABSORPTION
U.S. Environmental Protection Agency (EPA)
Office of Pesticides and Toxic Substances
401 M St., SW, MS-TS799
Washington, DC 20460   Phone: (202) 554-1404
General Description: Provides data on toxic effects, absorption, distribution, metabolism, and excretion relating to the dermal absorption of 655 chemicals. Includes data on the effects of other exposure, such as oral or inhalation, if such information is included in the article with the dermal data. **Language of Database:** English. **Subject Coverage:** Toxic effects, absorption, distribution, metabolism, and excretion data for chemicals absorbed through the skin.

★6867★ DEVELOPMENTAL AND REPRODUCTIVE TOXICOLOGY (DART)
U.S. National Library of Medicine
Toxicology Information Program
8600 Rockville Pike
Bethesda, MD 20894   Phone: (301) 496-1131
General Description: Provides citations and abstracts to literature on biological, physical or chemical agents that may cause birth defects. **Language of Database:** English. **Subject Coverage:** Physical, biological, and chemical agents that may cause birth defects, including some reproductive and developmental toxicology data dealing with infertility, paternal exposure, and neonatal exposure.

★6868★ DHSS-DATA
Great Britain Departments of Health and Social Security Library
Hannibal House
Elephant and Castle
London SE1 6TE, England
General Description: Contains full bibliographic descriptions of the holdings of the Departments of Health and Social Security Library. Covers primarily U.K. literature in the areas of health and social services. Includes citations and location information for official DHSS publications. **Language of Database:** English. **Subject Coverage:** Social policy issues, including all aspects of personal social services, social problems, social security, and health service administration and planning; related areas such as design and construction of health service buildings, medical equipment and supplies, public health and nursing, safety of medicines, occupational pensions, computers, industrial injuries, and psychology.

★6869★ DHSS-MEDTEH
Great Britain Departments of Health and Social Security Library
Hannibal House
Elephant and Castle
London SE1 6TE, England
General Description: Contains citations and abstracts of periodical and other literature covering the scientific and medical aspects of medical toxicology and environmental health issues. **Also Known as:** Medical Toxicology and Environmental Health. **Language of Database:** English. **Subject Coverage:** Medical toxicology and environmental health issues, including chemicals in food; consumer products and the environment; pesticides; industrial chemicals; health consequences of smoking, radiation, and noise; air and water pollution; radiation biology; veterinary medicines; good laboratory practices; cosmetics; and general toxicology.

★6870★ DIABETES DATABASE
U.S. National Diabetes Information Clearinghouse
PO Box NDIC
Bethesda, MD 20892   Phone: (301) 468-2162
General Description: Provides citations and abstracts of published materials dealing with diabetes mellitus and related patient education and health information programs and materials. **Language of Database:** English. **Subject Coverage:** Diabetes mellitus and related patient education and health information programs and materials.

★6871★ DIGESTIVE DISEASES DATABASE
U.S. National Digestive Diseases Information Clearinghouse
PO Box NDDIC
Bethesda, MD 20892   Phone: (301) 468-6344
General Description: Provides citations and abstracts of materials dealing with digestive health and disease, with emphasis on educating the public, patients and their families, physicians, and other health care providers about the prevention and management of digestive diseases. **Language of Database:** English. **Subject Coverage:** Digestive health and disease.

★6872★ DIGS
Korea Institute of Industry and Technology Information
PO Box 205, Cheongryangri
Seoul, Republic of Korea
General Description: Indexes articles from Korean periodicals acquired by the National Assembly Library. **Also Known as:** Domestic Information on the General Subjects; Korean Periodicals Index. **Language of Database:** Korean. **Subject Coverage:** All subject areas, including science, engineering, medical science and technology, and social science.

★6873★ DIOGENES: WASHINGTON NEWS AND DOCUMENT RETRIEVAL NETWORK
FOI Services, Inc.
12315 Wilkins Ave.
Rockville, MD 20852   Phone: (301) 881-0410
General Description: Contains the complete text of published and unpublished materials dealing with U.S. Food and Drug Administration (FDA) regulatory actions. **Language of Database:** English. **Subject Coverage:** The regulation of drugs and medical devices.

★6874★ DIRECTORY OF BIOTECHNOLOGY INFORMATION RESOURCES (DBIR)
American Type Culture Collection
Bioinformatics Department
12301 Parklawn Dr.
Rockville, MD 20852-1776   Phone: (301) 881-2600
General Description: Contains descriptions of international sources of publicly available biotechnology information with applications in medi-

cine, agriculture, pharmaceuticals, food technology, microbiology, and molecular biology. **Language of Database:** English. **Subject Coverage:** Biotechnology information resources, including computer-readable databases, database vendors, electronic bulletin boards and networks; culture collections and specimen banks; biotechnology centers and related organizations; periodicals, directories, and selected monographs, reviews, and compilations; and nomenclature committees.

★6875★ **DIRECTORY OF MEDICAL AND HEALTH CARE LIBRARIES IN THE UNITED KINGDOM AND REPUBLIC OF IRELAND**
Library Association Publishing Ltd.
7 Ridgmount St.
London WC1E 7AE, England
General Description: Contains information on approximately 650 medical and health care libraries in the United Kingdom and Republic of Ireland. Includes a geographical listing of names and addresses of the 16 members of the British National Health Services Librarians Group. **Language of Database:** English. **Subject Coverage:** Medical libraries in the United Kingdom and Ireland.

★6876★ **DIRECTORY OF MEDICAL REHABILITATION FACILITIES**
Oryx Press
4041 N. Central Ave.
Phoenix, AZ 85012-3399   Phone: (602) 265-2651
General Description: Provides information on more than 1800 physical rehabilitation centers for persons disabled because of injury or debilitating disease. Coverage includes services found in hospital-sponsored rehabilitation departments, private hospitals, and free-standing clinics. **Language of Database:** English. **Subject Coverage:** Rehabilitation facilities.

★6877★ **DIRECTORY OF ON-GOING RESEARCH IN CANCER EPIDEMIOLOGY**
World Health Organization
International Agency for Research on Cancer
150, cours Albert Thomas
F-69372 Lyon Cedex 08, France
General Description: Provides references and abstracts of current research projects dealing with cancer epidemiology. **Subject Coverage:** Current studies in cancer epidemiology.

★6878★ **DIRLINE**
U.S. National Library of Medicine
MEDLARS Management Section
8600 Rockville Pike
Bethesda, MD 20894   Phone: (301) 496-6193
General Description: Contains listings for organizations that provide information in specific subject areas. Includes Poison Control Centers and Drug Abuse Communications Network (DRA) subfiles. Intended as an alternative resource for answering information needs not met by bibliographic or factual databases. **Also Known as:** Directory of Information Resources Online. **Language of Database:** English. **Subject Coverage:** Information on health and biomedical organizations, including federal, state, and local government agencies; information and referral centers; professional societies; self-help, support groups, and voluntary associations; academic and research institutions; hospitals; libraries; and museums.

★6879★ **DISABILITIES FORUM**
Clarke School for the Deaf
The Mainstream Center
46 Round Hill Rd.
Northampton, MA 01060-2199   Phone: (413) 584-3450
General Description: Provides disabled people, parents and families of the disabled, and professionals, employers, and others who work with the disabled the opportunity to share information, ideas, and experiences relating to any handicapping condition through its online conferencing and public electronic bulletin board facilities. Also includes the complete text of The Mainstream News, a monthly newsletter about mainstreaming hearing impaired students, and Data Libraries that contain relevant articles, computer programs, and lists of organizations and publications. **Language of Database:** English. **Subject Coverage:** Issues relating to all handicapping conditions.

★6880★ **DISABILITY SOLUTIONS**
GE Information Services
GEnie
401 N. Washington Blvd.
Rockville, MD 20850   Phone: (301) 340-4000
General Description: Provides a forum enabling persons with disabilities as well as persons interested in disability education and rehabilitation to share information, concerns, ideas, and solutions for disability issues. **Language of Database:** English. **Subject Coverage:** Disability issues, including hearing impaired issues, vision impaired issues, physically impaired issues, and education, employment, and leisure for disabled people.

★6881★ **DISABILITY STATISTICS DATABASE (DISSTAT)**
United Nations Statistical Office
Rm. DC2-1620
New York, NY 10017   Phone: (212) 963-4996
General Description: Contains information on sources and availability of statistics on disability for 95 countries or areas and detailed statistics for 55 countries on disabled persons. **Language of Database:** English. **Subject Coverage:** worldwide statistics on the handicapped.

★6882★ **DISEASE PREVENTION/HEALTH PROMOTION DATABASE**
U.S. Office of Disease Prevention and Health Promotion
ODPHP National Health Information Center
PO Box 1133
Washington, DC 20013-1133   Phone: (301) 565-4167
General Description: Contains information on organizations providing health-related information in a variety of subject areas. Covers federal and state government agencies, voluntary associations, support groups, and information centers. **Language of Database:** English. **Subject Coverage:** Health information resources covering such topics as health statistics, vitamins, adolescent health, health risk appraisals, and other frequently requested subjects.

★6883★ **DOCUSEARCH**
FOI Services, Inc.
12315 Wilkins Ave.
Rockville, MD 20852   Phone: (301) 881-0410
General Description: Contains bibliographic descriptions and cataloging information for documents issued by the U.S. Food and Drug Administration (FDA). **Also Known as:** DA Document Data Base. **Language of Database:** English. **Subject Coverage:** U.S. Food and Drug Administration documents.

★6884★ **DOCUSER**
U.S. National Library of Medicine
MEDLARS Management Section
8600 Rockville Pike
Bethesda, MD 20894   Phone: (301) 496-6193
General Description: Contains current information on active users of the National Library of Medicine's DOCLINE automated interlibrary loan request and referral system. **Also Known as:** Document Delivery User. **Language of Database:** English. **Subject Coverage:** Interlibrary loan providers and users within the NLM network.

★6885★ **DRI HEALTH CARE COST FORECASTING**
DRI/McGraw-Hill
Data Products Division
24 Hartwell Ave.
Lexington, MA 02173   Phone: (617) 863-5100
General Description: Provides projections of operating cost indexes (market basket indexes) for health care facilities plus cost escalation forecasts for the individual expense items purchased by the facility. **Language of Database:** English. **Subject Coverage:** Operating costs for health care facilities, including the following factors: market baskets for hospitals, nursing homes, and home health agencies; wages and benefits for hospital, nursing and personal care facilities, and service workers; food and beverages at home; electricity, natural gas, fuel oil and coal, and residential water and sewerage; medical care commodities, pharmaceutical preparations, chemicals, rubber, textiles, and special machinery; physician fees and transportation; and short-term prime rate and yield on municipal bonds.

★6886★   DRUG INFO
University of Minnesota, College of Pharmacy
Drug Information Services
3-160 Health Sciences Unit F
308 Harvard St., SE
Minneapolis, MN 55455   Phone: (612) 624-6492
General Description: Provides citations and abstracts of journal articles, books, and other materials covering the educational, sociological, and psychological aspects of alcohol and drug use and abuse. **Language of Database:** English. **Subject Coverage:** Alcohol and drug use and abuse, including educational, sociological, and psychological aspects.

★6887★   DRUG INFORMATION FULLTEXT (DIF)
American Society of Hospital Pharmacists
4630 Montgomery Ave.
Bethesda, MD 20814   Phone: (301) 657-3000
General Description: Provides the complete text of evaluative monographs drawn from the American Hospital Formulary Service (AHFS) Drug Information and the Handbook on Injectable Drugs, discussing manufacturers, claims and actual clinical experience on approximately 60,000 marketed drug products as well as investigational drugs. **Language of Database:** English. **Subject Coverage:** Drugs marketed in the United States.

★6888★   DRUG PRODUCTS INFORMATION FILE (DPIF)
American Society of Hospital Pharmacists
4630 Montgomery Ave.
Bethesda, MD 20814   Phone: (301) 657-3000
General Description: Provides detailed descriptions of most commercially available drug products. Includes standard English-language descriptions and codes to facilitate automated processing of all types of drug data. **Language of Database:** English. **Subject Coverage:** Drug products in commercial distribution.

★6889★   DRUGDEX SYSTEM
Micromedex, Inc.
600 Grant St.
Denver, CO 80203-3527   Phone: (303) 831-1400
General Description: Provides current referenced drug information to support the prescribing, ordering, and administration of medicine. Comprises three sections: • Drug eval uations—contains references and summaries on pharmacokinetics, contraindications, precautions, adverse reactions, teratogenic effects in pregnancy, drug interactions, I.V. incompatibilities, therapeutic indications, and patient instructions. • Drug consults—contains case histories from drug information centers an d clinical pharmacology services. • Drugdex Index—contains 55,000 listings by generic drug name, brand names (U.S. and foreign), and disease state; secondary access is gained through such topics as interactions, adverse effects, and clinical applications. **Language of Database:** English. **Subject Coverage:** All aspects of drugs and their use, including investigational, FDA-approved, and OTC preparations.

★6890★   DRUGLINE
Huddinge University Hospital
Department of Clinical Pharmacology
Drug Information Center
S-141 86 Huddinge, Sweden
General Description: Contains drug information in the form of questions and answers concerning physicians' drug treatment problems handled by the Drug Information Center at the Huddinge Hospital. **Language of Database:** Swedish; English. **Subject Coverage:** Drugs and drug treatment.

★6891★   DRUGNEWS
ADIS International Ltd.
Private Bag, Mairangi Bay
Auckland 10, New Zealand
General Description: Provides summaries of current international clinical news on drugs. **Language of Database:** English. **Subject Coverage:** Clinical drug news.

★6892★   EMBASE PLUS
Excerpta Medica/EMBASE Publishing Group
Molenwerf 1
PO Box 1527
NL-1000 BM Amsterdam, Netherlands
General Description: Provides citations and abstracts of international literature dealing with the biomedical sciences as they relate to human medicine. **Also Known as:** Excerpta Medica. **Language of Database:** English. **Subject Coverage:** Biomedicine, human medicine, and related disciplines; drugs, pharmacy, environmental health and pollution control,

toxicology, cancer, forensic science, health economics and hospital management, occupational health, and public health. Excluded are veterinary medicine, nursing, dentistry, and paramedical professions such as podiatry, optometry, and chiropractic.

★6893★   EMCANCER
Excerpta Medica/EMBASE Publishing Group
Molenwerf 1
PO Box 1527
NL-1000 BM Amsterdam, Netherlands
General Description: Contains references and abstracts of international journal literature relating to cancer. **Language of Database:** English. **Subject Coverage:** Cancer, including general aspects of the cancer problem (such as different methods of diagnosis and therapy, multiple tumors, metastasis, cancer incidence, mortality, prevention and control); experimental cancer research (cancerogenesis, cytology, histopathology, transplantation, experimental therapy); and clinical aspects of cancer (including individual organs and parts of the body).

★6894★   EMDRUGS
Excerpta Medica/EMBASE Publishing Group
Molenwerf 1
PO Box 1527
NL-1000 BM Amsterdam, Netherlands
General Description: Provides references and abstracts of international journal literature relating to the biological effects of chemical compounds. **Language of Database:** English. **Subject Coverage:** The biological effects of drugs, related compounds, and naturally occurring substances on biological substrates (defined as human or animal tissues, bacteria, tissue cultures, mitochondrias); clinical studies on drug action; pharmacokinetic studies; structural analysis, synthesis, and determination methods of drugs, hormones, and other substances known to have an effect on a biological substrate; and other substances whose chemical structural formulas indicate that they may have an influence on a biological substrate.

★6895★   EMERGINDEX SYSTEM
Micromedex, Inc.
600 Grant St.
Denver, CO 80203-3527   Phone: (303) 831-1400
General Description: Provides current information on key issues in emergency medicine as well as references to the latest literature in emergency medicine and critical care. Contains 300 clinical reviews dealing with patient presentation and the treatment and disposition of problems in emergency medicine plus more than 17,000 clinical abstracts from the world's medical literature and 35 prehospital protocols. **Language of Database:** English. **Subject Coverage:** Emergency and critical care medicine.

★6896★   EMFORENSIC
Excerpta Medica/EMBASE Publishing Group
Molenwerf 1
PO Box 1527
NL-1000 BM Amsterdam, Netherlands
General Description: Provides citations and abstracts of international journal literature in the field of forensic science. **Language of Database:** English. **Subject Coverage:** Forensic science, including law, thanatology, odontology, identification, traffic medicine, toxicology, serology, microbiology, and physical anthropology; forensic aspects of sudden natural death, medical practice fatalities, injuries due to blunt trauma, bullets and missiles, heat or electricity, asphyxia, drowning, child abuse, abortion and infanticide, sexual problems, and suicide; crime investigation methods; alcohol and drug problems.

★6897★   EMHEALTH
Excerpta Medica/EMBASE Publishing Group
Molenwerf 1
PO Box 1527
NL-1000 BM Amsterdam, Netherlands
General Description: Contains citations and abstracts of international journal literature relating to public health, social medicine, and occupational health and safety. A subset of the EMBASE plus database (described in a separate entry). **Language of Database:** English. **Subject Coverage:** Public health, social medicine, and hygiene, including health education, forensic medicine, social insurance, mental hygiene, addiction, medical education, medical ethics, statistics, communicable diseases, birth control, maternal and child care, school and vocational hygiene, dental hygiene, sanitation, sports medicine, traffic medicine, chronic diseases, poisoning, military medicine, atomic warfare, nutrition, veterinary hygiene, and zoonoses and medical zoology; occupational health and industrial medi-

cine, including safety and health education, professional training, legislation, medical examination, sex and age as they affect the worker, working time and leisure, ergonomics, work load, absenteeism, accidents, rehabilitation, and the work environment.

★6898★ EMTOX
Excerpta Medica/EMBASE Publishing Group
Molenwerf 1
PO Box 1527
NL-1000 BM Amsterdam, Netherlands
General Description: Provides citations and abstracts of international journal literature dealing with toxicology. Language of Database: English. Subject Coverage: Toxicology, including general aspects and methods; pharmaceutical toxicology; foods, food additives and contaminants; cosmetics, toiletries, and household products; agricultural chemicals; trace elements; vitamins; toxins and venoms; occupational toxicology; industrial chemicals and materials; waste materials in the air, soil, and water; radionuclides; chemical teratogens, mutagens, and carcinogens; toxic mechanisms; therapy; laboratory hazards; and predictive toxicology.

★6899★ ENDOMETRIOSIS ASSOCIATION RESEARCH
REGISTRY
Endometriosis Association
8585 N. 76th Pl.
Milwaukee, WI 53223   Phone: (414) 355-2200
General Description: Contains detailed case histories of individuals diagnosed with endometriosis, a female disorder in which endometrial tissue, which lines the uterus, is found in other locations in the body, usually the abdomen. Provides coded and analyzed questionnaire responses that cover each respondent's experiences with the disease, including symptoms, diagnosis, treatment, and outcome of treatment. Language of Database: English. Subject Coverage: Endometriosis, including etiology, symptoms, treatment, psychosocial aspects, and coping methods.

★6900★ ENVIRONMENTAL HEALTH NEWS (EHN)
Occupational Health Services, Inc.
450 7th Ave., Ste. 2407
New York, NY 10123   Phone: (212) 967-1100
General Description: Provides news alerts on late-breaking events, court decisions, regulatory changes, and medical and scientific news related to hazardous substances. Language of Database: English. Subject Coverage: Hazardous substances.

★6901★ ENVIRONMENTAL MUTAGEN INFORMATION
CENTER DATA BASE
Oak Ridge National Laboratory
Biomedical and Environmental Information Analysis Section
Environmental Mutagen Information
PO Box 2008
Oak Ridge, TN 37831-6050   Phone: (615) 574-7871
General Description: Contains references to worldwide published literature reporting the testing of chemicals for genotoxicity. Includes CAS Registry Numbers for all chemicals covered. Language of Database: English. Subject Coverage: Chemical mutagenesis, including genetic effects of drugs, food additives, cosmetics, and industrial chemicals; mutagenicity of biological and some physical agents; test systems and organisms. Coverage excludes mutagenicity of ionizing or ultraviolet radiation.

★6902★ ENVIRONMENTAL TERATOLOGY INFORMATION
CENTER DATA BASE
Oak Ridge National Laboratory
Biomedical and Environmental Information Analysis Section
Environmental Teratology Information
PO Box 2008
Oak Ridge, TN 37831-6050   Phone: (615) 574-7871
General Description: Contains references to worldwide literature dealing with the chemical and drug effects on embryology of warm-blooded and cold-blooded animals. Also Known as: ETI Data Base. Language of Database: English. Subject Coverage: Experimental teratology in warm-blooded and cold-blooded animals.

★6903★ ESPECIALIDADES CONSUMIDAS POR LA
SEGURIDAD SOCIAL (ECOM)
Ministerio de Sanidad y Consumo de Espana
Direccion General de Farmacia y Productos Sanitarios
Servicio de Gestion del Banco de Datos de Medicamentos
Paseo del Prado, 18-20
28014 Madrid, Spain
General Description: Contains demographic data for pharmaceutical

expenditures related to drug consumption within the Social Security Services of Spain. Also Known as: Consumption of Pharmaceutical Specialties in the Social Security Services. Language of Database: Spanish. Subject Coverage: Pharmaceutical product data and related demographics for usage of drugs in Spain's Social Security Services.

★6904★ ESPECIALIDADES FARMACEUTICAS ESPANOLAS
(ESPES)
Ministerio de Sanidad y Consumo de Espana
Direccion General de Farmacia y Productos Sanitarios
Servicio de Gestion del Banco de Datos de Medicamentos
Paseo del Prado, 18-20
28014 Madrid, Spain
General Description: Contains current detailed composition and manufacturer data about pharmaceutical products and specialties registered in Spain. Prior to product description updates, the previous data are transferred to a backfile known as HESPES. Also Known as: Spanish Pharmaceutical Specialties. Language of Database: Spanish. Subject Coverage: Drugs registered in Spain, covering pharmaceutical and pharmacological, therapeutic, administrative, economic, technological, and management aspects.

★6905★ ESPECIALIDADES FARMACEUTICAS EN TRAMITE
DE REGISTRO (TRAMIT)
Ministerio de Sanidad y Consumo de Espana
Direccion General de Farmacia y Productos Sanitarios
Servicio de Gestion del Banco de Datos de Medicamentos
Paseo del Prado, 18-20
28014 Madrid, Spain
General Description: Contains information and data describing pharmaceutical products and specialties which are in the process of being authorized for marketing within Spain. Also Known as: Pharmaceutical Specialties in the Process of Authorization Marketing. Language of Database: Spanish. Subject Coverage: Pharmaceutical product data for drugs currently being authorized for use within Social Security Services of Spain.

★6906★ ESSENTIALS/REFERENCES ESSENTIELLES
Canadian Centre for Occupational Health and Safety (CCOHS)
250 Main St. E.
Hamilton, ON, Canada L8N 1H6   Phone: (416) 572-2981
General Description: Provides information on topics relating to occupational health and safety. Includes references to readings selected by CCOHS subject specialists as providing the most current information on the topic. Language of Database: English; French. Subject Coverage: Occupational health and safety and related topics.

★6907★ EXCEPTIONAL CHILD EDUCATION RESOURCES
(ECER)
Council for Exceptional Children
Department of Information Services
1920 Association Dr.
Reston, VA 22091   Phone: (703) 620-3660
General Description: Provides abstracts and citations to published and unpublished materials covering research, education, policy, and services for gifted and handicapped children. Language of Database: English. Subject Coverage: Gifted and handicapped children, including the visually, aurally, and mentally handicapped and children with learning disabilities, emotional disturbances, and speech handicaps.

★6908★ EXCERPTA MEDICA CD: DRUGS AND
PHARMACOLOGY
Excerpta Medica/EMBASE Publishing Group
Molenwerf 1
PO Box 1527
NL-1000 BM Amsterdam, Netherlands
General Description: Provides citations and abstracts of international literature dealing with drugs and pharmacology. Language of Database: English. Subject Coverage: Drugs and pharmacology, including the effects, side effects, and adverse effects of drugs, and the clinical and experimental aspects of pharmacokinetics and pharmacodynamics.

★6909★ EXCERPTA MEDICA CD: GASTROENTEROLOGY
Excerpta Medica/EMBASE Publishing Group
Molenwerf 1
PO Box 1527
NL-1000 BM Amsterdam, Netherlands
General Description: Provides citations and abstracts of international literature dealing with all aspects of gastroenterology. Language of Data-

base: English. **Subject Coverage:** All aspects of gastroenterology, including coverage of digestive system diseases and disorders, diseases and disorders of the mouth, the pharynx, the hepatobiliary system, the exocrine pancreas, the peritoneum, the mesentery, and the omentum.

★6910★ EXCERPTA MEDICA CD: IMMUNOLOGY AND AIDS
Excerpta Medica/EMBASE Publishing Group
Molenwerf 1
PO Box 1527
NL-1000 BM Amsterdam, Netherlands
General Description: Provides citations and abstracts of international literature dealing with immunology and Acquired Immune Deficiency Syndrome (AIDS). **Language of Database:** English. **Subject Coverage:** All aspects of clinical and experimental immunology, immunity, autoimmunity, hypersensitivity, histocompatibility, cancer immunology, immunotherapy, immunopharmacology, immunological aspects of transplantation, paraproteinemias, the lymphoreticular system, and AIDS.

★6911★ EXCERPTA MEDICA CD: NEUROSCIENCES
Excerpta Medica/EMBASE Publishing Group
Molenwerf 1
PO Box 1527
NL-1000 BM Amsterdam, Netherlands
General Description: Provides citations and abstracts of international literature dealing with clinical and other aspects of several neurosciences. **Language of Database:** English. **Subject Coverage:** Neuroscience, with emphasis on clinical neurology and neurosurgery, epilepsy, and neuromuscular disorders; neurophysiology, and animal models for human neuropharmacology.

★6912★ EXCERPTA MEDICA CD: PSYCHIATRY
Excerpta Medica/EMBASE Publishing Group
Molenwerf 1
PO Box 1527
NL-1000 BM Amsterdam, Netherlands
General Description: Provides citations and abstracts of international literature dealing with all aspects of psychology and psychiatry. **Language of Database:** English. **Subject Coverage:** All aspects of psychology and psychiatry, covering addiction, alcoholism, sexual behavior, suicide, mental deficiency, and the clinical use or abuse of psychotropic and psychomimetic substances.

★6913★ EXCERPTA MEDICA VOCABULARY (EVOC)
Excerpta Medica/EMBASE Publishing Group
Molenwerf 1
PO Box 1527
NL-1000 BM Amsterdam, Netherlands
General Description: Contains the complete text of the EMBASE Guide to EMTREE and Indexing Systems, the Master List of Medical Indexing Terms (MALIMET), the Item Index, and the EMBASE List of Journals Abstracted. **Language of Database:** English. **Subject Coverage:** Medical subject and indexing terms; medical journals.

★6914★ EXPERTNET
ExpertNet, Ltd.
225 W. Ohio St., Ste. 325
Chicago, IL 60610   Phone: (312) 527-0470
General Description: Contains biographical descriptions of more than 1000 experts willing to serve as consultants and trial witnesses for medical malpractice and personal injury cases. Provides information on expert specialties, education, area of the country, and typical hourly fees. **Language of Database:** English. **Subject Coverage:** Medical malpractice and personal injury expert witnesses.

★6915★ THE FAMILY DOCTOR
CMC ReSearch, Inc.
7150 SW Hampton, Ste. C-120
Portland, OR 97223   Phone: (503) 639-3395
General Description: Provides a full range of medical information organized and written for consumer use. Contains answers to more than 1500 commonly asked medical questions answered by Dr. Allen H. Bruckheim, author of the nationally syndicated "The Family Doctor" newspaper column; full color illustrations from Medical Times; health updates on such topics as the heart, aging, arthritis, diabetes, colon cancer, and cholestrol control; a directory of national and local support groups and education resources relating to medical topics; and Consumer Guide's Prescription Drugs, covering 1600 brand-name products. **Language of Database:** English. **Subject Coverage:** Consumer medical information, including prescription drugs, accidental poisoning, first aid, rare diseases,

ill-defined symptoms, pregnancy and childbirth, mental and emotional conditions, glands and metabolism, blood and blood-forming organs, tumors, infections or parasites, community and social problems, and diseases.

★6916★ FATALITY REPORTS
Canadian Centre for Occupational Health and Safety
250 Main St. E.
Hamilton, ON, Canada L8N 1H6   Phone: (416) 572-2981
General Description: Provides information about the circumstances surrounding occupationally related fatalities. **Language of Database:** English. **Subject Coverage:** Canadian occupational fatalities.

★6917★ FDA DRUG BULLETIN
U.S. Food and Drug Administration (FDA)
5600 Fishers Ln.
Rockville, MD 20857   Phone: (301) 443-3285
General Description: Reports news and developments relating to clinical drug testing, approvals of new drugs by the U.S. Food and Drug Administration (FDA), and information on food additives and food preparation processes. **Language of Database:** English. **Subject Coverage:** Drug testing, new drugs, food additives, and food preparation processes.

★6918★ FOOD/ANALYST
Hopkins Technology
421 Hazel Lane
Hopkins, MN 55343-7117   Phone: (612) 931-9376
General Description: Contains the complete U.S. Department of Agriculture's food database (Handbook 8), Home Economic Research Report 48 on sugar content, and Quaker Oats food data. Provides nutritional breakdowns for more than 80 nutrients found in nearly 5000 foods. **Language of Database:** English. **Subject Coverage:** Nutritional analysis of food ingredients, including protein, carbohydrates, fat, sugar, vitamins, minerals, and fiber, in the following food groups: dairy and egg products, spices and herbs, baby foods, fats and oils, poultry, soups, sauces and gravies, sausages and luncheon meats, breakfast cereals, fruits and fruit juices, pork products, vegetables and vegetable products, nut and seed products, beef products, beverages, fin and shellfish products, legumes and legume products, lamb, veal and game, baked products, snacks and sweets, cereal, grains and pastas, fast foods, and mixed dishes.

★6919★ FOODS ADLIBRA
FOODS ADLIBRA Publications
9000 Plymouth Ave., N.
Minneapolis, MN 55427   Phone: (612) 540-4759
General Description: Provides references and abstracts of worldwide food industry literature reporting developments in management, marketing, new food products, food-related patents, and other industry topics. **Language of Database:** English. **Subject Coverage:** The food industry, including new products, ingredient developments, management news, world food economics and international marketing, commodities, marketing statistics and market research, nutritional information and toxicology, research and technology, processing and engineering methods, patents, packaging developments, governmental information, and company and association news announcements.

★6920★ FORTHCOMING EVENTS
BIOSIS
2100 Arch St.
Philadelphia, PA 19103-1399   Phone: (215) 587-4800
General Description: Announces upcoming meetings, seminars, workshops, and special events of interest to life scientists. **Language of Database:** English. **Subject Coverage:** Meetings, seminars, workshops, and special events in the life sciences.

★6921★ 4-SIGHTS NETWORK
Greater Detroit Society for the Blind
16625 Grand River Ave.
Detroit, MI 48227   Phone: (313) 272-3900
General Description: Contains technology information, vocational information, and educational and rehabilitation resources for the blind and visually impaired. Comprises the following 15 files: • General Conference. • 4-Sights User Manual. • Reh abilitation Resources—research reports and other resources for rehabilitation teachers and counselors. • Multi-Handicapped Blind Resources—comments and re sources concerning multiply-impaired blind persons. • Software Exchange—pub lic domain programs and documentation. • Technology Conference—electronic d evices for use by the blind and visually impaired and general electronic applications. • Job Placement Exchange. • Calendar of Events—conferences, work shops,

and special programs at the national, regional, and local levels. • S pecialized Training Facilities—training programs for the blind, for those providing services to the blind, and college or university services for students with disabilities. • Low Vision Conferences—low vision conditions and related subjects. • Public Policy Issues—judicial, legislative, and government actions of import to blind people and programs. • Occupational Information - The Blind at Work—includes Occupational Information Library for the Blind, a directory of more than 500 jobs successfully performed by the blind or visually impaired. • Education Conference—trends and developments in education of the blind and visually impaired. • Michigan Occupational Information System—matches personal profiles to job descriptions. • Link-Up—bimonthly publication coveri ng online servies. **Language of Database:** English. **Subject Coverage:** Services for the blind and visually handicapped.

★6922★ **GASTROINTESTINAL ABSORPTION DATABASE (GIABS)**
U.S. Environmental Protection Agency
Office of Pesticides and Toxic Substances
401 M St., SW, MS-TS799
Washington, DC 20460   Phone: (202) 554-1404
General Description: Contains references and abstracts of articles in the scientific literature covering the absorption, distribution, metabolism, and excretion of 3100 chemicals in laboratory animals or humans. **Language of Database:** English. **Subject Coverage:** Absorption, distribution, metabolism, and excretion data for chemicals in laboratory animals and humans.

★6923★ **GENBANK (GENETIC SEQUENCES DATABANK)**
IntelliGenetics, Inc.
700 E. El Camino Real
Mountain View, CA 94040   Phone: (415) 962-7300
General Description: Provides all reported nucleic acid sequences, cataloged and annotated for sites of biological significance. **Subject Coverage:** Nucleic sequence data.

★6924★ **GENERAL PRACTITIONER**
Haymarket Medical Publications Ltd.
30 Lancaster Gate
London W2 3LP, England
General Description: Contains the complete text of the following three journals covering general practice medicine: • GP-General Practitioner—provides news on all aspects o f the general practitioner's work. Covers medico-political matters such as constraints on prescribing and the use of deputizing services. Also tracks scientific news and developments. • Mims Magazine—contains articles about medicines a nd their uses, developments in pharmaceuticals, and information on prescribing drugs and therapeutics. Features an article series which reviews the properties and uses of the 50 most commonly prescribed drugs in general practice. • Medeconomi cs—covers the business, financial, and organizational aspects of general practice within the British National Health Service. **Language of Database:** English. **Subject Coverage:** General practice medicine, including medico-political issues, scientific developments, pharmaceuticals, and financial and organizational aspects.

★6925★ **GENERAL SCIENCE INDEX**
H.W. Wilson Co.
950 University Ave.
Bronx, NY 10452   Phone: (212) 588-8400
General Description: Indexes articles appearing in English-language science periodicals of general interest published primarily in the United States. **Language of Database:** English. **Subject Coverage:** Science, including astronomy, atmospheric science, biology, botany, chemistry, earth science, environment and conservation, food and nutrition, genetics, mathematics, medicine and health, microbiology, oceanography, physics, physiology, and zoology.

★6926★ **GENETIC TECHNOLOGY NEWS (GTN)**
Technical Insights, Inc.
PO Box 1304
Fort Lee, NJ 07024-9967   Phone: (201) 568-4744
General Description: Covers advances in the field of molecular biology. Includes coverage of technical papers, meetings, new patents, industry news, and market forecasts for new products made by genetic engineering. **Language of Database:** English. **Subject Coverage:** Molecular biology and genetic engineering.

★6927★ **GENETIC TOXICITY (GENETOX)**
U.S. Environmental Protection Agency
Office of Pesticides and Toxic Substances
401 M St., SW, MS-TS799
Washington, DC 20460   Phone: (202) 554-1404
General Description: Provides mutagenicity information on more than 2600 chemicals tested on 38 biological systems. **Language of Database:** English. **Subject Coverage:** Chemical mutagens.

★6928★ **GENETICS ABSTRACTS**
Cambridge Scientific Abstracts
7200 Wisconsin Ave.
Bethesda, MD 20814   Phone: (301) 961-6750
General Description: Contains citations and abstracts of international periodical and other literature covering all aspects of molecular, viral, bacterial, fungal, algal, plant, animal, and human genetics. **Language of Database:** English. **Subject Coverage:** All aspects of molecular, viral, bacterial, fungal, algal, plant, animal, and human genetics. Specific topics covered include medical genetics, including oncology and hematological disorders; molecular genetics; chromosomes; extrachromosomal genetics; cell division; chemical mutagenesis; radiation genetics; immunogenetics; developmental, evolutionary, ecological, behavioral, theoretical, and population genetics; viral, bacterial, fungal, and algal genetics; plant genetics; vertebrate and invertebrate genetics; and human genetics.

★6929★ **HANDICAPPED EDUCATIONAL EXCHANGE (HEX)**
Amateur Radio Research and Development Corp.
11523 Charlton Dr.
Silver Spring, MD 20902   Phone: (301) 681-7372
General Description: Provides a forum for the exchange of information on the use of modern technology, such as computers, to aid the disabled. Lists sources of computer hardware and software, as well as conferences and seminars dealing with handicaps and special education, magazines and newsletters, user groups, and other sources of data. Includes a list of other bulletin boards dealing with disabilities. **Language of Database:** English. **Subject Coverage:** Modern technology designed to aid the handicapped, with emphasis on computer hardware and software.

★6930★ **HANDICAPPED USERS' DATABASE (HUD)**
CompuServe Information Service
5000 Arlington Centre Blvd.
PO Box 20212
Columbus, OH 43220   Phone: (614) 457-8600
General Description: Provides articles and information of interest both for and about the handicapped, including pertinent news and names and descriptions of service organizations. Also contains a reference library, lists of computer products specifically geared for use by handicapped individuals, and an online message board for the exchange of ideas. **Language of Database:** English. **Subject Coverage:** The handicapped.

★6931★ **THE HAZARD AWARENESS HEALTH AND SAFETY LIBRARY: HAZARD COMMUNICATION**
Online Computer Systems, Inc.
20251 Century Blvd.
Germantown, MD 20874   Phone: (301) 428-3700
General Description: Contains an integrated series of occupational safety and health presentations. Covers chemical labeling systems used by the U.S. Occupational Safety and Health Administration (OSHA), U.S. Department of Transportation (DOT), and U.S. National Fire Protection Agency (NFPA), as well as Material Safety Data Sheets (MSDS). Provides employee rights and employer responsibilities with regard to the OSHA Hazard Communication Standard, which requires employers to inform employees of hazardous chemicals in the workplace. **Language of Database:** English. **Subject Coverage:** Occupational safety and health.

★6932★ **THE HAZARD AWARENESS HEALTH AND SAFETY LIBRARY: HAZARD PROTECTION**
Online Computer Systems, Inc.
20251 Century Blvd.
Germantown, MD 20874   Phone: (301) 428-3700
General Description: Contains information on occupational health and safety, including basic human biology and toxicology, exposure to hazardous chemicals, exposure detection, and means of limiting exposure such as protective equipment and ventilation. **Language of Database:** English. **Subject Coverage:** Occupational health and safety.

★6933★   THE HAZARD AWARENESS HEALTH AND SAFETY LIBRARY: HEARING CONSERVATION
Online Computer Systems, Inc.
20251 Century Blvd.
Germantown, MD 20874   Phone: (301) 428-3700
General Description: Provides occupational safety and health information on workplace noise, including health effects, measurement, hearing protection, and hearing loss detection. **Language of Database:** English. **Subject Coverage:** Noise pollution, with emphasis on noise in the workplace.

★6934★   HAZARD COMMUNICATION COMPLIANCE MANUAL DATABASE
The Bureau of National Affairs, Inc. (BNA)
BNA ONLINE
1231 25th St., NW
Washington, DC 20037   Phone: (202) 452-4132
General Description: Provides information on establishing a hazard right-to-know program in the workplace. Includes instructions for obtaining Material Safety Data Sheets from chemical manufacturers, sample forms and handouts for training, the complete text of the Occupational Safety and Health Administration's Hazard Communication Standard, an explanation of related federal right-to-know programs, a summary of terms used in hazard communications, and a sample policy. **Language of Database:** English. **Subject Coverage:** The OSHA Hazard Communication Standard and instructions for developing right-to-know policies in the workplace.

★6935★   HAZARDLINE
Occupational Health Services, Inc.
450 7th Ave., Ste. 2407
New York, NY 10123   Phone: (212) 967-1100
General Description: Supplies identification, requirement, and recommendation information for more than 10,000 hazardous substances in the workplace. **Language of Database:** English. **Subject Coverage:** Hazardous chemical substances in the workplace; related federal and state regulations, court decisions, standards, and recommended procedures.

★6936★   HAZARDOUS SUBSTANCES DATA BANK (HSDB)
U.S. National Library of Medicine
Toxicology Information Program
8600 Rockville Pike
Bethesda, MD 20894   Phone: (301) 496-1131
General Description: Contains toxicological information on chemical substances augmented by data for such aspects as emergency handling procedures, environmental fate, human exposure, detection methods, and regulatory requirements. **Language of Database:** English. **Subject Coverage:** Toxicology of hazardous substances and the related areas of hazardous waste and occupational safety and health.

★6937★   HEALTH FOR ALL: PRIMARY CARE AND CONSUMER INFORMATION
CD Resources, Inc.
118 W. 74th St., Ste. 2A
New York, NY 10023   Phone: (212) 580-2263
General Description: Provides the complete text of documents, case studies, overviews, and training materials providing information on all aspects of health care. **Language of Database:** English. **Subject Coverage:** Health care, including legislation, health planning and management, primary health care, environmental and occupational health, maternal and child care, immunization, and health education and training materials.

★6938★   HEALTH CARE COMPETITION WEEK
Capitol Publications, Inc.
Capitol Publishing Group
PO Box 1453
Alexandria, VA 22313-2053   Phone: (703) 683-4100
General Description: Focuses on marketing strategies for health care providers. Includes a marketer's forum, industry statistics, cost-saving ideas, conference reports, market research data, Washington briefs, and earnings reports. Also covers trends in the field, including health maintenance organizations (HMOs), preferred-provider organizations (PPOs), and other alternative delivery services. **Language of Database:** English. **Subject Coverage:** Marketing strategies for health care providers.

★6939★   HEALTH CARE COSTS: WHERE'S THE BOTTOM LINE?
The Bureau of National Affairs, Inc. (BNA)
BNA ONLINE
1231 25th St., NW
Washington, DC 20037   Phone: (202) 452-4132
General Description: Focuses on initiatives that have been taken by private and public sector employers, welfare funds, unions, and health care providers in their attempts to bring down the rising costs of health care in the United States. Also covers various approaches to cost containment, legal issues, legislative developments in health care, and health care terminology. **Language of Database:** English. **Subject Coverage:** Health care cost containment approaches such as coalitions, HMOs, PPOs, wellness and health promotion programs, employee assistance programs, and hospitals; private sector case studies, public sector case studies, legal issues, health care terminology, and legislative developments.

★6940★   HEALTH CARE INDUSTRY COMPETITIVE INTELLIGENCE TRACKING SERVICE
SIS International
172 Madison Ave., Ste. 306
New York, NY 10016   Phone: (212) 725-4550
General Description: Provides comprehensive and up-to-date competitive intelligence on the health care industry. Contains citations and abstracts to periodical literature published worldwide. **Language of Database:** English. **Subject Coverage:** The health care industry, including industry trends and issues, consumer attitudes, market activity, legislation, competitor profiles, financial performance, mergers and acquisitions, new product development, technology, research, biotechnology, future trends, and the international scene.

★6941★   HEALTH CARE LITERATURE INFORMATION NETWORK (HECLINET)
Institut fur Krankenhausbau
Strasse des 17. Juni 135
D-1000 Berlin 12, Germany
General Description: Covers literature dealing with the nonclinical aspects of hospital management and health care delivery. **Language of Database:** German; English. **Subject Coverage:** Hospital administration; nonclinical aspects of health services; hospital design, construction, and maintenance; health insurance and economics; health policy and planning; personnel and training; and interdisciplinary areas.

★6942★   HEALTH CARE PURCHASING ORGANIZATIONS
McKnight Medical Communications, Inc.
1419 Lake Cook Rd.
Deerfield, IL 60015   Phone: (708) 945-0345
General Description: Provides listings for approximately 275 health care purchasing organizations representing more than 12,000 hospitals, health maintenance organizations (HMOs), preferred provider organizations (PPOs), nursing homes, and government institutions. **Language of Database:** English. **Subject Coverage:** Health care purchasing organizations in the United States.

★6943★   HEALTH DEVICES ALERTS
ECRI
5200 Butler Pike
Plymouth Meeting, PA 19462   Phone: (215) 825-6000
General Description: Reports on hazards, recalls, and problems with medical devices. Includes abstracts of articles, items that ECRI has investigated or verified, spontaneous problem reports submitted by health care professionals to the U.S. Food and Drug Administration (FDA), and mandatory medical device reports from the FDA. Includes recommended actions for remedying certain problems. **Language of Database:** English. **Subject Coverage:** Medical device defects and/or problems covering magnetic resonance imaging units, implanted devices and related accessories, disposable medical products, clinical laboratory reagents, hospital furniture, sutures, clinical cases, end-of-life failure, product misuse, and product recalls.

★6944★   HEALTH DEVICES SOURCEBOOK
ECRI
5200 Butler Pike
Plymouth Meeting, PA 19462   Phone: (215) 825-6000
General Description: Provides information on North American manufacturers, importers, and distributors of more than 5000 medical devices and equipment. Also covers medical equipment service companies. Includes trade names for products and an online thesaurus. **Language of Database:** English. **Subject Coverage:** Medical devices and materials, clinical laborato-

ry equipment and reagents, selected hospital furniture, casework, and systems and instruments used in testing medical equipment. Currently extends to U.S. manufacturers, products, and services with limited international coverage which is to be expanded in the future.

★6945★ HEALTH EDUCATION AND PROMOTION DATABASE
U.S. Centers for Disease Control
Center for Chronic Disease Prevention and Health Promotion
1600 Clifton Rd., MS K13
Atlanta, GA 30333   Phone: (404) 639-3492
General Description: Contains references and abstracts of published materials dealing with health education and promotion programs and risk reduction interventions. Language of Database: English. Subject Coverage: Health education and promotion.

★6946★ HEALTH AND FITNESS FORUM
CompuServe Information Service
5000 Arlington Centre Blvd.
PO Box 20212
Columbus, OH 43220   Phone: (614) 457-8600
General Description: Provides a forum for the discussion of physical fitness and stress management with members and health care professionals. Features online conferences held every Sunday evening. Language of Database: English. Subject Coverage: Health and stress management, including exercise equipment, fitness testing, health insurance, coping with stress, proper nutrition, and substance abuse.

★6947★ HEALTH GRANTS AND CONTRACTS WEEKLY
Capitol Publications, Inc.
Capitol Publishing Group
PO Box 1453
Alexandria, VA 22313-2053   Phone: (703) 683-4100
General Description: Lists medical and health grants available from the federal government. Reviews legislative actions and other developments affecting funding sources, and covers application deadlines and grants awarded, profiles on funding agencies, and regulatory and legislative events. Language of Database: English. Subject Coverage: Federal medical and health grants and contracts.

★6948★ HEALTH INDEX
Information Access Co.
362 Lakeside Dr.
Foster City, CA 94404   Phone: (415) 378-5000
General Description: Provides references to consumer health literature and health-related articles from more than 100 popular, business, and academic journals, and newspapers. Also covers selected articles from more than 3000 magazines and newspapers indexed in IAC's Academic Index, Business Index, Legal Resource Index, Magazine Index, and National Newspaper Index. Language of Database: English. Subject Coverage: Health, fitness, and nutrition, covering alcohol and drug abuse, health care delivery and politics, coping with chronic disease and disability, public health and nursing, nutrition policy/healthy lifestyles, occupational health and safety, pregnancy and childbirth, sports medicine and training, and law and medicine.

★6949★ HEALTH INDUSTRY RESEARCH REPORTS
Bowker Business Research
121 Chanlon Rd.
New Providence, NJ 07974   Phone: (908) 464-6800
General Description: Contains citations and abstracts of research reports covering the health industry and individual companies. Includes analyses of company financial information, philosophy, track record, management, research and development, product development, competitive position, projected strategies, and corporate and industry trends. Language of Database: English. Subject Coverage: Health industry analysis.

★6950★ HEALTH NEWS DAILY
FDC Reports, Inc.
5550 Friendship Blvd., Ste. 1
Chevy Chase, MD 20815   Phone: (301) 657-9830
General Description: Reports news and developments in the health industry in the United States and elsewhere. Covers corporate financial performance, mergers and acquisitions, new ventures and products, technological and scientific advancements, and the relationship between federal agencies and the hundreds of health industry and trade professional associations. Language of Database: English. Subject Coverage: The health industry in the United States and elsewhere.

★6951★ HEALTH PERIODICALS DATABASE
Information Access Co.
362 Lakeside Dr.
Foster City, CA 94404   Phone: (415) 378-5000
General Description: Provides citations to articles published in 600 health and medical periodicals. Includes the complete text of articles appearing in 120 core journals since January 1989. Language of Database: English. Subject Coverage: Health, medicine, fitness, and nutrition.

★6952★ HEALTH PLANNING AND ADMINISTRATION
U.S. National Library of Medicine
MEDLARS Management Section
8600 Rockville Pike
Bethesda, MD 20894   Phone: (301) 496-6193
General Description: Provides references to journal literature dealing with the nonclinical aspects of health care delivery, such as health care planning, organization, financing, management, and manpower. Also Known as: HEALTH. Language of Database: English. Subject Coverage: Administration and planning of health facilities; services and manpower; health insurance; health policy; aspects of financial management, regulation, personnel administration, quality assurance, and licensure and accreditation which apply to health care delivery.

★6953★ HEALTH PROMOTION RESOURCE CENTER (HPRC) DATABASE
United Nations Educational, Scientific and Cultural Organization
Documentation and Computer-Assisted Management Service
7, place de Fontenoy
F-75700 Paris, France
General Description: Provides references to published materials relating to education for AIDS prevention. Covers pedagogical materials such as audiovisual materials, leaflets, and posters. Language of Database: English; French; Spanish. Subject Coverage: Educational materials relating to the prevention of Acquired Immune Deficiency Syndrome (AIDS).

★6954★ HEALTH AND PSYCHOSOCIAL INSTRUMENTS (HAPI)
Behavioral Measurement Database Services
PO Box 110287
Pittsburgh, PA 15232-0787   Phone: (412) 687-6850
General Description: Contains citations to published materials providing information on instruments used in the fields of health, psychosocial sciences, organizational behavior, and human resources for research studies, grant proposals, client/patient assessment, class papers/projects, theses/dissertations, and program evaluation. Language of Database: English. Subject Coverage: Information gathering instruments, including questionnaires, interview schedules, observation checklists and manuals, index measures, coding schemes, scenarios, vignettes, rating scales, projective techniques, and tests used in health-related fields.

★6955★ HEALTH REFERENCE CENTER
Information Access Co.
362 Lakeside Dr.
Foster City, CA 94404   Phone: (415) 378-5000
General Description: Provides information on health, medical treatments, fitness, nutrition, and other health-related topics. Comprises the following sections: • Core health titles and general publications—contains citations and abstracts of articles published in more than 110 health publications and some 3000 general periodicals. Covers illnesses, prenatal care, dieting, drug abuse, mental health, sports medicine, cardiovascular disease, therapies, biotechnology, gerontology, treatments, drug side effects, and medical costs. Includes the complete text of selected publications. • Professional publications—provides summaries of articles fro m 40 technical journals. Include the complete text of selected journals. • R eference publications—contains the complete text of four publications geared towards the patient; includes selected information from USP Drug Information (described in a separate entry). • Patient Guided Access—contains tutorial information on 300 diseases and medical conditions. Includes detailed background information on causes, prevention, therapy, and questions patients should ask physicians. Language of Database: English. Subject Coverage: Health care and medicine.

★6956★ HEALTH AND SAFETY SCIENCE ABSTRACTS (HSSA)
Cambridge Scientific Abstracts
7200 Wisconsin Ave.
Bethesda, MD 20814   Phone: (301) 961-6750
General Description: Contains citations and abstracts of international literature on general health and safety science. Language of Database: English. Subject Coverage: General health and safety science. Topics

covered include industria l and occupational health and medical safety, including hospitals and medical research institutes, emergency medical services, epidemiology and public health, aviation and aerospace medicine, genetics, toxicology, radiology, immunology, and specific injuries/trauma and diseases.

★6957★   HEALTH WEEK
CMP Publications, Inc.
600 Community Dr.
Manhasset, NY 11030   Phone: (516) 562-5000
General Description: Covers the business side of the health care industry. Reports news and offers solutions relating to management issues and concerns faced by health care provider organizations. **Language of Database:** English. **Subject Coverage:** Business and management aspects of the health care industry.

★6958★   HEALTHCARE EVALUATION SYSTEM (HES)
National Planning Data Corp.
PO Box 610
Ithaca, NY 14851-0610   Phone: (607) 273-8208
General Description: Contains health care facilities utilization data for hospitals, nursing homes, and other health care institutions. **Language of Database:** English. **Subject Coverage:** Demographics of health care facilities for use in determining locations for new facilities.

★6959★   HEALTHCARE PRODUCT COMPARISON SYSTEMS
ECRI
5200 Butler Pike
Plymouth Meeting, PA 19462   Phone: (215) 825-6000
General Description: Provides descriptions of all types of equipment used in the healthcare professions. **Language of Database:** English. **Subject Coverage:** Healthcare equipment, including X-ray units, surgical lasers, and laboratory instrumentation.

★6960★   HEALTHWEEK
CMP Publications, Inc.
600 Community Dr.
Manhasset, NY 11030   Phone: (516) 562-5000
General Description: Contains the complete text of HealthWeek, a newspaper covering the health care industry. Covers legal and regulatory developments affecting health care financing, analyses of industry trends, information systems, patient care technology and business news, including contracts, mergers, and acquisitions. **Language of Database:** English. **Subject Coverage:** The health care industry, with emphasis on management and financial issues.

★6961★   HELMINTHOLOGICAL ABSTRACTS
C.A.B. International
Wallingford, Oxon. OX10 8DE, England
General Description: Indexes and abstracts current periodical and other published literature relating to medical and veterinary helminthology. **Language of Database:** English. **Subject Coverage:** Medical and veterinary helminthology; animal health; taxonomy; morphology; pathology; biochemistry; epidemiology; immunology and immunogenetics; control of pests, disease, and micro-organisms; and pesticides.

★6962★   HOSPITAL PERSONNEL DATABASE
Medical Device Register, Inc.
655 Washington Blvd.
Stamford, CT 06901   Phone: (203) 348-6319
General Description: Provides listings for key personnel working at some 7450 proprietary, government, teaching, nursing, and voluntary hospitals in the United States. **Language of Database:** English. **Subject Coverage:** U.S. hospital personnel in some 90 job title areas.

★6963★   HRAF DATA ARCHIVE
Human Relations Area Files, Inc.
755 Prospect St.
PO Box 2054, Yale Sta.
New Haven, CT 06520   Phone: (203) 777-2334
General Description: Contains the complete text of more than 1000 anthropological, sociological, and psychological books and articles dealing with life in 60 different societies worldwide during the 19th and 20th centuries. Consists of ten topical monographs in five volumes: • Human Sexuality and Marriage. • Family and Crime an d Social Problems. • Old Age and Death and Dying. • Childhood and Adolescence and Socialization and Education. • Religious Beliefs and Religious Practices. **Language of Database:** English. **Subject Coverage:** Sociological, anthropological, and

psychological studies of life in different cultures worldwide, including religion, education, social organization, demography, warfare, crime, social problems, cultural complexity, social change, birth, childhood, birth control, abortion, human sexuality, marriage, treatment of the aged, and death.

★6964★   HUMAN GENOME ABSTRACTS
Cambridge Scientific Abstracts
7200 Wisconsin Ave.
Bethesda, MD 20814   Phone: (301) 961-6750
General Description: Contains citations and abstracts of literature covering human genomes (chromosomes with the genes they contain). **Language of Database:** English. **Subject Coverage:** Human genomes.

★6965★   HUMAN NUTRITION DATABASE
Institut fur Ernaehrungswissenschaft
Abteilung Dokumentation
Goethestr. 55
D-6300 Giessen, Germany
General Description: Indexes and abstracts German journal literature in the field of food and nutrition. **Language of Database:** German. **Subject Coverage:** Food science and human nutrition.

★6966★   HUMAN RETROVIRUSES AND AIDS DATABASE
Los Alamos National Laboratory
Theoretical Division
Group T-10, Mail Stop K710
Los Alamos, NM 87545   Phone: (505) 665-0480
General Description: Provides fundamental molecular data pertaining to the nucleic acid and protein sequences for the immunodeficiency viruses HIV-1 and HIV-2, and related retroviruses. Includes references to source literature and other related literature. **Also Known as:** HIV Sequence Database. **Language of Database:** English. **Subject Coverage:** Sequence data for human immunodeficiency viruses and retroviruses.

★6967★   HUMAN SEXUALITY
Clinical Communications, Inc.
132 Hutchin Hill
Shady, NY 12409   Phone: (914) 679-2217
General Description: Provides information and advice on sexuality and sex-related topics as well as emotional support groups for participants. Organized into three basic sections: • The Hotline receives approximately 500 user messages each week; many ar e referred to the service's consulting medical editors. • The Information Se rvice contains more than 1500 replies to user questions and lists special features on major issues, online transcripts of conversations with experts, and a reader exchange on relationship experiences. • Support Groups enable users to sh are feelings through live conferencing and message boards; each group has a leader who serves as discussion facilitator. One group is geared toward specific relationship groups such as couples, parents, singles, women, and homosexuals; the other focuses on specific topics such as passages, breaking up, encounter groups, and bisexuality. **Language of Database:** English. **Subject Coverage:** Sexuality and sex-related topics, including relationships, contraception, homosexuality, sexual dysfunctions, and sexually transmitted diseases, as well as other areas of urology, gynecology, psychiatry, and pharmacology.

★6968★   ICBR DATA BANK
Institute for Child Behavior Research (ICBR)
4182 Adams Ave.
San Diego, CA 92116   Phone: (619) 281-7165
General Description: Contains detailed case and medical history records of more than 10,100 autistic-type children throughout the world. **Language of Database:** English. **Subject Coverage:** Children with autism, childhood schizophrenia, and other similar disorders.

★6969★   IDENTIDEX SYSTEM
Micromedex, Inc.
600 Grant St.
Denver, CO 80203-3527   Phone: (303) 831-1400
General Description: Provides identification of more than 40,000 drug tablets and capsules using the manufacturer's imprint coding and the tablet or capsule color and physical description. **Language of Database:** English. **Subject Coverage:** Drug identification of tablets and capsules from the ethical, prescription, OTC, and generic drug industries.

★6970★ IDIS DRUG FILE
University of Iowa
College of Pharmacy
Iowa Drug Information Service (IDIS)
Oakdale Hall
Oakdale, IA 52319   Phone: (319) 335-4800
General Description: Provides citations to more than 250,000 biomedical journal articles and other published literature dealing with drugs and drug therapy. Covers drugs by brand name, generic drug name, and clinical disease term. (The full text of the articles indexed are maintained on microfiche as the Drug Literature Microfilm File (DLMF) and made available by IDIS.). **Also Known as:** Iowa Drug Information Service Database. **Language of Database:** English. **Subject Coverage:** Drugs and drug therapy, including treatment efficacy, study population dosage, administration technique, pharmacokinetics, pharmaceutics, incompatibilities, drug interactions, toxicology, and side effects.

★6971★ IMMUNIZATION ALERT
93 Timber Dr.
Storrs, CT 06268   Phone: (203) 487-0611
General Description: Provides current information on foreign innoculation requirements and disease conditions in more than 200 countries. Includes general health warnings and tips on good health practices abroad. **Language of Database:** English. **Subject Coverage:** Health and innoculation information for travellers.

★6972★ THE IMMUNOCLONE DATABASE
Centre Europeen de Recherches Documentaires sur les Immunoclones
2eme C.A.I. Ave. des Maurettes
F-06270 Villeneuve-Loubet, France
General Description: Covers cells of immunological interest such as hybridomas, transfectomas, T-cell clones, and their products, monoclonal antibodies. Provides descriptions of hybridomas, monoclonal antibodies, and other immunocompetent cell clones, including such information as cell types, immunogen, immunocyte donors, immortal partners, and product information such as type and designation of the product and reactivities. Excludes information on polyclonal antibodies (e.g. serums) and kits. **Language of Database:** English. **Subject Coverage:** Cells of immunological interest, including hybridomas, monoclonal antibodies, and other immunocompetent cell clones.

★6973★ IMMUNOLOGY ABSTRACTS
Cambridge Scientific Abstracts
7200 Wisconsin Ave.
Bethesda, MD 20814   Phone: (301) 961-6750
General Description: Contains citations and abstracts of international periodical and other literature covering the immune systems of humans and animals. **Language of Database:** English. **Subject Coverage:** The immune systems of humans and animals, in normal functions and disorders, including AIDS, methodology, response to infections, tumors, transplantation, and genetic characteristics. Specific topics covered include molecular immunology and methodology; antigens, antibodies, and antigen-antibody interaction; complements; immune response (local and general), inflammation: biochemistry and function of lymphoid organs and tissues, macrophages, monocytes, lymphokines, and other mediators; genetics, ontogeny, and phylogeny; immunomodulation, stimulation, suppression, and immunopharmacology; immunity to infection: viruses, bacteria, fungi, protozoa, helminths, parasites, and passive and active immunization; tumor immunology, antigens, antitumor immune response, virus-associated tumors, and immunotherapy; histocompatibility and transplantation; immune disorders; cellular and molecular immunology; and immunogenetics.

★6974★ IMSPACT
IMS America Ltd.
PO Box 905
Plymouth Meeting, PA 19462-0905   Phone: (215) 834-5000
General Description: Provides sales and marketing research data, product management data, and corporate planning data for the pharmaceutical industry. Comprises nine major pharmaceutical audits: Drugstores, Pharmaceutical Market, Hospitals, National Disease & Therapeutic Index (NDTI), National Prescription Audit, National Journal Audit, National Mail Audit, National Detailing Audit, and Weekly Product Tracking Service. Enables the user to conduct interaudit linkages for cross-file searching by corporation, name, product, form, chemical, and product class. **Language of Database:** English. **Subject Coverage:** Pharmaceutical industry worldwide, including hospital and drugstore sales, drug prescriptions, pharmaceutical product characteristics, and promotions.

★6975★ INDEX VETERINARIUS
C.A.B. International
Wallingford, Oxon. OX10 8DE, England
General Description: Indexes the world's periodical and other published literature relating to veterinary science. Animals covered include cattle, horses, sheep, goats, pigs, poultry, cats, dogs, rabbits, cage birds, laboratory animals, wildlife, zoo animals, fish, and other domestic animals. **Language of Database:** English. **Subject Coverage:** Animal science, including animal physiology and biochemistry, animal health, medical and veterinary entomology, helminthology, mycology, protozoology.

★6976★ INDICE MEDICO ESPANOL
Universidad de Valencia
Centro de Documentacion e Informatica Biomedica
Avda. Biasco Ibanez, 17
10 Valencia, Spain
General Description: Provides citations to articles published in approximately 200 medical journals published in Spain. **Also Known as:** Spanish Medical Index. **Language of Database:** Spanish. **Subject Coverage:** Clinical and experimental medicine.

★6977★ INDUSTRIAL HEALTH AND HAZARDS UPDATE (IH&HU)
Merton Allen Associates
PO Box 15640
Plantation, FL 33318-5640   Phone: (305) 473-9560
General Description: Contains abstracts from reports on industrial health and hazards, covering topics such as regulations, legislation, litigation, industrial plant surveys, accident reports, toxicity of industrial materials and products, and diseases caused by occupational exposure. **Language of Database:** English. **Subject Coverage:** Industrial health and hazards.

★6978★ INTERNATIONAL DRUG INFORMATION SYSTEM (INTDIS)
World Health Organization
WHO Collaborating Centre for International Drug Monitoring
PO Box 26
S-751 03 Uppsala, Sweden
General Description: Contains information on drugs that cause adverse reactions. Comprises the following three subfiles: • The Case Report Register—consists of case reports describing the situation surrounding observed adverse drug reactions. • The Drug Register—contains approximately 25,000 proprietary and nonproprietary names of drugs; is divided into seven tables. • The Terminology Section—contai ns some 1200 preferred terms, as well as disease classifications. **Subject Coverage:** Adverse drug reactions, including death, neoplasms, fetal malformations, and drug dependence.

★6979★ INTERNATIONAL HEALTH PHYSICS DATA BASE (IHPD)
Creative Information Systems, Inc.
PO Box 30567
Portland, OR 97230   Phone: (503) 253-6812
General Description: Contains radiation exposure information on each employee at nuclear utilities. **Language of Database:** English. **Subject Coverage:** Radiation exposure information.

★6980★ INTERNATIONAL MEDICAL DISTRIBUTOR DATABASE
Medical Device Register, Inc.
655 Washington Blvd.
Stamford, CT 06901   Phone: (203) 348-6319
General Description: Provides listings for more than 19,000 worldwide and 15,000 U.S. distributors of medical equipment purchased by hospitals, clinics, and home healthcare organizations. Includes more than 30,000 key executives and 100,000 products. **Language of Database:** English. **Subject Coverage:** Distributors of medical equipment and supplies, lab equipment, test kits, dental products, pharmaceuticals, and other medical products.

★6981★ INTERNATIONAL MEDICAL TRIBUNE SYNDICATE
257 Park Ave. S., 19th Fl.
New York, NY 10010   Phone: (212) 674-8500
General Description: Reports news and developments in the U.S. medical and health sectors of interest to consumers. **Language of Database:** English. **Subject Coverage:** Consumer medical and health news, including AIDS, biotechnology, environmental health, fitness, new drugs, pediatrics, and preventive medicine.

★6982★   INTERNATIONAL PHARMACEUTICAL ABSTRACTS
(IPA)
American Society of Hospital Pharmacists
4630 Montgomery Ave.
Bethesda, MD 20814   Phone: (301) 657-3000
General Description: Indexes and abstracts the world's pharmaceutical, medical, and related journals. **Language of Database:** English. **Subject Coverage:** Pharmaceutical technology; institutional pharmacy practice; adverse drug reactions and toxicity; investigational drugs; drug evaluations and interactions; biopharmaceutics and pharmaceutics; drug stability; pharmacology and pharmaceutical chemistry; preliminary drug analysis; drug metabolism and body distribution; microbiology; pharmacognosy; environmental toxicity; legislation and regulations; history; sociology, economics, and ethics of drugs; pharmaceutical education; pharmacy practice; information processing; cosmetics; and related health topics.

★6983★   INTERNATIONAL RESEARCH AND EVALUATION-
INFORMATION AND TECHNOLOGY TRANSFER DATABASE
(IRE-ITTD)
International Research and Evaluation (IRE)
21098 IRE Control Center
Eagan, MN 55121   Phone: (612) 888-9635
General Description: Contains citations and abstracts of government, academic, and industrial sources of technical information. **Language of Database:** English. **Subject Coverage:** All aspects of science and technology, including waste management and resource recovery, fiber optics and lasers, earth sciences, agriculture and horticulture, transportation, medical science and health, law enforcement and justice, energy, construction and civil engineering, and infrastructures.

★6984★   IRIS
Merck, Sharp & Dohme/Chibret
Centre de Documentation de MSD/Chibret
200 blvd. E. Clementel
Clermont-Ferrand F-63018, France
General Description: Contains citations to worldwide literature on opthalmology. **Language of Database:** English. **Subject Coverage:** Opthalmology.

★6985★   ISST
Commission de la Sante et de la Securite du Travail du Quebec
1199, rue de Bleury
C.P. 6056, Succursale A
Montreal, PQ, Canada H3C 4E1   Phone: (514) 873-3160
General Description: Covers documents from the network of documentation centers of the Commission de la Sante et de la Securite du Travail du Quebec (CSST) and joint sector-based associations in medicine, engineering, and the humanities. **Language of Database:** French. **Subject Coverage:** Occupational health and safety and related topics.

★6986★   JAPIC DRUGS DATA BANK
Japan Pharmaceutical Information Center (JAPIC)
2F, Kyodo Bldg.
16 Ichiban-cho, Chiyoda-ku
Tokyo 102, Japan
General Description: Provides information on 16,000 over-the-counter and prescription drugs available in Japan. **Language of Database:** Japanese. **Subject Coverage:** Over-the-counter and prescription drugs in Japan.

★6987★   JAPICDOC
Japan Pharmaceutical Information Center (JAPIC)
2F, Kyodo Bldg.
16 Ichiban-cho, Chiyoda-ku
Tokyo 102, Japan
General Description: Indexes and abstracts drug package inserts and journal articles covering drugs, with emphasis on the regulation and safety of drugs in clinical use. **Language of Database:** Japanese. **Subject Coverage:** All aspects of drugs, especially their regulation and safety in clinical use.

★6988★   JICST FILE ON MEDICAL SCIENCE IN JAPAN
Japan Information Center of Science and Technology (JICST)
5-2, Nagatacho, 2-Chome, Chiyoda-ku
CPO Box 1478
Tokyo 100, Japan
General Description: Provides citations and abstracts of Japanese medical science literature. **Language of Database:** Japanese. **Subject Coverage:** Japanese medical science and related subjects.

★6989★   JICST FILE ON SCIENCE, TECHNOLOGY AND
MEDICINE IN JAPAN
Japan Information Center of Science and Technology (JICST)
5-2, Nagatacho, 2-Chome, Chiyoda-ku
CPO Box 1478
Tokyo 100, Japan
General Description: Provides English-language citations and abstracts of literature published in Japan in all fields of science, technology, and medicine. **Language of Database:** English. **Subject Coverage:** Japanese scientific and technological literature covering such topics as the pharmacology and medical sciences.

★6990★   JOB SAFETY AND HEALTH (JOSH)
The Bureau of National Affairs, Inc. (BNA)
BNA ONLINE
1231 25th St., N.W.
Washington, DC 20037   Phone: (202) 452-4132
General Description: Summarizes new industrial safety practices and trends in industry; examines difficult safety problems and their solutions; provides information on setting up and maintaining safety and health programs; and explains significant changes in the law, court and agency decisions, and important arbitration awards. **Language of Database:** English. **Subject Coverage:** Workplace safety and health issues, including right-to-know requirements; signs, labels, monitoring, and measuring; variances from standards; OSHA inspection policies; enforcement; safety programs; and training.

★6991★   JOURNAL WATCH
Massachusetts Medical Society
Medical Publishing Group
1440 Main St.
Waltham, MA 02254   Phone: (617) 890-0385
General Description: Provides summaries of important new clinical studies published in a core group of 20 biomedical journals. Physician-editors scan major medical journals, identify the articles that have the broadest relevance to practicing physicians, and prepare summaries of the articles. Not intended to replace the reading of the original documents. **Language of Database:** English. **Subject Coverage:** Current medical clinical studies.

★6992★   KIDNEY AND UROLOGIC DISEASE DATABASE
U.S. National Kidney and Urologic Diseases Information
   Clearinghouse
PO Box NKUDIC
Bethesda, MD 20892   Phone: (301) 468-6345
General Description: Provides citations and abstracts of materials dealing with kidney and urologic diseases. **Language of Database:** English. **Subject Coverage:** Kidney and urologic diseases.

★6993★   KINSEY INSTITUTE FOR RESEARCH IN SEX,
GENDER, AND REPRODUCTION BIBLIOGRAPHIC
DATABASE
Kinsey Institute for Research in Sex, Gender, and Reproduction
Information Services
Morrison Hall, 4th Fl.
Indiana University
Bloomington, IN 47405   Phone: (812) 855-7686
General Description: Provides full bibliographic descriptions of books received by the Kinsey Institute's library. **Language of Database:** English. **Subject Coverage:** Sex, gender, reproduction, and sexual behavior.

★6994★   KIRK-OTHMER ENCYCLOPEDIA OF CHEMICAL
TECHNOLOGY ONLINE
John Wiley & Sons, Inc.
Wiley Electronic Publishing
605 3rd Ave.
New York, NY 10158   Phone: (212) 850-6194
General Description: Contains the complete text, citations, tables, and abstracts of articles covering chemical technology in the areas of energy, health, safety, and new materials. **Language of Database:** English. **Subject Coverage:** Chemical technology, including agricultural chemicals; chemical engineering; coatings and inks; drugs, cosmetics, and biomaterials; ecology and industrial hygiene; food and animal nutrition; industrial organic and inorganic chemicals; and plastics and elastomers.

★6995★ KNMP DRUG FILE
Koninklijke Nederlandse Maatschappij ter bevordering der Pharmacia (KNMF)
PO Box 30460
Alexanderstr. 11
NL-2514 JL The Hague, Netherlands
General Description: Contains information on drugs available in the Netherlands. Covers 15,000 pharmaceutical products, 30,000 presentations, 1500 manufacturers. **Subject Coverage:** Pharmaceutical and related products and presentations available in the Netherlands.

★6996★ KNOW ABUSE DATABASE
Micromedex, Inc.
600 Grant St.
Denver, CO 80203-3527   Phone: (303) 831-1400
General Description: Provides information on urine drug testing in the workplace, including data on drugs most commonly tested. Contains descriptions of therapeutic uses, kinetics, toxicity of drug, and the likelihood of positive or false negative laboratory results. **Language of Database:** English. **Subject Coverage:** Drug testing in the workplace.

★6997★ LATIN AMERICAN AND CARIBBEAN HEALTH SCIENCES LITERATURE (LILACS)
Pan American Health Organization
Centro Latino-Americano e do Caribe de Informacao em Ciencias da Saude
Rua Botucatu, 862
C.P. 20381
04023 Sao Paulo, Brazil
General Description: Indexes and abstracts health sciences and health-related literature published in Latin American and Caribbean countries. **Language of Database:** Spanish; Portuguese. **Subject Coverage:** Health sciences and health-related environmental and legal issues, with emphasis on Latin American and Caribbean countries.

★6998★ LEXIS HEALTH LAW LIBRARY
Mead Data Central, Inc.
LEXIS
9393 Springboro Pike
PO Box 933
Dayton, OH 45401   Phone: (513) 865-6800
General Description: Provides the complete text of U.S. federal and state court decisions relating to health care issues, the U.S. Code Service, and such health-related periodicals as Hospital Law, Genetic Technology News, Hospital Admitting Monthly, Hospital Risk Management, Public Health Reports, and The Export and the Law, as well as newsletters and journals covering health-related legal issues. **Language of Database:** English. **Subject Coverage:** U.S. Health-related law.

★6999★ LEXIS MEDICAL MALPRACTICE LIBRARY
Mead Data Central, Inc.
LEXIS
9393 Springboro Pike
PO Box 933
Dayton, OH 45401   Phone: (513) 865-6800
General Description: Contains case law from 25 states, statutes and state bill tracking with summaries of new bills from 50 states, regulatory materials, and news about the health care industry, including the Journal of the American Medical Association. **Language of Database:** English. **Subject Coverage:** Medical malpractice law and the health care industry.

★7000★ LIBRARY AND INFORMATION NETWORK (LINK)
Planned Parenthood Federation of America, Inc.
Education Department
810 7th Ave.
New York, NY 10019   Phone: (212) 603-4637
General Description: Cites books, journal articles, and papers held in Planned Parenthood Federation's Katharine Dexter McCormick (KDM) Library covering 1973 to the present, as well as programs, program materials, curricula, audiovisual resources, and pamphlets held in the Federation's Clearinghouse of Educational Resources (CLH) covering 1980 to the present. **Language of Database:** English. **Subject Coverage:** Sexuality education, birth control, human sexuality, family planning, reproductive health, population, and related topics.

★7001★ LITHIUM LIBRARY
University of Wisconsin-Madison
Department of Psychiatry
Lithium Information Center
600 Highland Ave.
Madison, WI 53792   Phone: (608) 263-6171
General Description: Covers periodicals and other literature concerning the clinical and life science applications of lithium. **Language of Database:** English. **Subject Coverage:** Clinical and life sciences applications of lithium.

★7002★ MANAGED CARE LAW OUTLOOK
Capitol Publications, Inc.
Capitol Publishing Group
PO Box 1453
Alexandria, VA 22313-2053   Phone: (703) 683-4100
General Description: Provides briefs on the legal aspects of health maintenance organizations (HMOs), preferred-provider organizations (PPOs), and benefit options, including coverage of current court cases, decisions, trends, and legislation concerning managed care systems. **Language of Database:** English. **Subject Coverage:** Managed health care delivery law.

★7003★ MANAGED CARE OUTLOOK
Capitol Publications, Inc.
Capitol Publishing Group
PO Box 1453
Alexandria, VA 22313-2053   Phone: (703) 683-4100
General Description: Covers all aspects of managed health care, including health maintenance organizations (HMOs), preferred-provider organizations (PPOs), triple option plans, utilization reviews, information systems and contracting. Includes news on business, industry trends, regional events, legal and policy actions, conferences, and case studies. **Language of Database:** English. **Subject Coverage:** Managed health care delivery.

★7004★ MANAGED CARE REPORT
Key Communications
4350 E.W. Hwy., Ste. 1124
Bethesda, MD 20814   Phone: (301) 656-2923
General Description: Focuses on the prepaid health care movement, including HMOs, PPOs, IPAs, and other managed-care companies. Features inside news on cost-effective strategies in the industry. Reports developments concerning new laws, rules, and requirements emanating from Washington. **Language of Database:** English. **Subject Coverage:** Prepaid health care industry.

★7005★ MARTINDALE ONLINE
Royal Pharmaceutical Society of Great Britain
1 Lambeth High St.
London SE1 7JN, England
General Description: Contains evaluated data on 5400 drugs and ancillary substances used throughout the world. Includes manufacturer's names and addresses. Provides 50,000 drug names, synonyms, codes, and preparation names; 4600 manufacturer's names and addresses; and 35,000 references and abstracts of relevant scientific literature. **Language of Database:** English. **Subject Coverage:** Drugs and ancillary substances, including diagnostic agents, insecticides, coloring agents, preservatives, and toxic substances.

★7006★ MAXX: MAXIMUM ACCESS TO DIAGNOSIS AND THERAPY
Little, Brown and Co.
Medical Division
The Electronic Library of Medicine
34 Beacon St.
Boston, MA 02108   Phone: (617) 227-0730
General Description: Contains the complete text of 15 medical reference publications produced by Little, Brown and Company. Provides information on more than 500 diseases, including diagnostic evaluations and interpretations of laboratory tests, therapeutic recommendations, diagrams describing etiology for each disease and differential diagnoses, and schematic summaries of selected diseases containing relevant diagnostic and therapeutic data. Also covers information on prescription and nonprescription drugs contained in USP Drug Information (described in a separate entry). **Language of Database:** English. **Subject Coverage:** Biomedicine, including diseases, diagnoses, laboratory tests and procedures, and pharmaceutical information.

★7007★   MDR ON-LINE
Medical Device Register, Inc.
655 Washington Blvd.
Stamford, CT 06901   Phone: (203) 348-6319
General Description: Provides descriptions of 16,000 manufacturers of medical devices and clinical laboratory products, and 20,000 medical product distributors. **Language of Database:** English. **Subject Coverage:** Manufacturers and distributors of medical devices and clinical laboratory products.

★7008★   MDR WORLDWIDE MEDICAL DEVICE MANUFACTURERS
Medical Device Register, Inc. (MDR)
655 Washington Blvd.
Stamford, CT 06901   Phone: (203) 348-6319
General Description: Provides listings for more than 16,800 medical device manufacturers located in 75 countries; 10,000 United States manufacturers; 25,000 key executives; and 300,000 product listings. **Language of Database:** English. **Subject Coverage:** Medical device manufacturers.

★7009★   MDX HEALTH DIGEST
Medical Data Exchange
445 S. San Antonio Rd.
Los Altos, CA 94022   Phone: (415) 941-3600
General Description: Covers health information for the consumer. Provides references and abstracts of articles appearing in general and health-oriented magazines, newsletters, newspapers, and selected medical journals. **Language of Database:** English. **Subject Coverage:** Health information for the consumer.

★7010★   MEDIC
Finland Central Medical Library
Haartmaninkatu 4
SF-00290 Helsinki, Finland
General Description: Indexes the Finnish medical literature that is not covered by available international databases. **Language of Database:** Finnish. **Subject Coverage:** Finnish medical literature.

★7011★   MEDICAL ADVISORY SERVICES FOR TRAVELLERS ABROAD (MASTA)
London School of Hygiene and Tropical Medicine
Keppel St.
London WC1E 7HT, England
General Description: Provides information on 84 medical conditions and diseases that pose health risks for travellers in 230 countries. **Language of Database:** English. **Subject Coverage:** Health information for travellers.

★7012★   MEDICAL DEVICE DATABASE
Bradford Communications Corp.
Troiano Bldg., 2nd Fl.
Beltsville, MD 20705   Phone: (301) 345-0100
General Description: Provides health care purchasers and materials managers with an online information retrieval system for locating U.S. sources of medical devices and supplies available from more than 5000 manufacturers and over 12,000 supplier/dealers worldwide. **Language of Database:** English. **Subject Coverage:** Medical devices, supplies, drugs, durables, and capital equipment used by health care institutions of all types.

★7013★   MEDICAL AND HEALTH INFORMATION DIRECTORY (MHID)
Gale Research Inc.
835 Penobscot Bldg.
Detroit, MI 48226-4094   Phone: (313) 961-2242
General Description: Provides information on more than 48,000 medical organizations, services, and information sources. Includes more than 16,400 national, international, and state professional and voluntary associations, federal and state agencies, foundations and grant-awarding organizations, research centers, and medical and allied health schools; 9700 libraries, audiovisual producers and services, publications, publishers, and database services; and 23,000 clinics, treatment centers, care programs, counseling/diagnostic services, and other health services. **Language of Database:** English. **Subject Coverage:** Medical organizations, services, and information sources.

★7014★   THE MEDICAL LETTER ON DRUGS AND THERAPEUTICS
Medical Letter Inc.
1000 Main St.
New Rochelle, NY 10801   Phone: (914) 235-0500
General Description: Provides critical evaluations of drugs for physicians and other members of the health professions. **Language of Database:** English. **Subject Coverage:** Medicine and pharmacology, including drug effectiveness, toxicity, side effects, alternative medications, nondrug therapy, and new diagnostic aids.

★7015★   MEDICAL MALPRACTICE LAWSUIT FILINGS (MEDMAL)
Medical Malpractice Verdicts, Settlements & Experts
901 Church St.
Nashville, TN 37203   Phone: (615) 255-6288
General Description: Contains brief summaries of recently filed causes of action in medical malpractice complaints in non-insurance company hands in the United States. Provides medical specialty involved, plaintiff's allegations, and act of negligence. **Language of Database:** English. **Subject Coverage:** Medical malpractice lawsuits filed in U.S. courts.

★7016★   MEDICAL MALPRACTICE AND MUNICIPAL INSURANCE CLAIM FORMS AND HISTORY DATA BASE
Michigan State Department of Licensing and Regulation
Insurance Bureau
611 W. Ottawa
Lansing, MI 48909   Phone: (517) 373-2984
General Description: Contains information on plaintiffs and defendants involved in medical malpractice actions in the state of Michigan. **Language of Database:** English. **Subject Coverage:** Medical malpractice and liability in Michigan.

★7017★   MEDICAL AND PSYCHOLOGICAL PREVIEWS (PREV)
BRS Information Technologies
8000 Westpark Dr.
McLean, VA 22102   Phone: (703) 442-0900
General Description: Contains citations to articles, editorials, notes, and letters appearing in core medical and psychological journals published worldwide. Also covers key titles in psychiatry, nursing, and hospital administration. Citations are added within ten days of their receipt in United States libraries. **Language of Database:** English. **Subject Coverage:** Medicine and allied health fields such as nursing, psychology, psychiatry, and hospital administration.

★7018★   THE MEDICAL ROUNDTABLE
Michael P. Weinstein, M.D.
Nashua Medical Group
173 Daniel Webster Hwy.
Nashua, NH 03060   Phone: (603) 888-8800
General Description: A forum for the exchange of information among physicians, other health professionals, and the interested public. Features 15 data libraries providing current information on medical topics (including a graphics library); a bulletin board containing sections devoted to emergency medical care, pharmacy, nursing, and computers in medicine; and real-time conferences held at least twice monthly for the discussion of medical and health issues. **Language of Database:** English. **Subject Coverage:** Medical and health topics, including AIDS, pediatrics, internal medicine, surgery, obstetrics, psychiatry, dentistry, psychology, medical ethics, history, software designed for physicians and the public, emergency medical care, pharmacy, nursing, and computers in medicine.

★7019★   MEDICAL SCIENCE WEEKLY (MSW)
Excerpta Medica/EMBASE Publishing Group
Molenwerf 1
PO Box 1527
NL-1000 BM Amsterdam, Netherlands
General Description: Contains the complete text of more than 1000 major medical and biomedical journals published worldwide. **Language of Database:** English. **Subject Coverage:** Biomedicine, human medicine, and related disciplines.

★7020★   MEDICAL SUBJECT HEADINGS VOCABULARY FILE
U.S. National Library of Medicine
MEDLARS Management Section
8600 Rockville Pike
Bethesda, MD 20894   Phone: (301) 496-6193
General Description: Contains the controlled medical subject headings and vocabulary thesaurus terms used in compiling the databases of the

National Library of Medicine. Includes 16,000 medical subject headings and 54,000 chemical substances headings. **Also Known as:** MeSH Vocabulary File. **Language of Database:** English. **Subject Coverage:** Medical vocabulary thesaurus terms.

★7021★ MEDICAL WASTE NEWS
Business Publishers, Inc.
951 Pershing Dr.
Silver Spring, MD 20910-4464   Phone: (301) 587-6300
General Description: Covers U.S. regulation, legislation, and technological news and developments related to medical waste management and disposal. Reports on businesses involved in medical waste management as well as U.S. Environmental Protection Agency (EPA) efforts to control waste levels. **Language of Database:** English. **Subject Coverage:** Medical waste management and disposal, including regulations, legislation, and business practices.

★7022★ MEDIS
Mead Data Central, Inc.
9393 Springboro Pike
PO Box 933
Dayton, OH 45401   Phone: (513) 865-6800
General Description: Provides the complete text of selected journals, textbooks, and access to other databases covering all areas of medicine. **Language of Database:** English. **Subject Coverage:** Medicine, ranging from clinical procedures to medical practice management and including surgery, cardiology, rheumatology, psychiatry, pediatrics, oncology, hematology, public health, and general and internal medicine; pharmacy; hospital administration.

★7023★ MEDLINE
U.S. National Library of Medicine
MEDLARS Management Section
8600 Rockville Pike
Bethesda, MD 20894   Phone: (301) 496-6193
General Description: Contains references to the world's journal literature covering biomedicine, dentistry, nursing, and related topics. Includes English-language abstracts where possible. **Also Known as:** MEDLARS Online. **Language of Database:** English. **Subject Coverage:** Medicine (preclinical and clinical sciences), life sciences, and other health-sciences topics.

★7024★ MEDLINE CLINICAL COLLECTION
U.S. National Library of Medicine
MEDLARS Management Section
8600 Rockville Pike
Bethesda, MD 20894   Phone: (301) 496-6193
General Description: Contains citations and abstracts of articles on clinical medicine from journals covered by Abridged Index Medicus, Annals of Internal Medicine, and Bulletin of the Medical Library Association (United States). A subset of the MEDLINE database (described in a separate entry). **Language of Database:** English. **Subject Coverage:** Biomedicine.

★7025★ MEDLINE EXPRESS
U.S. National Library of Medicine
MEDLARS Management Section
8600 Rockville Pike
Bethesda, MD 20894   Phone: (301) 496-6193
General Description: Provides citations and abstracts to biomedical literature published worldwide. Includes coverage of chapters and articles from selected monographs from 1976 to 1981. A subset of the MEDLINE database (described in a separate entry). **Language of Database:** English. **Subject Coverage:** Biomedicine, including research, clinical practice, administration, policy issues, and health care.

★7026★ MEDLINE KNOWLEDGE FINDER
U.S. National Library of Medicine
MEDLARS Management Section
8600 Rockville Pike
Bethesda, MD 20894   Phone: (301) 496-6193
General Description: Covers the world's biomedical literature relating to research, clinical practice, administration, policy issues, and health care services. Comprises two files: • Unabridged MEDLINE—contains citations and abstracts of articles publi shed in some 3400 journals published in the United States and in 70 countries worldwide. • Core Journals—contains citations and abstracts of articles publi shed in some 270 primary biomedical journals as well as titles from the Brandon-Hill publications list recommended for nursing, small medical, and allied health sciences

libraries. **Language of Database:** English. **Subject Coverage:** Biomedicine, including research, clinical practice, administration, policy issues, and health care services.

★7027★ MEDLINE PROFESSIONAL
SilverPlatter Information, Inc.
River Ridge Office Park
100 River Ridge Rd.
Norwood, MA 02062   Phone: (617) 769-2599
General Description: Provides coverage of clinical medicine literature published worldwide. Comprises the following three files: • AIDSLINE—contains some 16,000 citations, some with abstracts, of published literature dealing with Acquired Immune Deficiency Syndrome (AIDS) and the biomedical, epidemiological, social, behavioral, clinical, and research aspects of the disease as well as health policy issues (described in a separate entry). • MEDLINE—contains citations to the world's li terature relating to clinical medicine (described in a separate entry). • Ye ar Book Series—contains the complete text of ten titles from the Year Book Series published by Mosby Year Book, Inc. **Language of Database:** English. **Subject Coverage:** Clinical medicine, including AIDS, anesthesiology, cardiology, critical care medicine, emergency medicine, orthopedics, pathology, radiology, surgery, and urology.

★7028★ MENTAL HEALTH ABSTRACTS
IFI/Plenum Data Corp.
302 Swann Ave.
Alexandria, VA 22301   Phone: (703) 683-1085
General Description: Provides citations and abstracts of worldwide journal articles, books, research reports, program data, and other materials on all aspects of mental health and mental illness. **Language of Database:** English. **Subject Coverage:** All aspects of mental health and mental illness, including psychology, psychiatry, aging, alcoholism, behavioral medicine, child psychology, drug abuse, education, ethics, family, genetics, geriatrics, legal aspects, mental health services, mental retardation, motivation, personality, prevention, psychopharmacology, schizophrenia, sexology, sleep, stress, suicide, treatment and therapy, and violence.

★7029★ THE MERCK INDEX ONLINE
Merck & Co. Inc.
Box 2000
Rahway, NJ 07065   Phone: (908) 594-4890
General Description: Contains more than 10,000 monographs describing approximately 30,000 substances of pharmaceutical, biological, chemical, and environmental interest. Covers isolation, preparation, synthesis, structure, chemical and physical properties, biological activity, toxicity, and medical and non-medical uses for these compounds and selected derivatives. **Language of Database:** English. **Subject Coverage:** Pharmaceuticals, chemicals, natural products, and veterinary and agricultural products.

★7030★ MICROBIAL CULTURE INFORMATION SERVICE (MICIS)
Information Centre for European Culture Collections
Mascheroder Weg 1b
D-3300 Braunschweig, Germany
General Description: Contains data on approximately 50,000 microorganisms held in European national and private culture collections and of interest to researchers in the biotechnology industry. **Language of Database:** English. **Subject Coverage:** Microorganisms, including bacteria, algae, protozoa, and fungi.

★7031★ MICROBIOLOGY ABSTRACTS, SECTION A: INDUSTRIAL AND APPLIED MICROBIOLOGY
Cambridge Scientific Abstracts
7200 Wisconsin Ave.
Bethesda, MD 20814   Phone: (301) 961-6750
General Description: Contains citations and abstracts of international periodical and other literature covering industrial and applied microbiology. **Language of Database:** English. **Subject Coverage:** The sciences of industrial and applied microbiology covering the agriculture, food, beverage, and chemical and pharmaceutical industries. Specific topics covered include antibiotics and antimicrobial agents, vaccines and serum production, drugs, hygiene, and quality control.

★7032★   MICROBIOLOGY ABSTRACTS, SECTION B:
   BACTERIOLOGY
Cambridge Scientific Abstracts
7200 Wisconsin Ave.
Bethesda, MD 20814   Phone: (301) 961-6750
General Description: Contains citations and abstracts of international periodical and other literature covering medically-oriented bacteriology topics. **Language of Database:** English. **Subject Coverage:** The sciences of bacteriology, including bacterial immunology and vaccinations, diseases in man and animals, pure bacteriology, biochemistry, and genetics. Specific topics covered include methodology; identification, taxonomy, and typing; cell structure and function; genetics and evolution; plasmids and gene manipulation; immunology; plant bacteriology; ecology; plasmids, antibiotics, antibacterial agents; and aggressins and toxins.

★7033★   MICROBIOLOGY ABSTRACTS, SECTION C:
   ALGOLOGY, MYCOLOGY AND PROTOZOOLOGY
Cambridge Scientific Abstracts
7200 Wisconsin Ave.
Bethesda, MD 20814   Phone: (301) 961-6750
General Description: Contains citations and abstracts of international periodical and other literature covering algology, mycology, and protozoology. **Language of Database:** English. **Subject Coverage:** Algae, fungi, protozoa, and lichens, including reproduction, growth, life cycles, biochemistry, genetics, and infection and immunity in man, other animals and plants. Specific topics covered include taxonomy, structure and function; growth, development and life cycles; ecology and distribution; biochemistry; effects of physical and chemical factors; methodology, media and cultures; nutrition; genetics, including yeast and fungal genetics; mycotoxins; immunology and vaccination; parasitism and diseases; viruses and bacteria of microorganisms; soil microbiology and mycorrhiza; food microbiology and fermentation; spoilage and biodegradation; and pollution.

★7034★   MULTIPLE SCLEROSIS RESEARCH PROJECTS
International Federation of Multiple Sclerosis Societies
3-9 Heddon St.
London W1R 7LE, England
General Description: Contains descriptions of ongoing research projects on multiple sclerosis. **Language of Database:** English. **Subject Coverage:** Multiple sclerosis research.

★7035★   NAIC AIDS EDUCATION MATERIALS DATABASE
U.S. National AIDS Information Clearinghouse
PO Box 6003
Rockville, MD 20850   Phone: (301) 251-5730
General Description: Provides references and abstracts of a wide variety of published and unpublished educational materials tailored to specific audiences and focusing on different aspects of AIDS (Acquired Immune Deficiency Syndrome). **Language of Database:** English. **Subject Coverage:** AIDS education, including testing and counseling, risk reduction and prevention, workplace policies and programs, health policies and programs, safe sex education, and educational programs.

★7036★   NAIC RESOURCES AND SERVICES DATABASE
U.S. National AIDS Information Clearinghouse (NAIC)
PO Box 6003
Rockville, MD 20850   Phone: (301) 251-5730
General Description: Provides descriptions of organizations that provide HIV (Human Immunodeficiency Virus) and AIDS (Acquired Immune Deficiency Syndrome) resources and services, including public health departments, community and social service organizations, hospitals, clinics, and professional organizations and associations. **Language of Database:** English. **Subject Coverage:** Providers of HIV and AIDS resources and services.

★7037★   NATIONAL CLEARINGHOUSE FOR ALCOHOL AND
   DRUG INFORMATION DATABASE
U.S. National Clearinghouse for Alcohol and Drug Information
Box 2345
Rockville, MD 20852   Phone: (301) 468-2600
General Description: Provides citations to published materials as well as general information on alcohol and drug use and related topics. **Also Known as:** NCADI Database. **Language of Database:** English. **Subject Coverage:** Alcohol and drug use and abuse, including the prevention, intervention, and treatment of substance abuse.

★7038★   NATIONAL DATABASE ON GERONTOLOGY IN
   HIGHER EDUCATION
Association for Gerontology in Higher Education
600 Maryland Ave., SW, West Wing 204
Washington, DC 20024   Phone: (202) 484-7505
General Description: Provides information on degrees, certificate programs, and courses offered in the field of gerontology by 3000 institutions of higher education. **Language of Database:** English. **Subject Coverage:** Courses, degrees, and certificate programs in gerontology; short-term instruction, including in-service training, institutes, and seminars; and offerings for older adults such as Elderhostel programs and special classes.

★7039★   NATIONAL DRUG CODE DATABASE
U.S. Food and Drug Administration (FDA)
Center for Drug Evaluation and Research
Drug Listing Branch
5600 Fishers Ln., HFD-334
Rockville, MD 20857   Phone: (301) 295-8077
General Description: Contains uniform classifications and codes that uniquely identify several hundred thousand individual drugs in commercial distribution in the United States by strength, dosage form, and trade package size. **Language of Database:** English. **Subject Coverage:** Chemical composition, active ingredients, dosage form, and other data for commercially marketed drug products in the United States, including human drugs, biologic drug products, and imported drugs.

★7040★   NATIONAL EYE HEALTH EDUCATION PROGRAM
   (NEHEP) DATABASE
U.S. National Eye Institute
National Eye Health Education Program
Bldg. 31, Rm. 6A32
Bethesda, MD 20892   Phone: (301) 496-5248
General Description: Contains references to published literature dealing with eye health education. **Language of Database:** English. **Subject Coverage:** Eye health education, with emphasis on such causes of blindness as glaucoma and diabetic retinopathy.

★7041★   NATIONAL HOSPITAL PANEL SURVEY
American Hospital Association (AHA)
Hospital Data Center
840 N. Lake Shore Dr.
Chicago, IL 60611   Phone: (312) 280-6000
General Description: Provides sample survey data on seasonal variations in health care delivery at more than 2000 AHA-registered hospitals in the United States. Contains 67 performance indicators for each hospital. **Language of Database:** English. **Subject Coverage:** National, regional, and state summary information on the number of beds regularly available, utilization, staffing, and finances for approximately 34 percent of the community hospitals registered with the AHA.

★7042★   NATIONAL MARROW DONOR PROGRAM (NMDP)
   DATABASE
National Marrow Donor Program
100 S. Robert St.
St. Paul, MN 55107
General Description: Contains a listing of more than 100,000 available tissue-typed bone marrow donors across the United States. Enables the efficient sharing and searching of information to join possible donors with patients in need of marrow transplants. **Language of Database:** English. **Subject Coverage:** Bone marrow donors.

★7043★   NATIONAL PEDIATRIC TRAUMA REGISTRY
New England Medical Center
Department of Rehabilitation Medicine
750 Washington St., No. 75 K/R
Boston, MA 02111   Phone: (617) 956-5031
General Description: Contains case histories of pediatric trauma. Includes demographic information, injury descriptions, and data on the management of injury at the scene and any referring hospitals. **Language of Database:** English. **Subject Coverage:** Pediatric trauma injury, with emphasis on emergency treatment management.

★7044★   NATIONAL PRACTITIONER DATA BANK (NPBD)
U.S. Public Health Service
Division of Quality Assurance and Liability Management
Parklawn Bldg., Rm. 815
5600 Fishers Ln.
Rockville, MD 20857   Phone: (301) 443-2300
General Description: Contains information on adverse actions taken

against physicians, dentists, and other licensed health care professionals in the United States. Includes information on malpractice payments made on behalf of any licensed health practitioner as the result of a judgment or settlement; disciplinary actions taken by the state medical and dental boards; adverse actions taken against a physician's or dentist's clinical privileges when such actions last more than 30 days; and adverse actions taken by professional societies against the membership of a physician or dentist when they have reached that action through peer review and when they have been assessing practitioner competency and/or professional conduct. Designed to act as an alert system by providing a means of identifying incompetent health practitioners. Hospitals will be required to consult the NPDB when granting privileges. **Language of Database:** English. **Subject Coverage:** Adverse actions taken against health professionals, including revocation, probation, suspension, and limitations of priviliges as well as judgements, settlements, reprimands, and other actions taken by state medical boards, courts, hospitals, medical societies, insurance companies, and peer review committees.

★7045★ **THE NATIONAL REPORT ON COMPUTERS AND HEALTH**
United Communications Group
11300 Rockville Pike, Ste. 1100
Rockville, MD 20852   Phone: (301) 816-8950
General Description: Provides news and information on data processing and clinical hospital information systems. Includes user comments on a variety of health care software. **Language of Database:** English. **Subject Coverage:** Computer hardware and software for the health care industry.

★7046★ **THE NATIONAL REPORT ON SUBSTANCE ABUSE**
The Bureau of National Affairs, Inc. (BNA)
BNA ONLINE
1231 25th St., NW
Washington, DC 20037   Phone: (202) 452-4132
General Description: Provides information for the establishment of substance abuse policies and implementation of employee assistance programs (EAPs) while minimizing the risk of lawsuits over privacy rights and liability issues. **Language of Database:** English. **Subject Coverage:** Substance abuse policies, including drug testing accuracy, types of tests available, legislation, government regulations, and evolving case law.

★7047★ **NATIONAL SAFETY COUNCIL LIBRARY DATABASE**
National Safety Council Library
444 N. Michigan Ave.
Chicago, IL 60611   Phone: (312) 527-4800
General Description: Furnishes citations to books, journals, and other materials dealing with health and safety. **Language of Database:** English. **Subject Coverage:** Health and safety, including accidents, injuries, hazards, occupational health, and traffic, home, industrial, farm, and public safety.

★7048★ **NATIONAL SPINAL CORD INJURY STATISTICAL CENTER DATABASE**
University of Alabama in Birmingham
Spain Rehabilitation Center
National Spinal Cord Injury Statistical Center
University Station
Birmingham, AL 35294   Phone: (205) 934-3334
General Description: Maintains spinal cord injury statistics submitted by federally sponsored Spinal Cord Injury Care Systems. **Subject Coverage:** Spinal cord injuries.

★7049★ **NCI CANCER WEEKLY**
CDC AIDS WEEKLY/NCI CANCER WEEKLY
206 Rogers St., NE, Ste. 104
PO Box 5528
Atlanta, GA 30307-0528   Phone: (404) 377-8895
General Description: Provides comprehensive coverage of world news and developments relating to cancer, with emphasis on research and clinical findings. **Language of Database:** English. **Subject Coverage:** Cancer research.

★7050★ **THE NEW ENGLAND JOURNAL OF MEDICINE**
Massachusetts Medical Society
Medical Publishing Group
1440 Main St.
Waltham, MA 02254   Phone: (617) 893-9800
General Description: Contains the complete text of The New England Journal of Medicine, a weekly journal covering current research in all areas of medicine. Includes articles, letters to the editor, editorials, and book reviews. **Language of Database:** English. **Subject Coverage:** All areas of medicine.

★7051★ **NIDR ONLINE**
U.S. National Institute of Dental Research (NIDR)
Office of Planning, Evaluation and Communications
Research Information Management and Analysis Information Section
Westwood Bldg., Rm. 537
Bethesda, MD 20892   Phone: (301) 496-7220
General Description: Contains abstracts of ongoing dental research projects which are supported by U.S. government agencies. **Language of Database:** English. **Subject Coverage:** Dentistry and dental research.

★7052★ **THE NIJ DRUGS AND CRIME CD-ROM LIBRARY**
U.S. National Institute of Justice
PO Box 6000
Rockville, MD 20850   Phone: (301) 251-5500
General Description: Contains information on drugs, drug-related crimes, and U.S. drug law. Provides research results with statistics and case histories from various government and private sector studies. Includes the complete text of some 328 current and out-of-print scholarly publications and references with abstracts to more than 4800 publications as well as approximately 650 images from publications. **Language of Database:** English. **Subject Coverage:** Drugs, drug-related crimes, and U.S. drug law, including the use and abuse of illegal drugs, drug cartels, international drug enforcement, U.S. state and federal drug enforcement, drug control policy, research, strategy, and types of prevention, treatment, and rehabilitation.

★7053★ **NORD SERVICES/RARE DISEASE DATABASE (RDB)**
National Organization for Rare Disorders (NORD)
PO Box 8923
New Fairfield, CT 06812   Phone: (203) 746-6518
General Description: Provides information on more than 2000 orphan diseases which are rare, debilitating illnesses each affecting fewer than 200,000 people in the United States. **Language of Database:** English. **Subject Coverage:** Orphan diseases; prevalent health conditions such as AIDS, Reye's Syndrome, and Toxic Shock Syndrome; orphan drugs and devices and medical foods.

★7054★ **NORDRUG**
Centralforbundet for Alkohol- och Narkotikaupplysning
PO Box 27302
S-102 54 Stockholm, Sweden
General Description: Provides references and abstracts of international research and primary literature dealing with alcohol and drug dependence. **Language of Database:** English. **Subject Coverage:** Alcohol and drug dependence and related topics.

★7055★ **NURSING AND ALLIED HEALTH DATABASE**
CINAHL Information Systems
1509 Wilson Terrace
PO Box 871
Glendale, CA 91209-0871   Phone: (818) 409-8005
General Description: Indexes and abstracts articles appearing in more than 330 current English-language nursing journals, publications of the American Nurses' Association and the National League for Nursing, and journals in more than a dozen allied health disciplines as well as nursing dissertations and selected articles appearing in 3200 biomedical journals, 20 journals in the field of health sciences librarianship, books from approximately 30 health care publishers, nursing dissertations, and education, psychological, management, and popular literature. **Language of Database:** English. **Subject Coverage:** Nursing and allied health professions, including cardiopulmonary technology, emergency services, health education, health sciences librarianship, medical and laboratory technology, medical assistance, medical records, occupational therapy, physician's assistant, physical therapy and rehabilitation, radiologic technology, respiratory therapy, social service in health care, and surgical technology.

★7056★ **NURSING HOMES DATABASE**
Oryx Press
4041 N. Central Ave.
Phoenix, AZ 85012-3399   Phone: (602) 265-2651
General Description: Provides information on more than 17,000 nursing homes located in the United States. **Language of Database:** English. **Subject Coverage:** U.S. nursing homes.

★7057★ NUTRITION ABSTRACTS AND REVIEWS, SERIES A: HUMAN AND EXPERIMENTAL
C.A.B. International
Wallingford, Oxon. OX10 8DE, England
General Description: Indexes and abstracts current periodical and other published literature relating to human nutrition and metabolism and allied topics. **Language of Database:** English. **Subject Coverage:** Human nutrition and metabolism, foods, microbiology, laboratory technique and equipment, immunology and immunogenetics, disease and therapeutic nutrition, and public health and hygiene.

★7058★ OBSTETRICS AND GYNECOLOGY ON DISC
Elsevier Science Publishing Co., Inc.
655 Avenue of the Americas
New York, NY 10010   Phone: (212) 989-5800
General Description: Contains the complete text of each issue of Obstetrics and Gynecology, the journal of the American College of Obstetricians and Gynecologists (ACOG). Includes all articles, tables, color and black & white images, and references cited. **Language of Database:** English. **Subject Coverage:** Obstetrics and gynecology, especially the medical and surgical treatment of female conditions, obstetrics management, and clinical evaluation of drugs and instruments.

★7059★ OCCUPATIONAL SAFETY AND HEALTH REPORTER
The Bureau of National Affairs, Inc. (BNA)
BNA ONLINE
1231 25th St., NW
Washington, DC 20037   Phone: (202) 452-4132
General Description: Covers legislative, regulatory, and judicial developments involving worker safety and health at both the federal and state levels. Includes proposed and final standards and regulations of the Occupational Safety and Health Administration (OSHA), enforcement activities, legal activities of the courts and the Occupational Safety and Health Review Commission, investigations, Congressional hearings, petitions for variances from OSHA standards and announcements of grants or denials, and news about worker safety and health conferences. Features coverage of worker right-to-know laws at the federal and state levels, and occasionally at the local level. **Language of Database:** English. **Subject Coverage:** Worker safety and health, including federal and state standards, regulations and policies, state and federal programs, enforcement efforts, research, and labor relations.

★7060★ ONCODISC
J.B. Lippincott Co.
E. Washington Sq.
Philadelphia, PA 19105   Phone: (215) 238-4443
General Description: Covers the world literature and persons and organizations involved in the diagnosis and treatment of cancer. Comprises the following six information resources: • Cancer Literature (CANCERLIT)—covers the world's literature relating to cancer for the most recent three years (for further information, see separate entry). • Physician Data Query (PDQ)—contains prognostic and treatment information for all major forms of cancer; a protocol file; a directory of physicians specializing in oncology; and a directory of health care organizations that have organized cancer care programs (for further information, see separate entries). • CANCER: Principles and Practice of Oncology—comprehensive textbook. • Manual for Staging of Cancer—issued by the American Joint Committee on Cancer. • Oncology Times—provides selected excerpts from the monthly news publication for cancer specialists. e. • Oncology Times—provides selected excerpts from the monthly news publication for cancer specialists. **Language of Database:** English. **Subject Coverage:** Cancer, including diagnosis, symptoms, stages, treatment, and protocols; cancer care programs; physicians specializing in oncology.

★7061★ ONCOGENES AND GROWTH FACTORS ABSTRACTS
Cambridge Scientific Abstracts
7200 Wisconsin Ave.
Bethesda, MD 20814   Phone: (301) 961-6750
General Description: Contains citations and abstracts of experimental and clinical literature covering oncogenes, the genetic mechanisms that cause cancerous cell growth. **Language of Database:** English. **Subject Coverage:** Cellular and viral oncogenes; growth factors and growth factor receptors associated with tyrosine kinase activity; oncogenes associated with serine-threonine kinase activity and other growth-factor-regulated serine-threonine kinases; nuclear oncogenes and DNA trans-acting binding factors; oncogenes and other growth factors associated with DNA tumor viruses; miscellaneous oncogenes and growth factors; human-related oncogenes and growth factors; and tumor suppressor genes and anti-oncogenes.

★7062★ OXFORD TEXTBOOK ON MEDICINE
Oxford University Press
Oxford Electronic Publishing
200 Madison Ave.
New York, NY 10016   Phone: (212) 679-7300
General Description: Contains the complete text of the Oxford Textbook of Medicine, a general medical reference book providing information on common and rare diseases. **Language of Database:** English. **Subject Coverage:** All fields of medicine.

★7063★ PASCAL
France Centre National de la Recherche Scientifique
Institut de l'Information Scientifique et Technique
2, allee du Parc de Brabois
F-54514 Vandoeuvre-les-Nancy Cedex, France
General Description: Provides citations and abstracts of worldwide journal and other published literature covering the numerous disciplines of science and technology. **Also Known as:** Programme Applique a la Selection et a la Compilation Automatiques de la Litterature (PASCAL). **Language of Database:** French. **Subject Coverage:** Science and technology, including physics, chemistry, biology, medicine (including tropical medicine), psychology, earth sciences, engineering, energy, food and agriculture, agronomy, biotechnology, zoology, metallurgy, welding, building construction, mathematics, and information science.

★7064★ PEDIATRIC INFECTIOUS DISEASE JOURNAL ON DISC
Williams & Wilkins
428 E. Preston St.
Baltimore, MD 21202   Phone: (301) 528-4000
General Description: Contains the complete text of all articles and supplements appearing in the bimonthly Pediatric Infectious Disease Journal. Includes text, tables, references cited, images, and radiographs. **Language of Database:** English. **Subject Coverage:** Pediatric infectious diseases.

★7065★ PEDIATRICS ON DISC
American Academy of Pediatrics
141 NW Point Blvd.
PO Box 927
Elk Grove Village, IL 60009-0927   Phone: (708) 228-5005
General Description: Contains the complete text of Pediatrics, the monthly journal of the American Academy of Pediatrics. **Language of Database:** English. **Subject Coverage:** Pediatric medicine.

★7066★ PHARMACEUTICAL AND HEALTHCARE INDUSTRIES NEWS DATABASE (PHIND)
PJB Publications Ltd.
18-20 Hill Rise
Richmond, Surrey TW10 6UA, England
General Description: Contains the complete text of all articles appearing in the following four PJB Publications newsletters: Scrip World Pharmaceutical News; Clinical World Medical Device and Diagnostic News; Animal Pharm World Animal Health; and Agrow World Crop Protection News. **Language of Database:** English. **Subject Coverage:** Pharmaceutical, medical device, veterinary, and crop protection industries.

★7067★ PHARMACEUTICAL LITERATURE DOCUMENTATION (RINGDOC)
Derwent Publications Ltd.
Rochdale House
128 Theobalds Rd.
London WC1X 8RP, England
General Description: Contains citations and abstracts of relevant papers found in the world's scientific journals on pharmaceuticals. **Language of Database:** English. **Subject Coverage:** Pharmaceuticals, including chemistry, biochemistry, pharmacology, therapeutics, and toxicology.

★7068★ PHARMACEUTICAL NEWS INDEX (PNI)
UMI/Data Courier
620 S. 3rd. St.
Louisville, KY 40202-2475   Phone: (502) 583-4111
General Description: Provides in-depth indexing of 20 leading pharmaceutical industry newsletters published in the United States, Great Britain, and Japan. **Language of Database:** English. **Subject Coverage:** The pharmaceutical, cosmetics, medical devices, biotechnology, and health care industries, including legislation and regulations, research progress, market analyses, future developments, and conference activities.

★7069★ PHARMACEUTICAL PROSPECTS
Healthcare Forecasting Inc.
110 National Dr.
Glastonbury, CT 06033 Phone: (203) 659-4077
General Description: Contains forecast data for time-series variables affecting the U.S. pharmaceutical industry. **Language of Database:** English. **Subject Coverage:** U.S. pharmaceutical industry, including industry characteristics, pharmaceutical sales, distribution, retailing, and national health and demographic data.

★7070★ PHARMACEUTICALS INDUSTRY COMPETITIVE INTELLIGENCE TRACKING SERVICE
SIS International
172 Madison Ave., Ste. 306
New York, NY 10016 Phone: (212) 725-4550
General Description: Provides comprehensive and up-to-date competitive intelligence on the pharmaceuticals industry. Contains citations and abstracts to periodical literature published worldwide. **Language of Database:** English. **Subject Coverage:** The pharmaceuticals industry, including industry trends and issues, consumer attitudes, market activity, legislation, competitor profiles, financial performance, mergers and acquisitions, new product development, technology, research, biotechnology, future trends, the international scene, and such product and market topics as FDA activities, pricing, distribution, generic drugs, and over-the-counter medications.

★7071★ PHARMAPROJECTS
PJB Publications Ltd.
18-20 Hill Rise
Richmond, Surrey TW10 6UA, England
General Description: Provides licensing and other information on some 5000 pharmaceutical products currently being developed by more than 800 companies worldwide. Covers novel formulations and combinations of therapeutic significance through the patent process from patenting to launching in all major markets. Includes descriptions of old projects, including those whose development has been discontinued, those for which there is no clear evidence of continuing development, and those which have been launched in all significant markets are removed from the database. Descriptions of those discontinuations which have been confirmed by their company are held in a companion file known as PHARMACEASED. **Language of Database:** English. **Subject Coverage:** Drug development and licensing worldwide.

★7072★ PHARMLINE
Regional Drug Information Service
The London Hospital
Whitechapel Rd.
London E1 1BB, England
General Description: Indexes and abstracts articles from major medical and pharmaceutical journals and other sources on all aspects of modern drug use. **Language of Database:** English. **Subject Coverage:** All aspects of drug use, including current drug therapy, adverse drug reactions, drug use in pregnancy, drugs for nursing mothers, drug interactions, drug stability, drugs in preventative medicine, and drugs for special patient groups.

★7073★ PHARMSEARCH
Institut National de la Propriete Industrielle
26 bis, rue de Leningrad
F-75800 Paris Cedex 8, France
General Description: Contains information on pharmaceutical patents published in France and the United States, and by the European Patent Office (EPO). Includes galenic, therapeutic, and generic structural aspects for patents, as well as the Markush structures used in the description of compound families, their graphic representation, and corresponding generic terms. **Language of Database:** French. **Subject Coverage:** Pharmaceutical patent information published in France, the United States, and by the European Patent Office (EPO), including new therapeutically active compounds and intermediates, compounds involved in novel preparation processes, compounds with novel therapeutic activities, and active ingredients of new pharmaceutical compounds.

★7074★ PHN AIDS NETWORK
Public Health Foundation
Public Health Network (PHN)
1220 L St., NW, Ste. 350
Washington, DC 20005 Phone: (202) 898-5600
General Description: Provides up-to-date information on the latest AIDS case statistics, treatment issues, AIDS education, U.S. federal and state AIDS policies statements, and a directory of all state AIDS coordinators.

Enables the user to exchange information and ask questions of more than 700 public health officials throughout the United States as well as access the following databases accessible through BRS Information Technologies (each is described in a separate entry): AIDS Knowledge Base; Comprehensive Core Medical Library; MEDLINE; AIDS Database (Bureau of Hygiene and Tropical Diseases); and AIDS School Health Education Database. **Also Known as:** AIDS-NET. **Language of Database:** English. **Subject Coverage:** Acquired Immune Deficiency Syndrome, including statistics, policy statements, diagnosis and treatment, and public education.

★7075★ PHYSICIAN DATA QUERY CANCER INFORMATION FILE
U.S. National Cancer Institute
International Cancer Information Center
Bldg. 82, Rm. 102
Bethesda, MD 20892 Phone: (301) 496-7403
General Description: Contains the complete text of prognostic and treatment information for more than 85 different cancers. Includes up-to-date information on prognosis, staging, cellular classification, and standard and investigational treatments. Provides references to relevant medical literature. **Also Known as:** PDQ Cancer Information File. **Language of Database:** English. **Subject Coverage:** Treatment and prognostic information for more than 85 different types of cancer.

★7076★ PHYSICIAN DATA QUERY DIRECTORY FILE
U.S. National Cancer Institute
International Cancer Information Center
Bldg. 82, Rm. 102
Bethesda, MD 20892 Phone: (301) 496-7403
General Description: Contains the names, addresses, and telephone numbers for more than 15,000 physicians and 1800 organizations devoted to the care of cancer patients. **Also Known as:** PDQ Directory File. **Language of Database:** English. **Subject Coverage:** Physicians and organizations devoted to the care of cancer patients.

★7077★ PHYSICIAN DATA QUERY PROTOCOL FILE
U.S. National Cancer Institute
International Cancer Information Center
Bldg. 82, Rm. 102
Bethesda, MD 20892 Phone: (301) 496-7403
General Description: Contains information on more than 1300 active cancer treatment protocols. Covers clinical trials supported directly by the National Cancer Institute as well as those voluntarily submitted by other investigators. **Also Known as:** PDQ Protocol File. **Language of Database:** English. **Subject Coverage:** Cancer treatment protocols.

★7078★ THE PHYSICIAN AND SPORTSMEDICINE
McGraw-Hill, Inc.
1221 Avenue of the Americas
New York, NY 10020-1095 Phone: (212) 512-2000
General Description: Contains the complete text of The Physician & Sportsmedicine, a magazine covering clinical articles on the recognition, treatment, and prevention of injury and disease caused by exercise and sports. **Language of Database:** English. **Subject Coverage:** Sportsmedicine, including training and conditioning principals such as nutrition, exercise methods, and fitness evaluations; fitness prevention and amelioration of chronic disease; and the use of sports and games for conditioning and rehabilitation of physically handicapped people.

★7079★ PHYSICIANS AND DENTISTS DATABASE
FIRSTMARK
34 Juniper Ln.
Newton Center, MA 02159 Phone: (617) 965-7989
General Description: Provides directory listings for more than 432,000 physicians and 151,000 dentists nationwide. **Language of Database:** English. **Subject Coverage:** U.S. physicians and dentists; coverage extends to all medical and dental specialties.

★7080★ PHYSICIANS' DESK REFERENCE (PDR)
Medical Economics Co., Inc.
5 Paragon Dr.
Oradell, NJ 07645 Phone: (201) 262-3030
General Description: Provides descriptions of more than 2750 commonly prescribed drug products as well as ophthalmological products and nonprescription (over-the-counter) drug products. Includes drug interaction and side effects data. **Language of Database:** English. **Subject Coverage:** Prescription, ophthalmological, and over-the-counter drugs, including uses, dosage, side effects, interaction, and other information.

★7081★ PLANTAS MEDICINALES (PLAMED)
Ministerio de Sanidad y Consumo de Espana
Direccion General de Farmacia y Productos Sanitarios
Servicio de Gestion del Banco de Datos de Medicamentos
Paseo del Prado, 18-20
28014 Madrid, Spain
General Description: Contains data describing herbal remedies registered and in the process of being authorized for marketing within Spain. **Also Known as:** Herbal Remedies. **Language of Database:** Spanish. **Subject Coverage:** Pharmaceutical product data for herbal remedies currently in the process of being authorized for use in Spain.

★7082★ POPLINE
U.S. National Library of Medicine
MEDLARS Management Section
8600 Rockville Pike
Bethesda, MD 20894   Phone: (301) 496-6193
General Description: Provides citations to worldwide published and unpublished biomedical and social science literature concerning family planning and population. **Also Known as:** Population Information Online. **Language of Database:** English. **Subject Coverage:** Family planning and population, including human fertility, contraceptive control, community-based services, program evaluation, demography, censuses, and related health, law, and policy issues.

★7083★ POSTGRADUATE MEDICINE
McGraw-Hill, Inc.
1221 Avenue of the Americas
New York, NY 10020-1095   Phone: (212) 512-2000
General Description: Contains the complete text of Postgraduate Medicine, a magazine covering the diagnosis and treatment of general medical problems. Includes clinical articles of articles to physicians, nurses, dentists, and other healthcare professionals. **Language of Database:** English. **Subject Coverage:** General medicine.

★7084★ PRINCIPOS ACTIVOS (PACTIV)
Ministerio de Sanidad y Consumo de Espana
Direccion General de Farmacia y Productos Sanitarios
Servicio de Gestion del Banco de Datos de Medicamentos
Paseo del Prado, 18-20
28014 Madrid, Spain
General Description: Contains information on the active chemical ingredients for drugs and pharmaceutical specialties registered and in the process of authorization for marketing in Spain. Includes therapeutical groups, pharmacological groups, CAS Registry Number, and other indicators. **Also Known as:** Active Ingredients. **Language of Database:** Spanish. **Subject Coverage:** Pharmaceutical products currently under development in Spain, including descriptive data, pharmaceutical data, effectiveness, and grave interactions with other factors.

★7085★ PROTOZOOLOGICAL ABSTRACTS
C.A.B. International
Wallingford, Oxon. OX10 8DE, England
General Description: Indexes and abstracts current periodical and other published literature relating to protozoan diseases affecting man and animals. Covers malaria, trypanosoma, amoebal, toxoplasma, babesia, coccidia, giardia, leishmania, and AIDS-opportunistic infections. **Language of Database:** English. **Subject Coverage:** Medical and veterinary protozoology, including taxonomy; pathology; biochemistry; microbiology; immunology and immunogenetics; epidemiology; treatment and control; animal health; control of pests, disease, and micro-organisms; taxonomy.

★7086★ PUBLIC HEALTH AND TROPICAL MEDICINE DATA BASE
Bureau of Hygiene and Tropical Diseases
Keppel St.
London WC1E 7HT, England
General Description: Contains citations and abstracts of published materials covering tropical medicine, communicable diseases, and occupational health. **Language of Database:** English. **Subject Coverage:** Tropical and communicable diseases, including causes, transmission, and control; occupational hygiene and medicine; environmental and community health; bacterial, viral, fungal, and protozoal infections and helminthiases (including AIDS and Legionnaires' disease); toxicology and industrial health; cancer epidemiology; medical entomology; and community health-primary health care.

★7087★ RADIOPHARMACEUTICAL INTERNAL DOSE DATABASE
Oak Ridge Associated Universities
Radiopharmaceutical Internal Dose Information Center
PO Box 117
Oak Ridge, TN 37831-0117   Phone: (615) 576-3450
General Description: Contains information on the characteristics of radiopharmaceuticals based on internal radiation doses received by patients at hospitals with nuclear medicine facilities. **Language of Database:** English. **Subject Coverage:** Nuclear medicine, including retention and distribution of radiopharmaceuticals in patients; health physics.

★7088★ READING MATERIAL FOR THE BLIND AND PHYSICALLY HANDICAPPED (BLND)
U.S. Library of Congress
National Library Service for the Blind and Physically Handicapped
1291 Taylor St., NW
Washington, DC 20542   Phone: (202) 707-5100
General Description: Contains complete MARC-format records describing reading material for the blind and physically handicapped available in braille and recorded formats. **Language of Database:** English. **Subject Coverage:** Fiction and nonfiction literature, including bestsellers, classics, mysteries, science fiction, history, biographies, poetry, religious works, juvenile and children's books, foreign language materials, music scores, textbooks, and instructional material; more than 70 popular magazines.

★7089★ RECAL OFFLINE
University of Strathclyde
National Centre for Training and Education in Prosthetics and Orthotics
Curran Bldg.
131 St. James Rd.
Glasgow G4 0LS, Scotland
General Description: Contains citations to periodical articles and other materials covering prosthetics, orthotics, and rehabilitation engineering. **Language of Database:** English. **Subject Coverage:** Prosthetics, orthotics, and rehabilitation engineering.

★7090★ REHABDATA
National Rehabilitation Information Center
Macro Systems, Inc.
8455 Colesville Rd., Ste. 935
Silver Spring, MD 20910-3319   Phone: (301) 588-9284
General Description: Contains citations to print and nonprint materials on the rehabilitation of most physical and mental disabilities. **Also Known as:** National Rehabilitation Information Center Data Base. **Language of Database:** English. **Subject Coverage:** All aspects of rehabilitation of persons with mental, physical, or developmental disabilities, including individuals who are blind, deaf, spinal cord injured, and emotionally disturbed, as well as relevant professional and administrative practices.

★7091★ RENAL TUMORS OF CHILDREN
CMC ReSearch, Inc.
7150 SW Hampton, Ste. C-120
Portland, OR 97223   Phone: (503) 639-3395
General Description: Contains the complete text of the lectures on the subject of renal tumors of children as given by Dr. J. Bruce. **Language of Database:** English. **Subject Coverage:** Pediatric renal tumors.

★7092★ REPRORISK
Micromedex, Inc.
600 Grant St.
Denver, CO 80203-3527   Phone: (303) 831-1400
General Description: Provides information on the reproductive risks of drugs, chemicals, and physical and environmental agents for males and females with emphasis on the unborn child. **Also Known as:** Reproductive Risk Information System. **Language of Database:** English. **Subject Coverage:** Teratology, including drug effects, industrial chemicals, food additives, household products, radiation, carcinogenic and genetic effects, and hazard ratings.

★7093★ REPROTOX
Columbia Hospital for Women
Reproductive Toxicology Center
2440 M St., NW, Ste. 217
Washington, DC 20037-1404   Phone: (202) 293-5137
General Description: Provides up-to-date information and summaries of relevant articles dealing with industrial and environmental chemicals and their effects on human fertility, pregnancy, and fetal development.

Language of Database: English. Subject Coverage: Reproductive toxicology (the effects of chemicals on human reproduction). Covers fertility, pregnancy, development, male exposures, and lactation; industrial and environmental chemicals, including prescription, over-the-counter, and recreational drugs, nutritional agents, pesticides, radiation, and water and air pollutants.

★7094★ RESEAU DOCUMENTAIRE EN SCIENCES HUMAINES DE LA SANTE (RESHUS)
France Centre National de la Recherche Scientifique
Institut de l'Information Scientifique et Technique
2, allee du Parc de Brabois
F-54514 Vandoeuvre-lens-Nancy Cedex, France
General Description: Contains references and abstracts of journal articles and other published literature relating to the social and human aspects of health. Also Known as: Network for Documentation in the Human Sciences of Health. Language of Database: French. Subject Coverage: Social and human aspects of health sciences, including methodology, teaching, and research; birth rate, mortality rate, and disease; health and development; risk factors for health deterioration; health organizations and policies; health education; medical ethics; status, management, and structure of hospitals and preventive care facilities; health system facilities; risk coverage system; medical expenditures; evaluation of treatment; absenteeism; and health insurance.

★7095★ RESOURCE ORGANIZATIONS/ORGANISMES RESSOURCES
Canadian Centre for Occupational Health and Safety
250 Main St. E.
Hamilton, ON, Canada L8N 1H6   Phone: (416) 572-2981
General Description: Provides information on Canadian organizations involved in the field of occupational health and safety. Includes information on the organization's areas of responsibility, name, location and working language. Language of Database: English; French. Subject Coverage: Canadian occupational health and safety organizations.

★7096★ RESOURCE PEOPLE/PERSONNES RESSOURCES
Canadian Centre for Occupational Health and Safety
250 Main St. E.
Hamilton, ON, Canada L8N 1H6   Phone: (416) 572-2981
General Description: Provides information on Canadians involved in the field of occupational health and safety. Includes information on the person's type of activity, name, location, working language, and employing organization. Language of Database: English; French. Subject Coverage: Canadian occupational health and safety professionals.

★7097★ REVIEW OF MEDICAL AND VETERINARY ENTOMOLOGY
C.A.B. International
Wallingford, Oxon. OX10 8DE, England
General Description: Indexes and abstracts current periodical and other published literature relating to medical and veterinary entomology. Covers insects and other arthropods which transmit diseases or are otherwise injurious to man and to animals of significance to man, including blattaria, mallophaga, anoplura, hemiptera, siphonaptera, dipters, acari, and arachnida. Language of Database: English. Subject Coverage: Medical and veterinary entomology, including control of pests, disease, and micro-organisms; pesticides; animal health; morphology; physiology; ecology; geographical distribution; public health and hygiene; and taxonomy.

★7098★ REVIEW OF MEDICAL AND VETERINARY MYCOLOGY
C.A.B. International
Wallingford, Oxon. OX10 8DE, England
General Description: Indexes and abstracts current periodical and other published literature relating to medical and veterinary mycology. Covers mycoses of man and domestic, farm, and wild animals as well as allergic disorders associated with fungi and poisoning by fungi or mold-contaminated food. Language of Database: English. Subject Coverage: Medical and veterinary mycology, including control of pests, disease, and micro-organisms; immunology and immunogenetics; food contaminants and additives; animal health; taxonomy; antifungal agents; asthma and allergy; yeast infections; actinomycete infections; mycotoxins; dermatomycoses; aspergillosis; candidosis; cryptococcosis; coccidiodomycosis; and histoplasmosis.

★7099★ RHEO
Deutsche Bundesanstalt fur Materialforschung und -prufung
Unter den Eichen 87
D-1000 Berlin 45, Germany
General Description: Provides citations to literature covering rheology. Emphasis is on materials which do not react the way the Hookean body or a Newtonian fluid does. Language of Database: English; German. Subject Coverage: Rheology, covering the deformation and flow of materials and biological systems, including liquids, solids, gases, and dispersed and granular systems.

★7100★ SCIENTIFIC AMERICAN MEDICINE (SAM)
Scientific American, Inc.
415 Madison Ave.
New York, NY 10017   Phone: (212) 754-0563
General Description: Contains the complete text of reports providing information on current developments in clinical medicine, broken down into the 15 subspecialties of internal medicine. Covers developments in patient management, diagnostic techniques, basic medical science, and drug regimens. Language of Database: English. Subject Coverage: Current developments in the 15 subspecialties of clinical medicine: cardiovascular medicine, dermatology, endocrinology, gastroenterology, hematology, immunology, infectious disease, interdisciplinary medicine, metabolism, nephrology, neurology, oncology, psychiatry, respiratory medicine, and rheumatology.

★7101★ SCISCAN
Institute for Scientific Information
3501 Market St.
Philadelphia, PA 19104   Phone: (215) 386-0100
General Description: Contains citations to current international literature covering the natural, physical, and biomedical sciences. Corresponds to the four most recent weeks of coverage in SciSearch (described in a separate entry). Language of Database: English. Subject Coverage: Natural, physical, earth, environmental, biomedical, and life sciences; chemistry, agriculture, clinical medicine, engineering, technology and applied sciences, and computer and information science.

★7102★ SCISEARCH
Institute for Scientific Information
3501 Market St.
Philadelphia, PA 19104   Phone: (215) 386-0100
General Description: Contains citations to international literature covering the natural, physical, and biomedical sciences. Includes all references cited within a covered article. Language of Database: English. Subject Coverage: Natural, physical, earth, environmental, biomedical, and life sciences; chemistry, agriculture, clinical medicine, engineering, technology and applied sciences, and computer and information science.

★7103★ SEDBASE
Excerpta Medica/EMBASE Publishing Group
Molenwerf 1
PO Box 1527
NL-1000 BM Amsterdam, Netherlands
General Description: Contains critical analyses of published drug side effects and adverse reactions to drugs currently in use. Analyses are prepared by recognized authorities. Includes citations to articles describing drug side effects and adverse reactions as covered in EMBASE plus (described in a separate entry). Also Known as: Side Effects of Drugs (SED) Database. Language of Database: English. Subject Coverage: Adverse drug reactions, drug interactions, drug toxicity, special risk situations, and pharmacological or patient-dependent factors associated with the occurrence of side effects.

★7104★ SEGURIDAD E HIGIENE EN EL TRABAJO
Ministerio de Trabajo de Espana
Instituto Nacional de Seguridad e Higiene en el Trabajo
Programa de Informacion y Documentacion
Calle Dulcet s/n
08034 Barcelona, Spain
General Description: Cites published literature dealing with all aspects of occupational health and safety. Also Known as: BIBLIOG. Language of Database: Spanish. Subject Coverage: Occupational health and safety, occupational medicine, industrial hygiene, industrial toxicology, ergonomics, and safety education.

★7105★ SEIBT
Seibt Verlag GmbH
Leopoldstr, 208
D-8000 Munich 40, Germany
General Description: Provides descriptions of German manufacturers, wholesalers, importers, exporters, and service firms that supply products for industry and international trade. Also covers German companies involved in manufacturing and supply of medical equipment and supplies, pharmaceutical equipment and supplies, and surface technological equipment and suppplies. **Language of Database:** German; English. **Subject Coverage:** German companies involved in the manufacturing, sales, import and export, and supply of industrial products, including those for the pharmaceutical, medical, and surface technology sectors.

★7106★ SERLINE
U.S. National Library of Medicine
MEDLARS Management Section
8600 Rockville Pike
Bethesda, MD 20894   Phone: (301) 496-6193
General Description: Provides bibliographic descriptions of all journals currently cataloged or on order for the National Library of Medicine's collection as well as titles selectively indexed for MEDLINE, POPLINE, or HEALTH which do not meet NLM scope and coverage requirements or are held by libraries participating in the NLM National Biomedical Serials Holdings Database (SERHOLD). Includes locator information for approximately one-half of the journals cited, enabling the user to determine which U.S. medical libraries own a particular journal. **Also Known as:** Serials Online. **Language of Database:** English. **Subject Coverage:** Biomedical serials.

★7107★ SIRS SOCIAL ISSUES AND CRITICAL ISSUES CD-ROM
Social Issues Resources Series, Inc. (SIRS)
PO Box 2348
Boca Raton, FL 33427-2348   Phone: (407) 994-0079
General Description: Contains the complete text of articles providing current information on the latest issues affecting the general citizenry, changing behavior, and threatening society with impending disaster. **Language of Database:** English. **Subject Coverage:** Social issues, including aging, alcoholism, communications, consumerism, corrections, crime, death and dying, defense, drugs, energy, ethics, ethnic groups, family, food, habitat, health, human rights, mental health, money, pollution, population, privacy, religion, school, sexuality, sports, technology, Third World, transportation, women, work, and youth; and the critical issues of AIDS and the atmosphere.

★7108★ SMALL ANIMALS
C.A.B. International
Wallingford, Oxon. OX10 8DE, England
General Description: Indexes and abstracts current periodical and other published literature related to dogs, cats, and other domestic animals. **Language of Database:** English. **Subject Coverage:** Small animals, including bacterial diseases, viral diseases, mycoses, parasites, helminths and protozoa, organic diseases, neoplasms, toxicology, immunology, pharmacology, anesthesia, physiology, breeding, genetics, nutrition, nutritional and metabolic disorders, biochemistry, hematology, anatomy, welfare, radiology, and surgery.

★7109★ SMOKING AND HEALTH
U.S. Centers for Disease Control
Office on Smoking and Health
Rhodes Bldg., Mailstop K12
1600 Clifton Rd., NE
Atlanta, GA 30333   Phone: (404) 488-5080
General Description: Provides references and abstracts of worldwide scientific and technical literature covering all aspects of smoking, tobacco, and tobacco use. **Language of Database:** English. **Subject Coverage:** Smoking, tobacco, and health, including cancer, respiratory ailments and heart disease, chemical by-products of tobacco and tobacco smoke, behavioral aspects of smoking, and statistics on smoking.

★7110★ SOMED
Institut fur Dokumentation und Information, Sozialmedizin und Offentliches Gesundheitswesen
Postfach 20 10 12
Westerfeldstr. 35-37
D-4800 Bielefeld 1, Germany
General Description: Contains citations and abstracts of published literature on social medicine and related fields. **Also Known as:** Sozialmedizin

Language of Database: German; English. **Subject Coverage:** Nonclinical medicine, including occupational medicine and industrial toxicology, community medicine, public health, health education, dependence problems (drugs, narcotics, alcoholism, smoking and other dependencies), epidemiology and medical statistics, environmental medicine and hygiene, environmental toxicology, and related fields.

★7111★ SOUTH AFRICAN MEDICAL LITERATURE (SAMED)
South African Medical Research Council
Institute for Biomedical Communication
PO Box 19070
Tygerberg, Republic of South Africa
General Description: Provides references to biomedical literature published in South Africa. **Language of Database:** English. **Subject Coverage:** Medicine, biology, and health care.

★7112★ SPORT DATABASE
Sport Information Resource Centre (SIRC)
1600 James Naismith Dr.
Gloucester, ON, Canada K1B 5N4   Phone: (613) 748-5658
General Description: Provides citations to the world's literature dealing with sports, fitness, and recreation, including both practical and scientific aspects. Includes abstracts for selected items. **Also Known as:** SIRC Database. **Language of Database:** English. **Subject Coverage:** Physical education; physical fitness; exercise physiology; sports medicine; coaching; officiating; sports administration; sport and the humanities/social sciences; handicapped sport and recreation, including such areas as etiology and treatment of sport injuries; drills; techniques; administration of physical education programs and facilities; health; and leisure and recreation. Excludes news items and information on competition results.

★7113★ SPRILINE
Sjukvardens och Socialvardens Planerings- och Rationaliserings-institut
SPRI Biblioteket och Utredningsbanken
PO Box 27310
S-102 54 Stockholm, Sweden
General Description: Provides citations to Swedish and international literature covering research in the field of health care planning. Excludes purely medical literature. **Also Known as:** SPRI Research Report Bank. **Language of Database:** Swedish. **Subject Coverage:** International health care planning.

★7114★ STANDARD DRUG FILE (SDF)
Derwent Publications Ltd.
Rochdale House
128 Theobalds Rd.
London WC1X 8RP, England
General Description: Lists drugs and other commonly occurring compounds that are indexed in RINGDOC. **Language of Database:** English. **Subject Coverage:** Pharmaceuticals, including chemistry, biochemistry, pharmacology, therapeutics, and toxicology.

★7115★ STANDARDS AND DIRECTORIES/NORMES ET REPERTOIRES
Canadian Centre for Occupational Health and Safety
250 Main St. E.
Hamilton, ON, Canada L8N 1H6   Phone: (416) 572-2981
General Description: Provides information from the Canadian Standards Association (CSA) standards, certified product directories, and other miscellaneous publications dealing with occupational safety and health. Includes the preface, scope, and table of contents. Records are in English. **Language of Database:** English; French. **Subject Coverage:** Standards, directories, and publications covering occupational health and safety, electrical, mechanical, and mine safety, and environmental sciences.

★7116★ STAT!-REF
Teton Data Systems
PO Box 3082
Jackson, WY 83001   Phone: (307) 733-5494
General Description: Contains the complete text of 12 medical reference publications dealing with primary care. Provides information on basic and clinical immunology, diagnosis and treatments for surgery, pediatrics, and obstetrics and gynecology, emergency diagnosis and treatment, general psychiatry, and medical physiology. Also provides information on prescription and nonprescription drugs covered in USP Drug Information (described in a separate entry). **Language of Database:** English. **Subject Coverage:** Primary care medicine, including diagnoses and treatment, pediatrics, emergency medicine, immunology, obstetrics and gynecology, urology, and pharmaceutical information.

★7117★ STEDMAN'S MEDICAL DICTIONARY
Williams & Wilkins
428 E. Preston St.
Baltimore, MD 21202   Phone: (301) 528-4000
General Description: Contains complete text of Stedman's Medical Dictionary, a medical terminology reference guide containing 100,000 definitions pertaining to the field of medicine. Features the Random House Concise Dictionary comprising an additional 51,000 definitions. **Language of Database:** English. **Subject Coverage:** Medical terminology.

★7118★ SUBIDEX
Sheffield University Biomedical Information Service
Sheffield S10 2TN, England
General Description: Provides references to periodical articles covering specific aspects of cell biology, physiology, immunobiology, neurobiology, and biotechnology. Includes notices of forthcoming books and conferences. **Language of Database:** English. **Subject Coverage:** Biomedicine, including adrenergic receptors, atrial natriuretic factors, bio-electronic and bio-sensors, biological rhythms, blood coagulation factors, cell calcium, cell contact phenomena, cell membranes, clinical cyto-genetics, cyclic AMP, cytoskeleton, DNA probes, drug targeting, erythrocytes, extracellular matrix, gastric secretion, gastrointestinal hormones, growth factors, high performance liquid chromatography, immunoassay, immunohistochemistry, intestinal function, invertebrate neurobiology, leucocytes, liposomes, lymphokines, macrophages, mitochondria, monoclonal antibodies, nerve cell biology, neuropeptides, neuro-physiology, oncogenes, oxygen radicals, pancreatic and salivary secretion, peptide hormone receptors, plant biotechnology, platelets, prostaglandins, proteins, recombinant DNA, renal physiology, signal transduction, steroid receptors, thyroid hormones, tissue culture, transmitters, receptors and synapses, and vision.

★7119★ SUICIDE INFORMATION AND EDUCATION (SIE)
Suicide Information and Education Center
1615 10th Ave., SW, Ste. 201
Calgary, AB, Canada T3C 0J7   Phone: (403) 245-3900
General Description: Contains references and abstracts of published materials on the topic of suicidal behaviors and suicide prevention and education. **Language of Database:** English. **Subject Coverage:** Suicide and suicidal behaviors, including such aspects as biomedicine, psychosociology, epidemiology, community education, research, theoretical perspectives, legal aspects, and suicide in literature.

★7120★ SWEDISH DRUG INFORMATION SYSTEM (SWEDIS)
Sweden National Board of Health and Welfare
Department of Drugs
PO Box 607
S-751 25 Uppsala, Sweden
General Description: Contains comprehensive descriptions of all drugs on the Swedish market. **Subject Coverage:** Drugs available in Sweden.

★7121★ SWEMED
Karolinska Institutets Bibliotek och Informationscentral
Medical Information Center
Doktorsringen 21D
Box 60201
S-104 01 Stockholm, Sweden
General Description: Contains references to biomedical journal articles and reports published in Sweden, and to all medical dissertations at Swedish universities. **Language of Database:** English. **Subject Coverage:** All areas of medicine.

★7122★ TOXICOLOGY ABSTRACTS
Cambridge Scientific Abstracts
7200 Wisconsin Ave.
Bethesda, MD 20814   Phone: (301) 961-6750
General Description: Contains citations and abstracts of international periodical and other literature covering toxicology. **Language of Database:** English. **Subject Coverage:** Toxicological studies of industrial chemicals, pharmaceuticals, food, agricultural chemicals, natural toxins, household products, and other substances. Specific topics covered include food additives and contaminants; social poisons and drug abuse; agrochemicals; metals; industrial chemicals; toxins and other natural substances; cosmetics, toiletries, and household products; polycyclic hydrocarbons; radiation and radioactive materials; nitrosamines and related compounds; and legislation and recommended standards.

★7123★ TOXLINE
U.S. National Library of Medicine
Toxicology Information Program
8600 Rockville Pike
Bethesda, MD 20894   Phone: (301) 496-1131
General Description: Provides citations to published sources of information on the pharmacological, biochemical, physiological, and toxicological effects of drugs and other chemicals. Comprises the following four files: • TOXLINE—covers the period 1981 to the present. • TOXLINE—covers the period 1965 through 1980. • TOX LIT (Toxicology Literature from Special Sources). • TOXLIT65—covers the period 1965 through 1980. TOXLINE files contain references collected from sources that do not require royalty charges; TOXLIT files contain references from sources with royalty charges. **Also Known as:** Toxicology Information Online. **Language of Database:** English. **Subject Coverage:** Biological and adverse effects of drugs; human and animal toxicity; pesticides; environmental chemicals and pollutants; food additives; industrial and household chemicals; radioactive materials.

★7124★ UK NATIONAL FOOD NUTRIENT DATABANK
Royal Society of Chemistry
Information Services
Thomas Graham House
Science Park
Cambridge CB4 4WF, England
General Description: Contains data on the nutrient content of foods. Updates and expands "The Composition of Foods" (4th edition) by Drs. McCance and Widdowson. Calculates recipes, meals, 7-day dietary records, and comparisons. **Language of Database:** English. **Subject Coverage:** Nutrient composition of foods, including cereals and cereal products, milk products, eggs, fruits, and vegetables.

★7125★ UNION CATALOGUE OF SERIALS IN SWISS LIBRARIES
Academie Suisse des Sciences Medicales
c/o Redaction RPM
Bibliotheque de la Faculte de Medecine, CMU
CH-1211 Geneva 4, Switzerland
General Description: Contains full bibliographic descriptions of periodical titles held by 650 Swiss scientific, industrial, and public libraries. Covers serials published outside Swizerland after 1945 excluding titles that ceased before 1946 and titles published outside Switzerland, and covers all biomedical titles regardless of their place or year of publication. Includes the names and addresses of Swiss libraries providing photocopies of articles from the periodicals. **Subject Coverage:** Serials published worldwide, with special focus on biomedical periodicals.

★7126★ USP DRUG INFORMATION (USP DI)
U.S. Pharmacopeial Convention, Inc. (USP)
12601 Twinbrook Pkwy.
Rockville, MD 20852   Phone: (301) 881-0666
General Description: Contains the complete text of drug monographs for health care professionals and consumers relating to the prescription, dispensation, and administration of prescription and nonprescription drug products. Provides information on drug chemistry, pharmacology, precautions to consider, side effects, adverse effects, patient consultation, and general dosing information. **Language of Database:** English. **Subject Coverage:** Drugs and pharmacology.

★7127★ USP DRUG INFORMATION PATIENT DRUG EDUCATION LEAFLETS (USP DI PDEL'S)
U.S. Pharmacopeial Convention, Inc. (USP)
12601 Twinbrook Pkwy.
Rockville, MD 20852   Phone: (301) 881-0666
General Description: Contains the complete text of some 350 patient drug monographs covering 5000 of the most widely used brand name and generic drug products. Provides lay-language information on the use of prescription and nonprescription medications. **Language of Database:** English. **Subject Coverage:** Drugs and pharmacology.

★7128★ VA PATIENT EDUCATION DATABASE
U.S. Department of Veterans Affairs (VA)
VA Patient Health Education Clearinghouse
810 Vermont Ave., NW
Washington, DC 20420   Phone: (202) 233-3842
General Description: Contains references and abstracts of published literature dealing with the health education programs for patients in Veterans Administration hospitals. **Language of Database:** English. **Subject**

Coverage: Health education programs for Veterans Administration patients.

★7129★ VA REHABILITATION DATABASE
U.S. Department of Veterans Affairs (VA)
Office of Technology Transfer
Prosthetics Research & Development Center
103 S. Gay St.
Baltimore, MD 21202   Phone: (301) 962-1800
General Description: Provides access to rehabilitation research and technology information. **Language of Database:** English. **Subject Coverage:** Rehabilitation research and technology, including bioengineering; biomechanics; neuroscience; orthopedic implants; orthotics; prosthetics; hearing, speech, and vision sensory aids; spinal cord injuries; and surgery.

★7130★ VETERINARY BULLETIN
C.A.B. International
Wallingford, Oxon. OX10 8DE, England
General Description: Indexes and abstracts current periodical and other published literature relating to the field of animal health. Animals covered include cattle, horses, sheep, goats, pigs, poultry, cats, dogs, rabbits, cage birds, other small animals, loboratory animals, wildlife, zoo animals, fish, and other domestic animals. **Language of Database:** English. **Subject Coverage:** Veterinary science, including animal physiology and biochemistry; animal health; medical and veterinary entomology, helminthology, mycology, and protozoology.

★7131★ VETERINARY LITERATURE DOCUMENTATION (VETDOC)
Derwent Publications Ltd.
Rochdale House
128 Theobalds Rd.
London WC1X 8RP, England
General Description: Covers relevant papers found in the world's veterinary scientific journals. **Language of Database:** English. **Subject Coverage:** Veterinary drugs, vaccines, growth promotants, toxicology, hormonal control of breeding, and related topics.

★7132★ VIROLOGY AND AIDS ABSTRACTS
Cambridge Scientific Abstracts
7200 Wisconsin Ave.
Bethesda, MD 20814   Phone: (301) 961-6750
General Description: Contains citations and abstracts of international periodical and other literature covering virology, with particular emphasis on Acquired Immune Deficiency Syndrome (AIDS). **Language of Database:** English. **Subject Coverage:** Virology, including effects of viruses on humans, animals and plants. Specific topics covered include Acquired Immune Deficiency Syndrome (AIDS); virus taxonomy and classification;

tissue culture studies and methodology; physico-chemical properties, structure and morphology; replication cycle; viral genetics; phage-host interactions; immunology; interferon and other antiviral agents; oncogenic viruses; viral infections of man; diseases associated with slow viruses; animal models and experimentally-induced viral infections; and viral infections of fungi, plants, and invertebrates.

★7133★ WESTLAW HEALTH SERVICES LIBRARY
West Publishing Co.
50 W. Kellogg Blvd.
PO Box 64526
St. Paul, MN 55164-0526   Phone: (612) 228-2500
General Description: Contains the complete text of U.S. federal court decisions, statutes and regulations, state court decisions, and law reviews, texts, bar journals, and specialized legal sources covering health services and medical malpractice. Includes relevant cases decided by the U.S. Supreme Court (1790 to the present), U.S. Courts of Appeal (1891 to the present), and U.S. District Courts (1789 to the present); relevant statutes and regulations from the U.S. Code (current), the Federal Register (1980 to the present), and the U.S. Code of Federal Regulations (current); relevant state court decisions from all 50 states and the District of Columbia; specialized health-related sources; and relevant law reviews, texts, and bar journals. **Language of Database:** English. **Subject Coverage:** U.S. law relating to health services and medical malpractice.

★7134★ WORLD HEALTH STATISTICS DATA BASE (WHS)
World Health Organization
Division of Epidemiological Surveillance and Health Situation and
  Trend Assessment
20, ave. Appia
CH-1211 Geneva 27, Switzerland
General Description: Contains a full range of health and demographic statistics on a worldwide basis. **Subject Coverage:** Health and demographic statistics, including mortality, cancer, and global indicators.

★7135★ YEAR BOOKS ON DISC
Year Book Medical Publishers, Inc.
200 N. LaSalle St.
Chicago, IL 60601   Phone: (312) 726-9733
General Description: Contains the complete text of the preceeding year's Year Books reporting developments in popular fields of medicine: Cardiology, Dermatology, Diagnostic Radiology, Drug Therapy, Emergency Medinice, Family Practice, Medicine, Neurology and Neurosurgery, Obstetrics and Gynecology, Oncology, Pediatrics, and Psychiatry and Applied Mental Health, as well as selected articles from other Year Books. **Language of Database:** English. **Subject Coverage:** Medicine, especially caridology, dermatology, drug therapy, emergency medicine, family practice, neurology and neurosurgery, obstetrics and gynecology, oncology, pediatrics, psychiatry and applied mental health, and radiology.

(9) Libraries and Information Centers

Chapter 9 lists, in separate sections, U.S. and Canadian libraries. Within each country, entries are arranged alphabetically by states or provinces, then by cities, then by library names. For additional information, consult the User's Guide located at the front of this directory.

United States

Alabama

★7136★ NORTHEAST ALABAMA REGIONAL MEDICAL CENTER
MEDICAL LIBRARY
400 E. 10th St.
Box 2208
Anniston, AL 36202   Phone: (205) 235-5877
Kathy Bishop, Libn.
Subjects: Medicine, allied health sciences. **Holdings:** 360 books; 850 bound periodical volumes. **Subscriptions:** 77 journals and other serials.

★7137★ AUBURN UNIVERSITY
VETERINARY MEDICAL LIBRARY
Veterinary Medical Complex
Greene Hall
Auburn University, AL 36849   Phone: (205) 844-1749
Tamera P. Lee, Hd.
Subjects: Veterinary medicine. **Holdings:** 33,000 volumes. **Subscriptions:** 600 journals and other serials.

★7138★ BAPTIST MEDICAL CENTER, PRINCETON
MEDICAL LIBRARY
701 Princeton Ave., SW
Birmingham, AL 35211   Phone: (205) 783-3078
Maureen S. Battistella, Med.Libn.
Subjects: Medicine, surgery, nursing. **Holdings:** 2058 books; 6200 bound periodical volumes. **Subscriptions:** 165 journals.

★7139★ BAPTIST MEDICAL CENTERS-SAMFORD UNIVERSITY
IDA V. MOFFETT SCHOOL OF NURSING
L.R. JORDAN LIBRARY
820 Montclair Rd.
Birmingham, AL 35213   Phone: (205) 592-5103
Jewell Alexander Carter, Lib.Dir.
Subjects: Nursing, allied health sciences. **Holdings:** 8951 books; 2169 bound periodical volumes; 420 VF folders; 1718 AV programs. **Subscriptions:** 139 journals and other serials.

★7140★ CARRAWAY METHODIST MEDICAL CENTER
MEDICAL LIBRARY
1600 N. 26th St.
Birmingham, AL 35234   Phone: (205) 226-6265
Mrs. Bobby H. Powell, Med.Libn.
Subjects: Medicine, surgery, nursing, allied health sciences. **Holdings:** 1293 books; 7805 bound periodical volumes. **Subscriptions:** 235 journals and other serials.

★7141★ EYE FOUNDATION HOSPITAL
JOHN E. MEYER EYE FOUNDATION LIBRARY
1720 University Blvd.
Birmingham, AL 35233-1895   Phone: (205) 325-8505
Hugh Thomas, Med.Libn.
Subjects: Ophthalmology, otolaryngology, medicine, plastic surgery, hospital administration. **Holdings:** 1000 books; 1100 bound periodical volumes; 500 slides and cassettes. **Subscriptions:** 81 journals and other serials.

★7142★ ST. VINCENT'S HOSPITAL
CUNNINGHAM WILSON LIBRARY
Box 12407
Birmingham, AL 35202-2407   Phone: (205) 320-7830
Subjects: Medicine, nursing, hospital administration. **Holdings:** 2537 books; 1316 bound periodical volumes; 335 vertical files; 20 videotapes; 240 audiotapes. **Subscriptions:** 158 journals and other serials.

★7143★ SOUTHERN RESEARCH INSTITUTE
THOMAS W. MARTIN MEMORIAL LIBRARY
PO Box 55305
Birmingham, AL 35255-5305   Phone: (205) 581-2518
Mary L. Pullen, Lib.Mgr.
Subjects: Chemistry, biology, biomaterials, virology, AIDS research, microbiology, mechanical and materials engineering, energy, pollution, metallurgy, physics. **Holdings:** 13,000 books; 34,000 bound periodical volumes. **Subscriptions:** 850 journals and other serials.

★7144★ U.S. DEPARTMENT OF VETERANS AFFAIRS
MEDICAL CENTER LIBRARY
700 S. 19th St.
Birmingham, AL 35233   Phone: (205) 933-8101
Mary Ann Knotts, Chf., Lib.Serv.
Subjects: Medicine, dentistry, nursing, hospital administration. **Holdings:** 1000 books; 2487 bound periodical volumes; 1000 AV programs. **Subscriptions:** 300 journals and other serials.

★7145★ UNIVERSITY OF ALABAMA IN BIRMINGHAM
LISTER HILL LIBRARY OF THE HEALTH SCIENCES
UAB Sta.
Birmingham, AL 35294   Phone: (205) 934-5460
Virginia Algermissen, Dir.
Subjects: Medicine, dentistry, nursing, public health, optometry, allied health fields. **Holdings:** 96,609 books; 132,003 bound periodical volumes;

120.5 linear feet of archival material; 24,867 microforms; 2346 AV programs. **Subscriptions:** 2872 journals and other serials; 5 newspapers.

★7146★ UNIVERSITY OF ALABAMA IN BIRMINGHAM
SCHOOL OF MEDICINE
ANESTHESIOLOGY LIBRARY
Department of Anesthesiology
619 19th St., S.
Birmingham, AL 35233-1924   Phone: (205) 934-6500
A.J. Wright, Clin.Libn.
Subjects: Anesthesia, pain management. **Holdings:** 1161 books; 865 bound periodical volumes; 100 cassettes; 110 videotapes. **Subscriptions:** 105 journals and other serials.

★7147★ UNITED STATES SPORTS ACADEMY
LIBRARY
1 Academy Dr.
Daphne, AL 36526   Phone: (205) 626-3303
Jeff Calametti, Hd.Libn.
Subjects: Sports, including medicine, research and management; fitness; coaching. **Holdings:** 3064 books; 8 VF drawers of clippings; 271 cassette tapes; films; slides; 100 videotapes; periodicals on microfiche. **Subscriptions:** 390 journals and other serials.

★7148★ SOUTHEAST ALABAMA MEDICAL CENTER
MEDICAL LIBRARY
Drawer 6987
Dothan, AL 36302   Phone: (205) 793-8102
Pat McGee, Libn.
Subjects: General medicine, nursing, hospital administration. **Holdings:** 700 books; 2400 bound periodical volumes. **Subscriptions:** 112 journals and other serials.

★7149★ LLOYD NOLAND HOSPITAL
DAVID KNOX MCKAMY MEDICAL LIBRARY
701 Lloyd Noland Pkwy.
Fairfield, AL 35064   Phone: (205) 783-5121
Barbara Estep, Dir., Med.Rec.
Subjects: Medicine, allied health sciences. **Holdings:** 1500 volumes. **Subscriptions:** 147 journals and other serials.

★7150★ U.S. ARMY HOSPITALS
NOBLE ARMY HOSPITAL
MEDICAL LIBRARY
HSXQ-DCS
Fort McClellan, AL 36205   Phone: (205) 848-2411
Kathryn S. Aide, Lib.Techn.
Subjects: Medicine and allied health sciences. **Holdings:** 2100 books; 604 bound periodical volumes. **Subscriptions:** 120 journals and other serials.

★7151★ U.S. ARMY
MEDICAL RESEARCH AND DEVELOPMENT COMMAND
AEROMEDICAL RESEARCH LABORATORY
SCIENTIFIC INFORMATION CENTER
Box 577
Fort Rucker, AL 36362-5292   Phone: (205) 255-6907
Diana L. Hemphill, Libn.
Subjects: Aviation medicine, medicine, vision, audiology, aviation psychology, acoustics, optics. **Holdings:** 15,000 books; 5000 bound periodical volumes; 15,000 documents; 2500 reels of microfilm; 1500 VF items; 50 magnetic tapes. **Subscriptions:** 425 journals and other serials.

★7152★ U.S. ARMY HOSPITALS
LYSTER ARMY COMMUNITY HOSPITAL
MEDICAL LIBRARY
Bldg. 301
U.S. Army Aeromedical Center
Fort Rucker, AL 36362-5333   Phone: (205) 255-7350
Mary Fran Prottsman, Med.Libn.
Subjects: Medicine, nursing, veterinary medicine, aviation medicine, dentistry. **Holdings:** 2500 books; 2500 bound and microform periodical volumes. **Subscriptions:** 150 journals and other serials.

★7153★ BAPTIST MEMORIAL HOSPITAL
MEDICAL LIBRARY
1007 Goodyear Ave.
Gadsden, AL 35903   Phone: (205) 494-4128
Paula G. Davis, Med.Libn.
Subjects: Medicine, nursing, surgery, obstetrics, gynecology, management. **Holdings:** 1750 books; 900 bound periodical volumes. **Subscriptions:** 131 journals and other serials.

★7154★ HOLY NAME OF JESUS HOSPITAL
LIBRARY
Box 268
Gadsden, AL 35902   Phone: (205) 547-4911
Jean F. Bonds, Supv.
Subjects: Medicine, medical specialties, surgery, surgical specialties. **Holdings:** 615 books; 586 bound periodical volumes. **Subscriptions:** 60 journals and other serials.

★7155★ PROVIDENCE HOSPITAL
HEALTH SCIENCE LIBRARY
Box 850724
Mobile, AL 36685   Phone: (205) 633-1373
Mary Ann Donnell, Libn.
Subjects: Nursing, medicine, hospital administration, allied health sciences. **Holdings:** 1800 books; bound periodical volumes. **Subscriptions:** 111 journals and other serials.

★7156★ UNIVERSITY OF SOUTH ALABAMA
COLLEGE OF MEDICINE
BIOMEDICAL LIBRARY
Library 312
Mobile, AL 36688   Phone: (205) 460-7043
Spencer Marsh, Dir.
Subjects: Medicine, nursing, and allied health sciences. **Holdings:** 30,960 books; 51,495 bound periodical volumes; 613 reels of microfilm of periodicals; 7958 microfiche; AV programs. **Subscriptions:** 1963 journals and other serials.

★7157★ ALABAMA DEPARTMENT OF PUBLIC HEALTH
HEALTH RESOURCE CENTER
434 Monroe St., Rm. 557
Montgomery, AL 36130   Phone: (205) 242-5095
Fran Edwards, Lib.Techn.
Subjects: Preventable diseases, smoking, injury prevention, health education. **Holdings:** 500 books; 1000 bound periodical volumes; 807 films. **Subscriptions:** 22 journals.

★7158★ ALABAMA PUBLIC LIBRARY SERVICE
REGIONAL LIBRARY FOR THE BLIND AND PHYSICALLY
  HANDICAPPED
6030 Monticello Dr.
Montgomery, AL 36130   Phone: (205) 277-7330
Fara L. Zaleski, Hd.
Subjects: Recorded and braille fiction and nonfiction. **Holdings:** 225,900 books. **Subscriptions:** 10 journals and other serials.

★7159★ BAPTIST MEDICAL CENTER
MEDICAL LIBRARY
2105 E. South Blvd.
Box 11010
Montgomery, AL 36198   Phone: (205) 286-2952
Jerrie Burton, Libn.
Subjects: Medicine, nursing, allied health sciences. **Holdings:** 1029 books; 1060 bound periodical volumes. **Subscriptions:** 99 journals and other serials.

★7160★ JACKSON HOSPITAL AND CLINIC, INC.
MEDICAL LIBRARY
1235 Forest Ave.
Montgomery, AL 36106   Phone: (205) 298-8898
Cindy Musso, Med.Libn.
Subjects: Medicine, surgery, pediatrics. **Holdings:** 342 books; 663 bound periodical volumes. **Subscriptions:** 42 journals and other serials.

★7161★ **U.S. AIR FORCE HOSPITAL**
AIR UNIVERSITY REGIONAL HOSPITAL
HEALTH SCIENCES LIBRARY
Maxwell AFB
Montgomery, AL 36112-5304   Phone: (205) 293-5852
Patricia A. Kuther, Med.Lib.Techn.
Subjects: General medicine, surgery, pathology, dentistry, nursing, veterinary medicine. **Holdings:** 4000 books and bound periodical volumes. **Subscriptions:** 200 journals and other serials.

★7162★ **U.S. DEPARTMENT OF VETERANS AFFAIRS**
MEDICAL CENTER LIBRARY
215 Perry Hill Rd.
Montgomery, AL 36193   Phone: (205) 272-4670
Steven F. Toepper
Subjects: Medicine, allied health sciences. **Holdings:** 600 books; 175 video cassettes (restricted use); unbound periodicals. **Subscriptions:** 100 journals.

★7163★ **ALABAMA INSTITUTE FOR THE DEAF AND BLIND**
LIBRARY AND RESOURCE CENTER FOR THE BLIND AND
PHYSICALLY HANDICAPPED
Box 698
Talladega, AL 35160   Phone: (205) 761-3288
Teresa Lacy, Libn.
Subjects: General collection. **Holdings:** 28,000 books. **Subscriptions:** 35 journals and other serials.

★7164★ **U.S. DEPARTMENT OF VETERANS AFFAIRS**
MEDICAL CENTER LIBRARY
Loop Rd.
Tuscaloosa, AL 35404   Phone: (205) 553-3760
Olivia S. Maniece, Chf.Libn.
Subjects: Psychiatry, nursing, geriatrics and gerontology, community mental health. **Holdings:** 1751 books; 981 bound periodical volumes; 150 other cataloged items; 200 manuscripts, reports, clippings. **Subscriptions:** 24 newspapers.

★7165★ **UNIVERSITY OF ALABAMA**
COLLEGE OF COMMUNITY HEALTH SCIENCES
HEALTH SCIENCES LIBRARY
PO Box 870378
Tuscaloosa, AL 35487-0378   Phone: (205) 348-1360
Lisa Rains Russell, Chf.Med.Libn.
Subjects: Medicine, nursing, pharmacy, medical sociology. **Holdings:** 9000 books; 16,000 bound periodical volumes; 16 VF drawers of pamphlets and clippings. **Subscriptions:** 475 journals and other serials.

★7166★ **TUSKEGEE UNIVERSITY**
VETERINARY MEDICINE LIBRARY
Patterson Hall
Tuskegee, AL 36088   Phone: (205) 727-8307
Margaret D. Alexander, Libn.
Subjects: Anatomy, physiology, pathology, pharmacology, microbiology, radiology. **Holdings:** 15,565 volumes; 194 reels of microfilm; 447 slide programs; 478 video programs; 49 filmstrips; 20 tape programs. **Subscriptions:** 420 journals and other serials.

★7167★ **U.S. DEPARTMENT OF VETERANS AFFAIRS**
MEDICAL CENTER LIBRARY
Tuskegee, AL 36083   Phone: (205) 727-0550
Artemisia J. Junier, Chf., Lib.Serv.
Subjects: Medicine, patient education. **Holdings:** 28,000 books; 9500 bound periodical volumes; 2800 AV programs. **Subscriptions:** 586 journals and other serials.

Alaska

★7168★ **ALASKA AIR NATIONAL GUARD**
176TH TACTICAL CLINIC MEDICAL LIBRARY
Kulis Air National Guard Base
6000 Air Guard Rd.
Anchorage, AK 99502-1998   Phone: (907) 249-1416
Rosa Williams, Med.Libn.
Subjects: Emergency medicine, dentistry, pharmacy, bioenvironmental and environmental health, nursing, optometry. **Holdings:** 80 books.

★7169★ **ALASKA COUNCIL ON PREVENTION OF ALCOHOL**
AND DRUG ABUSE
LIBRARY
3333 Daniels St., Ste. 201
Anchorage, AK 99503   Phone: (907) 258-6021
Joyce Paulus
Subjects: Alcohol and other drugs. **Holdings:** 1000 books; 120 videotapes. **Subscriptions:** 180 journals and other serials.

★7170★ **ALASKA HEALTH SCIENCES LIBRARY**
ALASKA STATE LIBRARY
3211 Providence Dr.
Anchorage, AK 99508   Phone: (907) 786-1870
Jeraldine Jo Van Den Top, MLS
Subjects: Medicine, dentistry, nursing. **Holdings:** Figurers not available.

★7171★ **U.S. AIR FORCE HOSPITAL**
MEDICAL LIBRARY
Elmendorf AFB, AK 99506-5300   Phone: (907) 552-3383
Donna M. Hudson, Libn.
Subjects: General and military medicine. **Holdings:** 4600 books;. **Subscriptions:** 251 journals and other serials.

★7172★ **UNIVERSITY OF ALASKA, FAIRBANKS**
BIO-MEDICAL LIBRARY
Fairbanks, AK 99775-0300   Phone: (907) 474-7442
Dwight Ittner, Libn.
Subjects: Health sciences, veterinary medicine, fish biology and fisheries, animal physiology, microbiology, plant pathology, ocean sciences, molecular biology. **Holdings:** 48,783 books; 21,638 bound periodical volumes; 2315 volumes in microform. **Subscriptions:** 550 journals and other serials.

★7173★ **U.S. ARMY HOSPITALS**
BASSETT ARMY COMMUNITY HOSPITAL
MEDICAL LIBRARY
Commander USA MEDDAC
Fort Wainwright, AK 99703-7300   Phone: (907) 353-5194
George P. Kimmell, Lib.Techn.
Subjects: Surgery, obstetrics/gynecology, pediatrics, nursing, internal medicine, radiology. **Holdings:** 2450 books; 50 bound periodical volumes. **Subscriptions:** 110 journals and other serials.

Arizona

★7174★ **BULLHEAD COMMUNITY HOSPITAL**
MEDICAL LIBRARY
2735 Silver Creek Rd.
Bullhead City, AZ 86442   Phone: (602) 763-2273
Kathleen Stanley, Med.Libn.
Subjects: Medicine, nursing, and allied health sciences. **Holdings:** 500 books. **Subscriptions:** 25 journals and other serials.

★7175★ **ARIZONA DEPARTMENT OF ECONOMIC SECURITY**
ARIZONA TRAINING PROGRAM AT COOLIDGE
ADMINISTRATION LIBRARY
Box 1467
Coolidge, AZ 85228-1467   Phone: (602) 723-4151
Subjects: Developmental disabilities, psychology, behavioral management, medicine, teaching, social work. **Holdings:** 1200 books; 300 other cataloged items. **Subscriptions:** 10 journals and other serials.

★7176★ **U.S. ARMY HOSPITALS**
BLISS ARMY HOSPITAL
MEDICAL LIBRARY
Fort Huachuca, AZ 85613-7040   Phone: (602) 533-5668
Richard A. Sajac, Lib.Off.
Subjects: Clinical medicine, nursing, hospital administration. **Holdings:** 1354 books; 951 bound and unbound periodical volumes; 112 audio cassettes. **Subscriptions:** 102 journals and other serials.

★7177★ **U.S. AIR FORCE BASE**
LUKE BASE MEDICAL LIBRARY
58th Medical Group/SQQL
Luke AFB, AZ 85309-5300   Phone: (602) 856-7585
Sharon A. Primus, Med.Libn.
Subjects: Medicine, dentistry. **Holdings:** 2200 books; 439 bound periodical volumes. **Subscriptions:** 75 journals and other serials.

★7178★ MESA LUTHERAN HOSPITAL
MEDICAL LIBRARY
525 W. Brown Rd.
Mesa, AZ 85201   Phone: (602) 834-1211
Angela Blahak, Med.Lib.Techn.
Subjects: Medicine. **Holdings:** 3000 books; journal titles on microfilm.
Subscriptions: 290 journals.

★7179★ ARIZONA DEPARTMENT OF HEALTH SERVICES
PUBLIC HEALTH LIBRARY
1740 W. Adams
Phoenix, AZ 85007   Phone: (602) 542-1013
Patricia L. Aiken, Lib.Mgr.
Subjects: Public health, environmental health, medical statistics, epidemiology, nursing, medicine. **Holdings:** 5000 books; 600 state documents.
Subscriptions: 225 journals.

★7180★ ARIZONA STATE HOSPITAL
MEDICAL LIBRARY
2500 E. Van Buren
Phoenix, AZ 85008   Phone: (602) 220-6045
Donna Gerometta, Med.Libn.
Subjects: Psychiatry, psychiatric nursing, psychology, psychotherapy and psychoanalysis, social case work, child psychiatry, addictive behaviors.
Holdings: 7850 books; 3700 bound periodical volumes; 650 cassettes and tapes. **Subscriptions:** 110 journals and other serials.

★7181★ ARIZONA STATE LIBRARY FOR THE BLIND AND
PHYSICALLY HANDICAPPED
1030 N. 32nd St.
Phoenix, AZ 85008   Phone: (602) 225-5578
Richard C. Peel, Adm.Libn.
Subjects: Fiction, nonfiction, blindness, physical handicaps. **Holdings:** 275,000 talking books. **Subscriptions:** 90 journals and other serials.

★7182★ CENTER FOR NEURODEVELOPMENTAL STUDIES,
INC.
LIBRARY
8434 N. 39th Ave.
Phoenix, AZ 85051-4778   Phone: (602) 433-1400
Subjects: Autism, sensory systems, neurodevelopment, special education.
Holdings: 350 volumes.

★7183★ GATEWAY COMMUNITY COLLEGE
LIBRARY
108 N. 40th St.
Phoenix, AZ 85034   Phone: (602) 392-5147
Peg Smith, Dir.
Subjects: Business, graphic communications, computer technology, pharmacy technology, nursing, electronics, robotics, respiratory therapy, radiography. **Holdings:** 42,000 books; 7000 programmed materials and media kits; 6873 microfiche; 395 reels of microfilm; 1393 titles on cassette tapes; 864 titles of filmstrips and film loops; computer software. **Subscriptions:** 350 journals and other serials; 10 newspapers.

★7184★ GOOD SAMARITAN REGIONAL MEDICAL CENTER
HEALTH SCIENCE LIBRARY
1111 E. McDowell St.
Box 2989
Phoenix, AZ 85062   Phone: (602) 239-4353
Jacqueline D. Doyle, Dir.
Subjects: Medicine, nursing, health administration. **Holdings:** 6500 books; 8000 bound periodical volumes; 8 drawers of pamphlets; 200 AV programs. **Subscriptions:** 600 journals and other serials.

★7185★ JOHN C. LINCOLN HOSPITAL
LIBRARY
205 E. Dunlap St.
Phoenix, AZ 85020   Phone: (602) 870-6328
Edith M. Hart, Med.Libn.
Subjects: Medicine, nursing. **Holdings:** 1000 books. **Subscriptions:** 125 journals and other serials.

★7186★ MARICOPA COUNTY MEDICAL SOCIETY
ROBERT S. FLINN MEDICAL LIBRARY
326 E. Coronado, Ste. 104
Phoenix, AZ 85004-1576   Phone: (602) 252-2451
Patricia K. Sullivan, Hd.Libn.
Subjects: Medicine, surgery, allied health sciences. **Holdings:** 75,000 volumes. **Subscriptions:** 180 journals and other serials.

★7187★ MARICOPA MEDICAL CENTER
MEDICAL LIBRARY
2601 E. Roosevelt St.
Phoenix, AZ 85008   Phone: (602) 267-5197
Fernande Hebert, Med.Libn.
Subjects: Medicine, surgery, nursing, hospital administration. **Holdings:** 3775 books; 6660 bound periodical volumes. **Subscriptions:** 275 journals and other serials.

★7188★ MARICOPA MENTAL HEALTH ANNEX
LIBRARY
2601 E. Roosevelt
PO Box 5099
Phoenix, AZ 85008   Phone: (602) 267-5990
Connie Thompson
Subjects: Psychiatry. **Holdings:** 750 books; 44 bound periodical volumes.
Subscriptions: 44 journals and other serials.

★7189★ MILTON ERICKSON FOUNDATION, INC.
ARCHIVES
3606 N. 24th St.
Phoenix, AZ 85016   Phone: (602) 956-6196
Subjects: Hypnotherapy, pain control. **Holdings:** 100 books; 160 videotapes; 702 audiotapes; memorabilia.

★7190★ O'CONNOR, CAVANAGH, ANDERSON,
KILLINGSWORTH & BESHEARS, P.A.
LAW LIBRARY
1 E. Camelback Rd., Ste. 900
Phoenix, AZ 85012-1656   Phone: (602) 263-2488
Kathy Shimpock-Vieweg, Dir., Lib.Serv.
Subjects: Law - medical, insurance, corporate, tax, labor, real estate, bond, employment practice, workers compensation. **Holdings:** 24,000 books.

★7191★ PHOENIX CHIDREN'S HOSPITAL
FAMILY LEARNING CENTER
LIBRARY
909 E. Brill St.
Phoenix, AZ 85006   Phone: (602) 239-2567
Kathy Werner
Subjects: Medicine, health, abuse, family life issues, parenting, safety.
Holdings: 179 books; 19 audiotapes; 39 videotapes; pamphlets. **Subscriptions:** 51 journals and other serials.

★7192★ PHOENIX DAY SCHOOL FOR THE DEAF
LIBRARY/MEDIA CENTER
1935 W. Hayward Ave.
Phoenix, AZ 85021   Phone: (602) 255-3448
Donna L. Farman, Libn.
Subjects: Juvenile fiction, signed English. **Holdings:** 8000 books. **Subscriptions:** 28 journals and other serials.

★7193★ PHOENIX INDIAN MEDICAL CENTER
LIBRARY
4212 N. 16th St.
Phoenix, AZ 85016   Phone: (602) 263-1200
Jean Crosier, Adm.Libn.
Subjects: Medicine, nursing, dentistry. **Holdings:** 1800 books; 2000 bound periodical volumes; 524 medical tapes; 3000 unbound journals; 5 VF drawers of pamphlets and reprints. **Subscriptions:** 180 journals and other serials.

★7194★ PHOENIX PUBLIC LIBRARY
BUSINESS & SCIENCES DEPARTMENT
12 E. McDowell Rd.
Phoenix, AZ 85004   Phone: (602) 262-6451
Shera Farnham, Hd.
Subjects: Business and economics, technology, social sciences, sciences, medicine, psychology. **Holdings:** 200,000 books; government documents.
Subscriptions: 900 journals and other serials.

★7195★ PHOENIX PUBLIC LIBRARY
SPECIAL NEEDS CENTER
12 E. McDowell Rd.
Phoenix, AZ 85004　　　　　　　　　Phone: (602) 261-8690
Cynthia R. Holt, Supv.
Subjects: Special education, rehabilitation, blindness and visual impairment, deafness and speech impairment, physical disability, mental disability. **Holdings:** 5800 books; 6000 large type books; 105 videotapes; 200 toys in toybrary. **Subscriptions:** 180 journals and other serials.

★7196★ ST. JOSEPH'S HOSPITAL
HEALTH SCIENCES LIBRARY
350 W. Thomas Rd.
Box 2071
Phoenix, AZ 85001　　　　　　　　　Phone: (602) 285-3299
Kay E. Wellik, Mgr., Lib.Serv.
Subjects: Medicine. **Holdings:** 4500 books; 8500 bound periodical volumes. **Subscriptions:** 380 journals and other serials.

★7197★ ST. LUKE'S MEDICAL CENTER
ROSENZWEIG HEALTH SCIENCES LIBRARY
1800 E. Van Buren St.
Phoenix, AZ 85006　　　　　　　　　Phone: (602) 251-8100
Barbara Hasan, Dir.
Subjects: Cardiology, nursing, behavioral health. **Holdings:** 1000 books; 2050 bound periodical volumes; 500 videotapes. **Subscriptions:** 217 journals.

★7198★ SEMANTODONTICS, INC.
LIBRARY
3400 E. McDowell
PO Box 29222
Phoenix, AZ 85038　　　　　　　　　Phone: (602) 225-9090
Jim Rhode, Pres.
Subjects: Dentistry, patient care, dental staff training, psychology, communications, transactional analysis, motivation. **Holdings:** 400 books; 50 bound periodical volumes; 200 magnetic tapes; 100 patient education pamphlets. **Subscriptions:** 43 journals and other serials; 8 newspapers.

★7199★ U.S. DEPARTMENT OF VETERANS AFFAIRS
MEDICAL CENTER LIBRARY
650 E. Indian School Rd.
Phoenix, AZ 85012　　　　　　　　　Phone: (602) 222-6411
Susan Harker, Chf., Lib.Serv.
Subjects: Medicine, nursing, allied health sciences. **Holdings:** 2081 books; 3560 bound periodical volumes; AV programs. **Subscriptions:** 396 journals.

★7200★ U.S. DEPARTMENT OF VETERANS AFFAIRS
HEALTH SCIENCES LIBRARY
Prescott, AZ 86313　　　　　　　　　Phone: (602) 445-4860
Carol Clark, Chf., Lib.Serv.
Subjects: Medicine, nursing, surgery, dentistry, allied health sciences, administration. **Holdings:** 600 books; 300 AV programs; 30 titles on microfilm. **Subscriptions:** 140 journals and other serials; 10 newspapers.

★7201★ FOUNDATION FOR BLIND CHILDREN
ARIZONA INSTRUCTIONAL RESOURCE CENTER
1201 N. 85th Pl.
Scottsdale, AZ 85257　　　　　　　　Phone: (602) 947-3744
Jodene L. Ludden, Mtls.Coord.
Subjects: Educational material for visually impaired students. **Holdings:** 28,828 large-type textbooks, braille books, supplemental reading materials (10,719 titles). **Subscriptions:** 12 journals and other serials.

★7202★ SCOTTSDALE MEMORIAL HOSPITAL
DR. ROBERT C. FOREMAN HEALTH SCIENCES LIBRARY
7400 E. Osborn Rd.
Scottsdale, AZ 85251　　　　　　　　Phone: (602) 481-4870
Marihelen O'Connor, Med.Libn.
Subjects: Family practice, medicine, surgery, pediatrics, cardiology, orthopedics, radiology, nursing. **Holdings:** 2500 books; 5000 bound periodical volumes; 40 VF items; videotapes. **Subscriptions:** 235 journals and other serials.

★7203★ SCOTTSDALE MEMORIAL HOSPITAL, NORTH
HEALTH SCIENCES LIBRARY
10450 N. 92nd. St.
Scottsdale, AZ 85258-4514　　　　　Phone: (602) 860-3870
Mary Lou Goldstein, Libn.
Subjects: Cardiology, nursing, anesthesiology. **Holdings:** 100 books; 150 bound periodical volumes. **Subscriptions:** 175 journals and other serials.

★7204★ BOSWELL MEMORIAL MEDICAL CENTER
LIBRARY
10401 Thunderbird Blvd.
Sun City, AZ 85351　　　　　　　　　Phone: (602) 977-7211
Thelma Wheeler, Libn.
Subjects: Geriatrics. **Holdings:** 550 books; 20 bound periodical volumes titles. **Subscriptions:** 101 journals and other serials.

★7205★ ARIZONA HOSPITAL ASSOCIATION
LIBRARY
Park Bridge at Fountainhead
1501 W. Fountainhead Pkwy., Ste. 650
Tempe, AZ 85282　　　　　　　　　　Phone: (602) 968-1083
Thomas D. Misch
Subjects: Health care, hospitals, nursing. **Holdings:** 30 books; 400 bound periodical volumes; 500 newsletters and newspapers. **Subscriptions:** 7 newspapers.

★7206★ AHEC RURAL HEALTH OFFICE
LIBRARY
2501 E. Elm St.
Tucson, AZ 85716　　　　　　　　　　Phone: (602) 606-7946
Patricia A. Auflick, LRS Coord.
Subjects: Rural health, health policy, health statistics, consumer health information. **Holdings:** 600 books. **Subscriptions:** 20 journals and other serials.

★7207★ ARIZONA STATE SCHOOL FOR THE DEAF AND
BLIND
LIBRARY
1200 W. Speedway
Tucson, AZ 85703　　　　　　　　　　Phone: (602) 628-5732
Janet Miller, Libn.
Subjects: Education, professional development. **Holdings:** 15,000 volumes; other cataloged items. **Subscriptions:** 14 journals and other serials.

★7208★ KINO COMMUNITY HOSPITAL
LIBRARY
2800 E. Ajo Way
Tucson, AZ 85713　　　　　　　　　　Phone: (602) 294-4471
Barbara Edwards, Act.Libn.
Subjects: Human anatomy, physiology, biochemistry, pharmacology, bacteriology and immunology, pathology, psychiatry, nursing, radiology, obstetrics/gynecology, geriatrics, gastrointerology. **Holdings:** 1344 books. **Subscriptions:** 55 journals and other serials.

★7209★ PIMA COUNCIL ON AGING
LIBRARY
2919 E. Broadway
Tucson, AZ 85716-5311　　　　　　　Phone: (602) 795-5800
Mary C. Guilbert, Libn.
Subjects: Aging programs and services, gerontology, longterm care. **Holdings:** 100 books; 24 VF drawers; 5000 other cataloged items. **Subscriptions:** 30 journals and other serials; 350 newsletters; 6 newspapers.

★7210★ PIMA COUNTY JUVENILE COURT CENTER
LIBRARY
2225 E. Ajo Way
Tucson, AZ 85713　　　　　　　　　　Phone: (602) 740-2082
Gwen Reid, Ct.Libn.
Subjects: Juvenile crime, penal institutions, adolescent problems, drug addiction, status offenses, sexual and child abuse. **Holdings:** 800 books. **Subscriptions:** 30 journals and other serials.

★7211★ ST. JOSEPH'S HOSPITAL AND HEALTH CENTER
BRUCE M. COLE MEMORIAL LIBRARY
350 N. Wilmot
Tucson, AZ 85711　　　　　　　　　　Phone: (602) 721-3925
Marcia Arsenault, Libn.
Subjects: Surgery, internal medicine, infection control, ophthalmology,

nursing. **Holdings:** 800 books; 1100 bound periodical volumes; 50 other cataloged items. **Subscriptions:** 144 journals and other serials.

★7212★ ST. MARY'S HOSPITAL AND HEALTH CENTER
RALPH FULLER MEDICAL LIBRARY
1601 W. St. Mary's Rd.
Box 5386
Tucson, AZ 85703   Phone: (602) 622-5833
Jeffrey W. St. Clair, Libn.
Subjects: Medicine, nursing, hospital administration, allied health sciences. **Holdings:** 900 books; 3000 bound periodical volumes; 166 videotapes; 4 VF drawers of pamphlets and reprints. **Subscriptions:** 133 journals and other serials.

★7213★ TUCSON GENERAL HOSPITAL
MEDICAL LIBRARY
3838 N. Campbell Ave.
Tucson, AZ 85717   Phone: (602) 327-5431
Judy Snow
Subjects: Medicine, nursing, and allied health sciences. **Holdings:** 630 books; 122 bound periodical volumes; 283 videotapes; 140 audiotapes; 41 slide/tape sets. **Subscriptions:** 67 journals and other serials.

★7214★ TUCSON MEDICAL CENTER
MEDICAL LIBRARY
Box 42195
Tucson, AZ 85733   Phone: (602) 327-5461
Lynn Flance, Mgr., Lib.Serv.
Subjects: Clinical medicine and related sciences. **Holdings:** 1200 books; 10,000 bound periodical volumes; 400 AV programs. **Subscriptions:** 300 journals and other serials.

★7215★ U.S. DEPARTMENT OF VETERANS AFFAIRS
MEDICAL CENTER LIBRARY
3601 S. 6th Ave.
Tucson, AZ 85723   Phone: (602) 792-1450
William E. Azevedo, Chf., Lib.Serv.
Subjects: Medicine, nursing, surgery, neurology, psychiatry, radiology, management, patient health education. **Holdings:** 3204 books; 7802 bound periodical volumes; 968 volumes on microfilm. **Subscriptions:** 320 journals and other serials.

★7216★ UNIVERSITY OF ARIZONA
ARIZONA HEALTH SCIENCES CENTER LIBRARY
1501 N. Campbell Ave.
Tucson, AZ 85724   Phone: (602) 626-6121
Thomas D. Higdon, Dir.
Subjects: Medicine and allied health sciences; preclinical sciences. **Holdings:** 73,280 books; 96,485 bound periodical volumes; 3253 AV program titles; 20 drawers of microforms. **Subscriptions:** 3590 journals and other serials.

Arkansas

★7217★ BENTON SERVICES CENTER
MEDICAL LIBRARY
Hwy. 67
Benton, AR 72015   Phone: (501) 778-1111
Susan Carson
Subjects: Psychiatry, geriatrics, psychology, medicine, nursing, social work. **Holdings:** 4259 books; 604 bound periodical volumes; 86 article files on mental health; 200 pamphlets and documents (uncataloged). **Subscriptions:** 55 journals and other serials.

★7218★ LUTHERANS FOR LIFE
LIBRARY
PO Box 819
Benton, AR 72015   Phone: (501) 794-2212
Subjects: Abortion, infanticide, euthanasia, theology. **Holdings:** 50 books; 10 filing drawers; newsletters; clippings. **Subscriptions:** 30 journals and other serials; 10 newspapers.

★7219★ U.S. DEPARTMENT OF VETERANS AFFAIRS
MEDICAL CENTER LIBRARY SERVICE
1100 N. College Ave.
Fayetteville, AR 72701   Phone: (501) 444-5096
Kimberly Megginson, Chf., Lib.Serv.
Subjects: Medicine, nursing, allied health sciences. **Holdings:** 3125 books; 1900 microfilm and unbound periodical volumes; 604 AV items. **Subscriptions:** 211 journals and other serials.

★7220★ UNIVERSITY OF ARKANSAS FOR MEDICAL SCIENCES
NORTHWEST AREA HEALTH EDUCATION CENTER LIBRARY
1125 N. College
Fayetteville, AR 72703   Phone: (501) 521-7615
Connie M. Wilson, Libn.
Subjects: Medicine, nursing, and allied health sciences. **Holdings:** 1500 books; 3260 bound periodical volumes. **Subscriptions:** 168 journals and other serials.

★7221★ SPARKS REGIONAL MEDICAL CENTER
REGIONAL HEALTH SCIENCES LIBRARY
1311 S. I St.
Box 17006
Fort Smith, AR 72917-7006   Phone: (501) 441-4035
Grace Anderson, Dir.
Subjects: Medicine and biological sciences. **Holdings:** 2000 books; 3000 bound periodical volumes. **Subscriptions:** 237 journals and other serials.

★7222★ U.S. FOOD AND DRUG ADMINISTRATION
NATIONAL CENTER FOR TOXICOLOGICAL RESEARCH LIBRARY
Jefferson, AR 87102
Billie Gough, Supv.Libn.
Subjects: Toxicology, chemistry, teratogenesis, carcinogenesis, mutagenesis, biochemistry. **Holdings:** 15,000 books; 500 bound periodical volumes. **Subscriptions:** 250 journals and other serials.

★7223★ ARKANSAS STATE HOSPITAL
MEDICAL LIBRARY
4313 W. Markham St.
Little Rock, AR 72205   Phone: (501) 686-9040
Bernadine F. Zerr, Libn.
Subjects: Psychiatry, psychology, social work, mental health. **Holdings:** 5100 books; 100 bound periodical volumes; 113 other cataloged items; 19 drawers of cassette tapes. **Subscriptions:** 113 journals and other serials.

★7224★ ARKANSAS STATE WORKERS' COMPENSATION COMMISSION
LIBRARY
Justice Bldg.
State Capitol Grounds
Little Rock, AR 72201   Phone: (501) 682-3930
Pat Capps, Libn.
Subjects: Arkansas law, workers' compensation law, medicine, rehabilitation. **Holdings:** 3200 books. **Subscriptions:** 16 journals and other serials.

★7225★ BAPTIST MEDICAL CENTER
MARGARET CLARK GILBREATH MEMORIAL LIBRARY
9601 Interstate 630
Little Rock, AR 72205   Phone: (501) 227-2671
Auburn Steward, Libn.
Subjects: Nursing, medicine. **Holdings:** 1900 books; 2400 bound periodical volumes. **Subscriptions:** 197 journals and other serials.

★7226★ ST. VINCENT INFIRMARY
MEDICAL LIBRARY
2 St. Vincent Circle
Little Rock, AR 72205   Phone: (501) 660-3000
Sr. Jean B. Roberts, S.C.N., Med.Libn.
Subjects: Medicine, medical specialties. **Holdings:** 4935 books; 3500 bound periodical volumes. **Subscriptions:** 200 journals and other serials.

★7227★ U.S. DEPARTMENT OF VETERANS AFFAIRS
HOSPITAL LIBRARIES
4300 W. 7th St.
Little Rock, AR 72205   Phone: (501) 660-2044
George M. Zumwalt, Chf., Lib.Serv.
Subjects: Medicine, surgery, nursing, psychiatry, psychology, social work, dietetics. Holdings: 3985 books; 6500 bound periodical volumes; 2 16mm motion pictures; 527 video cassettes; 14 audio cassettes; 50 slide programs. Subscriptions: 306 journals and other serials.

★7228★ UNIVERSITY OF ARKANSAS FOR MEDICAL
SCIENCES
LIBRARY
Slot 586
4301 W. Markham
Little Rock, AR 72205-7186   Phone: (501) 686-5980
Rose Hogan, Dir.
Subjects: Medical sciences. Holdings: 151,448 books and bound periodical volumes; 2200 AV programs. Subscriptions: 1545 journals and other serials.

California

★7229★ CALIFORNIA SCHOOL OF PROFESSIONAL
PSYCHOLOGY
BERKELEY/ALAMEDA CAMPUS
RUDOLPH HARWICH LIBRARY
1005 Atlantic Ave.
Alameda, CA 94501   Phone: (510) 523-2300
Harry Hosel, Dir. of Lib.Serv.
Subjects: Clinical psychology, psychoanalysis, organizational behavior. Holdings: 15,000 books; 5000 bound periodical volumes; 350 tapes; 900 dissertations. Subscriptions: 275 journals and other serials.

★7230★ ENSR HEALTH SCIENCES
LIBRARY/INFORMATION CENTER
1320 Harbor Bay Pkwy., Ste. 100
Alameda, CA 94501   Phone: (510) 865-1888
Glenn London, Mgr., Info.Serv.
Subjects: Occupational medicine, industrial hygiene, epidemiology, environment, risk assessment, consulting, engineering, environmental health. Holdings: 1500 books; 1000 reports. Subscriptions: 100 journals and other serials.

★7231★ TRITON BIOSCIENCES INC.
LIBRARY
1501 Harbor Bay Pkwy.
Alameda, CA 94501   Phone: (510) 769-5216
Margaret N. Burnett, Supv., Lib. & Info.Serv.
Subjects: Molecular biology, immunology, biochemistry, virology, genetics. Holdings: 2500 books; 150 bound periodical volumes. Subscriptions: 234 journals and other serials.

★7232★ DANNY FOUNDATION
LIBRARY
3160F Danville Blvd.
PO Box 680
Alamo, CA 94507   Phone: (415) 833-2669
Jack Walsh
Subjects: Crib safety, juvenile products. Holdings: 170 bound periodical volumes. Subscriptions: 7 journals and other serials; 2 newspapers.

★7233★ CALIFORNIA SCHOOL OF PROFESSIONAL
PSYCHOLOGY
LOS ANGELES LIBRARY
1000 S. Fremont Ave.
Alhambra, CA 91803-1360   Phone: (818) 284-2777
Tobeylynn Birch, Hd.Libn.
Subjects: Psychology - clinical, industrial/organizational, health, community; public policy; women's issues; homosexuality and lesbianism; minority mental health. Holdings: 20,000 books; 1700 bound periodical volumes; 4000 microfiche; 1600 dissertations; 75 reels of microfilm; 450 audiotapes; 60 video cassettes; 7 films. Subscriptions: 330 journals and other serials.

★7234★ ANAHEIM MEMORIAL HOSPITAL
MEDICAL LIBRARY
1111 W. LaPalma Ave.
PO Box 3005
Anaheim, CA 92803   Phone: (714) 999-6020
Veena N. Vyas, Dir., Med.Libn.
Subjects: Medicine. Holdings: 1200 books. Subscriptions: 136 journals and other serials.

★7235★ ATASCADERO STATE HOSPITAL
PROFESSIONAL LIBRARY
Box 7001
Atascadero, CA 93423-7001   Phone: (805) 461-2491
Beverly J. Clayman, Sr.Libn.
Subjects: Sex pathology, forensic psychiatry, criminal insanity, psychotherapy, nursing and nursing education, medicine. Holdings: 11,266 books; 4500 bound periodical volumes; 984 AV programs; 5 VF drawers. Subscriptions: 155 journals and other serials.

★7236★ KERN MEDICAL CENTER
KERN HEALTH SCIENCES LIBRARY
1830 Flower St.
Bakersfield, CA 93305-4197   Phone: (805) 326-2227
Pat Hamlett, Lib.Techn.
Subjects: Clinical medicine, nursing, allied health sciences, hospital administration. Holdings: 3000 books; 11,000 bound periodical volumes; 300 audiotapes; 3500 slides. Subscriptions: 325 journals and other serials.

★7237★ MERCY HOSPITAL
MEDICAL LIBRARY
Box 119
Bakersfield, CA 93302-0119   Phone: (805) 327-3371
Brooke Lilly, Med.Libn.
Subjects: Medicine, gastroenterology, pediatrics, surgery, physical therapy, internal medicine, oncology. Holdings: 368 books; 451 bound periodical volumes. Subscriptions: 135 journals and other serials.

★7238★ SAN GORGONIO MEMORIAL HOSPITAL
MEDICAL LIBRARY
600 N. Highland Springs Ave.
Banning, CA 92220   Phone: (714) 845-1121
Linda Rubin, Med.Lib.Cons.
Subjects: Medicine. Holdings: 100 volumes. Subscriptions: 20 journals and other serials.

★7239★ KAISER PERMANENTE MEDICAL CARE PROGRAM
HEALTH SCIENCES LIBRARY/MEDIA CENTER
9400 E. Rosecrans Ave.
Bellflower, CA 90706   Phone: (213) 920-4938
Geraldine N. Graves, Lib./Media Oper.
Subjects: Medicine and medical specialties, nursing, hospital administration. Holdings: 4828 books; 5093 bound periodical volumes; 1350 Audio-Digest tapes; 2 VF drawers of pamphlets; 2471 AV programs; videotapes; 15 trays microfiche; 325 other cataloged items. Subscriptions: 325 journals and other serials.

★7240★ ALCOHOL RESEARCH GROUP
LIBRARY
2000 Hearst
Berkeley, CA 94709-2176   Phone: (510) 642-5208
Andrea L. Mitchell, Dir.
Subjects: Alcohol use and abuse, epidemiology of alcohol use and allied problems, drug use and abuse. Holdings: 6000 books; 50,000 reprints, reports, dissertations. Subscriptions: 180 journals and other serials.

★7241★ ALTA BATES-HERRICK HOSPITALS
ALTA BATES HOSPITAL
STUART MEMORIAL LIBRARY
3001 Colby at Ashby
Berkeley, CA 94705   Phone: (510) 540-1696
Kay Kammerer, Hea.Sci.Libn.
Subjects: Medicine. Holdings: 1800 books; 2500 bound periodical volumes; 500 reprints. Subscriptions: 240 journals and other serials.

★7242★ ALTA BATES-HERRICK HOSPITALS
HERRICK HEALTH SCIENCES LIBRARY
2001 Dwight Way
Berkeley, CA 94704   Phone: (510) 540-4517
Dorrie Slutsker, Libn.
Subjects: Psychoanalysis, psychiatry, psychology, neurology, psychosomatic medicine, rehabilitation. **Holdings:** 7000 volumes. **Subscriptions:** 150 journals and other serials.

★7243★ ALTA BATES-HERRICK HOSPITALS
VINTAGE HEALTH LIBRARY AND RESOURCE CENTER
2484 Shattuck Ave.
Berkeley, CA 94704   Phone: (510) 540-4475
Sandy Dennett, Mgr.
Subjects: Aging and health, gerontology, geriatrics. **Holdings:** 950 books; 60 AV programs. **Subscriptions:** 22 journals and other serials.

★7244★ INTERNATIONAL CHILD RESOURCE INSTITUTE
INFORMATION CLEARINGHOUSE
1810 Hopkins
Berkeley, CA 94707   Phone: (510) 644-1000
Susan Gordon, Off.Mgr.
Subjects: Children - health, abuse, care, advocacy. **Holdings:** 10,000 pieces of information.

★7245★ MILES, INC.
CUTTER LIBRARY AND INFORMATION SERVICES
4th & Parker Sts.
Box 1986
Berkeley, CA 94701   Phone: (510) 420-5187
H. Wen Ng, Libn.
Subjects: Biomedicine, biotechnology, pharmaceutical sciences. **Holdings:** 16,000 volumes. **Subscriptions:** 440 journals and other serials.

★7246★ NATIONAL CLEARINGHOUSE ON MARITAL AND DATE RAPE
2325 Oak St.
Berkeley, CA 94708   Phone: (510) 524-1582
Laura X, Exec.Dir.
Subjects: Rape - marital, date, cohabitation, legislation; marital rape legislation and prosecution. **Holdings:** 20 books; 1000 files of briefs, testimony, clippings, reports, newsletters, studies, research, dissertations. **Subscriptions:** 10 journals and other serials.

★7247★ PREVENTION RESEARCH CENTER
LIBRARY
2532 Durant Ave.
Berkeley, CA 94704   Phone: (510) 486-1111
Subjects: Alcohol and drug abuse prevention research. **Holdings:** 700 books; 4000 reprints. **Subscriptions:** 85 journals and other serials.

★7248★ UNIVERSITY OF CALIFORNIA, BERKELEY
OPTOMETRY LIBRARY
490 Minor Hall
Berkeley, CA 94720   Phone: (510) 642-1020
Alison Howard, Hd.
Subjects: Optometry, physiological optics, ophthalmology. **Holdings:** 8041 volumes; 668 pamphlets; 414 microforms; 251 sound recordings; 3300 slides; 120 video recordings; 30 motion pictures. **Subscriptions:** 188 journals and other serials.

★7249★ UNIVERSITY OF CALIFORNIA, BERKELEY
PUBLIC HEALTH LIBRARY
42 Earl Warren Hall
Berkeley, CA 94720   Phone: (510) 642-2511
Thomas J. Alexander, Libn.
Subjects: Public health, epidemiology, biostatistics, hospital administration, environmental health, maternal and child health, biomedical science (laboratory), occupational health, toxicology. **Holdings:** 80,121 volumes; 10,000 pamphlets; 1100 microforms. **Subscriptions:** 2151 journals and other serials.

★7250★ UNIVERSITY OF CALIFORNIA, BERKELEY
SCHOOL OF PUBLIC HEALTH
LABOR OCCUPATIONAL HEALTH PROGRAM LIBRARY
2521 Channing Way
Berkeley, CA 94720   Phone: (510) 642-5507
Donna Jarvis
Subjects: Chemical and physical occupational hazards, medical and industrial hygiene, standards and regulations, workers' compensation and education. **Holdings:** 2200 books; 180 unbound periodicals; newspaper clipping file. **Subscriptions:** 50 journals and other serials; 110 newspapers.

★7251★ WOMEN'S HISTORY RESEARCH CENTER
WOMEN'S HISTORY LIBRARY
2325 Oak St.
Berkeley, CA 94708   Phone: (510) 524-1582
Laura X, Dir.
Subjects: Women's health and mental health, women and law, Black and Third World women, female artists, children, films by and/or about women, Soviet women. **Holdings:** 2000 books; 300 tapes; 54 reels of microfilm on health and law; 90 reels of microfilm of women's periodicals in Herstory Collection.

★7252★ INSTITUTE FOR CANCER AND BLOOD RESEARCH
LIBRARY
150 N. Robertson Blvd., Ste. 350 N.
Beverly Hills, CA 90211-9951   Phone: (213) 655-4706
Belle Gould, Libn.
Subjects: Hematology, oncology. **Holdings:** 300 books; 30 bound periodical volumes. **Subscriptions:** 35 journals and other serials.

★7253★ SOUTHERN CALIFORNIA PSYCHOANALYTIC INSTITUTE
FRANZ ALEXANDER LIBRARY
9024 Olympic Blvd.
Beverly Hills, CA 90211   Phone: (213) 276-2455
Lena Pincus, Libn.
Subjects: Psychoanalysis, psychiatry, psychology. **Holdings:** 4000 volumes; 2200 reprints. **Subscriptions:** 45 journals and other serials.

★7254★ BURBANK COMMUNITY HOSPITAL
HEALTH SCIENCES LIBRARY
466 E. Olive Ave.
Burbank, CA 91501   Phone: (818) 953-6516
Jeanne S. Dawes, Cons.Libn.
Subjects: Medicine, nursing, pharmacy, administration, allied health sciences. **Holdings:** 900 books; Audio-Digest tapes; vertical files. **Subscriptions:** 50 journals and other serials.

★7255★ ST. JOSEPH MEDICAL CENTER
HEALTH SCIENCE LIBRARY
501 S. Buena Vista St.
Burbank, CA 91505-4866   Phone: (818) 843-5111
Sr. Naomi Hurd, S.P., Libn.
Subjects: Medicine, nursing, hospital administration. **Holdings:** 3258 books; 5000 bound periodical volumes; 1200 audio cassettes; 245 video cassettes; 25 16mm films; 40 filmstrips; 65 slide programs; 4 transparency programs; 36 items of miscellanea. **Subscriptions:** 623 journals and other serials.

★7256★ MILLS-PENINSULA HOSPITALS
HEALTH SCIENCES LIBRARY
1783 El Camino Real
Burlingame, CA 94010   Phone: (415) 696-5621
Sally C. Chu, Chf., Lib.Serv.
Subjects: Medicine. **Holdings:** 1400 books; 3000 bound periodical volumes. **Subscriptions:** 289 journals and other serials.

★7257★ WOODVIEW-CALABASAS PSYCHIATRIC HOSPITAL
LIBRARY
25100 Calabasas Rd.
Calabasas, CA 91302   Phone: (818) 888-7500
Ching-Fen Wu Tsiang, Libn.
Subjects: Psychiatry, nursing, general medicine. **Holdings:** 2000 books; 500 bound periodical volumes. **Subscriptions:** 25 journals and other serials.

★7258★ CAMARILLO STATE HOSPITAL AND DEVELOPMENTAL CENTER
PROFESSIONAL LIBRARY
1878 S. Lewis Rd.
Box 6022
Camarillo, CA 93011-6022   Phone: (805) 484-3661
Mrs. Nagiko Sato Kiser, Sr.Libn.
Subjects: Psychiatric and psychological treatment, neurology, internal medicine, nursing services, public health, behavioral science. **Holdings:** 8250 books; 910 bound periodical volumes; 6080 unbound volumes of periodicals; 21 linear feet of journals; 2 VF drawers. **Subscriptions:** 131 journals and other serials.

★7259★ U.S. NAVY
NAVAL HOSPITAL
MEDICAL LIBRARY
Camp Pendleton, CA 92055-5008   Phone: (619) 725-1322
Christina D. Bell, Med.Libn.
Subjects: General medicine, nursing, family practice. **Holdings:** 1000 books; 4800 bound periodical volumes; 1100 AV programs. **Subscriptions:** 200 journals and other serials.

★7260★ AMERICAN RIVER HOSPITAL
ERLE M. BLUNDEN, M.D. MEMORIAL LIBRARY
4747 Engle Rd.
Carmichael, CA 95608   Phone: (916) 484-2452
Maryjane Trujillo, Med.Libn.
Subjects: Medicine, nursing, psychiatry, hospital administration. **Holdings:** 400 books. **Subscriptions:** 100 journals and other serials.

★7261★ COUNTY OF LOS ANGELES PUBLIC LIBRARY
CONSUMER HEALTH INFORMATION PROGRAM AND SERVICES
151 E. Carson St.
Carson, CA 90745   Phone: (213) 830-0909
Ellen Mulkern, CHIPS Libn.
Subjects: Health, medicine. **Holdings:** 6500 books; 350 video cassettes; 150 films; 24 VF drawers of pamphlets. **Subscriptions:** 35 journals and other serials.

★7262★ EDEN HOSPITAL MEDICAL CENTER
MEDICAL AND DENTAL STAFF LIBRARY
19933 Lake Chabot Rd.
Castro Valley, CA 94546
Subjects: Medicine. **Holdings:** Figures not available.

★7263★ IOLAB CORPORATION
RESEARCH INFORMATION SERVICES
500 Iolab Dr.
Claremont, CA 91711   Phone: (714) 399-1571
Ardis Weiss, Sr.Res.Info.Sci.
Subjects: Ophthalmology, pharmaceuticals, polymer chemistry. **Holdings:** 600 books; 561 periodical volumes. **Subscriptions:** 182 journals and other serials.

★7264★ MEXICAN-AMERICAN OPPORTUNITY FOUNDATION
RESOURCE AND REFERRAL SERVICE
LENDING LIBRARY
6252 E. Telegraph Rd.
Commerce, CA 90040   Phone: (213) 722-7842
Yolanda Franco, Prog.Coord.
Subjects: Infant development, parenting, domestic and child abuse, self-esteem, emotional and physical handicaps; displaced homemakers. **Holdings:** 2500 volumes; filmstrips; cassettes; records; audiophonic media cards; arts and crafts materials.

★7265★ FAIRVIEW DEVELOPMENTAL CENTER
STAFF LIBRARY
2501 Harbor Blvd.
Costa Mesa, CA 92626   Phone: (714) 957-5394
Barbara Rycroft, Sr.Libn.
Subjects: Mental retardation, developmental disabilities, psychology, special education, medicine. **Holdings:** 2654 books; 3120 bound periodical volumes; 45 staff research reports; 5 VF drawers of pamphlets. **Subscriptions:** 103 journals and other serials.

★7266★ SETON MEDICAL CENTER
LIBRARY
1900 Sullivan Ave.
Daly City, CA 94015   Phone: (415) 991-6700
Janice Perlman-Stites, Libn.
Subjects: Medicine, nursing, hospital administration. **Holdings:** 1000 books; 2000 bound periodical volumes; 4 shelves of audio cassettes and tapes. **Subscriptions:** 130 journals and other serials.

★7267★ FREEDOM FROM HUNGER FOUNDATION
LIBRARY
Box 2000
Davis, CA 95617   Phone: (916) 758-6200
Judy Vulliet, Dir., Rsrc.Ctr.
Subjects: International agriculture, health, nurtrition, and development. **Holdings:** 1600 books; 12 VF drawers of reports and articles; 4 VF drawers of annual reports and pamphlets. **Subscriptions:** 200 journals and other serials.

★7268★ UNIVERSITY OF CALIFORNIA, DAVIS
LOREN D. CARLSON HEALTH SCIENCES LIBRARY
Davis, CA 95616   Phone: (916) 752-1214
Jo Anne Boorkman, Hd.Libn.
Subjects: Medicine, veterinary medicine, primatology. **Holdings:** 52,031 books; 164,766 bound periodical volumes; 12,586 microforms; 4157 foreign veterinary theses; 430 AV programs; 5384 government documents. **Subscriptions:** 4096 journals and other serials.

★7269★ RANCHO LOS AMIGOS MEDICAL CENTER
HEALTH SCIENCES LIBRARY
7601 E. Imperial Hwy.
Downey, CA 90242-3456   Phone: (213) 940-7696
Subjects: Rehabilitation medicine, orthopedics, nursing, diabetes, pulmonary disease, rheumatology. **Holdings:** 6500 books; 15,000 bound periodical volumes; 250 Rancho resident papers; 650 audio cassettes. **Subscriptions:** 634 journals and other serials.

★7270★ BAXTER HYLAND DIVISION
RESEARCH LIBRARY
1710 Flower Ave.
Duarte, CA 91010   Phone: (818) 303-2491
Emily L. Giustino, Libn.
Subjects: Immunology, biochemistry, hematology, virology, microbiology. **Holdings:** 2000 books; 5000 bound periodical volumes. **Subscriptions:** 250 journals and other serials.

★7271★ CITY OF HOPE NATIONAL MEDICAL CENTER
GRAFF MEDICAL AND SCIENTIFIC LIBRARY
1500 E. Duarte Rd.
Duarte, CA 91010   Phone: (818) 301-8497
Anne Dillibe, Dir., Lib.Serv.
Subjects: Neuroscience, immunology, biomedicine, medical genetics, biochemistry, biology, pediatrics, cancer pathology. **Holdings:** 5000 books; 45,000 bound periodical volumes. **Subscriptions:** 1000 journals and other serials.

★7272★ NASA
AMES RESEARCH CENTER
DRYDEN FLIGHT RESEARCH FACILITY
LIBRARY
Box 273
Edwards AFB, CA 93523   Phone: (805) 258-3702
Karen Puffer, Libn.
Subjects: Flight research, aerodynamics, flight testing and systems, aerospace medicine and human factors, instrumentation, aerostructures, propulsion, data systems. **Holdings:** 3500 books; 2400 bound periodical volumes; microfiche; reports. **Subscriptions:** 120 journals and other serials.

★7273★ SONOMA DEVELOPMENTAL CENTER
STAFF LIBRARY
Box 1493
Eldridge, CA 95431   Phone: (707) 938-6244
Angela Brunton, Sr.Libn.
Subjects: Mental retardation, psychology, nursing, social work, rehabilitation therapy, medicine. **Holdings:** 9000 books; 8417 bound periodical volumes; 70 AV programs. **Subscriptions:** 91 journals and other serials.

★7274★   AGE WAVE, INC.
LIBRARY
1900 Powell St., Ste. 800
Emeryville, CA 94608   Phone: (415) 652-9099
Judith Peck, Res.Dir.
Subjects: Aging, health, stress management, communications, marketing to older adults. **Holdings:** 1300 books; 20 VF drawers; periodicals; pamphlets. **Subscriptions:** 60 journals and other serials.

★7275★   KAISER FOUNDATION HOSPITAL
MEDICAL LIBRARY
9961 Sierra Ave.
Fontana, CA 92335   Phone: (714) 829-5085
Sue D. Layvas, Chf.Med.Libn.
Subjects: Orthopedics, dermatology, surgery, ophthalmology, pediatrics, internal medicine. **Holdings:** 3500 books; 4000 bound periodical volumes. **Subscriptions:** 400 journals and other serials.

★7276★   U.S. ARMY HOSPITALS
COMMANDER SILAS B. HAYS ARMY COMMUNITY
   HOSPITAL
MEDICAL LIBRARY
Commander
USA MEDDAC
Attn: HSXT-CSD (Medical Library)
Fort Ord, CA 93941-5800   Phone: (408) 242-2023
Dustin Miller, Med.Libn.
Subjects: Medicine and allied health sciences. **Holdings:** 3000 books; 3500 bound periodical volumes. **Subscriptions:** 300 journals and other serials.

★7277★   U.S. NAVY
NAVAL HOSPITAL
MEDICAL LIBRARY
Box 7747
FPO San Francisco, CA 96630-1649   Phone: (671) 344-9250
Alice E. Hadley, Med.Libn.
Subjects: Medicine, nursing, dentistry, surgery, obstetrics. **Holdings:** 1800 books; 1300 bound periodical volumes. **Subscriptions:** 115 journals and other serials.

★7278★   CALIFORNIA SCHOOL FOR THE BLIND
LIBRARY MEDIA CENTER
500 Walnut Ave.
Fremont, CA 94536   Phone: (510) 794-3854
Marjorie Carpenter, Libn.
Subjects: Educational and recreational books and media for pre-kindergarten and high school level blind and multi-handicapped children. **Holdings:** 4700 braille and print books; 200 professional books; 2200 records and tapes; 200 models, realia, maps, charts, kits; 51 boxes of pamphlets; specialized equipment for the handicapped. **Subscriptions:** 20 journals and other serials.

★7279★   CALIFORNIA SCHOOL OF PROFESSIONAL
   PSYCHOLOGY
INGEBORG S. KAUFFMAN LIBRARY
1350 M St.
Fresno, CA 93721   Phone: (209) 486-8424
Dorothy A. Spencer, Ph.D., Dir.
Subjects: Psychology, organizational behavior. **Holdings:** 10,000 books; 4000 bound periodical volumes; 16 VF drawers of documents and reprints; 1334 microforms; 315 audio cassettes. **Subscriptions:** 250 journals and other serials.

★7280★   COMMUNITY HOSPITALS OF CENTRAL
   CALIFORNIA
MEDICAL LIBRARY
Box 1232
Fresno, CA 93715   Phone: (209) 442-3968
Penny Ward, Mgr., Lib.Serv.
Subjects: Medicine, nursing, and allied health sciences. **Holdings:** 7000 books; 2500 bound periodical volumes; 12 VF drawers of pamphlets and clippings; microfilm backfiles. **Subscriptions:** 700 journals and other serials.

★7281★   ST. AGNES MEDICAL CENTER
MEDICAL LIBRARY
1303 E. Herndon Ave.
Fresno, CA 93720   Phone: (209) 449-3322
Sr. Louise Lovely, C.H.M., Med.Libn.
Subjects: Nursing, cardiovascular system, hospitals, medicine, surgery, pharmocology. **Holdings:** 868 books; 4000 bound periodical volumes; 800 reports; 6315 microfiche.

★7282★   U.S. DEPARTMENT OF VETERANS AFFAIRS
HOSPITAL MEDICAL LIBRARY
2615 E. Clinton Ave.
Fresno, CA 93703   Phone: (209) 228-5341
Cynthia K. Meyer, Chf., Lib.Serv.
Subjects: Medicine, nursing, allied health sciences. **Holdings:** 4250 books; 7527 bound periodical volumes. **Subscriptions:** 362 journals and other serials.

★7283★   VALLEY MEDICAL CENTER OF FRESNO
MEDICAL LIBRARY
445 S. Cedar Ave.
Fresno, CA 93702   Phone: (209) 453-5030
Vicky Christianson, Hosp.Libn.
Subjects: Medicine, dentistry, nursing, hospital administration. **Holdings:** 5000 volumes. **Subscriptions:** 150 journals and other serials.

★7284★   BECKMAN INSTRUMENTS, INC.
RESEARCH LIBRARY
2500 Harbor Blvd.
Fullerton, CA 92634   Phone: (714) 773-8906
Jean R. Miller, Mgr., Info. & Lib.Serv.
Subjects: Electrochemistry, scientific instrumentation, spectroscopy, chemistry, chromatography, medical electronics, clinical chemistry. **Holdings:** 8000 books; 8200 bound periodical volumes; 1200 reports, papers, pamphlets; 10 VF drawers of cataloged pamphlets; 2550 reels of microfilm; 4050 microfiche. **Subscriptions:** 425 journals and other serials.

★7285★   ST. JUDE MEDICAL CENTER
MEDICAL LIBRARY
101 E. Valencia Mesa Dr.
Fullerton, CA 92635   Phone: (714) 871-3280
Carol Bondurant, Lib.Techn.
Subjects: Medicine, nursing. **Holdings:** 500 books; 20 sound-slide sets; 100 video cassettes. **Subscriptions:** 105 journals and other serials.

★7286★   SOUTHERN CALIFORNIA COLLEGE OF
   OPTOMETRY
M.B. KETCHUM MEMORIAL LIBRARY
2565 Yorba Linda Blvd.
Fullerton, CA 92631-1699   Phone: (714) 449-7440
Mrs. Pat Carlson, Dir. of Lib.Serv.
Subjects: Optometry, optics, ophthalmology; vision. **Holdings:** 8400 books; 5700 bound periodical volumes; 450 theses; 400 AV programs. **Subscriptions:** 350 serials.

★7287★   GLENDALE ADVENTIST MEDICAL CENTER
LIBRARY
1509 Wilson Terr.
Glendale, CA 91206   Phone: (818) 409-8034
Marcia Arado, Lib.Dir.
Subjects: Medicine, nursing, paramedical sciences, health education. **Holdings:** 6724 books; 9400 bound periodical volumes; 1126 AV programs; 50 microcomputer software programs; Cumulative Index to Nursing and Allied Health Literature. **Subscriptions:** 600 journals and other serials.

★7288★   BAY HARBOR HOSPITAL
MEDICAL LIBRARY
1437 W. Lomita Blvd.
Harbor City, CA 90710   Phone: (213) 325-1221
James H. Harlan, Libn.
Subjects: Medicine, allied health sciences, nursing, hospital administration. **Holdings:** 902 books; Audio-Digest tapes. **Subscriptions:** 68 journals.

★7289★ KAISER FOUNDATION HOSPITAL
MEDICAL LIBRARY
25825 S. Vermont Ave.
Harbor City, CA 90710   Phone: (213) 517-2090
Lily Yang, Act.Med.Libn.
Subjects: Health sciences. **Holdings:** 3840 books; 4560 bound periodical volumes. **Subscriptions:** 317 journals and other serials.

★7290★ KAISER-PERMANENTE MEDICAL CENTER
HEALTH EDUCATION CENTER
27400 Hesprian Blvd.
Hayward, CA 94545   Phone: (510) 784-4531
Marilyn Libresco, Hea.Educ.Dir.
Subjects: Health information for the layperson. **Holdings:** Medical reference texts; pamphlets; AV programs.

★7291★ KAISER-PERMANENTE MEDICAL CENTER
HEALTH SCIENCES LIBRARY
27400 Hesperian Blvd.
Hayward, CA 94545   Phone: (510) 784-4420
Marsha Mielke, Med.Libn.
Subjects: Medicine and medical specialties, nursing, allied health sciences. **Holdings:** 1970 volumes. **Subscriptions:** 210 journals and other serials.

★7292★ HEMET VALLEY HOSPITAL DISTRICT
DR. LESLIE J. CLARK MEMORIAL LIBRARY
1116 E. Latham Ave.
Hemet, CA 92343   Phone: (714) 652-2811
Dixie Cirocco, Med.Libn.
Subjects: Clinical medicine, nursing, psychiatry. **Holdings:** 1136 books; 918 bound periodical volumes. **Subscriptions:** 106 journals and other serials.

★7293★ HOLLYWOOD COMMUNITY HOSPITAL
MEDICAL STAFF LIBRARY
6245 DeLongpre Ave.
Hollywood, CA 90028   Phone: (213) 462-2271
Betsey Beamish, Med.Lib.Cons.
Subjects: Clinical medicine, nursing. **Holdings:** 320 books; 80 Audio-Digest tapes; 188 NCME video cassettes. **Subscriptions:** 58 journals and other serials.

★7294★ JOHN F. KENNEDY MEMORIAL HOSPITAL
MEDICAL AND NURSING LIBRARIES
47-111 Monroe St.
Indio, CA 92201   Phone: (619) 347-6191
Dan Dickinson, Med.Libn.
Subjects: Medicine, nursing. **Holdings:** 1000 books; 100 bound periodical volumes; 100 pamphlets. **Subscriptions:** 130 journals.

★7295★ CENTINELA HOSPITAL MEDICAL CENTER
EDWIN W. DEAN MEMORIAL LIBRARY
555 E. Hardy St.
Box 720
Inglewood, CA 90307   Phone: (213) 673-4660
Marilyn K. Slater, Ph.D., Hea.Sci.Libn.
Subjects: Sports medicine, orthopedics, clinical medicine, nursing. **Holdings:** 6000 books; 8200 bound periodical volumes. **Subscriptions:** 250 journals and other serials.

★7296★ DANIEL FREEMAN HOSPITALS
HEALTH SCIENCES LIBRARY
333 N. Prairie Ave.
Inglewood, CA 90301   Phone: (213) 674-7050
Tracie Thomas, Lib.Asst.
Subjects: Medicine, nursing, hospital administration. **Holdings:** 2012 books; 4305 bound periodical volumes; 998 cassette tapes; 8 audiotape titles; 15 videotape titles; 25 video cassettes. **Subscriptions:** 420 journals and other serials.

★7297★ ALLERGAN, INC.
CORPORATE INFORMATION CENTER
2525 Dupont Dr.
Irvine, CA 92715-1599   Phone: (714) 752-4314
Heidemarie B. von Tilsit, Mgr.
Subjects: Ophthalmology, dermatology, contact lenses, pharmacology, chemistry, business and management, general medicine and science.

Holdings: 6000 books; 3800 bound periodical volumes; 300 technical reports. **Subscriptions:** 717 journals and other serials.

★7298★ UNIVERSITY OF CALIFORNIA, IRVINE
BIOMEDICAL LIBRARY
Box 19556
Irvine, CA 92713   Phone: (714) 856-6652
J. Michael Homan, Asst.Univ.Libn. for the Sci.
Subjects: Medicine. **Holdings:** 152,000 volumes; 5635 audio cassettes; 1245 microfiche; pamphlet file. **Subscriptions:** 2555 journals and other serials.

★7299★ CALBIOCHEM CORPORATION
LIBRARY
10933 N. Torrey Pines Rd.
La Jolla, CA 92037   Phone: (619) 450-5701
Sue Wright, Libn.
Subjects: Biochemistry, microbiology, enzymology, fermentation technology, organic and bio-organic chemistry, immunochemistry. **Holdings:** 500 books; 1000 bound periodical volumes. **Subscriptions:** 30 journals and other serials; 5 newspapers.

★7300★ SCRIPPS CLINIC AND RESEARCH FOUNDATION
KRESGE MEDICAL LIBRARY
10666 N. Torrey Pines Rd.
La Jolla, CA 92037   Phone: (619) 544-8705
Subjects: Immunology, medicine, molecular and cellular biology, biochemistry, psychiatry, chemistry. **Holdings:** 4600 books; 45,000 bound periodical volumes. **Subscriptions:** 685 journals and other serials.

★7301★ UNIVERSITY OF CALIFORNIA, SAN DIEGO
BIOMEDICAL LIBRARY
La Jolla, CA 92093-0175   Phone: (619) 534-3253
Mary Horres, Libn.
Subjects: Clinical and pre-clinical medicine, biology. **Holdings:** 182,359 volumes. **Subscriptions:** 3417 journals and other serials.

★7302★ AMERICAN FITNESS ASSOCIATION
LIBRARY
PO Box 700
Lakewood, CA 90714   Phone: (213) 596-0977
Ms. Brooks, Libn./Media Dir.
Subjects: Fitness, sports medicine. **Holdings:** 2500 books; tapes.

★7303★ LOS ANGELES COUNTY/HIGH DESERT HOSPITAL
RICHARD E. OSGOOD, M.D. MEDICAL LIBRARY
44900 N. 60th St., W.
Lancaster, CA 93536   Phone: (805) 945-8350
Dorothy Schoeppner, Lib.Asst. II
Subjects: Medicine, nursing, administration, management. **Holdings:** 903 books; 810 bound periodical volumes; 79 code books; 56 telephone directories. **Subscriptions:** 160 journals and other serials.

★7304★ U.S. DEPARTMENT OF VETERANS AFFAIRS
MEDICAL LIBRARY
4951 Arroyo Rd.
Livermore, CA 94550   Phone: (510) 447-2560
Sandra Lynch, Libn.
Subjects: Medicine, nursing, allied health sciences. **Holdings:** 1300 books; 2365 bound periodical volumes; 128 AV programs; 204 boxes of microfilm. **Subscriptions:** 188 journals and other serials.

★7305★ LOMA LINDA UNIVERSITY
DEL E. WEBB MEMORIAL LIBRARY
Loma Linda, CA 92350-0001   Phone: (714) 824-4550
David W. Rios, Dir.
Subjects: Medicine, nursing, dentistry, religion, health, allied health professions. **Holdings:** 175,540 books; 101,815 bound periodical volumes; 49,856 microforms; 6633 tapes and phonograph records; 1108 filmstrips, films, slides; 1069 feet of archival materials. **Subscriptions:** 2795 journals and other serials; 13 newspapers.

★7306★ LOMA LINDA UNIVERSITY
JORGENSEN LEARNING RESOURCE CENTER
Del E. Webb Memorial Library
Loma Linda, CA 92350   Phone: (714) 824-4585
John Morovati, Act.Chm.
Subjects: Dentistry; dental anesthesiology and pain control; national, regional, state board review materials. **Holdings:** 264 volumes; 160 video cassettes; 55 self-study units; 25 boxes of archival materials. **Subscriptions:** 120 journals and other serials.

★7307★ LOMA LINDA UNIVERSITY MEDICAL CENTER
MEDICAL LIBRARY & INFORMATION CENTER
11234 Anderson St.
PO Box 2000
Loma Linda, CA 92354   Phone: (714) 824-4620
Paul W. Kittle
Subjects: Internal medicine, pediatrics, cardiology, radiation oncology, oncology, nephrology. **Holdings:** 3000 books. **Subscriptions:** 360 journals and other serials.

★7308★ NATIONAL COUNCIL AGAINST HEALTH FRAUD
LIBRARY
PO Box 1276
Loma Linda, CA 92354   Phone: (714) 824-4690
Subjects: Consumer protection in health marketplace; health - fraud, misinformation, quackery.

★7309★ U.S. DEPARTMENT OF VETERANS AFFAIRS
HOSPITAL LIBRARY SERVICE
11201 Benton St.
Loma Linda, CA 92357   Phone: (714) 422-3063
Kathleen M. Puffer, Chf.
Subjects: Medicine. **Holdings:** 2500 books. **Subscriptions:** 500 journals and other serials.

★7310★ LONG BEACH COMMUNITY HOSPITAL
JOHNSON HEALTH SCIENCES LIBRARY
1720 Termino Ave.
Box 2587
Long Beach, CA 90801   Phone: (213) 494-0751
Lois O. Clark, Med.Libn.
Subjects: Medicine, nursing, hospital administration. **Holdings:** 1950 books; 1500 bound periodical volumes; Audio-Digest tapes. **Subscriptions:** 289 journals and other serials.

★7311★ LONG BEACH MEMORIAL MEDICAL CENTER
MEDICAL LIBRARY
2801 Atlantic Ave.
Box 1428
Long Beach, CA 90801-1428   Phone: (213) 595-3841
Marion Sabella, Dir.
Subjects: Medicine, hospitals, nursing, allied health sciences. **Holdings:** 24,165 books; 27,707 bound periodical volumes. **Subscriptions:** 1000 journals and other serials.

★7312★ PACIFIC HOSPITAL OF LONG BEACH
MEDICAL STAFF LIBRARY
2776 Pacific Ave.
Box 1268
Long Beach, CA 90801   Phone: (213) 595-1911
Lois E. Harris, Dir., Lib.Serv.
Subjects: General medicine, surgery, osteopathy, nursing. **Holdings:** 2000 volumes. **Subscriptions:** 200 journals and other serials.

★7313★ ST. MARY MEDICAL CENTER
BELLIS MEDICAL LIBRARY
1050 Linden Ave.
Box 887
Long Beach, CA 90801-0887   Phone: (213) 491-9295
Lorraine B. Attarian, Mgr.
Subjects: Medicine, nursing. **Holdings:** 30,000 volumes; pamphlet files; historical collection. **Subscriptions:** 500 journals and other serials.

★7314★ U.S. DEPARTMENT OF VETERANS AFFAIRS
MEDICAL CENTER LIBRARY
5901 E. 7th St., 142B
Long Beach, CA 90822   Phone: (213) 494-5529
Betty F. Connolly, Chf., Lib.Serv.
Subjects: Medicine and allied health sciences, patient education. **Holdings:** 6100 books; 9000 bound periodical volumes; 1141 other volumes; AV programs. **Subscriptions:** 650 journals and other serials.

★7315★ AMERICAN ACADEMY OF REFLEXOLOGY
LIBRARY
4070 W. 3rd St.
Los Angeles, CA 90020   Phone: (213) 389-4424
Subjects: Reflexology. **Holdings:** 200 volumes.

★7316★ BARLOW HOSPITAL
ELKS LIBRARY
2000 Stadium Way
Los Angeles, CA 90026-2696   Phone: (213) 250-4200
Rose Thompson, Libn.
Subjects: Tuberculosis and diseases of the chest. **Holdings:** 3500 volumes; 12,000 medical reprints. **Subscriptions:** 70 journals and other serials.

★7317★ BRAILLE INSTITUTE OF AMERICA
LIBRARY SERVICES
741 N. Vermont Ave.
Los Angeles, CA 90029   Phone: (213) 660-3880
Dr. Henry Chang, Lib.Dir.
Subjects: General collection of books for the blind and physically handicapped. **Holdings:** 20,443 braille volumes; 124,930 talking books; 506,766 cassette tapes. **Subscriptions:** 54 talking book periodicals; 36 braille periodicals.

★7318★ CEDARS-SINAI MEDICAL CENTER
HEALTH SCIENCES INFORMATION CENTER
8700 Beverly Blvd.
Box 48956
Los Angeles, CA 90048   Phone: (213) 855-3751
Ellen Wilson Green, Dir. of Libs.
Subjects: Clinical medicine. **Holdings:** 10,000 books; microfilm. **Subscriptions:** 561 journals and other serials.

★7319★ CHIER INFORMATION CENTER
320 W. 15th St.
Los Angeles, CA 90015   Phone: (213) 742-5872
Cynthia Perkins, Dir., Lib. & Info.Serv.
Subjects: Clinical medicine, oncology, hospital management, nursing. **Holdings:** 3180 books; 3500 bound periodical volumes; 500 audio cassettes. **Subscriptions:** 282 journals and other serials.

★7320★ CHILDREN'S HOSPITAL OF LOS ANGELES
MEDICAL LIBRARY
4650 Sunset Blvd.
Los Angeles, CA 90027   Phone: (213) 669-2254
Doreen B. Keough, Med.Libn.
Subjects: Pediatrics. **Holdings:** 5000 books; 4000 bound periodical volumes; 1250 reels of microfilm. **Subscriptions:** 350 journals and other serials.

★7321★ CLEVELAND CHIROPRACTIC COLLEGE
LEARNING RESOURCE CENTERS
590 N. Vermont
Los Angeles, CA 90004   Phone: (213) 660-6166
Donna Gerometta, Dir.
Subjects: Chiropractic and manipulative medicine, basic human life sciences, diagnosis, physical therapy, orthopedics. **Holdings:** 14,000 books; 3582 bound periodical volumes; 13 periodicals on microfiche; 3332 x-rays; 1114 slide sets; 580 video cassettes; 3731 audio cassettes; 16 16mm films. **Subscriptions:** 314 journals and other serials.

★7322★ CURE FOUNDATION
LIBRARY
11661 San Vicente Blvd., Ste. 300
Los Angeles, CA 90049   Phone: (213) 825-5091
Subjects: Gastrointestinal diseases, peptic ulcers. **Holdings:** Books; 500 bound periodical volumes; 1000 original manuscripts and research reports.

★7323★ ESTELLE DOHENY EYE INSTITUTE
KENNETH T. NORRIS, JR. VISUAL SCIENCE LIBRARY
1355 San Pablo St.
Los Angeles, CA 90033   Phone: (213) 342-6644
Ann Dawson, Act.Libn.
Subjects: Ophthalmology. **Holdings:** 1500 books; 1000 bound periodical volumes. **Subscriptions:** 95 journals and other serials.

★7324★ GATEWAYS HOSPITAL AND COMMUNITY MENTAL
HEALTH CENTER
PROFESSIONAL LIBRARY
1891 Effie St.
Los Angeles, CA 90026   Phone: (213) 666-0171
Celia A. Palant, Libn.
Subjects: Psychiatry, community mental health, penology. **Holdings:** 1000 books; 100 unbound periodical volumes; 500 pamphlets and government documents; 200 tape cassettes. **Subscriptions:** 25 journals and other serials.

★7325★ HOSPITAL OF THE GOOD SAMARITAN
MEDICAL LIBRARY
616 S. Witmer St.
Los Angeles, CA 90017-2395   Phone: (213) 977-2326
Susan Efteland, Lib.Dir.
Subjects: Preclinical and clinical medicine, nursing, hospital administration. **Holdings:** 3000 books; 5300 bound periodical volumes. **Subscriptions:** 170 journals and other serials.

★7326★ HOUSE EAR INSTITUTE
GEORGE KELEMEN LIBRARY
2100 W. 3rd St.
Los Angeles, CA 90057   Phone: (213) 483-4431
Liz Gnerre, Libn.
Subjects: Otology, otolaryngology, psychoacoustics, audiology, hearing rehabilitation, neurosurgery, biomedical engineering. **Holdings:** 2200 books; 1615 bound periodical volumes; 3700 reprints; 20 dissertations; 200 audio cassettes; 500 slides. **Subscriptions:** 180 journals and other serials.

★7327★ HOUSE EAR INSTITUTE
SAM AND ROSE STEIN CHILDREN'S CENTER
PARENT RESOURCE LIBRARY
2100 W. 3rd St.
Los Angeles, CA 90057   Phone: (213) 483-4431
Liz Gnerre, Libn.
Subjects: Deafness - social problems, special education, sign language, communication, child rearing. **Holdings:** 550 books; 9 VF drawers of reprints, manuscripts, reports, graduate projects, clippings, brochures, special studies, documents pertaining to hearing-impaired children and adults and family relationships.

★7328★ KAISER-PERMANENTE MEDICAL CENTER
KAISER FOUNDATION HOSPITAL MEDICAL LIBRARY
4867 Sunset Blvd.
Los Angeles, CA 90027   Phone: (213) 667-8568
Judith A. Dowd, Dept.Hd.
Subjects: Clinical medicine, nursing, health media. **Holdings:** 6300 books; 6000 bound periodical volumes; 1000 audiotapes. **Subscriptions:** 400 journals and other serials.

★7329★ KAISER-PERMANENTE MENTAL HEALTH CENTER
PROFESSIONAL LIBRARY
765 College St.
Los Angeles, CA 90012   Phone: (213) 580-7260
L.A. Ravenswood, MALS, MA, Libn.
Subjects: Psychology, psychiatry, clinical social work, psychopharmacology, psychoanalysis, women's studies, body/mind interface. **Holdings:** 6000 books; 4500 bound periodical volumes. **Subscriptions:** 152 journals and other serials; 6 newspapers.

★7330★ LOS ANGELES COUNTY DEPARTMENT OF HEALTH
SERVICES-PREVENTIVE/PUBLIC HEALTH
HEALTH ADMINISTRATION/MANAGEMENT LIBRARY
313 N. Figueroa St., Rm. Mz1
Los Angeles, CA 90012   Phone: (213) 974-7780
Sharon Pruhs, Med.Libn. II
Subjects: Public health, preventive medicine, environmental toxicology, administration, management. **Holdings:** 1200 books; 2000 bound periodical volumes. **Subscriptions:** 421 journals and other serials.

★7331★ LOS ANGELES COUNTY/KING/DREW MEDICAL
CENTER
HEALTH SCIENCES LIBRARY
1621 E. 120th St., MP 36
Los Angeles, CA 90059   Phone: (213) 563-4869
Ms. M. Moss Humphrey, Dir.
Subjects: Medicine. **Holdings:** 9500 books; 33,000 bound periodical volumes; 16 drawers of audio cassettes; 200 videotapes. **Subscriptions:** 825 journals and other serials.

★7332★ LOS ANGELES COUNTY MEDICAL ASSOCIATION
LIBRARY
634 S. Westlake Ave.
Los Angeles, CA 90057   Phone: (213) 483-1581
Joyce Crump, Ref.
Subjects: Medicine, history of medicine. **Holdings:** 87,000 books; 55,000 bound periodical volumes; 1 room of AV programs; 2 rooms of medical artifacts; boxed archival material; 12 VF drawers of pamphlets. **Subscriptions:** 60 journals and other serials.

★7333★ LOS ANGELES COUNTY/UNIVERSITY OF
SOUTHERN CALIFORNIA MEDICAL CENTER
MEDICAL LIBRARIES
General Hospital, Rm. 2050
1200 N. State St.
Los Angeles, CA 90033-1084   Phone: (213) 226-7006
Alice Reinhardt, Chf., Lib.Serv.
Subjects: Medicine, nursing, allied health sciences. **Holdings:** 24,000 books; 29,500 bound periodical volumes; 1000 audio cassettes; 55 slide sets; 697 transparencies and filmstrips. **Subscriptions:** 1100 journals and other serials.

★7334★ LOS ANGELES PSYCHOANALYTIC SOCIETY AND
INSTITUTE
SIMMEL-FENICHEL LIBRARY
2014 Sawtelle Blvd.
Los Angeles, CA 90025   Phone: (213) 478-6541
Subjects: Psychoanalysis and psychiatry, the behavioral sciences. **Holdings:** 5500 books; 800 bound periodical volumes; 1500 unbound periodicals; 14 VF drawers of reprints and pamphlets; 550 unpublished papers; 600 tapes; 18 videotapes. **Subscriptions:** 40 journals and other serials.

★7335★ LOS ANGELES PUBLIC LIBRARY
SCIENCE, TECHNOLOGY AND PATENTS DEPARTMENT
630 W. 5th St.
Los Angeles, CA 90071   Phone: (213) 612-3270
Billie M. Connor, Dept.Mgr.
Subjects: Physical and biological sciences, consumer health, medicine and drugs, alternative medicine, earth and natural sciences, applied technology, ecology, astronomy, foods and beverages, computer sciences, natural history, climatology, oceanography, motor vehicles. **Holdings:** 250,000 volumes; 50,000 documents. **Subscriptions:** 1700 journals; 1500 serials.

★7336★ LOS ANGELES REGIONAL FAMILY PLANNING
COUNCIL
LIBRARY
3600 Wilshire Blvd., Ste. 600
Los Angeles, CA 90010-0605   Phone: (213) 386-5614
Selda Roth, Libn.
Subjects: Family planning, education for professionals in reproductive health, family life education, prevention of teenage pregnancy, birth control, reproductive health. **Holdings:** 1500 books; 400 AV programs. **Subscriptions:** 70 journals and other serials.

★7337★ LOS ANGELES TRADE-TECHNICAL COLLEGE
LIBRARY
400 W. Washington Blvd.
Los Angeles, CA 90015   Phone: (213) 746-0800
Doris W. Ramey, Chm., Lib.Serv.
Subjects: Trades - apparel, commercial art, automotive, building, cosmetology, culinary arts, drafting, electricity, electronics, metal, office administration, plastics, printing, vocational nursing, registered nursing, business administration. **Holdings:** 65,000 volumes. **Subscriptions:** 363 journals and other serials; 14 newspapers.

★7338★ ORTHOPAEDIC HOSPITAL
RUBEL MEMORIAL LIBRARY
2400 S. Flower St.
Box 60132, Terminal Annex
Los Angeles, CA 90060-0132   Phone: (213) 742-1530
Mina R. Mandal, Dir., Med.Lib.
Subjects: Orthopedics. **Holdings:** 3030 books; 3290 bound periodical volumes. **Subscriptions:** 143 journals and other serials.

★7339★ QUEEN OF ANGELS
HOLLYWOOD PRESBYTERIAN MEDICAL CENTER
HEALTH SCIENCES LIBRARY
1300 N. Vermont Ave.
Los Angeles, CA 90027   Phone: (213) 413-3000
Pacita Estepa, Hea.Sci.Libn.
Subjects: Medicine, nursing, allied health sciences, patient education, hospital administration, health care. **Holdings:** 5700 books; 3000 bound periodical volumes; 900 AV programs. **Subscriptions:** 182 journals and other serials.

★7340★ REISS-DAVIS CHILD STUDY CENTER
RESEARCH LIBRARY
3200 Motor Ave.
Los Angeles, CA 90034   Phone: (213) 204-1666
Leonore W. Freehling, Libn.
Subjects: Child psychology, child psychiatry, child development, psychiatric social work, educational psychology, child analysis, psychoanalysis. **Holdings:** 12,500 books; 3500 bound periodical volumes; 10 VF drawers of information files; 25 films; 500 audiotapes; 25 videotapes. **Subscriptions:** 125 journals and other serials.

★7341★ ST. VINCENT MEDICAL CENTER
HEALTH SCIENCES LIBRARY
2131 W. 3rd St.
Los Angeles, CA 90057   Phone: (213) 484-5530
Marsha Gelman-Kmec, Dir., Lib.Serv.
Subjects: Medicine, nursing, administration, cardiology, heart and kidney transplantation. **Holdings:** 1200 books; 400 bound periodical volumes. **Subscriptions:** 202 journals and other serials.

★7342★ U.S. DEPARTMENT OF VETERANS AFFAIRS
MEDICAL RESEARCH LIBRARY
691/W142-D
Wilshire & Sawtelle Sts.
Los Angeles, CA 90073   Phone: (213) 478-3711
Merianne Davis, Chf., Med.Res.Lib.Sect.
Subjects: Biochemistry, immunology, microbiology, molecular biology, physiology, ultrastructural research, metabolism. **Holdings:** 3400 books; 6200 bound periodical volumes. **Subscriptions:** 125 journals and other serials.

★7343★ U.S. DEPARTMENT OF VETERANS AFFAIRS
WADSWORTH MEDICAL LIBRARY
Wilshire & Sawtelle Blvds.
Los Angeles, CA 90073   Phone: (213) 478-3711
Subjects: Clinical medicine, surgery, dentistry, nursing, epilepsy, geriatrics, nutrition, social work. **Holdings:** 6044 books; 12,557 bound periodical volumes; pamphlet file of monographs. **Subscriptions:** 480 journals and other serials; 12 newspapers.

★7344★ UNIVERSITY OF CALIFORNIA, LOS ANGELES
BRAIN INFORMATION SERVICE
Center for Health Sciences, No. 43-367
Los Angeles, CA 90024   Phone: (213) 825-3417
Michael H. Chase, Dir.
Subjects: Neurosciences, alcohol and driving, sleep. **Holdings:** Figures not available.

★7345★ UNIVERSITY OF CALIFORNIA, LOS ANGELES
EDUCATION AND PSYCHOLOGY LIBRARY
390 Powell Library Bldg.
Los Angeles, CA 90024-1516   Phone: (213) 825-4081
Barbara Duke, Hd.
Subjects: Education; psychology - general, experimental, cognitive, abnormal, social, developmental; English as a second language; applied linguistics. **Holdings:** 154,151 volumes; 597,688 microfiche (including ERIC); 337 audiotapes; 2221 reels of microfilm. **Subscriptions:** 2672 journals and other serials.

★7346★ UNIVERSITY OF CALIFORNIA, LOS ANGELES
LABORATORY OF BIOMEDICAL AND ENVIRONMENTAL
   SCIENCES
LIBRARY
900 Veteran Ave.
Los Angeles, CA 90024-1786   Phone: (213) 825-8741
Janet D. Carter, Libn.
Subjects: Biochemistry, nuclear medicine, environmental science, cell biology. **Holdings:** 37,650 bound volumes (books and journals); 100,000 reports on microfiche; 1550 technical reports. **Subscriptions:** 166 journals and other serials.

★7347★ UNIVERSITY OF CALIFORNIA, LOS ANGELES
LOUISE DARLING BIOMEDICAL LIBRARY
Center for Health Sciences
10833 Le Conte Blvd.
Los Angeles, CA 90024-1798   Phone: (213) 825-5781
Alison Bunting, Biomed.Libn.
Subjects: Medicine, dentistry, nursing, public health, biology, microbiology, botany, zoology. **Holdings:** 486,184 volumes; 334 manuscripts; 472 maps; 1556 reels of microfilm; 35,553 microfiche; 3602 sound recordings; 6917 pamphlets; 31,191 slides; 9496 pictorial items; 5 filmstrips; 5 motion pictures; 1914 video recordings; 13 videodiscs; 15 machine-readable data files. **Subscriptions:** 5956 journals and other serials.

★7348★ UNIVERSITY OF SOUTHERN CALIFORNIA
DENTISTRY LIBRARY
DEN 201
University Park - MC 0641
Los Angeles, CA 90089-0641   Phone: (213) 740-6476
Frank O. Mason, Dental Libn.
Subjects: Dentistry, medicine, allied sciences. **Holdings:** 17,325 books; 11,500 bound periodical volumes; 2300 test files; 2519 AV programs and filmstrips; 1142 reading files. **Subscriptions:** 645 journals and other serials.

★7349★ UNIVERSITY OF SOUTHERN CALIFORNIA
GERONTOLOGY LIBRARY
120 Gerontology - MC 0191
Los Angeles, CA 90089-0191   Phone: (213) 740-5990
Stella Fu, Act.Hd.Libn.
Subjects: Gerontology. **Holdings:** 10,000 books; 750 bound periodical volumes; 1500 reels of microfilm of dissertations. **Subscriptions:** 105 journals; 200 newsletters and other serials.

★7350★ UNIVERSITY OF SOUTHERN CALIFORNIA
HEALTH SCIENCES CAMPUS
NORRIS MEDICAL LIBRARY
2003 Zonal Ave.
Los Angeles, CA 90033-4582   Phone: (213) 342-1116
Nelson J. Gilman, Libn./Dir.
Subjects: Medicine, pharmacy, occupational therapy, physical therapy. **Holdings:** 44,214 books; 92,809 bound periodical volumes; 40,540 slides; 9000 microfiche; 105 reels of microfilm; 2396 audio cassettes; 1042 video cassettes; 107 films; 48 filmstrips; 26 phonograph discs; 729 floppy discs; 12 compact discs; 29 video discs. **Subscriptions:** 2585 journals and other serials.

★7351★ WHITE MEMORIAL MEDICAL CENTER
COURVILLE-ABBOTT MEMORIAL LIBRARY
1720 Brooklyn Ave.
Los Angeles, CA 90033   Phone: (213) 260-5715
Joyce Marson, Libn.
Subjects: Medicine, nursing, dietetics, paramedical sciences. **Holdings:** 45,000 volumes; 8 VF drawers of pamphlets; tapes; phonograph records; filmstrips. **Subscriptions:** 350 journals and other serials.

★7352★ ST. FRANCIS MEDICAL CENTER
MOTHER MACARIA HEALTH SCIENCE LIBRARY
3630 E. Imperial Hwy.
Lynwood, CA 90262   Phone: (213) 603-6045
Eva Kratz, Dir. of Lib.Serv.
Subjects: Medicine, nursing, hospital administration, paramedical sciences. **Holdings:** 3000 books; 4000 bound periodical volumes; 120 other cataloged items; 800 audiotapes; 90 boxes of peripheral material; 175 archival materials; 48 videotapes. **Subscriptions:** 300 journals and other serials.

★7353★ MEDICAL PLANNING ASSOCIATES
LIBRARY
1601 Rambla Pacifico
Malibu, CA 90265   Phone: (213) 456-2084
Subjects: Hospital design and planning, health care delivery systems, computer technology, architecture. Holdings: 2100 books; 6000 unbound periodicals; 8000 monographs; architectural records; 4800 cataloged journal articles and newspaper clippings. Subscriptions: 265 journals and other serials.

★7354★ DANIEL FREEMAN HOSPITAL
MEDICAL LIBRARY & RESOURCE CENTER
4650 Lincoln Blvd.
Marina Del Rey, CA 90292   Phone: (213) 823-8911
Gillian Olechno, Lib.Dir.
Subjects: Medicine, nursing, allied health sciences. Holdings: 154 books; 198 audiotapes. Subscriptions: 57 journals and other serials.

★7355★ U.S. DEPARTMENT OF VETERANS AFFAIRS
MEDICAL CENTER STAFF LIBRARY
150 Muir Rd.
Martinez, CA 94553   Phone: (415) 372-2000
Dorothea E. Bennett (142D), Chf., Lib.Serv.
Subjects: Medicine. Holdings: 6127 books; 8550 bound periodical volumes; 945 audiotapes. Subscriptions: 530 journals and other serials.

★7356★ U.S. AIR FORCE HOSPITAL
MEDICAL LIBRARY
Mather AFB, CA 95655-5000   Phone: (916) 364-3179
Willis J. Collick, Med.Libn.
Subjects: Medicine. Holdings: 960 books. Subscriptions: 91 journals and other serials.

★7357★ MERCED COMMUNITY MEDICAL CENTER
WILLIAM E. FOUNTAIN HEALTH SCIENCES LIBRARY
301 E. 13th St.
Box 231
Merced, CA 95340   Phone: (209) 385-7058
Betty Maddalena, Libn.
Subjects: Medicine, nursing. Holdings: 1715 books; 2560 bound periodical volumes; 301 Audio-Digest tapes. Subscriptions: 179 journals and other serials.

★7358★ HOLY CROSS MEDICAL CENTER
HEALTH SCIENCES LIBRARY
15031 Rinaldi St.
Mission Hills, CA 91345-9986   Phone: (818) 898-4545
Lucille R. Moss, Mgr.
Subjects: Clinical medicine, nursing, hospital administration. Holdings: 1200 books; 3200 bound periodical volumes. Subscriptions: 250 journals and other serials.

★7359★ DOCTORS' MEDICAL CENTER
PROFESSIONAL LIBRARY
1441 Florida Ave.
Box 4138
Modesto, CA 95352   Phone: (209) 578-1211
Margaret F. Luebke, Med.Libn.
Subjects: Medicine, nursing. Holdings: 600 books; 400 bound periodical volumes. Subscriptions: 160 journals and other serials.

★7360★ MEMORIAL HOSPITALS ASSOCIATION
HEALTH SCIENCES LIBRARY
Box 942
Modesto, CA 95353   Phone: (209) 526-4500
S.A. Hammett, Dir.
Subjects: Medicine, nursing, hospital administration. Holdings: 1000 books; 300 pamphlet files. Subscriptions: 200 journals and other serials.

★7361★ SCENIC GENERAL HOSPITAL
STANISLAUS COUNTY MEDICAL LIBRARY
830 Scenic Dr.
Modesto, CA 95350   Phone: (209) 526-6926
Margie A. Felt, Med.Lib.Asst.
Subjects: General and family practice, orthopedics, surgery, pediatrics, radiology, nursing, psychiatry. Holdings: 3563 books; 4330 bound periodical volumes; 931 other cataloged items; 97 slides; Audio-Digest tapes. Subscriptions: 162 journals and other serials.

★7362★ PHARMACIA OPHTHALMICS
LIBRARY
PO Box 5036
605 E. Huntington Dr.
Monrovia, CA 91017   Phone: (818) 301-8500
Subjects: Ophthalmology, biomaterials, polymer science. Holdings: 500 books; 75 bound periodical volumes. Subscriptions: 71 journals and other serials.

★7363★ BEVERLY HOSPITAL
BREITMAN MEMORIAL LIBRARY
309 W. Beverly Blvd.
Montebello, CA 90640   Phone: (213) 726-1222
Margot D. Jensen, Libn.
Subjects: Medicine. Holdings: 750 books; 718 bound periodical volumes. Subscriptions: 123 journals and other serials; 2 newspapers.

★7364★ COMMUNITY HOSPITAL OF THE MONTEREY
PENINSULA
MEDICAL LIBRARY
Box HH
Monterey, CA 93942   Phone: (408) 625-4550
Julia Richardson
Subjects: Medicine, allied health sciences. Holdings: 1030 books; 1700 bound periodical volumes; 650 audiotapes. Subscriptions: 130 journals and other serials.

★7365★ WOMEN EXPLOITED BY ABORTION
LIBRARY
24823 Nogal St.
Moreno Valley, CA 92388   Phone: (714) 924-4164
Kathy Walker, Pres.
Subjects: Abortion, post abortion syndrome (PAS) counseling, physical and psychological aftereffects of abortion. Holdings: 10 books; 1000 pamphlets and other items.

★7366★ NAPA STATE HOSPITAL
WRENSHALL A. OLIVER PROFESSIONAL LIBRARY
2100 Napa-Vallejo Hwy.
Napa, CA 94558   Phone: (707) 253-5477
Barbara Fetesoff, Sr.Libn.
Subjects: Psychiatry, psychiatric social work, psychiatric nursing, neurology, clinical psychology. Holdings: 9000 books; 901 bound periodical volumes; 800 tape cassettes. Subscriptions: 128 journals and other serials.

★7367★ PARADISE VALLEY HOSPITAL
MEDICAL LIBRARY
2400 E. 4th St.
National City, CA 92050   Phone: (619) 470-4155
Valeria Bouchard, CMSC, Libn.
Subjects: Medicine, nursing, hospital administration. Holdings: 600 books; 50 other cataloged items. Subscriptions: 60 journals and other serials.

★7368★ ACNE RESEARCH INSTITUTE, INC.
LIBRARY
1236 Somerset Ln.
Newport Beach, CA 92660   Phone: (714) 722-1805
Dr. James E. Fulton, Jr.
Subjects: Acne - pathogenesis, aggravating factors, available treatments; cosmetic surgery. Holdings: Figures not available.

★7369★ HOAG MEMORIAL HOSPITAL-PRESBYTERIAN
MEDICAL LIBRARY
301 Newport Blvd.
Box Y
Newport Beach, CA 92658   Phone: (714) 760-2308
Mrs. Ute Schultz, Med.Libn.
Subjects: Medicine, nursing, psychiatry. Holdings: 5000 books; 9000 bound periodical volumes; 1500 audio cassettes and other AV programs. Subscriptions: 300 journals and other serials.

★7370★ CALIFORNIA STATE UNIVERSITY, NORTHRIDGE
LIBRARY
HEALTH SCIENCE COLLECTION
18111 Nordhoff St.
Northridge, CA 91330   Phone: (818) 885-3012
Marcia Henry, Sci.Ref.Libn.
Subjects: Health education, nutrition, occupational health, sanitation,

child and maternity care, medical statistics, preventive medicine, public health administration, physiology, communicative disorders. **Holdings:** 45,000 books; 13,000 bound periodical volumes. **Subscriptions:** 520 journals and other serials.

★7371★   NORTHRIDGE HOSPITAL MEDICAL CENTER
ATCHERLEY MEDICAL LIBRARY
18300 Roscoe Blvd.
Northridge, CA 91328   Phone: (818) 885-8500
Theresa Sase, M.L.S
Subjects: Medicine, health sciences. **Holdings:** 3000 books; 7 VF drawers; pamphlet file. **Subscriptions:** 376 journals and other serials.

★7372★   METROPOLITAN STATE HOSPITAL
STAFF LIBRARY
11400 Norwalk Blvd.
Norwalk, CA 90650   Phone: (213) 863-7011
Beni Santa Maria, Dir.
Subjects: Psychiatry, psychology, psychiatric social work, psychiatric nursing. **Holdings:** 8050 books; 1705 bound periodical volumes; 1100 audiotapes; 510 videotapes. **Subscriptions:** 91 journals and other serials.

★7373★   ALAMEDA-CONTRA COSTA MEDICAL
ASSOCIATION/HIGHLAND HOSPITAL
LIBRARY
1411 E. 31st St.
Oakland, CA 94602   Phone: (510) 536-3331
Linda M. Morgan, Med.Libn.
Subjects: Medicine, surgery, orthopedics. **Holdings:** 2000 books; 16,500 bound periodical volumes; 700 cassettes. **Subscriptions:** 248 journals and other serials.

★7374★   BERKELEY PLANNING ASSOCIATES
LIBRARY
440 Grand Ave., Ste. 500
Oakland, CA 94610   Phone: (510) 465-7884
Linda Tom Barker, V.Pres.
Subjects: Housing, disability, child welfare, labor, social services, health care financing. **Holdings:** 500 books; 1000 reports. **Subscriptions:** 12 journals and other serials.

★7375★   CALIFORNIA DEPARTMENT OF ALCOHOL AND
DRUG PROGRAMS
PREVENTION RESOURCE CENTER
440 Grand Ave., Ste. 401
Oakland, CA 94610   Phone: (510) 839-9151
Janet Coles, Libn.
Subjects: Alcohol and drug abuse, prevention. **Holdings:** 500 books; 1000 bound periodical volumes; 3500 reprints, clippings, reports; 200 films; 90 titles on microfilm. **Subscriptions:** 25 journals and other serials.

★7376★   CHILDREN'S HOSPITAL MEDICAL CENTER OF
NORTHERN CALIFORNIA
MEDICAL LIBRARY
747 52nd St.
Oakland, CA 94609   Phone: (510) 428-3448
Leonard P. Shapiro, Med.Libn.
Subjects: Pediatrics, neonatology, adolescent medicine, pediatric nursing, child development, child psychology. **Holdings:** 2800 books; 7200 bound periodical volumes; 250 Audio-Digest tapes; 400 videotapes. **Subscriptions:** 300 journals and other serials.

★7377★   CROSBY, HEAFEY, ROACH & MAY
LAW LIBRARY
1999 Harrison St.
Oakland, CA 94612   Phone: (510) 763-2000
Nora L. Skrukrud, Libn.
Subjects: Civil litigation, taxation, labor law, medical jurisprudence, environmental law, intellectual property, products liability. **Holdings:** 20,000 books; 150 bound periodical volumes. **Subscriptions:** 400 journals and other serials; 13 newspapers.

★7378★   EVERETT A. GLADMAN MEMORIAL HOSPITAL
MEDICAL LIBRARY
2633 E. 27th St.
Oakland, CA 94601   Phone: (510) 536-8111
Lee Vares, Dir.Med.Rec.
Subjects: Psychiatry, psychology, medicine. **Holdings:** 500 books. **Subscriptions:** 50 journals and other serials.

★7379★   KAISER-PERMANENTE MEDICAL CENTER
HEALTH EDUCATION CENTER
3772 Howe St.
Oakland, CA 94611   Phone: (510) 596-6204
Subjects: Health maintenance, prenatal care, nutrition, family planning, child care, cancer, medicine. **Holdings:** 1000 books; 226 pamphlet titles; 52 audio cassettes; 200 video cassettes; AV programs. **Subscriptions:** 12 journals and other serials.

★7380★   KAISER-PERMANENTE MEDICAL CENTER
MEDICAL LIBRARY
280 W. MacArthur Blvd.
Oakland, CA 94611   Phone: (510) 596-6158
Ysabel R. Bertolucci, Libn.
Subjects: Medicine, surgery. **Holdings:** 3400 books; 8000 bound periodical volumes. **Subscriptions:** 300 journals and other serials.

★7381★   MERRITT PERALTA MEDICAL CENTER
JOHN A. GRAZIANO MEMORIAL LIBRARY
400 Hawthorne Ave.
Oakland, CA 94609   Phone: (510) 420-6180
Sharon Wosnick, Dir.
Subjects: Nursing, medicine, allied health sciences. **Holdings:** 4500 books; 600 bound periodical volumes; 4 VF drawers of pamphlets. **Subscriptions:** 350 journals and other serials.

★7382★   NATIONAL HISPANIC UNIVERSITY
NATIONAL HISPANIC CENTER FOR ADVANCED STUDIES
AND POLICY
LIBRARY
262 Grand Ave.
Oakland, CA 94806   Phone: (510) 451-0511
Barbara Fukai, Libn.
Subjects: Bilingual education, general education, business administration, health sciences, liberal arts. **Holdings:** 5000 books; 1000 bound periodical volumes. **Subscriptions:** 20 journals and other serials.

★7383★   U.S. NAVY
NAVAL HOSPITAL
MEDICAL LIBRARY
8750 Mountain Blvd.
Oakland, CA 94627-5000   Phone: (510) 639-2031
Harriet V. Cohen, Adm.Libn.
Subjects: Medicine, nursing, paramedical sciences, psychiatry. **Holdings:** 8000 books; 10,000 bound periodical volumes. **Subscriptions:** 400 journals and other serials.

★7384★   ST. JOSEPH HOSPITAL
BURLEW MEDICAL LIBRARY
1100 Stewart Dr.
Orange, CA 92668   Phone: (714) 771-8291
Julie Smith, Lib.Mgr.
Subjects: Medicine, nursing, hospital administration. **Holdings:** 10,000 books; 4798 bound periodical volumes; 7800 AV programs. **Subscriptions:** 713 journals and other serials.

★7385★   UNIVERSITY OF CALIFORNIA, IRVINE
MEDICAL CENTER LIBRARY
Rte. 82
101 City Dr., S.
Orange, CA 92668   Phone: (714) 634-5585
Susan Russell, Hd.Libn.
Subjects: Clinical medicine. **Holdings:** 28,000 volumes; 4 VF drawers; 10 filmstrips; 100 slide and cassette programs; 130 videotapes; 200 software diskettes. **Subscriptions:** 825 journals and other serials.

★7386★ OROVILLE HOSPITAL
EDWARD P. GODDARD, M.D., MEMORIAL LIBRARY
2767 Olive Hwy.
Oroville, CA 95966   Phone: (916) 533-8500
Gertrude N. Bartley, Libn.
Subjects: Medicine. **Holdings:** 150 books. **Subscriptions:** 46 journals and other serials.

★7387★ ST. JOHN'S REGIONAL MEDICAL CENTER
HEALTH SCIENCE LIBRARY
333 N. F St.
Oxnard, CA 93030   Phone: (805) 988-2820
Joanne Kennedy, Libn.
Subjects: Clinical medicine, nursing, health management. **Holdings:** 3200 volumes. **Subscriptions:** 200 journals and other serials.

★7388★ ALZA CORPORATION
RESEARCH LIBRARY
950 Page Mill Rd.
Palo Alto, CA 94304   Phone: (415) 494-5548
Helen T. Rolen, Mgr., Lib.Serv.
Subjects: Pharmacology, biochemistry, medicine, dermatology, veterinary medicine, pharmaceuticals, obstetrics, gynecology, physiology, polymer science, analytical chemistry, chemical engineering. **Holdings:** 20,000 books; 20,000 bound periodical volumes; 5000 reels of microfilm; 500 microfiche; 20 VF drawers. **Subscriptions:** 550 journals and other serials; 6 newspapers.

★7389★ CELTRIX LABORATORIES, INC.
LIBRARY
2500 Faber Pl.
Palo Alto, CA 94303   Phone: (415) 354-4920
Maria Hylkema, Tech.Info.Spec.
Subjects: Biochemistry, chemical engineering, dermatology, plastic surgery, immunology, dentistry, orthopedics. **Holdings:** 2500 books; 750 other cataloged items. **Subscriptions:** 160 journals and other serials.

★7390★ DNAX RESEARCH INSTITUTE
LIBRARY
901 California Ave.
Palo Alto, CA 94304-1104   Phone: (415) 496-1285
Nancy S. Fadis, Lib.Mgr.
Subjects: Immunology, molecular biology, genetic engineering, patents, parasitology, virology. **Holdings:** 1000 books. **Subscriptions:** 168 journals and other serials.

★7391★ PACIFIC GRADUATE SCHOOL OF PSYCHOLOGY
RESEARCH LIBRARY
935 E. Meadow Dr.
Palo Alto, CA 94303-4233   Phone: (415) 494-7477
Christine Dassoff, Res.Libn.
Subjects: Clinical psychology, psychological assessment, psychopathology, psychotherapy, neuropsychology, developmental psychology, child psychiatry, research methodology and statistics. **Holdings:** 5200 books; 2500 bound periodical volumes; 75 psychological tests; 93 dissertations; 350 audio cassettes. **Subscriptions:** 175 journals and other serials.

★7392★ PALO ALTO MEDICAL FOUNDATION
BARNETT-HALL LIBRARY
860 Bryant St.
Palo Alto, CA 94301   Phone: (415) 321-4121
Judith M. Cummings, Hd.Libn.
Subjects: Medicine, medical research, basic sciences, nursing, pharmacology. **Holdings:** 11,631 volumes; 13 VF drawers of pamphlets. **Subscriptions:** 330 journals and other serials.

★7393★ SYNTEX U.S.A. INC.
CORPORATE LIBRARY/INFORMATION SERVICES
3401 Hillview Ave.
Palo Alto, CA 94304   Phone: (415) 855-5431
Caren A. Cavanaugh, Mgr.
Subjects: Organic chemistry, biochemistry, pharmacology, clinical medicine, veterinary medicine, physiology. **Holdings:** 8000 books; 16,000 bound periodical volumes; 1400 microfilm cartridges; 22 volumes of bound reprints of papers authored by Syntex personnel. **Subscriptions:** 600 journals and other serials.

★7394★ SYVA COMPANY
LIBRARY/INFORMATION CENTER
900 Arastradero
Palo Alto, CA 94304   Phone: (415) 493-2200
Meaghan Wheeler, Mgr.
Subjects: Organic chemistry, biochemistry, microbiology, medicine. **Holdings:** 6000 books. **Subscriptions:** 300 journals and other serials.

★7395★ U.S. DEPARTMENT OF VETERANS AFFAIRS
MEDICAL CENTER
MEDICAL LIBRARIES
3801 Miranda Ave.
Palo Alto, CA 94304   Phone: (415) 493-5000
C.R. Gallimore, Chf., Lib.Serv.
Subjects: Medicine, behavioral sciences. **Holdings:** 13,000 books; 13,000 bound periodical volumes; 5000 recreational books. **Subscriptions:** 690 journals and other serials; 6 newspapers.

★7396★ KAISER-PERMANENTE MEDICAL CENTER
PANORAMA CITY HEALTH SCIENCE LIBRARY
13652 Cantara St.
Panorama City, CA 91402   Phone: (818) 908-2239
Winnie Yu, Hd.Libn.
Subjects: Medicine. **Holdings:** 1800 books; 2500 bound periodical volumes; 200 cassettes. **Subscriptions:** 225 journals and other serials.

★7397★ HUNTINGTON MEMORIAL HOSPITAL
HEALTH SCIENCES LIBRARY
100 W. California Blvd.
Box 7013
Pasadena, CA 91109-7013   Phone: (818) 397-5161
Samir Maurice Zeind, Mgr.
Subjects: Medicine, surgery, nursing, radiology, psychiatry, hospital administration, patient information and resources. **Holdings:** 5000 books; 20,000 bound periodical volumes; 1000 audiotapes. **Subscriptions:** 617 journals and other serials.

★7398★ KAISER FOUNDATION HOSPITALS
MANAGEMENT EFFECTIVENESS LIBRARY
393 E. Walnut St.
Pasadena, CA 91188   Phone: (818) 405-3089
Henri Mondschein, Mgr.
Subjects: Hospital administration, management. **Holdings:** 4600 books; 1050 bound periodical volumes. **Subscriptions:** 250 journals and other serials.

★7399★ RIGHT TO LIFE LEAGUE OF SOUTHERN CALIFORNIA
LIBRARY
50 N. Hill Ave., Ste. 306
Pasadena, CA 91106   Phone: (818) 449-8408
Lori Hougens, Dir., Educ.
Subjects: Abortion, pre-natal development, euthanasia, genetic engineering, infanticide, human experimentation. **Holdings:** Books; periodicals; clippings; pamphlets; cassettes; videotapes.

★7400★ ST. LUKE MEDICAL CENTER
WILLIAM P. LONG MEDICAL LIBRARY
2632 E. Washington Blvd., Bin 7021
Pasadena, CA 91109-7021   Phone: (818) 797-1141
Christine De Cicco, Cons.Libn.
Subjects: Clinical medicine, surgery, nursing. **Holdings:** 690 books; 87 bound periodical volumes; 2 cassettes. **Subscriptions:** 97 journals and other serials.

★7401★ PATTON STATE HOSPITAL
STAFF LIBRARY
3102 E. Highland Ave.
Patton, CA 92369   Phone: (714) 862-8121
Laurie Piccolotti, Sr.Libn.
Subjects: Psychiatry, psychology, psychiatric nursing, forensic psychiatry. **Holdings:** 3600 books; 2025 bound periodical volumes; 1100 unbound periodical volumes; 2 VF drawers of unbound reports; 2 VF drawers of documents. **Subscriptions:** 101 journals and other serials.

★7402★ SOUTHERN CALIFORNIA COLLEGE OF CHIROPRACTIC
LIBRARY
8420 Beverly Rd.
Pico Rivera, CA 90660   Phone: (213) 692-0331
Rodney M. Vliet, Ph.D./Dir.
Subjects: Chiropractic. **Holdings:** 8000 books; 900 bound periodical volumes; 5000 unbound periodicals. **Subscriptions:** 106 journals and other serials.

★7403★ LANTERMAN DEVELOPMENTAL CENTER
LIBRARY
3530 W. Pomona Blvd.
Box 100
Pomona, CA 91769   Phone: (714) 595-1221
Kathryn Pudlock, Libn.
Subjects: Mental retardation, child psychology, neurology, special education, medicine. **Holdings:** 12,000 volumes; 15 VF drawers of pamphlets. **Subscriptions:** 202 journals and other serials.

★7404★ POMONA VALLEY COMMUNITY HOSPITAL
MEDICAL LIBRARY
1798 N. Garey Ave.
Pomona, CA 91767   Phone: (714) 865-9878
Deborah Klein, Libn.
Subjects: Clinical medicine, nursing, bioethics. **Holdings:** 1400 books; 5000 bound periodical volumes; 600 audiotapes. **Subscriptions:** 180 journals and other serials; 10 audiotape subscriptions.

★7405★ PORTERVILLE DEVELOPMENTAL CENTER
PROFESSIONAL LIBRARY
Box 2000
Porterville, CA 93258   Phone: (209) 782-2609
Mary Jane Berry, Libn.
Subjects: Mental retardation - psychology, medical aspects, education, social welfare. **Holdings:** 6000 books; 3800 bound periodical volumes. **Subscriptions:** 125 journals and other serials.

★7406★ SIERRA VIEW DISTRICT HOSPITAL
MEDICAL LIBRARY
465 W. Putnam Ave.
Porterville, CA 93257   Phone: (209) 784-1110
Marilyn R. Pankey, Dir., Med.Rec.
Subjects: Anatomy, physiology, medicine, surgery. **Holdings:** 150 books. **Subscriptions:** 22 journals and other serials.

★7407★ EISENHOWER MEDICAL CENTER
DEL E. WEBB MEMORIAL MEDICAL INFORMATION CENTER
39000 Bob Hope Dr.
Rancho Mirage, CA 92270   Phone: (619) 773-1400
Barbara E. Potts, MLS
Subjects: Medicine, health sciences. **Holdings:** 6500 books; 4000 bound periodical volumes; 250 AV program titles. **Subscriptions:** 300 journals and other serials.

★7408★ CANADA COLLEGE
RUSSELL L. STIMSON OPHTHALMIC REFERENCE LIBRARY
4200 Farm Hill Blvd.
Redwood City, CA 94061   Phone: (415) 306-3293
Anne L. Nicholls, Coord.
Subjects: Ophthalmology, ophthalmic dispensing and optics, geometrical optics, eye examination, refraction. **Holdings:** 800 books; 30 bound periodical volumes.

★7409★ CHEVRON ENVIRONMENTAL HEALTH CENTER, INC.
INFORMATION SERVICES
15299 San Pablo Ave.
PO Box 4054
Richmond, CA 94804-0054   Phone: (510) 231-6049
Sharon L. Modrick, Supv., Info.Serv.
Subjects: Toxicology, environmental health, chemical regulation, risk assessment. **Holdings:** 3500 books. **Subscriptions:** 100 journals and other serials.

★7410★ RIVERSIDE GENERAL HOSPITAL
MEDICAL LIBRARY
9851 Magnolia Ave.
Riverside, CA 92503   Phone: (714) 358-7066
Rosalie Reed, Med.Lib.Coord.
Subjects: Medicine, surgery, nursing, allied health sciences. **Holdings:** 1189 books; 5616 bound periodical volumes. **Subscriptions:** 216 journals and other serials.

★7411★ ROSEVILLE HOSPITAL
MEDICAL LIBRARY
333 Sunrise Ave.
Roseville, CA 95661   Phone: (916) 781-1580
Subjects: Medicine, nursing, surgery. **Holdings:** 1560 books; 90 bound periodical volumes; 8 VF drawers of pamphlets. **Subscriptions:** 174 journals and other serials.

★7412★ AMERICAN AMBULANCE ASSOCIATION
RESOURCE LIBRARY
3814 Auburn Blvd., Ste. 70
Sacramento, CA 95821   Phone: (916) 483-3827
Brenda Staffan, Dir. of Pubns.
Subjects: Emergency medical services - personnel training, regulatory control, state information and public education; legislation; Medicare. **Holdings:** 220 books; 10 VF drawers of unbound reports; 3 VF drawers of manuscripts; 28 boxes of archival material. **Subscriptions:** 30 journals and other serials.

★7413★ CALIFORNIA STATE UNIVERSITY, SACRAMENTO
LIBRARY
SCIENCE & TECHNOLOGY REFERENCE DEPARTMENT
2000 Jed Smith Dr.
Sacramento, CA 95819-2695   Phone: (916) 278-6373
Joseph Kramer, Hd.
Subjects: Biology and environment, engineering, geology, chemistry, physics, mathematics, computer science, nursing, speech pathology, home economics. **Holdings:** 171,938 books; 63,528 bound periodical volumes; 23,000 microforms and AV programs; 11,100 geologic maps of California and neighboring states; 5800 pamphlets; 8800 clippings. **Subscriptions:** 3114 journals.

★7414★ KAISER-PERMANENTE MEDICAL CENTER
HEALTH SCIENCES LIBRARY
2025 Morse Ave.
Sacramento, CA 95825   Phone: (916) 973-6944
Michael W. Bennett, Hea.Sci.Libn.
Subjects: Medicine, nursing, allied health sciences, health care administration. **Holdings:** 3000 books; 3000 bound periodical volumes; 780 Audio-Digest tapes; 200 videotapes. **Subscriptions:** 305 journals and other serials.

★7415★ SACRAMENTO-EL DORADO MEDICAL SOCIETY
GUTTMAN LIBRARY AND INFORMATION CENTER
5380 Elvas Ave.
Sacramento, CA 95819   Phone: (916) 456-2687
Dorothy Thurmond, Libn.
Subjects: Clinical medicine. **Holdings:** 1500 books; 1200 bound periodical volumes. **Subscriptions:** 110 journals and other serials.

★7416★ UNIVERSITY OF CALIFORNIA, DAVIS
MEDICAL CENTER LIBRARY
4301 X St., Rm. 1005
Sacramento, CA 95817   Phone: (916) 734-3529
Terri L. Malmgren, Hd.Libn.
Subjects: Medicine, nursing, and allied health sciences. **Holdings:** 9500 books; 14,423 bound periodical volumes; 2565 AV programs 3883 microforms. **Subscriptions:** 791 journals and other serials.

★7417★ ST. BERNARDINE MEDICAL CENTER
NORMAN F. FELDHEYM LIBRARY
2101 N. Waterman Ave.
San Bernardino, CA 92404   Phone: (714) 883-8711
Kathy Crumpacker, Lib.Asst.
Subjects: Medicine, paramedical fields, nursing, surgery. **Holdings:** 1500 books. **Subscriptions:** 155 journals and other serials.

★7418★ SAN BERNARDINO COMMUNITY HOSPITAL
MEDICAL LIBRARY
1500 W. 17th St.
San Bernardino, CA 92411   Phone: (714) 887-6333
V. Neil Goodwin
Subjects: Medicine. Holdings: 1500 books; 5000 bound periodical volumes. Subscriptions: 139 journals and other serials.

★7419★ SAN BERNARDINO COUNTY MEDICAL CENTER
MEDICAL LIBRARY
780 E. Gilbert St.
San Bernardino, CA 92415-0935   Phone: (714) 387-7996
Marlene E. Nourok, Med.Libn.
Subjects: Medicine. Holdings: 2000 volumes; 1020 Audio-Digest tapes; 4 VF drawers of pamphlets. Subscriptions: 212 journals and other serials.

★7420★ KRAMES COMMUNICATIONS
LIBRARY AND RESOURCE CENTER
1100 Grundy Ln.
San Bruno, CA 94066-3030   Phone: (415) 742-0400
Susan Prather, Libn.
Subjects: Health, wellness, patient information. Holdings: Figures not available. Subscriptions: 300 journals and other serials.

★7421★ PSORIASIS RESEARCH ASSOCIATION
LIBRARY
107 Vista del Grande
San Carlos, CA 94070   Phone: (415) 593-1394
Subjects: Psoriasis - cause, cure, related subspecialties. Holdings: 1500 volumes.

★7422★ AUTISM RESEARCH INSTITUTE
LIBRARY AND INFORMATION REFERRAL
4182 Adams Ave.
San Diego, CA 92113   Phone: (619) 281-7165
Mollie Odle
Subjects: Autism, nutrition. Holdings: 1000 books; archival materials.

★7423★ CALIFORNIA SCHOOL OF PROFESSIONAL
PSYCHOLOGY
SAN DIEGO LIBRARY
6212 Ferris Sq.
San Diego, CA 92121-3205   Phone: (619) 452-1664
Ada Burns, Libn.
Subjects: Psychology. Holdings: 18,000 books; 1110 bound periodical volumes; 1100 cassette tapes. Subscriptions: 293 journals and other serials.

★7424★ CHILDREN'S HOSPITAL AND HEALTH CENTER
HEALTH SCIENCES LIBRARY
8001 Frost St.
San Diego, CA 92123   Phone: (619) 576-1700
Paula K. Turley, Mgr.
Subjects: Pediatrics. Holdings: 2300 books; 2631 bound periodical volumes; 676 audiotapes; 128 videotapes. Subscriptions: 200 journals and other serials.

★7425★ HELICON FOUNDATION
LIBRARY
4622 Santa Fe St.
San Diego, CA 92109   Phone: (619) 272-3884
Dr. Charles A. Thomas, Jr.
Subjects: Health promotion, human defense/repair systems assessment, nutritional/neural enhancement. Holdings: 25 contemporary scientific journals on biochemistry and molecular biology.

★7426★ IMED CORPORATION
LIBRARY
9775 Businesspark Ave.
San Diego, CA 92131   Phone: (619) 566-9000
Sue R. Albright, Libn.
Subjects: Medicine, electronics, thermoplastics, assembly, engineering, medical instrumentation, clinical medicine. Holdings: 1200 books; 7 VF drawers of patents; 4 VF drawers of manuals. Subscriptions: 200 journals and other serials.

★7427★ KAISER-PERMANENTE MEDICAL CENTER
HEALTH SCIENCES LIBRARY
4647 Zion Ave.
San Diego, CA 92120   Phone: (619) 528-READ
Sheila E. Latus, Med.Libn.
Subjects: Medicine, nursing, allied health professions. Holdings: 6050 books; 7700 bound periodical volumes; 2000 audiotapes. Subscriptions: 450 journals and other serials.

★7428★ MERCY HOSPITAL AND MEDICAL CENTER
JEAN FARB MEMORIAL MEDICAL LIBRARY
4077 5th Ave.
San Diego, CA 92103   Phone: (619) 260-7024
Anna M. Habetler, Lib.Dir.
Subjects: Medicine, nursing, basic sciences, hospital management, psychology and psychiatry. Holdings: 2600 books; 9150 bound periodical volumes. Subscriptions: 300 journals and other serials.

★7429★ SHARP MEMORIAL HOSPITAL
HEALTH SCIENCES LIBRARY
7901 Frost St.
San Diego, CA 92123   Phone: (619) 541-3242
A. Peri Worthington, Mgr.
Subjects: Clinical medicine, nursing, management. Holdings: 1382 books; 2957 bound periodical volumes. Subscriptions: 215 journals and other serials; 5 newspapers.

★7430★ U.S. DEPARTMENT OF VETERANS AFFAIRS
MEDICAL CENTER LIBRARY
3350 La Jolla Village Dr.
San Diego, CA 92161   Phone: (619) 552-8585
Deborah G. Batey, Chf., Lib.Serv.
Subjects: Medicine, patient education, management, self development. Holdings: 11,000 bound periodical volumes; 500 reels of microfilm; 700 AV programs. Subscriptions: 520 journals and other serials.

★7431★ U.S. NAVY
NAVAL HEALTH RESEARCH CENTER
WALTER L. WILKINS BIO-MEDICAL LIBRARY
Box 85122
San Diego, CA 92186-5122   Phone: (619) 553-8425
Mary Aldous, Libn.
Subjects: Environmental and stress medicine, psychiatry, medical information systems, work physiology, biological sciences, social medicine, enhanced performance, sleep research, military medicine, sustained operations, sports medicine. Holdings: 10,000 books; 6944 bound periodical volumes; 10,000 technical reports; 410 audiotapes. Subscriptions: 350 journals and other serials.

★7432★ U.S. NAVY
NAVAL HOSPITAL
MEDICAL AND GENERAL LIBRARIES
San Diego, CA 92134   Phone: (619) 532-7950
Marilyn Schwartz, Chf.Libn.
Subjects: Medicine, nursing, dentistry, hospital administration. Holdings: 13,792 books; 15,204 bound periodical volumes. Subscriptions: 724 journals.

★7433★ UNIVERSITY OF CALIFORNIA, SAN DIEGO
MEDICAL CENTER LIBRARY
225 Dickinson St.
San Diego, CA 92103   Phone: (619) 543-6520
Christine Chapman, Hd.Libn.
Subjects: Medicine, nursing. Holdings: 26,523 volumes. Subscriptions: 757 journals and other serials.

★7434★ ALS AND NEUROMUSCULAR RESEARCH
FOUNDATION
BRIAN POLSLEY MEMORIAL AUDIO/VIDEO LIBRARY
2351 Clay St., No. 416
San Francisco, CA 94115   Phone: (415) 923-3604
Dolores Holden, Dir.
Subjects: ALS (amyotrophic lateral sclerosis). Holdings: AV programs.

★7435★ AMERICAN ACADEMY OF OPHTHALMOLOGY LIBRARY
PO Box 7424
San Francisco, CA 94966   Phone: (415) 561-8500
Beverly Taugher, Info.Coord.
Subjects: Ophthalmology. **Holdings:** 2000 books; 1000 bound periodical volumes; 5000 artifacts (instruments, visual aids, memorabilia, art, photography). **Subscriptions:** 60 journals and other serials; 2 newspapers.

★7436★ AMERICAN HYPNOTISTS' ASSOCIATION HYPNOSIS TECHNICAL CENTER
Glanworth Bldg., Ste. 6
1159 Green St.
San Francisco, CA 94109   Phone: (415) 775-6130
Dr. Angela Bertuccelli, Libn.
Subjects: Hypnosis - medical, psychological, surgical; methods of hypnotism; history and practice of hypnosis. **Holdings:** 3800 books; 304 bound periodical volumes; International Association of Hypnotists' reports.

★7437★ AMERICAN SOCIETY FOR SURGERY OF THE HAND MUSEUM AND LIBRARY
Box 7999
San Francisco, CA 94120   Phone: (415) 923-3240
Harold R. Gibson, Libn.
Subjects: Hand surgery. **Holdings:** 282 books; 453 bound periodical volumes; 62 audiovisual tapes. **Subscriptions:** 19 journals and other serials.

★7438★ CALIFORNIA COLLEGE OF PODIATRIC MEDICINE SCHMIDT MEDICAL LIBRARY
Rincon Annex, Box 7855
San Francisco, CA 94120   Phone: (415) 292-0409
Ronald E. Schultz, Lib.Dir.
Subjects: Clinical medicine, basic science. **Holdings:** 6500 books; 15,000 bound periodical volumes; 200 AV programs; 5 VF drawers of reprints; 6 VF drawers of city state file. **Subscriptions:** 195 journals and other serials.

★7439★ CALIFORNIA DEPARTMENT OF INDUSTRIAL RELATIONS DIVISION OF LABOR STATISTICS & RESEARCH RESEARCH LIBRARY
PO Box 603
San Francisco, CA 94101
Subjects: Wage settlements, work stoppages, work injuries and illnesses, and occupational diseases in California; work injuries in selected industries. **Holdings:** Figures not available.

★7440★ CALIFORNIA MEDICAL ASSOCIATION SOCIOECONOMIC LIBRARY
Box 7690
San Francisco, CA 94120-7690   Phone: (415) 882-5133
Susan Salisbury, Adm., Info.Serv.
Subjects: Medical socioeconomics, health insurance, public assistance. **Holdings:** 3600 books and pamphlets. **Subscriptions:** 195 journals and other serials.

★7441★ CARTWRIGHT, SLOBODIN LAW LIBRARY
101 California St., 26th Fl.
San Francisco, CA 94114   Phone: (415) 433-0440
Mary Kissinger, Law Libn.
Subjects: Law, product safety, medicine. **Holdings:** 7000 books and nonbook items. **Subscriptions:** 30 journals and other serials; 5 newspapers.

★7442★ DAVIES MEDICAL CENTER O.W. JONES MEDICAL LIBRARY
Castro & Duboce St.
San Francisco, CA 94114   Phone: (415) 565-6352
Anne Shew, Med.Libn.
Subjects: Biomedical sciences. **Holdings:** 1200 books; 4600 bound periodical volumes; 208 audio cassettes; 135 videotapes. **Subscriptions:** 145 journals and other serials.

★7443★ GUEDEL MEMORIAL ANESTHESIA CENTER LIBRARY
2395 Sacramento St.
Box 7999
San Francisco, CA 94120
Harold R. Gibson, Libn.
Subjects: Anesthesiology. **Holdings:** 1228 books; 863 bound periodical volumes; 813 cassette tapes; 36 videotapes; exhibits; artifacts. **Subscriptions:** 53 journals and other serials.

★7444★ HASSARD BONNINGTON ROGERS & HUBER LIBRARY
50 Fremont St., Ste. 3400
San Francisco, CA 94105   Phone: (415) 543-6444
Jeanne Shea
Subjects: Law, medical law. **Holdings:** 7000 books; 700 other cataloged items. **Subscriptions:** 209 journals and other serials.

★7445★ INSTITUTE FOR ADVANCED STUDY OF HUMAN SEXUALITY RESEARCH LIBRARY
1523 Franklin St.
San Francisco, CA 94109   Phone: (415) 928-1133
Dr. Ted McIlvenna, Dir.
Subjects: Human sexuality. **Holdings:** 45,000 books; 8000 bound periodical volumes; 61,000 films; 200,000 slides; 8000 videotapes; 8000 periodicals; 22,000 magazines, special photographs; videotapes of all lectures given at the institute; 10 unbound volumes of American and European journals on homosexuality. **Subscriptions:** 15 journals and other serials; 5 newspapers.

★7446★ KAISER-PERMANENTE MEDICAL CENTER HEALTH SCIENCES LIBRARY
2425 Geary Blvd.
San Francisco, CA 94115   Phone: (415) 929-4101
Vincent Lagano, Med.Libn.
Subjects: Clinical sciences. **Holdings:** 3800 books; 12,000 bound periodical volumes; 200 pamphlets; 2 file boxes of staff reprints. **Subscriptions:** 197 journals.

★7447★ LANGLEY PORTER PSYCHIATRIC INSTITUTE PROFESSIONAL LIBRARY
University of California
401 Parnassus Ave.
Box 13-B/C
San Francisco, CA 94143-0984   Phone: (415) 476-7380
Lisa M. Dunkel, Libn.
Subjects: Psychiatry, psychoanalysis, clinical psychology, allied mental health sciences. **Holdings:** 6575 books; 4145 bound periodical volumes; pamphlets. **Subscriptions:** 160 journals and other serials.

★7448★ LIGHTHOUSE FOR THE BLIND AND VISUALLY IMPAIRED LIBRARY
20 10th St.
San Francisco, CA 94103   Phone: (415) 431-1481
Dorothy M. Allen
Subjects: General collection. **Holdings:** 2200 braille volumes.

★7449★ NORTHERN CALIFORNIA HEALTH CENTER EMGE MEDICAL LIBRARY
Box 3805
San Francisco, CA 94119   Phone: (415) 750-6072
Peggy Tahir, Med.Libn.
Subjects: Medicine, allied health sciences. **Holdings:** 5000 books; 7500 bound periodical volumes; 600 audiotapes. **Subscriptions:** 451 journals and other serials.

★7450★ PACIFIC PRESBYTERIAN MEDICAL CENTER/UNIVERSITY OF THE PACIFIC HEALTH SCIENCES LIBRARY
2395 Sacramento St.
Box 7999
San Francisco, CA 94120   Phone: (415) 923-3240
Harold R. Gibson, Lib.Dir.
Subjects: Medicine, dentistry, ophthalmology. **Holdings:** 10,824 books; 62,913 bound periodical volumes; 1039 audiotapes; 251 videotapes. **Subscriptions:** 840 journals and other serials.

★7451★ PLANETREE HEALTH RESOURCE CENTER
2040 Webster St.
San Francisco, CA 94115   Phone: (415) 923-3680
Tracey Cosgrove, Med.Libn.
Subjects: Consumer health information, preventive medicine, self-care, holistic health, body systems and diseases, nutrition, fitness, pharmaceutical drugs. **Holdings:** 2000 books; 24 VF drawers of clippings; 2000 entries in Information and Reference System. **Subscriptions:** 58 journals and other serials.

★7452★ PROFESSIONAL SCHOOL OF PSYCHOLOGY
LIBRARY
2190 Sutter
San Francisco, CA 94115   Phone: (415) 563-9289
Alan Schut, Libn.
Subjects: Psychology - general, clinical, organizational. **Holdings:** 2800 books; dissertations. **Subscriptions:** 44 journals and other serials.

★7453★ ST. FRANCIS MEMORIAL HOSPITAL
WALTER F. SCHALLER MEMORIAL LIBRARY
Box 7726
San Francisco, CA 94120   Phone: (415) 775-4321
Maryann Zaremska, Dir., Lib.Serv.
Subjects: Medicine, nursing. **Holdings:** 6300 volumes; 650 audiotapes. **Subscriptions:** 145 journals and other serials and newspapers.

★7454★ ST. LUKE'S HOSPITAL
MEDICAL LIBRARY
3555 Army St.
San Francisco, CA 94110   Phone: (415) 647-8600
Laurie Bagley, Med.Libn.
Subjects: Medicine and nursing. **Holdings:** 2000 books; 4319 bound periodical volumes. **Subscriptions:** 106 journals and other serials.

★7455★ ST. MARY'S HOSPITAL AND MEDICAL CENTER
MEDICAL LIBRARY
450 Stanyan St.
San Francisco, CA 94117   Phone: (415) 750-5784
Rochelle Perrine Schmalz, Dir., Lib.Serv.
Subjects: Medicine, psychiatry, nursing, orthopedics, patient information. **Holdings:** 5250 books; 7800 bound periodical volumes; surgical, psychiatry, orthopedics, patient information audio and video cassettes. **Subscriptions:** 350 journals and other serials.

★7456★ SAN FRANCISCO GENERAL HOSPITAL MEDICAL
CENTER
BARNETT-BRIGGS LIBRARY
1001 Potrero Ave.
San Francisco, CA 94110   Phone: (415) 821-3113
Miriam Hirsch, Med.Libn.
Subjects: Medicine. **Holdings:** 13,985 books; 20,346 bound periodical volumes. **Subscriptions:** 420 journals and other serials.

★7457★ SMITH-KETTLEWELL EYE RESEARCH INSTITUTE
IN-HOUSE LIBRARY
2232 Webster St.
San Francisco, CA 94115   Phone: (415) 561-1620
Dr. Alex Cogan, Sci.
Subjects: Vision research and rehabilitation engineering. **Holdings:** 2000 volumes.

★7458★ STONE, MARRACCINI & PATTERSON
LIBRARY
1 Market Plaza
Spear St. Tower, Ste. 400
San Francisco, CA 94105   Phone: (415) 227-0100
Judy Borthwick, Libn.
Subjects: Health planning, health care facilities design, medical facility planning, architecture, population statistics, urban planning. **Holdings:** 7280 books; 2100 manufacturers' catalogs; codes; project specifications; 24 drawers of brochures, articles, clippings, reports. **Subscriptions:** 84 journals and other serials.

★7459★ U.S. ARMY
LETTERMAN ARMY INSTITUTE OF RESEARCH
HERMAN MEMORIAL LIBRARY
Bldg. 1110
Presidio of San Francisco
San Francisco, CA 94129-6800   Phone: (415) 561-2600
Richard Kempton
Subjects: Biomedicine, nutrition. **Holdings:** 5400 books; 20,000 bound periodical volumes; 2000 reports. **Subscriptions:** 410 journals and other serials.

★7460★ U.S. ARMY HOSPITALS
LETTERMAN ARMY MEDICAL CENTER
MEDICAL LIBRARY
Bldg. 1100, Rm. 338
Presidio of San Francisco
San Francisco, CA 94129-6700   Phone: (415) 561-2465
Dixie Meagher, Adm.Libn.
Subjects: Medicine, nursing, psychology, hospital administration, military medical history. **Holdings:** 5000 books; 30,000 bound periodical volumes. **Subscriptions:** 500 journals and other serials.

★7461★ U.S. DEPARTMENT OF VETERANS AFFAIRS
MEDICAL CENTER LIBRARY SERVICE
4150 Clement St., Bldg. 6
Rm. 209 E
San Francisco, CA 94121   Phone: (415) 221-4810
William Koch, Chf., Lib.Serv.
Subjects: Health sciences. **Holdings:** 5500 books; 20,000 bound periodical volumes. **Subscriptions:** 400 journals and other serials.

★7462★ U.S. ENVIRONMENTAL PROTECTION AGENCY
REGION 9 LIBRARY
75 Hawthorne St., 13th Fl.
San Francisco, CA 94105   Phone: (415) 774-1510
Linda Vida-Sunnen, Hd.Libn.
Subjects: Environment; water and air pollution; pesticides; hazardous waste; environmental health and law for California, Arizona, Nevada, Hawaii, and the Pacific Islands. **Holdings:** 4000 books; 250,000 reports; 300,000 reports on microfiche. **Subscriptions:** 250 journals and other serials.

★7463★ UNIVERSITY OF CALIFORNIA, SAN FRANCISCO
LIBRARY
530 Parnassus Ave.
San Francisco, CA 94143-0840   Phone: (415) 476-2334
Richard S. Cooper, Act.Univ.Libn.
Subjects: Health sciences, medicine, dentistry, pharmacy, nursing. **Holdings:** 687,069 volumes. **Subscriptions:** 5611 journals and other serials.

★7464★ UNIVERSITY OF CALIFORNIA, SAN FRANCISCO
MEDICAL LIBRARY
ORIENTAL COLLECTION
San Francisco, CA 94143-0840   Phone: (415) 476-8101
Atsumi Minami, Libn./Hd., Oriental Med.Coll.
Subjects: History of medicine in Japan and China; Chinese medicine; development of Western medicine in China and Japan. **Holdings:** 13,984 volumes; 1260 bound periodical volumes; 309 nonbook items. **Subscriptions:** 51 journals and other serials.

★7465★ UNIVERSITY OF CALIFORNIA, SAN FRANCISCO
MOUNT ZION MEDICAL CENTER
HARRIS M. FISHBON MEMORIAL LIBRARY
Box 7921
San Francisco, CA 94120   Phone: (415) 885-7378
Gail Sorrough, Dir.
Subjects: Medicine, geriatrics, cardiology, pediatrics, psychiatry. **Holdings:** 15,000 books; 30,000 bound periodical volumes; 1300 AV programs. **Subscriptions:** 350 journals and other serials.

★7466★ AMERICAN OTOLOGICAL SOCIETY
LIBRARY
2120 Forest Ave.
San Jose, CA 95128   Phone: (408) 288-7777
Mansfield F.W. Smith, M.D., Ed.-Libn.
Subjects: Otology. **Holdings:** 114 books; transactions of the American Otological Society.

★7467★ CALIFORNIA DEPARTMENT OF DEVELOPMENTAL SERVICES
STAFF LIBRARY
Agnews Developmental Center
3500 Zanker Rd.
San Jose, CA 95134   Phone: (408) 432-8500
Subjects: Mental retardation, developmental disabilities, neurology, psychology, psychiatric nursing, rehabilitation therapies. **Holdings:** 4000 books; 1020 bound periodical volumes; 125 videotapes. **Subscriptions:** 40 journals and other serials.

★7468★ O'CONNOR HOSPITAL
LIBRARY MEDIA CENTER
2105 Forest Ave.
San Jose, CA 95128   Phone: (408) 947-2950
Linda Hayes, Med.Libn.
Subjects: Medicine, nursing, administration. **Holdings:** 800 books; 234 bound periodical volumes; 200 audio cassettes; 40 filmstrips; 15 films; 77 slide cassettes; 240 video cassettes. **Subscriptions:** 128 journals and other serials.

★7469★ PARENTS HELPING PARENTS
SPECIAL CHILDREN'S RESOURCE CENTER
535 Race St., Ste. 220
San Jose, CA 95126   Phone: (408) 288-5010
June Wright, Libn.
Subjects: The welfare of children with physical, mental, emotional, or learning disabilities. **Holdings:** 800 volumes. **Subscriptions:** 80 journals and other serials.

★7470★ PLANETREE HEALTH RESOURCE CENTER
98 N. 17th St.
San Jose, CA 95112   Phone: (408) 977-4549
Candace Ford, Med.Dir./Libn.
Subjects: Consumer health information. **Holdings:** 2000 books; 18 VF drawers of clippings. **Subscriptions:** 25 journals and other serials.

★7471★ SAN JOSE MEDICAL CENTER
HEALTH SCIENCES LIBRARY
675 E. Santa Clara St.
San Jose, CA 95114   Phone: (408) 998-3212
Deloris Osby, Dir.
Subjects: Medicine, nursing, health care administration, family practice, allied health sciences, wellness. **Holdings:** 39,932 books; 12,000 bound periodical volumes; 12 VF drawers of pamphlets and clippings; 150 AV programs; 80 filmstrips; 19 films; 200 archival items. **Subscriptions:** 450 journals and other serials; 6 newspapers.

★7472★ SANTA CLARA COUNTY HEALTH DEPARTMENT
LIBRARY
2220 Moorpark Ave.
San Jose, CA 95128   Phone: (408) 299-6021
Felicia Angeles, Lib.Supv.
Subjects: Public health, psychology, nutrition, environmental health, medicine, alcoholism and drug abuse, AIDS, toxic substances, hazardous wastes. **Holdings:** 7000 books; 1200 bound periodical volumes; pamphlets; reprints; hearing reports; clippings. **Subscriptions:** 300 journals and other serials.

★7473★ SANTA CLARA VALLEY MEDICAL CENTER
MILTON J. CHATTON MEDICAL LIBRARY
751 S. Bascom Ave.
San Jose, CA 95128   Phone: (408) 299-5650
Shirley Kinoshita, Med.Libn.(Act.Dir.)
Subjects: Clinical medicine, nursing, pathology, physical medicine. **Holdings:** 4000 books; 25,000 bound periodical volumes. **Subscriptions:** 650 journals and other serials.

★7474★ TDS HEALTHCARE SYSTEMS CORPORATION
TECHNICAL LIBRARY
160 E. Tasman Dr.
San Jose, CA 95134   Phone: (408) 943-5619
Cheryl Caccialanza, Tech.Libn.
Subjects: Hospital information systems, physicians and computers. **Holdings:** 1300 books; 50 other cataloged items. **Subscriptions:** 98 journals and other serials.

★7475★ J2CP INFORMATION SERVICES
Box 184
San Juan Capistrano, CA 92693-0184   Phone: (714) 248-0443
Sr. Mary Elizabeth, SSE, Dir.
Subjects: Transsexualism, gender dysphoria syndrome. **Holdings:** 800 books.

★7476★ LIFE CHIROPRACTIC COLLEGE WEST
LIBRARY
2005 Via Barrett
San Lorenzo, CA 94580   Phone: (415) 276-9345
Marda Woodbury, Lib.Dir.
Subjects: Chiropractic, basic sciences, roentgenology, manipulative and physical therapy, medicine, health, musculoskeletal system. **Holdings:** 10,500 books; 2366 bound periodical volumes; 800 AV programs; 6000 vertical files. **Subscriptions:** 280 journals and other serials.

★7477★ MILLS-PENINSULA HOSPITALS
MILLS HOSPITAL
MEDICAL LIBRARY
100 S. San Mateo Dr.
San Mateo, CA 94401   Phone: (415) 696-4621
Sally Chu, Chf. of Lib.Serv.
Subjects: Medicine, nursing. **Holdings:** 1000 books; 2000 bound periodical volumes. **Subscriptions:** 152 journals and other serials.

★7478★ BROOKSIDE HOSPITAL
MEDICAL STAFF LIBRARY
2000 Vale Rd.
San Pablo, CA 94806   Phone: (415) 235-7000
Barbara T. Dorham, Libn.
Subjects: Medicine. **Holdings:** 500 books; 100 bound periodical volumes. **Subscriptions:** 152 journals and other serials.

★7479★ SAN PEDRO PENINSULA HOSPITAL
JOHN T. BURCH, M.D. MEMORIAL LIBRARY
1300 W. 7th St.
San Pedro, CA 90732-3593   Phone: (213) 832-3311
James H. Harlan, Lib.Cons.
Subjects: Clinical medicine, nursing. **Holdings:** 500 books; 1550 bound periodical volumes; 250 Audio-Digest tapes; 22 videotapes; 8 reels of microfilm. **Subscriptions:** 90 journals and other serials.

★7480★ MARIN GENERAL HOSPITAL
LIBRARY
Box 2129
San Rafael, CA 94912   Phone: (415) 925-7000
Katherine Renick, Libn.
Subjects: Medicine, psychiatry, nursing. **Holdings:** 1500 books; 2800 bound periodical volumes; 1 VF cabinet of pamphlets; 8 shelves of documents. **Subscriptions:** 130 journals and other serials.

★7481★ HUMAN FACTOR PROGRAMS
LIBRARY
1125 E. 17th St., Ste. E-209
Santa Ana, CA 92701   Phone: (714) 972-0117
Linda Garcia, Dir. of Res.
Subjects: Behavioral medicine, biofeedback, forensic psychology, hypnosis, medical psychology, stress, allied health sciences. **Holdings:** 8000 books, reprints, bound journals.

★7482★ ORANGE COUNTY SHERIFF/CORONER
FORENSIC SCIENCE SERVICES LIBRARY
550 N. Flower St.
Box 449
Santa Ana, CA 92702   Phone: (714) 834-4540
Mr. Frank Fitzpatrick, Lab.Dir.
Subjects: Chemistry, criminalistics, toxicology, forensic medicine, investigation. **Holdings:** 2600 books; 4 VF drawers of catalogs and brochures; 2 VF drawers of lab equipment manuals; 3200 reprints; 22 videotapes; 3 boxes of microfiche and microfilm. **Subscriptions:** 71 journals and other serials.

★7483★ WESTERN MEDICAL CENTER
MEDICAL LIBRARY
1001 N. Tustin Ave.
Santa Ana, CA 92705   Phone: (714) 835-3555
Phyllis Dowling, Dir.
Subjects: Medicine, nursing, surgery. **Holdings:** 4800 books; 5000 bound periodical volumes; 2300 Audio-Digest tapes (9 specialties); video cassettes. **Subscriptions:** 260 journals and other serials.

★7484★ COTTAGE HOSPITAL
DAVID L. REEVES MEDICAL LIBRARY
Box 689
Santa Barbara, CA 93102   Phone: (805) 569-7240
Lucy Thomas, Lib.Dir.
Subjects: Medicine, surgery. **Holdings:** 4000 books; 6800 bound periodical volumes; 1000 other cataloged items. **Subscriptions:** 200 journals and other serials.

★7485★ INFOMART RESEARCH SERVICES
LIBRARY
PO Box 629
Santa Barbara, CA 93102   Phone: (805) 965-5555
Subjects: Medicine, technology. **Holdings:** 200 volumes; 4000 microfiche.

★7486★ ST. FRANCIS HOSPITAL
MEDICAL LIBRARY
601 E. Micheltorena
Santa Barbara, CA 93103   Phone: (805) 962-7661
Marilyn Shearer, Dir.
Subjects: Medicine and medical specialties. **Holdings:** 1020 books; 469 bound periodical volumes; videotapes; cassettes. **Subscriptions:** 38 journals and other serials.

★7487★ BAXTER HEALTHCARE CORPORATION
PHARMASEAL DIVISION
INFORMATION CENTER
27200 N. Tourney Rd.
Box 5900
Santa Clarita, CA 91355   Phone: (805) 253-1300
Eloise A. Richer, Mgr., Info./Trng.Serv.
Subjects: Medicine, applied technology, business, basic sciences. **Holdings:** 2300 books; 1100 reports and pamphlets; 21,000 patents; 27 periodicals in microform. **Subscriptions:** 240 journals and other serials.

★7488★ DOMINICAN SANTA CRUZ HOSPITAL
MEDICAL LIBRARY
1555 Soquel Dr.
Santa Cruz, CA 95065   Phone: (408) 462-7738
Candace Walker, Med.Libn.
Subjects: Medicine, nursing, health. **Holdings:** 1000 books; 2500 bound periodical volumes; 500 videotapes. **Subscriptions:** 75 journals and other serials.

★7489★ ST. JOHN'S HOSPITAL AND HEALTH CENTER
HOSPITAL LIBRARY
1328 22nd St.
Santa Monica, CA 90404   Phone: (213) 829-8494
Cathey L. Pinckney, Libn.
Subjects: Medicine, nursing, and hospital administration. **Holdings:** 5878 books; 2706 bound periodical volumes; 3142 unbound journal volumes. **Subscriptions:** 321 journals and other serials.

★7490★ SANTA MONICA HOSPITAL MEDICAL CENTER
LIBRARY
1250 16th St.
Santa Monica, CA 90404   Phone: (213) 319-4000
Lenore F. Orfirer, Libn.
Subjects: Medicine. **Holdings:** 1600 books; 1025 bound periodical volumes; 2250 unbound periodical volumes; 275 video cassettes. **Subscriptions:** 125 journals and other serials.

★7491★ COMMUNITY HOSPITAL
MEDICAL LIBRARY
3325 Chanate Rd.
Santa Rosa, CA 95404   Phone: (707) 576-4675
Joan Chilton, Med.Libn.
Subjects: Medicine. **Holdings:** 3000 books; 6500 bound periodical vol-

umes; Audio-Digest tapes; video cassettes. **Subscriptions:** 215 journals and other serials.

★7492★ HEALTH OCCUPATIONS CENTER
LIBRARY
8756 Mast Blvd.
Santee, CA 92071   Phone: (619) 579-4793
Kathleen A. Johnson
Subjects: Nursing, medicine, dentistry. **Holdings:** 2100 books. **Subscriptions:** 40 journals and other serials.

★7493★ INSTITUTE OF NOETIC SCIENCES
LIBRARY
475 Gate Five Rd., Ste. 300
Sausalito, CA 94965   Phone: (415) 331-5650
Nola D. Lewis, Res.Asst.
Subjects: Psychology and cognitive sciences, health and biomedical sciences, neurosciences, social issues, futures studies, religion and philosophy, education and training. **Holdings:** 1200 books; 12 VF drawers of unbound reports, manuscripts, clippings, documents. **Subscriptions:** 50 journals and other serials.

★7494★ WORLD RESEARCH FOUNDATION
LIBRARY
15300 Ventura Blvd., Ste. 405
Sherman Oaks, CA 91403   Phone: (818) 907-5483
Subjects: Health and the environment, health tools and technologies available outside the United States. **Holdings:** 10,000 volumes.

★7495★ INSPIRATION UNIVERSITY
LIBRARY
1 Campbell Hot Springs Rd.
Sierraville, CA 96126-0234   Phone: (916) 994-3737
Leonard Orr, Owner
Subjects: Physical immortality, rebirthing, prosperity, gentle childbirth, energy breathing. **Holdings:** 500 books; 20 cassette tapes; 3 videotapes; 33 other cataloged items. **Subscriptions:** 10 journals and other serials; 5 newspapers.

★7496★ ISLAMIC LIBRARY ASSOCIATION
LIBRARY
6304 Cory St.
Simi Valley, CA 93063   Phone: (805) 526-3999
Rasheed H. Moinuddin, Sec.
Subjects: Medicine, engineering, technology, science, pure and applied sciences. **Holdings:** Figures not available.

★7497★ GEOSCIENCE, LTD.
LIBRARY
410 S. Cedros Ave.
Solana Beach, CA 92075   Phone: (619) 755-9396
Subjects: Mathematics, physics, medicine. **Holdings:** 700 volumes.

★7498★ KAISER-PERMANENTE MEDICAL CENTER
SOUTH SAN FRANCISCO HEALTH SCIENCES LIBRARY
1200 El Camino Real
South San Francisco, CA 94080   Phone: (415) 742-2540
Sara Pimental, Health Sci.Libn.
Subjects: Medicine and nursing. **Holdings:** 1000 books; 2000 bound periodical volumes. **Subscriptions:** 160 journals and other serials.

★7499★ STANFORD UNIVERSITY
LANE MEDICAL LIBRARY
Stanford University Medical Center
Stanford, CA 94305-5323   Phone: (415) 723-6831
Peter Stangl, Dir.
Subjects: Clinical medicine and its specialties, preclinical and basic sciences, public health, nursing and allied fields. **Holdings:** 308,503 volumes; 28,648 pamphlets and theses; 1816 audio recordings; 687 videotapes and cassettes; 165 computer materials. **Subscriptions:** 3272 journals and other serials; 6 newspapers.

★7500★ ST. JOSEPH'S MEDICAL CENTER
LIBRARY
1800 N. California St.
Stockton, CA 95204   Phone: (209) 467-6332
Colleen Lamkin, Lib.Coord.
Subjects: Medicine, nursing, hospital administration, human relations.
Holdings: 400 books; 840 bound periodical volumes; 50 video cassettes.
Subscriptions: 140 journals and other serials.

★7501★ STOCKTON DEVELOPMENTAL CENTER
STAFF LIBRARY
510 E. Magnolia St.
Stockton, CA 95202   Phone: (209) 948-7181
Walter Greening, Sr.Libn.
Subjects: Mentally handicapped, mentally ill, behavior therapy, child psychiatry, community mental health, psychiatric nursing. **Holdings:** 6700 books; 1200 bound periodical volumes; 158 reels of microfilm of periodicals; 300 audiotapes. **Subscriptions:** 100 journals and other serials.

★7502★ UNIVERSITY OF THE PACIFIC
SCIENCE LIBRARY
Stockton, CA 95211   Phone: (209) 946-2940
Judith K. Andrews, Sci.Libn.
Subjects: Pharmacy and pharmacology, medicine, chemistry, drug information. **Holdings:** 17,770 books; 23,000 bound periodical volumes; 82,745 index cards; 1600 reels of microfilm; 9478 microcards; 12,000 microfiche. **Subscriptions:** 371 journals and other serials.

★7503★ PALMER COLLEGE OF CHIROPRACTIC, WEST
LIBRARY
1095 Dunford Way
Sunnyvale, CA 94087   Phone: (408) 983-4142
Patricia McGrew, Dir.
Subjects: Chiropractic, health sciences, medicine, basic sciences, education. **Holdings:** 6300 books; 2750 bound periodical volumes; 600 AV programs; 30,000 microfiche; periodicals. **Subscriptions:** 200 journals and other serials.

★7504★ SOLA/BARNES-HIND
TECHNICAL LIBRARY AND INFORMATION CENTER
810 Kifer Rd.
Sunnyvale, CA 94086   Phone: (408) 991-6435
Sidney C. Frederick, Tech.Libn.
Subjects: Contact lens products, glaucoma drug research, cataract drug research, polymer science, ophthalmology. **Holdings:** 1400 books; 65,000 bound periodical volumes; 1000 internal reports; 800 lab notebooks; 4000 patents; 200 reels of microfilm. **Subscriptions:** 311 journals and other serials.

★7505★ LOS ANGELES COUNTY/OLIVE VIEW MEDICAL
 HEALTH CENTER
HEALTH SCIENCES LIBRARY
14445 Olive View Dr., 2C 160
Sylmar, CA 91343   Phone: (818) 364-4241
Miriam Kafka, Act.Libn.
Subjects: Dentistry, internal medicine, ophthalmology, emergency medicine, obstetrics/gynecology, pathology, pediatrics, psychiatry, perinatology, radiology/nuclear medicine, surgery. **Holdings:** 3000 books; 7000 bound periodical volumes. **Subscriptions:** 480 journals and other serials.

★7506★ LOS ANGELES COUNTY/HARBOR-UCLA MEDICAL
 CENTER
A.F. PARLOW LIBRARY OF THE HEALTH SCIENCES
1000 W. Carson St.
Box 18
Torrance, CA 90509   Phone: (213) 533-2373
Mary Ann Berliner, Dir., Lib.Serv.
Subjects: Medicine, nursing, dentistry, patient education, administration. **Holdings:** 21,653 books; 24,268 bound periodical volumes; 3000 pamphlet titles; 453 reels of microfilm; 850 AV programs. **Subscriptions:** 866 journals and other serials.

★7507★ TORRANCE MEMORIAL MEDICAL CENTER
MEDICAL LIBRARY
3330 W. Lomita Blvd.
Torrance, CA 90509   Phone: (213) 517-4720
Anita N. Klecker, Med.Libn.
Subjects: Medicine, surgery, cardiology, pediatrics, nursing, psychiatry,

oncology. **Holdings:** 433 books; 221 Audio-Digest tapes; 27 videotapes. **Subscriptions:** 116 journals and other serials.

★7508★ U.S. AIR FORCE HOSPITAL
DAVID GRANT MEDICAL CENTER
MEDICAL LIBRARY
Travis AFB, CA 94535   Phone: (707) 423-7963
V. Kay Hafner, Med.Libn./Dir.
Subjects: Medicine, family practice, dentistry, nursing. **Holdings:** 4615 books; 12,836 bound periodical volumes. **Subscriptions:** 500 journals and other serials.

★7509★ EMANUEL MEDICAL CENTER
MEDICAL LIBRARY
825 Delbon Ave.
Box 2120
Turlock, CA 95381-2120   Phone: (209) 667-4200
Donna Cardoza, Lib.Ck.
Subjects: Medicine, allied health sciences. **Holdings:** 836 books; 210 bound periodical volumes. **Subscriptions:** 115 journals and other serials.

★7510★ MEDIC ALERT FOUNDATION INTERNATIONAL
CENTRAL REFERENCE FILE OF MEMBERSHIP
2323 Colorado
Turlock, CA 95380   Phone: (209) 668-3333
Kenneth W. Harms, Pres.
Holdings: Figures not available.

★7511★ SAN ANTONIO COMMUNITY HOSPITAL
WEBER MEMORIAL LIBRARY
999 San Bernardino Rd.
Upland, CA 91786   Phone: (714) 920-4972
Francena Johnston, Med.Libn.
Subjects: Medicine, health services management, allied health sciences. **Holdings:** 4800 books; 3150 bound periodical volumes; 1715 other cataloged items; 1031 audio cassettes; 550 Audio-Digest tapes; 450 videotapes; 100 filmstrip/cassette sets; 15 films. **Subscriptions:** 620 journals and other serials; 17 newspapers.

★7512★ CALIFORNIA STATE MEDICAL FACILITY
MEDICAL STAFF LIBRARY
1600 California Dr.
Vacaville, CA 95696   Phone: (707) 448-6841
Victoria Bayubay, Libn.
Subjects: Psychiatry, medicine, surgery, penology, criminology, psychology, social work, nursing, hospital administration. **Holdings:** 6000 books; 130 bound periodical volumes; research materials relating to criminology and case work; reports from other state and national agencies; releases from federal, state, local agencies interested in inmate care and welfare and community adjustment. **Subscriptions:** 149 journals and other serials.

★7513★ CALRECO, INC.
LIBRARY
8015 Van Nuys Blvd.
Van Nuys, CA 91412   Phone: (818) 376-4217
Kathryn A. Stewart, Sr.Libn.
Subjects: Food science, nutrition, chemistry, biological science. **Holdings:** 5000 books; 5170 bound periodical volumes; 27,000 reprints, government reports, pieces of miscellanea; 7200 patents. **Subscriptions:** 300 journals and other serials.

★7514★ SMITHKLINE BEECHAM CLINICAL LABORATORIES
LIBRARY
7600 Tyrone Ave.
Van Nuys, CA 91405   Phone: (818) 376-6270
Edward Kaufman, Info.Spec.
Subjects: Clinical chemistry, microbiology, endocrinology and immunology, business management. **Holdings:** 2000 books; 5000 bound periodical volumes; 200 doctors' papers written at laboratories. **Subscriptions:** 125 journals and other serials.

★7515★ VALLEY PRESBYTERIAN HOSPITAL
RICHARD O. MYERS LIBRARY
15107 Vanowen St.
Box 9102
Van Nuys, CA 91409-9102   Phone: (818) 902-2973
Francine Kubrin, Dir.Lib.Serv.
Subjects: General medicine, general surgery, nursing, hospital administra-

tion. **Holdings:** 5000 volumes; 500 audio cassettes; 1 VF drawer of pamphlets, bibliographies, and reprints; 1 VF drawer of AV catalogs. **Subscriptions:** 365 journals and other serials.

★7516★ **KAWEAH DELTA DISTRICT HOSPITAL**
LIBRARY
400 W. Mineral King Ave.
Visalia, CA 93291   Phone: (209) 625-7216
Jeannine M. Hinkel, Lib.Dir.
Subjects: Clinical medicine, nursing, hospital administration. **Holdings:** 2000 books. **Subscriptions:** 250 journals and other serials.

★7517★ **JOHN MUIR MEDICAL CENTER**
MEDICAL LIBRARY
1601 Ygnacio Valley Rd.
Walnut Creek, CA 94598   Phone: (510) 939-3000
Helen M. Reyes, Med.Libn.
Subjects: Health sciences, medicine, dentistry, nursing, pharmacy, hospital administration, psychiatry, allied health sciences. **Holdings:** 3280 books; 5200 bound periodical volumes. **Subscriptions:** 380 journals and other serials.

★7518★ **LOS ANGELES COLLEGE OF CHIROPRACTIC**
SEABURY MCCOY LIBRARY
16200 E. Amber Valley Dr.
Whittier, CA 90604   Phone: (213) 947-8755
Nehmat Ghandour Saab, Dir., Lib.Serv.
Subjects: Human spine and allied structures, chiropractic medicine, basic and clinical sciences, naturopathy. **Holdings:** 12,500 books; 3000 bound periodical volumes; 28,200 microfiche; VF materials. **Subscriptions:** 500 journals and other serials.

★7519★ **VETERANS HOME OF CALIFORNIA**
WILLIAM K. MURPHY MEMORIAL HEALTH SCIENCE
LIBRARY
Yountville, CA 94599   Phone: (707) 944-4715
Cynthia Hegedus, Libn.
Subjects: Medicine. **Holdings:** 1197 books; 118 bound periodical volumes. **Subscriptions:** 128 journals and other serials.

Colorado

★7520★ **U.S. ARMY HOSPITALS**
FITZSIMONS ARMY MEDICAL CENTER
MEDICAL-TECHNICAL LIBRARY HSHG-ZBM
Aurora, CO 80045-5000   Phone: (303) 361-3378
Alfreda H. Hanna, Adm.Libn.
Subjects: Medicine and allied health sciences. **Holdings:** 12,000 books; 27,000 bound periodical volumes. **Subscriptions:** 830 journals and other serials.

★7521★ **DORMANT BRAIN RESEARCH AND DEVELOPMENT**
LABORATORY
LIBRARY
Laughing Coyote Mountain
Box 10
Black Hawk, CO 80422
Mr. T.D. Lingo, Dir.
Subjects: Neural cybernetics. **Holdings:** 5000 volumes.

★7522★ **BOULDER COMMUNITY HOSPITAL**
MEDICAL LIBRARY
PO Box 9019
Boulder, CO 80301   Phone: (303) 440-2273
Teri Manzanares, Med.Libn.
Subjects: Clinical medicine. **Holdings:** 400 books; 1200 bound periodical volumes. **Subscriptions:** 98 journals and other serials.

★7523★ **CENTER FOR APPLIED PREVENTION RESEARCH**
LIBRARY
4760 Walnut St., Ste. 106
Boulder, CO 80301   Phone: (303) 443-5696
Tessa Davis
Subjects: Substance abuse prevention. **Holdings:** 2500 books; 500 reports. **Subscriptions:** 100 journals and other serials.

★7524★ **CHEYENNE MOUNTAIN ZOOLOGICAL PARK**
LIBRARY
4250 Cheyenne Mt. Zoo Rd.
Colorado Springs, CO 80906   Phone: (719) 633-9927
Kevin P. Tanski, Educ.Cur.
Subjects: Zoology, biology, veterinary medicine, botany. **Holdings:** 550 books; zoo publications. **Subscriptions:** 16 journals and other serials.

★7525★ **COLORADO SCHOOL FOR THE DEAF AND THE**
BLIND
MEDIA CENTER
33 N. Institute St.
Colorado Springs, CO 80903   Phone: (719) 578-2206
Janet L. Fleharty, Media Spec.
Subjects: Books of interest to deaf and blind children; professional books on deafness and blindness for staff and parents. **Holdings:** 10,000 books; 200 periodical volumes. **Subscriptions:** 51 journals and other serials.

★7526★ **MEMORIAL HOSPITAL**
HEALTH SCIENCES LIBRARY
1400 E. Boulder
Colorado Springs, CO 80909   Phone: (719) 475-5182
Rebecca Berg, Dir.
Subjects: Medicine, nursing, allied health. **Holdings:** 3000 books; 25,000 bound periodical volumes. **Subscriptions:** 300 journals and other serials.

★7527★ **PENROSE HOSPITAL**
WEBB MEMORIAL LIBRARY
2215 N. Cascade Ave.
Box 7021
Colorado Springs, CO 80933   Phone: (719) 630-5288
Nina Janes, Dir.
Subjects: Medicine, hospital administration. **Holdings:** 1000 books; 12,000 bound periodical volumes. **Subscriptions:** 500 journals and other serials.

★7528★ **U.S. OLYMPIC COMMITTEE**
OLYMPIC RESOURCE AND INFORMATION CENTER
Dept. Information Resources
1750 E. Boulder St.
Colorado Springs, CO 80909   Phone: (719) 578-4622
Cindy Slater, Mgr., Dept.Info.Rsrcs.
Subjects: Sports medicine - exercise physiology, biomechanics, sports psychology, vision and dental screening, athletic training, injury prevention and treatment, health maintenance and conditioning, coaching science. **Holdings:** 3500 books; unbound periodicals; 2000 reprints; sports rulebooks; U.S. Olympic Committee central files of photographs, slides, and 16mm films; N.G.B. constitutions and by-laws. **Subscriptions:** 400 journals and other serials; 5 newspapers.

★7529★ **AMC CANCER RESEARCH CENTER**
MEDICAL LIBRARY
1600 Pierce St.
Denver, CO 80214   Phone: (303) 239-3368
Eleanor Krakauer, Libn.
Subjects: Cancer - research, prevention, control. **Holdings:** 4000 books; 5500 bound periodical volumes; 8 VF drawers of pamphlets. **Subscriptions:** 180 journals and other serials.

★7530★ **ASSOCIATION OF OPERATING ROOM NURSES**
LIBRARY
10170 E. Mississippi Ave.
Denver, CO 80231   Phone: (303) 755-6300
Sara Katsh, Hd.Libn.
Subjects: Nursing, surgery. **Holdings:** 3300 books; 1500 bound periodical volumes. **Subscriptions:** 300 journals and other serials.

★7531★ **BETHESDA PSYCHEALTH SYSTEM**
PROFESSIONAL LIBRARY
4400 E. Iliff Ave.
Denver, CO 80222   Phone: (303) 758-1514
Nancy L. Jones, Staff Dev.Coord.
Subjects: Medicine, psychiatry, psychology, nursing, management. **Holdings:** 800 books. **Subscriptions:** 18 journals and other serials.

★7532★ C. HENRY KEMPE NATIONAL CENTER FOR THE PREVENTION AND TREATMENT OF CHILD ABUSE AND NEGLECT
LIBRARY
University of Colorado Health Sciences Center
Department of Pediatrics
1205 Oneida
Denver, CO 80220-2944   Phone: (303) 321-3963
Subjects: Child abuse - diagnosis, prevention, treatment, intervention; sexual abuse; parenting. **Holdings:** Books; bound periodical volumes; reports; files. **Subscriptions:** 6 journals and other serials.

★7533★ CHILDREN'S HOSPITAL
FORBES MEDICAL LIBRARY
1056 E. 19th Ave.
Denver, CO 80218   Phone: (303) 861-6400
Anne S. Klenk, Med.Libn.
Subjects: Pediatrics, nursing with emphasis on pediatrics, nonprofessional information on child care and common childhood diseases. **Holdings:** 3500 books; 5000 bound periodical volumes. **Subscriptions:** 320 journals and other serials.

★7534★ COLORADO DEPARTMENT OF EDUCATION
INSTRUCTIONAL MATERIALS CENTER FOR THE VISUALLY HANDICAPPED
201 E. Colfax Ave.
Denver, CO 80203   Phone: (303) 866-6860
W. Buck Schrotberger, Sr.Cons.
Holdings: Figures not available.

★7535★ COLORADO DEPARTMENT OF SOCIAL SERVICE
LIBRARY
1575 Sherman St.
Denver, CO 80203-1714   Phone: (303) 866-4086
Dorothy B. Shaughnessy, Libn.
Subjects: Social work, public and social welfare, psychology, sociology, child welfare, adoption, foster care, aged, child development, handicapped, crime and juvenile delinquency, group work and community organizations. **Holdings:** 9235 volumes; 3 VF drawers of pamphlets; 259 AV software programs. **Subscriptions:** 82 journals and other serials.

★7536★ DENVER GENERAL HOSPITAL
MEDICAL LIBRARY
777 Bannock St.
Denver, CO 80204-4507   Phone: (303) 893-7422
Anita F. Westwood, Dir., Med.Lib.
Subjects: Clinical medicine, nursing, surgery. **Holdings:** 2500 books; 10,500 bound periodical volumes. **Subscriptions:** 204 journals.

★7537★ DENVER MEDICAL LIBRARY
1719 E. 19th Ave.
Denver, CO 80218   Phone: (303) 839-6670
Mary De Mund, Lib.Dir.
Subjects: Medicine, dentistry, history of medicine, nursing, socioeconomics, health administration. **Holdings:** 7272 books; 27,200 bound periodical volumes. **Subscriptions:** 400 journals and other serials.

★7538★ DENVER ZOOLOGICAL GARDEN
LIBRARY
2300 E. 23rd Ave.
Denver, CO 80205   Phone: (303) 331-4114
John Wortman, Gen.Cur.
Subjects: Animal husbandry, endangered species, natural history, veterinary medicine, business. **Holdings:** 1500 books; 150 bound periodical volumes; 2000 annual reports, guidebooks from other zoos, other cataloged items. **Subscriptions:** 150 journals and other serials.

★7539★ FORT LOGAN MENTAL HEALTH CENTER
MEDICAL LIBRARY
3520 W. Oxford Ave.
Denver, CO 80236   Phone: (303) 762-4388
Kathleen Elder, Dir., Lib.Serv.
Subjects: Social psychiatry - social work, therapeutic community work, day hospital care; psychiatry; psychology; behavioral sciences. **Holdings:** 5000 books; 3213 bound periodical volumes. **Subscriptions:** 97 journals and other serials.

★7540★ MANVILLE CORPORATION
HS & E/TECHNICAL INFORMATION CENTER
PO Box 5108
Denver, CO 80217   Phone: (303) 978-5200
Barbara Norton, Dir.
Subjects: Occupational health, toxicology, industrial hygiene and safety, pollution, carcinogens. **Holdings:** 1000 books. **Subscriptions:** 164 journals and other serials.

★7541★ MERCY MEDICAL CENTER
HOSPITAL LIBRARY
1650 Fillmore St.
Denver, CO 80206   Phone: (303) 393-3296
Peggy Edwards, Libn.
Subjects: Medicine, nursing, hospital administration. **Holdings:** 2000 books; 4000 bound periodical volumes. **Subscriptions:** 250 journals and other serials.

★7542★ NATIONAL ENVIRONMENTAL HEALTH ASSOCIATION
LIBRARY
720 S. Colorado Blvd., Ste. 970, S. Tower
Denver, CO 80222   Phone: (303) 756-9090
Subjects: Environmental health concerns, environmental protection. **Holdings:** 1000 volumes.

★7543★ NATIONAL JEWISH CENTER FOR IMMUNOLOGY AND RESPIRATORY MEDICINE
GERALD TUCKER MEMORIAL MEDICAL LIBRARY
1400 Jackson St.
Denver, CO 80206   Phone: (303) 398-1483
Rosalind F. Dudden, Libn.
Subjects: Respiratory diseases, molecular and cellular biology, immunology, allergy, asthma, tuberculosis. **Holdings:** 3000 books; 10,500 bound periodical volumes. **Subscriptions:** 340 journals and other serials.

★7544★ PORTER MEMORIAL HOSPITAL
HARLEY E. RICE MEMORIAL LIBRARY
2525 S. Downing St.
Denver, CO 80210   Phone: (303) 778-5656
W. Robin Waters, Dir.
Subjects: Medicine. **Holdings:** 2250 books; 6500 bound periodical volumes; 125 audiotapes; 4 VF drawers. **Subscriptions:** 395 journals and other serials.

★7545★ ROSE MEDICAL CENTER
LIBRARY
4567 E. 9th Ave.
Denver, CO 80220   Phone: (303) 320-2160
Nancy Simon, Med.Libn.
Subjects: Medicine. **Holdings:** 1000 books; 2989 bound periodical volumes; 257 Audio-Digest tapes. **Subscriptions:** 197 journals and other serials.

★7546★ ST. ANTHONY HOSPITAL SYSTEMS
MEMORIAL MEDICAL LIBRARY
4231 W. 16th Ave.
Denver, CO 80204   Phone: (303) 629-3790
Christine Yolanda Crespin, Supv.Libn.
Subjects: Emergency medicine, trauma, critical care, allied health sciences. **Holdings:** 1000 books; 3500 bound periodical volumes; 50 pamphlets. **Subscriptions:** 254 journals and other serials.

★7547★ ST. JOSEPH HOSPITAL
HEALTH REACH PATIENT AND COMMUNITY LIBRARY
1835 Franklin St.
Denver, CO 80218   Phone: (303) 837-7188
Margaret Bandy, Libn.
Subjects: Consumer health. **Holdings:** 600 books. **Subscriptions:** 15 journals and other serials.

★7548★ ST. JOSEPH HOSPITAL
HEALTH SCIENCES LIBRARY
1835 Franklin St.
Denver, CO 80218   Phone: (303) 837-7188
Margaret Bandy, Libn.
Subjects: Medicine, nursing, hospital management. **Holdings:** 2800 books; pamphlets. **Subscriptions:** 208 journals and other serials.

★7549★ ST. LUKE'S HOSPITAL
HEALTH SCIENCES LIBRARY
601 E. 19th Ave.
Denver, CO 80203   Phone: (303) 869-2395
Lisa Traditi, Dir.
Subjects: Medicine, nursing, oncology, geriatrics, womens' health, cardiology, pediatrics, neonatology, transplantation. **Holdings:** 2599 books; 5815 bound periodical volumes. **Subscriptions:** 247 journals and other serials.

★7550★ U.S. DEPARTMENT OF VETERANS AFFAIRS
LIBRARY SERVICE
1055 Clermont St.
Denver, CO 80220   Phone: (303) 393-2821
Deborah A. Thompson, Chf., Lib.Serv.
Subjects: Medicine and allied clinical sciences. **Holdings:** 3000 books; 5000 bound periodical volumes; 200 pamphlets. **Subscriptions:** 250 journals and other serials.

★7551★ UNIVERSITY OF COLORADO HEALTH SCIENCES
CENTER
DENISON MEMORIAL LIBRARY
4200 E. 9th Ave.
Denver, CO 80262   Phone: (303) 270-5125
Charles Bandy, Dir.
Subjects: Medicine, nursing, dentistry, allied health sciences. **Holdings:** 85,698 books; 131,945 bound periodical volumes; 3505 AV programs; 194 computer software titles. **Subscriptions:** 2112 journals and other serials.

★7552★ UNIVERSITY OF COLORADO HEALTH SCIENCES
CENTER
RENE A. SPITZ PSYCHIATRIC LIBRARY
4200 E. 9th Ave., C-249
Denver, CO 80262   Phone: (303) 394-7039
Irwin Berry, Libn.
Subjects: Psychiatry, psychoanalysis. **Holdings:** 2900 books; 350 bound periodical volumes; 2550 unbound journals; 100 cassettes. **Subscriptions:** 15 journals and other serials.

★7553★ AMERICAN HUMANE ASSOCIATION
AMERICAN ASSOCIATION FOR PROTECTING CHILDREN
NATIONAL RESOURCE CENTER ON CHILD ABUSE AND
NEGLECT
63 Inverness Dr., E.
Englewood, CO 80112-5117   Phone: (303) 792-9900
Robyn Alsop, Coord.Info.Serv.
Subjects: Children - abuse, neglect, sexual abuse; risk assessment; case decisionmaking; staffing; caseload management; community resource integration; reasonable efforts. **Holdings:** 1000 books; 5 VF drawers of subject files; 5 VF drawers of organizations; 50 state child protective service newsletters. **Subscriptions:** 100 journals and other serials.

★7554★ MEDICAL GROUP MANAGEMENT ASSOCIATION
LIBRARY RESOURCE CENTER
104 Inverness Terr., E.
Englewood, CO 80112-5306   Phone: (303) 799-1111
Barbara U. Hamilton, Dir.
Subjects: Group practice administration and statistics; health maintenance organizations; ambulatory care administration; medical clinic architectural design and construction; managed care. **Holdings:** 5000 books; 900 folders of VF material. **Subscriptions:** 200 journals and other serials.

★7555★ MORRIS ANIMAL FOUNDATION
LIBRARY
45 Inverness Dr., E.
Englewood, CO 80112   Phone: (303) 790-2345
Jack Carpenter, Dev.Coord.
Subjects: Veterinary medicine, zoo medicine. **Holdings:** 500 books. **Subscriptions:** 75 journals and other serials; 5 newspapers.

★7556★ NATIONAL STROKE ASSOCIATION
STROKE INFORMATION AND REFERRAL CENTER
300 E. Hampden Ave., Ste. 240
Englewood, CO 80110-2622   Phone: (303) 762-9922
Thelma Edwards, RN, Dir., Prog.Dev.
Subjects: Stroke - prevention, medical care, rehabilitation, research, resocialization. **Holdings:** 100 books; 10 videotapes; 85 booklets, brochures, articles; 20 VF drawers. **Subscriptions:** 100 newspapers and newsletters.

★7557★ PAUL DE HAEN INTERNATIONAL, INC.
DRUG INFORMATION SYSTEMS AND SERVICES
2750 S. Shoshone St.
Englewood, CO 80110   Phone: (303) 781-6683
Harold L. Bober, Pres.
Subjects: Drug and biomedical information. **Holdings:** 500 books; 200,000 scientific reports from international biomedical literature. **Subscriptions:** 1250 journals and other serials.

★7558★ SWEDISH MEDICAL CENTER
LIBRARY
501 E. Hampden Ave., Dept. 8640
Box 2901
Englewood, CO 80110-0101   Phone: (303) 788-6616
Sandra Parker, Dir., Lib.Serv.
Subjects: Neurosciences, medicine, nursing, health administration, rehabilitation, spinal cord/head injuries. **Holdings:** 1500 books; 2500 bound periodical volumes; 1110 unbound periodicals. **Subscriptions:** 350 journals and other serials.

★7559★ U.S. ARMY HOSPITALS
EVANS ARMY COMMUNITY HOSPITAL
MEDICAL LIBRARY
Bldg. 7500
Fort Carson, CO 80913   Phone: (719) 579-7286
Roma A. Marcum, Act.Med.Libn.
Subjects: Medicine, nursing, allied health sciences, patient health education. **Holdings:** 4000 books; 13,000 bound periodical volumes; 360 AV programs; 9964 audiotapes. **Subscriptions:** 390 journals and other serials.

★7560★ COLORADO STATE UNIVERSITY
VETERINARY TEACHING HOSPITAL
BRANCH LIBRARY
300 W. Drake Rd.
Fort Collins, CO 80523   Phone: (303) 491-1213
Elizabeth A. Fuseler-McDowell, Hd., Sci./Tech.Dept.
Subjects: Veterinary medicine. **Holdings:** 1463 books; 3000 bound periodical volumes. **Subscriptions:** 175 journals and other serials.

★7561★ POUDRE VALLEY HOSPITAL
MEDICAL LIBRARY
1024 Lemay Ave.
Fort Collins, CO 80524   Phone: (303) 490-4155
Jerry Carlson, Med.Libn.
Subjects: Medicine, nursing. **Holdings:** 3000 books; 3500 bound periodical volumes. **Subscriptions:** 225 journals and other serials.

★7562★ U.S. DEPARTMENT OF VETERANS AFFAIRS
MEDICAL LIBRARY
VA Medical Center
Fort Lyon, CO 81038   Phone: (303) 456-1260
Helen S. Bradley, Chf., Lib.Serv.
Subjects: Psychiatry, nursing, geriatrics. **Holdings:** Figures not available.

★7563★ DR. E.H. MUNRO MEDICAL LIBRARY
St. Mary's Hospital & Medical Center
PO Box 1628
Grand Junction, CO 81502-1628   Phone: (303) 244-2171
Joan E. Paine, Dir.
Subjects: Medicine, nursing. **Holdings:** 1000 books. **Subscriptions:** 202 journals and other serials.

★7564★ U.S. DEPARTMENT OF VETERANS AFFAIRS
MEDICAL CENTER MEDICAL LIBRARY
2121 North Ave.
Grand Junction, CO 81501   Phone: (303) 242-0731
Lynn L. Bragdon, Chf., Lib.Serv.
Subjects: Medicine, surgery. **Holdings:** 1200 books; 900 bound periodical volumes. **Subscriptions:** 130 journals and other serials.

★7565★ COLORADO STATE HOSPITAL
PROFESSIONAL LIBRARY
1600 W. 24th St.
Pueblo, CO 81003   Phone: (719) 546-4677
Laura Penny Hulslander, Lib.Dir.
Subjects: Psychiatry, mental health, psychology, surgery, internal medicine, social work. **Holdings:** 6000 books. **Subscriptions:** 150 journals and other serials.

★7566★ PARKVIEW EPISCOPAL MEDICAL CENTER
MEDICAL LIBRARY
400 W. 16th St.
Pueblo, CO 81003   Phone: (719) 584-4582
Alma Williams, Lib.Coord.
Subjects: Medicine, nursing, surgery, hospital administration, allied health sciences. **Holdings:** 2119 books; 1648 bound periodical volumes; pamphlet file. **Subscriptions:** 120 journals and other serials.

★7567★ ST. MARY-CORWIN HOSPITAL
FINNEY MEMORIAL LIBRARY
1008 Minnequa Ave.
Pueblo, CO 81004-9988   Phone: (719) 560-5598
Shirley Chun-Harper, Med.Libn.
Subjects: Internal medicine, surgery, pediatrics, pathology, allied health sciences. **Holdings:** 2568 volumes; 66 video cassettes; 1154 Audio-Digest tapes. **Subscriptions:** 125 journals and other serials.

★7568★ U.S. AIR FORCE ACADEMY
MEDICAL LIBRARY
U.S. Air Force Academy, CO 80840-5300   Phone: (719) 472-5107
Jeanne Entze, Libn.
Subjects: Medicine. **Holdings:** 4636 books. **Subscriptions:** 324 journals and other serials.

★7569★ LUTHERAN MEDICAL CENTER
MEDICAL LIBRARY
8300 W. 38th Ave.
Wheat Ridge, CO 80033   Phone: (303) 425-8662
Susan Brandes, Mgr. & Med.Libn.
Subjects: Medicine, nursing, health management. **Holdings:** 1000 books; 3000 bound periodical volumes; 500 audiotapes; 200 videotapes. **Subscriptions:** 230 journals and other serials.

★7570★ WHEAT RIDGE REGIONAL CENTER
EMPLOYEE'S LIBRARY
10285 Ridge Rd.
Wheat Ridge, CO 80033   Phone: (303) 424-7791
Carl Schutter, Sup.Serv.Dir.
Subjects: Mental retardation, behavior modification, developmental disabilities, child development, psychology, sociology, medicine. **Holdings:** 1145 books; 200 pamphlets. **Subscriptions:** 28 journals and other serials.

Connecticut

★7571★ BRIDGEPORT HOSPITAL
REEVES MEMORIAL LIBRARY
267 Grant St.
Box 5000
Bridgeport, CT 06610   Phone: (203) 384-3254
Katherine Stemmer, Dir.
Subjects: Medicine, allied health sciences. **Holdings:** 3675 books; 4513 bound periodical volumes; 872 AV programs. **Subscriptions:** 300 journals and other serials; 5 newspapers.

★7572★ PARK CITY HOSPITAL
CARLSON FOUNDATION MEMORIAL LIBRARY
695 Park Ave.
Bridgeport, CT 06604   Phone: (203) 579-5097
Subjects: Medicine, nursing, dentistry, allied health sciences. **Holdings:** 2013 books; 2850 bound periodical volumes; 350 videotapes; 2 VF drawers. **Subscriptions:** 177 journals and other serials.

★7573★ ST. VINCENT'S MEDICAL CENTER
DANIEL T. BANKS HEALTH SCIENCE LIBRARY
2800 Main St.
Bridgeport, CT 06606   Phone: (203) 576-5336
Janet Goerig, Dir., Lib.Serv.
Subjects: Medicine, nursing, and allied health sciences. **Holdings:** 4246 books; 4614 bound periodical volumes; 40 VF drawers of reprints and pamphlets; 5978 AV programs. **Subscriptions:** 303 journals and other serials.

★7574★ DANBURY HOSPITAL
HEALTH SCIENCES LIBRARY
24 Hospital Ave.
Danbury, CT 06810   Phone: (203) 797-7279
Michael J. Schott, Dir.
Subjects: Medicine, nursing, hospitals, allied health sciences. **Holdings:** 3720 books; 5060 bound periodical volumes; 781 AV programs; 2 VF drawers of reports; 40 cases of pamphlets; 12 VF drawers of clippings. **Subscriptions:** 432 journals and other serials.

★7575★ GRIFFIN HOSPITAL
HEALTH SCIENCES
LIBRARY
130 Division St.
Derby, CT 06418   Phone: (203) 732-7399
Katerini Giotsas, Libn./Mgr.
Subjects: Medicine, nursing, and allied health sciences. **Holdings:** 800 journals and other serials; 2000 bound periodical volumes. **Subscriptions:** 225 journals and other serials; 4 newspapers.

★7576★ CIBA-GEIGY CORPORATION
TECHNICAL INFORMATION CENTER
400 Farmington Ave.
Farmington, CT 06032   Phone: (203) 674-6312
Joanna W. Eickenhorst, Supv., Info.Serv.
Subjects: Toxicology, environmental health, mutagenicity, metabolism, pharmacokinetics. **Holdings:** 4000 books. **Subscriptions:** 140 journals and other serials.

★7577★ CONNECTICUT DEPARTMENT OF MENTAL
RETARDATION, REGION 2
PROBUS CLUB RESOURCE CENTER
270 Farmington Ave., Ste. 260
Farmington, CT 06032-1909   Phone: (203) 679-8373
Donald N. Miller, Ph.D., Dir.Comm. & Staff Dev.
Subjects: Mental retardation, developmental disabilities, behavior modification, team functioning, emotional disturbance, physical handicaps. **Holdings:** 1000 books; 200 bound periodical volumes; 300 other cataloged items; 20 AV programs. **Subscriptions:** 3 journals and other serials.

★7578★ UNIVERSITY OF CONNECTICUT
HEALTH CENTER
LYMAN MAYNARD STOWE LIBRARY
PO Box 4003
Farmington, CT 06034-4003   Phone: (203) 679-2839
Ralph Arcari, Dir.
Subjects: Medicine, dentistry, nursing, allied health sciences. **Holdings:** 53,261 books; 103,652 bound periodical volumes; 303 computer software programs; 5 drawers of pamphlets. **Subscriptions:** 2379 journals and other serials.

★7579★ CADMIUM COUNCIL, INC.
LIBRARY
PO Box 2664
Greenwich, CT 06836   Phone: (203) 625-0911
Hugh Morrow, Exec.Dir.
Subjects: Cadmium - metal, compounds, industry, markets and applications, health effects, recycling and recovery, regulations. **Holdings:** Figures not available.

★7580★ GREENWICH HOSPITAL ASSOCIATION
GRAY CARTER LIBRARY
Perryridge Rd.
Greenwich, CT 06830   Phone: (203) 863-3284
Carmel Fedors, Lib.Dir.
Subjects: Medicine, allied health sciences, nursing, hospital administration. **Holdings:** 1617 books; 1949 bound periodical volumes. **Subscriptions:** 150 journals and other serials.

★7581★ PFIZER, INC.
CENTRAL RESEARCH
RESEARCH LIBRARY
Eastern Point Rd.
Groton, CT 06340   Phone: (203) 441-3687
Dr. Roger P. Nelson, Dir.
Subjects: Organic and pharmaceutical chemistry, pharmacology, antibiotics. **Holdings:** 7000 books; 30,000 bound periodical volumes; 2500 reels of

microfilm of patent specifications. **Subscriptions:** 1000 journals and other serials.

★7582★ U.S. NAVY
NAVAL SUBMARINE MEDICAL RESEARCH LABORATORY
MEDICAL LIBRARY
Naval Submarine Base New London
Box 900
Groton, CT 06340   Phone: (203) 449-3629
Elaine M. Gaucher, Libn.
Subjects: Submarine medicine, diving, physiology, psychology. **Holdings:** 4343 books; 8468 bound periodical volumes; 7000 documents; 1400 microforms; 1200 internal reports. **Subscriptions:** 175 journals and other serials.

★7583★ AETNA LIFE & CASUALTY
MP&P MEDICAL LIBRARY
LIBRARY
151 Farmington Ave.
Hartford, CT 06156   Phone: (203) 636-1087
Deborah Beauvais
Subjects: Medical reference. **Holdings:** 50 books. **Subscriptions:** 71 journals and other serials.

★7584★ CONNECTICUT DEPARTMENT OF HEALTH
SERVICES
STANLEY H. OSBORN MEDICAL LIBRARY
150 Washington St.
Hartford, CT 06106   Phone: (203) 566-2198
Margery A. Cohen, Libn.
Subjects: Public health, medicine. **Holdings:** 2610 books; 5126 pamphlets; 450 Children's Bureau publications; 2000 Public Health Service publications. **Subscriptions:** 150 journals and other serials.

★7585★ HARTFORD HOSPITAL
HEALTH SCIENCE LIBRARIES
80 Seymour St.
Hartford, CT 06115-0729   Phone: (203) 524-2971
Gertrude Lamb, Ph.D., Dir.
Subjects: Clinical medicine, nursing, education, administration, gerontology, allied health specialties. **Holdings:** 10,586 books; 15,109 bound periodical volumes; 30 VF drawers of pamphlets; 11 audio cassettes; 400 video cassettes; 450 slide sets and kits; 20 16mm films. **Subscriptions:** 817 journals and other serials.

★7586★ HARTFORD MEDICAL SOCIETY
WALTER STEINER MEMORIAL LIBRARY
230 Scarborough St.
Hartford, CT 06105   Phone: (203) 236-5613
H. David Crombie, M.D., Libn.
Subjects: Medicine, history of medicine, anesthesiology. **Holdings:** 34,342 volumes. **Subscriptions:** 100 journals and other serials.

★7587★ INSTITUTE OF LIVING
MEDICAL LIBRARY
400 Washington St.
Hartford, CT 06106   Phone: (203) 241-6824
Harriet E. Rosenfeld, Dir.
Subjects: Neurology, psychiatry, psychoanalysis, social sciences. **Holdings:** 24,000 books; 11,000 bound periodical volumes; 1200 pamphlets; 30 boxes of hospital archives; 60 shelf feet of asylum reports; 500 audio cassettes; 40 video cassettes. **Subscriptions:** 200 journals and other serials.

★7588★ MOUNT SINAI HOSPITAL
HEALTH SCIENCES LIBRARY
500 Blue Hills Ave.
Hartford, CT 06112   Phone: (203) 286-4617
Mary Pat Wilhem, Dir.
Subjects: Clinical medicine, nursing, allied health sciences. **Holdings:** 1000 books; 2500 bound periodical volumes; AV programs; microfilm. **Subscriptions:** 220 journals and other serials.

★7589★ ST. FRANCIS HOSPITAL AND MEDICAL CENTER
SCHOOL OF NURSING LIBRARY
338 Asylum St.
Hartford, CT 06103   Phone: (203) 247-4411
Ruth Carroll, Dir. of Libs.
Subjects: Nursing, psychiatry, psychology, pre-clinical medicine. **Holdings:**

6000 books; 400 bound periodical volumes; 15 VF drawers. **Subscriptions:** 150 journals and other serials.

★7590★ ST. FRANCIS HOSPITAL AND MEDICAL CENTER
WILSON C. JAINSEN LIBRARY
114 Woodland St.
Hartford, CT 06105   Phone: (203) 548-4746
Ruth Carroll, Dir. of Libs.
Subjects: Medicine, nursing, management, psychiatry, psychology. **Holdings:** 13,000 books; 450 periodical titles on microfilm. **Subscriptions:** 850 journals and other serials.

★7591★ MANCHESTER MEMORIAL HOSPITAL
MEDICAL LIBRARY
71 Haynes St.
Manchester, CT 06040   Phone: (203) 646-1222
Jeannine Cyr Gluck, Med.Libn.
Subjects: Medicine. **Holdings:** 400 books; 300 bound periodical volumes; audio cassettes; back volumes of periodicals on microfiche. **Subscriptions:** 85 journals and other serials.

★7592★ MERIDEN-WALLINGFORD HOSPITAL
HEALTH SCIENCES LIBRARY
181 Cook Ave.
Meriden, CT 06450   Phone: (203) 238-0771
Ellen C. Sheehan, Libn.
Subjects: Medicine, nursing. **Holdings:** 1000 books; 300 bound periodical volumes. **Subscriptions:** 125 journals and other serials.

★7593★ CONNECTICUT VALLEY HOSPITAL
HALLOCK MEDICAL LIBRARY
Box 351
Middletown, CT 06457   Phone: (203) 344-2304
Pauline Kruk, Med.Libn.
Subjects: Psychiatry, neurology, medicine. **Holdings:** 4500 books; 2500 bound periodical volumes. **Subscriptions:** 77 journals and other serials.

★7594★ CONNECTICUT VALLEY HOSPITAL
WILLIS ROYALE VALLEY
Merrit Hall
Tynan Dr.
Middletown, CT 06457   Phone: (203) 344-2449
Storm Somers
Subjects: Self-improvement, recreation, life skills. **Holdings:** 3000 books. **Subscriptions:** 25 journals and other serials; 3 newspapers.

★7595★ MIDDLESEX MEMORIAL HOSPITAL
HEALTH SCIENCES LIBRARY
28 Crescent St.
Middletown, CT 06457   Phone: (203) 344-6286
Evelyn M. Breck, Dir.
Subjects: Medicine, nursing. **Holdings:** 2000 books; 1400 bound periodical volumes; 6 VF drawers of clippings and catalogs. **Subscriptions:** 200 journals and other serials.

★7596★ SPECIAL EDUCATION RESOURCE CENTER
25 Industrial Park Rd.
Middletown, CT 06457-1520   Phone: (203) 632-1485
Marianne Kirner, Dir.
Subjects: Special education, education and training of handicapped people (birth to 21 years). **Holdings:** 3250 books; 16 VF drawers of material; 350 tests; 240 inservice training materials; 41 newsletters; 3385 instructional materials; 300 literature searches; 70 computer search reprints; 220 computer software packages. **Subscriptions:** 145 journals and other serials.

★7597★ WESLEYAN UNIVERSITY
PSYCHOLOGY LIBRARY
Judd Hall
Middletown, CT 06457   Phone: (203) 347-9411
Shirley Schmottlach, Lib.Asst.
Subjects: Psychology, psychoanalysis, behavioral sciences, neurosciences, cognitive sciences, women's studies. **Holdings:** 18,000 books; 8475 bound periodical volumes; 275 bound theses. **Subscriptions:** 200 journals and other serials.

★7598★ MILFORD HOSPITAL
HEALTH SCIENCES LIBRARY
2047 Bridgeport Ave.
Milford, CT 06460   Phone: (203) 876-4006
Patricia Westbrook, Libn.
Subjects: Medicine, nursing, and allied health sciences. **Holdings:** 1280 books; 2100 periodical volumes; 800 AV items. **Subscriptions:** 97 journals and other serials.

★7599★ NEW BRITAIN GENERAL HOSPITAL
HEALTH SCIENCE LIBRARY
100 Grand St.
New Britain, CT 06050   Phone: (203) 224-5011
Linda A. LaRue, Lib.Dir.
Subjects: Medicine, surgery, obstetrics and gynecology, pediatrics, cardiology. **Holdings:** 3000 books; 9000 bound periodical volumes; pamphlets; videotapes; films; slides; Audio-Digest tapes. **Subscriptions:** 240 journals and other serials.

★7600★ HOSPITAL OF ST. RAPHAEL
HEALTH SCIENCES LIBRARY
1450 Chapel St.
New Haven, CT 06511   Phone: (203) 789-3330
Patricia L. Wales, Dir., Lib.Serv.
Subjects: Medicine, nursing, and allied health sciences. **Holdings:** 2000 books; 4000 bound periodical volumes; 4 VF drawers; AV programs. **Subscriptions:** 460 journals and other serials.

★7601★ PLANNED PARENTHOOD OF CONNECTICUT
LIBRARY
129 Whitney Ave.
New Haven, CT 06510   Phone: (203) 865-5158
Susan Killheffer
Subjects: Reproductive health, sexuality curricula, teen sexuality and pregnancy, contraception, abortion, pregnancy, childbirth, rape, sexual abuse. **Holdings:** 2500 books; 300 videotapes. **Subscriptions:** 55 journals and other serials.

★7602★ YALE UNIVERSITY
HARVEY CUSHING/JOHN HAY WHITNEY MEDICAL LIBRARY
333 Cedar St.
Box 3333
New Haven, CT 06510   Phone: (203) 785-5354
Regina Kenny Fryer, Act.Dir.
Subjects: Medicine, nursing, public health, allied health sciences. **Holdings:** 369,649 volumes; 50 manuscript codices before 1600. **Subscriptions:** 2511 journals and other serials.

★7603★ YALE UNIVERSITY
IRA V. HISCOCK EPIDEMIOLOGY AND PUBLIC HEALTH
  LIBRARY
PO Box 3333
60 College St.
New Haven, CT 06520   Phone: (203) 785-5680
Carole A. Colter, Libn.
Subjects: Biostatistics, environmental health, epidemiology, health services administration, public health. **Holdings:** 20,000 books and bound journals. **Subscriptions:** 217 journals and other serials.

★7604★ NEW MILFORD HOSPITAL
HEALTH SCIENCES LIBRARY
21 Elm St.
New Milford, CT 06776   Phone: (203) 355-2611
Susan E. Hays, Libn.
Subjects: Medicine, nursing, allied health sciences. **Holdings:** 1200 books; 878 bound periodical volumes; 75 periodical titles on microfiche. **Subscriptions:** 106 journals and other serials.

★7605★ CEDARCREST REGIONAL HOSPITAL
MEDICAL LIBRARY
525 Russell Rd.
Newington, CT 06111   Phone: (203) 666-7638
Mary L. Conlon, Libn.
Subjects: Psychiatry, psychology, psychiatric nursing, medicine, mental health, pharmacology. **Holdings:** 1000 books; 800 bound periodical volumes; 200 cassettes; 166 pamphlets and reports. **Subscriptions:** 30 journals and other serials.

★7606★ HARTFORD HOSPITAL
JEFFERSON HOUSE GERONTOLOGY RESOURCE CENTER
1 John H. Stewart Dr.
Newington, CT 06111   Phone: (203) 667-4453
Virginia H. Corcoran, Dir.
Subjects: Geriatrics, gerontology. **Holdings:** 500 books; 360 bound periodical volumes; unpublished reports and news clippings (online). **Subscriptions:** 46 journals and other serials.

★7607★ NEWINGTON CHILDREN'S HOSPITAL
PROFESSIONAL LIBRARY
181 E. Cedar St.
Newington, CT 06111   Phone: (203) 667-5380
Julie Lueders, Dir.
Subjects: Orthopedics, pediatrics, nursing. **Holdings:** 2600 books; 3100 bound periodical volumes. **Subscriptions:** 125 journals and other serials.

★7608★ U.S. DEPARTMENT OF VETERANS AFFAIRS
HEALTH SCIENCES LIBRARY
555 Willard Ave.
Newington, CT 06111   Phone: (203) 666-6951
Lynn A. Lloyd
Subjects: Medicine, geriatrics. **Holdings:** 2279 books; 1700 bound periodical volumes. **Subscriptions:** 180 journals and other serials.

★7609★ FAIRFIELD HILLS HOSPITAL
HEALTH SCIENCES LIBRARY
Box 5525
Newtown, CT 06470   Phone: (203) 270-3083
Mark J. Sosnowski, Libn.
Subjects: Psychiatry, psychology, social service, rehabilitation. **Holdings:** 6000 books; 2000 bound periodical volumes; 150 cataloged reference materials; 350 pamphlets and periodicals; AV programs. **Subscriptions:** 149 journals and other serials.

★7610★ DUNLAP AND ASSOCIATES INC.
LIBRARY
17 Washington St.
Norwalk, CT 06854   Phone: (203) 866-8464
Frances Maloon, Dir.
Subjects: Psychology, human factors, statistics, military science, drug abuse, accidents, alcohol-related accidents. **Holdings:** 2500 books; 100 bound periodical volumes; 80 VF drawers of reports, government documents, pamphlets. **Subscriptions:** 50 journals and other serials; 5 newspapers.

★7611★ NORWALK HOSPITAL
WIGGANS HEALTH SCIENCES LIBRARY
Maple St.
Norwalk, CT 06856   Phone: (203) 852-2793
Jill Golrick, Dir.
Subjects: Medicine, allied health sciences. **Holdings:** 1300 books; 6500 bound periodical volumes; 6 indices; 6 VF drawers. **Subscriptions:** 165 journals and other serials.

★7612★ PURDUE FREDERICK COMPANY
CORPORATE LIBRARY
100 Connecticut Ave.
Norwalk, CT 06856   Phone: (203) 853-0123
Kathryn Walsh, Mgr., Lib.Serv.
Subjects: Pharmacology, chemistry, medicine, business. **Holdings:** 2500 books; 7000 bound periodical volumes; patent file. **Subscriptions:** 450 journals and other serials.

★7613★ NORWICH HOSPITAL
HEALTH SCIENCES LIBRARY
Box 508
Norwich, CT 06360   Phone: (203) 823-5697
Julia M. Traver, Libn. II
Subjects: Psychiatry, neurology, psychology, general medicine, nursing, occupational therapy, social service. **Holdings:** 4000 books; 5750 bound periodical volumes. **Subscriptions:** 125 journals and other serials.

★7614★ WILLIAM W. BACKUS HOSPITAL
MEDICAL/NURSING LIBRARY
326 Washington St.
Norwich, CT 06360
Elaine Spalding, Med.Libn. Phone: (203) 823-6327
Subjects: Anesthesiology, surgery, obstetrics, gynecology, internal medicine, pediatrics. **Holdings:** 500 books; 1700 bound periodical volumes. **Subscriptions:** 100 journals and other serials.

★7615★ COMMUNITY ASSOCIATES OF CONNECTICUT, INC.
PROFESSIONAL RESOURCE CENTER
25 Hillside Ave.
Oakville, CT 06779-1735 Phone: (203) 274-9241
Thomas R. Briggs, Ph.D., Pres./C.E.O.
Subjects: Physically and severely handicapped, communication training, special education, parent training, therapeutic training. **Holdings:** 150 books; 100 other cataloged items.

★7616★ LAPALME MEMORIAL HOSPITAL
LIBRARY
320 Pomfret St.
Putnam, CT 06260 Phone: (203) 928-6541
Elaine Davis, Libn.
Subjects: Medicine. **Holdings:** 500 books; 800 bound periodical volumes. **Subscriptions:** 56 journals and other serials; 3 newspapers.

★7617★ BOEHRINGER INGELHEIM LTD.
SCIENTIFIC INFORMATION SERVICES
90 E. Ridge
Ridgefield, CT 06877 Phone: (203) 798-5156
Margaret Norman, Mgr.
Subjects: Pharmacology, chemistry, biochemistry, clinical medicine, pharmaceutical trade and industry, business. **Holdings:** 7,500 books; 16,000 bound periodical volumes; 35,000 items in product files. **Subscriptions:** 1400 journals and other serials.

★7618★ ROCKVILLE GENERAL HOSPITAL
MEDICAL LIBRARY/RESOURCE ROOM
31 Union St.
Rockville, CT 06066 Phone: (203) 872-0501
Laurie S. Fornes, Dir., Lib.Serv.
Subjects: Medicine. **Holdings:** 600 books; 300 bound periodical volumes; Audio-Digest tapes, 1960 to present. **Subscriptions:** 118 journals and other serials.

★7619★ SHARON HOSPITAL
HEALTH SCIENCES LIBRARY
W. Main St.
Sharon, CT 06069 Phone: (203) 364-4095
Jackie Rorke, Libn.
Subjects: Medicine. **Holdings:** 400 books; 1440 bound periodical volumes. **Subscriptions:** 107 journals and other serials.

★7620★ RICHARDSON VICKS U.S.A. RESEARCH CENTER
LIBRARY
1 Far Mill Crossing
Shelton, CT 06484 Phone: (203) 929-2500
Mary Lou Wells, Libn.
Subjects: Drugs and pharmaceuticals, medicine, cosmetics and cosmetic science, analytical and physical chemistry, microbiology, biochemistry, biology, nutrition. **Holdings:** 6500 books; 7000 bound periodical volumes. **Subscriptions:** 275 journals and other serials.

★7621★ EASTER SEAL REHABILITATION CENTER OF
SOUTHWESTERN CONNECTICUT
FRANCIS M. HARRISON MEMORIAL LIBRARY
26 Palmer's Hill Rd.
Stamford, CT 06902 Phone: (203) 325-1544
Deborah Menchek
Subjects: Rehabilitation. **Holdings:** 500 books; 240 bound periodical volumes; 6 VF drawers of pamphlets and brochures; 3 shelves of reports and catalogs. **Subscriptions:** 18 journals and other serials.

★7622★ ST. JOSEPH MEDICAL CENTER
HEALTH SCIENCES LIBRARY
128 Strawberry Hill Ave.
Box 1222
Stamford, CT 06904-1222 Phone: (203) 353-2095
Lucille Lieberman, Dir.
Subjects: Medicine, nursing, and allied health sciences. **Holdings:** 1412 books; 160 bound periodical volumes; 106 video cassettes. **Subscriptions:** 160 journals and other serials.

★7623★ THE STAMFORD HOSPITAL
HEALTH SCIENCES LIBRARY
Shelburne Rd.
Box 9317
Stamford, CT 06904-7523 Phone: (203) 325-7523
Lynn Sabol, Dir.
Subjects: Clinical medicine, nursing. **Holdings:** 2376 books; 5174 bound periodical volumes; 1177 tapes; 3607 slides. **Subscriptions:** 353 journals and other serials.

★7624★ UNIVERSITY OF CONNECTICUT
PHARMACY LIBRARY AND LEARNING CENTER
Box U-92
Storrs, CT 06269-1092 Phone: (203) 486-2218
Sharon Giovenale, Dir.
Subjects: Pharmaceutics, pharmacology, pharmacognosy, pharmaceutical chemistry, health care services. **Holdings:** 5000 books; 14,000 bound periodical volumes; 5 VF drawers of pamphlets and clippings; 300 AV programs; 299 reels of microfilm of periodicals. **Subscriptions:** 282 journals and other serials.

★7625★ CHESEBROUGH-POND'S, INC.
RESEARCH LIBRARY
40 Merritt Blvd.
Trumbull, CT 06611 Phone: (203) 381-4312
Mary Suprynowicz, Res.Libn.
Subjects: Chemistry, cosmetic science, pharmacology, dentistry. **Holdings:** 5000 books; 2000 bound periodical volumes; 20 lateral file drawers of patents, reprints, pamphlets; 40 cartridges of microfilm; 20 boxes of microfiche. **Subscriptions:** 250 journals and other serials.

★7626★ BRISTOL-MYERS SQUIBB COMPANY
SCIENTIFIC INFORMATION DEPARTMENT
RESEARCH LIBRARY/809
5 Research Pkwy.
Box 5103
Wallingford, CT 06492-7663 Phone: (203) 284-6221
John E. MacNintch, Dir.
Subjects: Pharmacology, organic chemistry, microbiology, medicine, oncology, cardiovascular/central nervous system. **Holdings:** 24,000 bound periodical volumes; 6600 reels of microfilm; statistics. **Subscriptions:** 600 journals and other serials.

★7627★ GAYLORD HOSPITAL
MEDICAL LIBRARY
Box 400
Wallingford, CT 06492 Phone: (203) 284-2800
Meada G. Ebinger, Med.Libn.
Subjects: Rehabilitation, psychology, social service, medicine, nursing. **Holdings:** 1250 books; 100 video cassettes on rehabilitation. **Subscriptions:** 110 journals and other serials.

★7628★ ST. MARY'S HOSPITAL
FINKELSTEIN LIBRARY
56 Franklin St.
Waterbury, CT 06702 Phone: (203) 574-6408
Jean Fuller, Libn.
Subjects: Medicine and nursing. **Holdings:** 1200 books; 2240 bound periodical volumes. **Subscriptions:** 291 journals and other serials.

★7629★ WATERBURY HOSPITAL
HEALTH CENTER LIBRARY
64 Robbins St.
Waterbury, CT 06721 Phone: (203) 573-6136
Joan Ruszkowski, Dir.
Subjects: Medicine, nursing, and allied health sciences. **Holdings:** 3196 books; 8332 bound periodical volumes; 4 VF drawers of pamphlets; 800

videotapes; 5 drawers of audiotapes. **Subscriptions:** 281 journals and other serials.

★7630★ MILES, INC.
PHARMACEUTICAL DIVISION
LIBRARY
400 Morgan Ln.
West Haven, CT 06516   Phone: (203) 937-2594
Cecilia Scully, Assoc.Info.Sci.
Subjects: Medicine, pharmacology; business; statistics. **Holdings:** 1500 books; 6500 bound periodical volumes; 115 reels of microfilm. **Subscriptions:** 249 journals and other serials.

★7631★ MILES, INC.
RESEARCH CENTER
LIBRARY
400 Morgan Ln.
West Haven, CT 06516   Phone: (203) 937-2844
Georgia Scura, Supv., Sci.Info.
Subjects: Biotechnology, genetics, medicine, biochemistry. **Holdings:** 500 books; 1500 bound periodical volumes; 206 reels of microfilm. **Subscriptions:** 163 journals and other serials.

★7632★ U.S. DEPARTMENT OF VETERANS AFFAIRS
MEDICAL CENTER LIBRARY
950 Campbell Ave.
West Haven, CT 06516   Phone: (203) 932-5711
Joan McGinnis, Chf., Lib.Serv.
Subjects: Medicine, psychiatry, psychology. **Holdings:** 6500 books; 9000 bound periodical volumes; AV programs. **Subscriptions:** 360 journals and other serials.

★7633★ HALL-BROOKE HOSPITAL
PROFESSIONAL LIBRARY
47 Long Lots Rd.
Westport, CT 06880   Phone: (203) 227-1251
Sharon Rerak, Coord., Educ.
Subjects: Psychiatry, psychology, mental health, psychiatric nursing, family therapy. **Holdings:** 1800 books; 500 bound periodical volumes. **Subscriptions:** 120 journals and other serials.

★7634★ HUMAN LACTATION CENTER, LTD.
LIBRARY
666 Sturges Hwy.
Westport, CT 06880   Phone: (203) 259-5995
Dana Raphael, Ph.D., Dir.
Subjects: Breastfeeding, maternal and infant nutrition, social science, demography, childbirth, women in development, supportive behavior, mammalian reproduction, incest and child sexual abuse. **Holdings:** 4000 volumes; 7 VF drawers of reports, manuscripts, dissertations; 40 tapes; 4 films. **Subscriptions:** 70 journals and other serials; 5 newspapers.

★7635★ NORTHWESTERN CONNECTICUT COMMUNITY
    COLLEGE
LIBRARY
Park Place East
Winsted, CT 06098   Phone: (203) 738-6480
Anne Gifford, Dir. of Lib.Serv.
Subjects: Deaf education, recreation management. **Holdings:** 49,624 books; 2000 phonograph records; 2071 microforms. **Subscriptions:** 243 journals and other serials; 12 newspapers.

Delaware

★7636★ DELAWARE DEPARTMENT OF HEALTH AND
    SOCIAL SERVICES
DIVISION OF PUBLIC HEALTH
LIBRARY
PO Box 637
Dover, DE 19903   Phone: (302) 736-4754
Ellen Cavins, Libn.
Subjects: Medicine. **Holdings:** 5462 books; 65 bound periodical volumes. **Subscriptions:** 119 journals and other serials.

★7637★ KENT GENERAL HOSPITAL
MEDICAL LIBRARY
640 S. State St.
Dover, DE 19901   Phone: (302) 674-7357
Jane Irving, Circuit Libn.
Remarks: No further information was supplied by the respondent.

★7638★ MILFORD MEMORIAL HOSPITAL
MEDICAL LIBRARY
Clark Ave.
PO Box 199
Milford, DE 19963   Phone: (302) 424-5623
Gwendolyn Elliott
Subjects: Clinical medicine, clinical nursing. **Holdings:** 450 books. **Subscriptions:** 59 journals and other serials.

★7639★ DELAWARE STATE HOSPITAL
MEDICAL LIBRARY
1920 N. Dupont Hwy.
New Castle, DE 19720   Phone: (302) 421-6368
James M. McCloskey, Sr.Libn.
Subjects: Psychiatry, psychology, medicine, social work, nursing, pastoral care. **Holdings:** 4000 books; 1240 bound periodical volumes. **Subscriptions:** 125 journals and other serials.

★7640★ E.I. DU PONT DE NEMOURS & COMPANY, INC.
HASKELL LABORATORY FOR TOXICOLOGY AND
    INDUSTRIAL MEDICINE
LIBRARY
Elkton Rd.
Box 50
Newark, DE 19714   Phone: (302) 366-5225
Nancy S. Selzer, Site Libn.
Subjects: Industrial medicine and toxicology. **Holdings:** 5500 books; 15,500 bound periodical volumes. **Subscriptions:** 265 journals and other serials.

★7641★ E.I. DU PONT DE NEMOURS & COMPANY, INC.
STINE LABORATORY LIBRARY
Elkton Rd.
Box 30
Newark, DE 19714   Phone: (302) 366-5353
Nancy S. Selzer, Site Libn.
Subjects: Pharmacology, drug metabolism, biochemistry, agriculture, biology. **Holdings:** 1000 books; 2000 bound periodical volumes. **Subscriptions:** 265 journals and other serials.

★7642★ MEDICAL CENTER OF DELAWARE
CHRISTIANA HOSPITAL
LIBRARY
4755 Ogletown-Stanton Rd.
Box 6001
Newark, DE 19718   Phone: (302) 733-1115
Christine Chastain-Warheit, Dir. of Libs.
Subjects: Clinical medicine, nursing. **Holdings:** 7000 books; 7000 bound periodical volumes. **Subscriptions:** 423 journals and other serials.

★7643★ ALFRED I. DU PONT INSTITUTE
MEDICAL LIBRARY
Box 269
Wilmington, DE 19899   Phone: (302) 651-5821
Carl Nolting, Med.Libn.
Subjects: Orthopedics, pediatrics, biochemistry, genetics. **Holdings:** 5000 books; 16,000 bound periodical volumes. **Subscriptions:** 300 journals and other serials.

★7644★ DELAWARE ACADEMY OF MEDICINE, INC.
LEWIS B. FLINN LIBRARY
1925 Lovering Ave.
Wilmington, DE 19806   Phone: (302) 656-1629
Gail P. Gill, Libn., Dir.
Subjects: Medicine. **Holdings:** 4000 books; 9800 bound periodical volumes. **Subscriptions:** 245 journals and other serials.

★7645★ DU PONT MERCK PHARMACEUTICAL COMPANY
INFORMATION SERVICES CENTER
Information Center, Rm. 2202
Wilmington, DE 19880-0027   Phone: (312) 892-1713
Terri Licari, Mgr., Info.Serv.Ctr.
Subjects: Pharmacology, biomedicine, chemistry, computer science, information science, business, patents. **Holdings:** 3500 books; 2500 bound periodical volumes. **Subscriptions:** 500 journals and other serials.

★7646★ E.I. DU PONT DE NEMOURS & COMPANY, INC.
TECHNICAL LIBRARY NETWORK
PO Box 80014
Wilmington, DE 19880-0014   Phone: (302) 992-2666
Lois H. Bronstein, Supv., TLN
Subjects: Agricultural chemicals, business and economics, chemistry, biomedicine, electronics, engineering, fibers, films, imaging, industrial relations, management, marketing, pigments, plastics, polymers. **Holdings:** 97,000 books; 35,000 bound periodical volumes; journals in microform; 235 shelves of pamphlets. **Subscriptions:** 4181 journals and other serials.

★7647★ EMILY P. BISSELL HOSPITAL
MEDICAL LIBRARY
3000 Newport Gap Pike
Wilmington, DE 19808   Phone: (302) 995-8435
Margaret A. Lacy, Med.Serv.Sec.
Subjects: Pulmonary tuberculosis, medicine, geriatrics. **Holdings:** 250 books.

★7648★ ICI AMERICAS INC.
ATLAS LIBRARY
PO Box 15365
Wilmington, DE 19897   Phone: (302) 886-8232
Frieda S. Mecray, Libn.
Subjects: Biomedicine, chemistry, chemical technology, business economics, pharmaceuticals. **Holdings:** 15,000 volumes; 25 VF drawers of trade catalogs; U.S. patents, 1964 to present, on microfilm; 108 titles on microfilm. **Subscriptions:** 1400 journals and other serials; 6 newspapers.

★7649★ MEDICAL CENTER OF DELAWARE
WILMINGTON HOSPITAL
MEDICAL LIBRARY
501 W. 14th St.
Box 1668
Wilmington, DE 19899   Phone: (302) 428-2201
Christine Chastain-Warheit, Dir. of Libs.
Subjects: Medicine, dentistry. **Holdings:** 895 books; 1560 bound periodical volumes. **Subscriptions:** 115 journals and other serials.

★7650★ RIVERSIDE HOSPITAL
MEDICAL LIBRARY
Box 845
Wilmington, DE 19899   Phone: (302) 764-6120
Roxanne Walston, Libn.
Subjects: Osteopathic medicine, internal medicine, nursing. **Holdings:** 500 books. **Subscriptions:** 60 journals and other serials.

★7651★ ST. FRANCIS HOSPITAL
MEDICAL LIBRARY
7th & Clayton Sts.
Wilmington, DE 19805   Phone: (302) 421-4834
Marga Hirsch, Libn.
Subjects: Medicine, nursing. **Holdings:** 1400 books; 123 bound periodical volumes; 12 VF drawers of reprints, original articles, ephemera. **Subscriptions:** 150 journals and other serials.

★7652★ U.S. DEPARTMENT OF VETERANS AFFAIRS
CENTER MEDICAL LIBRARY
1601 Kirkwood Hwy.
Wilmington, DE 19805   Phone: (302) 994-2511
Donald A. Passidomo, Chf.Libn.
Subjects: General medicine, surgery, dentistry, nursing. **Holdings:** 5000 books; 6000 bound periodical volumes; 2000 AV programs; medical journals on microfilm. **Subscriptions:** 325 journals and other serials.

District of Columbia

★7653★ ALEXANDER GRAHAM BELL ASSOCIATION FOR
THE DEAF
VOLTA BUREAU LIBRARY
3417 Volta Pl., NW
Washington, DC 20007   Phone: (202) 337-5220
Judith A. Anderson, Libn.
Subjects: Deafness, hearing, speech. **Holdings:** 28,000 books; 2500 bound periodical volumes; photographs; 640 shelf feet of pamphlets, reports of schools for the deaf; 30 VF drawers of clippings and reprints. **Subscriptions:** 190 journals and other serials.

★7654★ AMERICAN BAR ASSOCIATION
CENTER ON CHILDREN AND THE LAW
1800 M. St., NW
Washington, DC 20036   Phone: (202) 331-2250
Sally Inada, Dir. of Pubns.
Subjects: Child abuse and neglect, foster care, adoption, parental kidnapping of children, child support, grandparents' rights, developmentally disabled children's rights, child exploitation. **Holdings:** 5000 books, periodicals, reports, and training and conference materials. **Subscriptions:** 12 journals and other serials.

★7655★ AMERICAN COLLEGE OF OBSTETRICIANS AND
GYNECOLOGISTS
RESOURCE CENTER
409 12th St., SW
Washington, DC 20024   Phone: (202) 638-5577
Pamela Van Hine, Assoc.Dir.
Subjects: Obstetrics, gynecology, medical socioeconomics, medical education, women's health care, abortion, contraception, venereal disease, sex education, patient education. **Holdings:** 8000 books; reprints. **Subscriptions:** 300 journals and other serials.

★7656★ AMERICAN MEDICAL ASSOCIATION
WASHINGTON OFFICE LIBRARY
1101 Vermont Ave., NW
Washington, DC 20005   Phone: (202) 789-7448
Subjects: Medical socioeconomics, health statistics, health policy. **Holdings:** 10,000 books. **Subscriptions:** 197 journals and other serials; 5 newspapers.

★7657★ AMERICAN PHARMACEUTICAL ASSOCIATION
FOUNDATION LIBRARY
2215 Constitution Ave., NW
Washington, DC 20037   Phone: (202) 429-7524
Subjects: Pharmacy, pharmacology, medicine. **Holdings:** 6000 books; 2000 bound periodical volumes; 45 VF drawers of pharmacy and association materials. **Subscriptions:** 225 journals and other serials.

★7658★ AMERICAN PSYCHIATRIC ASSOCIATION
LIBRARY AND ARCHIVES
1400 K St., NW
Washington, DC 20005   Phone: (202) 682-6080
William E. Baxter, Dir.
Subjects: Psychiatry - community and social, child and adolescent, forensic, history in America; psychoanalysis; psychosomatic medicine. **Holdings:** 17,000 volumes. **Subscriptions:** 302 journals and other serials.

★7659★ AMERICAN PSYCHOLOGICAL ASSOCIATION
ARTHUR W. MELTON LIBRARY
1200 17th St., NW
Washington, DC 20036   Phone: (703) 247-7747
Rick A. Sample, Hd.Libn.
Subjects: Psychology, mental health, and allied disciplines. **Holdings:** 1400 books and journals. **Subscriptions:** 35 journals and other serials; 4 newspapers.

★7660★ AMERICAN PUBLIC HEALTH ASSOCIATION
INTERNATIONAL HEALTH PROGRAMS
RESOURCE CENTER
1015 15th St., NW
Washington, DC 20005   Phone: (202) 789-5600
Gayle Gibbons, Info.Spec.
Subjects: Developing countries - health delivery systems, nutrition, development, water and sanitation, family planning, maternal and child health.

Holdings: 1000 books; 130 newsletters; 120 pamphlet boxes; reports; monographs. **Subscriptions:** 110 journals and other serials.

★7661★ AMERICAN SOCIETY FOR MEDICAL TECHNOLOGY
LIBRARY
2021 L St., NW, Ste. 400
Washington, DC 20036   Phone: (202) 785-3311
Greg D. Goss, Coord., Member Oper.
Subjects: Cytology, histology, microbiology, hematology, biochemistry.

★7662★ AMERICAN YOUTH WORK CENTER
1751 N St., NW, Ste. 302
Washington, DC 20036   Phone: (202) 785-0764
William Treanor, Exec.Dir.
Subjects: Youth programs and problems, juvenile justice, youth alcohol and drug abuse, youth employment, missing children, exchange programs. **Holdings:** Figures not available.

★7663★ ASSOCIATION FOR GERONTOLOGY IN HIGHER
EDUCATION
RESOURCE LIBRARY
600 Maryland Ave., SW, W. Wing 204
Washington, DC 20024   Phone: (202) 484-7505
Elizabeth Douglass, Exec.Dir.
Subjects: Aging - education, training programs, courses. **Holdings:** Brochures and information for 300 schools offering programs and courses in aging.

★7664★ CARNEGIE INSTITUTION OF WASHINGTON
LIBRARY
1530 P St., NW
Washington, DC 20005   Phone: (202) 387-6411
Ray Bowers, Ed./Pub.Off.
Subjects: Astronomy, geophysics, botany, embryology, genetics, archeology. **Holdings:** 1000 books; 195 bound periodical volumes of SCIENCE and NATURE.

★7665★ CATHOLIC UNIVERSITY OF AMERICA
NURSING/BIOLOGY LIBRARY
Washington, DC 20064   Phone: (202) 319-5411
N.L. Powell, Libn.
Subjects: Nursing, medicine, social and physical sciences, biological and botanical sciences. **Holdings:** 37,284 books; 14,501 bound periodical volumes; 3004 reels of microfilm; 2727 theses. **Subscriptions:** 460 journals and other serials.

★7666★ CENTER FOR POPULATION OPTIONS
LIBRARY
1012 14th St., NW, Ste. 1200
Washington, DC 20005   Phone: (202) 347-5700
Subjects: Adolescent fertility issues - sexuality education, birth control, teenage pregnancy and child bearing, health, human immunodeficiency virus (HIV) among adolescents. **Holdings:** 2500 volumes.

★7667★ CHILD TRENDS, INC.
LIBRARY
2100 M St., NW, Rm. 610
Washington, DC 20037-1207   Phone: (202) 223-6288
Dr. Nicholas Zill, Exec.Dir.
Subjects: Physical, social, emotional, and psychological development of children; influence of family, school, peers, neighborhood, religion, media on children; teen pregnancy; family strengths; statistics. **Holdings:** Statistics and reports from U.S. Bureau of the Census, National Center for Health Statistics, National Center for Education Statistics.

★7668★ CHILD WELFARE LEAGUE OF AMERICA
INFORMATION SERVICE
DOROTHY L. BERNHARD LIBRARY
440 1st St., NW
Washington, DC 20001   Phone: (202) 638-2952
Mary Suarez, Libn.
Subjects: Child welfare, social work, social welfare, child development. **Holdings:** 3500 books; 30 VF drawers of USHHS publications on child welfare; 600 research reports; 70 VF drawers. **Subscriptions:** 90 journals and other serials.

★7669★ CHILDREN'S HOSPITAL/NATIONAL MEDICAL
CENTER
HOSPITAL LIBRARY
111 Michigan Ave., NW
Washington, DC 20010   Phone: (202) 745-3195
Deborah D. Gilbert, Dir.
Subjects: Pediatrics, child development, nursing, dentistry, psychiatry, ophthalmology. **Holdings:** 2953 books; 8254 bound periodical volumes; 300 AV programs. **Subscriptions:** 550 journals and other serials.

★7670★ CLEARINGHOUSE ON CHILD ABUSE AND NEGLECT
INFORMATION
PO Box 1182
Washington, DC 20013   Phone: (703) 821-2086
Subjects: Child abuse and neglect, child protective services. **Holdings:** 12,000 books, articles, and reports. **Subscriptions:** 30 journals and other serials.

★7671★ CLEARINGHOUSE ON FAMILY VIOLENCE
INFORMATION
PO Box 1182
Washington, DC 20013   Phone: (703) 821-2086
Subjects: Spouse abuse, elder abuse, sibling abuse, parent abuse. **Holdings:** 700 books, articles, and reports. **Subscriptions:** 10 journals and other serials.

★7672★ COLUMBIA HOSPITAL FOR WOMEN
MEDICAL LIBRARY
2425 L St., NW
Washington, DC 20037   Phone: (202) 293-6560
Elizabeth M. Haggart, Libn.
Subjects: Gynecology, obstetrics. **Holdings:** 1800 books. **Subscriptions:** 280 journals and other serials.

★7673★ DHS/CMHS
HEALTH SCIENCES LIBRARY
Administration Bldg., Rm. 100
St. Elizabeths Campus
2700 Martin Luther King, Jr. Ave., SE
Washington, DC 20032   Phone: (202) 373-7175
Subjects: Psychiatry, occupational therapy, general medicine, Protestant and Catholic chaplaincy, neurology, dance therapy, dentistry, therapeutic recreation, clinical psychology, social work, speech pathology and audiology, psychiatric nursing, psychoanalysis, psychodrama. **Holdings:** 20,000 books; 18,000 bound periodical volumes. **Subscriptions:** 300 journals and other serials.

★7674★ DISTILLED SPIRITS COUNCIL OF THE U.S.
LIBRARY
1250 Eye St., NW, 8th Fl.
Washington, DC 20005   Phone: (202) 628-3544
Matthew J. Vellucci, Lib.Dir.
Subjects: Distilled spirits industry, prohibition, temperance movement, alcoholism, liquor laws, alcohol and health/safety issues, moderate drinking, drinking customs. **Holdings:** 3000 volumes; 72 VF drawers of information on subjects and organizations. **Subscriptions:** 225 journals and other serials.

★7675★ DISTRICT OF COLUMBIA GENERAL HOSPITAL
MEDICAL LIBRARY
19th St. & Massachusetts Ave., SE
Washington, DC 20003   Phone: (202) 675-5348
Lavonda K. Broadnax, Chf.Libn.
Subjects: Medicine, nursing, allied health sciences. **Holdings:** 11,000 books; 12,000 bound periodical volumes. **Subscriptions:** 599 journals and other serials.

★7676★ DISTRICT OF COLUMBIA PUBLIC LIBRARY
LIBRARY FOR THE BLIND AND PHYSICALLY HANDICAPPED
Martin Luther King Memorial Library
901 G St., NW
Washington, DC 20001   Phone: (202) 727-2142
Grace Lyons, Chf.
Subjects: Popular and general material in special formats; information on legislation and services for the disabled; volunteer production of graduate and post-secondary school and work-related materials in recorded formats; reference material on aging and the handicapped. **Holdings:** 6400 books; 2700 phonograph records; 172,000 recorded books; 11,560 large-print

books; 7000 books in braille. **Subscriptions:** 109 journals and other serials (55 print and braille, 54 recorded).

★7677★ DISTRICT OF COLUMBIA PUBLIC LIBRARY
TECHNOLOGY AND SCIENCE DIVISION
Martin Luther King Memorial Library
901 G St., NW
Washington, DC 20001   Phone: (202) 727-1175
Lessie O. Mtewa, Chf.
Subjects: Mathematics, computer science, biology, domestic arts, earth science, chemistry, physics, engineering, agriculture, gardening, medicine, psychiatry, astronomy, consumer information, health, veterinary science. **Holdings:** 77,000 books; 2500 bound periodical volumes; 5300 microforms; 65 VF drawers. **Subscriptions:** 300 journals and other serials.

★7678★ FAMILY LIFE INFORMATION EXCHANGE
PO Box 37299
Washington, DC 20013-7299   Phone: (301) 585-6636
Florence Lehr, Proj.Mgr.
Subjects: Family planning, sexually transmitted diseases, adolescent pregnancy, adoption, contraception, reproductive health. **Holdings:** 5000 monographs. **Subscriptions:** 60 journals and other serials.

★7679★ GALLAUDET UNIVERSITY
LIBRARY
SPECIAL COLLECTION ON DEAFNESS
800 Florida Ave., NE
Washington, DC 20002   Phone: (202) 651-5220
John Day, Univ.Libn.
Subjects: Deafness and the deaf, audiology and hearing. **Holdings:** 34,583 books; 360 AV programs; 100 VF drawers; 4748 linear feet of archival materials; 3291 theses and dissertations on microfilm; ERIC microfiche; films. **Subscriptions:** 550 journals and other serials.

★7680★ GENERAL SERVICES ADMINISTRATION
CONSUMER INFORMATION CENTER
18th & F St., NW, Rm. G-142
Washington, DC 20405   Phone: (202) 501-1794
Teresa Nasif, Dir.
Subjects: Federal benefits, money management, child care, careers, education, health, food, diet and nutrition, travel, housing and home maintenance. **Holdings:** 200 pamphlets.

★7681★ GEORGE WASHINGTON UNIVERSITY
MEDICAL CENTER
PAUL HIMMELFARB HEALTH SCIENCES LIBRARY
2300 Eye St., NW
Washington, DC 20037   Phone: (202) 994-3528
Shelley A. Bader, Dir.
Subjects: Medicine and allied health sciences. **Holdings:** 25,000 books; 95,000 bound periodical volumes; 1500 titles of AV programs. **Subscriptions:** 2500 journals and other serials.

★7682★ GEORGETOWN UNIVERSITY
MEDICAL CENTER
DAHLGREN MEMORIAL LIBRARY
3900 Reservoir Rd., NW
Washington, DC 20007   Phone: (202) 687-1176
Naomi C. Broering, Dir./Med.Ctr.Libn.
Subjects: Medicine, dentistry, nursing, basic sciences, hospital management, health care administration. **Holdings:** 42,742 books; 95,520 bound periodical volumes; 747 archival materials; 1257 dissertations; 2936 AV programs; 441 microcomputer software programs; 6602 microforms. **Subscriptions:** 1739 journals and other serials.

★7683★ GRAY PANTHERS
NATIONAL OFFICE LIBRARY
1424 16th St., NW, No.602
Washington, DC 20036   Phone: (202) 387-3111
James S. Beasley, Jr., Info.Spec.
Subjects: Aging - housing, health care, retirement and alternative work patterns, education, consciousness-raising; intergenerational programs in housing and education. **Holdings:** 15 VF drawers of clippings, pamphlets, and government publications; 100 tapes and cassettes. **Subscriptions:** 100 journals and other serials.

★7684★ GREATER SOUTHEAST COMMUNITY HOSPITAL
LURA HEALTH SCIENCES LIBRARY
1310 Southern Ave., SE
Washington, DC 20032   Phone: (202) 574-6793
Sally F. Reyes, Libn.
Subjects: Medicine, nursing, and allied health sciences; general management. **Holdings:** 2335 books; AV tapes (756 titles). **Subscriptions:** 197 journals and other serials.

★7685★ GROUP HEALTH ASSOCIATION OF AMERICA
GERTRUDE STURGES MEMORIAL LIBRARY
1129 20th St., NW
Washington, DC 20036   Phone: (202) 778-3200
Nina M. Lane, Lib.Dir.
Subjects: Health maintenance organizations, health insurance and administration, medical economics. **Holdings:** 3000 books. **Subscriptions:** 200 journals and other serials.

★7686★ HOWARD UNIVERSITY
HEALTH SCIENCES LIBRARY
600 W St., NW
Washington, DC 20059   Phone: (202) 806-6433
Salvador Waller, Assoc.Dir.
Subjects: Medicine, dentistry, nursing, and allied health sciences. **Holdings:** 204,558 books; 79,257 bound periodical volumes; 515 bibliographies; 121 shelves of AV programs; 20 VF drawers of disease, health, medicine files; 6 VF drawers of biographical files; 115 drawers of microfilm. **Subscriptions:** 5026 journals and other serials.

★7687★ HOWARD UNIVERSITY
HEALTH SCIENCES LIBRARY
PHARMACY ANNEX
2300 4th St.
Washington, DC 20059   Phone: (202) 806-6545
Mr. Jei Whan Kim, Libn.
Subjects: Pharmacy, pharmacology, pharmacognosy, biomedicinal chemistry. **Holdings:** 16,337 books; 4943 bound periodical volumes; 974 reels of microfilm; 415 cassettes; 4001 slides; 31,480 microfiche. **Subscriptions:** 448 journals and other serials.

★7688★ HOWARD UNIVERSITY
SCHOOL OF BUSINESS AND PUBLIC ADMINISTRATION
LIBRARY
2600 6th St., NW, Rm. 120
Washington, DC 20059   Phone: (202) 806-1561
Lucille B. Smiley, Libn.
Subjects: Business administration, public administration, health services administration, management, accounting, real estate, insurance, marketing, finance, computer-based management information systems, hotel/motel management, international business. **Holdings:** 60,991 books; 5780 bound periodical volumes; 82 technical assistance reports; 17,633 reels of microfilm; 308,814 10K reports on microfiche. **Subscriptions:** 3139 journals and other serials; 75 newspapers.

★7689★ INTERGOVERNMENTAL HEALTH POLICY PROJECT
CLEARINGHOUSE
2011 I St., NW, Ste. 200
Washington, DC 20006   Phone: (202) 872-1445
Molly Stauffer
Subjects: Medicaid, AIDS, longterm care, mental health, certificate of need, homelessness. **Holdings:** 10,000 books; 10,000 bound periodical volumes. **Subscriptions:** 30 journals and other serials.

★7690★ INTERNATIONAL FEDERATION OF FAMILY LIFE
**   PROMOTION**
LIBRARY
1511 K St., NW, Ste. 326
Washington, DC 20005   Phone: (202) 783-0137
Richard Sevigny
Subjects: Natural family planning, sexuality. **Holdings:** 1000 books; 5 bound periodical volumes; 250 reports. **Subscriptions:** 20 journals and other serials; 4 newspapers.

★7691★ LEAGUE FOR INTERNATIONAL FOOD EDUCATION
LIBRARY
1126 16th St., NW, Ste. 404
Washington, DC 20036
Brenda C. Higgins, Exec.Dir.
Subjects: Nutrition, food science and technology, agriculture, health.
Holdings: 650 books; 10,000 reprints and reports. **Subscriptions:** 302
journals and other serials.

★7692★ NATIONAL ABORTION FEDERATION
LIBRARY
1436 U St., NW, Ste. 103
Washington, DC 20009   Phone: (202) 667-5881
Subjects: Abortion, contraception, sexuality, sociology, health, medicine.
Holdings: 225 volumes.

★7693★ NATIONAL BIOMEDICAL RESEARCH FOUNDATION
LIBRARY
Georgetown University Medical Center
3900 Reservoir Rd., NW
Washington, DC 20007   Phone: (202) 687-2121
JoAnn Ahern, Adm.
Subjects: Biochemistry, evolution, proteins, nucleic acids, origins of life,
pattern recognition, biomedical engineering and instrumentation, mathe-
matics, computer technology, computerized radiology, computers in
biology and medicine, health operations research. **Holdings:** 4000 books; 8
VF drawers of staff publications reprints. **Subscriptions:** 130 journals and
other serials.

★7694★ NATIONAL COALITION AGAINST THE MISUSE OF
PESTICIDES
LIBRARY
530 7th St., SE
Washington, DC 20003   Phone: (202) 543-5450
Subjects: Pesticides - public health and safety, environmental problems,
economic problems. **Holdings:** 2000 volumes.

★7695★ NATIONAL COMMITTEE FOR ADOPTION
LIBRARY
1930 17th St., NW
Washington, DC 20009-6207   Phone: (202) 328-1200
Subjects: Adoption - voluntary agencies, adoptive parents, adoptees,
birthparents, maternity services; legislation for the adoption process;
infertility. **Holdings:** 2000 volumes and files; statistics.

★7696★ THE NATIONAL COUNCIL ON THE AGING
OLLIE A. RANDALL LIBRARY
600 Maryland Ave., SW, W. Wing 100
Washington, DC 20024   Phone: (202) 479-1665
Subjects: Aging, retirement, economics, employment, community organi-
zation, legislation, nursing homes, senior centers, health care. **Holdings:**
12,000 volumes; 30 VF drawers; 32 VF drawers of archival materials.
Subscriptions: 300 journals and other serials.

★7697★ NATIONAL COUNCIL OF SENIOR CITIZENS
INFORMATION CENTER
925 15th St., NW
Washington, DC 20005   Phone: (202) 347-8800
Brien Kinkel, Info.Spec.
Subjects: Gerontology. **Holdings:** 2000 books; 24 VF cabinets. **Subscrip-
tions:** 150 journals and other serials.

★7698★ NATIONAL INFORMATION CENTER FOR CHILDREN
AND YOUTH WITH HANDICAPS
Box 1492
Washington, DC 20013   Phone: (703) 893-6061
Lana Ambler, Info.Serv.Coord.
Subjects: Disabilities and special education. **Holdings:** 1000 books; vertical
files. **Subscriptions:** 400 journals and other serials.

★7699★ NATIONAL INFORMATION CENTER ON DEAFNESS
Gallaudet University
800 Florida Ave., NE
Washington, DC 20002   Phone: (202) 651-5051
Loraine DiPietro, Dir.
Subjects: Deafness, hearing loss, Gallaudet University. **Holdings:** 75 books;
5 VF drawers of subject files; 6 VF drawers of deafness agen-
cies/organizations files.

★7700★ NATIONAL INJURY INFORMATION
CLEARINGHOUSE
Westwood Towers Bldg., Rm. 625
5401 Westbard Ave.
Washington, DC 20207   Phone: (301) 492-6424
Joel I. Friedman, Dir.
Subjects: Injury data from accidents associated with consumer products;
epidemiology of accidents. **Holdings:** 100 staff studies and special reports
on consumer product-associated injuries.

★7701★ NATIONAL INSTITUTE ON ALCOHOL ABUSE AND
ALCOHOLISM
NIAAA RESEARCH LIBRARY
1400 Eye St., NW, C/CSR, Inc.
Washington, DC 22208   Phone: (202) 842-7600
June Picciano, Info.Serv.Mgr.
Subjects: Biomedical and psychosocial aspects of alcohol research. **Hold-
ings:** 2000 books; 70,000 accessioned items. **Subscriptions:** 122 journals
and other serials.

★7702★ NATIONAL INSTITUTE OF MENTAL HEALTH
NEUROSCIENCE RESEARCH CENTER/NEUROPSYCHIATRIC
RESEARCH HOSPITAL
LIBRARY
W.A.W. Bldg., Rm. 115
St. Elizabeth's Hospital
Washington, DC 20032   Phone: (202) 373-6071
LaVerne Corum, Hd.Libn.
Subjects: Neuroscience, psychopharmacology, psychiatry, pharmacology,
biochemistry, psychology. **Holdings:** 5700 books; 11,000 bound periodical
volumes; 18 drawers of journals on microfilm and microfiche; 5 drawers of
audio cassettes. **Subscriptions:** 301 journals and other serials.

★7703★ NATIONAL MINORITY AIDS COUNCIL
LIBRARY
300 I St., NE, Ste. 400
Washington, DC 20002   Phone: (202) 544-1076
Tomas Gomez
Subjects: AIDS issues relating to minorities population. **Holdings:** 30
books; 40 reports. **Subscriptions:** 20 journals and other serials; 5 newspa-
pers.

★7704★ NATIONAL REHABILITATION HOSPITAL
LEARNING RESOURCE CENTER
102 Irving St., NW
Washington, DC 20010   Phone: (202) 877-1995
Lynne Siemerr, Dir.
Subjects: Rehabilitation. **Holdings:** 350 books. **Subscriptions:** 76 journals
and other serials.

★7705★ NATIONAL RESTAURANT ASSOCIATION
INFORMATION SERVICE AND LIBRARY
1200 17th St., NW
Washington, DC 20036   Phone: (202) 331-5900
Larry Himelfarb, Lib.Mgr.
Subjects: Foodservice industry, restaurants, cookery, public health. **Hold-
ings:** 4000 books; 1300 subject clipping files; annual reports. **Subscriptions:**
250 journals and other serials.

★7706★ NATIONAL RIGHT TO LIFE COMMITTEE
LIBRARY
419 7th St., NW, Ste. 500
Washington, DC 20004   Phone: (202) 626-8800
Subjects: Abortion, euthanasia, and infanticide. **Holdings:** 430 books,
pamphlets, brochures, and audiovisual materials; vertical file containing
1650 items.

★7707★ NATIONAL WOMEN'S HEALTH NETWORK
WOMEN'S HEALTH INFORMATION SERVICE
LIBRARY
1325 G St., NW
Washington, DC 20005   Phone: (202) 347-1140
Subjects: Women's health issues - general, abortion, breast cancer, cervical
cancer, childbirth, contraceptives, menopause, occupational and environmental health, osteoporosis, pregnancy, premenstrual syndrome, sexually
transmitted diseases, teen pregnancy, toxic shock syndrome, women and
alcohol. **Holdings:** Figures not available.

★7708★ NONPRESCRIPTION DRUG MANUFACTURERS ASSOCIATION
LIBRARY
1150 Connecticut Ave., NW, Ste. 1200
Washington, DC 20036   Phone: (202) 429-9260
Phyllis M. Taylor, Libn.
Subjects: Medicines - nonprescription, limited prescription, allied-type groups; regulations affecting over-the-counter medicine. **Holdings:** 1000 volumes; U.S. Food and Drug Administration monographs and reports; AV programs. **Subscriptions:** 78 journals and other serials.

★7709★ PAN AMERICAN HEALTH ORGANIZATION
LIBRARY
525 23rd St., NW
Mail Code HBL
Washington, DC 20037   Phone: (202) 861-3305
Maria Theresa Astroza, Hd.
Subjects: Health sciences. **Holdings:** 15,000 books; 5000 bound periodical volumes; 25 file drawers of microfilm. **Subscriptions:** 130 journals and other serials.

★7710★ PROVIDENCE HOSPITAL
HEALTH SCIENCES LIBRARY
1150 Varnum St., NE
Washington, DC 20017   Phone: (202) 269-7144
RoseMarie G. Leone, Dir.
Subjects: Medicine, nursing, hospital administration, allied health sciences. **Holdings:** 1905 books; 5040 bound periodical volumes. **Subscriptions:** 200 journals and other serials.

★7711★ SCIENCE SERVICE, INC.
LIBRARY
1719 N St., NW
Washington, DC 20036   Phone: (202) 785-2255
Liz Marshall, Libn.
Subjects: Science, medicine, technology. **Holdings:** 3600 books; 1500 unbound periodicals. **Subscriptions:** 246 journals and other serials.

★7712★ SIBLEY MEMORIAL HOSPITAL
MEDICAL LIBRARY
5255 Loughboro Rd., NW
Washington, DC 20016   Phone: (202) 537-4110
Annie B. Footman, Libn.
Subjects: Medicine. **Holdings:** 1950 books; 913 bound periodical volumes; 4 VF drawers of clippings, reports, and documents. **Subscriptions:** 152 journals and other serials.

★7713★ THE SUGAR ASSOCIATION, INC.
LIBRARY
1101 15th St., NW, No. 600
Washington, DC 20005   Phone: (202) 785-1122
Suzanne Arnold, Libn.
Subjects: Sugar, nutrition and health, food technology. **Holdings:** 1500 books; 1000 bound periodical volumes; 50 VF drawers of pamphlets, clippings, patents, miscellaneous documents. **Subscriptions:** 100 journals and other serials; 7 newspapers.

★7714★ TOBACCO INSTITUTE
INFORMATION CENTER
1875 Eye St., NW, Ste. 800
Washington, DC 20006   Phone: (202) 457-9325
Maureen Booth, Res./Ref.Libn.
Subjects: Tobacco history, smoking/health controversy. **Holdings:** 2500 books; clippings; manuscripts; reports. **Subscriptions:** 200 journals and other serials; 10 newspapers.

★7715★ U.S. AIR FORCE HOSPITAL
MALCOLM GROW MEDICAL CENTER
MEDICAL LIBRARY/SGEL
Andrews AFB
Washington, DC 20331-5300   Phone: (202) 981-2354
Carol J. Davidson
Subjects: Internal medicine, nursing, cardiology, surgery, dentistry, food service, psychology. **Holdings:** 8000 books; 4000 bound periodical volumes; clippings; maps; bibliographies; dissertations; reprints; pamphlets; tapes. **Subscriptions:** 300 journals and other serials.

★7716★ U.S. ARMED FORCES INSTITUTE OF PATHOLOGY
ASH LIBRARY
Walter Reed Army Medical Center
Bldg. 54, Rm. 4077
Washington, DC 20306-6000   Phone: (202) 576-2983
Judith Paige, Libn.
Subjects: Pathology, medicine. **Holdings:** 6500 books; 18,000 bound periodical volumes; 2270 2x2's; 2425 glass slides; 3000 Massachusetts General Hospital sets. **Subscriptions:** 450 journals and other serials.

★7717★ U.S. ARMY
MEDICAL RESEARCH AND DEVELOPMENT COMMAND
WALTER REED ARMY INSTITUTE OF RESEARCH
LIBRARY
Walter Reed Army Medical Center
Washington, DC 20307-5100   Phone: (202) 576-3314
V. Lynn Gera, Dir., Info.Rsrcs.Ctr./Lib.
Subjects: Communicable diseases, immunology, dentistry, veterinary sciences, biochemistry, internal medicine, physiology, psychiatry, surgery, auto-immune deficiency syndrome. **Holdings:** 22,000 books; 11,000 bound periodical volumes. **Subscriptions:** 1000 journals and other serials.

★7718★ U.S. ARMY HOSPITALS
WALTER REED ARMY MEDICAL CENTER
WRAMC MEDICAL LIBRARY
Bldg. 2, Rm. 2G01
Washington, DC 20307-5001   Phone: (202) 576-1238
Hoyt W. Galloway, Lib.Dir.
Subjects: Clinical medicine, research, allied health sciences, history of medicine. **Holdings:** 10,000 books; 18,000 bound periodical volumes. **Subscriptions:** 750 journals and other serials.

★7719★ U.S. DEPARTMENT OF HEALTH AND HUMAN SERVICES
LIBRARY AND INFORMATION CENTER
330 Independence Ave., SW, Rm. G-619
Washington, DC 20201   Phone: (202) 619-0257
John R. Boyle, Dir.
Subjects: Social welfare, social sciences, education, health, medicine, law and legislation, administration and management. **Holdings:** 85,000 books; 40,000 archives; 450,000 microforms. **Subscriptions:** 1000 journals and other serials.

★7720★ U.S. DEPARTMENT OF HEALTH AND HUMAN SERVICES
POLICY INFORMATION CENTER
200 Independence Ave., SW, 438 F
Washington, DC 20201   Phone: (202) 245-6445
Carolyn Solomon, Tech.Info.Spec.
Subjects: Health, income maintenance and support, social services. **Holdings:** 4000 reports and executive summaries.

★7721★ U.S. DEPARTMENT OF LABOR
OSHA
TECHNICAL DATA CENTER
200 Constitution Ave., NW
Rm. N-2625
Washington, DC 20210   Phone: (202) 523-9700
Thomas A. Towers, Dir.
Subjects: Occupational safety, industrial hygiene, toxicology, control technology, hazardous materials, fire safety, electrical safety, noise, carcinogens, material safety, farm safety, process safety, ergonomics, occupational health nursing. **Holdings:** 12,000 books and bound periodical volumes; 250,000 microfiche; 2000 technical documents; 3000 standards and codes. **Subscriptions:** 250 journals and other serials.

★7722★ U.S. DEPARTMENT OF VETERANS AFFAIRS
HEADQUARTERS CENTRAL OFFICE LIBRARY
810 Vermont Ave., NW
Washington, DC 20420   Phone: (202) 233-2430
Wendy Carter, Chf., Pub.Serv.
Subjects: Medicine, health care administration, veterans affairs, management. **Holdings:** 13,000 books; 11,000 bound periodical volumes; 600 AV programs; slides. **Subscriptions:** 700 journals and other serials; 6 newspapers.

★7723★ U.S. DEPARTMENT OF VETERANS AFFAIRS
HEADQUARTERS LIBRARY DIVISION
810 Vermont Ave., NW
Washington, DC 20420   Phone: (202) 233-2711
Wendy Carter, Chf.Pub.Serv.
Subjects: Medicine, allied health sciences, health care administration, veterans affairs, management, medical education. **Holdings:** 695,000 books; 155,000 AV programs; pamphlets; microforms; government documents. **Subscriptions:** 3400 journals and other serials.

★7724★ U.S. DEPARTMENT OF VETERANS AFFAIRS
MEDICAL CENTER LIBRARY
50 Irving St., NW
Washington, DC 20422   Phone: (202) 745-8262
Mary Netzow, Chf.Libn.
Subjects: General medicine, surgery. **Holdings:** 2000 books; 4300 bound periodical volumes. **Subscriptions:** 200 journals and other serials.

★7725★ U.S. FOOD AND DRUG ADMINISTRATION
CENTER FOR FOOD SAFETY AND APPLIED NUTRITION
LIBRARY
200 C St., SW, Rm. 3321, HFF-37
Washington, DC 20204   Phone: (202) 245-1235
Michele R. Chatfield, Dir.
Subjects: Chemistry, analytical chemistry, toxicology, food technology, nutrition, medicine, biology, cosmetics. **Holdings:** 12,000 books; 1500 reports, documents, pamphlets; 18,000 cartridges of microfilm. **Subscriptions:** 900 journals and other serials.

★7726★ U.S. PUBLIC HEALTH SERVICE
HEALTH RESOURCES AND SERVICES ADMINISTRATION
BUREAU OF MATERNAL AND CHILD HEALTH AND
  RESOURCES DEVELOPMENT
NATIONAL CENTER FOR EDUCATION IN MATERNAL AND
  CHILD HEALTH LIBRARY
38th & R St., NW
Washington, DC 20057   Phone: (202) 625-8400
Rochelle Mayer, Prog.Dir.
Subjects: Maternal and child health - genetics, prenatal care, adolescent health, chronic illness/disability, developmental disabilities, infant mortality, nutrition. **Holdings:** 2000 books; ephemeral literature; organization files. **Subscriptions:** 50 journals and other serials.

★7727★ U.S. PUBLIC HEALTH SERVICE
OFFICE OF DISEASE PREVENTION AND HEALTH
  PROMOTION
ODPHP NATIONAL HEALTH INFORMATION CENTER
Box 1133
Washington, DC 20013-1133   Phone: (301) 565-4167
Patricia Lynch, Proj.Dir.
Subjects: Health, nutrition, health promotion. **Holdings:** 800 books; 50 bound periodical volumes; 44 VF drawers of pamphlets and clippings. **Subscriptions:** 75 journals and other serials.

★7728★ U.S. SOCIAL SECURITY ADMINISTRATION
BRANCH LIBRARY
Van Ness Centre, Rm. 206
4301 Connecticut Ave., NW
Washington, DC 20008   Phone: (202) 282-7000
Linda Del Bene, Libn.
Subjects: Social Security programs, retirement, disability insurance, income maintenance, pension benefits, health insurance, medical care. **Holdings:** 9000 books; 100 bound periodical volumes; 200 pamphlets; 500 microforms. **Subscriptions:** 260 journals and other serials.

★7729★ WASHINGTON HOSPITAL CENTER
MEDICAL LIBRARY
110 Irving St., NW, Rm. 2A-21
Washington, DC 20010   Phone: (202) 877-6221
Lynne Siemers, Dir.
Subjects: Medicine, nursing, health administration, allied health sciences. **Holdings:** 12,000 books; 18,000 bound periodical volumes; 1100 volumes on microfilm; 700 AV programs; 1 file drawer of pamphlets. **Subscriptions:** 960 journals and other serials.

★7730★ WASHINGTON PSYCHOANALYTIC SOCIETY
HADLEY MEMORIAL LIBRARY
4925 MacArthur Blvd., NW
Washington, DC 20007   Phone: (202) 338-5453
Joyce P. Burke
Subjects: Psychoanalysis, psychiatry, psychology. **Holdings:** 3200 books; 950 bound periodical volumes; 1200 unbound journals. **Subscriptions:** 50 journals and other serials.

Florida

★7731★ GORGAS ARMY COMMUNITY HOSPITAL
SAMUEL TAYLOR DARLING MEMORIAL LIBRARY
USA MEDDAC Panama
APO Miami, FL 34004
Fawn Walker, Libn.
Subjects: Medicine, allied health sciences. **Holdings:** 3000 books; 20,000 bound periodical volumes; 1000 videotapes; 300 AV programs. **Subscriptions:** 195 journals and other serials.

★7732★ ADVENTIST HEALTH SYSTEMS SUNBELT
WALKER MEMORIAL HOSPITAL
S.C. PARDEE MEDICAL LIBRARY
Hwy. 27, N.
Avon Park, FL 33825-1200   Phone: (813) 453-7511
Monica Lescay, Dir., Med.Rec. & Lib.
Subjects: Medicine and allied health sciences. **Holdings:** Figures not available.

★7733★ U.S. DEPARTMENT OF VETERANS AFFAIRS
MEDICAL LIBRARY
Bay Pines, FL 33504   Phone: (813) 398-9366
Ann A. Conlan, Chf., Lib.Serv.
Subjects: Medicine, surgery, psychiatry, nursing, radiology, dentistry. **Holdings:** 6000 books; 2000 bound periodical volumes. **Subscriptions:** 475 journals and other serials.

★7734★ BOCA RATON COMMUNITY HOSPITAL
HEALTH SCIENCES LIBRARY
800 Meadows Rd.
Boca Raton, FL 33486   Phone: (407) 393-4070
Carolyn F. Hill, Med.Libn.
Subjects: Medicine, nursing. **Holdings:** 1325 books; 2500 bound periodical volumes; 1 VF drawer of medical material. **Subscriptions:** 210 journals and other serials.

★7735★ HUXLEY INSTITUTE FOR BIOSOCIAL RESEARCH
LIBRARY AND RESOURCE CENTER
900 N. Federal Hwy., Ste. 330
Boca Raton, FL 33432   Phone: (407) 393-6167
Mary Roddy Haggerty, Dir.
Subjects: Orthomolecular medicine. **Holdings:** Figures not available.

★7736★ BETHESDA MEMORIAL HOSPITAL
MEDICAL LIBRARY
2815 S. Seacrest Blvd.
Boynton Beach, FL 33435   Phone: (407) 737-7733
Catherine J. Greene, Med.Libn.
Subjects: Medicine, nursing, hospital administration, allied health sciences. **Holdings:** 1800 books; 3218 bound periodical volumes; 253 unbound volumes; 6 VF drawers of clippings and pamphlets; 600 video cassettes. **Subscriptions:** 205 journals and other serials.

★7737★ MANATEE MEMORIAL HOSPITAL
WENTZEL MEDICAL LIBRARY
206 2nd St., E.
Bradenton, FL 34208   Phone: (813) 746-5111
Jeanette Mosher, Med.Libn.
Subjects: Medicine, nursing. **Holdings:** 2500 volumes. **Subscriptions:** 70 journals and other serials.

★7738★ FLORIDA STATE HOSPITAL
HEALTH SCIENCE LIBRARY
Chattahoochee, FL 32324   Phone: (904) 663-7205
Linda R. Hatcher, Lib.Asst.
Subjects: Psychiatry, medicine, psychology, nursing, social service. **Hold-**

ings: 2000 books; 75 bound periodical volumes. **Subscriptions:** 50 journals and other serials; 5 newspapers.

★7739★ **FLORIDA STATE HOSPITAL**
LIBRARY SERVICES
Chattahoochee, FL 32324   Phone: (904) 663-7671
Jane Marie Hamilton, Dir.
Subjects: General and mental health topics. **Holdings:** 15,000 volumes; 1200 films and filmstrips; 600 compact discs; photographs; toys; games; models. **Subscriptions:** 108 journals and other serials; 5 newspapers.

★7740★ **MORTON F. PLANT HOSPITAL**
MEDICAL LIBRARY
323 Jeffords St.
Box 210
Clearwater, FL 34617   Phone: (813) 462-7889
Cynthia Kisby, Med.Libn.
Subjects: Medicine, nursing, hospital administration. **Holdings:** 1200 books; 925 bound periodical volumes; 450 volumes on microfiche. **Subscriptions:** 143 journals and other serials.

★7741★ **DOCTORS' HOSPITAL**
MEDICAL LIBRARY
5000 University Dr.
Coral Gables, FL 33146   Phone: (305) 669-2334
Sandra E. Poston, Lib.Dir.
Subjects: Medicine, surgery, neurology and neurosurgery, ophthalmology. **Holdings:** 1156 books; 852 bound periodical volumes; video and audio cassettes. **Subscriptions:** 79 journals and other serials.

★7742★ **FLORIDA DEPARTMENT OF EDUCATION**
FLORIDA DIVISION OF BLIND SERVICES
BUREAU OF LIBRARY SERVICES FOR THE BLIND AND
  PHYSICALLY HANDICAPPED
420 Platt St.
Daytona Beach, FL 32114   Phone: (904) 254-3824
Donald John Weber, Dir.
Subjects: Recreational reading material for the print handicapped, blindness, physical handicaps, rehabilitation. **Holdings:** 600,000 books recorded on disc and cassette; 50,000 books in braille. **Subscriptions:** 100 journals and other serials.

★7743★ **HALIFAX HOSPITAL MEDICAL CENTER**
MEDICAL LIBRARY
Box 2830
Daytona Beach, FL 32115   Phone: (904) 254-4051
Addajane L. Wallace, Med.Libn.
Subjects: Medicine, nursing, hospital administration. **Holdings:** 2788 books; 2312 bound periodical volumes; 7 subscriptions for cassette tapes. **Subscriptions:** 200 journals and other serials.

★7744★ **FISH MEMORIAL HOSPITAL**
MEDICAL LIBRARY
245 E. New York Ave.
Box 167
De Land, FL 32721-0167   Phone: (904) 734-2323
Carolyn E. Creeron, Circuit Libn.
Subjects: Medicine, nursing, and allied health sciences. **Holdings:** 100 books; 20 unbound periodicals. **Subscriptions:** 10 journals and other serials.

★7745★ **WEST VOLUSIA MEMORIAL HOSPITAL**
MEDICAL LIBRARY
Box 509
De Land, FL 32721-0509   Phone: (904) 734-3320
Marjorie E. Cook, Lib.Mgr.
Subjects: Medicine and allied health sciences. **Holdings:** 800 books; 150 bound periodical volumes; 2 Audio-Digest subscriptions. **Subscriptions:** 50 journals and other serials.

★7746★ **FLORIDA OPHTHALMIC INSTITUTE**
LIBRARY
7106 NW 11th Pl.
Gainesville, FL 32605-3140   Phone: (904) 331-2020
Norman S. Levy
Subjects: Opthalmology, visual sciences. **Holdings:** 104 books; 14 bound periodical volumes. **Subscriptions:** 14 journals and other serials.

★7747★ **SUNLAND CENTER AT GAINESVILLE**
TACACHALE LIBRARY
Box 1150
Gainesville, FL 32602   Phone: (904) 395-1650
Subjects: Mental retardation, exceptional education. **Holdings:** 6800 volumes; 3500 AV programs; high interest-low vocabulary picture books; professional materials. **Subscriptions:** 25 journals and other serials.

★7748★ **TREE OF LIFE PRESS**
LIBRARY AND ARCHIVES
420 NE Blvd.
Gainesville, FL 32601
Reva Pachefsky, Libn.
Subjects: Infant language development, child development, graphic arts.

★7749★ **U.S. DEPARTMENT OF VETERANS AFFAIRS**
HOSPITAL LIBRARY
Archer Rd.
Gainesville, FL 32602   Phone: (904) 376-1611
Marylyn E. Gresser, Chf., Lib.Serv.
Subjects: Health education, neurology, surgery, internal medicine, nursing, pathology, pharmacology, ophthalmology, psychiatry, radiology. **Holdings:** 6657 books; 2500 periodical volumes; journal volumes on microfilm. **Subscriptions:** 358 journals and other serials; 9 newspapers.

★7750★ **UNIVERSITY OF FLORIDA**
HEALTH SCIENCE LIBRARY
Box J-206
Gainesville, FL 32611   Phone: (904) 392-4016
Ted F. Srygley, Dir.
Subjects: Medicine, basic medical sciences, nursing, pharmacy, veterinary medicine, allied health sciences, dentistry. **Holdings:** 239,061 volumes; 2400 films and tapes; 4117 microfiche; Ciba collection of slides. **Subscriptions:** 2355 journals and other serials.

★7751★ **HIALEAH HOSPITAL**
GEORGE H. WESSEL MEMORIAL LIBRARY
651 E. 25th St.
Hialeah, FL 33013   Phone: (305) 835-4635
Yvonne Barkman, Libn.
Subjects: Medicine, nursing, paramedical sciences, hospital administration. **Holdings:** 1300 books; 600 bound periodical volumes; 3 VF drawers of pamphlets and clippings; AV programs. **Subscriptions:** 105 journals and other serials.

★7752★ **SOUTH FLORIDA STATE HOSPITAL**
MEDICAL LIBRARY
1000 SW 84th Ave.
Hollywood, FL 33025   Phone: (305) 983-4321
Mabel E. Randall, Med.Libn.
Subjects: Psychiatry, neurology, psychology, nursing, social work. **Holdings:** 2650 books; 230 bound periodical volumes; cassettes; 3 masters' theses; tape cassettes. **Subscriptions:** 63 journals and other serials.

★7753★ **BLUE CROSS AND BLUE SHIELD OF FLORIDA**
CORPORATE RESEARCH LIBRARY
532 Riverside Ave.
Box 1798
Jacksonville, FL 32231   Phone: (904) 791-6937
William J. Condon, Lib.Mgr.
Subjects: Health insurance, health care, insurance, demographics, management, employee benefits. **Holdings:** 4000 books. **Subscriptions:** 220 journals and other serials.

★7754★ **MEDICAL CYBERNETICS FOUNDATION**
LIBRARY
Medical Design Center
PO Box 57333
Jacksonville, FL 32241   Phone: (904) 262-9248
Subjects: Medical machinery, cybernetics, engineering and medicine. **Holdings:** 5000 volumes; statistical materials.

★7755★ ST. LUKE'S HOSPITAL ASSOCIATION
MEDICAL, NURSING AND ALLIED HELP LIBRARY
4201 Belfort Rd.
Jacksonville, FL 32216   Phone: (904) 739-3735
Margarette Wally, Libn.
Subjects: Medicine, nursing. **Holdings:** 1155 books; 2128 bound periodical
volumes. **Subscriptions:** 77 journals and other serials.

★7756★ U.S. NAVY
NAVAL HOSPITAL
MEDICAL LIBRARY
Jacksonville, FL 32214   Phone: (904) 777-7583
Bettye W. Stilley, Med.Libn.
Subjects: Medicine. **Holdings:** 1500 books; 2400 bound periodical vol-
umes; 500 other cataloged items. **Subscriptions:** 162 journals and other
serials.

★7757★ UNIVERSITY OF FLORIDA
BORLAND HEALTH SCIENCES LIBRARY
PO Box 4426
Jacksonville, FL 32231   Phone: (904) 359-6516
Carolyn G. Hall, Dir.
Subjects: Medicine, public health, nursing, allied health sciences, dentistry.
Holdings: 3400 books; 24,400 bound periodical volumes. **Subscriptions:**
575 journals and other serials.

★7758★ U.S. DEPARTMENT OF VETERANS AFFAIRS
MEDICAL CENTER
LEARNING RESOURCE CENTER
801 S. Marion St.
Lake City, FL 32055-5898   Phone: (904) 755-3016
Shirley Mabry, Chf., Lib.Serv.
Subjects: Medicine, surgery, nursing, and allied health sciences; hospital
administration; patient education. **Holdings:** 4120 books; 2800 bound
periodical volumes; 1007 AV programs; 1100 patient health education
pamphlets and handouts; 300 talking books; 10 VF drawers; 2500 volumes
on microfilm; 30 software programs. **Subscriptions:** 506 journals and other
serials; 15 newspapers.

★7759★ LAKE WALES HOSPITAL
MEDICAL LIBRARY
410 S. 11th St.
Box 3460
Lake Wales, FL 33853   Phone: (813) 676-1433
Ada Leigh Byrd, Mgr.
Subjects: Medicine, pediatrics, obstetrics/gynecology, geriatrics. **Holdings:**
150 books; 15 bound periodical volumes. **Subscriptions:** 65 journals and
other serials; 6 newspapers.

★7760★ J.F.K. MEMORIAL HOSPITAL
MEDICAL LIBRARY
S. Congress Ave.
Box 1489
Lake Worth, FL 33460   Phone: (407) 965-7300
Nancy M. Adams, Dir.
Subjects: Medicine. **Holdings:** 450 books; 300 bound periodical volumes.
Subscriptions: 175 journals and other serials.

★7761★ LAKELAND REGIONAL MEDICAL CENTER
MEDICAL LIBRARY
1324 Lakeland Hills Blvd.
Drawer 95448
Lakeland, FL 33804-0448   Phone: (813) 687-1176
Jan Booker, Lib.Serv.Coord.
Subjects: Medicine, nursing, medical administration. **Holdings:** 1000
books; 5000 bound periodical volumes; AV programs; 300 other cataloged
items. **Subscriptions:** 166 journals and other serials.

★7762★ WATSON CLINIC
MEDICAL LIBRARY
Box 95000
Lakeland, FL 33804-5000   Phone: (813) 680-7098
Cheryl Dee, Lib.Dir.
Subjects: Medicine. **Holdings:** 1800 books; 3000 bound periodical vol-
umes; 550 cassettes. **Subscriptions:** 400 journals and other serials.

★7763★ A.G. HOLLEY STATE HOSPITAL
BENJAMIN L. BROCK MEDICAL LIBRARY
Box 3084
Lantana, FL 33462   Phone: (407) 582-5666
Andree D. Sweek, Dir., Med.Rec.
Subjects: Medicine. **Holdings:** 1325 books; 2100 bound periodical vol-
umes. **Subscriptions:** 27 journals and other serials.

★7764★ BAPTIST HOSPITAL OF MIAMI
HEALTH SCIENCES LIBRARY
8900 N. Kendall Dr.
Miami, FL 33176   Phone: (305) 596-6506
Diane F. Ream, Dir.
Subjects: Medicine, nursing, allied health sciences, hospital administration, consumer health. **Holdings:** 550 books; 1800 bound periodical
volumes; 4 VF drawers of pamphlets, reprints, clippings; 5500 slides; 500
audio cassettes. **Subscriptions:** 200 journals and other serials.

★7765★ BAXTER HEALTHCARE CORPORATION
BAXTER DADE DIVISION
RESEARCH LIBRARY
1851 Delaware Pkwy.
Box 520672
Miami, FL 33152   Phone: (305) 633-6461
Bernadene A. Chang, Res.Lib.Supv.
Subjects: Clinical chemistry, chemical abstracts, biochemistry, immunolo-
gy, medicine, pathology. **Holdings:** 1000 books; 1200 bound periodical
volumes; 2000 unbound journals; 20 directories; 2000 patents; 75 journal
titles on microfilm. **Subscriptions:** 200 journals and other serials.

★7766★ BLACKWELL & WALKER, P.A.
LAW LIBRARY
2400 Amerifirst Bldg.
One SE 3rd Ave.
Miami, FL 33131   Phone: (305) 995-5717
Angela Marie Speranza, Law Libn.
Subjects: Law - business, insurance, medical, litigation. **Holdings:** 25,000
volumes. **Subscriptions:** 20 journals and other serials.

★7767★ JACKSON MEMORIAL HOSPITAL
SCHOOL OF NURSING LIBRARY
1755 NW 12th Ave.
Miami, FL 33136-1094   Phone: (305) 549-6833
Lynn MacAuley, Libn.
Subjects: Nursing, medicine, health. **Holdings:** 2500 books; 150 bound
periodical volumes; 230 National League for Nursing reports and pam-
phlets; 80 video cassettes. **Subscriptions:** 67 journals and other serials.

★7768★ MERCY HOSPITAL
MEDICAL LIBRARY
3663 S. Miami Ave.
Miami, FL 33133   Phone: (305) 285-2160
David M. Olson, Dir.
Subjects: Cardiology, internal medicine, nursing. **Holdings:** 1300 books;
4800 bound periodical volumes; 250 video cassettes; 1200 audio cassettes.
Subscriptions: 130 journals and other serials.

★7769★ MIAMI-DADE COMMUNITY COLLEGE
MEDICAL CENTER CAMPUS LIBRARY
950 NW 20th St.
Miami, FL 33127   Phone: (305) 347-4129
Sally Ream, Dir.
Subjects: Allied health, nursing. **Holdings:** 12,000 books; 2054 bound
periodical volumes. **Subscriptions:** 279 journals and other serials.

★7770★ MIAMI-DADE PUBLIC LIBRARY
BUSINESS, SCIENCE AND TECHNOLOGY DEPARTMENT
101 W. Flagler St.
Miami, FL 33130-1504   Phone: (305) 375-2665
John Heim
Subjects: Business, economics, international trade, investments, layperson's medical reference, pure and applied sciences. **Holdings:** 45,000
volumes; 80 VF drawers of pamphlets. **Subscriptions:** 700 journals and
other serials.

★7771★ NORTH SHORE MEDICAL CENTER
MEDICAL LIBRARY
1100 NW 95th St.
Miami, FL 33150   Phone: (305) 835-6000
Stephanie Thomas, Supr.
Subjects: Surgery, pathology, thoracic medicine, cancer, dermatology, pharmacology. **Holdings:** 250 books; 44 bound periodical volumes; 30 pamphlets; 47 films. **Subscriptions:** 26 journals and other serials.

★7772★ SYLVESTER COMPREHENSIVE CANCER CENTER
THE CANCER INFORMATION SERVICE
Jackson Towers, Rm. 1015
Miami, FL 33136   Phone: (305) 548-4821
Jo Beth Speyer, Dir.
Subjects: Cancer, nutrition. **Holdings:** Figures not available.

★7773★ U.S. DEPARTMENT OF VETERANS AFFAIRS
MEDICAL LIBRARY
1201 NW 16th St.
Miami, FL 33125   Phone: (305) 324-3187
Mark A. Petersen, Chf.Libn.
Subjects: Medicine, nursing, psychology, allied health sciences. **Holdings:** 3032 books; 5328 bound periodical volumes; 392 AV programs. **Subscriptions:** 650 journals and other serials.

★7774★ UNIVERSITY OF MIAMI
SCHOOL OF MEDICINE
BASCOM PALMER EYE INSTITUTE
MARY AND EDWARD NORTON LIBRARY OF
    OPHTHALMOLOGY
Anne Bates Leach Eye Hospital
900 NW 17th St.
Box 016880
Miami, FL 33101   Phone: (305) 326-6078
Reva Hurtes, Libn.
Subjects: Ophthalmology, visual optics, visual physiology and anatomy. **Holdings:** 15,000 volumes; AV programs. **Subscriptions:** 200 journals and other serials.

★7775★ UNIVERSITY OF MIAMI
SCHOOL OF MEDICINE
LOUIS CALDER MEMORIAL LIBRARY
Box 016950
Miami, FL 33101   Phone: (305) 547-6441
Henry L. Lemkau, Jr., Dir.
Subjects: Medicine, nursing. **Holdings:** 63,674 books; 103,469 bound periodical volumes; 620 Florida pamphlets; 261 linear feet of archives; 20 linear feet of clipping files; 1821 illustrations; 212 medallions; 1226 portraits; 347 dissertations; 353 volumes of faculty publications. **Subscriptions:** 2405 journals and other serials.

★7776★ UP FRONT DRUG INFORMATION
LIBRARY
5701 Biscayne Blvd., Ste. 602
Miami, FL 33137   Phone: (305) 757-2566
James N. Hall, Exec.Dir.
Subjects: Drug information. **Holdings:** 1000 books; 900 unbound periodicals; 12 VF drawers and 100 pamphlet files of drug information. **Subscriptions:** 27 journals and other serials; 5 newspapers.

★7777★ MIAMI HEART INSTITUTE HOSPITAL
MEDICAL LIBRARY
4701 Meridian Ave.
Miami Beach, FL 33140   Phone: (305) 674-3108
Irene Bohlmann, Dir.
Subjects: Medicine, cardiovascular research. **Holdings:** 500 books; 7000 bound periodical volumes. **Subscriptions:** 150 journals and other serials.

★7778★ MOUNT SINAI MEDICAL CENTER OF GREATER
    MIAMI
MEDICAL LIBRARY
4300 Alton Rd.
Miami Beach, FL 33140   Phone: (305) 674-2840
Mildred Karukin, Chf.Med.Libn.
Subjects: Medicine, nursing, hospital administration, allied health sciences. **Holdings:** 5000 books; 9000 bound periodical volumes; 400 audiotapes; 200 videotapes; 3000 slides. **Subscriptions:** 450 journals and other serials.

★7779★ NATIONAL NETWORK OF YOUTH ADVISORY
    BOARDS, INC.
TECHNICAL ASSISTANCE LIBRARY
Ocean View Branch
PO Box 402036
Miami Beach, FL 33140   Phone: (305) 532-2607
Stuart Alan Rado, Dir.
Subjects: Youth involvement and employment, child abuse, juvenile justice, substance abuse, education. **Holdings:** 500 books; manuals.

★7780★ ST. FRANCIS HOSPITAL
BIOETHICS INSTITUTE
LIBRARY
250 W. 63rd St.
Miami Beach, FL 33141   Phone: (305) 868-5000
Wilma S. Grover, Libn.
Subjects: Judeo-Christian medical ethics, withholding treatment, living wills, allocation of health care resources, ethics committees, nursing ethics. **Holdings:** Figures not available. **Subscriptions:** 25 journals and other serials.

★7781★ ST. FRANCIS HOSPITAL
MEDICAL LIBRARY
250 W. 63rd St.
Miami Beach, FL 33141   Phone: (305) 868-5000
Wilma S. Grover, Libn.
Subjects: Medicine and allied health sciences. **Holdings:** 700 books; 2750 bound periodical volumes; 856 audiotapes; 12 phonograph records; 576 slides; videotapes. **Subscriptions:** 100 journals and other serials.

★7782★ SOUTHEASTERN UNIVERSITY OF THE HEALTH
    SCIENCES
HEALTH SCIENCES LIBRARY
1750 NE 168th St.
North Miami Beach, FL 33162   Phone: (305) 949-4000
Erica L. Moon, Act.Dir.
Subjects: Clinical medicine, basic sciences, osteopathy, pharmacy, optometry. **Holdings:** 8500 books; 5453 bound periodical volumes; 118 state osteopathic journals and newsletters. **Subscriptions:** 475 journals and other serials.

★7783★ FLORIDA HOSPITAL
MEDICAL LIBRARY
601 E. Rollins St.
Orlando, FL 32803   Phone: (407) 897-1860
Barbara Beckner, Libn.
Subjects: Medicine, surgery. **Holdings:** 1000 books; 6000 bound periodical volumes; 1 VF drawer; 25 titles on microfiche. **Subscriptions:** 320 journals and other serials.

★7784★ ORLANDO REGIONAL MEDICAL CENTER
MEDICAL LIBRARY
1414 S. Kuhl Ave.
Orlando, FL 32806   Phone: (407) 841-5111
Naomi F. Elia, Lib.Mgr.
Subjects: Medicine. **Holdings:** 2500 books; 15,325 bound periodical volumes. **Subscriptions:** 320 journals and other serials.

★7785★ U.S. NAVY
NAVAL HOSPITAL
MEDICAL LIBRARY
Orlando, FL 32813   Phone: (407) 646-4959
Nancy B. Toole, Med.Libn.
Subjects: Clinical medicine. **Holdings:** 1032 books; 500 bound periodical volumes; 625 video cassettes. **Subscriptions:** 86 journals and other serials.

★7786★ U.S. AIR FORCE HOSPITAL
MEDICAL LIBRARY
Patrick AFB, FL 32925-5300   Phone: (407) 494-8105
Arlene S. Bilsky, Med.Lib.Techn.
Subjects: Medicine, surgery, nursing. **Holdings:** 774 books. **Subscriptions:** 50 journals and other serials.

★7787★ BAPTIST HOSPITAL
MEDICAL LIBRARY
1000 W. Moreno
Pensacola, FL 32501   Phone: (904) 434-4877
Ellen Richbourg, Libn.
Subjects: Medicine. **Holdings:** 600 books; 5000 bound periodical volumes.
Subscriptions: 150 journals and other serials.

★7788★ ESCAMBIA COUNTY HEALTH DEPARTMENT
LIBRARY
Box 12604
Pensacola, FL 32574-2604   Phone: (904) 435-6550
Linda Mills, Hea.Educ.Supv.
Subjects: Health, public health. **Holdings:** Vertical files.

★7789★ LAKEVIEW CENTER, INC.
LIBRARY
1221 W. Lakeview Ave.
Pensacola, FL 32501-1857   Phone: (904) 432-1222
Dr. Susan Seabury Smith, Ctr.Libn.
Subjects: Psychiatry, psychology, alcoholism, drug addiction, children's and young adult's problems, management. **Holdings:** 1587 books; 213 audio cassettes; 52 video cassettes; 56 kits; 13 films; 219 government documents; 5 games. **Subscriptions:** 36 journals and other serials.

★7790★ SACRED HEART HOSPITAL
MEDICAL LIBRARY
5151 N. 9th Ave.
Pensacola, FL 32504   Phone: (904) 476-7851
Florence V. Ruby, Hosp.Libn.
Subjects: Medicine, pediatrics, nursing, management. **Holdings:** 918 books; 3520 bound periodical volumes. **Subscriptions:** 142 journals and other serials.

★7791★ U.S. NAVY
NAVAL AEROSPACE MEDICAL INSTITUTE
LIBRARY
Bldg. 1953, Code 03L
Pensacola, FL 32508-5600   Phone: (904) 452-2256
Ruth T. Rogers, Adm.Libn.
Subjects: Aviation and aerospace medicine, medical specialties, basic sciences. **Holdings:** 10,000 books; 10,000 bound periodical volumes. **Subscriptions:** 300 journals and other serials.

★7792★ U.S. NAVY
NAVAL HOSPITAL
MEDICAL LIBRARY
Pensacola, FL 32512-5000   Phone: (904) 452-6635
Mrs. Connie C. Walker, Med.Libn.
Subjects: Medicine, allied health sciences. **Holdings:** 5000 books; 15,000 bound periodical volumes. **Subscriptions:** 228 journals and other serials.

★7793★ UNIVERSITY HOSPITAL AND CLINIC
HERBERT L. BRYANS MEMORIAL LIBRARY
1200 W. Leonard St.
Pensacola, FL 32501   Phone: (904) 436-9187
Ms. Sammie Campbell, Libn.
Subjects: Medicine, dentistry, nursing, dietetics, hospital administration.
Holdings: 200 books. **Subscriptions:** 37 journals and other serials.

★7794★ UNIVERSITY OF WEST FLORIDA
HUMAN RESOURCE VIDEOTAPE LIBRARY
Dept. of Social Work
College of Arts & Sciences
11000 University Pkwy.
Pensacola, FL 32514-5751   Phone: (904) 474-2381
Prof. Bonnie Bedics
Subjects: Addiction, child abuse, mental illness and therapy. **Holdings:** 200 videotapes.

★7795★ WEST FLORIDA REGIONAL MEDICAL CENTER
MEDICAL LIBRARY
8383 N. Davis Hwy.
Box 18900
Pensacola, FL 32523-8900   Phone: (904) 478-4460
Kay Franklin, Dir./Med.Libn.
Subjects: Clinical medicine, oncology. **Holdings:** 1400 books. **Subscriptions:** 307 journals and other serials.

★7796★ METROPOLITAN GENERAL HOSPITAL
MEDICAL LIBRARY
7950 66th St., N.
Pinellas Park, FL 33565   Phone: (813) 546-9871
Jeanna Burchick, Rec.Adm.
Subjects: Medicine, family practice, osteopathy. **Holdings:** 520 books; 554 audiotapes. **Subscriptions:** 22 journals and other serials.

★7797★ WUESTHOFF MEMORIAL HOSPITAL
HOSPITAL LIBRARY
110 Longwood Ave.
Box 560006
Rockledge, FL 32956   Phone: (407) 636-2211
Subjects: Medicine, surgery, nursing, allied health sciences. **Holdings:** 1936 books; 620 bound periodical volumes; 480 audio cassettes; 49 slide carousels; 4 VF drawers of pamphlets. **Subscriptions:** 126 journals and other serials.

★7798★ FLORIDA SCHOOL FOR THE DEAF AND BLIND
LIBRARY FOR THE DEAF
207 San Marco Ave.
St. Augustine, FL 32084   Phone: (904) 823-4470
Linda L. Zimmerman, Hd.Libn.
Subjects: Education of the deaf (pre-kindergarden through high school), sign language and the deaf, fiction and nonfiction (low level, high interest). **Holdings:** 12,000 books; 5 bound periodical volumes; pamphlets; filmstrips; captioned films; film loops. **Subscriptions:** 68 journals and other serials.

★7799★ BAYFRONT MEDICAL CENTER
HEALTH SCIENCES LIBRARY
701 6th St., S.
St. Petersburg, FL 33701   Phone: (813) 893-6136
Sylvia Cesanek, Hea.Sci.Libn.
Subjects: Medicine, family practice, geriatrics, nursing, obstetrics, gynecology, oncology, physical rehabilitation. **Holdings:** 1500 books; 6000 bound periodical volumes; 200 Audio-Digest tapes; 300 video cassettes. **Subscriptions:** 180 journals.

★7800★ PINELLAS COUNTY JUVENILE WELFARE BOARD
MAILANDE W. HOLLAND LIBRARY
4140 49th St., N.
St. Petersburg, FL 33709   Phone: (813) 521-1853
Alison R. Birmingham, Libn.
Subjects: Child welfare, marriage and family therapy, juvenile delinquency, substance abuse, child abuse and neglect, day care and early childhood education, primary prevention, adolescent health, mental health, advocacy for economically disadvantaged, legislation, administration, funding and grant writing, community planning and development, community education. **Holdings:** 2000 books; 300 government documents; 300 AV programs. **Subscriptions:** 120 journals and other serials.

★7801★ ST. ANTHONY'S HOSPITAL
MEDICAL LIBRARY
1200 7th Ave. N.
St. Petersburg, FL 33705   Phone: (813) 825-1286
Grace DeWald, Med.Libn.
Subjects: Internal medicine, surgery, radiology, psychiatry, oncology, nursing. **Holdings:** 2248 books; 4412 bound periodical volumes; 240 unbound reports; 33 archival materials. **Subscriptions:** 141 journals and other serials; 6 newspapers.

★7802★ SARASOTA MEMORIAL HOSPITAL
MEDICAL LIBRARY
1700 S. Tamiami Trail
Sarasota, FL 34239-3555   Phone: (813) 953-1730
Subjects: Medicine, nursing. **Holdings:** 3000 books; 6000 bound periodical volumes; 1400 audio- and videotapes. **Subscriptions:** 175 journals.

★7803★ FLORIDA A&M UNIVERSITY
PHARMACY LIBRARY
Box 367
Tallahassee, FL 32307   Phone: (904) 599-3753
Pauline E. Hicks, Univ.Libn.
Subjects: Pharmacy, pharmaceutical chemistry, pharmacology, pharmacognosy, clinical pharmacy, environmental toxicology, medicinal chemistry. **Holdings:** 9935 books; 6800 bound periodical volumes; AV programs. **Subscriptions:** 525 journals and other serials.

★7804★ FLORIDA A&M UNIVERSITY
SCHOOLS OF NURSING LIBRARY/ALLIED HEALTH
 SCIENCES LIBRARY
Box 136
Florida A&M University
Tallahassee, FL 32307
Julita C. Awkard, Libn.   Phone: (904) 599-3872
Subjects: Nursing, allied health sciences, respiratory therapy, physical
therapy, health care management, medical records administration. Hold-
ings: 6000 books; 5194 software and hardware programs; 400 microfilm;
3000 microfiche; 150 films and AV materials. Subscriptions: 178 journals
and other serials.

★7805★ FLORIDA STATE UNIVERSITY
SCHOOL OF NURSING
LEARNING RESOURCE CENTER
310 School of Nursing
Tallahassee, FL 32306
Leonard N. Barnes, Sr., Lrng.Rsrcs.Spec.   Phone: (904) 644-1291
Subjects: Community health, mental health, maternal and child care,
surgery, pediatrics, anatomy, physiology. Holdings: 4820 books; 153 bound
periodical volumes; 108 nursing films; 325 slides; 378 videotapes; 103
filmstrips; 30 anatomical models; federal and state documents; newsletters.
Subscriptions: 76 journals and other serials.

★7806★ AMERICAN NATURAL HYGIENE SOCIETY
HERBERT SHELTON LIBRARY
Box 30630
Tampa, FL 33630
Barbara A. Bishop, Libn.   Phone: (813) 855-6607
Subjects: Natural hygiene, health, fasting, diet and nutrition, physical
culture. Holdings: 2000 books; 500 bound periodical volumes.

★7807★ CENTURION HOSPITAL OF CARROLLWOOD
MEDICAL LIBRARY
7171 N. Dale Mabry Hwy.
Tampa, FL 33614
Janna Cluxton, Libn.   Phone: (813) 935-1191
Subjects: Medicine, nursing, and allied health sciences. Holdings: 150
books; 27 bound periodical volumes. Subscriptions: 41 journals and other
serials.

★7808★ CHRISTIAN MEDICAL FOUNDATION
 INTERNATIONAL
LIBRARY
7522 N. Hines Ave.
Tampa, FL 33614
Lyn Thornton, Asst.Dir.   Phone: (813) 932-3688
Subjects: Christian medical and ethical principles, spiritual care of the ill.
Holdings: 2500 volumes; biographical archives.

★7809★ CRITIKON, INC.
R & D INFORMATION SERVICES LIBRARY
4110 George Rd.
Tampa, FL 33634-7498
Jeffrey A. Baker, Supv., Info.Serv.   Phone: (813) 887-2000
Subjects: Biomedical engineering, medicine, electronics, chemistry, bio-
chemistry. Holdings: 2600 books. Subscriptions: 100 journals and other
serials.

★7810★ ST. JOSEPH'S HOSPITAL
MEDICAL LIBRARY
3000 W. Buffalo Ave.
Box 4227
Tampa, FL 33677
Adelia P. Seglin, Dir., Med.Lib.   Phone: (813) 870-4658
Subjects: Medicine, nursing, cancer, pharmacology, management, cardiolo-
gy. Holdings: 1500 books; 5800 bound periodical volumes. Subscriptions:
257 journals and other serials.

★7811★ TAMPA GENERAL HOSPITAL
MEDICAL/CORPORATE INFORMATION CENTER
Box 1289
Tampa, FL 33601
Margaret Henry Petro, MLS, Libn.   Phone: (813) 251-7328
Subjects: Medicine, nursing, pharmacy, otorhinolaryngology, anesthesiolo-
gy, neurology, opthalmology, orthopedics, pathology, psychiatry, radiolo-
gy, urology, rehabilitation, pediatrics, obstetrics, gynecology, surgery.

Holdings: 3100 books; 3600 bound serial volumes; 12 drawers of microfiche. Subscriptions: 400 journals and other serials.

★7812★ U.S. DEPARTMENT OF VETERANS AFFAIRS
MEDICAL LIBRARY
James A. Haley Veterans Hospital
13000 N. Bruce B. Downs Blvd.
Tampa, FL 33612   Phone: (813) 972-2000
Subjects: Internal medicine, psychiatry, nursing, geriatrics. Holdings: 3508
books; 2281 bound periodical volumes. Subscriptions: 383 journals and
other serials.

★7813★ UNIVERSITY COMMUNITY HOSPITAL
MEDICAL LIBRARY
3100 E. Fletcher Ave.
Tampa, FL 33613   Phone: (813) 972-7236
Gwen E. Walters, Lib.Dir.
Subjects: Medicine, nursing, allied health sciences, health care delivery and
administration. Holdings: 1740 books; 715 bound periodical volumes; 168
periodicals in microform; 28 file drawers of microfilm; 12 file drawers of
microfiche; slides; audiotapes. Subscriptions: 439 journals and other
serials.

★7814★ UNIVERSITY OF SOUTH FLORIDA
FLORIDA MENTAL HEALTH INSTITUTE
LIBRARY
13301 Bruce B. Downs Blvd.
Tampa, FL 33612   Phone: (813) 974-4471
Josephine King Evans, Assoc.Univ.Libn./Dir.
Subjects: Psychology and psychiatry; epidemiology; aging, child, and
family programs; forensics; community mental health; social work. Holdings: 9574 books; 62 bound periodical volumes; 3000 unbound periodicals;
689 state and government documents; 60 microforms; 280 audio and video
cassettes; 74 kits; 82 computer diskettes. Subscriptions: 167 journals and
other serials.

★7815★ UNIVERSITY OF SOUTH FLORIDA
HEALTH SCIENCES CENTER LIBRARY
12901 Bruce B. Downs Blvd.
Box 31
Tampa, FL 33612   Phone: (813) 974-2399
Beverly Shattuck, Dir.
Subjects: Medicine, nursing, public health, allied health sciences. Holdings:
106,021 volumes. Subscriptions: 1504 journals and other serials.

★7816★ INDIAN RIVER MEMORIAL HOSPITAL
J.C. ROBERTSON MEMORIAL LIBRARY
1000 36th St.
Vero Beach, FL 32960   Phone: (407) 567-4311
E.W. Knowles, Aux.Libn.
Subjects: Medicine, medical specialties, surgery. Holdings: 616 books; 512
bound periodical volumes. Subscriptions: 62 journals and other serials.

★7817★ GOOD SAMARITAN HEALTH SYSTEMS
RICHARD S. BEINECKE MEDICAL LIBRARY
PO Box 3166
West Palm Beach, FL 33402   Phone: (407) 650-6315
Linda O'Callaghan, Dir.
Subjects: Clinical medicine, nursing, hospital management, management.
Holdings: 2500 books; 7690 bound periodical volumes; 150 rare books;
971 videotapes; 139 audiotapes; 92 slides. Subscriptions: 232 journals and
other serials.

★7818★ ST. MARY'S HOSPITAL
HEALTH SCIENCES LIBRARY
901 45th St.
West Palm Beach, FL 33407   Phone: (407) 881-2724
Christine M. McMahon, Libn.
Subjects: Medicine, nursing, allied health sciences. Holdings: 464 books;
6416 bound periodical volumes. Subscriptions: 150 journals and other
serials.

★7819★ WINTER HAVEN HOSPITAL
J.G. CONVERSE MEMORIAL MEDICAL LIBRARY
200 Ave. F., NE
Winter Haven, FL 33881   Phone: (813) 293-1121
Henry Hasse, Media Mgr.
Subjects: Medicine, nursing, allied health sciences, community mental

health. **Holdings:** 760 books; 1300 bound periodical volumes; 400 video cassettes. **Subscriptions:** 110 journals and other serials.

★7820★ WINTER PARK MEMORIAL HOSPITAL
MEDICAL STAFF LIBRARY
200 N. Lakemont Ave.
Winter Park, FL 32792   Phone: (407) 646-7049
Patricia N. Cole, Med.Libn.
Subjects: Medicine, surgery, nursing. **Holdings:** 2815 books; 8717 bound periodical volumes; 150 feet of unbound periodicals; 1450 tapes; 1 VF cabinet of pamphlets. **Subscriptions:** 250 journals and other serials.

Georgia

★7821★ SUMTER REGIONAL HOSPITAL
MEDICAL LIBRARY
100 Wheatley Dr.
Americus, GA 31709   Phone: (912) 924-6011
Claudia LeSueur
Subjects: Medicine, nursing, and allied health sciences. **Holdings:** Figures not available.

★7822★ AMERICAN ASSOCIATION OF OCCUPATIONAL
      HEALTH NURSES
LIBRARY
50 Lenox Pointe
Atlanta, GA 30324-3176   Phone: (404) 262-1162
Marcie Bates, Libn.
Subjects: Occupational health nursing, occupational medicine. **Holdings:** 1200 books; 24 bound periodical volumes; 1050 pamphlets. **Subscriptions:** 54 journals and other serials; 6 newspapers.

★7823★ AMERICAN CANCER SOCIETY
AUDIO VISUAL LIBRARIES
1599 Clifton Rd.
Atlanta, GA 30329   Phone: (404) 329-7914
Joni Zeccola, Proj.Coord.
Subjects: Cancer - diagnosis, treatment, rehabilitation, prevention, protection. **Holdings:** 16mm films; video cassettes; filmstrips; slide sets; audio cassettes.

★7824★ AMERICAN CANCER SOCIETY
MEDICAL LIBRARY
1599 Clifton Rd.
Atlanta, GA 30329   Phone: (404) 320-3333
Kathie Thodeson, Libn.
Subjects: Oncology, biochemistry, cytology, public health, rehabilitation of the cancer patient, smoking, radiobiology, general medicine. **Holdings:** 18,000 books; 7000 bound periodical volumes; 30 file holders of reports from foundations, institutes, and laboratories. **Subscriptions:** 620 journals and other serials.

★7825★ CRAWFORD LONG HOSPITAL OF EMORY
      UNIVERSITY
MEDICAL LIBRARY
550 Peachtree St., NE
Atlanta, GA 30365-2225   Phone: (404) 686-2678
Mrs. Girija Vijay, Dir.
Subjects: Medicine, nursing, allied health sciences. **Holdings:** 4811 books; 7959 bound periodical volumes; 710 VF folders; 448 audio cassettes; 14 slide sets; 12 phonograph records; 83 charts and pictures; 16 teaching aids; 9 maps; 11 microfiche sets; 786 videotapes. **Subscriptions:** 318 journals and other serials.

★7826★ EMORY UNIVERSITY
SCHOOL OF MEDICINE
HEALTH SCIENCES LIBRARY
Atlanta, GA 30322   Phone: (404) 727-5820
Carol A. Burns, Dir.
Subjects: Medicine, dentistry, nursing, public health. **Holdings:** 66,506 books; 113,804 bound periodical volumes; 4143 AV programs. **Subscriptions:** 3095 journals and other serials.

★7827★ EMORY UNIVERSITY
SCIENCE LIBRARY
Woodruff Library
Atlanta, GA 30322   Phone: (404) 727-6885
Elaine Wagner, Science Ref.Libn.
Subjects: Biology, psychology, physics, geology, mathematics, computer science, sociology of medicine. **Holdings:** 58,000 books. **Subscriptions:** 2000 journals and other serials.

★7828★ GEORGIA BAPTIST MEDICAL CENTER
MEDICAL LIBRARY
300 Boulevard, NE
Box 415
Atlanta, GA 30312   Phone: (404) 653-4603
Fay E. Evatt, Dir.
Subjects: Medicine, allied health sciences. **Holdings:** 3000 books; 12,000 bound periodical volumes. **Subscriptions:** 258 journals and other serials; 15 newspapers; 12 AV subscriptions.

★7829★ GEORGIA DEPARTMENT OF EDUCATION
LIBRARY FOR THE BLIND AND PHYSICALLY HANDICAPPED
1150 Murphy Ave., SW
Atlanta, GA 30310   Phone: (404) 756-4619
Dale S. Snair, Dir.
Holdings: 180,000 talking books; books in braille and large print; tapes and cassettes. **Subscriptions:** 4 journals and other serials.

★7830★ GEORGIA DEPARTMENT OF HUMAN RESOURCES
GEORGIA MENTAL HEALTH INSTITUTE
ADDISON M. DUVAL LIBRARY
1256 Briarcliff Rd., NE
Atlanta, GA 30306-2694   Phone: (404) 894-5663
Rosalind Lett, Lib.Dir.
Subjects: Psychiatry, nursing, social work, chaplaincy, activities therapy, psychology, substance abuse, forensic psychiatry. **Holdings:** 15,000 books; 3400 bound periodical volumes. **Subscriptions:** 152 journals and other serials.

★7831★ GEORGIA DEPARTMENT OF HUMAN RESOURCES
GEORGIA RETARDATION CENTER
PROFESSIONAL LIBRARY
4770 N. Peachtree Rd.
Atlanta, GA 30338   Phone: (404) 551-7076
Jane F. Clark, Sr.Libn.
Subjects: Mental retardation, behavior therapy, education of the mentally retarded, special education. **Holdings:** 9000 books; 500 bound periodical volumes; 3 VF drawers of pamphlets. **Subscriptions:** 202 journals and other serials.

★7832★ GEORGIA DEPARTMENT OF HUMAN RESOURCES
PUBLIC HEALTH DIVISION
LIBRARY
878 Peachtree St., NE, Rm. 115
Atlanta, GA 30309   Phone: (404) 894-6442
Shirley H. Bozeman, Lib.Asst.
Subjects: Public health, social services, science, sociology. **Holdings:** 3000 books; 5000 bound periodical volumes. **Subscriptions:** 61 journals and other serials.

★7833★ GEORGIA STATE HEALTH PLANNING AGENCY
LIBRARY
4 Executive Park Dr., NE, Ste. 2100
Atlanta, GA 30329   Phone: (404) 320-4829
Sharon Scott, Libn.
Subjects: Health planning, health and medical service delivery, health administration. **Holdings:** 3250 volumes; Federal Register, 1982-1983, on microfiche. **Subscriptions:** 72 journals, newsletters, and other serials.

★7834★ MERCER UNIVERSITY
SOUTHERN COLLEGE OF PHARMACY
H. CUSTER NAYLOR LIBRARY
345 Boulevard, NE
Atlanta, GA 30312   Phone: (404) 653-8881
Elizabeth Christian Jackson, Libn.
Subjects: Pharmacy, medicine, chemistry, biological sciences. **Holdings:** 3500 books; 3500 bound periodical volumes; Iowa Drug Information Service (microfiche). **Subscriptions:** 150 journals and other serials.

★7835★ MOREHOUSE SCHOOL OF MEDICINE
MULTI-MEDIA CENTER
720 Westview Dr., SW
Atlanta, GA 30310-1495   Phone: (404) 752-1530
Beverly E. Allen, Dir.
Subjects: Medical and life sciences. **Holdings:** 17,832 books; 26,649 bound periodical volumes. **Subscriptions:** 1020 journals and other serials.

★7836★ NATIONAL PARENTS' RESOURCE INSTITUTE FOR
DRUG EDUCATION, INC.
The Hurt Bldg., Ste. 210
50 Hurt Plaza
Atlanta, GA 30303   Phone: (404) 577-4500
Rebecca Lewis
Subjects: Drug abuse prevention, drug education and research, drug treatment centers, parent groups. **Holdings:** Archival materials. **Subscriptions:** 30 journals and other serials.

★7837★ PIEDMONT HOSPITAL
SAULS MEMORIAL LIBRARY
1968 Peachtree Rd., NW
Atlanta, GA 30309   Phone: (404) 350-3305
Alice DeVierno, Med.Libn.
Subjects: Clinical medicine, nursing. **Holdings:** 2500 books; 3500 bound periodical volumes; 200 video cassettes. **Subscriptions:** 300 journals and other serials.

★7838★ ST. JOSEPH'S HOSPITAL OF ATLANTA
RUSSELL BELLMAN MEMORIAL LIBRARY
5665 Peachtree Dunwoody Rd., NE
Atlanta, GA 30342   Phone: (404) 851-7040
Beth Poisson, Hea.Sci.Libn.
Subjects: Medicine, nursing, hospital administration, allied health sciences. **Holdings:** 2000 books; 2000 bound periodical volumes; videotapes. **Subscriptions:** 260 journals and other serials.

★7839★ U.S. CENTERS FOR DISEASE CONTROL
CDC INFORMATION CENTER
1600 Clifton Rd., NE
Atlanta, GA 30333   Phone: (404) 639-3396
Joan U. Kennedy, Chf.
Subjects: Infectious diseases, epidemiology, laboratory medicine, medical entomology, microbiology, biochemistry, public health, preventive medicine, virology. **Holdings:** 12,000 books; 130 theses; 2600 U.S. Department of Health and Human Services publications. **Subscriptions:** 370 journals and other serials.

★7840★ U.S. CENTERS FOR DISEASE CONTROL
CDC INFORMATION CENTER-CHAMBLEE
1600 Clifton Rd., NE, 30/1321
Atlanta, GA 30333   Phone: (404) 488-4167
Joan A. Redmond-Leonard, Tech.Info.Spec.
Subjects: Toxicology, clinical chemistry, vector biology and control, parasitic diseases. **Holdings:** 2000 books. **Subscriptions:** 180 journals and other serials.

★7841★ GEORGIA REGIONAL HOSPITAL AT AUGUSTA
HOSPITAL LIBRARY
3405 Old Savannah Rd.
Augusta, GA 30906   Phone: (404) 790-2699
Joyce Fears, Libn.
Subjects: Psychiatry, nursing, psychology, social work, chaplaincy, recreation. **Holdings:** 2961 books; 925 cassettes; 28 games; 3 VF drawers; 103 phonograph records; 55 maps; 63 slides; 2 filmstrips. **Subscriptions:** 102 journals and other serials.

★7842★ MEDICAL COLLEGE OF GEORGIA
ROBERT B. GREENBLATT, MD LIBRARY
Augusta, GA 30912-4400   Phone: (404) 721-3441
Thomas G. Basler, Dir. of Libs.
Subjects: Medicine, dentistry, nursing, allied health sciences. **Holdings:** 155,000 volumes. **Subscriptions:** 1700 journals and other serials; 7 newspapers.

★7843★ U.S. DEPARTMENT OF VETERANS AFFAIRS
HOSPITAL LIBRARY
2460 Wrightsboro Rd.
Augusta, GA 30910   Phone: (404) 724-5116
Elizabeth Northington, Chf., Lib.Serv.
Subjects: Medicine, nursing, psychiatry, allied health sciences. **Holdings:** 4801 books; 2497 bound periodical volumes; 3 VF drawers. **Subscriptions:** 299 journals and other serials; 30 newspapers.

★7844★ UNIVERSITY HOSPITAL
HEALTH SCIENCES LIBRARY
1350 Walton Way
Augusta, GA 30910-3599   Phone: (404) 722-9011
Jane B. Wells, Libn.
Subjects: Medicine, nursing, allied health sciences. **Holdings:** 5000 books; 450 bound periodical volumes. **Subscriptions:** 300 journals and other serials.

★7845★ MEDICAL CENTER
SIMON SCHWOB MEDICAL LIBRARY
710 Center St.
Columbus, GA 31902   Phone: (404) 571-1178
Opal Bartlett, Libn.
Subjects: Medicine, surgery, nursing. **Holdings:** 3474 books; 8077 bound periodical volumes; 275 tapes. **Subscriptions:** 195 journals.

★7846★ WEST CENTRAL GEORGIA REGIONAL HOSPITAL
LIBRARY
3000 Schatulga Rd.
Box 12435
Columbus, GA 31995-7499   Phone: (404) 568-5236
Linda Venuto, Sr.Libn.
Subjects: Alcohol and drug abuse, bibliotherapy, brief and short-term therapy/counseling, consumer/patient education, forensic psychiatry, psychiatric nursing, psychiatric social work, psychology. **Holdings:** 4200 books; 246 bound periodical volumes; 724 AV programs. **Subscriptions:** 100 journals and other serials.

★7847★ HAMILTON MEDICAL CENTER
MEDICAL LIBRARY
Memorial Dr.
PO Box 1168
Dalton, GA 30720   Phone: (404) 272-6056
Susan Seay
Subjects: Medicine, nursing, and allied health sciences. **Holdings:** 500 books; 1200 bound periodical volumes. **Subscriptions:** 79 journals and other serials.

★7848★ DE KALB MEDICAL CENTER
HEALTH SCIENCES LIBRARY
2701 N. Decatur Rd.
Decatur, GA 30033   Phone: (404) 501-5638
Marilyn Barry, Dir.
Subjects: Clinical medicine, nursing, allied health. **Holdings:** 900 books; 4500 periodical volumes. **Subscriptions:** 200 journals.

★7849★ U.S. DEPARTMENT OF VETERANS AFFAIRS
MEDICAL CENTER
MEDICAL LIBRARY
1670 Clairmont Rd.
Decatur, GA 30033   Phone: (404) 321-6111
Eugenia H. Abbey, Chf.Libn.
Subjects: Medicine, health and social sciences. **Holdings:** 3733 books; 7000 bound periodical volumes; 278 AV programs. **Subscriptions:** 454 journals and other serials.

★7850★ U.S. DEPARTMENT OF VETERANS AFFAIRS
CENTER LIBRARY
Carl Vinson VA Medical Center
Dublin, GA 31021   Phone: (912) 272-1210
Mrs. Kodell M. Thomas, Chf., Lib.Serv.
Subjects: Medicine, nursing and allied health sciences. **Holdings:** 3708 books; AV programs; microfilm. **Subscriptions:** 280 journals and other serials.

★7851★ U.S. ARMY HOSPITALS
MARTIN ARMY COMMUNITY HOSPITAL
MEDICAL LIBRARY
Bldg. 9200 HSXB-CSD-L
Fort Benning, GA 31905-6100   Phone: (404) 544-1341
Hugh Thomas, Med.Libn.
Subjects: Medicine, allied health sciences. **Holdings:** 2300 books; 6008 bound periodical volumes; 500 audio cassette tapes. **Subscriptions:** 317 journals and other serials.

★7852★ U.S. ARMY HOSPITALS
D.D. EISENHOWER ARMY MEDICAL CENTER
MEDICAL LIBRARY
Fort Gordon, GA 30905-5650   Phone: (404) 791-6765
Judy M. Krivanek, Med.Libn.
Subjects: Surgery, psychiatry, internal medicine, dentistry, nursing. **Holdings:** 6114 books; 8969 bound periodical volumes. **Subscriptions:** 500 journals and other serials.

★7853★ NORTHEAST GEORGIA MEDICAL CENTER AND
**   HALL SCHOOL OF NURSING/BRENAU COLLEGE**
LIBRARY
741 Spring St.
Gainesville, GA 30505   Phone: (404) 534-6219
Caroline E. Alday, Libn.
Subjects: Nursing, medicine. **Holdings:** 5900 books; 2500 bound periodical volumes; 4 VF drawers; 170 videotapes; 448 filmstrip/tape sets. **Subscriptions:** 112 journals and other serials.

★7854★ GRACEWOOD STATE SCHOOL AND HOSPITAL
LIBRARY
Gracewood, GA 30812-1299   Phone: (404) 790-2183
Linda D. Lawal, Libn.
Subjects: Mental retardation, pediatrics, psychology, medicine, dentistry, nursing. **Holdings:** 3600 books; 810 bound periodical volumes; 2100 cassette tapes; 2333 reprints; 703 pamphlets; 3 films. **Subscriptions:** 62 journals and other serials.

★7855★ MERCER UNIVERSITY
MEDICAL SCHOOL LIBRARY
Macon, GA 31207   Phone: (912) 752-2515
Jocelyn A. Rankin, Dir.
Subjects: Medicine. **Holdings:** 15,513 books; 53,538 bound periodical volumes; 3693 microfiche; 9214 government documents; 2589 AV programs. **Subscriptions:** 710 journals and other serials.

★7856★ CENTRAL STATE HOSPITAL
LIBRARIES
Milledgeville, GA 31062-9989   Phone: (912) 453-6889
Susan Lemme, Dir. of Libs.
Subjects: Psychiatry, neurology, medicine, nursing, psychology, social work, allied health sciences, religion. **Holdings:** 8100 volumes. **Subscriptions:** 90 journals and other serials.

★7857★ COLQUITT REGIONAL MEDICAL CENTER
HEALTH SCIENCES LIBRARY
PO Box 40
Moultrie, GA 31776   Phone: (912) 890-3460
Susan Statom, Med.Libn.
Subjects: Medicine, nursing, and allied health sciences. **Holdings:** 200 books; 350 bound periodical volumes. **Subscriptions:** 57 journals and other serials.

★7858★ FLOYD MEDICAL CENTER
MEDICAL LIBRARY
Turner McCall Blvd.
Box 233
Rome, GA 30162   Phone: (404) 295-5500
Dee Anna Ward, Libn.
Subjects: Medicine, nursing, hospital administration. **Holdings:** 1115 books; 3000 bound periodical volumes. **Subscriptions:** 100 journals and other serials.

★7859★ NORTHWEST GEORGIA REGIONAL HOSPITAL AT
**   ROME**
MEDICAL LIBRARY
1305 Redmond Rd.
Rome, GA 30161   Phone: (404) 295-6060
James R. Fletcher, Lib.Ck.
Subjects: Chest, tuberculosis, psychiatry, psychology, mental retardation, alcoholism. **Holdings:** 916 books; 1003 bound periodical volumes; 659 audiotapes; 4 VF drawers; 13 videotapes. **Subscriptions:** 64 journals and other serials.

★7860★ KIMBERLY-CLARK CORPORATION
TECHNICAL LIBRARY
1400 Holcomb Bridge Rd.
Roswell, GA 30201   Phone: (404) 587-7878
Jaye Peklo, Tech.Libn.
Subjects: Nonwoven textiles, polymers, pulp and paper, health care, engineering, chemistry. **Holdings:** 3000 books. **Subscriptions:** 400 journals.

★7861★ CANDLER GENERAL HOSPITAL
MEDICAL LIBRARY
5353 Reynolds St.
Savannah, GA 31412   Phone: (912) 356-6011
Mary V. Fielder, Libn.
Subjects: Medicine, nursing, hospital administration, rehabilitation. **Holdings:** 1150 books; 1700 bound periodical volumes; 2 VF drawers of subject files. **Subscriptions:** 178 journals and other serials.

★7862★ ST. JOSEPH'S HOSPITAL
MEDICAL LIBRARY
11705 Mercy Blvd.
Savannah, GA 31419   Phone: (912) 925-4100
Judy G. Henry, Libn.
Subjects: Medicine, surgery, nursing, allied health sciences. **Holdings:** 750 books; 150 bound periodical volumes; 100 pamphlets; 80 filmstrips with records; 4 VF drawers. **Subscriptions:** 104 journals and other serials.

★7863★ JOHN D. ARCHBOLD MEMORIAL HOSPITAL
RALPH PERKINS MEMORIAL LIBRARY
Gordon Ave. & Mimosa Dr.
Thomasville, GA 31792   Phone: (912) 228-2795
Susan Statom, Med.Libn.
Subjects: Medicine, nursing, allied health sciences. **Holdings:** 120 books; 2000 bound periodical volumes; 40 video cassettes. **Subscriptions:** 60 journals and other serials.

★7864★ SOUTH GEORGIA MEDICAL CENTER
MEDICAL LIBRARY
Box 1727
Valdosta, GA 31603-1727   Phone: (912) 333-1160
Susan T. Statom, Med.Libn.
Subjects: Medicine, nursing, and allied health sciences. **Holdings:** 200 books; 300 bound periodical volumes. **Subscriptions:** 70 journals and other serials.

★7865★ ROOSEVELT WARM SPRINGS INSTITUTE FOR
**   REHABILITATION**
Professional Library
Warm Springs, GA 31830-0268   Phone: (404) 655-2707
Michael D. Shadix
Subjects: Medical rehabilitation, physical therapy, occupational therapy, nursing, medicine, speech rehabilitation. **Holdings:** 2000 books. **Subscriptions:** 140 journals and other serials.

★7866★ NORTHEAST GEORGIA REGIONAL EDUCATION
**   SERVICE AGENCY**
NORTHEAST GEORGIA LEARNING RESOURCE SYSTEM
375 Winter St.
Winterville, GA 30683   Phone: (404) 742-8292
Gloria E. Frankum, Spec.Educ.Dir.
Subjects: Handicapped education and training, handicapped children. **Holdings:** 2000 books.

Guam

★7867★ GUAM MEMORIAL HOSPITAL AUTHORITY
MEDICAL LIBRARY
850 Gov. Carlos Camacho Rd.
Tamuning, GU 96911   Phone: (671) 646-5801
Juliana S. Torres, Med.Libn.
Subjects: Medicine, nursing, hospital administration. **Holdings:** 1519 books. **Subscriptions:** 75 journals and other serials.

Hawaii

★7868★ HILO HOSPITAL
MEDICAL LIBRARY
1190 Waianuenue Ave.
Hilo, HI 96720   Phone: (808) 969-4125
Lorna Nekoba, Libn.
Subjects: Medicine, allied health sciences. **Holdings:** 700 books; 1296 cassettes. **Subscriptions:** 60 journals and other serials.

★7869★ AMERICAN LUNG ASSOCIATION OF HAWAII
LEARNING CENTER FOR LUNG HEALTH
245 N. Kukui St.
Honolulu, HI 96817   Phone: (808) 537-5966
Rosemary Respicio, Dir.
Subjects: Lung health, asthma education, smoking prevention, air pollution, adult patient health care. **Holdings:** 100 books; 40 bound periodical volumes; 100 air pollution materials; 50 smoking prevention educational items; 25 marijuana and health education materials.

★7870★ HAWAII DEPARTMENT OF HEALTH
HASTINGS H. WALKER MEDICAL LIBRARY
3675 Kilauea Ave.
Honolulu, HI 96816   Phone: (808) 734-0221
Subjects: Clinical medicine, tuberculosis and respiratory diseases, tropical medicine, psychiatry, nursing, leprosy, hospital administration. **Holdings:** 6053 books; 1500 bound periodical volumes; 57 pamphlets. **Subscriptions:** 194 journals and other serials.

★7871★ HAWAII MEDICAL LIBRARY, INC.
1221 Punchbowl St.
Honolulu, HI 96813   Phone: (808) 536-9302
John A. Breinich, Exec.Dir.
Subjects: Medicine, nursing, tropical diseases. **Holdings:** 20,000 books; 50,000 bound periodical volumes; 500 pamphlets; 500 audio cassettes. **Subscriptions:** 1400 journals and other serials.

★7872★ KAISER-PERMANENTE MEDICAL CENTER
MEDICAL LIBRARY
3288 Moanalua Rd.
Honolulu, HI 96819   Phone: (808) 834-9420
Georgia Howton, Libn.
Subjects: Medicine, surgery, allied health sciences. **Holdings:** 1500 books; audio- and videotapes. **Subscriptions:** 190 journals and other serials.

★7873★ KAPIOLANI MEDICAL CENTER
KMC LIBRARY
1319 Punahou St.
Honolulu, HI 96816   Phone: (808) 973-8332
Ikuo Uesato, Libn.
Subjects: Obstetrics and gynecology, pediatrics, child psychiatry. **Holdings:** 1000 books; 600 bound periodical volumes. **Subscriptions:** 100 journals and other serials.

★7874★ LEGAL AID SOCIETY OF HAWAII
LIBRARY
1108 Nuuanu Ave.
Honolulu, HI 96817   Phone: (808) 536-4302
Mr. Kelly R. Madraisao, Lib.Techn.
Subjects: Law - public assistance, family, health, employment, housing, education, consumer. **Holdings:** Figures not available.

★7875★ ST. FRANCIS HOSPITAL
MEDICAL LIBRARY
2230 Liliha St.
Honolulu, HI 96817   Phone: (808) 547-6481
Julie J. Sirois, Libn.
Subjects: Nursing, medicine, hospital administration, sociology, psychology, pre-clinical sciences. **Holdings:** 5000 books; 1600 bound periodical volumes; 500 slides and tapes; 6 VF drawers of pamphlets. **Subscriptions:** 394 journals and other serials.

★7876★ STRAUB CLINIC AND HOSPITAL
ARNOLD LIBRARY
888 S. King St.
Honolulu, HI 96813   Phone: (808) 544-0317
Frances P. Smith, Hd.Libn.
Subjects: Medicine - internal, nuclear, pediatric, adolescent, dermatology, surgery. **Holdings:** 2500 books; 100 bound periodical volumes. **Subscriptions:** 280 journals and other serials.

★7877★ U.S. ARMY HOSPITALS
TRIPLER ARMY MEDICAL CENTER
MEDICAL LIBRARY
Honolulu, HI 96859-5000   Phone: (808) 433-6391
Linda Requena, Chf., Med.Lib.
Subjects: Medicine, paramedical sciences, dentistry, nursing. **Holdings:** 15,000 books; 25,000 bound periodical volumes. **Subscriptions:** 500 journals and other serials.

★7878★ UNIVERSITY OF HAWAII
JOHN A. BURNS SCHOOL OF MEDICINE
PACIFIC BASIN REHABILITATION RESEARCH AND
  TRAINING CENTER LIBRARY
Rehabilitation Hospital of the Pacific
226 N. Kuakini St., Rm. 233
Honolulu, HI 96817   Phone: (808) 537-5986
Joanne Yamada, Commun.Spec.
Subjects: Rehabilitation, disabled/disability, Pacific Basin, low-technology (orthotics, prosthetics), research, manpower development training, communications. **Holdings:** 140 books; 64 bound periodical volumes. **Subscriptions:** 35 journals and other serials; 106 serial newsletters.

★7879★ UNIVERSITY OF HAWAII
SCHOOL OF PUBLIC HEALTH
LIBRARY
1960 East-West Rd., Rm. D 206
Honolulu, HI 96822   Phone: (808) 956-8666
Virginia (Ginny) Tanji, Hd.Libn.
Subjects: Public health, health services planning and administration, environmental health, population studies, quantitative health sciences, health education, maternal and child health, public health nutrition, international health, population and family planning studies, gerontology. **Holdings:** 14,100 books; 1200 bound periodical volumes; 1500 theses and dissertations. **Subscriptions:** 200 journals and other serials.

★7880★ HAWAII STATE HOSPITAL
MEDICAL LIBRARY
45-710 Keaahala Rd.
Kaneohe, HI 96744   Phone: (808) 247-2191
Sandra L. Okubo, Med.Libn.
Subjects: Behavioral sciences, psychiatry, psychology, neuropsychology, psychiatric nursing, mental health. **Holdings:** 5000 books; 1400 bound periodical volumes; 8 VF drawers of unbound materials; 200 magnetic tapes; 100 cassette tapes; current and historic collection of Hawaii State Mental Health Division publications. **Subscriptions:** 98 journals and other serials.

★7881★ WILCOX MEMORIAL HOSPITAL
MEDICAL LIBRARY
3420 Kuhio Hwy.
Lihue, HI 96766   Phone: (808) 245-1173
Sylvia J. Duarte, Coord., Med. Staff Serv.
Subjects: General medicine. **Holdings:** Figures not available.

Idaho

★7882★ BINGHAM MEMORIAL HOSPITAL
MEDICAL LIBRARY
98 Poplar St.
Blackfoot, ID 83221   Phone: (208) 785-4100
Margaret Davis, Med.Libn.
Subjects: Medicine, nursing, hospital management, allied health sciences. **Holdings:** 400 books; 20 bound periodical volumes; 22 boxes of audiotapes; 80 videotapes. **Subscriptions:** 25 journals and other serials.

★7883★ IDAHO STATE LIBRARY
REGIONAL LIBRARY FOR THE BLIND AND PHYSICALLY
    HANDICAPPED
325 W. State St.
Boise, ID 83702   Phone: (208) 334-2117
Kay Salmon, Reg.Libn.
Holdings: 184,000 talking books.

★7884★ ST. ALPHONSUS REGIONAL MEDICAL CENTER
HEALTH SCIENCES LIBRARY
1055 N. Curtis Rd.
Boise, ID 83706   Phone: (208) 378-2271
Judy A. Balcerzak, Libn.
Subjects: Medicine, nursing, and allied health sciences. **Holdings:** 1000 books; 2 VF drawers of pamphlets (uncataloged). **Subscriptions:** 224 journals and other serials.

★7885★ ST. LUKE'S REGIONAL MEDICAL CENTER
MEDICAL LIBRARY
190 E. Bannock
Boise, ID 83712   Phone: (208) 386-2277
Pamela S. Spickelmier, Dir.
Subjects: Medicine, nursing, administration. **Holdings:** 1200 volumes. **Subscriptions:** 200 journals and other serials.

★7886★ U.S. DEPARTMENT OF VETERANS AFFAIRS
MEDICAL CENTER LIBRARY
500 W. Fort St.
Boise, ID 83702-4598   Phone: (208) 338-7206
Gordon Carlson, Chf.Libn.
Subjects: Clinical medicine. **Holdings:** 1800 books; 2894 bound periodical volumes; 450 AV programs. **Subscriptions:** 210 journals and other serials.

★7887★ WEST VALLEY MEDICAL CENTER
HEALTH INFORMATION CENTER
1717 Arlington
Caldwell, ID 83605   Phone: (208) 459-4641
Lynda Krun, Libn.
Subjects: Medicine, consumer health. **Holdings:** 276 books; 60 bound periodical volumes; 200 pamphlets; 300 other cataloged items. **Subscriptions:** 55 journals and other serials; 5 newspapers.

★7888★ EASTERN IDAHO REGIONAL MEDICAL CENTER
HEALTH SCIENCES LIBRARY
Box 2077
Idaho Falls, ID 83403-2077   Phone: (208) 529-6077
Coleen C. Winward, Med.Libn.
Subjects: Clinical medicine, nursing, hospital administration. **Holdings:** 500 books; 100 videotapes. **Subscriptions:** 200 journals and other serials; 5 newspapers.

★7889★ ST. BENEDICTS FAMILY MEDICAL CENTER
LIBRARY
709 N. Lincoln
Jerome, ID 83338   Phone: (208) 324-4301
Priscilla Malone, Libn.
Subjects: Medicine, nursing. **Holdings:** 100 books. **Subscriptions:** 25 journals and other serials.

★7890★ MORITZ COMMUNITY HOSPITAL
DEAN PIEROSE MEMORIAL HEALTH SCIENCES LIBRARY
Box 86
Sun Valley, ID 83353   Phone: (208) 622-3323
Subjects: Orthopedics, emergency medicine, general surgery and medicine, allied health professions. **Holdings:** 200 books; 800 bound periodical volumes; 24 pamphlets.

Illinois

★7891★ ABBOTT LABORATORIES
ABBOTT INFORMATION SERVICES
PPRD-0441, AP6B
1 Abbott Park Rd.
Abbott Park, IL 60064-3500   Phone: (708) 937-8698
John D. Opem, Mgr.
Subjects: Chemistry, pharmacology, medicine, pharmacy, microbiology. **Holdings:** 11,000 volumes. **Subscriptions:** 1100 journals and other serials.

★7892★ ALTON MENTAL HEALTH CENTER
PROFESSIONAL LIBRARY
4500 College Ave.
Alton, IL 62002   Phone: (618) 465-5593
Thomas M. McConahey, Dir. of Training
Subjects: Psychiatry, psychology, nursing, activity therapy, social work, mental retardation, medicine. **Holdings:** 2127 books; 495 bound periodical volumes. **Subscriptions:** 42 journals and other serials.

★7893★ ST. ANTHONY'S HEALTH CENTER
ST. ANTHONY'S HOSPITAL
MEDICAL LIBRARY
St. Anthony's Way
Alton, IL 62002   Phone: (618) 465-2571
Darla Ann Reif, Libn.Asst.
Subjects: Medicine, nursing. **Holdings:** 800 books. **Subscriptions:** 109 journals and other serials.

★7894★ ST. ANTHONY'S HEALTH CENTER
ST. CLAIRE HOSPITAL
MEDICAL LIBRARY
915 E. 5th St.
Alton, IL 62002   Phone: (618) 463-5645
Darla Rief, Libn.
Subjects: Medicine, nursing. **Holdings:** 1106 volumes. **Subscriptions:** 115 journals and other serials.

★7895★ NORTHWEST COMMUNITY HOSPITAL
MEDICAL LIBRARY
800 W. Central Rd.
Arlington Heights, IL 60005   Phone: (708) 259-1000
Ching-Ching Liang, Hosp.Libn.
Subjects: Medicine, nursing. **Holdings:** 2100 books; 4 VF drawers of pamphlets; AV programs; journal backfiles on microfiche, 1985-1989. **Subscriptions:** 250 journals and other serials.

★7896★ MERCY CENTER FOR HEALTH CARE SERVICES
MEDICAL LIBRARY
1325 N. Highland Ave.
Aurora, IL 60506   Phone: (708) 801-2686
Mary M. Howrey, Lib.Mgr.
Subjects: Medicine, psychiatry, nursing, hospital administration. **Holdings:** 5000 books; 480 periodical back titles; 4 VF drawers of pamphlets; 1000 AV programs. **Subscriptions:** 240 journals and other serials.

★7897★ MEMORIAL HOSPITAL
LIBRARY
4501 N. Park Dr.
Belleville, IL 62223   Phone: (618) 233-7750
Barbara Grout, Dir., Lib.Serv.
Subjects: Health sciences, hospital administration, nursing. **Holdings:** 2500 books; 4000 bound periodical volumes. **Subscriptions:** 430 journals and other serials.

★7898★ ST. ELIZABETH'S HOSPITAL
HEALTH SCIENCE LIBRARY
211 S. 3rd St.
Belleville, IL 62221   Phone: (618) 234-2120
Michael A. Campese, Lib.Dir.
Subjects: Medicine, nursing, hospital administration. **Holdings:** 2000 books; 1200 bound periodical volumes. **Subscriptions:** 323 journals and other serials.

★7899★ MACNEAL HOSPITAL
HEALTH SCIENCES RESOURCE CENTER
3249 S. Oak Park Ave.
Berwyn, IL 60402   Phone: (708) 795-3089
Rya Ben-Shir, MLS, Mgr.
Subjects: Medicine, nursing, hospital administration. **Holdings:** 3000
books; 1827 bound periodical volumes; cassette tapes. **Subscriptions:** 191
journals and other serials.

★7900★ GRAHAM HOSPITAL
MEDICAL STAFF LIBRARY
210 W. Walnut St.
Canton, IL 61520   Phone: (309) 647-5240
Mrs. Moneta Bedwell, Libn.
Subjects: Surgery, internal medicine. **Holdings:** 500 books; 40 bound
periodical volumes; Audio-Digest tapes. **Subscriptions:** 25 journals and
other serials.

★7901★ GRAHAM HOSPITAL
SCHOOL OF NURSING LIBRARY
210 W. Walnut St.
Canton, IL 61520   Phone: (309) 647-5240
Mrs. Moneta Bedwell, Libn.
Subjects: Nursing and medicine, chemistry, social sciences, psychology,
nutrition. **Holdings:** 3600 books; 170 bound periodical volumes; 3 VF
drawers of pamphlets and clippings; 400 AV program titles. **Subscriptions:**
60 journals and other serials.

★7902★ SOUTHERN ILLINOIS UNIVERSITY, CARBONDALE
SCIENCE DIVISION LIBRARY
Morris Library
Carbondale, IL 62901   Phone: (618) 453-2700
Kathy Fahey, Act.Sci.Libn.
Subjects: Agriculture, science, medicine, engineering. **Holdings:** 212,000
books; 190,000 bound periodical volumes; 2600 theses; 249,000 maps and
aerial photographs; 10,000 serial reports on microfilm; 1800 books on
microfilm. **Subscriptions:** 4600 journals and other serials.

★7903★ WARREN G. MURRAY DEVELOPMENTAL CENTER
LIBRARY
1717 W. Broadway
Centralia, IL 62801   Phone: (618) 532-1811
John Mannino, Libn.
Subjects: Mental retardation, medicine, nursing, psychology, special education, speech pathology. **Holdings:** 1000 volumes; 550 phonograph records;
2100 slides, filmstrips, cassette tapes, prints. **Subscriptions:** 15 journals and
other serials.

★7904★ COVENANT MEDICAL CENTER
CHAMPAIGN CAMPUS LIBRARY
407 S. 4th St.
Box 4003
Champaign, IL 61820   Phone: (217) 337-2591
April Bennington, Hd.Libn.
Subjects: Clinical medicine, nursing, allied health sciences, health care
administration. **Holdings:** 1000 books. **Subscriptions:** 240 journals and
other serials.

★7905★ NATIONAL PUBLICATIONS LIBRARY
1207 S. Oak St.
Champaign, IL 61820   Phone: (217) 333-4600
M. Jocelyn Armstrong, Supv.
Subjects: Physical and sensory impairments, rehabilitation concerning
persons with physical and sensory impairments. **Holdings:** 300 volumes.
Subscriptions: 50 serials and newsletters.

★7906★ U.S. AIR FORCE HOSPITAL
CHANUTE TECHNICAL TRAINING CENTER
MEDICAL LIBRARY
Chanute AFB, IL 61868-5300   Phone: (217) 495-3068
Gordon P. Laumer, Libn.
Subjects: Medicine. **Holdings:** 1600 books. **Subscriptions:** 60 journals and
other serials.

★7907★ AMERICAN COLLEGE OF HEALTHCARE
EXECUTIVES
RICHARD J. STULL MEMORIAL LEARNING RESOURCES
CENTER
840 N. Lake Shore Dr.
Chicago, IL 60611   Phone: (312) 943-0544
Arthur Strobeck, Lrng.Rsrcs.Coord./Libn.
Subjects: Health services administration, management. **Holdings:** 1000
books; 8 drawers of AV cassettes. **Subscriptions:** 100 journals and other
serials; 6 newspapers.

★7908★ AMERICAN DENTAL ASSOCIATION
BUREAU OF LIBRARY SERVICES
211 E. Chicago Ave.
Chicago, IL 60611   Phone: (312) 440-2642
Aletha A. Kowitz, Dir.
Subjects: Dentistry. **Holdings:** 20,000 books; 35,000 bound periodical
volumes; 3500 package libraries on 2200 topics. **Subscriptions:** 1050
journals and other serials.

★7909★ AMERICAN HOSPITAL ASSOCIATION
RESOURCE CENTER
840 N. Lake Shore Dr.
Chicago, IL 60611   Phone: (312) 280-6263
Eloise C. Foster, Dir.
Subjects: Administration, planning, and financing of health care facilities;
administrative aspects of medical, nursing, paramedical, and prepayment
fields. **Holdings:** 55,000 volumes; 36,000 microfiche; 2 VF drawers of
hospital annual reports; 219 cassettes. **Subscriptions:** 1000 journals and
other serials.

★7910★ AMERICAN MEDICAL ASSOCIATION
DIVISION OF LIBRARY AND INFORMATION MANAGEMENT
515 N. State St.
Chicago, IL 60610   Phone: (312) 464-4818
Arthur W. Hafner, Ph.D., Dir.
Subjects: Clinical medicine, medical socioeconomics, U.S. medical history,
international health. **Holdings:** 21,575 volumes; 62,790 items in medical
socioeconomics file; 165,290 documents and artifacts; 170 linear feet of
general medical and pamphlet material; 350 linear feet of biographical data
in Physician File; 145,575 volumes on microfilm. **Subscriptions:** 2255
journals and other serials.

★7911★ AMERICAN MEDICAL RECORD ASSOCIATION
FORE RESOURCE CENTER
919 N. Michigan Ave., Ste. 1400
Chicago, IL 60611   Phone: (312) 787-2672
Kay Walsh, Libn.
Subjects: Medical records. **Holdings:** 2500 books. **Subscriptions:** 185
journals and other serials.

★7912★ AMERICAN OSTEOPATHIC ASSOCIATION
A.T. STILL OSTEOPATHIC LIBRARY AND RESEARCH CENTER
142 E. Ontario St.
Chicago, IL 60611   Phone: (312) 280-5800
Subjects: Medicine, osteopathic medicine. **Holdings:** 1700 books; 540
bound periodical volumes. **Subscriptions:** 250 journals and other serials.

★7913★ AMERICANS UNITED FOR LIFE
LIBRARY
343 S. Dearborn St., Ste. 1804
Chicago, IL 60604   Phone: (312) 786-9494
Jeanette M. O'Connor, Pubns.Mgr.
Subjects: Abortion, euthanasia, infanticide. **Holdings:** Books, articles,
government publications.

★7914★ BLUE CROSS AND BLUE SHIELD ASSOCIATION
LIBRARY
676 N. St. Clair
Chicago, IL 60611   Phone: (312) 440-5510
Jan Ahrensfeld, Hd.Libn.
Subjects: Health - insurance, economics, services; business. **Holdings:**
15,000 books; 3000 congressional documents; Federal Register, 1965 to
present, on microfilm. **Subscriptions:** 180 journals and other serials.

★7915★ CENTRAL STATES INSTITUTE OF ADDICTIONS
ADDICTION MATERIAL CENTER
LIBRARY
721 N. LaSalle St.
Chicago, IL 60610   Phone: (312) 266-1056
Dr. Dan Hendershott, Libn.
Subjects: Alcohol and alcoholism, alcohol safety education, addictions, drug abuse education, drugs and driving. **Holdings:** 3500 books; 500 government publications; 600 pamphlets; 200 films on alcohol and drug abuse; abstract files. **Subscriptions:** 76 journals and other serials.

★7916★ CHICAGO CITY-WIDE COLLEGE
DAWSON TECHNICAL INSTITUTE LIBRARY
3901 S. State St.
Chicago, IL 60609   Phone: (312) 624-7300
Robert Palagi, LRC Mgr.
Subjects: Nursing, industrial arts, business. **Holdings:** 11,000 books. **Subscriptions:** 110 journals and other serials; 5 newspapers.

★7917★ CHICAGO COLLEGE OF OSTEOPATHIC MEDICINE
ALUMNI MEMORIAL LIBRARY
5200 S. Ellis Ave.
Chicago, IL 60615   Phone: (312) 947-4380
Sandra A. Worley, Dir. of Lib.Serv.
Subjects: Medicine, allied health sciences, osteopathy. **Holdings:** 20,207 books; 31,260 bound periodical volumes; 9176 audiotapes; 1014 videotapes; 40,410 slides; 15 videodiscs. **Subscriptions:** 850 journals and other serials; 5 newspapers.

★7918★ CHICAGO INSTITUTE FOR PSYCHOANALYSIS
MCLEAN LIBRARY
180 N. Michigan Ave.
Chicago, IL 60601   Phone: (312) 726-6300
Heidi Rosenberg, Libn.
Subjects: Psychoanalysis, psychosomatic medicine, psychiatry, allied social and behavioral sciences. **Holdings:** 13,000 books; 2000 bound periodical volumes; 6 VF drawers of psychoanalytic society meeting archives; 8 VF drawers of staff writing archives; 30 VF drawers of reprints and pamphlets; 2000 reels of microfilm. **Subscriptions:** 200 journals and other serials.

★7919★ CHICAGO SCHOOL OF PROFESSIONAL
  PSYCHOLOGY
LIBRARY
806 S. Plymouth Ct., 2nd Fl.
Chicago, IL 60605   Phone: (312) 786-9444
Phyllis Schub, Libn.
Subjects: Psychology - clinical, theoretical; psychotherapy; psychoanalysis; sociology. **Holdings:** 8200 books; 150 bound periodical volumes; 5300 cards of microfiche. **Subscriptions:** 200 journals and other serials.

★7920★ CHICAGO-READ MENTAL HEALTH CENTER
PROFESSIONAL LIBRARY
4200 N. Oak Park Ave.
Chicago, IL 60634   Phone: (312) 794-3746
Ruth Greenberg, Libn.
Subjects: Psychiatry, psychology, medicine, mental retardation, mental health, crisis intervention. **Holdings:** 6000 books; 6000 bound periodical volumes; 2000 unbound materials; 150 bibliographies. **Subscriptions:** 134 journals and other serials.

★7921★ CHILDREN'S MEMORIAL HOSPITAL
JOSEPH BRENNEMANN LIBRARY
2300 Children's Plaza
Chicago, IL 60614   Phone: (312) 880-4505
Meg Ward, Dir.
Subjects: Pediatrics, surgery, genetics, child psychiatry. **Holdings:** 5400 books; 25,000 bound periodical volumes. **Subscriptions:** 500 journals and other serials.

★7922★ COLUMBUS-CABRINI MEDICAL CENTER
COLUMBUS HOSPITAL MEDICAL LIBRARY
2520 N. Lakeview Ave.
Chicago, IL 60614   Phone: (312) 883-7341
James L. Finnerty, Ph.D., Dir., Lib.
Subjects: Clinical medicine, medical research, basic sciences in medicine. **Holdings:** 3600 books; 2200 bound periodical volumes; 250 videotapes. **Subscriptions:** 200 journals and other serials; 5 newspapers.

★7923★ COOK COUNTY HOSPITAL
HEALTH SCIENCE LIBRARY
1900 W. Polk St.
Chicago, IL 60612   Phone: (312) 633-7787
Grace Auer, Coord., Libs.
Subjects: Nursing, allied health sciences, management. **Holdings:** 3582 books. **Subscriptions:** 74 journals and other serials.

★7924★ COOK COUNTY HOSPITAL
TICE MEMORIAL LIBRARY
720 S. Wolcott St.
Chicago, IL 60612   Phone: (312) 633-6724
Estela B. Escudero, Lib.Coord.
Subjects: Medicine, surgery. **Holdings:** 3500 books; 6500 bound periodical volumes; AV programs. **Subscriptions:** 365 journals and other serials.

★7925★ DR. WILLIAM M. SCHOLL COLLEGE OF PODIATRIC
  MEDICINE
LIBRARY
1001 N. Dearborn St.
Chicago, IL 60610   Phone: (312) 280-2891
Richard S. Klein, Dir., Lib.Serv./Instr. Media
Subjects: Podiatric medicine, orthopedics, dermatology, anatomy, neurology, sports medicine, biomechanics. **Holdings:** 18,000 books and bound periodical volumes; AV programs. **Subscriptions:** 270 journals and other serials.

★7926★ EDGEWATER HOSPITAL
MEDICAL LIBRARY
5700 N. Ashland Ave.
Chicago, IL 60660   Phone: (312) 878-6000
Cathleen Collett, Med.Libn.
Subjects: Internal medicine, cardiology, surgery, orthopedics, obstetrics, oncology. **Holdings:** 1000 books; 4500 bound periodical volumes; 200 Audio-Digest tapes. **Subscriptions:** 130 journals and other serials.

★7927★ THE FAMILY INSTITUTE
CROWLEY LIBRARY
680 N. Lake Shore Dr., Ste. 1306
Chicago, IL 60611   Phone: (312) 908-7854
Phyllis Anne Miller, Libn.
Subjects: Therapy - family, marital, divorce, step-family, adolescent; adoption issues; death and mourning; anorexia; schizophrenia; dysfunctional families; ethnic issues. **Holdings:** 2500 books; 5000 reprints; 60 videotapes; 200 audio cassettes. **Subscriptions:** 25 journals and other serials.

★7928★ GRANT HOSPITAL OF CHICAGO
LINDON SEED LIBRARY
550 W. Webster Ave.
Chicago, IL 60614   Phone: (312) 883-3580
Donna Foley, Lib.Dir.
Subjects: Medicine, nursing, hospital administration. **Holdings:** 2400 books; 3600 bound periodical volumes. **Subscriptions:** 388 journals and other serials.

★7929★ HELENE CURTIS INDUSTRIES, INC.
CORPORATE LIBRARY
401 W. North Ave.
Chicago, IL 60639   Phone: (312) 292-2285
Jacquelyn B. Becker, Mgr.
Subjects: Cosmetics, chemistry, textiles, dermatology, toxicology, marketing, management, computers. **Holdings:** 4000 books; 20 reels of microfilm; 2 microfiche; annual and 10K reports; 3600 patents; 3 VF drawers of pamphlets. **Subscriptions:** 450 journals and other serials; 6 newspapers.

★7930★ HERMAN SMITH ASSOCIATES/COOPERS &
  LYBRAND
HEALTHCARE LIBRARY
203 N. LaSalle St., 22nd Fl.
Chicago, IL 60601   Phone: (312) 701-6412
Gail M. Langer, Libn.
Subjects: Hospital planning, design and construction, administration, regional health planning. **Holdings:** 1500 books; 7000 documents and reports; 55 VF drawers. **Subscriptions:** 200 journals and other serials.

★7931★ HOLY CROSS HOSPITAL
HEALTH SCIENCES LIBRARY
2701 W. 68th St.
Chicago, IL 60629   Phone: (312) 471-5643
Warren Albert, Med.Libn.
Subjects: Medicine, nursing, management. **Holdings:** 2500 books; 4600 bound periodical volumes; 7 audiotape title series; 7 VF drawers; 2 video cassette title series, 1987 to present; CIM microfiche, 1980 to present. **Subscriptions:** 170 journals and serials; 10 newspapers.

★7932★ ILLINOIS COLLEGE OF OPTOMETRY
CARL F. SHEPARD MEMORIAL LIBRARY
3241 S. Michigan Ave.
Chicago, IL 60616   Phone: (312) 225-1700
Gerald Dujsik, Dir., Lrng.Rsrcs.
Subjects: Optometry, vision, vision malfunctions, optics, perception, eye diseases. **Holdings:** 18,000 books; 4695 bound periodical volumes; 2129 pamphlets and theses; 700 AV programs; 750 microforms. **Subscriptions:** 225 journals and other serials.

★7933★ ILLINOIS INSTITUTE OF TECHNOLOGY
PRITZKER INSTITUTE OF MEDICAL ENGINEERING
LIBRARY
10 W. 32nd St.
Chicago, IL 60616   Phone: (312) 567-5324
Cathie D'Amico, Dept.Adm.
Subjects: Engineering, physiology, medicine. **Holdings:** 500 volumes.

★7934★ ILLINOIS MASONIC MEDICAL CENTER
MEDICAL LIBRARY
836 W. Wellington Ave., Rm. 7501
Chicago, IL 60657   Phone: (312) 975-1600
Ann Markham, Mgr., Lib.Serv.
Subjects: Health sciences. **Holdings:** 4500 books; bound periodical volumes. **Subscriptions:** 301 journals and other serials.

★7935★ ILLINOIS STATE PSYCHIATRIC INSTITUTE
JACK WEINBERG LIBRARY
1601 W. Taylor St.
Chicago, IL 60612   Phone: (312) 413-1320
Margo McClelland, Hd.Libn.
Subjects: Psychiatry, psychology, psychopharmacology. **Holdings:** 15,500 books; 380 audio cassettes; 294 videotapes. **Subscriptions:** 170 journals and other serials.

★7936★ INSTITUTE FOR CLINICAL SOCIAL WORK
LIBRARY
30 N. Michigan Ave., Ste. 420
Chicago, IL 60602   Phone: (312) 726-8480
Marylin Menchin, Libn.
Subjects: Clinical social work, psychology. **Holdings:** 4000 books; 300 professional articles. **Subscriptions:** 35 journals and other serials.

★7937★ INTERNATIONAL MUSEUM OF SURGICAL SCIENCE
LIBRARY
1524 N. Lake Shore Dr.
Chicago, IL 60610   Phone: (312) 642-6502
Louise L'Heureux-Giliberti, Cur.
Subjects: History of medicine and surgery. **Holdings:** 7000 volumes; 250 manuscripts and letters. **Subscriptions:** 30 journals and other serials.

★7938★ JACKSON PARK HOSPITAL
MEDICAL LIBRARY
7531 S. Stony Island Ave.
Chicago, IL 60649   Phone: (312) 947-7653
Syed A. Maghrabi, Med.Ref.Libn.
Subjects: Medicine. **Holdings:** 2300 books. **Subscriptions:** 190 journals and other serials.

★7939★ LARABIDA CHILDREN'S HOSPITAL AND RESEARCH
CENTER
LAWRENCE MERCER PICK MEMORIAL LIBRARY
E. 65th St. at Lake Michigan
Chicago, IL 60649   Phone: (312) 363-6700
Paula Jaudes, Chf. of Med. Staff
Subjects: Biomedical research, medicine, dentistry, nursing. **Holdings:** 920 books; 508 bound periodical volumes. **Subscriptions:** 49 journals and other serials.

★7940★ LORETTO HOSPITAL
HEALTH SCIENCES LIBRARY
645 S. Central Ave.
Chicago, IL 60644   Phone: (312) 626-4300
Sr. M. Cyril, Libn.
Subjects: Medicine, nursing, health administration. **Holdings:** 950 books. **Subscriptions:** 110 journals and other serials.

★7941★ LOUIS A. WEISS MEMORIAL HOSPITAL
L. LEWIS COHEN MEMORIAL MEDICAL LIBRARY
4646 N. Marine Dr.
Chicago, IL 60640   Phone: (312) 878-8700
Iris Sachs, Med.Libn.
Subjects: Medicine, pre-clinical sciences. **Holdings:** 1100 books; 800 bound periodical volumes. **Subscriptions:** 131 journals and other serials.

★7942★ MERCY HOSPITAL AND MEDICAL CENTER
MEDICAL LIBRARY
Stevenson Expy. at King Dr.
Chicago, IL 60616   Phone: (312) 567-2363
Timothy T. Oh, Dir. of Lib.
Subjects: Medicine, surgery, pediatrics, obstetrics-gynecology, radiology, pathology. **Holdings:** 5200 books; 8000 bound periodical volumes; 620 AV programs. **Subscriptions:** 360 journals and other serials.

★7943★ MICHAEL REESE HOSPITAL AND MEDICAL
CENTER
DEPARTMENT OF LIBRARY AND MEDIA RESOURCES
2908 S. Ellis Ave.
Chicago, IL 60616   Phone: (312) 791-2474
Dr. George Mozes, Dir.
Subjects: Medicine, dentistry, nursing. **Holdings:** 5725 books; 12,785 bound periodical volumes; 800 audio- and videotapes. **Subscriptions:** 331 journals and other serials.

★7944★ MOUNT SINAI HOSPITAL MEDICAL CENTER
LEWISON MEMORIAL LIBRARY
California Ave. at 15th St.
Chicago, IL 60608   Phone: (312) 542-2000
Emily Sobkowiak, Med./Nurs.Libn.
Subjects: Medicine, surgery, nursing. **Holdings:** 7500 books; 7500 bound periodical volumes. **Subscriptions:** 350 journals and other serials.

★7945★ MUSEUM OF SCIENCE AND INDUSTRY
LIBRARY
57th St. & Lake Shore Dr.
Chicago, IL 60637   Phone: (312) 684-1414
Pam Nelson, Lib.Hd.
Subjects: Science, technology, museology, health, science education, children's nonfiction. **Holdings:** 17,000 books; 900 bound periodical volumes; 1500 AV programs; 3500 software programs. **Subscriptions:** 60 journals and other serials.

★7946★ NATIONAL SAFETY COUNCIL
LIBRARY
444 N. Michigan Ave.
Chicago, IL 60611   Phone: (312) 527-4800
Robert J. Marecek, Mgr.
Subjects: Accident prevention, traffic safety, industrial health, all aspects of safety and safety research. **Holdings:** 4000 books; 700 bound periodical volumes; 67,000 other cataloged items; 20,000 research reports; 700 reels of microfilm; 5000 microfiche. **Subscriptions:** 250 journals and other serials.

★7947★ NORTHWESTERN MEMORIAL HOSPITAL
HEALTH LEARNING CENTER
333 E. Superior St., Rm. 467
Chicago, IL 60611   Phone: (312) 908-7503
Melinda Noonan, R.N.
Subjects: Health - general, women's. **Holdings:** 1400 books; 180 video-tapes; 525 pamphlets.

★7948★ NORTHWESTERN UNIVERSITY
DENTAL SCHOOL LIBRARY
311 E. Chicago Ave.
Chicago, IL 60611-3008   Phone: (312) 503-6896
Mary Kreinbring, Hd.Libn.
Subjects: Oral hygiene, operative dentistry, prosthetics, orthodontics,

endodontics, dental ethics and jurisprudence, dental office practice, oral surgery, pedodontics, periodontics, cleft palate, forensic dentistry, history of dentistry. **Holdings:** 68,899 volumes; 14,589 pamphlets; 63 manuscripts; 433 reels of microfilm; 67 moving pictures; 2425 photographs and prints; 7 discs; 497 tapes; 4627 slides. **Subscriptions:** 557 journals and other serials.

★7949★ NORTHWESTERN UNIVERSITY
GALTER HEALTH SCIENCES LIBRARY
303 E. Chicago Ave.
Chicago, IL 60611   Phone: (312) 503-8133
Cecile E. Kramer, Dir.
Subjects: All basic and clinical medical sciences, nursing, behavioral sciences, allied health sciences. **Holdings:** 245,000 volumes; slide sets; videotapes; 16mm films; audiotapes; models. **Subscriptions:** 2589 journals and other serials.

★7950★ NORWEGIAN-AMERICAN HOSPITAL
SEUFERT MEMORIAL LIBRARY
1044 N. Francisco Ave.
Chicago, IL 60622   Phone: (312) 278-8800
Subjects: Medicine, surgery, obstetrics, pediatrics. **Holdings:** 811 books; 173 bound periodical volumes; 200 Audio-Digest tapes. **Subscriptions:** 65 journals and other serials.

★7951★ OUR LADY OF THE RESURRECTION MEDICAL
CENTER
MEDICAL LIBRARY
5645 W. Addison St.
Chicago, IL 60634   Phone: (312) 282-7000
Sr. Joan McGovern, SSND, Med.Libn.
Subjects: Medicine, nursing, hospital administration, allied health sciences. **Holdings:** 1000 books; 5000 bound periodical volumes; 5 drawers of patient education pamphlets. **Subscriptions:** 150 journals and other serials.

★7952★ RAVENSWOOD HOSPITAL MEDICAL CENTER
MEDICAL-NURSING LIBRARY
4550 N. Winchester at Wilson
Chicago, IL 60640   Phone: (312) 878-4300
Mr. Zia Solomon Gilliana, Med.Libn.
Subjects: Medicine, nursing. **Holdings:** 4588 books; 6300 bound periodical volumes. **Subscriptions:** 252 journals and other serials.

★7953★ REHABILITATION INSTITUTE OF CHICAGO
LEARNING RESOURCES CENTER
345 E. Superior, Rms. 1671 and 1679
Chicago, IL 60611   Phone: (312) 908-2859
Karen Kaluzsa, Med.Libn.
Subjects: Physical rehabilitation, spinal cord injury, stroke, vocational rehabilitation, brain trauma. **Holdings:** 1400 books; 20 bound periodical volumes; 200 films and videotapes; 50 slide/sound sets and filmstrips; 7 VF drawers. **Subscriptions:** 145 journals and other serials.

★7954★ RESURRECTION MEDICAL CENTER
MEDICAL LIBRARY
7435 W. Talcott Rd.
Chicago, IL 60631   Phone: (312) 774-8000
Laura M. Wimmer, Med.Libn.
Subjects: Medicine, administration. **Holdings:** 1307 books; 3671 bound periodical volumes; 624 cassettes. **Subscriptions:** 120 journals and other serials.

★7955★ ROSELAND COMMUNITY HOSPITAL
HEALTH SCIENCE LIBRARY
45 W. 111th St.
Chicago, IL 60628   Phone: (312) 995-3191
Mary T. Hanlon, Libn.
Subjects: Medicine and nursing. **Holdings:** 900 books; 2 VF drawers of pamphlets. **Subscriptions:** 39 journals and other serials.

★7956★ ROSS & HARDIES
LIBRARY
150 N. Michigan Ave., 24th Fl.
Chicago, IL 60601   Phone: (312) 558-1000
Monice M. Kaczorowski, Dir. of Libs.
Subjects: Law, health. **Holdings:** 26,196 volumes. **Subscriptions:** 200 journals and other serials.

★7957★ RUSH UNIVERSITY
CENTER FOR HEALTH MANAGEMENT STUDIES
LIBRARY
202 Academic Facility
600 S. Paulina
Chicago, IL 60612   Phone: (312) 942-5402
Dr. Michael Counte, Assoc.Dir.
Subjects: Health care organizations and management. **Holdings:** 1000 books and professional journals.

★7958★ RUSH-PRESBYTERIAN-ST. LUKE'S MEDICAL
CENTER
LIBRARY OF RUSH UNIVERSITY
600 S. Paulina St.
Chicago, IL 60612-3874   Phone: (312) 942-5950
Trudy A. Gardner, Ph.D., Dir.
Subjects: Biomedical sciences, nursing, hospital administration, allied health fields, health care delivery. **Holdings:** 50,912 books; 54,420 bound periodical volumes; 112 microforms; 6898 AV programs. **Subscriptions:** 2271 journals and other serials; 6 newspapers.

★7959★ ST. ANTHONY HOSPITAL
MEDICAL LIBRARY
2875 W. 19th St.
Chicago, IL 60623   Phone: (312) 521-1710
Subjects: Medicine, nursing, administration. **Holdings:** Figures not available.

★7960★ ST. ELIZABETH'S HOSPITAL
LUKEN HEALTH SCIENCES LIBRARY
1431 N. Claremont Ave.
Chicago, IL 60622   Phone: (312) 278-2000
Subjects: Medicine, nursing and allied health sciences. **Holdings:** 1500 books; 722 bound periodical volumes; 309 volumes of unbound medical journals; 160 cassette tapes; 81 filmstrips. **Subscriptions:** 101 journals and other serials.

★7961★ ST. JOSEPH HOSPITAL AND HEALTH CARE
CENTER
LIBRARY
2900 N. Lake Shore
Chicago, IL 60657   Phone: (312) 975-3038
Gwen Jones, Libn.
Subjects: Medicine, nursing. **Holdings:** 5500 books; 8000 bound periodical volumes; 2500 audiotapes; 48 sets of slides and filmstrips; 10 VF drawers; 200 videotapes. **Subscriptions:** 170 journals and other serials.

★7962★ ST. MARY OF NAZARETH HOSPITAL CENTER
SISTER STELLA LOUISE HEALTH SCIENCES LIBRARY
2233 W. Division St.
Chicago, IL 60622   Phone: (312) 770-2219
Ms. Olivija Fistrovic, Med.Libn.
Subjects: Medicine. **Holdings:** 1400 books; 2200 bound periodical volumes; 65 slide sets; 200 video cassettes. **Subscriptions:** 216 journals and other serials.

★7963★ SHRINERS' HOSPITAL
MEDICAL LIBRARY
2211 N. Oak Park Ave.
Chicago, IL 60635   Phone: (312) 622-5400
Laura Mueller
Subjects: Orthopedics, pediatrics. **Holdings:** 1000 books. **Subscriptions:** 100 journals and other serials; 2 newspapers.

★7964★ SOUTH CHICAGO COMMUNITY HOSPITAL
DEPARTMENT OF LIBRARY SERVICES
2320 E. 93rd St.
Chicago, IL 60617   Phone: (312) 978-2000
Ronald Rayman, Dir.
Subjects: Clinical medicine, nursing, chemical dependency. **Holdings:** 3500 books; 3000 bound periodical volumes. **Subscriptions:** 250 journals and other serials.

★7965★ SWEDISH COVENANT HOSPITAL
JOSEPH G. STROMBERG LIBRARY OF THE HEALTH SCIENCES
5145 N. California Ave.
Chicago, IL 60625   Phone: (312) 878-8200
Alexander D. Trakas, Lib.Coord.
Subjects: Family practice, medicine, nursing. **Holdings:** 2000 books; 3100 bound periodical volumes; AV programs. **Subscriptions:** 103 journals.

★7966★ UKRAINIAN MEDICAL ASSOCIATION OF NORTH AMERICA
UKRAINIAN MEDICAL ARCHIVES AND LIBRARY
2247 W. Chicago Ave.
Chicago, IL 60632-4828   Phone: (312) 278-6262
Dr. Paul Pundy, Dir.
Subjects: Medicine. **Holdings:** 1800 books; 200 bound periodical volumes; 8 VF drawers of clippings, pamphlets, unbound reports, photograph albums.

★7967★ U.S. DEPARTMENT OF VETERANS AFFAIRS
LAKESIDE HOSPITAL MEDICAL LIBRARY
333 E. Huron St.
Chicago, IL 60611   Phone: (312) 943-6600
Lydia Tkaczuk, Chf., Lib.Serv.
Subjects: Medicine and allied health sciences. **Holdings:** 5000 books; 3500 bound periodical volumes; 200 other cataloged items; 2 VF drawers of pamphlets. **Subscriptions:** 250 journals and other serials.

★7968★ U.S. DEPARTMENT OF VETERANS AFFAIRS
WEST SIDE MEDICAL CENTER LIBRARY SERVICE
820 S. Damen Ave.
Chicago, IL 60612   Phone: (312) 633-2116
Susan L. Thompson, Chf., Lib.Serv.
Subjects: Medicine and allied health sciences. **Holdings:** 5300 books; 4275 unbound periodical volumes; 12 linear feet of VF materials; 2400 AV programs. **Subscriptions:** 473 journals and other serials.

★7969★ UNITED STATES LIFESAVING ASSOCIATION
LIBRARY AND INFORMATION CENTER
425 E. McFridge Dr.
Chicago, IL 60605   Phone: (312) 294-2332
Joe Pecoraro, Pres.
Subjects: Open-water lifeguarding, rescue procedures, first aid and resuscitation, ocean environment, marine safety, flood rescue procedures. **Holdings:** 1000 U.S. Lifesaving Magazines; 1000 lifesaving photographs.

★7970★ UNIVERSITY OF CHICAGO
JOHN CRERAR LIBRARY
5730 S. Ellis
Chicago, IL 60637   Phone: (312) 702-7715
Patricia K. Swanson, Asst.Dir. for Sci.Libs.
Subjects: Astronomy; astrophysics; biological sciences, including botany, physiology, and zoology; chemistry; clinical medicine; computer science; engineering; geophysical sciences, including geology, meteorology, and oceanography; history of medicine; history of science; mathematics; physics; statistics; technology. **Holdings:** 441,100 books; 663,785 bound periodical volumes. **Subscriptions:** 7072 journals and other serials.

★7971★ UNIVERSITY OF CHICAGO
SOCIAL SERVICES ADMINISTRATION LIBRARY
969 E. 60th St.
Chicago, IL 60637   Phone: (312) 702-1199
Eileen Libby, Libn.
Subjects: Social services, American and foreign social work, public welfare, mental health, urban policy, social problems, child welfare, health care, aged, psychotherapy. **Holdings:** 25,000 books; 1800 bound periodical volumes; 6500 pamphlets; 6510 microforms. **Subscriptions:** 400 journals and other serials.

★7972★ UNIVERSITY OF CHICAGO HOSPITALS
PHARMACEUTICAL SERVICES
DRUG INFORMATION SERVICE
5841 S. Maryland Ave.
Chicago, IL 60637   Phone: (312) 702-1388
Lora L. Armstrong, R.Ph., Dir.
Subjects: Pharmacy, biopharmaceutics, clinical pharmacology. **Holdings:** 300 books; 50 bound periodical volumes; 100 boxes of journals; MICRO-

MEDEX; Drug Information System. **Subscriptions:** 28 journals and other serials.

★7973★ UNIVERSITY OF ILLINOIS AT CHICAGO
LIBRARY OF THE HEALTH SCIENCES
1750 W. Polk St.
Chicago, IL 60612   Phone: (312) 996-8974
Frieda O. Weise
Subjects: Medicine, dentistry, nursing, pharmacy, public health, behavioral sciences, allied health professions. **Holdings:** 669,048 volumes; 35,030 document titles; 813 linear feet of archives. **Subscriptions:** 6043 journals and other serials.

★7974★ VISITING NURSE ASSOCIATION OF CHICAGO
MARJORIE MONTGOMERY WARD BAKER LIBRARY
322 S. Green St.
Chicago, IL 60607-3599   Phone: (312) 738-8622
Sarah Redinger, Libn.
Subjects: Nursing, medicine. **Holdings:** 2000 books; unbound periodicals; 100 archival items. **Subscriptions:** 100 journals and other serials.

★7975★ YOUTH NETWORK COUNCIL, INC.
CLEARINGHOUSE
506 S. Wabash Ave.
Chicago, IL 60605   Phone: (312) 427-2710
Denis Murstein, Adm.Dir.
Subjects: Alternative youth services, runaway youth, adolescent sexuality, youth employment, substance abuse, grantsmanship, juvenile justice, community development, public relations. **Holdings:** 500 books; 80 VF drawers of pamphlets; Federal Register, 1978 to present; videotapes. **Subscriptions:** 60 journals and other serials; 10 newspapers.

★7976★ ST. JAMES HOSPITAL AND MEDICAL CENTERS
DR. HUGO LONG LIBRARY
Chicago Rd. at Lincoln Hwy.
Chicago Heights, IL 60411   Phone: (708) 756-1000
Margaret A. Lindstrand, Libn.
Subjects: Medicine and related subjects. **Holdings:** 800 books; 800 bound periodical volumes. **Subscriptions:** 61 journals and other serials.

★7977★ UNITED SAMARITANS MEDICAL CENTER
LIBRARY
812 N. Logan Ave.
Danville, IL 61832   Phone: (217) 443-5270
Ann V. Mills, Libn.
Subjects: Nursing, medicine, clinical pathology, pharmacy, physical therapy, radiology. **Holdings:** 3939 books. **Subscriptions:** 110 journals and other serials.

★7978★ U.S. DEPARTMENT OF VETERANS AFFAIRS
MEDICAL CENTER LIBRARY
Danville, IL 61832   Phone: (217) 442-8000
Edward J. Poletti, Chf., Lib.Serv.
Subjects: Psychiatry, psychology, medicine, allied health sciences. **Holdings:** 2900 books; 2275 bound periodical volumes; 342 reels of microfilm. **Subscriptions:** 250 journals and other serials.

★7979★ DECATUR MEMORIAL HOSPITAL
HEALTH SCIENCE LIBRARY
2300 N. Edward St.
Decatur, IL 62526   Phone: (217) 877-8121
Karen J. Stoner, Libn.
Subjects: Nursing, general medicine. **Holdings:** 2500 books; 2800 bound periodical volumes; AV programs. **Subscriptions:** 140 journals and other serials.

★7980★ ST. MARY'S HOSPITAL
HEALTH SCIENCES LIBRARY
1800 E. Lake Shore Dr.
Decatur, IL 62525   Phone: (217) 464-2182
Laura L. Brosamer, Libn.
Subjects: Medicine, nursing, hospital administration. **Holdings:** 2200 books; 1700 bound periodical volumes; 184 slide/tape programs; 9 linear feet of vertical files; 200 video cassettes. **Subscriptions:** 300 journals and other serials.

★7981★ HOLY FAMILY HOSPITAL
HEALTH SCIENCES LIBRARY
100 N. River Rd.
Des Plaines, IL 60016   Phone: (708) 297-1800
Val Baker, Libn.
Subjects: Medicine, nursing, hospital administration. **Holdings:** 3000 books. **Subscriptions:** 295 journals and other serials; 2 newspapers.

★7982★ U.S. DEPARTMENT OF LABOR
OSHA
OFFICE OF TRAINING AND EDUCATION
LIBRARY
1555 Times Dr.
Des Plaines, IL 60018   Phone: (708) 297-4810
Linda Vosburgh
Subjects: Industrial hygiene, occupational safety, industrial toxicology. **Holdings:** 2200 books; 1200 government documents; 1082 standards. **Subscriptions:** 46 journals and other serials.

★7983★ JACK MABLEY DEVELOPMENT CENTER
PROFESSIONAL LIBRARY
1120 Washington Ave.
Dixon, IL 61021   Phone: (815) 288-8300
Charles Padgett, Trng.Coord.
Subjects: Mental retardation, psychology, psychiatry, medicine, special education. **Holdings:** 100 books. **Subscriptions:** 15 journals and other serials.

★7984★ ST. ANTHONY'S MEMORIAL HOSPITAL
HEALTH SCIENCE LIBRARY
503 N. Maple St.
Effingham, IL 62401   Phone: (217) 342-2121
Sr. M. Angelus Gardiner, Libn.
Subjects: Health, medicine, nursing. **Holdings:** 1444 books; 636 tapes; 73 video cassettes; archives; 12 VF drawers of other cataloged items. **Subscriptions:** 191 journals and other serials.

★7985★ ELGIN MENTAL HEALTH CENTER
ANTON BOISEN PROFESSIONAL LIBRARY
750 S. State St.
Elgin, IL 60123   Phone: (708) 742-1040
Jennifer Ford, Lib.Dir.
Subjects: Psychology, psychiatry, medicine, social work, nursing. **Holdings:** 7000 books; 700 bound periodical volumes; 500 audio cassettes; 16 VF drawers; 4 VF drawers of bibliographies. **Subscriptions:** 140 journals and other serials; 12 newspapers.

★7986★ ALEXIAN BROTHERS MEDICAL CENTER
MEDICAL LIBRARY
800 W. Biesterfield Rd.
Elk Grove Village, IL 60007   Phone: (708) 981-3657
Elizabeth Clausen, Med.Libn.
Subjects: Medicine, nursing, allied health sciences. **Holdings:** 2700 books; 5500 bound periodical volumes; 6 VF drawers of pamphlets; 300 videotapes; 470 audiotapes; 47 slide/tape sets. **Subscriptions:** 132 journals and other serials.

★7987★ AMERICAN ACADEMY OF PEDIATRICS
BAKWIN LIBRARY
141 Northwest Point Blvd.
Elk Grove Village, IL 60009-0927   Phone: (708) 981-4722
Virginia S. King, Academy Libn.
Subjects: Academy policy, health care advocacy for children. **Holdings:** 1500 books; 650 bound periodical volumes. **Subscriptions:** 225 journals and other serials.

★7988★ ELMHURST MEMORIAL HOSPITAL
MARQUARDT MEMORIAL LIBRARY
200 Berteau Ave.
Elmhurst, IL 60126   Phone: (708) 833-1400
Pauline Ng, Dir.
Subjects: Medicine, allied health sciences. **Holdings:** 2400 books; 2425 audiotapes; 385 videotapes; 735 files of pamphlets. **Subscriptions:** 240 journals and other serials.

★7989★ EVANSTON HOSPITAL
J.L. AND HELEN KELLOGG CANCER CARE CENTER
LIBRARY
2650 Ridge Ave.
Evanston, IL 60201   Phone: (708) 570-2108
K. Bauman, Med.Sec.
Subjects: Oncology. **Holdings:** 750 volumes.

★7990★ EVANSTON HOSPITAL
WEBSTER LIBRARY
2650 Ridge Ave.
Evanston, IL 60201   Phone: (708) 570-2665
Dalia S. Kleinmuntz, Dir.
Subjects: Medicine, nursing, allied health sciences. **Holdings:** 5000 books; 14,000 bound periodical volumes. **Subscriptions:** 400 journals and other serials.

★7991★ NATIONAL FOUNDATION OF FUNERAL SERVICE
BERYL L. BOYER LIBRARY
1614 Central St.
Evanston, IL 60201   Phone: (708) 328-6545
Subjects: Funeral service, mortuary management, death customs, burial, bereavement, embalming, mortuary science, restorative art. **Holdings:** 3100 books; 300 bound periodical volumes; 300 prints and pamphlets. **Subscriptions:** 48 journals and other serials.

★7992★ NATIONAL LEKOTEK CENTER
LIBRARY
2100 Ridge Ave.
Evanston, IL 60204   Phone: (708) 328-0001
Therese Wehman, Dir.
Subjects: Infant stimulation, fine motor coordination and development, language development, reading, mathematics, visual perception, musical play. **Holdings:** 3500 toys, books, computer materials, and other items. **Subscriptions:** 10 journals and other serials.

★7993★ ST. FRANCIS HOSPITAL
SCHOOL OF NURSING LIBRARY
319 Ridge Ave.
Evanston, IL 60202   Phone: (708) 492-6268
Patricia Gibson, Libn.
Subjects: Medicine, nursing, allied health sciences. **Holdings:** 3000 books; 420 bound periodical volumes; 6 VF drawers of clippings and pamphlets; 234 filmstrip programs; 160 film loops; 60 audio cassettes; 150 video cassettes; 6 16mm films. **Subscriptions:** 60 journals and other serials.

★7994★ FRONTIER COMMUNITY COLLEGE
LEARNING RESOURCE CENTER
SPECIAL COLLECTIONS
2 Frontier Dr.
Fairfield, IL 62837   Phone: (618) 842-3711
Ted Davis, Dir. of LRC
Subjects: Nursing. **Holdings:** 8000 books; 20,000 microfiche; 6 reels of microfilm. **Subscriptions:** 125 journals and other serials; 12 newspapers.

★7995★ LA LECHE LEAGUE INTERNATIONAL
LIBRARY
9616 Minneapolis Ave.
PO Box 1209
Franklin Park, IL 60131   Phone: (708) 455-7730
Subjects: Breast-feeding, parenting. **Holdings:** 200 books and monographs.

★7996★ FREEPORT MEMORIAL HOSPITAL
MEDICAL LIBRARY
1045 W. Stephenson St.
Freeport, IL 61032   Phone: (815) 235-0132
Jan Stilson, MLS
Subjects: Medicine, immediate care, surgery, rehabilitation. **Holdings:** 600 books; 1500 bound periodical volumes; 200 videotapes. **Subscriptions:** 75 journals and other serials; 3 newspapers.

★7997★ GALESBURG COTTAGE HOSPITAL
HEALTH SCIENCES LIBRARY
695 N. Kellogg St.
Galesburg, IL 61401   Phone: (309) 345-4237
Michael Wold, Hea.Sci.Libn.
Subjects: Medicine, nursing, allied health sciences. **Holdings:** 1200 books. **Subscriptions:** 175 journals and other serials.

★7998★   U.S. NAVY
NAVAL DENTAL RESEARCH INSTITUTE
THOMAS S. MEYER MEMORIAL LIBRARY
Bldg. 1-H
Great Lakes, IL 60088-5259   Phone: (708) 688-5647
Cheryl J.M. Lemley, Lib.Tech.
Subjects: Clinical dentistry, basic sciences, oral biology, dental research. **Holdings:** 1800 books; 3800 bound periodical volumes. **Subscriptions:** 85 journals and other serials.

★7999★   U.S. NAVY
NAVAL HOSPITAL
MEDICAL LIBRARY
Bldg. 200-H
Great Lakes, IL 60088-5230   Phone: (708) 688-4601
Bryan Parhad, Med.Libn.
Subjects: Medicine, surgery, dentistry, nursing. **Holdings:** 2100 books; 5260 bound periodical volumes. **Subscriptions:** 195 journals and other serials.

★8000★   INGALLS MEMORIAL HOSPITAL
MEDICAL LIBRARY
1 Ingalls Dr.
Harvey, IL 60426   Phone: (708) 333-2300
Donna L. Foley, Libn.
Subjects: Medicine, nursing, health sciences. **Holdings:** 2000 books; 3000 bound periodical volumes; 1000 cassette tapes; 2000 slides, videotapes, films. **Subscriptions:** 200 journals and other serials; 5 newspapers.

★8001★   HIGHLAND PARK HOSPITAL
MEDICAL LIBRARY
718 Glenview Ave.
Highland Park, IL 60035   Phone: (708) 432-8000
Susan Frissell, Med.Libn.
Subjects: Medicine. **Holdings:** 1400 books; microfiche. **Subscriptions:** 154 journals and other serials.

★8002★   NATIONAL ASSOCIATION OF ANOREXIA NERVOSA
AND ASSOCIATED DISORDERS
LIBRARY
Box 7
Highland Park, IL 60035   Phone: (708) 831-3438
Vivian Meehan, Adm.Dir.
Subjects: Anorexia nervosa, bulimia, bulimarexia, other eating disorders. **Holdings:** Figures not available.

★8003★   JOHN J. MADDEN MENTAL HEALTH CENTER
PROFESSIONAL LIBRARY
PO Box 7000
Hines, IL 60141-7000   Phone: (708) 531-7000
Kathryn Carlquist, Dir., Staff Dev.
Subjects: Psychiatry, psychology, administration, nursing, medicine, mental health, social work. **Holdings:** 3200 books; 50 bound periodical volumes; 60 videotapes. **Subscriptions:** 25 journals and other serials.

★8004★   U.S. DEPARTMENT OF VETERANS AFFAIRS
LIBRARY SERVICES
Edward Hines, Jr. Medical Center
Hines, IL 60141   Phone: (708) 216-2000
Christine M. Mitchell, Chf., Lib.Serv.
Subjects: Hospital administration, medicine, nursing, allied health sciences. **Holdings:** 8000 books; 23,000 bound periodical volumes. **Subscriptions:** 950 journals and other serials.

★8005★   HINSDALE HOSPITAL
HEALTH SCIENCES LIBRARY
120 N. Oak St.
Hinsdale, IL 60521   Phone: (708) 887-2868
Hilda J. Smith, MLS, Libn.
Subjects: Nursing, religion, medicine, clinical medicine. **Holdings:** 7000 books; 1000 bound periodical volumes; 19 VF drawers of pamphlets; 5 films; 200 pieces of miscellanea. **Subscriptions:** 246 journals and other serials.

★8006★   Y-ME NATIONAL ORGANIZATION FOR BREAST
CANCER INFORMATION AND SUPPORT
LIBRARY
18220 Harwood Ave.
Homewood, IL 60430   Phone: (708) 799-8338
Kay Mueller
Subjects: Breast cancer - medicine, personal narratives, psychology. **Holdings:** 140 books; clippings. **Subscriptions:** 15 journals and other serials; 15 newsletters.

★8007★   HOPEDALE MEDICAL COMPLEX
MEDICAL LIBRARY
Hopedale, IL 61747   Phone: (309) 449-3321
Mrs. Bobby Murphy, Libn.
Subjects: Geriatrics, substance abuse, rehabilitation. **Holdings:** 200 books; 200 bound periodical volumes. **Subscriptions:** 25 journals and other serials.

★8008★   ILLINOIS SCHOOL FOR THE DEAF
MEDIA CENTER
125 Webster
Jacksonville, IL 62650   Phone: (217) 245-5141
Randy Burge, Media Ctr.Dir.
Subjects: Deafness and deaf education, curriculum supporting AV programs, high interest/low vocabulary materials, audiology, children's and adult books. **Holdings:** 15,000 books; 560 bound periodical volumes; 21,500 nonprint materials; 42 boxes of pamphlets. **Subscriptions:** 51 journals and other serials; 8 newspapers.

★8009★   ILLINOIS SCHOOL FOR THE VISUALLY IMPAIRED
LIBRARY
658 E. State St.
Jacksonville, IL 62650   Phone: (217) 245-4101
Barbara J. Jenkins, Libn.Assoc.
Subjects: Blindness, education, child psychology, exceptional children, medicine, social work. **Holdings:** 15,290 books; 166 bound periodical volumes; 192 filmstrips; 96 video cassettes; 450 tactile items; pamphlets; unbound periodicals; tapes; scrapbooks; braille, talking, large print, cassette books; phonograph records. **Subscriptions:** 96 journals and other serials.

★8010★   MACMURRAY COLLEGE
HENRY PFEIFFER LIBRARY
Jacksonville, IL 62650   Phone: (217) 479-7111
Ronald B. Daniels
Subjects: Education - special, deaf; American history; nursing. **Holdings:** 145,000 books; 8000 microfiche; 7000 reels of microfilm. **Subscriptions:** 450 journals and other serials; 5 newspapers.

★8011★   PASSAVANT AREA HOSPITAL
SIBERT LIBRARY
1600 W. Walnut St.
Jacksonville, IL 62650   Phone: (217) 245-9541
Dorothy H. Knight, Libn.
Subjects: Nursing, medicine. **Holdings:** 3040 books; 140 bound periodical volumes; AV programs. **Subscriptions:** 315 journals and other serials.

★8012★   ST. JOSEPH MEDICAL CENTER
HEALTH SCIENCE LIBRARY
333 N. Madison St.
Joliet, IL 60435   Phone: (815) 725-7133
Catherine Siron, Mgr., Lib.Serv.
Subjects: Clinical medicine and nursing. **Holdings:** 2000 books; 5200 bound periodical volumes. **Subscriptions:** 300 journals and other serials.

★8013★   SILVER CROSS HOSPITAL
LLOYD W. JESSEN HEALTH SCIENCE LIBRARY
1200 Maple Rd.
Joliet, IL 60432   Phone: (815) 740-1100
Mary Ingmire, Libn.
Subjects: Medicine, nursing, hospital administration, social science. **Holdings:** 750 books; 1500 bound periodical volumes; 8 VF drawers of articles and pamphlets. **Subscriptions:** 102 journals and other serials.

★8014★ RHONE-POULENC RORER
ARMOUR PHARMACEUTICAL COMPANY
LIBRARY
Box 511
Kankakee, IL 60901   Phone: (815) 932-6771
Mary Blunk, Libn.
Subjects: Chemistry, biology, medicine, pharmacy. **Holdings:** 1000 books;
2000 bound periodical volumes. **Subscriptions:** 200 journals and other
serials.

★8015★ RIVERSIDE MEDICAL CENTER
MEDICAL LIBRARY
350 N. Wall St.
Kankakee, IL 60901   Phone: (815) 933-1671
Brenda Brower, Libn.
Subjects: Medicine, nursing, hospital administration, mental health, substance abuse. **Holdings:** 300 books; 200 bound periodical volumes; 110
cassettes; 120 slide/cassette sets. **Subscriptions:** 230 journals and other
serials; 10 newspapers.

★8016★ SAMUEL H. SHAPIRO DEVELOPMENTAL CENTER
PROFESSIONAL LIBRARY
100 E. Jeffery St.
Kankakee, IL 60901   Phone: (815) 939-8505
Juanita Licht, Br.Libn.
Subjects: Developmental disabilities, mental retardation. **Holdings:** 2200
volumes; videotapes; educational games. **Subscriptions:** 62 journals and
other serials.

★8017★ LA GRANGE MEMORIAL HOSPITAL
ZITEK MEDICAL LIBRARY
5101 Willow Springs Rd.
La Grange, IL 60525   Phone: (708) 579-4040
Patricia J. Grundke, Dir., Lib.Rsrcs.
Subjects: Medicine, nursing, and allied health sciences. **Holdings:** 1200
books; 3500 bound periodical volumes. **Subscriptions:** 160 journals and
other serials.

★8018★ LAKE FOREST HOSPITAL
MEDICAL STAFF LIBRARY
660 N. Westmoreland Rd.
Lake Forest, IL 60045   Phone: (708) 234-5600
Judy Curtis, Med.Libn.
Subjects: Medicine. **Holdings:** 1000 books; unbound periodicals. **Subscrip-
tions:** 41 journals and other serials.

★8019★ CONDELL MEMORIAL HOSPITAL
FOHRMAN LIBRARY
900 S. Garfield Ave.
Libertyville, IL 60048   Phone: (708) 362-2900
Subjects: Medicine, surgery. **Holdings:** 1000 volumes. **Subscriptions:** 100
journals and other serials.

★8020★ NATIONAL COLLEGE OF CHIROPRACTIC
LEARNING RESOURCE CENTER
200 E. Roosevelt Rd.
Lombard, IL 60148   Phone: (708) 629-2000
Joyce Whitehead, Dir.
Subjects: Chiropractic, manipulation, anatomy, radiology, neurology,
physiology, orthopedics. **Holdings:** 16,000 books; 8600 bound periodical
volumes; 600 AV program titles; 2000 reels of microfilm. **Subscriptions:**
525 journals and other serials.

★8021★ NATIONAL LOUIS UNIVERSITY
BRANCH LIBRARY
IS331 Grace St.
Lombard, IL 60148   Phone: (708) 691-9390
Jane Wilson Adickes
Subjects: Education, health and human services, business education.
Holdings: 10,000 books. **Subscriptions:** 5 newspapers.

★8022★ U.S. DEPARTMENT OF VETERANS AFFAIRS
HOSPITAL LIBRARY
W. Main St., 142-D
Marion, IL 62959   Phone: (618) 993-4114
Arlene M. Dueker, Chf., Lib.Serv.
Subjects: Medicine, surgery. **Holdings:** 956 books. **Subscriptions:** 156
journals and other serials.

★8023★ LOYOLA UNIVERSITY OF CHICAGO
MEDICAL CENTER LIBRARY
2160 S. 1st Ave.
Maywood, IL 60153   Phone: (708) 216-9192
Ludwig Logan, Ph.D., Dir.
Subjects: Biomedicine, dentistry, nursing, health sciences. **Holdings:**
47,000 books; 89,000 bound periodical volumes; 840 theses; 3844 AV
programs. **Subscriptions:** 2700 journals and other serials; 7 newspapers.

★8024★ GOTTLIEB MEMORIAL HOSPITAL
MEDICAL LIBRARY
701 W. North Ave.
Melrose Park, IL 60160   Phone: (708) 450-4526
Julie Mueller
Subjects: Clinical medicine, patient information. **Holdings:** 300 books; 200
bound periodical volumes; pamphlets. **Subscriptions:** 200 journals and
other serials; 2 newspapers.

★8025★ WESTLAKE COMMUNITY HOSPITAL
LIBRARY
1225 Lake St.
Melrose Park, IL 60160   Phone: (708) 681-3000
Christina E. Rudawski, Libn.
Subjects: Medicine, nursing, hospitals, health administration. **Holdings:**
750 books; 6 VF drawers of pamphlets. **Subscriptions:** 90 journals and
other serials.

★8026★ LUTHERAN HOSPITAL AND SCHOOL FOR NURSES
   LIBRARY
UNITED MEDICAL CENTER
501 10th Ave.
Moline, IL 61265   Phone: (309) 757-2912
Connie M. Santarelli, Coord., Lib.Serv.
Subjects: Medicine, nursing. **Holdings:** 4400 books; AV programs. **Sub-
scriptions:** 155 journals and other serials.

★8027★ GOOD SAMARITAN REGIONAL HEALTH CENTER
HEALTH SCIENCE LIBRARY
605 N. 12th St.
Mt. Vernon, IL 62864   Phone: (618) 242-4600
Linda Welch, Libn.
Subjects: Hospital administration, medicine, nursing. **Holdings:** 900 books;
500 periodical volumes. **Subscriptions:** 200 journals and other serials.

★8028★ EDWARD HOSPITAL
MEDICAL LIBRARY
801 S. Washington St.
Naperville, IL 60566   Phone: (708) 527-3937
Janette Trofimuk, Dir.
Subjects: Medicine, allied health, nursing. **Holdings:** 2000 books; 170
bound periodical volumes. **Subscriptions:** 170 journals and other serials.

★8029★ BROMENN HEALTHCARE
A.E. LIVINGSTON HEALTH SCIENCES LIBRARY
Virginia and Franklin Ave.
Normal, IL 61761   Phone: (309) 454-1400
Toni Tucker, Dir.
Subjects: Health sciences, nursing. **Holdings:** 9000 books; 232 bound
periodical volumes. **Subscriptions:** 491 journals and other serials.

★8030★ U.S. DEPARTMENT OF VETERANS AFFAIRS
MEDICAL LIBRARY
3001 Green Bay Rd.
North Chicago, IL 60064   Phone: (708) 688-3757
William E. Nielsen, Chf., Lib.Serv.
Subjects: Psychiatry, psychology, medicine, allied health sciences. **Hold-
ings:** 4600 books; 2 VF drawers; 700 AV programs. **Subscriptions:** 450
journals and other serials.

★8031★ UNIVERSITY OF HEALTH SCIENCES/CHICAGO
   MEDICAL SCHOOL
LEARNING RESOURCES CENTER
3333 Green Bay Rd.
North Chicago, IL 60064   Phone: (708) 578-3242
Nancy W. Garn, Dir. & Asst. Dean
Subjects: Medicine, psychology, and allied health sciences. **Holdings:**
19,775 books; 72,076 bound periodical volumes; 20,000 volumes on 2800
reels of microfilm; 3 drawers of residency catalogs; 150 dissertations; 3

drawers of elective catalogs; 8 drawers of pamphlets. **Subscriptions:** 1301 journals and other serials; 7 newspapers.

★8032★ **IRENE JOSSELYN CLINIC**
MENTAL HEALTH LIBRARY
405 Central
Northfield, IL 60093 Phone: (708) 441-5600
Jean M. Peterson, Libn.
Subjects: Child development, adolescence, parenting, divorce, psychoanalysis, psychotheraphy. **Holdings:** Figures not available.

★8033★ **RADIOLOGICAL SOCIETY OF NORTH AMERICA**
LIBRARY
2021 Spring Rd., Ste. 600
Oak Brook, IL 60521 Phone: (708) 571-2670
Subjects: Clinical radiology, allied health sciences. **Holdings:** 800 volumes; records of manuscripts received annually. **Subscriptions:** 120 journals and other serials.

★8034★ **OAK FOREST HOSPITAL**
PROFESSIONAL LIBRARY
15900 S. Cicero Ave.
Oak Forest, IL 60452 Phone: (708) 928-4200
Delores I. Quinn, Libn.
Subjects: Medicine, nursing, paramedical sciences. **Holdings:** 2000 books. **Subscriptions:** 250 journals and other serials.

★8035★ **EVANGELICAL HEALTH SYSTEMS**
CHRIST HOSPITAL
HEALTH SCIENCES LIBRARY
4440 W. 95th St.
Oak Lawn, IL 60453 Phone: (708) 857-5127
Janice E. Kelly, Chf.Libn.
Subjects: Medicine. **Holdings:** 7000 books; 5000 bound periodical volumes; 150 video cassettes; 475 audio cassettes. **Subscriptions:** 310 journals and other serials.

★8036★ **WEST SUBURBAN HOSPITAL MEDICAL CENTER**
HEALTH INFORMATION CENTER
Erie at Austin
Oak Park, IL 60302 Phone: (708) 383-6200
Constance M. Gibbon, Libn.
Subjects: Consumer health. **Holdings:** 900 books; 350 videotapes; pamphlets. **Subscriptions:** 25 journals and other serials.

★8037★ **WEST SUBURBAN HOSPITAL MEDICAL CENTER**
WALTER LAWRENCE MEMORIAL LIBRARY
Erie at Austin
Oak Park, IL 60302 Phone: (708) 383-6200
Carol Scherrer, Dir. of Lib. & Info.Serv.
Subjects: Clinical medicine, nursing. **Holdings:** 4000 books; 10 microfiche drawers of journal titles; 400 videotapes. **Subscriptions:** 350 journals and other serials; 5 newspapers.

★8038★ **WORLD FEDERATION OF DOCTORS WHO RESPECT**
HUMAN LIFE
LIBRARY
PO Box 508
Oak Park, IL 60303 Phone: (708) 383-8766
Subjects: Medical opposition to abortion, suicide, and direct euthanasia. **Holdings:** 700 volumes.

★8039★ **RICHLAND MEMORIAL HOSPITAL**
STAFF LIBRARY
800 E. Locust
Olney, IL 62450 Phone: (618) 395-2131
Beverly Keyth, Dir., Med.Rec.
Subjects: Internal medicine, surgery, oncology, hematology, orthopedics, obstetrics-gynecology. **Holdings:** 448 books. **Subscriptions:** 12 journals and other serials.

★8040★ **CHICAGO COLLEGE OF OSTEOPATHIC MEDICINE**
OLYMPIA FIELDS OSTEOPATHIC MEDICAL CENTER
LIBRARY
20201 S. Crawford
Olympia Fields, IL 60461 Phone: (708) 747-4000
Sandra A. Worley, Dir.
Subjects: Medicine, nursing. **Holdings:** 2500 books; 4800 bound periodical volumes; 225 videotapes. **Subscriptions:** 200 journals and other serials.

★8041★ **PALOS COMMUNITY HOSPITAL**
MEDICAL LIBRARY
80th Ave. & McCarthy Rd.
Palos Heights, IL 60463 Phone: (708) 361-4500
Gail Lahti, Libn.
Subjects: Medicine, allied health sciences. **Holdings:** 1000 books. **Subscriptions:** 100 journals and other serials.

★8042★ **AMERICAN SOCIETY OF ANESTHESIOLOGISTS**
WOOD LIBRARY-MUSEUM OF ANESTHESIOLOGY
515 Busse Hwy.
Park Ridge, IL 60068-3189 Phone: (708) 825-5586
Patrick Sim, Libn.
Subjects: Anesthesiology, resuscitation, shock, medical applications for hypnotism, inhalation therapy, history of anesthesiology. **Holdings:** 8000 books; 1000 bound periodical volumes; 40 VF drawers of pamphlets, photographs, clippings; 20 shelf feet of manuscripts. **Subscriptions:** 85 journals and other serials.

★8043★ **LUTHERAN GENERAL HOSPITAL**
MEDICAL LIBRARY
1775 Dempster St.
Park Ridge, IL 60068 Phone: (708) 696-5494
Marie T. Burns, Dir.
Subjects: Clinical medicine, nursing, pastoral psychology, social work, nutrition, physical rehabilitation. **Holdings:** 22,000 books; 12,700 bound periodical volumes; 6300 AV programs; current journals on microfilm. **Subscriptions:** 490 journals and other serials.

★8044★ **NATIONAL ASSOCIATION OF BOARDS OF**
PHARMACY
LIBRARY
1300 Higgins Rd., Ste. 103
Park Ridge, IL 60068-5743 Phone: (708) 698-6227
Carmen A. Catizone, Exec.Dir.
Subjects: Pharmacy - law and regulation, education, licensure. **Holdings:** Figures not available.

★8045★ **GEORGE A. ZELLER MENTAL HEALTH CENTER**
PROFESSIONAL LIBRARY
5407 N. University
Peoria, IL 61614 Phone: (309) 693-5272
Barbara Haun, Libn.
Subjects: Psychiatry, psychology, community mental health, geriatrics, sociology. **Holdings:** 3200 books; 300 bound periodical volumes; 4 VF drawers. **Subscriptions:** 25 journals and other serials.

★8046★ **METHODIST MEDICAL CENTER OF ILLINOIS**
HEALTH SCIENCE RESOURCE CENTER
221 NE Glen Oak
Peoria, IL 61636 Phone: (309) 672-4937
Royden R. Jones, HSRC Mgr.
Subjects: Medicine. **Holdings:** 3800 books; 5500 bound periodical volumes. **Subscriptions:** 353 journals and other serials.

★8047★ **METHODIST MEDICAL CENTER OF ILLINOIS**
SCHOOL OF NURSING LIBRARY
LEARNING RESOURCE CENTER
221 NE Glen Oak
Peoria, IL 61636 Phone: (309) 671-2794
Ms. Leslie Menz, Libn.
Subjects: Nursing, nursing education. **Holdings:** 4000 books; 204 bound periodical volumes; 6 VF drawers of pamphlets; 8000 unbound periodicals; 280 AV programs. **Subscriptions:** 55 journals and other serials.

★8048★   PROCTOR COMMUNITY HOSPITAL
MEDICAL LIBRARY
5409 N. Knoxville Ave.
Peoria, IL 61614   Phone: (309) 691-1000
Melody Reed, Lib.Ck.
Subjects: Medicine, nursing, allied health sciences. **Holdings:** 500 books; 210 bound periodical volumes; 550 unbound journal volumes. **Subscriptions:** 120 journals and other serials.

★8049★   ST. FRANCIS MEDICAL CENTER
MEDICAL LIBRARY
530 NE Glen Oak Ave.
Peoria, IL 61637   Phone: (309) 655-2210
Carol Galganski, Med.Libn.
Subjects: Surgery, internal medicine, neurology, orthopedics, family practice, pediatrics. **Holdings:** 2600 books; 9649 bound periodical volumes; 300 slide sets; 550 video cassettes; 1000 audio cassettes. **Subscriptions:** 525 journals and other serials.

★8050★   UNIVERSITY OF ILLINOIS AT CHICAGO
COLLEGE OF MEDICINE AT PEORIA
LIBRARY OF THE HEALTH SCIENCES
PO Box 1649
Peoria, IL 61656   Phone: (309) 671-8490
Trudy Landwirth, Hea.Sci.Libn., Peoria
Subjects: Medicine, basic sciences, nursing. **Holdings:** 25,862 books; 24,397 bound periodical volumes; 1884 AV programs; 5500 government documents; 1269 microfiche. **Subscriptions:** 502 journals and other serials.

★8051★   ST. JAMES HOSPITAL
MEDICAL LIBRARY
610 E. Water St.
Pontiac, IL 61764   Phone: (815) 842-2828
Patty Wolf, Lib.Ck.
Subjects: Medicine and allied health sciences. **Holdings:** 137 volumes; 13 video cassettes. **Subscriptions:** 21 journals and other serials.

★8052★   PERRY MEMORIAL HOSPITAL
DR. KENNETH O. NELSON LIBRARY OF THE HEALTH
  SCIENCES
530 Park Ave., E.
Princeton, IL 61356   Phone: (815) 875-2811
Linda Litherland, Dir.Med.Rec.
Subjects: Medicine. **Holdings:** 750 books. **Subscriptions:** 31 journals and other serials.

★8053★   BLESSING-RIEMAN COLLEGE OF NURSING
LIBRARY
Broadway at 11th St.
Quincy, IL 62301   Phone: (217) 223-8400
Arlis Dittmer, Libn.
Subjects: Nursing, medicine. **Holdings:** 4000 books; 720 bound periodical volumes; 230 reports; 520 AV programs. **Subscriptions:** 76 journals and other serials.

★8054★   ST. MARY HOSPITAL
STAFF LIBRARY
1415 Vermont
Quincy, IL 62301   Phone: (217) 223-1200
Dorcas Recks, Libn.
Subjects: Medicine, consumer health information. **Holdings:** 950 books; 650 bound periodical volumes. **Subscriptions:** 46 journals and other serials.

★8055★   FRANCISCAN MEDICAL CENTER
JORDAN LIBRARY
2701 17th St.
Rock Island, IL 61201   Phone: (309) 793-2069
Priscilla Swatos, Coord., Hea.Info.Serv.
Subjects: Clinical medicine, mental health. **Holdings:** 957 books. **Subscriptions:** 321 journals and other serials; 4 newspapers.

★8056★   WESTERN ILLINOIS AREA AGENCY ON AGING
SENIOR RESOURCE CENTER
729 34th Ave.
Rock Island, IL 61201   Phone: (309) 793-6800
Erma Dalton, Libn.
Subjects: Nursing home information, family caregiving, Medicare, Medicaid Social Security, retirement planning, intergenerational programs,

housing alternatives. **Holdings:** 1000 books; AV materials. **Subscriptions:** 40 journals and other serials.

★8057★   H. DOUGLAS SINGER MENTAL HEALTH AND
  DEVELOPMENTAL CENTER
LIBRARY
4402 N. Main St.
Rockford, IL 61103-1278   Phone: (815) 987-7092
Pat Ellison, Lib.Assoc.
Subjects: Mental health, psychology, psychiatry, psychotherapy, sociology. **Holdings:** 2000 books. **Subscriptions:** 100 journals and other serials.

★8058★   ROCKFORD MEMORIAL HOSPITAL
HEALTH SCIENCE LIBRARY
2400 N. Rockton Ave.
Rockford, IL 61101   Phone: (815) 968-6861
Phyllis Nathan, Coord., Lib.Serv.
Subjects: Clinical medicine, nursing, health care administration. **Holdings:** 2000 books; 2000 bound periodical volumes; 2 VF drawers; 100 nonprint items. **Subscriptions:** 240 journals and other serials.

★8059★   ST. ANTHONY COLLEGE OF NURSING
BISHOP LANE LIBRARY
5658 E. State St.
Rockford, IL 61108-2468   Phone: (815) 395-5091
Sr. Mary Linus, OSF, M.S.N.E.
Subjects: Nursing. **Holdings:** 4000 books; 600 bound periodical volumes. **Subscriptions:** 43 journals and 100 other serials.

★8060★   ST. ANTHONY MEDICAL CENTER
HEALTH INFORMATION RESOURCE CENTER
5666 E. State St.
Rockford, IL 61108   Phone: (815) 395-5191
Nancy Dale, Med.Libn.
Subjects: Clinical medicine. **Holdings:** 800 books; 2000 bound periodical volumes. **Subscriptions:** 200 journals and other serials.

★8061★   SWEDISH AMERICAN HOSPITAL
HEALTH CARE LIBRARY
1400 Charles St.
Rockford, IL 61104-2298   Phone: (815) 968-4400
Sharon Montana, Mgr., Educ.Serv.
Subjects: Clinical medicine, hospital administration. **Holdings:** 2500 books; 2000 video cassettes; 7 year backlog of periodicals. **Subscriptions:** 300 journals and other serials.

★8062★   UNIVERSITY OF ILLINOIS AT CHICAGO
COLLEGE OF MEDICINE AT ROCKFORD
WOODRUFF L. CRAWFORD BRANCH LIBRARY OF THE
  HEALTH SCIENCES
1601 Parkview Ave.
Rockford, IL 61107   Phone: (815) 395-5650
Don Lanier, Hea.Sci.Libn., Rockford
Subjects: Medicine, biomedical sciences. **Holdings:** 22,419 books; 26,437 bound periodical volumes; 358 pamphlets; 11,768 slides. **Subscriptions:** 414 journals and other serials; 7 newspapers.

★8063★   LEWIS UNIVERSITY
LIBRARY
Rte. 53
Romeoville, IL 60441   Phone: (815) 838-0500
Ms. F.A. Moskal, Lib.Dir.
Subjects: Business and economics, political science, mathematics, nursing, English and American literature. **Holdings:** 113,000 books; 20,503 bound periodical volumes; 50,000 federal government documents; 1252 records; 24,708 books on microfiche; 7000 microfiche; 5036 boxes of periodicals and newspapers on microfilm. **Subscriptions:** 550 journals and other serials; 5 newspapers.

★8064★   BAXTER HEALTHCARE CORPORATION
INFORMATION RESOURCE CENTER
Rte. 120 & Wilson Rd., WGI-IN
Box 490
Round Lake, IL 60073   Phone: (708) 270-5361
David Anderson, Mgr., Info.Rsrc.Ctr.
Subjects: Medicine, parenteral nutrition, hematology, pharmaceuticals, plastics, biomedical engineering, engineering, business and management, sales and management, corporate and patent law, international business

and law, health care administration, human resources. **Holdings:** 30,000 titles. **Subscriptions:** 600 journals and other serials.

★8065★ AMERICAN VETERINARY MEDICAL ASSOCIATION LIBRARY
930 N. Meacham Rd.
Schaumburg, IL 60196   Phone: (708) 605-8070
Liane Lenski, Libn.
Subjects: Veterinary medicine and allied fields. **Holdings:** 5000 books; 300 bound periodical volumes. **Subscriptions:** 35 journals and other serials; 185 exchanges.

★8066★ NATIONAL SOCIETY TO PREVENT BLINDNESS CONRAD BERENS LIBRARY
500 E. Remington Rd.
Schaumburg, IL 60173   Phone: (708) 843-2020
Glory Tenney Kosmatka, Assoc.Dir., Info.Serv.
Subjects: Ophthalmology, optometry, eye health and safety; association management. **Holdings:** 3000 volumes; 21 VF drawers of reports, pamphlets, clippings, association reports, bulletins, state health reports. **Subscriptions:** 100 journals and other serials.

★8067★ U.S. AIR FORCE HOSPITAL MEDICAL CENTER MEDICAL LIBRARY
Scott AFB, IL 62225   Phone: (618) 256-7437
Blanche A. Savage, Dir.
Subjects: Medicine, nursing, dentistry, allied health sciences. **Holdings:** 8000 books; 4633 bound periodical volumes; 1500 pamphlets and tapes. **Subscriptions:** 325 journals and other serials; 5 newspapers.

★8068★ ILLINI HOSPITAL HEALTH SCIENCES LIBRARY
801 Hospital Rd.
Silvis, IL 61282-1804   Phone: (309) 792-4360
Priscilla Swatos, Coord., Hea.Info.Serv.
Subjects: Clinical medicine, health care management. **Holdings:** 1571 books. **Subscriptions:** 325 journals and other serials; 2 newspapers.

★8069★ SEARLE RESEARCH LIBRARY
4901 Searle Pkwy.
Skokie, IL 60077   Phone: (708) 982-8285
Anthony Petrone, Mgr.
Subjects: Chemistry, biology, gastroenterology, gynecology and contraception, hypertension, pharmacology. **Holdings:** 6500 books. **Subscriptions:** 700 journals and other serials; 35 newsletters.

★8070★ ILLINOIS DEPARTMENT OF REHABILITATION SERVICES RESOURCE CENTER LIBRARY
623 E. Adams St.
Springfield, IL 62794-9429   Phone: (217) 524-0706
Jan Perone, Libn.
Subjects: Rehabilitation. **Holdings:** 600 books; 200 microfiche. **Subscriptions:** 200 journals and other serials; 10 newspapers.

★8071★ ILLINOIS EARLY CHILDHOOD INTERVENTION CLEARINGHOUSE
830 S. Spring St.
Springfield, IL 62704   Phone: (217) 785-1364
Chet Brandt, Proj.Dir.
Subjects: Early childhood, at-risk children, developmental disabilities. **Holdings:** 2100 books; 120 video cassettes. **Subscriptions:** 200 journals and other serials.

★8072★ ILLINOIS ENVIRONMENTAL PROTECTION AGENCY LIBRARY
2200 Churchill Rd.
Springfield, IL 62794-9276   Phone: (217) 782-9691
Nancy Simpson, Libn.
Subjects: Environmental pollution and protection, environmental law, environmental health. **Holdings:** 25,000 books; 300 bound periodical volumes; 1500 legal documents; 25,000 EPA technical reports on microfiche. **Subscriptions:** 350 journals and other serials.

★8073★ MCFARLAND MENTAL HEALTH CENTER STAFF LIBRARY
901 Southwind Rd.
Springfield, IL 62703   Phone: (217) 786-6851
Wanda Beck, Lib.Coord.
Subjects: Behavior therapy, psychology, psychiatry, psychotherapy, social psychiatry, family psychodynamics, addiction, mental retardation, psychiatric nursing. **Holdings:** 12,000 books; 250 bound periodical volumes; 3 drawers of journal reprints; 3 drawers of Department of Mental Health documents; 8 shelves of special education textbooks. **Subscriptions:** 30 journals and other serials.

★8074★ MEMORIAL MEDICAL CENTER KENNETH H. SCHNEPP MEDICAL LIBRARY
800 N. Rutledge St.
Springfield, IL 62781   Phone: (217) 788-3336
Myrtle Smarjesse, Libn.
Subjects: Medicine, nursing, allied health sciences. **Holdings:** 1342 books; 3745 bound periodical volumes; 3 VF drawers of medical and paramedical pamphlets; audio and video cassettes. **Subscriptions:** 174 journals and other serials.

★8075★ ST. JOHN'S HOSPITAL HEALTH SCIENCE LIBRARY
800 E. Carpenter
Springfield, IL 62769   Phone: (217) 544-6464
Kathryn Wrigley, Dir.
Subjects: Cardiovascular system, surgery, pediatrics, emergency medicine, nursing, pathology, psychiatry. **Holdings:** 4307 books; 295 AV programs; pamphlets. **Subscriptions:** 367 journals and other serials.

★8076★ SOUTHERN ILLINOIS UNIVERSITY SCHOOL OF MEDICINE MEDICAL LIBRARY
801 N. Rutledge
Box 19231
Springfield, IL 62794   Phone: (217) 782-2658
Robert Berk, Ph.D., Dir.
Subjects: Medical sciences. **Holdings:** 55,800 books; 66,800 bound periodical volumes; 1600 reels of microfilm; 3040 AV programs. **Subscriptions:** 1908 journals and other serials.

★8077★ SPRINGFIELD COLLEGE IN ILLINOIS BECKER LIBRARY
1521 N. 6th St.
Springfield, IL 62702   Phone: (217) 525-1420
Stephen Iden
Subjects: Religion, humanities, medicine, business. **Holdings:** 23,000 books; 3171 bound periodical volumes; 22 microfiche titles. **Subscriptions:** 121 journals and other serials.

★8078★ CARLE FOUNDATION HOSPITAL LIBRARY
611 W. Park St.
Urbana, IL 61801   Phone: (217) 337-3011
Anita D. Johnson, Lib.Mgr.
Subjects: Medicine, medical specialties. **Holdings:** 1020 books; 9000 bound periodical volumes. **Subscriptions:** 245 journals and other serials.

★8079★ COVENANT MEDICAL CENTER LIBRARY
1400 W. Park St.
Urbana, IL 61801   Phone: (217) 337-2283
Harriet Williamson, Mgr.
Subjects: Clinical medicine, nursing, allied health sciences. **Holdings:** 1000 books; 500 bound periodical volumes; 10 boxes of archival materials. **Subscriptions:** 175 journals and other serials.

★8080★ UNIVERSITY OF ILLINOIS VETERINARY MEDICINE LIBRARY
1257 Vet. Med. Basic Sciences Bldg.
2001 S. Lincoln Ave.
Urbana, IL 61801   Phone: (217) 333-2193
Mitsuko Williams, Hd.
Subjects: Pathology, physiology, pharmacology, bacteriology, veterinary science, parasitology, toxicology. **Holdings:** 33,746 volumes; 4 VF drawers of pamphlets. **Subscriptions:** 838 journals and other serials.

★8081★ UNIVERSITY OF ILLINOIS AT CHICAGO
LIBRARY OF THE HEALTH SCIENCES, URBANA
102 Medical Sciences Bldg.
506 S. Matthews
Urbana, IL 61801   Phone: (217) 333-4893
Ruth E. Fenske
Subjects: Medicine, nursing, medical applications of magnetic resonance imaging. **Holdings:** 27,096 books; 9907 bound periodical volumes; 1906 pamphlets; 3468 AV programs. **Subscriptions:** 650 journals and other serials.

★8082★ VICTORY MEMORIAL HOSPITAL
MEDICAL LIBRARY
1324 N. Sheridan Rd.
Waukegan, IL 60085   Phone: (708) 360-3000
Janet Cole, Med.Lib.Techn.
Subjects: Medicine, nursing, hospitals. **Holdings:** 514 volumes. **Subscriptions:** 45 journals and other serials.

★8083★ NATIONAL EMPLOYEE SERVICES AND
** RECREATION ASSOCIATION**
INFORMATION CENTER
2400 S. Downing Ave.
Westchester, IL 60154   Phone: (708) 562-8130
Patrick B. Stinson, Exec.Dir.
Subjects: Employees - activities, sports, recreation, facilities, travel, fitness, wellness, preretirement planning, assistance programs, productivity, day care. **Holdings:** 50 volumes.

★8084★ TRI BROOK GROUP, INC.
LIBRARY
999 Oakmont Plaza Dr., Ste. 600
Westmont, IL 60559-5504   Phone: (708) 990-8070
Sandra Rumbyrt, Libn.
Subjects: Health care management, health statistics. **Holdings:** 4000 volumes including government publications and reports. **Subscriptions:** 85 journals and other serials.

★8085★ MARIANJOY REHABILITATION CENTER
HEALTH SCIENCES LIBRARY
26W171 Roosevelt Rd.
Box 795
Wheaton, IL 60189-0795   Phone: (708) 462-4000
Nalini Mahajan, Med.Libn.
Subjects: Physical rehabilitation, neurology, orthopedics, pain, sports medicine. **Holdings:** 1500 books. **Subscriptions:** 150 journals and other serials.

★8086★ FOREST INSTITUTE OF PROFESSIONAL
** PSYCHOLOGY**
LIBRARY
200 Glendale St.
Wheeling, IL 60090   Phone: (708) 215-7870
Janan Lundgren, Dir., Lib.Serv.
Subjects: Psychology, psychiatry, health, medicine, family therapy, drugs, alcoholism, aging. **Holdings:** 9000 books; 2200 bound periodical volumes; 800 pamphlets and reprints; 2000 unbound periodicals; 5 drawers of microfiche; 120 dissertations. **Subscriptions:** 145 journals and other serials.

★8087★ CENTRAL DUPAGE HOSPITAL
MEDICAL LIBRARY
25 N. Winfield Rd.
Winfield, IL 60190   Phone: (708) 682-1600
Dorothy B. Rowe, Libn.
Subjects: Medicine, nursing, allied health sciences. **Holdings:** 4000 books; unbound periodicals; 8 VF drawers. **Subscriptions:** 400 journals and other serials.

Indiana

★8088★ CENTER FOR MENTAL HEALTH
LIBRARY
2020 Brown St.
Box 1258
Anderson, IN 46015   Phone: (317) 649-8161
Cindy Stafford, Libn.
Subjects: Family therapy, violence, stress management, psychiatry, psy-

chology, social work. **Holdings:** 500 books. **Subscriptions:** 15 journals and other serials; 7 newspapers.

★8089★ ST. JOHN'S HEALTH CARE CORPORATION
HEALTH SCIENCES LIBRARY
2015 Jackson St.
Anderson, IN 46016   Phone: (317) 646-8262
Scott S. Loman, Hea.Sci.Libn.
Subjects: Medicine, nursing, allied health sciences, health administration, marketing. **Holdings:** 2000 books; 4000 bound periodical volumes; 150 audio cassettes; 400 video cassettes. **Subscriptions:** 200 journals and other serials; 7 newspapers.

★8090★ INDIANA UNIVERSITY
HEALTH, PHYSICAL EDUCATION AND RECREATION
** LIBRARY**
HPER Bldg. 031
Bloomington, IN 47401   Phone: (812) 855-4420
Julie Bobay, Hd.
Subjects: Physical education, recreation and park administration, health and safety, coaching, adapted physical education and therapeutic recreation, sports medicine and psychology. **Holdings:** 14,000 volumes; 8100 microforms. **Subscriptions:** 200 journals and other serials.

★8091★ INDIANA UNIVERSITY
INSTITUTE FOR THE STUDY OF DEVELOPMENTAL
** DISABILITIES**
LIBRARY
2853 E. 10th St.
Bloomington, IN 47405   Phone: (812) 855-6508
Marilyn Irwin, Info. Dissemination Spec.
Subjects: Developmental disabilities; curriculum materials for the developmentally disabled; early childhood intervention programs; assistance for parents of the developmentally disabled; parenting; community integration of handicapped persons. **Holdings:** 6000 books; 10 VF drawers of information files; 2 drawers of bibliographies; 3 drawers of test files; 2 drawers of organization files; 15 drawers of periodical files; 10 drawers of publishers' catalogs. **Subscriptions:** 25 journals and other serials.

★8092★ INDIANA UNIVERSITY
MEDICAL SCIENCES LIBRARY
251 Myers Hall
Bloomington, IN 47405   Phone: (812) 855-3347
Doug Freeman, Hd.
Subjects: Anatomy, physiology, pharmacology, pathology, medicine, biomedical computer science, biochemistry, immunology. **Holdings:** 27,000 bound volumes; 3100 microforms. **Subscriptions:** 184 journals and other serials.

★8093★ INDIANA UNIVERSITY
OPTOMETRY LIBRARY
Optometry Bldg.
Bloomington, IN 47405   Phone: (812) 855-8629
Doug Freeman, Hd.
Subjects: Vision. **Holdings:** 16,000 volumes; 4100 microforms. **Subscriptions:** 265 journals and other serials.

★8094★ KINSEY INSTITUTE FOR RESEARCH IN SEX,
** GENDER AND REPRODUCTION**
LIBRARY AND INFORMATION SERVICE
313 Morrison Hall
Indiana University
Bloomington, IN 47405   Phone: (812) 855-7686
Subjects: Sexual behavior and attitudes, erotic literature and art, gender, reproduction. **Holdings:** 75,000 books, reprints, bound periodical volumes; 39 VF drawers; 209 reels of microfilm; 105 tapes; 108 phonograph records; 3500 objects; 55,000 photographs; 5000 slides; 6500 films. **Subscriptions:** 100 journals and other serials.

★8095★ CAYLOR-NICKEL MEDICAL CENTER
LIBRARY
1 Caylor-Nickel Sq.
Bluffton, IN 46714   Phone: (219) 824-3500
Patricia Niblick, Med.Libn.
Subjects: Surgery, internal medicine, pathology, radiology, pediatrics, obstetrics, gynecology, urology, nursing, pharmacology, endocrinology. **Holdings:** 9782 books; 5126 bound periodical volumes; 1 VF drawer of

staff reprints; 902 tapes; 10 films. **Subscriptions:** 417 journals and other serials.

★8096★ **MUSCATATUCK STATE DEVELOPMENTAL CENTER RESIDENT AND STAFF DEVELOPMENT LIBRARY**
Box 77
Butlerville, IN 47223   Phone: (812) 346-4401
Barbara Carter, Libn.
Subjects: Medicine, staff development, nursing, behavior modification, supervision and management, mental retardation. **Holdings:** 3200 books; 200 filmstrips, phonograph records, transparencies; videotapes. **Subscriptions:** 23 journals and other serials.

★8097★ **CENTRAL SOYA COMPANY, INC.**
FEED RESEARCH LIBRARY
1200 N. 2nd St.
Decatur, IN 46733   Phone: (219) 724-1304
Dr. R.L. Schoelkopf
Subjects: Animal nutrition and health. **Holdings:** 800 books; 21 journals and other serials; 40 titles of conference proceedings; 9 drawers of agribusiness documents; 2 cabinets of university/Agriculture Extension Service files; 18 reels of microfilm of Central Soya Feed Research reports. **Subscriptions:** 123 journals and other serials.

★8098★ **ST. CATHERINE HOSPITAL**
REGIONAL EDUCATIONAL SERVICES
MCGUIRE MEMORIAL LIBRARY
4321 Fir St.
East Chicago, IN 46312   Phone: (219) 392-7230
Madeline E. Downen, Coord., Lib.Serv.
Subjects: Medicine and allied health sciences. **Holdings:** 7600 volumes. **Subscriptions:** 300 journals and other serials.

★8099★ **MILES INC.**
SCIENCE AND BUSINESS INFORMATION SERVICES
1127 Myrtle St.
Elkhart, IN 46514-2282   Phone: (219) 264-6705
James L. Mucha, Mgr.
Subjects: Biotechnology, clinical medicine, chemistry, microbiology, business and management. **Holdings:** 15,000 books; 30,000 bound periodical volumes; 25 shelves of product literature; 8 drawers of microfilm; 13 VF drawers of company reports. **Subscriptions:** 533 journals and other serials; 7 newspapers.

★8100★ **OAKLAWN PSYCHIATRIC CENTER**
STAFF LIBRARY
2600 Oakland Ave.
Elkhart, IN 46507   Phone: (219) 533-1234
Nancy P. Price, Libn.
Subjects: Psychiatry, mental health, psychology, social work, addictions, pastoral counseling. **Holdings:** 2059 books; 1300 unbound periodical volumes; 24 VF drawers; 634 cassettes. **Subscriptions:** 101 journals and other serials.

★8101★ **BRISTOL MYERS SQUIBB COMPANY**
U.S. PHARMACEUTICAL AND NUTRITION GROUP
LIBRARY AND INFORMATION SERVICES
2400 Lloyd Expy.
Evansville, IN 47721-0001   Phone: (812) 426-8679
Alice M. Weisling, Libn.
Subjects: Chemistry, pharmaceuticals, marketing, nutrition, medicine, pediatrics, sales, human resources, management, finance, economics, psychology, law. **Holdings:** 50,000 books; 10,000 bound periodical volumes; 8 VF drawers of patents; 10,000 reels of microfilm of journals and patents. **Subscriptions:** 700 journals and other serials.

★8102★ **DEACONESS HOSPITAL**
HEALTH SCIENCE LIBRARY
600 Mary St.
Evansville, IN 47747   Phone: (812) 426-3385
Jean Weir, Med.Libn.
Subjects: Nursing education, clinical medicine, allied health sciences. **Holdings:** 11,000 books; 2000 AV programs. **Subscriptions:** 300 journals and other serials; 5 newspapers.

★8103★ **EVANSVILLE PSYCHIATRIC CHILDREN'S CENTER**
STAFF LIBRARY
3330 E. Morgan Ave.
Evansville, IN 47715   Phone: (812) 477-6436
Michele Haynes, Med.Rec.Adm./Libn.
Subjects: Psychotherapy, child development, recreation therapy, psychopathology, education, nursing. **Holdings:** Figures not available. **Subscriptions:** 4 journals and other serials.

★8104★ **PLANNED PARENTHOOD OF SOUTHWESTERN**
INDIANA
RESOURCE CENTER
Hebron Plaza
971 Kenmore Dr.
Evansville, IN 47715-7503   Phone: (812) 473-8800
Toni Godeke, Dir. of Educ.
Subjects: Contraceptives, sexuality, family life education curriculum, women's health, infertility, population. **Holdings:** 300 books; 5 VF drawers. **Subscriptions:** 6 journals and other serials.

★8105★ **ST. MARY'S MEDICAL CENTER**
HERMAN M. BAKER, M.D. MEMORIAL LIBRARY
3700 Washington Ave.
Evansville, IN 47750   Phone: (812) 479-4151
E. Jane Saltzman, Mgr.
Subjects: Medicine, nursing, health administration. **Holdings:** 1200 volumes; 300 AV programs. **Subscriptions:** 140 journals and other serials; 10 newspapers.

★8106★ **SOUTHWESTERN INDIANA MENTAL HEALTH**
CENTER
LIBRARY
415 Mulberry St.
Evansville, IN 47713   Phone: (812) 423-7791
Ina Freeman, Libn.
Subjects: Psychology, psychiatry, social work, child development, sexuality, therapeutic recreation, drug abuse. **Holdings:** 1000 books; 700 pamphlets; 125 AV programs. **Subscriptions:** 80 journals and other serials.

★8107★ **CENTRAL SOYA COMPANY, INC.**
FOOD RESEARCH LIBRARY
Fort Wayne National Bank Bldg.
PO Box 1400
Fort Wayne, IN 46801-1400   Phone: (219) 425-5906
Valesca Wilson, Jr., Res.Libn.
Subjects: Soybeans, nutrition, proteins, chemistry, food science. **Holdings:** 6500 books; 5067 bound periodical volumes; 3 VF drawers of pamphlets; 119 reels of microfilm. **Subscriptions:** 100 journals and other serials.

★8108★ **FRIENDS OF THE THIRD WORLD INC.**
WHOLE WORLD BOOKS
611 W. Wayne St.
Fort Wayne, IN 46802   Phone: (219) 422-6821
Marian R. Waltz, Rsrc.Coord.
Subjects: Hunger, population, international politics and economics, U.S. minorities, food and nutrition, international and national poverty issues, American lifestyles and the environment. **Holdings:** 800 books; 2000 pamphlets and periodicals; 24 VF drawers. **Subscriptions:** 30 journals and other serials.

★8109★ **LUTHERAN HOSPITAL OF INDIANA**
HEALTH SCIENCES LIBRARY
3024 Fairfield Ave.
Fort Wayne, IN 46807-1697   Phone: (219) 458-2277
Lauralee Aven, Dir.
Subjects: Nursing, medicine, hospital administration, health subjects. **Holdings:** 2500 books; 60 titles of audio cassettes on management; 5 years of audio cassette series in cardiology, internal medicine, pediatrics. **Subscriptions:** 200 journals and other serials; 5 newspapers.

★8110★ **PARKVIEW MEMORIAL HOSPITAL**
HEALTH SCIENCE LIBRARY
2200 Randallia Dr.
Fort Wayne, IN 46805   Phone: (219) 484-6636
Shannon Clever, Lib.Mgr.
Subjects: Medicine, nursing, and allied health sciences, hospital administration. **Holdings:** 3500 books. **Subscriptions:** 180 journals and other serials.

★8111★   ST. JOSEPH'S MEDICAL CENTER
MEDICAL LIBRARY
700 Broadway
Fort Wayne, IN 46802   Phone: (219) 425-3094
Ellen Schellhause, Med.Libn.
Subjects: Medical and health sciences. **Holdings:** 850 books; 300 periodical
volumes; 100 reels of microfilm; 106,000 microfiche. **Subscriptions:** 391
journals and other serials.

★8112★   JOHNSON COUNTY MEMORIAL HOSPITAL
LIBRARY
1125 W. Jefferson
Franklin, IN 46131   Phone: (317) 736-3456
Kathryn Jester, Libn.
Subjects: Medicine, nursing. **Holdings:** 300 books. **Subscriptions:** 51
journals and other serials.

★8113★   ELI LILLY AND COMPANY
GREENFIELD LABORATORIES
LIBRARY AGRICULTURAL SERVICE
Box 708
Greenfield, IN 46140   Phone: (317) 277-4000
Marta White, Sr.Libn.
Subjects: Plant science, animal nutrition, veterinary medicine, toxicology,
chemistry. **Holdings:** 5500 books; 6300 bound periodical volumes. **Sub-
scriptions:** 650 journals and other serials.

★8114★   ST. MARGARET HOSPITAL
SALLIE M. TYRRELL, M.D. MEMORIAL LIBRARY
5454 Hohman Ave.
Hammond, IN 46320   Phone: (219) 932-2300
Laurie Broadus, Lib.Coord.
Subjects: Medicine, nursing. **Holdings:** 2000 books; 1500 bound periodical
volumes; Audio-Digest tapes. **Subscriptions:** 150 journals and other serials.

★8115★   BUTLER UNIVERSITY
IRWIN LIBRARY
HUGH THOMAS MILLER RARE BOOK ROOM
46th & Sunset
Indianapolis, IN 46208   Phone: (317) 283-9265
Gisela S. Terrell, Rare Bks. & Spec.Coll.Libn.
Subjects: Liberal arts and sciences, pharmacy, education, fine and performing arts, athletics. **Holdings:** 32,000 book titles; 312 serial titles; 60 pieces
of sheet and bound music; 302 manuscripts; 209 phonograph records; 250
prints; 2445 photographs; 172 pieces of original art. **Subscriptions:** 36
journals and other serials.

★8116★   BUTLER UNIVERSITY
SCIENCE LIBRARY
46th & Sunset
Indianapolis, IN 46208   Phone: (317) 283-9401
Barbara Howes, Sci.Libn.
Subjects: Botany, chemistry, environmental sciences, mathematics, pharmacy, physics, zoology. **Holdings:** 21,000 books; 26,500 bound periodical
volumes; 36 VF drawers; 750 AV programs. **Subscriptions:** 600 journals
and other serials.

★8117★   CENTRAL STATE HOSPITAL
MEDICAL LIBRARY
3000 W. Washington St.
Indianapolis, IN 46222   Phone: (317) 639-3927
Bette A. Kinsley, Libn.
Subjects: Psychiatry, psychology, nursing, business and management,
geriatrics, mental retardation, social work. **Holdings:** 7500 books; 3000
bound periodical volumes; 300 archival materials; 116 video cassettes; 450
audio cassettes; 22 VF drawers. **Subscriptions:** 152 journals and other
serials.

★8118★   COMMUNITY HOSPITAL INDIANAPOLIS
LIBRARY
1500 N. Ritter Ave.
Indianapolis, IN 46219   Phone: (317) 353-5591
Sheila Hofstetter, Mgr.
Subjects: Medicine, nursing, allied health sciences. **Holdings:** 2000 books;
3000 bound periodical volumes. **Subscriptions:** 360 journals and other
serials.

★8119★   ELI LILLY AND COMPANY
SCIENTIFIC LIBRARY
Lilly Corporate Center
Indianapolis, IN 46285   Phone: (317) 276-4452
Adele Hoskin, Dept.Hd.
Subjects: Chemistry, medicine, biological sciences, pharmacy. **Holdings:**
35,000 volumes; 1.7 million drug product information cards. **Subscrip-
tions:** 1600 journals and other serials.

★8120★   INDIANA BOARD OF HEALTH
JACOB T. OLIPHANT LIBRARY
1330 W. Michigan St.
Indianapolis, IN 46202-2874   Phone: (317) 633-8585
Billy Smith, Libn.
Subjects: Communicable disease, chronic disease, nursing, public health,
health education, sanitation, pollution, drugs. **Holdings:** 3000 books; 3000
bound periodical volumes; 2 VF drawers of Board of Health archives.
Subscriptions: 150 journals and other serials.

★8121★   INDIANA HAND CENTER
LIBRARY
PO Box 80434
Indianapolis, IN 46280-0434   Phone: (317) 875-9105
Subjects: Surgery - hand, plastic, micro; general orthopedics. **Holdings:** 700
books; 100 videotapes. **Subscriptions:** 11 journals and other serials.

★8122★   INDIANA MEDICAL HISTORY MUSEUM
LIBRARY
3000 W. Washington St.
Old Pathology Bldg.
Indianapolis, IN 46222   Phone: (317) 635-7329
Katherine Mandusic McDonell, Dir.
Subjects: Historical medicine; late 19th to early 20th century medicine,
pathology, and psychiatry. **Holdings:** 3000 books; 3 boxes of manuscripts.
Subscriptions: 3 journals and other serials.

★8123★   INDIANA SCHOOL FOR THE DEAF
LIBRARY
1200 E. 42nd St.
Indianapolis, IN 46205   Phone: (317) 924-4374
Linda Canty
Subjects: Audiology, psychology of deafness, multiple-handicapped, spe-
cial education. **Holdings:** 25,455 volumes; 1000 other cataloged items.
Subscriptions: 140 journals and other serials.

★8124★   INDIANA UNIVERSITY, INDIANAPOLIS
SCHOOL OF DENTISTRY LIBRARY
1121 W. Michigan St.
Indianapolis, IN 46202   Phone: (317) 274-7204
Sara Hook-Shelton, Lib.Dir.
Subjects: Dentistry and allied health sciences, basic sciences, education.
Holdings: 51,921 volumes; 5148 other cataloged items; 12,943 uncataloged
items. **Subscriptions:** 670 journals and other serials.

★8125★   INDIANA UNIVERSITY, INDIANAPOLIS
SCHOOL OF MEDICINE LIBRARY
975 W. Walnut
Indianapolis, IN 46202   Phone: (317) 274-7182
Dana McDonald, Hd.
Subjects: Medicine, nursing, allied health sciences. **Holdings:** 169,376
volumes. **Subscriptions:** 1978 journals and other serials; 6 newspapers.

★8126★   LARUE D. CARTER MEMORIAL HOSPITAL
MEDICAL LIBRARY
1315 W. 10th St.
Indianapolis, IN 46202   Phone: (317) 634-8401
Philip I. Enz, Adm.Libn.
Subjects: Psychiatry, psychology, social work, psychiatric nursing, rehabilitation therapies, mental health. **Holdings:** 18,000 volumes; 200 audiotapes;
4 drawers of staff publications. **Subscriptions:** 236 journals and other
serials.

★8127★ MARION MERRELL DOW, INC.
RESEARCH CENTER LIBRARY
9550 Zionsville Rd.
Box 68470
Indianapolis, IN 46268-0470   Phone: (317) 873-7147
Pamela Pickens Kubiak, Res.Libn.
Subjects: Pharmacology, toxicology, pharmacokinetics, pharmacy research, chemistry, analytical chemistry. **Holdings:** 7000 books; 20,000 bound periodical volumes; abstract services; research notebooks on microfilm. **Subscriptions:** 525 journals and other serials.

★8128★ METHODIST HOSPITAL OF INDIANA
LIBRARY SERVICES
1701 N. Senate Blvd.
PO Box 1367
Indianapolis, IN 46206   Phone: (317) 929-8021
Joyce S. Allen, Lib.Mgr.
Subjects: Medicine, nursing, medical ethics, administration, health education, psychology, allied health sciences. **Holdings:** 6558 books; 3531 bound periodical volumes; 800 AV programs; 8 VF drawers of pamphlets. **Subscriptions:** 360 journals and other serials; 18 audiotape journals.

★8129★ NATIONAL LEGAL CENTER FOR THE MEDICALLY DEPENDENT AND DISABLED
LIBRARY AND INFORMATION CENTER
50 S. Meridian St., Ste. 605
Indianapolis, IN 46204-3541   Phone: (317) 632-6245
Tom Marzen
Subjects: Persons with disabilities, Baby Doe, death and dying, euthanasia, discrimination based on disability. **Holdings:** 400 books. **Subscriptions:** 20 journals and other serials.

★8130★ ORTHOPAEDICS INDIANAPOLIS, INC.
LIBRARY
1801 Senate Blvd., No. 200
Indianapolis, IN 46202   Phone: (317) 923-5352
Jean Bonner
Subjects: Clinical orthopaedics. **Holdings:** 400 books. **Subscriptions:** 21 journals and other serials.

★8131★ PLANNED PARENTHOOD OF CENTRAL INDIANA
RESOURCE CENTER
3209 N. Meridian St.
Indianapolis, IN 46208   Phone: (317) 925-6686
Betsy Lambie, Libn.
Subjects: Birth control, human sexuality, teen pregnancy, human reproduction, abortion, sex education, women's health, STDs, AIDS. **Holdings:** 1200 books; 130 films and videotapes; vertical files; poster collection. **Subscriptions:** 55 journals and other serials.

★8132★ ST. VINCENT'S HOSPITAL
GARCEAU LIBRARY
2001 W. 86th St.
Indianapolis, IN 46260   Phone: (317) 871-2095
Virginia Durkin, Mgr., Lib.Serv.
Subjects: Medicine, paramedical sciences, nursing, hospital administration. **Holdings:** 6980 volumes; 420 audiotapes; 4 VF drawers of pamphlets; 600 AV programs; microfiche. **Subscriptions:** 200 journals and other serials.

★8133★ SIGMA THETA TAU INTERNATIONAL
INTERNATIONAL NURSING LIBRARY
550 W. North St.
Indianapolis, IN 46202   Phone: (317) 634-8171
Carole Hudgings, Dir.
Subjects: Nursing. **Holdings:** 800 books; 160 bound periodical volumes; 183 videotapes; 425 audio cassettes. **Subscriptions:** 141 journals and other serials.

★8134★ U.S. DEPARTMENT OF VETERANS AFFAIRS
MEDICAL CENTER LIBRARY
1481 W. 10th St.
Indianapolis, IN 46202   Phone: (317) 635-7401
Lori L. Klein, Chf., Lib.Serv.
Subjects: General medicine, surgery, nursing, psychiatry, allied health sciences. **Holdings:** 4000 books; 4400 bound periodical volumes; 3000 reels of microfilm; 800 AV programs. **Subscriptions:** 400 journals and other serials.

★8135★ WILLIAM N. WISHARD MEMORIAL HOSPITAL
PROFESSIONAL LIBRARY/MEDIA SERVICES
1001 W. 10th St.
Indianapolis, IN 46202   Phone: (317) 630-7028
Kirsten Quam, Mgr., Lib./Media Serv.Dept.
Subjects: Medicine, nursing, health care administration. **Holdings:** 4500 books; 600 bound periodical volumes; 2800 AV programs. **Subscriptions:** 125 journals and other serials.

★8136★ WINONA MEMORIAL HOSPITAL
HEALTH SCIENCES LIBRARY
3232 N. Meridian
Indianapolis, IN 46208   Phone: (317) 927-2248
Susan Kent, Med.Libn.
Subjects: Medicine, nursing, hospital administration, allied health sciences. **Holdings:** 1000 books; 600 bound periodical volumes. **Subscriptions:** 75 journals and other serials.

★8137★ CLARK MEMORIAL HOSPITAL
MEDICAL LIBRARY
1220 Missouri Ave.
Jeffersonville, IN 47131-0069   Phone: (812) 283-2358
Kathleen Lynn, Libn.
Subjects: Medicine, nursing. **Holdings:** 300 books; 100 bound periodical volumes; 2 VF drawers of pamphlet material; 200 video cassettes; 1 video cassette series; 2 audio cassette series. **Subscriptions:** 57 journals and other serials.

★8138★ ST. JOSEPH MEMORIAL HOSPITAL
HEALTH SCIENCE LIBRARY
1907 W. Sycamore St.
Kokomo, IN 46901   Phone: (317) 452-5611
Jean Romack, Personnel Asst.
Subjects: Medicine, nursing, hospital administration and management. **Holdings:** 1609 books; 736 bound periodical volumes; 348 AV programs; 4 VF drawers. **Subscriptions:** 129 journals and other serials.

★8139★ ST. ELIZABETH HOSPITAL MEDICAL CENTER
BANNON HEALTH SCIENCE LIBRARY
1501 Hartford St.
Box 7501
Lafayette, IN 47903   Phone: (317) 423-6143
Ruth Pestalozzi Pape, Dir., Prof.Lib.Serv.
Subjects: Medicine, health care management, allied subjects. **Holdings:** 1500 books; 6000 bound periodical volumes; 1102 other books in departmental libraries; 700 audio cassettes; 300 video cassettes. **Subscriptions:** 300 journals and other serials.

★8140★ ST. ELIZABETH MEDICAL CENTER
ST. ELIZABETH HOSPITAL SCHOOL OF NURSING
LIBRARY
1508 Tippecanoe St.
Lafayette, IN 47904   Phone: (317) 423-6125
Lorraine Rund, Libn.
Subjects: Nursing, medicine, psychiatry. **Holdings:** 4000 books; 302 filmstrips; 6 16mm films; 50 charts; 300 videotapes. **Subscriptions:** 160 journals and other serials; 10 newspapers.

★8141★ LOGANSPORT STATE HOSPITAL
STAFF LIBRARY
R.R. 2
Logansport, IN 46947   Phone: (219) 722-4141
Pam Kindem, Rehabilitation Supv.
Subjects: Medicine, psychiatry, psychology, social service, drug abuse, nursing, alcoholism, geriatrics. **Holdings:** 1500 books. **Subscriptions:** 70 journals and other serials.

★8142★ MADISON STATE HOSPITAL
CRAGMONT MEDICAL LIBRARY
Lanier Dr.
Madison, IN 47250   Phone: (812) 265-2611
Lloyd Roberts, Libn.
Subjects: Medicine, psychiatry, psychology, social work. **Holdings:** 3824 volumes; 1750 clippings; 56 boxes of pamphlets. **Subscriptions:** 58 journals and other serials.

★8143★ MARION GENERAL HOSPITAL
LIBRARY
Wabash & Euclid Ave.
Marion, IN 46952   Phone: (317) 662-4607
Kay Lake, Dir., Educ.Serv.
Subjects: Medicine, nursing, management. **Holdings:** 1892 books; 194 bound periodical volumes; 237 video cassettes. **Subscriptions:** 196 journals and other serials.

★8144★ U.S. DEPARTMENT OF VETERANS AFFAIRS
HOSPITAL MEDICAL LIBRARY
E. 38th St. at Home Ave.
Marion, IN 46952   Phone: (317) 674-3321
Karen A. Davis, Chf., Lib.Serv.
Subjects: Medicine, with special emphasis on psychiatry and psychology. **Holdings:** 3799 books; 7243 bound periodical volumes (also in microform); government documents; slides; audio and video cassettes; microforms. **Subscriptions:** 190 journals and other serials; 40 newspapers.

★8145★ BALL MEMORIAL HOSPITAL
HEALTH SCIENCE LIBRARY
2401 University Ave.
Muncie, IN 47303-0137   Phone: (317) 747-3204
Jane A. Potee, Dir. of Lib.Serv.
Subjects: Clinical medicine, nursing, allied health sciences, health administration, medical education, business management. **Holdings:** 3500 books; 6000 bound periodical volumes; 15 files of subject headings; VF drawers. **Subscriptions:** 800 journals and other serials.

★8146★ BALL STATE UNIVERSITY
DEPARTMENT OF LIBRARY SERVICE
GOVERNMENT PUBLICATIONS
Bracken Library, Rm. 224
Muncie, IN 47306   Phone: (317) 285-1110
Diane Calvin, Govt.Pubns.Libn.
Subjects: Education, health and human services, U.S. Congress. **Holdings:** 87,294 federal government documents; 2550 Indiana state documents; 24,536 microfiche.

★8147★ NEW CASTLE STATE DEVELOPMENTAL CENTER
LIBRARY
100 Van Nuys Rd.
New Castle, IN 47362   Phone: (317) 529-0900
Subjects: Psychiatry, neurology, general medicine, physiology, nursing. **Holdings:** 600 books. **Subscriptions:** 25 journals and other serials.

★8148★ INLOW CLINIC
LIBRARY
Box 370
Shelbyville, IN 46176   Phone: (317) 392-3651
Subjects: History and philosophy of medicine, medicine, social sciences, history. **Holdings:** 3500 books; 2500 bound periodical volumes; 4 VF drawers of pamphlets.

★8149★ MEMORIAL HOSPITAL
LIBRARY SERVICES
615 N. Michigan
South Bend, IN 46601   Phone: (219) 284-7491
Jeanne M. Larson, Lib.Mgr.
Subjects: Medicine, nursing, health care administration, allied health sciences. **Holdings:** 3500 books; 5 VF drawers of pamphlets and reprints; 120 subscriptions on microfiche. **Subscriptions:** 300 journals and other serials.

★8150★ MICHIANA COMMUNITY HOSPITAL
LIBRARY
2515 E. Jefferson Blvd.
South Bend, IN 46615   Phone: (219) 288-8311
Mary Jo Tompos
Subjects: Medicine. **Holdings:** 1136 books; 160 bound periodical volumes; 50 video cassettes; Audio-Digest tapes. **Subscriptions:** 42 journals and other serials.

★8151★ ST. JOSEPH'S MEDICAL CENTER
MEDICAL LIBRARY
801 E. Lasalle
Box 1935
South Bend, IN 46634-1935   Phone: (219) 237-7228
Jennifer N. Helmen, Libn.
Subjects: Medicine, nursing, pharmacy, health administration, pastoral care, social work. **Holdings:** 2955 books; 13,170 unbound periodicals; 580 documents, pamphlets, brochures, and clippings; 50 video cassettes; 13 drawers of microfiche. **Subscriptions:** 280 journals and other serials.

★8152★ PURDUE UNIVERSITY
PHARMACY, NURSING AND HEALTH SCIENCES LIBRARY
Pharmacy Bldg.
West Lafayette, IN 47907   Phone: (317) 494-1416
Theodora Andrews, Libn.
Subjects: Pharmaceutical sciences, pharmacy, clinical medicine, nursing, bionucleonics, environmental sciences. **Holdings:** 41,071 volumes; 24 VF drawers of pamphlets; 150 audio cassettes; 102,461 microforms. **Subscriptions:** 622 journals and other serials.

★8153★ PURDUE UNIVERSITY
VETERINARY MEDICAL LIBRARY
C.V. Lynn Hall, Rm. 108
West Lafayette, IN 47907   Phone: (317) 494-2852
Gretchen Stephens, Libn.
Subjects: Comparative and veterinary medicine, animal behavior, comparative anatomy, neuroanatomy, pathology, laboratory animal medicine. **Holdings:** 24,599 volumes. **Subscriptions:** 758 journals and other serials.

Iowa

★8154★ IOWA STATE UNIVERSITY
VETERINARY MEDICAL LIBRARY
Ames, IA 50011   Phone: (515) 294-2225
Sara R. Peterson, Vet.Med.Libn.
Subjects: Veterinary and comparative medicine, anatomy, biomedical engineering, physiology, toxicology, clinical sciences, microbiology, preventive medicine, pathology, pharmacology. **Holdings:** 14,000 books; 14,000 bound periodical volumes. **Subscriptions:** 652 journals and other serials.

★8155★ U.S.D.A.
AGRICULTURAL RESEARCH SERVICE
NATIONAL ANIMAL DISEASE CENTER
LIBRARY
2300 Dayton Ave.
PO Box 70
Ames, IA 50010   Phone: (515) 239-8271
Janice K. Eifling, Libn.
Subjects: Biomedicine, microbiology, veterinary science. **Holdings:** 8000 books; 18,000 bound periodical volumes. **Subscriptions:** 350 journals and other serials.

★8156★ BURLINGTON MEDICAL CENTER
LIBRARY
602 N. 3rd
Burlington, IA 52601   Phone: (319) 753-3631
Sylvia Poe, Libn.
Subjects: Nursing, medicine. **Holdings:** 1000 books. **Subscriptions:** 250 journals and other serials.

★8157★ MERCY MEDICAL CENTER
HEALTH SERVICES LIBRARY
701 10th St., SE
Cedar Rapids, IA 52403   Phone: (319) 398-6165
Linda Roberts Armitage, Libn.
Subjects: Medicine, nursing, hospital administration. **Holdings:** 4000 books; 3000 bound periodical volumes. **Subscriptions:** 403 journals and other serials.

★8158★ ST. LUKE'S HOSPITAL
HEALTH SCIENCE LIBRARY
1026 A Ave., NE
Cedar Rapids, IA 52402   Phone: (319) 369-7358
Donald Pohnl, Dir.
Subjects: Medicine, nursing, allied health sciences, health administration,

child abuse. **Holdings:** 5000 books; 11,000 bound periodical volumes; 1500 AV programs. **Subscriptions:** 500 journals and other serials.

★8159★ MENTAL HEALTH INSTITUTE
HEALTH SCIENCE LIBRARY
1200 W. Cedar St.
Cherokee, IA 51012   Phone: (712) 225-2594
Tom Folkes, Hea.Sci.Libn.
Subjects: Psychiatry, psychology, neurology, nursing, social service, medicine. **Holdings:** 2599 books; 793 audio cassettes; 182 video cassettes; 5000 back issues of journals; 8 linear feet of vertical files. **Subscriptions:** 51 journals and other serials.

★8160★ IOWA STATE MENTAL HEALTH INSTITUTE
CLARINDA TREATMENT COMPLEX
PROFESSIONAL LIBRARY
Box 338
Clarinda, IA 51632   Phone: (712) 542-2161
Dorothy Horton, Libn.
Subjects: Psychiatry, psychology, psychiatric nursing, social services education, pastoral counseling, maintenance and dietary services. **Holdings:** 2800 books; 3 VF drawers; 190 cassette tapes. **Subscriptions:** 44 journals and other serials; 35 newspapers.

★8161★ JENNIE EDMUNDSON MEMORIAL HOSPITAL
SCHOOL OF NURSING
LIBRARY
933 E. Pierce St.
Council Bluffs, IA 51501   Phone: (712) 328-6130
Christine Kirby, Libn.
Subjects: Nursing, medicine, paramedical sciences. **Holdings:** 10,195 books; 2710 bound periodical volumes; 19 VF drawers of pamphlets and clippings; government documents; AV and computer-aided instruction programs. **Subscriptions:** 250 journals and other serials; 7 newspapers.

★8162★ DAVENPORT MEDICAL CENTER
MEDICAL STAFF LIBRARY
1111 W. Kimberly Rd.
Davenport, IA 52806   Phone: (319) 383-0295
J. Sue Ebel
Subjects: Medicine, nursing, hospital administration. **Holdings:** 350 books; 250 bound periodical volumes; 200 AV titles. **Subscriptions:** 53 journals and other serials.

★8163★ MARYCREST COLLEGE
CONE LIBRARY
1607 W. 12th St.
Davenport, IA 52804   Phone: (319) 326-9254
Sr. Joan Sheil, Dir.
Subjects: Education, social sciences, nursing, language and literature, art, music, computer science. **Holdings:** 105,000 books; 47,000 curriculum guides and textbooks, microforms, films, records, slides, tapes, transparencies, kits. **Subscriptions:** 770 journals and other serials; 7 newspapers.

★8164★ PALMER COLLEGE OF CHIROPRACTIC
DAVID D. PALMER HEALTH SCIENCES LIBRARY
1000 Brady St.
Davenport, IA 52803   Phone: (319) 326-9641
Dennis Peterson, Dir.
Subjects: Chiropractic, health sciences. **Holdings:** 26,062 books; 15,679 bound periodical volumes; 9145 microfiche; 1138 reels of microfilm; 1465 audiotapes; 1066 videotapes; 19,800 slides; 910 biological specimens and models; 1534 x-ray sets. **Subscriptions:** 900 journals and other serials; 14 newspapers.

★8165★ BROADLAWNS MEDICAL CENTER
HEALTH SCIENCES LIBRARY
18th & Hickman Rd.
Des Moines, IA 50314   Phone: (515) 282-2394
Phyllis A. Anderson, Libn.
Subjects: Medicine, nursing, psychiatry. **Holdings:** 800 books. **Subscriptions:** 110 journals and other serials.

★8166★ IOWA DEPARTMENT OF HUMAN SERVICES
LIBRARY
Hoover Bldg.
Des Moines, IA 50319   Phone: (515) 281-6033
Kay M. Elliott, Chf.Libn.
Subjects: Social casework, public assistance, mental health and retardation, child abuse, child support. **Holdings:** 8000 books; 100 bound periodical volumes; 1250 VF materials; 360 AV programs. **Subscriptions:** 127 journals and other serials.

★8167★ IOWA DEPARTMENT OF PUBLIC HEALTH
STATISTICAL SERVICES
Lucas State Office Bldg.
Des Moines, IA 50319-0075   Phone: (515) 281-4945
Mike Dare, Stat.Res.Anl.
Subjects: Vital statistics; statistical tabulations - Iowa births, marriages, divorces, deaths; health manpower statistics; statistical tabulations - location of Iowa dentists, dental hygienists, chiropractors, optometrists, physical therapists, physicians, podiatrists, nursing home administrators.

★8168★ IOWA HOSPITAL ASSOCIATION
LIBRARY
100 E. Grand
Des Moines, IA 50309   Phone: (515) 288-1955
Roxanna Tovrea, Lib.Dir.
Subjects: Hospital administration, rural health, nursing, inservice training and education, standards and regulations. **Holdings:** 3000 books; 180 AV programs; 5 lateral file drawers of pamphlet material, educational material, publications, bibliographies. **Subscriptions:** 200 journals and other serials.

★8169★ IOWA LUTHERAN HOSPITAL
DEPARTMENT OF MEDICAL EDUCATION SERVICES
LEVITT HEALTH SCIENCES LIBRARY
University at Penn
Des Moines, IA 50316   Phone: (515) 263-5181
Molly H. Yapp, Dir.
Subjects: Medicine, nursing, health care administration, practice management, patient education. **Holdings:** 2125 books; periodicals; 6 16mm films; 250 video cassettes; 591 audiotapes; 25 slide/tape kits; 2 VF drawers of pamphlets. **Subscriptions:** 160 journals and other serials.

★8170★ IOWA METHODIST MEDICAL CENTER
MARJORIE GERTRUDE MORROW LIBRARY
1117 Pleasant St.
Des Moines, IA 50309   Phone: (515) 283-6453
Nancy O'Brien, Libn.
Subjects: Nursing, nutrition. **Holdings:** 2919 books; 272 bound periodical volumes; brochures; pamphlets. **Subscriptions:** 118 journals and other serials.

★8171★ IOWA METHODIST MEDICAL CENTER
OLIVER J. FAY LIBRARY
1200 Pleasant St.
Des Moines, IA 50309   Phone: (515) 283-6490
Mary Wegner, Dir., Med.Lib.
Subjects: Medicine, allied health sciences. **Holdings:** 3800 books; 2900 bound periodical volumes; 650 cassette tapes. **Subscriptions:** 350 journals and other serials.

★8172★ MERCY HOSPITAL MEDICAL CENTER
LEVITT LEARNING RESOURCE CENTER
1165 5th Ave.
Des Moines, IA 50314   Phone: (515) 247-4189
Lenetta Atkins, Lib.Mgr.
Subjects: Medicine, religion, nursing, management. **Holdings:** 4785 books; 1662 bound periodical volumes; 96 filmstrips; 61 slides, tapes, film loops; 8 16mm sound filmstrips; 213 microfiche. **Subscriptions:** 146 journals and other serials.

★8173★ U.S. DEPARTMENT OF VETERANS AFFAIRS
MEDICAL CENTER LIBRARY
30th & Euclid Ave.
Des Moines, IA 50310   Phone: (515) 271-5824
Clare M. Jergens, Chf., Lib.Serv.
Subjects: Medicine, nursing, psychiatry, radiology, psychology, audiology, surgery, patient education, dentistry. **Holdings:** 3824 books; 4227 bound periodical volumes; Network for Continuing Medical Education video cassettes. **Subscriptions:** 405 journals and other serials.

★8174★ UNIVERSITY OF OSTEOPATHIC MEDICINE AND
HEALTH SCIENCES
LIBRARY
3200 Grand Ave.
Des Moines, IA 50312   Phone: (515) 271-1430
Larry D. Marquardt, Lib.Dir.
Subjects: Osteopathic and podiatric medicine, allied health sciences,
physical therapy. **Holdings:** 30,382 volumes. **Subscriptions:** 489 journals
and other serials.

★8175★ MERCY HEALTH CENTER
ANTHONY C. PFOHL HEALTH SCIENCE LIBRARY
Mercy Dr.
Dubuque, IA 52001   Phone: (319) 589-9620
James H. Lander, Hea.Sci.Libn.
Subjects: Medicine, patient education, management. **Holdings:** 6800
monographs; 250 bound periodical volumes; 1500 pamphlets (65 titles);
AV programs. **Subscriptions:** 320 journals and other serials.

★8176★ GLENWOOD STATE HOSPITAL
SCHOOL OF MEDICINE
STAFF LIBRARY
711 S. Vine
Glenwood, IA 51534   Phone: (712) 527-4811
Renee Pape, Temp.Libn.
Subjects: Mental retardation, psychiatry, psychology, social work, medi-
cine, nursing, special education. **Holdings:** 3540 books; 500 bound
periodical volumes. **Subscriptions:** 155 journals and other serials; 5
newspapers.

★8177★ INDEPENDENCE MENTAL HEALTH INSTITUTE
MEDICAL LIBRARY
Box 111
Independence, IA 50644   Phone: (319) 334-2583
Lois J. Samek, Med.Libn.
Subjects: Psychiatry, medicine, psychiatric nursing. **Holdings:** 3500 books;
650 bound periodical volumes; 200 cassette tapes. **Subscriptions:** 48
journals and other serials.

★8178★ U.S. DEPARTMENT OF VETERANS AFFAIRS
MEDICAL CENTER LIBRARY
Iowa City, IA 52246   Phone: (319) 339-7163
Helene Petty, Chf., Lib.Serv.
Subjects: Medicine, allied health sciences. **Holdings:** 2415 books; 455 AV
programs. **Subscriptions:** 209 journals and other serials.

★8179★ UNIVERSITY OF IOWA
HEALTH SCIENCES LIBRARY
Health Sciences Library Bldg.
Iowa City, IA 52242   Phone: (319) 335-9871
David S. Curry, Libn.
Subjects: Medicine, speech pathology, dentistry, nursing, pharmacy. **Hold-
ings:** 229,752 volumes.

★8180★ U.S. DEPARTMENT OF VETERANS AFFAIRS
MEDICAL CENTER LIBRARY
Knoxville, IA 50138   Phone: (515) 842-3101
R.B. Sayers, Chf.Libn.
Subjects: Psychiatry, psychology, medicine, nursing. **Holdings:** 10,500
books; 3000 bound periodical volumes; 400 other cataloged items.
Subscriptions: 400 journals and other serials; 20 newspapers.

★8181★ ST. JOSEPH MERCY HOSPITAL
MEDICAL LIBRARY
84 Beaumont Dr.
Mason City, IA 50401   Phone: (515) 424-7699
Judy I. Madson, Dir.
Subjects: Medicine, nursing, hospital administration. **Holdings:** 5300
volumes. **Subscriptions:** 250 journals and other serials.

★8182★ MOUNT PLEASANT MENTAL HEALTH INSTITUTE
PROFESSIONAL LIBRARY
1200 E. Washington St.
Mount Pleasant, IA 52641   Phone: (319) 385-7231
Georgia Kay Houseman, Libn.
Subjects: Psychiatry, nursing, psychology, social work, pharmacology,
nutrition, medicine. **Holdings:** 1600 books; 500 periodical volumes.
Subscriptions: 39 professional journals.

★8183★ IOWA DRUG INFORMATION SERVICE
Oakdale Hall
Oakdale, IA 52319   Phone: (319) 335-4800
C. David Butler, Pharm.D., Dir.
Subjects: Drugs and human drug therapy. **Holdings:** 275,000 articles on
microfilm; Drug and Disease Indexes with internal descriptor-index, 1966
to present, on microfilm. **Subscriptions:** 160 journals and other serials.

★8184★ OTTUMWA REGIONAL HEALTH CENTER
LIBRARY
1001 Pennsylvania Ave.
Ottumwa, IA 52501   Phone: (515) 682-7511
Bette Pope, Libn.
Subjects: Nursing, medicine, allied health sciences, religion, literature,
management. **Holdings:** 3520 books; 700 bound periodical volumes; 1712
pamphlets; 155 maps; 1542 AV programs; 14 VF drawers of reprints,
clippings, diagrams; 4 VF drawers of archival materials; 2 dissertations.
Subscriptions: 93 journals and other serials.

★8185★ ST. LUKE'S REGIONAL MEDICAL CENTER
INSTRUCTIONAL TECHNOLOGY CENTER
2720 Stone Park Blvd.
Sioux City, IA 51104   Phone: (712) 279-3156
Cathy Perley, Instr.Tech.Mgr.
Subjects: Medicine, nursing. **Holdings:** 2000 books; 200 filmstrips; 1200
video cassettes. **Subscriptions:** 90 journals and other serials.

★8186★ ALLEN MEMORIAL HOSPITAL
LIBRARIES
1825 Logan Ave.
Waterloo, IA 50703   Phone: (319) 235-3681
Risa Lumley, Libn.
Subjects: Nursing, medicine, hospital administration. **Holdings:** 3500
books; 600 bound periodical volumes. **Subscriptions:** 153 journals and
other serials.

★8187★ WOODWARD STATE HOSPITAL SCHOOL
STAFF LIBRARY
Woodward, IA 50276   Phone: (515) 438-2600
Joy Averill, Libn.
Subjects: Mental retardation, special education, psychology, training,
social services, medicine, nursing, leisure services. **Holdings:** 6000 books; 8
VF drawers of pamphlets and reprints; 250 video cassettes. **Subscriptions:**
70 journals and other serials; 5 newspapers.

Kansas

★8188★ U.S. ARMY HOSPITALS
IRWIN ARMY HOSPITAL
MEDICAL LIBRARY
Bldg. 600
Fort Riley, KS 66442-5036   Phone: (913) 239-7874
Phyllis J. Whiteside, Med.Libn.
Subjects: Medicine, surgery, dentistry, nursing. **Holdings:** 1500 books;
1146 bound periodical volumes; 455 reels of microfilm; 1049 microfiche.
Subscriptions: 250 journals and other serials.

★8189★ HERTZLER RESEARCH FOUNDATION
LIBRARY
4th & Chestnut
Halstead, KS 67056   Phone: (316) 835-2241
Teresa R. Coady, Med.Libn.
Subjects: Cardiology, oncology, thoracic and cardiovascular surgery, ortho-
paedics, pathology, gastroenterology. **Holdings:** 4000 books; 6662 periodi-
cal volumes. **Subscriptions:** 150 journals and other serials.

★8190★ BETHANY MEDICAL CENTER
W.W. SUMMERVILLE MEDICAL LIBRARY
51 N. 12th St.
Kansas City, KS 66102   Phone: (913) 281-8770
Kathleen McClure, Med.Libn.
Subjects: Medicine, nursing, and allied health sciences. **Holdings:** 1750
books; 3000 bound periodical volumes. **Subscriptions:** 300 journals and
other serials; 5 newspapers.

★8191★ PROVIDENCE-ST. MARGARET HEALTH CENTER LIBRARY
8929 Parallel Pkwy.
Kansas City, KS 66112　　　　　Phone: (913) 596-4795
Paul Nixon, Med.Libn.
Subjects: Medicine, surgery, nursing, health sciences. **Holdings:** 1000 books; 773 bound periodical volumes; AV programs; video cassettes; cassette tapes; 6 VF drawers. **Subscriptions:** 130 journals and other serials.

★8192★ UNIVERSITY OF KANSAS MEDICAL CENTER
ARCHIE R. DYKES LIBRARY OF THE HEALTH SCIENCES
2100 W. 39th St.
Kansas City, KS 66103　　　　　Phone: (913) 588-7166
James L. Bingham, Dir.
Subjects: Basic sciences, clinical medicine, allied health sciences, nursing, social work. **Holdings:** 55,947 books; 84,902 bound periodical volumes. **Subscriptions:** 1750 journals and other serials.

★8193★ UNIVERSITY OF KANSAS MEDICAL CENTER
CLENDENING HISTORY OF MEDICINE LIBRARY
History of Medicine Dept.
39th & Rainbow Blvd.
Kansas City, KS 66103　　　　　Phone: (913) 588-7040
Susan B. Case, Rare Bks.Libn.
Subjects: Medicine - history, philosophy, ethics; history of science. **Holdings:** 26,000 books; 2000 bound periodical volumes; 50 AV programs; 2000 artifacts; 2000 photograph/etched portraits; 500 manuscripts. **Subscriptions:** 58 journals and other serials.

★8194★ LARNED STATE HOSPITAL
J.T. NARAMORE LIBRARY
Rte. 3, Box 89
Larned, KS 67550-9365　　　　　Phone: (316) 285-2131
Rita Renfrow, Off.Asst. III
Subjects: Psychiatry, psychiatric nursing, psychology, mental health, medicine. **Holdings:** 5867 books; 80 journal titles, 1976-1991. **Subscriptions:** 68 journals and other serials.

★8195★ U.S. DEPARTMENT OF VETERANS AFFAIRS
CENTER MEDICAL LIBRARY
Leavenworth, KS 66048　　　　　Phone: (913) 682-2000
Bennett F. Lawson, Chf., Lib.Serv.
Subjects: Medicine, allied health sciences. **Holdings:** 3535 books; 4743 bound periodical volumes; 1400 periodical volumes on microfilm. **Subscriptions:** 230 journals and other serials.

★8196★ KANSAS STATE UNIVERSITY
FARRELL LIBRARY
Manhattan, KS 66506　　　　　Phone: (913) 532-7400
Brice G. Hobrock, Dean of Libs.
Subjects: Physical sciences, farming systems, agriculture, engineering, applied science and technology, natural sciences, veterinary medicine, home economics. **Holdings:** 1.16 million volumes; 680,000 government documents; 20,000 maps; 3.3 million microforms; 13,500 sound recordings; 29,500 slides; 650 tapes; 650 filmstrips; 350 films; 8662 scores; 2380 audio cassettes; 650 video cassettes. **Subscriptions:** 9170 journals and other serials; 195 newspapers.

★8197★ KANSAS STATE UNIVERSITY
VETERINARY MEDICAL LIBRARY
Manhattan, KS 66506　　　　　Phone: (913) 532-6006
Gayle K. Willard, Vet.Med.Libn.
Subjects: Veterinary medicine, comparative medicine, preclinical science, internal medicine, pharmacology, toxicology. **Holdings:** 32,400 volumes; 1700 AV programs; 8 VF drawers of pamphlets. **Subscriptions:** 950 journals and other serials.

★8198★ JOHNSON COUNTY MENTAL HEALTH CENTER
JOHN R. KEACH MEMORIAL LIBRARY
6000 Lamar Ave.
Mission, KS 66202　　　　　Phone: (913) 831-2550
Subjects: Mental health, psychology, psychiatry, social work. **Holdings:** 1722 books; 199 bound periodical volumes; 8 VF drawers. **Subscriptions:** 25 journals and other serials.

★8199★ OSAWATOMIE STATE HOSPITAL
RAPAPORT PROFESSIONAL LIBRARY
MENTAL HEALTH LIBRARY
Osawatomie, KS 66064　　　　　Phone: (913) 755-3151
Connie Park, Dir., Lib.Serv.
Subjects: Psychiatry, psychology, social sciences, medicine, nursing, special education. **Holdings:** 6045 books; 1704 bound periodical volumes; 624 audiotapes; 120 videotapes; 30 VF drawers of dissertations, reprints, pamphlets, documents. **Subscriptions:** 50 journals and other serials.

★8200★ PARSONS STATE HOSPITAL AND TRAINING CENTER
MEDICAL LIBRARY
2601 Gabriel
Box 738
Parsons, KS 67357-0738　　　　　Phone: (316) 421-6550
Linda Lee Stahlman, Staff Libn.
Subjects: Mental retardation, developmental disabilities, psychology, speech pathology, audiology, behavioral science. **Holdings:** 5200 books; 4 VF drawers of pamphlets; 282 working papers. **Subscriptions:** 75 journals and other serials.

★8201★ MOBAY CORPORATION
ANIMAL HEALTH DIVISION
MOBAY ANIMAL HEALTH LIBRARY
Box 390
Shawnee Mission, KS 66201-0390　　　　　Phone: (913) 268-2761
Ruth Lehman, Res. Data Asst.
Subjects: Veterinary medicine, animal health, pharmaceuticals. **Holdings:** 1000 books; 5000 bound periodical volumes; 12,000 technical reports; 100 company brochures; 50 annual reports. **Subscriptions:** 81 journals and other serials.

★8202★ SHAWNEE MISSION MEDICAL CENTER
MEDICAL LIBRARY
9100 W. 74th
Box 2923
Shawnee Mission, KS 66201　　　　　Phone: (913) 676-2101
Clifford L. Nestell, Lib.Dir.
Subjects: Medicine. **Holdings:** 8070 books; 7671 bound periodical volumes; 2943 audiotapes; 491 videotapes; 71 software packages. **Subscriptions:** 628 journals and other serials.

★8203★ AMERICAN LUNG ASSOCIATION OF KANSAS
INFORMATION CENTER
4300 Drury Ln.
Box 4426
Topeka, KS 66604-2419　　　　　Phone: (913) 272-9290
Steve Berndsen, Exec.Dir.
Subjects: Lung diseases - emphysema, tuberculosis, asthma; air pollution; smoking and health. **Holdings:** Books; pamphlets; filmstrips; films; videotapes.

★8204★ KANSAS DEPARTMENT OF HEALTH AND ENVIRONMENT
LIBRARY
Landon State Office Bldg., 10th Fl.
900 Jackson
Topeka, KS 66612　　　　　Phone: (913) 296-7901
Janet L. Weber, MLS
Subjects: Health, environment, health education. **Holdings:** 1300 books; 200 bound periodical volumes; 3000 reports; 400 archival items.

★8205★ MENNINGER FOUNDATION
ARCHIVES
Box 829
Topeka, KS 66601　　　　　Phone: (913) 273-7500
Kelly E. Burket, Archv.
Subjects: Psychiatry, psychoanalysis, clinical psychology, psychiatric social work, medical history. **Holdings:** 1800 pamphlets; 700 manuscript boxes; 400 VF drawers; 30,000 clippings; 12,000 photographs; 2500 tapes.

★8206★   MENNINGER FOUNDATION
DEPARTMENT OF RESEARCH
PROFESSIONAL LIBRARY
Box 829
Topeka, KS 66601   Phone: (913) 273-7500
Alice Brand Bartlett, Chf.Libn.
Subjects: Clinical psychiatry, psychoanalysis, clinical psychology, family therapy, forensic psychiatry, allied mental health sciences. **Holdings:** 27,000 books; 14,100 bound periodical volumes. **Subscriptions:** 420 journals and other serials.

★8207★   STORMONT-VAIL REGIONAL MEDICAL CENTER
STAUFFER HEALTH SCIENCES LIBRARY
1500 SW 10th St.
Topeka, KS 66604-1353   Phone: (913) 354-5800
Shirley Borglund, Dir.
Subjects: Medicine, nursing. **Holdings:** 8500 books; 15,000 unbound periodicals. **Subscriptions:** 400 journals and other serials.

★8208★   TOPEKA STATE HOSPITAL
STAFF LIBRARY
2700 W. 6th St.
Topeka, KS 66606-1898   Phone: (913) 296-4411
Laura E. Schafer, Libn.
Subjects: Psychiatry, psychology, psychiatric nursing, social work, chaplaincy training. **Holdings:** 7000 books; 3000 bound periodical volumes. **Subscriptions:** 50 journals and other serials.

★8209★   U.S. DEPARTMENT OF VETERANS AFFAIRS
DR. KARL A. MENNINGER MEDICAL LIBRARY
2200 SW Gage Blvd.
Topeka, KS 66622   Phone: (913) 272-3111
Eris R. Kirby, Chf., Lib.Serv.
Subjects: Psychiatry, internal medicine, pathology, neurology, surgery, rehabilitation medicine, psychology, social service, fine arts. **Holdings:** 19,000 books; 5800 bound periodical volumes; 13 VF drawers of clippings, reprints, original papers. **Subscriptions:** 340 journals and other serials.

★8210★   INSTITUTE OF LOGOPEDICS
CLYDE C. BERGER RESOURCE CENTER
2400 Jardine Dr.
Wichita, KS 67219   Phone: (316) 262-8271
Valorie Thaw, Libn.
Subjects: Speech pathology, audiology, neurology, psychology, special education. **Holdings:** 3000 books; 20,000 reprints of scientific articles, government documents, pamphlets, other ephemera. **Subscriptions:** 20 journals and other serials.

★8211★   INTERNATIONAL REFERENCE ORGANIZATION IN
**   FORENSIC MEDICINE AND SCIENCES**
LIBRARY AND REFERENCE CENTER
PO Box 8282
Wichita, KS 67208   Phone: (316) 685-7612
Dr. William G. Eckert, Dir.
Subjects: Abortion, accidents, alcohol, alcoholism, drugs and drug abuse, forensic sciences, medicolegal history, homicide, iatrogenic problems, legal medicine, pediatric medicine, poisoning, suicidology, sex problems, thanatology, toxicology, trauma, war crimes, war wounds. **Holdings:** 1700 books; 1500 bound periodical volumes; 2000 papers; 2000 miscellaneous reports; 100 bibliographies; 500 hours of videotapes; 1000 hours of magnetic tapes; AV programs; microfilm. **Subscriptions:** 30 journals and other serials.

★8212★   ROBERT C. TINKER LIBRARY
3600 E. Harry
Wichita, KS 67218   Phone: (316) 689-5377
Carol Matulka, Med.Libn.
Subjects: Medicine, nursing, and allied health sciences, administration. **Holdings:** 4198 books; 1355 bound periodical volumes; 4247 books and journals in storage for recall; cassettes; records; AV programs and video cassettes. **Subscriptions:** 200 journals and other serials.

★8213★   ST. FRANCIS REGIONAL MEDICAL CENTER
MARCUS HEALTH EDUCATION CENTER
929 N. St. Francis
Wichita, KS 67214   Phone: (316) 268-6080
Betty B. Wood, Libn.
Subjects: Patient education, consumer education, wellness, prevention. **Holdings:** 190 books; pamphlet collection.

★8214★   ST. FRANCIS REGIONAL MEDICAL CENTER
PROFESSIONAL LIBRARY
929 N. St. Francis
Wichita, KS 67214   Phone: (316) 268-5979
Betty B. Wood, Libn.
Subjects: Medicine, nursing, surgery, orthopedics, management. **Holdings:** 6000 books; 10,000 bound periodical volumes. **Subscriptions:** 550 journals and other serials.

★8215★   U.S. DEPARTMENT OF VETERANS AFFAIRS
MEDICAL AND REGIONAL OFFICE CENTER
LIBRARY SERVICE
5500 E. Kellogg
Wichita, KS 67218   Phone: (316) 651-3612
Alice H. Schad, Chf., Lib.Serv.
Subjects: Medicine, nursing, allied health sciences, social sciences, patient health education, veterans affairs. **Holdings:** 2000 books; 1155 bound periodical volumes; 1306 reels of microfilm; 4 VF drawers of pamphlets; 414 AV programs. **Subscriptions:** 427 journals and other serials.

★8216★   WESLEY MEDICAL CENTER
H.B. MCKIBBIN HEALTH SCIENCE LIBRARY
550 N. Hillside
Wichita, KS 67214   Phone: (316) 688-2715
Subjects: Medicine and nursing. **Holdings:** 10,000 books; 21,000 bound periodical volumes. **Subscriptions:** 500 journals and other serials.

★8217★   H.L. SNYDER MEMORIAL RESEARCH FOUNDATION
LIBRARY
1407 Wheat Rd.
PO Box 745
Winfield, KS 67156   Phone: (316) 221-4080
Darla Clark, Libn.
Subjects: Biochemistry, medicine, clinical chemistry. **Holdings:** 2000 books; 1000 bound periodical volumes. **Subscriptions:** 20 journals and other serials.

★8218★   WINFIELD STATE HOSPITAL AND TRAINING
**   CENTER**
PROFESSIONAL LIBRARY
Winfield, KS 67156   Phone: (316) 221-1200
Janis McGlasson, Lib.Ck.
Subjects: Mental retardation, psychology, medicine, social work and welfare, education and special education, nursing. **Holdings:** 2200 books; 189 bound periodical volumes; 259 AV programs; 476 unbound periodical volumes; 398 indexes and abstracts in volumes; 15 theses; 2500 pamphlets and clippings. **Subscriptions:** 56 journals and other serials.

Kentucky

★8219★   ST. THOMAS INSTITUTE
LIBRARY
6714 Sperti Ln.
Burlington, KY 41005-9640
Sr. M. Virgil Ghering, O.P., Libn.
Subjects: Biology, experimental medicine, physics, biophysics, chemistry, biochemistry. **Holdings:** 8200 books; 21,400 bound periodical volumes; 45 boxes and 4 VF drawers of reprints; 10 volumes of press clippings; 14 boxes of dissertation summaries. **Subscriptions:** 173 journals and other serials.

★8220★   KENTUCKY SCHOOL FOR THE DEAF
LEARNING RESOURCE CENTER
S. 2nd St.
Danville, KY 40422-0027   Phone: (606) 236-5132
Duane L. Belcher, Dir., Media Serv.
Subjects: K-12 educational materials. **Holdings:** 11,000 books; 75 bound periodical volumes; 5000 nonprint materials; Captioned Films for the Deaf depository. **Subscriptions:** 68 journals and other serials.

★8221★   ST. ELIZABETH MEDICAL CENTER
ALLNUTT HEALTH SCIENCES LIBRARY
1 Medical Village Dr.
Edgewood, KY 41017   Phone: (606) 344-2248
Donald R. Smith, Libn.
Subjects: Health sciences. **Holdings:** 2450 books; 4000 bound periodical volumes. **Subscriptions:** 200 journals and other serials; 5 newspapers.

★8222★ U.S. ARMY HOSPITALS
BLANCHFIELD ARMY COMMUNITY HOSPITAL
MEDICAL LIBRARY
Fort Campbell, KY 42223-1498   Phone: (502) 798-8014
Lillian G. Graham, Med.Libn.
Subjects: Medicine, allied health sciences. Holdings: 5700 books; 2400 bound periodical volumes; video and audio cassettes. Subscriptions: 396 journals and other serials.

★8223★ KENTUCKY COUNCIL ON HIGHER EDUCATION
INFORMATION SERVICES CENTER
1050 U.S. 127 S.
Frankfort, KY 40601-4395   Phone: (502) 564-3553
Elizabeth M. Harrod, Supv., Rec.Proc.
Subjects: Higher and health education. Holdings: 2500 books. Subscriptions: 70 journals and other serials; 5 newspapers.

★8224★ KENTUCKY DEPARTMENT FOR HUMAN
  RESOURCES
LIBRARY
275 E. Main St.
Frankfort, KY 40621   Phone: (502) 564-4530
Douglas Raisor, Supv.
Subjects: Public health, social welfare, social work, child welfare, mental health. Holdings: 27,500 books; 10,000 unbound periodicals; 3000 pamphlets. Subscriptions: 223 journals and other serials.

★8225★ KENTUCKY DEPARTMENT FOR LIBRARIES AND
  ARCHIVES
PUBLIC RECORDS DIVISION
ARCHIVES
300 Coffee Tree Rd.
Box 537
Frankfort, KY 40602   Phone: (502) 875-7000
Richard N. Belding, Dir./State Archv.
Subjects: Kentucky - history, genealogy, government, politics, health services. Holdings: 91,000 cubic feet of state and local documents; 26,000 reels of microfilm; 1000 microfiche; 100 video cassettes; 200 audio cassettes; 25,000 photographic negatives.

★8226★ WESTERN STATE HOSPITAL
PROFESSIONAL LIBRARY
Russellville Rd.
Box 2200
Hopkinsville, KY 42240   Phone: (502) 886-4431
Elizabeth W. Nelson, Staff Libn.
Subjects: Psychiatry, psychology, nursing, medicine, social work, management. Holdings: 2500 books; 240 bound periodical volumes. Subscriptions: 58 journals and other serials.

★8227★ EASTERN STATE HOSPITAL
RESOURCE LIBRARY
627 W. 4th St.
Lexington, KY 40508-9990   Phone: (606) 355-1431
Sonja Zaumeyer, Dir. of Staff Dev.
Subjects: Psychiatry, psychology, mental illness, nursing. Holdings: 1050 volumes. Subscriptions: 20 journals and other serials.

★8228★ GOOD SAMARITAN HOSPITAL
MEDICAL LIBRARY
310 S. Limestone
Lexington, KY 40508   Phone: (606) 252-6612
John Calk, M.D., MSLS, Knowledge Spec.
Subjects: Medicine, allied health sciences. Holdings: 250 books; 105 bound periodical volumes; 20 pamphlets; 80 cassettes. Subscriptions: 45 journals and other serials.

★8229★ LEXINGTON COMMUNITY COLLEGE
LIBRARY
Oswald Bldg.
Cooper Dr.
Lexington, KY 40506   Phone: (606) 258-4919
Martha J. Birchfield, Hd.Libn.
Subjects: Associated health technologies, engineering, data processing, business technology, statistical process control. Holdings: 20,000 volumes. Subscriptions: 180 journals and other serials.

★8230★ NATIONAL ASSOCIATION OF STATE EMERGENCY
  MEDICAL SERVICES DIRECTORS
SAM CHANNELL NATIONAL EMS CLEARINGHOUSE
PO Box 11910
Iron Works Pike
Lexington, KY 40578   Phone: (606) 252-2291
Subjects: Emergency medical services. Holdings: Reports; state statutes; regulations; comparative state studies; articles.

★8231★ ST. JOSEPH HOSPITAL
MEDICAL LIBRARY
1 St. Joseph Dr.
Lexington, KY 40504   Phone: (606) 278-3436
Jerri Trimble, Libn.
Subjects: Medicine, nursing, and allied health sciences. Holdings: 1115 books; 2935 bound periodical volumes; 10 directories; 818 audiotapes; 55 AV programs. Subscriptions: 177 journals and other serials.

★8232★ U.S. DEPARTMENT OF VETERANS AFFAIRS
MEDICAL CENTER LIBRARIES
142D
Leestown Rd. and Cooper Dr. Divisions
Lexington, KY 40511   Phone: (606) 281-4916
Deborah Kessler
Subjects: Psychology, psychiatry, nursing, medicine, surgery, social sciences, patient health education. Holdings: 7000 books; 5000 bound periodical volumes. Subscriptions: 260 journals and other serials; 60 newspapers.

★8233★ UNIVERSITY OF KENTUCKY
AGRICULTURE LIBRARY
N 24 Agricultural Science Ctr., N.
Lexington, KY 40546-0091   Phone: (606) 257-2758
Antoinette P. Powell, Dir.
Subjects: Agriculture, forestry, veterinary medicine, food, nutrition, entomology, horticulture, botany, landscape architecture. Holdings: 34,267 books; 56,386 bound periodical volumes; 3169 reels of microfilm; 82,099 microfiche; 10,070 U.S. Department of Agriculture publications; 3907 unbound materials. Subscriptions: 2118 journals and other serials; 10 newspapers.

★8234★ UNIVERSITY OF KENTUCKY
MEDICAL CENTER LIBRARY
Lexington, KY 40536-0084   Phone: (606) 233-5726
Omer Hamlin, Jr., Dir.
Subjects: Medicine, dentistry, nursing, pharmacy, allied health sciences. Holdings: 76,811 books; 97,010 bound periodical volumes; 1084 reels of microfilm; 2372 AV programs. Subscriptions: 1884 journals and other serials.

★8235★ UNIVERSITY OF KENTUCKY
TOBACCO AND HEALTH RESEARCH INSTITUTE
LIBRARY
Cooper and University Drs.
Lexington, KY 40546-0236   Phone: (606) 257-2877
Laura McIlwain
Subjects: Tobacco products, diseases, passive smoking, cessation of smoking, maternal smoking, legislation.

★8236★ ALLIANT HEALTH SYSTEM
LIBRARY/MEDIA SERVICES
Box 35070
Louisville, KY 40232   Phone: (502) 562-8125
Wenda Webster Fischer, Dir.
Subjects: Medicine, nursing, hospital administration, psychiatry, pediatrics, women's health, othopedics. Holdings: 5000 books; pamphlets; audio and video cassettes. Subscriptions: 330 journals and other serials.

★8237★ AMERICAN PRINTING HOUSE FOR THE BLIND
LIBRARY
1839 Frankfort Ave.
PO Box 6085
Louisville, KY 40206   Phone: (502) 895-2405
Subjects: Publishing for the blind and visually impaired - braille, large print, recorded; educational aids for visually impaired. Holdings: 3500 volumes.

**★8238★ BAPTIST HOSPITAL EAST
HAGAN-PEDIGO LIBRARY**
4000 Kresge Way
Louisville, KY 40207   Phone: (502) 897-8183
Kay Goldberg, Dir., Lib.Serv.
Subjects: Medicine, nursing, hospital administration. **Holdings:** 1200 books. **Subscriptions:** 222 journals and other serials.

**★8239★ HUMANA HOSPITAL AUDUBON
MEDICAL LIBRARY**
1 Audubon Plaza
Louisville, KY 40217   Phone: (502) 636-7296
Elizabeth Fischer, Libn.
Subjects: Medicine and nursing. **Holdings:** 450 books; 1300 bound periodical volumes; 400 Audio-Digest tapes. **Subscriptions:** 59 journals and other serials.

**★8240★ HUMANA HOSPITAL UNIVERSITY
GRADIE R. ROWNTREE MEDICAL LIBRARY**
530 S. Jackson St.
Louisville, KY 40202   Phone: (502) 562-3947
Jody Branson, Med.Libn.
Subjects: Medicine, surgery, allied health sciences, nursing. **Holdings:** 1000 books; 1000 bound periodical volumes. **Subscriptions:** 160 journals and other serials.

**★8241★ JEWISH HOSPITAL
MEDICAL LIBRARY**
217 E. Chestnut St.
Louisville, KY 40202   Phone: (502) 587-4280
Gene Haynes, Dir.
Subjects: Medicine. **Holdings:** 1500 books; 700 bound periodical volumes. **Subscriptions:** 270 journals and other serials.

**★8242★ KENTUCKY SCHOOL FOR THE BLIND
CAROL J. FREY LIBRARY**
1867 Frankfort Ave.
Louisville, KY 40206   Phone: (502) 897-1583
Cathy Hicks, Libn.
Subjects: Blind and physically handicapped, adult and juvenile fiction, nonfiction. **Holdings:** 4100 books; 6903 recorded books; 5087 braille volumes; 600 recordings; 300 filmstrips; 1116 tapes. **Subscriptions:** 49 journals and other serials.

**★8243★ OUR LADY OF PEACE HOSPITAL
MEDICAL LIBRARY**
PO Box 32690
Louisville, KY 40232   Phone: (502) 451-3330
Irene Satory, S.C.N., Dir.
Subjects: Psychiatry, alcoholism and substance abuse, nursing, pediatrics. **Holdings:** 1480 books; 836 bound periodical volumes; 500 cassettes (psychiatric series); 12 VF drawers of pamphlets, clippings, archives. **Subscriptions:** 84 journals and other serials.

**★8244★ ST. ANTHONY HOSPITAL
SISTER M. FRANCIS MEDICAL LIBRARY**
1313 St. Anthony Pl.
Louisville, KY 40204   Phone: (502) 587-1161
Alma Hall Berry, Libn.
Subjects: Medicine. **Holdings:** 500 books; 100 bound periodical volumes. **Subscriptions:** 25 journals and other serials.

**★8245★ STS. MARY AND ELIZABETH HOSPITAL
HEALTH SCIENCES LIBRARY**
1850 Bluegrass Ave.
Louisville, KY 40215   Phone: (502) 361-6428
Wanda Polley, Libn.
Subjects: Medicine and nursing. **Holdings:** 1800 books; 1600 bound periodical volumes; 2 VF drawers of clippings and pamphlets. **Subscriptions:** 200 journals and other serials.

**★8246★ U.S. DEPARTMENT OF VETERANS AFFAIRS
HOSPITAL LIBRARY**
800 Zorn Ave.
Louisville, KY 40206-1499   Phone: (502) 895-3401
James F. Kastner, Chf.Libn.
Subjects: Clinical medicine, surgery, nursing, psychiatry, social work. **Holdings:** 3250 books; 8000 bound periodical volumes; 20,000 volumes of journals in microform; 1325 AV programs. **Subscriptions:** 510 journals and other serials.

**★8247★ UNIVERSITY OF LOUISVILLE
KORNHAUSER HEALTH SCIENCES LIBRARY**
Louisville, KY 40292   Phone: (502) 588-5771
Leonard M. Eddy, Dir.
Subjects: Medicine, dentistry, nursing, allied health sciences, medical history. **Holdings:** 57,500 books; 103,985 bound periodical volumes; 3820 AV programs. **Subscriptions:** 1715 journals.

**★8248★ REGIONAL MEDICAL CENTER
MEDICAL LIBRARY**
900 Hospital Dr.
Madisonville, KY 42431   Phone: (502) 825-5252
Nadia E. Ingram, Med.Libn.
Subjects: Medicine, surgery. **Holdings:** 820 books; 1765 bound periodical volumes; 840 audio cassettes; 4000 unbound journals; films; AV programs. **Subscriptions:** 173 journals and other serials.

**★8249★ OUR LADY OF THE WAY HOSPITAL
MEDICAL LIBRARY**
Box 910
Martin, KY 41649   Phone: (606) 285-5181
Sonya Bergman, Act.Libn.
Subjects: Medicine, nursing. **Holdings:** 100 books. **Subscriptions:** 25 journals and other serials.

**★8250★ ST. CLAIRE MEDICAL CENTER
MEDICAL LIBRARY**
222 Medical Circle
Morehead, KY 40351   Phone: (606) 784-6661
Betty Ison, Med.Libn.
Subjects: Medicine, nursing, pharmacy, allied health sciences, health administration. **Holdings:** 2115 books; 910 bound periodical volumes; 300 videotapes; filmstrips; audio cassettes. **Subscriptions:** 160 journals and other serials; 12 newspapers.

**★8251★ LOURDES HOSPITAL
HEALTH SCIENCES LIBRARY**
1530 Lone Oak Rd.
Paducah, KY 42001   Phone: (502) 444-2138
Trudi A. Patterson, Libn.
Subjects: Medicine, nursing, allied health sciences. **Holdings:** 600 books. **Subscriptions:** 100 journals and other serials.

Louisiana

**★8252★ RAPIDES GENERAL HOSPITAL
MEDICAL LIBRARY**
Box 30101
Alexandria, LA 71301   Phone: (318) 473-3563
Janet Dawkins, Libn.
Subjects: Medicine. **Holdings:** 1800 books; 1112 bound periodical volumes. **Subscriptions:** 65 journals and other serials.

**★8253★ ST. FRANCES CABRINI HOSPITAL
MEDICAL LIBRARY**
3330 Masonic Dr.
Alexandria, LA 71301   Phone: (318) 487-1122
Carol Holloway, Act.Libn.
Subjects: Medicine, nursing, and allied health sciences. **Holdings:** 3471 books and bound periodical volumes; 900 tapes; 157 unbound journals. **Subscriptions:** 60 journals and other serials.

**★8254★ U.S. DEPARTMENT OF VETERANS AFFAIRS
MEDICAL CENTER MEDICAL LIBRARY**
Alexandria, LA 71301   Phone: (318) 473-0010
Nancy M. Guillet, Chf., Lib.Serv.
Subjects: Medicine, employee development, patient education and recreation. **Holdings:** 1568 books; 2475 bound periodical volumes; 61 maps and atlases; 481 AV programs. **Subscriptions:** 226 journals and other serials; 7 newspapers.

★8255★ EARL K. LONG MEMORIAL HOSPITAL
MEDICAL LIBRARY
5825 Airline Hwy.
Baton Rouge, LA 70805-2498   Phone: (504) 358-1089
Jean B. Finley, Dir., Lib.Serv.
Subjects: Clinical medicine. Holdings: 2200 books; 2600 bound periodical volumes; 750 AV programs; 20 VF drawers of articles. Subscriptions: 290 journals and other serials.

★8256★ LOUISIANA STATE UNIVERSITY
SCHOOL OF VETERINARY MEDICINE
LIBRARY
Baton Rouge, LA 70803   Phone: (504) 346-3173
Sue Loubiere, Libn.
Subjects: Veterinary medicine, medicine. Holdings: 13,252 books; 31,265 bound periodical volumes. Subscriptions: 1583 journals and other serials.

★8257★ OUR LADY OF THE LAKE REGIONAL MEDICAL
CENTER
HEALTH SCIENCES LIBRARY
5000 Hennessy Blvd.
Baton Rouge, LA 70808   Phone: (504) 765-8756
Diane D. Whited, Libn.
Subjects: Medicine, nursing. Holdings: 5000 volumes. Subscriptions: 101 journals and other serials.

★8258★ HOMOSEXUAL INFORMATION CENTER
LIBRARY
115 Monroe St.
Bossier City, LA 71111   Phone: (318) 742-4709
Leslie Colfax, Libn.
Subjects: Homosexuality, civil liberties, censorship, sexual freedom, lesbiana, prostitution, abortion. Holdings: 9800 books and bound periodical volumes; 32 VF drawers of manuscripts, clippings, pamphlets, documents; 86 legal briefs and court opinions; 30 boxes. Subscriptions: 32 journals and other serials; 21 newspapers.

★8259★ U.S. PUBLIC HEALTH SERVICE HOSPITAL
GILLIS W. LONG HANSEN'S DISEASE CENTER
MEDICAL LIBRARY
Carville, LA 70721   Phone: (504) 642-4748
Marilyn P. McManus, Med.Libn.
Subjects: Hansen's disease, dermatology, ophthalmology, bone and joint surgery, plastic surgery, rehabilitation, physical therapy, dentistry, nursing. Holdings: 8000 books; 10,000 unbound items; films; slides; tapes. Subscriptions: 130 journals and other serials.

★8260★ TULANE UNIVERSITY OF LOUISIANA
DELTA REGIONAL PRIMATE RESEARCH CENTER
SCIENCE INFORMATION SERVICE
3 Rivers Rd.
Covington, LA 70433   Phone: (504) 892-2040
Mercedes M. Fussell, Adm.Asst.
Subjects: Infectious disease - acquired immunodeficiency syndrome (AIDS), leprosy, filariasis, malaria, pyelonephritis, prostatitis, treatment of viral infections with antiviral substances; neurobiology, reproductive physiology, urology, veterinary science, immunology, parasitology, primatology. Holdings: 4608 books; 4480 bound periodical volumes; 6 dissertations; 175 microfiche. Subscriptions: 64 journals and other serials.

★8261★ U.S. ARMY HOSPITALS
BAYNE-JONES ARMY COMMUNITY HOSPITAL
MEDICAL LIBRARY
Fort Polk, LA 71459-6000   Phone: (318) 531-3725
Cecelia B. Higginbotham, Med.Libn.
Subjects: Medicine, pathology, hospital administration, dentistry. Holdings: 2300 monographs; 4000 bound periodical volumes. Subscriptions: 122 serials.

★8262★ OUR LADY OF LOURDES REGIONAL MEDICAL
CENTER
LEARNING RESOURCE CENTER
PO Box 4027C
Lafayette, LA 70502   Phone: (318) 231-2141
Annette Tremie, Med.Libn.
Subjects: Medicine, nursing, pastoral care. Holdings: 2500 books; unbound periodicals. Subscriptions: 128 journals and other serials.

★8263★ SOUTHEAST LOUISIANA HOSPITAL
PROFESSIONAL LIBRARY
Box 3850
Mandeville, LA 70448   Phone: (504) 626-8161
Janet D. Landrum, Libn.
Subjects: Psychiatry, psychology, sociology, psychiatric nursing, human physiology, biochemistry, philosophy. Holdings: 3000 books; 2800 periodical volumes; 70 other cataloged items; 3 VF drawers of doctoral dissertations, pamphlets, state vital statistics reports; 10 newsletters; 216 cassette tapes. Subscriptions: 103 journals and other serials.

★8264★ E.A. CONWAY MEMORIAL HOSPITAL
MEDICAL LIBRARY
Box 1881
Monroe, LA 71201   Phone: (318) 388-7644
Pamela D. Ashley, Med.Libn.
Subjects: Medicine and allied health sciences. Holdings: 650 volumes; 120 AV items. Subscriptions: 69 journals and other serials.

★8265★ ALTON OCHSNER MEDICAL FOUNDATION
MEDICAL LIBRARY
1516 Jefferson Hwy.
New Orleans, LA 70121   Phone: (504) 838-3760
Carol M. Liardon, Dir./Med.Libn.
Subjects: Medicine, nursing, allied health sciences, research. Holdings: 3000 books; 22,500 bound periodical volumes. Subscriptions: 565 journals and other serials.

★8266★ CHARITY-DELGADO SCHOOL OF NURSING
LIBRARY
450 S. Claiborne Ave.
New Orleans, LA 70112   Phone: (504) 568-6430
Anne B. Howard, Lib.Coord.
Subjects: Nursing. Holdings: 7500 books; 2000 bound periodical volumes. Subscriptions: 110 journals and other serials.

★8267★ HOTEL DIEU HOSPITAL
LIBRARY
Box 61262
New Orleans, LA 70161   Phone: (504) 588-3470
Sr. Agnes Caffarel, Hea.Sci.Libn.
Subjects: Medicine, surgery, hospital administration, nursing. Holdings: 1434 books; 1270 bound periodical volumes; 42 volumes of hospital archives. Subscriptions: 49 journals and other serials.

★8268★ LOUISIANA STATE UNIVERSITY MEDICAL CENTER
LIBRARY
433 Bolivar St.
New Orleans, LA 70112-2223   Phone: (504) 568-6105
Judith Caruthers, Dir.
Subjects: Medicine, dentistry, nursing, allied health sciences. Holdings: 58,410 books; 99,903 bound periodical volumes; 2461 volumes in microform; 3821 AV programs; 14 Audio-Digest titles. Subscriptions: 2134 journals and other serials.

★8269★ MERCY HOSPITAL OF NEW ORLEANS
MEDICAL LIBRARY
301 N. Jefferson Davis Pkwy.
New Orleans, LA 70119   Phone: (504) 486-7361
Jean Leonard, Med.Libn.
Subjects: Medicine, nursing, management. Holdings: 907 books; 500 bound periodical volumes. Subscriptions: 55 journals and other serials.

★8270★ NEW ORLEANS PSYCHOANALYTIC INSTITUTE
LIBRARY
3624 Coliseum St.
New Orleans, LA 70115   Phone: (504) 899-5815
Dr. Denise Dorsey, Chm.
Subjects: Psychoanalysis. Holdings: 650 books; 500 bound periodical volumes. Subscriptions: 13 journals and other serials.

★8271★ SOUTHERN BAPTIST HOSPITAL
LEARNING RESOURCE CENTER
2700 Napoleon Ave.
New Orleans, LA 70115   Phone: (504) 897-5825
Pauline Fulda, Dir.
Subjects: Medicine, nursing, allied health sciences, pastoral care and

counseling. **Holdings:** 7113 books; 2785 bound periodical volumes; 714 AV programs. **Subscriptions:** 203 journals and other serials.

★8272★   TOURO INFIRMARY
HOSPITAL LIBRARY SERVICES
1401 Foucher St., 10th Fl., M Bldg.
New Orleans, LA 70115   Phone: (504) 897-8102
Patricia J. Greenfield, Lib.Mgr.
Subjects: Clinical medicine, nursing. **Holdings:** 2000 books; 5000 bound periodical volumes; 300 videotapes; 100 Audio-Digest tapes. **Subscriptions:** 200 journals and other serials.

★8273★   TULANE UNIVERSITY OF LOUISIANA
SCHOOL OF MEDICINE
RUDOLPH MATAS MEDICAL LIBRARY
1430 Tulane Ave.
New Orleans, LA 70112   Phone: (504) 588-5155
William D. Postell, Jr., Med.Libn.
Subjects: Medicine, public health. **Holdings:** 145,000 volumes. **Subscriptions:** 1200 journals.

★8274★   U.S. DEPARTMENT OF VETERANS AFFAIRS
MEDICAL CENTER LIBRARY
1601 Perdido St.
New Orleans, LA 70146   Phone: (504) 589-5272
Donna L. Patsfield, Chf., Lib.Serv.
Subjects: Medicine, nursing, dentistry, surgery, allied health sciences. **Holdings:** 2100 books; 2482 bound periodical volumes. **Subscriptions:** 220 journals and other serials; 12 newspapers.

★8275★   XAVIER UNIVERSITY OF LOUISIANA
COLLEGE OF PHARMACY
LIBRARY
7325 Palmetto & Pine Sts.
New Orleans, LA 70125   Phone: (504) 486-7411
Yvonne C. Hull, Libn.
Subjects: Pharmacy, pharmacology, medicinal chemistry, pharmacognosy, clinical pathology, toxicology, drug interaction, public health, history of pharmacy. **Holdings:** 4000 books; 2800 bound periodical volumes; 250 audio cassettes; 10 records; 3 films. **Subscriptions:** 100 journals and other serials.

★8276★   CENTRAL LOUISIANA STATE HOSPITAL
MEDICAL AND PROFESSIONAL LIBRARY
Box 5031
Pineville, LA 71361-5031   Phone: (318) 484-6363
Benton Carol McGee, Med.Libn.
Subjects: Psychiatry, psychology, social work, occupational therapy, psychiatric nursing, psychiatric hospital administration. **Holdings:** 4000 books; 3500 bound periodical volumes; 12 VF drawers of pamphlets and reports. **Subscriptions:** 182 journals and other serials.

★8277★   GREEN CLINIC
LIBRARY
1200 S. Farmerville St.
Ruston, LA 71270   Phone: (318) 255-3690
Sara Sharp, Libn.
Subjects: Internal medicine, surgery, pediatrics, obstetrics and gynecology, ophthalmology, orthopaedics, otolaryngology, adolescent medicine, urology, family practice. **Holdings:** 850 books; 1500 bound periodical volumes; 500 bound single issues of medical journals and yearbooks; 50 volumes of unbound medical journals; 4 VF drawers. **Subscriptions:** 110 journals and other serials.

★8278★   LOUISIANA STATE UNIVERSITY MEDICAL CENTER
LIBRARY
Box 33932
Shreveport, LA 71130-3932   Phone: (318) 674-5448
James Pat Craig, Lib.Dir.
Subjects: Medicine, nursing, allied health, biomedical studies. **Holdings:** 35,143 books; 63,450 bound periodical volumes; 676 reels of microfilm; 5 VF drawers of pamphlets; 1100 video cassettes. **Subscriptions:** 1261 journals and other serials.

★8279★   NORTHWESTERN STATE UNIVERSITY OF
LOUISIANA
EUGENE P. WATSON LIBRARY
SHREVEPORT DIVISION
1800 Line Ave.
Shreveport, LA 71101   Phone: (318) 677-3007
Dorcas M.C. McCormick, Hd.
Subjects: Nursing, education. **Holdings:** 7200 books; 7200 bound periodical volumes; 186 reports and theses; 4000 microfiche; 1075 reels of microfilm; pamphlets; 1 VF drawer; 98 titles on microfilm. **Subscriptions:** 137 journals and other serials.

★8280★   SCHUMPERT MEDICAL CENTER
MEDICAL LIBRARY
915 Margaret Pl.
Box 21976
Shreveport, LA 71120-1976   Phone: (318) 227-4501
Marilyn Willis, Med.Libn.
Subjects: Medicine, surgery, and allied health sciences. **Holdings:** 1200 books; 3400 bound periodical volumes. **Subscriptions:** 140 journals and other serials.

★8281★   U.S. DEPARTMENT OF VETERANS AFFAIRS
OVERTON BROOKS MEDICAL CENTER LIBRARY
510 E. Stoner
Shreveport, LA 71101-4295   Phone: (318) 424-6036
Dixie A. Jones, Chf., Lib.Serv.
Subjects: General medicine. **Holdings:** 1920 books; 1497 bound periodical volumes. **Subscriptions:** 213 journals and other serials; 4 newspapers.

Maine

★8282★   KENNEBEC VALLEY MEDICAL CENTER
MEDICAL LIBRARY
6 E. Chestnut St.
Augusta, ME 04330   Phone: (207) 626-1000
Nancy Greenier, Med.Libn.
Subjects: Medicine, surgery, nursing, health sciences. **Holdings:** 3100 volumes; 6 VF drawers of reprints; 4 VF drawers of pamphlets; 2600 audiotapes; 320 filmstrips; 700 video cassettes; 350 slide sets; 64 16mm films. **Subscriptions:** 162 journals and other serials.

★8283★   MAINE STATE AUDIOVISUAL ALCOHOL/DRUG
RESOURCE CENTER
Stevens School Complex
State House Sta. 57
Augusta, ME 04333   Phone: (207) 289-2511
Gail Mazzaro, Rsrc.Cons.
Subjects: Alcohol and drugs - use, abuse, dependency, education, prevention, and training. **Holdings:** 1500 books; 1000 16mm films and videotapes. **Subscriptions:** 22 journals and other serials.

★8284★   MAINE STATE DEPARTMENT OF HUMAN
SERVICES
DEPARTMENTAL LIBRARY
State House, Sta. No. 11
Augusta, ME 04333   Phone: (207) 289-3055
Maryellen Fleming, Dept.Libn.
Subjects: Nuclear power and radiation, water sanitation, health promotion, disease prevention, AIDS, child health. **Holdings:** 3000 books. **Subscriptions:** 320 journals and other serials.

★8285★   MEDICAL CARE DEVELOPMENT, INC.
LIBRARY
11 Parkwood Dr.
Augusta, ME 04330   Phone: (207) 622-7566
Maryann Spindler, Libn.
Subjects: Health - planning, policy, manpower; rural health. **Holdings:** 300 books. **Subscriptions:** 30 journals and other serials.

★8286★   BANGOR MENTAL HEALTH INSTITUTE
HEALTH SCIENCES MEDIA CENTER
PO Box 926
Bangor, ME 04401   Phone: (207) 941-4226
Daphne Crocker, Libn. II
Subjects: Psychiatry, psychology, mental health services, medicine, psychiatric nursing, geriatrics, social work. **Holdings:** 3000 books; 12 drawers of

pamphlets; 170 AV programs. **Subscriptions:** 125 journals and other serials.

★8287★ EASTERN MAINE MEDICAL CENTER
PARROT HEALTH SCIENCES LIBRARY
489 State St.
Bangor, ME 04401   Phone: (207) 945-8228
Suellen Jagels, Lib.Dir.
Subjects: Medicine, surgery, obstetrics, gynecology, pediatrics, orthopedics, neurology. **Holdings:** 7417 book titles; 11,065 bound periodical volumes; 8 VF drawers of archival material. **Subscriptions:** 500 journals and other serials.

★8288★ JACKSON LABORATORY
JOAN STAATS LIBRARY
600 Main St.
Bar Harbor, ME 04609   Phone: (207) 288-3371
Douglas T. Macbeth, Libn.
Subjects: Inbred strains of mice, genetics, cancer, growth, animal health and husbandry, immunology, aging, cell biology, molecular genetics. **Holdings:** 3000 books; 20,000 bound periodical volumes; 46,000 reprints. **Subscriptions:** 350 journals and other serials.

★8289★ BATH MEMORIAL HOSPITAL
HEALTH SCIENCE LIBRARY
1356 Washington St. at Davenport Circle
Bath, ME 04530   Phone: (207) 443-5524
Joan M. Barnes, Libn.
Subjects: Medicine, allied health sciences. **Holdings:** 260 books. **Subscriptions:** 75 journals and other serials.

★8290★ WALDO COUNTY GENERAL HOSPITAL
MARX LIBRARY
Box 287
Belfast, ME 04915   Phone: (207) 338-2500
Lois Dutch, Educ.Asst./Libn.
Subjects: Medicine. **Holdings:** 152 books. **Subscriptions:** 44 journals and other serials.

★8291★ SOUTHERN MAINE MEDICAL CENTER
HEALTH SCIENCES LIBRARY
1 Medical Center Dr.
Box 626
Biddeford, ME 04005   Phone: (207) 283-7000
Patricia Goodwin, Libn.
Subjects: Medicine and allied health sciences. **Holdings:** 500 books; 30 bound periodical volumes. **Subscriptions:** 90 journals and other serials.

★8292★ ST. ANDREWS HOSPITAL
MEDICAL LIBRARY
3 St. Andrews Ln.
Boothbay Harbor, ME 04538   Phone: (207) 633-2121
Margaret Pinkham, R.N., Educ.Dir.
Subjects: Medicine, surgery, orthopedics, obstetrics/gynecology, pediatrics, urology, ophthalmology. **Holdings:** 100 books.

★8293★ NORTHERN CUMBERLAND MEMORIAL HOSPITAL
FREDERICK W. SKILLIN HEALTH SCIENCES LIBRARY
Box 230
Bridgton, ME 04009   Phone: (207) 647-8841
Sally M. MacAuslan, Hea.Sci.Libn.
Subjects: Medicine, nursing, hospital administration, patient education, health sciences. **Holdings:** 280 books; 140 videotapes; 8 films; 8 slide/tape sets; 18 audio cassettes. **Subscriptions:** 52 journals and other serials.

★8294★ REGIONAL MEMORIAL HOSPITAL
HEALTH SCIENCES LIBRARY
58 Baribeau Dr.
Brunswick, ME 04011   Phone: (207) 729-0181
Joan M. Barnes, Libn.
Subjects: Internal medicine, orthopedics, surgery, pediatrics, psychiatry, nursing. **Holdings:** 800 books; 2000 bound periodical volumes; 100 audio cassettes; 50 videotapes. **Subscriptions:** 146 journals and other serials.

★8295★ CALAIS REGIONAL HOSPITAL
HEALTH SCIENCE LIBRARY
50 Franklin St.
Calais, ME 04619   Phone: (207) 454-7521
Janet Barnes, Ck.
Subjects: Internal medicine, pediatrics, surgery, gynecology, nursing, anesthesia. **Holdings:** 1000 books. **Subscriptions:** 43 journals and other serials.

★8296★ CARY MEDICAL CENTER
HEALTH SCIENCE LIBRARY
Van Buren Rd.
MRA Box 37
Caribou, ME 04736   Phone: (207) 498-3111
Donna E. Cote-Thibodeau, Libn.
Subjects: Medicine. **Holdings:** 700 volumes. **Subscriptions:** 90 journals and other serials.

★8297★ FRANKLIN MEMORIAL HOSPITAL
TURNER MEMORIAL LIBRARY
1 Hospital Dr.
Farmington, ME 04938   Phone: (207) 778-6031
Betty Gensel, Lib.Mgr.
Subjects: Medicine. **Holdings:** 450 books. **Subscriptions:** 45 journals and other serials.

★8298★ HOULTON REGIONAL HOSPITAL
LIBRARY
20 Hartford St.
Houlton, ME 04730   Phone: (207) 532-9471
Sue Blake, Dir., Med.Rec.
Subjects: Medicine, nursing. **Holdings:** 150 books. **Subscriptions:** 40 journals and other serials.

★8299★ CENTRAL MAINE MEDICAL CENTER
HEALTH SCIENCE LIBRARY
300 Main St.
Box 4500
Lewiston, ME 04240-0309   Phone: (207) 795-2560
Maryanne Greven, Lib.Dir.
Subjects: Biomedicine, health care administration. **Holdings:** 1500 books; 3300 bound periodical volumes. **Subscriptions:** 425 journals and other serials; 8 newspapers.

★8300★ ST. MARY'S HOSPITAL
HEALTH SCIENCES LIBRARY
PO Box 291
Lewiston, ME 04243-0291   Phone: (207) 786-2901
Debra G. Warner, Dir.
Subjects: Medicine, nursing, hospital administration. **Holdings:** 970 books; 510 bound periodical volumes. **Subscriptions:** 145 journals and other serials.

★8301★ LEARNING INCORPORATED
LIBRARY
Learning Place
Manset-Seawall, ME 04656   Phone: (207) 244-5015
A.L. Welles, Dir.
Subjects: Learning handicaps, teaching spelling and reading, teaching those with learning disabilities and dyslexia. **Holdings:** 15,000 volumes.

★8302★ GOVERNOR BAXTER SCHOOL FOR THE DEAF
LIBRARY
Box 799
Portland, ME 04104-0799   Phone: (207) 781-3165
Robin Chibroski, Dir., Lib./Media Serv.
Subjects: Deafness, sign language, special education, professional education. **Holdings:** 7000 books; 100 bound periodical volumes; 300 unbound reports; 500 nonprint materials; American Annals of the Deaf, 1878-1984 (incomplete); 1100 Captioned Films for the Deaf (depository library). **Subscriptions:** 74 journals and other serials; 6 newspapers.

★8303★ MAINE MEDICAL CENTER
LIBRARY
22 Bramhall St.
Portland, ME 04102   Phone: (207) 871-2201
Robin M. Rand, Dir., Lib.Serv.
Subjects: Medicine, public health, nursing, medical education, hospital

administration. **Holdings:** 6376 books; 14,563 bound periodical volumes; 1348 AV titles. **Subscriptions:** 658 journals and other serials.

★8304★ MERCY HOSPITAL
HEALTH SCIENCES LIBRARY
144 State St.
Portland, ME 04101   Phone: (207) 879-3365
Marj Anderson, Lib./Mgr.Lib.Serv.
Subjects: Medicine, surgery, nursing. **Holdings:** 1700 books. **Subscriptions:** 100 journals and other serials.

★8305★ PINELAND CENTER
LIBRARY
Box E
Pownal, ME 04069-0902   Phone: (207) 688-4811
Margaret Greenlaw, SDS III, Staff Dev.
Subjects: Developmental disabilities, mental retardation, epilepsy, autism, cerebral palsy, medicine. **Holdings:** 1200 books; 80 videotapes. **Subscriptions:** 40 journals and other serials.

★8306★ AROOSTOOK MEDICAL CENTER
A.R. GOULD DIVISION
HEALTH SCIENCES LIBRARY
PO Box 151
Presque Isle, ME 04769-0151   Phone: (207) 768-4173
Marilyn W. Dean, Lib.Supv.
Subjects: Medicine, surgery, nursing. **Holdings:** 300 books; 94 periodicals.

★8307★ MID-COAST MENTAL HEALTH CENTER
VINCENT LATHBURY LIBRARY
12 Union St.
Box 526
Rockland, ME 04841   Phone: (207) 594-2541
Elisabeth Slagle, Libn.
Subjects: Psychology, counseling, psychiatric treatment. **Holdings:** Figures not available. **Subscriptions:** 10 journals and other serials.

★8308★ FOUNDATION FOR BLOOD RESEARCH
LIBRARY
Box 190
Scarborough, ME 04074   Phone: (207) 883-4131
Dawn E. Adams, Libn.
Subjects: Immunology, genetics, pediatrics, rheumatology, prenatal diagnosis. **Holdings:** 550 books; 1030 bound periodical volumes. **Subscriptions:** 64 journals and other serials.

★8309★ U.S. DEPARTMENT OF VETERANS AFFAIRS
MEDICAL AND REGIONAL OFFICE CENTER
LEARNING RESOURCES SERVICES
Togus, ME 04330   Phone: (207) 623-5743
Melda W. Page, Chf.Libn.
Subjects: Social sciences/psychiatry, medicine, alcoholism, nursing, dentistry, hospital administration. **Holdings:** 4000 books; 3800 bound periodical volumes; 2000 AV programs; 400 serial titles in microform; 3100 other cataloged items. **Subscriptions:** 570 journals and other serials; 50 newspapers.

★8310★ MID-MAINE MEDICAL CENTER
CLARA HODGKINS MEMORIAL HEALTH SCIENCES LIBRARY
North St.
Waterville, ME 04901   Phone: (207) 872-1224
Cora M. Damon, Libn.
Subjects: Medicine, allied health sciences. **Holdings:** 1000 books; 1000 bound periodical volumes. **Subscriptions:** 200 journals and other serials.

★8311★ WATERVILLE OSTEOPATHIC HOSPITAL
M.J. GERRIE, SR. MEDICAL LIBRARY
Kennedy Memorial Dr.
Waterville, ME 04901   Phone: (207) 873-0731
Subjects: Medicine, surgery, osteopathy. **Holdings:** 150 books. **Subscriptions:** 40 journals and other serials.

★8312★ YORK HOSPITAL
HEALTH SCIENCES LIBRARY
15 Hospital Dr.
York, ME 03909   Phone: (207) 363-4321
Darryl Hamson, Libn.
Subjects: Medicine, nursing, hospital administration. **Holdings:** 320 books; 480 bound periodical volumes. **Subscriptions:** 90 journals and other serials.

Maryland

★8313★ U.S. ARMY
HEALTH SERVICES COMMAND
ENVIRONMENTAL HYGIENE AGENCY
LIBRARY
Bldg. E1570
Aberdeen Proving Ground, MD 21010   Phone: (301) 671-4236
Krishan S. Goel, Libn.
Subjects: Occupational medicine, safety and health; chemistry and toxicology; audiology; medical entomology; laser, microwave, and radiological safety and health; air and water pollution; sanitary engineering. **Holdings:** 12,000 books; 8,000 bound periodical volumes; 8400 R&D reports; 3000 microfiche. **Subscriptions:** 400 journals and other serials.

★8314★ U.S. ARMY
MEDICAL RESEARCH & DEVELOPMENT COMMAND
MEDICAL RESEARCH INSTITUTE OF CHEMICAL DEFENSE
WOOD TECHNICAL LIBRARY
Bldg. E3100
Aberdeen Proving Ground, MD 21010-5425   Phone: (301) 671-4135
Diane Sherry, Supv.Libn.
Subjects: Pharmacology, biomedicine, psychology, biochemistry, medicine, toxicology. **Holdings:** 4000 books; 4416 bound periodical volumes; 10,956 reels of microfilm. **Subscriptions:** 832 journals and other serials.

★8315★ ANNE ARUNDEL MEDICAL CENTER
MEMORIAL LIBRARY
Franklin & Cathedral Sts.
Annapolis, MD 21401   Phone: (301) 267-1562
Joyce Richmond, Libn.
Subjects: Medicine, nursing. **Holdings:** 1200 books; 600 bound periodical volumes; 80 AV programs. **Subscriptions:** 248 journals and other serials.

★8316★ AMERICAN COUNCIL ON ALCOHOLISM
WALKER LIBRARY
5024 Campbell Blvd., No. H
Baltimore, MD 21236-5974   Phone: (301) 931-9393
Laura Krouse, Membership Mgr.
Subjects: Alcoholism. **Holdings:** 1,500 books; 200 bound periodical volumes. **Subscriptions:** 20 journals and other serials; 5 newspapers.

★8317★ BON SECOURS HOSPITAL
HEALTH SCIENCE LIBRARY
2000 W. Baltimore St.
Baltimore, MD 21223   Phone: (301) 362-3000
Sheila Oliveira, R.N.
Subjects: Medicine, surgery, obstetrics and gynecology, cardiovascular diseases, pathology, nursing. **Holdings:** 1908 books; 1876 bound periodical volumes; 2985 Audio-Digest tapes. **Subscriptions:** 81 journals and other serials; 7 newspapers.

★8318★ CARNEGIE INSTITUTION OF WASHINGTON
DEPARTMENT OF EMBRYOLOGY
LIBRARY
115 W. University Pkwy.
Baltimore, MD 21210   Phone: (301) 467-1414
John Watt, Libn.
Subjects: Embryology, biochemistry. **Holdings:** 1275 books; 1800 bound periodical volumes; 775 periodicals. **Subscriptions:** 55 journals and other serials.

★8319★ CHILDREN'S HOSPITAL
MEDICAL LIBRARY
3825 Greenspring Ave.
Baltimore, MD 21211   Phone: (301) 462-6800
Rita Billstone, Volunteer Libn.
Subjects: Orthopedics, plastic surgery, pediatrics, medicine. **Holdings:** 745

books; 260 bound periodical volumes. **Subscriptions:** 7 journals and other serials.

★8320★ FRANCIS SCOTT KEY MEDICAL CENTER
HAROLD E. HARRISON LIBRARY
4940 Eastern Ave.
Baltimore, MD 21224   Phone: (301) 955-0678
Rebecca A. Charton, Libn.
Subjects: Medicine. **Holdings:** 3503 books; 16,750 bound periodical volumes. **Subscriptions:** 364 journals and other serials.

★8321★ GREATER BALTIMORE MEDICAL CENTER
JOHN E. SAVAGE MEDICAL LIBRARY
6701 N. Charles St.
Baltimore, MD 21204   Phone: (301) 828-2530
Deborah Thomas, Lib. & AV Serv.Mgr.
Subjects: Medicine, nursing. **Holdings:** 1500 books; 12,000 bound periodical volumes; 200 AV programs. **Subscriptions:** 155 journals and other serials.

★8322★ HARBOR HOSPITAL CENTER
MEDICAL LIBRARY
3001 S. Hanover St.
Baltimore, MD 21230   Phone: (301) 347-3419
Shirley Lay, Libn.
Subjects: Internal medicine, nursing. **Holdings:** 1558 books; 3717 bound periodical volumes; 250 Network for Continuing Medical Education programs; 545 other AV programs. **Subscriptions:** 150 journals and other serials.

★8323★ HEALTH AND WELFARE COUNCIL, INC.
STAFF REFERENCE LIBRARY
22 Light St.
Baltimore, MD 21202-1075   Phone: (301) 752-4146
John G. Geist, Exec.Dir.
Subjects: Regional planning, personnel practices and agency management, census, employment and manpower, child welfare and day care, health, welfare, education, social service delivery systems, information and referral services. **Holdings:** 300 books; 500 other cataloged items; 42 loose-leaf binders of Health and Welfare Council Studies and Reports.

★8324★ JOHNS HOPKINS HOSPITAL
DEPARTMENT OF RADIOLOGY
LIBRARY
600 N. Wolfe St.
Baltimore, MD 21205   Phone: (301) 955-6029
Elaine Pinkney, Libn.
Subjects: Radiology, sonography, computed tomography, nuclear medicine, magnetic resonance imaging. **Holdings:** 1700 books; 5000 bound periodical volumes; 10,000 X-ray films. **Subscriptions:** 54 journals and other serials.

★8325★ JOHNS HOPKINS HOSPITAL
WILMER OPHTHALMOLOGICAL INSTITUTE
JONAS S. FRIEDENWALD LIBRARY
3/B 50 Woods Bldg.
601 N. Broadway
Baltimore, MD 21205   Phone: (301) 955-3127
Michael Piorunski, Dept.Libn.
Subjects: Ophthalmology. **Holdings:** 9500 books; 12,000 bound periodical volumes; 1000 AV programs. **Subscriptions:** 143 journals and other serials.

★8326★ JOHNS HOPKINS UNIVERSITY
POPULATION INFORMATION PROGRAM
527 St. Paul Pl.
Baltimore, MD 21202   Phone: (301) 659-6300
Dr. Phyllis T. Piotrow, Dir.
Subjects: Population, family planning, human fertility, contraception, allied health, law, and policy issues. **Holdings:** 1000 books; 110,000 documents. **Subscriptions:** 500 journals and other serials.

★8327★ JOHNS HOPKINS UNIVERSITY
SCHOOL OF HYGIENE AND PUBLIC HEALTH
ABRAHAM M. LILIENFELD MEMORIAL LIBRARY
624 N. Broadway, 9th Fl.
Baltimore, MD 21205-1901   Phone: (301) 955-3028
Edward S. Terry, Dir.
Subjects: Health policy and management, epidemiolgy, maternal and child

health, mental hygiene, international health, behavioral sciences, sociology, environmental health sciences, immunology, infectious diseases. **Holdings:** 30,000 volumes. **Subscriptions:** 250 journals and other serials.

★8328★ JOHNS HOPKINS UNIVERSITY
SCHOOL OF HYGIENE AND PUBLIC HEALTH
POPULATION DYNAMICS LIBRARY
615 N. Wolfe St.
Baltimore, MD 21205   Phone: (301) 955-3573
L. Terri Singer, Libn.
Subjects: Population dynamics, demography, family planning, physiology of reproduction, statistics. **Holdings:** 16,000 books; 700 bound periodical volumes; 175 theses; 675 National Center for Health Statistics pamphlets; 600 Population Association of America documents. **Subscriptions:** 157 journals and other serials.

★8329★ JOHNS HOPKINS UNIVERSITY
SCHOOL OF MEDICINE
DEPARTMENT OF PEDIATRICS
BAETJER MEMORIAL LIBRARY
CMSC 2-104 Johns Hopkins Hospital
Baltimore, MD 21205   Phone: (301) 955-3124
Sheila A. Kuhn, Libn.
Subjects: Pediatrics, general medicine. **Holdings:** 450 books; 2500 bound periodical volumes. **Subscriptions:** 53 journals and other serials.

★8330★ JOHNS HOPKINS UNIVERSITY
SCHOOL OF MEDICINE
JOSEPH L. LILIENTHAL LIBRARY
400 Halsted
600 N. Wolfe St.
Baltimore, MD 21205   Phone: (301) 955-7911
L. Robin Armstrong, Libn.
Subjects: Internal medicine. **Holdings:** 1000 books; 3000 bound periodical volumes; slide/tape Postgraduate Course in Internal Medicine. **Subscriptions:** 45 journals and other serials.

★8331★ JOHNS HOPKINS UNIVERSITY
WILLIAM H. WELCH MEDICAL LIBRARY
1900 E. Monument St.
Baltimore, MD 21205   Phone: (301) 955-3411
Nina W. Matheson, Dir./Libn.
Subjects: Medicine, clinical medicine, history of medicine, life sciences, nursing, public health, psychiatry, neurology, neurosurgery. **Holdings:** 354,773 volumes; 3966 AV programs. **Subscriptions:** 2947 journals and other serials.

★8332★ THE KENNEDY INSTITUTE
LIBRARY/MEDIA CENTER
707 N. Broadway, Rm. 512
Baltimore, MD 21205   Phone: (301) 550-9447
Bettea J. Hoofnagle, Hd., Info.Serv.
Subjects: Mental retardation, birth defects, cerebral palsy, epilepsy, developmental disabilities, special education, audiology, child psychology. **Holdings:** 3000 books; 1726 bound periodical volumes; 15 VF drawers; 300 videotapes; 370 audio cassettes; 15 teaching packages. **Subscriptions:** 102 journals and other serials.

★8333★ LIBERTY MEDICAL CENTER
REIGNER MEDICAL LIBRARY
2600 Liberty Heights Ave.
Baltimore, MD 21215   Phone: (301) 383-4351
Ellen Lindenbaum, Dir., Lib.Serv.
Subjects: Internal medicine, surgery, gynecology, podiatry, hospital administration. **Holdings:** 1500 books; 3800 bound periodical volumes. **Subscriptions:** 170 journals and other serials.

★8334★ MARYLAND COMMITTEE FOR CHILDREN
MCC RESOURCE CENTER
608 Water St.
Baltimore, MD 21202   Phone: (301) 752-7588
Sandra Skolnik, Exec.Dir.
Subjects: Day care, early childhood growth and development, child advocacy. **Holdings:** 1450 books; 115 file boxes. **Subscriptions:** 38 journals and other serials.

★8335★ MARYLAND DEPARTMENT OF HEALTH AND MENTAL HYGIENE
MEDIA SERVICES
300 W. Preston St.
Baltimore, MD 21201   Phone: (301) 225-5668
Julia Davidson-Randall, Chf.
Subjects: Public health policy and regulation, health, mental health, mental retardation, addictions, allied health sciences. **Holdings:** 16mm films; audio cassettes; videotapes.

★8336★ MARYLAND DEPARTMENT OF LICENSING AND REGULATION
OCCUPATIONAL SAFETY AND HEALTH LIBRARY
501 St. Paul Pl., 11th Fl.
Baltimore, MD 21202-2272   Phone: (301) 333-4164
David Murray, Lib.Hd.
Subjects: General reference, industrial hygiene, construction and industrial processes, occupational medicine and diseases, safety hazards, hazardous occupations, environmental pollution, toxicology. **Holdings:** 600 books; 30 bound periodical volumes; 30 other cataloged items. **Subscriptions:** 30.

★8337★ MARYLAND GENERAL HOSPITAL
MEDICAL STAFF LIBRARY
827 Linden Ave.
Baltimore, MD 21201   Phone: (301) 225-8383
Monica Yang, Coord., Lib.Serv.
Subjects: Medicine, nursing. **Holdings:** 1500 books; 800 bound periodical volumes; 5 Audio-Digest subscriptions; 500 tapes; 3000 slides; slide/tape sets; video-discs; video cassettes. **Subscriptions:** 100 journals and other serials.

★8338★ MARYLAND PHARMACISTS ASSOCIATION
LIBRARY
Kelly Memorial Bldg.
650 W. Lombard St.
Baltimore, MD 21201   Phone: (301) 727-0746
David Miller, Exec.Dir.
Subjects: Pharmacy, allied health sciences. **Holdings:** 1000 volumes.

★8339★ MARYLAND REHABILITATION CENTER
R.C. THOMPSON LIBRARY
2301 Argonne Dr.
Baltimore, MD 21218   Phone: (301) 554-3125
Jack Prial, Libn.
Subjects: Disability; vocational and physical rehabilitation; independent living; job placement of the disabled; physical, legal, and social barriers; substance abuse. **Holdings:** 2500 books; 8500 other cataloged items; 60 16mm films; 320 video cassettes. **Subscriptions:** 145 journals and other serials; 8 newspapers.

★8340★ MARYLAND STATE MEDICAL SOCIETY
MEDICAL AND CHIRURGICAL FACULTY
MUSIC MEDICINE CLEARINGHOUSE
1211 Cathedral St.
Baltimore, MD 21201   Phone: (301) 539-0872
Susan E. Harman, Clghse.Coord.
Subjects: Medical problems of performing musicians; music-making - physiology, anatomy. **Holdings:** 20 books; 600 journal article reprints (past 100 years, from medical, musical, and popular press); 5 AV programs; conference transcripts; arts medicine clinics brochures; arts medicine organizations information; subtopic bibliographies; other ephemeral material. **Subscriptions:** 3 journals and other serials.

★8341★ MEDICAL AND CHIRURGICAL FACULTY OF THE STATE OF MARYLAND
LIBRARY
1211 Cathedral St.
Baltimore, MD 21201   Phone: (301) 539-0872
Adam Szczepaniak, Lib.Dir.
Subjects: Medicine, allied health sciences, medical history. **Holdings:** 120,000 volumes; 750 manuscripts. **Subscriptions:** 600 journals and other serials.

★8342★ MERCY MEDICAL CENTER
McGLANNAN MEMORIAL LIBRARY
301 St. Paul Pl.
Baltimore, MD 21202   Phone: (301) 332-9189
Dolores H. Kaisler, Libn.
Subjects: Medicine, nursing, and allied health sciences. **Holdings:** 9818 books; 9464 bound periodical volumes; 12 VF drawers of pamphlets and reprints. **Subscriptions:** 276 journals and other serials.

★8343★ NATIONAL INSTITUTE ON AGING
GERONTOLOGY RESEARCH CENTER LIBRARY
4940 Eastern Ave.
Baltimore, MD 21224-2137   Phone: (301) 550-1730
Joanna Chen Lin, Hd., Lib. Unit
Subjects: Aging research, gerontology and geriatrics, psychology, biochemistry, biomedical research, genetics. **Holdings:** 9000 books; 10,000 bound periodical volumes; 500 unbound reports and statistics. **Subscriptions:** 500 journals and other serials.

★8344★ NATIONAL INSTITUTE ON DRUG ABUSE
ADDICTION RESEARCH CENTER LIBRARY
Box 5180
Baltimore, MD 21224   Phone: (301) 550-1488
Mary Pfeiffer, Libn.
Subjects: Pharmacology, psychology, psychiatry, biochemistry, neurochemistry, psychopathology, chemistry. **Holdings:** 7000 books; 2500 bound periodical volumes; 21,000 reprint articles. **Subscriptions:** 450 journals and other serials.

★8345★ ST. AGNES HOSPITAL
L.P. GUNDRY HEALTH SCIENCES LIBRARY
900 S. Caton Ave.
Baltimore, MD 21229   Phone: (301) 368-3123
Joanne Sullivan, Dir.
Subjects: Medicine, surgery, pediatrics, obstetrics, gynecology, pathology, nursing, psychiatry, management, health care careers. **Holdings:** 2500 books; 6000 bound periodical volumes. **Subscriptions:** 275 journals and other serials.

★8346★ SINAI HOSPITAL OF BALTIMORE
EISENBERG MEDICAL STAFF LIBRARY
Belvedere & Greenspring
Baltimore, MD 21215   Phone: (301) 578-5015
Rita Matcher, Dir., Lib.Serv.
Subjects: Medicine, nursing, Jewish medicine, management, thanatology. **Holdings:** 4300 books; 12,000 bound periodical volumes. **Subscriptions:** 275 journals and other serials.

★8347★ UNION MEMORIAL HOSPITAL
LIBRARY AND INFORMATION RESOURCES
201 E. University Pkwy.
Baltimore, MD 21218-2895   Phone: (301) 554-2294
Beverly Gresehover, Mgr.
Subjects: Medicine, orthopedics, nursing. **Holdings:** 5000 books; 6600 bound periodical volumes; 1656 AV programs. **Subscriptions:** 390 journals and other serials.

★8348★ UNION MEMORIAL HOSPITAL
NURSING LIBRARY
201 University Pkwy.
Baltimore, MD 21218   Phone: (301) 554-2296
Beverly Gresehover, Lib.Mgr.
Subjects: Nursing, medicine, sociology, psychology, life sciences. **Holdings:** 3000 books; 807 bound periodical volumes; 4 VF drawers of articles; 35 file boxes; 20 tapes; 50 cassettes. **Subscriptions:** 120 journals and other serials.

★8349★ U.S. DEPARTMENT OF VETERANS AFFAIRS
MEDICAL CENTER LIBRARY SERVICE
3900 Loch Raven Blvd.
Baltimore, MD 21218   Phone: (301) 467-9932
Deborah A. Stout, Chf., Lib.Serv.
Subjects: Medicine, surgery, nursing. **Holdings:** 2000 books; 4000 bound periodical volumes; 200 AV programs; staff and VA publications; pamphlets. **Subscriptions:** 300 journals and other serials.

★8350★ U.S. DEPARTMENT OF VETERANS AFFAIRS
OFFICE OF TECHNOLOGY TRANSFER
RESOURCE CENTER
VA Prosthetics Research & Development Center
103 S. Gay St.
Baltimore, MD 21202   Phone: (301) 962-1800
Helen Nowotarski, Med.Libn.
Subjects: Prosthetics, sensory aids, orthotics, spinal cord injury, rehabilitation, bioengineering. **Holdings:** 3600 books; 2500 technical and contractor reports. **Subscriptions:** 150 journals and other serials.

★8351★ U.S. SOCIAL SECURITY ADMINISTRATION
INFORMATION RESOURCES BRANCH
LIBRARY SERVICES SECTION
Altmeyer Bldg., Rm. 570
PO Box 17330
Baltimore, MD 21235   Phone: (301) 965-6107
M. Joyce Donohue
Subjects: Social insurance, medical and hospital economics, operations research, management, personnel administration, supervision and training, electronic data processing, law, health insurance, business and management. **Holdings:** 83,280 books; 1250 bound periodical volumes; 600,000 microfiche; 4700 ultrafiche. **Subscriptions:** 1447 journals and other serials.

★8352★ UNIVERSITY OF MARYLAND, BALTIMORE
HEALTH SCIENCES LIBRARY
111 S. Greene St.
Baltimore, MD 21201   Phone: (301) 328-7545
Diana Cunningham, Act.Dir.
Subjects: Medicine, dentistry, pharmacy, nursing, social work. **Holdings:** 146,739 books; 149,893 bound periodical volumes; University of Maryland archives. **Subscriptions:** 2913 journals and other serials.

★8353★ U.S.D.A.
NATIONAL AGRICULTURAL LIBRARY
FOOD AND NUTRITION INFORMATION CENTER
10301 Baltimore Blvd., Rm. 304
Beltsville, MD 20705   Phone: (301) 344-3719
Sandra L. Facinoli, Coord.
Subjects: Human nutrition research and education, food service management and food technology. **Holdings:** 50,000 books; VF drawers. **Subscriptions:** 200 journals and other serials.

★8354★ AMERICAN COLLEGE OF CARDIOLOGY
GRIFFITH RESOURCE LIBRARY
9111 Old Georgetown Rd.
Bethesda, MD 20814   Phone: (301) 897-5400
Helene Goldstein, Dir.
Subjects: Cardiovascular disease and surgery. **Holdings:** 1500 books; 350 bound periodical volumes; 250 AV programs. **Subscriptions:** 160 journals and other serials.

★8355★ HOWARD HUGHES MEDICAL INSTITUTE
LIBRARY
6701 Rockledge Dr.
Bethesda, MD 20817   Phone: (301) 571-0217
Cathy Harbert, Libn.
Subjects: Investments; medical research - genetics, immunology, cellular biology, structural biology, neurosciences. **Holdings:** 300 books. **Subscriptions:** 250 journals and other serials; 8 newspapers.

★8356★ MONTGOMERY COUNTY DEPARTMENT OF PUBLIC
LIBRARIES
SPECIAL NEEDS LIBRARY
6400 Democracy Blvd.
Bethesda, MD 20817   Phone: (301) 493-2555
Devon Liner, Sr.Libn.
Subjects: Handicapping conditions. **Holdings:** 8000 talking books; 4241 large print volumes; toys; computer programs.

★8357★ NATIONAL ARTHRITIS AND MUSCULOSKELETAL
AND SKIN DISEASES INFORMATION CLEARINGHOUSE
9000 Rockville Pike
Box AMS
Bethesda, MD 20892   Phone: (301) 495-4484
Peggy McCauley, Info.Spec.
Subjects: Arthritis; rheumatic, skin, and musculoskeletal diseases; sports

medicine. **Holdings:** 9000 database records. **Subscriptions:** 30 journals and other serials; 50 newspapers.

★8358★ NATIONAL DIGESTIVE DISEASES INFORMATION
CLEARINGHOUSE
Box NDDIC
Bethesda, MD 20892   Phone: (301) 468-6344
Subjects: Digestive diseases. **Holdings:** 100 books; 500 patient education booklets and pamphlets. **Subscriptions:** 15 journals and other serials.

★8359★ NATIONAL HEART, LUNG, AND BLOOD INSTITUTE
EDUCATION PROGRAMS' INFORMATION CENTER
University Research Corp.
4733 Bethesda Ave., Ste. 530
Bethesda, MD 20814   Phone: (301) 951-3260
Jory Barone, Ctr.Mgr.
Subjects: High blood pressure, cholesterol, smoking, health education, cardiovascular risk reduction, blood resources, asthma. **Holdings:** 2050 books; 235 periodicals; 8000 periodical articles; 1000 pamphlets; 2000 documents. **Subscriptions:** 190 journals and other serials.

★8360★ NATIONAL INSTITUTE OF ARTHRITIS AND
MUSCULOSKELETAL AND SKIN DISEASES
OFFICE OF SCIENTIFIC AND HEALTH COMMUNICATION
Bldg. 31, Rm. 4C05
NIH/NIAMS
9000 Rockville Pike
Bethesda, MD 20892   Phone: (301) 496-8188
Constance Raab, Dir.
Subjects: Clinical and laboratory research dealing with the various arthritic, rheumatic, and collagen diseases, the metabolic diseases including diabetes, digestive diseases, orthopedics, dermatology, hematology, nutrition, endocrine disorders, urology, and renal disease including research and development of the artificial kidney. Basic research includes biochemistry, nutrition, pathology, histochemistry, chemistry, pharmacology, toxicology, and physical, chemical, and molecular biology. **Holdings:** Figures not available.

★8361★ NATIONAL INSTITUTE OF DENTAL RESEARCH
RESEARCH DATA AND MANAGEMENT INFORMATION
5333 Westbard Ave.
Bethesda, MD 20016   Phone: (301) 496-7220
Carla Flora, Chf.
Subjects: Dental research. **Holdings:** 10,000 project summaries; 1500 technical reports on microfiche.

★8362★ U.S. ARMED FORCES RADIOBIOLOGY RESEARCH
INSTITUTE
LIBRARY SERVICES
National Naval Medical Ctr., Bldg. 42
Bethesda, MD 20814   Phone: (301) 295-1330
Ilse Vada, Adm.Libn.
Subjects: Radiobiology, radiation physics, neurobiology, nuclear medicine, behavioral science, veterinary medicine. **Holdings:** 10,000 books; 20,000 bound periodical volumes; 6000 technical reports; Atomic Bomb Casualty Commission technical reports; 50,000 microfiche of U.S. Government-funded technical reports. **Subscriptions:** 200 journals and other serials; 6 newspapers.

★8363★ U.S. NATIONAL INSTITUTES OF HEALTH
LIBRARY
9000 Rockville Pike
Bldg. 10, Rm. 1L-25
Bethesda, MD 20892   Phone: (301) 496-2447
Carolyn P. Brown, Chf.Libn.
Subjects: Medicine, health sciences, chemistry, pathology, physiology, biology. **Holdings:** 85,000 books; 152,000 bound periodical volumes; 17,000 microforms. **Subscriptions:** 6000 journals and other serials.

★8364★ U.S. NATIONAL LIBRARY OF MEDICINE
8600 Rockville Pike
Bethesda, MD 20894   Phone: (301) 496-6308
Donald A.B. Lindberg, M.D., Dir.
Subjects: Medicine, health sciences, dentistry, public health, nursing, biomedical research. **Holdings:** 650,000 books; 892,000 bound periodical volumes; 2.2 million manuscripts; 78,000 pictures; 272,000 microforms; 282,000 theses; 172,000 pamphlets; 49,000 AV programs; microfilm. **Subscriptions:** 21,800 journals and other serials.

★8365★   U.S. NAVY
NATIONAL NAVAL MEDICAL CENTER
EDWARD RHODES STITT LIBRARY
Bethesda, MD 20889-5000   Phone: (202) 295-1184
Jerry Meyer, Lib.Dir.
Subjects: Medicine and allied health sciences. **Holdings:** 70,000 volumes; 2000 audiotapes. **Subscriptions:** 890 journals.

★8366★   U.S. NAVY
NATIONAL NAVAL MEDICAL COMMAND
NAVAL DENTAL SCHOOL
NATIONAL NAVAL DENTAL CLINIC
WILLIAM L. DARNALL LIBRARY
Bethesda, MD 20889-5077   Phone: (202) 295-0080
Patricia A. Evans, Chf., Lrng.Rsrc.Div.
Subjects: Dentistry, medicine. **Holdings:** 8500 books. **Subscriptions:** 85 journals and other serials.

★8367★   U.S. NAVY
NAVAL MEDICAL RESEARCH INSTITUTE
INFORMATION SERVICES DIVISION
Bethesda, MD 20814-5055   Phone: (202) 295-2186
Phyllis R. Blum, Adm.Libn.
Subjects: Infectious diseases, casualty care, hyperbaric medicine, experimental surgery, transplantation, military medicine. **Holdings:** 5000 books. **Subscriptions:** 250 journals and other serials.

★8368★   U.S. UNIFORMED SERVICES UNIVERSITY OF THE
**   HEALTH SCIENCES**
LEARNING RESOURCE CENTER
4301 Jones Bridge Rd.
Bethesda, MD 20814-4799   Phone: (301) 295-3350
Chester J. Pletzke, Assoc.Prof. & Dir.
Subjects: Medicine, military medicine. **Holdings:** 114,450 books and journals. **Subscriptions:** 1640 journals and other serials.

★8369★   UNIVERSITY RESEARCH CORPORATION
LIBRARY
7200 Wisconsin Ave., Ste. 600
Bethesda, MD 20814   Phone: (301) 654-8338
Subjects: International health, health education, criminal justice, housing rehabilitation, management and evaluation. **Holdings:** 1000 books; 3500 other cataloged items; 30 VF drawers. **Subscriptions:** 25 journals and other serials; 20 newspapers.

★8370★   EASTERN SHORE HOSPITAL CENTER
PROFESSIONAL LIBRARY
Box 800
Cambridge, MD 21613   Phone: (301) 228-0800
Estella C. Clendaniel, Supv., Lib. & Files
Subjects: Psychiatry, medicine, nursing. **Holdings:** 2638 books; 361 bound periodical volumes; 4 VF drawers of pamphlets. **Subscriptions:** 39 journals and other serials.

★8371★   NATIONAL ARCHIVES AND RECORDS
**   ADMINISTRATION**
NATIONAL AUDIOVISUAL CENTER
CUSTOMER SERVICES
8700 Edgeworth Dr.
Capitol Heights, MD 20743-3701   Phone: (301) 763-1896
George H. Ziener, Dir.
Subjects: Alcohol, drugs, business and government management, career education, environment, energy conservation, foreign language instruction, industrial safety, information science, nursing, science, special and vocational education, consumer education, engineering, dentistry, medicine, emergency medical services, fire/law enforcement, flight/meteorology, social sciences, space. **Holdings:** 10,000 titles of slide sets, audiotapes, filmstrips, multimedia kits, video cassettes, 16mm films. **Subscriptions:** 30 journals and other serials.

★8372★   SPRING GROVE HOSPITAL CENTER
SULZBACHER MEMORIAL LIBRARY
Isidore Tuerk Bldg.
Wade Ave.
Catonsville, MD 21228   Phone: (301) 455-7824
Subjects: Psychiatry, psychology, psychotherapy, pharmacology, sociology, social work, neurology, pastoral care, nursing education, therapy. **Holdings:** 2835 books; 1000 bound periodical volumes; 954 cassettes; 10 films;

15 phonograph records; 2045 pamphlets; 13 AV programs; 20 archives; 30 dissertations; 25 reels of microfilm. **Subscriptions:** 297 journals and other serials; 10 newspapers.

★8373★   UNIVERSITY OF MARYLAND
SCHOOL OF MEDICINE
DEPARTMENT OF PSYCHIATRY
HELEN C. TINGLEY MEMORIAL LIBRARY
Maryland Psychiatric Research Ctr.
Box 21247
Catonsville, MD 21228   Phone: (301) 455-7667
Nancy Flowers, Libn.
Subjects: Psychiatry, allied health sciences. **Holdings:** 400 volumes; 50 bound periodical volumes; 50 audio cassettes; 50 reference works. **Subscriptions:** 15 journals and other serials.

★8374★   PRINCE GEORGE'S COUNTY HEALTH
**   DEPARTMENT**
PUBLIC HEALTH RESOURCE CENTER
Cheverly, MD 20785   Phone: (301) 386-0264
Peggy H. Bullock, Mgr.
Subjects: Public health, health education, nursing, mental health, administration, geriatrics. **Holdings:** 1500 books; educational pamphlets. **Subscriptions:** 100 journals and other serials.

★8375★   PRINCE GEORGE'S HOSPITAL CENTER
SAUL SCHWARTZBACH MEMORIAL LIBRARY
Cheverly, MD 20785   Phone: (301) 618-2000
Eleanor Kleman, Med.Libn.
Subjects: Medicine. **Holdings:** 1000 books; 2500 bound periodical volumes; 2350 AV programs. **Subscriptions:** 180 journals and other serials.

★8376★   AMERICAN ACADEMY OF OPTOMETRY
LIBRARY
5530 Wisconsin Ave., NW, Ste. 1149
Chevy Chase, MD 20815   Phone: (301) 652-0905
David Lewis, Exec.Dir.
Subjects: Optometry, physiological optics, ocular pathology. **Holdings:** Optometry & Vision Science (formerly the American Journal of Optometry & Physiological Optics). **Subscriptions:** 12 journals and other serials.

★8377★   HOWARD COUNTY GENERAL HOSPITAL
HEALTH SCIENCES LIBRARY
5755 Cedar Ln.
Columbia, MD 21044   Phone: (301) 740-7860
Marian G. Czajkowski, Med.Libn.
Subjects: Medicine. **Holdings:** 632 books; 1021 bound periodical volumes. **Subscriptions:** 140 journals and other serials.

★8378★   CROWNSVILLE HOSPITAL CENTER
STAFF LIBRARY
Crownsville, MD 21032   Phone: (301) 987-6200
Susan S. Merrill, Libn.
Subjects: Psychiatry, psychology, behavior therapy, family therapy, nursing, social services. **Holdings:** 1200 books; 15 file boxes; 250 VF items; 33 audio- and videotapes; unbound periodicals. **Subscriptions:** 25 journals and other serials.

★8379★   MEMORIAL HOSPITAL AND MEDICAL CENTER
MEDICAL AND NURSING LIBRARY
600 Memorial Ave.
Cumberland, MD 21502   Phone: (301) 777-4027
Mary E. Courtney, Libn.
Subjects: Medicine, surgery, nursing. **Holdings:** 1146 books; 40 bound periodical volumes. **Subscriptions:** 60 journals and other serials.

★8380★   SACRED HEART HOSPITAL
SISTER MARTHA MALLOY MEMORIAL LIBRARY
900 Seton Dr.
Cumberland, MD 21502   Phone: (301) 759-5229
Betty Ramsey, Libn.
Subjects: Medicine, nursing, allied health sciences. **Holdings:** 2100 books; 50 bound periodical volumes. **Subscriptions:** 63 journals and other serials.

★8381★ MEMORIAL HOSPITAL
HEALTH SCIENCES LIBRARY
S. Washington St.
Easton, MD 21601   Phone: (301) 822-1000
Lois Sanger, Libn.
Subjects: Medicine, nursing, allied health sciences. **Holdings:** 5000 books; 1900 bound periodical volumes; microfilm; AV programs. **Subscriptions:** 250 journals and other serials.

★8382★ FEDERAL EMERGENCY MANAGEMENT AGENCY
NATIONAL EMERGENCY TRAINING CENTER
LEARNING RESOURCE CENTER
16825 S. Seton Ave.
Emmitsburg, MD 21727   Phone: (301) 447-1032
Adele M. Chiesa, Chf.
Subjects: Emergency management, fire science, civil defense, natural hazards, hazardous materials, arson, disasters, emergency medical services. **Holdings:** 20,000 books; 1500 bound periodical volumes; 14,000 research reports; 3000 AV programs; 3500 titles in microform; 55 VF drawers. **Subscriptions:** 400 journals and other serials; 9 newspapers.

★8383★ U.S. DEPARTMENT OF VETERANS AFFAIRS
HOSPITAL LIBRARY
9600 N. Point Rd.
Fort Howard, MD 21052-3035   Phone: (301) 687-8729
Joanne M. Bennett, Chf.Libn.
Subjects: Medicine. **Holdings:** 1800 books; 2262 bound periodical volumes. **Subscriptions:** 160 journals and other serials.

★8384★ FREDERICK MEMORIAL HOSPITAL
WALTER F. PRIOR MEDICAL LIBRARY
Park Place & W. 7th St.
Frederick, MD 21701   Phone: (301) 698-3459
Linda A. Collenberg Bisaccia, Med.Libn.
Subjects: Clinical medicine. **Holdings:** 1500 volumes. **Subscriptions:** 75 journals and other serials.

★8385★ U.S. ARMY
MEDICAL RESEARCH AND DEVELOPMENT COMMAND
BIOMEDICAL RESEARCH AND DEVELOPMENT LABORATORY
TECHNICAL LIBRARY
Fort Detrick, Bldg. 568
Frederick, MD 21702-5010   Phone: (301) 663-2502
Al Reynolds, Libn.
Subjects: Biomedical engineering; pest management systems; entomology; environmental protection: air, land, and water pollution; solid waste and pesticide disposal; aquatic toxicology; occupational health. **Holdings:** 5500 books; 1500 bound periodical volumes; 6100 technical reprints, patents, reports; 1000 photographs; 2200 slides. **Subscriptions:** 220 journals and other serials.

★8386★ U.S. ARMY
MEDICAL RESEARCH AND DEVELOPMENT COMMAND
MEDICAL RESEARCH INSTITUTE OF INFECTIOUS DISEASES
MEDICAL LIBRARY
Fort Detrick
Frederick, MD 21702-5011   Phone: (301) 663-2717
Denise M. Lupp, Libn.
Subjects: Medicine, microbiology, biochemistry. **Holdings:** 7600 books; 6500 bound periodical volumes; 6 shelves of contract reports; 22 shelves of miscellaneous reports. **Subscriptions:** 250 journals and other serials.

★8387★ U.S. NATIONAL INSTITUTES OF HEALTH
NATIONAL CANCER INSTITUTE
FREDERICK CANCER RESEARCH AND DEVELOPMENT
   CENTER
SCIENTIFIC LIBRARY
Box B - Bldg. 549
Frederick, MD 21702-1013   Phone: (301) 846-1093
Susan W. Wilson, Dir.
Subjects: Cancer biology, biological and chemical carcinogenesis, acquired immunodeficiency syndrome, biomedical research. **Holdings:** 16,000 books; 24,000 bound periodical volumes; 2600 reels of microfilm of periodicals. **Subscriptions:** 718 journals and other serials.

★8388★ GILLETTE MEDICAL EVALUATION LABORATORIES
INFORMATION CENTER
401 Professional Dr.
Gaithersburg, MD 20879   Phone: (301) 590-1545
Colleen A. Pritchard, Info.Ctr.Supv.
Subjects: Toxicology, cosmetics, dermatology, organic and surface chemistry, biology. **Holdings:** 6500 books; 4200 bound periodical volumes; 1100 government documents; 13,000 reprints; 30 notebooks of OTC meeting minutes. **Subscriptions:** 312 journals and other serials.

★8389★ GEOMET TECHNOLOGIES INC.
INFORMATION CENTER
20251 Century Blvd.
Germantown, MD 20874   Phone: (301) 428-9898
Kris Hinkley, Libn.
Subjects: Toxicology, environmental health, industrial and occupational medicine, hazardous waste. **Holdings:** 400 books. **Subscriptions:** 30 journals and other serials; 5 newspapers.

★8390★ BROOK LANE PSYCHIATRIC CENTER
MEDICAL LIBRARY
Box 1945
Hagerstown, MD 21740   Phone: (301) 733-0330
Curtis E. Miller, Libn.
Subjects: Psychiatry, child psychiatry, social work, psychiatric nursing. **Holdings:** 700 books; 5 other cataloged items. **Subscriptions:** 48 journals and other serials.

★8391★ WASHINGTON COUNTY HOSPITAL
WROTH MEMORIAL LIBRARY
251 E. Antietam St.
Hagerstown, MD 21740   Phone: (301) 790-8801
Myra Binau, Coord., Lib.Serv.
Subjects: Medicine, nursing, and allied health sciences. **Holdings:** 5000 volumes; 8 VF drawers of pamphlets and clippings. **Subscriptions:** 178 journals and other serials.

★8392★ NATIONAL CENTER FOR HEALTH STATISTICS
CLEARINGHOUSE ON HEALTH INDEXES
6525 Belcrest Rd.
Hyattsville, MD 20782-2003   Phone: (301) 436-7035
Pennifer Erickson, Chf.
Subjects: Health statistics, quality of life assessment, cost of illness studies. **Holdings:** 3000 reprints and original manuscripts.

★8393★ NATIONAL EPILEPSY LIBRARY
4351 Garden City Dr., Ste. 406
Landover, MD 20785   Phone: (301) 459-3700
Bonnie Kessler, Dir.
Subjects: Social, psychological, medical aspects of epilepsy; neurology. **Holdings:** 1000 books; 60,000 microfiche; 200 reports. **Subscriptions:** 125 journals and other serials.

★8394★ ROSEWOOD CENTER
MIRIAM LODGE PROFESSIONAL LIBRARY
Owings Mills, MD 21117   Phone: (301) 363-0300
Thelma W. Newton, Supv., Lib. & Files
Subjects: Mental retardation, special education, social work, learning disorders, pediatrics, psychology. **Holdings:** 3000 books; 1000 bound periodical volumes; 6 VF drawers of pamphlets; 7 VF drawers of staff papers; 30 manuscripts. **Subscriptions:** 69 journals and other serials.

★8395★ U.S. DEPARTMENT OF VETERANS AFFAIRS
MEDICAL CENTER MEDICAL LIBRARY
Perry Point, MD 21902   Phone: (301) 642-2411
Barbara A. Schultz, Chf., Lib.Serv.
Subjects: Psychiatry, nursing, geriatrics. **Holdings:** 3800 books; 4000 bound periodical volumes; 660 cassettes; 12 VF drawers of clippings, pamphlets, reprints. **Subscriptions:** 200 journals and other serials.

★8396★ BALTIMORE COUNTY GENERAL HOSPITAL
HEALTH SCIENCES LIBRARY
5401 Old Court Rd.
Randallstown, MD 21133   Phone: (301) 521-2200
Betty Myers, Hea.Sci.Libn.
Subjects: Medicine, surgery, cardiology, orthopedics, management, nursing process. **Holdings:** 1475 books; college catalogs; Audio-Digest tapes (5

years of internal medicine and surgery, 5 years of opthalmology). **Subscriptions:** 72 journals and other serials.

**★8397★ AMERICAN OCCUPATIONAL THERAPY
FOUNDATION AND ASSOCIATION**
WILMA L. WEST LIBRARY
1383 Piccard Dr.
Box 1725
Rockville, MD 20850-4375   Phone: (301) 948-9626
Mary S. Binderman, Libn.
Subjects: Occupational therapy - physical, developmental, and psychosocial disabilities, human occupation, perceptual motor disabilities, child development, geriatrics, leisure time, work and rehabilitation. **Holdings:** 3500 books; 200 bound periodical volumes; 3 VF drawers of pamphlets. **Subscriptions:** 63 journals and other serials; 14 newsletters.

**★8398★ AMERICAN SPEECH-LANGUAGE-HEARING
ASSOCIATION**
ASHA LIBRARY
10801 Rockville Pike
Rockville, MD 20852   Phone: (301) 897-5700
Subjects: Speech, hearing, language, management, government affairs. **Holdings:** 1630 books; 60 bound periodical volumes; workshop and conference reports.

★8399★ AMERICAN TYPE CULTURE COLLECTION
DONOVICK LIBRARY
12301 Parklawn Dr.
Rockville, MD 20852   Phone: (301) 881-2600
Mary Jane Edwards, Sr.Ed.Info.Spec.
Subjects: Microbiology, bacteriology, protistology, virology, tissue culture, mycology, molecular biology, plasmids, biotechnology. **Holdings:** 3500 books; 2500 bound periodical volumes. **Subscriptions:** 200 journals and other serials.

**★8400★ NATIONAL CLEARINGHOUSE FOR ALCOHOL AND
DRUG INFORMATION**
LIBRARY
Box 2345
Rockville, MD 20852   Phone: (301) 468-2600
Lisa Swanberg, Dir., Lib. & Info.Serv.
Subjects: Alcohol and other drug abuse prevention. **Holdings:** 900 books; 19,000 cataloged items; 93,000 accessioned items. **Subscriptions:** 90 journals and other serials; 8 newspapers.

★8401★ U.S. CENTERS FOR DISEASE CONTROL
OFFICE ON SMOKING AND HEALTH
TECHNICAL INFORMATION CENTER
Park Bldg., Rm. 1-16
5600 Fishers Ln.
Rockville, MD 20857   Phone: (301) 443-1690
Susan Hawk, Tech.Info.Off.
Subjects: Smoking and health, tobacco, nicotine, behavioral aspects of smoking, cessation techniques. **Holdings:** 55,000 books, reprints, journal articles, and technical reports. **Subscriptions:** 40 journals and other serials.

★8402★ U.S. FOOD AND DRUG ADMINISTRATION
CENTER FOR DEVICES AND RADIOLOGICAL HEALTH
LIBRARY HFZ-46
1390 Piccard Dr.
Rockville, MD 20850   Phone: (301) 427-1235
Harriet Albersheim, Chf.Libn.
Subjects: Radiology, radiobiology, radiation, nuclear medicine, radiological health, radiation hazards, emission, microwaves, ultrasonics, lasers, medical devices, artificial organs, biomedical engineering, biomaterials. **Holdings:** 7000 books; periodical titles (bound and microfilm). **Subscriptions:** 700 journals and other serials.

★8403★ U.S. PUBLIC HEALTH SERVICE
PARKLAWN HEALTH LIBRARY
5600 Fishers Ln., Rm. 13-12
Rockville, MD 20857   Phone: (301) 443-2665
Bruce N. Yamasaki, Lib.Dir.
Subjects: Delivery of health services, drug abuse, health planning, health care statistics, health services research, mental health, social aspects of health care, emergency medical services. **Holdings:** 20,000 books; 2000 bound periodical volumes; 10,000 NTIS reports on microfiche. **Subscriptions:** 1100 journals and other serials.

★8404★ AUTISM SOCIETY OF AMERICA
INFORMATION AND REFERRAL SERVICE
8601 Georgia Ave., Ste. 503
Silver Spring, MD 20910
Subjects: Autism and allied subjects. **Holdings:** 200 books; 500 bound periodical volumes; 40 VF drawers of articles, lists, pamphlets, reports, bibliographies.

★8405★ HOLY CROSS HOSPITAL OF SILVER SPRING
MEDICAL LIBRARY
1500 Forest Glen Rd.
Silver Spring, MD 20910   Phone: (301) 565-1211
Bernetta Payne, Libn.
Subjects: Medicine, allied health sciences. **Holdings:** 1400 books; 525 bound periodical volumes; 500 Audio-Digest tapes. **Subscriptions:** 165 journals and other serials.

**★8406★ INTERNATIONAL HEALTH AND TEMPERANCE
ASSOCIATION**
LIBRARY
12501 Old Columbia Pike
Silver Spring, MD 20904   Phone: (301) 680-6719
Subjects: Social problems - alcohol, tobacco, narcotics; health and temperance - general, history. **Holdings:** 3200 volumes.

**★8407★ NATIONAL REHABILITATION INFORMATION
CENTER**
8455 Colesville Rd., Ste. 935
Silver Spring, MD 20910-3319   Phone: (301) 588-9284
Mark Odum, Dir.
Subjects: Rehabilitation of persons with mental or physical disabilities. **Holdings:** 30,000 listings. **Subscriptions:** 350 journals and other serials.

★8408★ RII-TRITON
LIBRARY
1010 Wayne Ave., Ste. 300
Silver Spring, MD 20910   Phone: (301) 565-4020
Richard Salvatierra, Chm.
Subjects: Health promotion, disease prevention. **Holdings:** 400 books; 1000 bound periodical volumes.

**★8409★ EA ENGINEERING, SCIENCE, AND TECHNOLOGY,
INC.**
LIBRARY
15 Loveton Circle
Sparks, MD 21152   Phone: (301) 771-4950
Kathleen E. Cohen, Mgr., Lib.Serv.
Subjects: Environmental science, health sciences, biology. **Holdings:** 15,000 books; 50 bound periodical volumes; 25,000 other cataloged items. **Subscriptions:** 65 journals and other serials; 5 newspapers.

★8410★ SPRINGFIELD HOSPITAL CENTER
MEDICAL LIBRARY
Sykesville, MD 21784   Phone: (301) 795-2100
Elizabeth D. Mercer, Libn.
Subjects: Psychiatry, neurology, clinical psychology, psychotherapy, psychiatric nursing, psychiatric social work, medicine, practical nursing. **Holdings:** 2000 books; 1000 bound periodical volumes. **Subscriptions:** 84 journals and other serials.

★8411★ WASHINGTON ADVENTIST HOSPITAL
HEALTH SCIENCES LIBRARY
7600 Carroll Ave.
Takoma Park, MD 20912   Phone: (301) 891-5261
Cathy Cumbo, Libn.
Subjects: Medicine, nursing, hospital administration. **Holdings:** 2700 volumes. **Subscriptions:** 260 journals and other serials; 5 newspapers.

★8412★ ST. JOSEPH HOSPITAL
OTTO C. BRANTIGAN, M.D. MEDICAL LIBRARY
7620 York Rd.
Towson, MD 21204   Phone: (301) 337-1210
Marianne Prenger, Med.Libn.
Subjects: Medicine, surgery, obstetrics, gynecology, pediatrics, nursing. **Holdings:** 1445 books; 404 bound periodical volumes; Audio-Digest tapes; audio and video cassette tapes. **Subscriptions:** 151 journals and other serials.

Massachusetts

★8413★ STURDY MEMORIAL HOSPITAL
HEALTH SCIENCES LIBRARY
211 Park St.
Attleboro, MA 02703   Phone: (508) 222-5200
Juliet I. Mansfield, Libn.
Subjects: Medicine, nursing. **Holdings:** 866 books; 584 bound periodical volumes; 8 VF drawers of articles, clippings, pamphlets. **Subscriptions:** 132 journals and other serials.

★8414★ BLIND CHILDREN'S FUND
PARENT RESOURCE CENTER
LIBRARY
230 Central St.
Auburndale, MA 02166-2399   Phone: (617) 332-4014
Sherry Raynor, Dir.
Subjects: Blind infants and toddlers - pre-braille skills, assessment tools, home teaching, preschool curriculums, special toys and equipment; premature infants; multihandicapped children. **Holdings:** Figures not available.

★8415★ NASHOBA COMMUNITY HOSPITAL
MEDICAL LIBRARY
200 Groton Rd.
Ayer, MA 01432   Phone: (508) 772-0200
Mary Ann Finnegan, Libn.
Subjects: Medicine, nursing. **Holdings:** 500 books; 400 bound periodical volumes. **Subscriptions:** 35 journals and other serials.

★8416★ U.S. DEPARTMENT OF VETERANS AFFAIRS
EDITH NOURSE ROGERS MEMORIAL VETERANS HOSPITAL
MEDICAL LIBRARY
200 Springs Rd.
Bedford, MA 01730   Phone: (617) 275-7500
Sanford S. Yagendorf, Chf., Lib.Serv.
Subjects: Psychiatry, geriatrics. **Holdings:** 6855 books; 3488 bound periodical volumes; 1702 boxes of microfilm; 776 tapes. **Subscriptions:** 270 journals and other serials.

★8417★ MCLEAN HOSPITAL
MENTAL HEALTH SCIENCES LIBRARY
115 Mill St.
Belmont, MA 02178   Phone: (617) 855-2460
Rosanne Labree, Dir.
Subjects: Mental health, behavioral sciences, alcoholism, drug abuse, psychiatry, psychoanalysis, psychology, psychosomatics, neurology, psychopharmacology, psychotherapy, schizophrenia, psychobiology, child and adolescent psychiatry, forensic psychiatry, neuroscience, social work. **Holdings:** 13,000 books; 17,000 bound periodical volumes. **Subscriptions:** 344 journals and other serials.

★8418★ BEVERLY HOSPITAL
LIBRARY
Herrick St.
Beverly, MA 01915   Phone: (508) 922-3000
Ann M. Tomes, Libn.
Subjects: Medicine. **Holdings:** 6000 volumes. **Subscriptions:** 125 journals and other serials.

★8419★ BETH ISRAEL HOSPITAL
AGOOS MEDICAL LIBRARY
330 Brookline Ave.
Boston, MA 02215   Phone: (617) 735-4225
Subjects: Medicine and allied health sciences. **Holdings:** 3200 books; 3800 bound periodical volumes. **Subscriptions:** 221 journals and other serials.

★8420★ BOSTON CITY HOSPITAL
MEDICAL LIBRARY
818 Harrison Ave.
Boston, MA 02118   Phone: (617) 534-4198
Margi Dempsey, Dir. of Med.Lib.
Subjects: Medicine, health sciences, Boston medical history. **Holdings:** 3239 books; 11,614 bound periodical volumes; 504 pictures; 123 microforms; 592 audiotapes; 16 slide sets. **Subscriptions:** 259 journals and other serials.

★8421★ BOSTON CITY HOSPITAL
NURSING DEPARTMENT
MORSE-SLANGER LIBRARY
818 Harrison Ave.
Boston, MA 02118   Phone: (617) 424-4926
Margi Dempsey, Dir.
Subjects: Nursing - medical, surgical, maternal, infant; pediatrics; paramedical sciences; psychology; sociology. **Holdings:** 1892 books; 723 bound periodical volumes. **Subscriptions:** 82 journals and other serials.

★8422★ BOSTON PSYCHOANALYTIC SOCIETY AND
    INSTITUTE
LIBRARY
15 Commonwealth Ave.
Boston, MA 02116   Phone: (617) 266-0953
Sanford Gifford, Dir. of Lib.
Subjects: Psychoanalysis. **Holdings:** 4800 books; 2000 bound periodical volumes; reports; reprints. **Subscriptions:** 85 journals and other serials.

★8423★ BOSTON STATE HOSPITAL
MEDICAL LIBRARY
591 Morton St.
Boston, MA 02124   Phone: (617) 436-6000
John B. Picott, Libn.
Subjects: Psychiatry, neurology, community mental health, psychiatric nursing, social service. **Holdings:** 2300 books; 1000 unbound and bound periodical volumes. **Subscriptions:** 199 journals and other serials.

★8424★ BOSTON UNIVERSITY
DEPARTMENT OF SPECIAL COLLECTIONS
NURSING ARCHIVES
771 Commonwealth Ave.
Boston, MA 02215   Phone: (617) 353-3696
Margaret R. Goostray, Asst.Dir., Spec.Coll.
Subjects: History - nursing education, nursing organizations and institutions, individual nurses. **Holdings:** 1800 volumes; 3000 manuscript boxes; 30 oral histories.

★8425★ BOSTON UNIVERSITY
GERONTOLOGY CENTER
LOUIS LOWY LIBRARY
67 Bay State Rd.
Boston, MA 02215   Phone: (617) 353-5045
Nan Genger, Act.Lib.Chf.
Subjects: Aging - health, housing, training, education, policy, House and Senate hearings, international aspects. **Holdings:** 1000 books; 2000 published and unpublished reports, papers, directories, articles, newsletters, and national conference notices. **Subscriptions:** 54 journals and other serials.

★8426★ BOSTON UNIVERSITY
LABORATORY OF NEUROPSYCHOLOGY
LIBRARY
Dept. of Behavioral Neuroscience
M-9, 85 E. Newton St.
Boston, MA 02118   Phone: (617) 638-4803
Subjects: Neuropsychology. **Holdings:** 300 books; 50 reports. **Subscriptions:** 10 journals and other serials.

★8427★ BOSTON UNIVERSITY
SCHOOL OF MEDICINE
ALUMNI MEDICAL LIBRARY
80 E. Concord St.
Boston, MA 02118-2394   Phone: (617) 638-4230
Irene Christopher, Chf.Libn.
Subjects: Medicine, dentistry, public health. **Holdings:** 101,790 volumes. **Subscriptions:** 1437 journals and other serials.

★8428★ CARNEY HOSPITAL
COLPOYS LIBRARY
2100 Dorchester Ave.
Boston, MA 02124-5666   Phone: (617) 296-4000
Catherine I. Moore, Med.Libn.
Subjects: Medicine. **Holdings:** 2000 books; 6000 bound periodical volumes; tapes. **Subscriptions:** 230 journals and other serials; 10 newspapers.

★8429★ DANA-FARBER CANCER INSTITUTE
PROFESSIONAL STAFF LIBRARY
44 Binney St.
Boston, MA 02115   Phone: (617) 732-3508
Christine W. Fleuriel, Libn.
Subjects: Cancer research. **Holdings:** 1400 books; 1500 bound periodical volumes. **Subscriptions:** 110 journals and other serials.

★8430★ E.I. DU PONT DE NEMOURS & COMPANY, INC.
NEN PRODUCTS
LIBRARY
549 Albany St.
Boston, MA 02118   Phone: (617) 350-9699
Pauline R. Leeds, Supv., Lib.Serv.
Subjects: Chemistry, nuclear medicine, pharmacology. **Holdings:** 15,000 books; 20,000 bound periodical volumes; 3000 reports. **Subscriptions:** 310 journals and other serials.

★8431★ ERICH LINDEMANN MENTAL HEALTH CENTER
LIBRARY
Government Center
25 Staniford St.
Boston, MA 02114   Phone: (617) 727-7100
Vishakha Menta, Lib.Dir.
Subjects: Psychology, psychiatry, community mental health, mental retardation, drug rehabilitation. **Holdings:** 3000 books; 300 bound periodical volumes; 500 documents; 16 VF drawers of pamphlets. **Subscriptions:** 20 journals and other serials.

★8432★ EYE RESEARCH INSTITUTE OF RETINA
FOUNDATION
LIBRARY
20 Staniford St.
Boston, MA 02114   Phone: (617) 742-3140
Subjects: Eye research. **Holdings:** 200 books; 1500 bound periodical volumes. **Subscriptions:** 38 journals and other serials.

★8433★ FAULKNER HOSPITAL
INGERSOLL BOWDITCH LIBRARY
Allandale at Centre St.
Boston, MA 02130   Phone: (617) 522-5800
Barbara P. Pastan, Dir., Lib.Serv.
Subjects: Medicine, surgery, nursing, administration. **Holdings:** 800 books; 4000 bound periodical volumes; 350 audiotapes; 50 videotapes; 25 slide/tape sets; hospital reports; microfiche. **Subscriptions:** 195 journals and other serials.

★8434★ FORSYTH DENTAL CENTER
PERCY HOWE MEMORIAL LIBRARY
140 The Fenway
Boston, MA 02115   Phone: (617) 262-5200
Roberta Oppenheim, Lib.Dir.
Subjects: Dentistry, dental hygiene, biochemistry, microbiology, molecular biology, anthropology, anatomy, immunology. **Holdings:** 6200 books; 14,575 bound periodical volumes; pamphlets; photographs; staff reprints. **Subscriptions:** 230 journals and other serials.

★8435★ HARVARD UNIVERSITY
SCHOOL OF MEDICINE
THE LIBRARIES OF THE MASSACHUSETTS EYE AND EAR
INFIRMARY
243 Charles St.
Boston, MA 02114   Phone: (617) 573-3196
Chris Nims, Lib.Dir.
Subjects: Ophthalmology, otolaryngology. **Holdings:** 16,000 books, bound periodical volumes, pamphlets; 300 stereophotographs of diseases of the eye; 130 cubic feet of archival materials; 40 cubic feet of manuscripts; 1500 rare books. **Subscriptions:** 212 journals and other serials.

★8436★ HARVARD UNIVERSITY
SCHOOL OF MEDICINE
SCHERING FOUNDATION LIBRARY OF HEALTH CARE
643 Huntington Ave.
Boston, MA 02115   Phone: (617) 432-2103
Anne L. Alach, Libn.
Subjects: Community health care, preventive and social medicine. **Holdings:** 5000 volumes. **Subscriptions:** 38 journals and other serials.

★8437★ HARVARD UNIVERSITY
SCHOOL OF PUBLIC HEALTH
KRESGE CENTER LIBRARY
665 Huntington Ave., Rm. 1306
Boston, MA 02115   Phone: (617) 432-3488
Betty Hauser, Libn.
Subjects: Physiology of the lung, environmental health. **Holdings:** 225 books; 225 bound periodical volumes; 120 dissertations. **Subscriptions:** 34 journals and other serials.

★8438★ HARVARD UNIVERSITY
SCHOOL OF PUBLIC HEALTH
POPULATION SCIENCES LIBRARY
665 Huntington Ave.
Boston, MA 02115   Phone: (617) 432-1234
Hannah Doress, Lib.Coord.
Subjects: Population studies and international health. **Holdings:** 22,000 volumes. **Subscriptions:** 235 journals and other serials.

★8439★ HARVARD UNIVERSITY
SCHOOLS OF MEDICINE, DENTAL MEDICINE AND PUBLIC
HEALTH
BOSTON MEDICAL LIBRARY
FRANCIS A. COUNTWAY LIBRARY
10 Shattuck St.
Boston, MA 02115   Phone: (617) 432-2142
Judith Messerle
Subjects: Anatomy, biochemistry, dentistry, history of medicine, legal medicine, microbiology, parasitology, physiology, public health. **Holdings:** 545,464 volumes. **Subscriptions:** 5346 journals and other serials.

★8440★ JOSLIN DIABETES CENTER
DOOLEY LIBRARY
1 Joslin Pl.
Boston, MA 02215   Phone: (617) 732-2573
Richard Kitch, Libn.
Subjects: Diabetes mellitus, physiology, pathology, biochemistry. **Holdings:** 7000 volumes; 80 VF folders. **Subscriptions:** 108 journals and other serials.

★8441★ LIBERTY MUTUAL INSURANCE COMPANY
LAW LIBRARY
175 Berkeley St.
Boston, MA 02117   Phone: (617) 357-9500
W. Leslie Peat, Dir. of Law Libs.
Subjects: Insurance, law, medicine. **Holdings:** 30,000 volumes. **Subscriptions:** 87 journals and other serials.

★8442★ MASSACHUSETTS COLLEGE OF PHARMACY AND
ALLIED HEALTH SCIENCES
SHEPPARD LIBRARY
179 Longwood Ave.
Boston, MA 02115   Phone: (617) 732-2810
Anne M. Pascarelli, Lib.Dir.
Subjects: Pharmacy, biological sciences, chemistry, medical botany, drug abuse, drug interactions, nursing, nuclear medicine, health psychology. **Holdings:** 64,278 volumes; 28 VF drawers of pamphlets, clippings, documents, advertising materials, reprints; audio and video cassettes; microfilm; slides. **Subscriptions:** 700 journals and other serials.

★8443★ MASSACHUSETTS DEPARTMENT OF PUBLIC
HEALTH
CENTRAL LIBRARY
150 Tremont St.
Boston, MA 02111   Phone: (617) 727-7022
Ann Collins, Dir., Lib.Serv.
Subjects: Public health, health care planning and administration, environmental health. **Holdings:** 550 books; 2640 unbound periodicals; 250 U.S. Government documents; 250 state government documents. **Subscriptions:** 70 journals and other serials.

★8444★ MASSACHUSETTS GENERAL HOSPITAL
MGH HEALTH SCIENCES LIBRARY
Fruit St.
Boston, MA 02114   Phone: (617) 726-8600
Jacqueline Bastille, Dir.
Subjects: Medicine, biochemistry, health care, nursing, allied health

sciences. **Holdings:** 13,471 books; 34,421 bound periodical volumes. **Subscriptions:** 913 journals and other serials.

★8445★ MASSACHUSETTS MENTAL HEALTH CENTER
CHARLES MACFIE CAMPBELL MEMORIAL LIBRARY
74 Fenwood Rd.
Boston, MA 02115-6196   Phone: (617) 734-1300
Elizabeth Banov, Libn.
Subjects: Psychiatry, neurology, occupational therapy, law, nursing, psychology. **Holdings:** 13,500 volumes; reprints. **Subscriptions:** 82 journals and other serials.

★8446★ MASSACHUSETTS REHABILITATION COMMISSION
LIBRARY
Fort Point Pl.
27-43 Wormwood St.
Boston, MA 02210-1606   Phone: (617) 727-1140
June C. Holt, Lib.Dir.
Subjects: Physical impairments, mental problems, accessibility (buildings, transportation, accomodation), legal rights of disabled, Rehabilitation Act & amendments, employment of disabled persons, severely disabled, counseling techniques, vocational rehabilitation, social problems, disability and disabilities, independent living, psychological rehabilitation, staff development, disability statistics. **Holdings:** 30,000 books; 1200 microfiche; 69 VF drawers; 13 16mm films; 10 videotapes; 34 audiotapes; Institute on Rehabilitation Issues Series. **Subscriptions:** 118 journals and other serials.

★8447★ MENTAL HEALTH LEGAL ADVISORS COMMITTEE
FLASCHNER DISABILITIES LIBRARY
11 Beacon St., Ste. 925
Boston, MA 21218   Phone: (617) 723-9130
Stan Goldman
Subjects: Law - disabilities, mental health. **Holdings:** 300 books; 200 bound periodical volumes; 50 reports. **Subscriptions:** 11 journals and other serials.

★8448★ NEW ENGLAND BAPTIST HOSPITAL
HEALTH SCIENCES LIBRARY
125 Parker Hill Ave.
Boston, MA 02120   Phone: (617) 738-5155
Paul Esty Woodard, Ph.D., Chf.Med.Libn.
Subjects: Medicine, orthopedics, history of medicine, nursing, history of nursing. **Holdings:** 6717 books; 3500 bound periodical volumes. **Subscriptions:** 153 journals and other serials.

★8449★ NEW ENGLAND COLLEGE OF OPTOMETRY
LIBRARY
420 Beacon St.
Boston, MA 02115   Phone: (617) 266-2030
Lynne A. Silvers, Lib.Dir.
Subjects: Optometry, ophthalmology. **Holdings:** 10,000 books; 2800 bound periodical volumes; 4 VF drawers of pamphlets; 8 VF drawers of reprints; 500 35mm color slides; 450 audiotape cassettes; 97 video cassettes; 82 slide/tape sets; 18 slide sets; 15 realia. **Subscriptions:** 275 journals and other serials.

★8450★ NEW ENGLAND DEACONESS HOSPITAL
HORRAX LIBRARY
185 Pilgrim Rd.
Boston, MA 02215   Phone: (617) 732-8311
Paul Vaiginas, Libn.
Subjects: General medicine, diabetes, cancer, renal disease, cardiology, surgery. **Holdings:** 3300 books; 3500 bound periodical volumes; 850 audio cassettes. **Subscriptions:** 252 journals and other serials.

★8451★ NEW ENGLAND MEDICAL CENTER
ELIZABETH S. MAKKAY LIBRARY
750 Washington St.
Box 395
Boston, MA 02111   Phone: (617) 956-5497
Nancy B. Duggan, Libn.
Subjects: Psychiatry, psychology, social work. **Holdings:** 1500 books; 500 bound periodical volumes; 100 AV programs; 1000 reprints. **Subscriptions:** 38 journals and other serials.

★8452★ NORTH CONWAY INSTITUTE
RESOURCE CENTER
ALCOHOL AND DRUGS
14 Beacon St.
Boston, MA 02108   Phone: (617) 742-0424
Rev. David A. Works, Pres.
Subjects: Alcohol, drugs. **Holdings:** Figures not available. **Subscriptions:** 50 journals and other serials.

★8453★ TUFTS UNIVERSITY
CENTER FOR THE STUDY OF DRUG DEVELOPMENT
LIBRARY
136 Harrison Ave.
Boston, MA 02111   Phone: (617) 956-0185
Drusilla Raiford, Res.Assoc.
Subjects: Drug development and regulation, pharmaceutical industry. **Holdings:** 2200 books; 160 bound periodical volumes; 13,000 reports, manuscripts, reprints. **Subscriptions:** 25 journals and other serials.

★8454★ TUFTS UNIVERSITY
HEALTH SCIENCES LIBRARY
145 Harrison Ave.
Boston, MA 02111   Phone: (617) 956-7481
Elizabeth K. Eaton, Ph.D., Dir.
Subjects: Medicine, dentistry, veterinary medicine, nutrition. **Holdings:** 34,673 books; 78,035 bound periodical volumes; 260 audiotapes; 222 slide titles; 3511 reels of microfilm; 7072 microcards; 717 videotapes; 11 phonograph records; 7 video discs. **Subscriptions:** 1532 journals and other serials; 6 newspapers.

★8455★ U.S. DEPARTMENT OF VETERANS AFFAIRS
HOSPITAL MEDICAL LIBRARY
150 S. Huntington Ave.
Boston, MA 02130   Phone: (617) 739-3434
John F. Connors, Chf., Lib.Serv.
Subjects: General medicine, surgery, allied health sciences, patient education. **Holdings:** 3000 books; 12,000 bound periodical volumes. **Subscriptions:** 450 journals and other serials.

★8456★ U.S.D.A.
HUMAN NUTRITION RESEARCH CENTER ON AGING
LIBRARY
711 Washington St.
Boston, MA 02111   Phone: (617) 556-3173
Kathleen L. Capellano, M.S., R.D.
Subjects: Nutrition, biomedical sciences, aging. **Holdings:** 500 books; 60 bound periodical volumes; 30 reports; 1200 publication archive s. **Subscriptions:** 115 journals and other serials.

★8457★ U.S. DEPARTMENT OF VETERANS AFFAIRS
OUTPATIENT CLINIC LIBRARY SERVICE
251 Causeway St.
Boston, MA 02114   Phone: (617) 248-1170
John F. Connors, Chf., Lib.Serv.
Subjects: Health sciences, patient health education. **Holdings:** 2000 books; 1836 periodical volumes on microfilm; 1000 patient education pamphlets. **Subscriptions:** 145 journals and other serials.

★8458★ FRANCISCAN CHILDREN'S HOSPITAL AND
REHABILITATION CENTER
MEDICAL LIBRARY
30 Warren St.
Brighton, MA 02135   Phone: (617) 254-3800
Anne Brasier, Med.Libn.
Subjects: Pediatrics, child development, developmental disorders, nursing, therapies, handicapped children, rehabilitation, birth defects. **Holdings:** 900 books; 1600 unbound and bound periodical volumes; 13 annuals. **Subscriptions:** 100 journals and other serials.

★8459★ ST. ELIZABETH'S HOSPITAL
SCHOOL OF NURSING
LIBRARY
159 Washington St.
Brighton, MA 02135   Phone: (617) 789-2304
Robert L. Loud, Libn.
Subjects: Nursing, medicine. **Holdings:** 2245 books; 1100 bound periodical volumes. **Subscriptions:** 90 journals and other serials.

★8460★   ST. ELIZABETH'S HOSPITAL
STOHLMAN LIBRARY
736 Cambridge St.
Brighton, MA 02135   Phone: (617) 789-2177
Robin E. Braun, Dir.
Subjects: Medicine. **Holdings:** 1500 books; 5135 bound periodical volumes. **Subscriptions:** 172 journals and other serials.

★8461★   VALUE OF LIFE COMMITTEE
LIBRARY
637 Cambridge St.
Brighton, MA 02135   Phone: (617) 787-4400
Subjects: Medical and legal aspects of abortion, euthanasia, ethics, and genetics. **Holdings:** 300 books, newspaper clippings, and other items.

★8462★   BROCKTON HOSPITAL
LIBRARY
680 Centre St.
Brockton, MA 02402   Phone: (508) 586-2600
Lovisa Kamenoff, Mgr., Lib.Serv.
Subjects: Medicine, nursing, hospital administration. **Holdings:** 2575 books; 6000 bound periodical volumes; 28 VF drawers of health sciences bibliographies. **Subscriptions:** 260 journals and other serials.

★8463★   CARDINAL CUSHING GENERAL HOSPITAL
STAFF LIBRARY
235 N. Pearl St.
Brockton, MA 02401   Phone: (617) 588-4000
Nancy Sezak, Med.Libn.
Subjects: Medicine. **Holdings:** 864 books; 1060 bound periodical volumes; 434 unbound journals; 2 drawers of pamphlets and reprints. **Subscriptions:** 108 journals and other serials.

★8464★   U.S. DEPARTMENT OF VETERANS AFFAIRS
MEDICAL CENTER LIBRARY
940 Belmont St.
Brockton, MA 02401   Phone: (508) 583-4500
Suzanne N. Noyes, Chf., Lib.Serv.
Subjects: Psychiatry, psychology, hospital administration, nursing, medicine, alcoholism, drug abuse. **Holdings:** 5200 books; 7000 bound periodical volumes; 400 other cataloged items. **Subscriptions:** 450 journals and other serials.

★8465★   LAHEY CLINIC MEDICAL CENTER
RICHARD B. CATTELL MEMORIAL LIBRARY
41 Mall Rd.
Burlington, MA 01805   Phone: (617) 273-8253
Carol Spencer, Libn.
Subjects: Medicine. **Holdings:** 1500 books; 7500 bound periodical volumes. **Subscriptions:** 300 journals and other serials.

★8466★   ARTHUR D. LITTLE, INC.
LIFE SCIENCES LIBRARY
25 Acorn Park
Cambridge, MA 02140   Phone: (617) 864-5770
Subjects: Biomedical sciences, toxicology, carcinogenesis, environmental health, bioassay. **Holdings:** 1900 books; 1135 bound periodical volumes. **Subscriptions:** 154 journals and other serials.

★8467★   CAMBRIDGE HOSPITAL
MEDICAL LIBRARY
1493 Cambridge St.
Cambridge, MA 02139   Phone: (617) 498-1439
Gina Chen, Med.Libn.
Subjects: Medicine, surgery, health sciences. **Holdings:** 550 books; 2000 bound periodical volumes. **Subscriptions:** 70 journals and other serials.

★8468★   MASSACHUSETTS INSTITUTE OF TECHNOLOGY
DEPARTMENT OF BRAIN AND COGNITIVE SCIENCES
TEUBER LIBRARY
Rm. E10-030
Cambridge, MA 02139   Phone: (617) 253-5755
Patricia Claffey, Libn.
Subjects: Cognitive psychology, cognitive science, developmental psychology, perception, psycholinguistics (especially language acquisition). **Holdings:** 5000 books; 3500 bound periodical volumes; 120 bound doctoral theses of psychology department graduates; masters' theses. **Subscriptions:** 50 journals and other serials.

★8469★   MASSACHUSETTS INSTITUTE OF TECHNOLOGY
SCHERING-PLOUGH LIBRARY
Rm. E25-131
Cambridge, MA 02139   Phone: (617) 253-6366
Subjects: Health sciences, technology, and management. **Holdings:** 3367 volumes; 1108 bound periodical volumes; 1338 bound serial volumes; 892 microfiche. **Subscriptions:** 175 journals and other serials.

★8470★   MOUNT AUBURN HOSPITAL
HEALTH SCIENCES LIBRARY
330 Mt. Auburn St.
Cambridge, MA 02138   Phone: (617) 492-3500
M. Cherie Haitz, Dir.
Subjects: Medicine, nursing, pathology, administration, consumer health, allied health sciences. **Holdings:** 2000 books; 3000 bound periodical volumes; AV programs; 4 VF drawers of pamphlets. **Subscriptions:** 273 journals and other serials.

★8471★   MASSACHUSETTS HOSPITAL SCHOOL
PAUL NORTON MEDICAL LIBRARY
3 Randolph St.
Canton, MA 02021   Phone: (617) 828-2440
Sylvia K. Gerhard, Libn.
Subjects: Orthopedics, pediatrics. **Holdings:** 500 books. **Subscriptions:** 65 journals.

★8472★   WHIDDEN MEMORIAL HOSPITAL
MEDICAL LIBRARY
103 Garland St.
Everett, MA 02149   Phone: (617) 389-6270
Phyllis Perlo, R.N./Educ.Dept.
Subjects: Medicine, nursing, allied health sciences. **Holdings:** 1000 books; 4 shelves of clippings and pamphlets. **Subscriptions:** 69 journals and other serials.

★8473★   ST. ANNE'S HOSPITAL
SULLIVAN MEDICAL LIBRARY
795 Middle St.
Fall River, MA 02721   Phone: (508) 674-5741
Elaine M. Crites, Med.Libn.
Subjects: Oncology, medicine, surgery, allied health sciences. **Holdings:** 100 books; 4000 bound periodical volumes. **Subscriptions:** 80 journals and other serials.

★8474★   FITCHBURG STATE COLLEGE
LIBRARY
160 Pearl St.
Fitchburg, MA 01420   Phone: (508) 345-2151
Robert Foley, Dir.
Subjects: Education, special education, nursing, industrial technology, liberal arts, business administration, computer science. **Holdings:** 140,400 books, 30,000 on microfiche; 29,457 bound periodical volumes; 12,826 pamphlets; 315,040 ERIC microfiche; 350 ultrafiche. **Subscriptions:** 1346 journals; 7 newspapers.

★8475★   U.S. ARMY HOSPITALS
CUTLER ARMY HOSPITAL
MEDICAL LIBRARY
Fort Devens, MA 01433-6401   Phone: (508) 796-6750
Debra S. Martin, Med.Libn.
Subjects: Medicine, surgery, nursing. **Holdings:** 1800 books; 1500 bound periodical volumes. **Subscriptions:** 130 journals and other serials.

★8476★   FRAMINGHAM UNION HOSPITAL
TEDESCHI LIBRARY AND INFORMATION CENTER
115 Lincoln St.
Framingham, MA 01701   Phone: (508) 626-3595
Sandra Clevesy, Dir.
Subjects: Medicine, nursing, nursing education, health care delivery. **Holdings:** 5596 books; 5900 bound periodical volumes; 9 VF drawers of pamphlets. **Subscriptions:** 275 journals and other serials.

★8477★   CHARLES V. HOGAN REGIONAL CENTER
STAFF LIBRARY
Box A
Hathorne, MA 01937-9998   Phone: (508) 774-5000
Bonnie Stecher, Libn.
Subjects: Mental retardation, special education, medicine, rehabilitation,

behavioral psychology, psychiatry, psychology, community mental health services. **Holdings:** 2000 books; 19 VF drawers of pamphlets, articles, booklets. **Subscriptions:** 100 journals and other serials.

★8478★ **HAVERHILL MUNICIPAL HALE HOSPITAL**
MEDICAL LIBRARY
140 Lincoln Ave.
Haverhill, MA 01830   Phone: (508) 374-2000
Eleanor Howard, Libn.
Subjects: Medicine, nursing, allied health sciences. **Holdings:** 1200 books; 2000 bound periodical volumes; 300 unbound journals; 4 VF drawers of pamphlets. **Subscriptions:** 76 journals and other serials.

★8479★ **LEMUEL SHATTUCK HOSPITAL**
MEDICAL LIBRARY
170 Morton St.
Jamaica Plain, MA 02130   Phone: (617) 522-8110
Ann Collins, Libn.
Subjects: Medicine and allied health sciences. **Holdings:** 940 books; 4360 bound periodical volumes; 320 audio cassettes. **Subscriptions:** 185 journals and other serials.

★8480★ **LAKEVILLE HOSPITAL**
HEALTH SCIENCES LIBRARY
Main St.
Lakeville, MA 02347   Phone: (508) 947-1231
Anne S. Lima, Libn.
Subjects: Medicine, nursing education, rehabilitation, orthopedics and orthopedic surgery, birth defects and crippling conditions. **Holdings:** 1500 books; 1520 bound periodical volumes; pamphlet file; 125 AV programs. **Subscriptions:** 103 journals and other serials.

★8481★ **LAWRENCE GENERAL HOSPITAL**
HEALTH SCIENCE LIBRARY
1 General St.
Lawrence, MA 01842   Phone: (508) 683-4000
Carmel M. Gram, Libn. Consultant
Subjects: Clinical medicine, nursing. **Holdings:** 1500 books; 156 bound periodical volumes. **Subscriptions:** 113 journals and other serials.

★8482★ **INSTRUMENTATION LABORATORY**
LIBRARY-S-33
113 Hartwell Ave.
Lexington, MA 02173   Phone: (617) 861-4328
Janet R. Mierzykowski, Mgr., Lib.Serv.
Subjects: Medicine, chemistry, biotechnology. **Holdings:** 6600 volumes; 400 technical reports, hardcopy and microfiche. **Subscriptions:** 200 journals and other serials.

★8483★ **WOMEN'S INTERNATIONAL NETWORK**
187 Grant St.
Lexington, MA 02173   Phone: (617) 862-9431
Fran P. Hosken, Ed.
Subjects: Women's development and health, women's economic development, property rights of women worldwide. **Holdings:** Books; Network publications; foreign journals; uncataloged items. **Subscriptions:** 40 journals and other serials; 10 newspapers.

★8484★ **LOWELL GENERAL HOSPITAL**
HEALTH SCIENCE LIBRARY
295 Varnum Ave.
Lowell, MA 01854   Phone: (508) 937-6247
Martha Bedard, Dir., Med.Lib.
Subjects: Basic sciences, nutrition, medicine, nursing, psychology, psychiatry, sociology. **Holdings:** 3000 books; AV programs. **Subscriptions:** 100 journals and other serials.

★8485★ **ST. JOHN'S HOSPITAL**
HEALTH SCIENCE LIBRARY
PO Box 30
Lowell, MA 01853   Phone: (508) 458-1411
Gale Cogan, Dir.
Subjects: Medicine and allied health sciences, hospital administration. **Holdings:** 1500 books. **Subscriptions:** 450 journals and other serials.

★8486★ **ST. JOSEPH'S HOSPITAL**
HEALTH SCIENCE LIBRARY
220 Pawtucket St.
Lowell, MA 01854   Phone: (508) 453-1761
Anne C. Dick, Lib.Dir.
Subjects: Medicine and nursing. **Holdings:** 3050 volumes. **Subscriptions:** 200 journals and other serials.

★8487★ **ATLANTICARE MEDICAL CENTER**
HEALTH SCIENCES LIBRARY
212 Boston St.
Lynn, MA 01904   Phone: (617) 599-4884
Deborah T. Almquist, Dir., Lib.Serv.
Subjects: Medicine, nursing, and allied health sciences. **Holdings:** 1365 books; 3000 bound periodical volumes; 128 video cassettes; 125 audio cassettes; 6 16mm films; 12 filmstrips and slide/tape programs. **Subscriptions:** 197 journals and other serials.

★8488★ **MALDEN HOSPITAL**
MEDICAL LIBRARY
Hospital Rd.
Malden, MA 02148   Phone: (617) 322-7560
Elizabeth F. Fitzpayne, Libn.
Subjects: Medicine, allied health sciences. **Holdings:** 732 books; 2100 bound periodical volumes; 125 pamphlets; 2 boxes of AV catalogs. **Subscriptions:** 109 journals and other serials.

★8489★ **MARLBOROUGH HOSPITAL**
HEALTH SCIENCE LIBRARY
57 Union St.
Marlborough, MA 01752   Phone: (508) 485-1121
Virginia Ferrara, Lib.Coord.
Subjects: Medicine, nursing, allied health sciences. **Holdings:** 900 books; 1200 bound periodical volumes; AV programs. **Subscriptions:** 153 journals and other serials.

★8490★ **CIBA CORNING DIAGNOSTICS CORPORATION**
STEINBERG INFORMATION CENTER
63 North St.
Medfield, MA 02052   Phone: (508) 359-3606
Kathleen E. McCabe, Supv.Info.Ctr.
Subjects: Clinical medicine, market research, engineering, biotechnology, business. **Holdings:** 3000 books; 2200 bound periodical volumes; 24,000 patents; 850 internal research reports. **Subscriptions:** 181 journals and other serials.

★8491★ **MEDFIELD STATE HOSPITAL**
MEDICAL LIBRARY
Hospital Rd.
Medfield, MA 02052   Phone: (617) 359-7312
Jeanne Migliacci, Sr.Libn.
Subjects: Psychiatry, nursing, neurology, psychology. **Holdings:** 2398 books; 1946 bound periodical volumes; 300 pamphlets; 105 cassettes; 3 drawers of pamphlets (uncataloged). **Subscriptions:** 37 journals and other serials; 5 newspapers.

★8492★ **LAWRENCE MEMORIAL HOSPITAL OF MEDFORD**
HEALTH SCIENCES LIBRARY
170 Governors Ave.
Medford, MA 02155   Phone: (617) 396-9250
John C. Harris, Hea.Sci.Libn.
Subjects: Nursing, medicine, hospital administration. **Holdings:** 4000 books; 1200 bound periodical volumes; 800 filmstrip cassettes and videotapes; 200 subject pamphlet file. **Subscriptions:** 161 journals and other serials.

★8493★ **AMERICAN SOCIETY OF ABDOMINAL SURGEONS**
DONALD COLLINS MEMORIAL LIBRARY
675 Main St.
Melrose, MA 02176   Phone: (617) 665-6102
Dr. Blaise F. Alfano, Hd.Libn.
Subjects: Surgery, medicine. **Holdings:** 900 books; 45 bound periodical volumes. **Subscriptions:** 52 journals and other serials; 10 newspapers.

★8494★   HOLY FAMILY HOSPITAL AND MEDICAL CENTER
HEALTH SCIENCE LIBRARY
70 East St.
Methuen, MA 01844   Phone: (508) 687-0151
Chin-Soon Han, Med.Libn.
Subjects: Medicine, nursing, hospital administration. **Holdings:** 1000 books; 1400 bound periodical volumes; 10 volumes of archival materials; 7 VF drawers on specific diseases. **Subscriptions:** 100 journals and other serials.

★8495★   ST. LUKE'S HOSPITAL OF MIDDLEBOROUGH
MEDICAL STAFF LIBRARY
52 Oak St.
Middleboro, MA 02346   Phone: (617) 947-6000
Gail Twomey, Med.Libn.
Subjects: Medicine and allied health sciences. **Holdings:** 112 volumes; 2000 unbound periodicals. **Subscriptions:** 45 journals and other serials.

★8496★   CURRY COLLEGE
LOUIS R. LEVIN MEMORIAL LIBRARY
SPECIAL COLLECTIONS
1071 Blue Hill Ave.
Milton, MA 02186   Phone: (617) 333-0500
Catharine King, Dir.
Subjects: Communication, learning disabilities. **Holdings:** 38,943 U.S. Government documents. **Subscriptions:** 700 journals and other serials.

★8497★   LEONARD MORSE HOSPITAL
MEDICAL LIBRARY
67 Union St.
Natick, MA 01760   Phone: (508) 653-3400
Subjects: Medicine, nursing, hospital administration. **Holdings:** 1200 books; 2600 bound periodical volumes; 147 AV programs. **Subscriptions:** 121 journals and other serials.

★8498★   GLOVER MEMORIAL HOSPITAL
MEDICAL LIBRARY
148 Chestnut St.
Needham, MA 02192   Phone: (617) 444-5600
Louisa Tseng, Dir., Med.Lib.
Subjects: Medicine, nursing, health care administration. **Holdings:** 650 books; 586 bound periodical volumes. **Subscriptions:** 75 journals and other serials.

★8499★   NATIONAL TAY-SACHS AND ALLIED DISEASES
     ASSOCIATION
LIBRARY
385 Elliot St.
Newton, MA 02164   Phone: (617) 964-5508
Marjorie Epstein
Subjects: Grief counseling, Tay-Sachs' disease, lysosomal storage diseases. **Holdings:** 100 books; 10,000 newspaper clippings.

★8500★   NEWTON-WELLESLEY HOSPITAL
PAUL TALBOT BABSON MEMORIAL LIBRARY
2014 Washington St.
Newton Lower Falls, MA 02162   Phone: (617) 243-6279
Christine L. Bell, Dir., Lib.Serv.
Subjects: Medicine, surgery, nursing, health care administration, psychiatry, allied health sciences. **Holdings:** 3500 books; 6000 bound periodical volumes; 7 VF drawers of pamphlets. **Subscriptions:** 317 journals and other serials; 7 newspapers.

★8501★   SOUTHWOOD COMMUNITY HOSPITAL
MEDICAL LIBRARY
111 Dedham St.
Norfolk, MA 02056   Phone: (508) 668-0385
Debbie MacDonald, Med.Libn.
Subjects: Oncology, medicine, surgery, nursing, radiology. **Holdings:** 1896 books and bound periodical volumes. **Subscriptions:** 94 journals and other serials.

★8502★   U.S. DEPARTMENT OF VETERANS AFFAIRS
MEDICAL CENTER LIBRARY
N. Main St.
Northampton, MA 01060   Phone: (413) 584-4040
Marjorie C. Dewey, Chf., Lib.Serv.
Subjects: Neurology, psychiatry, psychology, nursing, medicine. **Holdings:**
2600 books; 283 bound periodical volumes; 4039 volumes on microfilm; 1041 unbound periodical volumes. **Subscriptions:** 234 journals and other serials.

★8503★   BERKSHIRE MEDICAL CENTER
MEDICAL LIBRARY
725 North St.
Pittsfield, MA 01201   Phone: (413) 447-2000
Eleanor M. McNutt, Dir.
Subjects: Medicine, nursing, allied health sciences. **Holdings:** 8500 books; 6000 bound periodical volumes; 2 VF drawers. **Subscriptions:** 167 journals and other serials.

★8504★   SALEM HOSPITAL
HEALTH SCIENCES LIBRARY
81 Highland Ave.
Salem, MA 01970   Phone: (508) 741-1200
Nancy Fazzone, Dir., Lib.Serv.
Subjects: Medicine, nursing, and allied health sciences. **Holdings:** 3500 books; 7000 bound periodical volumes. **Subscriptions:** 275 journals and other serials.

★8505★   SOMERVILLE HOSPITAL
CARR HEALTH SCIENCES LIBRARY
230 Highland Ave.
Somerville, MA 02143   Phone: (617) 666-4400
Celeste F. Kozlowski, Med.Libn.
Subjects: Medicine, nursing. **Holdings:** 2678 books; 118 bound periodical volumes; 4 VF drawers pamphlets; 1 VF drawer of archives. **Subscriptions:** 139 journals and other serials.

★8506★   HARVARD UNIVERSITY
NEW ENGLAND REGIONAL PRIMATE RESEARCH CENTER
HENRY COE MEADOW LIBRARY
1 Pine Hill Dr.
Southborough, MA 01772-9102   Phone: (508) 481-0400
Sydney Ann Fingold, Libn.
Subjects: Primatology, veterinary research, cardiophysiology, reproductive physiology, pharmacology, immunology, pathology, behavioral biology. **Holdings:** 8000 books; 6000 bound periodical volumes. **Subscriptions:** 150 journals and other serials.

★8507★   AMERICAN INTERNATIONAL COLLEGE
JAMES J. SHEA MEMORIAL LIBRARY
ORAL HISTORY CENTER
1000 State St.
Springfield, MA 01109-3189   Phone: (413) 737-7000
Dr. F. Knowlton Utley, Dir. of Lib.
Subjects: Business, education, psychology, nursing. **Holdings:** 1350 tapes. **Subscriptions:** 489 journals and other serials; 8 newspapers.

★8508★   BAYSTATE MEDICAL CENTER
HEALTH SCIENCES LIBRARY
759 Chestnut St.
Springfield, MA 01199   Phone: (413) 784-5442
Isabel Hunter, Dir.
Subjects: Medicine, nursing, allied health sciences, health care administration. **Holdings:** 22,000 volumes. **Subscriptions:** 500 journals and other serials.

★8509★   MERCY HOSPITAL
HEALTH SCIENCES LIBRARY
Box 9012
Springfield, MA 01102-9012   Phone: (413) 781-9100
Roger S. Manahan, Hea.Sci.Libn.
Subjects: Medicine, nursing, allied health sciences. **Holdings:** 500 books; 800 bound periodical volumes. **Subscriptions:** 50 journals and other serials.

★8510★   AUSTEN RIGGS CENTER, INC.
AUSTEN FOX RIGGS LIBRARY
Main St.
Stockbridge, MA 01262   Phone: (413) 298-5511
Helen Linton, Libn.
Subjects: Psychoanalysis, psychiatry, psychology. **Holdings:** 9680 books; 2042 bound periodical volumes; 78 cassettes. **Subscriptions:** 154 journals and other serials.

★8511★ EUNICE KENNEDY SHRIVER CENTER FOR MENTAL RETARDATION
BIOCHEMISTRY LIBRARY
200 Trapelo Rd.
Waltham, MA 02254   Phone: (617) 642-0001
Dr. Peter Daniel, Libn.
Subjects: Biochemistry, chemistry, neurochemistry, neuroscience, genetics, cell biology. **Holdings:** 200 books; 400 bound periodical volumes; 50 pamphlets. **Subscriptions:** 30 journals and other serials.

★8512★ HEWLETT-PACKARD COMPANY
LIBRARY
175 Wyman St.
Waltham, MA 02254   Phone: (617) 890-6300
Susan Saraidaridis, Hd. Libn.
Subjects: Medicine, engineering, business. **Holdings:** 6500 books; 4000 bound periodical volumes. **Subscriptions:** 428 journals and other serials.

★8513★ WALTHAM WESTON HOSPITAL AND MEDICAL CENTER
MEDICAL LIBRARY
Hope Ave.
Waltham, MA 02254-9116   Phone: (617) 647-6261
Mr. Frank Landry, Med.Libn.
Subjects: Medicine, surgery, psychiatry, nursing, hospital administration. **Holdings:** 1000 books; 1600 bound periodical volumes; 2 VF drawers of pamphlets; 1200 volumes of unbound periodicals. **Subscriptions:** 153 journals and other serials.

★8514★ TOBEY HOSPITAL
STILLMAN LIBRARY
High St.
Wareham, MA 02571   Phone: (508) 295-0880
Athena Harvey, Libn.
Subjects: Medicine, surgery, nursing, hospital administration, basic sciences. **Holdings:** 1000 books; vertical files. **Subscriptions:** 50 journals and other serials; 5 newspapers.

★8515★ PERKINS SCHOOL FOR THE BLIND
SAMUEL P. HAYES RESEARCH LIBRARY
175 N. Beacon St.
Watertown, MA 02172   Phone: (617) 924-3434
Kenneth A. Stuckey, Res.Libn.
Subjects: Nonmedical aspects of blindness and deaf-blindness, including education, rehabilitation, welfare. **Holdings:** 18,000 volumes; bound newspaper clippings; Helen Keller material. **Subscriptions:** 125 journals and other serials.

★8516★ U.S. FOOD AND DRUG ADMINISTRATION
WINCHESTER ENGINEERING AND ANALYTICAL CENTER
LIBRARY
109 Holton St.
Winchester, MA 01890   Phone: (617) 729-5700
Subjects: Radiology, medical roentgenology, chemistry, physics, nuclear science, oceanography, statistics, medicine, electronics. **Holdings:** 1000 books; 710 bound periodical volumes; technical documents; miscellaneous reports; 20 VF drawers of unbound materials. **Subscriptions:** 109 journals and other serials.

★8517★ MEDICAL CENTER OF CENTRAL MASSACHUSETTS
MEDICAL CENTER LIBRARY SERVICES
119 Belmont St.
Worcester, MA 01605   Phone: (508) 793-6421
Terry Simeone, Dir., Lib.Serv.
Subjects: Medicine, nursing, dentistry. **Holdings:** 4000 books; 8000 bound periodical volumes. **Subscriptions:** 250 journals and other serials.

★8518★ ST. VINCENT HOSPITAL
JOHN J. DUMPHY MEMORIAL LIBRARY
25 Winthrop St.
Worcester, MA 01604   Phone: (508) 798-6117
Kris Benishek, Libn.
Subjects: Medicine, allied health sciences. **Holdings:** 1500 books; 5500 bound periodical volumes. **Subscriptions:** 162 journals and other serials.

★8519★ TSI
MASON RESEARCH INSTITUTE
LIBRARY
57 Union St.
Worcester, MA 01608   Phone: (508) 791-0931
H. Smith, Dir.
Subjects: Biomedical sciences, toxicology, pathology, immunobiology, endocrinology, reproductive physiology, biochemistry, tissue culture, veterinary medicine. **Holdings:** 1700 books, technical reports, directories, abstracts, indexes, reprints, bibliographies. **Subscriptions:** 35 journals and other serials.

★8520★ UNIVERSITY OF MASSACHUSETTS MEDICAL SCHOOL AND WORCESTER DISTRICT MEDICAL SOCIETY
LIBRARY
55 N. Lake Ave.
Worcester, MA 01655   Phone: (508) 856-2511
Donald J. Morton, Lib.Dir.
Subjects: Medicine, health sciences, human biology. **Holdings:** 38,426 books; 99,604 bound periodical volumes. **Subscriptions:** 2358 journals and other serials.

★8521★ WORCESTER CITY HOSPITAL
MEDICAL LIBRARY
26 Queen St.
Worcester, MA 01610   Phone: (508) 799-8186
Donrue M. Larson, Lib.Asst.
Subjects: Medicine and allied health sciences. **Holdings:** 1500 books; 4500 bound periodical volumes. **Subscriptions:** 200 journals and other serials.

Michigan

★8522★ EMMA L. BIXBY HOSPITAL
PATMOS/JONES MEMORIAL LIBRARY
818 Riverside Ave.
Adrian, MI 49221   Phone: (517) 263-0711
Cinda Walton, Dir. of Med.Rec.
Subjects: Medicine, surgery, obstetrics-gynecology, pediatrics. **Holdings:** 500 books; 150 bound periodical volumes. **Subscriptions:** 25 journals and other serials.

★8523★ U.S. DEPARTMENT OF VETERANS AFFAIRS
MEDICAL CENTER LIBRARY SERVICE
Southfield and Outer Dr.
Allen Park, MI 48101   Phone: (313) 562-3380
Arlene Devlin, Chf., Lib.Serv.
Subjects: Surgery, oncology, internal medicine, psychiatry, psychology, health management. **Holdings:** 8000 books; 10,000 bound periodical volumes; 1500 reels of microfilm. **Subscriptions:** 450 journals and other serials; 10 newspapers.

★8524★ CATHERINE MCAULEY HEALTH CENTER
RIECKER MEMORIAL LIBRARY
Box 995
Ann Arbor, MI 48106   Phone: (313) 572-3045
Metta T. Lansdale, Jr., Mgr., Lib.Serv.
Subjects: Surgery, medicine, nursing, health administration, patient health information, computers in health care. **Holdings:** 5000 books; 200 AV programs. **Subscriptions:** 600 journals and other serials.

★8525★ HERMAN MILLER RESEARCH CORPORATION
LIBRARY
3971 S. Research Park Dr.
Ann Arbor, MI 48108   Phone: (313) 994-0200
Dallas Moore, Libn.
Subjects: Gerontology, rehabilitation. **Holdings:** 200 books. **Subscriptions:** 82 journals and other serials.

★8526★ MICHIGAN DEPARTMENT OF MENTAL HEALTH
CENTER FOR FORENSIC PSYCHIATRY
STAFF LIBRARY
PO Box 2060
Ann Arbor, MI 48106   Phone: (313) 429-0862
Lois J. Staresina, Libn.
Subjects: Forensic psychiatry, psychiatry, medicine, psychology. **Holdings:** 2500 books; 400 audio- and videotapes. **Subscriptions:** 75 journals and other serials.

★8527★   U.S. DEPARTMENT OF VETERANS AFFAIRS
HOSPITAL LIBRARY
2215 Fuller Rd.
Ann Arbor, MI 48105   Phone: (313) 761-5385
Vickie Smith, Chf.Libn.
Subjects: Medicine, patient education. Holdings: 4610 books; 3610 bound
periodical volumes. Subscriptions: 345 journals and other serials.

★8528★   UNIVERSITY OF MICHIGAN
ALFRED TAUBMAN MEDICAL LIBRARY
1135 E. Catherine
Ann Arbor, MI 48109-0726   Phone: (313) 764-1210
Suzanne Grefsheim, Hd.Libn.
Subjects: Basic medical sciences, clinical medicine, nursing, pharmacy,
history of medicine. Holdings: 300,792 volumes. Subscriptions: 3413
journals and other serials.

★8529★   UNIVERSITY OF MICHIGAN
DENTISTRY LIBRARY
1100 Dental Bldg.
Ann Arbor, MI 48109-1078   Phone: (313) 764-1526
Susan I. Seger, Hd.Libn.
Subjects: Dentistry. Holdings: 48,400 volumes; 25 VF drawers of pam-
phlets. Subscriptions: 698 journals and other serials.

★8530★   UNIVERSITY OF MICHIGAN
SCHOOL OF PUBLIC HEALTH
DEPARTMENT OF POPULATION PLANNING AND
   INTERNATIONAL HEALTH
REFERENCE COLLECTION
Ann Arbor, MI 48109   Phone: (313) 763-5732
Subjects: National and international population policy and family plan-
ning; educational and medical aspects of family planning; family planning
systems; demography. Holdings: 500 books; 6000 unbound reports and
documents; 1000 country files representing 70 countries; family planning
program data; reprints; documents; conference proceedings. Subscriptions:
100 journals and other serials.

★8531★   UNIVERSITY OF MICHIGAN
SCHOOL OF PUBLIC HEALTH
PUBLIC HEALTH LIBRARY
M2030 School of Public Health
Ann Arbor, MI 48109   Phone: (313) 764-5473
Sandra C. Dow, Hd.Libn.
Subjects: Public health, environmental and industrial health, epidemiolo-
gy, population planning, health services management and policy, biostatis-
tics, health behavior, health education. Holdings: 64,000 volumes; 581
pamphlet boxes. Subscriptions: 420 journals and other serials.

★8532★   WARNER-LAMBERT/PARKE-DAVIS
RESEARCH LIBRARY
2800 Plymouth Rd.
Ann Arbor, MI 48105   Phone: (313) 996-7860
Sharon Lehman, Dir.
Subjects: Chemistry, pharmacology, medicine, toxicology, microbiology,
pathology. Holdings: 17,203 books; 13,532 bound periodical volumes;
7900 microfilm cassettes; 98,000 computerized and indexed product
documents; 3767 reprints. Subscriptions: 1000 journals and other serials.

★8533★   BATTLE CREEK ADVENTIST HOSPITAL
PROFESSIONAL LIBRARY
165 N. Washington Ave.
Battle Creek, MI 49016   Phone: (616) 964-7121
Lanette J. Penrod, Libn.
Subjects: Psychiatry, psychology, social work, substance abuse. Holdings:
540 books; 253 AV programs. Subscriptions: 55 journals and other serials.

★8534★   BATTLE CREEK HEALTH SYSTEM
PROFESSIONAL LIBRARY
300 North Ave.
Battle Creek, MI 49016   Phone: (616) 966-8331
Robin Alanen Mosher, Libn.
Subjects: Medicine, nursing. Holdings: 2758 volumes; 400 audio cassettes;
25 video cassettes. Subscriptions: 500 journals and other serials.

★8535★   U.S. DEPARTMENT OF VETERANS AFFAIRS
MEDICAL CENTER LIBRARY
Battle Creek, MI 49016   Phone: (616) 966-5600
Subjects: Psychiatry, neurology, psychology. Holdings: 2554 books; 913
bound periodical volumes; 1856 volumes of journals on microfilm.
Subscriptions: 423 journals and other serials; 21 newspapers.

★8536★   BAY MEDICAL CENTER
HEALTH SCIENCES LIBRARY
1900 Columbus Ave.
Bay City, MI 48708-6880   Phone: (517) 894-3782
Barbara Kormelink, Hea.Sci.Libn.
Subjects: Medicine, nursing, hospital administration, allied health sciences. Holdings: 2500 books; 5210 bound periodical volumes; 200 slide
sets; 110 titles on microfilm; 355 AV programs; 12 VF drawers of
pamphlets. Subscriptions: 285 journals and other serials.

★8537★   FERRIS STATE UNIVERSITY
ABIGAIL SMITH TIMME LIBRARY
901 S. State St.
Big Rapids, MI 49307   Phone: (616) 592-3602
Dr. Lawrence J. McCrank, Dean
Subjects: Pharmacy, optometry, allied health sciences, business, occupational education, criminal justice, engineering technology. Holdings:
309,352 volumes; 188,650 titles; 94,244 periodicals; 56,198 pamphlets and
documents; 39,597 titles in microform; 13,270 phonograph records, tapes,
and slides; 135 films. Subscriptions: 2099 journals and other serials; 22
newspapers.

★8538★   FERRIS STATE UNIVERSITY
SCHOOL OF PHARMACY
PHARMACY READING ROOM
901 S. State St.
Big Rapids, MI 49307   Phone: (616) 592-2338
Pat Hoek, Libn.
Subjects: Pharmacy, pharmaceutical sciences. Holdings: 1700 books;
pamphlets; reprints; 150 tapes, slides, filmstrips; Iowa Drug Information
Service, 1966 to present, on microfiche; DRUGDEX. Subscriptions: 160
journals and other serials.

★8539★   MICHIGAN DEPARTMENT OF MENTAL HEALTH
COLDWATER REGIONAL MENTAL HEALTH CENTER
MEDICAL STAFF LIBRARY
620 Marshall Rd.
Coldwater, MI 49036   Phone: (517) 278-3423
Eileen VanVleet, Libn.
Subjects: Mental health, mental illness, mental retardation. Holdings: 3000
books. Subscriptions: 100 journals and other serials.

★8540★   OAKWOOD HOSPITAL
HEALTH SCIENCE LIBRARY
18101 Oakwood Blvd.
Box 2500
Dearborn, MI 48123-2500   Phone: (313) 593-7685
Sharon A. Phillips, Dir.
Subjects: Medicine, allied health sciences. Holdings: 13,000 volumes; AV
programs. Subscriptions: 615 journals and other serials; 8 newspapers.

★8541★   ASH STEVENS, INC.
LIBRARY
5861 John C. Lodge Fwy.
Detroit, MI 48202   Phone: (313) 872-6400
Dr. Arthur B. Ash, Chf.Exec.Off.
Subjects: Experimental and clinical drug research and development.
Holdings: 800 books; 600 bound periodical volumes; 500 reports.

★8542★   CHARFOOS & CHRISTENSEN, P.C.
LIBRARY
4000 Penobscot Bldg.
Detroit, MI 48226   Phone: (313) 963-8080
Nora L.M. Shumake, Dir. of Libs.
Subjects: Law, medicine. Holdings: 560 books; 51 bound periodical
volumes; 65 other cataloged items. Subscriptions: 44 journals and other
serials.

★8543★ CHILDREN'S HOSPITAL OF MICHIGAN
MEDICAL LIBRARY
3901 Beaubien
Detroit, MI 48201   Phone: (313) 745-5322
Michele S. Klein, Dir., Lib.Serv.
Subjects: Pediatrics, growth and development, genetics, pediatric clinical research. **Holdings:** 3000 books; 8000 bound periodical volumes; 40 audiotapes. **Subscriptions:** 305 journals and other serials.

★8544★ DETROIT MACOMB HOSPITAL CORPORATION
DETROIT RIVERVIEW HOSPITAL
HOSPITAL LIBRARY
7733 E. Jefferson
Detroit, MI 48214   Phone: (313) 499-4123
Donna Marshall, Corp.Dir. of Libs.
Subjects: Medicine. **Holdings:** 2600 books; 2000 bound periodical volumes. **Subscriptions:** 290 journals and other serials.

★8545★ DETROIT PSYCHIATRIC INSTITUTE
LIBRARY
1151 Taylor
Detroit, MI 48202   Phone: (313) 876-4170
Rita H. Bigman, Libn.
Subjects: Psychiatry, psychoanalysis, social work, psychology, psychiatric nursing, general medicine. **Holdings:** 3300 books; 350 bound periodical volumes; 9 VF drawers of psychoanalysis and psychiatry articles. **Subscriptions:** 89 journals and other serials.

★8546★ DETROIT RECEIVING HOSPITAL AND UNIVERSITY
 HEALTH CENTER
LIBRARY
4201 St. Antoine
Detroit, MI 48201   Phone: (313) 745-4475
Cherrie M. Mudloff, Libn.
Subjects: Medicine. **Holdings:** 3000 books. **Subscriptions:** 286 journals and other serials.

★8547★ HARPER HOSPITAL
DEPARTMENT OF LIBRARIES
3990 John R St.
Detroit, MI 48201-2097   Phone: (313) 745-1443
Sandra I. Martin, Supv., Lib./AV Serv.
Subjects: Medicine, nursing, allied health sciences, hospital and business administration. **Holdings:** 9000 book titles; 19,000 bound periodical volumes; 8 VF drawers of pamphlets; audio- and videotapes; AV programs. **Subscriptions:** 720 journals and other serials.

★8548★ HARPER-GRACE HOSPITALS
GRACE HOSPITAL DIVISION
OSCAR LE SEURE PROFESSIONAL LIBRARY
18700 Meyers Rd.
Detroit, MI 48235   Phone: (313) 966-3276
Frances M. Phillips, Dir., Lib. & AV Serv.
Subjects: Medicine, medical specialties, nursing. **Holdings:** 3500 books; 6500 bound periodical volumes; 391 AV programs. **Subscriptions:** 251 journals and other serials.

★8549★ HENRY FORD HOSPITAL
FRANK J. SLADEN LIBRARY
2799 W. Grand Blvd.
Detroit, MI 48202   Phone: (313) 876-2550
Nardina L. Nameth, Dir., Lib.Serv.
Subjects: Medicine, nursing, administration and management, allied health and basic sciences. **Holdings:** 18,000 books; 70,000 bound periodical volumes. **Subscriptions:** 1100 journals and other serials.

★8550★ HUTZEL HOSPITAL
MEDICAL LIBRARY
4707 St. Antoine Blvd.
Detroit, MI 48201   Phone: (313) 745-7178
Jean M. Brennan, Dir., Lib.Serv.
Subjects: Obstetrics and gynecology, orthopedics, ophthalmology, substance abuse, arthritis/rheumatology. **Holdings:** 2500 books; 10,000 bound periodical volumes; 6 VF drawers; Audio-Digest tapes in surgery, internal medicine, obstetrics, gynecology; state medical association journals. **Subscriptions:** 656 journals and other serials.

★8551★ LAFAYETTE CLINIC
LIBRARY
951 E. Lafayette
Detroit, MI 48207   Phone: (313) 256-9596
Nancy E. Ward, Libn.
Subjects: Psychiatry, psychology, psychopharmacology, geriatrics, neurology, movement disorders, affective disorders, Alzheimer's Disease, memory disorders, Parkinsonism. **Holdings:** 4897 books; 1473 bound periodical volumes; 10 years of unbound periodicals. **Subscriptions:** 146 journals and other serials.

★8552★ METRO MEDICAL GROUP
DETROIT NORTHWEST
MEDICAL LIBRARY
1800 Tuxedo Ave.
Detroit, MI 48206   Phone: (313) 252-1204
Jerry Stuenkel, Med.Libn.
Subjects: Medicine, nursing, health maintenance organizations, allied health. **Holdings:** 2010 books; 5000 bound periodical volumes. **Subscriptions:** 350 journals and other serials.

★8553★ MICHIGAN CANCER FOUNDATION
LEONARD N. SIMONS RESEARCH LIBRARY
110 E. Warren
Detroit, MI 48201   Phone: (313) 833-0710
C.J. Glodek, Dir.
Subjects: Cancer research, allied health sciences. **Holdings:** 3000 books; 700 bound periodical volumes; 500 pamphlets and reprints; institutional archives. **Subscriptions:** 80 journals and other serials.

★8554★ MICHIGAN HEALTH CENTER
HEALTH SCIENCE LIBRARY
2700 Martin Luther King Jr. Blvd.
Detroit, MI 48208   Phone: (313) 361-8071
Carolyn A. Hough, Dir.
Subjects: Medicine, osteopathy, psychiatry. **Holdings:** 3000 books; 1200 bound periodical volumes; 350 video cassettes; 600 audio cassettes. **Subscriptions:** 300 journals and other serials.

★8555★ MOUNT CARMEL MERCY HOSPITAL
MEDICAL LIBRARY
6071 W. Outer Dr.
Detroit, MI 48235   Phone: (313) 927-7073
Jill Van Buskirk, Dir.
Subjects: Medicine, surgery, obstetrics, gynecology, radiology, pathology, pediatrics, nursing. **Holdings:** 5000 books; 8500 bound periodical volumes; 900 Audio-Digest tapes. **Subscriptions:** 450 journals and other serials.

★8556★ NORTH DETROIT GENERAL HOSPITAL
MEDICAL LIBRARY
3105 Carpenter
Detroit, MI 48212   Phone: (313) 369-3000
Subjects: Clinical medicine, surgery, nursing, allied health sciences. **Holdings:** 400 books; 100 bound periodical volumes. **Subscriptions:** 65 journals and other serials.

★8557★ PLUNKETT & COONEY
LAW LIBRARY
900 Marquette Bldg.
Detroit, MI 48226   Phone: (313) 983-4877
Melanie J. Dunshee, Hd.Libn.
Subjects: Medical liability; products liability; insurance; municipal liability; corporate law. **Holdings:** 13,000 volumes; microfiche.

★8558★ REHABILITATION INSTITUTE, INC.
LEARNING RESOURCES CENTER
261 Mack Blvd.
Detroit, MI 48201   Phone: (313) 745-9860
Daria Shackelford, Med.Libn./Dir.
Subjects: Physical medicine, rehabilitation, general medicine, physical therapy, occupational therapy, social service, patient education. **Holdings:** 3200 books; 3200 bound periodical volumes; 6 VF drawers of pamphlets; 5 boxes of reports; 1 VF drawer of reprints; 15 16mm films; 1000 35mm slides; 400 videotapes. **Subscriptions:** 125 journals and other serials.

★8559★   ST. JOHN HOSPITAL
MEDICAL LIBRARY
22101 Moross Rd.
Detroit, MI 48236   Phone: (313) 343-3733
Ellen E. O'Donnell, Dir.
Subjects: Medicine, nursing, allied health sciences, health care administration and management. **Holdings:** 5000 books; 5900 bound periodical volumes; 600 AV programs; 10 VF drawers of pamphlets, documents; 7 series of medical audiotapes; 245 journal titles on microfiche. **Subscriptions:** 525 journals and other serials.

★8560★   SARATOGA COMMUNITY HOSPITAL
HEALTH SCIENCE LIBRARY
15000 Gratiot Ave.
Detroit, MI 48205   Phone: (313) 245-1200
Viju Karnik, Med.Libn.
Subjects: Medicine, nursing, hospital administration. **Holdings:** 1100 books; 300 bound periodical volumes. **Subscriptions:** 137 journals and other serials.

★8561★   SINAI HOSPITAL OF DETROIT
SAMUEL FRANK MEDICAL LIBRARY
6767 W. Outer Dr.
Detroit, MI 48235   Phone: (313) 493-5140
Barbara L. Finn, Dir., Med.Lib.
Subjects: Medicine, nursing, and allied health sciences. **Holdings:** 9600 books; 15,135 bound periodical volumes; 9 VF drawers of reprints and pamphlets; cassettes; Audio-Digest tapes. **Subscriptions:** 571 journals and other serials.

★8562★   UNIVERSITY OF DETROIT
SCHOOL OF DENTISTRY LIBRARY
2931 E. Jefferson Ave.
Detroit, MI 48207   Phone: (313) 446-1817
M. Agnes Shoup, Dir.
Subjects: Dentistry. **Holdings:** 13,000 books; 15,000 bound periodical volumes. **Subscriptions:** 450 journals and other serials.

★8563★   WAYNE STATE UNIVERSITY
VERA PARSHALL SHIFFMAN MEDICAL LIBRARY
4325 Brush St.
Detroit, MI 48201   Phone: (313) 577-1088
Faith Van Toll, Dir.
Subjects: Clinical medicine, pharmacy, and allied health sciences. **Holdings:** 79,015 books; 123,648 bound periodical volumes. **Subscriptions:** 2924 journals and other serials.

★8564★   MICHIGAN STATE UNIVERSITY
CLINICAL CENTER LIBRARY
A-137, Clinical Center
East Lansing, MI 48823-1313   Phone: (517) 353-3037
Leslie M. Behm, Libn. II
Subjects: Clinical and osteopathic medicine, nursing. **Holdings:** 7004 volumes. **Subscriptions:** 157 journals and other serials.

★8565★   MICHIGAN STATE UNIVERSITY
HUMAN ECOLOGY LIBRARY
Human Ecology Bldg., Rm. 2
East Lansing, MI 48824-1030   Phone: (517) 355-7737
Stephanie C. Perentesis, Libn.
Subjects: Human ecology and environmental design, family/child ecology, human nutrition. **Holdings:** 4200 books; 800 bound periodical volumes; 860 theses and dissertations; AV materials; pictures; pamphlets; educational testing instruments. **Subscriptions:** 100 journals and other serials; 5 newspapers.

★8566★   MICHIGAN STATE UNIVERSITY
SCIENCE LIBRARY
East Lansing, MI 48824-1048   Phone: (517) 355-2347
Carole S. Armstrong, Hd., Sci.Libs.
Subjects: Medicine, biological sciences, agriculture, veterinary medicine, nursing, technology, human ecology, history of science. **Holdings:** 410,000 volumes. **Subscriptions:** 6000 journals and other serials.

★8567★   MICHIGAN STATE UNIVERSITY
VETERINARY CLINICAL CENTER LIBRARY
A 57 Veterinary Clinical Center
East Lansing, MI 48823-1314   Phone: (517) 353-5099
Leslie M. Behm, Libn. II
Subjects: Clinical veterinary medicine. **Holdings:** 2624 volumes. **Subscriptions:** 71 journals and other serials.

★8568★   BOTSFORD GENERAL HOSPITAL
HOSPITAL LIBRARY AND MEDIA CENTER
28050 Grand River Ave.
Farmington Hills, MI 48336-5933   Phone: (313) 471-8515
Deborah L. Adams, Dir.
Subjects: Medicine, nursing, health administration. **Holdings:** 2600 books; 260 journal titles on microfilm; AV programs. **Subscriptions:** 260 journals and other serials.

★8569★   MERCY HEALTH SERVICES
RESOURCE CENTER
34605 12 Mile Rd.
Farmington Hills, MI 48331   Phone: (313) 489-6754
Bonnie Tanase-Cairns
Subjects: Health administration, medicine, management. **Holdings:** 2500 books. **Subscriptions:** 150 journals and other serials; 2 newspapers.

★8570★   FLINT OSTEOPATHIC HOSPITAL
DR. E. HERZOG MEMORIAL MEDICAL LIBRARY
3921 Beecher Rd.
Flint, MI 48532-3699   Phone: (313) 762-4587
Doris M. Blauet, Dir.
Subjects: Clinical medicine. **Holdings:** 2000 books; 7000 bound periodical volumes. **Subscriptions:** 260 journals and other serials.

★8571★   HURLEY MEDICAL CENTER
COMMUNITY HEALTH INFORMATION LIBRARY
1 Hurley Plaza
Flint, MI 48502
Martha Studaker, Dir.
Subjects: Health. **Holdings:** 1200 books.

★8572★   HURLEY MEDICAL CENTER
HAMADY HEALTH SCIENCES LIBRARY
1 Hurley Plaza
Flint, MI 48502   Phone: (313) 257-9427
Martha Studaker, Dir.
Subjects: Medicine, nursing, hospital administration, health. **Holdings:** 8000 books; 1065 AV programs; pamphlet files. **Subscriptions:** 650 journals and other serials.

★8573★   MCLAREN GENERAL HOSPITAL
MEDICAL LIBRARY
401 Ballenger Hwy.
Flint, MI 48532   Phone: (313) 762-2141
Lea Ann McGaugh, Med.Lib.Mgr.
Subjects: Medicine, nursing, allied health sciences. **Holdings:** 3000 books; 4000 bound periodical volumes. **Subscriptions:** 300 journals and other serials.

★8574★   ST. JOSEPH HOSPITAL
HEALTH SCIENCES LIBRARY
302 Kensington Ave.
Flint, MI 48503-2000   Phone: (313) 762-8519
Ria Brown Lukes, Med.Libn.
Subjects: Medicine, nursing. **Holdings:** 3000 books; 8500 bound periodical volumes; 1227 audio cassettes; 250 video cassettes. **Subscriptions:** 245 journals and other serials.

★8575★   GERBER PRODUCTS COMPANY
CORPORATE LIBRARY
445 State St.
Fremont, MI 49413   Phone: (616) 928-2631
Sherrie Harris, Corp.Libn.
Subjects: Food processing, infant nutrition and development, pediatrics, business administration, international marketing, chemistry, microbiology, agriculture, quality control. **Holdings:** 6500 books; 2800 bound periodical volumes; 125 AV programs; 2000 patents on microfiche; 10,000 photoprints and pamphlets in hardcopy and on microfiche. **Subscriptions:** 1000 journals and other serials; 20 newspapers.

★8576★ GARDEN CITY OSTEOPATHIC HOSPITAL
MEDICAL/STAFF LIBRARY
6245 Inkster Rd.
Garden City, MI 48135   Phone: (313) 458-4311
A.J. Brabant
Subjects: Medicine, surgery, nursing, orthopedics, pathology, laboratory sciences. **Holdings:** 2500 books; 5000 bound periodical volumes; journals on microfiche; AV items. **Subscriptions:** 169 journals and other serials; 6 newspapers.

★8577★ BLODGETT MEMORIAL MEDICAL CENTER
RICHARD ROOT SMITH LIBRARY
1840 Wealthy St., SE
Grand Rapids, MI 49506   Phone: (616) 774-7624
Brian Simmons, Med.Libn.
Subjects: Medicine, surgery, allied health sciences. **Holdings:** 1800 books; 7100 bound periodical volumes; 500 audiotape cassettes; 3000 anatomical slides; 3000 unbound periodicals. **Subscriptions:** 250 journals and other serials.

★8578★ BUTTERWORTH HOSPITAL
BUTTERWORTH NURSING LIBRARY
100 Michigan, NE
Grand Rapids, MI 49503   Phone: (616) 774-1779
Diane Hummel, Nurs.Libn.
Subjects: Nursing and nursing education, psychology. **Holdings:** 2564 books; 1702 bound periodical volumes; 580 AV programs. **Subscriptions:** 106 journals and other serials.

★8579★ BUTTERWORTH HOSPITAL
HEALTH SCIENCES LIBRARY
100 Michigan, NE
Grand Rapids, MI 49503-9979   Phone: (616) 774-1655
Eileen M. Dechow, Dir.
Subjects: Medicine, surgery, medical/surgical specialties. **Holdings:** 3000 books; 6500 bound periodical volumes; pamphlets; 1500 audio and video cassettes. **Subscriptions:** 230 periodicals.

★8580★ PINE REST CHRISTIAN HOSPITAL
WEST MICHIGAN MENTAL HEALTH INFORMATION CENTER
PO Box 165
Grand Rapids, MI 49501-0165   Phone: (616) 455-5000
Thomas Van Dam, Libn.
Subjects: Psychiatry, psychiatric nursing, psychiatric social work, clinical psychology. **Holdings:** 4000 books; cassette tapes. **Subscriptions:** 140 journals and other serials.

★8581★ RIGHT TO LIFE OF MICHIGAN
STATE CENTRAL RESOURCE CENTER
920 Cherry, SE
Grand Rapids, MI 49506   Phone: (616) 451-0225
Sheri Hicks, Dir.
Subjects: Abortion, euthanasia, infanticide, legislation. **Holdings:** Books; videotapes; 16mm films; audio cassettes; slides; VF files; booklets; newspaper clippings; pamphlets.

★8582★ ST. MARY'S HOSPITAL
LIBRARY
200 Jefferson, SE
Grand Rapids, MI 49503   Phone: (616) 774-6243
Mary A. Hanson, Med.Libn.
Subjects: Medicine, nursing. **Holdings:** 3500 books; 8000 bound periodical volumes; 12 VF drawers. **Subscriptions:** 230 journals and other serials.

★8583★ BON SECOURS HOSPITAL
HEALTH SCIENCE LIBRARY
468 Cadieux Rd.
Grosse Pointe, MI 48230   Phone: (313) 343-1619
Beth S. Navalta, Lib.Supv.
Subjects: Medicine, nursing, hospital administration, pharmacology. **Holdings:** 4500 books; 3300 bound periodical volumes; 170 slide/tape sets; 220 videotapes; 628 AV programs; 200 government documents; 8 VF drawers of clippings, pamphlets, and newspaper articles. **Subscriptions:** 470 journals and other serials; 5 newspapers.

★8584★ COTTAGE HOSPITAL OF GROSSE POINTE
MEDICAL LIBRARY
159 Kercheval Ave.
Grosse Pointe Farms, MI 48236   Phone: (313) 884-8600
Carol Attar, Lib.Dir.
Subjects: Medicine, nursing, and allied health sciences. **Holdings:** 1272 books; 4 VF drawers of clippings and pamphlets; video cassettes; audio cassettes. **Subscriptions:** 145 journals and other serials.

★8585★ PENNOCK HOSPITAL
MEDICAL LIBRARY
1009 W. Green St.
Hastings, MI 49058   Phone: (616) 945-3451
Pam Noffke, Info.Spec.
Subjects: Medicine, nursing, pharmacy, allied health sciences. **Holdings:** 750 books. **Subscriptions:** 125 journals and other serials.

★8586★ DETROIT OSTEOPATHIC HOSPITAL
LIBRARY
12523 3rd Ave.
Highland Park, MI 48203   Phone: (313) 252-4830
Gayle A. Williams, Dir.
Subjects: Internal medicine, orthopedics, surgery, nephrology, cardiology, oncology. **Holdings:** 1700 books; 4200 bound periodical volumes; 400 audio cassettes. **Subscriptions:** 188 journals and other serials.

★8587★ HOLLAND COMMUNITY HOSPITAL
HOSPITAL AND MEDICAL STAFF LIBRARY
602 Michigan Ave.
Holland, MI 49423   Phone: (616) 394-3107
Eleanor Lopez, Libn.
Subjects: Medicine, hospital administration, nursing. **Holdings:** 1600 books; 1500 bound periodical volumes. **Subscriptions:** 220 journals and other serials.

★8588★ U.S. DEPARTMENT OF VETERANS AFFAIRS
MEDICAL CENTER LIBRARY
E. H St.
Iron Mountain, MI 49801   Phone: (906) 774-3300
Jeanne M. Durocher, Chf., Lib.Serv.
Subjects: Medicine, surgery, nursing, patient education. **Holdings:** 900 books; 1553 bound periodical volumes; 15 files of patient education materials; 550 video cassettes; 50 audio cassettes; 77 filmstrips and slide/tape kits. **Subscriptions:** 253 journals and other serials; 29 newspapers.

★8589★ W.A. FOOTE MEMORIAL HOSPITAL
MEDICAL LIBRARY
205 N. East Ave.
Jackson, MI 49201   Phone: (517) 788-4705
Janet Zimmerman
Subjects: Medicine, nursing, and allied health sciences. **Holdings:** 1200 books. **Subscriptions:** 250 journals and other serials.

★8590★ BORGESS MEDICAL CENTER
HEALTH INFORMATION LIBRARY
1521 Gull Rd.
Kalamazoo, MI 49001   Phone: (616) 383-7360
Sr. Norma Harvey, Lib.Mgr.
Subjects: Medicine, nursing, pharmacology, allied health sciences. **Holdings:** 4500 books; 6500 periodical volumes, hardcopy or microform; AV programs; models; 12 drawers of pamphlets and information files. **Subscriptions:** 400 journals and other serials.

★8591★ BRONSON METHODIST HOSPITAL
HEALTH SCIENCES LIBRARY
252 Lovell St., E.
Kalamazoo, MI 49007   Phone: (616) 341-6318
Marge Kars, Dir., Lib.Serv.
Subjects: Medicine, nursing, and allied health sciences. **Holdings:** 11,000 volumes; 9 VF drawers of information files. **Subscriptions:** 500 journals and other serials.

★8592★   MICHIGAN DEPARTMENT OF MENTAL HEALTH
KALAMAZOO REGIONAL PSYCHIATRIC HOSPITAL
STAFF LIBRARY
1312 Oakland Dr.
Box A
Kalamazoo, MI 49008   Phone: (616) 385-1265
Carol Aebli, Lib.Dir.
Subjects: Psychiatry, nursing, psychiatric nursing, psychology, social services. **Holdings:** 1780 books; 830 bound periodical volumes. **Subscriptions:** 90 journals and other serials.

★8593★   UPJOHN COMPANY
CORPORATE BUSINESS LIBRARY
Kalamazoo, MI 49001   Phone: (616) 323-6352
Valerie Noble, Mgr.
Subjects: Business and finance, management and supervision, marketing, self-improvement, microcomputer applications, pharmaceuticals and drugs. **Holdings:** 5000 books; SRI-BIP reports; annual reports; microforms; audio cassettes; video cassettes; IBM PC-compatible software; road maps to major U.S. cities. **Subscriptions:** 250 journals and other serials.

★8594★   UPJOHN COMPANY
CORPORATE TECHNICAL LIBRARY
7284-267-21
Kalamazoo, MI 49001   Phone: (616) 385-6414
Lorraine Schulte, Dir.
Subjects: Chemistry, biotechnology, biochemistry, pharmacology, biomedical and pharmaceutical sciences, statistics, computer science. **Holdings:** 23,500 books; 58,000 bound periodical volumes. **Subscriptions:** 1300 journals and other serials.

★8595★   UPJOHN COMPANY
MEDICAL LIBRARY SERVICES
Upjohn Laboratories
9184-298-04D
Kalamazoo, MI 49001   Phone: (616) 329-8086
L. Pauline Sattler, Mgr.
Subjects: Clinical medicine, drug information, clinical trials. **Holdings:** 700 books; 550 microfilm cartridges. **Subscriptions:** 325 journals and other serials.

★8596★   EDWARD W. SPARROW HOSPITAL
MEDICAL LIBRARY
1215 E. Michigan Ave.
Box 30480
Lansing, MI 48909-7980   Phone: (517) 483-2274
Doris H. Asher, Med.Libn.
Subjects: Medicine, nursing. **Holdings:** 3300 books. **Subscriptions:** 310 journals and other serials.

★8597★   INGHAM MEDICAL CENTER CORPORATION
JOHN W. CHI MEMORIAL MEDICAL LIBRARY
401 W. Greenlawn Ave.
Lansing, MI 48910-2819   Phone: (517) 334-2270
David G. Keddle, Dir.
Subjects: Medicine, nursing, pharmacology, hospital administration, allied health management, consumer health. **Holdings:** 10,500 books; 10,000 bound periodical volumes; 1000 audio cassettes. **Subscriptions:** 850 journals and other serials; 7 newspapers.

★8598★   LANSING GENERAL HOSPITAL, OSTEOPATHIC
K.M. BAKER MEMORIAL LIBRARY
2727 S. Pennsylvania
Lansing, MI 48910-3490   Phone: (517) 377-8389
Judith A. Barnes, Med.Libn.
Subjects: Medicine, sports medicine, nursing, substance abuse, rehabilitation, osteopathy, orthodpedics, geriatric psychiatry. **Holdings:** 2800 books; 2800 bound periodical volumes; 1000 microfiche of journals; 800 Audio-Digest tapes; 75 slide/tape programs. **Subscriptions:** 387 journals and other serials.

★8599★   MICHIGAN DEPARTMENT OF PUBLIC HEALTH
LIBRARY RESOURCE CENTER
3423 N. Logan St.
Box 30195
Lansing, MI 48909   Phone: (517) 335-8394
Bill Nelton, Libn.
Subjects: Public health. **Holdings:** 7000 bound periodical volumes. **Subscriptions:** 300 journals and other serials.

★8600★   MICHIGAN PROTECTION AND ADVOCACY SERVICE
LIBRARY
109 W. Michigan Ave., Ste. 900
Lansing, MI 48933   Phone: (517) 487-1755
Maureen MacLaughlin
Subjects: Developmental disabilities, human services, mental health, advocacy, special education. **Holdings:** 2000 books; 700 reports. **Subscriptions:** 15 journals and other serials; 215 newsletters.

★8601★   MICHIGAN SOCIETY FOR AUTISTIC CITIZENS
LIBRARY
530 W. Ionia, Ste. C
Lansing, MI 48933   Phone: (517) 487-9260
Subjects: Autism, developmental disabilities. **Holdings:** 1000 books.

★8602★   RIGHT TO LIFE OF MICHIGAN
RESOURCE CENTER
Knapp's Centre, Ste. 588
300 S. Washington Sq.
Lansing, MI 48933   Phone: (517) 487-3376
Malika Abdur-Rashid
Subjects: Abortion, euthanasia, infanticide, legislation. **Holdings:** Books; videotapes; 16mm films; audio cassettes; slides; VF files; booklets; newspaper clippings; pamphlets.

★8603★   ST. LAWRENCE HOSPITAL
MEDICAL LIBRARY
1210 W. Saginaw
Lansing, MI 48915   Phone: (515) 377-0354
Jane B. Claytor, Mgr.
Subjects: Medicine, nursing, mental health, hospital management, allied health science. **Holdings:** 2800 books; 7800 bound periodical volumes. **Subscriptions:** 360 journals and other serials.

★8604★   OAKDALE REGIONAL CENTER
STAFF LIBRARY
2995 W. Genesee St.
Lapeer, MI 48446   Phone: (313) 664-2951
Rollin Hill, Lib.Coord.
Subjects: Mental retardation, medicine, education, management, nursing, psychiatry. **Holdings:** 2700 books; 1 vertical file collection. **Subscriptions:** 80 journals and other serials.

★8605★   RIGHT TO LIFE OF MICHIGAN
RESOURCE CENTER
1574 Fort St.
Lincoln Park, MI 48146   Phone: (313) 381-2180
Betty Pevovar, Region 4 Dir. & Off.Mgr.
Subjects: Abortion, euthanasia, infanticide, legislation. **Holdings:** Books; videotapes; 16mm films; audio cassettes; slides; VF files; booklets; newspaper clippings; pamphlets.

★8606★   ST. MARY HOSPITAL
MEDICAL LIBRARY
36475 5 Mile Rd.
Livonia, MI 48154   Phone: (313) 464-4800
Shirley Welch, Asst.Libn.
Subjects: Medicine, surgery, radiology, nursing, obstetrics and gynecology, pediatrics, mental health. **Holdings:** 2143 books; 1230 bound periodical volumes; 800 tapes; 7 16mm films; 8 35mm filmstrips; Audio-Digest tapes; filmstrip/tape sets. **Subscriptions:** 40 journals and other serials.

★8607★ MEMORIAL MEDICAL CENTER OF WEST MICHIGAN
LIBRARY
1 Atkinson Dr.
Ludington, MI 49431   Phone: (616) 843-2591
Dr. James Larson
Subjects: Medicine. **Holdings:** 400 books; 500 bound periodical volumes. **Subscriptions:** 72 journals and other serials.

★8608★ OAKLAND GENERAL HOSPITAL
MEDICAL LIBRARY
27351 Dequindre
Madison Heights, MI 48071   Phone: (313) 967-7575
Geraldine A. Bard, Libn.
Subjects: Medicine. **Holdings:** 4000 books; 5500 bound periodical volumes. **Subscriptions:** 300 journals and other serials.

★8609★ MARQUETTE GENERAL HOSPITAL
KEVIN F. O'BRIEN HEALTH SCIENCES LIBRARY
420 W. Magnetic St.
Marquette, MI 49855-2000   Phone: (906) 228-9440
Mildred E. Kingsbury, Lib.Dir.
Subjects: Medicine, nursing, allied health sciences. **Holdings:** 7000 books; 675 bound periodical volumes; 3000 slides. **Subscriptions:** 250 journals and other serials.

★8610★ MIDMICHIGAN REGIONAL MEDICAL CENTER
HEALTH SCIENCES LIBRARY
4005 Orchard Dr.
Midland, MI 48670   Phone: (517) 839-3262
Patricia Wolfgram, Mgr.
Subjects: Medicine, nursing, family practice, allied health, management. **Holdings:** 2500 books; 9000 bound periodical volumes. **Subscriptions:** 400 journals and other serials.

★8611★ MOUNT CLEMENS GENERAL HOSPITAL
STUCK MEDICAL LIBRARY
1000 Harrington Blvd.
Mt. Clemens, MI 48043   Phone: (313) 466-8147
Lynne L. Coles, Libn.
Subjects: Medicine, nursing. **Holdings:** 2900 books; 2000 bound periodical volumes; 1600 audio cassettes; 1050 videotapes; 170 slide/tape sets; 4 VF drawers of pamphlets. **Subscriptions:** 120 journals and other serials.

★8612★ ST. JOHN HOSPITAL
MACOMB CENTER
MEDICAL LIBRARY
26755 Ballard Rd.
Mt. Clemens, MI 48045   Phone: (313) 465-5501
Deborah R. Cicchini, Lib.Tech.Asst.
Subjects: Podiatry, orthopedics, physical and emergency medicine, neurotrauma, alcoholism. **Holdings:** 427 books; 879 bound periodical volumes. **Subscriptions:** 104 journals and other serials.

★8613★ ST. JOSEPH'S HOSPITAL CENTERS
MEDICAL LIBRARY
215 North Ave.
Mt. Clemens, MI 48043   Phone: (313) 466-9485
Sandra A. Studebaker, Hd.Med.Libn.
Subjects: Medicine, nursing, allied health sciences, consumer health, healthcare management. **Holdings:** 3650 titles; 3500 bound periodical volumes. **Subscriptions:** 485 journals and other serials.

★8614★ HACKLEY HOSPITAL
LIBRARY
1700 Clinton St.
Muskegon, MI 49442   Phone: (616) 728-4766
Betty Marshall, Libn.
Subjects: Medicine, nursing, allied health sciences. **Holdings:** 1500 books; 3296 bound periodical volumes. **Subscriptions:** 155 journals and other serials.

★8615★ MERCY HOSPITAL
DAVID A. AMOS HEALTH SCIENCES LIBRARY
1500 E. Sherman Blvd.
Box 358
Muskegon, MI 49443   Phone: (616) 739-3972
Mary Jo Wyels, Libn.
Subjects: Medicine, nursing, allied health sciences. **Holdings:** 500 books; 3700 bound periodical volumes. **Subscriptions:** 165 journals and other serials.

★8616★ NORTHVILLE REGIONAL PSYCHIATRIC HOSPITAL
PROFESSIONAL LIBRARY
41001 W. 7 Mile Rd.
Northville, MI 48167   Phone: (313) 349-1800
Raman N. Bhavsar, Ch., Lib.Comm.
Subjects: Medicine, psychiatry, psychology, social service, nursing. **Holdings:** 3057 volumes; 100 reprints. **Subscriptions:** 66 journals and other serials.

★8617★ RIGHT TO LIFE OF MICHIGAN
RESOURCE CENTER
43000 9 Mile Rd., Ste. 213
Novi, MI 48375   Phone: (313) 347-1601
Barbara Lowman
Subjects: Abortion, euthanasia, infanticide, legislation. **Holdings:** Books; videotapes; 16mm films; audio cassettes; slides; VF files; booklets; newspaper clippings; pamphlets.

★8618★ THE DEAN C. BURNS HEALTH SCIENCES LIBRARY
560 W. Mitchell
Petoskey, MI 49770   Phone: (616) 348-4500
Kay Kelly, Dir.
Subjects: Health sciences. **Holdings:** 2240 books; 4500 bound periodical volumes; slides; audio- and videotapes. **Subscriptions:** 400 journals and other serials.

★8619★ EDUCATIONAL CENTER FOR LIFE
Professional Bldg., Ste. 19
909 Woodward Ave.
Pontiac, MI 48053   Phone: (313) 338-1910
Phyllis Sullivan, R.N., B.S.N., Dir.
Subjects: Abortion, infanticide, euthanasia, chastity, medical ethics, alternatives to abortion. **Holdings:** 220 books; 12 bound periodical volumes; 9 VF drawers; films; videotapes; audiotapes. **Subscriptions:** 20 journals and other serials.

★8620★ PONTIAC GENERAL HOSPITAL
LIBRARY/MEDIA DEPARTMENT
Seminole & W. Huron
Pontiac, MI 48053   Phone: (313) 857-7412
Naim K. Sahyoun, Dir. of Libs.
Subjects: Medicine, health care administration, nursing. **Holdings:** 3000 books; 10,000 bound periodical volumes; Audio-Digest tapes. **Subscriptions:** 400 journals and other serials.

★8621★ PONTIAC OSTEOPATHIC HOSPITAL
MEDICAL LIBRARY
50 N. Perry St.
Pontiac, MI 48342   Phone: (313) 338-5000
Janis M. Fox-Heroux, Libn.
Subjects: Medicine. **Holdings:** 2586 books; 3100 bound periodical volumes; AV programs; Audio-Digest tapes; slide/tape sets. **Subscriptions:** 149 journals and other serials.

★8622★ ST. JOSEPH MERCY HOSPITAL
LIBRARY
900 Woodward
Pontiac, MI 48341-2985   Phone: (313) 858-3495
Mollie S. Lynch, Lib.Mgr.
Subjects: Medicine, nursing, health care administration, allied health sciences. **Holdings:** 5000 books; 8000 bound periodical volumes; 300 media programs. **Subscriptions:** 500 journals and other serials.

★8623★ ST. CLAIR COUNTY MENTAL HEALTH SERVICE
MEDICAL/STAFF LIBRARY
1011 Military
Port Huron, MI 48060   Phone: (313) 985-8900
Tim Wittstock
Subjects: Mental illness, developmental disabilities, mental health treatment. Holdings: 346 books; 192 videotapes. Subscriptions: 15 journals and other serials.

★8624★ WILLIAM BEAUMONT HOSPITAL
MEDICAL LIBRARY
3601 W. 13 Mile Rd.
Royal Oak, MI 48072   Phone: (313) 551-1750
Joan M.B. Smith, Dir.
Subjects: Medicine, nursing. Holdings: 9500 books; 17,000 bound periodical volumes. Subscriptions: 740 journals and other serials.

★8625★ SAGINAW HEALTH SCIENCES LIBRARY
1000 Houghton St., Ste. 2000
Saginaw, MI 48602   Phone: (517) 771-6846
Stephanie John, Dir.
Subjects: Medicine, nursing, allied health sciences, dentistry, health care administration, behaviorial health. Holdings: 10,500 books; 14,750 bound periodical volumes; 1448 AV programs; 6 VF drawers of pamphlets. Subscriptions: 494 journals and other serials.

★8626★ U.S. DEPARTMENT OF VETERANS AFFAIRS
ALEDA E. LUTZ VA MEDICAL CENTER LIBRARY
1500 Weiss St.
Saginaw, MI 48602   Phone: (517) 793-2340
Nancy R. Dingman, Chf., Lib.Serv.
Subjects: Medicine, surgery, nursing, health education. Holdings: 2000 books; periodicals in microform; 300 AV programs; health education pamphlets. Subscriptions: 150 journals and other serials.

★8627★ RIGHT TO LIFE OF MICHIGAN
MACOMB COUNTY EDUCATION/RESOURCE CENTER
27417 Harper
St. Clair Shores, MI 48081   Phone: (313) 774-6050
Andrea Treall
Subjects: Abortion, euthanasia, infanticide, legislation. Holdings: 37 books; 30 videotapes; 12 16mm films; 125 audio cassettes; slides; booklets; pamphlets.

★8628★ AREA AGENCY ON AGING
REGION IB
LIBRARY
29508 Southfield Rd.
Southfield, MI 48076   Phone: (313) 569-0333
Colleen Blaesing, Dir. of Commun.
Subjects: Older adult issues. Holdings: 1310 books. Subscriptions: 18 journals and other serials; 9 newspapers.

★8629★ MICHIGAN PSYCHOANALYTIC INSTITUTE
IRA MILLER MEMORIAL LIBRARY
16310 W. 12 Mile Rd., Ste. 204
Southfield, MI 48076
Phyllis Kaplan, Libn.
Subjects: Psychoanalysis, psychotherapy, psychiatry. Holdings: 1000 books; 400 bound periodical volumes.

★8630★ PROVIDENCE HOSPITAL
HELEN L. DEROY MEDICAL LIBRARY
16001 W. 9 Mile Rd.
Box 2043
Southfield, MI 48037   Phone: (313) 424-3294
Carole M. Gilbert, Dir., Lib.Serv.
Subjects: Medicine, nursing, allied health sciences, hospitals. Holdings: 3000 books; 8500 bound periodical volumes; 700 audio-visuals and computer-assisted instruction programs. Subscriptions: 400 journals and other serials.

★8631★ RIVERSIDE OSTEOPATHIC HOSPITAL
MEDICAL LIBRARY
150 Truax St.
Trenton, MI 48183   Phone: (313) 676-4200
Susan E. Skoglund, Dir. of Lib.Serv.
Subjects: Medicine, nursing. Holdings: 1212 books; 1523 bound periodical volumes; 4 VF drawers of pamphlets; 576 Audio-Digest tapes. Subscriptions: 125 journals and other serials.

★8632★ OAKLAND COMMUNITY COLLEGE, HIGHLAND LAKES CAMPUS
LEARNING RESOURCE CENTER
SPECIAL COLLECTIONS
7350 Cooley Lake Rd.
Union Lake, MI 48387   Phone: (313) 360-3080
Laura Kolehmainen, Libn.
Subjects: Allied health special collection (nursing, dental). Holdings: 3000 titles.

★8633★ BI-COUNTY COMMUNITY HOSPITAL
LIBRARY
13355 E. 10 Mile Rd.
Warren, MI 48089   Phone: (313) 759-7345
Gayle A. Williams, Dir.
Subjects: Medicine, nursing, health care management, allied health sciences. Holdings: 2200 books; 3500 bound periodical volumes. Subscriptions: 200 journals and other serials.

★8634★ DETROIT MACOMB HOSPITAL CORPORATION
MACOMB HOSPITAL CENTER LIBRARY
11800 12 Mile Rd.
Warren, MI 48093   Phone: (313) 573-5117
Donna Marshall, Corp.Dir. of Libs.
Subjects: Medicine, surgery, obstetrics and gynecology, oral surgery, respiratory medicine. Holdings: 2600 books; 2000 bound periodical volumes; 5 VF drawers. Subscriptions: 290 journals and other serials.

★8635★ WAYNE COUNTY REGIONAL LIBRARY FOR THE BLIND AND PHYSICALLY HANDICAPPED
33030 Van Born Rd.
Wayne, MI 48184   Phone: (313) 274-2600
Pat Klemans, Reg.Libn.
Holdings: 110,000 talking books.

★8636★ WYANDOTTE HOSPITAL AND MEDICAL CENTER
MEDICAL/STAFF LIBRARY
2333 Biddle
Wyandotte, MI 48192   Phone: (313) 284-2400
Diane M. O'Keefe, Libn.
Subjects: Medicine, nursing, psychology, management, and allied subjects. Holdings: 1200 books; 1500 bound periodical volumes; 500 microfiche. Subscriptions: 130 journals and other serials; 3 newspapers.

★8637★ YPSILANTI REGIONAL PSYCHIATRIC HOSPITAL
STAFF LIBRARY
3501 Willis Rd.
Ypsilanti, MI 48197   Phone: (313) 434-3400
Bonnie A. Gasperini, Dir., Lib.Serv.
Subjects: Activity therapy, psychiatry, nursing, psychology, social work, medicine, neurology. Holdings: 800 books. Subscriptions: 75 journals and other serials.

Minnesota

★8638★ DOUGLAS COUNTY HOSPITAL
HEALTH SCIENCES LIBRARY
111 17th Ave., E.
Alexandria, MN 56308   Phone: (612) 762-6090
Mary Johnson, Lib.Mgr.
Subjects: Medicine, nursing. Holdings: 300 books. Subscriptions: 90 journals and other serials.

★8639★ ANOKA TECHNICAL COLLEGE
MEDIA CENTER
1355 W. Hwy. 10
Anoka, MN 55303   Phone: (612) 427-1880
Deborah J. Brude, Media Serv.Coord.
Subjects: Nursing and allied health fields; electronics; business; technology; horticulture. Holdings: 25,000 books; 1355 bound periodical volumes; 1816 AV programs. Subscriptions: 366 journals and other serials; 10 newspapers.

★8640★ ANOKA-METRO REGIONAL TREATMENT CENTER
LIBRARY
3300 4th Ave., N.
Anoka, MN 55303-1119   Phone: (612) 422-4330
Betty Palfalvi, Libn.
Subjects: Medicine, psychiatry, psychology, social science, nursing. **Holdings:** 3300 books. **Subscriptions:** 46 journals and other serials.

★8641★ NORTHWESTERN COLLEGE OF CHIROPRACTIC
LIBRARY
2501 W. 84th St.
Bloomington, MN 55431   Phone: (612) 888-4777
Marcia Stephens, Dir., Lib.Serv.
Subjects: Chiropractic, neurology, roentgenology, orthopedics, nutrition, allied medical and basic sciences. **Holdings:** 8304 books; 1497 bound periodical volumes; 16 VF drawers of clippings, reprints, pamphlets; 1276 audiotapes; 70 models; 126 video cassettes; 351 slide sets; 1300 microfiche of chiropractic journals. **Subscriptions:** 256 journals and other serials.

★8642★ BRAINERD STATE REGIONAL HUMAN SERVICES
CENTER
LIBRARY
177 E. Oak St., Hwy. 18
Brainerd, MN 56401   Phone: (218) 828-2357
Rod Brixius, Libn.
Subjects: Mental retardation, psychiatry and psychotherapy, alcoholism. **Holdings:** 2560 volumes. **Subscriptions:** 52 journals and other serials.

★8643★ ST. FRANCIS MEDICAL CENTER
COMMUNITY HEALTH SCIENCE LIBRARY
415 Oak St.
Breckenridge, MN 56520
Geralyn Terfehr
Subjects: Medicine, nursing, and allied health sciences. **Holdings:** 416 books; 4 VF drawers of pamphlets; 23 AV programs. **Subscriptions:** 168 journals and other serials.

★8644★ FAIRVIEW-RIDGES HOSPITAL
MEDICAL STAFF LIBRARY
201 E. Nicollet Blvd.
Burnsville, MN 55337   Phone: (612) 892-3013
Mary B. Femal, Med.Libn.
Subjects: Medicine, nursing, and allied health sciences. **Holdings:** 350 books. **Subscriptions:** 61 journals and other serials.

★8645★ CANBY COMMUNITY HEALTH SERVICES
MEDICAL LIBRARY
112 St. Olaf Ave., S.
Canby, MN 56220   Phone: (507) 223-7277
Subjects: Medicine, health, hospitals. **Holdings:** 900 books. **Subscriptions:** 10 journals and other serials; 4 newspapers.

★8646★ HAZELDEN FOUNDATION
STAFF LIBRARY
Box 11
Center City, MN 55012   Phone: (612) 257-4010
Joan A. Frederickson, Staff Libn.
Subjects: Chemical dependency. **Holdings:** 7000 books; 300 cassette tapes. **Subscriptions:** 130 journals and other serials; 15 newspapers.

★8647★ MILLER-DWAN MEDICAL CENTER
TILDERQUIST MEMORIAL MEDICAL LIBRARY
502 E. 2nd St.
Duluth, MN 55805   Phone: (218) 720-1362
Annelie Sober, Dir., Med.Lib.
Subjects: Medicine, allied health sciences. **Holdings:** 790 books; 2070 bound periodical volumes. **Subscriptions:** 165 journals and other serials.

★8648★ ST. LUKE'S HOSPITAL
HILDING MEDICAL LIBRARY
915 E. 1st St.
Duluth, MN 55805   Phone: (218) 726-5320
Doreen Roberts, Libn.
Subjects: Clinical medicine, nursing. **Holdings:** 1100 books; 8000 bound periodical volumes; 300 videotapes. **Subscriptions:** 270 journals and other serials.

★8649★ UNIVERSITY OF MINNESOTA, DULUTH
HEALTH SCIENCE LIBRARY
10 University Dr.
Duluth, MN 55812   Phone: (218) 726-8587
Diane C.P. Ebro, Dir.
Subjects: Medicine, allied clinical health, veterinary medicine, forensic medicine, nursing, biochemistry, behavioral science. **Holdings:** 21,782 books; 46,835 bound periodical volumes; 3000 pamphlets; 3784 reels of microfilm. **Subscriptions:** 691 journals and other serials.

★8650★ FAIRVIEW SOUTHDALE HOSPITAL
MARY ANN KING HEALTH SCIENCES LIBRARY
6401 France Ave., S.
Edina, MN 55435   Phone: (612) 924-5005
Mary B. Femal, Med.Libn.
Subjects: Medicine, nursing, allied health sciences, hospital administration and management. **Holdings:** 2000 books; 200 bound and unbound periodicals; vertical files. **Subscriptions:** 160 journals and other serials.

★8651★ FARIBAULT REGIONAL CENTER
LIBRARY
Faribault, MN 55021   Phone: (507) 332-3274
Mary K. Heltsley, Libn.
Subjects: Mental retardation. **Holdings:** 2550 books; 285 bound periodical volumes; 11 VF drawers of pamphlets; 275 pamphlet boxes of unbound periodicals. **Subscriptions:** 50 journals and other serials.

★8652★ FERGUS FALLS REGIONAL TREATMENT CENTER
LIBRARY
Corner of Fir & Union
Box 157
Fergus Falls, MN 56537   Phone: (218) 739-7327
Thomas Shubitz, Libn.
Subjects: Medicine, nursing, psychiatry, special education, drug abuse. **Holdings:** 6500 books; 800 other professional materials; 2000 articles. **Subscriptions:** 55 journals and other serials; 60 newspapers.

★8653★ UNITY MEDICAL CENTER
LIBRARY
550 Osborne Rd.
Fridley, MN 55432   Phone: (612) 780-6774
Aggie Koutroupas, Libn.
Subjects: Medicine, nursing, and allied health sciences. **Holdings:** 800 books; 3000 bound periodical volumes. **Subscriptions:** 108 journals and other serials.

★8654★ GOLDEN VALLEY HEALTH CENTER
MEDICAL LIBRARY AND RESEARCH CENTER
4101 Golden Valley Rd.
Golden Valley, MN 55422   Phone: (612) 588-2771
Ruth Edwards, Dir., Educ.
Subjects: Medicine, nursing, psychiatry. **Holdings:** 700 books; 65 bound periodical volumes; 200 cassette tapes. **Subscriptions:** 85 journals and other serials.

★8655★ ST. GABRIEL'S HOSPITAL
LIBRARY
815 SE 2nd St.
Little Falls, MN 56345   Phone: (612) 632-5441
Peggy Martin, Dir., Educ.
Subjects: Nursing, medicine, science. **Holdings:** Figures not available.

★8656★ ST. JOHN'S NORTHEAST HOSPITAL
MEMORIAL MEDICAL LIBRARY
1575 Beam Ave.
Maplewood, MN 55109   Phone: (612) 779-4276
Sherry Oleson, Lib.Serv.Dir.
Subjects: Medicine, nursing, allied health sciences. **Holdings:** 1200 books; 40 bound periodical volumes; 150 AV programs. **Subscriptions:** 170 journals and other serials.

★8657★ ABBOTT-NORTHWESTERN HOSPITAL
CORPORATION
LIBRARY/MEDIA SERVICES
800 E. 28th St.
Minneapolis, MN 55407   Phone: (612) 863-4312
Donna Johnson, Dir.
Subjects: Medicine, nursing, health care administration, psychology.

Holdings: 7000 books; 25,000 bound periodical volumes; 2 VF drawers of clippings and pamphlets; 140 filmstrip/record sets; 250 videotapes. **Subscriptions:** 625 journals and other serials.

★8658★ A CHANCE TO GROW
KRETSCH BRAIN INJURY RESOURCE LIBRARY
5034 Oliver Ave., N.
Minneapolis, MN 55430   Phone: (612) 521-2266
Emmett Davis, Lib.Dir.
Subjects: Brain injury, cerebral palsy, autism, learning disabilities, Down syndrome/genetics, brain allergy. **Holdings:** 2000 volumes.

★8659★ HAMILTON/KSA
LIBRARY
2021 E. Hennepin, Ste. 450
Minneapolis, MN 55413   Phone: (612) 378-1700
Subjects: Hospital and health care planning and administration; nursing administration; hospital financial management; hospitals - architecture, design, engineering, and construction. **Holdings:** 846 volumes; 14 shelves of documents and reports; 5 VF drawers; 2 VF drawers of maps; 20 shelves of government publications. **Subscriptions:** 61 journals and other serials.

★8660★ HENNEPIN COUNTY MEDICAL CENTER
THOMAS LOWRY HEALTH SCIENCES LIBRARY
701 Park Ave.
Minneapolis, MN 55415   Phone: (612) 347-2710
Barbara Brian, Dir.
Subjects: Clinical medicine, nursing, allied health sciences. **Holdings:** 60,000 books and bound periodical volumes; 900 video cassettes; AV programs. **Subscriptions:** 550 journals and other serials.

★8661★ INTERNATIONAL DIABETES CENTER
LIBRARY
5000 W. 39th St.
Minneapolis, MN 55416   Phone: (612) 927-3393
Helen R. Bowlin, Dir., Sys.Dev.
Subjects: Diabetes mellitus, patient education. **Holdings:** 500 books. **Subscriptions:** 15 journals and other serials.

★8662★ MEDTRONIC, INC.
LIBRARY
7000 Central Ave., NE
Minneapolis, MN 55432   Phone: (612) 574-3496
Steve Rasmussen, Mgr., Info.Rsrcs.
Subjects: Biomedical engineering, cardiac pacemaking, medical electronics, electrical stimulation, cardiology. **Holdings:** 6000 books; 5000 bound periodical volumes; 17,000 pacemaker papers. **Subscriptions:** 500 journals and other serials; 5 newspapers.

★8663★ MINNESOTA DEPARTMENT OF HEALTH
ROBERT N. BARR PUBLIC HEALTH LIBRARY
717 Delaware St., SE
Box 9441
Minneapolis, MN 55440   Phone: (612) 623-5090
Diane Jordan, Lib.Supv.
Subjects: Public health; health planning, promotion, statistics, administration; disease prevention; epidemiology. **Holdings:** 15,000 books; 5000 bound periodical volumes; 48 VF drawers of pamphlets. **Subscriptions:** 275 journals and other serials.

★8664★ NWNL COMPANIES, INC.
LIBRARY
20 Washington Ave., S.
Minneapolis, MN 55440   Phone: (612) 372-5606
Laurinda C. Dahl, Libn.
Subjects: Medical care, alternative health delivery systems, individual and group life and health insurance, law, taxes, business management, health statistics. **Holdings:** 10,000 books; 200 bound periodical volumes; 20 VF drawers. **Subscriptions:** 250 journals and other serials; 7 newspapers.

★8665★ PARK-NICOLLET MEDICAL FOUNDATION
ARNESON LIBRARY
5000 W. 39th St.
Minneapolis, MN 55416   Phone: (612) 927-3097
Barbara K. Latta, Dir.
Subjects: Medicine, nursing, allied health sciences. **Holdings:** 1212 books; 4206 bound periodical volumes; 5 boxes of pamphlets and reprints; 4 drawers of microfiche. **Subscriptions:** 159 journals and other serials.

★8666★ RIVERSIDE MEDICAL CENTER
HEALTH SCIENCES LIBRARY
Riverside at 25th Ave., S.
Minneapolis, MN 55454   Phone: (612) 371-6545
Mary Finnegan, Lib.Mgr.
Subjects: Medicine, orthopedics, nursing. **Holdings:** 3067 books; 4500 bound periodical volumes; 233 audiotapes. **Subscriptions:** 300 journals and other serials.

★8667★ U.S. DEPARTMENT OF VETERANS AFFAIRS
MEDICAL CENTER LIBRARY SERVICE
1 Veterans Dr.
Minneapolis, MN 55417   Phone: (612) 725-2000
Dorothy P. Sinha, Act.Chf.
Subjects: General medicine, psychology, pre-clinical sciences, biomedical research. **Holdings:** 5500 books; 11,000 bound periodical volumes; 1500 volumes on microfilm; 1000 AV programs. **Subscriptions:** 450 journals and other serials; 5 newspapers.

★8668★ UNIVERSITY OF MINNESOTA
BIO-MEDICAL LIBRARY
450 Diehl Hall
505 Essex St., SE
Minneapolis, MN 55455   Phone: (612) 626-3260
Ellen Nagle, Dir.
Subjects: Medicine and allied health sciences, nursing, dentistry, pharmacy, public health, biology. **Holdings:** 360,981 volumes; 2098 AV programs; 51 manuscripts; 53,230 microforms. **Subscriptions:** 4718 journals and other serials.

★8669★ UNIVERSITY OF MINNESOTA
BIO-MEDICAL LIBRARY
OWEN H. WANGENSTEEN HISTORICAL LIBRARY OF
** BIOLOGY AND MEDICINE**
568 Diehl Hall
505 Essex St., SE
Minneapolis, MN 55455   Phone: (612) 626-6881
Elaine Challacombe, Cur.
Subjects: Health sciences, surgery, nursing, tuberculosis, pharmacy, medicine. **Holdings:** 46,145 books; 51 feet of manuscripts; 790 microforms. **Subscriptions:** 14 journals and other serials.

★8670★ UNIVERSITY OF MINNESOTA
DRUG INFORMATION SERVICES
3-106 Health Science Unit F
308 Harvard St., SE
Minneapolis, MN 55455   Phone: (612) 624-6492
Gail Weinberg
Subjects: Psychosocial aspects and research findings of drugs of abuse, alternatives to drug abuse, school curricula, drug abuse in business, treatment and prevention of drug abuse, alcoholism. **Holdings:** 28,000 books, bound periodical volumes, reprints; pamphlets. **Subscriptions:** 90 journals and other serials.

★8671★ UNIVERSITY OF MINNESOTA
LITZENBERG-LUND LIBRARY
PO Box 395, Mayo Memorial Bldg.
420 Delaware St., SE
Minneapolis, MN 55455   Phone: (612) 626-2645
Sarah Birger, Lib.Mgr.
Subjects: Obstetrics, gynecology, endocrinology, oncology. **Holdings:** 450 books; 530 bound periodical volumes. **Subscriptions:** 14 journals and other serials.

★8672★ UNIVERSITY OF MINNESOTA
SOCIAL AND ADMINISTRATIVE PHARMACY READING
** ROOM**
7-159 Health Sciences Unit F
308 Harvard St., SE
Minneapolis, MN 55455   Phone: (612) 624-5900
Ronald S. Hadsall, Ph.D, Dir.
Subjects: Pharmacy, drugs, health service. **Holdings:** 340 books; 425 bound periodical volumes; 4000 NTIS reports on microfiche; government publications; Ph.D. dissertations. **Subscriptions:** 75 journals and other serials.

★8673★ **MINNESOTA DEPARTMENT OF HUMAN SERVICES**
DHS INFORMATION CENTER
Oak Terrace Nursing Home
14500 County Rd. 62
Minnetonka, MN 55345   Phone: (612) 934-4100
Colleen Spadaccini, Libn.
Subjects: Psychiatry, geriatrics, social issues. **Holdings:** 4000 volumes.
Subscriptions: 177 journals and other serials.

★8674★ **MOOSE LAKE REGIONAL TREATMENT CENTER**
STAFF LIBRARY
1000 Lake Shore Dr.
Moose Lake, MN 55767   Phone: (218) 485-4411
John C. Flynn, Lib.Supv.
Subjects: Psychiatry, mental retardation, chemical dependency, psycho-geriatrics. **Holdings:** 500 books. **Subscriptions:** 15 journals and other serials.

★8675★ **NORTH MEMORIAL MEDICAL CENTER**
MEDICAL LIBRARY
3300 Oakdale, N.
Robbinsdale, MN 55422   Phone: (612) 520-5673
Donna Barbour-Talley, Mgr., Med.Lib.
Subjects: Medicine, nursing, dentistry, paramedical sciences. **Holdings:** 2300 books; 5100 bound periodical volumes; 700 audiotape cassettes; 350 pamphlets; 500 journal volumes on microfiche. **Subscriptions:** 525 journals and other serials; 5 newspapers.

★8676★ **MAYO BIOMEDICAL IMAGING COMPUTER**
RESOURCES
LIBRARY
Mayo Clinic
200 1st St. SW
Rochester, MN 55901   Phone: (507) 284-4937
Richard A. Robb, Ph.D.
Subjects: Biomedical imaging, visualization science, software systems, workstations, networks, computer graphics. **Holdings:** 100 books; 200 bound periodical volumes; 100 reports. **Subscriptions:** 20 journals and other serials; 5 newspapers.

★8677★ **MAYO FOUNDATION**
MAYO CLINIC LIBRARY
200 1st St., SW
Rochester, MN 55905   Phone: (507) 284-2061
Jack D. Key, Libn.
Subjects: Medicine, basic sciences. **Holdings:** 94,167 books; 212,536 bound periodical volumes; 4300 dissertations, translations, pamphlets. **Subscriptions:** 4273 journals and other serials.

★8678★ **ROCHESTER METHODIST HOSPITAL**
METHODIST KAHLER LIBRARY
Rochester, MN 55902   Phone: (507) 286-7425
Karen Larsen, Hd.Libn.
Subjects: Nursing services and education, hospital administration and management. **Holdings:** 11,500 books; 500 bound periodical volumes; 1000 AV programs; 12 VF drawers of newspaper clippings and pamphlets. **Subscriptions:** 350 journals and other serials.

★8679★ **ST. MARY'S HOSPITAL**
LIBRARY
1216 2nd St., SW
Rochester, MN 55902   Phone: (507) 255-5647
Mona Stevermer, Libn.
Subjects: Nursing, allied health sciences, nutrition, hospital administration, medicine. **Holdings:** 5000 books. **Subscriptions:** 300 journals and other serials.

★8680★ **ST. CLOUD HOSPITAL**
HEALTH SCIENCES LIBRARY
1406 6th Ave., N.
St. Cloud, MN 56301   Phone: (612) 251-2700
Judith Heeter, Libn.
Subjects: Medicine, nursing, hospital management. **Holdings:** 1000 books; 800 bound periodical volumes; 120 videotapes; 25 16mm films; 50 audio cassettes; 20 AV programs. **Subscriptions:** 100 journals and other serials.

★8681★ **U.S. DEPARTMENT OF VETERANS AFFAIRS**
MEDICAL CENTER LIBRARY
4801 8th St., N.
St. Cloud, MN 56303   Phone: (612) 255-6342
Marjorie Hammer, Chf., Lib.Serv.
Subjects: General medicine, psychiatry, nursing, geriatrics. **Holdings:** 2200 books; 1000 bound periodical volumes; microfilm. **Subscriptions:** 250 journals and other serials.

★8682★ **METHODIST HOSPITAL**
MEDICAL LIBRARY
PO Box 650
St. Louis Park, MN 55440   Phone: (612) 932-5451
Pearly Rudin, Med.Libn.
Subjects: Clinical medicine, nursing. **Holdings:** 1500 volumes. **Subscriptions:** 100 journals and other serials.

★8683★ **CHILDREN'S HOSPITAL**
MEDICAL-NURSING LIBRARY
345 N. Smith Ave.
St. Paul, MN 55102   Phone: (612) 227-6521
Nancy W. Battaglia, Dir.
Subjects: Pediatrics, pediatric endocrinology, pediatric nursing, growth and development. **Holdings:** 1000 books; 600 bound periodical volumes; 2 VF drawers of reprints and photoduplicated articles; 100 Audio-Digest tapes on pediatrics. **Subscriptions:** 100 journals and other serials.

★8684★ **GILLETTE CHILDREN'S HOSPITAL**
PROFESSIONAL LIBRARY
200 E. University
St. Paul, MN 55101   Phone: (612) 229-3840
Barbara Carlson, Med. Staff Asst.
Subjects: Orthopedics, pediatrics, autistic children. **Holdings:** 2584 books; 54 bound periodical volumes. **Subscriptions:** 48 journals and other serials.

★8685★ **MIDWAY HOSPITAL**
HEALTH SCIENCES LIBRARY
1700 University Ave.
St. Paul, MN 55104   Phone: (612) 641-5607
Carol Windham, Libn.
Subjects: Medicine, nursing. **Holdings:** 1300 books; 72 bound periodical volumes; 25 films and filmstrips; 3500 slides; 65 transparencies; 75 audiotapes; 250 video cassettes. **Subscriptions:** 300 journals and other serials.

★8686★ **PLANNED PARENTHOOD OF MINNESOTA**
PHYLLIS COOKSEY RESOURCE CENTER
1965 Ford Pkwy.
St. Paul, MN 55116   Phone: (612) 698-2401
Debra Bauer, Rsrc.Ctr.Coord.
Subjects: Family planning, population growth, human sexuality, abortion, sex education. **Holdings:** 1500 books; 12 VF drawers of pamphlets and ephemera; 100 films, video- and audio cassettes. **Subscriptions:** 100 journals and other serials.

★8687★ **RAMSEY COUNTY MEDICAL SOCIETY**
BOECKMANN LIBRARY
345 N. Smith Ave.
St. Paul, MN 55102   Phone: (612) 224-3346
Mary Sandra Tarman, Libn.
Subjects: Medicine, nursing, hospital administration. **Holdings:** 15,000 books; 28,500 bound periodical volumes; 6500 unbound periodical volumes; 18 VF drawers of pamphlets and clippings; 800 medical instruments and memorabilia. **Subscriptions:** 650 journals and other serials; 8 newspapers.

★8688★ **ST. JOSEPH'S HOSPITAL**
JEROME MEDICAL LIBRARY
69 W. Exchange St.
St. Paul, MN 55102   Phone: (612) 291-3193
Karen Brudvig, Med.Libn.
Subjects: Medicine, hospital administration, nursing. **Holdings:** 2500 books; 2900 bound periodical volumes. **Subscriptions:** 200 journals and other serials.

★8689★ ST. PAUL RAMSEY MEDICAL CENTER
MEDICAL LIBRARY
640 Jackson St.
St. Paul, MN 55101   Phone: (612) 221-3607
Mary Dwyer, Hd.Libn.
Subjects: Medicine and nursing. **Holdings:** 4000 books; 6000 bound periodical volumes. **Subscriptions:** 390 journals and other serials.

★8690★ 3M COMPANY
270 TECHNICAL LIBRARY
3M Center, 270-4A-06
St. Paul, MN 55144   Phone: (612) 733-1703
Eloise M. Jasken, Tech.Libn.
Subjects: Biochemistry, medicine, physiology, chemistry, pharmacology, biomaterials. **Holdings:** 6500 books; 7200 bound periodical volumes. **Subscriptions:** 417 journals and other serials.

★8691★ UNIVERSITY OF MINNESOTA, ST. PAUL
VETERINARY MEDICAL LIBRARY
450 Veterinary Science Bldg.
1971 Commonwealth Ave.
St. Paul, MN 55108   Phone: (612) 624-4281
Livija Carlson, Hd.
Subjects: Veterinary medicine. **Holdings:** 44,009 books and bound periodical volumes; 18,056 documents; 83 AV programs; 731 microforms; dissertations. **Subscriptions:** 1019 journals and other serials.

★8692★ ST. PETER REGIONAL TREATMENT CENTER
BURTON P. GRIMES STAFF LIBRARY
100 Freeman Dr.
St. Peter, MN 56082   Phone: (507) 931-7720
Subjects: Medicine, nursing, drug addiction, mental retardation, and allied health sciences. **Holdings:** 1300 books; 650 bound periodical volumes; 3 VF drawers; 400 audiotapes; 200 microfiche; clippings. **Subscriptions:** 30 journals and other serials; 10 newspapers.

★8693★ PREGNANCY AND INFANT LOSS CENTER
LENDING LIBRARY
1415 E. Wayzata Blvd., No. 105
Wayzata, MN 55391   Phone: (612) 473-9372
Sherokee Ilse, Pres.
Subjects: Perinatal bereavement, coping with grief, children and death. **Holdings:** 100 books. **Subscriptions:** 30 newspapers.

★8694★ WHEATON COMMUNITY HOSPITAL
MEDICAL LIBRARY
401 12th St., N.
Wheaton, MN 56296   Phone: (612) 563-8226
Diane Zelka, Med.Libn., ART
Subjects: Medicine. **Holdings:** Figures not available. **Subscriptions:** 90 journals and other serials.

★8695★ RICE MEMORIAL HOSPITAL
HEALTH SCIENCE LIBRARY
301 Becker Ave., SW
Willmar, MN 56201   Phone: (612) 235-4543
Carol Conradi, Libn.
Subjects: Clinical medicine. **Holdings:** 1200 books; 925 bound periodical volumes. **Subscriptions:** 120 journals and other serials.

★8696★ WILLMAR REGIONAL TREATMENT CENTER
LIBRARY
Box 1128
Willmar, MN 56201   Phone: (612) 231-5934
Henry L. Wagener, Libn.
Subjects: Alcoholism, psychiatric nursing, mental retardation. **Holdings:** 2200 books. **Subscriptions:** 75 journals and other serials.

Mississippi

★8697★ FORREST GENERAL HOSPITAL
MEDICAL LIBRARY
Drawer 16389
Hattiesburg, MS 39402   Phone: (601) 288-4260
Bettye M. Duncan, Med.Libn.
Subjects: Medicine, renal medicine, gynecology and obstetrics, gastroenter-

ology, surgery. **Holdings:** 500 books; 1000 bound periodical volumes. **Subscriptions:** 31 journals and other serials.

★8698★ HINDS GENERAL HOSPITAL
WILLIAM M. SUTTLE MEDICAL LIBRARY
1850 Chadwick Dr.
Jackson, MS 39204   Phone: (601) 376-1148
Wanda W. King, Med.Libn.
Subjects: Medicine, nursing, dentistry, hospital administration. **Holdings:** 1500 books; 2500 bound periodical volumes. **Subscriptions:** 148 journals and other serials.

★8699★ MISSISSIPPI BAPTIST MEDICAL CENTER
LIBRARY
1225 N. State St.
Jackson, MS 39202-2002   Phone: (601) 968-4187
Cecelia Bell, Hea.Sci.Libn.
Subjects: Medicine, nursing. **Holdings:** 1500 books; 6000 bound periodical volumes. **Subscriptions:** 151 journals and other serials.

★8700★ MISSISSIPPI DEPARTMENT OF HEALTH
AUDIOVISUAL LIBRARY
2343 N. State St.
Box 1700
Jackson, MS 39205   Phone: (601) 960-7675
Nancy Kay Sullivan, Dir., P.R.
Subjects: Alcohol, dental health, diseases, drug addiction and narcotics, family planning, nursing, nutrition. **Holdings:** 1800 16mm films; 300 35mm filmstrips; 250 videotapes.

★8701★ MISSISSIPPI DEPARTMENT OF MENTAL HEALTH
LIBRARY
1101 Robert E. Lee Bldg.
Jackson, MS 39201   Phone: (601) 359-1288
Margueritte D. Ransom, Libn.
Subjects: Mental health and illness; mental retardation; child and adolescent mental health; alcohol and drug abuse. **Holdings:** 2500 books; 24 linear feet of departmental reports; 12 VF drawers of other cataloged items. **Subscriptions:** 7 journals and other serials.

★8702★ ST. DOMINIC-JACKSON MEMORIAL HOSPITAL
LUTHER MANSHIP MEDICAL LIBRARY
969 Lakeland Dr.
Jackson, MS 39216   Phone: (601) 982-0121
Nyla Stevens, Libn.
Subjects: Medicine, nursing, mental health. **Holdings:** 1911 books; 439 bound periodical volumes. **Subscriptions:** 127 journals and other serials.

★8703★ U.S. DEPARTMENT OF VETERANS AFFAIRS
MEDICAL CENTER LIBRARY
1500 E. Woodrow Wilson Dr.
Jackson, MS 39216   Phone: (601) 364-1273
Carol Sistrunk, Chf.Libn.
Subjects: Medicine and allied health sciences. **Holdings:** 1800 books; 2750 bound periodical volumes; 2000 volumes of journals on microfilm; 275 AV software programs. **Subscriptions:** 200 journals and other serials; 5 newspapers.

★8704★ UNIVERSITY OF MISSISSIPPI
MEDICAL CENTER
ROWLAND MEDICAL LIBRARY
2500 W. State St.
Jackson, MS 39216   Phone: (601) 984-1290
Ada M. Seltzer
Subjects: Medicine, nursing, allied health, dentistry. **Holdings:** 33,084 books; 103,852 bound periodical volumes; 12,516 microfiche; 535 reels of microfilm. **Subscriptions:** 2205 journals and other serials; 4 newspapers.

★8705★ U.S. AIR FORCE MEDICAL CENTER
MEDICAL LIBRARY
SGEL
Keesler AFB, MS 39534-5300   Phone: (601) 377-6249
Sherry N. Nave, Med.Libn.
Subjects: Medicine, surgery, nursing, dentistry, allied health sciences. **Holdings:** 5000 books; 4000 bound periodical volumes; 1100 volumes on microfilm. **Subscriptions:** 500 journals and other serials.

★8706★ MISSISSIPPI STATE UNIVERSITY
COLLEGE OF VETERINARY MEDICINE
BRANCH LIBRARY
Drawer V
Mississippi State, MS 39762   Phone: (601) 325-1240
June Breland, Br.Libn.
Subjects: Veterinary medicine, medicine, allied health sciences, animal husbandry, agriculture, science and technology. **Holdings:** 8381 books; 5959 bound periodical volumes; 181 resource and vertical files; 1275 reference monographs; 1268 16mm films, videotapes, and slide programs. **Subscriptions:** 259 journals and other serials.

★8707★ SINGING RIVER HOSPITAL
MEDICAL LIBRARY
2809 Denny Ave.
Pascagoula, MS 39567   Phone: (601) 938-5040
Mary Evelyn Dowell, Dir., Med.Lib.
Subjects: Medicine, nursing, allied health sciences, hospital administration, consumer health. **Holdings:** 4000 books; 10,000 bound periodical volumes. **Subscriptions:** 250 journals and other serials.

★8708★ NORTH MISSISSIPPI MEDICAL CENTER
RESOURCE CENTER
830 S. Gloster St.
Tupelo, MS 38801   Phone: (601) 841-4399
Mary Lillian Randle, Educ.Res.Coord.
Subjects: Medicine, nursing, health care administration. **Holdings:** 1150 books; 1000 periodical volumes. **Subscriptions:** 137 journals and other serials.

★8709★ UNIVERSITY OF MISSISSIPPI
JOHN DAVIS WILLIAMS LIBRARY
AUSTIN A. DODGE PHARMACY LIBRARY
215A Faser Hall
University, MS 38677   Phone: (601) 232-7381
Nancy F. Fuller, Libn.
Subjects: Pharmacy, medicine, organic chemistry, health care administration, botany (pharmacognosy). **Holdings:** 31,616 books, bound periodical volumes, reels of microfilm, AV programs; 34 VF drawers of pamphlets; 127 dissertations and graduate theses from School of Pharmacy. **Subscriptions:** 425 journals and other serials; 5 newspapers.

★8710★ PARKVIEW REGIONAL MEDICAL CENTER
MEDICAL LIBRARY
100 McAuley Dr.
PO Box 509
Vicksburg, MS 39180   Phone: (601) 631-2131
Subjects: Medicine, surgery, obstetrics, gynecology, allied health sciences. **Holdings:** 2400 books; 3532 unbound and bound periodical volumes. **Subscriptions:** 66 journals and other serials.

★8711★ VICKSBURG MEDICAL CENTER
MEDICAL LIBRARY
3311 I-20 Frontage Rd.
Vicksburg, MS 39180   Phone: (601) 636-2611
Linda Stephenson, Med.Rec.Mgr.
Subjects: Medicine, surgery, nursing, patient education. **Holdings:** 534 books; 1610 bound periodical volumes; 60 VF folders; 45 cassettes; 9 slide sets; 20 microforms; 2 video cassettes. **Subscriptions:** 70 journals and other serials.

Missouri

★8712★ DE PAUL HEALTH CENTER
MEDICAL LIBRARY
12303 DePaul Dr.
Bridgeton, MO 63044   Phone: (314) 344-6397
Joan A. Laneman, Lib.Dir.
Subjects: Medicine, nursing, psychiatry, management, staff and patient education. **Holdings:** 9500 books; 4000 bound periodical volumes; 300 other cataloged items; videotapes. **Subscriptions:** 262 journals and other serials.

★8713★ ST. FRANCIS MEDICAL CENTER
MEDICAL LIBRARY
211 St. Francis Dr.
Cape Girardeau, MO 63701   Phone: (314) 339-6859
Kilja Israel, Libn.
Subjects: Medicine, nursing, health care administration. **Holdings:** 1000 books; 325 bound periodical volumes; 85 volumes on microfilm. **Subscriptions:** 25 journals and other serials; 3 newspapers.

★8714★ LOGAN COLLEGE OF CHIROPRACTIC
LEARNING RESOURCES CENTER
1851 Schoettler Rd.
Box 1065
Chesterfield, MO 63006-1065   Phone: (314) 227-2100
Rosemary E. Buhr, Dir.
Subjects: Chiropractic, orthopedics, body mechanics, radiology, anatomy, nutrition, neurology, sports medicine, physical therapy. **Holdings:** 10,000 books; 950 slide/tape programs; videotapes. **Subscriptions:** 220 journals and other serials.

★8715★ ORTHOPEDIC FOUNDATION FOR ANIMALS
OFA HIP DYSPLASIA REGISTRY
2300 Nifong Rd.
Columbia, MO 65201   Phone: (314) 442-0418
Dr. E. A. Corley, Proj.Dir.
Subjects: Veterinary medicine. **Holdings:** 120,000 radiographs - Hip Registry X-Ray, evaluated for canine hip dysplasia in purebred dogs.

★8716★ U.S. DEPARTMENT OF VETERANS AFFAIRS
HOSPITAL LIBRARY
800 Stadium Rd.
Columbia, MO 65201   Phone: (314) 443-2511
Mark Fleetwood, Act.Chf., Lib.Serv.
Subjects: Medicine, surgery. **Holdings:** 4400 books; 2000 bound periodical volumes. **Subscriptions:** 300 journals and other serials; 14 newspapers.

★8717★ UNIVERSITY OF MISSOURI, COLUMBIA
J. OTTO LOTTES HEALTH SCIENCES LIBRARY
Health Sciences Center
Columbia, MO 65212   Phone: (314) 882-7033
Dean Schmidt, Dir.
Subjects: Medicine, nursing, hospital administration. **Holdings:** 184,003 volumes; 230 microforms; 500 tapes; 150 motion pictures; 400 AV programs; 25 phonograph records; 2000 slides. **Subscriptions:** 1891 journals and other serials.

★8718★ UNIVERSITY OF MISSOURI, COLUMBIA
VETERINARY MEDICAL LIBRARY
W218 Veterinary Medicine
Columbia, MO 65211   Phone: (314) 882-2461
Trenton Boyd, Libn.
Subjects: Veterinary medicine. **Holdings:** 20,046 books; 21,260 bound periodical volumes; 740 microforms. **Subscriptions:** 495 journals and other serials; 5 newspapers.

★8719★ SOUTHEAST MISSOURI MENTAL HEALTH CENTER
PROFESSIONAL LIBRARY
1010 W. Columbia
Farmington, MO 63640   Phone: (314) 756-6792
Anita Kellogg
Subjects: Psychiatry, psychology, nursing. **Holdings:** 1200 books. **Subscriptions:** 38 journals and other serials.

★8720★ U.S. ARMY HOSPITALS
GENERAL LEONARD WOOD ARMY COMMUNITY HOSPITAL
MEDICAL LIBRARY
Fort Leonard Wood, MO 65473-5700   Phone: (314) 596-9110
Linda Prokey, Med.Libn.
Subjects: Medicine. **Holdings:** 3500 books; 200 bound periodical volumes. **Subscriptions:** 200 journals and other serials.

★8721★ FULTON STATE HOSPITAL
PROFESSIONAL LIBRARY
600 E. 5th St., No. 102
Fulton, MO 65251   Phone: (314) 592-2262
Berneice Deloney, Libn.
Subjects: Psychiatry, pyschotherapy, medicine, nursing, social work, psy-

chology. **Holdings:** 700 books; 20 bound periodical volumes. **Subscriptions:** 60 journals and other serials.

★8722★   MISSOURI SCHOOL FOR THE DEAF
GROVER C. FARQUHAR LIBRARY
505 E. 5th St.
Fulton, MO 65251   Phone: (314) 592-2513
Patsy Craghead, Libn.
Subjects: Deafness, education, general collection (K-12). **Holdings:** 13,000 books; 171 bound periodical volumes; 1300 captioned films; Missouri Record on microfilm. **Subscriptions:** 35 journals and other serials; 6 newspapers.

★8723★   INDEPENDENCE REGIONAL HEALTH CENTER
DR. CHARLES F. GRABSKE, SR. LIBRARY
1509 W. Truman Rd.
Independence, MO 64050   Phone: (816) 836-6639
Katie Voss, Libn.
Subjects: Nursing. **Holdings:** 7000 books; 100 bound periodical volumes. **Subscriptions:** 178 journals and other serials.

★8724★   LINCOLN UNIVERSITY OF MISSOURI
INMAN E. PAGE LIBRARY
Jefferson City, MO 65101   Phone: (314) 681-5512
Elizabeth A. Wilson, Dir.
Subjects: Liberal arts; elementary and secondary education; nursing; corrections and law enforcement. **Holdings:** 134,169 books; 9000 bound periodical volumes; 74,670 government documents; 230 theses and dissertations; 30 VF drawers; 4 VF drawers of pictures; 91,945 titles in microform. **Subscriptions:** 705 journals and other serials; 53 newspapers.

★8725★   AMERICAN ACADEMY OF FAMILY PHYSICIANS
HUFFINGTON LIBRARY
8880 Ward Pkwy.
PO Box 8418
Kansas City, MO 64114-0418   Phone: (816) 333-9700
Patricia A. Gibson, Ph.D.
Subjects: Current clinical medicine, family practice. **Holdings:** 1415 books; 50 archival items; 1250 microfiche. **Subscriptions:** 507 journals and other serials.

★8726★   BAPTIST MEDICAL CENTER
LIBRARY
6601 Rockhill Rd.
Kansas City, MO 64131   Phone: (816) 276-7863
Richard Dalton, Dir.
Subjects: Health sciences. **Holdings:** 5500 books; 3500 bound periodical volumes; 10 VF drawers of pamphlets. **Subscriptions:** 283 journals and other serials.

★8727★   CHILDREN'S MERCY HOSPITAL
MEDICAL LIBRARY
24th at Gillham Rd.
Kansas City, MO 64108   Phone: (816) 234-3800
Naomi R. Adelman, Mgr., Lib.Serv.
Subjects: Pediatrics. **Holdings:** 1300 books; 8100 bound periodical volumes. **Subscriptions:** 215 journals and other serials.

★8728★   CLEVELAND CHIROPRACTIC COLLEGE
RUTH R. CLEVELAND MEMORIAL LIBRARY
6401 Rockhill Rd.
Kansas City, MO 64131   Phone: (816) 333-8230
Marcia M. Thomas, Lib.Dir.
Subjects: Health sciences, roentgenology, chiropractic, orthopedics, diagnosis, acupuncture. **Holdings:** 8600 books; 350 bound periodical volumes; 4100 radiographic films; 5000 radiographic slides; 8000 slides and tapes; 14 drawers of journals on microfiche. **Subscriptions:** 210 journals and other serials.

★8729★   LINDA HALL LIBRARY
5109 Cherry St.
Kansas City, MO 64110   Phone: (816) 363-4600
Louis E. Martin, Dir.
Subjects: Mathematics, astronomy, physics, chemistry, geology, biology, pharmacy, pharmacology, engineering, agriculture. **Holdings:** 627,000 volumes; U.S. patent specifications, July 1946 to present; 1.02 million microforms. **Subscriptions:** 16,500 journals and other serials.

★8730★   MEDICAL INFORMATION RETRIEVAL CENTER
CONSUMER HEALTH INFORMATION RESEARCH INSTITUTE
3521 Broadway
Kansas City, MO 64111   Phone: (816) 753-8850
Dr. George X. Trimble, Dir.
Subjects: Clinical medicine, health fraud and quackery, patient education, toxicology, history of medicine. **Holdings:** 575 volumes; 1050 monographs; 505,000 medical literature reprints. **Subscriptions:** 150 journals and other serials.

★8731★   MENORAH MEDICAL CENTER
ROBERT UHLMANN MEDICAL LIBRARY
4949 Rockhill Rd.
Kansas City, MO 64110   Phone: (816) 276-8157
Kitty Serling, Med.Lib.Mgr.
Subjects: Medicine, surgery, psychiatry, nursing, cardiology, lasers, pediatrics, neurology. **Holdings:** 2000 books; 20,000 bound periodical volumes. **Subscriptions:** 160 journals and other serials; 6 newspapers.

★8732★   QUINCY RESEARCH CENTER
INFORMATION SERVICES
5100 E. 24th St.
Kansas City, MO 64127   Phone: (816) 483-1850
Mona Bosch, Info.Serv.
Subjects: Pharmaceutical research, pharmacology, medicine. **Holdings:** 600 books; 100 bound periodical volumes. **Subscriptions:** 80 journals and other serials.

★8733★   RESEARCH MEDICAL CENTER
CARL R. FERRIS, M.D. MEDICAL LIBRARY
2316 E. Meyer Blvd.
Kansas City, MO 64132-1199   Phone: (816) 276-4310
Gerald R. Kruse, Lib.Dir.
Subjects: Medicine, nursing. **Holdings:** 8500 books; 10,000 bound periodical volumes; 350 reels of microfilm; 900 tapes; 150 filmstrips. **Subscriptions:** 404 journals and other serials.

★8734★   ST. JOSEPH HEALTH CENTER
HEALTH SCIENCE LIBRARY
1000 Carondelet Dr.
Kansas City, MO 64114   Phone: (816) 943-2160
Janice Foster, Libn.
Subjects: Medicine, nursing, and allied health sciences. **Holdings:** 1000 books; 1200 bound periodical volumes. **Subscriptions:** 156 journals and other serials.

★8735★   ST. LUKE'S HOSPITAL OF KANSAS CITY
MEDICAL LIBRARY
Spencer Center for Education
44th & Wornall Rd.
Kansas City, MO 64111   Phone: (816) 932-2333
Karen Wiederaenders, Dir. of Lib.Serv.
Subjects: Cardiology, nursing, sports medicine, medicine. **Holdings:** 5000 books; 10,000 bound periodical volumes; 1000 other cataloged items. **Subscriptions:** 624 journals and other serials.

★8736★   TRINITY LUTHERAN HOSPITAL
FLORENCE L. NELSON MEMORIAL LIBRARY
3030 Baltimore Ave.
Kansas City, MO 64108   Phone: (816) 751-2270
Cami L. Loucks, Dir.
Subjects: Clinical medicine, preclinical medicine, nursing, hospital administration. **Holdings:** 4500 books; 2600 bound periodical volumes; 12 VF drawers of pamphlets; 800 reels of microfilm; 180 filmstrips; 4000 slides; 450 audio cassettes; 10 16mm films; 450 video cassettes. **Subscriptions:** 375 journals and other serials; 8 newspapers.

★8737★   U.S. DEPARTMENT OF VETERANS AFFAIRS
MEDICAL CENTER LIBRARY
4801 Linwood Blvd.
Kansas City, MO 64128   Phone: (816) 861-4700
Shirley C. Ting, Chf., Lib.Serv.
Subjects: Medicine, surgery, neurology, nursing, psychology, psychiatry. **Holdings:** 3051 books; 6278 bound periodical volumes; 1077 AV programs. **Subscriptions:** 415 journals and other serials.

★8738★ UNIVERSITY OF HEALTH SCIENCES
MAZZACANO HALL LIBRARY
2105 Independence Blvd.
Kansas City, MO 64124   Phone: (816) 283-2290
Marilyn J. DeGeus, Dir. of Lib.
Subjects: Medicine, osteopathy. **Holdings:** 49,506 books; 17,546 bound periodical volumes; 198 cassette tape titles; 2553 slide titles; 2242 videotapes; 1 microfiche; 2 transparencies; 24 teaching models; 24 three-dimensional disc titles; 160 computer programs; 891 x-ray radiographs; 64 16mm films. **Subscriptions:** 450 journals and other serials.

★8739★ UNIVERSITY OF MISSOURI, KANSAS CITY
HEALTH SCIENCES LIBRARY
2411 Holmes
Kansas City, MO 64108   Phone: (816) 235-1880
Marilyn Sullivan, Chf.Libn.
Subjects: Medicine, nursing. **Holdings:** 15,693 books; 54,032 serial volumes; 3019 AV titles; 43,000 items in microform. **Subscriptions:** 789 journals and other serials.

★8740★ UNIVERSITY OF MISSOURI, KANSAS CITY
SCHOOL OF DENTISTRY LIBRARY
650 E. 25th St.
Kansas City, MO 64108   Phone: (816) 235-2030
Ann Marie Corry, Dental Libn.
Subjects: Dentistry. **Holdings:** 12,723 books; 10,388 bibliographic volumes of periodicals. **Subscriptions:** 833 journals and other serials.

★8741★ WESTERN MISSOURI MENTAL HEALTH CENTER
LIBRARY
600 E. 22nd St.
Kansas City, MO 64108   Phone: (816) 471-3000
Tyron Emerick, Med.Libn.
Subjects: Psychiatry, psychology, social science, psychological testing, psychoanalysis, drugs and alcohol. **Holdings:** 3400 books; 110 unbound periodical titles; 410 cassette tapes. **Subscriptions:** 90 journals and other serials.

★8742★ KIRKSVILLE COLLEGE OF OSTEOPATHIC
  MEDICINE
A.T. STILL MEMORIAL LIBRARY
Kirksville, MO 63501   Phone: (816) 626-2345
Lawrence W. Onsager, Dir. of Lib.
Subjects: Osteopathic medicine, medicine, psychology, basic sciences. **Holdings:** 38,223 books; 31,201 bound periodical volumes; 8508 AV programs; 600 osteopathic materials; 8 VF drawers of osteopathic pamphlets; 120 reels of microfilm; 35 linear feet of archives and manuscripts. **Subscriptions:** 840 journals and other serials; 5 newspapers.

★8743★ MISSOURI REHABILITATION CENTER
MEDICAL LIBRARY
Mount Vernon, MO 65712-1099   Phone: (417) 466-3711
Mary Ann Swearingen, Libn.Asst.
Subjects: Rehabilitation - respiratory, cardiac, head injury; stroke and spinal cord injuries; other disabilities. **Holdings:** 992 books; 892 periodical volumes; 91 articles by staff physicians; 212 magnetic tapes; 277 slides; 22 microfiche. **Subscriptions:** 54 journals and other serials.

★8744★ NEVADA HABILITATION CENTER
LIBRARY
Ashland at Highland
Nevada, MO 64772   Phone: (417) 448-2232
Mary Kralicek
Subjects: Mental retardation. **Holdings:** 1000 books. **Subscriptions:** 26 journals and other serials; 3 newspapers.

★8745★ NORTH KANSAS CITY HOSPITAL
MEDICAL LIBRARY
2800 Hospital Dr.
North Kansas City, MO 64116   Phone: (816) 346-7792
Anne Palmer, Med.Libn.
Subjects: Clinical medicine, nursing, pharmacy, allied health sciences, mental health. **Holdings:** 2200 books; 1700 reels of microfilm. **Subscriptions:** 220 journals and other serials.

★8746★ U.S. DEPARTMENT OF VETERANS AFFAIRS
LIBRARY SERVICE
John J. Pershing Veterans Administration Medical Center
1500 N. Westwood Blvd.
Poplar Bluff, MO 63901   Phone: (314) 686-4151
Genise E. Denton, Chf., Lib.Serv.
Subjects: Medicine. **Holdings:** 1305 books; AV equipment and programs. **Subscriptions:** 170 journals and other serials; 19 newspapers.

★8747★ ST. JOSEPH HEALTH CENTER
HEALTH SCIENCE LIBRARY
300 First Capitol Dr.
St. Charles, MO 63301   Phone: (314) 724-2810
Lucille Dykas, Lib.Mgr.
Subjects: Medicine. **Holdings:** 500 books; 320 bound periodical volumes. **Subscriptions:** 80 journals and other serials.

★8748★ BOEHRINGER INGELHEIM ANIMAL HEALTH, INC.
LIBRARY
2621 N. Belt Hwy.
St. Joseph, MO 64506   Phone: (816) 233-2571
Judy Heinje, Libn.
Subjects: Veterinary medicine, bacteriology, virology, pharmaceuticals, immunology, parasitology. **Holdings:** 5000 books; 15,000 bound periodical volumes; 750 documents and dissertations. **Subscriptions:** 165 journals and other serials.

★8749★ HEARTLAND HEALTH SYSTEMS
HEARTLAND HOSPITAL EAST
HEALTH SCIENCES LIBRARY
5325 Faraon St.
St. Joseph, MO 64506   Phone: (816) 271-6075
Joan Hughes, Hea.Sci.Libn.
Subjects: Medicine. **Holdings:** 350 books; 300 bound periodical volumes. **Subscriptions:** 64 journals and other serials.

★8750★ ST. JOSEPH STATE HOSPITAL
PROFESSIONAL LIBRARY
3400 Frederick Ave.
St. Joseph, MO 64506   Phone: (816) 387-2300
Judith L. Moore, Lib.Dir.
Subjects: Psychiatry, psychology, social service, nursing, education, alcoholism, therapy, dietetics, pharmacy. **Holdings:** 1400 books; 15 periodical titles; 200 Audio-Digest tapes; 200 video cassettes. **Subscriptions:** 70 journals and other serials.

★8751★ AMERICAN ASSOCIATION OF ORTHODONTISTS
CHARLES R. BAKER MEMORIAL LIBRARY
460 Lindbergh Rd.
St. Louis, MO 63141   Phone: (314) 993-1700
Celia Giltinan, Ref.Libn.
Subjects: Orthodontics. **Holdings:** 800 books; 600 bound periodical volumes; 10,000 microforms and nonbook items; 1050 manuscripts.

★8752★ BARNES COLLEGE
NURSING LIBRARY AND INSTRUCTIONAL RESOURCE
  LABORATORY
416 S. Kingshighway Blvd.
St. Louis, MO 63110   Phone: (314) 362-1566
Beth G. Carlin, Libn.
Subjects: Nursing. **Holdings:** 4000 books; 300 bound periodical volumes; AV programs; computer software; 12 VF drawers. **Subscriptions:** 90 journals and other serials.

★8753★ BLUE CROSS AND BLUE SHIELD OF MISSOURI
LIBRARY
4444 Forest Park Blvd.
St. Louis, MO 63108   Phone: (314) 658-4774
Mary Hebert, Libn.
Subjects: Health care, insurance, economics, business. **Holdings:** 6000 books; 210 bound periodical volumes; 9 VF drawers of pamphlets and clippings; 2 VF drawer of speeches and reports. **Subscriptions:** 228 journals and other serials.

★8754★ CATHOLIC HEALTH ASSOCIATION OF THE UNITED STATES
INFORMATION RESOURCE CENTER
4455 Woodson Rd.
St. Louis, MO 63134   Phone: (314) 427-2500
Mark Unger, Dir.
Subjects: Administrative aspects of health care facilities, advocacy, statistics, surveys, Catholic religion, business. **Holdings:** Figures not available. **Subscriptions:** 181 journals and other serials; 37 newspapers.

★8755★ CENTRAL INSTITUTE FOR THE DEAF
PROFESSIONAL LIBRARY
818 S. Euclid
St. Louis, MO 63110   Phone: (314) 652-3200
Mary M. Sicking, Libn.
Subjects: Audiology, early childhood education, behavioral sciences, speech pathology, physiology, otolaryngology, education of the deaf, noise control, electroacoustics, digital instrumentation, aural rehabilitation, neurophysiology. **Holdings:** 9000 books; 1015 bound periodical volumes; 135 dissertations; 109 drawers of clippings; 12 reels of microfilm; 20 videotapes. **Subscriptions:** 78 journals.

★8756★ DEACONESS HOSPITAL
DRUSCH PROFESSIONAL LIBRARY
6150 Oakland Ave.
St. Louis, MO 63139   Phone: (314) 768-3137
Carol Iglauer, Chf.Libn.
Subjects: Nursing, medicine. **Holdings:** 2812 books; 2824 bound periodical volumes; 188 videotapes; 416 audio cassettes; 66 instructional computer diskettes; 252 filmstrips; 2123 slides; 806 microfiche. **Subscriptions:** 202 journals and other serials.

★8757★ GAZETTE INTERNATIONAL NETWORKING INSTITUTE
LIBRARY
4502 Maryland Ave.
St. Louis, MO 63108   Phone: (314) 361-0475
Subjects: Disabled - education, employment, equipment, family, hobbies and sports, housing, independent living; ventilator-assisted living. **Holdings:** 3000 research monographs, reports, proceedings, case histories, and other volumes; 300 bound periodical volumes; archival items.

★8758★ INCARNATE WORD HOSPITAL
MEDICAL LIBRARY
3545 Lafayette Ave.
St. Louis, MO 63104   Phone: (314) 664-6500
Karen L. Launsby, Med.Libn.
Subjects: Medicine, allied health sciences, staff development. **Holdings:** 1000 books; 1000 bound periodical volumes; 50 pamphlets; reports and medical papers. **Subscriptions:** 70 journals and other serials.

★8759★ INTERNATIONAL LIBRARY, ARCHIVES AND MUSEUM OF OPTOMETRY
243 N. Lindbergh Blvd.
St. Louis, MO 63141   Phone: (314) 991-0324
Bridget Kowalczyk, Libn.
Subjects: Vision, optometry, ophthalmology. **Holdings:** 6000 books; 400 feet of archives. **Subscriptions:** 500 journals and other serials.

★8760★ JEWISH HOSPITAL
SCHOOL OF NURSING
MOSES SHOENBERG MEMORIAL LIBRARY
306 S. Kingshighway
St. Louis, MO 63110   Phone: (314) 454-8474
Betsy Mueth, Libn.
Subjects: Nursing, nursing education, medicine. **Holdings:** 2000 books; VF materials; AV collection; software; anatomical models. **Subscriptions:** 100 journals and other serials.

★8761★ JEWISH HOSPITAL AT WASHINGTON UNIVERSITY MEDICAL CENTER
ROTHSCHILD MEDICAL LIBRARY
216 S. Kingshighway
St. Louis, MO 63110   Phone: (314) 454-7208
Kathleen Mullen, Lib.Dir.
Subjects: Medicine. **Holdings:** 2262 books; 5634 bound periodical volumes. **Subscriptions:** 95 journals and other serials.

★8762★ LUTHERAN MEDICAL CENTER
MEDICAL LIBRARY
2639 Miami St.
St. Louis, MO 63118   Phone: (314) 772-1456
Chidi C. Ukabam, Med.Libn.
Subjects: Medicine. **Holdings:** 310 books; 1134 bound periodical volumes; 200 cassette tapes. **Subscriptions:** 49 journals and other serials.

★8763★ MALLINCKRODT INC.
LIBRARY
3600 2nd St.
Box 5439
St. Louis, MO 63147   Phone: (314) 539-1514
Juanita M. McCarthy, Mgr., Lib.Serv.
Subjects: Chemistry, pharmacology. **Holdings:** 7000 books; 15,000 bound periodical volumes. **Subscriptions:** 400 journals and other serials.

★8764★ MISSOURI BAPTIST MEDICAL CENTER
MEDICAL LIBRARY
3015 N. Ballas Rd.
St. Louis, MO 63131   Phone: (314) 432-1212
Subjects: Medicine, allied health sciences. **Holdings:** 645 books; 1900 bound periodical volumes. **Subscriptions:** 86 journals and other serials.

★8765★ MISSOURI BAPTIST MEDICAL CENTER
SCHOOL OF NURSING LIBRARY
3015 N. Ballas Rd.
St. Louis, MO 63131   Phone: (314) 569-5193
Carolyn McGinty, Libn.
Subjects: Nursing, medicine, psychology. **Holdings:** 2500 books; AV programs. **Subscriptions:** 55 journals and other serials.

★8766★ MISSOURI SCHOOL FOR THE BLIND
LIBRARY
3815 Magnolia Ave.
St. Louis, MO 63110   Phone: (314) 776-4320
Mary Dingus
Subjects: General collection, special education, blind education. **Holdings:** 4000 Braille books and magazines; 4700 audio books and magazines; 900 large-print books and magazine. **Subscriptions:** 100 journals and other serials; 2 newspapers.

★8767★ NATIONAL ARCHIVES AND RECORDS ADMINISTRATION
NATIONAL PERSONNEL RECORDS CENTER
9700 Page Blvd.
St. Louis, MO 63132-5100   Phone: (314) 263-7201
David L. Petree, Dir.
Subjects: Service and medical records of persons who have served in the Armed Forces, noncurrent records of organizations which have been a part of the military establishment, personnel and medical records of former federal civilian employees. **Holdings:** 1.8 million cubic feet of military and personnel records (MPR) and organizational records; 1.9 million cubic feet of civilian personnel records (CPR) and agency organizational records.

★8768★ PLANNED PARENTHOOD OF THE ST. LOUIS REGION
EDUCATION DEPARTMENT
LIBRARY
7415 Manchester Rd.
St. Louis, MO 63143   Phone: (314) 781-3800
Denise Page, Dir. of Pub.Educ.
Subjects: Family planning, human reproduction, sexually transmitted diseases, pregnancy, homosexuality, human sexuality, abortion, parenting. **Holdings:** 500 books; 20 bound periodical volumes; clippings and articles. **Subscriptions:** 11 journals and other serials.

★8769★ RALSTON PURINA COMPANY
INFORMATION CENTER
Checkerboard Sq.
St. Louis, MO 63164-0001   Phone: (314) 982-1000
Linda S. Lincks, Mgr.
Subjects: Animal and human nutrition, veterinary medicine, food processing, food sanitation. **Holdings:** 13,000 volumes; 20 VF drawers of proceedings; 69 VF drawers of government reports. **Subscriptions:** 392 journals and other serials.

★8770★ ST. JOHN'S MERCY MEDICAL CENTER
JOHN YOUNG BROWN MEMORIAL LIBRARY
621 S. New Ballas Rd.
St. Louis, MO 63141-8221   Phone: (314) 569-6340
Saundra H. Brenner, Dir.
Subjects: Medicine, nursing. **Holdings:** 1391 books; 10,000 bound periodical volumes. **Subscriptions:** 600 journals and other serials.

★8771★ ST. LOUIS COLLEGE OF PHARMACY
O.J. CLOUGHLY ALUMNI LIBRARY
4588 Parkview Pl.
St. Louis, MO 63110   Phone: (314) 367-8700
Judith A. Longstreth, Lib.Dir.
Subjects: Pharmacy, pharmacology, medicine, drug information. **Holdings:** 35,000 volumes; 500 audiotapes; 12,700 microforms. **Subscriptions:** 442 journals and other serials; 8 newspapers.

★8772★ ST. LOUIS HEARING AND SPEECH CENTERS
LIBRARY
9526 Manchester
St. Louis, MO 63119-1313   Phone: (314) 968-4710
Peggy Thompson, Exec.Dir.
Subjects: Audiology, speech pathology, sign language, industrial hearing conservation, accent reduction, stutterers, preschool language. **Holdings:** 600 volumes.

★8773★ ST. LOUIS PSYCHOANALYTIC INSTITUTE
BETTY GOLDE SMITH MEMORIAL LIBRARY
4524 Forest Park Ave.
St. Louis, MO 63108   Phone: (314) 361-7075
Celia D. Bouchard
Subjects: Psychoanalysis and related subjects. **Holdings:** 6000 volumes. **Subscriptions:** 33 journals and other serials.

★8774★ ST. LOUIS REGIONAL MEDICAL CENTER
MEDICAL LIBRARY
5535 Delmar Blvd.
St. Louis, MO 63112   Phone: (314) 879-6272
Mrs. Bernie Ferrell, Med.Libn.
Subjects: Medicine, surgery, pediatrics, orthopedics, obstetrics and gynecology, neurology, neonatology. **Holdings:** 1000 books; 10,000 bound periodical volumes. **Subscriptions:** 125 journals and other serials.

★8775★ ST. LOUIS UNIVERSITY
MEDICAL CENTER LIBRARY
1402 S. Grand Blvd.
St. Louis, MO 63104   Phone: (314) 577-8605
T. Scott Plutchak, Libn.
Subjects: Medicine, nursing, allied health sciences, hospital administration. **Holdings:** 47,278 books; 72,932 bound periodical volumes; 15 VF drawers of pamphlets; 400 pictures; 500 historical volumes; 3000 microfiche; 26,000 slides; 700 video cassettes; instrument collection. **Subscriptions:** 1728 journals and other serials; 4 newspapers.

★8776★ ST. MARY'S HEALTH CENTER
HEALTH SCIENCES LIBRARY
6420 Clayton Rd.
St. Louis, MO 63117   Phone: (314) 768-8112
Candace W. Thayer, Libn.
Subjects: Clinical medicine, nursing, allied health sciences. **Holdings:** 1000 books; 12,000 bound periodical volumes. **Subscriptions:** 200 journals and other serials.

★8777★ U.S. DEPARTMENT OF VETERANS AFFAIRS
LIBRARY SERVICE
Jefferson Barracks Division
St. Louis, MO 63125   Phone: (314) 894-6630
Larry Weitkemper, Chf., Lib.Serv.
Subjects: Medicine and allied health sciences. **Holdings:** 5500 books; 9000 bound periodical volumes; 9000 reels of microfilm; 1200 AV programs. **Subscriptions:** 750 journals and other serials.

★8778★ UNIVERSITY OF MISSOURI, COLUMBIA
MISSOURI INSTITUTE OF PSYCHIATRY LIBRARY
5400 Arsenal St.
St. Louis, MO 63139-1494   Phone: (314) 644-8838
Mary E. Johnson, Lib.Dir.
Subjects: Psychiatry, neurology, psychology, biochemistry, nursing. **Hold-ings:** 10,000 books; 14,000 bound periodical volumes; 7 VF drawers; 250 films and video cassettes; 650 audio cassettes; 50 microforms. **Subscriptions:** 400 journals and other serials.

★8779★ UNIVERSITY OF MISSOURI, ST. LOUIS
HEALTH SCIENCES LIBRARY
8001 Natural Bridge Rd.
St. Louis, MO 63121   Phone: (314) 553-5909
Cheryle J. Cann, Hd.Libn.
Subjects: Nursing science, vision science. **Holdings:** 5893 books; 3635 bound periodical volumes; 798 AV programs; 223 reels of microfilm; 4132 microfiche. **Subscriptions:** 200 journals and other serials.

★8780★ WASHINGTON UNIVERSITY
GEORGE WARREN BROWN SCHOOL OF SOCIAL WORK
LIBRARY AND LEARNING RESOURCES CENTER
Campus Box 1196
St. Louis, MO 63130   Phone: (314) 889-6633
Michael E, Powell, Dir.
Subjects: Alcoholism, women, women's issues, social work, gerontology, mental health, health, aging, gerontology, minorities, children and youth services, social and economic development, family therapy, management, special populations. **Holdings:** 39,126 volumes; 5000 government documents; 250 theses; 4122 pamphlets; 113 reels of microfilm; 11 films, filmstrips, slides; 843 videotapes; 162 audiotapes. **Subscriptions:** 519 journals and other serials; 7 newspapers.

★8781★ WASHINGTON UNIVERSITY
SCHOOL OF MEDICINE
DEPARTMENT OF PSYCHIATRY LIBRARY
4940 Audubon Ave.
St. Louis, MO 63110   Phone: (314) 362-2454
Subjects: Psychiatry, biochemistry, neurochemical pharmacology, epidemiology, genetics. **Holdings:** 1000 books; 20,000 bound periodical volumes; 3 VF drawers of department reprints. **Subscriptions:** 99 journals and other serials.

★8782★ WASHINGTON UNIVERSITY
SCHOOL OF MEDICINE
MALLINCKRODT INSTITUTE OF RADIOLOGY LIBRARY
510 S. Kingshighway Blvd.
St. Louis, MO 63110   Phone: (314) 362-2978
William Totty, M.D., Lib.Dir.
Subjects: Radiology. **Holdings:** 1402 books; 1534 bound periodical volumes; 365 videotapes; 106 slide lectures; 6 AV journals. **Subscriptions:** 69 journals and other serials.

★8783★ WASHINGTON UNIVERSITY
SCHOOL OF MEDICINE LIBRARY
660 S. Euclid Ave.
Campus Box 8132
St. Louis, MO 63110   Phone: (314) 362-7080
Prof. Susan Y. Crawford, Dir.
Subjects: Medicine. **Holdings:** 85,327 books; 146,944 bound periodical volumes; 1780 feet of archives; 2248 nonprint items. **Subscriptions:** 3123 journals and other serials.

★8784★ WASHINGTON UNIVERSITY MEDICAL CENTER
ST. LOUIS CHILDREN'S HOSPITAL LIBRARY
400 S. Kingshighway Blvd.
St. Louis, MO 63110   Phone: (314) 454-2767
Ileen R. Kendall, Libn.
Subjects: Medicine, pediatrics, nursing. **Holdings:** 1607 books; 1825 bound periodical volumes; 15 dissertations; 43 volumes of staff publications, 1920-1987; AV equipment. **Subscriptions:** 105 journals and other serials.

★8785★ COX MEDICAL CENTERS
LIBRARIES
1423 N. Jefferson Ave.
Springfield, MO 65802   Phone: (417) 836-3460
Paula Morrow, Supv., Lib.Serv.
Subjects: Medicine, nursing, allied health. **Holdings:** 2757 titles; 3684 volumes. **Subscriptions:** 220 journals and other serials.

★8786★   ST. JOHN'S REGIONAL HEALTH CENTER
MEDICAL LIBRARY
1235 E. Cherokee
Springfield, MO 65804-2263   Phone: (417) 885-2795
Anna Beth Crabtree, Dir., Med.Lib.Serv.
Subjects: Medicine, nursing, and allied health sciences, management.
Holdings: 2200 books; 6500 bound periodical volumes; 200 videotapes;
200 audiotapes; 125 microforms. **Subscriptions:** 400 journals and other
serials; 20 newspapers.

★8787★   ST. JOHN'S REGIONAL HEALTH CENTER
SCHOOL OF NURSING LIBRARY
4431 S. Fremont
Springfield, MO 65804   Phone: (417) 885-2104
Sandy J. Anderson, Libn.
Subjects: Nursing, medicine, and allied health sciences. **Holdings:** 5000
books; 155 reels of microfilm; 8 VF drawers of pamphlets; charts; models;
pictures; cassette tapes; video tapes; filmstrips. **Subscriptions:** 70 journals
and other serials.

★8788★   SPRINGFIELD REGIONAL CENTER FOR THE
DEVELOPMENTALLY DISABLED
LIBRARY
1515 E. Pythian
PO Box 5030
Springfield, MO 65801-5030   Phone: (417) 836-0400
Lyle Smith, Libn.
Subjects: Developmentally disabled.

Montana

★8789★   MENTAL HEALTH CENTER
LIBRARY
1245 N. 29th St.
Billings, MT 59101   Phone: (406) 252-5658
Lizbeth Barnea, Libn.
Subjects: Psychiatry, psychology, substance abuse, psychiatric nursing.
Holdings: 700 books; vertical files. **Subscriptions:** 29 journals and other
serials.

★8790★   U.S. DEPARTMENT OF LABOR
OSHA
BILLINGS AREA OFFICE LIBRARY
19 N. 25th St.
Billings, MT 59101   Phone: (406) 657-6649
Bonnie Albright, Ck.
Subjects: Safety and health in the workplace. **Holdings:** 500 books;
microfilm.

★8791★   MONTANA STATE UNIVERSITY
VETERINARY MOLECULAR BIOLOGY LABORATORY
HUIDEKOPER LIBRARY
S. 19th & Lincoln
Bozeman, MT 59717   Phone: (406) 994-4705
C.A. Speer, Dir.
Subjects: Veterinary science. **Holdings:** 3400 books; 3100 bound periodical
volumes; 6000 pamphlets and reprints. **Subscriptions:** 120 journals and
other serials.

★8792★   ST. JAMES COMMUNITY HOSPITAL
HEALTH SCIENCES LIBRARY
400 S. Clark
Butte, MT 59702   Phone: (406) 782-8361
Carole Ann Clark, Med.Libn.
Subjects: Oncology, nursing, medicine, ethics, pediatrics, obstetrics, gyne-
cology. **Holdings:** 750 books; 600 bound periodical volumes; 400 video
cassettes. **Subscriptions:** 159 journals and other serials.

★8793★   U.S. DEPARTMENT OF VETERANS AFFAIRS
MEDICAL CENTER LIBRARY
Fort Harrison, MT 59636   Phone: (406) 442-6410
Charles Grasmick, Chf., Lib.Serv.
Subjects: Medicine, internal medicine, surgery. **Holdings:** 1484 books.
Subscriptions: 268 journals and other serials; 10 newspapers.

★8794★   COLUMBUS HOSPITAL
HEALTH SCIENCES LIBRARY
Box 5013
Great Falls, MT 59403   Phone: (406) 771-5631
Katherine V. Chew, Dir.
Subjects: Medicine, nursing, science. **Holdings:** 8580 books; 10,000 bound
periodical volumes; 6 VF drawers of pamphlets; 6 catalog drawers of drug
description slips. **Subscriptions:** 550 journals and other serials.

★8795★   GREAT FALLS CLINIC
LIBRARY
1400 29th St., S.
Great Falls, MT 59405   Phone: (406) 454-2171
Ms. B.J. Vinson, Lib.Dir.
Subjects: Medicine, allied health sciences. **Holdings:** 3500 volumes.
Subscriptions: 125 journals and other serials.

★8796★   U.S. NATIONAL INSTITUTES OF HEALTH
NATIONAL INSTITUTE OF ALLERGY AND INFECTIOUS
DISEASES
ROCKY MOUNTAIN LABORATORY LIBRARY
Hamilton, MT 59840   Phone: (406) 363-3211
Leza Serha Hamby, Med.Libn.
Subjects: Medicine, virology, bacteriology, immunology, entomology,
chemistry, parasitology, pathology, microbiology, biochemistry, biology,
sexually transmitted disease. **Holdings:** 6000 books; 22,000 bound periodi-
cal volumes. **Subscriptions:** 287 journals and other serials.

★8797★   SHODAIR CHILDREN'S HOSPITAL
MEDICAL INFORMATION AND LIBRARY SERVICES
Box 5539
Helena, MT 59604   Phone: (406) 444-7534
Suzy Holt, Info.Spec.
Subjects: Clinical genetics, genetic disorders, prenatal diagnosis, genetic
counseling, cytogenetics, child psychiatry. **Holdings:** 2000 books; 1000
bound periodical volumes. **Subscriptions:** 65 journals and other serials.

★8798★   KALISPELL REGIONAL HOSPITAL
MEDICAL LIBRARY
310 Sunny View Ln.
Kalispell, MT 59901   Phone: (406) 752-5111
Susan Long, Med.Libn.
Subjects: Medicine, surgery, nursing. **Holdings:** 450 books; 742 bound
periodical volumes; 400 video cassettes. **Subscriptions:** 100 journals and
other serials.

★8799★   U.S. DEPARTMENT OF VETERANS AFFAIRS
MEDICAL CENTER LIBRARY
Miles City, MT 59301   Phone: (406) 232-3060
Gail Shaw Wilkerson, Chf., Lib.Serv.
Subjects: Medicine. **Holdings:** 1000 volumes. **Subscriptions:** 100 journals
and other serials.

★8800★   ST. PATRICK HOSPITAL
LIBRARY
500 W. Broadway
Box 4587
Missoula, MT 59806   Phone: (406) 543-7271
Kimberly M. Granath, Libn.
Subjects: Nursing, medicine, hospital administration, patient education.
Holdings: 2000 books; 24 VF drawers of pamphlets; 900 video cassettes.
Subscriptions: 250 journals and other serials.

★8801★   WESTERN MONTANA CLINIC
LIBRARY
515 W. Front St.
Box 7609
Missoula, MT 59807   Phone: (406) 721-5600
Tod A. Gregoire, Libn.
Subjects: Medicine. **Holdings:** 500 books; 165 bound periodical volumes.
Subscriptions: 165 journals and other serials.

Nebraska

★8802★ BEATRICE STATE DEVELOPMENTAL CENTER
LIBRARY/MEDIA CENTER
3000 Lincoln Blvd.
Beatrice, NE 68310   Phone: (402) 223-2302
Donald G. Robertson, Libn./Media Spec.
Subjects: Mental retardation, behavior modification, psychiatry, psychology. Holdings: 1500 books; 110 periodical titles; 350 other cataloged items. Subscriptions: 40 journals and other serials.

★8803★ U.S. DEPARTMENT OF VETERANS AFFAIRS
HOSPITAL LIBRARY
2201 N. Broadwell St.
Grand Island, NE 68803   Phone: (308) 382-3660
Shirley J. Barthelman, Chf., Lib.Serv.
Subjects: Medicine, surgery, nursing. Holdings: 1074 books. Subscriptions: 110 journals and other serials.

★8804★ HASTINGS REGIONAL CENTER
MEDICAL LIBRARY
Box 579
Hastings, NE 68902   Phone: (402) 463-2471
Ruth Swingle, Libn.
Subjects: Psychiatry, psychiatric nursing, psychiatric social work, medicine, patient education, mental health. Holdings: 4000 books; 500 bound periodical volumes; 12 VF drawers of pamphlets and reprints. Subscriptions: 47 journals and other serials.

★8805★ BRYAN MEMORIAL HOSPITAL
MEDICAL LIBRARY
1600 S. 48th
Lincoln, NE 68506   Phone: (402) 483-3030
Christina Hugly, Med.Lib.Spec.
Subjects: Clinical medicine, cardiovascular medicine. Holdings: 300 books. Subscriptions: 62 journals and other serials.

★8806★ BRYAN MEMORIAL HOSPITAL
SCHOOL OF NURSING
HELENE FULD MEMORIAL LEARNING RESOURCE CENTER
5000 Sumner St.
Lincoln, NE 68506   Phone: (402) 483-3908
Susan P. Echols, Libn.
Subjects: Nursing, nursing education. Holdings: 4500 books; 100 bound periodical volumes; journals on microfiche. Subscriptions: 75 journals and other serials.

★8807★ LINCOLN GENERAL HOSPITAL
HOSPITAL LIBRARY
2300 S. 16th St.
Lincoln, NE 68502   Phone: (402) 473-5637
Lucille Rosenberg, Hosp.Libn.
Subjects: Medicine, oncology, orthopedics, psychiatry, nursing, trauma, allied health sciences and professions. Holdings: 1000 books; 90 bound periodical volumes. Subscriptions: 100 journals and other serials.

★8808★ MADONNA CENTERS, INC.
MEDICAL LIBRARY
5401 South St.
Lincoln, NE 68506-2134   Phone: (402) 483-9595
Jean M. Powers, Dir. of Educ.
Subjects: Rehabilitation, gerontology, medical sciences, burn care, respiratory care. Holdings: 621 books; 17 bound periodical volumes; 4 file drawers of pamphlets. Subscriptions: 64 journals and other serials.

★8809★ ST. ELIZABETH COMMUNITY HEALTH CENTER
MEDICAL LIBRARY
555 S. 70th St.
Lincoln, NE 68510   Phone: (402) 486-7306
Beth Goble, Med.Libn.
Subjects: Medicine, nursing. Holdings: 2000 books; 1400 bound periodical volumes; 500 AV programs; 2524 unbound journals; 12 file drawers of pamphlets. Subscriptions: 130 journals and other serials.

★8810★ U.S. DEPARTMENT OF VETERANS AFFAIRS
MEDICAL CENTER LIBRARY
600 S. 70th St.
Lincoln, NE 68510   Phone: (402) 489-3802
Mrs. Svoboda, Libn.
Subjects: Medicine and allied health sciences. Holdings: 2511 titles; 1028 bound periodical volumes; 1436 boxes of microfilm (periodicals); 700 AV programs. Subscriptions: 280 journals and other serials; 5 newspapers.

★8811★ NORFOLK REGIONAL CENTER
STAFF LIBRARY
Box 1209
Norfolk, NE 68701   Phone: (402) 371-4343
Dolores E. Hartman, Libn. I
Subjects: Clinical psychology, psychiatry, medicine, social work. Holdings: 1500 books. Subscriptions: 20 journals and other serials.

★8812★ U.S. AIR FORCE HOSPITAL
EHRLING BERGQUIST STRATEGIC HOSPITAL
MEDICAL LIBRARY
Offutt AFB, NE 68113-5300   Phone: (402) 294-5499
Jan Hatcher, Lib.Mgr.
Subjects: Surgery and allied health sciences. Holdings: 2200 books. Subscriptions: 260 journals and other serials.

★8813★ BERGAN MERCY HOSPITAL
MEDICAL LIBRARY
7500 Mercy Rd.
Omaha, NE 68124   Phone: (402) 398-6092
Ken Oyer, Libn.
Subjects: Medicine, nursing, management, health care administration. Holdings: 2000 books; 25,000 microfiche; 234 reels of microfilm. Subscriptions: 168 journals and other serials.

★8814★ BISHOP CLARKSON MEMORIAL HOSPITAL
PATHOLOGY/MEDICAL STAFF LIBRARY
Dewey & 44th
Omaha, NE 68105   Phone: (402) 559-2058
Subjects: Medicine, pathology, laboratory diagnosis. Holdings: 450 books; 1200 bound periodical volumes. Subscriptions: 115 journals and other serials.

★8815★ CREIGHTON UNIVERSITY
HEALTH SCIENCES LIBRARY
California at 24th St.
Omaha, NE 68178   Phone: (402) 280-5108
Marjorie Wannarka, Dir.
Subjects: Medicine, pharmacy, dentistry, nursing, and allied health sciences. Holdings: 31,830 books; 58,623 bound periodical volumes; 4338 AV programs; 63,179 microforms. Subscriptions: 1443 journals and other serials; 6 newspapers.

★8816★ IMMANUEL MEDICAL CENTER
PROFESSIONAL LIBRARY
6901 N. 72nd St.
Omaha, NE 68122-1799   Phone: (402) 572-2345
Joy A. Winkler, Libn.
Subjects: Medicine, nursing, and allied health sciences. Holdings: 500 books; 189 bound periodical volumes. Subscriptions: 225 journals and other serials.

★8817★ NEBRASKA METHODIST HOSPITAL
JOHN MORITZ LIBRARY
8303 Dodge St.
Omaha, NE 68114   Phone: (402) 390-4611
Angela Armer, Lrng.Rsrcs.Mgr.
Subjects: Medicine, nursing, and allied health sciences. Holdings: 7649 books; 3586 bound periodical volumes; 10 VF drawers of pamphlets and reprints. Subscriptions: 535 journals and other serials.

★8818★ OMAHA PUBLIC LIBRARY
BUSINESS, SCIENCE AND TECHNOLOGY DEPARTMENT
215 S. 15th St.
Omaha, NE 68102   Phone: (402) 444-4817
Janet Davenport, Hd.
Subjects: Economics, insurance, mathematics, physics, investments, chemistry, engineering, agriculture, medicine, health, biology, botany. Holdings: 39,212 books; 6358 bound periodical volumes; 75 VF drawers of pam-

phlets, clippings, house organs, corporate annual reports; 350,603 U.S. Government documents; 56,240 topographic maps; microfilm. **Subscriptions:** 525 journals and other serials.

★8819★   U.S. DEPARTMENT OF VETERANS AFFAIRS
HOSPITAL LIBRARY
4101 Woolworth Ave.
Omaha, NE 68105   Phone: (402) 449-0652
Ronald L. Fingerson, Chf., Lib.Serv.
Subjects: Medicine and allied health sciences. **Holdings:** 872 books; 300 bound periodical volumes; 1014 AV programs. **Subscriptions:** 259 journals and other serials; 25 newspapers.

★8820★   UNIVERSITY OF NEBRASKA MEDICAL CENTER
MCGOOGAN LIBRARY OF MEDICINE
600 S. 42nd St.
Omaha, NE 68198-6705   Phone: (402) 559-4006
Nancy N. Woelfl, Ph.D., Dir.
Subjects: Medicine, nursing, pharmacy, psychiatry, allied health sciences. **Holdings:** 79,594 books; 144,549 bound periodical volumes; 681 microforms; 25 VF drawers of archives. **Subscriptions:** 2336 journals and other serials.

Nevada

★8821★   CARSON-TAHOE HOSPITAL
LAHONTAN BASIN MEDICAL LIBRARY
775 Fleischmann Way
Box 2168
Carson City, NV 89702-2168   Phone: (702) 882-1361
Elaine L. Laessle, Libn.
Subjects: Clinical medicine, health care. **Holdings:** 1000 books; unbound periodicals; 202 folders of medical files. **Subscriptions:** 190 journals and other serials.

★8822★   ELKO MEDICAL CLINIC
LIBRARY
762 14th St.
Elko, NV 89801   Phone: (702) 738-3111
Jeanette Tognini
Subjects: Medicine, allied health sciences. **Holdings:** 1025 books; 1950 bound periodical volumes; 50 unbound medical volumes; 721 postgraduate tapes. **Subscriptions:** 118 journals and other serials.

★8823★   CLARK COUNTY DISTRICT HEALTH DEPARTMENT
HEALTH EDUCATION RESOURCE CENTER
625 Shadow Ln.
Box 4426
Las Vegas, NV 89127   Phone: (702) 383-1218
Subjects: Environmental health, emergency medical service, public health nursing, air pollution control, epidemiology. **Holdings:** 3 VF drawers of health reprints; health pamphlets; news clippings; filmstrips; videotapes; 16mm films.

★8824★   HUMANA HOSPITAL SUNRISE
MEDICAL LIBRARY
3186 Maryland Pkwy.
Las Vegas, NV 89108   Phone: (702) 731-8210
Subjects: Medicine, allied health sciences. **Holdings:** 1600 books; 2500 bound periodical volumes; 400 reels of microfilm; 100 videotapes. **Subscriptions:** 160 journals.

★8825★   UNIVERSITY MEDICAL CENTER OF SOUTHERN
   NEVADA
MEDICAL LIBRARY
2040 W. Charleston Blvd., Ste. 500
Las Vegas, NV 89102   Phone: (702) 383-2368
Aldona Jonynas, Dir., Lib.Serv.
Subjects: Medicine, nursing. **Holdings:** 6000 books; 8200 bound periodical volumes; 320 bound indexes; 95 vertical files; 5 boxes of staff publications; 600 symposia; 700 audio cassettes and videotapes. **Subscriptions:** 250 journals and other serials.

★8826★   ST. MARY'S REGIONAL MEDICAL CENTER
MAX C. FLEISCHMANN MEDICAL LIBRARY
235 W. 6th St.
Reno, NV 89520-0108   Phone: (702) 789-3108
Kathleen L. Davis, Lib.Coord.
Subjects: Medicine, nursing, management. **Holdings:** 1564 books; 1244 bound periodical volumes. **Subscriptions:** 152 journals and other serials.

★8827★   U.S. DEPARTMENT OF VETERANS AFFAIRS
MEDICAL CENTER
LIBRARY SERVICES
1000 Locust St.
Reno, NV 89520   Phone: (702) 328-1471
Christine J. Camp, Chf., Lib.Serv.
Subjects: Clinical medicine, gerontology. **Holdings:** 2850 books; 500 AV items. **Subscriptions:** 350 journals and other serials.

★8828★   UNIVERSITY OF NEVADA, RENO
LIFE AND HEALTH SCIENCES LIBRARY
Fleischmann College of Agriculture Bldg./206
Reno, NV 89557   Phone: (702) 784-6616
Susan Stewart, Libn.
Subjects: Biology, agriculture, nursing, health resources, speech pathology and audiology, medical technology. **Holdings:** 28,187 books; 23,270 bound periodical volumes; 8013 bound government reports; 66,501 unbound government reports; 417 reels of microfilm; 12,283 microfiche. **Subscriptions:** 598 journals.

★8829★   UNIVERSITY OF NEVADA, RENO
SAVITT MEDICAL LIBRARY
Savitt Medical Sciences Bldg./306
Reno, NV 89557   Phone: (702) 784-4625
Joan S. Zenan, Dir.
Subjects: Medicine and allied health sciences. **Holdings:** 39,000 volumes. **Subscriptions:** 500 journals and other serials.

★8830★   WASHOE MEDICAL CENTER
MEDICAL LIBRARY
77 Pringle Way
Reno, NV 89520   Phone: (702) 328-5693
Sherry A. McGee, Dir., Med.Lib.
Subjects: Medicine, nursing, allied health sciences. **Holdings:** 2256 books; 4432 bound periodical volumes. **Subscriptions:** 265 journals and other serials.

★8831★   NEVADA MENTAL HEALTH INSTITUTE
LIBRARY
480 Galletti Way
Sparks, NV 89431-5574   Phone: (702) 688-2055
Robert D. Armstrong, Libn.
Subjects: Psychiatry, psychology, mental health, psychiatric nursing. **Holdings:** 5500 books; 500 government documents; 2000 pamphlets and reports; 450 audio cassettes. **Subscriptions:** 40 journals and other serials.

New Hampshire

★8832★   ANDROSCOGGIN VALLEY HOSPITAL
MEDICAL LIBRARY
59 Page Hill Rd.
Berlin, NH 03570   Phone: (603) 752-2200
Donna Adams, ART
Subjects: Medicine. **Holdings:** 450 volumes. **Subscriptions:** 18 journals and other serials.

★8833★   NEW HAMPSHIRE TECHNICAL COLLEGE
LIBRARY
1 College Dr.
Claremont, NH 03743   Phone: (603) 542-7744
Phil Prever, Libn.
Subjects: Technology, basic health sciences. **Holdings:** 11,000 books; film loops; filmstrips; records; cassettes. **Subscriptions:** 85 journals and other serials; 10 newspapers.

★8834★ VALLEY REGIONAL HOSPITAL
EDUCATION DEPARTMENT
HEALTH SCIENCE LIBRARY
Claremont, NH 03743   Phone: (603) 542-7771
Theresa Strickland
Subjects: Medicine. **Holdings:** 150 books. **Subscriptions:** 12 journals and other serials.

★8835★ NEW HAMPSHIRE HOSPITAL
PROFESSIONAL LIBRARY
105 Pleasant St.
Concord, NH 03301   Phone: (603) 271-5391
Linda McCracken, Libn.
Subjects: Psychiatry, psychology, geriatrics, nursing, neurology, social work. **Holdings:** 4000 books; 1000 bound periodical volumes; reports of the hospital to the governor and council, 1843-1956; 225 videotapes; 31 filmstrip/tape sets; 15 16mm films; 8 cassettes; 3 slide sets; 8 microfiche. **Subscriptions:** 131 journals and other serials.

★8836★ ORR AND RENO
LAW LIBRARY
1 Eagle Sq.
Box 709
Concord, NH 03302-0709   Phone: (603) 224-2381
David E. Selden, Libn.
Subjects: Law - corporate, estate, medical malpractice, tort. **Holdings:** 1000 volumes. **Subscriptions:** 36 journals and other serials.

★8837★ PARKLAND HOSPITAL
INFORMATION CENTER/LIBRARY
Derry, NH 03038   Phone: (603) 432-1500
Holly Eddy, Libn.
Subjects: Medicine.

★8838★ DARTMOUTH COLLEGE
DANA BIOMEDICAL LIBRARY
Dartmouth-Hitchcock Medical Ctr.
Hanover, NH 03756   Phone: (603) 646-7658
Shirley J. Grainger, Libn.
Subjects: Medicine, life sciences, nursing, agriculture. **Holdings:** 189,717 volumes; Dartmouth Medical School faculty reprints; 6289 AV programs; microforms; subject pamphlets; dissertations. **Subscriptions:** 3012 journals and other serials.

★8839★ CHESHIRE HOSPITAL
MACGRATH FAMILY MEDICAL LIBRARY
580 Court St.
Keene, NH 03431   Phone: (603) 352-4111
Jean Slepian, Libn.
Subjects: Medicine, nursing, and allied health sciences. **Holdings:** 1000 books; 1600 bound periodical volumes; 165 indices; 8 VF drawers of pamphlets. **Subscriptions:** 160 journals and other serials; 5 newspapers.

★8840★ CATHOLIC MEDICAL CENTER
HEALTH SCIENCE LIBRARY
100 McGregor St.
Manchester, NH 03102   Phone: (603) 668-3545
Marcia K. Allen, Dir., Lib.Serv.
Subjects: Medicine, nursing, allied health sciences, health care management. **Holdings:** 3160 books; 480 bound periodical volumes. **Subscriptions:** 240 journals and other serials.

★8841★ ELLIOT HOSPITAL
MEDICAL LIBRARY
Manchester, NH 30103   Phone: (603) 669-5300
Judy Reingold, Dir.
Subjects: Medicine, nursing, health administration. **Holdings:** 1500 books; 5000 bound periodical volumes; 1000 microfiche. **Subscriptions:** 250 journals and other serials.

★8842★ U.S. DEPARTMENT OF VETERANS AFFAIRS
MEDICAL CENTER LIBRARY
718 Smyth Rd.
Manchester, NH 03104   Phone: (603) 624-4366
Martha Roberts, Chf., Lib.Serv.
Subjects: Medicine, surgery, nursing. **Holdings:** 1650 books. **Subscriptions:** 168 journals and other serials; 7 newspapers.

★8843★ BROOKSIDE HOSPITAL
PROFESSIONAL LIBRARY
11 Northwest Blvd.
Nashua, NH 03063   Phone: (603) 886-5000
Laurie Smith, Libn.
Subjects: Psychiatry, mental health, chemical dependency. **Holdings:** 400 books. **Subscriptions:** 50 journals and other serials.

★8844★ NASHUA MEMORIAL HOSPITAL
HEALTH SCIENCES LIBRARY
8 Prospect St.
PO Box 2014
Nashua, NH 03061-2014   Phone: (603) 883-5521
Janis Isaacson Silver, Libn.
Subjects: Medicine, nursing, and allied health sciences. **Holdings:** 1000 books; 1920 bound periodical volumes; 30 videotapes; 600 VF items. **Subscriptions:** 131 journals and other serials.

★8845★ MONADNOCK COMMUNITY HOSPITAL
ECKFELDT MEMORIAL MEDICAL LIBRARY
452 Old Street Rd.
Peterborough, NH 03458   Phone: (603) 924-7191
Lesley Cass, Med.Libn.
Subjects: Clinical medicine, nursing, allied health, hospital administration. **Holdings:** 100 books; unbound medical journals. **Subscriptions:** 83 journals and other serials.

New Jersey

★8846★ ATLANTIC CITY MEDICAL CENTER
ATLANTIC CITY DIVISION
HEALTH SCIENCE LIBRARY
1925 Pacific Ave.
Atlantic City, NJ 08401   Phone: (609) 652-1000
John P. Doesburgh, Dir., Hea.Sci.Libs.
Subjects: Medicine, nursing, and allied health sciences. **Holdings:** 955 books; 2300 bound periodical volumes; Audio-Digest tapes in surgery and internal medicine. **Subscriptions:** 223 journals and other serials.

★8847★ CARRIER FOUNDATION
NOLAN D.C. LEWIS LIBRARY
Box 147
Belle Mead, NJ 08502   Phone: (201) 874-4000
Lynne Cohn, Dir.
Subjects: Psychiatry, psychotherapy, psychiatric nursing, family therapy, psychology, adjunctive therapies. **Holdings:** 3000 books; 600 audio and video cassettes. **Subscriptions:** 150 journals and other serials.

★8848★ CLARA MAASS MEDICAL CENTER
MEDICAL LIBRARY
Franklin Ave.
Belleville, NJ 07109   Phone: (201) 450-2294
Arlene Mangino, Libn.
Subjects: Medicine, surgery. **Holdings:** 827 books; 2704 bound periodical volumes; 360 audio cassettes; 15 video cassettes. **Subscriptions:** 81 journals and other serials.

★8849★ ASSOCIATION OF TONGUE DEPRESSORS
LIBRARY
c/o Dr. Matthew Schorr
12 Westminster Ave.
Bergenfield, NJ 07621   Phone: (201) 387-6969
Dr. Matthew Schorr, Sec.
Subjects: Health care, medical products, marketing. **Holdings:** 280 volumes.

★8850★ BLOOMFIELD COLLEGE
GEORGE TALBOTT HALL LIBRARY
467 Franklin St.
Bloomfield, NJ 07003   Phone: (201) 748-9000
Danilo Figueredo, Hd.Libn.
Subjects: Business administration, nursing, social and behavioral sciences, humanities, physical science, fine arts. **Holdings:** 59,000 books; 2361 bound periodical volumes; 4500 reels of microfilm. **Subscriptions:** 300 journals and other serials.

★8851★   CLARA MAASS MEDICAL CENTER
SCHOOL OF NURSING
LIBRARY
236 Hoover Ave.
Bloomfield, NJ 07003   Phone: (201) 680-4400
Arlene Mangino, Libn.
Subjects: Nursing. **Holdings:** 3300 books; 117 bound periodical volumes; 60 video cassettes. **Subscriptions:** 70 journals and other serials.

★8852★   SCHERING-PLOUGH CORPORATION
LIBRARY INFORMATION CENTER
60 Orange St.
Bloomfield, NJ 07003   Phone: (201) 429-3737
Gerald Wagman, Mgr.
Subjects: Pharmacy, biomedicine, microbiology, organic chemistry. **Holdings:** 30,000 volumes. **Subscriptions:** 1400 journals and other serials.

★8853★   E.R. JOHNSTONE TRAINING AND RESEARCH
** CENTER**
PROFESSIONAL LIBRARY
Burlington St.
Bordentown, NJ 08505   Phone: (609) 298-2500
Patricia Conlow-Scully, Act.Libn.
Subjects: Mental retardation, psychology. **Holdings:** 3350 books; 1450 bound periodical volumes; 110 Johnstone bulletins; 85 research reports; 60 microfiche. **Subscriptions:** 80 journals and other serials.

★8854★   SOUTH JERSEY HOSPITAL SYSTEM
HEALTH SCIENCES LIBRARY
Irving & Manheim Aves.
Bridgeton, NJ 08302   Phone: (609) 451-6600
Sue Dolbow, Med.Libn.
Subjects: Medicine, nursing. **Holdings:** 1000 books; AV catalogs; 260 AV programs; 8 VF drawers of articles and pamphlets. **Subscriptions:** 65 journals and other serials.

★8855★   DEBORAH HEART AND LUNG CENTER
MEDICAL LIBRARY
200 Trenton Rd.
Browns Mills, NJ 08015   Phone: (609) 893-6611
Carol A. Harris, Med.Libn.
Subjects: Cardiology, respiratory diseases, cardiothoracic surgery, medicine, pathology, nursing. **Holdings:** 3500 books; 2000 bound periodical volumes; AV programs. **Subscriptions:** 175 journals and other serials.

★8856★   COOPER HOSPITAL/UNIVERSITY MEDICAL CENTER
REUBEN L. SHARP HEALTH SCIENCE LIBRARY
1 Cooper Plaza
Camden, NJ 08103   Phone: (609) 342-2525
Joan Fierberg, Dir.
Subjects: Medicine, nursing, allied health sciences, patient education. **Holdings:** 4466 books; 13,500 periodicals, bound and on microfiche; 120 journal titles, 1976 to present; filmstrips; slide shows; video and audio cassettes. **Subscriptions:** 421 journals and other serials.

★8857★   HELENE FULD SCHOOL OF NURSING IN CAMDEN
** COUNTY**
LIBRARY
Mt. Ephraim & Atlantic Aves.
Camden, NJ 08104   Phone: (609) 342-4599
David A. Cohen, Libn.
Subjects: Nursing. **Holdings:** 2527 books; 500 bound periodical volumes; microfiche. **Subscriptions:** 117 journals and other serials.

★8858★   OUR LADY OF LOURDES MEDICAL CENTER
MEDICAL LIBRARY
1600 Haddon Ave.
Camden, NJ 08103   Phone: (609) 757-3548
Fred Kafes, Dir.
Subjects: Medicine, nursing, allied health sciences, hospital administration. **Holdings:** 900 books; 891 audio cassettes; 101 video cassettes; 5 slide/sound sets. **Subscriptions:** 290 journals and other serials.

★8859★   OUR LADY OF LOURDES MEDICAL CENTER
SCHOOL OF NURSING LIBRARY
1565 Vesper Blvd.
Camden, NJ 08103   Phone: (609) 757-3722
Eleanor M. Kelly, Libn.
Subjects: Medicine, nursing, allied health sciences. **Holdings:** 2617 books; 71 bound periodical volumes; 294 AV programs; 4 VF drawers of clippings, reports, pamphlets. **Subscriptions:** 52 journals and other serials.

★8860★   UMDNJ AND CORIELL RESEARCH
LIBRARY
401 Hadbon
Camden, NJ 08103   Phone: (609) 757-7740
Betty Jean Swartz, Libn.
Subjects: Cancer, immunology, genetics, pediatrics, microbiology, cell biology, cytogenetics, molecular biology, environmental mutagenesis, aging. **Holdings:** 9000 volumes. **Subscriptions:** 143 journals and other serials.

★8861★   ESSEX COUNTY HOSPITAL CENTER
HAMILTON MEMORIAL LIBRARY
Box 500
Cedar Grove, NJ 07009   Phone: (201) 228-8002
Elizabeth B. Guarducci, Med.Libn.
Subjects: Psychiatry, psychology, mental health, psychotherapy, medicine, social work. **Holdings:** 2500 books. **Subscriptions:** 100 journals and other serials; 7 newspapers.

★8862★   BERLEX LABORATORIES, INC.
RESEARCH AND DEVELOPMENT DIVISION LIBRARY
110 E. Hanover Ave.
Cedar Knolls, NJ 07927   Phone: (201) 292-8075
Lorene Lingelbach, Mgr., Lib.Serv.
Subjects: Pharmacology and the pharmaceutical industry, chemistry, internal medicine. **Holdings:** 7000 books; 7000 bound periodical volumes; 16,000 reels of microfilm of periodicals; 2500 reels of microfilm of patents. **Subscriptions:** 600 journals and other serials.

★8863★   PHARMACO-MEDICAL DOCUMENTATION INC.
LIBRARY
PO Box 429
Chatham, NJ 07928   Phone: (201) 822-9200
Dr. Boris R. Anzlowar, Tech.Dir.
Subjects: Pharmaceuticals, pharmacology, drug marketing. **Holdings:** 3500 volumes; machine-readable tapes; and other cataloged items. **Subscriptions:** 400 journals and other serials.

★8864★   KENNEDY MEMORIAL HOSPITALS
CHERRY HILL DIVISION
DR. BARNEY A. SLOTKIN MEMORIAL LIBRARY
Chapel Ave. & Cooper Landing Rd.
Box 5009
Cherry Hill, NJ 08034   Phone: (609) 488-6865
Sharon Sobel, Libn.
Subjects: Medicine, nursing, osteopathy. **Holdings:** 1148 books; 1710 bound periodical volumes. **Subscriptions:** 130 journals and other serials.

★8865★   HUNTERDON DEVELOPMENTAL CENTER
ADAPTIVE LEARNING CENTER
LIBRARY
Pittstown Rd.
CN 4220
Clinton, NJ 08809   Phone: (201) 735-4031
Roger Schumacher, Dir.
Subjects: Mental retardation, psychology, psychiatry, nursing, education. **Holdings:** 1700 professional books; 2000 children's books; AV programs and adapted materials for children. **Subscriptions:** 70 journals and other serials.

★8866★   CARTER-WALLACE, INC.
LIBRARY
Half-Acre Rd.
Cranbury, NJ 08512-0000   Phone: (609) 655-6000
Arthur Hilscher, Dir.
Subjects: Pharmacology, experimental medicine, organic chemistry, medicine, toiletries, diagnostics. **Holdings:** 3500 books; 1800 bound periodical volumes; 47,000 reports, pamphlets, documents. **Subscriptions:** 350 journals and other serials.

★8867★ JOHNSON AND JOHNSON
CHICOPEE RESEARCH LIBRARY
2351 Rte. 130
Box 940
Dayton, NJ 08810-0940   Phone: (908) 274-3126
Bryan Young, Libn.
Subjects: Textiles - medical, nonwoven, polymers. **Holdings:** 2000 books.
Subscriptions: 102 journals and other serials.

★8868★ ST. CLARES-RIVERSIDE MEDICAL CENTER
HEALTH SCIENCES LIBRARY
Pocono Rd.
Denville, NJ 07834   Phone: (201) 625-6547
Mildred E. Schaeffer, Libn.
Subjects: Medicine, surgery, dentistry, mental health, allied health sciences. **Holdings:** 300 books; 300 unbound periodicals; microfiche. **Subscriptions:** 81 journals and other serials.

★8869★ SANDOZ, INC.
LIBRARY
Rte. 10
East Hanover, NJ 07936   Phone: (201) 503-8306
Carol Bekar, Assoc.Dir.
Subjects: Medicine, chemistry, pharmacology, toxicology, biochemistry. **Holdings:** 8304 books; 26,285 bound periodical volumes; 20 drawers of microfilm; 2 drawers of annual reports. **Subscriptions:** 682 journals and other serials; 5 newspapers.

★8870★ SANDOZ PHARMACEUTICALS
MEDICAL INFORMATION SERVICES
Rte. 10
East Hanover, NJ 07936   Phone: (201) 503-8105
Joyce G. Koelle, Assoc.Dir.
Subjects: Corporation products, biomedicine, business. **Holdings:** Figures not available.

★8871★ EXXON BIOMEDICAL SCIENCES, INC.
LIBRARY
Mettlers Rd.
CN 2350
East Millstone, NJ 08875-2350   Phone: (201) 873-6091
Janice R. Seager, Libn.
Subjects: Toxicology, industrial hygiene, epidemiology, occupational medicine. **Holdings:** 5000 books; 8000 bound periodical volumes; 6000 government reports; clippings; pamphlets; reprints. **Subscriptions:** 250 journals and other serials.

★8872★ EAST ORANGE GENERAL HOSPITAL
MEDICAL LIBRARY
300 Central Ave.
East Orange, NJ 07018-2819   Phone: (201) 266-8520
Cindy Santamaria, Mgr. of Lib.Serv.
Subjects: Medicine, mental health, allied health sciences. **Holdings:** 1200 books. **Subscriptions:** 85 journals and other serials.

★8873★ U.S. DEPARTMENT OF VETERANS AFFAIRS
MEDICAL CENTER LIBRARY
385 Tremont Ave.
East Orange, NJ 07019   Phone: (201) 676-1000
Calvin A. Zamarelli, Chf., Lib.Serv.
Subjects: General medicine. **Holdings:** 11,000 books; 16,000 bound periodical volumes; 900 AV programs. **Subscriptions:** 400 journals and other serials.

★8874★ JOHN F. KENNEDY MEDICAL CENTER
MEDICAL LIBRARY
65 James St.
PO Box 3059
Edison, NJ 08818-3059   Phone: (201) 321-7181
Maria C. Daly, Med.Libn.
Subjects: Internal medicine, family practice, rehabilitation. **Holdings:** 600 books; 1000 bound periodical volumes; Audio-Digest tapes; NCME videotapes. **Subscriptions:** 200 journals and other serials.

★8875★ REVLON GROUP, INC.
REVLON RESEARCH CENTER
INFORMATION SERVICES
2121 Rte. 27
Edison, NJ 08818   Phone: (201) 287-7650
Lee J. Tanen, Mgr., Lib./Info.Serv.
Subjects: Cosmetics, soaps, chemistry, perfumery, dermatology, pharmacology, microbiology, aerosols. **Holdings:** 11,000 books; 4000 bound periodical volumes; central files; research notebooks. **Subscriptions:** 300 journals and other serials.

★8876★ ELIZABETH GENERAL MEDICAL CENTER
CHARLES H. SCHLICHTER, M.D. HEALTH SCIENCE LIBRARY
925 E. Jersey St.
Elizabeth, NJ 07201   Phone: (201) 558-8092
Catherine M. Boss, Dir.
Subjects: Nursing, medicine. **Holdings:** 4332 books; 3023 microfilm and bound periodical volumes. **Subscriptions:** 216 journals and other serials.

★8877★ ST. ELIZABETH HOSPITAL
HEALTH SCIENCES LIBRARY
225 Williamson St.
Elizabeth, NJ 07207   Phone: (201) 527-5371
Sally Holdorf, Libn.
Subjects: Medicine, nursing, and allied health fields. **Holdings:** 1000 books; 1200 bound periodical volumes. **Subscriptions:** 117 journals and other serials.

★8878★ ENGLEWOOD HOSPITAL
LEARNING CENTER LIBRARY
350 Engle St.
Englewood, NJ 07631   Phone: (201) 894-3070
Katherine L. Lindner, Dir.
Subjects: Medicine, allied health sciences. **Holdings:** 3000 books; 10,000 bound periodical volumes. **Subscriptions:** 400 journals and other serials.

★8879★ ENGLEWOOD HOSPITAL
SCHOOL OF NURSING LIBRARY
350 Engle St.
Englewood, NJ 07631   Phone: (201) 894-3145
Lia Sabbagh, Libn.
Subjects: Nursing, history of nursing. **Holdings:** 6000 books; 328 bound periodical volumes; 325 cassette and filmstrip titles; 50 film titles; 20 slides and cassettes; 60 other cataloged items. **Subscriptions:** 70 journals and other serials.

★8880★ PAT GUIDA ASSOCIATES
LIBRARY
24 Spielman Rd.
Fairfield, NJ 07004-3412   Phone: (201) 227-7418
Pat Guida, Pres.
Subjects: Food chemistry, chemistry, medicine, pharmacology, technology, nutrition, toxicology, environmental sciences. **Holdings:** 1400 books; 1000 bound periodical volumes; unbound periodicals. **Subscriptions:** 55 journals and other serials.

★8881★ HUNTERDON MEDICAL CENTER
MEDICAL LIBRARY
Rte. 31
Flemington, NJ 08822   Phone: (201) 788-6100
Jeanne L. Dutka, Med.Libn.
Subjects: Medicine, family practice. **Holdings:** 2000 books; 1500 bound periodical volumes; 200 Audio-Digest tapes. **Subscriptions:** 66 journals and other serials.

★8882★ U.S. ARMY HOSPITALS
WALSON ARMY HOSPITAL
MEDICAL LIBRARY
Fort Dix, NJ 08640-6734   Phone: (609) 562-5741
Subjects: Medicine, dentistry, nursing, psychiatry. **Holdings:** Figures not available.

★8883★ BECTON, DICKINSON & COMPANY
CORPORATE INFORMATION CENTER
1 Becton Dr.
Franklin Lakes, NJ 07417-1880   Phone: (201) 848-7230
Faina Menzul, Mgr.
Subjects: Medicine, science and technology, law, business, marketing.

Holdings: 2000 books; 220 periodicals. **Subscriptions:** 133 journals and other serials.

★8884★ GREYSTONE PARK PSYCHIATRIC HOSPITAL
HEALTH SCIENCE LIBRARY
Box A
Greystone Park, NJ 07950   Phone: (201) 538-1800
Brian C. Hamilton, Libn.
Subjects: Psychiatry, psychiatric nursing, psychology, medicine. **Holdings:** 1570 books; 60 bound periodical volumes. **Subscriptions:** 109 journals and other serials.

★8885★ BERGEN COUNTY DIVISION ON AGING
LIBRARY
Court Plaza S.
21 Main St., Rm. 109 W. Wing
Hackensack, NJ 07601-7000   Phone: (201) 646-2625
Gloria Layne, Div.Dir.
Subjects: Geriatrics, gerontology, health care and human services for the elderly, statistics. **Holdings:** 275 books; 500 bound periodical volumes; 1500 clippings and manuscripts. **Subscriptions:** 500 journals and other serials.

★8886★ HACKENSACK MEDICAL CENTER
MEDICAL LIBRARY
30 Prospect Ave.
Hackensack, NJ 07601   Phone: (201) 441-2326
Duressa Pujat, Libn.
Subjects: Medicine, surgery, nursing, hospital administration. **Holdings:** 5200 books; 15,000 bound periodical volumes; vertical files; pamphlets; 500 tapes. **Subscriptions:** 272 journals and other serials.

★8887★ HACKETTSTOWN COMMUNITY HOSPITAL
MEDICAL STAFF LIBRARY
651 Willow Grove St.
Hackettstown, NJ 07840   Phone: (908) 852-5100
Ruth E. Scarborough, Libn.
Subjects: Medicine, nursing. **Holdings:** 1000 books; 300 bound periodical volumes; 95 reports. **Subscriptions:** 106 journals and other serials.

★8888★ ANCORA PSYCHIATRIC HOSPITAL
HEALTH SCIENCES LIBRARY
Hammonton, NJ 08037   Phone: (609) 561-1700
Lorraine L. Chudomelka, Libn.
Subjects: Psychiatry, psychology, medicine, occupational therapy. **Holdings:** 3500 books; 600 bound periodical volumes; 289 audio cassettes; 24 video cassettes; 16 films. **Subscriptions:** 72 journals and other serials.

★8889★ BRISTOL-MYERS PRODUCTS
TECHNICAL INFORMATION CENTER
1350 Liberty Ave.
Hillside, NJ 07205   Phone: (201) 851-6053
Subjects: Biology, pharmacology, chemistry, pharmaceutical science, toiletries. **Holdings:** 12,000 books; 11,000 bound periodical volumes; 7500 reels of microfilm of periodicals; 5 drawers of patents, microfiche and hardcopy; 40 drawers of documents and reports, microfiche and hardcopy. **Subscriptions:** 350 journals and other serials; 2 newspapers.

★8890★ BLOCK DRUG COMPANY
RESEARCH AND DEVELOPMENT LIBRARY
257 Cornelison Ave.
Jersey City, NJ 07302   Phone: (201) 424-3000
Karen Berryman, Tech.Libn.
Subjects: Dentistry, medicine, pharmacology, dermatology. **Holdings:** Figures not available.

★8891★ CHRIST HOSPITAL
SCHOOL OF NURSING LIBRARY
176 Palisade Ave.
Jersey City, NJ 07306   Phone: (201) 795-8200
Katherine Vargo, Libn.
Subjects: Nursing. **Holdings:** 2343 volumes. **Subscriptions:** 52 journals and other serials.

★8892★ JERSEY CITY MEDICAL CENTER
MEDICAL LIBRARY
50 Baldwin Ave.
Jersey City, NJ 07304   Phone: (201) 915-2009
Judith Wilkinson
Subjects: Medicine. **Holdings:** 1000 books; 10,000 bound periodical volumes. **Subscriptions:** 200 journals and other serials; 3 newspapers.

★8893★ ST. BARNABAS MEDICAL CENTER
MEDICAL LIBRARY
Old Short Hills Rd.
Livingston, NJ 07039   Phone: (201) 533-5050
A. Christine Connor, Lib.Dir.
Subjects: Medicine, nursing. **Holdings:** 5000 books; 15,000 bound periodical volumes. **Subscriptions:** 365 journals and other serials.

★8894★ MONMOUTH MEDICAL CENTER
ALTSCHUL MEDICAL LIBRARY
300 2nd Ave.
Long Branch, NJ 07740   Phone: (908) 870-5170
Frederic C. Pachman, Dir.
Subjects: Medicine, nursing, dentistry, pediatrics, geriatrics, obstetrics, neurology. **Holdings:** 3000 books; 1700 bound periodical volumes; 4200 reels of microfilm. **Subscriptions:** 400 journals and other serials.

★8895★ U.S. DEPARTMENT OF VETERANS AFFAIRS
HOSPITAL LIBRARY
Knollcroft Rd.
Lyons, NJ 07939   Phone: (908) 604-5822
James G. Delo, Chf., Lib.Serv.
Subjects: Psychiatry, neurology, psychology, medicine, nursing, patient health education. **Holdings:** 7500 books; 5200 bound periodical volumes; 500 AV programs; 14 newspapers. **Subscriptions:** 300 journals and other serials; 5 newspapers.

★8896★ MARLBORO PSYCHIATRIC HOSPITAL
STAFF LIBRARY
Rte. 520, Newman Springs Rd.
Marlboro, NJ 07746   Phone: (908) 946-8100
Carla Zimmerman
Subjects: Psychiatry, psychology, clinical medicine, nursing, social work. **Holdings:** 2500 books. **Subscriptions:** 90 journals and other serials; 4 newspapers.

★8897★ ROOSEVELT HOSPITAL
HEALTH SCIENCE LIBRARY
Box 151
Metuchen, NJ 08840   Phone: (201) 321-6800
Karen Rubin, Libn.
Subjects: Medicine, nursing. **Holdings:** 1000 books. **Subscriptions:** 65 journals and other serials.

★8898★ MOUNTAINSIDE HOSPITAL
ASSMANN HEALTH SCIENCES LIBRARY
Bay & Highland Aves.
Montclair, NJ 07042   Phone: (201) 429-6240
Patricia Regenberg, Dir.
Subjects: Clinical medicine. **Holdings:** 3000 books; 12,000 bound periodical volumes. **Subscriptions:** 304 journals and other serials.

★8899★ MOUNTAINSIDE HOSPITAL
SCHOOL OF NURSING LIBRARY
Bay & Highland Aves.
Montclair, NJ 07042   Phone: (201) 429-6063
Juliette Ratner, Libn.
Subjects: Nursing, allied health sciences. **Holdings:** 1850 books; 7 bound periodical volumes. **Subscriptions:** 130 journals and other serials.

★8900★ WARNER-LAMBERT COMPANY
CORPORATE LIBRARY
182 Tabor Rd.
Morris Plains, NJ 07950   Phone: (201) 540-2875
Nedra Behringer, Dir., Corp.Lib. and Lit.Serv.
Subjects: Pharmaceuticals, medicine, chemistry, business, marketing, finance, competitive intelligence, confectionery. **Holdings:** 17,000 books; 25,000 bound periodical volumes; 7200 reels of microfilm. **Subscriptions:** 550 journals and other serials.

★8901★ MORRISTOWN MEMORIAL HOSPITAL
LATHROPE HEALTH SCIENCES LIBRARY
100 Madison Ave.
PO Box 1956
Morristown, NJ 07962-1956   Phone: (201) 540-5657
JoAnne M. Searle, Dir.
Subjects: Medicine, dentistry, nursing. **Holdings:** 3500 books; 7000 bound periodical volumes; 55 slide/tape sets; 127 video cassettes. **Subscriptions:** 540 journals and other serials.

★8902★ MEMORIAL HOSPITAL OF BURLINGTON COUNTY
LINDLEY B. REAGAN HEALTH SCIENCES LIBRARY
175 Madison Ave.
Mt. Holly, NJ 08060   Phone: (609) 267-0700
Betsy O'Connor, Dir.
Subjects: Health sciences. **Holdings:** 1100 books; 5000 bound periodical volumes; 80 other cataloged items; 5 drawers of slides; articles published by staff; 10 drawers of audio programs; 500 video cassettes. **Subscriptions:** 301 journals and other serials.

★8903★ CHILDREN'S SPECIALIZED HOSPITAL
MEDICAL LIBRARY
150 New Providence Rd.
Mountainside, NJ 07091   Phone: (201) 233-3720
Anne Glasser, Med.Libn.
Subjects: Pediatrics, rehabilitation, nursing. **Holdings:** 3000 books; 14 VF drawers; 320 audio cassettes; 105 filmstrip kits; 450 slides. **Subscriptions:** 150 journals and other serials.

★8904★ THE BOC GROUP INC.
TECHNICAL CENTER
INFORMATION CENTER
100 Mountain Ave.
Murray Hill, NJ 07974   Phone: (201) 665-2400
Robert N. Yeager, Mgr.
Subjects: Chemical engineering, cryogenics, metallurgy, ceramics, engineering, anesthesiology, health care, industrial gases. **Holdings:** 25,000 volumes; 4000 volumes on microfilm; AV programs. **Subscriptions:** 550 journals and other serials.

★8905★ JERSEY SHORE MEDICAL CENTER
ANN MAY SCHOOL OF NURSING LIBRARY AND MEDIA
CENTER
1945 Rte. 33
Neptune, NJ 07754   Phone: (201) 776-4195
Darlene Robertelli, Lib.Serv.Coord.
Subjects: Nursing, women's health, consumer education and health, allied health sciences. **Holdings:** 4000 books; 650 bound periodical volumes; 20 VF drawers; computer programs; 500 AV programs; National League for Nurses' and American Nursing Association publications. **Subscriptions:** 175 journals and other serials.

★8906★ JERSEY SHORE MEDICAL CENTER
MEDICAL LIBRARY
1945 Rte. 33
Neptune, NJ 07753   Phone: (201) 776-4265
Mr. Gian C. Hasija, Lib.Supv.
Subjects: Medicine. **Holdings:** 1200 books; 6500 bound periodical volumes; 1500 AV programs. **Subscriptions:** 205 journals.

★8907★ BRISTOL-MYERS SQUIBB COMPANY
NEW BRUNSWICK LIBRARY
Rte. 1 & College Farm Rd., Bldg. 100
New Brunswick, NJ 08903   Phone: (201) 519-2269
Phyllis J. Minicuci, Supv., Lib.Oper.
Subjects: Analytical chemistry, pharmaceutics, pharmacology, quality control, biochemistry. **Holdings:** 4000 books; 6600 bound periodical volumes. **Subscriptions:** 350 journals and other serials.

★8908★ JOHNSON AND JOHNSON
COSAT INFORMATION SERVICES
410 George St.
New Brunswick, NJ 08901-2021   Phone: (201) 524-2555
Anne D. Stark, Info.Spec.
Subjects: Science, medicine, biotechnology. **Holdings:** 1000 books. **Subscriptions:** 100 journals and other serials.

★8909★ ST. PETER'S MEDICAL CENTER
LIBRARY
254 Easton Ave.
New Brunswick, NJ 08903   Phone: (201) 745-8545
Subjects: Medicine, nursing. **Holdings:** 10,000 books; 20,000 bound periodical volumes; 3600 AV programs. **Subscriptions:** 550 journals and other serials.

★8910★ UNIVERSITY OF MEDICINE AND DENTISTRY OF
NEW JERSEY
ROBERT WOOD JOHNSON LIBRARY OF THE HEALTH
SCIENCES
CN 19
New Brunswick, NJ 08903   Phone: (201) 937-7606
Mary R. Scanlon, Lib.Dir.
Subjects: Clinical medicine, hospital administration, nursing. **Holdings:** 6133 books; 14,266 bound periodical volumes; 310 AV programs. **Subscriptions:** 601 journals and other serials.

★8911★ BLUME, VAZQUEZ, GOLDFADEN, BERKOWITZ, ET
AL.
LIBRARY
5 Commerce St.
Newark, NJ 07102   Phone: (201) 622-1881
June Beckford-Smith, Libn.
Subjects: Law, medical malpractice, products liability. **Holdings:** 3000 books; 100 standards; 600 pamphlets; 1500 internal documents. **Subscriptions:** 40 journals and other serials.

★8912★ COLUMBUS HOSPITAL
MEDICAL LIBRARY
495 N. 13th St.
Newark, NJ 07107-1397   Phone: (201) 268-1400
Paula Fuseli
Subjects: Medicine, nursing. **Holdings:** 745 books; 1186 bound periodical volumes; 36 boxes of American College of Physicians-Self Learning Series materials; tapes; microfiche. **Subscriptions:** 75 journals and other serials.

★8913★ NEWARK BETH ISRAEL MEDICAL CENTER
DR. VICTOR PARSONNET MEMORIAL LIBRARY
201 Lyons Ave.
Newark, NJ 07112   Phone: (201) 926-7233
Betty L. Garrison, Chf.Libn.
Subjects: Medicine, surgery, cardiology, oncology, pediatrics, dentistry. **Holdings:** 1200 books; 5500 bound periodical volumes; 180 video cassettes; 540 cassettes. **Subscriptions:** 225 journals and other serials.

★8914★ ST. MICHAEL MEDICAL CENTER
AQUINAS MEDICAL LIBRARY
268 Dr. Martin Luther King Jr. Blvd.
Newark, NJ 07102   Phone: (201) 877-5471
Joann Mehalick, Dir., Med.Lib.
Subjects: Medicine, pediatrics, obstetrics and gynecology, surgery, infectious diseases. **Holdings:** 2000 books; 4500 bound periodical volumes; 1 VF drawer of clippings. **Subscriptions:** 95 journals and other serials.

★8915★ UNITED HOSPITALS MEDICAL CENTER
LIBRARY
15 S. 9th St.
Newark, NJ 07107   Phone: (201) 268-8774
Linda De Muro, Dir., Lib.Serv.
Subjects: Medicine, nursing, ophthalmology, otorhinolaryngology, pediatrics, orthopedics, hospital administration. **Holdings:** 5000 books; 8000 bound periodical volumes; tapes; 6 VF drawers of pamphlets, clippings, reprints; 2 VF drawers and 3 shelves of archival materials; 1883 AV programs; 7 audio cassette subscriptions. **Subscriptions:** 250 journals and other serials.

★8916★ UNIVERSITY OF MEDICINE AND DENTISTRY OF
NEW JERSEY
GEORGE F. SMITH LIBRARY
30 12th Ave.
Newark, NJ 07103-2706   Phone: (201) 456-4580
Madeline Taylor, Dir.
Subjects: Health sciences. **Holdings:** 66,500 books; 77,500 bound periodical volumes; AV programs. **Subscriptions:** 2500 journals and other serials.

★8917★ HOFFMANN-LA ROCHE, INC.
LIBRARY
340 Kingsland St.
Nutley, NJ 07110   Phone: (201) 235-3091
Phyllis Deline, Mgr.
Subjects: Pharmaceutical industry, medicinal chemistry, business, vitamins, pharmacology, marketing. **Holdings:** 22,000 books; 19,200 bound periodical volumes; 414 pamphlets; 350 annual reports; 2000 reels of microfilm of journals; 85,000 microfiche of Roche product reprint file. **Subscriptions:** 500 journals and other serials; 4 newspapers.

★8918★ PATIENT CARE
LIBRARY
690 Kinderkamack Rd.
Oradell, NJ 07649-1506   Phone: (201) 599-8029
Christine T. O'Connor, Libn.
Subjects: Medicine, family practice, medical marketing. **Holdings:** 600 books; 100 audio cassettes; 30 VF drawers. **Subscriptions:** 152 journals and other serials.

★8919★ HOSPITAL CENTER AT ORANGE
WILLIAM PIERSON MEDICAL LIBRARY
188 S. Essex Ave.
Orange, NJ 07051-3421   Phone: (201) 266-2000
Jeanette Merkl, Libn.
Subjects: Medicine. **Holdings:** 1016 books; 1120 bound periodical volumes. **Subscriptions:** 78 journals and other serials.

★8920★ BERGEN COMMUNITY COLLEGE
LIBRARY AND LEARNING RESOURCES CENTER
SPECIAL COLLECTIONS
400 Paramus Rd.
Paramus, NJ 07652   Phone: (201) 447-7131
Prof. Marilyn Gilray
Subjects: Nursing.

★8921★ BERGEN PINES COUNTY HOSPITAL
MEDICAL LIBRARY
E. Ridgewood Ave.
Paramus, NJ 07652   Phone: (201) 967-4000
Victoria E. Gonzalez, Med.Libn.
Subjects: Medicine. **Holdings:** 1400 books; 1824 bound periodical volumes. **Subscriptions:** 180 journals and other serials.

★8922★ ST. MARY'S HOSPITAL
MEDICAL ALLIED HEALTH LIBRARY
211 Pennington Ave.
Passaic, NJ 07055   Phone: (201) 470-3055
Sr. Gertrude Doremus, S.C., Dir.
Subjects: Medicine, surgery, orthopedics, vascular surgery, psychiatry, urology, gastrointestinal diseases, cardiovascular systems, hematology, gynecology and obstetrics. **Holdings:** 450 books; 1900 bound periodical volumes. **Subscriptions:** 120 journals and other serials.

★8923★ ST. JOSEPH'S HOSPITAL AND MEDICAL CENTER
HEALTH SCIENCES LIBRARY
703 Main St.
Paterson, NJ 07503   Phone: (201) 977-2104
Patricia May, Lib.Serv.
Subjects: Medicine, biological sciences, dentistry, psychology, nursing. **Holdings:** 4500 books; 4800 bound periodical volumes. **Subscriptions:** 275 journals and other serials.

★8924★ RARITAN BAY MEDICAL CENTER
HEALTH SCIENCE LIBRARY
530 New Brunswick Ave.
Perth Amboy, NJ 08861   Phone: (201) 442-3700
Catherine A. Hilman, Hea.Sci.Libn.
Subjects: Medicine, nursing, allied health sciences. **Holdings:** 1800 books; 770 bound periodical volumes. **Subscriptions:** 140 journals and other serials.

★8925★ WARREN HOSPITAL
MEDICAL LIBRARY
185 Roseberry St.
Phillipsburg, NJ 08865   Phone: (201) 859-6728
Esther Tews, Dir., Volunteer Serv.
Subjects: Medicine. **Holdings:** 700 books. **Subscriptions:** 47 journals and other serials.

★8926★ RUTGERS UNIVERSITY, THE STATE UNIVERSITY
OF NEW JERSEY
LIBRARY OF SCIENCE AND MEDICINE
Box 1029
Piscataway, NJ 08855-1029   Phone: (908) 932-3850
Jeanne E. Boyle, Dir.
Subjects: Medicine, agriculture, biology and biochemistry, engineering, geology, pharmacy, pharmacology, psychology. **Holdings:** 190,725 books; 175,220 bound periodical volumes; 448,456 government documents; 486,289 microforms. **Subscriptions:** 5627 periodicals.

★8927★ RUTGERS UNIVERSITY, THE STATE UNIVERSITY
OF NEW JERSEY
RUTGERS CENTER OF ALCOHOL STUDIES
LIBRARY
Busch Campus
Smithers Hall
Piscataway, NJ 08855-0969   Phone: (908) 932-4442
Penny B. Page, Hd.Libn.
Subjects: Alcohol, drinking, alcoholism. **Holdings:** 8600 books; 2800 bound periodical volumes; 150 boxes of archival materials; 20,000 abstracts on 6x7 edge notched cards (Classified Abstract Archive of the Alcohol Literature); 1750 doctoral dissertations on microfilm; 120 alcohol-related bibliographies; 500 questionnaires, interview schedules, survey forms. **Subscriptions:** 200 journals and other serials.

★8928★ RUTGERS UNIVERSITY, THE STATE UNIVERSITY
OF NEW JERSEY
RUTGERS CENTER OF ALCOHOL STUDIES
NEW JERSEY ALCOHOL/DRUG RESOURCE CENTER AND
CLEARINGHOUSE
Box 518
Piscataway, NJ 08855-0518   Phone: (201) 932-5528
Penny B. Page, Co-Dir.
Subjects: Alcohol and drug use, alcohol and drug education, substance abuse prevention. **Holdings:** 2000 books and pamphlets. **Subscriptions:** 220 journals and other serials.

★8929★ UNIVERSITY OF MEDICINE AND DENTISTRY OF
NEW JERSEY
ROBERT WOOD JOHNSON MEDICAL SCHOOL
MEDIA LIBRARY
675 Hoes Ln.
Piscataway, NJ 08854-5635   Phone: (908) 463-4671
Zana Etter, Media Libn.
Subjects: Medicine, allied health sciences. **Holdings:** 750 books; 2200 AV programs; 400 tapes of lectures; 18 VF drawers; 35 software programs.

★8930★ MUHLENBERG REGIONAL MEDICAL CENTER
E. GORDON GLASS, M.D., MEMORIAL LIBRARY
Park Ave. & Randolph Rd.
Plainfield, NJ 07061   Phone: (201) 668-2005
Jane McCarthy, Libn.
Subjects: Medicine, nursing, hospital management. **Holdings:** 6050 books; 3000 bound periodical volumes. **Subscriptions:** 200 journals and other serials.

★8931★ ATLANTIC CITY MEDICAL CENTER
MAINLAND DIVISION
HEALTH SCIENCE LIBRARY
Jim Leeds Rd.
Pomona, NJ 08240   Phone: (609) 652-1000
John P. Doesburgh, Dir., Hea.Sci.Libs.
Subjects: Medicine, nursing, and allied health sciences. **Holdings:** 180 books; 189 bound periodical volumes. **Subscriptions:** 42 journals and other serials.

★8932★ BETTY BACHARACH REHABILITATION HOSPITAL LIBRARY
Jim Leeds Rd.
Pomona, NJ 08240   Phone: (609) 652-7000
Catherine Curran, Libn.
Subjects: Physical therapy, audiology, respiratory therapy, physical medicine, clinical psychology, rehabilitative nursing. **Holdings:** 271 books; 57 bound periodical volumes; 50 documents. **Subscriptions:** 38 journals and other serials.

★8933★ CHILTON MEMORIAL HOSPITAL MEDICAL LIBRARY
97 West Parkway
Pompton Plains, NJ 07444   Phone: (201) 831-5058
Janice Sweeton, Mgr.
Subjects: Medicine, allied health sciences. **Holdings:** 2500 books; 3000 bound periodical volumes; 165 video cassettes. **Subscriptions:** 120 journals and other serials.

★8934★ BRISTOL-MYERS SQUIBB COMPANY PHARMACEUTICAL RESEARCH INSTITUTE SCIENCE INFORMATION DEPARTMENT
Box 4000
Princeton, NJ 08540   Phone: (609) 921-4844
Subjects: Pharmacology, chemistry, medicine, pharmacy. **Holdings:** 30,000 books; 60,000 bound periodical volumes; 30,000 volumes on microfilm; 100 VF drawers. **Subscriptions:** 1600 journals and other serials.

★8935★ CYTOGEN CORPORATION R & D LIBRARY
Princeton Forrestal Ctr.
201 College Rd., E.
Princeton, NJ 08540   Phone: (609) 987-8237
Bonnie Myers
Subjects: Cancer research, biotechnology. **Holdings:** 600 books. **Subscriptions:** 189 journals and other serials.

★8936★ HEALTH RESEARCH AND EDUCATIONAL TRUST OF NEW JERSEY CORPORATE INFORMATION CENTER
760 Alexander Rd. (CN-1)
Princeton, NJ 08543-0001   Phone: (609) 275-4230
Michelle Volesko, Dir.
Subjects: Hospital and health care administration, consumer health education, hospital and in-service education, business and management. **Holdings:** 2300 books; 720 bound periodical volumes; 2500 serial volumes; 1900 vertical files; 200 videotape and film titles; 200 audio cassettes; 4 drawers of microfiche; 26 internal newsletters. **Subscriptions:** 400 journals and other serials; 5 newspapers.

★8937★ HOSPITAL ENGINEERING LOGISTICS AND PLANNING, INC. LIBRARY
PO Box 7059
Princeton, NJ 08540   Phone: (609) 683-1990
Subjects: Hospital and biomedical engineering, electromechanical techniques in medicine. **Holdings:** 160 volumes.

★8938★ MEDICAL CENTER AT PRINCETON MEDICAL CENTER LIBRARY
253 Witherspoon St.
Princeton, NJ 08540   Phone: (609) 497-4488
Louise M. Yorke, Med.Libn.
Subjects: Medicine, surgery, nursing, allied health sciences. **Holdings:** 3000 books; 4500 bound periodical volumes; 4 drawers of pamphlets; 500 video cassettes; 450 audio cassettes; 100 slide sets and filmstrips. **Subscriptions:** 216 journals and other serials.

★8939★ MOBIL CORPORATION TOXICOLOGY INFORMATION CENTER
Box 1029
Princeton, NJ 08543   Phone: (609) 737-5583
Sharon Smith, Info.Spec.
Subjects: Toxicology, environmental health, biomedicine, analytical chemistry. **Holdings:** 6000 books. **Subscriptions:** 550 journals and other serials; 7 newspapers.

★8940★ NORTH PRINCETON DEVELOPMENTAL CENTER HEALTH SERVICES LIBRARY
Gerry Bldg.
Box 1000
Princeton, NJ 08543-1000   Phone: (609) 466-0400
W.R. Thompson, MD, Med.Dir.
Subjects: Psychiatry, psychology, mental retardation, medicine. **Holdings:** 945 books. **Subscriptions:** 30 journals and other serials.

★8941★ PRINCETON UNIVERSITY PSYCHOLOGY LIBRARY
Green Hall
Princeton, NJ 08544   Phone: (609) 258-3239
Mary C. Chaikin, Psych.Libn.
Subjects: Psychology - cognitive, developmental, social, experimental, health, physiological; neuropsychology; perception; personality; psychotherapy; psycholinguistics; artificial intelligence. **Holdings:** 18,425 books; 14,282 bound periodical volumes; 4882 microfiche. **Subscriptions:** 400 journals and other serials.

★8942★ ROBERT WOOD JOHNSON FOUNDATION LIBRARY
Rte. 1 and College Rd.
Box 2316
Princeton, NJ 08543-2316   Phone: (609) 243-5897
Philip J. Gallagher, Libn.
Subjects: Health policy, health economics, health manpower, medical education, philanthropy. **Holdings:** 5500 books; 80 bound periodical volumes; 200 annual reports of foundations; 9 films; 105 cassettes; 170 health school catalogs. **Subscriptions:** 165 journals and other serials; 6 newspapers.

★8943★ WYETH-AYERST RESEARCH RESEARCH LIBRARY
CN 8000
Princeton, NJ 08543-8000   Phone: (908) 274-4268
Barbara Boyajian, Libn.
Subjects: Chemistry, biological sciences, medical sciences. **Holdings:** 4000 books; 25,000 bound periodical volumes; 1500 reels of microfilm. **Subscriptions:** 450 journals and other serials.

★8944★ MERCK & COMPANY, INC. MERCK SHARP & DOHME RESEARCH LABORATORIES LITERATURE RESOURCES, RAHWAY
R86-240
Box 2000
Rahway, NJ 07065   Phone: (908) 594-6754
Evelyn Armstrong, Dir.
Subjects: Chemistry, biochemistry, pharmacology, immunology, veterinary science, biomedical sciences, science and technology. **Holdings:** 25,000 books; 25,000 bound periodical volumes; 1000 reels of microfilm of U.S. chemical patents; 115 periodicals on microfilm. **Subscriptions:** 2000 journals and other serials.

★8945★ MERCK & COMPANY, INC. MERCK SHARP & DOHME RESEARCH LABORATORIES RESEARCH INFORMATION SYSTEMS
Box 2000
Rahway, NJ 07065   Phone: (201) 574-4726
Dr. Marcia Zweerink, Dir.
Subjects: Chemistry, biology, medicine, pharmaceuticals, veterinary medicine. **Holdings:** Unpublished research reports; manuscripts.

★8946★ ROBERT WOOD JOHNSON PHARMACEUTICAL RESEARCH INSTITUTE HARTMAN LIBRARY
Rte. 202, Box 300
Raritan, NJ 08869-0602   Phone: (908) 704-4109
June Bente, Mgr., Lib.Serv.
Subjects: Medicine, pharmacy, endocrinology, biological sciences, chemistry. **Holdings:** 8000 books; 15,000 bound periodical volumes. **Subscriptions:** 1000 journals and other serials.

★8947★ RIVERVIEW MEDICAL CENTER
CLINICAL LIBRARY
1 Riverview Plaza
Red Bank, NJ 07701   Phone: (908) 530-2275
Cheryl Newman, Med.Libn.
Subjects: Clinical medicine. **Holdings:** 2500 books; 900 audio cassettes; microfilm. **Subscriptions:** 250 journals and other serials.

★8948★ VALLEY HOSPITAL
MEDICAL LIBRARY
223 N. Van Dien Ave.
Ridgewood, NJ 07450   Phone: (201) 447-8285
Claudia Allocco, Dir., Lib.Serv.
Subjects: Medicine, nursing, hospital management, allied health sciences. **Holdings:** 1000 books; 3000 bound periodical volumes; 2 VF drawers of pamphlets. **Subscriptions:** 175 journals and other serials.

★8949★ LEBERCO TESTING, INC.
LIBRARY
123 Hawthorne St.
Roselle Park, NJ 07204   Phone: (201) 245-1933
Anthony Lo Pinto
Subjects: Toxicology, microbiology, analytic chemistry, in regard to pharmaceutical and medical devices, cosmetics, toiletries, household products, food, industrial chemicals, and drinking and waste water. **Holdings:** 3500 volumes. **Subscriptions:** 37 journals and other serials; 2 newspapers.

★8950★ MEMORIAL HOSPITAL OF SALEM COUNTY
DAVID W. GREEN MEDICAL LIBRARY
Salem Woodstown Rd.
Salem, NJ 08079   Phone: (609) 935-1000
Subjects: Medicine, allied health sciences. **Holdings:** 726 books; 750 bound periodical volumes. **Subscriptions:** 31 journals and other serials.

★8951★ PW COMMUNICATIONS INTERNATIONAL
CORPORATE LIBRARY
400 Plaza Dr.
Secaucus, NJ 07096   Phone: (201) 865-7500
Leila M. Hover, Corp.Libn.
Subjects: Medicine, pharmaceuticals. **Holdings:** 900 books; 919 bound periodical volumes. **Subscriptions:** 100 journals and other serials.

★8952★ JOHNSON AND JOHNSON CONSUMER PRODUCTS INC.
BUSINESS AND TECHNICAL INFORMATION CENTER
Grandview Rd.
Skillman, NJ 08558   Phone: (201) 874-1439
Marilyn H. Faulkner, Mgr.
Subjects: Infant care, health and beauty aids, toiletries, chemistry, pharmaceuticals, oral care, wound care. **Holdings:** 1000 books; 1500 bound periodical volumes. **Subscriptions:** 200 journals and other serials.

★8953★ ETHICON, INC.
SCIENTIFIC INFORMATION SERVICES
PO Box 151
Somerville, NJ 08876-0151   Phone: (201) 218-3272
Dr. Charles G. Fritz, Dir.
Subjects: Biological and physical sciences, sterilization, polymer chemistry, surgery, controlled drug delivery. **Holdings:** 7000 books; 20,500 bound periodical volumes; 10 VF drawers of U.S. and foreign patents. **Subscriptions:** 400 journals and other serials.

★8954★ HOECHST-ROUSSEL PHARMACEUTICALS, INC.
LIBRARY
Rte. 202-206, N.
Somerville, NJ 08876   Phone: (201) 231-2394
Loretta F. Stangs, Gp.Mgr.
Subjects: Chemistry, pharmacology, toxicology, medicine, pharmaceutical marketing, pesticides, psychopharmacology, industrial management. **Holdings:** 72,000 books; 7500 bound periodical volumes; 5000 reels of microfilm of journals and patents; 1000 AV programs. **Subscriptions:** 1000 journals and other serials.

★8955★ SOMERSET MEDICAL CENTER
MEDICAL LIBRARY
110 Rehill Ave.
Somerville, NJ 08876   Phone: (201) 685-2200
Kenneth Whitmore, Lib.Coord.
Subjects: Medicine, nursing. **Holdings:** 2100 books; 1200 bound periodical volumes. **Subscriptions:** 155 journals and other serials.

★8956★ SOUTH MOUNTAIN LABORATORIES, INC.
LIBRARY
380 Lackawanna Pl.
South Orange, NJ 07079   Phone: (201) 762-0045
David Reifsnyder, Dir.
Subjects: Biology, chemistry, medicine, pharmaceutics. **Holdings:** 1000 books; 500 bound periodical volumes. **Subscriptions:** 14 journals and other serials.

★8957★ UNIVERSITY OF MEDICINE AND DENTISTRY OF NEW JERSEY
SCHOOL OF OSTEOPATHIC MEDICINE
HEALTH SCIENCES LIBRARY
Ambulatory Health Care Ctr.
301 S. Central Plaza, Ste. 1100
Laurel Rd.
Stratford, NJ 08084   Phone: (609) 346-6800
Judith Schuback Cohn, Lib.Dir.
Subjects: Medicine, nursing, hospital administration, allied health sciences. **Holdings:** 6500 books; 12,000 bound periodical volumes; 300 AV programs; 2 vertical files; 200 reels of microfilm. **Subscriptions:** 610 journals and other serials.

★8958★ CIBA-GEIGY CORPORATION
PHARMACEUTICALS DIVISION
SCIENTIFIC INFORMATION CENTER
566 Morris Ave.
Summit, NJ 07901   Phone: (201) 277-4826
Lynette C. Schneider, Dir.
Subjects: Medicine, chemistry, pharmacology, pharmacy, business. **Holdings:** 5000 books; 24,000 bound periodical volumes; 2260 reels of microfilm of journal holdings; 500,000 unpublished proprietary documents. **Subscriptions:** 900 journals and other serials.

★8959★ FAIR OAKS HOSPITAL
MEDICAL LIBRARY
19 Prospect St.
Summit, NJ 07901   Phone: (908) 522-7000
JoAn Petersen, Libn.
Subjects: Psychiatry, psychopharmacology, psychobiology, neuropsychiatry, neuropsychology. **Holdings:** 500 books; 200 bound periodical volumes. **Subscriptions:** 90 journals and other serials.

★8960★ OVERLOOK HOSPITAL
HEALTH SCIENCES LIBRARY
99 Beauvoir Ave.
Summit, NJ 07902-0220   Phone: (201) 522-2119
Kathleen A. Moeller, Dir.
Subjects: Medicine, surgery, nursing, radiology, emergency medicine, psychiatry, pediatrics, orthopedics. **Holdings:** 6000 books; 12,000 bound periodical volumes; 2000 subject files for LATCH Program; 600 AV programs. **Subscriptions:** 550 journals and other serials.

★8961★ HOLY NAME HOSPITAL
LIBRARY
Teaneck Rd.
Teaneck, NJ 07666   Phone: (201) 833-3395
Ronald Rizio, Dir., Lib.Serv.
Subjects: Medicine, nursing, and allied health sciences. **Holdings:** 6000 books; 3000 bound periodical volumes; 250 video cassettes; 500 cassette tapes. **Subscriptions:** 200 journals and other serials; 3 newspapers.

★8962★ HAMILTON HOSPITAL
MEDICAL LIBRARY
1881 Whitehorse-Hamilton Square Rd.
Box H
Trenton, NJ 08690   Phone: (609) 584-6473
Patricia Kowalski, Coord.
Subjects: Medicine, sports medicine. **Holdings:** 382 books; 200 bound

periodical volumes; 3500 other cataloged items. **Subscriptions:** 67 journals and other serials.

★8963★ HELENE FULD MEDICAL CENTER
HEALTH SCIENCES LIBRARY
750 Brunswick Ave.
Trenton, NJ 08638   Phone: (609) 394-6065
Mary Anne Toner, Lib.Dir.
Subjects: Medicine, nursing, allied health sciences. **Holdings:** 3500 books; 2800 bound periodical volumes; 750 reels of microfilm of journals; 350 videotapes; 5000 slides; 850 audiocassettes. **Subscriptions:** 245 journals and other serials.

★8964★ MERCER MEDICAL CENTER
HEALTH SCIENCES LIBRARY
446 Bellevue Ave. - Box 1658
Trenton, NJ 08607   Phone: (609) 394-4125
Catherine W. Marchok, Dir.
Subjects: Medicine, nursing. **Holdings:** 3100 titles; 4064 bound periodical volumes; 5 VF drawers of clippings and pamphlets; 1 VF drawer of pictures; 400 audiotapes; 1455 slides. **Subscriptions:** 202 journals and other serials.

★8965★ NEW JERSEY DEPARTMENT OF ENVIRONMENTAL
PROTECTION
INFORMATION RESOURCE CENTER
CN-409
432 E. State St.
Trenton, NJ 08625   Phone: (609) 984-2249
Maria Baratta, Lib.Mgr.
Subjects: Toxic substances; hazardous waste; pollution - water, air, soil; carcinogens; mutagens; teratogens; water resources. **Holdings:** 2500 books; 4500 technical documents; 12 VF drawers of Chemical Reference Files; 5 VF drawers. **Subscriptions:** 125 journals and other serials.

★8966★ NEW JERSEY DEPARTMENT OF HEALTH
DIVISION OF OCCUPATIONAL/ENVIRONMENTAL HEALTH
INFORMATION CENTER
Health Agricultural Bldg. CN 360
John Fitch Plaza
Trenton, NJ 08625   Phone: (609) 633-2039
Suzanne Ficara, Res.Sci.
Subjects: Occupational health and safety; industrial hygiene; epidemiology; medicine - environmental, occupational; toxicology; pesticides; public health. **Holdings:** 500 books; 200 subject files; government documents. **Subscriptions:** 31 journals and other serials.

★8967★ ST. FRANCIS MEDICAL CENTER
HEALTH SCIENCES LIBRARY
601 Hamilton Ave.
Trenton, NJ 08629   Phone: (609) 599-5068
Donna Barlow, Dir.
Subjects: Medicine, nursing, allied health sciences. **Holdings:** 5000 books. **Subscriptions:** 300 journals and other serials.

★8968★ KENNEDY MEMORIAL HOSPITALS/UNIVERSITY
MEDICAL CENTER
WASHINGTON TOWNSHIP DIVISION
BARSKY MEMORIAL LIBRARY
Hurffville and Cross Keys Rds.
Turnersville, NJ 08012   Phone: (609) 582-2675
William Dobkowski, Med.Libn.
Subjects: Medicine. **Holdings:** 500 books; 700 bound periodical volumes. **Subscriptions:** 105 journals and other serials.

★8969★ UNION HOSPITAL
MEDICAL LIBRARY
1000 Galloping Hill Rd.
Union, NJ 07083   Phone: (201) 851-7234
Subjects: Medicine. **Holdings:** 800 monographs. **Subscriptions:** 121 journals and other serials.

★8970★ WEST JERSEY HEALTH SYSTEM, VOORHEES
DIVISION
STAFF MEDICAL LIBRARY
101 Carnie Blvd.
Voorhees, NJ 08043   Phone: (609) 772-5494
Susan E. Cleveland, Lib.Dir.
Subjects: Medicine, nursing, administration. **Holdings:** 1000 books; 3000 bound periodical volumes; 15 AV programs. **Subscriptions:** 165 journals and other serials.

★8971★ AMERICAN CYANAMID COMPANY
ENVIRONMENTAL HEALTH LIBRARY
1 Cyanamid Plaza
Wayne, NJ 07470   Phone: (201) 831-4379
Anita M. Jones, Supv./Info.Sci.
Subjects: Toxicology, occupational medicine, industrial hygiene and safety, clinical medicine, environmental protection, loss prevention. **Holdings:** 5000 books; 350 bound periodical volumes; 2000 pamphlets; 12 VF drawers of reprints. **Subscriptions:** 150 journals and other serials.

★8972★ TRENTON PSYCHIATRIC HOSPITAL
PROFESSIONAL LIBRARY
Box 7500
West Trenton, NJ 08628   Phone: (609) 633-1572
Elaine Scheuerer, Lib.Coord.
Subjects: Psychiatry, psychotherapy, medicine, psychoanalysis, nursing. **Holdings:** 3400 books; 2910 bound periodical volumes; 5 VF drawers of pamphlets; 585 audio cassettes; 3 16mm films; 27 video cassettes; manuscripts; reports; clippings; 1 cabinet of phonograph records, tapes, filmstrips. **Subscriptions:** 92 journals and other serials.

★8973★ PASCACK VALLEY HOSPITAL
DAVID GOLDBERG MEMORIAL MEDICAL LIBRARY
Old Hook Rd.
Westwood, NJ 07675   Phone: (201) 358-3240
Debbra Michaels, Dir.
Subjects: Medicine, surgery, nursing, allied health sciences, management. **Holdings:** 1200 books; 25 bound periodical volumes; 4 indexes; 9 audiotape subscriptions; 100 videotapes; pamphlets. **Subscriptions:** 208 journals and other serials.

★8974★ KNOLL PHARMACEUTICALS
SCIENCE INFORMATION CENTER
30 N. Jefferson Rd.
Whippany, NJ 07981   Phone: (201) 428-4199
Joanne Lustig, Mgr., Med./Sci.Info.
Subjects: Cardiovascular medicine, drug information, pharmacology, pharmaceutical industry. **Holdings:** 1500 books; 3000 bound periodical volumes; 30 VF drawers of unpublished reports and manuscripts; foreign and domestic patents. **Subscriptions:** 350 journals and other serials; 10 newspapers.

★8975★ RANCOCAS HOSPITAL
HEALTH SCIENCES LIBRARY
Sunset Rd.
Willingboro, NJ 08046   Phone: (609) 835-2900
Gary J. Christopher, Libn.
Subjects: Medicine, nursing, hospital administration. **Holdings:** 600 books; 2800 bound periodical volumes; 190 videotapes. **Subscriptions:** 101 journals and other serials; 2 newspapers.

★8976★ WOODBRIDGE DEVELOPMENTAL CENTER
LIBRARY
Rahway Ave.
PO Box 189
Woodbridge, NJ 07095   Phone: (201) 499-5596
Margaret DeRidder, Dir. of Educ.
Subjects: Retardation, medicine, education, developmental disabilities, recreation, management. **Holdings:** 1000 books; filmstrips. **Subscriptions:** 20 journals and other serials.

★8977★ UNDERWOOD-MEMORIAL HOSPITAL
ANTHONY J.D. MARINO, M.D. MEMORIAL LIBRARY
509 N. Broad St.
Woodbury, NJ 08096   Phone: (609) 845-0100
Ellen K. Tiedrich, Libn.
Subjects: Medicine, nursing, and allied health sciences. **Holdings:** 3500

books; 100 bound periodical volumes; 1500 reels of microfilm. **Subscriptions:** 125 journals and other serials.

★8978★   CHRISTIAN HEALTH CARE CENTER
PETER CARRAS LIBRARY
301 Sicomac Ave.
Wyckoff, NJ 07481   Phone: (201) 848-5200
Subjects: Medicine, nursing, psychiatry. **Holdings:** Figures not available.

New Mexico

★8979★   NEW MEXICO SCHOOL FOR THE VISUALLY
   HANDICAPPED
LIBRARY AND MEDIA CENTER
1900 White Sands Blvd.
Alamogordo, NM 88310   Phone: (505) 437-3505
Bill Davis, Media Coord.
Holdings: 10,000 books in braille and print; 3500 AV programs; 7500 textbooks in special media and instructional aids for the visually handicapped. **Subscriptions:** 46 journals and other serials.

★8980★   CARRIE TINGLEY HOSPITAL
MEDICAL LIBRARY
1127 University Blvd., NE
Albuquerque, NM 87102   Phone: (505) 272-5200
Subjects: Orthopedics - pediatric, general; pediatric dysmorphology; pediatrics; rehabilitation. **Holdings:** 760 books; 250 bound periodical volumes; 200 resident research papers. **Subscriptions:** 12 journals and other serials.

★8981★   LOVELACE BIOMEDICAL AND ENVIRONMENTAL
   RESEARCH INSTITUTE
INHALATION TOXICOLOGY RESEARCH INSTITUTE
LIBRARY
Box 5890
Albuquerque, NM 87185   Phone: (505) 844-2600
Judy C. Neff, Libn.
Subjects: Inhalation toxicology, aerosol physics, radiobiology, biophysics, veterinary medicine, comparative medicine. **Holdings:** 10,000 books; 10,500 bound periodical volumes; 15,000 documents in microform; 12,000 technical reports. **Subscriptions:** 311 journals and other serials.

★8982★   LOVELACE MEDICAL FOUNDATION
LIBRARY
5400 Gibson Blvd., SE
Albuquerque, NM 87108   Phone: (505) 262-7158
Sarah K. Morley, Med.Libn.
Subjects: Clinical medicine. **Holdings:** 2000 books; 7500 bound periodical volumes. **Subscriptions:** 198 journals and other serials.

★8983★   PRESBYTERIAN HOSPITAL
ROBERT SHAFER MEMORIAL LIBRARY
Box 26666
Albuquerque, NM 87125-6666   Phone: (505) 841-1516
Revathi A. Davidson, Dir.
Subjects: Medicine. **Holdings:** 2000 books; 1544 bound periodical volumes; 11,808 unbound materials; AV collection. **Subscriptions:** 160 journals and other serials.

★8984★   ST. JOSEPH MEDICAL CENTER
MEDICAL LIBRARY
601 Grand Ave., NE
Albuquerque, NM 87102   Phone: (505) 848-8291
Melba Clark, Med.Libn.
Subjects: Medicine, nursing, rehabilitation, orthopedics, neurology. **Holdings:** 700 books; 800 bound periodical volumes. **Subscriptions:** 90 journals and other serials.

★8985★   U.S. DEPARTMENT OF VETERANS AFFAIRS
MEDICAL CENTER LIBRARY
2100 Ridgecrest Dr., SE
Albuquerque, NM 87108   Phone: (505) 256-2786
Nancy Myer, Chf., Lib.Serv.
Subjects: Medicine, surgery, nursing, psychiatry. **Holdings:** 1530 books; 8537 bound periodical volumes; 500 reels of microfilm of journals. **Subscriptions:** 393 journals and other serials; 10 newspapers.

★8986★   UNIVERSITY OF NEW MEXICO
MEDICAL CENTER LIBRARY
North Campus
Albuquerque, NM 87131   Phone: (505) 277-2548
Erika Love, Dir.
Subjects: Medicine, basic sciences, nursing, pharmacy, Indian health, dental hygiene, allied health sciences. **Holdings:** 51,895 books; 83,004 bound periodical volumes; 1881 AV programs. **Subscriptions:** 1904 titles.

★8987★   GUADALUPE MEDICAL CENTER
MEDICAL STAFF LIBRARY
2430 W. Pierce St.
Carlsbad, NM 88220   Phone: (505) 887-6633
Lee Weeks, Med. Staff Libn.
Subjects: Medicine and allied health sciences. **Holdings:** 562 books; 212 bound periodical volumes; 5 VF drawers of Pediatric Notes; 51 VF drawers of medical journals. **Subscriptions:** 17 journals and other serials.

★8988★   GALLUP INDIAN MEDICAL CENTER
MEDICAL LIBRARY
E. Nizhoni Blvd.
Box 1337
Gallup, NM 87301   Phone: (505) 722-1119
Patricia V. Bradley, Med.Libn.
Subjects: Medicine, nursing, surgery, dentistry. **Holdings:** 2000 books. **Subscriptions:** 114 journals and other serials.

★8989★   NEW MEXICO DEPARTMENT OF HOSPITALS
LAS VEGAS MEDICAL CENTER
MEDICAL AND STAFF LIBRARY
Box 1388
Las Vegas, NM 87701   Phone: (505) 454-2111
Bonnie S. Hatch, Dir., Lib.Serv.
Subjects: Medicine, psychiatry, clinical psychology, psychoanalysis and therapy, hospital management. **Holdings:** 3000 volumes; 905 bound periodical volumes, 50 cassette tapes. **Subscriptions:** 100 journals and other serials.

★8990★   LOS LUNAS HOSPITAL AND TRAINING SCHOOL
LIBRARY
Box 1269
Los Lunas, NM 87031   Phone: (505) 841-5317
Subjects: Mental retardation, developmental disabilities, special education, psychology, medicine, nursing, social services. **Holdings:** 2000 books; 15 dissertations; 40 reports; 498 videotapes; 74 adapted switches and assistive devices. **Subscriptions:** 78 journals and other serials.

★8991★   MESCALERO PUBLIC HEALTH SERVICE HOSPITAL
LIBRARY
Box 210
Mescalero, NM 88340   Phone: (505) 671-4441
F. Bryant, M.D.
Subjects: Medicine. **Holdings:** 150 books; 25 bound periodical volumes. **Subscriptions:** 16 journals and other serials.

★8992★   NEW MEXICO SCHOOL FOR THE DEAF
LIBRARY
1060 Cerrillos Rd.
Santa Fe, NM 87503   Phone: (505) 827-6743
Carla Fenner, Libn.
Subjects: Deafness, sign language. **Holdings:** 10,000 books; 260 bound periodical volumes. **Subscriptions:** 48 journals and other serials.

★8993★   ST. VINCENT HOSPITAL
LIBRARY
455 St. Michael's Dr.
Santa Fe, NM 87501   Phone: (505) 989-5218
Jane Knowles, Libn.
Subjects: Clinical medicine, hospital problems, basic nursing. **Holdings:** 1000 books; 1600 periodical volumes. **Subscriptions:** 100 journals and other serials.

New York

★8994★ ALBANY COLLEGE OF PHARMACY
LIBRARY
106 New Scotland Ave.
Albany, NY 12208   Phone: (518) 445-7217
Irene Petzinger Kaplan, Libn.
Subjects: Pharmacy, medicine, chemistry, biology, technology. Holdings:
6000 books; 2000 bound periodical volumes; 155 periodicals; de Haen and
Iowa Drug Information Service; 25 linear feet of archival material.
Subscriptions: 155 journals and other serials.

★8995★ ALBANY MEDICAL COLLEGE
SCHAFFER LIBRARY OF HEALTH SCIENCES
47 New Scotland Ave.
Albany, NY 12208   Phone: (518) 445-5586
Sherry A. Hartman, Dir./Libn.
Subjects: Medicine, pre-clinical sciences, nursing, psychiatry. Holdings:
40,017 books; 112,616 bound periodical volumes; 1996 AV programs.
Subscriptions: 1248 journals and other serials.

★8996★ ALBANY MEMORIAL HOSPITAL
EDUCATION RESOURCE CENTER
Northern Blvd.
Albany, NY 12204   Phone: (518) 471-3264
Barbara Ost, Hosp.Libn.
Subjects: Medicine, nursing. Holdings: 4000 books; 300 bound periodical
volumes; tapes; films. Subscriptions: 100 journals and other serials.

★8997★ CAPITAL DISTRICT PSYCHIATRIC CENTER
LIBRARY
75 New Scotland Ave.
Albany, NY 12208   Phone: (518) 447-9611
Gail Botta, Libn.
Subjects: Psychiatry, psychology. Holdings: 5925 books; 5964 bound
periodical volumes. Subscriptions: 180 journals and other serials.

★8998★ CENTER FOR THE STUDY OF AGING
LIBRARY
706 Madison Ave.
Albany, NY 12208   Phone: (518) 465-6927
Sara Harris, Exec.Dir.
Subjects: Gerontology and geriatrics, physical activity and aging, mental
health and illness, environment, housing, medicine, social sciences.
Holdings: 4500 volumes. Subscriptions: 10 journals and other serials.

★8999★ HOSPITAL ASSOCIATION OF NEW YORK STATE
HOSPITAL EDUCATIONAL AND RESEARCH FUND
LILLIAN R. HAYT MEMORIAL LIBRARY
74 N. Pearl St.
Albany, NY 12207   Phone: (518) 434-7600
Elaine C. Rotman, Dir., Lib.Serv.
Subjects: Hospital and health care administration, management, health
economics. Holdings: 3000 books; 18 VF drawers of pamphlets and
reports. Subscriptions: 400 journals and other serials.

★9000★ NEW YORK STATE DEPARTMENT OF HEALTH
WADSWORTH CENTER FOR LABORATORIES AND RESEARCH
LIBRARY
Empire State Plaza
Albany, NY 12201   Phone: (518) 474-6172
Thomas Flynn, Lib.Dir.
Subjects: Public health, bacteriology, biochemistry, birth defects, child
health, clinical labs, communicable diseases, cytology, environmental
health, epidemiology, laboratory animals, mycology, pathology, radiology,
sanitary engineering, toxicology, veterinary medicine, virology, zoonoses.
Holdings: 20,500 books; 33,500 bound periodical volumes; 600 linear feet
of U.S. and New York State Government publications; 180 linear feet of
reference materials. Subscriptions: 1200 journals and other serials.

★9001★ NEW YORK STATE OFFICE OF MENTAL HEALTH
RESEARCH RESOURCE CENTER LIBRARY
44 Holland Ave.
Albany, NY 12229   Phone: (518) 474-7167
Paul G. Hillengas, Libn.
Subjects: Psychiatry, psychology, mental hygiene, sociology. Holdings:

4000 books; 8000 unbound periodicals; 2258 reprints. Subscriptions: 103
journals and other serials.

★9002★ NEW YORK STATE OFFICE OF MENTAL
RETARDATION AND DEVELOPMENTAL DISABILITIES
REFERENCE CENTER
800 N. Pearl St.
Albany, NY 12204   Phone: (518) 474-4613
Kathryn J. Jasenski, Sec.
Subjects: Mental retardation, developmental disabilities, community-
based services, foster care, residential services. Holdings: 1000 books; 1000
other cataloged items; archival materials; records; photographs. Subscrip-
tions: 66 journals and other serials.

★9003★ ST. PETER'S HOSPITAL
HEALTH SCIENCES LIBRARY
315 S. Manning Blvd.
Albany, NY 12208   Phone: (518) 454-1670
Phyllis Miyauchi, Dir.
Subjects: Medicine, surgery, nursing. Holdings: 1324 books; 1194 bound
periodical volumes; 162 audiotapes. Subscriptions: 185 journals and other
serials.

★9004★ U.S. DEPARTMENT OF VETERANS AFFAIRS
MEDICAL CENTER LIBRARY
113 Holland Ave.
Albany, NY 12208   Phone: (518) 462-3311
Subjects: Medicine, social services, nursing, mental health. Holdings: 2000
books; 2300 bound periodical volumes; 210 AV programs. Subscriptions:
302 journals and other serials.

★9005★ HUMAN RESOURCES SCHOOL
REHABILITATION RESEARCH LIBRARY
201 I.U. Willets Rd., W.
Albertson, NY 11507   Phone: (516) 747-5400
Gary Kishanuk, Lib.Hd.
Subjects: Rehabilitation, vocational rehabilitation of disabled, job placements, attitudes, career education, self sufficiency, recreation, special
education. Holdings: 2000 books; 45 VF drawers of pamphlets; 300
periodical volumes on microfilm. Subscriptions: 250 journals and other
serials.

★9006★ AUBURN MEMORIAL HOSPITAL
LIBRARY/RESOURCE CENTER
5-19 Lansing St.
Auburn, NY 13021   Phone: (315) 255-7231
Anne Costello Tomlin, Libn.
Subjects: Medicine, nursing, and allied health sciences. Holdings: 1850
books; 3500 bound periodical volumes. Subscriptions: 167 journals and
other serials.

★9007★ SAINT JEROME HOSPITAL
MEDICAL LIBRARY
16 Bank St.
Batavia, NY 14020   Phone: (716) 343-3131
Eleanor Randall, Libn.
Subjects: Medicine, nursing, and allied health sciences. Holdings: Figures
not available.

★9008★ U.S. DEPARTMENT OF VETERANS AFFAIRS
MEDICAL CENTER LIBRARY
Redfield Pkwy.
Batavia, NY 14020   Phone: (716) 343-7500
Madeline A. Coco, Chf.Libn.
Subjects: General medicine, surgery, nursing, pathology, radiology. Hold-
ings: 1700 books; 1700 bound periodical volumes. Subscriptions: 99
journals and other serials.

★9009★ U.S. DEPARTMENT OF VETERANS AFFAIRS
MEDICAL CENTER LIBRARY SERVICE
Bath, NY 14810   Phone: (607) 776-2111
Sally Ann Hillegas, Chf., Lib.Serv.
Subjects: Geriatrics, chronic diseases, general internal medicine, long term
care. Holdings: 1282 books; 125 video cassettes; 600 periodical volumes on
microfilm. Subscriptions: 116 journals and other serials; 12 newspapers.

★9010★   SOUTHSIDE HOSPITAL
MEDICAL LIBRARY
Montauk Hwy.
Bay Shore, NY 11706   Phone: (516) 968-3026
Caryl Kazen, Med.Libn.
Subjects: Family practice, internal medicine, surgery, nursing, dentistry, psychiatry. **Holdings:** 700 books; 100 bound periodical volumes; 5 VF drawers of pamphlets; 150 audio cassette programs. **Subscriptions:** 150 journals and other serials.

★9011★   QUEENS CHILDREN'S PSYCHIATRIC CENTER
LAURETTA BENDER STAFF LIBRARY
74-03 Commonwealth Blvd.
Bellerose, NY 11426   Phone: (718) 464-2900
Naomi Leiten, MD
Subjects: Psychiatry, psychology, social work. **Holdings:** 5000 books; 300 bound periodical volumes; 650 reprints and pamphlets; 300 reels of tape; Audio-Digest tapes on psychiatry. **Subscriptions:** 80 journals and other serials.

★9012★   ASSOCIATION FOR CHILDREN WITH DOWN
   SYNDROME
LIBRARY
2616 Martin Ave.
Bellmore, NY 11710   Phone: (516) 221-4700
Muriel Golieb
Subjects: Down's syndrome, mental retardation, early childhood education, special education, advocacy, families with special needs. **Holdings:** 1000 books; periodicals; audiotapes; videotapes; toys. **Subscriptions:** 10 journals and other serials.

★9013★   BROOME DEVELOPMENTAL SERVICES
STAFF LIBRARY
241 Glenwood Rd.
Binghamton, NY 13905-1695   Phone: (607) 770-0410
Mary Jeanne Perlmutter, Sr.Libn.
Subjects: Mental retardation, developmental disabilities. **Holdings:** 9923 books. **Subscriptions:** 131 journals and other serials.

★9014★   NEW YORK STATE OFFICE OF MENTAL HEALTH
BINGHAMTON PSYCHIATRIC CENTER
PROFESSIONAL LIBRARY
425 Robinson St.
Binghamton, NY 13901   Phone: (607) 773-4316
Martha A. Mason, Sr.Libn.
Subjects: Psychiatry, child psychiatry, community mental health, psychology, child psychology, group psychotherapy, mental illness, general medicine, psychoanalysis, social services. **Holdings:** 3200 books, bound periodicals, and pamphlets; 400 cassette tapes. **Subscriptions:** 63 journals and other serials.

★9015★   UNITED HEALTH SERVICES/BINGHAMTON
   GENERAL HOSPITAL
STUART B. BLAKELY MEMORIAL LIBRARY
Mitchell Ave.
Binghamton, NY 13903   Phone: (607) 771-2110
Maryanne Donnelly, Med.Libn.
Subjects: Medicine and nursing. **Holdings:** 11,000 volumes; 400 audiotapes; 200 videotapes; 10 films; 500 slides; 10 VF drawers of pamphlets. **Subscriptions:** 208 journals and other serials.

★9016★   THE HASTINGS CENTER
LIBRARY
255 Elm Rd.
Briarcliff Manor, NY 10510   Phone: (914) 762-8500
Marna Howarth, Libn.
Subjects: Medical ethics, ethics, ethics in life and social sciences, reproductive technologies, congressional ethics, teaching of ethics, abortion, death/dying, AIDS, genetics, public policy, health policy. **Holdings:** 6000 books; 40 VF drawers. **Subscriptions:** 120 journals and other serials.

★9017★   BRONX-LEBANON HOSPITAL CENTER
CONCOURSE DIVISION MEDICAL LIBRARY
1650 Grand Concourse
Bronx, NY 10457   Phone: (212) 588-7000
Gerardo Gomez, Libn.
Subjects: Medicine, allied health sciences. **Holdings:** 1200 books; 6497 bound periodical volumes. **Subscriptions:** 156 journals and other serials.

★9018★   CALVARY HOSPITAL
MEDICAL LIBRARY
1740 Eastchester Rd.
Bronx, NY 10461-9955   Phone: (212) 518-2229
Dorothy M. Maucione, Med.Libn.
Subjects: Medicine, cancer, nutrition, ethics, nursing. **Holdings:** 2079 books; medical journal articles; 100 microfiche, slides, audio- and video-tapes. **Subscriptions:** 265 journals and other serials.

★9019★   LINCOLN MEDICAL CENTER
HEALTH SCIENCES LIBRARY
234 E. 149th St.
Bronx, NY 10451   Phone: (212) 579-5745
Miss Milagros M. Paredes, Med.Libn.
Subjects: Medicine, surgery, pediatrics, obstetrics and gynecology, nursing. **Holdings:** 2265 books; 7677 bound periodical volumes. **Subscriptions:** 300 journals and other serials.

★9020★   MONTEFIORE MEDICAL CENTER
HEALTH SCIENCES LIBRARY/TISHMAN LEARNING CENTER
111 E. 210th St.
Bronx, NY 10467   Phone: (212) 920-4666
Josefina P. Lim, Dir.
Subjects: Medicine, health sciences administration, geriatrics, psychology, psychiatry, nursing. **Holdings:** 10,000 books; AV programs; software packages. **Subscriptions:** 800 journals.

★9021★   MONTEFIORE MEDICAL CENTER
KARL CHERKASKY SOCIAL MEDICINE LIBRARY
111 E. 210th St.
Bronx, NY 10467   Phone: (212) 920-5508
Michael Alderman, M.D.
Subjects: Social medicine, epidemiology, community and international health, occupational health. **Holdings:** 350 volumes.

★9022★   NEW YORK INSTITUTE FOR SPECIAL EDUCATION
WALTER BROOKS LIBRARY
999 Pelham Pkwy.
Bronx, NY 10469   Phone: (212) 519-7000
Harriet Rothstein, Hd.Libn.
Subjects: Special education. **Holdings:** 6600 ink-print books; 14,750 braille books; 650 talking books; 5000 pamphlets; 10 VF drawers; 205 filmstrips; 200 tapes. **Subscriptions:** 111 journals and other serials.

★9023★   NORTH CENTRAL BRONX HOSPITAL
J.L. AMSTER HEALTH SCIENCES LIBRARY
3424 Kossuth Ave., Rm. 14A-04
Bronx, NY 10467   Phone: (212) 519-4688
Wanda Perez, Asst.Libn.
Subjects: Internal medicine, obstetrics, gynecology, pediatrics, surgery, hospital administration. **Holdings:** 4000 books; 7000 bound periodical volumes; 1500 slides. **Subscriptions:** 263 journals and other serials; 6 newspapers.

★9024★   OUR LADY OF MERCY MEDICAL CENTER
MEDICAL LIBRARY
600 E. 233rd St., Rm. B-11
Bronx, NY 10466   Phone: (212) 920-9869
Sr. Jeanne Atkinson, Dir./Med.Libn.
Subjects: Medicine. **Holdings:** 2185 books; 7840 bound periodical volumes; 64 volumes of microforms. **Subscriptions:** 350 journals and other serials.

★9025★   U.S. DEPARTMENT OF VETERANS AFFAIRS
MEDICAL CENTER LIBRARY
130 W. Kingsbridge Rd.
Bronx, NY 10468   Phone: (212) 579-1631
Margaret M. Kinney, Chf.Libn.
Subjects: Medicine and allied health sciences. **Holdings:** 20,244 volumes. **Subscriptions:** 395 journals and other serials.

★9026★   YESHIVA UNIVERSITY
ALBERT EINSTEIN COLLEGE OF MEDICINE
D. SAMUEL GOTTESMAN LIBRARY
1300 Morris Park Ave.
Bronx, NY 10461   Phone: (212) 430-3108
Judie Malamud, Dir., Lib.
Subjects: Biochemistry, cell biology, psychology, medicine, molecular

biology, pharmacology, physiology, genetics, anatomy, oncology, pathology, psychiatry, immunology. **Holdings:** 72,768 books; 101,974 bound periodical volumes; 1401 theses; 50 VF drawers of archival materials; 541 dissertations; 10,433 microforms; 17,493 other cataloged items. **Subscriptions:** 2518 journals and other serials.

★9027★ **YESHIVA UNIVERSITY**
ALBERT EINSTEIN COLLEGE OF MEDICINE
DEPARTMENT OF ANESTHESIOLOGY
LIBRARY
Montefiore Medical Center
Jacobi, Rm. 1226
1300 Morris Park Ave.
Bronx, NY 10461   Phone: (212) 918-6865
Rosemary Vecchio
Subjects: Anesthesiology. **Holdings:** 200 books; 500 bound periodical volumes; 110 slide/tape sets. **Subscriptions:** 30 journals and other serials.

★9028★ **YESHIVA UNIVERSITY**
ALBERT EINSTEIN COLLEGE OF MEDICINE
DEPARTMENT OF PSYCHIATRY
J. THOMPSON PSYCHIATRY LIBRARY
Bronx Municipal Hospital Center
NR 2E7A
Bronx, NY 10461   Phone: (212) 918-4545
Mary Nahon Galgan, Libn.
Subjects: Psychiatry, psychoanalysis, social work. **Holdings:** 8000 books; 3700 bound periodical volumes; 9 VF drawers of reprints; 98 masters' dissertations. **Subscriptions:** 100 journals and other serials.

★9029★ **YESHIVA UNIVERSITY**
ALBERT EINSTEIN COLLEGE OF MEDICINE
SURGERY LIBRARY
Pelham Pkwy. & Eastchester Rd.
Bronx, NY 10461   Phone: (212) 918-5371
Subjects: Surgery, medicine. **Holdings:** 571 books; 1448 bound periodical volumes; 2 drawers of reprints. **Subscriptions:** 21 journals and other serials.

★9030★ **LAWRENCE HOSPITAL**
ASHLEY BAKER MORRILL LIBRARY
55 Palmer Ave.
Bronxville, NY 10708   Phone: (914) 337-7300
Virgil C. Larkin, Libn.
Subjects: Medicine, nursing, hospital administration. **Holdings:** 2220 books; 2184 bound periodical volumes; 9 VF drawers. **Subscriptions:** 210 journals and other serials.

★9031★ **BROOKDALE HOSPITAL MEDICAL CENTER**
MARIE SMITH SCHWARTZ MEDICAL LIBRARY
Linden Blvd. & Rockaway Pkwy.
Brooklyn, NY 11212   Phone: (718) 240-5312
Sophie Winston, Chf.Med.Libn.
Subjects: Medicine, health sciences, nursing. **Holdings:** 3000 books; 17,000 bound periodical volumes; 50 audiotapes; 40 slide programs; 80 videotapes; 7 CAI programs. **Subscriptions:** 365 journals and other serials.

★9032★ **BROOKLYN HOSPITAL**
MEDICAL LIBRARY
121 DeKalb Ave.
Brooklyn, NY 11201   Phone: (718) 403-6943
Narciso Rodriguez, Libn.
Subjects: Medicine, medical specialties. **Holdings:** 1200 books; 6000 bound periodical volumes; 250 AV programs. **Subscriptions:** 130 journals and other serials.

★9033★ **CENTER FOR THANATOLOGY RESEARCH**
LIBRARY
391 Atlantic Ave.
Brooklyn, NY 11217   Phone: (718) 858-3026
Roberta Halporn, Dir.
Subjects: Aging, dying, death, bereavement, gravestone studies. **Holdings:** 1000 books; 40 bound periodical volumes; videotapes; audio cassettes; photographs; rubbings. **Subscriptions:** 6 journals and other serials.

★9034★ **CONEY ISLAND HOSPITAL**
HAROLD FINK MEMORIAL LIBRARY
2601 Ocean Pkwy.
Brooklyn, NY 11235   Phone: (718) 615-4299
Munir U. Din, Dir.
Subjects: Medicine, nursing, pharmacy, psychiatry, podiatry, hospital administration. **Holdings:** 5700 books; 17,000 bound periodical volumes; 350 video cassettes; 200 slide/tape sets; 150 slide sets with pamphlets. **Subscriptions:** 325 journals and other serials.

★9035★ **DICYAN LIBRARY**
1486 E. 33rd St.
Brooklyn, NY 11234   Phone: (718) 252-8844
Subjects: Pharmacology, psychopharmacology, neuropharmacology, psychiatry, therapeutics, biochemistry, drugs. **Holdings:** 3000 volumes.

★9036★ **INTERFAITH MEDICAL CENTER**
BROOKLYN JEWISH DIVISION
MEDICAL AND NURSING LIBRARY
555 Prospect Pl.
Brooklyn, NY 11238   Phone: (718) 935-7085
Sharon Ruth Peterson, Med.Libn.
Subjects: Medicine, nursing, and allied health sciences. **Holdings:** 2500 books; 10,000 bound periodical volumes; 6 VF drawers. **Subscriptions:** 210 journals and other serials.

★9037★ **KINGSBORO PSYCHIATRIC CENTER**
HEALTH SCI LIBRARY
681 Clarkson Ave.
Brooklyn, NY 11203-2199   Phone: (718) 221-7273
Basheva Blokh, Dir., Hea.Sci.Lib.
Subjects: Psychiatry, medicine, psychology, rehabilitation, social service, nursing. **Holdings:** 3000 books; 4 VF files of pamphlets and clippings; 258 tape cassettes. **Subscriptions:** 144 journals and other serials.

★9038★ **KINGSBROOK JEWISH MEDICAL CENTER**
MEDICAL LIBRARY
585 Schenectady Ave.
Brooklyn, NY 11203-1891   Phone: (718) 604-5689
Mary E. Buchheit, Dir., Med.Lib.
Subjects: Pathology, neurology, orthopedics, rehabilitative medicine, clinical medicine. **Holdings:** 4900 books; 7200 bound periodical volumes. **Subscriptions:** 272 journals and other serials.

★9039★ **LONG ISLAND COLLEGE HOSPITAL**
MORGAN HEALTH SCIENCES LIBRARY
340 Henry St.
Brooklyn, NY 11201   Phone: (718) 780-1077
Gabriel Bakcsy, Dir.
Subjects: Medicine, nursing, basic sciences, social sciences, education. **Holdings:** 20,000 volumes; 60 linear feet of archival materials; 3 VF drawers of National League for Nursing pamphlets; 600 audio cassettes. **Subscriptions:** 377 journals and other serials.

★9040★ **LONG ISLAND UNIVERSITY**
ARNOLD AND MARIE SCHWARTZ COLLEGE OF PHARMACY
 AND HEALTH SCIENCES
PHARMACEUTICAL STUDY CENTER
75 DeKalb Ave.
Brooklyn, NY 11201   Phone: (718) 403-1060
Alisa Yalan, Media Dir.
Subjects: Pharmacy, pharmacology, pharmacy administration, biomedical communications, hospital pharmacy. **Holdings:** 30 books; 250 current periodicals; 500 AV programs. **Subscriptions:** 225 journals and other serials.

★9041★ **LUTHERAN MEDICAL CENTER**
MEDICAL LIBRARY
150 55th St.
Brooklyn, NY 11220   Phone: (718) 630-7200
Estela Longo, Med.Libn.
Subjects: Pathology, medicine, surgery, gynecology, obstetrics, pediatrics, radiology, family health, anesthesiology. **Holdings:** 7829 books; 2761 AV programs; 428 videotapes; 40 VF drawers; 270 other cataloged items. **Subscriptions:** 214 journals and other serials.

★9042★   MAIMONIDES MEDICAL CENTER
GEORGE A. DEGENSHEIN, M.D. MEMORIAL LIBRARY
4802 10th Ave.
Brooklyn, NY 11219   Phone: (718) 283-7406
Lydia Friedman, Chf.Med.Libn.
Subjects: Medicine, dentistry, gynecology, surgery, pediatrics, obstetrics, nursing, pharmacology, psychiatry, anatomy, physiology. **Holdings:** 4678 books; 10,639 bound periodical volumes; 8 Audio-Digest series; 886 video programs; 188 slide programs. **Subscriptions:** 271 journals and other serials.

★9043★   METHODIST HOSPITAL
HEALTH SCIENCES LIBRARY
506 6th St.
Brooklyn, NY 11215   Phone: (718) 780-3195
Robin L. Tannenbaum, Dir.
Subjects: Medicine, surgery, nursing, allied health sciences. **Holdings:** 3000 books; 4033 bound periodical volumes; 400 videotapes; 90 slide/tape sets; 5 audio cassette subject series. **Subscriptions:** 300 journals and other serials.

★9044★   NEW YORK CITY TECHNICAL COLLEGE OF THE
CITY UNIVERSITY OF NEW YORK
LIBRARY
300 Jay St.
Brooklyn, NY 11201   Phone: (718) 260-5470
Darrow Wood, Chf.Libn. & Dept.Chm.
Subjects: Paramedical sciences, graphic arts, hotel and restaurant management, Afro-American studies, engineering technology, business fields. **Holdings:** 158,372 books; 5156 bound periodical volumes; 108 VF drawers of pamphlet material; 3 VF drawers of menus; 15 VF drawers of pictures; 15 VF drawers of career material; 15 VF drawers of company history; 9051 reels of microfilm; 1934 phonograph records; 797 8mm film loops; 327 audio tapes; 743 video cassettes. **Subscriptions:** 934 journals and other serials; 15 newspapers.

★9045★   ST. JOHN'S EPISCOPAL HOSPITAL
INTERFAITH MEDICAL CENTER
NURSING AND MEDICAL LIBRARY
1545 Atlantic Ave.
Brooklyn, NY 11216   Phone: (718) 604-6030
Dallas C. Hopson, Dir.
Subjects: Pediatrics, obstetrics/gynecology. **Holdings:** 2500 books; 200 bound periodical volumes. **Subscriptions:** 105 journals and other serials.

★9046★   ST. MARY'S HOSPITAL OF BROOKLYN
MEDICAL LIBRARY
170 Buffalo Ave.
Brooklyn, NY 11213   Phone: (718) 774-3600
Elsa Sansaricq, Dir.
Subjects: Medicine, allied health sciences, nursing, sickle cell anemia, administration, drug addiction. **Holdings:** 1000 books; 100 administrative materials; Audio-Digest tapes. **Subscriptions:** 112 journals and other serials.

★9047★   SOCIETY FOR THE ADVANCEMENT OF TRAVEL
FOR THE HANDICAPPED
LIBRARY
26 Court St., Penthouse Ste.
Brooklyn, NY 11424   Phone: (718) 858-5483
Subjects: Travel facilities for the handicapped. **Holdings:** 300 volumes; literature provided by tourist offices, carriers, hotels, destinations, and car rental agencies; statistics.

★9048★   SUNY
HEALTH SCIENCE CENTER AT BROOKLYN
DEPARTMENT OF PSYCHIATRY LIBRARY
450 Clarkson Ave.
Brooklyn, NY 11203   Phone: (718) 245-3131
Subjects: Psychiatry, psychoanalysis, child psychiatry, psychology. **Holdings:** 2038 books; 1150 bound periodical volumes; 5 VF drawers of pamphlets and reprints. **Subscriptions:** 50 journals and other serials.

★9049★   SUNY
HEALTH SCIENCE CENTER AT BROOKLYN
LIBRARY
450 Clarkson Ave.
Box 14
Brooklyn, NY 11203   Phone: (718) 270-1038
Julie Semkow, Act.Lib.Dir.
Subjects: Medicine, nursing, and allied health sciences. **Holdings:** 252,752 volumes; archives and memorabilia of various Brooklyn hospitals and medical societies. **Subscriptions:** 1579 journals and other serials.

★9050★   U.S. DEPARTMENT OF VETERANS AFFAIRS
MEDICAL CENTER LIBRARY
800 Poly Pl.
Brooklyn, NY 11209   Phone: (718) 836-6600
Francine Tidona
Subjects: Medicine, surgery, psychiatry, psychology, nursing, social work. **Holdings:** 6685 books; 7226 bound periodical volumes; 106 video cassettes; 138 slide sets; 6 films. **Subscriptions:** 477 journals and other serials.

★9051★   WOODHULL MEDICAL AND MENTAL HEALTH
CENTER
HEALTH SCIENCES LIBRARY
760 Broadway, Rm. 3A160
Brooklyn, NY 11206   Phone: (718) 963-8397
Maria N. Perez, Sr.Dept.Libn.
Subjects: Medicine, allied health sciences. **Holdings:** 1300 books; 250 bound periodical volumes; 300 unbound journals. **Subscriptions:** 154 journals and other serials.

★9052★   BRISTOL-MYERS SQUIBB COMPANY
PHARMACEUTICAL RESEARCH INSTITUTE
RESEARCH LIBRARY
100 Forest Ave.
Buffalo, NY 14213   Phone: (716) 887-3637
Rose Ann Gubbins, Asst.Mgr., Lib.Oper.
Subjects: Dermatology, chemistry, pharmacology, pharmacy and pharmaceuticals, medicine, opthalmology. **Holdings:** 3000 books; 8000 bound periodical volumes; 2000 microfilm cartridges; 150 audio cassettes. **Subscriptions:** 500 journals and other serials.

★9053★   BUFFALO GENERAL HOSPITAL
A.H. AARON HEALTH SCIENCES LIBRARY
100 High St.
Buffalo, NY 14203   Phone: (716) 845-2878
Wentsing Liu, Lib.Dir.
Subjects: Medicine, surgery, dentistry, nursing, pharmacology. **Holdings:** 3200 books; 10,000 bound periodical volumes; Audio-Digest tapes on internal medicine and surgery; 950 AV programs. **Subscriptions:** 400 journals and other serials.

★9054★   BUFFALO PSYCHIATRIC CENTER
BPC LIBRARY
400 Forest Ave.
Buffalo, NY 14213   Phone: (716) 885-2261
Margaret Litzenberger, Asst.Libn.
Subjects: Psychiatry, psychology, psychiatric nursing. **Holdings:** 6000 books; 686 bound periodical volumes; 5000 reports, pamphlets, clippings. **Subscriptions:** 101 journals and other serials.

★9055★   CHILDREN'S HOSPITAL OF BUFFALO
MEDICAL LIBRARY
219 Bryant St.
Buffalo, NY 14222   Phone: (716) 878-7304
Lucy Wargo, Lib.Dir.
Subjects: Pediatrics, general medicine. **Holdings:** 1856 books; 10,393 bound periodical volumes. **Subscriptions:** 343 journals and other serials.

★9056★   ERIE COUNTY MEDICAL CENTER
MEDICAL LIBRARY
462 Grider St.
Buffalo, NY 14215   Phone: (716) 898-3939
Edward J. Leisner, Sr.Med.Libn.
Subjects: Medicine, orthopedics, cardiology, neurology, surgery, nursing. **Holdings:** 2300 books; 16,000 bound periodical volumes; 1150 AV programs; 4 VF drawers of reprints and pamphlets. **Subscriptions:** 382 journals and other serials.

★9057★   MEDICAL FOUNDATION OF BUFFALO
LIBRARY
73 High St.
Buffalo, NY 14203   Phone: (716) 856-9600
Dr. Vivian Cody, Sr.Res.Sci.
Subjects: Hormone-related disorders, including studies in cancer, heart disease, diabetes. **Holdings:** 2000 books and scientific journals.

★9058★   MERCY HOSPITAL
MEDICAL LIBRARY
565 Abbott Rd.
Buffalo, NY 14220   Phone: (716) 827-2323
Nancy A. Griffin, Libn.
Subjects: Medicine, nursing, allied health sciences. **Holdings:** 3000 books; 7000 bound periodical volumes; 300 slides, audio cassettes, video cassettes. **Subscriptions:** 215 journals and other serials.

★9059★   MILLARD FILLMORE HOSPITALS
KIDENEY HEALTH SCIENCES LIBRARY
3 Gates Circle
Buffalo, NY 14209   Phone: (716) 887-4845
Susan Grossman, Corp.Lib.Dir.
Subjects: Clinical medicine, nursing, surgery, health care administration, management. **Holdings:** 2570 books; 4861 bound periodical volumes; 4 VF drawers of pamphlets and articles; 1007 audio cassettes. **Subscriptions:** 349 journals and other serials.

★9060★   RESEARCH INSTITUTE ON ALCOHOLISM
LIBRARY
1021 Main St.
Buffalo, NY 14203   Phone: (716) 887-2511
Diane Augustino, Res.Sci. I
Subjects: Alcoholism, drug dependence, and alcohol and drug abuse - physiological, psychological, sociological, biochemical, pharmacological aspects. **Holdings:** 6300 books; 1450 bound periodical volumes; 8 VF drawers. **Subscriptions:** 120 journals and other serials.

★9061★   ROSWELL PARK MEMORIAL INSTITUTE
MEDICAL AND SCIENTIFIC LIBRARY
Carlton & Elm Sts.
Buffalo, NY 14263   Phone: (716) 845-5966
Ann P. Hutchinson, Lib.Dir.
Subjects: Cancer and allied diseases. **Holdings:** 73,000 books and bound periodical volumes; 400 AV programs. **Subscriptions:** 1200 journals and other serials.

★9062★   ST. MARY'S SCHOOL FOR THE DEAF
INFORMATION CENTER
2253 Main St.
Buffalo, NY 14214   Phone: (716) 834-7200
Jean Odien, Libn.
Subjects: Deafness, audiology, speech, special education. **Holdings:** 11,207 books; 683 bound periodical volumes; 436 microfiche. **Subscriptions:** 57 journals and other serials.

★9063★   SISTERS OF CHARITY HOSPITAL
MEDICAL STAFF LIBRARY
2157 Main St.
Buffalo, NY 14214   Phone: (716) 862-2846
Anne Cohen, Med.Libn.
Subjects: Medicine, surgery, obstetrics and gynecology, pediatrics. **Holdings:** 5974 books and bound periodical volumes. **Subscriptions:** 99 journals and other serials.

★9064★   SUNY AT BUFFALO
HEALTH SCIENCES LIBRARY
Main St. Campus
Buffalo, NY 14214   Phone: (716) 831-3337
Mr. C.K. Huang, Dir.
Subjects: Medicine, nursing, dentistry, pharmacy, allied health sciences, basic sciences. **Holdings:** 129,813 books; 148,060 bound periodical volumes; 1998 AV programs; 3000 pamphlets. **Subscriptions:** 2716 journals and other serials.

★9065★   SUNY AT BUFFALO
INDUSTRY/UNIVERSITY CENTER FOR BIOSURFACES
LIBRARY
110 Parker Hall
Buffalo, NY 14214   Phone: (716) 831-3560
Anne E. Meyer, Prog.Mgr.
Subjects: Biomaterials, biofouling, artificial organs. **Holdings:** 500 volumes.

★9066★   SUNY AT BUFFALO
SCHOOL OF PHARMACY
DRUG INFORMATION SERVICE
LIBRARY
Erie County Medical Center
462 Grider St.
Buffalo, NY 14215   Phone: (716) 898-3927
Dr. Susan L. Rozek, Dir.
Subjects: Medicinals, pharmacology, therapeutics. **Holdings:** 70 books; files; microfilm. **Subscriptions:** 25 journals and other serials.

★9067★   U.S. DEPARTMENT OF VETERANS AFFAIRS
MEDICAL CENTER LIBRARY SERVICE
3495 Bailey Ave.
Buffalo, NY 14215   Phone: (716) 834-9200
Betty A. Withrow, Chf.Libn.
Subjects: Medicine, surgery, nursing, management, patient education. **Holdings:** 2000 books; 9000 periodical volumes; 700 AV programs. **Subscriptions:** 400 journals and other serials.

★9068★   BEECH-NUT NUTRITION CORPORATION
LIBRARY
2 Church St.
Canajoharie, NY 13317   Phone: (518) 673-3251
Virginia A. San Fanandre-Russo, Libn.
Subjects: Nutrition, pediatrics, food chemistry. **Holdings:** 1000 books. **Subscriptions:** 31 journals and other serials.

★9069★   U.S. DEPARTMENT OF VETERANS AFFAIRS
MEDICAL CENTER LIBRARY
Canandaigua, NY 14424   Phone: (716) 396-3649
Peter Fleming, Chf., Lib.Serv.
Subjects: Psychiatry, psychology, medicine, nursing, alcoholism, geriatrics. **Holdings:** 4000 books; 612 bound periodical volumes; 2488 other volumes. **Subscriptions:** 240 journals and other serials.

★9070★   U.S. DEPARTMENT OF VETERANS AFFAIRS
DEPARTMENT OF MEDICINE AND SURGERY
LIBRARY SERVICE
Castle Point, NY 12511   Phone: (914) 831-2000
Jeffrey Nicholas, Chf., Lib.Serv.
Subjects: Spinal cord injuries, surgery, nursing education, geriatric medicine, dentistry. **Holdings:** 1966 books; 649 periodicals on microfilm; 286 audio cassettes; 129 video cassettes. **Subscriptions:** 130 journals and other serials; 5 newspapers.

★9071★   CENTRAL ISLIP PSYCHIATRIC CENTER
HEALTH SCIENCE LIBRARY
Carlton Ave., Med. Surg. Bldg.
Central Islip, NY 11722   Phone: (516) 234-6262
, Libn.
Subjects: Psychiatry, nursing, psychology, rehabilitation, retardation, developmental disabilities, geriatrics. **Holdings:** 9011 books; 1257 bound periodical volumes; 20 VF drawers; 28 AV programs. **Subscriptions:** 188 journals and other serials.

★9072★   ST. JOSEPH HOSPITAL
LIBRARY
2605 Harlem Rd.
Cheektowaga, NY 14225   Phone: (716) 891-2400
Subjects: Medicine. **Holdings:** 750 books; 57 bound periodical volumes. **Subscriptions:** 30 journals and other serials.

★9073★   COLD SPRING HARBOR LABORATORY
MAIN LIBRARY
Box 100
Cold Spring Harbor, NY 11724   Phone: (516) 367-8352
Susan Cooper, Dir., Libs./Dir, Pub.Aff.
Subjects: Biological sciences, genetics, cancer research, cell science, neuro-

biology, virology. **Holdings:** 8600 books; 23,000 bound periodical volumes; 24 VF drawers of archives, letters, clippings; 4 boxes of pamphlets. **Subscriptions:** 621 journals and other serials.

★9074★ MARY IMOGENE BASSETT HOSPITAL
MEDICAL LIBRARY
Atwell Rd.
Cooperstown, NY 13326   Phone: (607) 547-3115
Linda F. Muehl, Med.Libn.
Subjects: Clinical medicine, surgery. **Holdings:** 5000 books; 25,000 bound periodical volumes. **Subscriptions:** 524 journals and other serials.

★9075★ SUNY AT CORTLAND
MEMORIAL LIBRARY
Prospect Terr.
Box 2000
Cortland, NY 13045   Phone: (607) 753-2221
Selby U. Gration, Dir. of Libs.
Subjects: Education, recreation, physical education, health education. **Holdings:** 378,250 books; 42,691 bound periodical volumes; 575,587 microforms; 8,930 AV programs; 271 VF drawers; 10 files of pamphlets; 25,397 government documents. **Subscriptions:** 1527 journals and other serials; 8 newspapers.

★9076★ LINDSAY A. AND OLIVE B. O'CONNOR HOSPITAL
LIBRARY
Andes Road, Rte. 28
Box 205A
Delhi, NY 13753   Phone: (607) 746-2371
Barbara Green, Lib.Serv.
Subjects: Medicine, nursing. **Holdings:** 200 books. **Subscriptions:** 30 journals and other serials.

★9077★ NASSAU COUNTY MEDICAL CENTER
HEALTH SCIENCES LIBRARY
2201 Hempstead Tpke.
East Meadow, NY 11554   Phone: (516) 542-3542
William F. Casey, Lib.Dir.
Subjects: Medicine, nursing, and allied health sciences. **Holdings:** 9000 books; 6000 bound periodical volumes; 100 AV programs. **Subscriptions:** 700 journals and other serials.

★9078★ SUNY AT STONY BROOK
HEALTH SCIENCES LIBRARY
Box 66
East Setauket, NY 11733-0066   Phone: (516) 444-2512
Ruth Marcolina, Dir.
Subjects: Medicine, dentistry, nursing, allied health and basic medical sciences, social welfare. **Holdings:** 250,510 books and bound periodical volumes; microfilm. **Subscriptions:** 3244 journals and other serials.

★9079★ MOUNT SINAI SERVICES
ELMHURST HOSPITAL CENTER
MEDICAL LIBRARY
79-01 Broadway
Elmhurst, NY 11373   Phone: (718) 830-1538
Stacey Saley, Chf.Med.Libn.
Subjects: Basic sciences, health sciences. **Holdings:** 8000 books; 13,500 bound periodical volumes; pamphlets; AV programs. **Subscriptions:** 400 journals and other serials.

★9080★ ARNOT-OGDEN MEMORIAL HOSPITAL
WEY MEMORIAL LIBRARY
600 Roe Ave.
Elmira, NY 14905-1676   Phone: (607) 737-4101
Peggy Sleeth, Med.Libn.
Subjects: Medicine, nursing, and allied health sciences. **Holdings:** 4200 books; 3300 bound periodical volumes; 28 VF drawers; 300 cataloged items in historical collection; 600 AV programs. **Subscriptions:** 300 journals and other serials.

★9081★ ELMIRA PSYCHIATRIC CENTER
PROFESSIONAL LIBRARY
Caller 1527
Elmira, NY 14902   Phone: (607) 737-4769
Consuelo R. Madumba, Act.Dir., Educ. & Trng.
Subjects: Psychiatry, psychology, sociology. **Holdings:** 2416 books; 798 AV programs. **Subscriptions:** 58 journals and other serials.

★9082★ ST. JOSEPH'S HOSPITAL
HELENE FULD LEARNING RESOURCE CENTER
555 E. Market St.
Elmira, NY 14902   Phone: (607) 733-6541
Arlene C. Pien, Libn.
Subjects: Medicine, nursing. **Holdings:** 5000 books; 4000 bound periodical volumes; 1500 AV programs; 10 drawers of pamphlets. **Subscriptions:** 165 journals and other serials.

★9083★ EPISCOPAL HEALTH SERVICES OF LONG ISLAND
ST. JOHN'S EPISCOPAL HOSPITAL, SOUTH SHORE DIVISION
MEDICAL LIBRARY
327 Beach 19th St.
Far Rockaway, NY 11691   Phone: (718) 868-7699
Kalpana Desai, Chf.Med.Libn.
Subjects: Medicine, pediatrics, surgery, obstetrics/gynecology, psychiatry, nursing. **Holdings:** 800 books; 2000 bound periodical volumes; audio cassettes. **Subscriptions:** 124 journals and other serials.

★9084★ PENINSULA HOSPITAL CENTER
MEDICAL LIBRARY
51-15 Beach Channel Dr.
Far Rockaway, NY 11691   Phone: (718) 945-7100
Edith Rubinstein, Dir.
Subjects: Medicine, surgery, nursing, dentistry, podiatry, orthopedics. **Holdings:** 1182 books; 2150 bound periodical volumes; 75 video cassettes; 228 audio cassettes. **Subscriptions:** 105 journals and other serials.

★9085★ BOOTH MEMORIAL MEDICAL CENTER
HEALTH EDUCATION LIBRARY
Main St. at Booth Memorial Ave.
Flushing, NY 11355   Phone: (718) 670-1118
Rita S. Maier, Lib.Dir.
Subjects: Medicine, surgery, pediatrics, obstetrics and gynecology, nursing, dentistry. **Holdings:** 3200 books; 7800 bound periodical volumes; 350 AV programs. **Subscriptions:** 400 journals and other serials.

★9086★ FLUSHING HOSPITAL AND MEDICAL CENTER
MEDICAL LIBRARY
4500 Parsons Blvd. & 45th Ave.
Flushing, NY 11355-9980   Phone: (718) 670-5653
Vincent C. Notarstefano, Dir.
Subjects: Medicine and allied health sciences. **Holdings:** 3000 books; 2000 bound periodical volumes; 8 VF drawers of pamphlets and clippings; Audio-Digest tapes. **Subscriptions:** 190 journals and other serials.

★9087★ QUEENS COLLEGE OF THE CITY UNIVERSITY OF NEW YORK
BENJAMIN S. ROSENTHAL LIBRARY
REFERENCE DEPARTMENT
SCIENCE COLLECTION
65-30 Kissena Blvd.
Flushing, NY 11367   Phone: (718) 997-3700
Matthew J. Simon, Chf.Libn.
Subjects: Biology, psychology, chemistry, mathematics, physics, geology, computer science, home economics, speech pathology, audiology, sports physiology and medicine. **Holdings:** 68,000 books; 34,000 bound periodical volumes; microfilm. **Subscriptions:** 1850 journals and other serials.

★9088★ ST. JOSEPH'S HOSPITAL
MEDICAL LIBRARY
158-40 79th Ave.
Flushing, NY 11366   Phone: (718) 591-1000
Frances Taub, Libn.
Subjects: Medicine. **Holdings:** Figures not available.

★9089★ LA GUARDIA HOSPITAL
HEALTH SCIENCES LIBRARY
102-01 66 Rd.
Forest Hills, NY 11366   Phone: (718) 830-4188
Rosalyn Barth, Lib.Dir.
Subjects: Medicine, surgery, nursing. **Holdings:** 1589 books; 2900 bound periodical volumes. **Subscriptions:** 165 journals and other serials.

★9090★ NASSAU COMMUNITY COLLEGE
NEW YORK STATE HEALTH FILM COLLECTION
Garden City, NY 11530   Phone: (516) 222-7406
Arthur L. Friedman, Chm.
Subjects: Health. **Holdings:** 2334 16mm films; filmstrips; slides; overhead transparencies.

★9091★ NASSAU COUNTY MEDICAL SOCIETY
NASSAU ACADEMY OF MEDICINE
JOHN N. SHELL LIBRARY
1200 Stewart Ave.
Garden City, NY 11530   Phone: (516) 832-2320
Mary L. Westermann, Cons.
Subjects: Medicine, psychiatry, nursing. **Holdings:** 8000 books; 45,000 bound periodical volumes; 3 VF drawers. **Subscriptions:** 500 journals and other serials.

★9092★ COMMUNITY HOSPITAL AT GLEN COVE
MEDICAL LIBRARY
St. Andrews Ln.
Glen Cove, NY 11542   Phone: (516) 676-5000
Kathryn M. Gegan, Libn.
Subjects: Medicine. **Holdings:** Figures not available. **Subscriptions:** 89 journals and other serials.

★9093★ NEW YORK CHIROPRACTIC COLLEGE
LIBRARY
Box 167
Glen Head, NY 11545   Phone: (516) 626-3115
Marilyn Stern, Lib.Dir.
Subjects: Health sciences, basic sciences, chiropractic. **Holdings:** 9000 books. **Subscriptions:** 332 journals and other serials.

★9094★ LONG ISLAND JEWISH MEDICAL CENTER
HILLSIDE HOSPITAL
HEALTH SCIENCES LIBRARY
75-59 263rd St.
Box 38
Glen Oaks, NY 11004   Phone: (718) 470-8090
Joan L. Kauff, Asst.Dir., Hea.Sci.Libs.
Subjects: Psychiatry, psychoanalysis, psychology, nursing, social work, hospital administration. **Holdings:** 10,000 books; 5500 bound periodical volumes; 36 VF drawers of reprints and pamphlets; 800 audio cassettes. **Subscriptions:** 250 journals and other serials.

★9095★ U.S.D.A.
AGRICULTURAL RESEARCH SERVICE
PLUM ISLAND ANIMAL DISEASE CENTER
LIBRARY
Box 848
Greenport, NY 11944-0848   Phone: (516) 323-2500
Stephen Perlman, Libn.
Subjects: Virology, microbiology, immunology, molecular biology, veterinary medicine, laboratory animal sciences. **Holdings:** 14,000 books; 16,000 bound periodical volumes; 12,645 reprints; 85 VF drawers of pamphlets and reprints. **Subscriptions:** 166 journals and other serials.

★9096★ U.S. AIR FORCE HOSPITAL
416 STRATEGIC HOSPITAL
MEDICAL LIBRARY
Griffiss AFB, NY 13441-5300   Phone: (315) 330-7713
Patty Sbaraglia, Med.Libn.
Subjects: Nursing, dental services, mental and social health, surgery, internal medicine, food service. **Holdings:** 753 books. **Subscriptions:** 73 journals and other serials.

★9097★ NEW YORK STATE NURSES ASSOCIATION
LIBRARY
2113 Western Ave.
Guilderland, NY 12084   Phone: (518) 456-5371
Warren G. Hawkes, Lib.Dir.
Subjects: Nursing and allied health fields, labor, collective bargaining. **Holdings:** 7500 books; 695 bound periodical volumes; New York State nursing school catalogs (complete set); 6 VF drawers of pamphlets. **Subscriptions:** 275 journals and other serials.

★9098★ COMMUNITY GENERAL HOSPITAL OF SULLIVAN
COUNTY
HEALTH SCIENCES LIBRARY
Bushville Rd.
Box 800
Harris, NY 12742-0800   Phone: (914) 794-3300
Mary Jo Russell, Libn.
Subjects: Medicine, nursing, pharmacology, medical specialties, allied health sciences. **Holdings:** 550 books; 450 bound periodical volumes. **Subscriptions:** 75 journals and other serials.

★9099★ ST. VINCENT'S HOSPITAL AND MEDICAL CENTER
OF NEW YORK, WESTCHESTER BRANCH
MEDICAL LIBRARY
240 North St.
Harrison, NY 10528   Phone: (914) 967-6500
Ethel Eisenberg, Med.Libn.
Subjects: Psychiatry, psychology, alcoholism, drug abuse. **Holdings:** 3000 books; 2000 bound periodical volumes; cassettes. **Subscriptions:** 60 journals and other serials.

★9100★ SUFFOLK ACADEMY OF MEDICINE
LIBRARY
850 Veterans Memorial Hwy.
Hauppauge, NY 11788   Phone: (516) 724-7970
Joyce A. Bahr
Subjects: Medicine, dentistry, nursing, history. **Holdings:** 2500 books; 10,000 periodical volumes; 90 bulletin collections; 24 shelves of pamphlets. **Subscriptions:** 350 journals and other serials.

★9101★ GOWANDA PSYCHIATRIC CENTER
A. STEPHEN DUBOIS LIBRARY
Rte. 62
Helmuth, NY 14079   Phone: (716) 532-3311
Mark Wudyka, Libn.
Subjects: Psychiatry, psychology. **Holdings:** 4398 volumes. **Subscriptions:** 47 journals and other serials.

★9102★ NASSAU COUNTY DEPARTMENT OF HEALTH
DIVISION OF LABORATORIES AND RESEARCH
MEDICAL LIBRARY
209 Main St.
Hempstead, NY 11550   Phone: (516) 483-9158
Douglas S. Lieberman, Libn.
Subjects: Laboratory diagnosis, communicable diseases, environmental health. **Holdings:** 1000 books; 2500 bound periodical volumes; 1800 microfilm cartridges; microfiche of previous two years of journals. **Subscriptions:** 60 journals and other serials.

★9103★ ST. JAMES MERCY HOSPITAL
MEDICAL AND SCHOOL OF NURSING LIBRARY
440 Monroe Ave.
Hornell, NY 14843   Phone: (607) 324-0841
Brian Smith, Libn.
Subjects: Nursing. **Holdings:** 3500 books; 475 bound periodical volumes; 300 AV programs. **Subscriptions:** 65 journals and other serials.

★9104★ HUNTINGTON HOSPITAL
MEDICAL LIBRARY
270 Park Ave.
Huntington, NY 11743   Phone: (516) 351-2283
Ruth I. Glick, Dir.
Subjects: Medicine and surgery, nursing, pathology, radiology, nuclear medicine, sonography. **Holdings:** 900 books; 5325 bound periodical volumes; audiotapes. **Subscriptions:** 261 journals and other serials.

★9105★ CORNELL UNIVERSITY
FLOWER VETERINARY LIBRARY
Schurman Hall
Ithaca, NY 14853-6401   Phone: (607) 253-3510
Susanne K. Whitaker, Vet.Med.Libn.
Subjects: Veterinary medicine and supporting biomedical subjects. **Holdings:** 79,000 volumes; 35,000 AV items. **Subscriptions:** 1300 journals and other serials.

★9106★ TOMPKINS COMMUNITY HOSPITAL
ROBERT BROAD MEDICAL LIBRARY
101 Dates Dr.
Ithaca, NY 14850   Phone: (607) 274-4407
Sally Van Idistine, Libn.
Subjects: Surgery, medicine, nursing. **Holdings:** 500 books; 800 bound periodical volumes. **Subscriptions:** 70 journals and other serials.

★9107★ LEXINGTON SCHOOL FOR THE DEAF
LIBRARY MEDIA CENTER
30th Ave. & 25th St.
Jackson Heights, NY 11370   Phone: (718) 899-8800
Marie-Ann Marchese, Coord., Lib.Serv.
Subjects: Audiology, behavior modification, deafness, education, language, child study, exceptional children, psychology, reading, speech, parenting. **Holdings:** 16,788 books. **Subscriptions:** 59 journals and other serials; 6 newspapers.

★9108★ CATHOLIC MEDICAL CENTER OF BROOKLYN AND QUEENS
CENTRAL MEDICAL LIBRARY
88-25 153rd St.
Jamaica, NY 11432   Phone: (718) 657-6800
Joan A. Napolitano, Dir.
Subjects: Medicine, surgery, orthopedics, ophthalmology, family practice, dentistry. **Holdings:** 4000 books; 5400 bound periodical volumes; 24 VF drawers; 1100 Audio-Digest tapes; 100 MEDCOM slides; microforms; 200 video cassettes. **Subscriptions:** 250 journals and other serials.

★9109★ JAMAICA HOSPITAL
MEDICAL LIBRARY
89th Ave. & Van Wyck Expy.
Jamaica, NY 11418   Phone: (718) 262-6042
Carolyn Mansbach, Dir.
Subjects: Medicine. **Holdings:** 4000 books; 2500 bound periodical volumes; Audio-Digest tapes. **Subscriptions:** 275 journals and other serials.

★9110★ LONG ISLAND JEWISH MEDICAL CENTER
QUEENS HOSPITAL CENTER
HEALTH SCIENCE LIBRARY
82-68 164th St.
Jamaica, NY 11432   Phone: (718) 883-4019
Ruth Hoffenberg, Chf.Med.Libn., QHC
Subjects: Clinical medicine, health services administration, nursing. **Holdings:** 6000 books; 7000 bound periodical volumes. **Subscriptions:** 462 journals and other serials.

★9111★ ST. JOHN'S UNIVERSITY
COLLEGE OF PHARMACY AND ALLIED HEALTH PROFESSIONS
HEALTH EDUCATION RESOURCE CENTER
Grand Central & Utopia Pkwys.
Jamaica, NY 11439   Phone: (718) 990-6685
Mary A. Grant, Dir.
Subjects: Clinical pharmacy, pharmacology, pharmacy administration, toxicology, pharmacokinetics, industrial pharmacy. **Holdings:** 1840 volumes; 16 newsletters; 533 video cassettes; 120 audio slide programs; 16 drawers of article and pamphlet files; 279 transparencies; 41 Computer Assisted Learning programs; 106 slide programs. **Subscriptions:** 100 journals and other serials.

★9112★ UNITED HEALTH SERVICES/WILSON HOSPITAL
LEARNING RESOURCES DEPARTMENT
33-57 Harrison St.
Johnson City, NY 13790   Phone: (607) 763-6030
Maryanne Donnelly, Mgr., Lrng.Rsrcs.Dept.
Subjects: Medicine, nursing, health sciences administration. **Holdings:** 6000 books; 5400 bound periodical volumes; 1800 video cassettes, slide/tape programs, models, films, charts. **Subscriptions:** 305 journals and other serials.

★9113★ KENMORE MERCY HOSPITAL
HEALTH SCIENCES LEARNING RESOURCE CENTER
2950 Elmwood Ave.
Kenmore, NY 14217   Phone: (716) 879-6114
Brenda L. Cassoni, Libn.
Subjects: Medicine, nursing, allied health sciences. **Holdings:** 500 books; 10,000 unbound periodicals. **Subscriptions:** 115 journals and other serials.

★9114★ KINGS PARK PSYCHIATRIC CENTER
KPPC MEDICAL LIBRARY
Box 9000
Kings Park, NY 11754   Phone: (516) 544-3207
James W. Macinick, Sr.Libn.
Subjects: Psychiatry, nursing, medicine, allied health sciences. **Holdings:** 7000 books; 1000 bound periodical volumes; 15 VF drawers of pamphlets; 1000 audiotapes. **Subscriptions:** 70 journals and other serials.

★9115★ KINGSTON HOSPITAL
LIBRARY
396 Broadway
Kingston, NY 12401   Phone: (914) 331-3131
Ann Blish, Libn.
Subjects: Medicine, nursing. **Holdings:** 850 books; 4 VF drawers of articles and bibliographies. **Subscriptions:** 123 journals and other serials.

★9116★ OUR LADY OF VICTORY HOSPITAL
HOSPITAL LIBRARY
55 Melroy at Ridge Rd.
Lackawanna, NY 14218   Phone: (716) 825-8000
Judy Pacholec, Lib.Mgr.
Subjects: Medicine, surgery, head trauma rehabilitation, allied health sciences. **Holdings:** 650 books. **Subscriptions:** 70 journals and other serials.

★9117★ W. ALTON JONES CELL SCIENCE CENTER
GEORGE AND MARGARET GEY LIBRARY
10 Old Barn Rd.
Lake Placid, NY 12946   Phone: (518) 523-1267
Sallie B. Roberts, Libn.
Subjects: Cell culture, organ culture, cytology, cancer research, virology, biochemistry, immunology. **Holdings:** 5000 books; 4500 bound periodical volumes. **Subscriptions:** 125 journals and other serials.

★9118★ MEDICAL SOCIETY OF THE STATE OF NEW YORK
ALBION O. BERNSTEIN LIBRARY
420 Lakeville Rd.
Lake Success, NY 11042   Phone: (516) 488-6100
Ella Abney, Libn.
Subjects: Socioeconomic and clinical medicine. **Holdings:** 7000 books; 10,000 bound periodical volumes; 2000 other cataloged items. **Subscriptions:** 375 journals and other serials; 5 newspapers.

★9119★ LONG BEACH MEMORIAL HOSPITAL
LIBRARY
455 E. Bay Dr.
Long Beach, NY 11561   Phone: (516) 432-8000
Sharon Player
Subjects: Medicine, surgery, cardiology, psychiatry. **Holdings:** 240 books; 16 bound periodical volumes; 94 AV programs; 2 sets of microforms.

★9120★ ALICE HYDE HOSPITAL ASSOCIATION
MEDICAL/NURSING LIBRARY
Malone, NY 12953   Phone: (518) 483-3000
Lori Maloy, Lib.Mgr.
Subjects: Medicine, nursing. **Holdings:** 250 books. **Subscriptions:** 20 journals and other serials.

★9121★ THE NATUROPATHY INSTITUTE
LIBRARY
PO Box 56
Malverne, NY 11565
Dr. Edgar A. Kinon, N.D., Dir.
Subjects: Naturopathy, nutrition, natural healing sciences, radiesthesia/radionics, botanical medicine, anatomy, physiology. **Holdings:** 850 books; 1000 nonbook items. **Subscriptions:** 7 journals and other serials.

★9122★ NORTH SHORE UNIVERSITY HOSPITAL
DANIEL CARROLL PAYSON MEDICAL LIBRARY
300 Community Dr.
Manhasset, NY 11030   Phone: (516) 562-4324
Debra Eisenberg, Dir.
Subjects: Clinical medicine, nursing, psychiatry, allied health sciences. **Holdings:** 5359 books; 13,622 bound periodical volumes; 2418 AV programs. **Subscriptions:** 727 journals and other serials.

★9123★ MASSENA MEMORIAL HOSPITAL
MEDICAL LIBRARY
1 Hospital Dr.
Massena, NY 13662   Phone: (315) 764-1711
Shaylyn Frederick, Med.Lib.Mgr.
Subjects: Medicine, surgery, nursing, respiratory and physical therapy.
Holdings: 240 books. **Subscriptions:** 48 journals and other serials.

★9124★ ESTEE LAUDER INC.
INFORMATION CENTER
125 Pine Lawn Rd.
Melville, NY 11747   Phone: (516) 531-1174
Dr. Dorothy A. Kramer, Mgr. & Info.Sci.
Subjects: Cosmetics, dermatology, biochemistry, chemistry, computer science, engineering. **Holdings:** 4500 books; 1500 bound periodical volumes; supplier literature. **Subscriptions:** 250 journals and other serials; 6 newspapers.

★9125★ HORTON MEMORIAL HOSPITAL
MEDICAL LIBRARY
60 Prospect Ave.
Middletown, NY 10940   Phone: (914) 343-2424
Laura Leese, Med.Libn.
Subjects: Medicine, surgery, nursing, allied health sciences. **Holdings:** 1500 books; 2000 bound periodical volumes; 50 pamphlets; 25 pamphlets (uncataloged); vertical file of 1900 research topics; 200 audiotapes. **Subscriptions:** 100 journals and other serials.

★9126★ MIDDLETOWN PSYCHIATRIC CENTER
MEDICAL/PROFESSIONAL LIBRARY
141 Monhagen Ave.
Box 1453
Middletown, NY 10940   Phone: (914) 342-5511
Judith A. Mann, Sr.Libn.
Subjects: Psychiatry, medicine, nursing. **Holdings:** 7300 books; 862 bound periodical volumes. **Subscriptions:** 90 journals and other serials.

★9127★ NASSAU COUNTY DEPARTMENT OF HEALTH
LIBRARY
240 Old Country Rd., Rm. 613
Mineola, NY 11501   Phone: (516) 535-3470
Douglas S. Lieberman, Libn.
Subjects: Public health. **Holdings:** 1000 books; 259 reels of microfilm of journals; microfiche; Nassau County Department of Health publications, monthly and annual reports. **Subscriptions:** 60 journals and other serials.

★9128★ WINTHROP-UNIVERSITY HOSPITAL
HOLLIS HEALTH SCIENCES LIBRARY
259 1st St.
Mineola, NY 11501   Phone: (516) 663-2280
Virginia I. Cook, Med.Libn.
Subjects: Medicine, surgery, nursing, allied health sciences. **Holdings:** 3460 books; 8250 bound periodical volumes; 385 AV programs; 125 computer-assisted instruction programs; audiotapes; pamphlets. **Subscriptions:** 390 journals and other serials.

★9129★ NEW YORK STATE DEPARTMENT OF STATE
OFFICE OF FIRE PREVENTION AND CONTROL
ACADEMY OF FIRE SCIENCE
LIBRARY
600 College Ave.
Box 811
Montour Falls, NY 14865   Phone: (607) 535-7136
Diana Zell, Libn.
Subjects: Fire protection, prevention, and control; occupational safety; fire department administration and management; codes, standards, and regulations; emergency medical services; consumer safety; hazardous materials; arson prevention and control; history of fire service in New York State. **Holdings:** 5250 books; 175 bound periodical volumes; 16 VF drawers; 150 microfiche. **Subscriptions:** 130 journals and other serials.

★9130★ U.S. DEPARTMENT OF VETERANS AFFAIRS
MEDICAL LIBRARY
Franklin Delano Roosevelt Veterans Medical Ctr.
Montrose, NY 10548   Phone: (914) 737-4400
Bruce S. Delman, Ph.D., Chf., Lib.Serv.
Subjects: Psychiatry, psychology, medicine, social work, nursing, geriatrics.
Holdings: 7422 books; 1600 bound periodical volumes; 2800 boxes of microfilm; 1250 AV programs. **Subscriptions:** 615 journals and other serials; 8 newspapers.

★9131★ NORTHERN WESTCHESTER HOSPITAL CENTER
HEALTH SCIENCES LIBRARY
400 Main St.
Mount Kisco, NY 10549   Phone: (914) 666-1259
Nona C. Willoughby, Dir.
Subjects: Clinical medicine, nursing, nutrition, laboratory sciences, obstetrics and gynecology, hospital management. **Holdings:** 1900 books; 3500 bound periodical volumes; 300 audio cassettes; 3 VF cabinets of pamphlets and clippings. **Subscriptions:** 142 journals and other serials.

★9132★ MOUNT VERNON HOSPITAL
LIBRARY AND INFORMATION SERVICES
12 N. 7th Ave.
Mount Vernon, NY 10550   Phone: (914) 664-8000
Joan L. Riggs, Lib.Coord.
Subjects: Health sciences, medicine, nursing. **Holdings:** 3059 books; 323 bound periodical volumes; 12 VF drawers; 394 AV programs. **Subscriptions:** 119 journals and other serials.

★9133★ LONG ISLAND JEWISH MEDICAL CENTER
HEALTH SCIENCES LIBRARY
Lakeville Rd.
New Hyde Park, NY 11042   Phone: (718) 470-7070
Debra Cassel Rand, Dir.
Subjects: Medicine, dentistry, allied health sciences. **Holdings:** 9000 books; 15,000 bound periodical volumes. **Subscriptions:** 700 journals and other serials.

★9134★ MEDICAL LETTER
LIBRARY
1000 Main St.
New Rochelle, NY 10801   Phone: (914) 235-0500
Amy Faucard, Libn.
Subjects: Drugs, therapeutic agents. **Holdings:** Books; reprints; advertisements. **Subscriptions:** 180 journals and other serials.

★9135★ NEW ROCHELLE HOSPITAL MEDICAL CENTER
HEALTH SCIENCE LIBRARY
16 Guion Pl.
New Rochelle, NY 10802   Phone: (914) 632-5000
Mary F. Shanahan, Lib.Dir.
Subjects: Surgery, medicine, nursing, graphics. **Holdings:** 3000 books; 10,000 bound periodical volumes; 300 tapes; 100 AV programs; staff reprints. **Subscriptions:** 300 journals and other serials.

★9136★ A. FOSTER HIGGINS & COMPANY, INC.
RESEARCH LIBRARY
125 Broad St., 4th Fl.
New York, NY 10004   Phone: (212) 574-9022
Patrick Sweeney, Libn.
Subjects: Health care, pensions, Social Security, group insurance. **Holdings:** 3000 books; 15 VF drawers of annual reports; 32 VF drawers of clippings. **Subscriptions:** 200 journals and other serials.

★9137★ ALFRED ADLER INSTITUTE
LIBRARY
1841 Broadway, 4th Fl.
New York, NY 10023   Phone: (212) 974-0431
Leo Rattner, Ph.D., Exec.Dir.
Subjects: Psychotherapy, psychology, psychiatry, counseling. **Holdings:** 500 volumes.

★9138★ AMERICAN ARBITRATION ASSOCIATION
EASTMAN ARBITRATION LIBRARY
140 W. 51st St.
New York, NY 10020   Phone: (212) 484-4127
Laura Ferris Brown, Chf.Libn.
Subjects: Arbitration, mediation, and other forms of alternative dispute resolution - general, commercial, international, labor, environmental, compulsory, maritime, insurance, medical and health, public employment. **Holdings:** 16,000 volumes; arbitration awards; 19,500 microfiche. **Subscriptions:** 240 journals and other serials.

★9139★ AMERICAN BUREAU FOR MEDICAL ADVANCEMENT IN CHINA
LIBRARY
2 E. 103rd St.
New York, NY 10029   Phone: (212) 860-1990
Subjects: Taiwanese medical and health services, diseases prevalent in Southeast Asia. **Holdings:** 45,000 items of correspondence, memoranda, reports, photographs, posters, and printed materials.

★9140★ AMERICAN FOUNDATION FOR THE BLIND
HELEN KELLER ARCHIVES
15 W. 16th St.
New York, NY 10011   Phone: (212) 620-2157
Alberta J. Lonergan, Archv.
Subjects: Helen Keller; Anne Sullivan Macy; John Albert Macy; Polly Thomson; work on behalf of the blind, deaf-blind, and deaf; children and women in factories; planned parenthood; labor movements; peace; suffrage. **Holdings:** 65,000 manuscripts, sound recordings, photographs, films, slides, letters, speeches, literary manuscripts, legal and genealogical material.

★9141★ AMERICAN FOUNDATION FOR THE BLIND
M.C. MIGEL MEMORIAL LIBRARY
15 W. 16th St.
New York, NY 10011   Phone: (212) 620-2162
Leslie Rosen, Hd.Libn.
Subjects: Blindness - education, psychology, rehabilitation. **Holdings:** 40,000 volumes. **Subscriptions:** 150 journals and other serials.

★9142★ AMERICAN JOURNAL OF NURSING COMPANY
SOPHIA F. PALMER LIBRARY
555 W. 57th St.
New York, NY 10019   Phone: (212) 582-8820
Frederick W. Pattison, Libn.
Subjects: Nursing and allied fields. **Holdings:** 9000 books and bound periodical volumes. **Subscriptions:** 300 journals and other serials.

★9143★ ANIMAL MEDICAL CENTER
LIBRARY
510 E. 62nd St.
New York, NY 10021   Phone: (212) 838-8100
A. Christine MacMurray, Ed.
Subjects: Veterinary medicine, medicine. **Holdings:** 1000 books; 1000 bound periodical volumes; 500 periodical volumes on microfiche. **Subscriptions:** 50 journals and other serials.

★9144★ ARICA INSTITUTE, INC.
LIBRARY AND ARCHIVES
150 5th Ave., No. 912
New York, NY 10011-4311   Phone: (212) 807-9600
David J. Johnson, Libn./Archv.
Subjects: Psychology, medicine, creativity, organization, metaphysics, enlightenment. **Holdings:** Figures not available.

★9145★ ASSOCIATION FOR VOLUNTARY SURGICAL CONTRACEPTION
LIBRARY
122 E. 42nd St.
New York, NY 10168   Phone: (212) 351-2504
William J. Record, Libn.
Subjects: Sexual sterilization. **Holdings:** 3010 books; 80 feet of vertical files. **Subscriptions:** 118 journals and other serials.

★9146★ BARNARD COLLEGE
BARNARD CENTER FOR RESEARCH ON WOMEN
BIRDIE GOLDSMITH AST RESOURCE COLLECTION
101 Barnard Hall
3009 Broadway
New York, NY 10027   Phone: (212) 854-2067
Temma Kaplan, Dir., Women's Ctr.
Subjects: Feminist theory; sex roles and sex differences; women's movement; education; employment; legal status; health; violence and sexual exploitation; women in other countries, history, and the arts; women and development. **Holdings:** 1800 volumes; 5700 journal articles, reports, clippings, fact sheets, pamphlets, conference proceedings, unpublished papers, government documents; bibliographies; handbooks; directories; special issues of journals. **Subscriptions:** 160 periodicals, newspapers, and newsletters.

★9147★ BELLEVUE HOSPITAL
CLARENCE DE LA CHAPELLE MEDICAL LIBRARY
1st Ave. at 27th St.
New York, NY 10016   Phone: (212) 561-6535
Martha Lynch, Dir.
Subjects: Clinical medicine. **Holdings:** 3000 books; 20,000 bound periodical volumes. **Subscriptions:** 301 journals and other serials.

★9148★ BETH ISRAEL HOSPITAL NORTH
ECKMAN MEDICAL LIBRARY
170 E. End Ave. at 87th St.
New York, NY 10128   Phone: (212) 870-9470
Antoinette Drago, Libn.
Subjects: Medicine, surgery. **Holdings:** 3000 books; 300 bound periodical volumes. **Subscriptions:** 100 journals.

★9149★ BETH ISRAEL MEDICAL CENTER
HOSPITAL FOR JOINT DISEASES ORTHOPAEDIC INSTITUTE
SEYMOUR J. PHILLIPS HEALTH SCIENCES LIBRARY
1st Ave. at 16th St.
New York, NY 10003   Phone: (212) 420-2855
Ellen H. Poisson, Dir., Lib.Serv.
Subjects: Medicine, nursing, allied health sciences, social work, orthopedics, substance abuse. **Holdings:** 14,000 books; 16,000 bound periodical volumes. **Subscriptions:** 670 journals and other serials.

★9150★ CABRINI MEDICAL CENTER
DR. MASSIMO BAZZINI MEMORIAL LIBRARY
227 E. 19th St.
New York, NY 10003   Phone: (212) 995-6630
Judith M. Topper, Med.Libn.
Subjects: Medicine, surgery, nursing. **Holdings:** 2650 books; 3300 bound periodical volumes; 350 AV programs. **Subscriptions:** 290 journals and other serials.

★9151★ CENTER FOR MEDICAL CONSUMERS AND HEALTH INFORMATION
CONSUMER'S MEDICAL LIBRARY
237 Thompson St.
New York, NY 10012   Phone: (212) 674-7105
Arthur Levin, Dir.
Subjects: Medicine, health, nutrition. **Holdings:** 1500 books; subject files. **Subscriptions:** 58 journals and other serials.

★9152★ CENTER FOR MODERN PSYCHOANALYTIC STUDIES
LIBRARY
16 W. 10th St.
New York, NY 10011   Phone: (212) 260-7050
Cyril Z. Meadow, Dir.
Subjects: Psychoanalysis, psychology, psychiatry, sociology, anthropology. **Holdings:** 5000 books; 300 lecture tapes. **Subscriptions:** 16 journals and other serials.

★9153★ CLINICAL RESEARCH ASSOCIATES
LIBRARY
50 Madison Ave.
New York, NY 10010   Phone: (212) 685-8788
Carol Dorsey, Libn.
Subjects: Chemistry, pharmacology. **Holdings:** 15,000 books. **Subscriptions:** 25 journals and other serials.

★9154★ COLUMBIA UNIVERSITY
AUGUSTUS C. LONG HEALTH SCIENCES LIBRARY
701 W. 168th St.
New York, NY 10032   Phone: (212) 305-3692
Rachael K. Anderson, Libn.
Subjects: Anatomy; biochemistry; clinical medicine; dentistry; medical history and practice; microbiology; neurology; nursing; oncology; pathology; pharmacology; physiology; public health; surgery - general, orthopedic, plastic; thanatology. **Holdings:** 445,000 volumes; 2562 AV programs. **Subscriptions:** 4414 journals and other serials.

★9155★ COLUMBIA UNIVERSITY
BIOLOGICAL SCIENCES LIBRARY
601 Fairchild Bldg.
New York, NY 10027   Phone: (212) 854-4715
Kathleen Kehoe, Ref./Coll.Dev.Libn.
Subjects: Experimental zoology, neurosciences, genetics, molecular biolo-

gy, cytology, histology, animal and plant physiology, biochemistry, cell biology. **Holdings:** 46,000 volumes. **Subscriptions:** 330 journals and other serials.

★9156★ COLUMBIA UNIVERSITY
CENTER FOR POPULATION AND FAMILY HEALTH
LIBRARY/INFORMATION PROGRAM
60 Haven Ave.
New York, NY 10032   Phone: (212) 305-6960
Susan K. Pasquariella, Ph.D, Hd.Libn.
Subjects: Family planning, evaluative methodology, operations research, demography. **Holdings:** 7000 books; 30,000 published and unpublished reports, manuscripts, reprints, documents. **Subscriptions:** 200 journals and other serials.

★9157★ COLUMBIA UNIVERSITY
COMPREHENSIVE CANCER CENTER
LIBRARY
701 W. 168th St.
New York, NY 10032   Phone: (212) 305-6948
Betty Rose Moore, Lib.Serv.Coord.
Subjects: Cancer.

★9158★ COLUMBIA UNIVERSITY
WHITNEY M. YOUNG, JR. MEMORIAL LIBRARY OF SOCIAL
WORK
309 International Affairs Bldg.
New York, NY 10027   Phone: (212) 854-5159
Laura Delaney
Subjects: Social work; community organization; social policy development and administration; health, mental health, mental retardation; social services - family and children, homemaker, day care, legal; aging; corrections and court services - probation, parole, diversionary treatment; alcoholism and drug addiction; industrial social welfare and manpower programs; urban education; intergroup relations; social and physical rehabilitation. **Holdings:** 130,000 volumes; student projects; dissertations; agency reports. **Subscriptions:** 646 journals and other serials.

★9159★ CORNELL UNIVERSITY
MEDICAL COLLEGE
SAMUEL J. WOOD LIBRARY
C.V. STARR BIOMEDICAL INFORMATION CENTER
1300 York Ave.
New York, NY 10021   Phone: (212) 746-6050
Robert M. Braude, Ph.D., Dir.
Subjects: Medicine, nursing. **Holdings:** 51,015 books; 93,186 bound periodical volumes; 5119 microfiche; 470 audio recordings; 394 video cassettes; 37 reels of microfilm; 27,472 iconographic images, photographs, and prints. **Subscriptions:** 1684 journals and other serials.

★9160★ DEFENSE FOR CHILDREN INTERNATIONAL,
UNITED STATES OF AMERICA
LIBRARY
210 Forsyth St.
New York, NY 10002   Phone: (212) 353-0951
Subjects: Child maltreatment and abuse, children's rights legislation, children and war, refugees, juvenile justice. **Holdings:** 1000 volumes; statistical materials.

★9161★ EDWARD S. HARKNESS EYE INSTITUTE
JOHN M. WHEELER LIBRARY
635 W. 165th St.
New York, NY 10032   Phone: (212) 305-2916
Ilse B. Philleo, Dir.
Subjects: Ophthalmology. **Holdings:** 13,628 books; 4641 bound periodical volumes; 4250 reprints; 485 audiotapes. **Subscriptions:** 93 journals and other serials.

★9162★ EMPIRE BLUE CROSS BLUE SHIELD
ARCHIVES AND CORPORATE LIBRARY
3 Park Ave., Mezzanine
New York, NY 10016   Phone: (212) 251-2385
Christopher Moir, Dir.
Subjects: Health insurance, medical economics, health industry. **Holdings:** 5000 books; 15 bound periodical volumes; 2282 reels of microfilm; corporate archives. **Subscriptions:** 300 journals and other serials; 15 newspapers.

★9163★ FORDHAM UNIVERSITY
LIBRARY AT LINCOLN CENTER
W. 60th St. and Columbus Ave.
New York, NY 10023   Phone: (212) 841-5130
Clement J. Anzul, Libn.
Subjects: Education, educational testing and measurement, educational psychology, guidance, mental health, business, liberal arts, social work and casework, community organization, government and social welfare, delinquency and crime. **Holdings:** 340,349 volumes; Alcohol Abstracts; ERIC microfiche. **Subscriptions:** 1500 journals and other serials.

★9164★ HARLEM HOSPITAL MEDICAL CENTER
HEALTH SCIENCES LIBRARY
506 Lenox Ave., KP 6108
New York, NY 10037   Phone: (212) 491-8264
Vernon Bruette, Chf.Libn.
Subjects: Medicine, dentistry, nursing, allied health sciences. **Holdings:** 3500 books; 9000 bound periodical volumes. **Subscriptions:** 400 journals and other serials.

★9165★ HOME LIFE INSURANCE COMPANY
LIBRARY
75 Wall St.
New York, NY 10005   Phone: (212) 428-2142
Jennie Del Vecchio, Libn.
Subjects: Life insurance, health insurance, tax, securities. **Holdings:** 1350 volumes; 58 VF drawers of unbound materials. **Subscriptions:** 130 journals and other serials.

★9166★ HOSPITAL FOR SPECIAL SURGERY
KIM BARRETT MEMORIAL LIBRARY
535 E. 70th St., Rm. 212
New York, NY 10021   Phone: (212) 606-1210
Marshall J. Giannotti, Med.Libn.
Subjects: Orthopedic surgery and rheumatic diseases. **Holdings:** 3117 books; 2918 bound periodical volumes; 2924 reprints; 335 video cassettes, slide programs, films. **Subscriptions:** 94 journals and other serials.

★9167★ THE HUNGER PROJECT
LIBRARY
1 Madison Ave., 8A
New York, NY 10010   Phone: (212) 532-4255
Subjects: Hunger, starvation, elimination of both. **Holdings:** 1200 volumes.

★9168★ HUNTER COLLEGE OF THE CITY UNIVERSITY OF
NEW YORK
HEALTH PROFESSIONS LIBRARY
425 E. 25th St.
New York, NY 10010   Phone: (212) 481-5117
Barbara Charton, Assoc.Prof.
Subjects: Nursing, medicine, speech and hearing pathology, physical therapy, dance therapy, medical laboratory sciences, environmental health sciences, allied health services administration, community health education, nutrition, occupational health. **Holdings:** 20,000 books; 6200 bound periodical volumes; 1500 federal and state environmental reports on microfiche. **Subscriptions:** 400 journals and other serials.

★9169★ HUNTER COLLEGE OF THE CITY UNIVERSITY OF
NEW YORK
HUNTER COLLEGE SCHOOL OF SOCIAL WORK
LIBRARY
129 E. 79th St.
New York, NY 10021   Phone: (212) 452-7076
Tom Jennings, Hd.Libn.
Subjects: Social work, psychology, sociology, public administration, urban affairs, ethnology, education, law, health. **Holdings:** 25,000 books; 6000 bound periodical volumes; 480 volumes of masters' theses; 60 dissertations; 13 VF drawers; 2214 reels of microfilm; 1100 microfiche. **Subscriptions:** 276 journals and other serials.

★9170★ INSTITUTE FOR RESEARCH IN HYPNOSIS
BERNARD B. RAGINSKY RESEARCH LIBRARY
1991 Broadway, Suite 18B
New York, NY 10023   Phone: (212) 874-5290
Dr. Milton V. Kline, Dir.
Subjects: Clinical and experimental applications of hypnosis, hypnoanalysis, and hypnotherapy. **Holdings:** 1000 books; 2000 reprints; 500 tapes. **Subscriptions:** 15 journals and other serials; 3 newspapers.

★9171★ INSTITUTES OF RELIGION AND HEALTH
LIBRARY
3 W. 29th St.
New York, NY 10001   Phone: (212) 725-7850
Rob S. Coleman
Subjects: Psychiatry, psychology, pastoral counseling, marriage counseling, psychotherapy. **Holdings:** 5000 books; 4 VF drawers of reports, pamphlets, dissertations. **Subscriptions:** 23 journals and other serials.

★9172★ INTERNATIONAL CENTER FOR THE DISABLED
BRUCE BARTON MEMORIAL LIBRARY
340 E. 24th St.
New York, NY 10010   Phone: (212) 679-0100
Helen Stonehill, Dir., Lib./Info.Ctr.
Subjects: Rehabilitation, physical medicine, vocational training, psychology, psychiatry, psychopharmacology, job placement, speech and hearing, gerontology, chemical dependency. **Holdings:** 6000 books; 2000 bound periodical volumes; 78 VF drawers; 50 boxes of occupational materials; 4000 research reports on microfiche. **Subscriptions:** 150 journals and other serials.

★9173★ INTERNATIONAL PLANNED PARENTHOOD
FEDERATION
WESTERN HEMISPHERE REGION, INC.
LIBRARY
902 Broadway, 10th Fl.
New York, NY 10010   Phone: (212) 995-8800
Abigail Hourwich, Libn.
Subjects: Family planning, population, demography, maternal-child health. **Holdings:** 5000 books; AV programs. **Subscriptions:** 200 journals and other serials.

★9174★ INTERNATIONAL SOCIETY FOR REHABILITATION
OF THE DISABLED REHABILITATION INTERNATIONAL
LIBRARY
25 E. 21st St.
New York, NY 10010   Phone: (212) 420-1500
Barbara Duncan, Dir. of Info.
Subjects: International aspects of disability. **Holdings:** 2500 books; 5000 documents.

★9175★ JEWISH BOARD OF FAMILY AND CHILDREN
SERVICES
MARY AND LOUIS ROBINSON LIBRARY
120 W. 57th St.
New York, NY 10019   Phone: (212) 582-9100
Sue Weiland, Libn.
Subjects: Child and adolescent psychology and psychiatry, social work, family therapy, psychoanalysis, psychiatry. **Holdings:** 5000 books; 2000 bound periodical volumes; 8 VF drawers of manuscripts and dissertations. **Subscriptions:** 50 journals and other serials.

★9176★ JEWISH GUILD FOR THE BLIND
JGB CASSETTE LIBRARY INTERNATIONAL
15 W. 65th St.
New York, NY 10023   Phone: (212) 769-6331
Bruce E. Massis, Dir.
Subjects: Fiction, nonfiction, poetry. **Holdings:** 64,000 cassettes containing 1200 titles; periodicals.

★9177★ LENOX HILL HOSPITAL
JEROME S. LEOPOLD HEALTH SCIENCES LIBRARY
100 E. 77th St.
New York, NY 10021   Phone: (212) 439-2075
Shirley E. Dansker, Dir.
Subjects: Medicine and medical specialties, surgery, nursing, history of medicine. **Holdings:** 4500 books; 10,000 bound periodical volumes. **Subscriptions:** 380 journals and other serials.

★9178★ LEUKEMIA SOCIETY OF AMERICA
LIBRARY
733 3rd Ave.
New York, NY 10017   Phone: (212) 573-8484
Mariana Jordan, Pub.Info.Spec.
Subjects: Leukemia, lymphomas, multiple myeloma, Hodgkin's Disease, psychosocial aspects of leukemia and allied diseases, cancer. **Holdings:** 300 books; 3 drawers of clippings, unbound reports, resource organization materials. **Subscriptions:** 20 journals and other serials.

★9179★ MARGARET SANGER CENTER
PLANNED PARENTHOOD NEW YORK CITY
ABRAHAM STONE LIBRARY
380 Second Ave.
New York, NY 10010   Phone: (212) 677-6474
Subjects: Abortion, adolescent sexuality, infertility, sex, family living, demography, population, sexuality of the handicapped, women's health. **Holdings:** 6000 books; 3000 bound periodical volumes; 60 VF drawers of reprints and newspaper clippings. **Subscriptions:** 85 journals and other serials.

★9180★ MATERNITY CENTER ASSOCIATION
REFERENCE LIBRARY
48 E. 92nd St.
New York, NY 10028   Phone: (212) 369-7300
Esther Hanchett, Act.Libn.
Subjects: Obstetrics, maternal and infant care, family life, nurse-midwifery, preparation for child-bearing. **Holdings:** 2300 books. **Subscriptions:** 31 journals and other serials.

★9181★ MCADAMS, WILLIAM DOUGLAS, INC.
MEDICAL LIBRARY
425 W. 59th St.
New York, NY 10019   Phone: (212) 698-4011
Molly Garfin, Mgr.
Subjects: Medicine, pharmacology, biological sciences, drugs and therapeutics, advertising. **Holdings:** 1500 books; 10,000 bound periodicals; 50 VF drawers. **Subscriptions:** 500 journals and other serials.

★9182★ MEDICAL LIBRARY CENTER OF NEW YORK
5 E. 102nd St., 7th Fl.
New York, NY 10029   Phone: (212) 427-1630
Lois Weinstein, Dir.
Subjects: Medicine, allied health sciences, nursing, dentistry. **Holdings:** 102,000 bound periodical volumes; 160,156 unbound periodical issues; 150,000 dissertations; 11,000 government documents.

★9183★ MEMORIAL SLOAN-KETTERING CANCER CENTER
MEDICAL LIBRARY
NATHAN CUMMINGS CENTER
1275 York Ave.
New York, NY 10021   Phone: (212) 639-7439
Jeanne Becker, Dir.
Subjects: Cancer and allied diseases. **Holdings:** 11,624 books; 18,866 bound periodical volumes; 18 drawers of microforms. **Subscriptions:** 927 journals and other serials.

★9184★ METROPOLITAN HOSPITAL CENTER
DRAPER HALL LIBRARY
1901 1st Ave.
New York, NY 10029   Phone: (212) 230-6262
Walter Krivickas, Libn.
Subjects: Nursing, medicine. **Holdings:** 2050 books; 300 bound periodical volumes; 10 VF drawers of pamphlets; 103 envelopes of clippings.

★9185★ METROPOLITAN HOSPITAL CENTER
FREDERICK M. DEARBORN MEDICAL LIBRARY
1901 1st. Ave.
New York, NY 10029   Phone: (212) 230-6270
Vivienne Whitson, Chf.Libn.
Subjects: Medicine, allied health sciences. **Holdings:** 5340 books; 15,215 bound periodical volumes; 470 pamphlets; 1540 Audio-Digest tapes. **Subscriptions:** 412 journals and other serials.

★9186★ METROPOLITAN HOSPITAL CENTER
PSYCHIATRY LIBRARY
1901 1st Ave., Rm. 10M13
New York, NY 10029   Phone: (212) 230-7285
Lorna Macdonald, Libn.
Subjects: Psychiatry, psychoanalysis. **Holdings:** 7500 volumes; 3 VF drawers of reprints; 21 films. **Subscriptions:** 40 journals and other serials.

★9187★ METROPOLITAN LIFE INSURANCE COMPANY
CORPORATE INFORMATION CENTER AND LIBRARY
1 Madison Ave., 1 M-R
New York, NY 10010   Phone: (212) 578-3700
Rosemary Stevens, Mng.Libn.
Subjects: Insurance, management, medicine and medical economics.
Holdings: 88,000 volumes. **Subscriptions:** 500 journals and other serials.

★9188★ MOUNT SINAI SCHOOL OF MEDICINE OF THE
CITY UNIVERSITY OF NEW YORK
GUSTAVE L. AND JANET W. LEVY LIBRARY
1 Gustave L. Levy Pl., Box 1102
New York, NY 10029-6574   Phone: (212) 241-7793
Lynn Kasner Morgan, Dir.
Subjects: Clinical medicine, nursing, basic sciences. **Holdings:** 47,023
books; 103,739 bound periodical volumes; 2550 AV programs; 574 lateral
files of archival materials. **Subscriptions:** 2907 journals and other serials.

★9189★ MURIEL IVIMEY LIBRARY
329 E. 62nd St.
New York, NY 10021   Phone: (212) 838-8044
Frederick Burnett, CSW, Chm., Lib.Comm.
Subjects: Psychoanalysis. **Holdings:** 4000 books; 500 bound periodical
volumes. **Subscriptions:** 35 journals and other serials.

★9190★ MUTUAL LIFE INSURANCE COMPANY OF NEW
YORK
LAW LIBRARY
1740 Broadway
New York, NY 10019   Phone: (212) 708-2235
Marie Papandrea, Law Libn.
Subjects: Life insurance, accident and health insurance, pensions, law.
Holdings: 26,000 volumes. **Subscriptions:** 40 journals and other serials.

★9191★ NARCOTIC AND DRUG RESEARCH INC.
RESOURCE CENTER
11 Beach St., 2nd Fl.
New York, NY 10013-2429   Phone: (212) 966-8700
Betty Gee, Rsrc.Ctr.Coord.
Subjects: Drug abuse, addiction treatment, pharmacology, counseling,
training, AIDS. **Holdings:** 1500 books; 8000 VF materials; 150 computer
searches. **Subscriptions:** 75 journals and other serials.

★9192★ NATIONAL ASSOCIATION FOR VISUALLY
HANDICAPPED
LIBRARY
22 W. 21st St.
New York, NY 10010   Phone: (212) 889-3141
Ann Illuzi
Subjects: General collection for the visually impaired. **Holdings:** 1200
large-print books.

★9193★ NATIONAL CENTER ON WOMEN AND FAMILY LAW
INFORMATION CENTER
799 Broadway, Rm. 402
New York, NY 10003   Phone: (212) 674-8200
Laurie Woods, Dir.
Subjects: Battered women and law, marital rape, rape, single mothers,
divorce, custody, child snatching, child and wife support. **Holdings:** 500
books; 50 VF drawers; 100 resource packets. **Subscriptions:** 1500 newspapers.

★9194★ NATIONAL MULTIPLE SCLEROSIS SOCIETY
INFORMATION RESOURCE CENTER AND LIBRARY
205 E. 42nd St., 3rd Fl.
New York, NY 10017   Phone: (212) 986-3240
Margaret Calvano, Dir., Info. & Prof.Educ.
Subjects: Medical research; medical, psychosocial, socioeconomic aspects
of multiple sclerosis. **Holdings:** 700 books; 12,000 indexed reprints; client
service materials; professional and lay pamphlets. **Subscriptions:** 120
journals and other serials.

★9195★ NATIONAL PSYCHOLOGICAL ASSOCIATION FOR
PSYCHOANALYSIS
GEORGE LAWTON MEMORIAL LIBRARY
150 W. 13th St.
New York, NY 10011   Phone: (212) 924-7440
Subjects: Psychoanalysis, psychology. **Holdings:** 2000 volumes. **Subscriptions:** 25 journals and other serials.

★9196★ NEUROSCIENCES INSTITUTE OF THE
NEUROSCIENCES RESEARCH PROGRAM
LIBRARY
Smith Hall Annex
Rockefeller University
1230 York Ave.
New York, NY 10021-6399   Phone: (212) 570-8975
Stephanie Greggerman, Bibliog.
Subjects: Neurosciences, brain sciences, neurobiology. **Holdings:** 3000
books. **Subscriptions:** 50 journals and other serials.

★9197★ NEW YORK ACADEMY OF MEDICINE
LIBRARY
2 E. 103rd St.
New York, NY 10029   Phone: (212) 876-8200
Arthur Downing, Act.Libn.
Subjects: Medicine, allied health sciences, health statistics. **Holdings:**
507,000 bound volumes; 182,928 pamphlets; 141 incunabula; 2227
manuscripts; 494 reels of microfilm; 250,245 portraits; 25,543 illustrations; 14,429 separate portraits. **Subscriptions:** 4197 journals and other
serials.

★9198★ NEW YORK ASSOCIATION FOR THE BLIND
LIGHTHOUSE LIBRARY
111 E. 59th St.
New York, NY 10022   Phone: (212) 355-2200
Subjects: Blindness and visual impairment, handicaps. **Holdings:** 2000
books; 2000 volumes in braille; 400 large print books; 1700 talking books
on disc and cassette; 8 VF drawers. **Subscriptions:** 110 journals and other
serials.

★9199★ NEW YORK CITY HEALTH AND HOSPITALS
CORPORATION
COLER MEMORIAL HOSPITAL
MEDICAL LIBRARY
Roosevelt Island
New York, NY 10044   Phone: (212) 848-6071
Rosemary Ellis, Asst.Libn.
Subjects: Medical sciences, rehabilitation medicine, psychiatry, geriatrics
and gerontology, nursing, audiology and speech. **Holdings:** 1500 volumes;
Audio-Digest tapes; Network for Continuing Medical Education videotapes. **Subscriptions:** 112 journals and other serials.

★9200★ NEW YORK CITY HUMAN RESOURCES
ADMINISTRATION
MEDICAL ASSISTANCE PROGRAM
MAP LIBRARY
11-17 Beach St., 6th Fl. N.W.
New York, NY 10013   Phone: (212) 941-5134
Barry L. Cohen, MAP Libn.
Subjects: Medicaid, long-term care, health care management, HMOs
(Health Maintenance Organizations), social services, Medicare. **Holdings:**
200 books; 225 binders; VF drawers of reports, studies, documents,
pamphlets, and clippings. **Subscriptions:** 3 journals and other serials; 15
newsletters.

★9201★ NEW YORK CITY OFFICE OF CHIEF MEDICAL
EXAMINER
MILTON HELPERN LIBRARY OF LEGAL MEDICINE
520 First Ave.
New York, NY 10016   Phone: (212) 340-0102
Malvin Vitriol, Med.Libn.
Subjects: Legal medicine, forensic pathology, forensic toxicology, forensic
serology, criminology, forensic immunology. **Holdings:** 4500 books; 928
bound periodical volumes; 480 microfiche; 58 reels of microfilm; 16 VF
drawers; 136 tapes; vertical files. **Subscriptions:** 41 journals and other
serials.

★9202★ NEW YORK CITY PUBLIC HEALTH LABORATORIES
WILLIAM HALLOCK PARK MEMORIAL LIBRARY
455 1st Ave.
New York, NY 10016   Phone: (212) 340-4700
Shirley Chapin, Libn.
Subjects: Virology, applied immunology, biochemistry, bacteriology, genetics, laboratory diagnosis, microbiology, cytobiology, toxicology. **Holdings:** 28,000 books and bound periodical volumes; microcards; 5 VF drawers of archival materials. **Subscriptions:** 265 journals and other serials.

★9203★ NEW YORK COLLEGE OF PODIATRIC MEDICINE
MEDICAL LIBRARY
53-55 E. 124th St., 2nd Fl.
New York, NY 10035   Phone: (212) 410-8020
Bernice Kornegay, Act.Lib.Dir.
Subjects: Podiatry, medicine, orthopedics, physical medicine, basic sciences. **Holdings:** 10,000 volumes; reprints of journal articles; slides; audiotapes; video cassettes; microfilm; pamphlets. **Subscriptions:** 300 journals and other serials.

★9204★ NEW YORK EYE AND EAR INFIRMARY
BERNARD SAMUELS LIBRARY
310 E. 14th St.
New York, NY 10003   Phone: (212) 979-4431
Carolyn Stafford, Dir.
Subjects: Ophthalmology, otolaryngology, plastic surgery. **Holdings:** 1300 books; 1300 bound periodical volumes; pamphlets. **Subscriptions:** 52 journals and other serials.

★9205★ NEW YORK HOSPITAL-CORNELL MEDICAL CENTER
MEDICAL ARCHIVES
1300 York Ave.
New York, NY 10021   Phone: (212) 746-6072
Adele A. Lerner, Archv.
Subjects: Medical education; health care; history - medicine, nursing, psychiatry; women's history. **Holdings:** 4600 linear feet of archival materials and manuscripts; 217 films; 22 videotapes; 844 audiotapes and cassettes. **Subscriptions:** 8 journals and other serials (for archival reference).

★9206★ NEW YORK HOSPITAL-CORNELL MEDICAL CENTER
OSKAR DIETHELM HISTORICAL LIBRARY
525 E. 68th St.
New York, NY 10021   Phone: (212) 472-6434
Subjects: History of psychiatry, philosophy, psychology. **Holdings:** 17,000 books; 3850 bound periodical volumes; 673 philosophy and psychology materials; 254 cubic feet of archival materials and manuscripts; 123 reels of microfilm. **Subscriptions:** 55 journals and other serials.

★9207★ NEW YORK INFIRMARY BEEKMAN DOWNTOWN
HOSPITAL
ELISHA WALKER STAFF LIBRARY
170 William St.
New York, NY 10038   Phone: (212) 312-5229
Annette Leyden, Dir.
Subjects: Medicine, surgery, nursing. **Holdings:** 4500 volumes; 105 bound journals; reprints; catalogs; reports. **Subscriptions:** 125 journals and other serials.

★9208★ NEW YORK PSYCHOANALYTIC INSTITUTE
ABRAHAM A. BRILL LIBRARY
247 E. 82nd St.
New York, NY 10028   Phone: (212) 879-6900
Maria Astifidis, Libn.
Subjects: Psychoanalysis, psychiatry. **Holdings:** 50,000 volumes. **Subscriptions:** 35 journals and other serials.

★9209★ NEW YORK PUBLIC LIBRARY
ARENTS TOBACCO COLLECTION
Fifth Ave. & 42nd St., Rm. 324
New York, NY 10018   Phone: (212) 930-0801
Subjects: Tobacco, herbals, history, medicine, law. **Holdings:** 13,000 books and manuscripts; 150,000 cards and pieces of ephemera.

★9210★ NEW YORK PUBLIC LIBRARY
EARLY CHILDHOOD RESOURCE AND INFORMATION
CENTER
66 Leroy St., 2nd Fl.
New York, NY 10014   Phone: (212) 929-0815
Hannah Nuba, Supv.Libn.
Subjects: Early childhood and parent education, prenatal care, parent-child activities, language and intellectual development, multicultural and multilingual education, adoption and foster care. **Holdings:** 14,198 books; 72 noncirculating filmstrip kits; 52 noncirculating films; 345 sound recordings; 114 video cassettes; toys; pamphlets. **Subscriptions:** 125 journals and other serials.

★9211★ NEW YORK PUBLIC LIBRARY
MID-MANHATTAN LIBRARY
PROJECT ACCESS
455 Fifth Ave.
New York, NY 10016   Phone: (212) 340-0843
Lois O'Neill, Sr.Libn.
Subjects: The disabled - blind, deaf, learning and mobility impaired. **Holdings:** 200 books; 10 VF drawers of pamphlet material concerning the disabled.

★9212★ NEW YORK PUBLIC LIBRARY
REGIONAL LIBRARY FOR THE BLIND AND PHYSICALLY
HANDICAPPED
166 Ave. of the Americas
New York, NY 10013   Phone: (212) 925-1011
Barbara Nugent, Reg.Br.Libn.
Holdings: 14,523 braille books; 440,908 recorded books.

★9213★ NEW YORK STATE PSYCHIATRIC INSTITUTE
RESEARCH LIBRARY
722 W. 168th St.
New York, NY 10032   Phone: (212) 960-5670
David Lane, Lib.Dir.
Subjects: Psychiatry, neurology, psychology, neuropathology. **Holdings:** 20,000 books; 21,000 bound periodical volumes; 300 dissertations and theses; 500 dissertations on microfilm; 1000 microfiche reports and journal volumes. **Subscriptions:** 600 journals and other serials.

★9214★ NEW YORK UNIVERSITY
DAVID B. KRISER DENTAL CENTER
JOHN AND BERTHA E. WALDMANN MEMORIAL LIBRARY
345 E. 24th St.
New York, NY 10010   Phone: (212) 998-9794
Roy C. Johnson, Libn.
Subjects: Dentistry, allied health sciences. **Holdings:** 12,000 books; 22,000 bound periodical volumes; 88 volumes of masters' theses; 4 VF drawers of archival materials. **Subscriptions:** 449 journals and other serials.

★9215★ NEW YORK UNIVERSITY MEDICAL CENTER
FREDERICK L. EHRMAN MEDICAL LIBRARY
550 1st Ave.
New York, NY 10016   Phone: (212) 340-5393
Karen Brewer, Lib.Dir.
Subjects: Medicine, allied health sciences. **Holdings:** 162,000 volumes. **Subscriptions:** 2019 journals and other serials.

★9216★ NEW YORK UNIVERSITY MEDICAL CENTER
GOLDWATER MEMORIAL HOSPITAL
HEALTH SCIENCES LIBRARY
Franklin D. Roosevelt Island
New York, NY 10044   Phone: (212) 750-6749
Martin M. Leibovici, Lib.Dir.
Subjects: General medicine, rehabilitation medicine, geriatrics, chronic disease. **Holdings:** 3800 books; 6000 bound periodical volumes; 850 AV programs; 4 VF drawers. **Subscriptions:** 342 journals and other serials.

★9217★ NORTH GENERAL HOSPITAL
MEDICAL LIBRARY
1919 Madison Ave.
New York, NY 10035   Phone: (212) 650-4475
Robert Feinstein, Hd.Libn.
Subjects: Medicine. **Holdings:** 2500 books; 5400 bound periodical volumes; 3 VF drawers of clippings. **Subscriptions:** 125 journals and other serials.

**★9218★ PANNELL KERR FORSTER
LIBRARY**
420 Lexington Ave.
New York, NY 10170   Phone: (212) 867-8000
Leslie Slocum, Libn.
Subjects: Research on hospitality, tourism, health care, accounting, auditing, real estate. **Holdings:** 2000 volumes; pamphlets; clippings. **Subscriptions:** 300 journals and other serials.

★9219★ PAYNE WHITNEY PSYCHIATRIC CLINIC LIBRARY
New York Hospital-Cornell University Medical College
525 E. 68th St.
New York, NY 10021   Phone: (212) 746-3795
Patricia Tomasulo, Dept.Libn.
Subjects: Psychiatry, psychology, behavioral sciences. **Holdings:** 21,000 volumes; 125 video cassettes; 50 audio cassettes. **Subscriptions:** 140 journals and other serials.

**★9220★ PFIZER, INC.
N.Y.O. LIBRARY**
235 E. 42nd St.
New York, NY 10017   Phone: (212) 573-2966
Veronica Plucinski, Mgr., Lib.Serv.
Subjects: Pharmaceuticals, pharmacology, clinical medicine. **Holdings:** 15,000 volumes; 1500 reels of microfilm. **Subscriptions:** 630 journals and other serials.

**★9221★ PLANNED PARENTHOOD FEDERATION OF
AMERICA
KATHARINE DEXTER MCCORMICK LIBRARY**
810 7th Ave.
New York, NY 10019   Phone: (212) 541-7800
Gloria A. Roberts, Hd.Libn.
Subjects: Family planning in the U.S., contraceptives, abortion and sterilization, history of birth control, population, sexuality, sexuality education, reproductive rights, teen sexuality. **Holdings:** 4000 books; 35 VF drawers of journal articles, reprints, unpublished mimeographs. **Subscriptions:** 125 journals and other serials.

**★9222★ POPULATION COUNCIL
LIBRARY**
1 Dag Hammarskjold Plaza
New York, NY 10017   Phone: (212) 644-1620
Hue Neil Zimmerman, Libn.
Subjects: Population; demography; family planning; contraception; statistics; public health; development - economic, social, agricultural. **Holdings:** 20,000 books; 6,000 pamphlets, mimeographs, reprints, other cataloged items. **Subscriptions:** 350 journals and other serials.

**★9223★ POSTGRADUATE CENTER FOR MENTAL HEALTH
EMIL AND LILLY GUTHEIL MEMORIAL LIBRARY**
124 E. 28th St.
New York, NY 10016   Phone: (212) 689-7700
Leona Mackler, Dir.
Subjects: Psychiatry, psychology, psychoanalysis, psychotherapy, clinical social work, pastoral counseling. **Holdings:** 10,000 books; 150 bound periodical volumes; 7000 unbound journals; 2 VF cabinets of pamphlets. **Subscriptions:** 100 journals and other serials.

**★9224★ ROCKEFELLER UNIVERSITY
LIBRARY**
1230 York Ave.
RU Box 263
New York, NY 10021-6399   Phone: (212) 570-8914
Patricia E. Mackey, Libn.
Subjects: Biological sciences, medicine, chemistry, physics, mathematics. **Holdings:** 238,000 volumes. **Subscriptions:** 2470 journals and other serials.

**★9225★ ROOSEVELT HOSPITAL
MEDICAL LIBRARY**
428 W. 59th St.
New York, NY 10019   Phone: (212) 523-6100
Paul E. Barth, Libn.
Subjects: Medicine, surgery, gerontology, geriatrics, hospital administration, pediatrics, anesthesia. **Holdings:** 20,000 books and bound periodical volumes. **Subscriptions:** 500 journals and other serials.

**★9226★ ST. CLARE'S HOSPITAL AND HEALTH CENTER
MEDICAL LIBRARY**
415 W. 51st St.
New York, NY 10019   Phone: (212) 459-8221
Mitchell A. Bogen, Med.Libn.
Subjects: Medicine, surgery. **Holdings:** 1500 books; 6000 bound periodical volumes; tapes. **Subscriptions:** 81 journals and other serials.

**★9227★ ST. LUKE'S HOSPITAL CENTER
RICHARD WALKER BOLLING MEMORIAL MEDICAL LIBRARY**
Amsterdam Ave. & 114th St.
New York, NY 10025   Phone: (212) 523-4315
Nancy Mary Panella, Libn. & Dir.
Subjects: Medicine, surgery. **Holdings:** 10,000 books; 42,000 bound periodical volumes; 4 VF drawers. **Subscriptions:** 475 journals and other serials.

**★9228★ ST. VINCENT'S HOSPITAL
SCHOOL OF NURSING LIBRARY**
27 Christopher St.
New York, NY 10014   Phone: (212) 790-8486
Clare E. Higgins, Libn.
Subjects: Nursing and allied professional sciences, social sciences, medicine, religion, humanities. **Holdings:** 3000 books; 225 bound periodical volumes; 8 VF drawers of pamphlets; 825 AV programs. **Subscriptions:** 65 journals and other serials.

**★9229★ ST. VINCENT'S HOSPITAL AND MEDICAL CENTER
OF NEW YORK
MEDICAL LIBRARY**
153 W. 11th St.
New York, NY 10011   Phone: (212) 790-7811
Agnes T. Frank, Dir.
Subjects: Health sciences, psychology. **Holdings:** 8805 volumes. **Subscriptions:** 276 journals and other serials.

**★9230★ SEX INFORMATION AND EDUCATION COUNCIL OF
THE U.S.
MARY S. CALDERONE LIBRARY**
130 W. 42nd St., Ste. 2500
New York, NY 10036   Phone: (212) 819-9770
Daniel M. Donohue
Subjects: Sex education, behavior, and research; human sexuality; family life education. **Holdings:** 4000 books; 200 curriculum items; 15 VF drawers; 750 pamphlets and booklets; 350 curricula. **Subscriptions:** 100 journals and other serials.

**★9231★ STERLING DRUG, INC.
CORPORATE MEDICAL LIBRARY**
90 Park Ave.
New York, NY 10016   Phone: (212) 907-2504
Lynn Siegelman, Lib.Mgr.
Subjects: Pharmaceuticals, clinical medicine. **Holdings:** 3000 books and bound periodical volumes. **Subscriptions:** 260 journals and other serials.

**★9232★ SUNY
COLLEGE OF OPTOMETRY
HAROLD KOHN MEMORIAL VISUAL SCIENCE LIBRARY**
100 E. 24th St.
New York, NY 10010-3677   Phone: (212) 420-5086
Claudia Perry, Libn.
Subjects: Physiological optics, perception, developmental psychology, theory of optometry, public health, learning disabilities, ocular pathology, orthoptics. **Holdings:** 23,000 books; 7000 bound periodical volumes; 2000 tapes; 90 phonograph records; 30,000 slides; 400 reels of microfilm; 7000 pamphlets; 1200 indexed reprints on optics. **Subscriptions:** 540 journals and other serials.

**★9233★ TEACHERS COLLEGE
MILBANK MEMORIAL LIBRARY**
Columbia University
DB, Box 307
New York, NY 10027   Phone: (212) 678-3494
Jane P. Franck, Dir.
Subjects: Education, psychology, health sciences, nutrition, nursing, communications, computing, technology, speech and language pathology, audiology. **Holdings:** 522,053 monograph and serial volumes; 405,968 microforms; 14,898 nonprint materials; 4025 cubic feet of manuscript

material; 79,300 photographs; 9019 titles in microform; 910 software programs. **Subscriptions:** 2529 journals and other serials.

★9234★ UNITED CEREBRAL PALSY OF NEW YORK CITY LIBRARY
120 E. 23rd St.
New York, NY 10010   Phone: (212) 979-9700
Richard Gordon, Lib.Adm.
Subjects: Cerebral palsy and allied subjects. **Holdings:** 524 books; 19 bound periodical volumes. **Subscriptions:** 13 journals and other serials; 5 newspapers.

★9235★ UNITED CEREBRAL PALSY RESEARCH AND EDUCATIONAL FOUNDATION LIBRARY
7 Penn Plaza, Ste. 804
New York, NY 10001   Phone: (212) 268-5962
Subjects: Cerebral palsy.

★9236★ UNITED HOSPITAL FUND OF NEW YORK REFERENCE LIBRARY
55 5th Ave., 16th Fl.
New York, NY 10003   Phone: (212) 645-2500
Rochelle Yates, Libn.
Subjects: Hospital management, health services research, fund raising, volunteer services. **Holdings:** 5000 books; 90 VF drawers of reports, documents, pamphlets, clippings. **Subscriptions:** 100 journals and other serials.

★9237★ U.S. DEPARTMENT OF VETERANS AFFAIRS MEDICAL CENTER LIBRARY
423 E. 23rd St.
New York, NY 10010   Phone: (212) 686-7500
Karin Wiseman, Chf.Libn.
Subjects: Medicine, surgery, neurology, psychiatry, nursing. **Holdings:** 5000 books; 5684 bound periodical volumes. **Subscriptions:** 500 journals and other serials; 10 newspapers.

★9238★ A WELLNESS CENTER, INC. LIBRARY
15 E. 40th St., Ste. 704
New York, NY 10016   Phone: (212) 532-4286
Subjects: Preventive health care, psychology, psychotherapy, nutrition, exercise, medicine, naturopathy, substance abuse. **Holdings:** 5000 volumes.

★9239★ WOMEN'S ACTION ALLIANCE, INC. LIBRARY
370 Lexington Ave., Ste. 603
New York, NY 10017   Phone: (212) 532-8330
Paulette Brill, Info.Serv.
Subjects: Women's issues - child care, sex discrimination, marriage, divorce, family, health, employment, affirmative action, reproductive rights, legislation, organizations and centers, chemical dependency, AIDS, teenage pregancy. **Holdings:** 2000 books; 2000 bound periodical volumes; 40 VF drawers. **Subscriptions:** 200 journals and other serials.

★9240★ XAVIER SOCIETY FOR THE BLIND NATIONAL CATHOLIC PRESS AND LIBRARY FOR THE VISUALLY HANDICAPPED
154 E. 23rd St.
New York, NY 10010   Phone: (212) 473-7800
Rev. Thomas R. Fitzpatrick, S.J., Exec.Dir.
Subjects: Religion, inspirational. **Holdings:** 554 books in braille; 570 books in large type; 518 books on cassette. **Subscriptions:** 9 journals and other serials.

★9241★ U.S. DEPARTMENT OF VETERANS AFFAIRS HEALTH SCIENCE LIBRARY
Middleville Rd.
Northport, NY 11768   Phone: (516) 261-4400
Caryl Kazen, Chf., Lib.Sect.
Subjects: Medicine, allied health sciences, psychiatry, dentistry. **Holdings:** 5000 books; 2000 AV programs. **Subscriptions:** 530 journals and other serials.

★9242★ CHENANGO MEMORIAL HOSPITAL MEDICAL LIBRARY
179 N. Broad St.
Norwich, NY 13815-1097   Phone: (607) 335-4159
Ann L. Slocum, Lib.Serv.Mgr.
Subjects: Medicine, nursing, and allied health sciences. **Holdings:** 800 books; 570 bound periodical volumes. **Subscriptions:** 199 journals and other serials.

★9243★ NORWICH EATON PHARMACEUTICALS, INC. RESEARCH LIBRARY
PO Box 191
Norwich, NY 13815-1709   Phone: (607) 335-2678
Margaret W. DeBruine, Res.Libn.
Subjects: Pharmacy, medicine, chemistry, pharmacology, basic sciences. **Holdings:** Figures not available. **Subscriptions:** 510 journals and other serials.

★9244★ NYACK HOSPITAL MEMORIAL LIBRARY
N. Midland Ave.
Nyack, NY 10960   Phone: (914) 358-6200
Christine M. Giuricin, Mgr., Lib.Serv.
Subjects: Medicine, nursing. **Holdings:** 1400 books; 2500 bound periodical volumes; 50 video cassettes; 100 audiotapes. **Subscriptions:** 215 journals and other serials.

★9245★ STIEFEL LABORATORIES, INC. RESEARCH INSTITUTE LIBRARY
Oak Hill, NY 12460   Phone: (518) 239-6901
Joanne Fraser, Act.Libn.
Subjects: Dermatology. **Holdings:** 300 books; 10 bound periodical volumes. **Subscriptions:** 40 journals and other serials.

★9246★ SOUTH NASSAU COMMUNITIES HOSPITAL JULES REDISH MEMORIAL MEDICAL LIBRARY
Oceanside Rd.
Oceanside, NY 11572   Phone: (516) 763-2030
Claire Strelzoff, Med.Libn.
Subjects: Medicine, surgery, nursing. **Holdings:** 1000 books; 6000 bound periodical volumes. **Subscriptions:** 111 journals and other serials.

★9247★ A. BARTON HEPBURN HOSPITAL MEDICAL LIBRARY
214 King St.
Ogdensburg, NY 13669   Phone: (315) 393-3600
Ellen J. Darabaner, Circuit Rider Libn.
Subjects: Medicine, nursing, allied health sciences. **Holdings:** 300 books. **Subscriptions:** 32 journals and other serials.

★9248★ NEW YORK STATE OFFICE OF MENTAL HEALTH ST. LAWRENCE PSYCHIATRIC CENTER PROFESSIONAL LIBRARY
Sta. A
Ogdensburg, NY 13669   Phone: (315) 393-3000
Eleanor Cunningham, Lib.Techn.
Subjects: Nursing, psychiatry, general medicine. **Holdings:** 5493 volumes; 110 VF folders of clippings; 71 videotapes; 1100 nonprint materials. **Subscriptions:** 200 journals and other serials; 15 newspapers.

★9249★ NEW YORK COLLEGE OF OSTEOPATHIC MEDICINE MEDICAL LIBRARY
c/o New York Institute of Technology
Old Westbury, NY 11568   Phone: (516) 626-6943
G. Flanzraich, Chf.Med.Libn.
Subjects: Medicine. **Holdings:** 4000 books. **Subscriptions:** 250 journals and other serials.

★9250★ NEW YORK STATE OFFICE OF MENTAL HEALTH NATHAN S. KLINE INSTITUTE FOR PSYCHIATRIC RESEARCH HEALTH SCIENCES LIBRARY
Bldg. 37
Orangeburg, NY 10962   Phone: (914) 365-2000
Lois Cohan, Lib.Dir.
Subjects: Psychiatry, psychopharmacology, biomedical computers, psychology, biochemistry, mental health, neurochemistry, neuroscience. **Holdings:** 19,000 books; 21,000 bound periodical volumes; 18 VF drawers; 12

VF drawers of pamphlets, brochures, and catalogs. **Subscriptions:** 350 journals and other serials.

★9251★   OXFORD GERONTOLOGY CENTER
LIBRARY
New York State Veterans' Home
Oxford, NY 13830   Phone: (607) 843-6991
Raymond Vickers, M.D.
Subjects: Long-term care, gerontology. **Holdings:** 450 books; 130 bound periodical volumes; 112 reports.

★9252★   BROOKHAVEN MEMORIAL HOSPITAL MEDICAL
**   CENTER**
DR. JOSEPH D'AGROSA MEDICAL LIBRARY
101 Hospital Rd.
Patchogue, NY 11772   Phone: (516) 654-7774
Mrs. Freddie Borock, Med.Libn.
Subjects: Medicine, nursing, and allied health sciences. **Holdings:** 3000 books. **Subscriptions:** 325 journals and other serials.

★9253★   AMERICAN CYANAMID COMPANY
LEDERLE LABORATORIES DIVISION
SUBBAROW MEMORIAL LIBRARY
401 N. Middletown Rd.
Pearl River, NY 10965   Phone: (914) 732-5000
Dr. M. Gert Howell, Hd., Tech.Info.Serv.
Subjects: Biomedical sciences, pharmacology, organic chemistry, management. **Holdings:** 80,000 volumes; 10,000 reels of microfilm; 150 AV programs. **Subscriptions:** 1100 journals and other serials.

★9254★   CENTRAL GENERAL HOSPITAL
MEDICAL LIBRARY
888 Old Country Rd.
Plainview, NY 11803   Phone: (516) 681-8900
Paula Goldfader, Libn.
Remarks: No further information was supplied by the respondent.

★9255★   CVPH MEDICAL CENTER
MEDICAL LIBRARY
100 Beekman St.
Plattsburgh, NY 12901   Phone: (518) 562-7325
Christina Ransom, Med.Libn.
Subjects: Medicine, nursing, health care. **Holdings:** 550 books. **Subscriptions:** 149 journals and other serials.

★9256★   PORT JEFFERSON HOSPITAL
JOHN T. MATHER MEMORIAL HOSPITAL
MEDICAL LIBRARY
North Country Rd.
Port Jefferson, NY 11777   Phone: (516) 473-1320
Margaret Corrigan, Lib.Ck.
Remarks: No further information was supplied by the respondent.

★9257★   CANTON-POTSDAM HOSPITAL
MEDICAL LIBRARY
50 Leroy St.
Potsdam, NY 13676   Phone: (315) 265-3300
Mark Uebler, Libn.
Subjects: Medicine. **Holdings:** 243 books. **Subscriptions:** 21 journals and other serials.

★9258★   HUDSON RIVER PSYCHIATRIC CENTER
STAFF LIBRARY
Cheney Bldg. - H.R.P.C. Branch B
Poughkeepsie, NY 12601   Phone: (914) 452-8000
Norma Parkinson, Asst.
Subjects: Psychiatry, medicine, psychology, social services, mental health administration. **Holdings:** 4000 books; 12,000 bound periodical volumes; 65 computer searches; 80 tapes. **Subscriptions:** 101 journals and other serials.

★9259★   MENTAL HEALTH ASSOCIATION IN DUTCHESS
**   COUNTY**
DEPARTMENT OF MENTAL HYGIENE
LIBRARY
230 North Rd.
Poughkeepsie, NY 12601   Phone: (914) 485-9700
Janet Caruso, Libn.
Subjects: Psychiatry, child psychiatry, alcoholism, drug abuse, Alzheimers disease, psychology, mental retardation, the family. **Holdings:** 1850 books; 150 AV program titles; 75 audiotapes; 4 VF drawers of clippings, pamphlets, reprints. **Subscriptions:** 70 journals and other serials.

★9260★   ST. FRANCIS HOSPITAL
HEALTH SCIENCE LIBRARY
North Rd.
Poughkeepsie, NY 12601   Phone: (914) 431-8132
Linda Lee Paquin, Med.Libn.
Subjects: Internal medicine, surgery, health care administration. **Holdings:** 1200 books; 130 unbound journals. **Subscriptions:** 130 journals and other serials.

★9261★   VASSAR BROTHERS HOSPITAL
MEDICAL LIBRARY
Reade Place
Poughkeepsie, NY 12601   Phone: (914) 437-3121
Emily Arter, Libn.
Subjects: Internal medicine, surgery, cardiology, pulmonary medicine, orthopedics. **Holdings:** 1425 books; 450 bound periodical volumes; 8 VF drawers of pamphlets, flyers, and reports. **Subscriptions:** 60 journals and other serials.

★9262★   CREEDMOOR PSYCHIATRIC CENTER
HEALTH SCIENCES LIBRARY
80-45 Winchester Blvd.
Queens Village, NY 11427   Phone: (718) 464-7500
Pushpa Bhati, Sr.Libn.
Subjects: Psychiatry, psychology, medicine, sociology, hospital administration. **Holdings:** 14,550 books; 2210 bound periodical volumes; 2409 other cataloged items; 3298 pamphlets. **Subscriptions:** 175 journals and other serials.

★9263★   STERLING DRUG, INC.
STERLING RESEARCH GROUP
LIBRARY
81 Columbia Turnpike
Rensselaer, NY 12144-3493   Phone: (518) 445-8262
Patsy L. Schulenberg, Mgr., Lib. & Info.Serv.
Subjects: Biomedicine, chemistry, pharmacology, biology. **Holdings:** 20,000 books; 30,000 bound periodical volumes; 2600 reels of microfilm; 8300 microfiche. **Subscriptions:** 800 journals and other serials.

★9264★   ASTOR HOME FOR CHILDREN
PROFESSIONAL LIBRARY
36 Mill St., PO Box 5005
Rhinebeck, NY 12572   Phone: (914) 876-4081
Theresa Brettschneider, Libn.
Subjects: Child psychology and allied sciences; residential treatment centers; foster child care; adoption. **Holdings:** 3000 books; 872 bound periodical volumes; 2 VF drawers of staff papers and theses. **Subscriptions:** 40 journals and other serials.

★9265★   SHARON LONG
PRIVATE COLLECTION
104-06 85th Ave.
Richmond Hill, NY 11418   Phone: (718) 441-8917
Sharon Long
Subjects: Abortion. **Holdings:** 25 books; 50 bound periodical volumes; 5 VF drawers of articles and pamphlets.

★9266★   CENTRAL SUFFOLK HOSPITAL
MEDICAL LIBRARY
1300 Roanoke Ave.
Riverhead, NY 11901   Phone: (516) 548-6445
Anne Kirsch, Med.Libn.
Subjects: Medicine, nursing, surgery, allied health and hospital fields. **Holdings:** 700 books; 275 bound periodical volumes; 200 cassettes; 4 VF drawers of pamphlets. **Subscriptions:** 125 journals and other serials.

★9267★ BAUSCH & LOMB
INFORMATION RESOURCE CENTER
Optics Center
1400 N. Goodman St.
Rochester, NY 14692   Phone: (716) 338-6053
Adwoa Boateng, Mgr.
Subjects: Ophthalmology, optics, chemistry, pharmacology, business, management. **Holdings:** 4000 books. **Subscriptions:** 300 journals and other serials.

★9268★ CONVALESCENT HOSPITAL FOR CHILDREN
ARTHUR M. LOWENTHAL LIBRARY
2075 Scottsville Rd.
Rochester, NY 14623   Phone: (716) 436-4442
Marilyn Kalmbacher, Libn.
Subjects: Child psychiatry, clinical psychology, community and child mental health, psychiatric social work. **Holdings:** 2050 books; 500 bound periodical volumes. **Subscriptions:** 70 journals and other serials.

★9269★ EASTMAN DENTAL CENTER
BASIL G. BIBBY LIBRARY
625 Elmwood Ave.
Rochester, NY 14620   Phone: (716) 275-5010
June Glaser, Libn.
Subjects: Dentistry. **Holdings:** 3150 books; 5600 bound periodical volumes. **Subscriptions:** 150 journals and other serials.

★9270★ EASTMAN KODAK COMPANY
INFOSOURCE HEALTH AND ENVIRONMENT
LIBRARY
Kodak Park Division, Bldg. 320
Rochester, NY 14652-3615   Phone: (716) 588-3619
Richard Bartl, Libn., InfoSource Res.Lib.
Subjects: Toxicology, occupational medicine, environmental sciences, biosciences, ergonomics. **Holdings:** 5000 books and government publications; 5000 bound periodical volumes. **Subscriptions:** 300 journals and other serials.

★9271★ FISONS PHARMACEUTICALS
LIBRARY AND INFORMATION SERVICES
755 Jefferson Rd.
Box 1710
Rochester, NY 14603   Phone: (716) 475-9000
Angela M. Scarfia, Mgr., Lib. & Info.Serv.
Subjects: Pharmacology, pharmacy, chemistry, bioscience, medicine. **Holdings:** 3500 books; 4750 bound periodical volumes. **Subscriptions:** 400 journals and other serials.

★9272★ GENESEE HOSPITAL
SAMUEL J. STABINS, M.D. MEDICAL LIBRARY
224 Alexander St.
Rochester, NY 14607   Phone: (716) 263-6305
Sally M. Gerling, Chf.Libn.
Subjects: Medicine, nursing, allied health sciences. **Holdings:** 4000 books; 4700 bound periodical volumes; slide/tape sets; audio- and videotapes. **Subscriptions:** 250 journals and other serials.

★9273★ HIGHLAND HOSPITAL
JOHN R. WILLIAMS, SR. HEALTH SCIENCES LIBRARY
1000 South Ave.
Rochester, NY 14620   Phone: (716) 461-6761
Diane Dayton Robbins, Lib.Dir.
Subjects: Medicine, surgery, family medicine, nursing, hematology/oncology, radiation therapy, obstetrics, gynecology. **Holdings:** 6000 books and bound periodical volumes; 7 VF drawers of archives; AV programs. **Subscriptions:** 170 journals and other serials.

★9274★ MONROE COMMUNITY HOSPITAL
T.F. WILLIAMS HEALTH SCIENCES LIBRARY
435 E. Henrietta Rd.
Rochester, NY 14620   Phone: (716) 274-7362
Elinor Reynolds, Lib.Dir.
Subjects: Geriatrics, gerontology, long-term care, medicine, nursing, administration. **Holdings:** 998 books; 2164 bound periodical volumes. **Subscriptions:** 164 journals and other serials.

★9275★ MONROE DEVELOPMENTAL CENTER
STAFF/PARENT LIBRARY
620 Westfall Rd.
Rochester, NY 14620   Phone: (716) 461-8975
Mary Ann Howie, Libn.
Subjects: Mental retardation, developmental disabilities. **Holdings:** 3100 books; 200 videos; 30 films; 50 slide shows; 300 subject packets. **Subscriptions:** 50 journals and other serials.

★9276★ NEW YORK OFFICE OF MENTAL HEALTH
ROCHESTER PSYCHIATRIC CENTER
PROFESSIONAL LIBRARY
1600 South Ave.
Rochester, NY 14620   Phone: (716) 473-3230
Subjects: Psychiatry, nursing. **Holdings:** 5320 books; 21 bound periodical volumes; 275 Audio-Digest tapes. **Subscriptions:** 33 journals and other serials.

★9277★ PARK RIDGE HOSPITAL
NATHANIEL J. HURST LIBRARY
1555 Long Pond Rd.
Rochester, NY 14626   Phone: (716) 723-7755
Kathleen A. Martin, Libn.
Subjects: Medicine, nursing, surgery, hospital administration, alcoholism and drug abuse. **Holdings:** 1500 books; 2840 bound periodical volumes; 880 audio cassettes; 430 videotapes. **Subscriptions:** 140 journals and other serials.

★9278★ ROCHESTER ACADEMY OF MEDICINE
LIBRARY
1441 East Ave.
Rochester, NY 14610   Phone: (716) 271-1313
Mrs. Stockweather, Libn.
Subjects: Medicine and allied health sciences. **Holdings:** 31,300 volumes. **Subscriptions:** 90 journals.

★9279★ ROCHESTER GENERAL HOSPITAL
LILLIE B. WERNER HEALTH SCIENCES LIBRARY
1425 Portland Ave.
Rochester, NY 14621   Phone: (716) 338-4743
Bernie Todd Smith, Lib.Dir.
Subjects: Medicine, psychiatry, nursing. **Holdings:** 6000 books; 6000 bound periodical volumes; 1500 AV programs. **Subscriptions:** 400 journals and other serials.

★9280★ ROCHESTER INSTITUTE OF TECHNOLOGY
NATIONAL TECHNICAL INSTITUTE FOR THE DEAF
STAFF RESOURCE CENTER
Lyndon Baines Johnson Bldg., Rm. 2490
1 Lomb Memorial Dr.
Rochester, NY 14623   Phone: (716) 475-6823
Gail Kovalik, Res.Spec.
Subjects: Deafness. **Holdings:** 800 books; 1100 videotapes; 300 AV programs; 3000 pamphlets. **Subscriptions:** 30 journals and other serials.

★9281★ SENECA ZOOLOGICAL SOCIETY
LIBRARY
2222 St. Paul St.
Rochester, NY 14621   Phone: (716) 342-2744
Subjects: Zoos, zoo animals, veterinary medicine, ecology, zoology, herpetology. **Holdings:** 2100 books; 7800 slides; 1900 photographs; 30 zoo guidebooks. **Subscriptions:** 55 journals and other serials.

★9282★ UNIVERSITY OF ROCHESTER
SCHOOL OF MEDICINE AND DENTISTRY
EDWARD G. MINER LIBRARY
601 Elmwood Ave.
Rochester, NY 14642   Phone: (716) 275-3364
Lucretia McClure, Med.Libn.
Subjects: Medicine, nursing, psychiatry, dental research. **Holdings:** 220,000 volumes. **Subscriptions:** 3074 journals and other serials.

★9283★ MERCY HOSPITAL
PROFESSIONAL LIBRARY SERVICES
1000 N. Village Ave.
Rockville Centre, NY 11570   Phone: (516) 255-2255
Carol L. Reid, Prof.Libn.
Subjects: Medicine, surgery, nursing. **Holdings:** 2450 books; 4000 bound

periodical volumes; 1000 audio cassette tapes. **Subscriptions:** 180 journals and other serials.

★9284★ ST. FRANCIS HOSPITAL
MEDICAL LIBRARY
100 Port Washington Blvd.
Roslyn, NY 11576   Phone: (516) 562-6673
Judith Weinstein, Med.Libn.
Subjects: Cardiology, pulmonary diseases, biomedical sciences, hospitals, management. **Holdings:** 2000 books; 1000 bound periodical volumes; 200 audio cassettes; pamphlets. **Subscriptions:** 70 journals and other serials.

★9285★ WYETH-AYERST RESEARCH
INFORMATION CENTER
64 Maple St.
Rouses Point, NY 12979-9985   Phone: (518) 297-8294
George L. Curran, III, Sr.Libn. & Info.Sci.
Subjects: Analytical and pharmaceutical chemistry, pharmacy, pharmacology, business management, quality control. **Holdings:** 5500 books; 3500 bound periodical volumes; chemical and world patents, 1970-1989, on microfilm; 1400 volumes on microfilm; 100 cassette programs. **Subscriptions:** 500 serials.

★9286★ INTERNATIONAL ASSOCIATION FOR PSYCHIATRIC
RESEARCH
LIBRARY
PO Box 457
St. James, NY 11780   Phone: (516) 862-6651
Max Fink, M.D.
Subjects: Electroconvulsive therapy. **Holdings:** 800 books; 600 bound periodical volumes. **Subscriptions:** 20 journals and other serials.

★9287★ TRUDEAU INSTITUTE IMMUNOBIOLOGICAL
RESEARCH LABORATORIES
LIBRARY
Algonquin Ave.
Box 59
Saranac Lake, NY 12983   Phone: (518) 891-3080
Helen Jarvis, Libn.
Subjects: Immunobiological research. **Holdings:** 13,000 books and bound periodical volumes. **Subscriptions:** 120 journals and other serials.

★9288★ SARATOGA HOSPITAL
MEDICAL STAFF LIBRARY
211 Church St.
Saratoga Springs, NY 12866   Phone: (518) 583-8301
Julie VanDussen, Mgr.
Subjects: Medicine, nursing, surgery, psychiatry. **Holdings:** 340 books. **Subscriptions:** 32 journals and other serials.

★9289★ ELLIS HOSPITAL
MACMILLAN LIBRARY
1101 Nott St.
Schenectady, NY 12308   Phone: (518) 382-4381
Christopher Stater, Dir.
Subjects: Medicine, nursing, hospital administration, allied health. **Holdings:** 2000 books; 5000 bound periodical volumes. **Subscriptions:** 180 journals and other serials.

★9290★ EPISCOPAL HEALTH SERVICES, INC.
ST. JOHN'S EPISCOPAL HOSPITAL
SMITHTOWN MEDICAL LIBRARY
Rte. 25A
Smithtown, NY 11785   Phone: (516) 862-3186
Laura Righter, Act.Adm.
Subjects: Medicine, health care administration. **Holdings:** 400 books. **Subscriptions:** 100 journals and other serials.

★9291★ BAYLEY SETON HOSPITAL
CHARLES FERGUSON MEDICAL LIBRARY
Bay St. & Vanderbilt Ave.
Staten Island, NY 10304   Phone: (718) 390-5525
Marie A. Sheldon, Libn.
Subjects: Medicine, surgery, radiology, urology, dermatology, pediatrics, nursing. **Holdings:** 4100 books; 7950 bound periodical volumes; 408 audiotapes; 126 cassette tapes; 110 video cassettes; 107 slide and cassette programs. **Subscriptions:** 243 journals and other serials.

★9292★ NEW YORK STATE INSTITUTE FOR BASIC
RESEARCH IN DEVELOPMENTAL DISABILITIES
LIBRARY
1050 Forest Hill Rd.
Staten Island, NY 10314   Phone: (718) 494-5407
Lawrence Black, Assoc.Libn.
Subjects: Neurology, neurophysiology, neurochemistry, neuropathology, genetics, virology, immunology. **Holdings:** Figures not available. **Subscriptions:** 200 journals and other serials.

★9293★ ST. VINCENT'S MEDICAL CENTER OF RICHMOND
MEDICAL LIBRARY
355 Bard Ave.
Staten Island, NY 10310   Phone: (718) 876-3117
Lucy DiMatteo, Dir.
Subjects: Medicine, nursing, health administration. **Holdings:** 5000 books; 3000 bound periodical volumes. **Subscriptions:** 180 journals and other serials.

★9294★ SEA VIEW HOSPITAL AND HOME
HEALTH SCIENCES LIBRARY
460 Brielle Ave.
Staten Island, NY 10314   Phone: (718) 317-3689
Lorraine Blank, Sr.Hea. Care Plan.
Subjects: Medicine, nursing, geriatrics, hospital administration, social service, rehabilitation, dentistry. **Holdings:** 3000 books; 4160 bound periodical volumes. **Subscriptions:** 150 journals and other serials.

★9295★ STATEN ISLAND UNIVERSITY HOSPITAL
MEDICAL STAFF LIBRARY
475 Seaview Ave.
Staten Island, NY 10305   Phone: (718) 226-9545
Song Ja Oh, Dir.
Subjects: Internal medicine, surgery, pediatrics, obstetrics, gynecology, dentistry, nursing, psychiatry, rehabilitation, pathology, pharmacy. **Holdings:** 2200 books; 15,000 bound periodical volumes; 1736 Audio-Digest tapes; videotapes. **Subscriptions:** 400 journals; 2207 other serials.

★9296★ AVON PRODUCTS, INC.
RESEARCH LIBRARY
Division St.
Suffern, NY 10901   Phone: (914) 357-2000
Sarah Boroson, Prog.Ldr.
Subjects: Cosmetics, packaging, toxicology, dermatology, pharmacology, chemistry, engineering, microbiology. **Holdings:** 6500 books; 5000 bound periodical volumes; 6000 U.S. and foreign patents. **Subscriptions:** 300 journals and other serials.

★9297★ BRISTOL-MYERS SQUIBB COMPANY
SCIENTIFIC INFORMATION DEPARTMENT
Box 4755
Syracuse, NY 13221-4755   Phone: (315) 432-2231
Dr. John E. MacNintch, Dir.
Subjects: Pharmacology, pharmacy, organic chemistry, microbiology, medicine, engineering. **Holdings:** 8200 books; 14,500 bound periodical volumes; 8 VF drawers; 73 VF drawers of reprints; 3100 microfilm cartridges. **Subscriptions:** 266 journals and other serials; 7 newspapers.

★9298★ COMMUNITY-GENERAL HOSPITAL OF GREATER
SYRACUSE
MEDICAL LIBRARY
Broad Rd.
Syracuse, NY 13215   Phone: (315) 492-5500
Diana Reinstein, Med. Staff Libn.
Subjects: General surgery and medicine, nursing. **Holdings:** 3000 books; 3000 bound periodical volumes; 2 drawers of microfiche; 5 VF drawers of pamphlets and clippings; video cassettes. **Subscriptions:** 305 journals and other serials.

★9299★ CROUSE-IRVING MEMORIAL HOSPITAL
LIBRARY
736 Irving Ave.
Syracuse, NY 13210   Phone: (315) 470-7380
Wendy Skinner, Dir., Lib.Serv.
Subjects: Nursing, medicine. **Holdings:** 3000 books; 650 bound periodical volumes; 1500 AV programs. **Subscriptions:** 228 journals and other serials.

★9300★   ST. JOSEPH'S HOSPITAL HEALTH CENTER
MEDICAL AND SCHOOL OF NURSING LIBRARIES
206-301 Prospect Ave.
Syracuse, NY 13203   Phone: (315) 424-5053
Mr. V. Juchimek, Hd.Libn.
Subjects: Nursing, medicine, psychology, social sciences, religion. **Holdings:** 10,000 books; 3000 bound periodical volumes; 30 VF drawers of pamphlets; 450 cassette programs; models; slides; filmstrips; recordings. **Subscriptions:** 195 journals and other serials.

★9301★   SUNY AT SYRACUSE
HEALTH SCIENCE CENTER
LIBRARY
766 Irving Ave.
Syracuse, NY 13210   Phone: (315) 464-4582
Suzanne H. Murray, Dir.
Subjects: Medicine, nursing, and allied health sciences. **Holdings:** 52,444 books; 108,899 bound periodical volumes; 2760 AV program titles. **Subscriptions:** 1830 journals and other serials.

★9302★   SYRACUSE UNIVERSITY
SCIENCE AND TECHNOLOGY LIBRARY
105 Carnegie
Syracuse, NY 13244-2010   Phone: (315) 443-2160
Lee M. Murray, Hd., Sci. & Tech.Dept.
Subjects: Engineering - chemical, civil, electrical, bio-industrial, mechanical, aerospace; computers and data processing; biology; botany; zoology; microbiology; biochemistry; chemistry; immunology; genetics; ecology; public health; general medicine; medicine and society; nursing; neuroscience; general science and technology; history and philosophy of science; nutrition; mining and metallurgy; physical geography. **Holdings:** 390,000 books and bound periodical volumes; 700,000 microforms. **Subscriptions:** 2100 journals and other serials.

★9303★   U.S. DEPARTMENT OF VETERANS AFFAIRS
MEDICAL CENTER LIBRARY
Irving Ave. & University Pl.
Syracuse, NY 13210   Phone: (315) 476-7461
June M. Mitchell, Chf., Lib./LRC Serv.
Subjects: Clinical medicine, surgery, nursing, psychology, social work. **Holdings:** 3000 books; 2625 bound and microform periodical volumes; 350 pamphlets. **Subscriptions:** 190 journals and other serials.

★9304★   TECHNICON INSTRUMENTS CORPORATION
LIBRARY
511 Benedict Ave.
Tarrytown, NY 10591   Phone: (914) 524-2338
Gitta Benglas, Mgr. of Lib Resources & Serv.
Subjects: Medicine, chemistry, computer science. **Holdings:** 15,000 books; laboratory notebooks; dissertations; reports; microfilm; microfiche; 30 VF drawers; 200 audiotapes. **Subscriptions:** 320 journals and other serials.

★9305★   LETCHWORTH DEVELOPMENTAL DISABILITIES
   SERVICES
ISAAC N. WOLFSON LIBRARY
Thiells, NY 10984   Phone: (914) 947-1000
Eleanor Flaherty, Sr.Ck./Lib.Asst.
Subjects: Mental retardation, special education, psychology. **Holdings:** 8000 books; 60 reports on microfiche; 125 cassettes and videotapes; 10 VF drawers of pamphlets. **Subscriptions:** 50 journals and other serials.

★9306★   ST. MARY'S HOSPITAL
MEDICAL STAFF LIBRARY
1300 Massachusetts Ave.
Troy, NY 12180   Phone: (518) 272-5000
Audna T. Clum, Libn.
Subjects: Medicine. **Holdings:** 450 books; 1300 bound periodical volumes; 719 other cataloged items. **Subscriptions:** 78 journals and other serials.

★9307★   SAMARITAN HOSPITAL
MEDICAL LIBRARY
2215 Burdett Ave.
Troy, NY 12180   Phone: (518) 271-3200
Annie J. Smith, Med.Libn.
Subjects: Medicine, allied health sciences. **Holdings:** 290 books; 1500 bound periodical volumes. **Subscriptions:** 64 journals and other serials.

★9308★   NEW YORK UNIVERSITY MEDICAL CENTER
DEPARTMENT OF ENVIRONMENTAL MEDICINE
LIBRARY
Long Meadow Rd.
Tuxedo, NY 10987   Phone: (914) 351-4232
Christine M. Singleton, Res.Libn.
Subjects: Environmental medicine and science, cancer research, air and water pollution, industrial health, radiobiology and toxicology. **Holdings:** 5500 books; 6500 bound periodical volumes. **Subscriptions:** 165 journals and other serials.

★9309★   BROOKHAVEN NATIONAL LABORATORY
TECHNICAL INFORMATION DIVISION
LIBRARY
Upton, NY 11973   Phone: (516) 282-3489
Diane C. Mirvis, Mgr.
Subjects: Physics, chemistry, mathematics, biology, medicine, environment, energy, instrumentation, nuclear science and engineering. **Holdings:** 60,000 books; 40,000 bound periodical volumes; 200,000 reports; 6000 reels of periodical volumes; 522,000 reports on microfiche. **Subscriptions:** 818 journals and other serials.

★9310★   FAXTON-CHILDREN'S HOSPITAL
MEDICAL LIBRARY
1676 Sunset Ave.
Utica, NY 13502   Phone: (315) 732-3101
Marilyn Rosen, Med.Libn.
Subjects: Oncology, chemotherapy, surgery, cardiology. **Holdings:** 815 books. **Subscriptions:** 132 journals and other serials.

★9311★   MASONIC MEDICAL RESEARCH LABORATORY
MAX L. KAMIEL LIBRARY
2150 Bleecker St.
Utica, NY 13501-1787   Phone: (315) 735-2217
Patricia M. Dugan, Libn.
Subjects: Cardiac arrhythmias, cardiovascular pharmacology, cancer research, aging, artificial blood. **Holdings:** 2200 books; 19,000 bound periodical volumes; 500 films; 300 microcards; 250 reels of microfilm; 8 other cataloged items. **Subscriptions:** 100 journals and other serials.

★9312★   MOHAWK VALLEY PSYCHIATRIC CENTER
GEORGE M. LEIN INFORMATION CENTER
1400 Noyes at York
Utica, NY 13502-3852   Phone: (315) 797-6800
Kay Sangani, Act.Libn.
Subjects: Psychiatry, neurology, medicine, nursing. **Holdings:** 3500 books; 1500 bound periodical volumes; 2500 unbound periodical volumes. **Subscriptions:** 75 journals and other serials.

★9313★   ST. ELIZABETH   HOSPITAL
NURSING SCHOOL LIBRARY
2215 Genesee St.
Utica, NY 13501   Phone: (315) 798-5209
Ann M. Kelly, Libn.
Subjects: Nursing, medicine, sociology, psychology. **Holdings:** 4991 books; 694 bound periodical volumes; 9 VF drawers; 220 phonograph records; 209 videotapes; 293 AV programs. **Subscriptions:** 83 journals and other serials.

★9314★   AMERICAN HEALTH FOUNDATION
NAYLOR DANA INSTITUTE FOR DISEASE PREVENTION
LIBRARY
Dana Rd.
Valhalla, NY 10595   Phone: (914) 592-2600
Noreen T. Sweeney, Libn.
Subjects: Medicine, science, social science. **Holdings:** 2000 books; 3000 bound periodical volumes. **Subscriptions:** 211 journals and other serials.

★9315★   NEW YORK MEDICAL COLLEGE
MEDICAL SCIENCES LIBRARY
Basic Sciences Bldg.
New York Medical College
Valhalla, NY 10595   Phone: (914) 993-4200
Donald E. Roy, Dir.
Subjects: Basic science, clinical medicine. **Holdings:** 34,000 books; 109,660 bound periodical volumes; 65 VF drawers; 616 microfiche; 410 reels of microfilm; 32 audiotapes; 702 videotapes. **Subscriptions:** 1306 journals and other serials.

★9316★ **WESTCHESTER COUNTY MEDICAL CENTER**
HEALTH SCIENCES LIBRARY
Eastview Hall
Valhalla, NY 10595   Phone: (914) 285-7033
Charlene Sikorski, Med.Libn.
Subjects: Medicine, nursing, psychiatry, psychology, dentistry. **Holdings:** 12,000 volumes. **Subscriptions:** 190 journals and other serials.

★9317★ **FRANKLIN HOSPITAL MEDICAL CENTER**
MEDICAL LIBRARY
900 Franklin Ave.
Valley Stream, NY 11582   Phone: (516) 825-8800
Kathryn A. Boccieri, Libn.
Subjects: Medicine. **Holdings:** 1500 books; 3000 bound periodical volumes; Audio-Digest tapes; slides. **Subscriptions:** 55 journals and other serials.

★9318★ **DELAWARE VALLEY HOSPITAL**
LIBRARY
1 Titus Pl.
Walton, NY 13856   Phone: (607) 865-4101
Marian Platt, Libn.
Subjects: Medicine, allied health sciences. **Holdings:** 257 volumes. **Subscriptions:** 40 journals and other serials.

★9319★ **MERCY HOSPITAL OF WATERTOWN**
HEALTH SCIENCE LIBRARY
218 Stone St.
Watertown, NY 13601   Phone: (315) 782-7400
Jeffrey M. Garvey, Libn.
Subjects: Medicine, nursing, mental health, hospital management. **Holdings:** 2200 books; 9200 bound periodical volumes; 140 AV programs; 87 reels of microfilm. **Subscriptions:** 125 journals and other serials.

★9320★ **PILGRIM PSYCHIATRIC CENTER**
HEALTH SCIENCES LIBRARY
Bldg. 23
Box A
West Brentwood, NY 11717   Phone: (516) 231-8000
Judy R. Sartori, Sr.Libn.
Subjects: Psychiatry, social sciences, psychology, medicine, nursing. **Holdings:** 6000 books; 120 bound periodical volumes; 8 VF drawers of pamphlets and clippings; 3 VF drawers of reports and manuscripts; 1 VF drawer of documents; 145 reels of microfilm; 260 cassette tapes. **Subscriptions:** 120 journals and other serials; 7 newspapers.

★9321★ **HELEN HAYES HOSPITAL**
LIBRARY
Route 9W
West Haverstraw, NY 10993   Phone: (914) 947-3000
Kathleen Fiola, Lib.Dir.
Subjects: Orthopedics, rehabilitation medicine, neurology, physical therapy, occupational therapy, biomedical engineering, rehabilitation technology, psychology, psychiatry, speech and hearing. **Holdings:** 5000 books; 5000 bound periodical volumes. **Subscriptions:** 200 journals and other serials.

★9322★ **GOOD SAMARITAN HOSPITAL**
MEDICAL LIBRARY
1000 Montauk Hwy.
West Islip, NY 11795   Phone: (516) 661-3000
Karen Tubolino, Med.Libn.
Subjects: Medicine, surgery, obstetrics, pediatrics. **Holdings:** 500 books; 4000 bound periodical volumes; yearbooks. **Subscriptions:** 80 journals.

★9323★ **U.S. ARMY HOSPITALS**
KELLER ARMY COMMUNITY HOSPITAL
MEDDAC LIBRARY
Bldg. 900
West Point, NY 10996-1197   Phone: (914) 938-2722
Linda Wooster, Libn.
Subjects: Orthopedics, medicine, nursing. **Holdings:** 2500 books; 2800 bound periodical volumes. **Subscriptions:** 212 journals and other serials.

★9324★ **MARCH OF DIMES BIRTH DEFECTS FOUNDATION**
REFERENCE ROOM
1275 Mamaroneck Ave.
White Plains, NY 10605   Phone: (914) 428-7100
Subjects: Birth defects, pediatrics, obstetrics, maternal and child health. **Holdings:** 2500 books; 1722 bound periodical volumes; 5 VF drawers. **Subscriptions:** 108 journals and other serials.

★9325★ **MENTAL HEALTH ASSOCIATION OF WESTCHESTER**
LIBRARY
29 Sterling Ave.
White Plains, NY 10606   Phone: (914) 949-6741
Phyllis Getlan, Ombudsman
Subjects: Mental health, psychiatry, psychology, drugs, graduate social work. **Holdings:** 3150 volumes; 150 VF drawers of pamphlets and clippings; 50 films and videotapes. **Subscriptions:** 25 journals and other serials.

★9326★ **NEW YORK HOSPITAL**
CORNELL MEDICAL CENTER, WESTCHESTER DIVISION
MEDICAL LIBRARY
21 Bloomingdale Rd.
White Plains, NY 10605   Phone: (914) 997-5897
Marcia A. Miller, Med.Libn.
Subjects: Psychiatry, clinical psychology, psychoanalysis, psychiatric nursing. **Holdings:** 7000 books; 5000 bound periodical volumes; 19 VF drawers of reprints and pamphlets; 800 audiotapes; 39 videotapes. **Subscriptions:** 163 journals and other serials.

★9327★ **WHITE PLAINS HOSPITAL**
MEDICAL LIBRARY
E. Post Rd. at Davis Ave.
White Plains, NY 10601   Phone: (914) 681-1231
Rachel Dwyer, Mgr., Med.Lib.
Subjects: Medicine, nursing, allied health fields. **Holdings:** 1000 books; 2900 bound periodical volumes; VF of allied health subjects. **Subscriptions:** 160 journals and other serials.

★9328★ **WILLARD PSYCHIATRIC CENTER**
HATCH LIBRARY
Hatch Bldg.
Willard, NY 14588   Phone: (607) 869-3111
Helen Bunting, Sr.Libn.
Subjects: Psychiatry, medicine, psychology, health sciences, nursing, rehabilitative geriatrics. **Holdings:** 3300 books; 1200 bound periodical volumes; 12 cubic feet of medical files. **Subscriptions:** 80 journals and other serials; 8 newspapers.

★9329★ **HARLEM VALLEY PSYCHIATRIC CENTER**
E.W. WIMBLE MEMORIAL LIBRARY
Sta. A
Wingdale, NY 12594-0330   Phone: (914) 832-6611
Virginia Lewandowski, Sr.Libn.
Subjects: Psychology, psychiatry, medicine, nursing, social work. **Holdings:** 3500 books; 800 bound periodical volumes; AV programs. **Subscriptions:** 60 journals and other serials.

★9330★ **ST. JOHN'S RIVERSIDE HOSPITAL**
LIBRARY
967 N. Broadway
Yonkers, NY 10701   Phone: (914) 964-4281
Margaret Haag, Lib.Hd.
Subjects: Nursing, medicine. **Holdings:** 2539 books. **Subscriptions:** 95 journals and other serials.

★9331★ **ST. JOSEPH'S MEDICAL CENTER**
MEDICAL LIBRARY
127 S. Broadway
Yonkers, NY 10701   Phone: (914) 738-7539
Virginia Gregory, Libn.
Subjects: Medicine, psychiatry, geriatrics, rehabilitation, family medicine. **Holdings:** 1600 volumes; 125 bound periodical volumes. **Subscriptions:** 125 journals and other serials.

★9332★   YONKERS GENERAL HOSPITAL
MEDICAL LIBRARY
2 Park Ave.
Yonkers, NY 10701   Phone: (914) 964-7300
M. Danber, Libn.
Subjects: Internal medicine, surgery, gynecology, pathology, psychiatry. **Holdings:** 150 books; 250 bound periodical volumes. **Subscriptions:** 42 journals and other serials.

North Carolina

★9333★   MOUNTAIN AREA HEALTH EDUCATION CENTER
INFORMATION AND MEDIA SERVICES
501 Biltmore Ave.
Asheville, NC 28801   Phone: (704) 257-4444
Patricia L. Thibodeau, Dir.
Subjects: Health sciences, health care administration. **Holdings:** 6600 books; 10,050 bound and unbound periodicals; 820 AV programs; slides; filmstrips; videotapes. **Subscriptions:** 400 journals and other serials.

★9334★   U.S. DEPARTMENT OF VETERANS AFFAIRS
MEDICAL CENTER LIBRARY
Riceville & Tunnel Rds.
Asheville, NC 28805   Phone: (704) 298-7911
Jane Lambremont, Chf., Lib.Serv.
Subjects: General and cardiopulmonary medicine, thoracic surgery, nursing. **Holdings:** 2000 books; 3000 bound periodical volumes. **Subscriptions:** 334 journals and other serials.

★9335★   COUNTRY DOCTOR MUSEUM
LIBRARY
Vance St.
Box 34
Bailey, NC 27807   Phone: (919) 235-4165
Subjects: Medicine, pharmacy. **Holdings:** 800 volumes.

★9336★   NORTHWEST AREA HEALTH EDUCATION CENTER
NW AHEC LIBRARY
Watauga County Hospital
Deerfield Rd.
Boone, NC 28607   Phone: (704) 262-4101
Jill Byerly, AHEC Libn./Coord.
Subjects: Medicine, nursing, allied health sciences. **Holdings:** 910 books; 1058 unbound periodicals; 150 clippings; 80 special bibliographies. **Subscriptions:** 155 journals and other serials.

★9337★   ALAMANCE HEALTH SERVICES, INC.
MEDICAL LIBRARY
PO Box 202
Burlington, NC 27216-0202   Phone: (919) 570-5027
Virginia Marshall, Educ.Dir.
Subjects: Medicine, nursing, pharmacology, hospital administration, biomedical engineering. **Holdings:** 350 books; 85 audio cassettes; 50 videotapes. **Subscriptions:** 72 journals and other serials.

★9338★   JOHN UMSTEAD HOSPITAL
LEARNING RESOURCE CENTER
12th St.
Butner, NC 27509   Phone: (919) 575-7259
Brenda M. Ellis, Libn.
Subjects: Psychiatry, neurology, nursing, medicine, sociology, psychology, geriatrics, child psychiatry. **Holdings:** 3000 books; 3175 bound periodical volumes; 350 other cataloged items. **Subscriptions:** 45 journals and other serials.

★9339★   U.S. NAVY
NAVAL HOSPITAL
MEDICAL LIBRARY
Camp Lejeune, NC 28542   Phone: (919) 451-4076
Gladys Dixon, Lib.Techn.
Subjects: Medicine and allied health sciences. **Holdings:** 2124 books; 4936 bound periodical volumes. **Subscriptions:** 151 journals and other serials.

★9340★   CAROLINA LIBRARY SERVICES, INC.
209 N. Columbia St.
Chapel Hill, NC 27514   Phone: (919) 929-4870
Kate Millard, Dir.
Subjects: Biotechnology, medicine, information science. **Holdings:** 1000 books; 500 government reports; 50 dissertations on microfilm. **Subscriptions:** 20 journals and other serials.

★9341★   CAROLINA POPULATION CENTER
LIBRARY
University of North Carolina at Chapel Hill
CB No. 8120
Chapel Hill, NC 27516-3997   Phone: (919) 962-3081
Patricia E. Shipman, Hd.Libn.
Subjects: Population dynamics, policy, education; abortion; family planning; fertility. **Holdings:** 9000 books; 1500 bound periodical volumes; 40,000 analytics; 15,000 documents, technical reports, manuscripts; 90 documents on microfiche. **Subscriptions:** 375 journals and other serials.

★9342★   UNIVERSITY OF NORTH CAROLINA, CHAPEL HILL
CENTER FOR ALCOHOL STUDIES
LIBRARY
CB 7175 UNC School of Medicine, Bldg. A
Chapel Hill, NC 27514   Phone: (919) 966-5678
Dr. Amir Rezvani, Asst.Dir.
Subjects: Alcohol research, alcoholism. **Holdings:** 250 books; 3000 reprints; clippings. **Subscriptions:** 5 journals and other serials.

★9343★   UNIVERSITY OF NORTH CAROLINA, CHAPEL HILL
HEALTH SCIENCES LIBRARY
Chapel Hill, NC 27599-7585   Phone: (919) 966-2111
Carol G. Jenkins, Dir.
Subjects: Medicine, nursing, dentistry, public health, pharmacy, allied health sciences. **Holdings:** 82,000 books; 165,000 bound periodical volumes; 4400 AV programs. **Subscriptions:** 4797 journals and other serials.

★9344★   UNIVERSITY OF NORTH CAROLINA, CHAPEL HILL
OCCUPATIONAL SAFETY AND HEALTH EDUCATIONAL
    RESOURCE CENTER
OSHERC LIBRARY
311 Pittsboro St., C.B. No. 7410
Chapel Hill, NC 27599-7410   Phone: (919) 966-5001
Mary Ellen Tucker, Libn.
Subjects: Industrial hygiene; occupational medicine, occupational health nursing, and safety. **Holdings:** 2500 books. **Subscriptions:** 18 journals and other serials.

★9345★   MEDICAL LIBRARY OF MECKLENBURG COUNTY
BRYANT L. GALUSHA, M.D. LRC OF CHARLOTTE AHEC
Box 32861
Charlotte, NC 28232-2861   Phone: (704) 355-3129
Constance M. Wallace, Dir., Lib.Serv.
Subjects: Clinical medicine, allied health sciences. **Holdings:** 5000 books; 30,000 bound periodical volumes; 3 VF drawers of pamphlets; 1200 video cassettes. **Subscriptions:** 400 journals and other serials.

★9346★   MERCY SCHOOL OF NURSING
LIBRARY
1921 Vail Ave.
Charlotte, NC 28207   Phone: (704) 379-5845
Carol Liu, Libn.
Subjects: Nursing, medicine. **Holdings:** 4327 books; 436 bound periodical volumes; 201 AV titles; 4 VF drawers. **Subscriptions:** 49 journals and other serials.

★9347★   PRESBYTERIAN HOSPITAL
LEARNING RESOURCE CENTER
Box 33549
Charlotte, NC 28233-3549   Phone: (704) 384-4258
Mary Wallace Berry, Libn.
Subjects: Nursing, medicine, allied health education. **Holdings:** 6000 books; 3 VF drawers; AV programs. **Subscriptions:** 200 journals and other serials.

★9348★ SUNHEALTH, INC.
SUNHEALTH RESOURCE CENTER
Box 668800
Charlotte, NC 28266-8800   Phone: (704) 529-3324
T. Joan Crouze, Mgr., Res.Ctr.
Subjects: Hospitals, health care, safety, marketing. Holdings: 4000 books; 210 bound periodical volumes; 3750 confidential reports; 30 magazine volumes on microfiche; 10 sound slide sets; 125 audio cassettes; 50 video cassettes. Subscriptions: 477 journals and other serials.

★9349★ BLUE CROSS AND BLUE SHIELD OF NORTH
  CAROLINA
INFORMATION CENTER
Box 2291
Durham, NC 27702   Phone: (919) 490-4176
Elizabeth J. Turner, Mgr., Corp.Info.Ctr.
Subjects: Health insurance, health economics, management, North Carolina population and economy. Holdings: 2000 books; 130 bound periodical volumes; 50,500 reports; 10,000 microfiche. Subscriptions: 175 journals and other serials; 7 newspapers.

★9350★ DUKE UNIVERSITY
MEDICAL CENTER LIBRARY
Durham, NC 27710   Phone: (919) 684-2092
Warren Bird, Dir.
Subjects: Medicine, allied health sciences. Holdings: 246,310 volumes. Subscriptions: 4789 journals and other serials.

★9351★ DURHAM COUNTY HOSPITAL CORPORATION
WATTS SCHOOL OF NURSING
LIBRARY
3643 N. Roxboro Rd.
Durham, NC 27704   Phone: (919) 470-7346
Priscilla W. Hoover, Libn.
Subjects: Nursing and nursing education, pediatrics, obstetrics and gynecology, sociology and psychology. Holdings: 5333 books; 249 bound periodical volumes; 4 VF drawers; 20 boxes of pamphlets. Subscriptions: 59 journals and other serials.

★9352★ U.S. DEPARTMENT OF VETERANS AFFAIRS
MEDICAL CENTER LIBRARY
508 Fulton St.
Durham, NC 27705   Phone: (919) 286-6929
Jeffrey F. Kager, Chf., Lib.Serv.
Subjects: Clinical medicine, pre-clinical sciences, allied health sciences, management, research, patient health education. Holdings: 1600 books; 9000 bound periodical volumes; 2600 reels of microfilm; 70 microfiche; 927 AV programs. Subscriptions: 360 journals and other serials; 13 newspapers.

★9353★ CAPE FEAR VALLEY MEDICAL CENTER
LIBRARY SERVICES
Box 2000
Fayetteville, NC 28302   Phone: (919) 323-6601
Jane Moore, Lib.Dir.
Subjects: Medicine, surgery, nursing, rehabilitation, allied health sciences, consumer health. Holdings: 1500 books. Subscriptions: 200 journals and other serials.

★9354★ FAYETTEVILLE AREA HEALTH EDUCATION
  CENTER
LIBRARY/INFORMATION SERVICES
1601 Owen Dr.
Fayetteville, NC 28304   Phone: (919) 678-7276
Barbara A. Wright, Dir.
Subjects: Medicine, nursing, mental health, allied health sciences. Holdings: 5000 books; 2000 bound periodical volumes; 1500 AV programs; 3 drawers of clippings and pamphlets. Subscriptions: 302 journals and other serials.

★9355★ U.S. DEPARTMENT OF VETERANS AFFAIRS
MEDICAL CENTER LIBRARY SERVICE
2300 Ramsey St.
Fayetteville, NC 28301   Phone: (919) 822-7072
Diana Akins, Chf., Lib.Serv.
Subjects: Medicine, nursing, dentistry, patient education, allied health sciences. Holdings: 2500 books; 3978 periodicals; 467 AV programs. Subscriptions: 400 journals and other serials.

★9356★ U.S. ARMY HOSPITALS
WOMACK ARMY COMMUNITY HOSPITAL
MEDICAL LIBRARY
Fort Bragg, NC 28307-5000   Phone: (919) 432-1819
Joan Hathaway, Med.Libn.
Subjects: Medicine, dentistry, allied health sciences, orthopedics. Holdings: 3381 books; 2995 bound periodical volumes; 2 VF drawers of clippings, pamphlets, documents. Subscriptions: 258 journals and other serials.

★9357★ CHERRY HOSPITAL
LEARNING RESOURCE CENTER
Box 8000
Goldsboro, NC 27530   Phone: (919) 731-3447
Maxim Tabory, Dir. of LRC
Subjects: Psychiatry, medicine, nursing, psychology, social work, allied health sciences. Holdings: 2000 books; 800 bound periodical volumes; 986 AV programs. Subscriptions: 95 journals and other serials.

★9358★ MOSES H. CONE MEMORIAL HOSPITAL
MEDICAL LIBRARY
1200 N. Elm St.
Greensboro, NC 27420   Phone: (919) 379-4484
Leslie G. Mackler, Dir., Med.Lib.
Subjects: Medicine, medical specialities. Holdings: 3800 books; 8000 bound periodical volumes; 1400 AV programs. Subscriptions: 200 journals and other serials.

★9359★ NORTH CAROLINA AGRICULTURAL AND
  TECHNICAL STATE UNIVERSITY
F.D. BLUFORD LIBRARY
Greensboro, NC 27411   Phone: (919) 334-7782
Alene C. Young, Dir., Lib.Serv.
Subjects: Agriculture, nursing, engineering, education. Holdings: 410,170 volumes; 271,590 microforms; archival materials; government documents; theses; pictures; maps; modules. Subscriptions: 1716 journals and other serials.

★9360★ BURROUGHS WELLCOME COMPANY
TECHNICAL INFORMATION DEPARTMENT
Box 1887
Greenville, NC 27834   Phone: (919) 758-3436
Hyder A. Zahed, Hd., Tech.Info./Lib.Serv.
Subjects: Pharmaceutical sciences and technology, chemistry, engineering, medicine. Holdings: 7000 books; 1650 bound periodical volumes. Subscriptions: 250 journals and other serials.

★9361★ EAST CAROLINA UNIVERSITY
HEALTH SCIENCES LIBRARY
Greenville, NC 27854-4354   Phone: (919) 551-2212
JoAnn Bell, Ph.D., Dir.
Subjects: Medicine, allied health sciences, social welfare. Holdings: 61,659 books; 62,587 bound periodical volumes; 16,682 reels of microfilm; 3795 nonprint materials. Subscriptions: 1990 journals and other serials.

★9362★ NORTHWEST AREA HEALTH EDUCATION CENTER
NW AHEC LIBRARY
Catawba Memorial Hospital
Hickory, NC 28602-9643   Phone: (704) 322-0662
Phyllis C. Gillikin, Dir.
Subjects: Medicine, nursing, health care administration, allied health sciences. Holdings: 2264 books. Subscriptions: 223 journals and other serials.

★9363★ NORTH AMERICAN YOUTH SPORT INSTITUTE
INFORMATION CENTER
4985 Oak Garden Dr., Ste. 91
Kernersville, NC 27284   Phone: (919) 784-4926
Jack Hutslar, Ph.D., Dir.
Subjects: Youth, sports, sport sociology and psychology, education, physical education, fitness, health, recreation and leisure, models, management. Holdings: 1000 books, manuscripts, clippings, reports, journals, newsletters, publications, and youth agency literature.

★9364★ SOUTHEASTERN GENERAL HOSPITAL
LIBRARY
300 W. 27th St.
Box 1408
Lumberton, NC 28358   Phone: (919) 671-5046
Ida Griffin, Libn.
Subjects: Medicine, surgery, nursing. **Holdings:** 600 books. **Subscriptions:** 120 journals and other serials.

★9365★ BROUGHTON HOSPITAL
JOHN S. MCKEE, JR., M.D. MEMORIAL LIBRARY
1000 S. Sterling St.
Morganton, NC 28655   Phone: (704) 433-2303
Mary E. Bush, Libn.
Subjects: Psychiatry, psychiatric social work, psychology, child psychiatry, geriatric psychiatry, medicine. **Holdings:** 3100 books; 2000 bound periodical volumes; clippings; archives; publications. **Subscriptions:** 27 journals and other serials.

★9366★ AMERICAN HOLISTIC NURSES ASSOCIATION
LIBRARY
4101 Lake Boome Trail, No. 201
Raleigh, NC 27607-6518   Phone: (919) 787-5181
Susan Rexer, Exec.Dir.
Subjects: Holistic health, nursing, communication. **Holdings:** 150 books; videotapes. **Subscriptions:** 15 journals and other serials.

★9367★ DOROTHEA DIX HOSPITAL
F.T. FULLER STAFF LIBRARY
S. Boylan Ave.
Box 7597
Raleigh, NC 27611   Phone: (919) 733-5111
Spanola M. Eubanks, Dir., Lib.Serv.
Subjects: Psychiatry, psychiatric nursing, social service, psychology, neurology. **Holdings:** 9450 books; 3536 bound periodical volumes; 350 reels of microfilm; 585 cassette tapes. **Subscriptions:** 142 journals and other serials.

★9368★ NORTH CAROLINA DEPARTMENT OF CULTURAL
RESOURCES
LIBRARY FOR THE BLIND AND PHYSICALLY HANDICAPPED
1811 Capital Blvd.
Raleigh, NC 27635   Phone: (919) 733-4376
Charles H. Fox, Reg.Libn.
Holdings: 180,000 books, including talking books on phonograph records and cassettes, braille books, large type books.

★9369★ NORTH CAROLINA DEPARTMENT OF
ENVIRONMENT, HEALTH, AND NATURAL RESOURCES
PUBLIC HEALTH PEST MANAGEMENT SECTION
ENVIRONMENTAL HEALTH DIVISION
LIBRARY
Box 27687
Raleigh, NC 27611-7687   Phone: (919) 733-6407
Dr. N.H. Newton, Chf.
Subjects: Vector-borne disease detection and control, integrated management for mosquito control, medical entomology, coastal ecology. **Holdings:** 200 volumes.

★9370★ NORTH CAROLINA DEPARTMENT OF LABOR
CHARLES H. LIVENGOOD, JR. MEMORIAL LABOR LAW
LIBRARY
4 W. Edenton St.
Raleigh, NC 27601   Phone: (919) 733-2799
Catherine Rubin, Libn.
Subjects: Labor law and history, occupational safety and health. **Holdings:** 4500 books; 60 bound periodical volumes; 2 vertical file cabinets; 1 box of microfiche; state government documents. **Subscriptions:** 45 journals and other serials.

★9371★ NORTH CAROLINA STATE UNIVERSITY
VETERINARY MEDICAL LIBRARY
College of Veterinary Medicine
Raleigh, NC 27606   Phone: (919) 829-4218
Subjects: Veterinary medicine, medicine, biology, biochemistry, pharmacology, toxicology. **Holdings:** 12,000 books; 15,000 bound periodical volumes; 250 autotutorial programs. **Subscriptions:** 1055 journals and other serials.

★9372★ REX HOSPITAL
LIBRARY
4420 Lake Boone Trail
Raleigh, NC 27607   Phone: (919) 783-3100
Dorothy T. McCallum, Libn.
Subjects: Medicine, nursing. **Holdings:** 1650 books; 2000 bound periodical volumes; 4 VF drawers of pamphlets, brochures, clippings. **Subscriptions:** 100 journals and other serials.

★9373★ WAKE COUNTY MEDICAL CENTER
MEDICAL LIBRARY
3000 New Bern Ave.
Raleigh, NC 27610   Phone: (919) 250-8528
Karen K. Grandage, Dir., Lib./Info.Serv.
Subjects: Medicine, pediatrics, orthopedics, nursing, hospital administration, allied health sciences. **Holdings:** 8000 books; 2988 bound periodical volumes; 1000 AV programs. **Subscriptions:** 300 journals and other serials.

★9374★ ANNIE PENN MEMORIAL HOSPITAL
MEDICAL LIBRARY
618 S. Main St.
Reidsville, NC 27320   Phone: (919) 349-8461
Sandra King, Libn.
Subjects: Medicine, nursing, allied health sciences. **Holdings:** 500 books. **Subscriptions:** 43 journals and other serials.

★9375★ BECTON DICKINSON RESEARCH CENTER
INFORMATION CENTER
Box 12016
Research Triangle Park, NC 27709   Phone: (919) 549-8641
Barbara K. Post, Hd., Info.Ctr.
Subjects: Biomedicine, organic chemistry, polymer chemistry, microbiology and immunology, materials science, business. **Holdings:** 1800 books; 150 bound periodical volumes; 350 microfiche; pamphlets. **Subscriptions:** 300 journals and other serials.

★9376★ BURROUGHS WELLCOME COMPANY
LIBRARY
3030 Cornwallis Rd.
Research Triangle Park, NC 27709   Phone: (919) 248-4908
Ildiko Trombitas, Mgr., Tech.Info.Dept.
Subjects: Organic chemistry, medicine, biochemistry, pharmacology, microbiology, toxicology, business. **Holdings:** 13,785 books; 30,539 bound periodical volumes; product literature files; 3 bookcases of archival materials. **Subscriptions:** 1581 journals and other serials; 9 newspapers.

★9377★ FAMILY HEALTH INTERNATIONAL
LIBRARY
PO Box 13950
Research Triangle Park, NC 27709   Phone: (919) 544-7040
William Barrows, Info.Serv.Mgr.
Subjects: Reproductive medicine, family planning, contraception, population, developing countries. **Holdings:** 4500 books; 800 unbound periodical volumes; 9000 reprints and unpublished documents; 330 patents. **Subscriptions:** 350 journals and other serials; 230 newsletters.

★9378★ GLAXO INC.
LIBRARY
5 Moore Dr.
Research Triangle Park, NC 27709   Phone: (919) 990-5382
Peggy F. Hull, Hd., Lib. & Info.Serv.
Subjects: Medicine, pharmacy and pharmacology, chemistry, biology, business, computer science. **Holdings:** 7636 books; 6000 bound periodical volumes; 200 annual reports. **Subscriptions:** 1404 journals and other serials; 6 newspapers.

★9379★ NATIONAL INSTITUTE OF ENVIRONMENTAL
HEALTH SCIENCES
LIBRARY
Box 12233
Research Triangle Park, NC 27709   Phone: (919) 541-3426
W. Davenport Robertson, Lib.Dir.
Subjects: Pharmacology, toxicology, mutagenesis, teratogenesis, cell biology, carcinogenesis. **Holdings:** 22,500 books; 2700 bound periodical volumes; 20,000 unbound periodical volumes; 2500 reels of microfilm; 3500 microfiche; 8 VF drawers of manuscripts; 200 reports on microfiche; 5 file drawers of internal reprints. **Subscriptions:** 800 journals and other serials.

★9380★ NORTHWEST AREA HEALTH EDUCATION CENTER
NW AHEC LIBRARY
Rowan Memorial Hospital
612 Mocksville Ave.
Salisbury, NC 28144   Phone: (704) 638-1069
Connie Schardt, AHEC Lib.Dir.
Subjects: Medicine, nursing, allied health sciences. Holdings: 900 books;
1734 bound periodical volumes. Subscriptions: 137 journals and other
serials.

★9381★ U.S. DEPARTMENT OF VETERANS AFFAIRS
MEDICAL CENTER LIBRARY
1601 Brenner Ave.
Salisbury, NC 28144   Phone: (704) 638-9000
Nancy Smith, Chf., Lib.Serv.
Subjects: Psychology, psychiatry, nursing, internal medicine, alcoholism,
surgery, gerontology, dentistry. Holdings: 2700 books; 1500 AV programs.
Subscriptions: 274 journals and other serials.

★9382★ WILMINGTON AREA HEALTH EDUCATION CENTER
LEARNING RESOURCE CENTER
LIBRARY
2131 S. 17th St.
Wilmington, NC 28402-9990   Phone: (919) 343-0161
Steve Owen, Dir.
Subjects: Internal medicine, nursing, oncology, cardiology, surgery, obstet-
rics and gynecology, allied health sciences. Holdings: 3000 books; 3000
bound periodical volumes; AV programs. Subscriptions: 250 journals and
other serials.

★9383★ WILSON MEMORIAL HOSPITAL
LEARNING CENTER/LIBRARY
1705 S. Tarboro St.
Wilson, NC 27893   Phone: (919) 399-8253
Rosa Edwards, Supv.
Subjects: Medicine, nursing, and allied health sciences. Holdings: 613
volumes; 730 video cassettes; 39 slide sets; 293 filmstrips; 269 audio
cassettes. Subscriptions: 90 journals and other serials.

★9384★ FORSYTH MEMORIAL HOSPITAL
JOHN C. WHITAKER LIBRARY
3333 Silas Creek Pkwy.
Winston-Salem, NC 27103-3090   Phone: (919) 760-5995
Margaret L. Cobb, Med.Libn.
Subjects: Medicine, allied health sciences. Holdings: 1000 books; 5330
bound periodical volumes; 300 videotapes. Subscriptions: 124 journals and
other serials.

★9385★ FORSYTH TECHNICAL COLLEGE
LIBRARY
2100 Silas Creek Pkwy.
Winston-Salem, NC 27103   Phone: (919) 723-0371
Audrey B. Zablocki, Dir.
Subjects: Technology, health, law, business, psychology, art. Holdings:
32,000 books; 1317 bound periodical volumes. Subscriptions: 303 journals
and other serials; 6 newspapers.

★9386★ WAKE FOREST UNIVERSITY
BOWMAN GRAY SCHOOL OF MEDICINE
COY C. CARPENTER LIBRARY
300 S. Hawthorne Rd.
Winston-Salem, NC 27103   Phone: (919) 748-4691
Michael D. Sprinkle, Dir.
Subjects: Medicine, nursing. Holdings: 31,143 books; 78,743 bound
periodical volumes; 1796 AV programs; 2028 microforms. Subscriptions:
3690 journals and other serials.

★9387★ WINSTON-SALEM STATE UNIVERSITY
C.G. O'KELLY LIBRARY
SPECIAL COLLECTIONS
Winston-Salem, NC 27110   Phone: (919) 750-2440
Vicki S. Miller, Ref.Libn.
Subjects: Nursing. Holdings: 5000 items.

North Dakota

★9388★ NORTH DAKOTA STATE DEPARTMENT OF HEALTH
DIVISION OF HEALTH PROMOTION AND EDUCATION
600 E. Boulevard Ave.
Bismarck, ND 58505-0200   Phone: (701) 224-2368
Lynette Pitzer, Film Libn.
Subjects: Health. Holdings: 1385 16mm films and videotapes; 800
pamphlet titles. Subscriptions: 25 journals and other serials.

★9389★ Q & R MEDCENTER ONE
HEALTH SCIENCES LIBRARY
622 Ave. A East
Bismarck, ND 58501   Phone: (701) 222-5390
Leeila Bina, Med.Libn.
Subjects: Clinical medicine, nursing, hospital administration. Holdings:
8000 books; 10,000 bound periodical volumes; 4 VF drawers of pamphlets
and reprints; 2000 AV items. Subscriptions: 300 journals and other serials.

★9390★ ST. JOSEPH'S HOSPITAL AND HEALTH CENTER
MEDICAL LIBRARY
30 W. 7th St.
Dickinson, ND 58601   Phone: (701) 225-7515
Sr. Salome Tlusty, Lib.Ck.
Subjects: Medicine, nursing, administration, life search (ADS and MHU),
womankind. Holdings: Figures not available. Subscriptions: 157 journals
and other serials; 4 newspapers.

★9391★ CENTER FOR THE RIGHTS OF THE TERMINALLY
ILL
RESOURCE LIBRARY
2319 18 Ave., S.
Fargo, ND 58103   Phone: (701) 237-5667
Julie A. Grimstad, Exec.Dir.
Subjects: Euthanasia and infanticide, "Right to Die" court cases, patients'
rights, suicide, death and dying, death education, care of the elderly.
Holdings: 50 books; 17 bound periodical volumes; 15,000 newspaper and
magazine articles; 10 AV programs. Subscriptions: 5 journals and other
serials; 4 newspapers.

★9392★ DAKOTA HOSPITAL
LIBRARY
1720 S. University Dr.
Box 6014
Fargo, ND 58108-6014   Phone: (701) 280-4187
Ardis Haaland, Med.Libn.
Subjects: Internal medicine, obstetrics and gynecology, physical medicine
and rehabilitation, nursing, surgery, pediatrics. Holdings: 2000 books;
3500 bound periodical volumes; 600 AV program titles. Subscriptions: 285
journals and other serials.

★9393★ LUTHERAN HOSPITALS AND HOMES SOCIETY
CORPORATE LIBRARY
1202 Westrac Dr.
Box 6200
Fargo, ND 58106-6200   Phone: (701) 293-9053
Subjects: Hospital management, hospital law, human resources develop-
ment, rehabilitation. Holdings: 400 books; 250 reports, manuals, pam-
phlets. Subscriptions: 102 journals and other serials.

★9394★ NEUROPSYCHIATRIC RESEARCH INSTITUTE
LIBRARY
700 1st Ave., S.
Fargo, ND 58103   Phone: (701) 239-1620
Diane Nordeng, Libn.
Subjects: Neurosurgery, neurology, psychiatry, neuropsychology. Holdings:
416 books; 1878 bound periodical volumes. Subscriptions: 52 journals and
other serials.

★9395★ NORTH DAKOTA STATE UNIVERSITY
PHARMACY LIBRARY
Sudro Hall
University Sta.
Fargo, ND 58105-5599   Phone: (701) 237-7748
Linda Schultz, Supv.
Subjects: Pharmacy, nursing. Holdings: 5276 books. Subscriptions: 367
journals and other serials.

★9396★ ST. LUKE'S HOSPITAL
MERITCARE LIBRARY
720 4th St., N.
Fargo, ND 58122   Phone: (701) 234-5571
Margaret Wagner, Lib.Mgr.
Subjects: Medicine, paramedicine, consumer medicine, nursing, hospital administration. **Holdings:** 3370 books; 3871 bound periodical volumes; 721 volumes on microfiche; 83 volumes on microfilm; 1080 AV programs. **Subscriptions:** 359 library journals and other serials; 309 hospital journals and other serials.

★9397★ SOUTHEAST HUMAN SERVICES CENTER
LIBRARY
700 1st Ave., S.
Fargo, ND 58103   Phone: (701) 239-1620
Diane Nordeng, Libn.
Subjects: Mental health, child growth and development, counseling.
Holdings: 210 books.

★9398★ U.S. DEPARTMENT OF VETERANS AFFAIRS
CENTER LIBRARY
2101 Elm St.
Fargo, ND 58102   Phone: (701) 232-3241
James Robbins, Chf., Lib.Serv.
Subjects: Medicine, dentistry, nursing, social work, hospital administration. **Holdings:** 2800 books; 5605 bound periodical volumes; 2 VF drawers of reprints, pamphlets, bibliographies. **Subscriptions:** 310 journals and other serials.

★9399★ UNITED HOSPITAL
LIBRARY
1200 S. Columbia Rd.
Grand Forks, ND 58201   Phone: (701) 780-5187
Patrice Conely, Med.Libn.
Subjects: Medicine, nursing, allied health sciences. **Holdings:** 1000 books; 3 VF drawers of pamphlets. **Subscriptions:** 257 journals and other serials.

★9400★ UNIVERSITY OF NORTH DAKOTA
SCHOOL OF MEDICINE
HARLEY E. FRENCH LIBRARY OF THE HEALTH SCIENCES
Grand Forks, ND 58202-9002   Phone: (701) 777-3993
David Boilard, Dir.
Subjects: Medicine, nursing, physical therapy. **Holdings:** 32,000 books; 40,000 bound periodical volumes; 1600 AV programs; 1450 volumes on microfiche. **Subscriptions:** 1113 journals and other serials.

★9401★ NORTH DAKOTA STATE HOSPITAL
HEALTH SCIENCE LIBRARY
Box 476
Jamestown, ND 58402-0476   Phone: (701) 253-3679
Denise K. Pahl, Act.Hd.
Subjects: Psychiatry, psychology, psychiatric rehabilitation, nursing, medicine, social work, alcoholism and addiction. **Holdings:** 6000 books; 3563 bound periodical volumes; 600 cassettes; 25 video cassettes; 44 biennial reports; 35 cases of pamphlets and miscellanea; 26 therapy films; 47 AV programs. **Subscriptions:** 103 journals and other serials.

★9402★ TRINITY MEDICAL CENTER
ANGUS L. CAMERON MEDICAL LIBRARY
Trinity Professional Bldg.
20 Burdick Expwy.
Minot, ND 58701   Phone: (701) 857-5435
Barb Knight, NW Campus Libn.
Subjects: Medicine, nursing. **Holdings:** 3000 books; 13.000 bound periodical volumes; 2000 AV programs. **Subscriptions:** 150 journals and other serials.

★9403★ MERCY HOSPITAL
MEDICAL LIBRARY
570 Chautauqua Blvd.
Valley City, ND 58072   Phone: (701) 845-0440
Pam Lacher, Lib.Mgr.
Subjects: Medicine. **Holdings:** 75 books. **Subscriptions:** 50 journals and other serials.

Ohio

★9404★ AKRON CITY HOSPITAL
MEDICAL LIBRARY
55 Arch St., Ste. 3-G
Akron, OH 44304   Phone: (216) 375-3260
Marilee S. Creelan, Dir., Hosp.Libs.
Subjects: Medicine, nursing, allied health sciences, social sciences, hospital administration. **Holdings:** 8200 books; 20,000 bound periodical volumes; 100 AV programs; 750 Audio-Digest tapes. **Subscriptions:** 370 journals and other serials.

★9405★ AKRON GENERAL MEDICAL CENTER
J.D. SMITH MEMORIAL LIBRARY
400 Wabash Ave.
Akron, OH 44307   Phone: (216) 384-6242
Christine J. Williams, Dir., Lib.Serv.
Subjects: Medicine. **Holdings:** 3200 books; 7000 bound periodical volumes; audiotapes. **Subscriptions:** 287 journals and other serials.

★9406★ CHILDREN'S HOSPITAL MEDICAL CENTER
MARY A. HOWER MEDICAL LIBRARY
281 Locust St.
Akron, OH 44308   Phone: (216) 379-8250
Julie Thom, Dir.
Subjects: Medicine, pediatrics. **Holdings:** 2833 books; 5000 bound periodical volumes. **Subscriptions:** 325 journals and other serials.

★9407★ ST. THOMAS MEDICAL CENTER
MEDICAL LIBRARY
444 N. Main St.
Akron, OH 44310   Phone: (216) 379-5505
Linda E. Bunyan, Med.Libn.
Subjects: Medicine, nursing, and allied health sciences. **Holdings:** 1758 books; 3381 bound periodical volumes; 400 cassette tapes; 600 slides; 1 file case of clippings and pamphlets; AV programs; computer software. **Subscriptions:** 170 journals and other serials.

★9408★ APPLE CREEK DEVELOPMENTAL CENTER
PROFESSIONAL LIBRARY/INFORMATION CENTER
2532 S. Apple Creek Rd.
Apple Creek, OH 44606   Phone: (216) 698-2411
John A. Kolarovsky, AV Spec.
Subjects: Mental retardation, behavior modification, psychology, medicine. **Holdings:** 1150 books. **Subscriptions:** 20 journals and other serials.

★9409★ ATHENS MENTAL HEALTH CENTER
STAFF LIBRARY
Richland Ave.
Athens, OH 45701   Phone: (614) 592-3031
Judy McGinn, Staff Libn.
Subjects: Psychology, psychiatry, medicine, nursing, sociology. **Holdings:** 3200 books; 675 bound periodical volumes; 150 indexes, directories, reference tools; 9 VF drawers of pamphlets and clippings; 150 audio cassette tapes. **Subscriptions:** 40 journals and other serials.

★9410★ OHIO UNIVERSITY
HEALTH SCIENCES LIBRARY
Athens, OH 45701   Phone: (614) 593-2680
Anne S. Goss, Dir.
Subjects: Medicine, nursing, psychology, basic sciences, allied health fields. **Holdings:** 36,172 books; 35,213 bound periodical volumes; 21,904 government documents; 14,012 microfiche. **Subscriptions:** 1489 journals and other serials.

★9411★ BARBERTON CITIZENS HOSPITAL
MEDICAL LIBRARY
155 5th St., NE
Barberton, OH 44203   Phone: (216) 745-1611
Subjects: Clinical medicine and nursing. **Holdings:** 962 books; 2487 bound periodical volumes. **Subscriptions:** 112 journals and other serials.

★9412★ U.S. DEPARTMENT OF VETERANS AFFAIRS
MEDICAL LIBRARY
10000 Brecksville Rd.
Brecksville, OH 44141   Phone: (216) 526-3030
Janet Monk Gillette, Chf., Reg.Lib.Serv.
Subjects: Psychology, nursing, psychiatry, social work, clinical medicine.
Holdings: 4807 volumes; 20 dissertations; 1900 AV programs. Subscriptions: 300 journals and other serials.

★9413★ NATIONAL REYE'S SYNDROME FOUNDATION
LIBRARY
426 N. Lewis
PO Box 829
Bryan, OH 43506   Phone: (419) 636-2679
Subjects: Reye's Syndrome - awareness, guidance, treatment, research.

★9414★ CAMBRIDGE MENTAL HEALTH AND
DEVELOPMENTAL CENTER
RESOURCE CENTER
County Rd. 35
Cambridge, OH 43725   Phone: (614) 439-1371
Noreen M. Kenney, Dir., Lib.Serv.
Subjects: Mental health, psychology, psychiatry, mental retardation. Holdings: 701 books; AV programs. Subscriptions: 70 journals and other serials.

★9415★ AULTMAN HOSPITAL
MEDICAL LIBRARY
2600 6th St., SW
Canton, OH 44710   Phone: (216) 452-9911
Leah R. Lloyd, Libn.
Subjects: Medicine. Holdings: 1657 books; 5661 bound periodical volumes; 90 AV programs. Subscriptions: 199 journals and other serials.

★9416★ AULTMAN HOSPITAL
SCHOOL OF NURSING LIBRARY
2614 6th St., SW
Canton, OH 44710   Phone: (216) 452-9911
Fay E. Rue, Lib.Asst.
Subjects: Nursing, medicine, education. Holdings: 5447 books; 470 bound periodical volumes; 8 VF drawers of pamphlets and clippings. Subscriptions: 94 journals and other serials.

★9417★ TIMKEN MERCY MEDICAL CENTER
MEDICAL LIBRARY
1320 Timken Mercy Dr.
Canton, OH 44708   Phone: (216) 489-1462
Nancy S. Erwin, Dir.
Subjects: Medicine, nursing, and allied health sciences. Holdings: 4000 books; 4100 bound periodical volumes; 400 AV programs. Subscriptions: 200 journals and other serials.

★9418★ U.S. DEPARTMENT OF VETERANS AFFAIRS
MEDICAL CENTER LIBRARY
Chillicothe, OH 45601   Phone: (614) 773-1141
John A. Package, Chf., Lib.Serv.
Subjects: Psychiatry, medicine, allied health sciences. Holdings: 2793 volumes. Subscriptions: 373 journals and other serials.

★9419★ BETHESDA OAK HOSPITAL
MEDICAL LIBRARY
619 Oak St.
Cincinnati, OH 45206   Phone: (513) 569-6176
Beth White, Med.Libn.
Subjects: Medicine, nursing, allied health sciences, health administration. Holdings: 1500 books. Subscriptions: 350 journals and other serials.

★9420★ CHILDREN'S HOSPITAL RESEARCH FOUNDATION
EDWARD L. PRATT LIBRARY
Elland & Bethesda Avenues
Cincinnati, OH 45229   Phone: (513) 559-4300
Barbarie F. Hill, Lib.Dir.
Subjects: Pediatrics, genetics, medicine. Holdings: 4500 books; 12,000 bound periodical volumes; 250 videotapes. Subscriptions: 280 journals and other serials.

★9421★ CINCINNATI COLLEGE OF MORTUARY SCIENCE
LIBRARY
Cohen Center
3860 Pacific Ave.
Cincinnati, OH 45207-1033   Phone: (513) 745-3631
Dan L. Flory, Pres.
Subjects: Mortuary science, funeral service, thanatology, death and dying, embalming, public health. Holdings: 5000 books; 1000 bound periodical volumes; filmstrips; cassettes. Subscriptions: 30 journals and other serials.

★9422★ CINCINNATI PSYCHOANALYTIC INSTITUTE
FREDERIC T. KAPP MEMORIAL LIBRARY
3001 Highland Ave.
Cincinnati, OH 45219   Phone: (513) 961-8886
Subjects: Psychoanalysis, psychiatry, mental health. Holdings: 3000 volumes; 300 reprints; 40 audio cassettes. Subscriptions: 45 journals and other serials.

★9423★ CITIZENS AGAINST TOBACCO SMOKE
LIBRARY
Box 36236
Cincinnati, OH 45236   Phone: (513) 984-8833
Ahron Leichtman, Pres.
Subjects: Smoking, health, nonsmokers' rights. Holdings: 300 volumes.

★9424★ COMMUNITY MUTUAL INSURANCE COMPANY
BLUE CROSS/BLUE SHIELD
COMMUNICATIONS RESOURCE CENTER
1351 William Howard Taft Rd., CK1-231
Cincinnati, OH 45206   Phone: (513) 872-8460
Maureen McKee, Rsrc.Ctr.Coord.
Subjects: Insurance, health care costs, health maintenance organizations, health education, management. Holdings: 900 books; 150 reports; 50 VF drawers of newspaper and magazine articles. Subscriptions: 120 journals and other serials; 8 newspapers.

★9425★ ELIZABETH GAMBLE DEACONESS HOME
ASSOCIATION
JAMES N. GAMBLE INSTITUTE OF MEDICAL RESEARCH
LIBRARY
2141 Auburn Ave.
Cincinnati, OH 45219   Phone: (513) 369-2540
Lisa L. McCormick, Res.Libn.
Subjects: Virology, oncology, immunology, cardiology, clinical medicine. Holdings: 4000 books; 5000 bound periodical volumes. Subscriptions: 282 journals and other serials.

★9426★ GOOD SAMARITAN HOSPITAL
HEALTH SCIENCES LIBRARY
3217 Clifton Ave.
Cincinnati, OH 45220-2489   Phone: (513) 872-2433
Rosalie V. Zajac, Dir.
Subjects: Clinical medicine, clinical surgery, nursing, neurosurgery, obstetrics, gynecology. Holdings: 7172 books; 13,747 bound periodical volumes; 120 AV programs; 1371 audio cassettes; 271 videotapes; 266 slide/tape sets. Subscriptions: 606 journals and other serials.

★9427★ JEWISH HOSPITAL OF CINCINNATI
MEDICAL LIBRARY
3200 Burnet Ave.
Cincinnati, OH 45229   Phone: (513) 569-2014
David Self, Med.Libn.
Subjects: Medicine. Holdings: 4000 books; 6000 bound periodical volumes; 280 video cassettes; 1000 audio cassettes. Subscriptions: 280 journals and other serials.

★9428★ LLOYD LIBRARY AND MUSEUM
917 Plum St.
Cincinnati, OH 45202   Phone: (513) 721-3707
Rebecca A. Perry, Libn.
Subjects: Botany, pharmacy, biology, chemistry, natural science, zoology, entomology, mycology. Holdings: 70,000 books; 120,000 bound periodical volumes; 120,000 pamphlets. Subscriptions: 500 journals and other serials.

★9429★ MARION MERRELL DOW PHARMACEUTICALS, INC.
MARION MERRELL DOW RESEARCH INSTITUTE LIBRARY
2110 E. Galbraith Rd.
Cincinnati, OH 45215   Phone: (513) 948-6300
Elaine Semancik, Mgr., Res.Lib.
Subjects: Chemistry, medicine, pharmacology, pharmacy. **Holdings:**
10,000 books; 20,500 bound periodical volumes; 2 VF drawers of
pamphlets; 4500 cartridges of microfilm of journals; 3500 microfiche.
Subscriptions: 750 journals and other serials.

★9430★ PROVIDENCE HOSPITAL
MEDICAL LIBRARY
2446 Kipling Ave.
Cincinnati, OH 45239   Phone: (513) 853-5806
Mary Lou Klapper
Subjects: Medicine, nursing, and allied health sciences. **Holdings:** 300
books; 4000 bound periodical volumes. **Subscriptions:** 179 journals and
other serials.

★9431★ PUBLIC LIBRARY OF CINCINNATI AND HAMILTON
COUNTY
LIBRARY FOR THE BLIND AND PHYSICALLY HANDICAPPED
Library Sq.
800 Vine St.
Cincinnati, OH 45202   Phone: (513) 369-6075
Donna Foust, Reg.Libn.
Subjects: Books for the blind and physically handicapped in braille, on
records and cassettes. **Holdings:** 19,054 volumes in braille; 67,815 record-
ed disc containers; 168,485 cassette containers. **Subscriptions:** 45 on
talking books; 40 in braille; 29 on cassettes.

★9432★ ST. FRANCIS-ST. GEORGE HOSPITAL
HEALTH SCIENCES LIBRARY
3131 Queen City Ave.
Cincinnati, OH 45238   Phone: (513) 389-5118
Carol Mayor, Libn.
Subjects: Medicine, nursing, hospital administration. **Holdings:** 830 books;
365 periodicals. **Subscriptions:** 143 journals and other serials.

★9433★ U.S. DEPARTMENT OF VETERANS AFFAIRS
MEDICAL CENTER LIBRARY
3200 Vine St.
Cincinnati, OH 45220   Phone: (513) 861-3100
Judith Alfred, Chf., Lib.Serv.
Subjects: Medicine, mental health, nursing, surgery. **Holdings:** 10,036
volumes. **Subscriptions:** 318 journals and other serials.

★9434★ U.S. NATIONAL INSTITUTE FOR OCCUPATIONAL
SAFETY AND HEALTH
TAFT CENTER C-21
LIBRARY
Robert A. Taft Laboratory
4676 Columbia Pkwy.
Cincinnati, OH 45226   Phone: (513) 533-8321
Janice Huy, Sect.Chf.
Subjects: Occupational safety and health, industrial hygiene and toxicolo-
gy. **Holdings:** 10,000 books; 10,000 bound periodical volumes. **Subscrip-
tions:** 400 journals and other serials.

★9435★ UNIVERSITY AFFILIATED CINCINNATI CENTER FOR
DEVELOPMENTAL DISORDERS
RESEARCH LIBRARY
Pavilion Bldg.
3300 Elland Ave.
Cincinnati, OH 45229   Phone: (513) 559-4626
Subjects: Developmental disabilities, mental retardation, learning disabilities, special education, pediatrics, neurology, nutrition, rehabilitation,
psychology, social work, vocational counseling. **Holdings:** 17,000 books;
2000 bound periodical volumes; 100 AV programs; 175,000 reprint articles
relating to developmental disorders and pediatrics; 4 VF drawers of staff
publications; 10,000 slides. **Subscriptions:** 250 journals and other serials.

★9436★ UNIVERSITY OF CINCINNATI
DEPARTMENT OF ENVIRONMENTAL HEALTH LIBRARY
Kettering Laboratory Library
3223 Eden Ave.
Cincinnati, OH 45267-0056   Phone: (513) 558-1721
Sherrie Kline, Sr.Res.Assoc./Libn.
Subjects: Environmental health, toxicology, physiology, analytical chemis-
try, statistics. **Holdings:** 6000 books; 4500 bound periodical volumes; 78
VF drawers of reprints, reports, translations; 400 microfiche; 565 unpubl-
ished reports. **Subscriptions:** 185 journals and other serials.

★9437★ UNIVERSITY OF CINCINNATI
MEDICAL CENTER INFORMATION AND COMMUNICATIONS
CINCINNATI MEDICAL HERITAGE CENTER
121 Wherry Hall
Eden & Bethesda Aves.
Cincinnati, OH 45267-0574   Phone: (513) 558-5120
Billie Broaddus, Dir.
Subjects: History of medicine and pharmacy. **Holdings:** 32,000 books;
3782 bound periodical volumes; 10,000 pamphlets; 3100 linear feet of
archives; 5000 photographs; 51 oral history videotapes; 150 diplomas and
certificates; 2000 medical instruments; 109 pharmacy jars (Cantagalli 15th
century replicas produced in 1890s). **Subscriptions:** 15 journals and other
serials.

★9438★ UNIVERSITY OF CINCINNATI
MEDICAL CENTER INFORMATION AND COMMUNICATIONS
HEALTH SCIENCES LIBRARY
231 Bethesda Ave.
Cincinnati, OH 45267-0574   Phone: (513) 558-5627
Phyllis Self, Ph.D.
Subjects: Medicine, biomedical sciences, pharmacy. **Holdings:** 53,701
books; 89,214 bound periodical volumes; 47,461 monographs. **Subscrip-
tions:** 3057 journals and other serials.

★9439★ UNIVERSITY OF CINCINNATI
MEDICAL CENTER INFORMATION AND COMMUNICATIONS
NURSING EDUCATIONAL RESOURCES
3110 Vine St.
Cincinnati, OH 45221-0038   Phone: (513) 558-8378
Leslie Schick, Dir., Lib.Serv.
Subjects: Nursing, clinical medicine, gerontology, education, sociology.
Holdings: 20,000 volumes; 500 AV programs. **Subscriptions:** 475 journals
and other serials.

★9440★ UNIVERSITY OF CINCINNATI
RAYMOND WALTERS COLLEGE
LIBRARY
9555 Plainfield Rd.
Cincinnati, OH 45236   Phone: (513) 745-5710
Lucy Wilson, Coll.Libn.
Holdings: 50,000 books; 12,000 microforms. **Subscriptions:** 671 journals
and other serials; 16 newspapers.

★9441★ BENJAMIN ROSE INSTITUTE
LIBRARY
500 Hanna Bldg.
1422 Euclid Ave.
Cleveland, OH 44115   Phone: (216) 621-7201
Karen McNally Bensing, Libn.
Subjects: Aged - research, home care, long-term care, nursing homes, social
work, nursing. **Holdings:** 3600 books; 116 bound periodical volumes; 7
lateral file drawers and 4 VF drawers of reports, papers, manuscripts.
Subscriptions: 76 journals and other serials.

★9442★ BRENTWOOD HOSPITAL
LIBRARY
4110 Warrensville Center Rd.
Cleveland, OH 44122   Phone: (216) 283-3458
Jean Dreifort, Dir., Educ.Info.Serv.
Subjects: Medicine, osteopathic medicine. **Holdings:** 5000 books; 1300
bound periodical volumes; 550 AV programs; 30 shelves of video cassettes;
28 drawers of audio cassettes. **Subscriptions:** 452 journals and other serials.

★9443★ CASE WESTERN RESERVE UNIVERSITY
ELDERLY CARE RESEARCH CENTER
LIBRARY
Mather Memorial, Rm. 226
Cleveland, OH 44106   Phone: (216) 368-2700
Eva Kahana, Ph.D., Dir., Res. Center
Subjects: Sociology of aging, gerontology, medical sociology, environmental psychology/sociology. **Holdings:** 500 books; 300 bound periodical volumes; 200 other cataloged items.

★9444★ CASE WESTERN RESERVE UNIVERSITY
FES INFORMATION CENTER
25100 Euclid Ave., Ste. 105
Cleveland, OH 44117   Phone: (216) 231-3257
Geoffrey Thrope, Dir.
Subjects: Electrical stimulation, rehabilitation. **Holdings:** 12 books; 24 bound periodical volumes; 20 reports. **Subscriptions:** 2 journals and other serials.

★9445★ CASE WESTERN RESERVE UNIVERSITY
LAW SCHOOL LIBRARY
11075 East Blvd.
Cleveland, OH 44106   Phone: (216) 368-2792
Kathleen M. Carrick, Dir.
Subjects: Law, international law, medical jurisprudence. **Holdings:** 225,000 books; 47,482 microcards; 126 reels of microfilm; 57,379 microfiche; 501 VF materials; 1700 unbound reports, pamphlets, documents. **Subscriptions:** 3610 journals and other serials; 12 newspapers.

★9446★ CASE WESTERN RESERVE UNIVERSITY
LILLIAN AND MILFORD HARRIS LIBRARY
Mandel School of Applied Social Sciences
11235 Bellflower Rd.
Cleveland, OH 44106   Phone: (216) 368-2302
Arthur S. Biagianti, Dir./Libn.
Subjects: Social work, social welfare, poverty, alcoholism, corrections, aging, child welfare, minority group relations, community organization, psychiatry and mental health. **Holdings:** 22,000 books; 1500 bound periodical volumes; 7000 pamphlets and monographs; 533 microforms; 274 AV programs. **Subscriptions:** 309 journals and other serials.

★9447★ CENTER FOR HEALTH AFFAIRS
GREATER CLEVELAND HOSPITAL ASSOCIATION LIBRARY
Playhouse Sq.
1226 Huron Rd.
Cleveland, OH 44115   Phone: (216) 696-6900
Dorothy R. Leicht, Asst.Libn.
Subjects: Administration of health care facilities; hospital administration; health services - planning, education, statistics, demographics; association management. **Holdings:** 5000 books; 70 bound periodical volumes; 50 shelves of other cataloged items; 10 VF drawers of reports and newsletters; annual reports. **Subscriptions:** 261 journals and other serials.

★9448★ CLEVELAND CLINIC FOUNDATION
LIBRARY SERVICES DEPARTMENT
9500 Euclid Ave.
Cleveland, OH 44195-5243   Phone: (216) 444-5697
Gretchen Hallerberg, Mgr., Lib.Serv.Dept.
Subjects: Medical sciences. **Holdings:** 7000 books; 28,000 bound periodical volumes. **Subscriptions:** 700 journals and other serials.

★9449★ CLEVELAND HEALTH SCIENCES LIBRARY
2119 Abington Rd.
Cleveland, OH 44106   Phone: (216) 368-3427
Robert G. Cheshier, Dir.
Subjects: Medicine, dentistry, nursing, biology, nutrition. **Holdings:** 133,067 books; 215,889 bound periodical volumes; 2048 AV programs; 100 microforms. **Subscriptions:** 2841 journals and other serials.

★9450★ CLEVELAND HEALTH SCIENCES LIBRARY
ALLEN MEMORIAL LIBRARY
11000 Euclid Ave.
Cleveland, OH 44106   Phone: (216) 368-3640
Lillian S. Levine, Asst.Dir.
Subjects: Medicine. **Holdings:** 76,356 books; 107,793 bound periodical volumes. **Subscriptions:** 1332 journals and other serials.

★9451★ CLEVELAND HEALTH SCIENCES LIBRARY
HEALTH CENTER LIBRARY
2119 Abington Rd.
Cleveland, OH 44106   Phone: (216) 368-4540
Marjorie Saunders, Assoc.Dir.
Subjects: Medicine, nursing, dentistry, nutrition, biology. **Holdings:** 108,096 serials; 56,711 monographs; 2048 AV programs. **Subscriptions:** 1509 journals and other serials.

★9452★ CLEVELAND HEALTH SCIENCES LIBRARY
MEDICAL HISTORY DIVISION
11000 Euclid Ave.
Cleveland, OH 44106   Phone: (216) 368-3648
Dr. Patsy A. Gerstner, Chf.Cur.
Subjects: History of medicine. **Holdings:** 35,000 books; 75,000 artifacts.

★9453★ CLEVELAND HEARING AND SPEECH CENTER
LUCILE DAUBY GRIES MEMORIAL LIBRARY
11206 Euclid Ave.
Cleveland, OH 44106   Phone: (216) 231-8787
Subjects: Audiology, speech, language, deafness, rehabilitation, psychology. **Holdings:** 1200 books; 490 bound periodical volumes; 90 dissertations; 4 VF drawers of reprints, abstracts, former comprehensive examinations. **Subscriptions:** 29 journals and other serials.

★9454★ CLEVELAND PSYCHIATRIC INSTITUTE
KARNOSH MEDICAL LIBRARY
1708 Aiken Ave.
Cleveland, OH 44109   Phone: (216) 661-6200
Michael Petit, Libn.
Subjects: Psychology, psychiatry, psychoanalysis, medicine, sociology, clinical neurology, psychological nursing, social work. **Holdings:** 5740 books; 1819 bound periodical volumes; 5 VF drawers of pamphlets; 301 cassette tapes; 16 reels of tape; 64 slides. **Subscriptions:** 60 journals and other serials.

★9455★ CLEVELAND PSYCHOANALYTIC INSTITUTE
LIBRARY
11328 Euclid Ave., No. 205
Cleveland, OH 44106   Phone: (216) 229-2111
Jane Zimring, Libn.
Subjects: Psychoanalysis, child therapy. **Holdings:** 1500 books; 440 bound periodical volumes; 170 tape recordings of scientific psychoanalytic meetings; 8 shelves of unbound periodicals; 10 boxes of reprints; 25 boxes of unpublished papers. **Subscriptions:** 15 journals and other serials.

★9456★ FAIRVIEW GENERAL HOSPITAL
MEDICAL LIBRARY
18101 Lorain Ave.
Cleveland, OH 44111   Phone: (216) 476-7118
Susan L. Favorite, Dir.
Subjects: Internal medicine, obstetrics, gynecology, surgery, pediatrics, nursing. **Holdings:** 8700 books; 3520 bound periodical volumes. **Subscriptions:** 442 journals and other serials.

★9457★ LUTHERAN MEDICAL CENTER
C.W. NEVEL MEMORIAL LIBRARY
2609 Franklin Blvd.
Cleveland, OH 44113   Phone: (216) 363-2143
Irene B. Szentkiralyi, Libn.
Subjects: Medicine, surgery, nursing, allied health sciences. **Holdings:** 2000 volumes; 300 cassettes and filmstrips. **Subscriptions:** 108 journals and other serials.

★9458★ MERIDIA HURON HOSPITAL
PROFESSIONAL LIBRARY
13951 Terrace Rd.
Cleveland, OH 44112   Phone: (216) 761-3300
Keith A. Stincic, Lib.Dir.
Subjects: Medicine, nursing, hospital administration, allied health sciences. **Holdings:** 2000 books; 1800 bound periodical volumes; 4 VF drawers; cassette tapes. **Subscriptions:** 150 journals and other serials.

★9459★   METROHEALTH MEDICAL CENTER
HAROLD H. BRITTINGHAM MEMORIAL LIBRARY
3395 Scranton Rd.
Cleveland, OH 44109-9990   Phone: (216) 459-5623
Christine A. Dziedzina, Chf.Libn.
Subjects: Medicine, nursing. **Holdings:** 9985 books; 24,448 bound periodical volumes; 4 VF drawers of pamphlets. **Subscriptions:** 485 journals and other serials.

★9460★   MOUNT SINAI MEDICAL CENTER OF CLEVELAND
GEORGE H. HAYS MEMORIAL LIBRARY
1 Mount Sinai Dr.
Cleveland, OH 44106-4198   Phone: (216) 421-5615
Pamela Alderman, Dir.
Subjects: Medicine, nursing, hospital administration, allied health sciences. **Holdings:** 6000 books; 3000 bound periodical volumes; 8 VF drawers of pamphlets. **Subscriptions:** 352 journals and other serials.

★9461★   OHIO COLLEGE OF PODIATRIC MEDICINE
LIBRARY/MEDIA CENTER
10515 Carnegie Ave.
Cleveland, OH 44106   Phone: (216) 231-3300
Judy Mehl Cowell, Dir.
Subjects: Podiatric medicine, orthopedics, dermatology, biomechanics, sports medicine. **Holdings:** 11,000 books; 2000 bound periodical volumes; 300 AV programs; VF drawers of pamphlet material; 800 reprints; School Papers File; state file. **Subscriptions:** 225 journals and other serials.

★9462★   PLANNED PARENTHOOD OF CLEVELAND
LIBRARY
3135 Euclid Ave., No. 101
Cleveland, OH 44115   Phone: (216) 881-7742
Betsey C. Kaufman, Exec.Dir.
Subjects: Birth control and contraceptives, family planning, population, sexuality, family life education. **Holdings:** 600 books; 10 films; 103 videotapes. **Subscriptions:** 10 journals and other serials.

★9463★   ST. ALEXIS HOSPITAL
HEALTH SCIENCES LIBRARY
5163 Broadway Ave.
Cleveland, OH 44127   Phone: (216) 429-8245
Verne Zach
Subjects: Medicine, allied health sciences, hospitals, nursing. **Holdings:** 2000 books; 1500 bound periodical volumes; 400 AV programs; pamphlets; reprints. **Subscriptions:** 175 journals and other serials.

★9464★   ST. LUKE'S HOSPITAL
TAYLOR FAMILY HEALTH SCIENCES LIBRARY
11311 Shaker Blvd.
Cleveland, OH 44104   Phone: (216) 368-7699
Pam Billick, Dir.
Subjects: Medicine, nursing, management. **Holdings:** 2500 books; 6300 bound periodical volumes. **Subscriptions:** 350 journals and other serials.

★9465★   ST. VINCENT CHARITY HOSPITAL
LIBRARY
2351 E. 22nd St.
Cleveland, OH 44115   Phone: (216) 861-6200
Joanne Billiar, Hd.Libn.
Subjects: Medicine, nursing, administration, allied health sciences. **Holdings:** 2500 titles; 3 audio cassette series. **Subscriptions:** 180 journals and other serials.

★9466★   UNIVERSITY HOSPITALS OF CLEVELAND AND
  CASE WESTERN RESERVE UNIVERSITY
DEPARTMENT OF PATHOLOGY
LIBRARY
2085 Adelbert Rd.
Cleveland, OH 44106   Phone: (216) 368-2482
Jeanette W. Nagy, Dir.
Subjects: Pathology, biochemistry, obstetrics, gynecology, surgery, neuropathology, immunology, histology, cytology. **Holdings:** 2000 books; 7000 bound periodical volumes; reprints; theses; dissertations. **Subscriptions:** 75 journals and other serials.

★9467★   CHILDREN'S HOSPITAL
LIBRARY
700 Children's Dr.
Columbus, OH 43205   Phone: (614) 461-2713
Susan Kroll, Act.Hd.Libn.
Subjects: Pediatrics, allied health sciences. **Holdings:** 4200 books; 8500 bound periodical volumes. **Subscriptions:** 300 journals and other serials.

★9468★   DOCTORS HOSPITAL
W.S. KONOLD MEMORIAL LIBRARY
1087 Dennison Ave., LIBID 43201B
Columbus, OH 43201   Phone: (614) 297-4113
Subjects: Osteopathy, medicine, nursing. **Holdings:** 3000 books; 10,000 bound periodical volumes; 300 slide sets; 500 videotapes; 900 audiotapes. **Subscriptions:** 225 journals and other serials.

★9469★   GRANT HOSPITAL
MEDICAL LIBRARY
111 S. Grant Ave.
Columbus, OH 43215   Phone: (614) 461-3467
Nancy E. Cohen, Libn.
Subjects: Medicine, nursing, allied health sciences. **Holdings:** 5500 books; 6500 bound periodical volumes; audiotapes; 9 VF drawers. **Subscriptions:** 250 journals and other serials.

★9470★   MOUNT CARMEL HEALTH
MOTHER M. CONSTANTINE MEMORIAL LIBRARY
793 W. State St.
Columbus, OH 43222   Phone: (614) 225-5214
Pamela M. Elwell, Dir.
Subjects: Medicine, nursing, allied health sciences, health administration. **Holdings:** 3500 books; 20,000 bound periodical volumes; kits; slides; audio cassettes. **Subscriptions:** 450 journals and other serials.

★9471★   OHIO BUREAU OF WORKERS' COMPENSATION
REHABILITATION DIVISION LIBRARY
2050 Kenny Rd.
Columbus, OH 43221   Phone: (614) 421-1150
Melissa Heilman
Subjects: Rehabilitation of the injured worker; back pain treatment; therapy - physical, psychological, occupational, vocational. **Holdings:** 1000 books. **Subscriptions:** 80 journals and other serials; 2 newspapers.

★9472★   OHIO DEPARTMENT OF AGING
RESOURCE CENTER
50 W. Broad St.
Columbus, OH 43266-0501   Phone: (614) 466-9086
Cheryl A. Canaday, Rsrc.Ctr.Coord.
Subjects: Aged and aging, social services, demographics. **Holdings:** 300 AV programs; government reports and other monographs; VF drawers. **Subscriptions:** 100 serials.

★9473★   OHIO DEPARTMENT OF DRUG AND ALCOHOL
  ADDICTION SERVICES
REGIONAL ALCOHOL AND DRUG AWARENESS
RESOURCE CENTER
170 N. High St., 3rd Fl.
Columbus, OH 43215   Phone: (614) 466-7893
Deborah Chambers, Prevention Spec.
Subjects: Drug abuse, alcohol, AIDS. **Holdings:** 1000 books. **Subscriptions:** 17 journals and other serials.

★9474★   OHIO DEPARTMENT OF MENTAL HEALTH
EDUCATIONAL MEDIA CENTER
2401 W. Walnut St.
Columbus, OH 43223   Phone: (614) 466-6013
Subjects: Mental health, prevention of mental illness, social issues, clinical issues. **Holdings:** 450 films.

★9475★   OHIO DIVISION OF SAFETY AND HYGIENE
RESOURCE CENTER
246 N. High St.
Columbus, OH 43215   Phone: (614) 466-7388
Rosemary Larkins, Mgr.
Subjects: Occupational safety, industrial hygiene. **Holdings:** 4000 books; 850 standards; 200 microfiche; 20 VF drawers of pamphlets; 650 subject headings; 2 VF drawers of clippings. **Subscriptions:** 280 journals and other serials.

★9476★ OHIO SCHOOL FOR THE DEAF
LIBRARY
500 Morse Rd.
Columbus, OH 43214   Phone: (614) 888-3221
Ada G. Kent, Libn., Media Spec.
Subjects: General collection, deafness, professional education. **Holdings:** 14,000 books; archival materials. **Subscriptions:** 42 journals and other serials.

★9477★ OHIO STATE SCHOOL FOR THE BLIND
LIBRARY
5220 N. High St.
Columbus, OH 43214   Phone: (614) 888-1122
Beverly Kessler, Libn.
Subjects: Special education with emphasis on blindness. **Holdings:** 9000 books; 1500 AV programs; 150 models. **Subscriptions:** 120 journals and other serials.

★9478★ OHIO STATE UNIVERSITY
JOHN A. PRIOR HEALTH SCIENCES LIBRARY
376 W. 10th Ave.
Columbus, OH 43210   Phone: (614) 292-9810
Susan Kroll, Interim Dir.
Subjects: Clinical medicine, dentistry, nursing, allied health sciences, experimental medicine, optometry. **Holdings:** 192,298 volumes; 4362 government documents. **Subscriptions:** 2169 journals and other serials.

★9479★ OHIO STATE UNIVERSITY
PHARMACY LIBRARY
207 Parks Hall
500 W. 12th Ave.
Columbus, OH 43210   Phone: (614) 292-8026
Hazel Benson, Hd.Libn.
Subjects: Pharmacy, pharmaceutical chemistry, pharmacology, pharmacognosy, pharmacy administration. **Holdings:** 33,089 volumes; 2100 pamphlets. **Subscriptions:** 440 journals and other serials.

★9480★ OHIO STATE UNIVERSITY
SOCIAL WORK LIBRARY
400 Stillman Hall
1947 College Rd.
Columbus, OH 43210   Phone: (614) 292-6627
Jennifer Kuehn, Hd.Libn.
Subjects: Social work education, criminology, social group work, family, social casework, mental health. **Holdings:** 41,534 volumes; 700 pamphlets. **Subscriptions:** 263 journals and other serials.

★9481★ OHIO STATE UNIVERSITY
VETERINARY MEDICINE LIBRARY
229 Sisson Hall
1900 Coffey Rd.
Columbus, OH 43210   Phone: (614) 292-6107
Norma Bruce
Subjects: Veterinary medicine, medicine, pharmacology, biochemistry, comparative medicine. **Holdings:** 41,066 volumes. **Subscriptions:** 507 journals and other serials.

★9482★ RIVERSIDE METHODIST HOSPITAL
D.J. VINCENT MEDICAL LIBRARY
3535 Olentangy River Rd.
Columbus, OH 43214   Phone: (614) 261-5230
Josephine W. Yeoh, Dir.
Subjects: Clinical medicine, nursing, hospital administration, microcomputers, management, patient education, fiction. **Holdings:** 22,000 books; 15,000 bound periodical volumes; 4 Audio-Digest tapes; NCME video cassettes; books, videotapes, and pamphlet files for patient education; professional reprints file; 500 archives of papers published by professionals connected with the hospital. **Subscriptions:** 500 journals and other serials.

★9483★ ROSS LABORATORIES
LIBRARY
625 Cleveland Ave.
Columbus, OH 43216   Phone: (614) 227-3503
Linda Mitro Hopkins, Mgr.
Subjects: Nutrition, food technology, business, analytical chemistry. **Holdings:** 3500 books; 6000 bound periodical volumes. **Subscriptions:** 550 journals and other serials.

★9484★ ST. ANTHONY MEDICAL CENTER
PHILIP B. HARDYMON LIBRARY
1492 E. Broad St.
Columbus, OH 43205   Phone: (614) 251-3248
Pamela L. Caruzzi, Chf.Med.Libn.
Subjects: Medicine, medical specialties. **Holdings:** 2800 books; 3500 bound periodical volumes; 92 pamphlets; 392 audio cassettes; holdings in various hospital departments. **Subscriptions:** 200 journals and other serials.

★9485★ FALLSVIEW PSYCHIATRIC HOSPITAL
STAFF LIBRARY
330 Broadway, E.
Cuyahoga Falls, OH 44221   Phone: (216) 929-8301
Joy Prichard, Libn.
Subjects: Psychology, psychiatry, psychiatric nursing, pastoral counseling. **Holdings:** 3000 books. **Subscriptions:** 40 journals and other serials.

★9486★ CHILDREN'S MEDICAL CENTER
LIBRARY
1 Children's Plaza
Dayton, OH 45404   Phone: (513) 226-8307
Jane R. Bottoms, Libn.
Subjects: Pediatrics, allied health sciences. **Holdings:** 2000 books; 5000 bound periodical volumes. **Subscriptions:** 240 journals and other serials.

★9487★ DAYTON MENTAL HEALTH CENTER
STAFF LIBRARY
2611 Wayne Ave.
Dayton, OH 45420   Phone: (513) 258-0440
Leonard Skonecki, Libn.
Subjects: Psychiatry, psychology, medicine, social work. **Holdings:** 660 books. **Subscriptions:** 17 journals and other serials.

★9488★ GOOD SAMARITAN HOSPITAL
SHANK MEMORIAL LIBRARY
2222 Philadelphia Dr.
Dayton, OH 45406   Phone: (513) 278-2612
Elizabeth A. Robinson, Libn.
Subjects: Medicine. **Holdings:** 6000 books; 14,000 bound periodical volumes; 1026 Audio-Digest tapes; 120 videotapes; 8 VF drawers of pamphlets. **Subscriptions:** 420 journals and other serials.

★9489★ GRANDVIEW HOSPITAL
MEDICAL LIBRARY
405 Grand Ave.
Dayton, OH 45405   Phone: (513) 226-3379
Candy Winteregg, Dir.
Subjects: Osteopathy, anesthesia, ophthalmology, orthopedics. **Holdings:** 4500 books; 3500 bound periodical volumes. **Subscriptions:** 406 journals and other serials.

★9490★ MIAMI VALLEY HOSPITAL
CRAIG MEMORIAL LIBRARY
1 Wyoming St.
Dayton, OH 45409   Phone: (513) 223-6192
Margaret C. Hardy, Dir.
Subjects: Medicine, nursing, allied health sciences. **Holdings:** 7745 books; 32,000 bound periodical volumes; 12 VF drawers of pamphlets; 12 VF drawers of hospital archives. **Subscriptions:** 600 journals and other serials.

★9491★ ST. ELIZABETH MEDICAL CENTER
HEALTH SCIENCES LIBRARY
601 Edwin Moses Blvd., W.
Dayton, OH 45408   Phone: (513) 229-6061
Ann L. Lewis, Med.Libn.
Subjects: Medicine, sports medicine, rehabilitation, physical medicine, family practice, gastroenterology. **Holdings:** 7239 books; 6752 bound periodical volumes; AV programs. **Subscriptions:** 450 journals and other serials.

★9492★ U.S. DEPARTMENT OF VETERANS AFFAIRS
CENTER LIBRARY SERVICE
4100 W. 3rd St.
Dayton, OH 45428   Phone: (513) 268-6511
Lendell Beverly, Chf., Lib.Serv.
Subjects: Medicine, nursing, hospital administration, patient education, military history. **Holdings:** 7000 books; 4840 bound periodical volumes. **Subscriptions:** 500 journals and other serials; 22 newspapers.

★9493★ WRIGHT STATE UNIVERSITY
SCHOOL OF MEDICINE
FORDHAM HEALTH SCIENCES LIBRARY
3640 Colonel Glenn Hwy.
Dayton, OH 45435   Phone: (513) 873-2266
Sarah S. Timmons, Act.Hea.Sci.Libn.
Subjects: Medicine, human anatomy, microbiology, physiology, psychology, biochemistry. **Holdings:** 44,871 books; 50,367 bound periodical volumes; 2678 AV programs; 191 computer software programs. **Subscriptions:** 1335 journals and other serials.

★9494★ ELYRIA MEMORIAL HOSPITAL
LIBRARY
630 E. River St.
Elyria, OH 44035   Phone: (216) 323-3221
Linda Masek, Hd.Libn.
Subjects: Orthopedics, nursing, pediatrics. **Holdings:** 3783 books; 3102 bound periodical volumes; 20 VF drawers of pamphlets, reports, clippings, bibliographies, AV programs. **Subscriptions:** 260 journals and other serials.

★9495★ HOLZER MEDICAL CENTER
MEDICAL LIBRARY
385 Jackson Pike
Gallipolis, OH 45631   Phone: (614) 446-5057
Beverly J. Jackson, Libn.
Subjects: Medicine, surgery, urology, pediatrics, diseases of the eye, ear, nose and throat, oncology, cardiology, radiation oncology. **Holdings:** 2500 books; 70 periodical titles.

★9496★ FORT HAMILTON-HUGHES MEMORIAL HOSPITAL
CENTER
SOHN MEMORIAL HEALTH SERVICES LIBRARY
630 Eaton Ave.
Hamilton, OH 45013   Phone: (513) 867-2310
Judy Leeds, Libn.
Subjects: Medicine. **Holdings:** 1000 books; 467 periodical volumes. **Subscriptions:** 50 journals and other serials.

★9497★ MERCY HOSPITAL
HEALTH SCIENCES LIBRARY
100 Riverfront Plaza
Hamilton, OH 45011   Phone: (513) 867-6458
Sr. Mary Annrita Mitchell, Libn.
Subjects: Medicine, nursing, hospital administration, allied health sciences. **Holdings:** 2000 books; 4 VF drawers of pamphlets and clippings. **Subscriptions:** 200 journals and other serials.

★9498★ CENTER FOR HUMANE OPTIONS IN CHILDBIRTH
EXPERIENCES
LIBRARY
5426 Madison St.
Hilliard, OH 43026
Abby Kinne, Founder
Subjects: Home birth, Lamaze method, natural childbirth, breast feeding, birth alternatives, nutrition, midwifery, Monitrice program for hospital coaches. **Holdings:** 400 books; films; pamphlets; statistical reports.

★9499★ KENT STATE UNIVERSITY
SPEECH AND HEARING CLINIC
LIBRARY
Kent, OH 44242   Phone: (213) 672-3150
Dr. Toliver
Subjects: Speech, language, communication disorders, psycholinguistics, audiology, language disorders, speech pathology. **Holdings:** Figures not available.

★9500★ KETTERING COLLEGE OF MEDICAL ARTS
LEARNING RESOURCES CENTER
3737 Southern Blvd.
Kettering, OH 45429   Phone: (513) 296-7201
Sheila Shellabarger, Dir.
Subjects: Nursing, allied health sciences. **Holdings:** 53,513 volumes; 6289 AV programs. **Subscriptions:** 507 journals and other serials.

★9501★ KETTERING MEDICAL CENTER HOSPITAL
MEDICAL LIBRARY
3535 Southern Blvd.
Kettering, OH 45429   Phone: (513) 298-4331
Dr. Joseph P. Stoia, Lib.Dir.
Subjects: Medicine, allied health sciences. **Holdings:** 8600 books; 16,500 bound periodical volumes; 3776 AV programs; 32,000 microfiche. **Subscriptions:** 672 journals and other serials; 6 newspapers.

★9502★ LAKEWOOD HOSPITAL
MEDICAL LIBRARY
14519 Detroit Ave.
Lakewood, OH 44107   Phone: (216) 521-4200
Jo Ann Hudson, Dir.
Subjects: Medicine, nursing, hospital administration, sciences. **Holdings:** 6605 books; 4787 bound periodical volumes; pamphlet files. **Subscriptions:** 352 journals and other serials; 5 newspapers.

★9503★ LIMA MEMORIAL HOSPITAL
HEALTH SCIENCES LIBRARY
Linden & Mobel Sts.
Lima, OH 45804   Phone: (419) 228-3335
Margaret S. Cutter, Hea.Sci.Libn.
Subjects: Medicine, nursing, pharmacology, hospital administration. **Holdings:** 1400 books; 682 bound periodical volumes; 1 drawer of clippings, pamphlets, documents. **Subscriptions:** 50 journals and other serials.

★9504★ LIMA STATE HOSPITAL
OAKWOOD FORENSIC CENTER
3200 N. West St.
Lima, OH 45801   Phone: (419) 225-8052
Mary Bice, Libn.
Subjects: Philosophy and psychology, religion, social service, science, psychiatry. **Holdings:** 14,000 books; 78 bound periodical volumes; 2500 tapes. **Subscriptions:** 32 journals and other serials; 14 newspapers.

★9505★ ST. RITA'S MEDICAL CENTER
MEDICAL LIBRARY
730 W. Market St.
Lima, OH 45801   Phone: (419) 227-3361
Sharon A. Bilopavlovich, Libn.
Subjects: Medicine. **Holdings:** 1552 volumes. **Subscriptions:** 59 journals and other serials.

★9506★ LORAIN COMMUNITY HOSPITAL
MEDICAL STAFF LIBRARY
3700 Kolbe Rd.
Lorain, OH 44053   Phone: (216) 960-3327
Patti Ryder, Med.Lib.Coord.
Subjects: Medicine, nursing, psychiatry, alcoholism. **Holdings:** 1200 books; 150 bound periodical volumes; 1500 unbound journals. **Subscriptions:** 140 journals and other serials.

★9507★ ST. JOSEPH HOSPITAL AND HEALTH CENTER
MEDICAL LIBRARY
205 W. 20th St.
Lorain, OH 44052   Phone: (216) 245-6851
John L. Reese, Libn.
Subjects: Medicine, nursing. **Holdings:** 1597 books; 1650 bound periodical volumes; 386 video cassettes. **Subscriptions:** 187 journals and other serials.

★9508★ MANSFIELD GENERAL HOSPITAL
MEDICAL LIBRARY
335 Glessner Ave.
Mansfield, OH 44903   Phone: (419) 526-8515
Marilyn J. Roe, Med.Libn.
Subjects: Nursing, medicine, and allied subjects. **Holdings:** 1700 books; 85 bound periodical volumes; 6 microfiche.

★9509★ FREDERICK C. SMITH CLINIC
MEDICAL LIBRARY
1040 Delaware Ave.
Marion, OH 43302   Phone: (614) 383-8098
B. Darlene Dyer, Libn.
Subjects: Medicine. **Holdings:** 750 books; 2000 bound periodical volumes. **Subscriptions:** 100 journals and other serials.

★9510★ MARION GENERAL HOSPITAL
MEDICAL LIBRARY
McKinley Park Dr.
Marion, OH 43302   Phone: (614) 383-8668
Marilyn J. Roe, Med.Libn.
Subjects: Medicine, nursing. **Holdings:** 500 books; 1800 bound periodical volumes. **Subscriptions:** 85 journals and other serials.

★9511★ DOCTORS HOSPITAL OF STARK COUNTY
MEDICAL LIBRARY
400 Austin Ave., NW
Massillon, OH 44646   Phone: (216) 837-7371
Valerie Haren, Chf.Med.Libn.
Subjects: Medicine, osteopathy. **Holdings:** 1500 books; 2900 bound periodical volumes. **Subscriptions:** 150 journals and other serials.

★9512★ MIDDLETOWN REGIONAL HOSPITAL
ADA I. LEONARD MEMORIAL LIBRARY
105 McKnight Dr.
Middletown, OH 45044-8787   Phone: (513) 422-2111
Catherine M. Nolte, Media Coord.
Subjects: Medicine, nursing, allied health sciences. **Holdings:** 1200 books; 150 periodical volumes; 500 AV programs; 500 health information pamphlets. **Subscriptions:** 150 journals and other serials.

★9513★ SOCIETY FOR THE STUDY OF MALE PSYCHOLOGY
AND PHYSIOLOGY
LIBRARY
321 Iuka
Montpelier, OH 43543   Phone: (419) 485-3602
Jerry Bergman, Ph.D., Dir.
Subjects: Male psychology and physiology. **Holdings:** 1900 books; 1200 bound periodical volumes; 1000 reports, 800 manuscripts, 80 microfiche, 40 reels of microfilm. **Subscriptions:** 40 journals and other serials.

★9514★ KNOX COMMUNITY HOSPITAL
MEDICAL LIBRARY
1330 Coshocton Rd.
Mount Vernon, OH 43050   Phone: (614) 393-9000
Havilah Phelps, Libn.
Subjects: Medicine, surgery, nursing. **Holdings:** 1250 books; 300 bound periodical volumes. **Subscriptions:** 30 journals and other serials.

★9515★ LICKING MEMORIAL HOSPITAL
RALPH E. PICKETT MEDICAL LIBRARY
1320 W. Main St.
Newark, OH 43055   Phone: (614) 344-0331
Lindsay J. Freytag, Libn.
Subjects: Clinical medicine. **Holdings:** 300 books; tapes. **Subscriptions:** 25 journals.

★9516★ SAGAMORE HILLS CHILDREN'S PSYCHIATRIC
HOSPITAL
STAFF MEDICAL LIBRARY
11910 Dunham Rd.
Northfield, OH 44067   Phone: (614) 467-7955
Subjects: Child psychology, institutional care, nursing, activity and educational therapy, psychiatry. **Holdings:** 950 books; tapes. **Subscriptions:** 15 journals and other serials.

★9517★ WESTERN RESERVE PSYCHIATRIC HABILITATION
CENTER
STAFF LIBRARY
1756 Sagamore Rd.
Box 305
Northfield, OH 44067   Phone: (216) 467-7131
Pearlie McAlpine, Libn.
Subjects: Psychiatry, psychiatric nursing, psychology, social service. **Holdings:** 500 books. **Subscriptions:** 55 journals and other serials.

★9518★ OBERLIN COLLEGE
CLASS OF 1904 SCIENCE LIBRARY
Kettering Hall
Oberlin, OH 44074   Phone: (216) 775-8310
Alison Scott Ricker, Sci.Libn.
Subjects: Biology, chemistry, earth sciences, medicine, technology. **Holdings:** 52,000 volumes; 90 loose-leaf binders of Thermodynamics Research Center Spectral and Thermodynamics Data; 1080 reels of microfilm. **Subscriptions:** 300 journals and other serials.

★9519★ MIAMI UNIVERSITY
BRILL SCIENCE LIBRARY
Oxford, OH 45056   Phone: (513) 529-7200
Barbara A. Galik, Act.Hd.Sci.Libn.
Subjects: Science - biological, physical, earth; mathematics; technology; medicine. **Holdings:** 129,903 books; 107,964 bound periodical volumes; 262,000 microforms; 20,500 specialized maps; 22,520 U.S. Defense Mapping Agency/Army Map Service maps; 48,900 U.S. Geological Survey maps; 9 VF drawers of pamphlets. **Subscriptions:** 2200 journals and other serials.

★9520★ LAKE HOSPITAL SYSTEM
MEDICAL LIBRARIES
Washington at Liberty
Painesville, OH 44077   Phone: (216) 354-2400
Holly S. Kimborowicz, Hea.Sci.Libn.
Subjects: Medicine, nursing, health administration. **Holdings:** 2185 books. **Subscriptions:** 270 journals and other serials.

★9521★ KAISER FOUNDATION HOSPITALS
MEDICAL LIBRARY
12301 Snow Rd.
Parma, OH 44130   Phone: (216) 362-2086
Bonita Rosen, Med.Libn.
Subjects: Medicine, nursing, ancillary health services. **Holdings:** Figures not available. **Subscriptions:** 136 journals and other serials.

★9522★ PORTSMOUTH RECEIVING HOSPITAL
MEDICAL LIBRARY
25th St. & Elmwood Dr.
Box 561
Portsmouth, OH 45662   Phone: (614) 354-2804
Marilyn Stafford, Educ.Dir.
Subjects: Psychiatry, psychology, allied health sciences. **Holdings:** 1509 books; 26 bound periodical volumes. **Subscriptions:** 24 journals and other serials.

★9523★ NORTHEASTERN OHIO UNIVERSITIES COLLEGE OF
MEDICINE
OLIVER OCASEK REGIONAL MEDICAL INFORMATION
CENTER
4209 State Rte. 44
Box 95
Rootstown, OH 44272   Phone: (216) 325-2511
Subjects: Basic life sciences, medicine. **Holdings:** 34,104 books; 34,159 bound periodical volumes; 2041 AV programs; 270 linear feet of archival material and manuscripts. **Subscriptions:** 1040 journals and other serials.

★9524★ PROVIDENCE HOSPITAL
SCHOOL OF NURSING LIBRARY
1912 Hayes Ave.
Sandusky, OH 44870   Phone: (419) 625-8450
Marie L. Paulson, Libn.
Subjects: Nurses and nursing, medicine, social sciences, natural science, philosophy, religion. **Holdings:** 3160 books; 600 bound periodical volumes; 12 VF drawers of pamphlets, leaflets, pictures, articles. **Subscriptions:** 81 journals and other serials.

★9525★ COMMUNITY HOSPITAL OF SPRINGFIELD AND
CLARK COUNTY
HEALTH SCIENCES LIBRARY
2615 E. High St.
Springfield, OH 45501   Phone: (513) 325-0531
Joyce Davis, Libn.
Subjects: Medicine, nursing. **Holdings:** 3900 books; 2100 bound periodical volumes. **Subscriptions:** 120 journals and other serials.

★9526★ MERCY MEDICAL CENTER
HEALTH SCIENCES LIBRARY
1343 Fountain
Springfield, OH 45501   Phone: (513) 390-5000
Marietta R. Wilson, Hea.Sci.Libn.
Subjects: Clinical medicine, allied health sciences. **Holdings:** 1200 books; 1000 bound periodical volumes. **Subscriptions:** 135 journals and other serials.

★9527★ HUMAN LIFE CENTER
LIBRARY
University of Steubenville
Steubenville, OH 43952   Phone: (614) 282-9953
Subjects: Abortion, euthanasia, and allied "sanctity of human life" issues; sexuality corresponding to Christian moral values; Catholic moral and social teachings; natural family planning; pro-life organizations. **Holdings:** 4000 volumes.

★9528★ OHIO VALLEY HOSPITAL
HEALTH SCIENCES LIBRARY
1 Ross Park
Steubenville, OH 43952   Phone: (614) 283-7400
Subjects: Medicine, nursing. **Holdings:** 1968 books; 2731 bound periodical volumes; 4 theses; 4 VF drawers of pamphlets; 277 filmstrip/tape sets and slide/tape sets; 35 slide sets; 16 overhead transparencies; 276 videotapes; 5 films; 14 charts; 29 audio cassettes; 45 models. **Subscriptions:** 68 journals and other serials.

★9529★ LOURDES COLLEGE
DUNS SCOTUS LIBRARY
6832 Convent Blvd.
Sylvania, OH 43560   Phone: (419) 885-3211
Sr. Mary Thomas More Ruffing, Hd.Libn.
Subjects: Religious studies, health sciences, psychology, occupational therapy, gerontology, art. **Holdings:** 41,336 books; 8375 bound periodical volumes; 8252 microforms. **Subscriptions:** 323 journals and other serials; 17 newspapers.

★9530★ MEDICAL COLLEGE OF OHIO AT TOLEDO
RAYMON H. MULFORD LIBRARY
3000 Arlington Ave.
Toledo, OH 43614   Phone: (419) 381-4225
R.M. Watterson, Libn.
Subjects: Medicine, dentistry, nursing, animal medicine, allied health sciences. **Holdings:** 43,505 books; 65,481 bound periodical volumes; 3439 microfiche; 99 reels of microfilm. **Subscriptions:** 1895 journals and other serials.

★9531★ MERCY HOSPITAL
EDWARD L. BURNS HEALTH SCIENCES LIBRARY
2200 Jefferson Ave.
Toledo, OH 43624   Phone: (419) 259-1327
Thomas R. Sink, Dir., Lib.Serv.
Subjects: Medicine, nursing, allied health sciences. **Holdings:** 6000 volumes; AV programs; VF materials. **Subscriptions:** 320 journals and other serials.

★9532★ PARKVIEW OSTEOPATHIC HOSPITAL
LIBRARY
1920 Parkwood Ave.
Toledo, OH 43624   Phone: (419) 242-8471
Mary Bracey, Libn.
Subjects: Osteopathy, orthopedics, radiology, surgery, anesthesiology, pediatrics, clinical and family medicine. **Holdings:** 1050 books; 1450 bound periodical volumes; Audio-Digest tapes. **Subscriptions:** 74 journals and other serials.

★9533★ RIVERSIDE HOSPITAL
SARAH AND JULIUS STEINBERG MEMORIAL LIBRARY
1600 N. Superior St.
Toledo, OH 43604   Phone: (419) 729-6198
Kathryn Maluchnik, Libn.
Subjects: Medicine, nursing, podiatry, sports medicine, health promotion, hospital management. **Holdings:** 900 books; 850 bound periodical volumes. **Subscriptions:** 55 journals and other serials.

★9534★ ST. VINCENT MEDICAL CENTER
HEALTH SCIENCE LIBRARY
2213 Cherry St.
Toledo, OH 43608   Phone: (419) 321-4329
Subjects: Clinical medicine and surgery, nursing, hospital administration. **Holdings:** 10,101 books; 8000 bound periodical volumes. **Subscriptions:** 704 journals and other serials.

★9535★ TOLEDO HOSPITAL
MEDICAL LIBRARY
2142 N. Cove Blvd.
Toledo, OH 43606   Phone: (419) 471-5437
Linda M. Tillman, Dir.
Subjects: Medicine, nursing, allied health sciences. **Holdings:** 6687 books; 24,399 bound periodical volumes; video cassettes; audio cassettes; slides; filmstrips. **Subscriptions:** 610 journals and other serials.

★9536★ TRUMBULL MEMORIAL HOSPITAL
WEAN MEDICAL LIBRARY
1350 E. Market St.
Warren, OH 44482   Phone: (216) 841-9379
Diane Richardson, Med.Libn.
Subjects: Medicine and allied health sciences. **Holdings:** 3500 books; 5500 bound periodical volumes. **Subscriptions:** 223 journals and other serials.

★9537★ WARREN GENERAL HOSPITAL
MEDICAL STAFF LIBRARY
667 Eastland Ave., SE
Warren, OH 44484   Phone: (216) 399-7541
Nancy L. Bindas, Med.Libn.
Subjects: Medicine, surgery, and allied health sciences. **Holdings:** 550 books; 500 bound periodical volumes; 480 Audio-Digest tapes and cassettes; 400 videotapes. **Subscriptions:** 48 journals and other serials.

★9538★ ST. JOHN AND WEST SHORE HOSPITAL
MEDIA CENTER
29000 Center Ridge Rd.
Westlake, OH 44145   Phone: (216) 835-6000
Jennifer Jung Gallant, Dir.
Subjects: Medicine, nursing, allied health sciences. **Holdings:** 2300 books; 2 drawers of pamphlets. **Subscriptions:** 130 journals and other serials.

★9539★ LAURELWOOD HOSPITAL
LIBRARY
35900 Euclid Ave.
Willoughby, OH 44094
Pamela Alderman, Dir.
Subjects: Psychiatry, substance abuse, geriatrics, adolescent health. **Holdings:** Figures not available.

★9540★ U.S. AIR FORCE MEDICAL CENTER
MEDICAL LIBRARY
SGEL/Bldg. 830A
Wright-Patterson AFB, OH 45433-5300   Phone: (513) 257-4506
Subjects: Clinical medicine, dentistry, veterinary medicine, hospital administration. **Holdings:** 9000 books; 11,000 bound periodical volumes; 4000 AV programs; 45,000 microfiche. **Subscriptions:** 800 journals and other serials.

★9541★ ST. ELIZABETH HOSPITAL MEDICAL CENTER
MEDICAL LIBRARY
1044 Belmont Ave.
Youngstown, OH 44501   Phone: (216) 746-7211
Barbara G. Rosenthal, Med.Libn.
Subjects: Medicine and related subjects. **Holdings:** 2500 books; 7300 bound periodical volumes; 720 reels of microfilm. **Subscriptions:** 305 journals and other serials.

★9542★ ST. ELIZABETH HOSPITAL MEDICAL CENTER
SCHOOL OF NURSING
LIBRARY
1044 Belmont Ave.
Youngstown, OH 44501   Phone: (216) 746-7211
Doris L. Crawford, Libn.
Subjects: Nursing, health education, medicine, allied health. **Holdings:** 8783 books; 2170 bound periodical volumes; 20 lateral file drawers of pamphlets; 10 drawers of microfiche; 1058 AV programs; 60 computer programs. **Subscriptions:** 350 journals and other serials.

★9543★ WESTERN RESERVE CARE SYSTEM
HEALTH SCIENCES LIBRARIES
345 Oak Hill Ave.
Youngstown, OH 44501   Phone: (216) 740-4689
Patricia L. Augustine, Dir., Hea.Sci.Lib.
Subjects: Clinical medicine, science and nursing. **Holdings:** 4214 books;

8338 bound periodical volumes; Audio-Digest tapes; AV slides. **Subscriptions:** 366 journals and other serials; 5 newspapers.

★9544★ **WOODSIDE RECEIVING HOSPITAL**
STAFF RESOURCE LIBRARY/PATIENTS' LIBRARY
800 E. Indianola Ave.
Youngstown, OH 44502   Phone: (216) 788-8712
Louise M. Mulderig, Libn.
Subjects: Psychiatry, psychiatric nursing, mental illness, mental health, social services, psychotherapy. **Holdings:** 6405 books; 31 bound periodical volumes; 300 boxes of archives; 200 reports; 2000 pamphlets; 22 documents; 200 phonograph records; 10 drawers of filmstrips and cassette tapes; 450 items in picture files; 260 dissertations. **Subscriptions:** 80 journals and other serials.

★9545★ **BETHESDA HOSPITAL**
LIBRARY AND EDUCATION SERVICES
2951 Maple Ave.
Zanesville, OH 43701   Phone: (614) 454-4624
Lea Craig, Mgr.
Subjects: Internal medicine, cardiology, surgery, pediatrics, oncology, psychiatry. **Holdings:** 800 volumes; 133 bound periodical volumes; pamphlets. **Subscriptions:** 121 journals and other serials.

Oklahoma

★9546★ **SAMUEL ROBERTS NOBLE FOUNDATION**
BIOMEDICAL DIVISION LIBRARY
2510 Hwy. 199 E.
Box 2180
Ardmore, OK 73402   Phone: (405) 223-5810
Jeanine Phipps, Biomed. & Plant Biol.Libn.
Subjects: Cancer research, biochemistry, plant biology, medicine, immunology, nutrition, cell biology, plant cell biology, biochemical pharmacology, science, chemistry, molecular plant pathology, applied molecular biology, molecular analysis. **Holdings:** 1525 books; 5500 bound periodical volumes; 1150 annual publications; 2710 reels of microfilm of journals. **Subscriptions:** 153 journals and other serials.

★9547★ **ST. MARY'S HOSPITAL**
MEDICAL LIBRARY
305 S. 5th St.
Box 232
Enid, OK 73701   Phone: (405) 249-3092
Janet Puckett, Med.Libn.
Subjects: Medicine, nursing, hospital administration. **Holdings:** 2364 books; 2052 bound periodical volumes; 350 videotapes. **Subscriptions:** 160 journals and other serials.

★9548★ **WESTERN STATE HOSPITAL**
LIBRARY
Box 1
Fort Supply, OK 73841   Phone: (405) 766-2311
Karen Putnam, Lib.Techn.
Subjects: Substance abuse, psychiatry, psychology. **Holdings:** 2778 books; 23 bound periodical volumes; 50 boxes of booklets, pamphlets, and reports; 43 slide sets; 43 audiotapes; 6 video recordings. **Subscriptions:** 20 journals and other serials; 18 newspapers.

★9549★ **OKLAHOMA SCHOOL FOR THE BLIND**
PARKVIEW LIBRARY
3300 Gibson St.
Box 309
Muskogee, OK 74402-0309   Phone: (918) 682-6641
Shonda Konemann, Lib.-Media Spec.
Subjects: Books in braille and talking books. **Holdings:** 8013 titles; 840 talking books. **Subscriptions:** 81 journals and other serials.

★9550★ **U.S. DEPARTMENT OF VETERANS AFFAIRS**
MEDICAL CENTER LIBRARY
1101 Honor Height Dr.
Muskogee, OK 74401   Phone: (918) 683-3261
Jenneane Brown, Chf., Lib.Serv.
Subjects: Medicine, nursing, allied health sciences. **Holdings:** 3269 books; 4584 bound periodical volumes; 737 AV programs. **Subscriptions:** 275 medical journals; 12 newspapers.

★9551★ **CENTRAL STATE HOSPITAL**
PROFESSIONAL LIBRARY
Box 151
Norman, OK 73070   Phone: (405) 321-4880
Shirley M. Pierce, Med.Libn.
Subjects: Psychiatry, psychology, medicine, nursing. **Holdings:** 7800 books; 140 bound periodical volumes; 4 VF drawers of clippings and dissertations; 3 shelves of government documents; 3 VF drawers of newsletters and nursing statements; 115 tapes; 20 films; 2 video cassettes; 200 filmstrips. **Subscriptions:** 106 journals and other serials.

★9552★ **NORMAN REGIONAL HOSPITAL**
HEALTH SCIENCES LIBRARY
901 N. Porter
Box 1308
Norman, OK 73070   Phone: (405) 321-1700
Michelynn McKnight, Dir.
Subjects: Medicine, nursing, and allied health sciences. **Holdings:** 1000 books; 300 reels of microfilm. **Subscriptions:** 150 journals and other serials.

★9553★ **BAPTIST MEDICAL CENTER**
WANN LANGSTON MEMORIAL LIBRARY
3300 Northwest Expy.
Oklahoma City, OK 73112   Phone: (405) 949-3766
Cheryl Suttles, Dir., Med.Lib.
Subjects: Geriatrics, medicine, nursing, hospital management. **Holdings:** 2186 books; 3654 bound periodical volumes. **Subscriptions:** 270 journals and other serials.

★9554★ **CHILDREN'S HOSPITAL OF OKLAHOMA**
CHO MEDICAL LIBRARY
Box 26307
Oklahoma City, OK 73126   Phone: (405) 271-5699
Jean Cavett, Dir.
Subjects: Pediatrics. **Holdings:** 900 books; 1750 bound periodical volumes. **Subscriptions:** 135 journals and other serials.

★9555★ **CHILDREN'S HOSPITAL OF OKLAHOMA**
FAMILY RESOURCE CENTER
940 NE 13th St., Rm. 3N 109
Box 26307
Oklahoma City, OK 73126   Phone: (405) 271-5525
Madalyn McCollom, Dir.
Subjects: Lay medical information, parenting/child care, community resource files, general health care, caring for the chronically ill, preparation/hospitalization. **Holdings:** 850 books; 1 vertical file; 70 videotapes; 30 audio cassettes. **Subscriptions:** 11 journals and other serials; 8 newsletters.

★9556★ **MERCY HEALTH CENTER**
MEDICAL LIBRARY
4300 W. Memorial Rd.
Oklahoma City, OK 73118   Phone: (405) 752-3390
May Cordry, Hd.Libn.
Subjects: Medicine, nursing, allied health sciences. **Holdings:** 852 books; 5003 bound periodical volumes. **Subscriptions:** 225 journals and other serials.

★9557★ **OKLAHOMA DEPARTMENT OF HEALTH**
INFORMATION AND REFERRAL HEALTHLINE
1000 NE 10th St.
Box 53551
Oklahoma City, OK 73152   Phone: (405) 271-5600
Janet Smith, Dir.
Subjects: Medicine, nursing, psychology, personal health, epidemiology, venereal disease. **Holdings:** 2500 volumes; 90,000 general health pamphlets covering approximately 300 areas. **Subscriptions:** 30 journals and other serials.

★9558★ **OKLAHOMA REGIONAL LIBRARY FOR THE BLIND**
AND PHYSICALLY HANDICAPPED
1108 NE 36th St.
Oklahoma City, OK 73111   Phone: (405) 521-3514
Geraldine Adams, Lib.Dir.
Subjects: Recreational and informational reading materials in special media collections. **Holdings:** 165,000 books; magnetic tapes; microfiche. **Subscriptions:** 56 journals and other serials.

★9559★   PRESBYTERIAN HOSPITAL
MEDICAL LIBRARY
NE 13th and Lincoln Blvd.
Oklahoma City, OK 73104   Phone: (405) 271-4266
Mary Lou Tremblay, Lib.Dir.
Subjects: Medicine, nursing, surgery, cardiology. **Holdings:** 4000 books; 6000 bound periodical volumes; 24 boxes of pamphlets; 175 file boxes of unbound periodicals; 2 VF drawers; 800 cassettes. **Subscriptions:** 257 journals and other serials.

★9560★   RAINBOW FLEET, INC.
LIBRARY
3016 Paseo
Oklahoma City, OK 73103   Phone: (405) 521-1426
Marti Nicholson, Exec.Dir.
Subjects: Child development; infant stimulation; preschool enhancement, including language and sensorial development, pre-math skills, and practical life skills. **Holdings:** 2500 books; 3000 toys and games.

★9561★   ST. ANTHONY HOSPITAL
O'DONOGHUE MEDICAL LIBRARY
1000 N. Lee St.
Box 205
Oklahoma City, OK 73102   Phone: (405) 272-6284
Sharon Jorski, Dir.
Subjects: Cardiovascular medicine, neurosurgery and neurology, general medicine, nursing, community health, allied health sciences, dentistry. **Holdings:** 4000 books; 3800 bound periodical volumes; 13 VF drawers of pamphlets, reports, clippings, illustrations, and reprints. **Subscriptions:** 185 journals and other serials.

★9562★   U.S. DEPARTMENT OF VETERANS AFFAIRS
MEDICAL CENTER LIBRARY
921 NE 13th St.
Oklahoma City, OK 73104   Phone: (405) 270-0501
Verlean Delaney, Chf.Libn.
Subjects: Medicine, patient health education. **Holdings:** 2243 books; 459 AV programs; talking books. **Subscriptions:** 310 journals and other serials.

★9563★   U.S. FEDERAL AVIATION ADMINISTRATION
CIVIL AEROMEDICAL INSTITUTE LIBRARY, AAM 400A
6500 S. MacArthur Blvd.
Box 25082
Oklahoma City, OK 73125   Phone: (405) 680-4398
Janice Varner Nakagawara, Med.Libn.
Subjects: Aviation medicine, biochemistry, psychology, human factors, toxicology, occupational hygiene. **Holdings:** 8000 books; 12,000 bound periodical volumes; 20,000 unbound reports. **Subscriptions:** 200 journals and other serials.

★9564★   UNIVERSITY OF OKLAHOMA
HEALTH SCIENCES CENTER
DEAN A. MCGEE EYE INSTITUTE
LIBRARY
Department of Ophthalmology
608 Stanton L. Young Blvd.
Oklahoma City, OK 73104   Phone: (405) 271-6085
Sheri Greenwood, Med.Libn.
Subjects: Ophthalmology. **Holdings:** 1200 books; 1000 bound periodical volumes; 30 slide sets; 84 video cassettes. **Subscriptions:** 34 journals and other serials.

★9565★   UNIVERSITY OF OKLAHOMA
HEALTH SCIENCES CENTER
DEPARTMENT OF SURGERY LIBRARY
PO Box 26901, RM 4SP305
Oklahoma City, OK 73190   Phone: (405) 271-5506
Linda R. O'Rourke, Med.Libn.
Subjects: Surgery - general, plastic, neurosurgery, thoracic and cardiovascular, oral; emergency medicine and trauma. **Holdings:** 3349 volumes. **Subscriptions:** 90 journals and other serials.

★9566★   UNIVERSITY OF OKLAHOMA
HEALTH SCIENCES CENTER
LIBRARY
1000 Stanton L. Young Blvd.
Box 26901
Oklahoma City, OK 73190   Phone: (405) 271-2285
C.M. Thompson, Jr., Dir.
Subjects: Medicine, dentistry, nursing, public health, pharmacy, allied health subjects. **Holdings:** 63,886 books; 124,541 bound periodical volumes. **Subscriptions:** 2500 journals and other serials.

★9567★   NATIONAL CLEARING HOUSE OF REHABILITATION
TRAINING MATERIALS
816 W. 6th St.
Oklahoma State University
Stillwater, OK 74078-0435   Phone: (405) 624-7650
Paul G. Gaines, Proj.Dir.
Subjects: Rehabilitation training and counselor skills, disabilities, special needs education, vocational rehabilitation, service delivery. **Holdings:** 3500 titles in hardcopy or microfiche; 2000 microfiche; AV programs.

★9568★   OKLAHOMA STATE UNIVERSITY
VETERINARY MEDICINE LIBRARY
University Library
Stillwater, OK 74078-0375   Phone: (405) 744-6655
Patricia Mullen, Hd.
Subjects: Veterinary medicine, health sciences, laboratory animal medicine. **Holdings:** 8819 books; 9427 bound periodical volumes; 775 tapes; 694 slides; 30 study guides; 25 films. **Subscriptions:** 307 journals and other serials.

★9569★   OKLAHOMA SCHOOL FOR THE DEAF
LIBRARY
E. 10th. and Tahlequah
Sulphur, OK 73086   Phone: (405) 622-3186
Helen Freeman, Libn.
Remarks: No further information was supplied by the respondent.

★9570★   U.S. AIR FORCE HOSPITAL
MEDICAL LIBRARY
Tinker AFB, OK 73145   Phone: (405) 734-8443
Mary B. Mills, Lib.Techn.
Subjects: Pediatrics, internal medicine, surgery, nursing. **Holdings:** 1263 books. **Subscriptions:** 93 journals and other serials.

★9571★   ATOCHEM NORTH AMERICA
RESEARCH LIBRARY
5101 W. 21st St.
Tulsa, OK 74107   Phone: (918) 583-0851
Subjects: Chemistry - general, fluorine, inorganic; chemicals for dental application. **Holdings:** 500 books; 300 bound periodical volumes; 50 volumes of unbound journals. **Subscriptions:** 24 journals and other serials.

★9572★   HILLCREST MEDICAL CENTER
LIBRARY
1120 S. Utica
Tulsa, OK 74104   Phone: (918) 587-1300
Peggy Cook, Libn.
Subjects: Medicine, nursing, aging and health. **Holdings:** 2604 books; 4409 bound periodical volumes; 1021 AV programs; 3 lateral file drawers drawers of pamphlets; 1 lateral file drawer of bibliographies; 1 lateral file drawer of newsletters. **Subscriptions:** 236 journals and other serials.

★9573★   OKLAHOMA STATE UNIVERSITY
COLLEGE OF OSTEOPATHIC MEDICINE
MEDICAL LIBRARY
1111 W. 17th St.
Tulsa, OK 74107-1898   Phone: (918) 582-1972
Linda L. Roberts, Coll.Libn.
Subjects: Medicine. **Holdings:** 21,109 books; 1682 bound periodical volumes; 3599 AV programs; 28,368 microfiche; 998 reels of microfilm. **Subscriptions:** 544 journals; 79 serials; 5 newspapers.

★9574★ ST. FRANCIS HOSPITAL
HEALTH SCIENCES LIBRARY
6161 S. Yale Ave.
Tulsa, OK 74316   Phone: (918) 494-1210
Darryl Logan, Med.Libn.
Subjects: Health sciences, nursing, hospital management. **Holdings:** 2002 books; 4904 bound periodical volumes; 278 government documents. **Subscriptions:** 250 journals and other serials.

★9575★ ST. JOHN MEDICAL CENTER
HEALTH SCIENCES LIBRARY
1923 S. Utica
Tulsa, OK 74104   Phone: (918) 744-2970
James M. Donovan, Libn.
Subjects: Medicine, nursing, and allied health sciences, management. **Holdings:** 3200 books; 8000 bound periodical volumes; Audio-Digest tapes. **Subscriptions:** 160 journals and other serials.

★9576★ TULSA REGIONAL MEDICAL CENTER
L.C. BAXTER MEDICAL LIBRARY
744 W. 9th
Tulsa, OK 74127   Phone: (918) 599-5297
S. Jane Cooper, Lib.Dir.
Subjects: General medicine, internal medicine, surgery, ophthalmology, allied health sciences. **Holdings:** 2500 books; 2200 bound periodical volumes; 1600 AV cassettes; 1900 slides. **Subscriptions:** 200 journals and other serials.

★9577★ UNIVERSITY OF OKLAHOMA
HEALTH SCIENCES CENTER
TULSA CAMPUS
LIBRARY
2808 S. Sheridan
Tulsa, OK 74129   Phone: (918) 838-4616
Janet Minnerath, Lib.Dir.
Subjects: Medicine. **Holdings:** 4000 books; 21,076 bound periodical volumes. **Subscriptions:** 674 journals and other serials.

★9578★ SOUTHWESTERN OKLAHOMA STATE UNIVERSITY
AL HARRIS LIBRARY
Weatherford, OK 73096   Phone: (405) 772-6611
Sheila Wilder Hoke, Lib.Dir.
Subjects: Pharmacy, education, psychology, business administration. **Holdings:** 236,656 bound books and periodicals; 16,458 reels of microfilm; 396,708 microfiche; 90,250 microcards; 32,632 government documents. **Subscriptions:** 1509 subscriptions.

Oregon

★9579★ ALBANY GENERAL HOSPITAL
STANLEY K. DAVIS LIBRARY
1046 W. 6th
Albany, OR 97321   Phone: (503) 926-9449
Roger Bonner, Libn.
Subjects: Clinical medicine, nursing, hospital administration, radiology. **Holdings:** 800 books; 300 bound periodical volumes. **Subscriptions:** 180 journals and other serials.

★9580★ KAISER SUNNYSIDE MEDICAL CENTER
HEALTH SCIENCES LIBRARY
10180 SE Sunnyside Rd.
Clackamas, OR 97015   Phone: (503) 652-2880
Ann H. Haines, Dir. of the Hea.Sci.Lib.
Subjects: Medicine, nursing. **Holdings:** 800 books. **Subscriptions:** 150 journals and other serials.

★9581★ CORVALLIS CLINIC
MEDICAL LIBRARY
3680 NW Samaritan Dr.
Corvallis, OR 97330   Phone: (503) 754-1150
Gail Drlica, Med.Libn.
Subjects: Clinical medicine. **Holdings:** 5000 books; 6000 bound periodical volumes; 2500 tapes; 4000 slides. **Subscriptions:** 200 journals and other serials.

★9582★ GOOD SAMARITAN HOSPITAL
HEALTH SCIENCES LIBRARY
3600 NW Samaritan Dr.
Corvallis, OR 97330   Phone: (503) 757-5007
Arleen Libertini, Libn.
Subjects: Medicine, nursing, and allied health sciences.

★9583★ HEMLOCK SOCIETY
LIBRARY
Box 11830
Eugene, OR 97440   Phone: (503) 342-5748
Diana Smith, Libn.
Subjects: Voluntary euthanasia. **Holdings:** 200 volumes.

★9584★ OREGON RESEARCH INSTITUTE
LIBRARY
1899 Willamette
Eugene, OR 97401   Phone: (503) 484-2123
Amy Greenwold, Lib.Mgr.
Subjects: Psychology, behavioral sciences, behavioral medicine, health psychology, depression, tobacco cessation, AIDS prevention, personality. **Holdings:** 1500 volumes; 6000 reprints of journal articles. **Subscriptions:** 150 journals and other serials.

★9585★ SACRED HEART GENERAL HOSPITAL
PROFESSIONAL LIBRARY SERVICES
1255 Hilyard St.
PO Box 10905
Eugene, OR 97440   Phone: (503) 686-6837
Kim E. Tyler, Dir.
Subjects: Medicine, nursing, paramedicine, hospital administration, patient education. **Holdings:** 4000 books; 7000 bound periodical volumes; 1000 video recordings. **Subscriptions:** 450 journals and other serials.

★9586★ TUALITY COMMUNITY HOSPITAL
HEALTH SCIENCES LIBRARY
335 SE 8th Ave.
Hillsboro, OR 97123   Phone: (503) 681-1121
Natalie Norcross, Med.Libn.
Subjects: Clinical medicine, pharmacology, nursing, therapeutics, cardiovascular medicine. **Holdings:** 460 books; 109 bound periodical volumes. **Subscriptions:** 175 journals and other serials.

★9587★ TUALITY HEALTHCARE FOUNDATION
TUALITY HEALTH INFORMATION RESOURCE CENTER
Box 309
334 SE 8th Ave.
Hillsboro, OR 97123   Phone: (503) 681-1702
Cindy Muller, Hea.Info.Spec.
Subjects: Health, fitness, nutrition, diseases, support groups. **Holdings:** 635 books; 4500 pamphlets; 25 anatomical models and charts; 80 videotapes. **Subscriptions:** 70 journals and other serials.

★9588★ WILLAMETTE FALLS HOSPITAL
MEDICAL LIBRARY
1500 Division St.
Oregon City, OR 97045   Phone: (503) 650-6757
Katherine R. Martin, Libn.
Subjects: Medicine, nursing, consumer health. **Holdings:** 400 books. **Subscriptions:** 86 journals and other serials.

★9589★ EASTERN OREGON PSYCHIATRIC CENTER
MEDICAL LIBRARY
2600 Westgate
Pendleton, OR 97801   Phone: (503) 276-0810
Pamela Swap, Libn.
Subjects: Mental health, allied health sciences. **Holdings:** 1700 volumes. **Subscriptions:** 10 journals and other serials.

★9590★ EASTMORELAND GENERAL HOSPITAL
HEALTH SCIENCES LIBRARY
2900 SE Steele St.
Portland, OR 97202   Phone: (503) 234-0411
Dolores Judkins, Libn.
Subjects: Osteopathic medicine, medicine, nursing. **Holdings:** 489 books; 510 cassette tapes; 17 slide/tape kits. **Subscriptions:** 50 journals and other serials.

★9591★ EMANUEL HOSPITAL AND HEALTH CENTER
LIBRARY SERVICES
2801 N. Gantenbein Ave.
Portland, OR 97227　　　　　Phone: (503) 280-3558
Katherine W. Rouzie, Dir.
Subjects: Medicine, nursing, allied health sciences. **Holdings:** 1500 books.
Subscriptions: 250 journals and other serials.

★9592★ GOOD SAMARITAN HOSPITAL AND MEDICAL
CENTER
LIBRARY
1015 NW 22nd Ave.
Portland, OR 97210　　　　　Phone: (503) 229-7336
Melvina Stell-Marble, Dir.
Subjects: Medicine, nursing. **Holdings:** 8900 books; 5600 bound periodical
volumes; 8 VF drawers of pamphlets; 505 AV cassettes, filmstrips, slide
sets. **Subscriptions:** 530 journals and other serials.

★9593★ HOLLADAY PARK MEDICAL CENTER
LIBRARY
1225 NE 2nd Ave.
Portland, OR 97232　　　　　Phone: (503) 233-3242
Carolyn T. Olson, Libn.
Subjects: Medicine, psychiatry. **Holdings:** 600 books. **Subscriptions:** 125
journals and other serials.

★9594★ KAISER FOUNDATION HOSPITALS
CENTER FOR HEALTH RESEARCH LIBRARY
4610 SE Belmont St.
Portland, OR 97215　　　　　Phone: (503) 233-5631
Mara Sani, Ph.D., Res.Libn.
Subjects: Health maintenance organizations (HMO), quality of care, health
care utilization, manpower, health behavior, group practice. **Holdings:**
3500 books; 27 VF drawers; 30,000 microfiche. **Subscriptions:** 175 journals
and other serials.

★9595★ KAISER-PERMANENTE MEDICAL CENTER
MEDICAL LIBRARY
5055 N. Greeley Ave.
Portland, OR 97217　　　　　Phone: (503) 285-9321
Daphne Plaut, Med.Libn.
Subjects: Medicine. **Holdings:** 700 books; 400 bound periodical volumes.
Subscriptions: 270 journals and other serials.

★9596★ NATIONAL COLLEGE OF NATUROPATHIC
MEDICINE
LIBRARY
11231 SE Market
Portland, OR 97216　　　　　Phone: (503) 255-4860
Friedhelm Kirchfeld, Libn.
Subjects: Naturopathy, homeopathy, nutrition, physiotherapy, botanical
medicine, acupuncture, clinical and basic sciences. **Holdings:** 7500 books;
600 bound periodical volumes. **Subscriptions:** 103 journals and other
serials.

★9597★ OREGON HEALTH SCIENCES UNIVERSITY
DENTAL BRANCH LIBRARY
611 SW Campus Dr.
Portland, OR 97201　　　　　Phone: (503) 494-8822
Dolores Judkins, Supv.Br.Libn.
Subjects: Dental and oral science. **Holdings:** 17,650 volumes; 500 AV
programs. **Subscriptions:** 350 journals and other serials.

★9598★ OREGON HEALTH SCIENCES UNIVERSITY
LIBRARY
3181 SW Sam Jackson Park Rd.
Box 573
Portland, OR 97207　　　　　Phone: (503) 494-5481
James E. Morgan, Dir. of Libs.
Subjects: Medicine, dentistry, nursing, allied health sciences. **Holdings:**
198,560 volumes; 2089 AV programs. **Subscriptions:** 2650 journals and
other serials.

★9599★ OREGON HEALTH SCIENCES UNIVERSITY
OREGON HEARING RESEARCH CENTER
LIBRARY
3181 SW Sam Jackson Park Rd.
Portland, OR 97201　　　　　Phone: (503) 494-8032
Jill Lilly
Subjects: Auditory science, hearing. **Holdings:** 200 books; 500 bound
periodical volumes. **Subscriptions:** 10 journals and other serials.

★9600★ PROVIDENCE MEDICAL CENTER
MEDICAL LIBRARY
4805 NE Glisan
Portland, OR 97213　　　　　Phone: (503) 230-6075
Peggy R. Burrell, Med.Lib.Dir.
Subjects: Nursing, medicine, administration. **Holdings:** 600 books. **Sub-
scriptions:** 214 journals and other serials.

★9601★ ST. VINCENT HOSPITAL AND MEDICAL CENTER
HEALTH SCIENCES LIBRARY
9205 SW Barnes Rd.
Portland, OR 97225
Ann M. von Segen
Subjects: Medicine, nursing, hospital administration. **Holdings:** 4200
books; 8000 bound periodical volumes. **Subscriptions:** 625 journals and
other serials.

★9602★ U.S. DEPARTMENT OF VETERANS AFFAIRS
MEDICAL LIBRARY
Box 1034
Portland, OR 97207　　　　　Phone: (503) 220-8262
Mara R. Wilhelm
Subjects: Medicine, nursing, allied health sciences, psychology, basic
sciences. **Holdings:** 7681 books; 6010 bound periodical volumes; journals
on microfilm. **Subscriptions:** 613 journals; 111 administrative serials.

★9603★ U.S. DEPARTMENT OF VETERANS AFFAIRS
VANCOUVER DIVISION
MEDICAL LIBRARY
Box 1035
Portland, OR 97207　　　　　Phone: (206) 696-4061
Mara R. Wilhelm
Subjects: Medicine. **Holdings:** Figures not available.

★9604★ WALLA WALLA COLLEGE
SCHOOL OF NURSING PROFESSIONAL LIBRARY
10345 SE Market
Portland, OR 97216　　　　　Phone: (503) 251-6115
Shirley A. Cody, Libn.
Subjects: Nursing - administration, medical-surgical, parent-child, public
health, psychiatric, mental health. **Holdings:** 8000 books; 1100 bound
periodical volumes; 74 tape cassettes; 6 VF drawers of clippings; 2000
pamphlets; 20 slide/tape sets; 91 video cassettes; 60 filmstrips; 10 30mm
films. **Subscriptions:** 125 journals and other serials.

★9605★ WASHINGTON PARK ZOO
ANIMAL MANAGEMENT DIVISION
LIBRARY
4001 SW Canyon Rd.
Portland, OR 97221　　　　　Phone: (503) 226-1561
Janice Hixson
Subjects: Zoology, animal husbandry, animal behavior, conservation,
veterinary medicine, biology. **Holdings:** 800 books. **Subscriptions:** 50
journals and other serials.

★9606★ WESTERN STATES CHIROPRACTIC COLLEGE
W.A. BUDDEN MEMORIAL LIBRARY
2900 NE 132nd Ave.
Portland, OR 97230　　　　　Phone: (503) 256-3180
Kay Irvine, Hd.Libn.
Subjects: Chiropractic, neurology, orthopedics, radiology, alternative heal-
ing. **Holdings:** 9000 books; 3500 bound periodical volumes. **Subscriptions:**
400 journals and other serials.

★9607★ U.S. DEPARTMENT OF VETERANS AFFAIRS
MEDICAL CENTER LIBRARY SERVICE
Garden Valley Blvd.
Roseburg, OR 97470　　　　　Phone: (503) 440-1000
Subjects: Medicine, patient education, management, nursing. **Holdings:**

4400 books; 500 AV programs; 60 journals on microfilm. large-print materials. **Subscriptions:** 340 journals and other serials; 15 newspapers.

★9608★ OREGON DEPARTMENT OF HUMAN RESOURCES
SENIOR AND DISABLED SERVICES DIVISION
LIBRARY
313 Public Service Bldg.
Salem, OR 97310   Phone: (503) 378-4728
Subjects: Aging and the elderly - abuse and crime, long term care and housing, health; management. **Holdings:** Figures not available.

★9609★ OREGON STATE HOSPITAL
STAFF LIBRARY
2600 Center St., NE
Salem, OR 97310-1319   Phone: (503) 378-4375
Carol Snyder, Libn.
Subjects: Psychiatry, psychology. **Holdings:** 1500 books. **Subscriptions:** 40 journals and other serials.

★9610★ OREGON STATE LIBRARY
TALKING BOOK AND BRAILLE SERVICES
State Library Bldg.
Salem, OR 97310-0645   Phone: (503) 378-3849
Nancy Stewart, Adm.
Subjects: General collection. **Holdings:** 171,606 volumes, including 38,100 volumes on records; 9075 braille volumes, 117,436 book volumes on cassette tapes; 6497 large print titles.

★9611★ OREGON STATE SCHOOL FOR THE BLIND
MEDIA CENTER
700 Church St., SE
Salem, OR 97310   Phone: (503) 378-8025
Margie C. Jordan, Media Spec.
Subjects: Visual and hearing impairment; multihandicapped. **Holdings:** 3000 books; 250 talking books. **Subscriptions:** 18 journals and other serials.

★9612★ OREGON STATE SCHOOL FOR THE DEAF
LIBRARY
999 Locust St., NE
Salem, OR 97310   Phone: (503) 378-6252
Adoracion A. Alvarez, Curric.Dir.
Subjects: Education of deaf children, lipreading, audiology, audio-visual education, vocational education, arts and crafts, science. **Holdings:** 9800 books; 340 bound periodical volumes; 2405 filmstrips. **Subscriptions:** 49 journals and other serials.

★9613★ SALEM HOSPITAL
HEALTH SCIENCES LIBRARY
665 Winter St., SE
Box 14001
Salem, OR 97309-5014   Phone: (503) 370-5377
Carol Jones, Dir., Lib.Serv.
Subjects: Clinical medicine, allied health sciences. **Holdings:** 4000 monographs. **Subscriptions:** 355 journals and other serials.

★9614★ U.S. DEPARTMENT OF VETERANS AFFAIRS
LIBRARY
VA Domiciliary
White City, OR 97503   Phone: (503) 826-2111
Sarah Fitzpatrick, Chf., Lib.Serv.
Subjects: Medicine. **Holdings:** 11,000 books; 762 bound periodical volumes. **Subscriptions:** 362 journals and other serials; 4 newspapers.

Pennsylvania

★9615★ ABINGTON MEMORIAL HOSPITAL
SCHOOL OF NURSING LIBRARY
1942 Horace Ave.
Abington, PA 19001   Phone: (215) 576-2598
Carol Paskowsky, Libn.
Subjects: Nursing. **Holdings:** 2000 books; 125 bound periodical volumes. **Subscriptions:** 75 journals and other serials.

★9616★ ABINGTON MEMORIAL HOSPITAL
WILMER MEMORIAL MEDICAL LIBRARY
1200 York Rd.
Abington, PA 19001   Phone: (215) 576-2096
Marion C. Chayes, Dir.
Subjects: Surgery, internal medicine, obstetrics/gynecology, nursing. **Holdings:** 1800 books; 10,000 bound periodical volumes. **Subscriptions:** 300 journals and other serials.

★9617★ THE ALLENTOWN HOSPITAL
LEHIGH VALLEY HOSPITAL CENTER
HEALTH SCIENCES LIBRARY
17th & Chew Sts.
Allentown, PA 18102   Phone: (215) 778-2263
Barbara J. Iobst, Dir., Lib.Serv.
Subjects: Medicine, surgery, basic sciences, obstetrics, gynecology, nursing, psychiatry, trauma, critical care. **Holdings:** 7000 books; 15,000 bound periodical volumes; 300 AV programs. **Subscriptions:** 504 journals and other serials.

★9618★ ALLENTOWN OSTEOPATHIC MEDICAL CENTER
LEARNING RESOURCE CENTER
1736 Hamilton St.
Allentown, PA 18104   Phone: (215) 770-8355
Linda Schwartz, Med.Libn.
Subjects: Medicine, nursing, osteopathic medicine. **Holdings:** 1700 books; 300 AV programs. **Subscriptions:** 118 journals and other serials; 2 newspapers.

★9619★ ALLENTOWN STATE HOSPITAL
HEIM MEMORIAL LIBRARY
1600 Hanover Ave.
Allentown, PA 18103-2498   Phone: (215) 740-3412
Subjects: Psychiatry, psychology, social work, religion. **Holdings:** 2000 books. **Subscriptions:** 82 journals and other serials.

★9620★ GOOD SHEPHERD REHABILITATION HOSPITAL
LIBRARY
6th & St. John Sts.
Allentown, PA 18103   Phone: (215) 776-3294
Cynthia Smith, Coord., Lib.Serv.
Subjects: Medicine, nursing, and allied health sciences.

★9621★ LEHIGH VALLEY COMMITTEE AGAINST HEALTH
FRAUD
LIBRARY
Box 1747
Allentown, PA 18105   Phone: (215) 437-1795
Dr. Stephen Barrett, Chm.
Subjects: Quackery and health frauds, consumer health, chiropractic, nutrition, health food industry, consumer protection, medical care. **Holdings:** 1550 books; 3500 unbound magazines and journals; 100 VF drawers of documents and clippings; 300 cassette tapes; 80 reprints. **Subscriptions:** 130 journals and other serials.

★9622★ LEHIGH VALLEY HOSPITAL CENTER
HEALTH SCIENCES LIBRARY
1200 S. Cedar Crest Blvd.
Allentown, PA 18103   Phone: (215) 776-8410
Barbara J. Iobst
Subjects: Medicine - general, trauma, surgery, burns. **Holdings:** 2000 books; 8000 bound periodical volumes. **Subscriptions:** 350 journals and other serials; 3 newspapers.

★9623★ SACRED HEART HOSPITAL
WILLIAM A. HAUSMAN MEDICAL LIBRARY
4th & Chew Sts.
Allentown, PA 18102   Phone: (215) 776-4747
Diane M. Horvath, Libn.
Subjects: Nursing, medicine. **Holdings:** 1438 books; 5290 bound periodical volumes; 804 Audio-Digest tapes; clippings of Sacred Heart Hospital and School of Nursing history. **Subscriptions:** 77 journals and other serials.

★9624★ ALTOONA HOSPITAL
GLOVER MEMORIAL LIBRARY
620 Howard Ave.
Altoona, PA 16601-4899   Phone: (814) 946-2318
Tracie L. Kahler, Supv., Lib.Serv.
Subjects: Medicine, nursing, oncology. **Holdings:** 7480 books; 1746 bound periodical volumes; 2 VF drawers; 33 films; 1785 slides; 138 filmstrips; 23 film loops; 55 sound film loops; 32 models; 500 audiotapes; 56 video cassettes. **Subscriptions:** 300 journals and other serials.

★9625★ MERCY HOSPITAL
MEDICAL LIBRARY
2500 7th Ave.
Altoona, PA 16603   Phone: (814) 949-4140
Sherri Noon, Lib.Hd.
Subjects: Nursing, medicine. **Holdings:** 800 books; 350 bound periodical volumes. **Subscriptions:** 30 journals and other serials.

★9626★ U.S. DEPARTMENT OF VETERANS AFFAIRS
JAMES E. VAN ZANDT MEDICAL CENTER
LIBRARY SERVICE
2907 Pleasant Valley Blvd.
Altoona, PA 16602-4377   Phone: (814) 943-8164
Judith Gottshall, Chf., Lib.Serv.
Subjects: Medicine, patient education, management. **Holdings:** 5089 books; 500 periodical volumes; 1355 reels of microfilm and AV programs. **Subscriptions:** 220 journals and other serials; 43 newspapers.

★9627★ HORSHAM CLINIC
ANGELO ZOSA MEMORIAL LIBRARY
722 E. Butler Pike
Ambler, PA 19002-2398   Phone: (215) 643-7800
Stanley Gorski, Dir.
Subjects: Psychiatry, mental health, psychotherapy, psychology, psychodrama, family therapy. **Holdings:** 600 books; 100 audiotapes; 2 VF drawers of reprints and pamphlets; 25 videotapes. **Subscriptions:** 76 journals and other serials.

★9628★ PHILADELPHIA ASSOCIATION FOR
PSYCHOANALYSIS
LOUIS KAPLAN MEMORIAL LIBRARY
15 St. Asaph's Rd., PO Box 36
Bala Cynwyd, PA 19004   Phone: (215) 839-3966
June M. Strickland, Libn.
Subjects: Psychoanalysis. **Holdings:** 2500 books; 2400 bound periodical volumes. **Subscriptions:** 10 journals and other serials.

★9629★ MEDICAL CENTER OF BEAVER COUNTY
HEALTH SCIENCES LIBRARY
1000 Dutch Ridge Rd.
Beaver, PA 15009   Phone: (412) 728-7000
Patricia M. Coghlan, Dir.
Subjects: Internal medicine, surgery, oncology, nursing, hospital administration. **Holdings:** 3500 books; 7000 bound periodical volumes; NCME video cassettes. **Subscriptions:** 303 journals and other serials.

★9630★ MUHLENBERG HOSPITAL CENTER
MEDICAL LIBRARY
Schoenersville Rd.
Bethlehem, PA 18017   Phone: (215) 861-2237
Carole A. Mazzeo, Med.Libn.
Subjects: Medicine, nursing, dentistry. **Holdings:** 920 books; unbound periodicals. **Subscriptions:** 105 journals and other serials.

★9631★ NORTHAMPTON COMMUNITY COLLEGE
LEARNING RESOURCES CENTER
SPECIAL COLLECTIONS
3835 Green Pond Rd.
Bethlehem, PA 18017-7599   Phone: (215) 861-5360
Sarah B. Jubinski
Subjects: Nursing, dental auxiliaries, funeral service. **Holdings:** 68,000 books; 78 microfilm titles. **Subscriptions:** 378 journals and other serials; 10 newspapers.

★9632★ ST. LUKE'S HOSPITAL OF BETHLEHEM,
PENNSYLVANIA
AUDIOVISUAL LIBRARY
801 Ostrum St.
Bethlehem, PA 18015   Phone: (215) 691-4341
Robert R. Fields, AV Coord.
Subjects: Medicine, nursing, allied health sciences, patient education. **Holdings:** 700 AV programs.

★9633★ ST. LUKE'S HOSPITAL OF BETHLEHEM,
PENNSYLVANIA
SCHOOL OF NURSING
TREXLER NURSES' LIBRARY
Bishopthorpe & Ostrum Sts.
Bethlehem, PA 18015   Phone: (215) 954-3407
Diane Frantz, Libn.
Subjects: Nursing and allied health sciences. **Holdings:** 4600 volumes; 15 VF drawers. **Subscriptions:** 63 journals and other serials.

★9634★ ST. LUKE'S HOSPITAL OF BETHLEHEM,
PENNSYLVANIA
W.L. ESTES, JR. MEMORIAL LIBRARY
801 Ostrum St.
Bethlehem, PA 18015   Phone: (215) 954-4650
Maria D. Collette, Libn.
Subjects: Medicine, medical specialities, allied health sciences. **Holdings:** 2150 books; 5250 bound periodical volumes; 164 folders of ephemeral file articles. **Subscriptions:** 465 journals and other serials; 4 newspapers.

★9635★ BRADFORD HOSPITAL
HUFF MEMORIAL LIBRARY
116-156 Interstate Pkwy.
Bradford, PA 16701   Phone: (814) 362-8254
Janet Stanek, RRA
Subjects: Medicine. **Holdings:** 460 books; 760 bound periodical volumes. **Subscriptions:** 37 journals and other serials.

★9636★ PENNSYLVANIA DEPARTMENT OF PUBLIC
WELFARE
MAYVIEW STATE HOSPITAL
MENTAL HEALTH AND MEDICAL LIBRARY
1601 Mayview Rd.
Bridgeville, PA 15017-1599   Phone: (412) 257-6496
William A. Suvak, Jr., Libn.Supv. I
Subjects: Psychiatry, psychoanalysis, psychiatric nursing, psychology, hospital administration, psychiatric social work, psychopharmacology. **Holdings:** 4000 books; 1200 bound periodical volumes. **Subscriptions:** 64 journals and other serials.

★9637★ BRYN MAWR HOSPITAL
CLOTHIER NURSING LIBRARY
130 S. Bryn Mawr Ave.
Bryn Mawr, PA 19010   Phone: (215) 526-3084
L.D. Gundry, Chf.Med.Libn.
Subjects: Nursing, medicine. **Holdings:** 3500 books; 1000 bound periodical volumes. **Subscriptions:** 90 journals and other serials.

★9638★ BRYN MAWR HOSPITAL
JOSEPH N. PEW, JR. MEDICAL LIBRARY
Bryn Mawr, PA 19010   Phone: (215) 526-3160
L.D. Gundry, Chf.Med.Libn.
Subjects: Medicine, surgery, allied health sciences. **Holdings:** 3000 books; 5000 bound periodical volumes. **Subscriptions:** 200 journals and other serials.

★9639★ BUTLER MEMORIAL HOSPITAL
ARMSTRONG MEMORIAL MEDICAL LIBRARY
911 E. Brady St.
Butler, PA 16001   Phone: (412) 284-4240
Rita V. Liebler, Med.Libn.
Subjects: Medicine, nursing, and allied health sciences. **Holdings:** 1100 books; 300 bound periodical volumes; 275 videotapes; 575 audiotapes. **Subscriptions:** 117 journals and other serials.

★9640★ U.S. DEPARTMENT OF VETERANS AFFAIRS
MEDICAL CENTER LIBRARY
325 New Castle Rd.
Butler, PA 16001   Phone: (412) 287-4781
Dianne Hohn, Chf., Lib.Serv.
Subjects: Nursing, general medicine. **Holdings:** 1200 books; 3000 periodical volumes, bound and in microform. **Subscriptions:** 100 journals and other serials; 10 newspapers.

★9641★ BRANDYWINE HOSPITAL AND TRAUMA CENTER
HEALTH SCIENCES LIBRARY
201 Reeceville Rd.
Caln Township, PA 19320   Phone: (215) 383-8147
Rosemary Conway, Dir.
Subjects: Nursing, nursing research and education, medicine, allied health sciences, radiology education. **Holdings:** 3000 books; 1500 bound periodical volumes; 500 AV programs; 15 VF drawers. **Subscriptions:** 298 journals and other serials.

★9642★ PENNSYLVANIA DEPARTMENT OF PUBLIC
WELFARE
WESTERN CENTER
LIBRARY SERVICES
333 Curry Hill Rd.
Canonsburg, PA 15317   Phone: (412) 873-3200
Nicholas L. Liguori, Libn.
Subjects: Medicine, psychology, special education. **Holdings:** 1080 volumes. **Subscriptions:** 41 journals and other serials.

★9643★ CARLISLE HOSPITAL
MEDICAL LIBRARY
246 Parker St.
PO Box 310
Carlisle, PA 17013-0310   Phone: (717) 245-5184
Judith Welch, Staff Libn.
Subjects: Medicine, nursing. **Holdings:** 600 books. **Subscriptions:** 120 journals and other serials; 2 newspapers.

★9644★ WOODVILLE STATE HOSPITAL
PROFESSIONAL LIBRARY
Carnegie, PA 15106-3793   Phone: (412) 645-6470
Elaine M. Gruber, Libn.
Subjects: Psychiatry, psychology, behavioral sciences, psychiatric nursing, medicine. **Holdings:** 3000 books and bound periodical volumes. **Subscriptions:** 110 journals and other serials.

★9645★ CROZER CHESTER MEDICAL CENTER
MEDICAL LIBRARY
15th St. & Upland Ave.
Chester, PA 19013   Phone: (215) 447-2600
Catherine A. Dalton, Libn.
Subjects: Medicine, nursing, allied health sciences. **Holdings:** 1449 books; 6500 bound periodical volumes. **Subscriptions:** 335 journals and other serials.

★9646★ SACRED HEART MEDICAL CENTER
HEALTH SCIENCES LIBRARY
9th & Wilson Sts.
Chester, PA 19013   Phone: (215) 494-0700
Wesley Sollenberger, Hea.Sci.Libn.
Subjects: Medicine, nursing, and allied health sciences. **Holdings:** 900 books. **Subscriptions:** 125 journals and other serials.

★9647★ U.S. DEPARTMENT OF VETERANS AFFAIRS
MEDICAL CENTER LIBRARY
Coatesville, PA 19320   Phone: (215) 383-0288
Mary Lou Burton, Chf., Lib.Serv.
Subjects: Psychiatry, neurology, medicine, nursing, psychology. **Holdings:** 7200 books; 8000 bound periodical volumes; 10 VF drawers of information files; 1500 AV programs. **Subscriptions:** 150 journals and other serials; 5 newspapers.

★9648★ GEISINGER MEDICAL CENTER
MEDICAL LIBRARY
N. Academy Ave.
Danville, PA 17822   Phone: (717) 271-6463
Britain G. Roth, Dir., Lrng.Rsrcs.
Subjects: Medicine, paramedical sciences. **Holdings:** 33,000 volumes; 138

audio cassettes; 150 slide sets; 1180 videotapes. **Subscriptions:** 1100 journals and other serials.

★9649★ GEISINGER MEDICAL CENTER
SCHOOL OF NURSING LIBRARY
Danville, PA 17822   Phone: (717) 271-6288
Claire A. Huntington, Lrng.Rsrcs.Coord.
Subjects: Nursing, allied health sciences. **Holdings:** 4401 books; 851 bound periodical volumes; 2 VF drawers of pamphlet material. **Subscriptions:** 91 journals and other serials; 4 newspapers.

★9650★ FITZGERALD MERCY HOSPITAL
HEALTH SCIENCES LIBRARY
Lansdowne Ave. & Baily Rd.
Darby, PA 19023   Phone: (215) 237-4150
Janet C. Clinton, Chf. of Lib.Serv.
Subjects: Medicine, nursing, surgery and allied health sciences, psychiatry, religion and medical ethics. **Holdings:** 3000 books; 3040 periodical volumes; pamphlets; microforms; video cassettes; audio cassettes; filmstrips; slides. **Subscriptions:** 292 journals and other serials; 5 newspapers.

★9651★ DEVEREUX FOUNDATION
PROFESSIONAL LIBRARY
19 S. Waterloo Rd.
Box 400
Devon, PA 19333   Phone: (215) 296-6901
Joyce Matheson, Libn.
Subjects: Clinical psychology, special education, psychiatry, child care, vocational rehabilitation, psychoanalysis. **Holdings:** 3500 books; 150 bound periodical volumes; 6 multimedia training programs. **Subscriptions:** 145 journals and other serials.

★9652★ EAGLEVILLE HOSPITAL
HENRY S. LOUCHHEIM LIBRARY
100 Eagleville Rd.
Eagleville, PA 19408   Phone: (215) 539-6000
Kathryn Dobbs, Mgr. of Lib.Serv.
Subjects: Alcoholism, drug addiction, psychology, psychiatry, sociology. **Holdings:** 5000 books; 10 drawers of archival materials and reprints; 750 audio cassettes. **Subscriptions:** 116 journals and other serials.

★9653★ EAST STROUDSBURG UNIVERSITY
KEMP LIBRARY
East Stroudsburg, PA 18301-2999   Phone: (717) 424-3465
George V. Summers, Dir. of Lib.
Subjects: Health and physical education, education, history, political science, sociology, biology. **Holdings:** 312,770 books; 57,356 bound periodical volumes; 66,996 government documents; 10,501 microcards; 293,297 microprints; 733,133 microfiche; 34,393 reels of microfilm; ERIC microfiche; early American imprints and early English books in microform. **Subscriptions:** 2200 journals and other serials; 26 newspapers.

★9654★ POCONO MEDICAL CENTER
MARSHALL R. METZGAR MEDICAL LIBRARY
206 E. Brown St.
East Stroudsburg, PA 18301   Phone: (717) 476-3515
Ellen P. Woodhead, Lib.Dir.
Subjects: Medicine, nursing. **Holdings:** 780 books; 1450 periodical volumes; 16 VF drawers and 1270 pamphlets of patient education materials and AV programs. **Subscriptions:** 138 journals and other serials.

★9655★ EASTON HOSPITAL
MEDICAL LIBRARY
21st & Lehigh Sts.
Easton, PA 18042   Phone: (215) 250-4130
Mary James, Libn.
Subjects: Internal medicine, surgery, obstetrics, pediatrics, geriatrics, physical therapy. **Holdings:** 2000 books; 5500 bound periodical volumes. **Subscriptions:** 214 journals and other serials.

★9656★ ELWYN INSTITUTES
STAFF LIBRARY
111 Elwyn Rd.
Elwyn, PA 19063   Phone: (215) 891-2084
Joyce Lentz, Libn.
Subjects: Mental retardation, special education, vocational rehabilitation, psychology, medicine. **Holdings:** 2500 volumes; 8 VF drawers of reprints,

reports, bibliographies, and brochures. **Subscriptions:** 50 journals and other serials.

★9657★   AMERICAN STERILIZER COMPANY
LIBRARY
2424 W. 23rd St.
Erie, PA 16514   Phone: (814) 870-8453
Janis M. Ruben, Info.Spec.
Subjects: Bacteriology, medicine, microbiology, engineering, industrial design, marketing, management. **Holdings:** 3500 books; 300 bound periodical volumes; 13 drawers of reprints; 8 drawers of patents; microforms. **Subscriptions:** 350 journals and other serials.

★9658★   HAMOT MEDICAL CENTER
LIBRARY SERVICES
201 State St.
Erie, PA 16550   Phone: (814) 870-6000
Jean A. Tauber, Dir.
Subjects: Medicine, hospital administration, nursing. **Holdings:** 2200 books; 4500 bound periodical volumes. **Subscriptions:** 378 journals and other serials.

★9659★   ST. VINCENT HEALTH CENTER
HEALTH SCIENCE LIBRARY
232 W. 25th St.
Erie, PA 16544   Phone: (814) 452-5740
Joni M. Alex, Med.Libn.
Subjects: Clinical medicine, nursing, dentistry. **Holdings:** 3500 books; 5000 bound periodical volumes; 8 filing drawers of pamphlets; 200 cassettes and slides. **Subscriptions:** 279 journals and other serials.

★9660★   U.S. DEPARTMENT OF VETERANS AFFAIRS
MEDICAL CENTER LIBRARY
135 E. 38th St.
Erie, PA 16504   Phone: (814) 868-6207
Robert M. Schnick, Chf., Lib.Serv.
Subjects: Medicine, nursing, geriatrics, quality assurance. **Holdings:** 3000 books; 4000 reels of periodical microfilm. **Subscriptions:** 220 journals and other serials; 15 newspapers.

★9661★   SHENANGO VALLEY MEDICAL CENTER
MEDICAL LIBRARY
2200 Memorial Dr. Extended
Farrell, PA 16121   Phone: (412) 981-3500
Ethelnel Baron, Staff Sec.
Subjects: Medicine. **Holdings:** 500 books; 200 video cassettes; 200 Audio-Digest tapes. **Subscriptions:** 40 journals and other serials.

★9662★   MCNEIL CONSUMER PRODUCTS COMPANY
INFORMATION CENTER
Camp Hill Rd.
Fort Washington, PA 19034   Phone: (215) 233-7603
Helen J. Hohman, Mgr.Info.Serv.
Subjects: Pharmaceutics, medicine, chemistry, marketing, finance. **Holdings:** 3000 books; 4000 bound periodical volumes. **Subscriptions:** 550 journals and other serials; 5 newspapers.

★9663★   FRANKLIN REGIONAL MEDICAL CENTER
MEDICAL LIBRARY
1 Spruce St.
Franklin, PA 16323   Phone: (814) 437-7000
Mr. L.P. Gilliland, Libn.
Subjects: Medicine, nursing. **Holdings:** 500 books; 700 unbound periodical volumes. **Subscriptions:** 85 journals and other serials.

★9664★   FAIR ACRES GERIATRIC CENTER
MEDICAL LIBRARY
Rte. 352
Glen Riddle-Lima, PA 19037   Phone: (215) 891-5717
Lisa A. Maffei, Dir., Med.Rec.
Subjects: Medicine, nursing, geriatrics, allied health sciences. **Holdings:** 124 books; 60 unbound periodicals. **Subscriptions:** 10 journals and other serials.

★9665★   CHILD CUSTODY SERVICES OF PHILADELPHIA
RESOURCE CENTER
PO Box 202
Glenside, PA 19038-0202   Phone: (215) 576-0177
Dr. Ken Lewis, Dir.
Subjects: Child custody, single-parent families, divorce, child-snatching, mental health and law. **Holdings:** 828 books; 50 bound periodical volumes; 16 dissertation abstracts; 25 special reports; 12 grant narratives; 28 television and radio news documentaries; 50 monographs. **Subscriptions:** 75 journals and other serials; 58 newspapers.

★9666★   WESTMORELAND HOSPITAL
LIBRARY AND HEALTH RESOURCE CENTER
532 W. Pittsburgh St.
Greensburg, PA 15601-2282   Phone: (412) 832-4088
Janet C. Petrak, Med.Libn.
Subjects: Medicine, nursing, surgery. **Holdings:** 4000 books; 1499 bound periodical volumes. **Subscriptions:** 348 journals and other serials.

★9667★   GWYNEDD-MERCY COLLEGE
LOURDES LIBRARY
Gwynedd Valley, PA 19437   Phone: (215) 646-7300
Sr. Berenice Marie Appel
Subjects: Health, religious studies. **Holdings:** 90,000 books; 738 bound periodical volumes; 28,004 microfiche; 2071 reels of microfilm; media programs. **Subscriptions:** 738 journals and other serials; 6 newspapers.

★9668★   HAMBURG CENTER FOR THE MENTALLY
RETARDED
STAFF TRAINING LIBRARY
Hamburg Ctr., Old Rte. 22
Hamburg, PA 19526   Phone: (215) 562-6051
Frederick Herman, Dir., Staff Dev. & Trng.
Subjects: Mental retardation, medicine, nursing, psychiatry, diagnosis, nutrition, habilitation, behavior management, anatomy. **Holdings:** 755 books. **Subscriptions:** 10 journals and other serials.

★9669★   HANOVER GENERAL HOSPITAL
NEWKIRK MEDICAL LIBRARY
Hanover, PA 17331   Phone: (717) 637-3711
Diane Milcoff, Lib.Dir.
Remarks: No further information was supplied by the respondent.

★9670★   HARRISBURG HOSPITAL-CAPITAL HEALTH SYSTEM
LIBRARY SERVICES
S. Front St.
Harrisburg, PA 17101-2099   Phone: (717) 782-5510
Cheryl A. Capitani, Mgr.
Subjects: Clinical medicine, nursing, hospital management, consumer health information. **Holdings:** 3452 monographs; 5219 bound periodical volumes; 875 AV programs; journals on microfilm. **Subscriptions:** 519 journals.

★9671★   HARRISBURG STATE HOSPITAL
LIBRARY SERVICES
Cameron & Maclay Sts.
Pouch A
Harrisburg, PA 17105-1300   Phone: (717) 257-7615
Martha E. Ruff, Libn.
Subjects: Psychiatry, psychology, nursing, social work, rehabilitation, hospital administration. **Holdings:** 2500 books; Dorothea Dix Library and Museum (housed in Building 09); 1977 Audio-Digest tapes on psychiatry. **Subscriptions:** 90 journals and other serials; 10 newspapers.

★9672★   HOSPITAL ASSOCIATION OF PENNSYLVANIA
LIBRARY SERVICES
4750 Lindle Rd.
PO Box 8600
Harrisburg, PA 17105-8600   Phone: (717) 564-9200
Fran Cohen, Libn.
Subjects: Hospital administration; health regulation, legislation, economics; hospital data. **Holdings:** 4000 volumes. **Subscriptions:** 183 journals and other serials.

★9673★ PENNSYLVANIA DEPARTMENT OF PUBLIC WELFARE
OFFICE OF CHILDREN, YOUTH AND FAMILIES
RESEARCH CENTER
Harrisburg State Hospital
Lanco Lodge Bldg.
Box 2675
Harrisburg, PA 17105-2675   Phone: (717) 257-7291
Richard Fiene, Ph.D, Res.Dir.
Subjects: Day care, program evaluation, child care research, child welfare, child abuse, youth services. **Holdings:** 5000 books; 500 bound periodical volumes; 2000 other cataloged items. **Subscriptions:** 10 journals and other serials.

★9674★ POLYCLINIC MEDICAL CENTER
MEDICAL LIBRARY
2601 N. 3rd St.
Harrisburg, PA 17110   Phone: (717) 782-4292
Suzanne M. Shultz, Libn.
Subjects: Medicine, medical specialities. **Holdings:** 2000 books; 8000 bound periodical volumes. **Subscriptions:** 200 journals and other serials.

★9675★ HAVERFORD STATE HOSPITAL
MEDICAL LIBRARY
3500 Darby Rd.
Haverford, PA 19041-1098   Phone: (215) 525-9620
Diane K. Smith, Libn. I
Subjects: Psychiatry, psychiatric nursing, medicine, psychology, pharmacology, geriatrics, gerontology. **Holdings:** 2000 books; 214 bound periodical volumes; 800 unbound periodicals; 200 cassette tapes. **Subscriptions:** 118 journals and other serials.

★9676★ HAZLETON GENERAL HOSPITAL
MEDICAL LIBRARY
E. Broad St.
Hazleton, PA 18201   Phone: (717) 450-4250
Elaine M. Curry, Libn.
Subjects: Medicine, nursing, and allied health sciences. **Holdings:** 1168 books; 1513 bound periodical volumes. **Subscriptions:** 248 journals and other serials.

★9677★ PENNSYLVANIA STATE UNIVERSITY
COLLEGE OF MEDICINE
GEORGE T. HARRELL LIBRARY
Milton S. Hershey Medical Center
Hershey, PA 17033   Phone: (717) 531-8629
Lois J. Lehman, Libn./Dir.
Subjects: Medicine. **Holdings:** 25,520 books; 85,031 bound periodical volumes; 271 motion pictures, videotapes, video discs, and cassettes; 950 phonograph records, audiotapes, and audio cassettes; 72 slide programs; 6 filmstrips. **Subscriptions:** 1885 journals and other serials.

★9678★ MONSOUR MEDICAL CENTER
HEALTH SERVICES LIBRARY
70 Lincoln Way, E.
Jeannette, PA 15644   Phone: (412) 527-1511
Edith Gross, Med.Libn.
Subjects: Medicine, nursing, hospital management, social work, pharmacology. **Holdings:** 868 books; 500 bound periodical volumes; 378 audiotapes; 26 slide/tape sets. **Subscriptions:** 120 journals and other serials.

★9679★ CONEMAUGH VALLEY MEMORIAL HOSPITAL
HEALTH SCIENCES LIBRARY
1086 Franklin St.
Johnstown, PA 15905-4398   Phone: (814) 533-9111
Fred L. Wilson, Jr., Dir., Hea.Sci.Lib.
Subjects: Medicine, nursing, allied health sciences. **Holdings:** 4500 books; 6620 bound periodical volumes; 450 Audio-Digest tapes; 136 videotapes. **Subscriptions:** 266 journals and other serials.

★9680★ RHONE-POULENC RORER CENTRAL RESEARCH
LIBRARY
640 Allendale Rd.
King of Prussia, PA 19406   Phone: (215) 962-3937
Cynthia Supeau, Mgr.
Subjects: Organic chemistry, biochemistry, pharmacology, medicine, pharmacy, biotechnology. **Holdings:** 13,000 books; 45,000 bound periodical

volumes; 1000 reels of microfilm. **Subscriptions:** 675 journals and other serials.

★9681★ SMITHKLINE BEECHAM PHARMACEUTICALS, U.S.
RESEARCH AND DEVELOPMENT INFORMATION CENTER
709 Swedeland Rd.
Box 1539
King of Prussia, PA 19406   Phone: (215) 270-6400
Jane Whittall, Info.Sci.Mgr.
Subjects: Medicine, chemistry, pharmacology, pharmacy, biological sciences. **Holdings:** 15,000 books; 15,000 bound periodical volumes; 10,000 reels of microfilm. **Subscriptions:** 1100 journals and other serials.

★9682★ NESBITT MEMORIAL HOSPITAL
LIBRARY
562 Wyoming Ave.
Kingston, PA 18704   Phone: (717) 288-1411
Katherine L. McCrea, Libn.
Subjects: Medicine, nursing, paramedical sciences. **Holdings:** 3000 books; 380 bound periodical volumes. **Subscriptions:** 150 journals and other serials.

★9683★ LANCASTER GENERAL HOSPITAL
MUELLER HEALTH SCIENCES LIBRARY
555 N. Duke St.
Box 3555
Lancaster, PA 17603   Phone: (717) 299-5511
Claudette Strohm, Libn.
Subjects: Medicine, allied health sciences, hospital administration. **Holdings:** 5000 books; 2000 bound periodical volumes. **Subscriptions:** 361 journals and other serials.

★9684★ ST. JOSEPH HOSPITAL
WILLIAM O. UMIKER MEDICAL LIBRARY
250 College Ave.
Box 3509
Lancaster, PA 17604   Phone: (717) 291-8119
Patricia Ruch Miller, Libn.
Subjects: Medicine, nursing, and allied health sciences. **Holdings:** 4000 books; 350 AV programs. **Subscriptions:** 250 journals and other serials.

★9685★ DELAWARE VALLEY MEDICAL CENTER
JOHN A. WHYTE MEDICAL LIBRARY
200 Oxford Valley Rd.
Langhorne, PA 19047   Phone: (215) 949-5160
Jennifer J. Naus, Med.Libn.
Subjects: Medicine. **Holdings:** 800 books; 15 bound periodical volumes; 400 cassettes and videotapes. **Subscriptions:** 115 journals and other serials.

★9686★ LATROBE AREA HOSPITAL
MEDICAL AND NURSING LIBRARIES
W. 2nd Ave.
Latrobe, PA 15650   Phone: (412) 537-1275
Subjects: Medicine, nursing, medical technology. **Holdings:** 1600 books; 420 bound periodical volumes; 12 VF drawers of pamphlets and clippings; 2 VF drawers of patient education materials. **Subscriptions:** 147 journals and other serials.

★9687★ LAURELTON CENTER
LIBRARY
Laurelton, PA 17835   Phone: (717) 922-5266
Jane G. Slack, Libn.
Subjects: Mental retardation, psychology, special education, social service. **Holdings:** 5079 volumes. **Subscriptions:** 84 journals and other serials.

★9688★ GOOD SAMARITAN HOSPITAL
KROHN MEMORIAL LIBRARY
4th & Walnut Sts.
Lebanon, PA 17042   Phone: (717) 270-7500
Meretta J. Marks, Med.Libn.
Subjects: Medicine, surgery, pediatrics. **Holdings:** 500 books. **Subscriptions:** 75 journals and other serials.

★9689★ U.S. DEPARTMENT OF VETERANS AFFAIRS
MEDICAL CENTER LIBRARY
State Dr.
Lebanon, PA 17042   Phone: (717) 272-6621
David E. Falger, Chf., Lib.Serv.
Subjects: Medicine, aging and geriatrics, psychiatry. **Holdings:** 2557 books; 1200 periodical volumes on microfilm. **Subscriptions:** 296 journals and other serials; 33 newspapers.

★9690★ LEWISTOWN HOSPITAL
MEDICAL LIBRARY
Highland Ave.
Lewistown, PA 17044   Phone: (717) 242-7242
Brenda S. Funk, Med.Libn.
Subjects: Medicine, nursing, hospital administration. **Holdings:** 1200 books. **Subscriptions:** 110 journals and other serials; 7 newspapers.

★9691★ PENNSYLVANIA DEPARTMENT OF HEALTH
BUREAU OF LABORATORIES
HERBERT FOX MEMORIAL LIBRARY
Pickering Way & Welsh Pool Rd.
Lionville, PA 19353   Phone: (215) 363-8500
Leonard Sideman, Libn.
Subjects: Clinical chemistry, microbiology and virology, toxicology, hematology, laboratory legislation. **Holdings:** 500 books. **Subscriptions:** 50 journals and other serials.

★9692★ STERLING DRUG, INC.
STERLING RESEARCH GROUP
LIBRARY AND INFORMATION SERVICES
9 Great Valley Pkwy.
Malvern, PA 19355   Phone: (215) 640-8654
Don Miles, Mgr.
Subjects: Biomedicine, biochemistry, clinical medicine, chemistry, pharmacology, toxicology. **Holdings:** 4000 books; 300 bound periodical volumes; 3000 nonbook items. **Subscriptions:** 450 journals and other serials.

★9693★ OHIO VALLEY GENERAL HOSPITAL
PROFESSIONAL LIBRARY
Heckel Rd.
McKee's Rock, PA 15136   Phone: (412) 777-6159
Diane Faust, Libn.
Subjects: Nursing, medicine. **Holdings:** 1925 volumes. **Subscriptions:** 101 journals and other serials.

★9694★ MCKEESPORT HOSPITAL
HEALTH SERVICES LIBRARY
1500 5th Ave.
McKeesport, PA 15132-2483   Phone: (412) 664-2363
Karen M. Zundel, Dir.
Subjects: Medicine, nursing, consumerism. **Holdings:** 1800 books; 5000 bound periodical volumes; 300 AV programs. **Subscriptions:** 156 journals and other serials.

★9695★ MEADVILLE MEDICAL CENTER
WINSLOW LIBRARY
1034 Grove St.
Meadville, PA 16335   Phone: (814) 333-5740
Barbara Ewing, Libn.
Subjects: Nursing, medicine, pre-medical sciences, allied health sciences, management. **Holdings:** 936 books; 318 bound periodical volumes; 114 audio cassette programs; 90 video cassettes. **Subscriptions:** 92 journals and other serials.

★9696★ FORBES HEALTH SYSTEM
FORBES REGIONAL HEALTH CENTER
MEDICAL LIBRARY
2570 Haymaker Rd.
Monroeville, PA 15146   Phone: (412) 858-2422
Elena Hartmann, Med.Libn.
Subjects: Medicine, nursing, family practice, obstetrics, gynecology, pediatrics, oncology. **Holdings:** 1614 books; 462 bound periodical volumes; Audio-Digest tapes. **Subscriptions:** 111 journals and other serials.

★9697★ PHILHAVEN HOSPITAL
LIBRARY
283 S. Butler Rd.
Mount Gretna, PA 17064   Phone: (717) 270-2419
Harriet Doll, Lib.Dir.
Subjects: Psychology, psychiatry, pastoral care. **Holdings:** 1900 books. **Subscriptions:** 83 journals and other serials.

★9698★ FRICK COMMUNITY HEALTH CENTER
JOSEPH F. BUCCI HEALTH SCIENCES LIBRARY
S. Church St.
Mount Pleasant, PA 15666   Phone: (412) 547-1352
Rosemary C. Panichella, Libn.
Subjects: Medicine, nursing, hospital administration, allied health sciences. **Holdings:** 700 books. **Subscriptions:** 111 journals and other serials.

★9699★ JAMESON MEMORIAL HOSPITAL
SCHOOL OF NURSING LIBRARY
1211 Wilmington Ave.
New Castle, PA 16105-2595   Phone: (412) 656-4050
Karen S. Cilli, Libn.
Subjects: Medicine, surgery, nursing. **Holdings:** 4648 books; 341 bound periodical volumes. **Subscriptions:** 120 journals and other serials.

★9700★ MONTGOMERY HOSPITAL
MEDICAL LIBRARY
Powell & Fornance St.
Norristown, PA 19401   Phone: (215) 270-2232
Alberta T. O'Brien, Med.Libn.
Subjects: Medicine, surgery, drugs, nursing, basic sciences. **Holdings:** 2283 books; 599 bound periodical volumes; 2 VF drawers; 500 AV programs. **Subscriptions:** 102 journals and other serials.

★9701★ PENNSYLVANIA DEPARTMENT OF PUBLIC
 WELFARE
NORRISTOWN STATE HOSPITAL
PROFESSIONAL/STAFF LIBRARY
Bldg. 11
Norristown, PA 19401-5397   Phone: (215) 270-1369
Frieda Liem, Libn.
Subjects: Psychiatry and neurology; clinical psychology; psychiatric nursing; psychiatric and clinical social work; activities therapy - recreational, music, occupational, vocational; aging; geriatrics; gerontology. **Holdings:** 8450 books; 2 VF drawers; pamphlets. **Subscriptions:** 160 journals and other serials.

★9702★ PENNSYLVANIA DEPARTMENT OF PUBLIC
 WELFARE
PHILADELPHIA STATE HOSPITAL
STAFF LIBRARY
Stanbridge Sterigere St.
Norristown, PA 19401-5315   Phone: (215) 671-4145
Greta Clark, Libn.
Subjects: Psychiatry, psychology, psychiatric nursing, social services, family therapy. **Holdings:** 4000 volumes; 40 dissertations; 4 VF drawers. **Subscriptions:** 185 journals and other serials.

★9703★ WARREN STATE HOSPITAL
MEDICAL LIBRARY
33 Main Dr.
N. Warren, PA 16365-5099   Phone: (814) 726-4223
Helen Sweitzer, Act.Lib.Dir.
Subjects: Psychiatry, neurology, psychology, medicine, nursing, occupational therapy, therapeutic activities, sociology. **Holdings:** 20,000 books; 1600 bound periodical volumes; 1400 audio cassettes. **Subscriptions:** 190 journals and other serials.

★9704★ BOIRON RESEARCH FOUNDATION
LIBRARY
1208 Amosland Rd.
Norwood, PA 19074   Phone: (215) 532-8288
Thierry R. Montfort, Libn.
Subjects: Homeopathy, autohemic therapy. **Holdings:** 100 volumes.

★9705★ PALMERTON HOSPITAL
LIBRARY
135 Lafayette Ave.
Palmerton, PA 18071   Phone: (215) 826-3141
Marie T. Krepicz, Lib.Dir.

★9706★ PAOLI MEMORIAL HOSPITAL
ROBERT M. WHITE MEMORIAL LIBRARY
Lancaster Pike
Paoli, PA 19301   Phone: (215) 648-1570
Frances G. DeMillion, Hea.Sci.Libn.
Subjects: Clinical and pre-clinical medicine. **Holdings:** 800 books; 110 publications of medical staff members; 4 VF drawers of pamphlets. **Subscriptions:** 159 journals and other serials.

★9707★ MID-VALLEY HOSPITAL
PHYSICIAN'S LIBRARY
1400 Main St.
Peckville, PA 18452   Phone: (717) 489-7546
Debra Hopkins, Dir., Med.Rec.
Subjects: Medicine, orthopedic medicine, emergency medicine, surgery, infectious diseases, therapy. **Holdings:** 900 books; 398 audiotapes; 154 manuals; 4 AV cassettes. **Subscriptions:** 41 journals and other serials.

★9708★ AIDS LIBRARY OF PHILADELPHIA
32 N. 3rd St.
Philadelphia, PA 19106   Phone: (215) 922-5120
Jean Hofacket
Subjects: AIDS. **Holdings:** 2200 books; 16,000 clippings. **Subscriptions:** 50 journals and other serials; 30 newspapers.

★9709★ ALBERT EINSTEIN MEDICAL CENTER
NORTHERN DIVISION
LURIA MEDICAL LIBRARY
York & Tabor Roads
Philadelphia, PA 19141   Phone: (215) 456-6345
Marion H. Silverman, Dir.
Subjects: Medicine. **Holdings:** 2000 books; 16,000 bound periodical volumes. **Subscriptions:** 300 journals and other serials.

★9710★ AMERICAN ASSOCIATION OF MEDICO-LEGAL
CONSULTANTS
LIBRARY
The Barclay
Rittenhouse Sq.
Philadelphia, PA 19103-6164   Phone: (215) 545-6363
Arlene Goldman, Adm.Asst.
Subjects: Medicine, law, pharmacology, malpractice, medicolegal subjects. **Holdings:** 350 books.

★9711★ AMERICAN HOME PRODUCTS CORPORATION
WYETH-AYERST LABORATORIES DIVISION
LIBRARY
Box 8299
Philadelphia, PA 19101-8299   Phone: (215) 341-2491
Beverly L. Cantor, Supv., Lib.Serv.
Subjects: Pharmacy, medicine, marketing. **Holdings:** 5000 books; 20,000 bound periodical volumes; 12,350 microforms; pharmaceutical patents. **Subscriptions:** 600 journals and other serials.

★9712★ BEASLEY, CASEY, COLLERAN
LIBRARY
21 S. 12th St., 5th Fl.
Philadelphia, PA 19107   Phone: (215) 665-1000
Jill Feldman
Subjects: Law, medicine. **Subscriptions:** 30 journals and other serials; 3 newspapers.

★9713★ BOCKUS RESEARCH INSTITUTE
LIBRARY
415 S. 19th St.
Philadelphia, PA 19146   Phone: (215) 893-2375
Subjects: Cardiovascular research, cardiology, physiology, cancer research, neurology, emphysema. **Holdings:** 1000 volumes. **Subscriptions:** 25 journals and other serials.

★9714★ CENTER FOR THE STUDY OF THE HISTORY OF
NURSING
SPECIAL COLLECTIONS
University of Pennsylvania
Nursing Education Bldg.
Philadelphia, PA 19104-6096   Phone: (215) 898-4502
David M. Weinberg, Cur.
Subjects: History of nursing, with emphasis on the Mid-Atlantic region. **Holdings:** records of hospitals, health care agencies, nursing schools, and nursing agencies; personal papers, diaries, correspondence, and notebooks of individuals who have been employed as nurses or in allied health care fields; photographs; three-dimensional artifacts; magnetic media.

★9715★ CHESTNUT HILL HOSPITAL
MEDICAL LIBRARY
8835 Germantown Ave.
Philadelphia, PA 19118-2767   Phone: (215) 248-8206
Susan G. Mowery, Med.Libn.
Subjects: Medicine, nursing, consumer health. **Holdings:** 3000 books; 500 bound periodical volumes; 153 filmstrips. **Subscriptions:** 152 journals and other serials.

★9716★ CHILDREN'S HOSPITAL OF PHILADELPHIA
MEDICAL LIBRARY
34th & Civic Center Blvd.
Philadelphia, PA 19104-4399   Phone: (215) 590-2317
Mrs. Swaran Lata Chopra, Adm.Supv./Dir.
Subjects: Pediatrics, medicine, nursing. **Holdings:** 4300 books; 7000 bound periodical volumes; 6 VF drawers of clippings and pamphlets; audio cassettes; video cassettes; slides. **Subscriptions:** 200 journals and other serials.

★9717★ COLLEGE OF PHYSICIANS OF PHILADELPHIA
LIBRARY
19 S. 22nd St.
Philadelphia, PA 19103   Phone: (215) 561-6050
Subjects: Medicine, medical specialties, consumer health, history of medicine. **Holdings:** 145,000 monographs; 190,000 bound periodical volumes; theses; dissertations; 1500 manuscript record groups; 10,000 portraits, engravings, pictures; 10,000 autographs. **Subscriptions:** 700 journals and other serials.

★9718★ EPISCOPAL HOSPITAL
MEDICAL LIBRARY
Front St. & Lehigh Ave.
Philadelphia, PA 19125   Phone: (215) 427-7487
Nina P. Long, Dir., Lib.Serv.
Subjects: Medicine, nursing, cardiology. **Holdings:** 3054 books; 4112 bound periodical volumes; AV programs, software programs. **Subscriptions:** 210 journals and other serials.

★9719★ FRANK C. FARNHAM COMPANY, INC.
LIBRARY
Box 8187
Philadelphia, PA 19101   Phone: (215) 567-1500
David M. Wentz, Gen.Mgr.
Subjects: Medicine, chemistry, electronics, metallurgy, mining, plastics, pharmaceutics, history and art of translation. **Holdings:** 1100 books; 25,000 translations from patent and periodical literature. **Subscriptions:** 10 journals and other serials.

★9720★ FRANKFORD HOSPITAL
HOSPITAL LIBRARIES
Frankford Ave. & Wakeling St.
Philadelphia, PA 19124   Phone: (215) 831-2182
Dianne E. Rose, Med.Libn.
Subjects: Medicine, surgery, nursing, nursing education, health care administration. **Holdings:** 5200 books. **Subscriptions:** 240 journals and other serials.

★9721★ FRANKFORD HOSPITAL
SCHOOL OF NURSING
STUDENT LIBRARY
4918 Penn St.
Philadelphia, PA 19124   Phone: (215) 831-2372
Dianne Rose, Lib.Dir.
Subjects: Nursing, sciences, medicine. **Holdings:** 5100 volumes; phonograph records; filmstrips. **Subscriptions:** 112 journals and other serials.

★9722★   FRIENDS HOSPITAL
NORMAN D. WEINER PROFESSIONAL LIBRARY
4641 Roosevelt Blvd.
Philadelphia, PA 19124-2399   Phone: (215) 831-4763
Donna M. Zoccola Soultoukis, Libn.
Subjects: Psychoanalysis, psychiatry, psychology, behavioral sciences, human life cycle, psychiatric nursing. **Holdings:** 5000 books; 5000 bound periodical volumes; VF drawers; 275 audiotapes, 75 video cassettes. **Subscriptions:** 105 journals and other serials.

★9723★   GERMANTOWN HOSPITAL AND MEDICAL CENTER
LIBRARY
1 Penn Blvd.
Philadelphia, PA 19144   Phone: (215) 951-8291
Kathleen A. Leigh, Libn.
Subjects: Medicine, nursing, consumer information. **Holdings:** 4000 books; 1500 bound periodical volumes; 9 VF drawers; 378 audio cassettes; 28 videotapes. **Subscriptions:** 215 journals and other serials.

★9724★   GRADUATE HOSPITAL
LIBRARY
1 Graduate Plaza
Philadelphia, PA 19146   Phone: (215) 893-2401
Diane M. Farny, Dir. of Lib.Serv.
Subjects: Medicine, nursing, patient health education. **Holdings:** 1000 books; 6000 bound periodical volumes. **Subscriptions:** 330 journals and other serials.

★9725★   HAHNEMANN UNIVERSITY
LIBRARY
245 N. 15th St, M.S. 449
Philadelphia, PA 19102-1192   Phone: (215) 448-7631
Carol Hansen Fenichel, Ph.D., Dir.
Subjects: Medicine, allied health professions, nursing, mental health. **Holdings:** 42,000 books; 46,000 bound periodical volumes; 1300 theses; 1000 government and miscellaneous reports; 26 VF drawers; 450 reels of microfilm; 304 audiotapes; 379 videotapes; 202 slide sets; 175 films and filmstrips; 550 linear feet of archives, manuscripts, photographs, memorabilia. **Subscriptions:** 1263 journals and other serials.

★9726★   HOSPITAL OF THE UNIVERSITY OF
PENNSYLVANIA
ROBERT DUNNING DRIPPS LIBRARY OF ANESTHESIA
Department of Anesthesia
3400 Spruce St.
Philadelphia, PA 19104   Phone: (215) 662-3784
Janet Stokes, M.A.
Subjects: Anesthesia. **Holdings:** 600 books; 44 bound periodical volumes; 70 videotape teaching cassettes. **Subscriptions:** 65 journals and other serials.

★9727★   IIMI
INFORMATION CENTER
4205 K St.
Philadelphia, PA 19124
Albert C. Vara, Libn.
Subjects: Marketing; food research; job location for ex-convicts, parolees, and former addicts; natural family planning; parenteral nutrition; population studies. **Holdings:** 1998 books; 46 bound periodical volumes; 998 reports; 6 VF drawers of documents and reports. **Subscriptions:** 12 journals and other serials.

★9728★   INDEPENDENCE BLUE CROSS
CORPORATE LIBRARY
1901 Market St., 25th Fl.
Philadelphia, PA 19103-1480   Phone: (215) 241-3300
Denise M. Dodd, Libn.
Subjects: Health care, insurance, management, business. **Holdings:** 1700 volumes. **Subscriptions:** 135 journals and other serials; 7 newspapers.

★9729★   INFORMATION VENTURES, INC.
LIBRARY
1500 Locust, Ste. 3216
Philadelphia, PA 19102   Phone: (215) 732-9083
Subjects: Carcinogenesis, cancer biology, cancer diagnosis and therapy, occupational safety and health, toxicology, non-ionizing radiation, water resources, environment, medicine. **Holdings:** 1000 bound volumes. **Subscriptions:** 150 journals and other serials.

★9730★   INSTITUTE FOR CANCER RESEARCH
TALBOT RESEARCH LIBRARY
Fox Chase Cancer Center
Philadelphia, PA 19111   Phone: (215) 728-2710
Karen M. Albert, Libn.
Subjects: Biochemistry, cancer, cell biology, chemistry, clinical research, experimental pathology. **Holdings:** 4250 books; 22,000 bound periodical volumes; 800 reels of microfilm; 529 reports. **Subscriptions:** 422 journals and other serials.

★9731★   INSTITUTE OF THE PENNSYLVANIA HOSPITAL
MEDICAL LIBRARY
111 N. 49th St.
Philadelphia, PA 19139   Phone: (215) 471-2013
June M. Strickland, Libn.
Subjects: Psychiatry, psychology, psychoanalysis, mental health, allied health sciences. **Holdings:** 8000 books; 6700 bound periodical volumes; 200 microfiche; 100 reels of microfilm; hospital reports; pamphlets. **Subscriptions:** 210 journals and other serials.

★9732★   INSTITUTE FOR SCIENTIFIC INFORMATION
CORPORATE COMMUNICATIONS DEPARTMENT LIBRARY
3501 Market St.
Philadelphia, PA 19104   Phone: (215) 386-0100
Judith E. Schaeffer, Mgr., Bibliog.Res.Dept.
Subjects: Life sciences; physical and chemical sciences; clinical medicine; engineering and technology; agriculture; environmental, social, behavioral sciences; arts and humanities. **Holdings:** Figures not available. **Subscriptions:** 8000 journals and other serials.

★9733★   INTENSIVE CARING UNLIMITED
LIBRARY
910 Bent Ln.
Philadelphia, PA 19118   Phone: (215) 233-4723
Subjects: Premature and high-risk infants, children with medical or developmental problems, high-risk pregnancy, infant and neonatal death. **Holdings:** 1200 volumes.

★9734★   LANKENAU HOSPITAL
MEDICAL LIBRARY
Lancaster & City Line Aves.
Philadelphia, PA 19151   Phone: (215) 645-2698
Kathleen A. Leigh, Dir., Med.Lib.
Subjects: Medicine, medical research. **Holdings:** 4000 books; 12,000 bound periodical volumes; 450 audio cassettes. **Subscriptions:** 400 journals and other serials.

★9735★   LANKENAU HOSPITAL
SCHOOL OF NURSING LIBRARY
City Ave. & 64th St.
Philadelphia, PA 19151   Phone: (215) 642-3931
Maude H. Meyerend, Libn.
Subjects: Nursing and nursing history, medicine, public health, microbiology, chemistry, psychology, sociology. **Holdings:** 3600 volumes; 8 VF drawers of illustrations, clippings, pamphlets, reports, archival materials. **Subscriptions:** 75 journals and other serials.

★9736★   LIBRARY COMPANY OF PHILADELPHIA
1314 Locust St.
Philadelphia, PA 19107   Phone: (215) 546-3181
John C. VanHorne, Libn.
Subjects: Pre-1860 Americana, Philadelphia and Pennsylvania, pre-1820 medical material, black history before 1906. **Holdings:** 450,000 books; 50,000 prints and photographs; 160,000 manuscripts. **Subscriptions:** 130 journals and other serials.

★9737★   MAGEE REHABILITATION HOSPITAL
MEDICAL LIBRARY
6 Franklin Plaza
Philadelphia, PA 19102   Phone: (215) 587-3423
Susan Couch, Dir., Lib.Serv.
Subjects: Physical medicine and rehabilitation; nursing; therapy - physical, vocational, occupational, speech. **Holdings:** 400 books; 70 bound periodical volumes; 600 unbound periodicals; 40 cassette tapes; 30 bulletins and newsletters; 100 videotapes. **Subscriptions:** 100 journals and other serials.

★9738★ MARRIAGE COUNCIL OF PHILADELPHIA
DIVISION OF FAMILY STUDY AND MARRIAGE COUNCIL
LIBRARY
4025 Chestnut St., 2nd Fl.
Philadelphia, PA 19104   Phone: (215) 382-6680
Martin Goldberg, M.D., Dir.
Subjects: Marriage and family relationships, marriage counseling, human sexuality and sex therapy, mental health, religion and marriage. **Holdings:** 2000 books. **Subscriptions:** 16 journals and other serials.

★9739★ MEDICAL COLLEGE OF PENNSYLVANIA
ARCHIVES AND SPECIAL COLLECTIONS ON WOMEN IN
MEDICINE
3300 Henry Ave.
Philadelphia, PA 19129   Phone: (215) 842-7124
Janet Miller, Dir./Archv.
Subjects: Women physicians, health care for women, Medical College of Pennsylvania, education, medicine. **Holdings:** 1000 books; 6000 reprints; 14,000 photographs; 1300 linear feet of archival materials and manuscripts; memorabilia.

★9740★ MEDICAL COLLEGE OF PENNSYLVANIA
EASTERN PENNSYLVANIA PSYCHIATRIC INSTITUTE
MENTAL HEALTH AND NEUROSCIENCES LIBRARY
3200 Henry Ave.
Philadelphia, PA 19129   Phone: (215) 842-4509
Etheldra Templeton, Dir.
Subjects: Psychiatry, psychoanalysis, behavioral sciences, neurosciences. **Holdings:** 15,000 books; 14,000 bound periodical volumes; 500 audiotapes. **Subscriptions:** 600 journals and other serials.

★9741★ MEDICAL COLLEGE OF PENNSYLVANIA
FLORENCE A. MOORE LIBRARY OF MEDICINE
3300 Henry Ave.
Philadelphia, PA 19129   Phone: (215) 842-6910
Etheldra Templeton, Lib.Dir.
Subjects: Biomedicine. **Holdings:** 28,709 books; 55,443 bound periodical volumes. **Subscriptions:** 1554 journals and other serials.

★9742★ MERCY CATHOLIC MEDICAL CENTER
MISERICORDIA HOSPITAL
MEDICAL LIBRARY
54th St. & Cedar Ave.
Philadelphia, PA 19143   Phone: (215) 748-9415
Ann Marie Zglinicki, Libn.
Subjects: Medicine, nursing, psychiatry. **Holdings:** 950 books; 522 bound periodical volumes. **Subscriptions:** 110 journals and other serials.

★9743★ METHODIST HOSPITAL
LIBRARY
2301 S. Broad St.
Philadelphia, PA 19148   Phone: (215) 952-9404
Sara J. Richardson, Libn.
Subjects: Nursing, medicine, hospital administration, pre-clinical sciences. **Holdings:** 2900 books; 100 bound periodical volumes; 6 VF drawers of pamphlets; 500 AV program titles. **Subscriptions:** 171 journals and other serials.

★9744★ MT. SINAI HOSPITAL
MEDICAL LIBRARY
5th & Reed Sts.
Philadelphia, PA 19147   Phone: (215) 339-3780
Susan Cleveland, Lib.Dir.
Subjects: Medicine, nursing. **Holdings:** 3000 books; 3500 bound periodical volumes. **Subscriptions:** 150 journals and other serials.

★9745★ NORTHEASTERN HOSPITAL
SCHOOL OF NURSING LIBRARY
2301 E. Allegheny Ave.
Philadelphia, PA 19134-4499   Phone: (215) 291-3168
Rae Greenberg, Libn.
Subjects: Nursing, medicine, natural sciences, psychology, sociology. **Holdings:** 2024 books; 160 bound periodical volumes; filmstrips; videotapes; cassettes; software programs; 6 VF boxes. **Subscriptions:** 75 journals and other serials.

★9746★ OVERBROOK SCHOOL FOR THE BLIND
LIBRARY
64th St. & Malvern Ave.
Philadelphia, PA 19151   Phone: (215) 877-0313
Julia A. Flinchbaugh, Libn.
Subjects: Standard, large print, and braille books for kindergarten through high school; general library of braille, talking book, tape, and print titles for primary, elementary, and high school; library of print for faculty members. **Holdings:** 12,500 braille books; 5000 printed books; 600 large print books; 3000 talking books, tapes, cassettes. **Subscriptions:** 75 journals and other serials in print and braille.

★9747★ PENNSYLVANIA COLLEGE OF OPTOMETRY
ALBERT FITCH MEMORIAL LIBRARY
1200 W. Godfrey Ave.
Philadelphia, PA 19141   Phone: (215) 276-6270
Marita J. Krivda, Lib.Dir.
Subjects: Optometry, ophthalmology, optics theory, ophthalmic optics, contact lenses, low vision rehabilitation. **Holdings:** 6112 books; 6500 bound periodical volumes; 2 VF drawers of old instruments pamphlets; 50 video cassettes; 800 audio cassettes; 6640 slides. **Subscriptions:** 320 journals and other serials.

★9748★ PENNSYLVANIA COLLEGE OF PODIATRIC
MEDICINE
CENTER FOR THE HISTORY OF FOOT CARE AND
FOOTWEAR
8th St. & Race
Philadelphia, PA 19107   Phone: (215) 629-0300
Lisabeth M. Holloway, Dir.
Subjects: Podiatric medicine, anatomy and diseases of the foot, podiatry/chiropody as a profession, ethnic footwear. **Holdings:** 1800 books; 200 bound periodical volumes; 130 linear feet of archival materials; 700 other cataloged items; 600-item footwear collection.

★9749★ PENNSYLVANIA COLLEGE OF PODIATRIC
MEDICINE
CHARLES E. KRAUSZ LIBRARY
8th St. & Race
Philadelphia, PA 19107   Phone: (215) 629-0300
Linda C. Stanley, Coll.Libn.
Subjects: Podiatry, foot diseases, orthopedics, sports medicine, dermatology, medicine. **Holdings:** 10,500 books; 10,000 bound periodical volumes; 16 VF drawers of reprints of articles pertaining to the foot; 2500 pamphlets on medical subjects; 325 reels of microfilm; 1000 video cassettes; 101 films; 1000 audio cassettes; 2000 slides. **Subscriptions:** 375 journals and other serials.

★9750★ PENNSYLVANIA HOSPITAL
DEPARTMENT FOR SICK AND INJURED
HISTORICAL LIBRARY
8th & Spruce Sts.
Philadelphia, PA 19107   Phone: (215) 829-3998
Caroline Morris, Dir. of Libs.
Subjects: Pre-1800 chemistry, physics, botany, zoology, natural history, materia medica; medicine and surgery prior to 1940. **Holdings:** 8500 books; 4464 bound periodical volumes.

★9751★ PENNSYLVANIA HOSPITAL
DEPARTMENT FOR SICK AND INJURED
MEDICAL LIBRARY
8th & Spruce Sts.
Philadelphia, PA 19107   Phone: (215) 829-3998
Caroline Morris, Dir. of Libs.
Subjects: Medicine, nursing, allied health sciences. **Holdings:** 2122 books; 9500 bound periodical volumes; 3700 other cataloged items; 2 VF drawers. **Subscriptions:** 595 journals and other serials.

★9752★ PENNSYLVANIA SCHOOL FOR THE DEAF
LIBRARY
100 W. School House Ln.
Philadelphia, PA 19144   Phone: (215) 951-4743
Judith Finestone, Libn.
Subjects: Deafness, children's literature. **Holdings:** 13,000 books; 90 bound periodical volumes. **Subscriptions:** 50 journals and other serials; 5 newspapers.

★9753★ PHILADELPHIA COLLEGE OF OSTEOPATHIC MEDICINE
HOSPITAL
MEDICAL LIBRARY
1331 E. Wyoming Ave.
Philadelphia, PA 19124   Phone: (215) 537-7449
Eileen Smith, Med.Lib.Coord.
Subjects: Osteopathic medicine, orthopedics, medicine, nursing. **Holdings:** 1220 books; 357 bound periodical volumes; 335 cassettes. **Subscriptions:** 135 journals and other serials.

★9754★ PHILADELPHIA COLLEGE OF OSTEOPATHIC MEDICINE
O.J. SNYDER MEMORIAL MEDICAL LIBRARY
4150 City Ave.
Philadelphia, PA 19131   Phone: (215) 871-2821
Dr. Shanker H. Vyas, Prof./Dir. of Libs.
Subjects: Osteopathy, medicine, surgery. **Holdings:** 63,553 volumes; 5239 audiotapes; 1536 videotapes; 112 reels of 35mm microfilm; 6255 slides; 323 view master reels; 946 filmstrips; 16 anatomy study wheels. **Subscriptions:** 676 journals; 109 osteopathic serials.

★9755★ PHILADELPHIA COLLEGE OF PHARMACY AND SCIENCE
JOSEPH W. ENGLAND LIBRARY
42nd St. & Woodland Ave.
Philadelphia, PA 19104-4491   Phone: (215) 596-8960
Mignon Adams, Dir., Lib.Serv.
Subjects: Pharmacy, pharmacology, biological sciences, chemistry, pharmacognosy, toxicology. **Holdings:** 59,582 volumes; 5000 reels of microfilm; 30,000 microfiche; 150 audio cassettes; 24 VF drawers of pamphlets; AV programs. **Subscriptions:** 771 journals and other serials.

★9756★ PHILADELPHIA CORPORATION FOR AGING
LIBRARY
642 N. Broad St.
Philadelphia, PA 19130   Phone: (215) 765-9000
Maureen Neville, Ref.Libn.
Subjects: Gerontology, gerontological literature, programs for the aging. **Holdings:** 2000 books; 127 periodical volumes on microfiche; 400 government publications; 6540 documents; 16 VF drawers of pamphlets and reports. **Subscriptions:** 70 journals and other serials; 5 newspapers.

★9757★ PHILADELPHIA GERIATRIC CENTER
LIBRARY
5301 Old York Rd.
Philadelphia, PA 19141   Phone: (215) 456-2971
Joyce A. Post, Libn.
Subjects: Gerontology, geriatrics, psychology, sociology, housing, long-term care administration, anthropology, research methods, death and dying. **Holdings:** 9000 books; 450 bound periodical volumes. **Subscriptions:** 200 journals and other serials.

★9758★ PHILADELPHIA PSYCHIATRIC CENTER
PROFESSIONAL LIBRARY
Ford Rd. & Monument Ave.
Philadelphia, PA 19131   Phone: (215) 877-2000
Ann Vosburgh, Libn.
Subjects: Psychiatry, psychology, psychoanalysis, family therapy. **Holdings:** 7500 volumes. **Subscriptions:** 90 journals and other serials.

★9759★ PLANNED PARENTHOOD SOUTHEASTERN PENNSYLVANIA
RESOURCE CENTER
1144 Locust St.
Philadelphia, PA 19107-5740   Phone: (215) 351-5590
Wanda Mial, Rsrc.Ctr.Coord.
Subjects: Family planning, reproductive health, venereal diseases, childbearing and pregnancy options, sex education. **Holdings:** 2500 books; 40 bound periodical volumes; 12 VF drawers; 100 slides, videotapes, films, filmstrips. **Subscriptions:** 65 journals and other serials.

★9760★ PRESBYTERIAN MEDICAL CENTER OF PHILADELPHIA
HEALTH SCIENCES LIBRARY
51 N. 39th St.
Philadelphia, PA 19104   Phone: (215) 662-9181
Julia Urwin, Lib.Dir.
Subjects: Clinical medicine and nursing. **Holdings:** 2200 books; 3500 bound periodical volumes; 300 archival materials; 70 AV programs; 3 VF drawers. **Subscriptions:** 246 journals and other serials.

★9761★ ROXBOROUGH MEMORIAL HOSPITAL
SCHOOL OF NURSING AND MEDICAL STAFF LIBRARIES
5800 Ridge Ave.
Philadelphia, PA 19128   Phone: (215) 487-4345
Jaroslaw Fedorijczuk, Libn.
Subjects: Nursing, medicine, psychology, sociology, science, history of nursing. **Holdings:** 2429 books; 1555 bound periodical volumes; 6 VF drawers of pamphlets; 3 VF drawers of National League of Nursing pamphlets; 371 AV programs; 23 computer programs. **Subscriptions:** 203 journals and other serials.

★9762★ ST. AGNES MEDICAL CENTER
HEALTH SCIENCE LIBRARY
1900 S. Broad St.
Philadelphia, PA 19145   Phone: (215) 339-4448
Marian Schaner, Dir.
Subjects: Medicine, nursing, and allied health sciences. **Holdings:** 4000 books; 2000 bound periodical volumes; 8 VF drawers. **Subscriptions:** 200 journals and other serials.

★9763★ ST. CHRISTOPHER'S HOSPITAL FOR CHILDREN
MARGERY H. NELSON MEDICAL LIBRARY
3601 A St.
Philadelphia, PA 19134   Phone: (215) 427-5374
Frances B. Pinnel, Med.Libn.
Subjects: Pediatrics. **Holdings:** 3790 books; 2284 bound periodical volumes. **Subscriptions:** 150 journals and other serials.

★9764★ SMITHKLINE BEECHAM PHARMACEUTICALS, U.S.
PRODUCT INFORMATION LIBRARY
1500 Spring Garden St.
Philadelphia, PA 19130   Phone: (215) 751-6334
Gary Grey, Info.Sci.
Subjects: Medicine, veterinary medicine, chemistry, biology, business. **Holdings:** 2600 books; 4765 bound periodical volumes; 2.5 VF drawers of Class 424 patents. **Subscriptions:** 170 journals and other serials.

★9765★ TEMPLE UNIVERSITY
HEALTH SCIENCES CENTER
HEALTH SCIENCES LIBRARIES
Kresge Hall
3400 N. Broad St.
Philadelphia, PA 19140   Phone: (215) 221-2665
Mark-Allen Taylor, Dir.
Subjects: Medicine, dentistry, pharmacy, basic sciences, nursing, allied health sciences. **Holdings:** 99,444 volumes; audiotapes. **Subscriptions:** 1155 journals and other serials.

★9766★ TEMPLE UNIVERSITY HOSPITAL
DIAGNOSTIC IMAGING DEPARTMENT
GUSTAVUS C. BIRD, III, M.D. LIBRARY OF DIAGNOSTIC IMAGING
3401 N. Broad St.
Philadelphia, PA 19140   Phone: (215) 221-4226
Nancy G. Washburne, Libn./Dir.
Subjects: Diagnostic imaging, radiology, nuclear medicine. **Holdings:** 1000 books; 900 bound periodical volumes; 9 volumes of departmental publications; 80 videotapes; 20 slide/tape sets; 50 uncataloged items. **Subscriptions:** 50 journals and other serials.

★9767★ THOMAS JEFFERSON UNIVERSITY
CARDEZA FOUNDATION
TOCANTINS MEMORIAL LIBRARY
1015 Walnut St.
Philadelphia, PA 19107   Phone: (215) 955-7714
Sandor S. Shapiro, M.D., Dir.
Subjects: Hematology and allied health sciences. **Holdings:** 200 books; 400 bound periodical volumes. **Subscriptions:** 30 journals and other serials.

★9768★ THOMAS JEFFERSON UNIVERSITY
SCOTT MEMORIAL LIBRARY
11th & Walnut Sts.
Philadelphia, PA 19107   Phone: (215) 955-6994
Edward Tawyea, Univ.Libn.
Subjects: Medicine and allied health sciences. Holdings: 72,230 monographs; 73,860 periodical volumes; 14,984 microforms containing 184 periodical titles; 608 audiotapes and cassettes; 1298 video cassettes, slide sets, multimedia kits. Subscriptions: 2595 journals and other serials.

★9769★ U.S. DEFENSE LOGISTICS AGENCY
DEFENSE PERSONNEL SUPPORT CENTER
DIRECTORATE OF MEDICAL MATERIEL
MEDICAL INFORMATION CENTER
2800 S. 20th St., Bldg. 9-3-F
Philadelphia, PA 19101-8419   Phone: (215) 952-2110
Ann Cline Tobin, Libn.
Subjects: Medicine, pharmacy, engineering. Holdings: 2500 books; 1500 unbound periodical volumes; military and federal specifications and industry standards on microfilm. Subscriptions: 62 journals and other serials.

★9770★ U.S. DEPARTMENT OF LABOR
OSHA
REGION III LIBRARY
3535 Market St., Ste. 2100
Philadelphia, PA 19104   Phone: (215) 596-1201
Barbara Goodman, Libn.
Subjects: Occupational health and safety, industrial hygiene, toxic substances. Holdings: 1500 books.

★9771★ U.S. DEPARTMENT OF VETERANS AFFAIRS
MEDICAL CENTER LIBRARY
University & Woodland Aves.
Philadelphia, PA 19104   Phone: (215) 823-5860
Carol R. Glatt, Chf., Lib.Serv.
Subjects: Medicine and allied health sciences. Holdings: 3010 books; 7100 bound periodical volumes. Subscriptions: 429 journals and other serials.

★9772★ U.S. NAVY
NAVAL HOSPITAL
MEDICAL LIBRARY
17th & Pattison Aves.
Philadelphia, PA 19145-5199   Phone: (215) 897-8038
Giovina Cavacini, Libn.
Subjects: Medicine, allied health sciences. Holdings: 6000 books; 8000 bound periodical volumes; Audio-Digest tapes. Subscriptions: 275 journals and other serials.

★9773★ UNIVERSITY OF PENNSYLVANIA
BIOMEDICAL LIBRARY
Johnson Pavilion
36th & Hamilton Walk
Philadelphia, PA 19104-6060   Phone: (215) 898-5817
Valerie A. Pena, Libn.
Subjects: Medicine, biology, nursing, health care, basic sciences. Holdings: 155,170 volumes; 919 AV programs. Subscriptions: 2626 journals and other serials.

★9774★ UNIVERSITY OF PENNSYLVANIA
EDGAR FAHS SMITH MEMORIAL COLLECTION IN THE
   HISTORY OF CHEMISTRY
Van Pelt Library
Philadelphia, PA 19104-6206   Phone: (215) 898-7088
Dr. Arnold W. Thackray, Cur.
Subjects: History of chemistry, alchemy, chemical biography, chemical engineering, chemical industry, early medicine, metallurgy, mineralogy, pharmacy, pyrotechnics. Holdings: 3000 portraits, prints, and engravings; Robert Boyle and Joseph Priestley collections of manuscripts and printed material; imprints; 300 late 19th century German chemical dissertations; 8 boxes of Archives of the Division of Chemical Education, American Chemical Society; assorted manuscript collections (inventories available upon request). Subscriptions: 18 journals and other serials.

★9775★ UNIVERSITY OF PENNSYLVANIA
SCHOOL OF DENTAL MEDICINE
LEON LEVY LIBRARY
4001 Spruce St.
Philadelphia, PA 19104-6041   Phone: (215) 898-8969
Patricia Heller, Libn.
Subjects: Dentistry, oral biology, history of dentistry. Holdings: 43,613 volumes. Subscriptions: 437 journals and other serials.

★9776★ UNIVERSITY OF PENNSYLVANIA
SCHOOL OF MEDICINE
CLINICAL EPIDEMIOLOGY UNIT
LIBRARY
2L NEB/S2
Philadelphia, PA 19104   Phone: (215) 898-4623
Subjects: Medicine, clinical epidemiology, public health, statistics. Holdings: Figures not available.

★9777★ UNIVERSITY OF PENNSYLVANIA
SCHOOL OF VETERINARY MEDICINE
C.J. MARSHALL MEMORIAL LIBRARY
3800 Spruce St.
Philadelphia, PA 19104-6008   Phone: (215) 898-8874
Lillian D. Bryant, Libn.
Subjects: Veterinary and comparative medicine, animal husbandry. Holdings: 30,690 volumes; 18 VF drawers of pamphlets, bulletins, and annual reports. Subscriptions: 332 journals and other serials.

★9778★ WILLS EYE HOSPITAL AND RESEARCH INSTITUTE
ARTHUR J. BEDELL MEMORIAL LIBRARY
9th & Walnut Sts.
Philadelphia, PA 19107   Phone: (215) 928-3288
Fleur Weinberg, Libn.
Subjects: Clinical and historical ophthalmology. Holdings: 2500 books; 7600 bound periodical volumes; 200 Wills Quarterly Conference Papers; 2 VF drawers of Wills staff reprints; 5 VF drawers; 250,000 audiotapes, cassettes, slides; 78 video cassettes. Subscriptions: 125 journals and other serials.

★9779★ WISTAR INSTITUTE OF ANATOMY AND BIOLOGY
LIBRARY
36th & Spruce Sts.
Philadelphia, PA 19104   Phone: (215) 898-3805
J.A. Hunter, Libn.
Subjects: Cancer, virus diseases, cytology, immunology, genetics, biochemistry. Holdings: 3000 books; 10,000 bound periodical volumes. Subscriptions: 192 journals and other serials.

★9780★ PENNSYLVANIA DEPARTMENT OF PUBLIC
   WELFARE
PHILIPSBURG STATE GENERAL HOSPITAL
LIBRARY
Loch Lomond Rd.
Philipsburg, PA 16866   Phone: (814) 342-3320
Subjects: Medicine, hospital administration, patient education. Holdings: 597 books; 92 bound periodical volumes; 88 videotapes; 39 film loops; 2 drawers of audio cassettes; 2 shelves of patient education materials. Subscriptions: 89 journals and other serials.

★9781★ ALLEGHENY COUNTY HEALTH DEPARTMENT
LIBRARY
301 39th St., Bldg. 7
Pittsburgh, PA 15201   Phone: (412) 578-8028
Lois Jackson, Dir.
Subjects: Public health. Holdings: 13,568 books. Subscriptions: 135 journals and other serials.

★9782★ ALLEGHENY GENERAL HOSPITAL
HEALTH SCIENCES LIBRARY
320 E. North Ave.
Pittsburgh, PA 15212-9986   Phone: (412) 359-3040
Susan B. Hoehl, Dir.
Subjects: Medicine, surgery, oral surgery, obstetrics, gynecology, neurosciences, musculoskeletal disorders, cardiology, nursing, oncology, health administration. Holdings: 5000 books; 8500 bound periodical volumes; 450 audiotapes; 600 videotapes. Subscriptions: 640 journals and other serials; 20 microfilm subscriptions.

★9783★   BLUE CROSS OF WESTERN PENNSYLVANIA
HEALTH EDUCATION CENTER LIBRARY
5th Avenue Pl., Ste. 313
Pittsburgh, PA 15222   Phone: (412) 255-7390
Tina Palaggo-Toy, Mgr.
Subjects: Health education and promotion, prevention, wellness, health
care delivery, disease, patient education. **Holdings:** 700 books; 10,000
newsletters, pamphlets, reports, preprints. **Subscriptions:** 52 journals and
newsletters.

★9784★   CENTER FOR EMERGENCY MEDICINE OF
        WESTERN PENNSYLVANIA
LIBRARY
230 McKee Pl., Ste. 500
Pittsburgh, PA 15213   Phone: (412) 578-3200
R.D. Stewart, M.D., Dir.
Subjects: Emergency medicine, pre-hospital care, critical care medicine.
Holdings: 300 books; 500 bound periodical volumes. **Subscriptions:** 50
journals and other serials.

★9785★   CENTER FOR SENILITY STUDIES
LIBRARY
161 N. Dithridge St.
Pittsburgh, PA 15213   Phone: (412) 683-7111
Subjects: Alzheimer's Disease, dementias, schizophrenia, brain circulation.
Holdings: Clippings; books; research correspondence.

★9786★   CHILDREN'S HOSPITAL OF PITTSBURGH
BLAXTER MEMORIAL LIBRARY
3705 5th Ave. at De Soto
Pittsburgh, PA 15213-2583   Phone: (412) 692-5288
Nancy Dunn, Libn.
Subjects: Pediatric medicine. **Holdings:** 1000 books; 2600 bound periodi-
cal volumes. **Subscriptions:** 200 journals and other serials.

★9787★   EYE AND EAR INSTITUTE PAVILION
BLAIR-LIPPINCOTT LIBRARY/LRC
230 Lothrop St.
Pittsburgh, PA 15213   Phone: (412) 647-2287
Bruce Johnston, Dir.
Subjects: Ophthalmology, otolaryngology, audiology, head and neck surgery, speech pathology. **Holdings:** 5500 books; 6000 bound periodical
volumes; 1700 microfiche; 175 video cassettes; 1500 audio cassettes; 3000
35mm slides. **Subscriptions:** 175 journals and other serials.

★9788★   FORBES HEALTH SYSTEM
CORPORATE OFFICE LIBRARY
500 Finley St.
Pittsburgh, PA 15206   Phone: (412) 665-3553
Susan V. Reber, Libn.
Subjects: Health care administration, medicine, law. **Holdings:** 1381
books; 26 bound periodical volumes; 69 tapes; 3 VF drawers of pamphlets
and clippings. **Subscriptions:** 40 journals and other serials.

★9789★   FORBES HEALTH SYSTEM
FORBES CENTER FOR GERONTOLOGY
LIBRARY
Frankstown Ave. & Washington Blvd.
Pittsburgh, PA 15206   Phone: (412) 665-3050
Susan V. Reber, Libn.
Subjects: Medicine, nursing, geriatrics. **Holdings:** 843 books; 121 bound
periodical volumes; reprints; clippings. **Subscriptions:** 75 journals and
other serials.

★9790★   FORBES HEALTH SYSTEM
FORBES METROPOLITAN HEALTH CENTER LIBRARY
225 Penn Ave.
Pittsburgh, PA 15221   Phone: (412) 247-2424
Susan V. Reber, Libn.
Subjects: Health sciences, administration. **Holdings:** 2471 books; 1252
bound periodical volumes; 4 VF drawers. **Subscriptions:** 126 journals and
other serials.

★9791★   HARMARVILLE REHABILITATION CENTER
STAFF LIBRARY
Guys Run Rd.
Box 11460
Pittsburgh, PA 15238-0460   Phone: (412) 826-2741
Susan L. Wertz, Dir.
Subjects: Rehabilitation of the physically handicapped adult, spinal cord
injuries, hemiplegia, paraplegia, architectural accessibility, sexual aspects
of disability. **Holdings:** 2600 books; 1000 bound periodical volumes; 525
nonprint materials; 410 videotapes; 32 films; 14 audio cassette albums; 54
slide/sound sets. **Subscriptions:** 188 journals and other serials.

★9792★   INDUSTRIAL HEALTH FOUNDATION
LIBRARY
34 Penn Circle, W.
Pittsburgh, PA 15206   Phone: (412) 363-6600
Marianne C. Kaschak, Dir., Info.Serv.
Subjects: Industrial hygiene, occupational safety and health, toxicology,
environmental issues. **Holdings:** 2000 books; 100 bound periodical vol-
umes; 60,000 abstracts; 20 VF drawers of pamphlets and reprints.
Subscriptions: 60 journals and other serials.

★9793★   MAGEE-WOMENS HOSPITAL
HOWARD ANDERSON POWER MEMORIAL LIBRARY
Forbes Ave. & Halket St.
Pittsburgh, PA 15213   Phone: (412) 647-4288
Bernadette Kaelin, Dir., Lib.Serv.
Subjects: Obstetrics, gynecology, gynecological oncology, neonatology,
perinatology, genetics. **Holdings:** 1000 books; 1000 bound periodical
volumes; 200 pamphlets and documents. **Subscriptions:** 201 journals and
other serials.

★9794★   MERCY HOSPITAL
SCHOOL OF NURSING LIBRARY
1401 Blvd. of the Allies
Pittsburgh, PA 15219   Phone: (412) 232-7963
Veronica C. Harrison, Libn.
Subjects: Nursing, medicine, religion, psychology, sociology, ethics. **Hold-
ings:** 5351 books; 2117 bound periodical volumes; 9 VF drawers of
archival material, history of the school and Mercy Hospital; AV programs.
Subscriptions: 72 journals and other serials.

★9795★   MERCY HOSPITAL
FRED C. BRADY, M.D. MEMORIAL LIBRARY
1400 Locust St.
Pittsburgh, PA 15219   Phone: (412) 232-7520
Suzanne A. Gabany, Libn.
Subjects: Internal medicine, surgery, surgical specialties, anesthesia, obstetrics, pediatrics. **Holdings:** 3500 books; 9000 bound periodical volumes;
video cassettes; Audio-Digest tapes; Continuing Medical Education Software. **Subscriptions:** 280 journals and other serials.

★9796★   MONTEFIORE HOSPITAL
MEDICAL LIBRARY
3459 5th Ave.
Pittsburgh, PA 15213   Phone: (412) 648-6090
Gloria K. Rosen, Lib.Dir.
Subjects: Medicine. **Holdings:** 300 books; 4000 bound periodical volumes.
Subscriptions: 300 journals and other serials; 2 newspapers.

★9797★   NORTH HILLS PASSAVANT HOSPITAL
MEDICAL LIBRARY
9100 Babcock Blvd.
Pittsburgh, PA 15237   Phone: (412) 367-6320
Margaret U. Trevanion, Dir., Lib.Serv.
Subjects: Medicine, nursing. **Holdings:** 2419 books; 4428 bound periodical
volumes; 7 VF drawers of pamphlets. **Subscriptions:** 192 journals and other
serials.

★9798★   THE REHABILITATION INSTITUTE
LIBRARY AND LEARNING RESOURCES
6301 Northumberland St.
Pittsburgh, PA 15217   Phone: (412) 521-9000
Nancy J. Sakino-Spears, Dir.
Subjects: Head injuries, pediatrics, diabetes, asthma, rehabilitation, spina
bifida, Prader-Willi Syndrome. **Holdings:** 256 bound periodical volumes;
25 titles on microfiche. **Subscriptions:** 155 journals and other serials.

★9799★ ST. MARGARET MEMORIAL HOSPITAL
PAUL TITUS MEMORIAL LIBRARY AND SCHOOL OF
 NURSING LIBRARY
4631 Davison St.
Pittsburgh, PA 15201   Phone: (412) 622-7075
Dorothy Schiff, Libn.
Subjects: Medicine, nursing, allied health sciences. **Holdings:** 3500 books;
3100 bound periodical volumes; 8 VF drawers of pamphlets; 3 shelves of
archives; videotapes; audiotapes; filmstrips; slides; AV programs. **Sub-
scriptions:** 265 journals and other serials.

★9800★ SHADYSIDE HOSPITAL
JAMES FRAZER HILLMAN HEALTH SCIENCES LIBRARY
5230 Centre Ave.
Pittsburgh, PA 15232   Phone: (412) 622-2415
Malinda Fetkovich, Dir.
Subjects: Thoracic medicine, cardiology, internal medicine, nursing. **Hold-
ings:** 3000 books; 7000 bound periodical volumes. **Subscriptions:** 275
journals and other serials.

★9801★ SOUTH HILLS HEALTH SYSTEM
BEHAN HEALTH SCIENCE LIBRARY
Coal Valley Rd.
Box 18119
Pittsburgh, PA 15236   Phone: (412) 469-5786
Barbara Palso, Libn.
Subjects: Medicine, nursing, and allied health sciences. **Holdings:** 300
books. **Subscriptions:** 117 journals and other serials.

★9802★ U.S. DEPARTMENT OF VETERANS AFFAIRS
MEDICAL CENTER LIBRARY SERVICE
Highland Dr.
Pittsburgh, PA 15206   Phone: (412) 363-4900
Sandra Mason, Chf.
Subjects: Psychiatry, general medicine, neurology, nursing, social work.
Holdings: 3319 books; 8 VF drawers of pamphlets; 458 video cassettes.
Subscriptions: 298 journals and other serials; 6 newspapers.

★9803★ U.S. DEPARTMENT OF VETERANS AFFAIRS
MEDICAL CENTER LIBRARY SERVICE
University Dr. C
Pittsburgh, PA 15240   Phone: (412) 692-3259
Subjects: Medicine and allied health sciences. **Holdings:** 2200 books;
12,400 bound periodical volumes. **Subscriptions:** 400 journals and other
serials.

★9804★ UNIVERSITY OF PITTSBURGH
BIOLOGICAL SCIENCES AND PSYCHOLOGY LIBRARY
A-217 Langley Hall
Pittsburgh, PA 15260   Phone: (412) 624-4490
Drynda L. Johnston, Hd.
Subjects: Biological sciences, biophysics, biochemistry, psychology, behav-
ioral neurosciences. **Holdings:** 59,976 volumes; 4300 microfiche. **Subscrip-
tions:** 822 journals and other serials.

★9805★ UNIVERSITY OF PITTSBURGH
FALK LIBRARY OF THE HEALTH SCIENCES
Scaife Hall, 2nd Fl.
Pittsburgh, PA 15261   Phone: (412) 648-8824
P. Mickelson, Dir.
Subjects: Medicine, biology, dentistry, nursing, pharmacy, public health,
allied health professions. **Holdings:** 265,414 volumes. **Subscriptions:** 2623
journals and other serials.

★9806★ UNIVERSITY OF PITTSBURGH
PRESBYTERIAN-UNIVERSITY HOSPITAL
MEDICAL STAFF LIBRARY
DeSoto at O'Hara Sts.
Pittsburgh, PA 15213   Phone: (412) 647-3287
Charles B. Wessel, Coord., Hosp.Lib.Serv.
Subjects: Clinical medicine, surgery. **Holdings:** 1500 books; 2875 bound
periodical volumes; 639 Audio-Digest tapes. **Subscriptions:** 120 journals
and other serials.

★9807★ UNIVERSITY OF PITTSBURGH
WESTERN PSYCHIATRIC INSTITUTE AND CLINIC
LIBRARY
3811 O'Hara St.
Pittsburgh, PA 15213   Phone: (412) 624-2378
Barbara A. Epstein, Dir.
Subjects: Psychiatry, behavioral science, mental health. **Holdings:** 59,000
volumes; 2400 audio- and videotapes. **Subscriptions:** 538 journals and
other serials.

★9808★ ECRI
LIBRARY
5200 Butler Pike
Plymouth Meeting, PA 19462   Phone: (215) 825-6000
Lillian A. Linton
Subjects: Medical devices, biomedical engineering, hospital safety. **Hold-
ings:** 2200 books; 470 VF drawers of technical reports and evaluation data.
Subscriptions: 800 journals and other serials.

★9809★ POTTSTOWN MEMORIAL MEDICAL CENTER
MEDICAL STAFF LIBRARY
1600 E. High St.
Pottstown, PA 19464   Phone: (215) 327-7468
Marilyn D. Chapis, Med. Staff Libn.
Subjects: Medical and surgical specialties. **Holdings:** 300 books; 1000
bound periodical volumes. **Subscriptions:** 50 journals and other serials.

★9810★ GOOD SAMARITAN HOSPITAL
MEDICAL LIBRARY
Pottsville, PA 17901   Phone: (717) 621-4466
Velma L. Sippie, Libn.
Subjects: Health science. **Holdings:** 1200 books.

★9811★ POTTSVILLE HOSPITAL AND WARNE CLINIC
MEDICAL LIBRARY
420 S. Jackson St.
Pottsville, PA 17901   Phone: (717) 621-5000
Diane Leinheiser, Libn.
Subjects: Medicine, surgery. **Holdings:** 255 books; 1700 bound periodical
volumes. **Subscriptions:** 21 journals and other serials.

★9812★ QUAKERTOWN COMMUNITY HOSPITAL
HEALTH SCIENCES LIBRARY
1021 Park Ave.
PO Box 9003
Quakertown, PA 18951-9003   Phone: (215) 538-4563
Subjects: Internal medicine, surgery, geriatrics, psychiatry. **Holdings:** 400
books; 300 bound periodical volumes. **Subscriptions:** 137 journals and
other serials.

★9813★ READING HOSPITAL AND MEDICAL CENTER
MEDICAL LIBRARY
PO Box 16052
Reading, PA 19612-6052   Phone: (215) 378-6418
Margaret Hsieh, Med.Libn.
Subjects: Medicine, medical specialties, medical ethics, consumer health
education. **Holdings:** 4000 books; 18,000 bound periodical volumes; 4 VF
drawers; 300 audiotapes. **Subscriptions:** 200 journals and other serials.

★9814★ READING HOSPITAL AND MEDICAL CENTER
READING HOSPITAL SCHOOL OF NURSING LIBRARY
Reading, PA 19603   Phone: (215) 378-6359
Cynthia J. Spayd, Libn.
Subjects: Nursing, psychiatry, psychology. **Holdings:** 8590 volumes. **Sub-
scriptions:** 63 journals and other serials.

★9815★ READING REHABILITATION HOSPITAL
MEDICAL LIBRARY
Rte. 1, Box 250
Reading, PA 19607-9727   Phone: (215) 775-8297
Frances A. Mozloom, Libn.
Subjects: Rehabilitation, physical medicine, neurology, diabetes, spinal
cord and head injuries, communication disorders. **Holdings:** 1000 books;
1100 bound periodical volumes; 200 videotapes; 114 audio cassettes; 82
filmstrips; 56 slide programs. **Subscriptions:** 102 journals and other serials.

★9816★   ST. JOSEPH HOSPITAL
HEALTH SCIENCES LIBRARY
12th & Walnut Sts.
Reading, PA 19603   Phone: (215) 378-2389
Kathleen A. Izzo, Libn.
Subjects: Medicine, nursing, patient education, allied health professions, hospital administration, public health. **Holdings:** 2982 books; 4526 bound periodical volumes; 4 VF drawers of pamphlets. **Subscriptions:** 214 journals and other serials.

★9817★   GUTHRIE MEDICAL CENTER
ROBERT PACKER HOSPITAL HEALTH SCIENCES LIBRARY
Guthrie Sq.
Sayre, PA 18840   Phone: (717) 882-4700
E. Jean Antes, Act.Dir.
Subjects: Medicine, surgery, ophthalmology, anesthesia, nursing, oncology. **Holdings:** 4907 books; 4210 bound periodical volumes. **Subscriptions:** 715 journals and other serials.

★9818★   COMMUNITY MEDICAL CENTER
HOSPITAL LIBRARY
1800 Mulberry St.
Scranton, PA 18510   Phone: (717) 969-8197
Ann Duesing, Hd.Libn.
Subjects: Internal medicine, neonatology, oncology, pulmonary medicine, perinatology, cardiology. **Holdings:** 1500 books; 3000 reels of microfilm. **Subscriptions:** 200 journals and other serials; 3 newspapers.

★9819★   COMMUNITY MEDICAL CENTER
SCHOOL OF NURSING LIBRARY
315 Colfax Ave.
Scranton, PA 18510   Phone: (717) 969-8973
Ann Duesing, Hd.Libn.
Subjects: Nursing, medicine, health administration. **Holdings:** 2500 books; 174 bound periodical volumes; periodicals on microfilm. **Subscriptions:** 125 journals and other serials.

★9820★   MERCY HOSPITAL
MEDICAL LIBRARY
746 Jefferson Ave.
Scranton, PA 18501   Phone: (717) 348-7800
Sr. Elizabeth Anne Brandreth, Libn.
Subjects: Medicine, allied health sciences. **Holdings:** 2034 books; 4750 bound periodical volumes; 6100 microfiche. **Subscriptions:** 159 journals and other serials.

★9821★   MOSES TAYLOR HOSPITAL
LIBRARY
745 Quincy Ave.
Scranton, PA 18510   Phone: (717) 963-2145
Jo-Ann M. Babish, Dir., Lib.Serv.
Subjects: Medicine, health administration, nursing. **Holdings:** 2000 books; journals on microfilm. **Subscriptions:** 250 journals and other serials.

★9822★   GRAND VIEW HOSPITAL
EDWARD F. BURROW MEMORIAL LIBRARY
700 Lawn Ave.
Sellersville, PA 18960   Phone: (215) 453-4632
Evelyn H. Kuserk, Med.Libn.
Subjects: Medicine, nursing, administration. **Holdings:** 500 volumes; 1000 bound periodical volumes; 2 VF drawers of pamphlets. **Subscriptions:** 80 journals and other serials.

★9823★   SHARON REGIONAL HEALTH SYSTEMS
MEDICAL STAFF LIBRARY
740 E. State St.
Sharon, PA 16146   Phone: (412) 983-3911
Jean Burke, Sec.
Subjects: Medicine and allied health sciences. **Holdings:** 283 books; 679 bound periodical volumes; 2422 unbound journals; 2 VF drawers of clip sheets and pamphlets. **Subscriptions:** 33 journals and other serials.

★9824★   SHARON REGIONAL HEALTH SYSTEMS
SCHOOL OF NURSING
LIBRARY
740 E. State St.
Sharon, PA 16146   Phone: (412) 983-3865
Eugenia Christenson, Libn.
Subjects: Nursing, medicine, nutrition, and allied health sciences. **Holdings:** 1500 books; 200 bound periodical volumes; 50 volumes of unbound journals; 4 VF drawers of clipsheets and pamphlets; 117 videotapes; 261 filmstrips and records; 14 slide cassette programs; 23 audio cassettes. **Subscriptions:** 25 journals and other serials.

★9825★   PENNSYLVANIA DEPARTMENT OF PUBLIC
     WELFARE
SOMERSET STATE HOSPITAL
LIBRARY
Box 631
Somerset, PA 15501   Phone: (814) 443-0231
Eve Kline, Dir., Lib.Serv.
Subjects: Psychiatry, psychology, mental retardation. **Holdings:** 9300 books; 500 filmstrips; 650 cassettes; 125 videotapes. **Subscriptions:** 150 journals and other serials; 7 newspapers.

★9826★   R.W. JOHNSON PHARMACEUTICAL RESEARCH
     INSTITUTE
LIBRARY
Spring House, PA 19477   Phone: (215) 628-5627
Diane C. Shaffer, Mgr., Lib. & Info.Serv.
Subjects: Chemistry, pharmacology, biochemistry, clinical medicine, toxicology, technology. **Holdings:** 8000 books; 12,000 bound periodical volumes. **Subscriptions:** 800 journals and other serials.

★9827★   SPRINGHOUSE CORPORATION
CORPORATE LIBRARY
1111 Bethlehem Pike
Spring House, PA 19477   Phone: (215) 646-8700
Nancy H. Lange, Libn.
Subjects: Nursing, health care, education, office systems, management. **Holdings:** 6000 books; company archives. **Subscriptions:** 360 journals and other serials.

★9828★   SPRINGFIELD HOSPITAL
MEDICAL LIBRARY
190 W. Sproul Rd.
Springfield, PA 19064   Phone: (215) 328-8749
June Katucki, Dir., Lib. & Info.Serv.
Subjects: Osteopathic medicine, medicine, nursing. **Holdings:** 1000 books; 2000 bound periodical volumes; 1 VF drawer; 900 cassette tapes; slides. **Subscriptions:** 120 journals and other serials.

★9829★   CENTRE COMMUNITY HOSPITAL
ESKER W. CULLEN HEALTH SCIENCES LIBRARY
1800 E. Park Ave.
State College, PA 16803-6797   Phone: (814) 234-6191
Gloria Durbin Venett, Libn.
Subjects: Medicine, nursing, management, health administration. **Holdings:** 2625 books; 90 bound periodical volumes; 236 cassettes; 19 films; 133 multimedia kits; 15 slides; 111 videotapes. **Subscriptions:** 111 journals and other serials.

★9830★   EASTERN STATE SCHOOL AND HOSPITAL
STAFF LIBRARY
3740 Lincoln Hwy.
Trevose, PA 19047   Phone: (215) 953-6122
Gretchen E. Clark, Libn.
Subjects: Child psychiatry, nursing, psychology, social services, special education. **Holdings:** 3344 volumes; 59 dissertations; 292 pamphlets. **Subscriptions:** 69 journals and other serials.

★9831★   UNIONTOWN HOSPITAL
PROFESSIONAL LIBRARY
500 W. Berkeley St.
Uniontown, PA 15401   Phone: (412) 430-5191
Marilyn D. Miller, Dir.
Subjects: Medicine and allied health sciences. **Holdings:** 550 books; 2500 bound periodical volumes. **Subscriptions:** 75 journals and other serials.

★9832★ UNIONTOWN HOSPITAL
SCHOOL OF NURSING
LIBRARY
Annette Home
500 W. Berkeley St.
Uniontown, PA 15401   Phone: (412) 430-5348
Elizabeth A. Johnson, Libn.
Subjects: Nursing. **Holdings:** 4476 books; 214 bound periodical volumes; 555 audio cassettes; 24 charts; 167 computer disks; 13 filmloops; 224 filmstrips; 24 models; 15 motion pictures; 45 phonograph records; 2613 slides; 135 transparencies; 102 video cassettes. **Subscriptions:** 38 journals and other serials.

★9833★ PENNSYLVANIA STATE UNIVERSITY
GERONTOLOGY CENTER
HUMAN DEVELOPMENT COLLECTION
S109 Henderson Human Development Bldg.
University Park, PA 16802   Phone: (814) 863-0776
Faye Wohlwill, Coll.Dir.
Subjects: Gerontology, adolescent and child psychology, marriage and family. **Holdings:** 3500 volumes. **Subscriptions:** 25 journals and other serials.

★9834★ PENNSYLVANIA STATE UNIVERSITY
LABORATORY FOR HUMAN PERFORMANCE RESEARCH
LIBRARY
Noll Laboratory Bldg.
University Park, PA 16802   Phone: (814) 865-3453
Subjects: Applied physiology. **Holdings:** 300 books; 500 bound periodical volumes; 100 reports. **Subscriptions:** 6 journals and other serials.

★9835★ PENNSYLVANIA STATE UNIVERSITY
LIFE SCIENCES LIBRARY
E205 Pattee Library
University Park, PA 16802   Phone: (814) 865-7056
Katharine Clark, Hd.
Subjects: Agriculture, biology, forestry, microbiology, biophysics, biochemistry, veterinary science, health planning and administration, nursing, food science, nutrition. **Holdings:** 275,000 books. **Subscriptions:** 4000 journals and other serials.

★9836★ WASHINGTON HOSPITAL
HEALTH SCIENCES LIBRARIES
155 Wilson Ave.
Washington, PA 15301   Phone: (412) 223-3143
Joan Holloway Frasier, Hea.Sci.Libn./CME Coord.
Subjects: Internal medicine, nursing, cardiology, oncology. **Holdings:** 7800 books; 1500 bound periodical volumes; 1500 AV programs. **Subscriptions:** 277 journals and other serials.

★9837★ SOLDIERS AND SAILORS MEMORIAL HOSPITAL
HEALTH SCIENCE LIBRARY
Central Ave.
Wellsboro, PA 16901   Phone: (717) 724-1631
Charlean Patterson, Libn.
Subjects: Clinical medicine, nursing, hospital administration, allied health sciences, patient education. **Holdings:** 900 books; 10,000 unbound periodical volumes; 100 NCME videotapes. **Subscriptions:** 115 journals and other serials.

★9838★ CHESTER COUNTY HOSPITAL
MEDICAL STAFF LIBRARY
701 E. Marshall St.
West Chester, PA 19380   Phone: (215) 431-5204
Anne W. Harrington, Med. Staff Libn.
Subjects: Medicine, surgery. **Holdings:** 221 books; 730 bound periodical volumes and other cataloged items. **Subscriptions:** 112 journals and other serials.

★9839★ CHESTER COUNTY HOSPITAL
SCHOOL OF NURSING LIBRARY
701 E. Marshall St.
West Chester, PA 19380   Phone: (215) 431-5222
Subjects: Nursing, medicine, natural science, education, nutrition, psychology, social science. **Holdings:** 1689 books; 147 bound periodical volumes; pamphlets; filmstrips; phonograph records; audio and video cassettes; CAI programs. **Subscriptions:** 50 journals and other serials.

★9840★ MERCK & COMPANY, INC.
MERCK SHARP & DOHME RESEARCH LABORATORIES
LITERATURE RESOURCES WP42-1
West Point, PA 19486   Phone: (215) 661-7804
Ann Jenkins, Assoc.Dir.
Subjects: Organic chemistry, biochemistry, immunology, physiology, microbiology, pharmacology, medicine, veterinary medicine. **Holdings:** 6000 books; 20,000 bound periodical volumes; 6000 reels of microfilm. **Subscriptions:** 2000 journals and other serials.

★9841★ WHITE HAVEN CENTER
STAFF LIBRARY
Oley Valley Rd.
White Haven, PA 18661   Phone: (717) 443-9564
Frances M. McSpedon, M.L.S., Libn.
Subjects: Mental retardation, developmental disabilities. **Holdings:** 1600 books; 1 vertical file. **Subscriptions:** 75 journals and other serials.

★9842★ MERCY HOSPITAL
MEDICAL LIBRARY
25 Church St.
Wilkes-Barre, PA 18765   Phone: (717) 826-3699
Barbara Nanstiel, Dir., Info.Serv.
Subjects: Medicine, nursing, hospital administration. **Holdings:** 1936 books; 2304 journal volumes on microfilm; 303 AV programs. **Subscriptions:** 164 journals and other serials.

★9843★ U.S. DEPARTMENT OF VETERANS AFFAIRS
MEDICAL CENTER LIBRARY
1111 E. End Blvd.
Wilkes-Barre, PA 18711   Phone: (717) 824-3521
Bruce D. Reid, Chf., Lib.Serv.
Subjects: Medicine, allied health sciences. **Holdings:** 4900 books; 2600 bound periodical volumes; journals on microfilm. **Subscriptions:** 234 journals and other serials.

★9844★ WILKES-BARRE GENERAL HOSPITAL
HOSPITAL LIBRARY
Auburn & River Sts.
Wilkes-Barre, PA 18764   Phone: (717) 820-2180
Rosemarie Kazda Taylor, Dir., Lib./Commun.
Subjects: Medicine, nursing, allied health sciences, hospital administration. **Holdings:** 3283 books; 250 titles on microfilm; AV programs; 5 VF drawers of pamphlets; periodicals. **Subscriptions:** 376 journals and other serials.

★9845★ DIVINE PROVIDENCE HOSPITAL
MEDICAL LIBRARY
1100 Grampian Blvd.
Williamsport, PA 17701   Phone: (717) 326-8153
Bobbi Masten, Dir., Med.Rec.
Subjects: Medicine. **Holdings:** 781 books; 1200 bound periodical volumes. **Subscriptions:** 40 journals and other serials.

★9846★ WILLIAMSPORT HOSPITAL AND MEDICAL CENTER
LEARNING RESOURCES CENTER
777 Rural Ave.
Williamsport, PA 17701-3198   Phone: (717) 321-2266
Michael Heyd, Dir.
Subjects: Medicine, nursing, allied health sciences. **Holdings:** 4726 books; 6044 bound periodical volumes; 329 filmstrip/cassette programs; 256 slide/cassette programs; 700 video cassette programs; 317 audio cassette programs; 5 16mm films. **Subscriptions:** 220 journals and other serials.

★9847★ MEMORIAL HOSPITAL
MEDICAL LIBRARY
325 S. Belmont St.
York, PA 17403   Phone: (717) 843-8623
Elaine Homick, Med.Libn.
Subjects: Medicine, nursing, osteopathy. **Holdings:** 1070 books; 169 bound periodical volumes. **Subscriptions:** 89 journals and other serials.

★9848★ YORK HOSPITAL
PHILIP A. HOOVER, M.D. LIBRARY
1001 S. George St.
York, PA 17405   Phone: (717) 771-2495
Beth A. Evitts, Dir., Lib.Serv.
Subjects: Medicine, nursing, health education. **Holdings:** 5735 books; 6479 bound periodical volumes. **Subscriptions:** 500 journals and other serials.

Puerto Rico

★9849★ PUERTO RICO DEPARTMENT OF HEALTH
RAMON EMETERIO BETANCES MEDICAL CENTER LIBRARY
Bo. Sabalos Ave., Carr. No. 2
Box 1868
Mayaguez, PR 00708   Phone: (809) 834-8686
Myrna Y. Ramirez, Libn.
Subjects: Medicine, surgery, pediatrics, obstetrics and gynecology, laboratory medicine, dentistry. **Holdings:** 2239 books; 1258 bound periodical volumes; 13 reports. **Subscriptions:** 74 journals and other serials.

★9850★ PONCE SCHOOL OF MEDICINE FOUNDATION
MEDICAL LIBRARY
University Ave. No. 1
Box 7004
Ponce, PR 00731   Phone: (809) 840-2549
Carmen G. Malavet, Dir.
Subjects: Clinical and basic sciences, anatomy, microbiology. **Holdings:** 7758 books; 7080 bound periodical volumes; 14,838 uncataloged items. **Subscriptions:** 250 journals and other serials.

★9851★ UNIVERSITY OF PUERTO RICO
LIBRARY SYSTEM
LIBRARY SERVICES FOR THE PHYSICALLY HANDICAPPED
Box 23302, UPR Sta.
Rio Piedras, PR 00931-3302   Phone: (809) 764-0000
Ludim Diaz, Hd.Libn.
Subjects: Blind - education, printing, writing systems, rehabilitation; literature; history; languages. **Holdings:** 389 books; 2882 unbound periodicals; 571 maps; 555 cassette tapes; 41 open reel tapes; 4 records. **Subscriptions:** 30 journals and other serials.

★9852★ PUERTO RICO DEPARTMENT OF HEALTH
MEDICAL LIBRARY
Ant. Hospital de Psiquiatria - Bo. Monacillos
Call Box 70184
San Juan, PR 00936   Phone: (809) 766-1616
Jose Sorer, Libn.
Subjects: Public health, emergency and ambulatory services, mental health services, planning and evaluation of hospital development, health services administration, continuing medical education, allied health professions. **Holdings:** 3500 books; 180 bound periodical volumes; 1110 monographs and pamphlets; 600 bound reports and documents; 260 state reports; 558 unbound periodical volumes; 14 VF drawers of leaflets. **Subscriptions:** 563 journals and other serials.

★9853★ PUERTO RICO DEPARTMENT OF HEALTH
MENTAL HEALTH LIBRARY
Asst. Secretariat for Mental Health
Box GPO 61
San Juan, PR 00936   Phone: (809) 781-5660
Dr. Gomez, Libn.
Subjects: Psychiatry, drugs, neurology, psychotherapy, alcoholism, psychology, psychoanalysis, hypnosis, T-groups. **Holdings:** 5665 books; 300 bound periodical volumes; 100 special theme materials; 200 annual reports of the Mental Health Program; 50 publications of the Division of Human Resources.

★9854★ PUERTO RICO DEPARTMENT OF SOCIAL SERVICES
LIBRARY
Box 11398, Fernandez Juncos Sta.
San Juan, PR 00910   Phone: (809) 722-7400
Lillian Valcarcel, Libn.
Subjects: Social services to families, child welfare, social and vocational rehabilitation, child abuse and delinquency, juvenile delinquency, public assistance, training and staff development, nutrition, adult affairs, budget, federal resources. **Holdings:** 987 books; 9092 pamphlets. **Subscriptions:** 41 journals and other serials; 28 newspapers.

★9855★ U.S. DEPARTMENT OF VETERANS AFFAIRS
HOSPITAL LIBRARY
VA Medical & Regional Office Ctr.
1 Veteran Plaza
San Juan, PR 00927-5800   Phone: (809) 758-7575
Raquel A. Walters, Chf., Lib.Serv.
Subjects: Medicine and specialties, nursing, surgery and specialties, dietetics and nutrition. **Holdings:** 8598 books and bound periodical volumes; AV programs. **Subscriptions:** 610 journals and other serials.

★9856★ UNIVERSITY OF PUERTO RICO
MEDICAL SCIENCES CAMPUS
LIBRARY
PO Box 365067
San Juan, PR 00936-5067   Phone: (809) 758-2525
Ana Isabel Moscoso, Dir.
Subjects: Medicine, dentistry, public health, pharmacy, allied health sciences, nursing. **Holdings:** 29,985 books; 70,720 bound periodical volumes; 5000 clippings; 700 reprints; 1000 pamphlets. **Subscriptions:** 1407 journals and other serials.

Rhode Island

★9857★ INSTITUTE OF MENTAL HEALTH
LEARNING RESOURCE CENTER
Adolph Meyer Bldg.
Box 8281
Cranston, RI 02920   Phone: (401) 464-2580
Deirdre Donohue, Lib.Coord.
Remarks: No further information was supplied by the respondent.

★9858★ EMMA PENDLETON BRADLEY HOSPITAL
AUSTIN T. AND JUNE ROCKWELL LEVY LIBRARY
1011 Veterans Memorial Pkwy.
East Providence, RI 02915   Phone: (401) 434-3400
Deborah Shea Porrazzo, Dir., Lib. & Info.Serv.
Subjects: Child psychiatry, child psychology, social work, special education, child neurology, pediatrics. **Holdings:** 3250 books; 1500 bound periodical volumes; 300 archival materials; 200 pamphlets; 400 audiotape cassettes. **Subscriptions:** 200 journals and other serials.

★9859★ NEWPORT HOSPITAL
INA MOSHER HEALTH SCIENCES LIBRARY
Friendship St.
Newport, RI 02840   Phone: (401) 846-6400
Tosca N. Carpenter, Hd.Libn.
Subjects: Medicine, nursing, allided health sciences. **Holdings:** 4500 volumes; 56 newsletters; 15 VF drawers; 10 tape journals. **Subscriptions:** 160 journals and other serials.

★9860★ U.S. NAVY
NAVAL HOSPITAL
MEDICAL LIBRARY
Cypress & 3rd Sts.
Newport, RI 02841-5003   Phone: (401) 841-4512
Winifred M. Jacome, Med.Lib.Techn.
Subjects: Medicine and allied health sciences, dentistry, orthopedics, ophthalmology. **Holdings:** 2100 books; Audio-Digest tapes, 1989 to present; 2938 journal volumes. **Subscriptions:** 170 journals and other serials.

★9861★ ST. JOSEPH HOSPITAL
FATIMA UNIT
HEALTH SCIENCE LIBRARY
200 High Service Ave.
North Providence, RI 02904   Phone: (401) 456-3036
Sylvia Raymond, Lib.Asst.
Subjects: Medicine, surgery, nursing, allied health sciences. **Holdings:** 1700 books; 3365 bound periodical volumes; 2 VF drawers. **Subscriptions:** 194 journals and other serials.

★9862★ PAWTUCKET MEMORIAL HOSPITAL
HEALTH SCIENCES LIBRARY
Prospect & Pond Sts.
Pawtucket, RI 02860   Phone: (401) 722-6000
Sylvia Hampton, Med.Lib.Coord.
Subjects: Medicine, family medicine. **Holdings:** 660 books; 7852 bound periodical volumes. **Subscriptions:** 150 journals and other serials.

★9863★ BROWN UNIVERSITY
CENTER FOR NEURAL SCIENCES
PO Box 1953
Providence, RI 02912   Phone: (401) 863-3548
Mary Ellen Flinn-Butera, Adm.Asst.
Subjects: Brain and cerebral cortex - models and mechanisms of learning, memory, plasticity. **Holdings:** Journals.

★9864★ BROWN UNIVERSITY
SCIENCES LIBRARY
Brown Univ. Library, Box I
Providence, RI 02912   Phone: (401) 863-2405
Florence Kell Doksansky, Asst.Univ.Libn.
Subjects: Health sciences, life sciences, physical sciences, engineering. **Holdings:** 500,000 volumes. **Subscriptions:** 6566 journals and other serials.

★9865★ BUTLER HOSPITAL
ISAAC RAY MEDICAL LIBRARY
345 Blackstone Blvd.
Providence, RI 02906   Phone: (401) 455-6248
Linda Walton, Libn.
Subjects: Psychiatry, psychology. **Holdings:** 3000 books; 5000 bound periodical volumes. **Subscriptions:** 100 journals and other serials.

★9866★ MIRIAM HOSPITAL
HEALTH SCIENCES LIBRARY
164 Summit Ave.
Providence, RI 02906   Phone: (401) 331-8500
MaryAnn Slocomb, Dir., Hea.Sci.Lib.
Subjects: Clinical medicine, surgery, biomedical research. **Holdings:** 4142 books; 9870 bound periodical volumes; 969 cassettes; 16 tapes. **Subscriptions:** 409 journals and other serials.

★9867★ THE PROVIDENCE CENTER
PRESEL MEMORIAL LIBRARY
520 Hope St.
Providence, RI 02906   Phone: (401) 274-2500
Patricia M. Vigorito
Subjects: Psychiatry, psychology, social work. **Holdings:** 600 books. **Subscriptions:** 40 journals and other serials.

★9868★ RHODE ISLAND DEPARTMENT OF ELDERLY
  AFFAIRS
EVE M. GOLDBERG LIBRARY AND RESOURCE CENTER
160 Pine St.
Providence, RI 02903
Will Speck, Act.Libn.
Subjects: Gerontology, geriatrics, retirement. **Holdings:** 600 volumes; 50 state studies on aging; 100 pamphlets; 10 films; 40 video cassettes. **Subscriptions:** 5 journals and other serials.

★9869★ RHODE ISLAND DEPARTMENT OF HEALTH
GERTRUDE E. STURGES MEMORIAL LIBRARY
3 Capitol Hill, Rm. 407
Providence, RI 02908   Phone: (401) 277-2506
Barry J. Levin, Libn.
Subjects: Public health, preventive medicine, nursing. **Holdings:** 9400 books and pamphlets; 1200 bound periodical volumes; 4 drawers of newsletters; 2 cabinets of vertical files. **Subscriptions:** 275 journals and other serials; 5 newspapers.

★9870★ RHODE ISLAND HOSPITAL
PETERS HEALTH SCIENCES LIBRARY
593 Eddy St.
Providence, RI 02902   Phone: (401) 277-4671
Irene M. Lathrop, Dir., Lib.Serv.
Subjects: Medicine, medical specialities, nursing, hospital administration. **Holdings:** 9000 books; 11,000 bound periodical volumes. **Subscriptions:** 602 journals and other serials.

★9871★ RHODE ISLAND SCHOOL FOR THE DEAF
LIBRARY
Corliss Park
Providence, RI 02908   Phone: (401) 277-3525
Gerry Dunn, Libn.
Remarks: No further information was supplied by the respondent.

★9872★ ROGER WILLIAMS GENERAL HOSPITAL
HEALTH SCIENCES LIBRARY
825 Chalkstone Ave.
Providence, RI 02908   Phone: (401) 456-2036
Hadassah Stein, Libn.
Subjects: Medicine, nursing, allied health sciences. **Holdings:** 2200 books; 2800 bound periodical volumes; 600 indexes, clinics. **Subscriptions:** 182 journals and other serials.

★9873★ ST. JOSEPH HOSPITAL
OUR LADY OF PROVIDENCE UNIT
HEALTH SCIENCE LIBRARY
21 Peace St.
Providence, RI 02907   Phone: (401) 456-4035
Mary Zammarelli, Dir., Lib.Serv.
Subjects: Medicine, nursing, and allied health sciences. **Holdings:** 1500 books; 8855 bound periodical volumes; 4 VF drawers of pamphlets, reports. **Subscriptions:** 141 journals and other serials.

★9874★ U.S. DEPTARTMENT OF VETERANS AFFAIRS
HEALTH SCIENCES LIBRARY
Davis Park
Providence, RI 02908   Phone: (401) 457-3001
Cheryl R. Banick, Lib.Techn.
Subjects: Medicine, nursing, and allied health sciences. **Holdings:** 2249 books; AV programs. **Subscriptions:** 261 journals and other serials.

★9875★ IN-SIGHT
TECHNICAL INFORMATION CENTER
43 Jefferson Blvd.
Warwick, RI 02888   Phone: (401) 941-3322
Paula G. Olivieri, Coord., Volunteer Serv.
Subjects: Blindness, vision, education and rehabilitation of the blind, aging, diabetes. **Holdings:** 250 books. **Subscriptions:** 10 journals and other serials.

★9876★ KENT COUNTY MEMORIAL HOSPITAL
HEALTH SCIENCES LIBRARY
455 Toll Gate Rd.
Warwick, RI 02886   Phone: (401) 737-7010
Jo-Anne M. Aspri, Libn.
Subjects: Surgery, medicine, nursing, drug therapy. **Holdings:** 1100 books; 1700 bound periodical volumes; 957 journal volumes in microform. **Subscriptions:** 180 journals and other serials.

★9877★ NATIONAL FOUNDATION FOR GIFTED AND
  CREATIVE CHILDREN
LIBRARY
395 Diamond Hill Rd.
Warwick, RI 02886   Phone: (401) 738-0937
Marie Friedel, Exec.Dir.
Subjects: Gifted children, creative children, misuse of prescription drugs, physical chemistry and biology, science, humanities, music, art, creative writing. **Holdings:** 2500 books; 1000 unbound periodicals; 45 notebooks of newspaper clippings, 1968 to present; test scores of 800 children; 200 records of prescription drugs given to children. **Subscriptions:** 10 journals and other serials.

★9878★ WESTERLY HOSPITAL
Z.T. TANG MEDICAL LIBRARY
Wells St.
Westerly, RI 02891   Phone: (401) 596-6000
Natalie V. Lawton, Libn.
Subjects: Medicine, surgery. **Holdings:** 686 books; 525 bound periodical volumes. **Subscriptions:** 61 journals and other serials.

South Carolina

★9879★ MEDICAL UNIVERSITY OF SOUTH CAROLINA
LIBRARY
171 Ashley Ave.
Charleston, SC 29425-3001   Phone: (803) 792-2371
Anne K. Robichaux, Act.Dir.
Subjects: Medicine, dentistry, nursing, pharmacy, health-related professions, pharmacology. **Holdings:** 82,357 books; 105,962 bound periodical volumes; 12 VF drawers of pamphlets, clippings, South Carolina material; 2089 titles of AV programs, self-instructional programs, videotapes, audio cassettes, slides. **Subscriptions:** 2939 journals and other serials; 9 newspapers.

★9880★ MEDICAL UNIVERSITY OF SOUTH CAROLINA
MULTIPURPOSE ARTHRITIS CENTER LIBRARY
Division of Rheumatology and Immunology
171 Ashley Ave., CSB 912
Charleston, SC 29425   Phone: (803) 792-2000
E.C. LeRoy, M.D., Dir.
Subjects: Rheumatology, immunology, internal and physical medicine. **Holdings:** 200 books; 100 bound periodical volumes. **Subscriptions:** 25 journals and other serials.

★9881★ SOUTH CAROLINA DEPARTMENT OF MENTAL
RETARDATION
WHITTEN CENTER LIBRARY AND MEDIA RESOURCE
SERVICES
Columbia Hwy.
Box 239
Clinton, SC 29325   Phone: (803) 833-2736
Mr. Hsiu Yun Keng, Dir.
Subjects: Mental retardation, services for mentally retarded, special education, special media for mentally retarded, psychology. **Holdings:** 6500 books; 170 bound periodical volumes; 13,500 AV programs; 650 educational toys, games, fish, birds, and other animals. **Subscriptions:** 14 journals and other serials.

★9882★ BAPTIST MEDICAL CENTER
PITTS MEMORIAL LIBRARY
Taylor at Marion St.
Columbia, SC 29220   Phone: (803) 771-5281
Pat Pavlick, Libn.
Subjects: Nursing, medicine, pharmacology, pastoral care, respiratory therapy, hospital administration. **Holdings:** 800 books; 150 bound periodical volumes; 12 VF drawers of clippings and pamphlets; masters' theses. **Subscriptions:** 100 journals and other serials.

★9883★ G. WERBER BRYAN PSYCHIATRIC HOSPITAL
PROFESSIONAL LIBRARY
220 Faison Dr.
Columbia, SC 29203   Phone: (803) 935-7851
Steven T. Leap, Libn.
Subjects: Psychiatry, social work, psychology, recreation therapy. **Holdings:** 600 books. **Subscriptions:** 21 journals and other serials.

★9884★ NATIONAL ASSOCIATION FOR SPORT AND
PHYSICAL EDUCATION
MEDIA RESOURCE CENTER
Dept. of Physical Education
University of South Carolina
Columbia, SC 29208   Phone: (803) 777-3172
Dr. Richard C. Hohn, Dir.
Subjects: Physical education, sports, physical fitness, intramurals, dance and career related information. **Holdings:** 200 audio- and videotapes.

★9885★ RICHLAND MEMORIAL HOSPITAL
JOSEY MEMORIAL HEALTH SCIENCES LIBRARY
5 Richland Medical Park
Columbia, SC 29203   Phone: (803) 765-6312
Kay F. Harwood, Dir.
Subjects: Medicine, medical specialities, nursing, hospital administration. **Holdings:** 3000 books; 5000 bound periodical volumes; 600 videotapes; 1000 audiotapes; 5400 slides. **Subscriptions:** 450 journals and other serials.

★9886★ SOUTH CAROLINA COMMISSION ON ALCOHOL
AND DRUG ABUSE
THE DRUGSTORE INFORMATION CLEARINGHOUSE
3700 Forest Dr., Ste. 204
Columbia, SC 29204   Phone: (803) 734-9559
Elizabeth G. Peters, Adm.
Subjects: Alcohol and drug abuse - education, prevention, intervention, treatment. **Holdings:** 1500 books; 150 bound periodical volumes; 16 VF drawers; 50 pamphlet titles; 212 16mm films. **Subscriptions:** 44 journals and other serials.

★9887★ SOUTH CAROLINA DEPARTMENT OF HEALTH AND
ENVIRONMENTAL CONTROL
LIBRARY
2600 Bull St.
Columbia, SC 29201   Phone: (803) 737-3945
Jane K. Olsgaard, Dir.
Subjects: Public health, medicine, nursing, epidemiology, environmental sciences, nutrition, toxicology, health education. **Holdings:** 3000 books; 3000 bound periodical volumes; 1500 films; 500 pamphlet and poster titles. **Subscriptions:** 250 journals and other serials.

★9888★ SOUTH CAROLINA DEPARTMENT OF MENTAL
HEALTH
CRAFTS-FARROW STATE HOSPITAL
LIBRARY
7901 Farrow Rd.
Columbia, SC 29203   Phone: (803) 935-7721
Elizabeth H. Bonniwell, Libn.
Subjects: Geriatrics, psychiatry, religion, nursing homes. **Holdings:** 2955 books; 18 bound periodical volumes; 4 VF drawers. **Subscriptions:** 26 journals; 34 periodicals; 16 newspapers.

★9889★ SOUTH CAROLINA DEPARTMENT OF MENTAL
HEALTH
EARLE E. MORRIS, JR. ALCOHOL AND DRUG ADDICTION
TREATMENT CENTER
LIBRARY
610 Faison Dr.
Columbia, SC 29203   Phone: (803) 935-7791
Alice Jonas, Libn.
Subjects: Alcoholism, drug addiction, group and family therapy. **Holdings:** 2000 books. **Subscriptions:** 31 journals and other serials.

★9890★ SOUTH CAROLINA DEPARTMENT OF MENTAL
RETARDATION
MIDLANDS CENTER LIBRARY
8301 Farrow Rd.
Columbia, SC 29203   Phone: (803) 935-7500
Shirley Mitchell, Libn.
Subjects: Mental retardation, special education. **Holdings:** 2500 books; 33 video cassettes; 10 16mm films; 295 slides. **Subscriptions:** 28 journals and other serials.

★9891★ SOUTH CAROLINA PROTECTION AND ADVOCACY
SYSTEM FOR THE HANDICAPPED
LIBRARY
3710 Landmark Dr., Ste. 208
Columbia, SC 29204   Phone: (803) 782-0639
Hazel Mengedoht
Subjects: Handicapped - issues, laws. **Holdings:** Figures not available.

★9892★ U.S. DEPARTMENT OF VETERANS AFFAIRS
WILLIAM JENNINGS BRYAN-DORN VETERANS HOSPITAL
LIBRARY
Garners Ferry Rd.
Columbia, SC 29201   Phone: (803) 776-4000
Charletta P. Felder, Chf., Lib.Serv.
Subjects: Medicine, surgery, nursing, dentistry, psychiatry. **Holdings:** 3817 books; 3200 bound periodical volumes; 15 drawers of microfilm; 800 AV programs. **Subscriptions:** 250 journals and other serials; 12 newspapers.

★9893★ UNIVERSITY OF SOUTH CAROLINA
SCHOOL OF MEDICINE LIBRARY
Columbia, SC 29208   Phone: (803) 733-3344
R. Thomas Lange, Dir.
Subjects: Medicine. **Holdings:** 20,000 books; 51,400 bound periodical

volumes; 900 AV programs; 4280 reels of microfilm. **Subscriptions:** 1120 journals and other serials.

★9894★ WILLIAM S. HALL PSYCHIATRIC INSTITUTE PROFESSIONAL LIBRARY
PO Box 202
Columbia, SC 29202   Phone: (803) 734-7136
Ms. Neeta N. Shah, Chf.Med.Libn.
Subjects: Psychiatry, psychology, sociology, neurology, pastoral counseling, genetics, psychopharmacology, nursing, occupational therapy. **Holdings:** 12,800 books; 8500 bound periodical volumes; 64 videotapes; 550 cassettes; 12 VF drawers of pamphlets and reprints. **Subscriptions:** 340 journals and other serials.

★9895★ FLORENCE-DARLINGTON TECHNICAL COLLEGE LIBRARY
Drawer 8000
Florence, SC 29501   Phone: (803) 661-8032
Subjects: Health, business, data processing, secretarial science, engineering, fashion merchandising. **Holdings:** 28,364 books; 747 bound periodical volumes; 1273 pamphlets; 10,338 microforms. **Subscriptions:** 385 journals and other serials; 20 newspapers.

★9896★ PEE DEE AREA HEALTH EDUCATION CENTER LIBRARY
McLeod Regional Medical Center
555 E. Cheves St.
Florence, SC 29501   Phone: (803) 667-2275
Lillian Fisher, Reg.Libn.
Subjects: Clinical medicine, nursing, allied health sciences, competency-based nursing orientation, management. **Holdings:** 1565 books; 1587 bound periodical volumes; 1181 AV programs. **Subscriptions:** 317 journals and other serials.

★9897★ AMERICAN LEPROSY MISSIONS LIBRARY
1 Alm Way
Greenville, SC 29601   Phone: (803) 271-7040
Lynda S. Parrish, Asst.Ed.
Subjects: Leprosy treatment, medical missionary efforts to overcome the disease, ALM history, reconstructive surgery, rehabilitation, village health care. **Holdings:** 1200 books; films; videotapes; ALM records; slides. **Subscriptions:** 20 journals and other serials.

★9898★ GREENVILLE HOSPITAL SYSTEM HEALTH SCIENCE LIBRARY
701 Grove Rd.
Greenville, SC 29605   Phone: (803) 242-7176
Fay Towell, Dir.
Subjects: Medicine, nursing, allied health sciences, hospital administration, management. **Holdings:** 5000 books; 10,000 bound periodical volumes; AV programs. **Subscriptions:** 400 serials.

★9899★ GREENVILLE MENTAL HEALTH CENTER LIBRARY
715 Grove Rd.
Greenville, SC 29605-4280   Phone: (803) 241-1040
Helen B. Hammett, Libn.
Subjects: Mental health, psychiatry, psychology, counseling and therapy, social work. **Holdings:** 3000 books; 337 bound periodical volumes; 250 pamphlets and unbound periodicals; 8 VF drawers of pamphlet material. **Subscriptions:** 69 journals and other serials.

★9900★ UPPER SAVANNAH AREA HEALTH EDUCATION CONSORTIUM LIBRARY
Self Memorial Hospital
1325 Spring St.
Greenwood, SC 29646   Phone: (803) 227-4851
Thomas W. Hill, Libn.
Subjects: Medicine, health sciences, nursing. **Holdings:** 2000 books; 1000 audio and video cassettes, 16mm films, sound recordings. **Subscriptions:** 300 journals and other serials.

★9901★ CATAWBA-WATEREE AHEC LIBRARY
1020 W. Meeting
Box 1045
Lancaster, SC 29720   Phone: (803) 286-4121
Eric Morgan, Libn.
Subjects: Medicine. **Holdings:** 300 books; 150 periodical volumes; 150 AV programs. **Subscriptions:** 125 journals and other serials.

★9902★ MARION COUNTY MEMORIAL HOSPITAL LIBRARY
1108 N. Main St.
Marion, SC 29571   Phone: (803) 423-3210
Ann Finney, Educ.Dir.
Subjects: Medicine, surgery, nursing. **Holdings:** 490 books. **Subscriptions:** 22 journals and other serials.

★9903★ REGIONAL MEDICAL CENTER OF ORANGEBURG AND CALHOUN COUNTIES LIBRARY
3000 St. Matthews Rd.
Orangeburg, SC 29115   Phone: (803) 533-2293
Barbara Sifly, Dir., Med. Staff Serv.
Holdings: 175 books. **Subscriptions:** 14 journals and other serials.

★9904★ SHERMAN COLLEGE OF STRAIGHT CHIROPRACTIC TOM AND MAE BAHAN LIBRARY
Box 1452
Spartanburg, SC 29304   Phone: (803) 578-8770
David M. Bowles, Lib.Dir.
Subjects: Chiropractic, clinical and basic sciences. **Holdings:** 8708 books; 1137 bound periodical volumes; 303 audiotapes; 165 videotapes; 4514 slides; 4 16mm films; 8 phonograph records; 4 VF drawers. **Subscriptions:** 157 journals and other serials; 3 newspapers.

★9905★ SOUTH CAROLINA SCHOOL FOR THE DEAF AND BLIND DEAF LIBRARY
Cedar Spring Sta.
Spartanburg, SC 29302   Phone: (803) 585-7711
Deborah Wright, Libn.
Holdings: 9138 books; 136 bound periodical volumes; 1965 braille volumes; 1535 talking books; 52 audio cassettes; 27 phonograph records; 1027 captioned films; 1322 filmstrips; 284 videotapes; 13 computer software packages; 68 games and puzzles.

★9906★ SPARTANBURG REGIONAL MEDICAL CENTER HEALTH SCIENCES LIBRARY
101 E. Wood St.
Spartanburg, SC 29303   Phone: (803) 591-6220
Mary Ann Camp, Dir., Lib.Serv.
Subjects: Medicine, nursing, allied health sciences, hospital administration. **Holdings:** 4000 books; 3200 bound periodical volumes; 200 AV programs. **Subscriptions:** 230 journals and other serials.

★9907★ LOW COUNTRY AREA HEALTH EDUCATION CENTER LOW COUNTRY AHEC LIBRARY
Box 1488
Walterboro, SC 29488   Phone: (803) 549-1466
Subjects: Medicine, nursing. **Holdings:** 255 books; 295 bound periodical volumes; AV programs. **Subscriptions:** 120 journals and other serials.

South Dakota

★9908★ PRESENTATION COLLEGE LIBRARY
1500 N. Main
Aberdeen, SD 57401   Phone: (605) 229-8468
Arvyce Burns, Lib.Dir.
Subjects: Nursing, theology. **Holdings:** 33,797 books; 2317 bound periodical volumes; 2577 recordings, filmstrips, reels of microfilm, cassettes; 8 VF drawers of pamphlets. **Subscriptions:** 210 journals and other serials; 9 newspapers.

★9909★   ST. LUKES MIDLAND REGIONAL MEDICAL CENTER
DR. PAUL G. BUNKER MEMORIAL MEDICAL LIBRARY
305 S. State St.
Aberdeen, SD 57401   Phone: (605) 229-3355
Jane Reich, Med.Libn.
Subjects: Medicine, nursing. **Holdings:** 1200 books. **Subscriptions:** 220 journals and other serials; 7 newspapers.

★9910★   BROOKINGS HOSPITAL
BROOKVIEW MANOR
LIBRARY
300 22nd Ave.
Brookings, SD 57006   Phone: (605) 692-6351
Judy Costar, Dept.Hd., Med.Rec.
Subjects: Medicine. **Holdings:** 381 volumes. **Subscriptions:** 21 journals and other serials.

★9911★   SOUTH DAKOTA STATE UNIVERSITY
HILTON M. BRIGGS LIBRARY
Box 2115
Brookings, SD 57007   Phone: (605) 688-5106
Dr. Leon Raney, Dean of Lib.
Subjects: Agriculture; pharmacy; engineering - civil, mechanical, electrical; chemistry; entomology; plant pathology; biological sciences; nursing; home economics. **Holdings:** 430,923 books and bound periodical volumes; 349,238 documents; 412,322 microforms. **Subscriptions:** 3527 journals and other serials; 87 newspapers.

★9912★   U.S. DEPARTMENT OF VETERANS AFFAIRS
MEDICAL CENTER LIBRARY SERVICE
113 Comanche Rd.
Fort Meade, SD 57741-1099   Phone: (605) 347-2511
Gene Stevens, Chf., Lib.Serv.
Subjects: Medicine and allied health sciences. **Holdings:** 1450 books; 800 volumes of journals on microfilm; 220 AV programs. **Subscriptions:** 135 journals and other serials.

★9913★   U.S. DEPARTMENT OF VETERANS AFFAIRS
CENTER LIBRARY
Hot Springs, SD 57747   Phone: (605) 745-4101
Carole W. Miles, Chf., Lib.Serv.
Subjects: Geriatrics, surgery. **Holdings:** 845 books; 781 bound periodical volumes. **Subscriptions:** 108 journals and other serials.

★9914★   MADISON COMMUNITY HOSPITAL
HEALTH-SCIENCE LIBRARY
917 N. Washington Ave.
Madison, SD 57042   Phone: (605) 256-6551
Donna Sullivan, Lib.Mgr.
Subjects: Nursing, medicine, paramedical sciences. **Holdings:** 50 books; 20 unbound periodicals. **Subscriptions:** 16 journals and other serials.

★9915★   ST. MARY'S HOSPITAL
MEDICAL LIBRARY
803 E. Dakota Ave.
Pierre, SD 57501   Phone: (605) 224-3178
DeAnn DeKay Hilmoe, Med.Libn.
Subjects: Medicine, nursing, allied health sciences. **Holdings:** 2100 books; 25 bound periodical volumes. **Subscriptions:** 195 journals and other serials.

★9916★   RAPID CITY REGIONAL HOSPITAL
HEALTH SCIENCES LIBRARY
353 Fairmont Blvd.
Rapid City, SD 57701-6000   Phone: (605) 341-7101
Patricia J. Hamilton, Dept.Mgr./Lib.Serv.
Subjects: Medicine, nursing. **Holdings:** 8695 books; 4480 unbound periodicals; 2300 government documents. **Subscriptions:** 500 journals and other serials.

★9917★   SOUTH DAKOTA DEVELOPMENTAL CENTER,
** REDFIELD**
MEDIA CENTER
Box 410
Redfield, SD 57469-0410   Phone: (605) 472-2400
Mr. Lynn Loveland, Libn.
Subjects: Mental retardation, developmentally disabled, special education. **Holdings:** 3292 books; 848 filmstrips; 28 films; 984 phonograph records;

314 cassettes; 44 compact disks; 1200 games and manipulative toys; 89 videotapes; 40 computer programs; 25 microfiche; 180 AV materials.

★9918★   MCKENNAN HOSPITAL
MEDICAL LIBRARY
800 E. 21st St.
PO Box 5045
Sioux Falls, SD 57117-5045   Phone: (605) 339-8088
Frances Ellis Rice, Dir., Lib.Serv.
Subjects: Medicine, nursing, allied health sciences. **Holdings:** 4000 books; 800 bound periodical volumes; 500 microforms; 2 VF drawers. **Subscriptions:** 600 journals and other serials.

★9919★   SIOUX VALLEY HOSPITAL
MEDICAL LIBRARY
1100 S. Euclid Ave.
Box 5039
Sioux Falls, SD 57117-5039   Phone: (605) 333-6330
Anna Gieschen, Libn.
Subjects: Medicine, nursing, allied health sciences. **Holdings:** 4195 books; 3925 unbound and bound periodical volumes; 4 VF drawers of pamphlets, reprints, articles, clippings. **Subscriptions:** 300 journals and other serials.

★9920★   U.S. DEPARTMENT OF VETERANS AFFAIRS
MEDICAL AND REGIONAL OFFICE CENTER
MEDICAL LIBRARY
2501 W. 22nd St.
Box 5046
Sioux Falls, SD 57117   Phone: (605) 336-3230
Raisa Cherniv, Chf., Lib.Serv.
Subjects: General medicine and allied health sciences. **Holdings:** 4600 books; 4631 bound periodical volumes; 4968 reels of microfilm; 1168 AV programs. **Subscriptions:** 400 journals and other serials; 50 newspapers.

★9921★   UNIVERSITY OF SOUTH DAKOTA
CHRISTIAN P. LOMMEN HEALTH SCIENCES LIBRARY
School of Medicine
414 E. Clark
Vermillion, SD 57069-2390   Phone: (605) 677-5347
David A. Hulkonen, Dir.
Subjects: Anatomy, physiology, pharmacology, microbiology, pathology, biochemistry, nursing, dental hygiene, medical technology, clinical medicine. **Holdings:** 37,000 books; 46,000 bound periodical volumes; 900 AV programs. **Subscriptions:** 1078 journals and other serials.

★9922★   BAPTIST HOSPITAL
MEDICAL LIBRARY
E. 8th St.
Box 745
Winner, SD 57580   Phone: (605) 842-2110
Kris Schwartz, Dir., Med.Rec.
Subjects: Medicine. **Holdings:** 200 books. **Subscriptions:** 15 journals and other serials.

★9923★   SACRED HEART HOSPITAL
MEDICAL LIBRARY
501 Summit
Yankton, SD 57078   Phone: (605) 665-9371
Roxie Olson, Med.Libn.
Subjects: Life and health sciences, nursing, hospital administration. **Holdings:** 2700 volumes; 300 AV programs; 5 VF drawers. **Subscriptions:** 200 journals and other serials.

★9924★   SOUTH DAKOTA HUMAN SERVICES CENTER
MEDICAL LIBRARY
Box 76
Yankton, SD 57078   Phone: (605) 668-3165
Mary Lou Kostel, Libn.
Subjects: Psychiatry, psychology, psychiatric nursing, gerontology, social work, medicine. **Holdings:** 3088 books; 158 bound periodical volumes; 541 audiotapes; VF drawers of pamphlets; manuscripts; historical clippings. **Subscriptions:** 61 journals and other serials.

Tennessee

★9925★ ERLANGER MEDICAL CENTER
MEDICAL LIBRARY
975 E. 3rd St.
Chattanooga, TN 37403   Phone: (615) 778-7246
Belva Jennings, Lib.Mgr.
Subjects: Surgery, obstetrics and gynecology, pediatrics, ophthalmology, internal medicine, plastic surgery, oncology, nursing. **Holdings:** 31,276 books; 24,668 bound periodical volumes; 4 VF drawers of archival materials; 10 VF drawers of pamphlets; 1345 cassette tapes. **Subscriptions:** 562 journals and other serials.

★9926★ REBOUND, INC.
CORPORATE LIBRARY
PO Box 2159
Hendersonville, TN 37077   Phone: (615) 822-8430
Virginia Collier, Libn.
Subjects: Head injuries, rehabilitation, medical management, administration. **Holdings:** 150 books; 85 audiotapes; 100 videotapes. **Subscriptions:** 40 journals and other serials.

★9927★ JACKSON-MADISON COUNTY GENERAL HOSPITAL
LEARNING CENTER
708 W. Forest Ave.
Jackson, TN 38301   Phone: (901) 425-6024
Linda G. Farmer, Dir.
Subjects: Medicine, nursing, health. **Holdings:** 1500 books; 600 bound periodical volumes. **Subscriptions:** 202 journals and other serials.

★9928★ EAST TENNESSEE STATE UNIVERSITY
MEDICAL LIBRARY
James H. Quillen College of Medicine
Box 23290A
Johnson City, TN 37614-0002   Phone: (615) 929-6252
Janet S. Fisher, Asst. Dean
Subjects: Medicine. **Holdings:** 38,121 books; 35,100 bound periodical volumes; 6885 AV programs; government documents; microforms; vertical files. **Subscriptions:** 816 journals and other serials.

★9929★ EASTMAN KODAK COMPANY
EASTMAN CHEMICAL COMPANY
TECHNICAL INFORMATION CENTER
MEDICAL LIBRARY
Bldg. 215, Box 1975
Kingsport, TN 37662-1975   Phone: (615) 229-2237
Lillian L. Lewis, Libn.
Subjects: Industrial medicine, industrial hygiene, employee assistance programs. **Holdings:** 2000 books. **Subscriptions:** 90 journals and other serials.

★9930★ HOLSTON VALLEY HOSPITAL AND MEDICAL CENTER
THE ROBERT D. DOTY HEALTH SCIENCES LIBRARY
W. Ravine St.
Box 238
Kingsport, TN 37662   Phone: (615) 229-7063
Patsy S. Ellis, Libn.
Subjects: Medicine, nursing, and allied health sciences. **Holdings:** 5059 books; 5196 bound periodical volumes. **Subscriptions:** 157 journals and other serials.

★9931★ EAST TENNESSEE BAPTIST HOSPITAL
HEALTH SCIENCES LIBRARY
Box 1788
Knoxville, TN 37901   Phone: (615) 632-5618
Mary C. Congleton, Libn.
Subjects: Nursing, allied health sciences, cardiology, gerontology, oncology. **Holdings:** 2300 books. **Subscriptions:** 368 journals and other serials.

★9932★ FORT SANDERS REGIONAL MEDICAL CENTER
MEDICAL/NURSING LIBRARY
1915 White Ave.
Knoxville, TN 37916-2399   Phone: (615) 541-1293
Nedra Cook, Libn.
Subjects: Nursing and nursing education, medicine. **Holdings:** 8000 books;

890 bound periodical volumes; 16 VF drawers. **Subscriptions:** 173 journals and other serials.

★9933★ ST. MARY'S MEDICAL CENTER
MEDICAL LIBRARY
Oak Hill Ave.
Knoxville, TN 37917   Phone: (615) 971-7916
Kenton O'Kane, Libn.
Subjects: Medicine, nursing, hospital administration. **Holdings:** 1500 books; 425 bound periodical volumes; 300 pamphlets. **Subscriptions:** 122 journals and other serials.

★9934★ UNIVERSITY OF TENNESSEE
AGRICULTURE-VETERINARY MEDICINE LIBRARY
Veterinary Medicine Teaching Hospital
Knoxville, TN 37996-4500   Phone: (615) 974-7338
Don Jett, Libn.
Subjects: Agriculture, veterinary medicine. **Holdings:** 111,000 volumes. **Subscriptions:** 2500 journals and other serials.

★9935★ UNIVERSITY OF TENNESSEE
MEDICAL CENTER, KNOXVILLE
PRESTON MEDICAL LIBRARY
1924 Alcoa Hwy.
Knoxville, TN 37920   Phone: (615) 544-9525
Lynne Y. Craver, Dir.
Subjects: Surgery and trauma, pediatrics, hematology, immunology, obstetrics, gynecology. **Holdings:** 3000 books; 26,000 bound periodical volumes. **Subscriptions:** 512 journals and other serials.

★9936★ BLOUNT MEMORIAL HOSPITAL
LESLIE R. LINGEMAN MEMORIAL MEDICAL LIBRARY
907 E. Lamar Alexander Hwy.
Maryville, TN 37801-5193   Phone: (615) 977-5520
Barbara H. Payne, Med.Libn.
Subjects: Internal medicine, pediatrics, nursing, psychiatry, surgery, dermatology, obstetrics, gynecology, urology, orthopedics, cardiology, and allied health subjects. **Holdings:** 773 books; 1511 bound periodical volumes; 6 VF drawers of pamphlets. **Subscriptions:** 85 journals and other serials.

★9937★ BAPTIST MEMORIAL HOSPITAL
JOHN L. MCGEHEE LIBRARY
899 Madison Ave.
Memphis, TN 38146   Phone: (901) 522-5140
Nancy N. Smith, Med.Libn.
Subjects: Medicine. **Holdings:** 1000 books; 3000 bound periodical volumes. **Subscriptions:** 161 journals and other serials.

★9938★ BAPTIST MEMORIAL HOSPITAL
SCHOOL OF NURSING
LIBRARY
999 Monroe
Memphis, TN 38104   Phone: (901) 522-4307
Sherry Young, Libn.
Subjects: Nursing, health care. **Holdings:** 6864 books; 245 bound periodical volumes; 1 VF drawer of clippings and pamphlets; 45 anatomical maps and charts; 225 slides. **Subscriptions:** 51 journals and other serials.

★9939★ LE BONHEUR CHILDREN'S MEDICAL CENTER
HEALTH SCIENCES LIBRARY
1 Children's Plaza
Memphis, TN 38103   Phone: (901) 522-3167
Jan LaBeause, Libn.
Subjects: Pediatrics. **Holdings:** 1200 books; 1500 bound periodical volumes; 1 shelf of faculty reprints. **Subscriptions:** 150 journals and other serials.

★9940★ MEMPHIS MENTAL HEALTH INSTITUTE
JAMES A. WALLACE LIBRARY
865 Poplar Ave.
Box 40966
Memphis, TN 38174-0966   Phone: (901) 524-1261
Josephine Maddry, Libn.
Subjects: Psychiatry, psychology, nursing, social work and activity therapy, medicine. **Holdings:** 2700 volumes; 103 tapes. **Subscriptions:** 135 journals and other serials.

★9941★ MEMPHIS STATE UNIVERSITY LIBRARIES
SPEECH AND HEARING CENTER LIBRARY
807 Jefferson Ave.
Memphis, TN 38104   Phone: (901) 678-5846
John Swearengen, Lib.Asst.
Subjects: Audiology, speech pathology. **Holdings:** 5964 volumes. **Subscriptions:** 90 journals and other serials.

★9942★ METHODIST HOSPITALS OF MEMPHIS
EDUCATIONAL RESOURCES DEPARTMENT
LESLIE M. STRATTON NURSING LIBRARY
251 S. Claybrook
Memphis, TN 38104-6499   Phone: (901) 726-8862
Joanne S. Guyton, Mgr.
Subjects: Nursing, medicine, psychology, sociology, education. **Holdings:** 6200 books; 339 periodical volumes; 462 volumes of journals on microfiche. **Subscriptions:** 107 journals and other serials.

★9943★ ST. JOSEPH HOSPITAL
HEALTH SCIENCE LIBRARY
220 Overton
Box 178
Memphis, TN 38105-0178   Phone: (901) 577-2828
Patricia Irby, Libn.
Subjects: Medicine, nursing, management. **Holdings:** 2735 books; 2834 bound periodical volumes. **Subscriptions:** 172 journals and other serials.

★9944★ ST. JUDE CHILDREN'S RESEARCH HOSPITAL
BIOMEDICAL LIBRARY
332 N. Lauderdale
Box 318
Memphis, TN 38101   Phone: (901) 525-0388
Mary Edith Walker, Lib.Dir.
Subjects: Medicine, biological sciences. **Holdings:** 2200 books; 11,000 bound periodical volumes; 17 dissertations; 300 audio cassettes; 120 AV programs. **Subscriptions:** 275 journals and other serials.

★9945★ SCHERING-PLOUGH HEALTH CARE
R & D LIBRARY
3030 Jackson Ave.
Box 377
Memphis, TN 38151   Phone: (901) 320-2702
Martha Hurst, Libn.
Subjects: Pharmacology, toxicology, medicine, chemistry, pharmaceutical technology. **Holdings:** 1600 books; 1800 bound periodical volumes; 3000 reprints. **Subscriptions:** 113 journals and other serials.

★9946★ SEMMES-MURPHEY CLINIC
LIBRARY
920 Madison Ave., Ste. 201
Memphis, TN 38103   Phone: (901) 522-7700
Patricia P. Irby, Libn.
Subjects: Neurosurgery, neurology. **Holdings:** 1327 books; 819 bound periodical volumes. **Subscriptions:** 38 journals and other serials.

★9947★ SOUTHERN COLLEGE OF OPTOMETRY
LIBRARY
1245 Madison Ave.
Memphis, TN 38104   Phone: (901) 722-3237
Nancy Gatlin, Dir.
Subjects: Optometry, optics, ophthalmology, psychology, exceptional education. **Holdings:** 15,019 books; 4701 bound periodical volumes; 12,302 slides; 376 microfiche; 153 reels of microfilm; 245 video cassettes. **Subscriptions:** 175 journals and other serials.

★9948★ U.S. DEPARTMENT OF VETERANS AFFAIRS
MEDICAL CENTER LIBRARY
1030 Jefferson Ave.
Memphis, TN 38104   Phone: (901) 523-8990
Mary Virginia Taylor, Chf., Lib.Serv.
Subjects: Medicine, dentistry, nursing. **Holdings:** 4650 books; 3377 bound periodical volumes; microfilm. **Subscriptions:** 250 journals and other serials.

★9949★ UNIVERSITY OF TENNESSEE, MEMPHIS
HEALTH SCIENCES LIBRARY
877 Madison Ave.
Memphis, TN 38163   Phone: (901) 528-5638
Susan A. Selig, Act.Dir.
Subjects: Medicine, dentistry, nursing, pharmacy, allied health sciences, social work. **Holdings:** 41,232 books; 120,857 bound periodical volumes; 130 microforms; 306 slide programs; 403 filmstrips; 220 films; 1185 video and audio cassettes. **Subscriptions:** 2111 journals and other serials.

★9950★ U.S. NAVY
NAVAL HOSPITAL
GENERAL AND MEDICAL LIBRARY
Millington, TN 38054   Phone: (901) 873-5846
G.R. Counts, Libn.
Subjects: Dentistry, medicine, nursing. **Holdings:** 5511 volumes. **Subscriptions:** 81 journals and other serials.

★9951★ U.S. DEPARTMENT OF VETERANS AFFAIRS
MEDICAL CENTER LIBRARY
Mountain Home, TN 37684   Phone: (615) 926-1171
Nancy Dougherty, Chf., Lib.Serv.
Subjects: Medicine and allied health sciences. **Holdings:** 2925 books; 3681 bound periodical volumes. **Subscriptions:** 315 journals and other serials.

★9952★ U.S. DEPARTMENT OF VETERANS AFFAIRS
MEDICAL CENTER LIBRARY SERVICE
Murfreesboro, TN 37130   Phone: (615) 893-1360
Joy W. Hunter, Chf., Lib.Serv.
Subjects: Psychiatry, medicine, nursing, geriatrics. **Holdings:** 2800 books; 1200 bound periodical volumes; 1200 AV programs. **Subscriptions:** 280 journals and other serials.

★9953★ BAPTIST HOSPITAL
MEDICAL LIBRARY
2000 Church St.
Nashville, TN 37236   Phone: (615) 329-5373
Lynne A. Wood, Chf.Med.Libn.
Subjects: Medicine, nursing, and allied health sciences. **Holdings:** 2793 books; 1550 bound periodical volumes; 980 pamphlets; clippings; anatomy charts and models; 12 AV items. **Subscriptions:** 140 journals and other serials.

★9954★ GEORGE PEABODY COLLEGE FOR TEACHERS OF
VANDERBILT UNIVERSITY
KENNEDY CENTER
MATERIALS CENTER
Box 62
Nashville, TN 37203   Phone: (615) 322-8184
Mrs. Jamesie Rodney, Mgr.
Subjects: Mental retardation, special education, psychology, remedial reading, educational and psychological tests. **Holdings:** 4000 volumes; 23 VF drawers and 50 shelves containing 560 tests; AV equipment. **Subscriptions:** 12 journals and other serials.

★9955★ MEHARRY MEDICAL COLLEGE
LIBRARY
1005 D.B. Todd
Nashville, TN 37208   Phone: (615) 327-6728
Cheryl Hamberg, Dir.
Subjects: Medicine, dentistry, public health, medical technology, health care administration. **Holdings:** 20,954 books; 51,889 bound periodical volumes; 514 audio cassettes; 559 video cassettes; 150 slide/tape sets. **Subscriptions:** 1607 journals and other serials.

★9956★ METROPOLITAN NASHVILLE GENERAL HOSPITAL
HEALTH SCIENCE LIBRARY
72 Hermitage Ave.
Nashville, TN 37210   Phone: (615) 862-4416
Glenda L. Perry, Libn.
Subjects: Medicine, surgery, nursing. **Holdings:** 500 books; 1000 bound periodical volumes. **Subscriptions:** 81 journals and other serials.

★9957★ NASHVILLE METROPOLITAN DEPARTMENT OF PUBLIC HEALTH
LENTZ HEALTH CENTER LIBRARY
311 23rd Ave., N.
Nashville, TN 37203   Phone: (615) 327-9313
Feli C. Propes, Libn.
Subjects: Internal medicine, public health, nursing, environmental health. **Holdings:** 2000 volumes. **Subscriptions:** 123 journals and other serials.

★9958★ QUORUM HEALTH RESOURCES
CORPORATE INFORMATION CENTER
1 Park Plaza
Box 24347
Nashville, TN 37203   Phone: (615) 340-5852
Ewa Griffin
Subjects: Health care industry, business management, hospital management, health care marketing. **Holdings:** 3000 volumes; 36 volumes of periodicals on microfiche; 30 VF drawers; 12 VF drawers of microfiche. **Subscriptions:** 200 journals and other serials; 4 newspapers.

★9959★ TENNESSEE DEPARTMENT OF HEALTH AND ENVIRONMENT
DIVISION OF INFORMATION RESOURCES
LIBRARY AND RESOURCE CENTER
419 Cordell Hull Bldg.
Nashville, TN 37247-0360   Phone: (615) 741-3752
Ann Hogan, Dir.
Subjects: Health and vital statistics, population, computers and personal computers, health care costs. **Holdings:** 1500 books. **Subscriptions:** 65 journals and other serials.

★9960★ TENNESSEE DEPARTMENT OF HEALTH AND ENVIRONMENT
HEALTH PROMOTION/DISEASE CONTROL SECTION
MEDIA RESOURCE CENTER
Cordell Hull Bldg., 5th Fl., Rm. 546
Nashville, TN 37219-5402   Phone: (615) 741-0380
Nancy Heaney, Dir., Media Rsrc.Ctr.
Subjects: Health, safety, nutrition, drug abuse, family life, allied health fields. **Holdings:** 450 films; 300 video cassettes; filmstrips; slide series.

★9961★ TENNESSEE STATE COMMISSION ON AGING
LIBRARY
706 Church St., Ste. 201
Nashville, TN 37243-0860   Phone: (615) 741-2056
Subjects: Aging, geriatric psychology and sociology, retirement planning, community based health and social services. **Holdings:** 500 books; VF drawers. **Subscriptions:** 10 journals and other serials.

★9962★ TENNESSEE STATE LIBRARY
LIBRARY FOR THE BLIND AND PHYSICALLY HANDICAPPED
403 7th Ave., N.
Nashville, TN 37243-0313   Phone: (615) 741-3915
Miss Francis H. Ezell, Dir.
Subjects: General reading material for the blind and physically handicapped. **Holdings:** 30,000 titles of books recorded on disc and cassette, transcribed into braille; large print books. **Subscriptions:** 83 journals and other serials (45 disc, 35 braille, 3 cassette).

★9963★ U.S. DEPARTMENT OF VETERANS AFFAIRS
MEDICAL CENTER LIBRARY SERVICE
1310 24th Ave., S.
Nashville, TN 37203   Phone: (615) 327-4751
Barbara A. Meadows, Chf., Lib.Serv.
Subjects: Medicine, nursing, dentistry, surgery. **Holdings:** 2843 books; 2600 bound periodical volumes; 775 AV programs; 2757 periodical volumes on microfilm. **Subscriptions:** 356 journals and other serials.

★9964★ VANDERBILT UNIVERSITY
MEDICAL CENTER LIBRARY
Nashville, TN 37232-2340   Phone: (615) 343-6454
T. Mark Hodges, Dir.
Subjects: Health sciences. **Holdings:** 56,966 books and theses; 96,594 bound periodical volumes; 6616 government publications; 6781 AV programs; 5757 microforms; 491 linear feet of manuscripts; 54 computer diskettes. **Subscriptions:** 2308 journals and other serials.

★9965★ OAK RIDGE ASSOCIATED UNIVERSITIES
MEDICAL LIBRARY
Box 117
Oak Ridge, TN 37831-0117   Phone: (615) 576-3490
Rana Yalcintas, Dir.
Subjects: Biochemistry, occupational medicine, cytogenetics, radiopharmacy, epidemiology, nuclear medicine. **Holdings:** 2300 books; 2849 bound periodical volumes; 9500 reports in microform; 1777 reels of microfilm. **Subscriptions:** 106 journals and other serials.

★9966★ OAK RIDGE ASSOCIATED UNIVERSITIES
RADIOPHARMACEUTICAL INTERNAL DOSE INFORMATION CENTER
Box 117
Oak Ridge, TN 37831-0117   Phone: (615) 576-3450
Evelyn E. Watson, Prog.Mgr.
Subjects: Internal dosimetry, radiation absorbed dose, radionuclide kinetics, nuclear medicine, health and medical physics, radiation protection.

★9967★ OAK RIDGE NATIONAL LABORATORY
BIOMEDICAL AND ENVIRONMENTAL INFORMATION ANALYSIS SECTION
LIBRARY
PO Box 2008, MS-6050
Oak Ridge, TN 37831-6050   Phone: (615) 574-7803
Dr. Po-Yung Lu, Sect.Hd.
Subjects: Information systems, health, energy, environmental research. **Holdings:** 1200 bound volumes; 18,000 reports. **Subscriptions:** 125 journals and other serials.

★9968★ OAK RIDGE NATIONAL LABORATORY
HEALTH AND SAFETY RESEARCH DIVISION
ENVIRONMENTAL MUTAGEN INFORMATION CENTER
Bldg. 2001
Box 2008
Oak Ridge, TN 37831-6050   Phone: (615) 574-7871
John S. Wassom, Dir.
Subjects: Genetic toxicology, chemical mutagenesis. **Holdings:** 75,000 references on the genotoxicity of chemicals.

★9969★ OAK RIDGE NATIONAL LABORATORY
TOXICOLOGY INFORMATION RESPONSE CENTER
Bldg. 2001, MS 6050
Box 2008
Oak Ridge, TN 37831-6050   Phone: (615) 576-1746
Kim Slusher, Dir.
Subjects: Toxicology, pharmacology, veterinary toxicology, heavy metals, pesticides, chemistry, biology, medicine, industrial hygiene. **Holdings:** 7700 search files; 250 microfiche of published bibliographies. **Subscriptions:** 50 journals and other serials.

Texas

★9970★ ABILENE STATE SCHOOL
SPECIAL LIBRARY
Box 451
Abilene, TX 79604   Phone: (915) 692-4053
Peggy G. Allen, Libn. I
Subjects: Mental retardation, psychology, education, behavior modification, social services, special education, child development. **Holdings:** 4500 books; 350 bound periodical volumes; 300 pamphlets; 8 VF drawers of dissertations, reports, articles, government documents. **Subscriptions:** 150 journals.

★9971★ HENDRICK MEDICAL CENTER
SELLERS LIBRARY
N. 19th and Hickory St.
Abilene, TX 79601   Phone: (915) 670-2375
Jean Snodgrass
Subjects: Medicine, health, nursing. **Holdings:** 1600 books; 150 microfilms. **Subscriptions:** 250 journals and other serials; 3 newspapers.

★9972★ U.S. DEPARTMENT OF VETERANS AFFAIRS
HOSPITAL LIBRARY
Amarillo, TX 79106   Phone: (806) 354-7877
Cheryl A. Latham, Chf., Lib.Serv.
Subjects: General medicine, surgery, nursing, dentistry. **Holdings:** 3894

books; periodicals on microfilm. **Subscriptions:** 235 journals and other serials.

★9973★   ASSOCIATION FOR RETARDED CITIZENS
LIBRARY
PO Box 6109
Arlington, TX 76005   Phone: (817) 640-0204
Subjects: Mental retardation. **Holdings:** 2000 volumes.

★9974★   JOHNSON AND JOHNSON MEDICAL
    CORPORATION
TECHNICAL INFORMATION CENTER
2500 Arbrook Blvd.
Box 130
Arlington, TX 76004-0130   Phone: (817) 465-3141
W.B. Scroggs, Tech.Info.Coord.
Subjects: Chemical and biological sciences. **Holdings:** 2400 books; 4500 bound periodical volumes. **Subscriptions:** 352 journals and other serials.

★9975★   AUSTIN COMMUNITY COLLEGE
HEALTH SCIENCES COLLECTION
1020 Grove Blvd.
Austin, TX 78741   Phone: (512) 389-4003
Margaret Peloquin, Hd.Libn.
Subjects: Medicine, surgery, nursing, public health, hospitals. **Holdings:** 8000 books; 1100 AV programs; 8 VF drawers of reprints, pamphlets, medical care materials. **Subscriptions:** 350 journals and other serials.

★9976★   AUSTIN STATE HOSPITAL
STAFF LIBRARY
4110 Guadalupe St.
Austin, TX 78751   Phone: (512) 371-6740
Nancy H. Dobson, Libn.
Subjects: Psychiatry, psychology, nursing, neurology, community mental health. **Holdings:** 4000 books; 1000 bound periodical volumes; 150 tape recordings. **Subscriptions:** 90 journals and other serials.

★9977★   CLARK, THOMAS, WINTERS, & NEWTON
LIBRARY
1200 Texas Commerce Bank Bldg.
700 Lavaca
Austin, TX 78701   Phone: (512) 472-8800
Deborah K. Meleski, Law Libn.
Subjects: Law, banking law, medicine. **Holdings:** 13,000 books; 500 bound periodical volumes. **Subscriptions:** 200 journals and other serials; 8 newspapers.

★9978★   TEXAS DEPARTMENT OF HEALTH
LIBRARY
1100 W. 49th St.
Austin, TX 78756   Phone: (512) 458-7559
John Burlinson, Libn.
Subjects: Public health, infectious diseases, laboratory methods, environmental health, dental health, pediatrics, nursing, hospitals and nursing homes, heart, cancer, health promotion, health funding. **Holdings:** 10,000 volumes; 2000 unbound items; 4787 AV materials. **Subscriptions:** 435 journals and other serials.

★9979★   TEXAS DEPARTMENT OF HUMAN SERVICES
LIBRARY AND REFERENCE SERVICES
Box 149030
MC W-211
Austin, TX 78714-9030   Phone: (512) 450-3530
Brenda Ziser, Lib.Adm./Cons.
Subjects: Social work, child welfare, management, geriatrics, health services, human services, nutrition. **Holdings:** 8000 books; 1500 AV programs. **Subscriptions:** 120 journals and other serials.

★9980★   TEXAS DEPARTMENT OF MENTAL HEALTH AND
    MENTAL RETARDATION
CENTRAL OFFICE LIBRARY
Box 12668
Austin, TX 78711   Phone: (512) 465-4621
Russlene Waukechon
Subjects: Mental health, mental retardation, alcoholism, drug abuse, rehabilitation. **Holdings:** 6000 books; 3000 bound periodical volumes; 20 file drawers of mental health files; 4 drawers of mental retardation files. **Subscriptions:** 50 journals and other serials.

★9981★   TEXAS MEDICAL ASSOCIATION
LIBRARY
1801 Lamar Blvd.
Austin, TX 78701   Phone: (512) 477-6704
Susan Brock, Lib.Dir.
Subjects: Clinical medicine. **Holdings:** 60,000 volumes; 5000 reprints; 300 motion pictures; 1300 lecture tapes; 300 slide/tape programs; 400 video cassettes. **Subscriptions:** 868 journals and other serials.

★9982★   TEXAS REHABILITATION COMMISSION
LIBRARY
4900 N. Lamar
Austin, TX 78751   Phone: (512) 483-4240
Terry Foster, Libn.
Subjects: Rehabilitation theory, disabilities, psychology of disability, caseload management, management skills, occupational therapy. **Holdings:** 12,000 books; 360 bound periodical volumes; videotapes; audio cassettes. **Subscriptions:** 52 journals and other serials.

★9983★   TEXAS SCHOOL FOR THE DEAF
LIBRARY
Box 3538
Austin, TX 78764   Phone: (512) 440-5364
Susan A. Anderson, Libn.
Subjects: Deafness. **Holdings:** 12,000 books; manuscripts; archives; microfilm. **Subscriptions:** 77 journals and other serials.

★9984★   TEXAS STATE LIBRARY
DIVISION FOR THE BLIND AND PHYSICALLY
    HANDICAPPED
Box 12927
Austin, TX 78711   Phone: (512) 463-5458
Dale W. Propp, Dir.
Subjects: Visual impairment, physical handicaps, Texana, Spanish language, learning disabilities. **Holdings:** 695,777 books; 135 bound periodical volumes; cassettes. **Subscriptions:** 63 journals and other serials.

★9985★   BAPTIST HOSPITAL OF SOUTHEAST TEXAS
MEDICAL LIBRARY
College & 11th
Box 1591
Beaumont, TX 77704   Phone: (409) 839-5160
Deloris Blake, Med.Libn.
Subjects: Nursing, health administration, medicine, surgery, obstetrics, pediatrics. **Holdings:** 5539 books; 1296 bound periodical volumes; 2 VF drawers of pamphlets; 569 Audio-Digest tapes; 13 films; 101 files of clippings. **Subscriptions:** 80 journals and other serials.

★9986★   ST. ELIZABETH HOSPITAL
HEALTH SCIENCES LIBRARY
2830 Calder Ave.
Box 5405
Beaumont, TX 77702   Phone: (409) 899-7189
Sue Martin, Libn.
Subjects: Medicine, dentistry, allied health sciences. **Holdings:** 900 books; 5400 bound periodical volumes; AV programs. **Subscriptions:** 307 journals and other serials.

★9987★   TEXAS DEPARTMENT OF MENTAL HEALTH AND
    MENTAL RETARDATION
BIG SPRING STATE HOSPITAL
PROFESSIONAL LIBRARY
Box 231
Big Spring, TX 79721-0231   Phone: (915) 264-4215
Anna Lou Bradberry, Libn.
Subjects: Medicine. **Holdings:** 5000 books. **Subscriptions:** 59 journals and other serials.

★9988★   U.S. DEPARTMENT OF VETERANS AFFAIRS
HOSPITAL LIBRARY
2400 S. Gregg St.
Big Spring, TX 79720   Phone: (915) 263-7361
Don Fortner
Subjects: General medicine, surgery. **Holdings:** 700 books;. **Subscriptions:** 40 journals and other serials.

★9989★ U.S. DEPARTMENT OF VETERANS AFFAIRS
SAM RAYBURN MEMORIAL VETERANS CENTER
MEDICAL LIBRARY
E. 9th & Lipscomb Sts.
Bonham, TX 75418   Phone: (903) 583-2111
Elizabeth J. Alme, Chf., Lib.Serv.
Subjects: Medicine and allied health sciences. Holdings: 713 books; 110
Audio-Digest tapes. Subscriptions: 152 journals and other serials.

★9990★ TEXAS DEPARTMENT OF MENTAL HEALTH AND
  MENTAL RETARDATION
BRENHAM STATE SCHOOL
STAFF LIBRARY
PO Box 161
Brenham, TX 77833   Phone: (409) 836-4511
Linda Kocian
Subjects: Special education, mental retardation. Holdings: 250 books.
Subscriptions: 5 journals and other serials.

★9991★ U.S. AIR FORCE
AIR FORCE SYSTEMS COMMAND
HUMAN SYSTEMS DIVISION
SCHOOL OF AEROSPACE MEDICINE
STRUGHOLD AEROMEDICAL LIBRARY
Brooks AFB, TX 78235-5301   Phone: (512) 536-3321
Fred W. Todd, Chf.Libn.
Subjects: Aerospace medicine, bioastronautics, bionucleonics, clinical
medicine, dentistry, life sciences. Holdings: 35,799 books; 109,891 bound
periodical volumes; 53,429 microfiche; 153,190 technical reports. Sub-
scriptions: 1636 journals and other serials; 11 newspapers.

★9992★ U.S. AIR FORCE HOSPITAL
ROBERT L. THOMPSON STRATEGIC HOSPITAL
MEDICAL LIBRARY/SGEL
Carswell AFB, TX 76127   Phone: (817) 782-4598
Jean Robbins, Med.Libn.
Subjects: Medicine, surgery, nursing, psychiatry, dentistry, orthopedics,
veterinary medicine. Holdings: 3014 books; 2751 bound periodical vol-
umes. Subscriptions: 240 journals and other serials; 9 newspapers.

★9993★ TEXAS A & M UNIVERSITY
MEDICAL SCIENCES LIBRARY
College Station, TX 77843-4462   Phone: (409) 845-7427
Dottie Eakin, Dir.
Subjects: Biomedical sciences, veterinary medicine. Holdings: 31,300
books; 86,160 bound periodical volumes; 27,450 microforms. Subscrip-
tions: 2100 journals and other serials.

★9994★ EAST TEXAS STATE UNIVERSITY
ORAL HISTORY PROGRAM
James Gilliam Gee Library
East Texas Sta.
Commerce, TX 75429-2953   Phone: (214) 886-5738
Dr. James Conrad, Coord. of Oral Hist.
Subjects: History of East Texas - railroad, cotton, blacks, medicine; Texas
social work; institutional history. Holdings: 205 volumes; 800 cassette
tapes of interviews. Subscriptions: 3 journals and other serials.

★9995★ DRISCOLL FOUNDATION CHILDREN'S HOSPITAL
MEDICAL LIBRARY
3533 Alameda
Box 6530
Corpus Christi, TX 78411   Phone: (512) 854-5341
Becky Melton, Med.Libn.
Subjects: General pediatrics, neonatology, pediatric surgery and cardiolo-
gy. Holdings: 330 books; 4000 bound periodical volumes. Subscriptions: 80
journals and other serials.

★9996★ MEMORIAL MEDICAL CENTER
HEALTH SCIENCES LIBRARY
2606 Hospital Blvd.
Box 5280
Corpus Christi, TX 78465-5280   Phone: (512) 881-4197
Leta Dannelley, Dir.
Subjects: Medicine, nursing, pre-clinical sciences. Holdings: 3000 books;
4000 bound periodical volumes; 1 VF drawer of pamphlets; 660 AV
programs; 500 audio cassettes; 35 video cassettes; 25 slide/tape sets.
Subscriptions: 270 journals and other serials.

★9997★ SPOHN HOSPITAL
MEDICAL LIBRARY
600 Elizabeth St.
Corpus Christi, TX 78404   Phone: (512) 881-3261
Sr. Julia Delaney, Libn.
Subjects: Medicine, nursing, medical technology, management, x-ray.
Holdings: 3500 books; 1200 bound periodical volumes; 8 VF drawers of
pamphlets; AV programs. Subscriptions: 50 journals and other serials.

★9998★ U.S. NAVY
NAVAL HOSPITAL
PATRICIA M. SESSIONS MEMORIAL LIBRARY
Corpus Christi, TX 78419   Phone: (512) 939-3863
Jolee M. Reinke, Hd., Educ. & Trng.Dept.
Subjects: Medicine, surgery, nursing, allied health sciences. Holdings:
Bound periodical volumes; reports; archives; other cataloged items.
Subscriptions: 110 journals and other serials.

★9999★ AESTHETICIANS INTERNATIONAL ASSOCIATION
LIBRARY
4447 Mc Kinney Ave.
Dallas, TX 75205   Phone: (214) 526-0752
Ron Renee, Pres.
Subjects: Skin care, makeup, body therapy, spa treatments. Holdings: 250
volumes; 50 AV programs.

★10000★ AMERICAN HEART ASSOCIATION
CORPORATE REFERENCE CENTER
7320 Greenville Ave.
Dallas, TX 75231   Phone: (214) 706-1408
Theresa W. Barasch, Mgr.
Subjects: Cardiovascular and cerebrovascular diseases. Holdings: 2000
books; 1000 bound periodical volumes; microforms. Subscriptions: 200
journals and other serials.

★10001★ BAYLOR HEALTH SCIENCES LIBRARY
3500 Gaston Ave.
Dallas, TX 75246   Phone: (214) 820-2372
Barbara A. Downey, Dir.
Subjects: Medicine, dentistry, nursing. Holdings: 8928 books; 27,436
bound periodical volumes; 1303 reels of microfilm; 1 drawer of microfiche;
4 VF drawers. Subscriptions: 614 journals and other serials.

★10002★ CHILDREN'S MEDICAL CENTER OF DALLAS
LAUREN TAYLOR REARDON FAMILY LIBRARY
1935 Amelia St.
Dallas, TX 75235   Phone: (214) 920-2280
Sally Francis, Dir., Ch. Life Dept.
Subjects: Health, cancer, child development, children's literature, medi-
cine, death and bereavement. Holdings: 1000 books; pamphlets; brochures.

★10003★ MARY KAY COSMETICS, INC.
TECHNICAL INFORMATION CENTER
1330 Regal Row
Dallas, TX 75247   Phone: (214) 905-6299
Paula L. Galbraith, Supv., Tech.Info.
Subjects: Cosmetics, dermatology, toxicology, chemistry, business. Hold-
ings: 1700 books; 450 bound periodical volumes. Subscriptions: 200
journals and other serials.

★10004★ METHODIST MEDICAL CENTER
MEDICAL LIBRARY
301 W. Colorado
Box 655999
Dallas, TX 75265-5999   Phone: (214) 944-8321
Janet L. Cowen, Med.Libn.
Subjects: Medicine, nursing. Holdings: 1900 books; 4000 bound periodical
volumes; 1150 cassette tapes; clippings; reports. Subscriptions: 200 jour-
nals and other serials.

★10005★ PRESBYTERIAN HEALTHCARE SYSTEM
GREEN LEARNING CENTER
LIBRARY
8200 Walnut Hill Ln.
Dallas, TX 75231   Phone: (214) 891-2310
Barbara D. Pace, Dir., Lib.Serv.
Subjects: Medicine, nursing, psychiatry. Holdings: 2450 books; 3465
bound periodical volumes. Subscriptions: 366 journals and other serials.

★10006★   ST. PAUL MEDICAL CENTER
C.B. SACHER MEDICAL LIBRARY
5909 Harry Hines Blvd.
Dallas, TX 75235   Phone: (214) 879-2390
Eva G. Osborn, Coord., Lib.Serv.
Subjects: Nursing, medicine, and allied health sciences. **Holdings:** 3000 books; 1100 bound periodical volumes; 750 audio cassettes. **Subscriptions:** 150 journals and other serials.

★10007★   TEXAS SCOTTISH RITE HOSPITAL FOR CRIPPLED CHILDREN
BRANDON CARRELL, M.D., MEDICAL LIBRARY
2222 Welborn St.
Dallas, TX 75219-0567   Phone: (214) 521-3168
Mary Peters, Med.Libn.
Subjects: Pediatric orthopedics and neurology. **Holdings:** 700 books; 525 bound periodical volumes. **Subscriptions:** 100 journals and other serials.

★10008★   TEXAS WOMAN'S UNIVERSITY, DALLAS CENTER
F.W. AND BESSIE DYE MEMORIAL LIBRARY
1810 Inwood Rd.
Dallas, TX 75235   Phone: (214) 689-6580
Patricia Jackson, Coord., Hea.Sci.Lib.
Subjects: Nursing, occupational therapy, medical records, health care administration, psychology, physical therapy. **Holdings:** 23,877 books; 10,903 bound periodical volumes; 1791 bound theses, dissertations, and professional papers; 1271 volumes on microfilm; 1735 volumes on microfiche; 172 volumes on microcard. **Subscriptions:** 298 journals and other serials.

★10009★   U.S. DEPARTMENT OF VETERANS AFFAIRS
LIBRARY SERVICE
4500 S. Lancaster Rd.
Dallas, TX 75216   Phone: (214) 372-7025
Nancy A. Clark, Chf., Lib.Serv.
Subjects: Medicine, surgery, allied health sciences, management. **Holdings:** 4500 books; 10,000 bound periodical volumes; 4500 volumes on microfilm; 1000 AV programs. **Subscriptions:** 480 journals and other serials.

★10010★   UNIVERSITY OF TEXAS SOUTHWESTERN MEDICAL CENTER, DALLAS
LIBRARY
5323 Harry Hines Blvd.
Dallas, TX 75235   Phone: (214) 688-3368
Helen Mayo, Act.Dir.
Subjects: Medicine, biochemistry, biological science, medical specialities. **Holdings:** 230,640 volumes; 3060 AV programs; 20,860 microforms. **Subscriptions:** 1997 journals and other serials; 5 newspapers.

★10011★   WADLEY INSTITUTES OF MOLECULAR MEDICINE
RESEARCH INSTITUTE LIBRARY
9000 Harry Hines Blvd.
Dallas, TX 75235   Phone: (214) 351-8648
Kathryn Manning, Libn.
Subjects: Cancer, microbiology, hematology, biochemistry, immunology, genetics, interferon. **Holdings:** 11,629 volumes; 73 dissertations; 225 reprints; 6 VF drawers of unbound material. **Subscriptions:** 235 journals and other serials.

★10012★   UNIVERSITY OF NORTH TEXAS LIBRARIES
MEDIA LIBRARY
Box 12898
Denton, TX 76203-2898   Phone: (817) 565-2691
George D. Mitchell, III, Media Lib.Dir.
Subjects: Gerontology, education, psychology, business, sciences, film studies. **Holdings:** 1989 reels of motion picture film; 1425 video cassettes; 79 laser discs; 2142 filmstrips; 2475 phonograph records; 3251 phonotapes; 36,096 slides; 231 transparencies; 65 kits; 428 microcomputer discs. **Subscriptions:** 12 journals and other serials.

★10013★   TEXAS TECH UNIVERSITY
HEALTH SCIENCES CENTER
REGIONAL ACADEMIC HEALTH CENTER LIBRARY
4800 Alberta Ave.
El Paso, TX 79905   Phone: (915) 545-6650
Teresa L. Knott, Assoc.Dir., El Paso
Subjects: Medicine. **Holdings:** 14,178 books; 17,471 bound periodical

volumes; 361 audiotapes; 65 slide/tape sets; 3 models; 2675 slides; 120 videotapes. **Subscriptions:** 402 journals and other serials.

★10014★   U.S. ARMY HOSPITALS
WILLIAM BEAUMONT ARMY MEDICAL CENTER
MEDICAL LIBRARY
Bldg. 7777, Rm. 2-246
El Paso, TX 79920-5001   Phone: (915) 569-2580
Carolyn J. Rymer, Chf.Med.Libn.
Subjects: Surgery, medicine, nursing, dentistry, trauma medicine. **Holdings:** 6000 books; 32,400 bound periodical volumes; 4000 periodical volumes on microfilm; 630 AV programs. **Subscriptions:** 750 journals and other serials.

★10015★   U.S. ARMY HOSPITALS
DARNALL ARMY HOSPITAL
MEDICAL LIBRARY
Bldg. 36000
Fort Hood, TX 76544-5063   Phone: (817) 288-8368
Frank M. Norton, Adm.Libn.
Subjects: Medicine and allied health sciences. **Holdings:** 2600 books; 3500 bound periodical volumes; 400 videotapes. **Subscriptions:** 750 journals and other serials.

★10016★   U.S. ARMY
HEALTH SERVICES COMMAND
ACADEMY OF HEALTH SCIENCES
STIMSON LIBRARY
Bldg. 2840, Rm. 106
Fort Sam Houston, TX 78234-6100   Phone: (512) 221-5932
Norma L. Sellers, Chf.Libn.
Subjects: Military medicine, nursing, health care administration, management, psychiatry, veterinary medicine. **Holdings:** 34,000 books; 13,397 bound periodical volumes; 5800 technical reports; 2500 archival materials; 3500 items on microfilm; 1557 AV programs. **Subscriptions:** 560 journals and other serials.

★10017★   U.S. ARMY
INSTITUTE OF SURGICAL RESEARCH ON BURNS
LIBRARY
Bldg. 2653
Fort Sam Houston, TX 78234-5012   Phone: (512) 221-4559
Subjects: Burns, scalds, surgical research. **Holdings:** 8800 volumes.

★10018★   U.S. ARMY HOSPITALS
BROOKE ARMY MEDICAL CENTER
MEDICAL LIBRARY
Bldg. 1001
Fort Sam Houston, TX 78234-6200   Phone: (512) 221-4119
Kimmie Yu, Med.Libn.
Subjects: Medicine, dentistry, nursing, allied health sciences, religion, social work. **Holdings:** 15,000 books; 22,500 bound periodical volumes. **Subscriptions:** 645 journals and other serials.

★10019★   ALCON LABORATORIES, INC.
RESEARCH LIBRARY
6201 S. Freeway
Fort Worth, TX 76134-2099   Phone: (817) 551-8319
Sharon L. McAllister, Sci.Libn.
Subjects: Ophthalmology, lens care, pharmaceutics. **Holdings:** 6500 books; 10,000 bound periodical volumes; 3450 patents. **Subscriptions:** 275 journals and other serials.

★10020★   HARRIS METHODIST FORT WORTH
MEDICAL LIBRARY
1301 Pennsylvania Ave.
Fort Worth, TX 76104   Phone: (817) 882-2118
Vaida Durham, Libn.
Subjects: Medicine, surgery. **Holdings:** 1800 books; 3500 bound periodical volumes; 2266 tapes and cassettes. **Subscriptions:** 161 journals and other serials.

★10021★   JOHN PETER SMITH HOSPITAL
MARIETTA MEMORIAL MEDICAL LIBRARY
1500 S. Main
Fort Worth, TX 76104   Phone: (817) 921-3431
M. June Bowman, Med.Libn.
Subjects: Medicine, nursing, and allied health sciences. **Holdings:** 4200

books; 12,000 bound periodical volumes; 800 audiotapes. **Subscriptions:** 325 journals and other serials.

★10022★ **NATIONAL VICTIM CENTER**
LIBRARY
307 W. 7th St., Ste. 1001
Fort Worth, TX 76107   Phone: (817) 877-3355
Cindy Lea Arbelbide, Libn.
Subjects: Victims of violent crimes, legislation, national and local victim organizations. **Holdings:** 10,000 books and articles. **Subscriptions:** 76 journals and other serials.

★10023★ **THE O.A. BATTISTA RESEARCH INSTITUTE**
LIBRARY
3863 Southwest Loop - 820, Ste. 100
Fort Worth, TX 76133-2076   Phone: (817) 292-4272
David M. Whitely, Libn.
Subjects: Polymer science and technology, chemistry, medicine. **Holdings:** 3000 books. **Subscriptions:** 102 journals and other serials.

★10024★ **TEXAS COLLEGE OF OSTEOPATHIC MEDICINE**
HEALTH SCIENCES LIBRARY
3500 Camp Bowie Blvd.
Fort Worth, TX 76107   Phone: (817) 735-2464
Bobby R. Carter, Dir., Lib.Serv.
Subjects: Health sciences, clinical and osteopathic medicine. **Holdings:** 43,909 books; 64,248 bound periodical volumes; 4282 AV programs; 4 VF drawers of pamphlets; 91 anatomical models. **Subscriptions:** 2212 journals and other serials.

★10025★ **INTERMEDICS, INC.**
LIBRARY INFORMATION SERVICES DEPARTMENT
240 W. 2nd St.
Box 617
Freeport, TX 77541   Phone: (409) 233-8611
Charlene P. Kanter, Mgr.
Subjects: Cardiology, biomedical engineering, electrical engineering. **Holdings:** 1000 books. **Subscriptions:** 50 journals and other serials.

★10026★ **UNIVERSITY OF TEXAS MEDICAL BRANCH**
MOODY MEDICAL LIBRARY
Galveston, TX 77550-2782   Phone: (409) 772-1971
Brett A. Kirkpatrick, Dir.
Subjects: Medicine, nursing, history of medicine, allied health sciences. **Holdings:** 91,212 books; 140,461 bound periodical volumes; 1814 AV programs. **Subscriptions:** 2883 journals and other serials.

★10027★ **DALLAS-FORT WORTH MEDICAL CENTER**
LIBRARY
2709 Hospital Blvd.
Grand Prairie, TX 75051   Phone: (214) 641-5000
Subjects: Medicine. **Holdings:** 532 books; 380 bound periodical volumes; 75 audiotapes. **Subscriptions:** 33 journals and other serials.

★10028★ **DEAF SMITH GENERAL HOSPITAL**
LIBRARY
801 E. 3rd St.
Hereford, TX 79045   Phone: (806) 364-2141
Debbie Foerster, Dir., Med.Rec.
Subjects: Medicine and allied health sciences. **Holdings:** 175 volumes.

★10029★ **BAYLOR COLLEGE OF MEDICINE**
DEPARTMENT OF OPHTHALMOLOGY
CULLEN EYE INSTITUTE LIBRARY
6501 Fannin
Houston, TX 77030   Phone: (713) 798-3035
Gylene Wilcox, Libn.
Subjects: Ophthalmology. **Holdings:** 1850 books; 2265 bound periodical volumes; 470 AV programs. **Subscriptions:** 55 journals and other serials.

★10030★ **BEN TAUB GENERAL HOSPITAL**
DOCTOR'S MEDICAL LIBRARY
1502 Taub Loop
Houston, TX 77030   Phone: (713) 791-7441
Angie Ortiz, Lib.Ck.
Subjects: Medicine. **Holdings:** 1100 books; 110 bound periodical volumes; 12 VF drawers. **Subscriptions:** 110 journals and other serials; 8 newspapers.

★10031★ **HOUSTON ACADEMY OF MEDICINE**
TEXAS MEDICAL CENTER LIBRARY
1133 M.D. Anderson Blvd.
Houston, TX 77030   Phone: (713) 797-1230
Richard Lyders, Exec.Dir.
Subjects: Medicine, nursing, psychology, psychiatry, biological sciences, pharmacology. **Holdings:** 237,237 volumes. **Subscriptions:** 2718 journals; 1766 other serials.

★10032★ **HOUSTON COMMUNITY COLLEGE**
EASTWOOD CAMPUS NURSING SCHOOL LIBRARY
3100 Shenandoah
Houston, TX 77021   Phone: (713) 748-8810
Oraida Padron Starr, Libn.
Subjects: Nursing, emergency medical technology, radiologic technology, respiratory therapy, animal health management, surgical technology, physical and occupational therapy, and other allied health occupation fields. **Holdings:** 13,500 books; 261 unbound titles; 2000 AV programs; 50,000 microform and nonbook items. **Subscriptions:** 78 journals and other serials.

★10033★ **THE INSTITUTE FOR REHABILITATION AND**
RESEARCH
INFORMATION SERVICES CENTER
1333 Moursund Ave.
Houston, TX 77030   Phone: (713) 797-5947
Dell M. Davis
Subjects: Rehabilitation medicine. **Holdings:** 2000 books; 590 bound periodical volumes. **Subscriptions:** 40 journals and other serials.

★10034★ **NASA**
LYNDON B. JOHNSON SPACE CENTER
TECHNICAL LIBRARY/JM2
Houston, TX 77058   Phone: (713) 483-4248
Laura Chiu, Lib.Supv.
Subjects: Space sciences, space vehicles, life sciences, space medicine, space shuttles, space station, astronomy, astrophysics, navigation and guidance, telemetry, mathematics, physics. **Holdings:** 69,033 books; 18,781 bound periodical volumes; 247,406 technical reports; 909,805 microfiche; 200 AV materials. **Subscriptions:** 463 journals and other serials.

★10035★ **PLANNED PARENTHOOD OF HOUSTON AND**
SOUTHEAST TEXAS
MARY ELIZABETH HUDSON LIBRARY
3601 Fannin St.
Houston, TX 77004   Phone: (713) 522-6363
Natalie H. Thrall, Volunteer Libn.
Subjects: Sexuality education, family planning, parenting, reproductive health, reproductive rights, population, women's issues. **Holdings:** 2500 books; 100 bound periodical volumes; 400 file folders of reprints and newspaper clippings. **Subscriptions:** 23 journals and other serials.

★10036★ **ST. JOSEPH HOSPITAL**
HEALTH SCIENCE LIBRARY
1919 LaBranch
Houston, TX 77002   Phone: (713) 757-1000
Shelley G. Mao, Dir.
Subjects: Medicine, sciences, management. **Holdings:** 3817 books; 4793 bound periodical volumes; 83 titles on Network for Continuing Medical Education (NCME) tapes; 83 volumes of Audio-Digest tapes. **Subscriptions:** 200 journals and other serials.

★10037★ **ST. LUKE'S EPISCOPAL AND TEXAS CHILDREN'S**
HOSPITALS
MEDICAL LIBRARY
6621 Fannin St.
Houston, TX 77030   Phone: (715) 791-3054
Robert C. Park, Dir. of Lib.Serv.
Subjects: Medicine and related fields. **Holdings:** 15,000 books. **Subscriptions:** 154 journals and other serials.

★10038★ **SHRINERS HOSPITAL FOR CRIPPLED CHILDREN**
ORTHOPEDIC LIBRARY
1402 N. MacGregor
Houston, TX 77030-1695   Phone: (713) 797-1616
Jean Rasmussen, Med. Staff Coord.
Subjects: Orthopedics. **Holdings:** 200 books; 668 bound periodical volumes. **Subscriptions:** 20 journals and other serials.

★10039★ TEXAS SOUTHERN UNIVERSITY
ROBERT JAMES TERRY LIBRARY
3201 Wheeler Ave.
Houston, TX 77004   Phone: (713) 527-7163
Norma Bean, Interim Dir.
Subjects: Pharmacology. **Holdings:** 4500 books; 2500 bound periodical volumes. **Subscriptions:** 177 journals and other serials.

★10040★ U.S. DEPARTMENT OF VETERANS AFFAIRS
MEDICAL CENTER LIBRARY
2002 Holcombe Blvd.
Houston, TX 77211   Phone: (713) 795-4411
Jerry E. Barrett
Subjects: Medicine. **Holdings:** 2864 books; 7500 periodical volumes. **Subscriptions:** 235 journals and other serials.

★10041★ UNIVERSITY OF HOUSTON
COLLEGE OF OPTOMETRY LIBRARY
Houston, TX 77204-6052   Phone: (713) 749-2411
Suzanne Ferimer, Dir., Lrng.Rsrcs.
Subjects: Ocular diagnosis, public health services, contact lenses, history of optometry, pediatric optometry, optics, physiological optics. **Holdings:** 6500 books and bound periodical volumes; 400 audio cassettes; 3 drawers of vertical files, bibliographies, reports; 140 video cassettes; 60 slide-tape presentations; 310 pamphlets. **Subscriptions:** 125 journals and other serials.

★10042★ UNIVERSITY OF HOUSTON
COLLEGE OF PHARMACY LIBRARY
Houston, TX 77204-5511   Phone: (713) 749-1566
Derral Parkin, Libn.
Subjects: Chemistry, pharmacy, pharmaceuticals, toxicology, pharmacognosy, pharmacology. **Holdings:** 15,487 books and bound periodical volumes; pharmaceutical catalogs. **Subscriptions:** 154 journals and other serials.

★10043★ UNIVERSITY OF TEXAS
M.D. ANDERSON CANCER CENTER
RESEARCH MEDICAL LIBRARY
Texas Medical Center
Houston, TX 77030   Phone: (713) 792-2282
Sara Jean Jackson, Dir.
Subjects: Cancer, radiological physics, cell biology. **Holdings:** 45,000 volumes. **Subscriptions:** 1200 journals and other serials.

★10044★ UNIVERSITY OF TEXAS HEALTH SCIENCE
CENTER, HOUSTON
DENTAL BRANCH LIBRARY
6516 John Freeman Ave.
Houston, TX 77225   Phone: (713) 792-4094
Leah Krevit, Dir.
Subjects: Dentistry. **Holdings:** 13,675 books; 12,856 bound periodical volumes; 525 videotapes; theses. **Subscriptions:** 340 journals and other serials.

★10045★ UNIVERSITY OF TEXAS MENTAL SCIENCES
INSTITUTE
UT PSYCHIATRY LIBRARY
1300 Moursund Ave.
Houston, TX 77030   Phone: (713) 792-7711
Felicia S. Chuang, Libn.
Subjects: Psychiatry, psychopharmacology, clinical psychology, gerontology, drug abuse. **Holdings:** 10,350 books; 4770 bound periodical volumes; 64 dissertations on microfilm; 735 journal volumes on microfilm. **Subscriptions:** 235 journals and other serials.

★10046★ HUNTSVILLE MEMORIAL HOSPITAL
MEDICAL LIBRARY
3000 Interstate 45
PO Box 4001
Huntsville, TX 77342-4001   Phone: (409) 291-4545
Darlene Burris, Libn.
Subjects: Professional and vocational nursing, medicine. **Holdings:** 750 books; 100 bound periodical volumes; 200 filmstrips; 1500 videotapes. **Subscriptions:** 20 journals and other serials.

★10047★ KERRVILLE STATE HOSPITAL
PROFESSIONAL LIBRARY
Box 1468
Kerrville, TX 78029-1468   Phone: (512) 896-2211
Dana L. White, Libn.
Subjects: Geriatrics, psychology, medicine, nursing. **Holdings:** 1800 books; audio cassettes. **Subscriptions:** 49 journals and other serials.

★10048★ U.S. DEPARTMENT OF VETERANS AFFAIRS
HEALTH SCIENCES LIBRARY
Memorial Blvd.
Kerrville, TX 78028   Phone: (512) 896-2020
Lois A. Johnson, Chf., Lib.Serv.
Subjects: Medicine and allied health sciences. **Holdings:** 2300 books; journals, 1967 to present, on microfilm; 400 video cassettes and 16mm films. **Subscriptions:** 125 journals and other serials.

★10049★ GOOD SHEPHERD MEDICAL CENTER
MEDICAL LIBRARY
621 N. 5th St.
Longview, TX 75601   Phone: (903) 236-2165
Laurie S. O'Neal, Med.Libn.
Subjects: Medicine, nursing, and allied health sciences. **Holdings:** Figures not available.

★10050★ HIGHLAND HOSPITAL
MEDICAL LIBRARY
2412 50th St.
Lubbock, TX 79412   Phone: (806) 795-8251
Jo Nell Wischkaemper, Dir.
Subjects: Medicine, allied health sciences. **Holdings:** 475 books; 250 bound periodical volumes; 324 audio cassettes. **Subscriptions:** 28 journals and other serials.

★10051★ METHODIST HOSPITAL
MEDICAL LIBRARY
3615 19th St.
Lubbock, TX 79410   Phone: (806) 793-4180
Mary Jarvis, Med.Libn.
Subjects: Medicine, nursing, allied health sciences. **Holdings:** 3500 books; 5000 bound periodical volumes; 25 boxes of pamphlets; 14 VF drawers. **Subscriptions:** 230 journals and other serials.

★10052★ TEXAS TECH UNIVERSITY
HEALTH SCIENCES CENTER
LIBRARY OF THE HEALTH SCIENCES
Lubbock, TX 79430-0001   Phone: (806) 743-2203
Richard Wood, Dir.
Subjects: Medicine, nursing, and allied health sciences. **Holdings:** 190,000 volumes; 100,000 slides, videotapes, and other AV programs. **Subscriptions:** 3000 journals and other serials.

★10053★ MEMORIAL HOSPITAL
MEDICAL LIBRARY
Box 1447
Lufkin, TX 75902   Phone: (409) 634-8111
Hilda Becerra, Dir., Med.Rec.
Subjects: Medicine, obstetrics and gynecology, surgery, pediatrics. **Holdings:** 500 books; 20 bound periodical volumes.

★10054★ U.S. DEPARTMENT OF VETERANS AFFAIRS
MEDICAL CENTER LIBRARY SERVICE
1016 Ward St.
Marlin, TX 76661   Phone: (817) 883-3511
Mavis Williams, Act.Chf.
Subjects: Medicine, nursing, allied health sciences, health care administration. **Holdings:** 780 books; 1031 periodical volumes on microfilm; unbound reports; pamphlets. **Subscriptions:** 112 journals and other serials.

★10055★ NORTH TEXAS MEDICAL CENTER
LIBRARY
1800 N. Graves St.
McKinney, TX 75069   Phone: (214) 548-3000
Patricia Gidney, Med. Staff Coord.
Subjects: Medicine. **Holdings:** 150 volumes.

★10056★ MEMORIAL HOSPITAL
MOLLIE SUBLETT TUCKER MEMORIAL MEDICAL LIBRARY
1204 Mound St.
Nacogdoches, TX 75961   Phone: (409) 564-4611
Carlie Howard, Libn.
Subjects: Medicine. **Holdings:** 758 books; 121 bound periodical volumes; 198 boxes of unbound periodicals. **Subscriptions:** 41 journals and other serials.

★10057★ CARSON COUNTY SQUARE HOUSE MUSEUM
INFORMATION CENTER
Box 276
Panhandle, TX 79068   Phone: (806) 537-3524
Don L. Markham, Dir.
Subjects: Carson County and Texas Panhandle history, pioneer health and medicine, museology, Texana, American Indians, art. **Holdings:** 908 books; 36 bound periodical volumes; 5200 documents; 9800 artifacts, including 5 photographs, maps, business and personal communications, postcards, legal and offical correspondence. **Subscriptions:** 25 journals and other serials; 6 newspapers.

★10058★ TEXAS CHIROPRACTIC COLLEGE
MAE HILTY MEMORIAL LIBRARY
5912 Spencer Hwy.
Pasadena, TX 77505   Phone: (713) 487-1170
Barbara Gordon Webb, Dir. of Lib.Serv.
Subjects: Chiropractic, basic sciences, diagnosis, x-ray, public health, clinical sciences. **Holdings:** 7000 books; 3094 bound periodical volumes; 60 titles in microform; 6 VF drawers of pamphlets; 542 AV programs. **Subscriptions:** 142 journals.

★10059★ ST. MARY HOSPITAL
HEALTH SCIENCE LIBRARY
3600 Gates Blvd.
Port Arthur, TX 77643-3696   Phone: (409) 985-7431
Ethel M. Granger, Libn.
Subjects: Allergic diseases, dermatology, radiology, pathology, genitourinary medicine, physicians and surgeons, family practice, hemodialysis, thoracic and cardiovascular surgery, internal medicine, obstetrics/gynecology, child specialists, dentistry, infection. **Holdings:** 3710 books; 839 bound periodical volumes; 400 unbound reports; 168 Audio-Digest tapes; 700 video cassettes. **Subscriptions:** 135 journals and other serials.

★10060★ U.S. AIR FORCE HOSPITAL
MEDICAL LIBRARY
SGQA/35
Reese AFB, TX 79489-5300   Phone: (806) 885-3543
Sgt. Ron Sircher, Libn.
Subjects: Medicine and medical specialties, dentistry. **Holdings:** 780 books. **Subscriptions:** 40 journals and other serials.

★10061★ TEXAS DEPARTMENT OF MENTAL HEALTH AND
MENTAL RETARDATION
RUSK STATE HOSPITAL
STAFF LIBRARY
Box 318
Rusk, TX 75785   Phone: (903) 683-3421
Judy Vermillion, Staff Libn.
Remarks: No further information was supplied by the respondent.

★10062★ BAPTIST MEMORIAL HOSPITAL SYSTEM
BRUCE A. GARRETT MEMORIAL LIBRARY AND MEDIA
CENTER
111 Dallas St.
San Antonio, TX 78286   Phone: (512) 222-8431
Ruth R. Libby, Chf.Libn.
Subjects: Medicine, nursing, hospital administration, counseling, religion. **Holdings:** 3120 books; 376 bound periodical volumes. **Subscriptions:** 144 journals and other serials.

★10063★ BEXAR COUNTY MEDICAL LIBRARY ASSOCIATION
202 W. French Pl.
Box 12678
San Antonio, TX 78212   Phone: (512) 734-6691
Laura Ibara, Libn.
Subjects: Medicine. **Holdings:** 7000 books; 150 bound periodical volumes; 10 VF drawers of clippings. **Subscriptions:** 17 journals and other serials.

★10064★ MIND SCIENCE FOUNDATION
LIBRARY
8301 Broadway, No. 100
San Antonio, TX 78209-2006   Phone: (512) 821-6094
Beverly Evenson Casey, Libn.
Subjects: Parapsychology, psychology, Alzheimer's disease, mind-made health, creativity, traditional healing, self-esteem. **Holdings:** 5000 books; 100 bound periodical volumes; 3 16mm films; 2 VF drawers; 20 journals on microfiche; 150 other cataloged items. **Subscriptions:** 33 journals and other serials.

★10065★ NORTHEAST BAPTIST HOSPITAL
BATES LIBRARY
8811 Village Dr.
San Antonio, TX 78217   Phone: (512) 653-2330
Carolyn Mueller, Libn.
Subjects: Medicine, nursing, and allied health sciences. **Holdings:** 100 books. **Subscriptions:** 4 journals and other serials.

★10066★ PLANNED PARENTHOOD OF SAN ANTONIO AND
SOUTH CENTRAL TEXAS
LIBRARY
104 Babcock Rd.
San Antonio, TX 78201   Phone: (512) 736-2244
Patricia Sidebottom, Exec.Dir.
Subjects: Birth control, population, human sexuality, sex education, family planning, AIDS, ecology, environment, women's health, teenage pregnancy. **Holdings:** 1500 books; 500 periodicals; pamphlets; vertical files; 100 films, filmstrips, slide sets. **Subscriptions:** 35 journals and other serials.

★10067★ SAN ANTONIO STATE CHEST HOSPITAL
HEALTH SCIENCE LIBRARY
Highland Hills Sta., Box 23340
San Antonio, TX 78223   Phone: (512) 534-8857
Patricia Beaman, Libn.
Subjects: Medicine, chest diseases, nursing. **Holdings:** 1800 books; 1500 bound periodical volumes; 450 AV programs. **Subscriptions:** 120 journals and other serials.

★10068★ SAN ANTONIO STATE HOSPITAL
STAFF LIBRARY
Box 23991, Highland Hills Sta.
San Antonio, TX 78223-0991   Phone: (512) 532-8811
Alma D. Guevara, Lib.Asst.
Subjects: Medical sciences, psychology, psychiatric medicine, theology, mental health, mental hospitals. **Holdings:** 4000 books and bound periodical volumes; 12 VF drawers of reports, pamphlets, and documents; cassette tapes. **Subscriptions:** 130 journals and other serials.

★10069★ SANTA ROSA HEALTH CARE CORPORATION
HEALTH SCIENCE LIBRARY
EDUCATIONAL RESOURCES DEPARTMENT
519 W. Houston St.
Sta. A, Box 7330
San Antonio, TX 78285   Phone: (512) 228-2284
Marjorie McFarland, Clinical Info.Spec.
Subjects: Medicine, nursing, pediatrics, cancer. **Holdings:** 2048 books; 5064 bound periodical volumes; 155 audio cassette tapes; 4 file drawers of pamphlets; 199 AV programs. **Subscriptions:** 112 journals and other serials.

★10070★ SOUTHWEST FOUNDATION FOR BIOMEDICAL
RESEARCH
PRESTON G. NORTHRUP MEMORIAL LIBRARY
Box 28147
San Antonio, TX 78228-0147   Phone: (512) 674-1410
Maureen D. Funnell, Libn.
Subjects: Biomedicine. **Holdings:** 9200 books; 38,000 bound periodical volumes. **Subscriptions:** 600 journals and other serials.

★10071★ SOUTHWEST TEXAS METHODIST HOSPITAL
LIBRARY
7700 Floyd Curl Dr.
San Antonio, TX 78229   Phone: (512) 692-4583
Christy Floerke, Libn.
Subjects: Medicine, nursing. **Holdings:** 1275 books; 195 bound periodical volumes. **Subscriptions:** 91 journals and other serials.

★10072★   U.S. AIR FORCE HOSPITAL
WILFORD HALL U.S.A.F. MEDICAL CENTER
MEDICAL LIBRARY
Lackland AFB
San Antonio, TX 78236-5300   Phone: (512) 670-7204
Rita F. Smith, Med.Libn.
Subjects: Medicine, nursing, dentistry, hospital administration, veterinary medicine. **Holdings:** 9800 books; 13,800 bound periodical volumes; 4900 AV programs; 1825 reels of microfilm of journals. **Subscriptions:** 900 journals and other serials.

★10073★   U.S. DEPARTMENT OF VETERANS AFFAIRS
MEDICAL CENTER LIBRARY SERVICE
7400 Merton Minter Blvd.
San Antonio, TX 78284   Phone: (512) 696-9660
Elosia Mitchell, Chf.
Subjects: Medicine, allied health sciences. **Holdings:** 4367 books; 5000 microfilm volumes; 503 AV programs. **Subscriptions:** 565 journals and other serials; 21 newspapers.

★10074★   UNIVERSITY OF TEXAS HEALTH SCIENCE
     CENTER, SAN ANTONIO
BRISCOE LIBRARY
7703 Floyd Curl Dr.
San Antonio, TX 78284-7940   Phone: (512) 567-2400
Virginia M. Bowden, Lib.Dir.
Subjects: Health related sciences, nursing, dentistry. **Holdings:** 100,000 books; 92,000 bound periodical volumes; 3000 AV programs. **Subscriptions:** 2500 journals and other serials.

★10075★   UNIVERSITY OF TEXAS HEALTH SCIENCE
     CENTER, SAN ANTONIO
BRISCOE LIBRARY
BRADY/GREEN LIBRARY
4502 Medical Dr.
San Antonio, TX 78284-4402   Phone: (512) 270-3938
Cathy McKinney, Brady/Green Libn.
Subjects: Obstetrics, pediatrics, family practice, ambulatory care, general medicine. **Holdings:** 1350 books; 4225 bound periodical volumes. **Subscriptions:** 121 journals.

★10076★   U.S. AIR FORCE
AIR TRAINING COMMAND
U.S. AIR FORCE 3790 MEDICAL SERVICE TRAINING WING
ACADEMIC LIBRARY
3790 MSTW/CCAAL
Sheppard AFB, TX 76311-5465   Phone: (817) 676-2736
Ms. Boyd, Supv.Libn.
Subjects: General medicine, biological science, nursing, dentistry, pharmacy, hospital administration, management. **Holdings:** 9000 books; 1200 technical reports; 2000 pamphlets. **Subscriptions:** 225 journals and other serials.

★10077★   U.S. AIR FORCE HOSPITAL
SHEPPARD TECHNICAL TRAINING CENTER HOSPITAL
HEALTH SCIENCES LIBRARY
Sheppard AFB, TX 76311-5300   Phone: (817) 676-6647
Marilyn Lucas, Lib.Techn.
Subjects: Medicine, nursing, dentistry, pharmacy, hospital administration. **Holdings:** 6000 books; 2308 bound periodical volumes; 90 video cassettes. **Subscriptions:** 185 journals and other serials.

★10078★   SCOTT AND WHITE MEMORIAL HOSPITAL
RICHARD D. HAINES MEDICAL LIBRARY
2401 S. 31st St.
Temple, TX 76508   Phone: (817) 774-2228
Penny Worley, Dir.
Subjects: Clinical medicine, nursing care and education, allied health sciences. **Holdings:** 8826 books; 23,266 bound periodical volumes. **Subscriptions:** 870 journals and other serials.

★10079★   U.S. DEPARTMENT OF VETERANS AFFAIRS
MEDICAL CENTER MEDICAL LIBRARY
Olin E. Teague Veterans Adm. Ctr.
1901 S. 1st St.
Temple, TX 76504   Phone: (817) 778-4811
Barbara A. Ward, Chf., Lib.Serv.
Subjects: Medicine, surgery, nursing, dentistry. **Holdings:** 3500 books;

9038 bound periodical volumes; 8 VF drawers of clippings and pamphlets; 17 VF drawers of audio cassettes; 260 video cassette tapes. **Subscriptions:** 500 journals and other serials; 12 newspapers.

★10080★   TERRELL STATE HOSPITAL
STAFF LIBRARY
Brin Ave.
Box 70
Terrell, TX 75160   Phone: (214) 563-6452
Josie Richardson, Libn.
Subjects: Psychiatry, neurology, medicine, nursing, psychology, mental health and allied sciences. **Holdings:** 6775 books; 260 bound periodical volumes; 2145 unbound journals; 2369 pamphlets and nonbook materials. **Subscriptions:** 145 journals and other serials.

★10081★   MEDICAL CENTER HOSPITAL
BELL-MARSH MEMORIAL LIBRARY
Box 6400
Tyler, TX 75711   Phone: (903) 531-8685
Ana Wright, Med. Staff Coord.
Subjects: Medicine. **Holdings:** 250 books; 500 bound periodical volumes. **Subscriptions:** 19 journals and other serials.

★10082★   UNIVERSITY OF TEXAS HEALTH CENTER, TYLER
WATSON W. WISE MEDICAL RESEARCH LIBRARY
Box 2003
Tyler, TX 75710   Phone: (903) 877-7354
Elaine Wells, Dir., Lib.Serv.
Subjects: Lung and heart diseases, biochemistry, oncology, nursing, surgery. **Holdings:** 3000 books; 7000 bound periodical volumes; 900 AV programs; 600 reels of microfilm. **Subscriptions:** 408 journals and other serials.

★10083★   U.S. DEPARTMENT OF VETERANS AFFAIRS
MEDICAL CENTER LIBRARY
4800 Memorial Dr.
Waco, TX 76711   Phone: (817) 752-6581
Barbara H. Hobbs, Chf., Lib.Serv.
Subjects: Psychiatry, neurology, psychology, nursing, gerontology, post-traumatic stress. **Holdings:** 3153 volumes; 1219 volumes on microfilm; 1046 AV programs; 8 VF drawers. **Subscriptions:** 320 journals and other serials.

★10084★   WICHITA FALLS STATE HOSPITAL
THOMAS J. GALVIN MEMORIAL MEDICAL LIBRARY
Box 300
Wichita Falls, TX 76307   Phone: (817) 692-1220
Judith A. Morris, Libn.
Subjects: Psychiatry, psychology, surgery and nursing, philosophy, anatomy, education, forensic medicine, history of medicine. **Holdings:** 3500 books; 120 bound periodical volumes; 1050 AV programs; 200 pamphlets; 100 medical reports. **Subscriptions:** 67 journals and other serials.

Utah

★10085★   UTAH STATE UNIVERSITY
DEVELOPMENTAL CENTER FOR HANDICAPPED PERSONS
FAMILY RESOURCE LIBRARY
UMC 9621
Logan, UT 84332   Phone: (801) 752-0238
Julia Burnham, Lib.Coord.
Subjects: Family resources about handicapping conditions and training of the handicapped. **Holdings:** 900 volumes.

★10086★   MCKAY DEE HOSPITAL CENTER
LIBRARY
3939 Harrison Blvd.
Ogden, UT 84409   Phone: (801) 625-2035
Mark Meldrum, Libn.
Subjects: Medicine, hospital administration, nursing. **Holdings:** 2000 books; Audio-Digest tapes. **Subscriptions:** 400 journals and other serials.

★10087★ ST. BENEDICT'S HOSPITAL
HEALTH SCIENCES LIBRARY
5475 S. 500 East
Ogden, UT 84405-6978   Phone: (801) 479-2055
Sandy Eckersley, Info.Spec.
Subjects: Medicine, nursing, and allied health sciences. **Holdings:** 2000
books; 125 videotapes. **Subscriptions:** 202 journals and other serials.

★10088★ UTAH STATE HOSPITAL
LIBRARY
1300 East Center St.
Box 270
Provo, UT 84601   Phone: (801) 373-4400
Janina Chilton, Libn.
Subjects: Medicine, psychology. **Holdings:** 900 volumes; records; tapes.
Subscriptions: 54 journals and other serials.

★10089★ UTAH VALLEY REGIONAL MEDICAL CENTER
MEDICAL LIBRARY
1034 N. 500 W.
Provo, UT 84603   Phone: (801) 371-7180
Alan Grosbeck, Media Spec.
Subjects: Medicine. **Holdings:** 1200 books; 135,000 periodicals; 88 drawers
of microfilm and microfiche. **Subscriptions:** 500 journals and other serials.

★10090★ HOLY CROSS HOSPITAL
MEDICAL LIBRARY
1050 E. South Temple
Salt Lake City, UT 84102   Phone: (801) 350-4060
Lynda Van Wagoner, Med.Libn.
Subjects: Medicine, surgery, nursing, allied health sciences. **Holdings:** 1000
books; 200 Audio-Digest tapes. **Subscriptions:** 125 journals and serials.

★10091★ L.D.S. HOSPITAL
LIBRARY
325 8th Ave.
Salt Lake City, UT 84143   Phone: (801) 321-1054
Mr. Terry L. Heyer, Lib.Dir.
Subjects: Medicine, nursing. **Holdings:** 3500 books; 7500 bound periodical
volumes; 175 pamphlets; 900 audiotape cassettes. **Subscriptions:** 400
journals and other serials; 12 newspapers.

★10092★ ST. MARK'S HOSPITAL
LIBRARY AND MEDIA SERVICES
1200 E. 3900 South St.
Salt Lake City, UT 84124   Phone: (801) 268-7004
Jane M. Errion, Libn.
Subjects: Medicine and allied health sciences. **Holdings:** 1200 books;
unbound periodicals; 1550 AV programs. **Subscriptions:** 400 journals and
other serials.

★10093★ U.S. DEPARTMENT OF VETERANS AFFAIRS
HOSPITAL MEDICAL LIBRARY
500 Foothill Dr.
Salt Lake City, UT 84148   Phone: (801) 584-1209
Carl Worstell, Chf.Libn.
Subjects: Medicine, surgery, psychiatry, emergency medicine, research,
allied health sciences. **Holdings:** 3000 books; 11,262 bound periodical
volumes; 1696 reels of microfilm; 85 video cassettes; 240 pamphlets; 1830
other cataloged items. **Subscriptions:** 325 journals and other serials.

★10094★ UNIVERSITY OF UTAH
SPENCER S. ECCLES HEALTH SCIENCES LIBRARY
Bldg. 89
10 N. Medical Dr.
Salt Lake City, UT 84112   Phone: (801) 581-8771
Wayne J. Peay, Dir.
Subjects: Medicine, pharmacy, nursing, basic sciences, health. **Holdings:**
43,121 books; 77,098 bound periodical volumes; 3376 AV programs.
Subscriptions: 1916 journals and other serials.

★10095★ UTAH STATE LIBRARY
BLIND AND PHYSICALLY HANDICAPPED PROGRAM
REGIONAL LIBRARY
2150 S. 300 West, Ste. 16
Salt Lake City, UT 84115   Phone: (801) 466-6363
Gerald A. Buttars, Prog.Dir.
Holdings: 384,771 talking books and braille books; cassettes; open reel
tapes; large print books. **Subscriptions:** 120 journals and other serials.

Vermont

★10096★ CENTRAL VERMONT HOSPITAL
MEDICAL LIBRARY
Box 547
Barre, VT 05641   Phone: (802) 229-9121
Betty-Jean Eastman, Med.Libn.
Subjects: Medicine, surgery, nursing, allied health sciences. **Holdings:** 500
books. **Subscriptions:** 60 journals and other serials.

★10097★ SOUTHWESTERN VERMONT MEDICAL CENTER
MEDICAL LIBRARY
100 Hospital Dr., E.
Bennington, VT 05201   Phone: (802) 442-6361
Alexandra Heintz, Lib.Coord.
Subjects: Medicine, surgery. **Holdings:** 1300 books; 400 volumes of bound
journals; 10 titles of Audio-Digest tapes; 200 video cassettes. **Subscriptions:**
120 journals and other serials.

★10098★ BRANDON TRAINING SCHOOL
LIBRARY
Brandon, VT 05733   Phone: (802) 247-5711
Sandi Sanderson, Lib.Ck.
Subjects: Mental retardation, education, psychology. **Holdings:** 1600
books; 60 bound periodical volumes; 80 AV programs. **Subscriptions:** 65
journals and other serials.

★10099★ AUSTINE SCHOOL
LIBRARY
120 Maple St.
Brattleboro, VT 05301   Phone: (802) 254-4571
John I. Enola, Libn.
Subjects: Education of the deaf. **Holdings:** 10,000 books; 350 bound
periodical volumes. **Subscriptions:** 40 journals and other serials.

★10100★ BRATTLEBORO MEMORIAL HOSPITAL
MEDICAL LIBRARY
9 Belmont Ave.
Brattleboro, VT 05301   Phone: (802) 257-0341
Martha J. Fenn, Libn.
Subjects: Medicine, nursing, hospitals, health. **Holdings:** 1700 books; 100
pamphlets and clippings. **Subscriptions:** 80 journals and other serials.

★10101★ BRATTLEBORO RETREAT
ASA KEYES MEDICAL LIBRARY
75 Linden St.
Box 803
Brattleboro, VT 05301   Phone: (802) 257-7785
Jane Rand, Dir. of Lib.Serv.
Subjects: Psychiatry, behavioral sciences. **Holdings:** 2700 books; 643
bound periodical volumes. **Subscriptions:** 60 journals and other serials.

★10102★ PLANNED PARENTHOOD OF NORTHERN NEW
    ENGLAND
PPNNE RESOURCE CENTER
23 Mansfield Ave.
Burlington, VT 05401   Phone: (802) 862-9637
Tracy Fisk, Res.Coord.
Subjects: Family life education, sexual development, parenting and child
care, women's health, infertility. **Holdings:** 2300 books; 4 VF drawers of
articles. **Subscriptions:** 30 journals and other serials; 30 newsletters.

★10103★ UNIVERSITY OF VERMONT
CHARLES A. DANA MEDICAL LIBRARY
Given Bldg.
Burlington, VT 05405   Phone: (802) 656-2200
Robert J. Sekerak, Interim Med.Libn.
Subjects: Medicine, nursing, and allied health sciences. **Holdings:** 26,822

books; 65,110 bound periodical volumes; 3144 AV programs. **Subscriptions:** 1649 journals and other serials.

★10104★ **FANNY ALLEN HOSPITAL**
HEALTH SCIENCE LIBRARY
101 College Pkwy.
Colchester, VT 05446   Phone: (802) 655-1234
Ann M. Bousquet, Med.Libn.
Subjects: Medicine, nursing, hospital administration, patient education. **Holdings:** 600 books; patient education pamphlets and AV programs. **Subscriptions:** 85 journals and other serials.

★10105★ **PORTER MEDICAL CENTER**
MEDICAL LIBRARY AND INFORMATION SERVICE
South St.
Middlebury, VT 05753   Phone: (802) 388-7901
Michaela Ledden, Libn.
Subjects: Medicine, nursing. **Holdings:** 500 books; 300 video cassettes. **Subscriptions:** 15 journals and other serials.

★10106★ **VERMONT CENTER FOR INDEPENDENT LIVING**
INFORMATION AND REFERRAL SYSTEM
174 River St.
Montpelier, VT 05602   Phone: (802) 229-0501
Erica Garfin, Dir.
Subjects: Disability, adaptive equipment. **Holdings:** 773 books; 24 VF drawers. **Subscriptions:** 25 journals and other serials; 274 newspapers and newsletters.

★10107★ **NORTH COUNTRY HOSPITAL AND HEALTH**
   CENTER
MEDICAL LIBRARY
Prouty Dr.
Newport, VT 05855   Phone: (802) 334-7331
Marika Szabo, Libn.
Subjects: Medicine, nursing. **Holdings:** 400 books. **Subscriptions:** 40 journals and other serials.

★10108★ **LANDMARK COLLEGE**
LIBRARY
SPECIAL COLLECTIONS
Putney, VT 05346   Phone: (802) 387-4767
Robert H. Rhodes
Subjects: Dyslexia, Specific Learning Disabilities Collection. **Holdings:** 725 books.

★10109★ **GIFFORD MEMORIAL HOSPITAL**
HEALTH INFORMATION CENTER
44 S. Main St.
Randolph, VT 05060   Phone: (802) 728-4441
Linda Minsinger, Inservice Dir.
Subjects: Medicine, nursing. **Holdings:** 532 books; 45 bound periodical volumes; 1 VF drawer of pamphlets; 4 drawers of journals on microfiche; 150 government publications; 50 tapes and filmstrips. **Subscriptions:** 42 journals and other serials.

★10110★ **RUTLAND REGIONAL MEDICAL CENTER**
HEALTH SCIENCES LIBRARY
160 Allen St.
Rutland, VT 05701   Phone: (802) 747-3777
Daphne S. Pringle, Dir.
Subjects: Medicine, nursing, and allied health sciences, hospital administration. **Holdings:** 1000 books; unbound reports, clippings; journal reprints. **Subscriptions:** 94 journals and other serials.

★10111★ **NORTHWESTERN MEDICAL CENTER**
INFORMATION CENTER
Fairfield St.
St. Albans, VT 05478   Phone: (802) 524-5911
DiAnne Bedard, Info.Ctr.Dir.
Subjects: Medicine, nursing, behavioral science. **Holdings:** 800 books; tapes. **Subscriptions:** 40 journals and other serials.

★10112★ **NORTHEASTERN VERMONT REGIONAL HOSPITAL**
INFORMATION CENTER/LIBRARY
Hospital Dr.
St. Johnsbury, VT 05819   Phone: (802) 748-8141
Eleanor B. Simons, Libn.
Subjects: Medicine, nursing, allied health sciences. **Holdings:** 1201 books; 4 filing drawers of pamphlets. **Subscriptions:** 87 journals and other serials.

★10113★ **SPRINGFIELD HOSPITAL**
MEDICAL LIBRARY
25 Ridgewood Rd.
Springfield, VT 05156   Phone: (802) 885-2151
Janet Constantine, Educ.Dir.
Subjects: Medicine, surgery, nursing. **Holdings:** 304 volumes. **Subscriptions:** 41 journals and other serials.

★10114★ **VERMONT STATE HOSPITAL**
AGENCY OF HUMAN SERVICES
RESEARCH LIBRARY
103 S. Main St.
Waterbury, VT 05676   Phone: (802) 241-2248
Jane Hull, Libn.
Subjects: Psychiatry, public health, psychology, medicine, alcohol and drug abuse, corrections. **Holdings:** 10,000 books; 2000 bound periodical volumes; 30 cassettes; 60 cases of pamphlets; 45 boxes of government documents. **Subscriptions:** 200 journals and other serials.

★10115★ **U.S. DEPARTMENT OF VETERANS AFFAIRS**
MEDICAL & REGIONAL OFFICE CENTER
LIBRARY SERVICE
White River Junction, VT 05001   Phone: (802) 295-9363
Richard Haver, Chf., Lib.Serv.
Subjects: Medicine, surgery, psychiatry, nursing. **Holdings:** 1000 books. **Subscriptions:** 240 journals and other serials.

Virginia

★10116★ **ALEXANDRIA HOSPITAL**
HEALTH SCIENCES LIBRARY
4320 Seminary Rd.
Alexandria, VA 22304   Phone: (703) 379-3126
Nina S. McCleskey, Med.Lib.Dir.
Subjects: Medicine, nursing, health care administration. **Holdings:** 2800 books; 2000 bound periodical volumes. **Subscriptions:** 200 journals and other serials.

★10117★ **AMERICAN ACADEMY OF PHYSICIAN ASSISTANTS**
INFORMATION CENTER
950 N. Washington St.
Alexandria, VA 22314   Phone: (703) 836-2272
F. Lynn May, Exec. V.P.
Subjects: Physician assistants, health manpower. **Holdings:** 200 books; 1000 journal articles and bibliographic research materials. **Subscriptions:** 45 journals and other serials.

★10118★ **AMERICAN COLLEGE OF HEALTH CARE**
   ADMINISTRATORS
INFORMATION CENTRAL
325 S. Patrick St.
Alexandria, VA 22314   Phone: (703) 739-7932
Laura R. Ellis, Info.Spec.
Subjects: Long-term care, gerontology. **Holdings:** 16,000 books; 65 bound periodical volumes. **Subscriptions:** 80 journals and other serials.

★10119★ **AMERICAN PHYSICAL THERAPY ASSOCIATION**
LIBRARY
1111 N. Fairfax St.
Alexandria, VA 22314   Phone: (703) 684-2782
Phyllis Quinn
Subjects: Physical therapy. **Holdings:** 500 books; 70 bound periodical volumes; 200 archival items.

★10120★ ASTRE CORPORATE GROUP
LIBRARY
809 Princess St.
Alexandria, VA 22314   Phone: (703) 739-0397
Roy A. Ackerman, Tech.Dir.
Subjects: Medicine, pharmaceuticals, biomedical and biochemical engineering, water pollution, hazardous wastes, chemical engineering, fermentation, strategic planning. **Holdings:** 600 books; 11,210 reports. **Subscriptions:** 320 journals and other serials; 5 newspapers.

★10121★ INSTITUTE FOR ALTERNATIVE FUTURES
LIBRARY
108 N. Alfred St.
Alexandria, VA 22314   Phone: (703) 684-5880
Clement Bezold, Ph.D., Exec.Dir.
Subjects: Health issues, futures, political science. **Holdings:** 1000 volumes; files on citizen goals and futures projects in the U.S.

★10122★ NATIONAL MENTAL HEALTH ASSOCIATION
CLIFFORD BEERS MEMORIAL LIBRARY
1021 Prince St.
Alexandria, VA 22314-2971   Phone: (703) 684-7722
Subjects: Mental health for laymen, voluntary public agencies. **Holdings:** 1500 books.

★10123★ ORTHOTICS AND PROSTHETICS NATIONAL
OFFICE
LIBRARY
1650 King St., 5th Fl.
Alexandria, VA 22314   Phone: (703) 836-7116
Dr. Ian R. Horen, Exec.Dir.
Subjects: Prosthetics and orthotics. **Holdings:** 200 books. **Subscriptions:** 10 journals and other serials.

★10124★ AMERICAN HEALTH RESEARCH INSTITUTE
LIBRARY
4111 Gallows Rd.
Annandale, VA 22003   Phone: (703) 256-4848
Karen Kelly
Subjects: Biomedicine, biology, anatomical sciences, injuries, malpractice, biotechnology, psychology and allied subjects. **Holdings:** 1520 books; 20,000 reports. **Subscriptions:** 15 journals and other serials; 4 newspapers.

★10125★ ARLINGTON HOSPITAL
DOCTORS' LIBRARY
1701 N. George Mason Dr.
Arlington, VA 22205   Phone: (703) 558-6524
Donna Giampa, Libn.
Subjects: Medicine. **Holdings:** 650 books; 2725 bound periodical volumes; 960 audiotapes; 130 video cassettes; 386 unbound volumes of journals. **Subscriptions:** 115 journals and other serials.

★10126★ ASBESTOS INFORMATION ASSOCIATION/NORTH
AMERICA
TECHNICAL AND MEDICAL FILES
1745 Jefferson Davis Hwy.
Crystal Sq. Four, Ste. 509
Arlington, VA 22202   Phone: (703) 979-1150
Kenneth Nyquist, Govt.Aff.Couns.
Subjects: Health and asbestos, asbestos regulation. **Holdings:** 300 books; 10 VF drawers of clippings and medical files. **Subscriptions:** 18 journals and other serials.

★10127★ ASSOCIATION OF UNIVERSITY PROGRAMS IN
HEALTH ADMINISTRATION
RESOURCE CENTER FOR HEALTH SERVICES
ADMINISTRATION EDUCATION
1911 N. Fort Myer Dr., Ste. 503
Arlington, VA 22209   Phone: (703) 524-5500
Karen Cutliff
Subjects: Health services administration, health services administration education, long-term care administration, international health, hospital administration, higher education, medical care, medical economics and public health. **Holdings:** 2000 books; 150 program information files; 55 accreditation self-survey reports; 75 geographic files; 200 files for allied organizations. **Subscriptions:** 100 journals and other serials.

★10128★ NATIONAL INSTITUTE OF VICTIMOLOGY
LIBRARY
2333 N. Vernon St.
Arlington, VA 22207   Phone: (703) 536-1750
Subjects: Victim/witness programs, victim/witness services, problems and needs of crime victims. **Holdings:** 3500 volumes; file collection of research, statistics, and publications.

★10129★ U.S. NAVY
OFFICE OF THE CHIEF OF NAVAL RESEARCH
LIBRARY
Code 01232L
800 N. Quincy St.
Arlington, VA 22217-5000   Phone: (202) 696-4415
W.F. Rettenmaier, Jr., Libn.
Subjects: Biological and medical sciences, physical and chemical sciences, naval and marine sciences, social sciences. **Holdings:** 150 reference books. **Subscriptions:** 260 journals and other serials; 5 newspapers.

★10130★ VIRGINIA POLYTECHNIC INSTITUTE AND STATE
UNIVERSITY
VIRGINIA-MARYLAND REGIONAL COLLEGE OF VETERINARY
MEDICINE
VETERINARY MEDICAL LIBRARY
CVM, Phase II
Blacksburg, VA 24061   Phone: (703) 231-6610
Victoria T. Kok, Vet.Med.Libn.
Subjects: Clinical and preclinical veterinary medicine, biomedicine. **Holdings:** 11,208 books; 3301 bound periodical volumes; 440 slide sets and video cassettes. **Subscriptions:** 575 journals and other serials.

★10131★ AMERICAN MEDICAL LABORATORIES, INC.
LIBRARY
14225 Newbrook Dr.
Chantilly, VA 22021   Phone: (703) 691-9100
Cecilia Durkin, Libn.
Subjects: Laboratory medicine, pathology, toxicology, immunology, industrial medicine, cytogenetics. **Holdings:** 1600 books; 2000 bound periodical volumes. **Subscriptions:** 150 journals and other serials; 5 newspapers.

★10132★ UNIVERSITY OF VIRGINIA
HEALTH SCIENCES CENTER
CLAUDE MOORE HEALTH SCIENCES LIBRARY
Box 234
Charlottesville, VA 22908   Phone: (804) 924-5464
Linda Watson, Dir.
Subjects: Biological and medical sciences, nursing, allied health sciences. **Holdings:** 159,786 volumes; 4895 AV programs. **Subscriptions:** 2897 journals and other serials.

★10133★ UNIVERSITY OF VIRGINIA
MEDICAL CENTER
DEPARTMENT OF NEUROLOGY
ELIZABETH J. OHRSTROM LIBRARY
PO Box 394
Charlottesville, VA 22908   Phone: (804) 924-5321
Barbara Wjite, Lib.Asst.
Subjects: General and pediatric neurology, cardiovascular systems, neuroscience. **Holdings:** 3000 books; 2000 bound periodical volumes. **Subscriptions:** 35 journals and other serials.

★10134★ MEMORIAL HOSPITAL
RALPH R. LANDES MEDICAL LIBRARY
142 S. Main St.
Danville, VA 24541   Phone: (804) 799-4418
Ann B. Sasser, Med.Libn.
Subjects: Medicine, surgery, basic and clinical sciences, hospital administration. **Holdings:** 992 books; bound periodical volumes. **Subscriptions:** 132 journals and other serials.

★10135★ MEMORIAL HOSPITAL
SCHOOL OF PROFESSIONAL NURSING
LIBRARY
142 S. Main St.
Danville, VA 24541   Phone: (804) 799-4510
Connie Quisenberry, Coord., Lib.Serv.
Subjects: Nursing. **Holdings:** 2100 books. **Subscriptions:** 36 journals and other serials.

★10136★   FAIRFAX HOSPITAL
JACOB D. ZYLMAN MEMORIAL LIBRARY
3300 Gallows Rd.
Falls Church, VA 22046   Phone: (703) 698-3234
Alice J. Sheridan, Lib.Dir.
Subjects: Medicine, nursing, hospital management. **Holdings:** 6500 books; 7500 bound periodical volumes; 500 AV programs. **Subscriptions:** 420 journals and other serials.

★10137★   U.S. ARMY/U.S. AIR FORCE
OFFICES OF THE SURGEONS GENERAL
JOINT MEDICAL LIBRARY
5109 Leesburg Pike, Rm. 670
Falls Church, VA 22041-3258   Phone: (703) 756-8028
Mary Ann Nowell, Lib.Dir.
Subjects: Military and general medicine, hospital administration. **Holdings:** 13,000 books; 8000 bound periodical volumes; 500 microfiche; 200 pamphlets. **Subscriptions:** 430 journals and other serials.

★10138★   U.S. ARMY HOSPITALS
MCDONALD ARMY COMMUNITY HOSPITAL
MEDICAL LIBRARY
Fort Eustis, VA 23604-5549   Phone: (804) 878-5800
Ruth E. Shepard, Libn.
Subjects: Medicine, dentistry, nursing. **Holdings:** 1500 books; 1100 bound periodical volumes. **Subscriptions:** 100 journals and other serials.

★10139★   U.S. ARMY HOSPITALS
KENNER ARMY COMMUNITY HOSPITAL
MEDICAL LIBRARY
Fort Lee, VA 23801-5260   Phone: (804) 734-1339
Betty K. Lewis, Libn.
Subjects: Medicine. **Holdings:** 2200 volumes.

★10140★   MARY WASHINGTON HOSPITAL
GORDON W. JONES MEDICAL LIBRARY
2300 Fall Hill Ave.
Fredericksburg, VA 22401   Phone: (703) 899-1597
Karen Nelson, Med.Libn.
Subjects: Medicine, nursing, biomedical sciences, administration, management. **Holdings:** 1000 books; 3000 bound periodical volumes. **Subscriptions:** 144 journals and other serials.

★10141★   RAPPAHANNOCK COMMUNITY COLLEGE
LIBRARY
Glenns Campus Library
Box 287
Glenns, VA 23149   Phone: (804) 758-5324
Carol L. Jones
Subjects: Nursing, business management, drafting, design, history, art. **Holdings:** 20,000 books; 500 microfiche; 1450 reels of microfilm. **Subscriptions:** 170 journals and other serials.

★10142★   SENTARA HAMPTON GENERAL HOSPITAL
MEDICAL LIBRARY
3120 Victoria Blvd.
Hampton, VA 23669   Phone: (804) 727-7102
Ms. Tonilee Moore-Wright, Med.Lib.Dir.
Subjects: Medical sciences, hospital administration, nursing. **Holdings:** 759 books; 2275 bound periodical volumes. **Subscriptions:** 75 journals and other serials.

★10143★   U.S. DEPARTMENT OF VETERANS AFFAIRS
MEDICAL CENTER LIBRARY
Hampton, VA 23667   Phone: (804) 722-9961
Jacqueline Bird, Chf., Lib.Serv.
Subjects: Surgery, medicine, nursing, psychology, patient education. **Holdings:** 4000 books; 800 bound periodical volumes; 7500 unbound periodicals. **Subscriptions:** 425 journals and other serials.

★10144★   ROCKINGHAM MEMORIAL HOSPITAL
HEALTH SCIENCES LIBRARY
235 Cantrell Ave.
Harrisonburg, VA 22801-3293   Phone: (703) 433-4166
Ilene N. Smith, Lib.Dir.
Subjects: Clinical medicine, nursing, allied health subjects. **Holdings:** 6000 books and bound periodical volumes; 337 AV programs. **Subscriptions:** 280 journals and other serials.

★10145★   CENTRAL VIRGINIA TRAINING CENTER
PROFESSIONAL LIBRARY
Box 1098
Lynchburg, VA 24505   Phone: (804) 528-6171
Helen Hester, Libn.
Subjects: Mental retardation, epilepsy, psychology, medicine, social work, special education. **Holdings:** 5000 books; 2200 bound periodical volumes; 85 audiotapes; 225 slides; reports; articles; clippings. **Subscriptions:** 130 journals and other serials.

★10146★   LYNCHBURG GENERAL MARSHALL LODGE
HOSPITAL
HEALTH SCIENCES LIBRARY
1901 Tate Springs Rd.
Lynchburg, VA 24501-1167   Phone: (804) 947-3147
Sybil A. Sturgis, Hea.Sci.Libn.
Subjects: Medicine, nursing, allied health, health administration, nursing and allied health education. **Holdings:** 2500 books; 4350 bound periodical volumes. **Subscriptions:** 57 journals and other serials.

★10147★   VIRGINIA BAPTIST HOSPITAL
BARKSDALE MEDICAL LIBRARY
3300 Rivermont Ave.
Lynchburg, VA 24503   Phone: (804) 522-4505
Anne M. Nurmi, Libn.
Subjects: Obstetrics and gynecology, pediatrics, internal medicine. **Holdings:** 300 books; 1000 bound periodical volumes; video cassettes. **Subscriptions:** 37 journals and other serials.

★10148★   SOUTHWESTERN VIRGINIA MENTAL HEALTH
INSTITUTE
PROFESSIONAL LIBRARY
502 E. Main St.
Marion, VA 24354   Phone: (703) 783-1200
Elizabeth Kent
Subjects: Psychiatry. **Holdings:** 900 volumes; 479 AV programs. **Subscriptions:** 35 journals and other serials.

★10149★   MEMORIAL HOSPITAL OF MARTINSVILLE
MEDICAL LIBRARY
320 Hospital Dr.
Martinsville, VA 24112   Phone: (703) 666-7467
Mary Alice Sherrard, Med.Libn.
Subjects: Medicine, nursing, allied health sciences. **Holdings:** 2000 books; 3000 bound periodical volumes; 600 videotapes. **Subscriptions:** 115 journals and other serials.

★10150★   NATIONAL SUDDEN INFANT DEATH SYNDROME
CLEARINGHOUSE
8201 Greensboro Dr., Ste. 600
McLean, VA 22102   Phone: (703) 821-8955
Liz Eckel, Info.Spec.
Subjects: Sudden Infant Death Syndrome, family grief, loss.

★10151★   RIVERSIDE REGIONAL MEDICAL CENTER
HEALTH SCIENCES LIBRARY
J. Clyde Morris Blvd.
Newport News, VA 23601   Phone: (804) 599-2175
Subjects: Family practice, medicine, pediatrics, obstetrics-gynecology, nursing, allied health sciences. **Holdings:** 4038 books; 6742 bound periodical volumes. **Subscriptions:** 203 journals and other serials.

★10152★   CHILDREN'S HOSPITAL OF THE KING'S
DAUGHTERS
MEDICAL LIBRARY
800 W. Olney Rd.
Norfolk, VA 23507   Phone: (804) 628-7232
Brenda L. Taylor, Libn.
Subjects: Pediatrics. **Holdings:** 432 books; 263 bound periodical volumes; 300 audio cassettes; 18 video cassettes; 5 slide collections on pediatric specialties. **Subscriptions:** 31 journals and other serials.

★10153★   DE PAUL MEDICAL CENTER
DR. HENRY BOONE MEMORIAL LIBRARY
150 Kingsley Ln.
Norfolk, VA 23505   Phone: (804) 489-5270
Ramona C. Parrish, Libn.
Subjects: Medicine. **Holdings:** 1809 books; 2948 bound periodical vol-

umes; 595 Audio-Digest tapes. **Subscriptions:** 136 journals and other serials.

★10154★ DE PAUL MEDICAL CENTER
SCHOOL OF NURSING LIBRARY
150 Kingsley Ln.
Norfolk, VA 23505   Phone: (804) 489-5386
Elinor B. Arsic, Libn.
Subjects: Medicine and religion. **Holdings:** 4317 books; 540 bound periodical volumes; 3724 AV programs; 9 VF drawers of clippings and pamphlets. **Subscriptions:** 80 journals and other serials.

★10155★ EASTERN VIRGINIA MEDICAL SCHOOL
MOORMAN MEMORIAL LIBRARY
700 W. Olney Rd.
Box 1980
Norfolk, VA 23501   Phone: (804) 446-5845
Anne O. Cramer, Dir./Asst. Dean
Subjects: Medicine, allied health sciences, behavioral sciences. **Holdings:** 19,438 books; 39,738 bound periodical volumes; 3557 microforms; 1964 media packages; 5300 unbound periodical volumes. **Subscriptions:** 1155 journals and other serials.

★10156★ CENTRAL STATE HOSPITAL
MEDICAL LIBRARY
Box 4030
Petersburg, VA 23803   Phone: (804) 524-7517
Mrs. Phyllis Mangum, Act.Libn.
Subjects: Psychiatry, psychiatric nursing, social work, clinical psychology, mental retardation. **Holdings:** 98,000 books; 2000 bound periodical volumes. **Subscriptions:** 150 journals and other serials.

★10157★ SOUTHSIDE REGIONAL MEDICAL CENTER
MEDICAL LIBRARY MEDIA SERVICES
801 S. Adams St.
Petersburg, VA 23803   Phone: (804) 732-7220
Joan B. Pollard, Med.Lib./Media Serv.Dir.
Subjects: Medicine, nursing. **Holdings:** 1002 books; 5230 bound periodical volumes; 4 VF drawers of reprints; 120 video cassettes; 1260 Audio-Digest tapes. **Subscriptions:** 125 journals and other serials.

★10158★ MARYVIEW HOSPITAL
HEALTH SCIENCES LIBRARY
3636 High St.
Portsmouth, VA 23707   Phone: (804) 398-2330
Rene L. Brown, Libn.
Subjects: Medicine. **Holdings:** 1000 books; 1065 bound periodical volumes. **Subscriptions:** 114 journals and other serials.

★10159★ PORTSMOUTH GENERAL HOSPITAL
MEDICAL LIBRARY
850 Crawford Pkwy.
Portsmouth, VA 23704   Phone: (804) 398-4217
Sallie B. Dellinger, Libn.
Subjects: Medicine, allied health sciences. **Holdings:** 900 books; 1325 bound periodical volumes; 60 other cataloged items. **Subscriptions:** 30 journals and other serials.

★10160★ PORTSMOUTH PSYCHIATRIC CENTER
MEDICAL LIBRARY
301 Fort Ln.
Portsmouth, VA 23704   Phone: (804) 393-0061
Virginia M. Kerstetter, Med.Libn.
Subjects: Psychiatry, psychology, clinical social work, adjunct therapies, nursing, alcoholism. **Holdings:** 1400 books; 700 bound periodical volumes; 298 audio cassettes. **Subscriptions:** 60 journals and other serials.

★10161★ U.S. NAVY
NAVAL HOSPITAL
MEDICAL LIBRARY
Portsmouth, VA 23708   Phone: (804) 398-5383
Suad Jones, Med.Libn.
Subjects: Medicine, dentistry, nursing, allied health sciences. **Holdings:** 7155 books; 15,997 bound periodical volumes; 1371 cartridges of microfilm. **Subscriptions:** 590 journals and other serials.

★10162★ HUNTON & WILLIAMS
LAW LIBRARY
Riverfront Plaza, East Tower
951 E. Byrd St.
Richmond, VA 23219   Phone: (804) 788-8245
Dale Owen, Dir.
Subjects: Law - corporate, real estate, antitrust, tax, labor, environmental, health care; litigation. **Holdings:** 60,000 volumes. **Subscriptions:** 500 journals and other serials; 6 newspapers.

★10163★ RICHMOND MEMORIAL HOSPITAL
MEDICAL AND NURSING SCHOOL LIBRARIES
1300 Westwood Ave.
Richmond, VA 23227   Phone: (804) 254-6008
Merle L. Colglazier, Libn.
Subjects: Medicine, nursing, health sciences. **Holdings:** 8000 books and bound periodical volumes; nursing AV programs. **Subscriptions:** 149 journals and other serials.

★10164★ ST. MARY'S HOSPITAL
HEALTH SCIENCES LIBRARY
5801 Bremo Rd.
Richmond, VA 23226   Phone: (804) 281-8247
Damon Persiani, Libn.
Subjects: Medicine, hospital administration, nursing. **Holdings:** 600 books; 1000 bound periodical volumes. **Subscriptions:** 115 journals and other serials.

★10165★ U.S. DEPARTMENT OF VETERANS AFFAIRS
HOSPITAL LIBRARY
1201 Broad Rock Blvd.
Richmond, VA 23249   Phone: (804) 230-0001
Eleanor Rollins, Chf., Lib.Serv.
Subjects: Medicine, psychology, sociology. **Holdings:** 4000 books; 6000 bound periodical volumes; 1000 AV programs; 1000 volumes on microfilm. **Subscriptions:** 830 journals and other serials.

★10166★ VIRGINIA COMMONWEALTH UNIVERSITY
MEDICAL COLLEGE OF VIRGINIA
TOMPKINS-MCCAW LIBRARY
509 N. 12th St.
PO Box 582
Richmond, VA 23298-0582   Phone: (804) 786-0633
Subjects: Medicine, dentistry, pharmacy, nursing, basic sciences, allied health sciences. **Holdings:** 247,591 bound volumes. **Subscriptions:** 3470 journals and other serials.

★10167★ VIRGINIA COMMONWEALTH UNIVERSITY
VIRGINIA CENTER ON AGING
PO Box 229, MCV Sta.
Richmond, VA 23298-0229   Phone: (804) 786-1525
Ruth B. Finley, IRC Hd.
Subjects: Gerontology, mental health, sociology and the politics of aging, geriatrics, family relationships, long-term care. **Holdings:** 1500 books; 100 reports; 4 archives; 50 AV items. **Subscriptions:** 3 journals and other serials.

★10168★ VIRGINIA DEPARTMENT OF CRIMINAL JUSTICE
SERVICES
LIBRARY
805 E. Broad St.
Richmond, VA 23219   Phone: (804) 786-8478
Stephen E. Squire, Libn.
Subjects: Criminal and juvenile justice planning and evaluation; crime prevention programs; domestic violence. **Holdings:** 7000 volumes; 10 VF drawers; 80 video cassettes. **Subscriptions:** 250 journals and other serials.

★10169★ VIRGINIA DEPARTMENT OF HEALTH
BUREAU OF TOXIC SUBSTANCES
LIBRARY
109 Governor St., Rm. 918
Richmond, VA 23219   Phone: (804) 786-1763
Vickie O'Dell, Info.Spec.
Subjects: Toxicology, occupational health. **Holdings:** 500 books. **Subscriptions:** 10 journals and other serials.

★10170★ VIRGINIA DEPARTMENT FOR RIGHTS OF VIRGINIANS WITH DISABILITIES
LIBRARY
James Monroe Bldg.
101 N. 14th St., 17th Fl.
Richmond, VA 23219   Phone: (804) 225-2042
Iris S. Judkins, Info. & Referral Mgr.
Subjects: Persons with disabilities - civil rights, education, training, housing, transportation. **Holdings:** Figures not available.

★10171★ COLLEGE OF HEALTH SCIENCES
LEARNING RESOURCES CENTER
920 S. Jefferson St., Rm. 611
Roanoke, VA 24016   Phone: (703) 985-8270
Nan Seamans, Dir.
Subjects: Nursing, allied health. **Holdings:** 4500 books; 600 bound periodical volumes. **Subscriptions:** 175 journals and other serials.

★10172★ ROANOKE MEMORIAL HOSPITALS
MEDICAL LIBRARY
Box 13367
Roanoke, VA 24033   Phone: (703) 981-7371
Lucy D. Glenn, Dir.
Subjects: Medicine, nursing, allied health sciences. **Holdings:** 3488 books; 3839 bound periodical volumes; 52 slide sets. **Subscriptions:** 209 journals and other serials.

★10173★ HCA/LEWIS-GALE HOSPITAL
MEDICAL LIBRARY
1900 Electric Rd.
Salem, VA 24153   Phone: (703) 989-4261
Roberta L. Miller, Med.Lib.Cons.
Subjects: Medicine, surgery. **Holdings:** 500 books; bound periodical volumes. **Subscriptions:** 150 journals and other serials.

★10174★ U.S. DEPARTMENT OF VETERANS AFFAIRS
MEDICAL CENTER LIBRARY
1970 Roanoke Blvd.
Salem, VA 24153   Phone: (703) 982-2463
Jean A. Kennedy, Chf.Libn.
Subjects: Medicine, psychiatry, nursing, allied health sciences. **Holdings:** 4891 books; 1220 AV programs. **Subscriptions:** 251 journals and other serials.

★10175★ LAW ENVIRONMENTAL
LIBRARY
7375 Boston Blvd., Ste. 200
Springfield, VA 22153   Phone: (703) 912-9400
Subjects: Water, wastewater, sanitary engineering, solid and hazardous wastes and their effects on health, environmental engineering. **Holdings:** 2000 books. **Subscriptions:** 39 journals and other serials.

★10176★ AMERICAN LIFE LOBBY
LIBRARY
PO Box 490
Stafford, VA 22554   Phone: (703) 659-4171
Subjects: Abortion; euthanasia; infanticide; opposition to tax-subsidized birth control organizations, population control in foreign countries; opposition to sex, violence, and profanity on television and radio; opposition to school and television sex education programs. **Holdings:** 17,000 flyers, leaflets, booklets, books, audiovisual materials, and other items.

★10177★ NATIONAL COUNCIL FOR MEDICAL RESEARCH
LIBRARY
PO Box 1105
Staunton, VA 24401
E.C. Mullins
Subjects: History of medicine; organized medicine in the United States; health care - alternative, government. **Holdings:** 800 books. **Subscriptions:** 8 journals and other serials; 3 newspapers.

★10178★ WESTERN STATE HOSPITAL
MEDICAL LIBRARY
Box 2500
Staunton, VA 24401-1405   Phone: (703) 332-8307
Richard D. Wills, Med.Libn.
Subjects: Psychology, psychiatry, general medicine, nursing. **Holdings:**

3600 books; 600 bound periodical volumes. **Subscriptions:** 117 journals and other serials.

★10179★ LOUISE OBICI MEMORIAL HOSPITAL
LIBRARY
1900 N. Main
Suffolk, VA 23434   Phone: (804) 934-4865
Janet B. Daum, Libn.
Subjects: Medicine, allied health. **Holdings:** 1000 books. **Subscriptions:** 190 journals and other serials.

★10180★ MATERNAL AND CHILD HEALTH STUDIES PROJECT
INFORMATION SCIENCES RESEARCH INSTITUTE
LIBRARY
8375 Leesburg Pike, Ste. 439
Vienna, VA 22182   Phone: (703) 255-1408
Margaret W. Pratt
Subjects: Infant mortality, child mortality, maternal mortality. **Holdings:** 100 books; 200 bound periodical volumes; 150 reports.

★10181★ EASTERN STATE HOSPITAL
LIBRARY SERVICES
STAFF LIBRARY
4601 Ironbound Rd.
Drawer A
Williamsburg, VA 23187   Phone: (804) 253-5457
R. Blanton McLean, Lib.Dir.
Subjects: Psychiatry, psychology, medicine, nursing. **Holdings:** 1883 books; 767 bound periodical volumes; 1016 AV programs. **Subscriptions:** 114 journals and other serials.

★10182★ WINCHESTER MEDICAL CENTER
HEALTH SCIENCES LIBRARY
Box 3340
Winchester, VA 22601-2540   Phone: (703) 722-8040
Mary A. Salem, Libn.
Subjects: Medicine, nursing, allied health sciences. **Holdings:** 600 books; 1500 bound periodical volumes. **Subscriptions:** 175 journals and other serials.

★10183★ POTOMAC HOSPITAL
RICHARD P. IMMERMAN MEMORIAL LIBRARY
2300 Opitz Blvd.
Woodbridge, VA 22191   Phone: (703) 670-1331
Debra G. Scarborough, Hea.Sci.Libn.
Subjects: Medicine, hospital administration, nursing. **Holdings:** 450 books; 1000 microfiche. **Subscriptions:** 200 journals and other serials.

Washington

★10184★ HUXLEY COLLEGE OF ENVIRONMENTAL STUDIES
ENVIRONMENTAL RESOURCE LIBRARY
ESC 535, Huxley College
Bellingham, WA 98225   Phone: (206) 676-3520
Diane Merrill, Asst. to the Dean
Subjects: Environmental education; human ecology; social science; environmental philosophy and ethics; environmental planning; terrestrial, fresh water, marine ecology; environmental health and toxicology; agriculture, nutrition, food supply; environmental technology and recycling; energy alternatives. **Holdings:** 2000 books; 3 files of pamphlets and clippings; 50 newsletters; 600 student reports; 12 tapes; Environmental Protection Agency documents. **Subscriptions:** 32 journals and other serials.

★10185★ ST. JOSEPH HOSPITAL
LIBRARY
2901 Squalicum Pkwy.
Bellingham, WA 98225   Phone: (206) 734-5400
Bea Dickerson, Libn.
Subjects: Medicine, nursing, and allied health sciences. **Holdings:** 800 books. **Subscriptions:** 150 journals and other serials.

★10186★ HARRISON MEMORIAL HOSPITAL
ROBERT S. FRECH, M.D., MEMORIAL HEALTH SCIENCES
  LIBRARY
2520 Cherry Ave.
Bremerton, WA 98310   Phone: (206) 377-3911
Selma Kannel, Dir., Lib.Serv.
Subjects: Clinical sciences, nursing, hospital administration. **Holdings:** 750 books; 900 unbound periodical volumes. **Subscriptions:** 122 journals and other serials.

★10187★ U.S. NAVY
NAVAL HOSPITAL
MEDICAL LIBRARY
Bremerton, WA 98314   Phone: (206) 478-9316
Jane Easley, Libn.
Subjects: Medicine, nursing, administration. **Holdings:** 1300 books; 2700 bound periodical volumes. **Subscriptions:** 185 journals and other serials.

★10188★ WASHINGTON STATE LIBRARY
RAINIER SCHOOL BRANCH LIBRARY
Box 600
Buckley, WA 98321   Phone: (206) 829-1111
Lynn Red, Module Supv.
Subjects: Mental retardation, developmental psychology, institutionalization, deaf/blind/retarded handicapped. **Holdings:** 3000 books; 1596 bound and unbound periodical volumes; 100 boxes of pamphlets; 15 boxes of periodical, book, and film catalogs in the field of retardation. **Subscriptions:** 163 journals and other serials; 30 newspapers.

★10189★ HEALTH INFORMATION NETWORK SERVICES
Pacific & Nassau
Box 1067
Everett, WA 98206   Phone: (206) 258-7558
Cheryl M. Goodwin, Dir.
Subjects: Medicine, nursing, hospital management. **Holdings:** 2000 books. **Subscriptions:** 500 journals and other serials.

★10190★ U.S. AIR FORCE HOSPITAL
MEDICAL LIBRARY
92 Strategic Hospital/SGASA
Fairchild AFB, WA 99011-5300   Phone: (509) 247-5353
Susan Coleman, Med.Libn.
Subjects: General internal medicine, pediatrics, orthopedics, obstetrics and gynecology, family practice. **Holdings:** 1260 books; 54 bound periodical volumes. **Subscriptions:** 48 journals and other serials; 6 newspapers.

★10191★ WASHINGTON STATE LIBRARY
WESTERN STATE HOSPITAL BRANCH LIBRARY
Fort Steilacoom, WA 98494   Phone: (206) 756-2715
Neal Van Der Voorn, Libn.
Subjects: Psychiatry, clinical psychology, mental health, psychiatric nursing, psychiatric social work, medicine, occupational therapy, recreational therapy. **Holdings:** 4500 books; 375 tapes. **Subscriptions:** 154 journals and other serials.

★10192★ ST. JOHN'S MEDICAL CENTER
HERBERT H. MINTHORN MEMORIAL LIBRARY
1614 E. Kessler Blvd.
Box 3002
Longview, WA 98632   Phone: (206) 423-1530
Barbara Sherry, Med.Libn.
Subjects: Medicine, nursing, and allied health sciences. **Holdings:** 1200 books. **Subscriptions:** 200 journals and other serials.

★10193★ WASHINGTON STATE LIBRARY
EASTERN STATE HOSPITAL LIBRARY
Box A
Medical Lake, WA 99022   Phone: (509) 299-4276
Nancy White, Libn.
Subjects: Psychiatry, nursing, medicine, mental health, social work. **Holdings:** 2283 books; 3 VF drawers. **Subscriptions:** 66 journals and other serials.

★10194★ WASHINGTON STATE LIBRARY
LAKELAND VILLAGE BRANCH LIBRARY
Box 200 B32-25
Medical Lake, WA 99022-0200   Phone: (509) 299-5089
Nancy P. White, Libn.
Subjects: Mental retardation, medicine. **Holdings:** 1698 books; back issues of unbound journals (latest 5 years). **Subscriptions:** 66 journals and other serials.

★10195★ ST. PETER HOSPITAL
LIBRARY SERVICES
413 Lilly Rd., NE
Olympia, WA 98506-5166   Phone: (206) 493-7222
Edean Berglund, Dir.
Subjects: Health care. **Holdings:** Figures not available. **Subscriptions:** 400 journals and other serials.

★10196★ WASHINGTON STATE UNIVERSITY
VETERINARY MEDICAL/PHARMACY LIBRARY
170 Wegner Hall
Pullman, WA 99164-6512   Phone: (509) 335-9556
Vicki F. Croft, Hd.
Subjects: Veterinary and human medicine, pharmacy and pharmacology. **Holdings:** 21,900 books; 30,500 bound periodical volumes. **Subscriptions:** 800 journals and other serials.

★10197★ GOOD SAMARITAN HOSPITAL
DR. THOMAS CLARK HEALTH SERVICES LIBRARY
407 14th Ave., SE
Puyallup, WA 98371   Phone: (206) 848-6661
Jade Trevere, Asst.Libn.
Subjects: Medicine, nursing, management. **Holdings:** 303 volumes. **Subscriptions:** 72 journals and other serials.

★10198★ VALLEY MEDICAL CENTER
LIBRARY
400 S. 43rd St.
Renton, WA 98055   Phone: (206) 251-5194
Subjects: Medicine, surgery, allied health sciences. **Holdings:** 1050 books; 200 bound periodical volumes. **Subscriptions:** 210 journals and other serials; 5 newspapers.

★10199★ WASHINGTON STATE DEPARTMENT OF
VETERANS AFFAIRS
STAFF & MEMBER LIBRARY
Washington Veterans' Home
PO Box 698
Retsil, WA 98378   Phone: (206) 895-4700
Velta Ashbrook, Libn.
Subjects: Geriatric medicine and nursing, long term care, autism, mental retardation, child welfare and abuse, gerontology. **Holdings:** 5200 books; 2000 large print books. **Subscriptions:** 100 journals and other serials.

★10200★ HANFORD ENVIRONMENTAL HEALTH
FOUNDATION
RESOURCE CENTER
Box 100
Richland, WA 99352   Phone: (509) 376-6125
Athena Bradham, Libn.
Subjects: Medicine, industrial hygiene, psychology. **Holdings:** 2500 volumes; 1500 other cataloged items. **Subscriptions:** 143 journals and other serials.

★10201★ CHILDREN'S HOSPITAL AND MEDICAL CENTER
HOSPITAL LIBRARY
4800 Sand Point Way NE
PO Box C-5371
Seattle, WA 98105   Phone: (206) 526-2118
Tamara A. Turner, Dir.
Subjects: Pediatrics. **Holdings:** 3500 books; 4500 bound periodical volumes. **Subscriptions:** 800 journals and other serials.

★10202★ FIFTH AVENUE HOSPITAL
MEDICAL LIBRARY
10560 5th, NE
Seattle, WA 98125   Phone: (206) 364-2050
Subjects: Medicine, osteopathy, podiatry, surgery. **Holdings:** 525 books. **Subscriptions:** 55 journals and other serials.

★10203★ FRED HUTCHINSON CANCER RESEARCH CENTER
LIBRARY
1124 Columbia St.
Seattle, WA 98104   Phone: (206) 667-4314
Eve Ruff, M.S.
Subjects: Leukemia, immunology, molecular biology, cancer research, genetics, cancer prevention. **Holdings:** 2000 books; 11,000 bound periodical volumes. **Subscriptions:** 250 journals and other serials; 2 newspapers.

★10204★ GROUP HEALTH COOPERATIVE OF PUGET
SOUND
MEDICAL LIBRARY
200 15th Ave., E.
Seattle, WA 98112   Phone: (206) 326-3393
Jackie Gagne, Dir., Med.Libs.
Subjects: Clinical medicine, group medical plans, family practice, nursing, pharmacy. **Holdings:** 1800 books; 2500 bound periodical volumes; 4000 audiotape cassettes; Audio-Digest tapes. **Subscriptions:** 410 journals and other serials.

★10205★ NATIONAL WRITERS GROUP
LIBRARY
PO Box 25678
Seattle, WA 98125-1178   Phone: (206) 365-1624
Mike Perry, Ed.
Subjects: German euthanasia program, medical ethics, resistance to Nazism, abortion, Holocaust. **Holdings:** 1000 books. **Subscriptions:** 15 journals and other serials.

★10206★ NORTHWEST GERIATRIC EDUCATION CENTER
CLEARINGHOUSE RESOURCE CENTER
University of Washington HL-23
Seattle, WA 98195   Phone: (206) 685-7478
Susan Guralnick, Clghse.Coord.
Subjects: Geriatrics. **Holdings:** Books, newsletters, curriculum guides, videotapes.

★10207★ NORTHWEST HOSPITAL
EFFIE M. STOREY LEARNING CENTER
1550 N. 115th
Seattle, WA 98133   Phone: (206) 368-1642
Edith Sutton, Libn.
Subjects: Medicine, nursing, management. **Holdings:** 700 books; 100 videotapes; 100 audiotapes; 15 slide sets. **Subscriptions:** 88 journals and other serials.

★10208★ PACIFIC MEDICAL CENTER
ELLEN GRIEP MEMORIAL LIBRARY
1200 12th Ave., S.
Seattle, WA 98144   Phone: (206) 326-4085
Seungja Song, Mgr., Med.Lib.
Subjects: Ambulatory care medicine, medicine, dentistry, hospital administration. **Holdings:** 1300 books; 5000 bound periodical volumes. **Subscriptions:** 165 journals and other serials.

★10209★ PROVIDENCE MEDICAL CENTER
HORTON HEALTH SCIENCES LIBRARY
500 17th Ave., C-34008
Seattle, WA 98124   Phone: (206) 320-2423
Kathleen Murray, Dir., Lib.Serv.
Subjects: Clinical medicine, surgery, cardiology, nursing, psychiatry. **Holdings:** 9000 volumes; 1 VF drawer. **Subscriptions:** 500 journals and other serials.

★10210★ PSYCHOANALYTIC SOCIETY OF SEATTLE
EDITH BUXBAUM LIBRARY
4027 E. Madison St.
Seattle, WA 98112   Phone: (206) 328-5315
Roger C. Eddy, M.D., Chm., Lib.Comm.
Subjects: Psychoanalysis, allied health sciences. **Holdings:** 1750 volumes; 24 pamphlet boxes of journal reprints; 811 unbound journals; videotapes. **Subscriptions:** 20 journals and other serials.

★10211★ SCHICK SHADEL HOSPITAL
MEDICAL LIBRARY
Box 48149
Seattle, WA 98148   Phone: (206) 244-8100
Pamela W. Miles, Med.Libn.
Subjects: Medicine, smoking, alcoholism and substance abuse, behavior modification. **Holdings:** 800 books; 60 unbound periodical volumes; 15 VF drawers of reports, reprints, clippings. **Subscriptions:** 60 journals and other serials.

★10212★ SEATTLE PUBLIC LIBRARY
EDUCATION, PSYCHOLOGY, SOCIOLOGY, SPORTS
DEPARTMENT
1000 4th Ave.
Seattle, WA 98104   Phone: (206) 386-4620
Lynn Daniel, Coord.Dir.
Subjects: Education, psychology, sociology, human relations, recreation, sports and games, vocations, occult, etiquette, childbirth, child care, criminology, sex, marriage and family. **Holdings:** 80,000 books; microforms; college catalogs.

★10213★ SISTERS OF PROVIDENCE HEALTHCARE
CORPORATION
CORPORATE LIBRARY
Box C11038
Seattle, WA 98111   Phone: (206) 464-3028
Keith Dahlgren, Lib.Coord.
Subjects: Health care - administration, planning, law, financing. **Holdings:** 1200 books. **Subscriptions:** 375 journals and other serials; 10 newspapers.

★10214★ SWEDISH HOSPITAL MEDICAL CENTER
REFERENCE LIBRARY
747 Summit Ave.
Seattle, WA 98104   Phone: (206) 386-2484
Jean C. Anderson, Chf.Libn.
Subjects: Surgery, medicine, nursing, hospital administration. **Holdings:** 2900 volumes; 40 videotapes; 6100 slides. **Subscriptions:** 375 journals and other serials.

★10215★ U.S. DEPARTMENT OF LABOR
OSHA
REGION X LIBRARY
1111 3rd Ave., Ste. 715
Seattle, WA 98101-3212   Phone: (206) 553-5930
Donna M. Hoffman, Libn.
Subjects: Industrial hygiene, toxic substances, industrial safety, toxicology, safety, engineering. **Holdings:** 1000 titles. **Subscriptions:** 10 journals and other serials.

★10216★ U.S. DEPARTMENT OF VETERANS AFFAIRS
HOSPITAL MEDICAL LIBRARY
1660 S. Columbian Way, 142-D
Seattle, WA 98108   Phone: (206) 764-2065
Maryanne Blake, Chf., Lib.Serv.
Subjects: Medicine. **Holdings:** 1620 books; 4000 bound periodical volumes; 570 AV programs. **Subscriptions:** 365 journals and other serials.

★10217★ UNIVERSITY OF WASHINGTON
ALCOHOL AND DRUG ABUSE INSTITUTE
LIBRARY
3937 15th Ave., NE, NL-15
Seattle, WA 98105   Phone: (206) 543-0937
Nancy Sutherland, Dir. of Lib.
Subjects: Alcohol and drug abuse. **Holdings:** 2000 books; 5000 reprints. **Subscriptions:** 80 journals and other serials.

★10218★ UNIVERSITY OF WASHINGTON
HEALTH SCIENCES LIBRARY AND INFORMATION CENTER
T-227 Health Sciences, SB-55
Seattle, WA 98195   Phone: (206) 543-5530
Sherrilynne Fuller, Dir.
Subjects: Medicine, dentistry, nursing, pharmacy, public health. **Holdings:** 87,396 books; 203,237 bound periodical volumes; 82,091 microfiche. **Subscriptions:** 4108 journals and other serials.

★10219★ UNIVERSITY OF WASHINGTON
HEALTH SCIENCES LIBRARY AND INFORMATION CENTER
K.K. SHERWOOD LIBRARY
Harborview Medical Center
325 9th Ave., ZA-43
Seattle, WA 98104   Phone: (206) 223-3360
Ellen Howard, Libn.
Subjects: Core medical collection. **Holdings:** 408 books; 4799 bound periodical volumes. **Subscriptions:** 179 journals and other serials.

★10220★ UNIVERSITY OF WASHINGTON
REGIONAL PRIMATE RESEARCH CENTER
PRIMATE INFORMATION CENTER
SJ-50
Seattle, WA 98195   Phone: (206) 543-4376
Jackie Lee Pritchard, Mgr.
Subjects: Nonhuman primates, biomedical research, behavioral sciences. **Holdings:** 800 books; 100 bound periodical volumes; 2000 microfiche; microfilm. **Subscriptions:** 60 journals and other serials.

★10221★ VIRGINIA MASON MEDICAL CENTER
MEDICAL LIBRARY
925 Seneca
Seattle, WA 98111   Phone: (206) 223-6733
Ann Robertson, Dir. of Lib.Serv.
Subjects: Biomedicine. **Holdings:** 3000 books; 5000 bound periodical volumes; videotapes; microfilms. **Subscriptions:** 750 journals and other serials.

★10222★ WASHINGTON LIBRARY FOR THE BLIND AND
PHYSICALLY HANDICAPPED
821 Lenora St.
Seattle, WA 98129   Phone: (206) 464-6930
Jan Ames, Dir.
Subjects: Blindness and disabilities. **Holdings:** 5800 braille books; 101,000 recorded books; 7500 ink print books. **Subscriptions:** 100 journals and other serials.

★10223★ WEST SEATTLE COMMUNITY HOSPITAL
LIBRARY
2600 S.W. Holden St.
Box C26002
Seattle, WA 98126   Phone: (206) 938-6000
Beverly D. Downing, Libn.
Subjects: Medicine, nursing, hospital administration. **Holdings:** 500 books; 166 bound periodical volumes; 150 AV programs. **Subscriptions:** 90 journals and other serials.

★10224★ EMPIRE HEALTH SERVICES
HEALTH INFORMATION CENTER
PO Box 288
Spokane, WA 99210   Phone: (509) 838-4771
Delores Brewer, Libn.
Subjects: Orthopedics, nursing, medicine, surgery, pathology, neurology, rehabilitation, outpatient surgery, oncology, family home care. **Holdings:** 200 books; 21 periodical volumes; 39 titles of Medcom slides; Audio-Digest tapes. **Subscriptions:** 35 journals and other serials.

★10225★ INTERCOLLEGIATE CENTER FOR NURSING
EDUCATION
BETTY M. ANDERSON LIBRARY
W. 2917 Ft. George Wright Dr.
Spokane, WA 99204-5290   Phone: (509) 325-6139
Robert M. Pringle, Jr., Hd.Libn.
Subjects: Nursing, allied health sciences. **Holdings:** 10,000 books; 500 bound periodical volumes; 25 VF drawers. **Subscriptions:** 300 journals and other serials.

★10226★ SACRED HEART MEDICAL CENTER
HEALTH SCIENCES LIBRARY
W. 101 8th Ave.
TAF-C9
Spokane, WA 99220-4045   Phone: (509) 455-3094
Sandra L. Keno, Libn.
Subjects: Medicine and surgery, nursing, dietetics, psychiatry, administration and management, clinical laboratory. **Holdings:** 2500 books; 3000 bound periodical volumes; 16 VF drawers of clippings, pamphlets,

pictures; slides; videotapes; cassettes; filmstrips. **Subscriptions:** 300 journals and other serials.

★10227★ SPOKANE MEDICAL LIBRARY
705 W. 1st
Spokane, WA 99204-0409   Phone: (509) 458-6251
Michelanne Adams, Lib.Spec. I
Subjects: Clinical medicine. **Holdings:** 3000 books; 10,000 bound periodical volumes. **Subscriptions:** 126 journals and other serials.

★10228★ U.S. DEPARTMENT OF VETERANS AFFAIRS
MEDICAL CENTER LIBRARY
N. 4815 Assembly St.
Spokane, WA 99205   Phone: (509) 328-4521
Mary Curtis-Kellett, Chf., Lib.Serv.
Subjects: Medicine and allied health sciences. **Holdings:** 1441 books; 978 bound periodical volumes; 502 video cassettes; 15 models; pamphlets; patient teaching charts. **Subscriptions:** 168 journals and other serials.

★10229★ AMERICAN INSTITUTE FOR BIOSOCIAL
RESEARCH
LIBRARY
PO Box 1174
Tacoma, WA 98401-1174   Phone: (206) 922-0448
Laura Babin, Libn.
Subjects: Behavioral science - eating disorders, abnormal behavior, learning disabilities, behavior disorders; mental illness; biochemistry; environmental health; nutrition; psychology; sociology; criminology; medicine; organic chemistry; photobiology; neurology; toxicology. **Holdings:** 5915 books; 95 periodicals. **Subscriptions:** 111 journals and other serials; 2 newspapers.

★10230★ MADIGAN ARMY MEDICAL CENTER
MADIGAN COMMUNITY LIBRARY
Box 263
Tacoma, WA 98431-5263   Phone: (206) 967-6198
Mary Magie, Libn.
Holdings: 20,000 books; 1800 phonograph records; 8 VF drawers of pamphlets. **Subscriptions:** 141 journals and other serials; 10 newspapers.

★10231★ MEDICAL LIBRARY OF PIERCE COUNTY
315 South K St.
Box 5299
Tacoma, WA 98405-0986   Phone: (206) 594-1075
Cathy Edelman, Exec.Dir./Hd.Libn.
Subjects: Medicine. **Holdings:** 2000 books; 1222 bound periodical volumes; 8 VF drawers. **Subscriptions:** 165 biomedical and administrative journals.

★10232★ ST. JOSEPH HOSPITAL AND HEALTH CARE
CENTER
HOSPITAL LIBRARY
1718 South I St.
Box 2197
Tacoma, WA 98401   Phone: (206) 591-6778
Brynn Beals, Libn.
Subjects: Medicine, nursing, health sciences, autism. **Holdings:** 2000 books; 150 bound periodical volumes. **Subscriptions:** 100 journals and other serials.

★10233★ U.S. ARMY HOSPITALS
MADIGAN ARMY MEDICAL CENTER
MEDICAL LIBRARY
Box 375
Tacoma, WA 98431   Phone: (206) 967-6782
Marcia I. Batchelor, Libn.
Subjects: Medicine, dentistry, nursing, hospital administration, pharmacology. **Holdings:** 12,000 books; 13,000 bound periodical volumes; 1000 reels of microfilm; 100 video cassettes; 4 VF drawers of pamphlets and reprints. **Subscriptions:** 750 journals and other serials.

★10234★ U.S. DEPARTMENT OF VETERANS AFFAIRS
MEDICAL CENTER LIBRARY SERVICE
American Lake
Tacoma, WA 98493   Phone: (206) 582-8440
Dennis L. Levi, Chf., Lib.Serv.
Subjects: Psychiatry, psychology, general medicine, nursing. **Holdings:**

1917 books; 2 VF drawers of pamphlets. **Subscriptions:** 258 journals and other serials; 33 newspapers.

★10235★ ST. JOSEPH COMMUNITY HOSPITAL
LIBRARY
600 NE 92nd Ave.
Box 1600
Vancouver, WA 98668   Phone: (206) 256-2045
Sylvia E. MacWilliams, Lib.Coord.
Subjects: Medicine, nursing. **Holdings:** 1054 books. **Subscriptions:** 354 journals and other serials.

★10236★ VANCOUVER MEMORIAL HOSPITAL
R.D. WISWALL MEMORIAL LIBRARY
3400 Main St.
Box 1600
Vancouver, WA 98668   Phone: (206) 696-5143
Sylvia E. MacWilliams, Dir., Lib.Serv.
Subjects: Medicine, nursing. **Holdings:** Figures not available.

★10237★ WASHINGTON STATE SCHOOL FOR THE DEAF
MCGILL LIBRARY
611 Grand Blvd.
Vancouver, WA 98661-4918   Phone: (206) 696-6223
James D. Randall, Dir.
Subjects: Elementary and secondary education. **Holdings:** 10,672 books; VF drawers; 226 videotapes; 2943 filmstrips; 545 film loops; 369 study prints; 250 microfiche; 44 charts. **Subscriptions:** 89 journals and other serials.

★10238★ U.S. DEPARTMENT OF VETERANS AFFAIRS
HOSPITAL LIBRARY
77 Wainwright Dr.
Walla Walla, WA 99362   Phone: (509) 525-5200
Max J. Merrell, Chf.Libn.
Subjects: Medicine, surgery, nursing, allied health sciences. **Holdings:** 1500 books; 700 volumes of journals. **Subscriptions:** 100 journals and other serials.

★10239★ CENTRAL WASHINGTON HOSPITAL
HEMINGER HEALTH SCIENCES LIBRARY
1300 Fuller St.
PO Box 1887
Wenatchee, WA 98807-1887   Phone: (509) 662-1511
Jane Belt, Med.Libn.
Subjects: Nursing, medicine, paramedical sciences, hospital administration and management. **Holdings:** 2000 books; 30 bound periodical volumes; 25 tapes. **Subscriptions:** 75 journals and other serials.

★10240★ ST. ELIZABETH MEDICAL CENTER
HEALTH SCIENCES LIBRARY
110 S. 9th Ave.
Yakima, WA 98902   Phone: (509) 575-5073
Marilyn Jardine, Med.Libn.
Subjects: Medicine, nursing, health sciences, hospital administration. **Holdings:** Figures not available. **Subscriptions:** 95 journals and other serials.

West Virginia

★10241★ APPALACHIAN REGIONAL HEALTHCARE
BECKLEY APPALACHIAN REGIONAL HOSPITAL
MEDICAL LIBRARY
306 Stanaford Rd.
Beckley, WV 25801   Phone: (304) 255-3420
Barbara Frame-Cook, Coord., Educ.
Subjects: Internal medicine, surgery, pediatrics, nursing, psychiatry and behavioral science, allied health sciences. **Holdings:** 1228 books; 425 bound periodical volumes. **Subscriptions:** 90 journals and other serials.

★10242★ U.S. DEPARTMENT OF VETERANS AFFAIRS
LIBRARY SERVICE
200 Veterans Ave.
Beckley, WV 25801   Phone: (304) 255-2121
Lois M. Watson, Chf., Lib.Serv.
Subjects: Medicine, nursing, surgery. **Holdings:** 1004 volumes; 973 journal

volumes; 2 VF drawers of patient education pamphlets; Audio-Digest tapes; microfilm. **Subscriptions:** 117 journals and other serials.

★10243★ WEST VIRGINIA LIBRARY COMMISSION
SERVICES FOR THE BLIND AND PHYSICALLY
     HANDICAPPED
Cultural Center
Charleston, WV 25305   Phone: (304) 348-4061
Shirley Smith, Act.Dept.Hd.
Subjects: General collection. **Holdings:** 15,563 large-print books; 80,022 nonbook materials. **Subscriptions:** 55 journals and other serials; 10 newspapers.

★10244★ WEST VIRGINIA STATE COMMISSION ON AGING
RESOURCE CENTER
State Capitol
Charleston, WV 25305   Phone: (304) 348-2917
Tom Dudley
Subjects: Gerontology. **Holdings:** 9063 books; 7 shelves of newsletters, reports, bulletins; 5 VF drawers of pamphlets; 5 VF drawers of clippings. **Subscriptions:** 25 journals and other serials.

★10245★ WEST VIRGINIA UNIVERSITY
HEALTH SCIENCES LIBRARY
3110 Maccorkle Ave., SE
Charleston, WV 25304   Phone: (304) 347-1285
Patricia Powell, Hd.Libn.
Subjects: Medicine, nursing. **Holdings:** 19,000 books; 15,000 bound periodical volumes; 1800 AV programs. **Subscriptions:** 525 journals and other serials.

★10246★ UNITED HOSPITAL CENTER INC.
INFORMATION CENTER
3 Hospital Plaza
Clarksburg, WV 26301   Phone: (304) 624-2230
Bruce Campbell, Med.Libn.
Subjects: Medicine, continuing education, health administration, health education. **Holdings:** 2600 books; 1400 bound periodical volumes; 260 microforms; 400 AV programs; 300 video cassettes; 500 audio cassettes. **Subscriptions:** 230 journals and other serials.

★10247★ U.S. DEPARTMENT OF VETERANS AFFAIRS
MEDICAL CENTER LIBRARY SERVICE
Clarksburg, WV 26301   Phone: (304) 623-3461
Wanda F. Kincaid, Chf.,Lib.Serv.
Subjects: Medicine. **Holdings:** 1415 books; 2330 bound periodical volumes. **Subscriptions:** 194 journals and other serials; 10 newspapers.

★10248★ CABELL HUNTINGTON HOSPITAL
HEALTH SCIENCE LIBRARY
1340 Hal Greer Blvd.
Huntington, WV 25701   Phone: (304) 526-2022
Deborah L. Woodburn, Hea.Sci.Libn.
Subjects: Medicine, surgery, neonatal care, pediatric intensive care, burns, kidney dialysis, allied health sciences. **Holdings:** 1466 books; 207 bound periodical volumes. **Subscriptions:** 102 journals and other serials.

★10249★ MARSHALL UNIVERSITY
JAMES E. MORROW LIBRARY
SPECIAL COLLECTIONS
Huntington, WV 25701   Phone: (304) 696-2343
Lisle G. Brown, Cur.
Subjects: West Virginiana, Civil War, Appalachian studies, history of medicine. **Holdings:** 18,000 books; 400 bound periodical volumes; 1300 linear feet of manuscripts; 25,000 West Virginia state documents; 600 cubic feet of university archives; 30 linear feet of miscellanea. **Subscriptions:** 130 journals and other serials; 10 newspapers.

★10250★ MARSHALL UNIVERSITY
SCHOOL OF MEDICINE
HEALTH SCIENCE LIBRARIES
Marshall University Campus
Huntington, WV 25701   Phone: (304) 696-6426
Edward Dzierzak, Dir.
Subjects: Clinical medicine, basic sciences, nursing, allied health sciences. **Holdings:** 19,670 books; 185 slide sets; 350 video cassettes; 45 audio cassettes. **Subscriptions:** 434 journals and other serials.

★10251★ ST. MARY'S HOSPITAL
MEDICAL LIBRARY
6-East
Huntington, WV 25702-1271   Phone: (304) 526-1314
Kay Gibson, Med.Libn.
Subjects: Medicine, surgery, allied health sciences. Holdings: 587 books;
1227 bound periodical volumes; 577 unbound periodicals; 90 pamphlets.
Subscriptions: 142 journals and other serials.

★10252★ U.S. DEPARTMENT OF VETERANS AFFAIRS
MEDICAL CENTER LIBRARY
1540 Spring Valley Dr.
Huntington, WV 25704   Phone: (304) 429-6741
Bruce Thornlow, Chf., Lib.Serv.
Subjects: Clinical medicine. Holdings: 1000 books; Audio-Digest tapes;
microfilm. Subscriptions: 189 journals and other serials.

★10253★ WEST VIRGINIA STATE BOARD OF
REHABILITATION
DIVISION OF REHABILITATION SERVICES
STAFF LIBRARY
Rehabilitation Center
Institute, WV 25112-1004   Phone: (304) 766-4644
Mrs. Jo Skiles, Staff Libn.
Subjects: Physical and vocational rehabilitation, behavioral sciences,
management, medicine. Holdings: 11,835 books; 5900 monographs, re-
ports, projects; 93 16mm films; 36 slides and cassettes; 471 videotapes.
Subscriptions: 56 journals and other serials.

★10254★ WEST VIRGINIA SCHOOL OF OSTEOPATHIC
MEDICINE
WVSOM LIBRARY
400 N. Lee St.
Lewisburg, WV 24901-0827   Phone: (304) 647-6261
Mary Frances Bodemuller, Dir., Educ.Rsrcs.
Subjects: Medicine. Holdings: 11,000 books; 3000 bound periodical
volumes; 4000 AV programs. Subscriptions: 470 journals and other serials;
5 newspapers.

★10255★ U.S. DEPARTMENT OF VETERANS AFFAIRS
CENTER MEDICAL LIBRARY
Martinsburg, WV 25401   Phone: (304) 263-0811
Barbara S. Adams, Chf.Libn.
Subjects: Medicine, surgery, allied health sciences. Holdings: 3000 books;
5435 bound periodical volumes; 996 AV programs; 53 titles on microfilm.
Subscriptions: 300 journals and other serials.

★10256★ WEST VIRGINIA UNIVERSITY
HEALTH SCIENCES LIBRARY
Health Sciences N.
Morgantown, WV 26506-6306   Phone: (304) 293-2113
Robert Murphy, Dir.
Subjects: Medicine, dentistry, pharmacy, nursing, hospital administration.
Holdings: 53,292 books; 140,192 bound periodical volumes; 879 disserta-
tions and theses; 6098 reels of microfilm containing 469 titles; 10,661
microfiche containing 550 titles; 3800 slides and films. Subscriptions: 2227
journals and other serials.

★10257★ WEST VIRGINIA UNIVERSITY
OFFICE OF HEALTH SERVICES RESEARCH
LIBRARY
Health Sciences South
Morgantown, WV 26506   Phone: (304) 293-2601
Stephanie Pratt, Res.Asst. III
Subjects: Census and vital statistics, hospital discharges, Medicaid and
Medicare, employment-related health insurance, small computer systems
development, adolescent pregnancy. Holdings: Books; reports; census
documents for West Virginia and contiguous states; tape files of vital
statistics for West Virginia.

★10258★ WEST VIRGINIA SCHOOLS FOR THE DEAF AND
BLIND
SCHOOL FOR THE BLIND LIBRARY
301 E. Main St.
Romney, WV 26757   Phone: (304) 822-3521
Leslie C. Durst, Coord., Lib.Serv.
Subjects: General collection. Holdings: 10,000 talking books; 220 magnetic

tapes; 2881 braille books; 3750 print books; 650 commercial sound
recordings. Subscriptions: 60 journals and other serials; 9 newspapers.

★10259★ THOMAS MEMORIAL HOSPITAL
MEDICAL/NURSING LIBRARY
4605 MacCorkle Ave., SW
South Charleston, WV 25309   Phone: (304) 766-3791
Drema A. Pierson, Dir., Ed. & Trng.
Subjects: Medicine, nursing. Holdings: 300 books; 80 bound periodical
volumes. Subscriptions: 80 journals and other serials.

★10260★ WEST VIRGINIA DEPARTMENT OF HEALTH
OFFICE OF LABORATORY SERVICES
LIBRARY
167 11th Ave.
South Charleston, WV 25303   Phone: (304) 348-3530
Jennifer J. Graley, Sec.
Subjects: Public health. Holdings: 500 books. Subscriptions: 12 journals
and other serials.

★10261★ STEVENS CLINIC HOSPITAL
LIBRARY
U.S. 52, E.
Welch, WV 24801   Phone: (304) 436-3161
Karen Peery, Libn.
Subjects: Medicine, surgery, allied health sciences. Holdings: 800 volumes.

★10262★ OHIO VALLEY MEDICAL CENTER
HUPP MEDICAL LIBRARY
2000 Eoff St.
Wheeling, WV 26003   Phone: (304) 234-8771
Janis Quinlisk, Med.Libn.
Subjects: Surgery, internal medicine, obstetrics, gynecology, radiology,
hospital administration, pediatrics. Holdings: 3382 books; 3737 bound
periodical volumes; 2231 unbound journals; 785 audio cassettes; 54 video
cassettes. Subscriptions: 233 journals and other serials.

★10263★ WHEELING HOSPITAL
HENRY G. JEPSON MEMORIAL LIBRARY
Medical Park
Wheeling, WV 26003   Phone: (304) 243-3308
Linda E. White
Subjects: Medicine, nursing, allied health sciences. Holdings: 2200 books;
118 bound periodical volumes; 612 cassettes; 5 VF drawers; pamphlet file.
Subscriptions: 113 journals and other serials.

Wisconsin

★10264★ ST. ELIZABETH HOSPITAL
HEALTH SCIENCE LIBRARY
1506 S. Oneida St.
Appleton, WI 54915   Phone: (414) 738-2324
Mary M. Bayorgeon, Dir., Lib.Serv.
Subjects: Medicine, nursing, hospital administration. Holdings: 3256
books; 3666 bound periodical volumes; 1536 audiotapes; 602 videotapes.
Subscriptions: 325 journals and other serials.

★10265★ ELMBROOK MEMORIAL HOSPITAL
MARY BETH CURTIS HEALTH SCIENCE LIBRARY
19333 W. North Ave.
Brookfield, WI 53005   Phone: (414) 785-2091
Mary Rheineck, Med.Libn.
Subjects: Medicine, nursing, hospital administration. Holdings: 1600
books; 35 boxes of pamphlets; 4 VF drawers; 200 reels of microfilm of
periodicals. Subscriptions: 130 journals and other serials.

★10266★ TRINITY MEMORIAL HOSPITAL
LIBRARY
5900 S. Lake Dr.
Cudahy, WI 53110   Phone: (414) 769-4028
Carl W. Baehr, Libn.
Subjects: Medicine, nursing. Holdings: 1050 books; 2100 bound periodical
volumes; 8 VF drawers of pamphlets; 4 VF drawers of news clippings.
Subscriptions: 140 journals and other serials.

★10267★ WISCONSIN SCHOOL FOR THE DEAF
EVELYN AND JOHN R. GANT LIBRARY
309 W. Walworth Ave.
Delavan, WI 53115   Phone: (414) 728-6477
Betty E. Watkins, Libn.
Subjects: Books of high interest-low vocabulary, professional library, K-12 general collection. **Holdings:** 6000 books; 1700 filmstrips; 150 film loops; 500 microfiche; 16 drawers of transparencies. **Subscriptions:** 89 journals and other serials.

★10268★ LUTHER HOSPITAL
LIBRARY SERVICES
1221 Whipple St.
Eau Claire, WI 54701   Phone: (715) 839-3248
Virginia L. Wright, Mgr., Lib.Serv.
Subjects: Nursing and clinical medicine, hospital administration. **Holdings:** 3000 books; 5000 bound periodical volumes; 6 VF drawers of pamphlets; 850 AV programs. **Subscriptions:** 200 journals and other serials.

★10269★ SACRED HEART HOSPITAL
MEDICAL LIBRARY
900 W. Clairemont Ave.
Eau Claire, WI 54701   Phone: (715) 839-4330
Bruno Warner, Libn.
Subjects: Medicine, nursing, dentistry, hospital administration, patient teaching. **Holdings:** 5000 books; 1000 bound periodical volumes; 2000 unbound periodicals; 4 VF drawers of pamphlets. **Subscriptions:** 286 journals and other serials.

★10270★ LAKELAND HOSPITAL
MEDICAL LIBRARY
Hwy. NN
Box 1002
Elkhorn, WI 53121   Phone: (414) 723-2960
Ann Sheehy, Libn.
Subjects: Medicine, nursing. **Holdings:** 554 books. **Subscriptions:** 70 journals and other serials.

★10271★ MORAINE PARK TECHNICAL COLLEGE
LEARNING RESOURCE CENTER
235 N. National Ave.
PO Box 1940
Fond du Lac, WI 54936-1940   Phone: (414) 929-2470
Judy Denor, LRC Mgr.
Subjects: Health occupations; business and marketing; trade, police, fire sciences; home economics; agribiotechnology. **Holdings:** 24,000 books; 650 bound periodical volumes; 2000 pamphlets; 600 microforms; 6000 AV program titles. **Subscriptions:** 500 journals and other serials; 25 newspapers.

★10272★ ST. AGNES HOSPITAL
HEALTH SCIENCES LIBRARY
430 E. Division St.
Fond du Lac, WI 54935-4597   Phone: (414) 929-1559
Sr. Sharon McEnery, C.S.A., Libn.
Subjects: Medicine, nursing, allied health, hospital management. **Holdings:** 961 books; 3835 bound periodical volumes. **Subscriptions:** 101 journals and other serials.

★10273★ BELLIN MEMORIAL HOSPITAL
HEALTH SCIENCES LIBRARY
744 S. Webster Ave.
Box 1700
Green Bay, WI 54305   Phone: (414) 433-3693
Cynthia M. Reinl, Hea.Sci.Libn.
Subjects: Nursing, medicine. **Holdings:** 2700 books; 1055 bound periodical volumes; 500 video cassettes; 400 filmstrip programs; 20 motion pictures; 6 VF drawers of pamphlets and clippings. **Subscriptions:** 210 journals and other serials.

★10274★ BROWN COUNTY MENTAL HEALTH CENTER
H.H. HUMPHREY MEMORIAL STAFF LIBRARY
2900 S. Anthony Dr.
Green Bay, WI 54311   Phone: (414) 468-1136
Cindy M. Ducat, Lib.Mgr.
Subjects: Psychiatry, psychology, social work, nursing, growth and development, geriatrics, mental retardation, developmental disability, alcohol and drug abuse. **Holdings:** 2000 books; 100 bound periodical volumes; 100 AV programs. **Subscriptions:** 45 journals and other serials.

★10275★ NORTHEAST WISCONSIN TECHNICAL COLLEGE
LEARNING RESOURCE CENTER
2740 W. Mason
Box 19042
Green Bay, WI 54307-9042   Phone: (414) 498-5490
Mary Parrott, Libn.
Subjects: Health occupations, trade and industry, business and marketing, education, police science, agriculture, home economics, fire science. **Holdings:** 21,650 books; 4700 AV programs; 5200 reels of microfilm; 170 microfiche; 2160 video cassettes. **Subscriptions:** 630 journals and other serials; 50 newspapers.

★10276★ ST. VINCENT HOSPITAL
HEALTH SCIENCE LIBRARY
835 S. VanBuren St.
Box 13508
Green Bay, WI 54305   Phone: (414) 433-8171
Subjects: Medicine, allied health sciences. **Holdings:** 3100 books; 525 bound periodical volumes. **Subscriptions:** 140 journals and other serials.

★10277★ MERCY HOSPITAL
MEDICAL LIBRARY
1000 Mineral Point
Janesville, WI 53545   Phone: (608) 756-6749
Doris Brewster, Libn.
Subjects: Medicine. **Holdings:** 702 books. **Subscriptions:** 61 journals and other serials.

★10278★ ROCK COUNTY HEALTH CARE CENTER
STAFF LIBRARY
Box 351
Janesville, WI 53547   Phone: (608) 755-2590
Louise Keating, Inserv.Dir.
Subjects: Psychiatry, psychiatric social work, geriatrics, nursing. **Holdings:** 1052 books; 29 bound periodical volumes; AV programs. **Subscriptions:** 63 journals and other serials.

★10279★ WISCONSIN DEPARTMENT OF PUBLIC INSTRUCTION
SCHOOL FOR THE VISUALLY HANDICAPPED
LIBRARY
1700 W. State St.
Janesville, WI 53545   Phone: (608) 755-2967
Jean Wolski, Libn.
Subjects: General collection. **Holdings:** 3000 print books; 280 tactile items; 3000 braille books; 5000 talking books; 3000 cassette books. **Subscriptions:** 60 journals and other serials.

★10280★ COUNTRYSIDE HOME
STAFF LIBRARY
1425 Wisconsin Dr.
Jefferson, WI 53549   Phone: (414) 674-3170
Catherine M. Rueth, Sec./Libn.
Subjects: Medicine, nursing, and allied health sciences. **Holdings:** 1011 books. **Subscriptions:** 28 journals and other serials.

★10281★ KENOSHA HOSPITAL AND MEDICAL CENTER
HEALTH SCIENCES LIBRARY
6308 8th Ave.
Kenosha, WI 53143   Phone: (414) 656-2120
Sue Freedman, Hea.Sci.Libn.
Subjects: Medicine, nursing. **Holdings:** 2000 books; 100 audio cassettes; 200 video cassettes. **Subscriptions:** 135 journals and other serials.

★10282★ ST. CATHERINE'S HOSPITAL
MEDICAL LIBRARY
3556 7th Ave.
Kenosha, WI 53140   Phone: (414) 656-3230
Rick Henning, Med.Libn.
Subjects: Medicine, family practice. **Holdings:** 1500 volumes; 300 video cassettes. **Subscriptions:** 120 journals and other serials.

★10283★ GUNDERSEN/LUTHERAN MEDICAL CENTER
HEALTH SCIENCES LIBRARY
1910 South Ave.
La Crosse, WI 54601   Phone: (608) 785-0530
Kathleen Cimpl Wagner, Dir.
Subjects: Medicine, nursing, allied health sciences, administration, pastoral care. **Holdings:** 7000 books; 14,000 bound periodical volumes; 250 software programs. **Subscriptions:** 650 journals and other serials.

★10284★ ST. FRANCIS MEDICAL CENTER
HEALTH SCIENCES LIBRARY
615 S. 10th St.
La Crosse, WI 54601   Phone: (608) 785-0940
Sr. Louise Therese Lotze, Lib.Supv.
Subjects: Medicine, dentistry, nursing, allied health sciences. **Holdings:** 3500 books; 5400 bound periodical volumes; 12 VF drawers of clippings and articles. **Subscriptions:** 300 journals and other serials.

★10285★ CENTRAL WISCONSIN CENTER FOR
DEVELOPMENTALLY DISABLED
LIBRARY INFORMATION CENTER
317 Knutson Dr.
Madison, WI 53704   Phone: (608) 249-2151
Geraldine Matthews, Libn.
Subjects: Developmental disabilities. **Holdings:** 12,000 books; 4000 bound periodical volumes; reports; manuscripts; archives; microfiche; microfilm. **Subscriptions:** 50 journals and other serials.

★10286★ MADISON PHARMACY ASSOCIATES
PMS ACCESS
LIBRARY
P.O. Box 9326
Madison, WI 53715   Phone: (608) 833-4PMS
Marla Ahlgrimm
Subjects: Premenstrual syndrome. **Holdings:** Current literature; audio cassettes; slide programs.

★10287★ MENDOTA MENTAL HEALTH INSTITUTE
LIBRARY MEDIA SERVICES
301 Troy Dr.
Madison, WI 53704   Phone: (608) 244-2411
Subjects: Clinical psychology and psychiatry; psychiatric nursing and social work; mental health - administration, training, research, prevention, consultation; psychiatry for the deaf; forensic psychiatry. **Holdings:** 22,416 books; 1945 bound periodical volumes; 12 VF drawers of specialized reprints and reports; 340 film and videotape titles; AV catalogs; 107 newsletters. **Subscriptions:** 162 journals and other serials.

★10288★ MERITER HOSPITAL LIBRARIES
309 W. Washington Ave.
Madison, WI 53703   Phone: (608) 251-2371
Robert Koehler, Libn.
Subjects: Medicine, nursing, health management. **Holdings:** 2000 books; 1400 bound periodical volumes. **Subscriptions:** 300 journals and other serials.

★10289★ MERITER HOSPITAL-PARK
MEDICAL LIBRARY
202 S. Park St.
Madison, WI 53715   Phone: (608) 267-6234
Robert Koehler, Med.Libn.
Subjects: Medicine, nursing, dentistry, health administration. **Holdings:** 3500 books; 2500 bound periodical volumes; 1000 other cataloged items. **Subscriptions:** 282 journals and other serials.

★10290★ PREVENTION AND INTERVENTION CENTER OF
ALCOHOL AND OTHER DRUG ABUSE
LIBRARY
2000 Fordham Ave.
Madison, WI 53704   Phone: (608) 246-7606
Martha Nicholson, Libn.
Remarks: No further information was supplied by the respondent.

★10291★ U.S. DEPARTMENT OF VETERANS AFFAIRS
WILLIAM S. MIDDLETON MEMORIAL VETERANS HOSPITAL
LIBRARY
2500 Overlook Terr.
Madison, WI 53705   Phone: (608) 256-1901
Phyllis E. Goetz, Chf., Lib.Serv.
Subjects: General medicine. **Holdings:** 6303 books; 15,700 bound periodical volumes; 2566 journal volumes on microfilm. **Subscriptions:** 268 journals and other serials.

★10292★ UNIVERSITY OF WISCONSIN, MADISON
CENTER FOR HEALTH SCIENCES LIBRARIES
1305 Linden Dr.
Madison, WI 53706   Phone: (608) 262-6594
Virginia Holtz, Dir.
Subjects: Health sciences and health care administration. **Holdings:** 119,000 books; 121,200 bound periodical volumes; 5000 AV programs; 3660 pamphlets and government documents. **Subscriptions:** 4000 journals and other serials.

★10293★ UNIVERSITY OF WISCONSIN, MADISON
CLINICAL RESEARCH LABORATORIES
THORNGATE LIBRARY
Clinical Science Center, Rm. B4/257
600 Highland Ave.
Madison, WI 53792   Phone: (608) 263-7507
Russell Tomar, Div.Dir.
Subjects: Clinical laboratories - instrument design and applications, test development and applications, quality control techniques, computer system design, clinical evaluation of cancer markers. **Holdings:** 450 books. **Subscriptions:** 80 journals and other serials.

★10294★ UNIVERSITY OF WISCONSIN, MADISON
CRIMINAL JUSTICE REFERENCE AND INFORMATION
CENTER
L140 Law Library
Madison, WI 53706   Phone: (608) 262-1499
Sue L. Center, Asst.Dir.
Subjects: Criminal justice system, police science, corrections, drug abuse, delinquency, alcoholism. **Holdings:** 29,000 volumes. **Subscriptions:** 200 journals and other serials.

★10295★ UNIVERSITY OF WISCONSIN, MADISON
DEPARTMENT OF PSYCHIATRY
LITHIUM INFORMATION CENTER
600 Highland Ave.
Madison, WI 53792   Phone: (608) 263-6171
Margaret G. Baudhuin, Libn./Info.Spec.
Subjects: Medical uses of lithium. **Holdings:** 20,000 articles, books, abstracts, miscellaneous items stored online.

★10296★ UNIVERSITY OF WISCONSIN, MADISON
F.B. POWER PHARMACEUTICAL LIBRARY
School of Pharmacy
425 N. Charter St.
Madison, WI 53706   Phone: (608) 262-2894
Dolores Nemec, Libn.
Subjects: Pharmacy and related subjects. **Holdings:** 13,266 books; 19,092 bound periodical volumes. **Subscriptions:** 404 journals; 311 serials.

★10297★ UNIVERSITY OF WISCONSIN, MADISON
MCARDLE LABORATORY FOR CANCER RESEARCH
LIBRARY
Madison, WI 53706   Phone: (608) 262-2177
Ilse L. Riegel
Subjects: Cancer, molecular biology, virology. **Holdings:** 500 books; 2000 bound periodical volumes. **Subscriptions:** 100 journals and other serials.

★10298★ UNIVERSITY OF WISCONSIN, MADISON
MEDICAL PHYSICS DEPARTMENT
LIBRARY
1530 Medical Sciences Center
1300 University Ave.
Madison, WI 53706   Phone: (608) 262-0878
Perry Pickhardt, Libn.
Subjects: Medical physics, biomedical engineering, physics, radiology. **Holdings:** 2500 books; 835 bound periodical volumes; 123 audio cassettes. **Subscriptions:** 60 journals and other serials.

★10299★ UNIVERSITY OF WISCONSIN, MADISON
STUDY IN HEALTH CARE FISCAL MANAGEMENT
  ORGANIZATION AND CONTROL
LIBRARY
1155 Observatory Dr., Rm. 301
Madison, WI 53706   Phone: (608) 262-1943
Prof. Roger Formisano, Dir.
Subjects: Health care fiscal management, financial management, accounting and internal auditing, sources of funding, reimbursement and related subjects, information systems. **Holdings:** 825 books; 17 bound periodical volumes. **Subscriptions:** 14 journals and other serials.

★10300★ UNIVERSITY OF WISCONSIN, MADISON
TRACE R & D CENTER
INFORMATION AREA
S157 Waisman Center
1500 Highland Ave.
Madison, WI 53705-2280   Phone: (608) 262-6966
Peter Borden, Proj.Dir.
Subjects: Nonvocal communication, computer access for the disabled, rehabilitation engineering, software/hardware for the disabled. **Holdings:** 12 linear feet and 2 filing cabinets of research materials; directories; newsletters; conference proceedings. **Subscriptions:** 10 journals and other serials.

★10301★ UNIVERSITY OF WISCONSIN, MADISON
WISCONSIN REGIONAL PRIMATE RESEARCH CENTER
PRIMATE CENTER LIBRARY
1223 Capitol Ct.
Madison, WI 53715-1299   Phone: (608) 263-3512
Lawrence Jacobsen, Hd.Libn.
Subjects: Primatology, neurosciences, reproductive physiology, ethology/ecology, conservation, ethics. **Holdings:** 5000 books; 10,000 bound periodical volumes; 500 unbound volumes; 12,000 topical reprints and bibliographies; 4000 AV programs; 100 masters' and Ph.D. theses. **Subscriptions:** 370 journals and other serials.

★10302★ WISCONSIN DEPARTMENT OF HEALTH AND
  SOCIAL SERVICES
LIBRARY
1 W. Wilson St., Rm. 630
Madison, WI 53702   Phone: (608) 266-7473
Elisabeth R. Boehnen, Libn.
Subjects: Public health and welfare, corrections, community services, mental health, vocational rehabilitation. **Holdings:** 10,000 books; 460 periodical titles; 75 pamphlet boxes. **Subscriptions:** 400 journals and other serials.

★10303★ WISCONSIN HOSPITAL ASSOCIATION
MEMORIAL LIBRARY
5721 Odana Rd.
Madison, WI 53719   Phone: (608) 274-1820
Ann C. Boyer, Libn.
Subjects: Health care, hospital administration, health careers, health insurance, hospital law and regulation. **Holdings:** 2100 books. **Subscriptions:** 90 journals and other serials.

★10304★ WISCONSIN STATE MEDICAL SOCIETY
LIBRARY
330 E. Lakeside St.
Box 1109
Madison, WI 53701   Phone: (608) 257-6781
Russell King, Pubns.Mgr.
Subjects: Medicine. **Holdings:** 125 volumes. **Subscriptions:** 158 journals and other serials.

★10305★ HOLY FAMILY MEDICAL CENTER
HEALTH SCIENCES LIBRARY
2300 Western Ave.
PO Box 1450
Manitowoc, WI 54221-1450   Phone: (414) 684-2260
Dan Eckert, Libn.
Subjects: Medicine and nursing. **Holdings:** 1500 books. **Subscriptions:** 128 journals and other serials.

★10306★ MARSHFIELD CLINIC
MEDICAL LIBRARY
1000 N. Oak
Marshfield, WI 54449   Phone: (715) 387-9183
Albert Zimmermann, Libn.
Subjects: Medicine, allied health sciences. **Holdings:** 2639 books; 15,177 bound periodical volumes. **Subscriptions:** 450 journals and other serials.

★10307★ ST. JOSEPH'S HOSPITAL
LEARNING RESOURCE CENTER
611 St. Joseph Ave.
Marshfield, WI 54449   Phone: (715) 387-7374
Ruth Wachter-Nelson, Libn.
Subjects: Nursing. **Holdings:** 7800 books; 881 bound periodical volumes; 10 VF drawers of pamphlets; school archives; 1054 AV programs. **Subscriptions:** 135 journals and other serials.

★10308★ COMMUNITY MEMORIAL HOSPITAL
MCKAY MEMORIAL LIBRARY
W180 N8085 Town Hall Rd.
Box 408
Menomonee Falls, WI 53051-0408   Phone: (414) 251-1000
B.J. Keppel, Med.Libn.
Subjects: Medicine, nursing, health care. **Holdings:** 375 books; 50 bound periodical volumes; 1859 slides; 156 microfiche; 217 video cassettes; 10 audio cassettes. **Subscriptions:** 225 journals and other serials.

★10309★ MEDICAL ASSOCIATES
HEALTH CENTER
LIBRARY
W180 N7950 Town Hall Rd.
Menomonee Falls, WI 53051   Phone: (414) 255-2500
Joyce Madsen, Libn.
Subjects: Medicine. **Holdings:** 350 books; 1000 bound periodical volumes; 5 VF drawers of pamphlets; 600 cassette tapes. **Subscriptions:** 98 journals and other serials.

★10310★ CHILDREN'S HOSPITAL OF WISCONSIN
HEALTH SCIENCES LIBRARY
9000 W. Wisconsin
Milwaukee, WI 53201   Phone: (414) 266-2000
Molly Youngkin, Br.Libn.
Subjects: Pediatrics, nursing, medicine. **Holdings:** 1300 books; 2300 bound periodical volumes. **Subscriptions:** 190 journals and other serials.

★10311★ COLUMBIA HOSPITAL
COLLEGE OF NURSING
LIBRARY
2121 E. Newport Ave.
Milwaukee, WI 53211   Phone: (414) 961-3533
Shirley S. Chan, Libn.
Subjects: Nurses and nursing, nursing education, pharmacology, community health, psychology, sociology, nutrition. **Holdings:** 4500 books; 511 bound periodical volumes; pamphlets on 129 subjects; 65 slide/tape sets; 65 filmstrip/record sets; 90 filmstrip/cassette sets; 60 audio cassettes; 388 slides; 15 faculty theses; 4 VF drawers of pamphlets; 3 VF drawers of book/AV catalogs; 139 transparencies; 11 videotapes; 19 anatomical models; 2 charts; 1 skeleton. **Subscriptions:** 100 journals and other serials.

★10312★ COLUMBIA HOSPITAL
MEDICAL LIBRARY
2025 E. Newport Ave.
Milwaukee, WI 53211   Phone: (414) 961-3858
Ruth Holst, Dir., Lib.Serv.
Subjects: Medicine, nursing, hospital administration, consumer health. **Holdings:** 2000 books; 8000 bound periodical volumes; 450 audio cassettes. **Subscriptions:** 300 journals and other serials.

★10313★ COMMUNITY RELATIONS-SOCIAL DEVELOPMENT
  COMMISSION
RESEARCH LIBRARY
231 W. Wisconsin Ave.
Milwaukee, WI 53203   Phone: (414) 272-5600
Signe Waller, Res.Spec.
Subjects: Poverty/social welfare, aging, employment and training, health, criminal justice, education. **Holdings:** 1000 books; 50 bound periodical volumes; 20 VF drawers; census and statistics collection; agency archives. **Subscriptions:** 40 journals and other serials; 6 newspapers.

★10314★ FIRST CALL FOR HELP, MILWAUKEE
231 W. Wisconsin Ave.
Milwaukee, WI 53203   Phone: (414) 272-5600
Subjects: Human services, especially health, social work, and older adults.
Holdings: Files on 1500 Milwaukee area human service agencies.

★10315★ MARQUETTE UNIVERSITY
SCIENCE LIBRARY
560 N. 16th St.
Milwaukee, WI 53233   Phone: (414) 288-3396
Jay Kirk, Hd., Sci.Lib.
Subjects: Human biology, dentistry, nursing, engineering, chemistry, mathematics, physics. **Holdings:** 75,000 books; 90,000 bound periodical volumes. **Subscriptions:** 2000 journals and other serials.

★10316★ MEDICAL COLLEGE OF WISCONSIN
LIBRARIES
8701 Watertown Plank Rd.
Milwaukee, WI 53226   Phone: (414) 257-8323
Patrick W. Brennen, Dir. of Libs.
Subjects: Medicine, allied health sciences. **Holdings:** 79,000 books; 130,000 bound periodical volumes; 1310 AV programs. **Subscriptions:** 2755 journals and other serials.

★10317★ MILWAUKEE ACADEMY OF MEDICINE
LIBRARY
8701 Watertown Plank Rd.
Box 26509
Milwaukee, WI 53226   Phone: (414) 257-8249
Warren Smirl, M.D., Libn.
Subjects: Medical history. **Holdings:** 1532 books.

★10318★ MILWAUKEE COUNTY MENTAL HEALTH
COMPLEX
MICHAEL KASAK LIBRARY
9455 Watertown Plank Rd.
Milwaukee, WI 53226   Phone: (414) 257-7381
Anna M. Green, Libn.
Subjects: Psychology, mental health, psychiatry, psychoanalysis. **Holdings:** 6650 books; 5600 bound periodical volumes; 250 video cassettes; 500 audio cassettes. **Subscriptions:** 303 journals and other serials.

★10319★ NATIONAL FUNERAL DIRECTORS ASSOCIATION
LEARNING RESOURCE CENTER
11121 W. Oklahoma Ave.
Milwaukee, WI 53227   Phone: (414) 541-2500
Debra Pass, Dir. of Educ.
Subjects: Dying and death, grief and mourning, funeral customs, embalming, business practices. **Holdings:** 500 books; films.

★10320★ NORTHWEST GENERAL HOSPITAL
MEDICAL LIBRARY
5310 W. Capitol Dr.
Milwaukee, WI 53216   Phone: (414) 447-8600
Coralyn Marks, Lib.Dir.
Subjects: Medicine, nursing. **Holdings:** 925 books; 300 bound periodical volumes. **Subscriptions:** 187 journals and other serials.

★10321★ NORTHWESTERN MUTUAL LIFE INSURANCE
COMPANY
CORPORATE INFORMATION CENTER/MEDICAL LIBRARY
720 E. Wisconsin Ave.
Milwaukee, WI 53202   Phone: (414) 271-1444
Carolyn Barloga, Spec.
Subjects: Medicine, medical insurance underwriting. **Holdings:** 300 books. **Subscriptions:** 40 journals and other serials.

★10322★ PLANNED PARENTHOOD OF WISCONSIN
MAURICE RITZ RESOURCE LIBRARY AND BOOKSTORE
302 N. Jackson St.
Milwaukee, WI 53202   Phone: (414) 271-7930
Ann H. McIntyre, Libn.
Subjects: Family planning, reproductive health, sexuality education, contraception, obstetrics/gynecology nursing education, population. **Holdings:** 3000 books; 12 VF drawers of clippings and reports; 100 pamphlets, booklets, reprints; 80 films, slides, tapes, filmstrip kits, videotapes. **Subscriptions:** 55 journals and other serials.

★10323★ SACRED HEART REHABILITATION HOSPITAL
STAFF LIBRARY
1545 S. Layton Blvd.
Milwaukee, WI 53215   Phone: (414) 383-4490
Patti Malmberg, Libn.
Remarks: No further information was supplied by the respondent.

★10324★ ST. FRANCIS HOSPITAL
LIBRARY/AV CENTER
3237 S. 16th St.
Milwaukee, WI 53215   Phone: (414) 647-5156
Joy Shong, Dir.
Subjects: Medicine, nursing, paramedicine. **Holdings:** 2000 books; 3200 bound periodical volumes; 1000 AV programs. **Subscriptions:** 245 journals and other serials.

★10325★ ST. JOSEPH'S HOSPITAL
SAMUEL ROSENTHAL MEMORIAL LIBRARY
5000 W. Chambers St.
Milwaukee, WI 53210   Phone: (414) 447-2194
Sunja Shaikh, Lib.Coord.
Subjects: Medicine, nursing, and allied health sciences, management. **Holdings:** 3000 books; 8000 bound periodical volumes; 150 Audio-Digest tapes. **Subscriptions:** 270 journals and other serials.

★10326★ ST. LUKE'S MEDICAL CENTER
MEDICAL LIBRARY
2900 W. Oklahoma Ave.
Milwaukee, WI 53215   Phone: (414) 649-7357
Midge Wos, Mgr.
Subjects: Medicine, nursing, paramedicine. **Holdings:** 23,621 books; 8259 bound periodical volumes; 100 filmstrips, records, transparencies, slides, film reels; 1080 cassettes; 2000 video cassettes; 1176 volumes on microfilm. **Subscriptions:** 1105 journals and other serials; 15 newspapers.

★10327★ ST. MARY'S HOSPITAL
HEALTH SCIENCES LIBRARY
2323 N. Lake Dr.
Box 503
Milwaukee, WI 53201   Phone: (414) 289-7000
Sharon A. Wochos, Libn.
Subjects: Nursing, medicine, management. **Holdings:** 2500 books; 3500 bound periodical volumes. **Subscriptions:** 260 journals and other serials.

★10328★ ST. MICHAEL HOSPITAL
REGNER HEALTH SCIENCES LIBRARY
2400 W. Villard Ave.
Milwaukee, WI 53209   Phone: (414) 527-8477
Vicki Schluge, Med.Libn.
Subjects: Medicine, nursing, allied health sciences, management. **Holdings:** 1700 books; 80 video cassettes. **Subscriptions:** 225 journals and other serials.

★10329★ SINAI SAMARITAN MEDICAL CENTER
HURWITZ MEMORIAL LIBRARY
Box 342
Milwaukee, WI 53201   Phone: (414) 289-8318
Janice A. Curnes, Dir.
Subjects: Clinical medicine, surgery, obstetrics and gynecology. **Holdings:** 1500 books; 5400 periodical volumes. **Subscriptions:** 385 journals and other serials.

★10330★ SINAI SAMARITAN MEDICAL CENTER
JAMRON HEALTH SCIENCE LIBRARY
2000 W. Kilbourn Ave.
Milwaukee, WI 53233   Phone: (414) 937-5412
Ann Towell, Libn.
Subjects: Medicine, nursing, hospital administration. **Holdings:** 900 volumes; 4 VF drawers of professional pamphlets. **Subscriptions:** 350 periodical titles.

★10331★ U.S. DEPARTMENT OF VETERANS AFFAIRS
MEDICAL CENTER LIBRARY
5000 W. National Ave.
Milwaukee, WI 53295   Phone: (414) 384-2000
Maureen L. Farmer, Chf., Lib.Serv.
Subjects: Medicine, nursing, dentistry, allied health sciences. **Holdings:**

5500 books; 5000 bound periodical volumes; 2000 AV programs. **Subscriptions:** 525 journals and other serials.

★10332★   ST. CLARE HOSPITAL
MEDICAL LIBRARY
515 22nd Ave.
Monroe, WI 53566   Phone: (608) 328-0244
Carol Hasse, Libn.
Subjects: Health science. **Holdings:** 700 books. **Subscriptions:** 150 journals and other serials.

★10333★   THEDA CLARK REGIONAL MEDICAL CENTER
HEALTH SCIENCES LIBRARY
130 2nd St.
Neenah, WI 54956   Phone: (414) 729-2190
Mary Horan, Libn.
Subjects: Medicine. **Holdings:** 1200 books; 1500 bound periodical volumes. **Subscriptions:** 350 journals and other serials.

★10334★   MEMORIAL HOSPITAL AT OCONOMOWOC
HEALTH SCIENCES LIBRARY
791 E. Summit Ave.
Oconomowoc, WI 53066   Phone: (414) 569-9400
Donna M. Dunham, Hea.Sci.Libn.
Subjects: Medicine, nursing, dentistry. **Holdings:** 1300 books and AV programs; 1268 bound periodical volumes; 6 VF drawers; 5 VF drawers of patient education pamphlets; 59 audiotapes; 150 videotapes; teaching materials. **Subscriptions:** 200 journals and other serials.

★10335★   OSSEO AREA MUNICIPAL HOSPITAL AND
** NURSING HOME**
MEDICAL LIBRARY
PO Box 70
Osseo, WI 54758   Phone: (715) 597-3121
Mary Gunderson, Libn.
Remarks: No further information was supplied by the respondent.

★10336★   WAUKESHA COUNTY TECHNICAL COLLEGE
WCTC LIBRARY
800 Main St.
Pewaukee, WI 53072   Phone: (414) 691-5316
Ruth Ahl, Lib.Dir.
Subjects: Nursing, allied health sciences, industrial technology, business, police and fire sciences, electronics, food service, automotive technology, accounting, data processing, financial planning, hospitality management, marketing, retailing, real estate, child care, international trade, interior design. **Holdings:** 33,893 books; 29,100 unbound periodicals; 918 reels of microfilm; 56 films; 355 videotapes; 789 audio cassettes; SAMS Photofact Service. **Subscriptions:** 459 periodicals; 13 newspapers.

★10337★   ST. MARY'S MEDICAL CENTER
LIBRARY
3801 Spring St.
Racine, WI 53405   Phone: (414) 636-4300
Subjects: Medicine, nursing, and allied health sciences. **Holdings:** 500 books. **Subscriptions:** 75 journals and other serials.

★10338★   ST. NICHOLAS HOSPITAL
HEALTH SCIENCES LIBRARY
1601 N. Taylor Dr.
Sheboygan, WI 53081   Phone: (414) 459-4713
Kathleen Blaser, Coord., Lib.Serv.
Subjects: Medicine, nursing, management, philosophy. **Holdings:** 850 books. **Subscriptions:** 125 journals and other serials.

★10339★   ST. MICHAEL'S HOSPITAL
HEALTH SCIENCES LIBRARY
900 Illinois Ave.
Stevens Point, WI 54481   Phone: (715) 346-5091
Jan Kraus, Libn.
Subjects: Medicine, nursing. **Holdings:** 900 books. **Subscriptions:** 95 journals and other serials.

★10340★   WISCONSIN INDIANHEAD TECHNICAL COLLEGE,
** SUPERIOR CAMPUS**
LIBRARY
600 N. 21st St.
Superior, WI 54880   Phone: (715) 394-6677
Donald Rantala, LRC Spec.
Subjects: Nursing, electronics, business, data processing, marketing and advertising. **Holdings:** 10,000 books; 1500 pamphlets; 50 maps; theses; microfilm; slides; cassettes. **Subscriptions:** 170 journals and other serials; 25 newspapers.

★10341★   U.S. DEPARTMENT OF VETERANS AFFAIRS
MEDICAL CENTER LIBRARY
Tomah, WI 54660   Phone: (608) 372-1716
Xena C. Kenyon, Chf., Lib.Serv.
Subjects: Psychiatry, neurology, general medicine, psychology, nursing, aging. **Holdings:** 2536 books; 117 bound periodical volumes; 2103 volumes of unbound journals; 515 AV programs. **Subscriptions:** 204 journals and other serials.

★10342★   SOUTHERN WISCONSIN CENTER FOR THE
** DEVELOPMENTALLY DISABLED**
MEDICAL STAFF LIBRARY
21425 Spring St.
Union Grove, WI 53182-9708   Phone: (414) 878-2411
Subjects: Medicine, mental retardation, medical specialties, current therapy, syndromes, malformations. **Holdings:** 124 books; 260 Audio-Digest tapes; statistical reports. **Subscriptions:** 15 journals and other serials.

★10343★   SOUTHERN WISCONSIN CENTER FOR THE
** DEVELOPMENTALLY DISABLED**
NURSING EDUCATION LIBRARY
21425 Spring St.
Union Grove, WI 53182-9708   Phone: (414) 878-2411
Subjects: Nursing, pharmacology, nutrition, mental retardation. **Holdings:** Books; AV programs. **Subscriptions:** 27 journals and other serials.

★10344★   BETHESDA LUTHERAN HOME
NATIONAL CHRISTIAN RESOURCE CENTER
700 Hoffmann Dr.
Watertown, WI 53094   Phone: (414) 261-3050
Linda A. Sires, Dir.
Subjects: Mental retardation, religious special education. **Holdings:** 3000 books. **Subscriptions:** 53 journals and other serials.

★10345★   WAUKESHA MEMORIAL HOSPITAL
MEDICAL LIBRARY
725 American Ave.
Waukesha, WI 53186   Phone: (414) 544-2150
Linda Oddan, Med.Libn.
Subjects: Medicine, nursing, hospital administration. **Holdings:** 2100 books; 2500 bound periodical volumes; 9 VF drawers of pamphlets. **Subscriptions:** 200 journals and other serials.

★10346★   RIVERSIDE MEDICAL CENTER
HEALTH SCIENCE LIBRARY
800 Riverside Dr.
Waupaca, WI 54981   Phone: (715) 258-1065
Andrea Crane, Libn.
Subjects: Medicine, nursing, health care administration, pathology. **Holdings:** 630 books. **Subscriptions:** 90 journals and other serials.

★10347★   CURATIVE REHABILITATION CENTER
LEARNING RESOURCE CENTER
1000 N. 92nd St.
Wauwatosa, WI 53226   Phone: (414) 259-1414
Terry Bochte, Libn.
Subjects: Physical medicine and rehabilitation, psychology, pediatrics, brain injury rehabilitation, orthopedics. **Holdings:** 1200 books; 800 bound periodical volumes. **Subscriptions:** 80 journals and other serials.

★10348★   WEST ALLIS MEMORIAL HOSPITAL
MEDICAL LIBRARY
8901 W. Lincoln Ave.
West Allis, WI 53227   Phone: (414) 546-6162
Joan A. Clausz, Med.Libn.
Subjects: Medicine. **Holdings:** 500 books; 900 bound periodical volumes. **Subscriptions:** 100 journals and other serials.

★10349★ WINNEBAGO MENTAL HEALTH INSTITUTE
MEDICAL LIBRARY
Box 9
Winnebago, WI 54985-0009   Phone: (414) 235-4910
Mary Kotschi, Dir. of Lib.Serv.
Subjects: Psychiatry, psychology, social service, counseling, hospital administration, nursing, sociology. **Holdings:** 6500 volumes; 8 VF drawers of pamphlets; 585 cassette tapes; 15 videotapes. **Subscriptions:** 183 journals and other serials.

★10350★ HOWARD YOUNG MEDICAL CENTER
HEALTH SCIENCE LIBRARY
Box 470
Woodruff, WI 54568   Phone: (715) 356-8070
Suzanne C. Miller, Med.Libn.
Subjects: Medicine, nursing. **Holdings:** 1200 volumes; 200 pamphlets; 250 video cassettes; 500 audio cassettes. **Subscriptions:** 150 journals and other serials.

Wyoming

★10351★ UNIVERSITY OF WYOMING
FAMILY PRACTICE RESIDENCY PROGRAM AT CASPER
LANGE LIBRARY
1522 East A St.
Casper, WY 82601   Phone: (307) 266-3076
Michael Watson, M.D., M.L.S., Med.Libn.
Subjects: Medicine - clinical, family practice, behavioral. **Holdings:** 800 books; 260 video cassettes; 500 audio cassettes; 42 slide/tape programs; 16 slide programs. **Subscriptions:** 38 journals and other serials.

★10352★ WYOMING MEDICAL CENTER
MEDICAL LIBRARY
1233 E. 2nd St.
Casper, WY 82601   Phone: (307) 577-2450
J. Wilbert, Dir.
Subjects: Medicine. **Holdings:** 810 books; 800 bound periodical volumes. **Subscriptions:** 111 journals and other serials.

★10353★ U.S. DEPARTMENT OF VETERANS AFFAIRS
MEDICAL AND REGIONAL OFFICE CENTER
LIBRARY
2360 E. Pershing Blvd.
Cheyenne, WY 82001   Phone: (307) 778-7550
Terry Skidmore, Chf., Lib.Serv.
Subjects: Medicine, nursing. **Holdings:** 759 books; 2063 volumes of journals, bound and on microfilm. **Subscriptions:** 119 journals and other serials; 15 newspapers.

★10354★ UNIVERSITY OF WYOMING
FAMILY PRACTICE RESIDENCY PROGRAM AT CHEYENNE
FAMILY PRACTICE LIBRARY AT CHEYENNE
821 E. 18th St.
Cheyenne, WY 82001-4797   Phone: (307) 777-7911
Carol McMurry, Libn.
Subjects: Clinical medicine. **Holdings:** 300 books; 1500 bound periodical volumes; 1500 current journals on microfilm. **Subscriptions:** 82 journals and other serials.

★10355★ WYOMING DEPARTMENT OF HEALTH
DIVISION OF PUBLIC HEALTH
FILM LIBRARY
Hathaway Bldg.
Cheyenne, WY 82002-0710   Phone: (307) 777-7363
Ramona L. Nelson, Film Libn.
Subjects: Nursing, mental health, childbirth education, venereal diseases, dental health, school health. **Holdings:** 431 16mm films; 353 videotape and filmstrip programs.

★10356★ CONVERSE COUNTY MEMORIAL HOSPITAL
WILLIAM A. HINRICHS MEDICAL LIBRARY
111 S. 5th St.
Douglas, WY 82633   Phone: (307) 358-2122
Karen A. Trohkimoinen, Med.Lib.Mgr.
Subjects: Medicine, surgery. **Holdings:** 220 books; 6 bound periodical volumes.

★10357★ WYOMING STATE HOSPITAL
MEDICAL LIBRARY
Box 177
Evanston, WY 82931-0177   Phone: (307) 789-3464
William L. Matchinski, Libn.
Subjects: Psychiatry, medicine, nursing, social work, psychology. **Holdings:** 2500 volumes. **Subscriptions:** 155 journals and other serials; 42 newspapers.

★10358★ LANDER VALLEY MEDICAL CENTER
MEDICAL LIBRARY
1320 Bishop Randall Dr.
Lander, WY 82520   Phone: (307) 332-4420
Jane Heuer, Med.Libn.
Subjects: Medicine, nursing, and allied health sciences. **Holdings:** 800 books. **Subscriptions:** 10 journals and other serials.

★10359★ PSYCHIATRIC INSTITUTE OF WYOMING
LIBRARY
150 Wyoming St.
Lander, WY 82520   Phone: (307) 332-5700
Jane Heuer, Libn.
Subjects: Alcohol and drug abuse, psychiatry, anorexia and bulimia. **Holdings:** 100 books. **Subscriptions:** 19 journals and other serials.

★10360★ WYOMING STATE TRAINING SCHOOL
MEDICAL LIBRARY
8204 State Hwy. 789
Lander, WY 82520   Phone: (307) 332-5302
Shirley J. Townsend, Libn.
Subjects: Mental retardation, epilepsy, neurological disorders, pediatric medicine, occupational and physical therapy. **Holdings:** 300 books. **Subscriptions:** 16 journals and other serials.

★10361★ IVINSON MEMORIAL HOSPITAL
MEDICAL LIBRARY
255 N. 30th St.
Laramie, WY 82070   Phone: (307) 742-2141
Connie Baker, Med.Libn.
Subjects: Medicine, patient care, nursing, health administration. **Holdings:** 350 books; 5 drawers of pamphlets. **Subscriptions:** 105 journals and other serials.

★10362★ HEALTHTRUST
RIVERTON MEMORIAL HOSPITAL
MEDICAL LIBRARY
2100 W. Sunset
Riverton, WY 82501   Phone: (307) 856-4161
Connie Krause, RN, Pt.Educ./Staff Dev.Coord.
Subjects: Medicine, nursing, management. **Holdings:** 200 books; 220 bound periodical volumes. **Subscriptions:** 34 journals and other serials.

★10363★ U.S. DEPARTMENT OF VETERANS AFFAIRS
MEDICAL CENTER LIBRARY
Sheridan, WY 82801   Phone: (307) 672-1661
Subjects: Psychiatry, psychology, medicine, nursing, administration. **Holdings:** 2250 books; 250 bound periodical volumes; 1620 periodical volumes on microfilm; 2000 AV programs. **Subscriptions:** 300 journals and other serials.

★10364★ WHEDON CANCER FOUNDATION
LIBRARY
30 S. Scott St.
Box 683
Sheridan, WY 82801-0683   Phone: (307) 672-2941
Nancy E. Peterson, Lib.Mgr.
Subjects: Cancer research, hospice care, medicine, cancer patient education materials. **Holdings:** 75 books. **Subscriptions:** 5 journals and other serials; 2 newspapers.

★10365★ TORRINGTON COMMUNITY HOSPITAL
MEDICAL LIBRARY
2000 Campbell Dr.
Torrington, WY 82240   Phone: (307) 532-4181
Valerie Lamb, ART, URDRG Coord./Libn.
Subjects: Medicine, nursing, patient care. **Holdings:** 150 books. **Subscriptions:** 25 journals and other serials.

Canada

Alberta

★10366★ MINERAL SPRINGS HOSPITAL
MEDICAL LIBRARY
Box 1050
Banff, AB, Canada T0L 0C0   Phone: (403) 762-2222
Mrs. E. Heikkila, Dir., Med.Rec.
Subjects: Medicine, administration. **Holdings:** 75 books. **Subscriptions:** 30 journals and other serials.

★10367★ ALBERTA CHILDREN'S HOSPITAL
LIBRARY
1820 Richmond Rd., SW
Calgary, AB, Canada T2T 5C7   Phone: (403) 229-7077
Barbara Hatt, Libn.
Subjects: Children's health care. **Holdings:** 2700 books. **Subscriptions:** 250 journals and other serials.

★10368★ ALBERTA EDUCATION
MATERIALS RESOURCE CENTRE FOR THE VISUALLY
IMPAIRED, SOUTH
575 28th St., SE, Rm. 15
Calgary, AB, Canada T2A 6X1   Phone: (403) 297-4378
Colleen Tobman, Mgr.
Holdings: 1460 books; 2662 braille titles; 2472 audiotape titles; 2695 large print titles; 340 kit titles. **Subscriptions:** 10 journals and other serials.

★10369★ ALBERTA OCCUPATIONAL HEALTH AND SAFETY
LIBRARY
1021 10th Ave., SW, 3rd Fl.
Calgary, AB, Canada T2R 0B7   Phone: (403) 297-7860
Marilyn Segall, Info.Spec.
Subjects: Occupational health and safety. **Holdings:** 1000 books. **Subscriptions:** 30 journals and other serials.

★10370★ CALGARY GENERAL HOSPITAL
LIBRARY SERVICES
841 Centre Ave., E.
Calgary, AB, Canada T2E 0A1   Phone: (403) 268-9234
Elizabeth Kirchner, Chf.Med.Libn.
Subjects: Medicine, dentistry, hospital administration, nursing, paramedical sciences, allied health sciences. **Holdings:** 8500 books; 9000 bound periodical volumes; 1400 tapes and slides. **Subscriptions:** 425 journals and other serials.

★10371★ CALGARY SOCIETY FOR STUDENTS WITH
LEARNING DIFFICULTIES
THE LEARNING CENTRE
LEARNING DIFFICULTIES LIBRARY AND RESOURCE CENTRE
2315 1st Ave., NW
Calgary, AB, Canada T2N 4N9   Phone: (403) 270-3711
Thelma M. Wager, Libn.
Subjects: Learning disabilities in children, adolescents, and adults. **Holdings:** 100 taped books; 1500 professional, teaching, and learning resources; 6 VF drawers of articles; 180 assessment tools; 2 VF drawers of transparencies and internal reports. **Subscriptions:** 10 journals and other serials.

★10372★ CALGARY ZOOLOGICAL SOCIETY
TECHNICAL SERVICES DEPARTMENT
PO Box 3036, Sta. B
Calgary, AB, Canada T2M 4R8   Phone: (403) 265-9310
Karen Almadi, Libn.
Subjects: Animals, zoology, captive animal management, veterinary medicine. **Holdings:** 1504 volumes. **Subscriptions:** 88 journals and other serials.

★10373★ CANADIAN MENTAL HEALTH ASSOCIATION,
ALBERTA DIVISION
SUICIDE INFORMATION AND EDUCATION CENTRE
No. 201 1615 10th Ave., SW
Calgary, AB, Canada T3C 0J7   Phone: (403) 245-3900
G.G. Harrington, Dir.
Subjects: Suicidal behaviors, suicide prevention, bereavement. **Holdings:**

15,000 articles, manuscripts, documents, films, tapes, theses, cassettes; information kits. **Subscriptions:** 14 journals and other serials.

★10374★ FOOTHILLS HOSPITAL
LIBRARY SERVICES
1403 29th St., NW
Calgary, AB, Canada T2N 2T9   Phone: (403) 270-4848
Ruth MacRae, Lib.Coord.
Subjects: Nursing and allied health. **Holdings:** 5000 volumes; 1000 AV programs. **Subscriptions:** 150 journals and other serials.

★10375★ HEART AND STROKE FOUNDATION OF ALBERTA
LIBRARY
1825 Park Rd., SE
Calgary, AB, Canada T2G 3Y6   Phone: (403) 264-5549
Tracey Ginn, Lib.Serv.Coord.
Subjects: Cardiovascular health and disease, treatment, prevention, rehabilitation, stress, smoking, high blood pressure, blood cholesterol, exercise, nutrition and heart health. **Holdings:** 600 volumes; 70 films; 12 slide/tape sets.

★10376★ HOLY CROSS HOSPITAL OF CALGARY
LIBRARY SERVICES
2210 2nd St., SW
Calgary, AB, Canada T2S 1S6   Phone: (403) 228-8142
Mumtaz Jivraj, Hd.Libn.
Subjects: Medicine, nursing, hospitals, allied health sciences. **Holdings:** 3300 books; 1200 bound periodical volumes; 700 cassette tapes; 275 video cassettes; 40 slide/tape programs. **Subscriptions:** 250 journals and other serials.

★10377★ SALVATION ARMY GRACE HOSPITAL
HOSPITAL LIBRARY
1402 8th Ave., NW
Calgary, AB, Canada T2N 1B9   Phone: (403) 284-1141
Subjects: Medicine, paramedicine, history and poetry of medicine. **Holdings:** 2000 books; 50 bound periodical volumes; 40 tapes. **Subscriptions:** 30 journals and other serials.

★10378★ SOCIETY FOR TECHNOLOGY AND
REHABILITATION
TECHNICAL RESOURCE CENTRE
200, 1201-5 St., SW
Calgary, AB, Canada T2R 0Y6   Phone: (403) 262-9445
Kathy Dilts, Dir., Lib. & Info.Rsrcs.
Subjects: Physical disabilities, rehabilitation technology. **Holdings:** 3000 books; vertical files; software and supplier catalogs; technical aids. **Subscriptions:** 89 journals and other serials.

★10379★ TOM BAKER CANCER CENTRE
LIBRARY
1331 29th St., NW
Calgary, AB, Canada T2N 4N2   Phone: (403) 270-1765
Judy Flax, Libn.
Subjects: Oncology. **Holdings:** 1300 books; 900 bound periodical volumes; 60 audio cassettes; 105 video cassettes; 6 slide/tape programs. **Subscriptions:** 87 journals and other serials.

★10380★ UNIVERSITY OF CALGARY
MEDICAL LIBRARY
Health Sciences Centre
3330 Hospital Dr., NW
Calgary, AB, Canada T2N 4N1   Phone: (403) 220-6858
Andras Kirchner, Med.Libn.
Subjects: Health sciences with special emphasis on family practice. **Holdings:** 95,345 volumes; 14,695 microforms; 67 films; 482 videotapes; 332 slide/tape programs; 3062 cassettes. **Subscriptions:** 1583 journals and other serials.

★10381★ THE VOCATIONAL AND REHABILITATION
RESEARCH INSTITUTE
RESOURCE CENTRE/LIBRARY
3304 33rd St., NW
Calgary, AB, Canada T2L 2A6   Phone: (403) 284-1121
Bob McGowan, Libn.
Subjects: Developmental disabilities, rehabilitation, vocational training, residential services. **Holdings:** 2600 books; 2000 manuscripts, reports, dissertations. **Subscriptions:** 80 serials.

**★10382★ ALBERTA ALCOHOL AND DRUG ABUSE
COMMISSION
LIBRARY**
10909 Jasper Ave., 7th Fl.
Edmonton, AB, Canada T5J 3M9   Phone: (403) 427-7303
Bette Reimer, Hd.Libn.
Subjects: Alcoholism, drug dependence, counseling. **Holdings:** 7000 books;
6000 reprints; 6 linear feet of news clippings. **Subscriptions:** 250 journals
and other serials.

**★10383★ ALBERTA ASSOCIATION OF REGISTERED NURSES
LIBRARY**
11620 168th St.
Edmonton, AB, Canada T5M 4A6   Phone: (403) 451-0043
Lloanne G. Walker, Libn.
Subjects: Nursing. **Holdings:** 4700 books. **Subscriptions:** 110 journals and
other serials.

**★10384★ ALBERTA EDUCATION
MATERIALS RESOURCE CENTRE FOR THE VISUALLY
IMPAIRED, NORTH**
Edwards Bldg., 1st Fl.
10053 111th St.
Edmonton, AB, Canada T5K 2H8   Phone: (403) 427-4681
Kathryn Ribeiro, Mgr.
Holdings: 1460 books; 2662 braille titles; 2472 audiotape titles; 2695 large
print titles; 340 kit titles. **Subscriptions:** 20 journals and other serials.

**★10385★ ALBERTA FAMILY AND SOCIAL SERVICES
LIBRARY**
7th St. Plaza, 6th Fl.
10035 108th St.
Edmonton, AB, Canada T5J 3E1   Phone: (403) 427-7272
Teresa Bendall, Lib.Adm.
Subjects: Family and social services, handicapped. **Holdings:** 10,000
volumes; 8 VF drawers; 20 shelves of Statistics Canada publications.
Subscriptions: 200 journals and other serials; 7 newspapers.

**★10386★ ALBERTA HEALTH
HOSPITALS AND MEDICAL CARE
LIBRARY**
10025 Jasper Ave., 24th Fl.
Box 2222
Edmonton, AB, Canada T5J 2P4   Phone: (403) 427-8720
Peggy Yeh, Libn.
Subjects: Health care, hospital administration, hospitals and nursing
homes, health and medical legislation, management, records management,
hospital architecture, health manpower, long-term care, physical and
occupational therapy, drug information, nursing management. **Holdings:**
10,000 books; 1000 microfiche; 30 videotapes; 100 audio cassettes.
Subscriptions: 350 journals and other serials.

**★10387★ ALBERTA HEALTH
LIBRARY AND INQUIRY SERVICES BRANCH**
10709 Jasper Ave., 6th Fl.
Edmonton, AB, Canada T5J 3N3   Phone: (403) 427-3530
Joanne Lavkulich, Act.Dir.
Subjects: Health - public, mental, environmental; hospitals and medical
care. **Holdings:** 14,000 books; 1100 films and videos. **Subscriptions:** 600
journals and other serials; 15 newspapers.

**★10388★ ALBERTA HOSPITAL ASSOCIATION
RESOURCE LIBRARY**
10009 108th St.
Edmonton, AB, Canada T5J 3C5   Phone: (403) 498-8400
Patricia Baxter, Libn.
Subjects: Health care management and research. **Holdings:** 2500 books;
400 bound periodical volumes; 400 briefs and studies. **Subscriptions:** 60
journals and other serials.

**★10389★ ALBERTA HOSPITAL EDMONTON
LIBRARY**
Box 307
Edmonton, AB, Canada T5J 2J7   Phone: (403) 472-5555
Margaret Pierre, Med.Lib.Techn.
Subjects: Psychiatry, psychiatric nursing, psychology, neuropsychology,
social service, occupational and recreational therapy, gerontology, forensic

psychiatry, hospital administration, rehabilitation. **Holdings:** 5000 books;
134 periodicals; 109 videotapes; 121 audio cassettes.

**★10390★ ALBERTA MENTAL HEALTH SERVICES
CLINIC LIBRARY**
9942 108th St., 5th Fl.
Edmonton, AB, Canada T5K 2J5   Phone: (403) 427-4444
Nirmala Koganty
Subjects: Psychiatry, psychology, nursing, occupational therapy, social
work, domestic science. **Holdings:** 1594 books. **Subscriptions:** 38 journals
and other serials.

**★10391★ ALBERTA OCCUPATIONAL HEALTH AND SAFETY
LIBRARY SERVICES**
10709 Jasper Ave., 6th Fl.
Edmonton, AB, Canada T5J 3N3   Phone: (403) 427-3530
Joanne Lavkulich, Act.Mgr.
Subjects: Occupational health and safety. **Holdings:** 8000 books; 600 films
and videos. **Subscriptions:** 350 journals and other serials.

**★10392★ ALBERTA PUBLIC AFFAIRS BUREAU
PROVINCIAL FILM LIBRARY**
11510 Kingsway Ave.
Edmonton, AB, Canada T5G 2Y5   Phone: (403) 427-4381
Mr. Ashley Daniel, Mgr.
Subjects: Health, hunter training, recreational activities, parenting of
children, consumer affairs, driver training, native issues, Alberta, teens and
adolescents. **Holdings:** 3000 16mm films; video cassettes; slide/tape sets;
filmstrips.

**★10393★ ALBERTA SCHOOL FOR THE DEAF
L.A. BROUGHTON LIBRARY**
6240 113th St.
Edmonton, AB, Canada T6H 3L2
Subjects: Deaf - teaching, psychology, research, educational technology.
Holdings: 1500 books; tapes; 50 periodicals.

**★10394★ CHARLES CAMSELL GENERAL HOSPITAL
PETER WILCOCK LIBRARY**
12815 115th Ave.
Edmonton, AB, Canada T5M 3A4   Phone: (403) 453-5581
Gail Moores
Subjects: Medicine, nursing, paramedical sciences, hospital administration. **Holdings:** 1500 books; 2300 bound periodical volumes; 1000 cassettes; 2 VF drawers of pamphlets and reports. **Subscriptions:** 250 journals
and other serials.

**★10395★ CROSS CANCER INSTITUTE
LIBRARY**
11560 University Ave.
Edmonton, AB, Canada T6G 1Z2   Phone: (403) 492-8593
Juliana Zia, Libn.
Subjects: Neoplastic diseases, cancer research. **Holdings:** 4000 books; 860
bound periodical volumes; 2 drawers of pamphlets; government docu-
ments. **Subscriptions:** 171 journals and other serials.

**★10396★ EASTER SEAL ABILITY COUNCIL
LIBRARY**
11010-101 St., No. 216
Edmonton, AB, Canada T5H 4B8   Phone: (403) 429-0137
Gwen Sanderson, Lib.Techn.
Subjects: Barrier-free design, disabilities, aids and devices for the disabled,
attitudes and awareness. **Holdings:** 800 books. **Subscriptions:** 20 journals
and other serials.

**★10397★ EDMONTON AUTISM SOCIETY
INFORMATION CENTRE**
7515A Mount Lawn Rd.
Edmonton, AB, Canada T5B 4J1   Phone: (403) 479-0088
Barbara Stewart, Pres.
Subjects: Autism, behavior management. **Holdings:** 200 items (books,
audio cassettes, video recordings, pamphlets). **Subscriptions:** 18 journals
and other serials.

★10398★   THE GENERAL HOSPITAL OF EDMONTON, GREY NUNS
HEALTH SCIENCES LIBRARY
1100 Youville Dr., W.
Edmonton, AB, Canada T6L 5X8   Phone: (403) 450-7301
John Bach, Lib.Mgr.
Subjects: Medicine and nursing. **Holdings:** 5500 books; 1900 bound periodical volumes. **Subscriptions:** 398 journals and other serials.

★10399★   THE GENERAL HOSPITAL OF EDMONTON, GREY NUNS
HEALTH SCIENCES LIBRARY
11111 Jasper Ave.
Edmonton, AB, Canada T6L 5X8   Phone: (403) 450-7301
John Bach
Subjects: Geriatrics, medicine, nursing. **Holdings:** 5000 books; 1200 bound periodical volumes. **Subscriptions:** 425 journals and other serials.

★10400★   GLENROSE REHABILITATION HOSPITAL
LIBRARY
Glen East 613
10230-111 Ave.
Edmonton, AB, Canada T5G 0B7   Phone: (403) 471-2262
Peter Schoenberg
Subjects: Rehabilitation, child development, occupational therapy, physical therapy, speech disorders. **Holdings:** 5000 books; 3500 bound periodical volumes; 200 reports; 40 boxes of archives; 200 videotapes. **Subscriptions:** 200 journals and other serials.

★10401★   GOOD SAMARITAN SOCIETY
LIBRARY
Good Samaritan Auxiliary Hospital
9649 71st Ave.
Edmonton, AB, Canada T6E 5J2   Phone: (403) 439-6381
Marion Sadauskas, Libn.
Subjects: Geriatrics, long-term care, nursing, rehabilitation, pastoral care; home and community services. **Holdings:** 2060 books; 5 16mm films; 23 filmstrip/cassette sets; 300 cassette tapes; 600 slides; 110 video cassettes. **Subscriptions:** 102 journals and other serials.

★10402★   HEALTH LAW INSTITUTE
LIBRARY
461 Law Centre
University of Alberta
Edmonton, AB, Canada T6G 2H5   Phone: (403) 432-2435
Prof. Gerald Robertson, Faculty Dir.
Subjects: Health law, medicolegal issues, medical malpractice. **Holdings:** Reported and unreported Canadian court cases dealing with health law, 1950 to present; English and Commonwealth health law cases, 1975 to present; United States health law court cases; Canadian, Commonwealth, and American journals and articles on medicolegal issues; Law Reform Commission of Canada reports.

★10403★   MISERICORDIA HOSPITAL
WEINLOS MEDICAL LIBRARY
16940 87th Ave.
Edmonton, AB, Canada T5R 4H5   Phone: (403) 486-8708
John Back, Libn.
Subjects: Medicine, surgery, nursing, allied health sciences. **Holdings:** 3800 books. **Subscriptions:** 300 journals and other serials.

★10404★   NORTHERN ALBERTA INSTITUTE OF TECHNOLOGY
LEARNING RESOURCE CENTRE
11762 106th St.
Edmonton, AB, Canada T5G 2R1   Phone: (403) 471-8844
Helga Kinnaird, Chf.Libn.
Subjects: Business, applied sciences, medical sciences, vocational education. **Holdings:** 45,000 books, pamphlets, documents. **Subscriptions:** 610 journals.

★10405★   ROYAL ALEXANDRA HOSPITAL
LIBRARY SERVICES
10240 Kingsway Ave.
Edmonton, AB, Canada T5H 3V9   Phone: (403) 477-4135
Donna Dryden, Supv.
Subjects: Medicine, allied health sciences. **Holdings:** 1600 books. **Subscriptions:** 180 journals and other serials.

★10406★   ROYAL ALEXANDRA HOSPITAL
SCHOOL OF NURSING LIBRARY
10415 111th Ave.
Edmonton, AB, Canada T5G 0B8   Phone: (403) 477-4939
Kay B. Walker, Libn.
Subjects: Nursing, medicine, social and behavioral sciences. **Holdings:** 13,073 books; 250 videotapes, 200 filmstrips, 30 models. **Subscriptions:** 120 journals and other serials.

★10407★   UNIVERSITY OF ALBERTA
DEVELOPMENTAL DISABILITIES CENTRE
LIBRARY
6-123A Education II
Edmonton, AB, Canada T6G 2G5   Phone: (403) 492-4439
Fran Russell, Adm.Asst.
Subjects: Biology, medicine, neurology, psychology, education. **Holdings:** 250 books and bound periodical volumes; 50 other cataloged items.

★10408★   UNIVERSITY OF ALBERTA
JOHN W. SCOTT HEALTH SCIENCES LIBRARY
Edmonton, AB, Canada T6G 2R7   Phone: (403) 492-3899
Sylvia R. Chetner, Area Coord.
Subjects: Medicine, nursing, dentistry, pharmacy, rehabilitation medicine, health services administration. **Holdings:** 177,425 books and bound periodical volumes; 7657 microfiche. **Subscriptions:** 2150 journals and other serials.

★10409★   FAIRVIEW VETERINARY LABORATORY
BRANCH LIBRARY
PO Box 197
Fairview, AB, Canada T0H 1L0   Phone: (403) 835-2238
Carol Kaip, Libn.
Subjects: Veterinary medicine.

★10410★   FORT MCMURRAY REGIONAL HOSPITAL
LIBRARY
7 Hospital St.
Fort McMurray, AB, Canada T9H 1P2   Phone: (403) 791-6084
Marianne E. Bruce, Libn.
Subjects: Medicine, nursing, and allied health. **Holdings:** 2800 books. **Subscriptions:** 165 journals and other serials.

★10411★   QUEEN ELIZABETH II HOSPITAL
STAFF LIBRARY
10409 98th St.
Postal Bag 2600
Grande Prairie, AB, Canada T8V 2E8   Phone: (403) 538-7186
Phyllis Brazeau, Lib.Techn.
Subjects: Medicine. **Holdings:** 4000 books; 220 bound periodical volumes; 385 videotapes. **Subscriptions:** 211 journals and other serials.

★10412★   ALBERTA HOSPITAL PONOKA
LIBRARY RESOURCES CENTRE
PO Box 1000
Ponoka, AB, Canada T0C 2H0   Phone: (403) 783-7691
Peter Managhan, Staff Libn.
Subjects: Psychiatry, psychology, nursing, social work, gerontology. **Holdings:** 3000 books; VF material; cassette tapes. **Subscriptions:** 163 journals and other serials.

★10413★   MICHENER CENTRE
STAFF LIBRARY
Box 5002
Red Deer, AB, Canada T4N 5Y5   Phone: (403) 340-5929
Margaret Hardy, Libn.
Subjects: Mental retardation, behavior modification, sociology, psychology, medicine. **Holdings:** 5000 volumes; 17 bound periodical volumes. **Subscriptions:** 100 journals and other serials.

★10414★   RED DEER REGIONAL HOSPITAL CENTRE
LEARNING RESOURCE CENTRE
3942 50A Ave.
Red Deer, AB, Canada T4N 4E7   Phone: (403) 343-4557
Elizabeth Kavanagh, Libn.
Subjects: Medicine, nursing, allied health sciences, hospital administration. **Holdings:** 850 books; 520 bound periodical volumes; 110 videotapes; 350 audiotapes; 120 filmstrips. **Subscriptions:** 115 journals and other serials.

★10415★ WAINWRIGHT GENERAL HOSPITAL
MEDICAL LIBRARY
Box 820
Wainwright, AB, Canada T0B 4P0   Phone: (403) 842-3324
Loretta Haire, Hea.Rec.Adm.
Subjects: Medicine, nursing, hospital administration, allied health sciences. Holdings: 500 books. Subscriptions: 20 journals and other serials.

British Columbia

★10416★ BRITISH COLUMBIA MINISTRY OF HEALTH
DR. KEN KAYE MEMORIAL LIBRARY
3405 Willingdon Ave.
Burnaby, BC, Canada V5G 3H4   Phone: (604) 660-5886
Joy Fourchalk, Lib.Techn.
Subjects: Forensic psychiatry, psychiatry, psychology, nursing, social sciences. Holdings: 3045 books; 1200 bound periodical volumes; 336 Audio-Digest tapes. Subscriptions: 53 journals.

★10417★ BURNABY HOSPITAL
DR. H.H.W. BROOKE MEMORIAL LIBRARY
3935 Kincaid St.
Burnaby, BC, Canada V5G 2X6   Phone: (604) 434-4211
Mr. Hoong Lim, Libn.
Subjects: Medicine, nursing, health care administration. Holdings: 800 books; 500 bound periodical volumes; 4000 pamphlets and clippings. Subscriptions: 85 journals and other serials.

★10418★ CANADA
HEALTH AND WELFARE CANADA
HEALTH PROTECTION BRANCH
REGIONAL LIBRARY
3155 Willingdon Green
Burnaby, BC, Canada V5G 4P2   Phone: (604) 666-3350
Elizabeth Hardacre, Libn.
Subjects: Food inspection and analysis, microbiology, pesticides, pharmaceuticals, illicit drug analysis. Holdings: 2500 books; 1000 bound periodical volumes. Subscriptions: 100 journals and other serials.

★10419★ ROYAL COLUMBIAN HOSPITAL
LIBRARY
330 E. Columbia St.
New Westminster, BC, Canada V3L 3W7   Phone: (604) 520-4255
Ms. S. Abzinger, Mgr.
Subjects: Medicine, allied health sciences. Holdings: 2300 books; 2200 bound periodical volumes. Subscriptions: 172 journals and other serials.

★10420★ LIONS GATE HOSPITAL
DR. H. CARSON GRAHAM MEMORIAL LIBRARY
231 E. 15th St.
North Vancouver, BC, Canada V7L 2L7   Phone: (604) 988-3131
Sharon M. Lyons, Libn.
Subjects: Medicine. Holdings: 2500 books. Subscriptions: 120 journals and other serials.

★10421★ RIVERVIEW HOSPITAL
LIBRARY SERVICES
500 Lougheed Hwy.
Port Coquitlam, BC, Canada V3C 4J2   Phone: (604) 524-7018
Min-Ja Laubental, Libn.
Subjects: Psychiatry, psychology, psychiatric nursing, social sciences, medicine, hospital administration, forensic psychiatry. Holdings: 10,000 books; 1510 bound periodical volumes; 160 staff publications; 50 annual reports; 580 pamphlets. Subscriptions: 150 journals and other serials.

★10422★ BRITISH COLUMBIA WORKER'S COMPENSATION
BOARD
LIBRARY
6951 Westminster Hwy.
Richmond, BC, Canada V7C 1C6   Phone: (604) 273-2266
Lance Nordstrom, Libn.
Subjects: Industrial hygiene and medicine, worker's compensation law, accident prevention, first aid and safety training, rehabilitation of the industrially injured. Holdings: 15,000 books; 5000 bound periodical volumes; 1500 government publications. Subscriptions: 850 journals and other serials.

★10423★ BRITISH COLUMBIA CANCER AGENCY
LIBRARY
600 W. 10th Ave.
Vancouver, BC, Canada V5Z 4E6   Phone: (604) 877-6000
David Noble, Hd.Libn.
Subjects: Radiotherapy, medical oncology, cancer nursing, immunology. Holdings: 3500 books; 3500 bound periodical volumes; 100 annual reports. Subscriptions: 213 journals and other serials.

★10424★ BRITISH COLUMBIA HEALTH ASSOCIATION
LIBRARY
1985 W. Broadway, Ste. 500
Vancouver, BC, Canada V6J 4Y3   Phone: (604) 734-2423
Carolyn Hall, Lib.Coord.
Subjects: Hospital and health care administration. Holdings: 2000 books; 4000 unbound periodicals; hospital annual reports; 60 films and videotapes; 200 pamphlets. Subscriptions: 75 journals and other serials.

★10425★ BRITISH COLUMBIA MEDICAL ASSOCIATION
ARCHIVES
1665 W. Broadway, Ste. 115
Vancouver, BC, Canada V6J 5A4   Phone: (604) 736-5551
Subjects: Medicine in British Columbia. Holdings: 80 boxes of documents.

★10426★ BRITISH COLUMBIA MINISTRY OF SOCIAL
SERVICES AND HOUSING
LIBRARY
800 Cassiar St.
Vancouver, BC, Canada V5K 4N6   Phone: (604) 660-7666
Robert D. Harvey, Libn.
Subjects: Social welfare, social work, sociology, psychology, child welfare, management. Holdings: 10,000 books; 1000 AV programs; archival materials. Subscriptions: 100 journals and other serials.

★10427★ BRITISH COLUMBIA REHABILITATION SOCIETY
G.F. STRONG CENTRE
STAFF MEDICAL LIBRARY
4255 Laurel St.
Vancouver, BC, Canada V5Z 2G9   Phone: (604) 734-1313
Robert Trowsdale, Chf.Libn.
Subjects: Physical medicine, rehabilitation, long term care, chronic disease. Holdings: 1200 books; 100 cassette tapes. Subscriptions: 110 journals and other serials.

★10428★ BRITISH COLUMBIA REHABILITATION SOCIETY
GEORGE PEARSON CENTRE
INFORMATION RESOURCE DEPARTMENT
700 W. 57th Ave.
Vancouver, BC, Canada V6A 1S1   Phone: (604) 321-3231
Robert Trowsdale, Chf.Libn.
Subjects: Physical medicine, rehabilitation, long term care, chronic disease. Holdings: 1200 books. Subscriptions: 110 journals and other serials.

★10429★ COLLEGE OF PHYSICIANS AND SURGEONS OF
BRITISH COLUMBIA
MEDICAL LIBRARY SERVICE
1383 W. 8th Ave.
Vancouver, BC, Canada V6H 4C4   Phone: (604) 733-6671
Jim Henderson, Dir.
Subjects: Medicine, medical history, medical biography. Holdings: 10,000 books; 50,000 bound periodical volumes; 1500 pamphlets; 8 VF drawers of archival materials; 3 shelves of reports; 1800 audiotapes; 100 video cassettes; 30 interactive computer discs. Subscriptions: 650 journals and other serials.

★10430★ JUSTICE INSTITUTE OF BRITISH COLUMBIA
LIBRARY
4198 W. 4th Ave.
Vancouver, BC, Canada V6R 4K1   Phone: (604) 222-7200
April Haddad, Libn.
Subjects: Police science, criminology, fire science, corrections, emergency medicine, management, disasters, search and rescue. Holdings: 10,000 books; 2000 AV items. Subscriptions: 150 journals and other serials.

★10431★ KINSMEN REHABILITATION FOUNDATION OF BRITISH COLUMBIA
LIBRARY
2256 W. 12th Ave.
Vancouver, BC, Canada V6K 2N5   Phone: (604) 736-8841
Katheleen M. Ellis, Libn.
Subjects: Physical disabilities, independent living, equipment and services for people with disabilities, accessibility, attitudes. **Holdings:** 2200 books; 121 equipment catalogs; 1200 equipment/service brochures, 3200 computer records; 90 AV programs; 15 multimedia kits. **Subscriptions:** 175 journals and other serials.

★10432★ REGISTERED NURSES' ASSOCIATION OF BRITISH COLUMBIA
HELEN RANDAL LIBRARY
2855 Arbutus St.
Vancouver, BC, Canada V6J 3Y8   Phone: (604) 736-7331
Joan I. Andrews, Libn.
Subjects: Nursing and allied health. **Holdings:** 3000 books; 450 bound periodical volumes; 30 shelves of pamphlets; 400 audiotapes; 150 videotapes. **Subscriptions:** 125 journals and other serials.

★10433★ UNITED WAY OF THE LOWER MAINLAND
SOCIAL PLANNING AND RESEARCH DEPARTMENT LIBRARY
1625 W. 8th Ave.
Vancouver, BC, Canada V6J 1T9   Phone: (604) 731-7781
Jennifer Cleathero, Libn.
Subjects: Family violence, income security, housing, social problems, child abuse and child sexual abuse, social services planning. **Holdings:** 3000 books and bound reports; 2500 unbound reports, pamphlets, and ephemera. **Subscriptions:** 75 journals and other serials.

★10434★ UNIVERSITY OF BRITISH COLUMBIA
BIOMEDICAL BRANCH LIBRARY
Vancouver General Hospital
700 W. 10th Ave.
Vancouver, BC, Canada V5Z 1L5   Phone: (604) 875-4505
George C. Freeman, Hd., Biomed.Br.
Subjects: Clinical medicine. **Holdings:** 12,860 books; 16,684 bound periodical volumes. **Subscriptions:** 562 journals and other serials.

★10435★ UNIVERSITY OF BRITISH COLUMBIA
CHARLES CRANE MEMORIAL LIBRARY
1874 E. Mall
Vancouver, BC, Canada V6T 1W5   Phone: (604) 228-6111
Paul E. Thiele, Hd.Libn.
Subjects: University and college texts, reference materials, literature, research, and reports for the blind, visually impaired, and handicapped nonprint readers. **Holdings:** 40,000 talking books on cassette and reel tapes; 25,000 braille volumes; 300 large print books; 500 printed books on blindness and disability. **Subscriptions:** 12 journals and other serials (recorded, braille, large print, and ordinary print).

★10436★ UNIVERSITY OF BRITISH COLUMBIA
ERIC W. HAMBER LIBRARY
Children's Hospital
4480 Oak St.
Vancouver, BC, Canada V6H 3V4   Phone: (604) 875-2154
Pat Lysyk, Libn.
Subjects: Clinical medicine, pediatrics, obstetrics and gynecology. **Holdings:** 6824 books; 4675 bound periodical volumes. **Subscriptions:** 404 journals and other serials.

★10437★ UNIVERSITY OF BRITISH COLUMBIA
ST. PAUL'S HOSPITAL HEALTH SCIENCES LIBRARY
1081 Burrard St.
Vancouver, BC, Canada V6Z 1Y6   Phone: (604) 682-2344
Barbara J. Saint, Hd.
Subjects: Health sciences. **Holdings:** 5000 books; 2 VF drawers of pamphlets. **Subscriptions:** 225 journals and other serials.

★10438★ UNIVERSITY OF BRITISH COLUMBIA
WOODWARD BIOMEDICAL LIBRARY
2198 Health Sciences Mall
Vancouver, BC, Canada V6T 1W5   Phone: (604) 228-2762
Douglas N. McInnes, Hd.
Subjects: Medicine, zoology, botany, dentistry, pharmacy, nursing, rehabilitation medicine, nutrition. **Holdings:** 180,208 books; 149,452 bound periodical volumes; 35,878 microforms. **Subscriptions:** 4044 journals and other serials.

★10439★ BRITISH COLUMBIA ALCOHOL AND DRUG PROGRAMS
LIBRARY
1019 Wharf St., 5th Fl.
Victoria, BC, Canada V8V 1X4   Phone: (604) 387-5870
Lee Peacock, Libn.
Subjects: Alcohol and other drugs, substance abuse, psychology, addictions. **Holdings:** 6100 books; 250 audio-visual titles; archival materials; vertical files. **Subscriptions:** 80 journals and other serials.

★10440★ BRITISH COLUMBIA CAPITAL REGIONAL DISTRICT
COMMUNITY HEALTH SERVICES LIBRARY
524 Yates St.
PO Box 1000
Victoria, BC, Canada V8W 2S6   Phone: (604) 388-4421
Patrick Lindsay, Mgr.
Holdings: 200 volumes.

★10441★ BRITISH COLUMBIA MINISTRY OF HEALTH
LIBRARY AND A-V LIBRARY
1515 Blanshard St., Main Fl.
Victoria, BC, Canada V8W 3C8   Phone: (604) 387-2337
Elizabeth M. Woodworth, Libn.
Subjects: Public health, medicine, hospital administration, nursing, mental health, nutrition, geriatrics, health education. **Holdings:** 12,000 books; 20,000 bound periodical volumes; 12 VF drawers of pamphlets; 2600 AV filmstrips and cassettes. **Subscriptions:** 400 journals and other serials.

★10442★ GREATER VICTORIA HOSPITAL SOCIETY
VICTORIA MEDICAL AND HOSPITAL LIBRARIES
1900 Fort St.
Victoria, BC, Canada V8R 1J8   Phone: (604) 595-9723
Cliff Cornish, Mgr.
Subjects: Clinical medicine, nursing, rehabilitation, long term care, hospital administration. **Holdings:** 10,000 books; 10,000 bound periodical volumes; 800 AV programs. **Subscriptions:** 553 journals and other serials.

Manitoba

★10443★ BRANDON GENERAL HOSPITAL
LIBRARY SERVICES
150 McTavish Ave., E.
Brandon, MB, Canada R7A 2B3   Phone: (204) 726-2257
Kathy Eagleton, Dir.
Subjects: Medicine, nursing, allied health sciences, hospital administration. **Holdings:** 7000 books; AV programs. **Subscriptions:** 250 journals and other serials.

★10444★ BRANDON MENTAL HEALTH CENTRE
REFERENCE AND LENDING LIBRARY
Box 420
Brandon, MB, Canada R7A 5Z5   Phone: (204) 726-2587
Marjorie G. McKinnon, Lib.Techn.
Subjects: Psychiatry, psychiatric treatment services, psychology, social work, hospital administration. **Holdings:** 7791 books; 217 bound periodical volumes; 1445 cassette tapes; 7 drawers of pamphlets; 43,751 journals; 28 reel-to-reel tapes; 49 VF drawers; 215 videotapes, films, and filmstrips. **Subscriptions:** 154 journals and other serials.

★10445★ MANITOBA COMMUNITY SERVICES
MANITOBA DEVELOPMENTAL CENTRE
LIBRARY
3rd St., NE
Box 1190
Portage La Prairie, MB, Canada R1N 3C6   Phone: (204) 239-6435
Jo-Anne Doan, Lib.Techn.
Subjects: Developmentally disabled, genetics, medicine, nursing, psychology, management. **Holdings:** 4000 books; 20 dissertations and theses; 1000 slides; 120 videotapes. **Subscriptions:** 100 journals and other serials and newspapers.

★10446★ SELKIRK MENTAL HEALTH CENTRE
CENTRAL LIBRARY
Box 9600
Selkirk, MB, Canada R1A 2B5   Phone: (204) 482-3810
B. Scarsbrook, Chm., Lib.Comm.
Subjects: Psychiatry, psychiatric nursing, psychology, social service, nursing, allied health sciences. **Holdings:** 4000 books; 1050 bound periodical volumes; AV programs. **Subscriptions:** 100 journals and other serials.

★10447★ ALCOHOLISM FOUNDATION OF MANITOBA
WILLIAM POTOROKA MEMORIAL LIBRARY
1031 Portage Ave.
Winnipeg, MB, Canada R3G 0R8   Phone: (204) 944-6233
Rita Shreiber, Mgr., Lib.Serv.
Subjects: Alcohol and drug use and abuse, psychology, education, treatment, counseling, values clarification. **Holdings:** 3200 books; 19 pamphlet titles; 150 16mm films; 80 filmstrips; 200 videotapes. **Subscriptions:** 45 journals and other serials.

★10448★ BETHANIA MENNONITE PERSONAL CARE HOME
LIBRARY
1045 Concordia Ave.
Winnipeg, MB, Canada R2K 3S7   Phone: (204) 667-0795
Esther Fransen
Subjects: Gerontology, nursing, medicine, psychology. **Holdings:** 500 books; 40 bound periodical volumes. **Subscriptions:** 35 journals and other serials.

★10449★ CANADA
NATIONAL FILM BOARD OF CANADA
FILM AND VIDEO LIBRARY
245 Main St.
Winnipeg, MB, Canada R3C 1A7   Phone: (204) 983-4131
Roberta Boily, Sr.Libn.
Subjects: Social issues, women's issues, health, nature and ecology, Native issues, history. **Holdings:** 3000 films; 1000 video cassettes.

★10450★ CANADIAN CANCER SOCIETY
LIBRARY
193 Sherbrook St.
Winnipeg, MB, Canada R3C 2B7   Phone: (204) 774-7483
Remarks: No further information was supplied by the respondent.

★10451★ CANADIAN PARAPLEGIC ASSOCIATION,
   MANITOBA
LIBRARY
825 Sherbrook St.
Winnipeg, MB, Canada R3A 1M5   Phone: (204) 786-4753
Lucy DeLuca, Libn.
Subjects: Spinal cord injury. **Holdings:** 500 books; reports; archives. **Subscriptions:** 52 journals and other serials.

★10452★ CONCORDIA HOSPITAL
LIBRARY
1095 Concordia Ave.
Winnipeg, MB, Canada R2K 3S8   Phone: (204) 661-7163
Edith Konoplenko, Lib.Techn.
Subjects: Medicine, nursing. **Holdings:** 2000 books. **Subscriptions:** 90 journals and other serials.

★10453★ J. W. CRANE MEMORIAL LIBRARY
2109 Portage Ave.
Winnipeg, MB, Canada R3J 0L3   Phone: (204) 831-2152
Judy Inglis, Dir.
Subjects: Geriatrics, long-term care. **Holdings:** 6000 books. **Subscriptions:** 185 journals and other serials.

★10454★ MANITOBA CANCER TREATMENT AND RESEARCH
   FOUNDATION
LIBRARY
100 Olivia St.
Winnipeg, MB, Canada R3E 0V9   Phone: (204) 787-2136
Donna G. Chornenki, Libn.
Subjects: Oncology, medicine, radiology, basic sciences, cell biology. **Holdings:** 3366 volumes; 3171 bound periodical volumes. **Subscriptions:** 108 journals and other serials.

★10455★ MANITOBA HEALTH
INFORMATION RESOURCES CENTRE
202-880 Portage Ave.
Winnipeg, MB, Canada R3G 0P1   Phone: (204) 945-8000
Marilyn R. Brooke, Chf.Libn.
Subjects: Public health, preventive medicine, public welfare, social service, health education, sociology, medicine, nursing, mental health. **Holdings:** 20,000 books; 1000 bound periodical volumes; 5000 pamphlets; 33,000 unbound periodicals; 10,000 government publications; 900 AV items; annual reports; statistics; statutes; calendars. **Subscriptions:** 235 journals and other serials.

★10456★ MANITOBA HEALTH SERVICES COMMISSION
LIBRARY
599 Empress St.
PO Box 925
Winnipeg, MB, Canada R3C 2T6   Phone: (204) 786-7398
Vera Ott, Libn.
Subjects: Medicine, health services administration, laboratory technology. **Holdings:** 2145 books; 180 hospital-related Statistics Canada materials; 240 annual reports of provincial medical plans; 450 pamphlets. **Subscriptions:** 181 journals and other serials; 6 newspapers.

★10457★ MANITOBA PHARMACEUTICAL ASSOCIATION
LIBRARY
187 St. Mary's Rd.
Winnipeg, MB, Canada R2H 1J2   Phone: (204) 233-1411
Janet McGillivray, Dir. of Cont.Educ.
Subjects: Therapeutics, pharmacy practice and history, business management. **Holdings:** 200 books. **Subscriptions:** 14 journals and other serials.

★10458★ MANITOBA SCHOOL FOR THE DEAF
LIBRARY
500 Shaftesbury Blvd.
Winnipeg, MB, Canada R3P 0M1   Phone: (204) 945-8934
Margaret Kovacs, Libn.
Subjects: Deafness. **Holdings:** 1500 books; 80 bound periodical volumes.

★10459★ MISERICORDIA GENERAL HOSPITAL
HOSPITAL LIBRARY
99 Cornish Ave.
Winnipeg, MB, Canada R3C 1A2   Phone: (204) 788-8109
Sharon Allentuck, Libn.
Subjects: Nursing, medicine, allied health sciences. **Holdings:** 5300 volumes. **Subscriptions:** 324 journals and other serials.

★10460★ ST. AMANT CENTRE INC.
MEDICAL LIBRARY
440 River Rd.
Winnipeg, MB, Canada R2M 3Z9   Phone: (204) 256-4301
Pauline Dufresne, Techn.
Subjects: Mental retardation, genetics. **Holdings:** 450 books. **Subscriptions:** 20 journals and other serials.

★10461★ SALVATION ARMY GRACE GENERAL HOSPITAL
LIBRARY
300 Booth Dr.
Winnipeg, MB, Canada R3J 3M7   Phone: (204) 837-0127
Mrs. J. Kochan, Dir.
Subjects: Medicine, nursing, and allied health sciences. **Holdings:** 10,054 books; 636 AV programs; 18 linear feet of pamphlets. **Subscriptions:** 175 journals and other serials.

★10462★ SOCIETY FOR MANITOBANS WITH DISABILITIES
STEPHEN SPARLING LIBRARY
825 Sherbrook St.
Winnipeg, MB, Canada R3A 1M5   Phone: (204) 786-5601
Cheryl Manness, Lib.Techn.
Subjects: Rehabilitation, social work, learning disorders, physical disabilities, therapy, psychology, special education, children's literature. **Holdings:** 2000 books and bound periodical volumes; 1000 monographs, reprints, and pamphlets. **Subscriptions:** 45 journals and other serials.

★10463★ UNIVERSITY OF MANITOBA
MEDICAL LIBRARY
Medical College Bldg.
770 Bannatyne Ave.
Winnipeg, MB, Canada R3T 0W3   Phone: (204) 788-6342
Audrey M. Kerr, Hd.Med.Libn.
Subjects: Medicine and basic medical sciences. **Holdings:** 106,000 volumes. **Subscriptions:** 1550 journals and other serials.

★10464★ UNIVERSITY OF MANITOBA
NEILSON DENTAL LIBRARY
780 Bannatyne Ave.
Winnipeg, MB, Canada R3E 0W3   Phone: (204) 788-6635
Anne Thornton-Trump, Hd.Libn.
Subjects: Dentistry. **Holdings:** 23,400 volumes; 1500 pamphlets. **Subscriptions:** 380 journals and other serials.

★10465★ WINNIPEG CLINIC
LIBRARY
425 St. Mary Ave.
Winnipeg, MB, Canada R3C 0N2   Phone: (204) 957-1900
S. Loeppky, Libn.
Subjects: Medicine. **Holdings:** Figures not available. **Subscriptions:** 78 journals and other serials.

★10466★ WINNIPEG HEALTH SCIENCES CENTRE
LIBRARY SERVICES
700 McDermot Ave.
Winnipeg, MB, Canada R3E 0T2   Phone: (204) 787-3416
Ada M. Ducas, Dir., Educ.Rsrcs. & Lib.Serv.
Subjects: Medicine, surgery, pediatrics, nursing, allied health sciences, hospital administration. **Holdings:** 5183 books; 4000 bound periodical volumes; 100 slides; 309 videotapes; 143 slidetapes; 32 audiotapes; 113 films. **Subscriptions:** 400 journals and other serials.

New Brunswick

★10467★ ALCOHOLISM AND DRUG DEPENDENCY
COMMISSION OF NEW BRUNSWICK
CHEMICAL DEPENDENCY LIBRARY
65 Brunswick St.
Fredericton, NB, Canada E3B 2H4   Phone: (506) 453-2136
Gwen Sedman, Libn.
Subjects: Alcoholism, drug addiction, mental health. **Holdings:** 1200 books; 16 VF drawers of reports, articles, pamphlets. **Subscriptions:** 45 journals and other serials; 5 newspapers.

★10468★ DR. EVERETT CHALMERS HOSPITAL
DR. GARFIELD MOFFATT HEALTH SCIENCES LIBRARY
PO Box 9000
Fredericton, NB, Canada E3B 5N5   Phone: (506) 452-5432
Paul Clark, Libn.
Subjects: Medicine, nursing, allied health sciences. **Holdings:** 1500 books; 700 bound periodical volumes. **Subscriptions:** 172 journals and other serials.

★10469★ NEW BRUNSWICK DEPARTMENT OF HEALTH AND
COMMUNITY SERVICES
LIBRARY
Carleton Pl., 3rd Fl.
PO Box 5100
Fredericton, NB, Canada E3B 5G8   Phone: (506) 453-2536
Subjects: Health, medicine, social services. **Holdings:** 1000 books; 100 bound periodical volumes. **Subscriptions:** 100 journals and other serials.

★10470★ NURSES ASSOCIATION OF NEW BRUNSWICK
LIBRARY
231 Saunders St.
Fredericton, NB, Canada E3B 1N6   Phone: (506) 458-8731
Barbara Thompson, Libn.
Subjects: Nursing - education, research, manpower, management; medicine; allied health sciences. **Holdings:** 900 books; 300 bound periodical volumes; 6 VF drawers; 2 drawers of bulletins; clinical textbooks. **Subscriptions:** 35 journals and other serials; 4 newspapers.

★10471★ MONCTON HOSPITAL
HEALTH SCIENCES LIBRARY
135 MacBeath Ave.
Moncton, NB, Canada E1C 6Z8   Phone: (506) 857-5447
Susan P. Libby, Hosp.Libn.
Subjects: Medicine, nursing, health sciences. **Holdings:** 2300 volumes. **Subscriptions:** 500 journals and other serials.

★10472★ MIRAMICHI HOSPITAL
HEALTH SCIENCES LIBRARY
PO Box 420
Newcastle, NB, Canada E1V 3M5   Phone: (506) 622-1340
Audrey D. Somers, Educ.Coord.
Subjects: Medicine, nursing, administration, patient education, allied health sciences. **Holdings:** 2000 books; 186 bound periodical volumes; 194 AV programs. **Subscriptions:** 146 journals and other serials.

★10473★ CANADA
AGRICULTURE CANADA
HEALTH OF ANIMALS LABORATORY
LIBRARY
4 College St.
Sackville, NB, Canada E0A 3C0   Phone: (506) 536-0135
Dr. R.A. Heckert, Lib.Hd.
Subjects: Veterinary medicine. **Holdings:** 500 volumes. **Subscriptions:** 61 journals and other serials.

★10474★ SAINT JOHN REGIONAL HOSPITAL
DR. CARL R. TRASK HEALTH SCIENCES LIBRARY
Box 2100
Saint John, NB, Canada E2L 4L2   Phone: (506) 648-6763
Anne Kilfoil, Mgr.
Subjects: Medicine, nursing, and allied health sciences. **Holdings:** 6000 books; 300 bound periodical volumes; 1000 AV items. **Subscriptions:** 402 journals and other serials.

★10475★ CARLETON MEMORIAL HOSPITAL
LIBRARY
Box 400
Woodstock, NB, Canada E0J 2B0   Phone: (506) 328-3341
Joanne E. Rosevear, Adm.
Subjects: Medicine, management, computers. **Holdings:** 3500 books; 90 cassettes. **Subscriptions:** 146 journals and other serials; 5 newspapers.

Newfoundland

★10476★ WESTERN MEMORIAL REGIONAL HOSPITAL
HEALTH SCIENCES LIBRARY
PO Box 2005
Corner Brook, NF, Canada A2H 6J7   Phone: (709) 637-5395
Patricia Tilley, Libn.
Subjects: Medicine, nursing, paramedical fields. **Holdings:** 2500 books; 1150 bound periodical volumes. **Subscriptions:** 167 journals and other serials.

★10477★ JAMES PATON MEMORIAL HOSPITAL
STAFF LIBRARY
Trans Canada Hwy.
Gander, NF, Canada A1V 1P7   Phone: (709) 256-5527
Teresita Hearn, Libn.
Subjects: Medicine, orthopedics, ophthalmology, pediatrics, obstetrics, gynecology, allied health sciences. **Holdings:** 700 books. **Subscriptions:** 130 journals and other serials.

★10478★ MELVILLE HOSPITAL
MEDICAL LIBRARY
Goose Bay, NF, Canada A0P 1C0   Phone: (709) 896-2417
Teresa O'Keefe
Remarks: No further information was supplied by the respondent.

★10479★ CENTRAL NEWFOUNDLAND REGIONAL HEALTH
CENTER
HOSPITAL LIBRARY
Union St.
Grand Falls, NF, Canada A2A 2E1   Phone: (709) 292-2228
Ellen Lewis, Libn.
Subjects: Medicine. **Holdings:** Figures not available.

★10480★ CHARLES S. CURTIS MEMORIAL HOSPITAL
MEDICAL LIBRARY
St. Anthony, NF, Canada A0K 4S0   Phone: (709) 454-3333
Joan Hillier, Libn.
Subjects: Medicine. **Holdings:** 200 books. **Subscriptions:** 70 journals and other serials.

★10481★ CABOT INSTITUTE OF APPLIED ARTS AND
TECHNOLOGY
TOPSAIL CAMPUS RESOURCE CENTER
PO Box 1693
St. John's, NF, Canada A1C 5P7   Phone: (709) 778-2320
Lillian Dawe, Lib.Techn.
Subjects: Medical laboratory and x-ray technology, nursing, food management, commercial art, hotel management, respiratory therapy, ultrasonography, biomedical technology. **Holdings:** 7000; 600 BPV; 300 AV programs; 300 volumes of periodicals on microfiche. **Subscriptions:** 175 journals and other serials.

★10482★ CHILDREN'S REHABILITATION CENTRE
MEDICAL LIBRARY
Box 1403
St. John's, NF, Canada A1C 5N5   Phone: (709) 754-1970
Kathleen Legge, Libn.
Holdings: 200 books. **Subscriptions:** 75 journals and other serials.

★10483★ DR. CHARLES A. JANEWAY CHILD HEALTH
CENTRE
JANEWAY MEDICAL LIBRARY
Pleasantville
St. John's, NF, Canada A1A 1R8   Phone: (709) 778-4344
Shaila Mensinkai, Hosp.Libn.
Subjects: Pediatrics, medicine, surgery. **Holdings:** 3000 books; 4500 bound periodical volumes; 857 Audio-Digest tapes; 390 pamphlets. **Subscriptions:** 170 journals and other serials.

★10484★ GRACE GENERAL HOSPITAL
SCHOOL OF NURSING LIBRARY
241 LeMarchant Rd.
St. John's, NF, Canada A1E 1P9   Phone: (709) 778-66425
Debbie O'Rielly, Libn.
Subjects: Nursing. **Holdings:** 2700 books; 130 bound periodical volumes; 20 boxes of pamphlets.

★10485★ THE HUB
PHYSICALLY DISABLED SERVICE CENTRE
INFORMATION CENTRE
21 Merrymeeting Rd.
PO Box 13788
St. John's, NF, Canada A1B 4G3   Phone: (709) 754-0352
Maureen Broderick, Info.Ctr.Coord.
Subjects: Physical disabilities, rehabilitation. **Holdings:** Figures not available. **Subscriptions:** 100 journals and other serials; 25 newspapers.

★10486★ MEMORIAL UNIVERSITY OF NEWFOUNDLAND
HEALTH SCIENCES LIBRARY
Health Science Centre
300 Prince Philip Dr.
St. John's, NF, Canada A1B 3V6   Phone: (709) 737-6672
Linda Barnett, Act.Assoc.Univ.Libn., Hea.Sci.
Subjects: Medicine, history of medicine, nursing, pharmacy, dentistry, allied health professions. **Holdings:** 40,024 books; 51,423 bound periodical volumes; 10,000 slides; 3400 audiotapes; 1257 reels of microfilm; 121 motion pictures; 113 microfilm sets; 545 slide/tape sets; 1174 microfiche; 2 models; 773 videotapes. **Subscriptions:** 1623 journals and other serials.

★10487★ NEWFOUNDLAND DEPARTMENT OF HEALTH
PUBLIC HEALTH NURSING DIVISION
LIBRARY
Forest Rd.
PO Box 8700
St. John's, NF, Canada A1B 4J6   Phone: (709) 576-3440
Linda Carter, Hea.Educ.
Subjects: Health. **Holdings:** 500 books. **Subscriptions:** 30 journals and other serials.

★10488★ ST. CLARE'S MERCY HOSPITAL
LIBRARY
St. Clare Ave.
St. John's, NF, Canada A1C 5B8   Phone: (709) 778-3414
Catherine Lawton, Libn.
Subjects: Medicine, nursing, hospital administration, allied health sciences. **Holdings:** 470 books; 100 AV tapes. **Subscriptions:** 121 journals and other serials.

★10489★ ST. CLARE'S MERCY HOSPITAL
SCHOOL OF NURSING LIBRARY
250 Waterford Bridge Rd.
St. John's, NF, Canada A1E 1E3   Phone: (709) 778-3577
Dora M. Braffet, Instr.Mtls.Spec.Libn.
Subjects: Nursing. **Holdings:** 3000 books; 26 bound periodical volumes; AV programs. **Subscriptions:** 31 journals and other serials.

★10490★ SALVATION ARMY GRACE GENERAL HOSPITAL
CHESLEY A. PIPPY, JR. MEDICAL LIBRARY
241 Lemarchant Rd.
St. John's, NF, Canada A1E 1P9   Phone: (709) 778-6796
Elizabeth Duggan, Med.Libn.
Subjects: Medicine. **Holdings:** 950 books; 1200 bound periodical volumes. **Subscriptions:** 110 journals and other serials.

★10491★ WATERFORD HOSPITAL
HEALTH SERVICES LIBRARY
Waterford Bridge Rd.
St. John's, NF, Canada A1E 4J8   Phone: (709) 364-0269
Maisie Young, Libn.
Subjects: Psychiatry, nursing, medicine, social work, psychology, pharmacology. **Holdings:** 2300 books; unbound periodicals; annual reports; manuscripts; pamphlets; AV programs. **Subscriptions:** 104 journals and other serials.

★10492★ NOTRE DAME BAY MEMORIAL HOSPITAL
LIBRARY
Twillingate, NF, Canada A0G 4M0   Phone: (709) 884-2131
Barbara Hamlyn, Libn.
Remarks: No further information was supplied by the respondent.

Northwest Territories

★10493★ NORTHWEST TERRITORIES DEPARTMENT OF
HEALTH
DR. OTTO SCHAEFER HEALTH RESOURCE CENTRE
The Centre Square Tower, 2nd Fl.
Yellowknife, NT, Canada X1A 2L9   Phone: (403) 873-7713
Florrie Cook, Libn.
Subjects: Public health, nursing, health care administration, Northern health care, hospital operations. **Holdings:** 4000 books. **Subscriptions:** 160 journals and other serials.

★10494★ NORTHWEST TERRITORIES SAFETY DIVISION
DEPARTMENT OF SAFETY AND PUBLIC SERVICES
SAFETY/EDUCATION RESOURCE CENTRE
Yellowknife, NT, Canada X1A 2L9   Phone: (403) 873-7470
Rita Denneron, Lib.Techn.
Subjects: Safety, industrial hygiene, law, legislation, occupational health and safety regulations. **Holdings:** 348 volumes; 97 microfiche; 4 topic files; 6 file cabinets; 120 reports on microfiche; 6 lateral file drawers of reports and clippings; 190 manufacture equipment catalogs; 290 films and videos; 120 posters; 97 pamphlets. **Subscriptions:** 22 journals and other serials; 53 newsletters.

Nova Scotia

★10495★ ST. MARTHA'S HOSPITAL
SCHOOL OF NURSING LIBRARY
25 Bay St.
Antigonish, NS, Canada B2G 2G5   Phone: (902) 863-2830
Sr. Mary Chisholm, Libn.
Subjects: Nursing. **Holdings:** 4152 books; 158 bound periodical volumes; 50 videotapes; AV programs. **Subscriptions:** 70 journals and other serials.

★10496★ NOVA SCOTIA HOSPITAL
HEALTH SCIENCE LIBRARY
PO Box 1004
Dartmouth, NS, Canada B2Y 3Z9   Phone: (902) 469-7500
Marjorie A. Cox
Subjects: Psychiatry, medicine, psychology, neurology, pre-clinical science. **Holdings:** 5500 books; 400 bound periodical volumes; 8000 psychiatric and medical reprints; 450 slides and cassettes; hospital archives. **Subscriptions:** 108 journals and other serials.

★10497★ CAMP HILL HOSPITAL
HEALTH SCIENCES LIBRARY
1763 Robie St.
Halifax, NS, Canada B3H 3G2   Phone: (902) 420-2287
Verona Leslie, Lib.Asst.
Subjects: Medicine, surgery, psychiatry, nursing, gerontology, psychology, pharmacology. **Holdings:** 2000 books; 100 bound periodical volumes; tapes. **Subscriptions:** 200 journals and other serials.

★10498★ CAMP HILL MEDICAL CENTRE
PROVINCIAL DRUG INFORMATION SERVICE
1763 Robie St.
Halifax, NS, Canada B3H 3G2   Phone: (902) 420-2211
C. Brian Tuttle, Dir.
Subjects: Therapeutics, pharmacology, toxicology, institutional and professional pharmacy practice. **Holdings:** 2000 files. **Subscriptions:** 18 journals and other serials.

★10499★ DALHOUSIE UNIVERSITY
W.K. KELLOGG HEALTH SCIENCES LIBRARY
Sir Charles Tupper Medical Bldg.
Halifax, NS, Canada B3H 4H7   Phone: (902) 494-2458
J. Elizabeth Sutherland, Hea.Sci.Libn.
Subjects: Medicine, dentistry, nursing, pharmacy, physiotherapy, health services administration, physical education, human communication disorders, occupational therapy. **Holdings:** 150,400 volumes; 2765 audiotapes, videotapes, slide-tape programs. **Subscriptions:** 2516 journals and other serials.

★10500★ GRACE MATERNITY HOSPITAL
MEDICAL LIBRARY
5821 University Ave.
Halifax, NS, Canada B3H 1W3   Phone: (902) 420-6600
Darlene A. Chapman, Libn.
Subjects: Obstetrics and gynecology, pediatrics, surgery, medicine. **Holdings:** 400 books. **Subscriptions:** 15 journals and other serials.

★10501★ HALIFAX INFIRMARY
HEALTH SERVICES LIBRARY
1335 Queen St.
Halifax, NS, Canada B3J 2H6   Phone: (902) 428-3058
Dr. Anitra Laycock, Libn.
Subjects: Medicine, nursing, allied health sciences, administration. **Holdings:** 1500 books; 5000 slides, archives, and videotapes. **Subscriptions:** 350 journals and other serials.

★10502★ IZAAK WALTON KILLAM HOSPITAL FOR
    CHILDREN
HEALTH SCIENCES LIBRARY
5850 University Ave.
Halifax, NS, Canada B3J 3G9   Phone: (902) 428-8238
Darlene Chapman, Libn.
Subjects: Medicine, allied health. **Holdings:** 900 books; 125 titles; 300 audiotapes. **Subscriptions:** 150 journals and other serials.

★10503★ NOVA SCOTIA COMMISSION ON DRUG
    DEPENDENCY
LIBRARY
Lord Nelson Bldg., 5th Fl.
5675 Spring Garden Rd.
Halifax, NS, Canada B3J 1H1   Phone: (902) 424-4270
Ruth Vaughan, Libn.
Subjects: Drug and alcohol use, sociology, social problems, psychology and psychiatry, highway safety, women's treatment issues. **Holdings:** 3000 books and documents; 150 video tapes. **Subscriptions:** 87 journals and other serials.

★10504★ NSCC INSTITUTE OF TECHNOLOGY
LIBRARY
5685 Leeds St.
PO Box 2210
Halifax, NS, Canada B3J 3C4   Phone: (902) 424-4224
Nola D. Brennan, Libn.
Subjects: Engineering, medical laboratory, dental, construction administration, and other resources technologies; automated manufacturing; computer technology; food services; nuclear medicine; dental assisting; business computer programming; mini/microcomputer systems; plant apprenticeship and trades. **Holdings:** 11,800 books; 1200 bound periodical volumes; 500 student reports; 35 school calendars. **Subscriptions:** 200 journals and other serials.

★10505★ VICTORIA GENERAL HOSPITAL
HEALTH SCIENCES LIBRARY
Halifax, NS, Canada B3H 2Y9   Phone: (902) 428-2641
Samuel B. King, Libn.
Subjects: Medicine, medical research, nursing, nursing education, allied health sciences, hospital administration and management. **Holdings:** 10,000 books; 5500 bound periodical volumes; 4000 pamphlets. **Subscriptions:** 550 journals and other serials; 10 newspapers.

★10506★ SYDNEY COMMUNITY HEALTH CENTRE
HEALTH SCIENCES LIBRARY
409 King's Rd.
Sydney, NS, Canada B1S 1B4   Phone: (902) 562-2322
Patricia Keough, Libn.
Subjects: Health sciences, medicine, nursing, obstetrics, gynecology, pediatrics, anatomy, physiology, nutrition, psychiatry. **Holdings:** 2466 books; 5 bound periodical volumes. **Subscriptions:** 84 journals and other serials.

Ontario

★10507★ LOYALIST COLLEGE OF APPLIED ARTS AND
    TECHNOLOGY
ANDERSON RESOURCE CENTRE
Loyalist-Wallbridge Rd.
Box 4200
Belleville, ON, Canada K8N 5B9   Phone: (613) 969-1913
Ronald H. Boyce, Mgr., Educ.Rsrcs.
Subjects: Science and technology, behavioral sciences, health sciences. **Holdings:** 55,000 books; 1100 bound periodical volumes; 12,000 AV programs. **Subscriptions:** 590 journals and other serials.

★10508★ CANADA
NATIONAL DEFENCE
CANADIAN FORCES MEDICAL SERVICES SCHOOL
LIBRARY
Canadian Forces Base
Borden, ON, Canada L0M 1C0   Phone: (705) 424-1200
Mrs. Marion Thomson, Libn.
Subjects: Nursing, preventive medicine, hospital administration, military science. **Holdings:** 16,000 volumes. **Subscriptions:** 80 journals and other serials.

★10509★ BROCKVILLE PSYCHIATRIC HOSPITAL
LIBRARY RESOURCES AND INFORMATION CENTRE
Box 1050
Brockville, ON, Canada K6V 5W7   Phone: (613) 345-1461
Michelle R. Lamarche, Staff Libn.
Subjects: Psychiatry, psychology, geriatrics, nursing, hospital administration, social work. **Holdings:** 2271 books; 3 VF drawers; 15,000 periodicals; Audio-Digest tapes. **Subscriptions:** 104 journals and other serials.

★10510★ JOSEPH BRANT MEMORIAL HOSPITAL
HOSPITAL LIBRARY
1230 Northshore Blvd.
Burlington, ON, Canada L7R 4C4   Phone: (416) 632-3730
Catherine Newman, Libn.
Subjects: Medicine, nursing, administration, paramedical sciences. **Holdings:** 500 books; videotapes. **Subscriptions:** 150 journals and other serials.

★10511★ NORWICH EATON
FILM LIBRARY
PO Box 819
210 Sheldon Dr.
Cambridge, ON, Canada N1R 5W6   Phone: (519) 622-3000
Maureen Chesney, Prof.Serv.Adm.
Subjects: Urology, nutrition, neurology, spasticity, plastic and reconstructive burn therapy, gynecology. **Holdings:** 45 films.

★10512★ CANADIAN PARAPLEGIC ASSOCIATION
LIBRARY
1500 Don Mills Rd.
Don Mills, ON, Canada M3B 3K4   Phone: (416) 391-0203
Greg Pyc, Coord., Info.Serv.
Subjects: Spinal cord injury and rehabilitation; social, political, technical concerns of the handicapped. **Holdings:** 1200 volumes; 1200 reprints. **Subscriptions:** 60 journals and newsletters.

★10513★ THE EASTER SEAL SOCIETY
RESOURCE CENTRE
200-250 Ferrand Dr.
Don Mills, ON, Canada M3C 3P2   Phone: (416) 421-8377
Georgina Westdyk
Subjects: Physical disabilities; housing, transportation, education, and special services for the disabled. **Holdings:** 1000 books; 30 other cataloged items. **Subscriptions:** 41 journals and other serials.

★10514★ ONTARIO HOSPITAL ASSOCIATION
LIBRARY
150 Ferrand Dr.
Don Mills, ON, Canada M3C 1H6   Phone: (416) 429-2661
John Tagg, Mgr.
Subjects: Hospital administration, health economics, health insurance, management. **Holdings:** 1500 books. **Subscriptions:** 102 journals and other serials.

★10515★ ORTHO PHARMACEUTICAL, LTD.
R.W. JOHNSON PHARMACEUTICAL RESEARCH INSTITUTE
LIBRARY
19 Green Belt Dr.
Don Mills, ON, Canada M3C 1L9   Phone: (416) 449-9444
Subjects: Contraception, family planning, immunology, business management, biotechnology. **Holdings:** 1565 books; 580 bound periodical volumes; microfiche. **Subscriptions:** 285 journals and other serials.

★10516★ CANADA
DEFENCE AND CIVIL INSTITUTE OF ENVIRONMENTAL
  MEDICINE
SCIENTIFIC INFORMATION CENTRE
1133 Sheppard Ave., W.
PO Box 2000
Downsview, ON, Canada M3M 3B9   Phone: (416) 635-2070
Anthony Cheung, Chf.Libn.
Subjects: Aviation medicine, environmental physiology, biochemistry, biophysics, biostatistics, human engineering, electronics, aircraft accident investigation, computer systems. **Holdings:** 8000 books; 8000 bound periodical volumes; 20,000 reports; 2000 microforms. **Subscriptions:** 150 journals and other serials.

★10517★ CONCORD ENVIRONMENTAL CORPORATION
LIBRARY
2 Tippett Rd.
Downsview, ON, Canada M3H 2V2   Phone: (416) 630-6331
Cathy Lindsey-King, Libn. & Info.Off.
Subjects: Air pollution, hazardous substances, atmospheric and environmental science, meteorology, occupational hygiene and health, risk assessment. **Holdings:** 100 books; 150 bound periodical volumes; 2000 reports; 650 microfiche. **Subscriptions:** 150 journals and other serials.

★10518★ G. ALLAN ROEHER INSTITUTE
LIBRARY
Kinsmen Bldg., York University
4700 Keele St.
Downsview, ON, Canada M3J 1P3   Phone: (416) 661-9611
Miriam Ticoll, Libn.
Subjects: Mental handicaps, developmental disabilities, deinstitutionalization, special education, community organization. **Holdings:** 10,000 books;

12 VF drawers of pamphlets and reprints; 75 films. **Subscriptions:** 100 journals and other serials.

★10519★ WYETH, LTD.
WYETH RESOURCE LIBRARY
1120 Finch Ave., W., 7th Fl.
Downsview, ON, Canada M3J 3H7   Phone: (416) 736-4056
Shamim Jamal-Rajan, Sci.Prod.Info.Off.
Subjects: Pharmacology - general, clinical, hormonal; psychiatry; gynecology; cardiovascular system. **Holdings:** 725 books; 765 bound periodical volumes; 4798 reprints; 10 reports and current awareness publications. **Subscriptions:** 62 journals and other serials.

★10520★ YORK-FINCH GENERAL HOSPITAL
THOMAS J. MALCHO MEMORIAL LIBRARY
2111 Finch Ave., W.
Downsview, ON, Canada M3N 1N1   Phone: (416) 744-2500
Mona Kakoschke, Med.Libn.
Subjects: Medicine, nursing, hospital administration. **Holdings:** 2000 books. **Subscriptions:** 210 journals.

★10521★ THISTLETOWN REGIONAL CENTRE
LIBRARY
Rexdale Campus
51 Panorama Court
Etobicoke, ON, Canada M9V 4L8   Phone: (416) 326-0717
Joy Shanfield, Supv., Libs.
Subjects: Child psychiatry and psychology, family therapy, special education, adolescent psychiatry and psychology, juvenile corrections. **Holdings:** 3150 books; 2200 bound periodical volumes; 300 audiotapes; 7 VF drawers; 2 drawers of legislation materials. **Subscriptions:** 104 journals and other serials.

★10522★ GUELPH GENERAL HOSPITAL
DR. WILLIAM HOWITT MEMORIAL LIBRARY
115 Delhi St.
Guelph, ON, Canada N1E 4J4   Phone: (519) 822-5350
Brenda Vegso, Libn.
Remarks: No further information was supplied by the respondent.

★10523★ CANADIAN CENTRE FOR OCCUPATIONAL HEALTH
  AND SAFETY
250 Main St., E.
Hamilton, ON, Canada L8N 1H6   Phone: (416) 572-2981
J. Arthur St. Aubin, Pres. & Chf. Exec. Off.
Subjects: Occupational health and safety. **Holdings:** 24,000 volumes; 222,000 microfiche. **Subscriptions:** 863 journals and other serials.

★10524★ CHEDOKE-MCMASTER HOSPITALS
CHEDOKE HOSPITAL LIBRARY
Box 2000, Sta. A
Hamilton, ON, Canada L8N 3Z5   Phone: (416) 521-2100
Lois M. Wyndham, Chf.Libn.
Subjects: Rehabilitation medicine, geriatrics, child psychology and psychiatry, alcohol and drug abuse. **Holdings:** 2500 books. **Subscriptions:** 251 journals and other serials.

★10525★ HAMILTON GENERAL DIVISION
MEDICAL LIBRARY
286 Victoria Ave. N.
Hamilton, ON, Canada L8L 5G4   Phone: (416) 527-0271
Candace A. Thacker, Hd,, HG Div. Med.Lib.
Subjects: Medicine, allied health, nursing. **Holdings:** 3500 books; 10,000 bound periodical volumes. **Subscriptions:** 140 journals and other serials.

★10526★ HAMILTON PSYCHIATRIC HOSPITAL
LIBRARY RESOURCE CENTRE
PO Box 585
Hamilton, ON, Canada L8N 3K7   Phone: (416) 388-2511
Anne Devries, Libn.
Subjects: Psychiatry, social work, psychiatric nursing, psychology, psychogeriatrics, occupational therapy, rehabilitation services, pastoral services. **Holdings:** 6000 books; 1000 bound periodical volumes; 60 slide/tape sets; 225 tapes; 9 VF drawers. **Subscriptions:** 175 journals and other serials.

★10527★   MCMASTER UNIVERSITY
HEALTH SCIENCES LIBRARY
1200 Main St., W.
Hamilton, ON, Canada L8N 3Z5   Phone: (416) 525-9140
Dorothy Fitzgerald, Hea.Sci.Libn.
Subjects: Basic medical sciences, clinical medicine, nursing, allied health sciences, history of medicine. **Holdings:** 57,179 books; 67,572 bound periodical volumes; 842 slide/tape programs; 149 16mm films; 779 videotapes; 181 audio cassettes; 89 computer software programs. **Subscriptions:** 1801 journals and other serials.

★10528★   MOHAWK COLLEGE OF APPLIED ARTS AND
**   TECHNOLOGY**
HEALTH SCIENCES EDUCATION CENTRE
LIBRARY RESOURCE CENTRE
PO Box 2034
Hamilton, ON, Canada L8N 3T2   Phone: (416) 575-1515
Maureen Price, Lib.Supv.
Subjects: Nursing, medical laboratory technology, radiography, physiotherapy, occupational therapy. **Holdings:** 17,900 books; 2650 bound periodical volumes; 2625 AV programs. **Subscriptions:** 180 journals and other serials.

★10529★   MOHAWK COLLEGE OF APPLIED ARTS AND
**   TECHNOLOGY**
SAM MITMINGER LIBRARY RESOURCE CENTRE
PO Box 2034
Hamilton, ON, Canada L8N 3T2   Phone: (416) 575-2077
Sandra M. Black, Dir., Lrng.Res.
Subjects: Business, technology, health sciences, early childhood education, academic upgrading. **Holdings:** 114,000 books; 8000 periodical volumes; 24,000 AV programs; 5500 microforms; 800 maps; 948 clipping file folders; 10,000 uncataloged items, including government documents. **Subscriptions:** 1030 journals and other serials; 15 newspapers.

★10530★   ONTARIO CANCER FOUNDATION
HAMILTON REGIONAL CENTRE
LIBRARY
711 Concession St.
Hamilton, ON, Canada L8V 1C3   Phone: (416) 387-9495
Michael Fraumeni, Libn.
Subjects: Cancer, medical physics. **Holdings:** 1000 books; 1000 bound periodical volumes. **Subscriptions:** 58 journals and other serials.

★10531★   ST. JOSEPH'S HOSPITAL
DRUG INFORMATION CENTRE
50 Charlton Ave., E.
Hamilton, ON, Canada L8N 4A6   Phone: (416) 522-4941
Miss N. Giovinazzo, Act.Dir., Pharm.Serv.
Subjects: Drugs, pharmacology, disease, clinical pharmacy services, pharmaceutical techniques. **Holdings:** 175 volumes; 125 cassette tapes; 50 videotapes; archives and teaching files. **Subscriptions:** 32 journals and other serials.

★10532★   ST. JOSEPH'S HOSPITAL
LIBRARY SERVICES
50 Charlton Ave., E.
Hamilton, ON, Canada L8N 1Y4   Phone: (416) 522-4941
Mrs. Gayle Fitzgerald, Hd., Lib.Serv.
Subjects: Medicine, nursing, hospital administration. **Holdings:** 2200 books; 7000 bound periodical volumes. **Subscriptions:** 200 journals and other serials.

★10533★   ST. PETER'S HOSPITAL
LIBRARY
88 Maplewood Ave.
Hamilton, ON, Canada L8M 1W9   Phone: (416) 549-6525
Peggy Ross, Libn.
Subjects: Geriatrics, nursing. **Holdings:** 1100 books. **Subscriptions:** 90 journals and other serials.

★10534★   NOTRE DAME HOSPITAL
LIBRARY
1405 Edward St.
PO Box 8000
Hearst, ON, Canada P0L 1N0   Phone: (705) 362-4291
Suzanne Allaire, Med.Rec.Supv.
Subjects: Medicine, nursing, paramedical sciences, hospital administra-

tion. **Holdings:** 1000 books; 675 bound periodical volumes. **Subscriptions:** 109 journals and other serials.

★10535★   ONTARIO MINISTRY OF AGRICULTURE AND
**   FOOD**
VETERINARY SERVICES LABORATORY LIBRARY
PO Box 2005
Kemptville, ON, Canada K0G 1J0   Phone: (613) 258-8320
Vivian Martineau, Libn.
Subjects: Veterinary medicine, pathology, animal science. **Holdings:** Figures not available. **Subscriptions:** 31 journals and other serials.

★10536★   HOTEL-DIEU HOSPITAL
STAFF LIBRARY
166 Brock St.
Kingston, ON, Canada K7L 5G2   Phone: (613) 544-3310
Lynda Silver, Dir., Staff Lib.
Remarks: No further information was supplied by the respondent.

★10537★   KINGSTON GENERAL HOSPITAL
HOSPITAL LIBRARY
76 Stuart St.
Kingston, ON, Canada K7L 2V7   Phone: (613) 548-3232
Margaret Darling, Lib.Mgr.
Subjects: Medicine, surgery, nursing, nutrition, laboratory technology, rehabilitative medicine, administration, respiratory technology. **Holdings:** 1400 books; 2000 bound periodical volumes. **Subscriptions:** 190 journals and other serials.

★10538★   KINGSTON PSYCHIATRIC HOSPITAL
STAFF LIBRARY
Bag 603
Kingston, ON, Canada K7L 4X3   Phone: (613) 546-1101
Karen Gagnon, Libn.
Subjects: Psychiatry, psychology, medicine, nursing, social sciences. **Holdings:** 2741 books; 4639 bound periodical volumes; 6 VF drawers of clippings and pamphlets; 418 audio cassettes; 40 videos. **Subscriptions:** 110 journals and other serials.

★10539★   ONGWANADA HOSPITAL
LIBRARY
191 Portsmouth Ave.
Kingston, ON, Canada K7L 1J9   Phone: (613) 544-9611
Rhoda McFarlane, Supv., Clin.Rec.
Subjects: Mental retardation. **Holdings:** 750 books; 1 VF drawer of reprints; 95 AV programs; 1 film; 5 pieces of training equipment. **Subscriptions:** 23 journals and other serials.

★10540★   QUEEN'S UNIVERSITY AT KINGSTON
BRACKEN LIBRARY
Kingston, ON, Canada K7L 3N6   Phone: (613) 545-2510
Mrs. V. Ludwin, Libn.
Subjects: Medicine, nursing, rehabilitation, life sciences. **Holdings:** 111,935 volumes. **Subscriptions:** 1411 journals and other serials.

★10541★   QUEEN'S UNIVERSITY AT KINGSTON
OCCUPATIONAL HEALTH AND SAFETY RESOURCE CENTRE
LIBRARY
Abramsky Hall, 2nd Fl.
Kingston, ON, Canada K7L 3N6   Phone: (613) 545-2909
Gloria Hetherington
Subjects: Occupational health, environmental health, occupational medicine, occupational safety, epidemiology, indoor air quality, ventilation. **Holdings:** 833 books; 39 reports. **Subscriptions:** 12 journals and other serials.

★10542★   ST. MARY'S OF THE LAKE HOSPITAL
GIBSON MEDICAL RESOURCE CENTRE
Box 3600
Kingston, ON, Canada K7L 5A2   Phone: (613) 544-5220
Penny G. Levi, Dir., Lib.Serv.
Subjects: Geriatrics and chronic care, rehabilitation, allied health sciences. **Holdings:** 2800 books; 600 bound periodical volumes. **Subscriptions:** 130 journals and other serials.

★10543★ KITCHENER-WATERLOO HOSPITAL
HEALTH SCIENCES LIBRARY
835 King St., W.
Kitchener, ON, Canada N2G 1G3   Phone: (519) 742-3611
Thelma Bisch, Libn.
Subjects: Medicine, nursing, hospital administration, paramedical sciences. **Holdings:** 2800 books; 4000 bound periodical volumes; 1000 AV programs. **Subscriptions:** 250 journals and other serials.

★10544★ ST. MARY'S HOSPITAL
MEDICAL LIBRARY
911 Queen St. N.
Kitchener, ON, Canada N2M 1B2   Phone: (519) 744-3311
Elaine Baldwin, Libn.
Subjects: Medicine, nursing, hospital administration. **Holdings:** 1000 books; 900 bound periodical volumes. **Subscriptions:** 100 journals and other serials.

★10545★ COLLEGE OF FAMILY PHYSICIANS OF CANADA
CANADIAN LIBRARY OF FAMILY MEDICINE
Natural Sciences Centre, Rm. 101
University of Western Ontario
London, ON, Canada N6A 5B7   Phone: (519) 661-3170
Lynn Dunikowski, Libn.
Subjects: Family medicine, general practice.

★10546★ LONDON PSYCHIATRIC HOSPITAL
LIBRARY
850 Highbury Ave.
Box 2532, Terminal A
London, ON, Canada N6A 4H1   Phone: (519) 455-5110
Subjects: Psychiatry. **Holdings:** 4000 books; 800 bound periodical volumes. **Subscriptions:** 175 journals and other serials.

★10547★ LONDON REGIONAL CANCER CENTRE
LIBRARY
790 Commissioners Rd. E
London, ON, Canada N6A 4L6   Phone: (519) 685-8626
Charlene Campbell
Subjects: Oncology - general, radiation, research, medical, nursing, radiotherapy. **Holdings:** 900 books; 1500 bound periodical volumes. **Subscriptions:** 125 journals and other serials.

★10548★ ST. JOSEPH'S HEALTH CENTRE OF LONDON
LIBRARY SERVICES
268 Grosvenor St.
London, ON, Canada N6A 4V2   Phone: (519) 439-3271
Louise Lin, Mgr., Lib.Serv.
Subjects: Clinical medicine, nursing, allied health sciences. **Holdings:** 3900 books; 5422 bound periodical volumes; 2000 physical diagnosis teaching slides; 2000 hematology teaching slides. **Subscriptions:** 415 journals and other serials.

★10549★ UNIVERSITY OF WESTERN ONTARIO
DR. JOSEPH POZSONYI MEMORIAL LIBRARY
CPRI
600 Sanatorium Rd.
London, ON, Canada N6H 3W7   Phone: (519) 471-2540
Alexander Lyubichanski, Lib.Supv.
Subjects: Administration; audiology; behavior modification; biochemistry; clinical chemistry; cytogenetics; electroencephalography; therapy - music, physical, occupational, speech; neurology; nursing; pathology; nutrition; pediatrics; psychiatry; psychology; public health; recreation; social work; sociology; special education. **Holdings:** 2800 books; 3800 bound periodical volumes; 400 staff papers; 6000 reprints; 60 government directories and acts. **Subscriptions:** 125 journals and other serials.

★10550★ UNIVERSITY OF WESTERN ONTARIO
OCCUPATIONAL HEALTH AND SAFETY RESOURCE CENTRE
LIBRARY
Bio Engineering Bldg.
London, ON, Canada N6A 5B9   Phone: (519) 661-3044
Martin J. Bracken
Subjects: Occupational health, occupational safety, air pollution. **Holdings:** 600 books; 35 bound periodical volumes; 115 reports. **Subscriptions:** 7 journals and other serials.

★10551★ UNIVERSITY OF WESTERN ONTARIO
SCIENCES LIBRARY
Natural Sciences Centre
London, ON, Canada N6A 5B7   Phone: (519) 679-2111
Lorraine Busby, Hd./Sci.Lib.
Subjects: Anesthesia, anatomy, applied mathematics, astronomy, biochemistry, biology, biophysics, chemistry, clinical neurological sciences, communicative disorders, computer science, dentistry, epidemiology, family medicine, genetics, geology, geophysics, history of medicine and science, mathematics, medicine, microbiology, nursing, obstetrics and gynecology, occupational therapy, ophthalmology, otolaryngology, pediatrics, pathology, pharmacology, physical medicine, physical therapy, physics, physiology, plant sciences, psychiatry, radiation oncology, radiology, statistics, surgery, zoology. **Holdings:** 162,409 books; 148,301 bound periodical volumes; 37,078 microforms; 9077 AV materials; 1192 pamphlets. **Subscriptions:** 4409 journals and other serials.

★10552★ UNIVERSITY OF WESTERN ONTARIO
SCIENCES LIBRARY
NORTHERN OUTREACH LIBRARY SERVICE
London, ON, Canada N6A 5B7   Phone: (519) 661-3169
Sylvia Katzer, Libn.
Subjects: Medicine, allied health sciences, nursing, biological sciences. **Holdings:** Figures not available.

★10553★ CANADIAN FILM INSTITUTE
NATIONAL SCIENCE FILM LIBRARY
115 Torbay Rd., Unit 9
Markham, ON, Canada L3R 2M9   Phone: (416) 475-3750
Eileen Laba, V.P.
Subjects: Health and medicine, earth sciences, physical and engineering sciences, behavioral and biological sciences, geography and history, arts, performing arts and film. **Holdings:** 6000 16mm film and videotape titles.

★10554★ CIBA-GEIGY LTD.
PHARMACEUTICAL LIBRARY
6860 Century Ave.
Mississauga, ON, Canada L5N 2W5   Phone: (416) 821-4420
Heather Dansereau, Med.Libn.
Subjects: Medicine, pharmacy, pharmacology, business. **Holdings:** 3000 volumes; 70,000 microfiche. **Subscriptions:** 260 journals and other serials.

★10555★ HOFFMANN-LA ROCHE, LTD.
CORPORATE LIBRARY
2455 Meadowpine Blvd.
Mississauga, ON, Canada L5N 6L7   Phone: (416) 542-5542
Colin G.D. Hoare, Mgr.
Subjects: Medicine, clinical pharmacology, toxicology, analytical chemistry, pharmaceutical technology, marketing. **Holdings:** 1200 books; 30 periodical titles on microfiche; 18 VF drawers of product literature catalogs; 25 drawers of microfiche; pamphlets; brochures. **Subscriptions:** 264 journals and other serials.

★10556★ MISSISSAUGA HOSPITAL
L.G. BRAYLEY HEALTH SCIENCES LIBRARY
100 Queensway, W.
Mississauga, ON, Canada L5B 1B8   Phone: (416) 848-7394
Tsai-o Wong, Mgr., Lib.Serv.
Subjects: Medicine, nursing, health, hospitals. **Holdings:** 3000 books; 300 bound periodical volumes; archives. **Subscriptions:** 171 journals and other serials.

★10557★ ALGONQUIN COLLEGE OF APPLIED ARTS AND
TECHNOLOGY
RESOURCE CENTRES
1385 Woodroffe Ave.
Nepean, ON, Canada K2G 1V8   Phone: (613) 727-7713
Jocelyne Chaperon-Beck, Dir.
Subjects: Business, trades and technology, social sciences, nursing and allied health sciences, applied arts. **Holdings:** 111,607 books; 3037 bound periodical volumes; 2231 reels of microfilm; 3330 microfiche; 1366 films; 595 filmstrips; 28,831 slides; 5727 phonograph records; 1863 video records. **Subscriptions:** 1501 journals and other serials; 41 newspapers.

★10558★ CANADA
AGRICULTURE CANADA
ANIMAL DISEASES RESEARCH INSTITUTE LIBRARY
801 Chemin Fallowfield Rd.
PO Box 11300, Sta. H
Nepean, ON, Canada K2H 8P9   Phone: (613) 998-9320
P. Atherton, Libn.
Subjects: Veterinary medicine, virology, immunology, bacteriology. **Holdings:** 10,500 volumes. **Subscriptions:** 255 journals and other serials.

★10559★ ONTARIO MINISTRY OF AGRICULTURE AND
     FOOD
VETERINARY SERVICES LABORATORY LIBRARY
Box 790
New Liskeard, ON, Canada P0J 1P0   Phone: (705) 647-6701
Mr. Veldhuis, Techn.
Subjects: Veterinary medicine and pathology. **Holdings:** 200 books; 340 bound periodical volumes. **Subscriptions:** 25 journals and other serials; 10 newspapers.

★10560★ GREATER NIAGARA GENERAL HOSPITAL
HEALTH SCIENCES LIBRARY
PO Box 1018
Niagara Falls, ON, Canada L2E 6X2   Phone: (416) 358-0171
John Dunn, Lib.Techn.
Subjects: Medicine, nursing, and allied health sciences. **Holdings:** 1000 books. **Subscriptions:** 176 journals and other serials.

★10561★ FOREST PRODUCTS ACCIDENT PREVENTION
     ASSOCIATION
LIBRARY
Box 270
North Bay, ON, Canada P1B 8H2   Phone: (705) 472-4120
V. Jones, Libn.
Subjects: Occupational safety and health, accident prevention, industrial and occupational diseases, forests and forestry, management, total loss control. **Holdings:** 600 books; 21 16mm films; 80 videotapes. **Subscriptions:** 30 journals and other serials.

★10562★ NORTH BAY COLLEGE EDUCATION CENTRE
LIBRARY
Gormanville Rd.
Box 5001
North Bay, ON, Canada P1B 8K9   Phone: (705) 474-7600
B.A. Nettlefold, Dir. of Lib.Serv.
Subjects: Education, nursing, arts, commerce, science, social work, technology. **Holdings:** 130,000 volumes; VF drawers; government documents; pictures. **Subscriptions:** 770 journals and other serials; 10 newspapers.

★10563★ NORTH BAY PSYCHIATRIC HOSPITAL
LIBRARY
Hwy. 11 North
PO Box 3010
North Bay, ON, Canada P1B 8L1   Phone: (705) 474-1200
Judy Elston, Libn.
Remarks: No further information was supplied by the respondent.

★10564★ SENECA COLLEGE OF APPLIED ARTS AND
     TECHNOLOGY
LESLIE CAMPUS LIBRARY/RESOURCE CENTRE
1255 Sheppard Ave., E.
North York, ON, Canada M2K 1E2   Phone: (416) 491-5050
Vinh P. Le, Campus Libn.
Subjects: Nursing, dentistry. **Holdings:** 14,016 books; 266 audiotapes; 803 videotapes; 103 films; 200 slide sets; 146 dental models. **Subscriptions:** 104 journals and other serials.

★10565★ SUNNYBROOK HEALTH SCIENCE CENTRE
HEALTH SCIENCES LIBRARY
2075 Bayview Ave.
North York, ON, Canada M4N 3M5   Phone: (416) 480-6100
Linda McFarlane, Dir., Hea.Sci.Lib.
Subjects: Medicine and nursing, hospital administration. **Holdings:** 8000 books; 19,000 bound periodical volumes; 2500 audiotapes; 260 videotapes; 15 drawers of pamphlets. **Subscriptions:** 535 journals and other serials.

★10566★ SEARLE CANADA INC.
CORPORATE INFORMATION RESEARCH SERVICES
400 Iroquois Shore Rd.
Oakville, ON, Canada L6H 1M5   Phone: (416) 844-1040
Alison J. Ball, Corp.Libn.
Subjects: Pharmacy and pharmacology, cardiology, gastroenterology, therapeutics. **Holdings:** 900 books; 8 drawers of microfiche. **Subscriptions:** 275 serials.

★10567★ SMITHKLINE BEECHAM, PHARMA CANADA
MEDICAL LIBRARY
2030 Bristle Circle
Oakville, ON, Canada L68 5V2   Phone: (416) 829-2030
Janet B. Hillis, Lib.Techn.
Subjects: Medicine - antibiotics, gastrointestinal, oncology, central nervous system, cardiology; pharmacy; pharmacology; biochemistry; microbiology. **Holdings:** 500 books; 650 bound periodical volumes; 600 volumes of reprints. **Subscriptions:** 100 journals and other serials.

★10568★ HURONIA REGIONAL CENTRE
LIBRARY
Box 1000
Orillia, ON, Canada L3V 6L2   Phone: (705) 326-7361
Maureen Maguire, Libn.
Subjects: Mental retardation. **Holdings:** 2500 books; 200 reports; 14 VF drawers of reports, pamphlets, articles. **Subscriptions:** 125 journals and other serials.

★10569★ OSHAWA GENERAL HOSPITAL
EDUCATION RESOURCE CENTRE
24 Alma St.
Oshawa, ON, Canada L1G 2B9   Phone: (416) 576-8711
Susan Hendricks, Med.Libn.
Subjects: Medicine, nursing, allied health sciences, telemedicine. **Holdings:** 1000 books; 3000 bound periodical volumes; VF drawers. **Subscriptions:** 155 journals and other serials.

★10570★ BREWERS ASSOCIATION OF CANADA
LIBRARY
Heritage Pl., Ste. 1200
155 Queen St.
Ottawa, ON, Canada K1P 6L1   Phone: (613) 232-9601
Edwin Gregory, Libn.
Subjects: Alcoholic beverages and their abuse, history of the brewing industry, taverns and inns. **Holdings:** 500 books; 500 papers on use and abuse of alcohol. **Subscriptions:** 60 journals and other serials; 19 newspapers.

★10571★ CANADA
AGRICULTURE CANADA
ANIMAL RESEARCH CENTRE LIBRARY
Genetics Bldg.
Ottawa, ON, Canada K1A 0C6   Phone: (613) 993-6002
J.P. Miska, Reg.Coord.
Subjects: Animal science and nutrition, genetics, physiology, biochemistry. **Holdings:** 3000 books; 4200 bound periodical volumes. **Subscriptions:** 200 journals and other serials.

★10572★ CANADA
AGRICULTURE CANADA
CANADIAN AGRICULTURE LIBRARY
Sir John Carling Bldg., Rm. 245
Ottawa, ON, Canada K1A 0C5   Phone: (613) 995-7829
M.L. Morton, Dir., CAL
Subjects: Agriculture and allied sciences, economics, veterinary medicine, chemistry, biochemistry, nutrition, management science. **Holdings:** 1 million volumes; 20,000 microforms; 7700 translations. **Subscriptions:** 22,600 journals and other serials.

★10573★ CANADA
HEALTH AND WELFARE CANADA
HEALTH PROTECTION BRANCH
LIBRARY SERVICES
Sir F.G. Banting Research Centre, 3rd Fl., W.
Ross Ave., Tunney's Pasture
Ottawa, ON, Canada K1A 0L2   Phone: (613) 957-1026
Susan Higgins, Chf., Lib.Serv.
Subjects: Pharmacology, pharmaceutical chemistry, food science, nutrition

research, microbiology, toxicology, medical sciences, public health, epidemiology, environmental health, radiation protection, drug abuse. **Holdings:** 15,000 books; 500 microforms. **Subscriptions:** 1500 journals.

★10574★ CANADA
HEALTH AND WELFARE CANADA
POLICY, PLANNING & INFORMATION BRANCH
LIBRARY
Brooke Claxton Bldg., 2nd Fl. N
Tunney's Pasture
Ottawa, ON, Canada K1A 0K9   Phone: (613) 957-1545
Ms. Marty H. Lovelock, Chf., Lib.Serv.
Subjects: Health policy, social welfare, income support, gerontology, demography, family violence, child care. **Holdings:** 25,000 titles. **Subscriptions:** 400 journals and other serials.

★10575★ CANADA
LABOUR CANADA
LIBRARY SERVICES
OCCUPATIONAL SAFETY AND HEALTH REFERENCE CENTRE
Ottawa, ON, Canada K1A 0J2   Phone: (819) 997-8458
Subjects: Occupational safety and health, industrial hygiene, safety engineering, ergonomics, fire prevention and protection. **Holdings:** 10,000 books; standards; VF; material safety data sheets. **Subscriptions:** 250 journals and other serials.

★10576★ CANADA
NATIONAL DEFENCE
NATIONAL DEFENCE MEDICAL CENTRE
MEDICAL LIBRARY
Alta Vista Dr.
Ottawa, ON, Canada K1A 0K6   Phone: (613) 738-5211
Philip B. Allan, Chf.Med.Libn.
Subjects: Medicine, nursing. **Holdings:** 4200 books; 9800 bound periodical volumes; 1250 video and audio cassettes. **Subscriptions:** 295 journals and other serials.

★10577★ CANADA
NATIONAL LIBRARY OF CANADA
CANADIAN BOOK EXCHANGE CENTRE
85 Bentley Ave.
Ottawa, ON, Canada K2E 6T7   Phone: (613) 952-8902
Ergun Camlioglu, Chf.
Subjects: Social sciences, humanities, science, technology, medicine, Canadian history and literature. **Holdings:** 140,000 books; 2.2 million periodical volumes; 730,000 government publications.

★10578★ CANADA
NATIONAL RESEARCH COUNCIL
CANADA INSTITUTE FOR SCIENTIFIC AND TECHNICAL INFORMATION
Montreal Rd.
Ottawa, ON, Canada K1A 0S2   Phone: (613) 993-1600
Elmer V. Smith, Dir.Gen.
Subjects: Science and technology, medicine. **Holdings:** 475,000 books; 2 million microfiche. **Subscriptions:** 55,000 journals and other serials.

★10579★ CANADIAN COUNCIL ON CHILDREN AND YOUTH
RESOURCE CENTRE
55 Parkdale Ave., 3rd Fl.
Ottawa, ON, Canada K1Y 1E5   Phone: (613) 722-0133
Elizabeth Bourque, Hd.
Subjects: Children and youth - health, law, education, culture, recreation, agencies, native, environment. **Holdings:** 200 books and bound periodical volumes; reports; briefs; essays; directories; statistics; inventory of programs. **Subscriptions:** 235 journals and other serials; 15 newspapers; list of subscriptions and topics available for a fee.

★10580★ CANADIAN DEAF AND HARD OF HEARING
FORUM
RESOURCE LIBRARY
2435 Holly Ln., Ste. 205
Ottawa, ON, Canada K1V 7P2   Phone: (613) 526-4867
Yvette Kereluk, Hd.
Subjects: Hearing impairment - legal rights, education, technical aids. **Holdings:** Figures not available.

★10581★ CANADIAN DENTAL ASSOCIATION
SYDNEY WOOD BRADLEY MEMORIAL LIBRARY
1815 Alta Vista Dr.
Ottawa, ON, Canada K1N 6E7   Phone: (613) 523-1770
Martha Vaughan, Libn.
Subjects: Dentistry, dental health, dental hygiene, dental research, business, medicine. **Holdings:** 5100 books; 1320 bound periodical volumes; internal documents; governmnet reports. **Subscriptions:** 207 journals and other serials.

★10582★ CANADIAN MEDICAL ASSOCIATION
LIBRARY
1867 Alta Vista Dr.
PO Box 8650
Ottawa, ON, Canada K1G 0G8   Phone: (613) 731-9331
Kathleen Beaudoin, Libn.
Subjects: Medicine. **Holdings:** 900 books; 1250 bound periodical volumes; 900 other cataloged items. **Subscriptions:** 400 journals and other serials.

★10583★ CANADIAN NURSES ASSOCIATION
HELEN K. MUSSALLEM LIBRARY
50 The Driveway
Ottawa, ON, Canada K2P 1E2   Phone: (613) 237-2133
Elizabeth Hawkins Brady, Lib.Mgr.
Subjects: Nursing. **Holdings:** 16,000 books and documents; photographs. **Subscriptions:** 500 journals and other serials.

★10584★ CANADIAN RED CROSS SOCIETY
NATIONAL OFFICE
LIBRARY
1800 Alta Vista Dr.
Ottawa, ON, Canada K1G 4J5   Phone: (613) 739-2371
Ann M. Butryn, Mgr., Off.Serv./Libn.
Subjects: Canadian Red Cross Society, International Committee of the Red Cross, League of Red Cross Societies, blood services collection. **Holdings:** 1500 books; 600 bound periodical volumes; 100 boxes of archival material; 50 boxes of pamphlets, clippings, press releases. **Subscriptions:** 200 journals and other serials.

★10585★ CHILDREN'S HOSPITAL OF EASTERN ONTARIO
MEDICAL LIBRARY
401 Smyth Rd.
Ottawa, ON, Canada K1H 8L1   Phone: (613) 737-2206
Patricia Johnston, Dir., Lib.Serv.
Subjects: Pediatrics, nursing, allied health sciences, general medicine, hospital management. **Holdings:** 8500 books; 3500 bound periodical volumes; 6 VF drawers of pamphlets and reprints; 850 AV programs. **Subscriptions:** 400 journals and other serials.

★10586★ HEALTH SERVICES AND PROMOTION
INFORMATION NETWORK
Jeanne Mance Bldg, Rm. 500
Tunney's Pasture
Ottawa, ON, Canada K1A 1B4   Phone: (613) 954-8590
Mrs. B.H. Garland, Chf., Lib.Serv.
Subjects: Health administration and policy; healthcare for special groups - children, women, handicapped, natives, elderly; substance abuse. **Holdings:** 30,000 books; 500 reports. **Subscriptions:** 1100 journals and other serials; 5 newspapers.

★10587★ OTTAWA CIVIC HOSPITAL
DR. GEORGE S. WILLIAMSON HEALTH SCIENCES LIBRARY
1053 Carling Ave.
Ottawa, ON, Canada K1Y 4E9   Phone: (613) 761-4450
Mabel C. Brown, Dir., Lib.Serv.
Subjects: Medicine, nursing, allied health sciences. **Holdings:** 3000 books; 5000 bound periodical volumes. **Subscriptions:** 300 journals and other serials.

★10588★ OTTAWA GENERAL HOSPITAL
MEDICAL LIBRARY
501 Smyth Rd.
Ottawa, ON, Canada K1H 8L6   Phone: (613) 737-8530
Francine Ryan, Supv.
Subjects: Medicine. **Holdings:** 994 books; 3000 bound periodical volumes. **Subscriptions:** 245 journals and other serials.

★10589★ OTTAWA REGIONAL CANCER CENTRE
LIBRARY
190 Melrose Ave.
Ottawa, ON, Canada K1Y 4K7   Phone: (613) 725-6277
Anne LeBrun, Libn.
Subjects: Cancer, palliative care. Holdings: 950 books, 1500 bound periodical volumes. Subscriptions: 325 journals and other serials.

★10590★ RIVERSIDE HOSPITAL
SCOBIE MEMORIAL LIBRARY
1967 Riverside Dr.
Ottawa, ON, Canada K1H 7W9   Phone: (613) 738-8230
Jean E. White, Libn.
Subjects: Medicine, nursing, hospital administration. Holdings: 1000 books; 500 bound periodical volumes; 200 videotapes and cassettes. Subscriptions: 175 journals and other serials.

★10591★ ST. VINCENT HOSPITAL
LIBRARY/AV SERVICES
60 Cambridge St.
Ottawa, ON, Canada K1R 7A5   Phone: (613) 233-4041
Anita Beausoleil, Dir.
Subjects: Gerontology, physiotherapy, occupational therapy, speech and hearing therapy, longterm care, rehabilitation, research, head injuries. Holdings: 4500 books; 50 unbound documents; 8 VF drawers; 118 video cassettes; 26 slide kits; 21 filmstrip kits; 95 audio cassettes; government documents, catalogs, and theses on microfiche. Subscriptions: 271 journals and other serials.

★10592★ TRAFFIC INJURY RESEARCH FOUNDATION OF CANADA
LIBRARY
171 Nepean St., 6th Fl.
Ottawa, ON, Canada K2P 0B4   Phone: (613) 238-5235
Subjects: Road safety - behavioral, medical, pharmacological, statistical. Holdings: 800 books; 100 bound periodical volumes; 4500 technical reports, statistics reports, government publications, newsletters. Subscriptions: 53 journals and other serials.

★10593★ UNIVERSITY OF OTTAWA
HEALTH SCIENCES LIBRARY
451 Smyth Rd., No. 1020
Ottawa, ON, Canada K1H 8M4   Phone: (613) 787-6431
Myra Owen, Dir.
Subjects: Medicine, nursing, kinanthropology, physiotherapy, human kinetics. Holdings: 46,151 books; 47,044 bound periodical volumes; 540 filmstrips; 250 video cassettes; 685 audio cassettes. Subscriptions: 1301 journals and other serials.

★10594★ THE GREY BRUCE REGIONAL HEALTH CENTRE
HEALTH SCIENCES LIBRARY
1400 8th St., E.
PO Box 1400
Owen Sound, ON, Canada N4K 6M9   Phone: (519) 376-2121
Vicky Duncan, Hea.Sci.Libn.
Subjects: Medicine, nursing, psychiatry, psychology, allied health sciences, patient education. Holdings: 2100 books; 77 government documents. Subscriptions: 210 journals and other serials.

★10595★ PRINCE EDWARD HEIGHTS
RESIDENT RECORDS LIBRARY
Box 440
Picton, ON, Canada K0K 2T0   Phone: (613) 476-2104
Cindy Renaud, Libn.
Subjects: Mental retardation, psychology, medicine, pharmacy, social work, management. Holdings: 730 volumes; 93 files of reference material; 2 educational kits. Subscriptions: 34 journals and other serials.

★10596★ ETOBICOKE GENERAL HOSPITAL
MEDICAL LIBRARY
101 Humber College Blvd.
Rexdale, ON, Canada M9V 1R8   Phone: (416) 744-3334
Joyce Gitt, Lib.Techn.
Subjects: Medicine, allied health sciences. Holdings: 3700 books; 178 bound periodical volumes. Subscriptions: 96 journals and other serials.

★10597★ HUMBER COLLEGE OF APPLIED ARTS AND TECHNOLOGY
LIBRARY
SPECIAL COLLECTIONS
205 Humber College Blvd.
Rexdale, ON, Canada M9W 5L7   Phone: (416) 675-3111
K.R. (Vihari) Hivale, Dir.
Subjects: Horsemanship, mortuary science, Canadiana, horticulture. Holdings: 134,650 volumes; 6231 AV items. Subscriptions: 1000 journals and other serials; 13 newspapers.

★10598★ YORK CENTRAL HOSPITAL
DOUGLAS STORMS MEMORIAL LIBRARY
10 Trench St.
Richmond Hill, ON, Canada L4C 4Z3   Phone: (416) 883-2018
Kathy Dedrick, Mgr.
Subjects: Medicine, nursing, and allied health sciences. Holdings: 1500 books. Subscriptions: 142 journals and other serials.

★10599★ NIAGARA COLLEGE OF APPLIED ARTS AND TECHNOLOGY
LEARNING RESOURCE CENTRE
178 Queenston St.
St. Catharines, ON, Canada L2R 2Z7   Phone: (416) 688-5310
Maria Edelman, Libn.
Subjects: Nursing, medicine, psychology, social sciences, anatomy and physiology, biological sciences. Holdings: 3200 books; 360 bound periodical volumes; 1300 AV programs. Subscriptions: 85 journals and other serials.

★10600★ ST. CATHARINES GENERAL HOSPITAL
HEALTH SCIENCES LIBRARY
142 Queenston St.
St. Catharines, ON, Canada L2R 7C6   Phone: (416) 684-7271
Susan P. Armbrust, Libn.
Subjects: Medicine, nursing, laboratory and business administration. Holdings: 1000 books; 100 bound periodical volumes; audiotapes; vertical files. Subscriptions: 152 journals and other serials.

★10601★ SHAVER HOSPITAL
HEALTH SCIENCES LIBRARY
541 Glenridge Ave.
St. Catharines, ON, Canada L2R 6S5   Phone: (416) 685-1381
Ruth Servos, Dir., Hea.Rec./Lib.
Subjects: Medicine, nursing, palliative care, geriatrics, and allied health sciences. Holdings: 3000 books; 300 bound periodical volumes; manuscripts; reports and clippings. Subscriptions: 52 journals and other serials.

★10602★ ST. THOMAS PSYCHIATRIC HOSPITAL
LIBRARY SERVICES
Box 2004
St. Thomas, ON, Canada N5P 3V9   Phone: (519) 631-8510
Jean Heriot, Libn.
Subjects: Psychiatry, psychology, medicine, nursing, allied health professions. Holdings: 6000 books; 4000 bound periodical volumes; 250 videotapes. Subscriptions: 175 journals and other serials; 5 newspapers.

★10603★ PLUMMER MEMORIAL PUBLIC HOSPITAL
LIBRARY
969 Queen St., E.
Sault Ste. Marie, ON, Canada P6A 2C4   Phone: (705) 759-3434
Kathy You, Dir., Lib.Serv.
Subjects: Medicine, nursing, allied health sciences, management, psychiatry, social work, sexual assault treatment, psychogeriatrics. Holdings: 1000 books. Subscriptions: 120 journals and other serials.

★10604★ SAULT STE. MARIE GENERAL HOSPITAL
HEALTH SCIENCES LIBRARY
941 Queen St., E.
Sault Ste. Marie, ON, Canada P6A 2B8   Phone: (705) 759-3333
Elizabeth Iles, Dir., Lib.Serv.
Subjects: Medicine, nursing, hospital administration. Holdings: 1000 books; unbound journals kept for 10 years. Subscriptions: 100 journals and other serials.

★10605★ CANADA
HEALTH AND WELFARE CANADA
HEALTH PROTECTION BRANCH
REGIONAL LIBRARY
2301 Midland Ave.
Scarborough, ON, Canada M1P 4R7   Phone: (604) 666-3350
S. Brockhurst, Lib.Techn.
Subjects: Food analysis, food and drug legislation, microbiology, chemistry, pharmacology, toxicology, cosmetics, pesticides, narcotics. **Holdings:** 2500 books; 212 bound periodical volumes. **Subscriptions:** 97 journals and other serials.

★10606★ CENTENARY HOSPITAL
C.D. FARQUHARSON HEALTH SCIENCES LIBRARY
2867 Ellesmere Rd.
Scarborough, ON, Canada M1E 4B9   Phone: (416) 284-8131
Vadla Poplak, Hd.Libn.
Subjects: Medicine, pediatrics, surgery, obstetrics, gynecology, anesthesia, psychology. **Holdings:** 1500 books. **Subscriptions:** 100 journals and other serials.

★10607★ CENTENNIAL COLLEGE OF APPLIED ARTS AND
     TECHNOLOGY
WARDEN WOODS CAMPUS RESOURCE CENTRE
Sta. A, PO Box 631
Scarborough, ON, Canada M1K 5E9   Phone: (416) 694-3241
Ron Wood, Dir.
Subjects: Nursing, social sciences and humanities, travel, fashion, early childhood education, social services. **Holdings:** 32,411 volumes. **Subscriptions:** 230 periodicals.

★10608★ SCARBOROUGH CITY HEALTH DEPARTMENT
HEALTH RESOURCE CENTRE
JEAN CREW DEEKS MEMORIAL LIBRARY
305 Milner Ave., Ste. 510
Scarborough, ON, Canada M1B 3V4   Phone: (416) 396-7453
Dianne Beal, Libn.
Subjects: Nursing; prenatal, maternal, and child care; psychology; geriatrics; nutrition. **Holdings:** 1500 books; 500 studies and reports; 100 posters; 700 pamphlet titles; 100 audio cassettes; 80 videotapes; 40 resource kits. **Subscriptions:** 82 journals and other serials.

★10609★ SCARBOROUGH GENERAL HOSPITAL
HEALTH SCIENCES LIBRARY
3050 Lawrence Ave., E.
Scarborough, ON, Canada M1P 2V5   Phone: (416) 431-8114
Helvi Thomas, Libn.
Subjects: Health sciences. **Holdings:** 1900 books; 85 bound periodical volumes. **Subscriptions:** 200 journals and other serials.

★10610★ ONTARIO MINISTRY OF COMMUNITY AND
     SOCIAL SERVICES
RIDEAU REGIONAL CENTRE
STAFF LIBRARY AND INFORMATION CENTRE
PO Box 2000
Smiths Falls, ON, Canada K7A 4T7   Phone: (613) 283-5533
Pat Kiteley, Lib.Techn.
Subjects: Mental retardation, psychology, social work, medicine. **Holdings:** 4000 books. **Subscriptions:** 127 journals and other serials.

★10611★ MCNEIL PHARMACEUTICAL LTD.
LIBRARY
PO Box 600
Stouffville, ON, Canada L4A 7X7   Phone: (416) 640-6900
Karen Connell, Libn.
Subjects: Medicine, pharmaceuticals, marketing, business, chemistry. **Holdings:** 1000 books; 20 VF drawers of documents. **Subscriptions:** 302 journals and other serials.

★10612★ CAMBRIAN COLLEGE OF APPLIED ARTS AND
     TECHNOLOGY
LEARNING RESOURCES CENTRE
1400 Barrydowne Rd., Sta. A
Sudbury, ON, Canada P3A 3V8   Phone: (705) 566-8101
Mr. Chris Bartlett, Dir., LRC
Subjects: Science, technology, business, health sciences, applied arts, industrial training, support programs. **Holdings:** 35,682 books; 4543 bound periodical volumes; 44 VF drawers of pamphlets and clippings; 4346

microfiche; 1775 recordings; 187 film loops; 450 films; 514 filmstrips; 221 kits; 115 reels of microfilm; 937 scores; 132 slide sets; 2032 videotapes; 4678 uncataloged government publications, including 3210 Statistics Canada publications. **Subscriptions:** 644 journals and other serials; 17 newspapers.

★10613★ LAURENTIAN HOSPITAL
MEDICAL LIBRARY
41 Ramsey Lake Rd.
Sudbury, ON, Canada P3E 5J1   Phone: (705) 522-2200
Rannah Brosseau, Libn.
Subjects: Medicine, allied health sciences. **Holdings:** 1000 books; 5000 bound periodical volumes; 250 cassettes; 35 video cassettes. **Subscriptions:** 120 journals and other serials.

★10614★ SUDBURY GENERAL HOSPITAL
HOSPITAL LIBRARY
700 Paris St., Sta. B
Sudbury, ON, Canada P3E 3B5   Phone: (705) 674-3181
D.M. Hawryliuk, Libn.
Subjects: Clinical medicine. **Holdings:** 1200 books; 1300 bound periodical volumes. **Subscriptions:** 145 journals and other serials.

★10615★ CONFEDERATION COLLEGE OF APPLIED ARTS
     AND TECHNOLOGY
CHALLIS RESOURCE CENTRE
Box 398, Sta. F
Thunder Bay, ON, Canada P7C 4W1   Phone: (807) 475-6241
Laraine Tapak, Dir.
Subjects: Applied arts, business, technology, health sciences, distance education. **Holdings:** 34,000 books; 10,000 AV programs. **Subscriptions:** 600 journals and other serials; 50 newspapers.

★10616★ HOGARTH-WESTMOUNT HOSPITAL
STAFF LIBRARY
300 N. Lillie St.
Thunder Bay, ON, Canada P7C 4Y7   Phone: (807) 625-1110
Kathy Deguns, Libn.
Subjects: Long term care, geriatrics, rehabilitation. **Holdings:** 800 books. **Subscriptions:** 112 journals and other serials.

★10617★ ONTARIO MINISTRY OF LABOUR
RESOURCE CENTRE FOR OCCUPATIONAL HEALTH AND
     SAFETY
Lakehead University
Oliver Rd.
Thunder Bay, ON, Canada P7B 5E1   Phone: (807) 343-8128
Shann Brown, Info/Educ.Off.
Subjects: Hazardous substances, occupational health, toxicology, radiation, noise, health services. **Holdings:** 800 books; 1500 reprints in 4 VF drawers; 25 videotapes; 4 slide programs. **Subscriptions:** 51 journals and other serials.

★10618★ ST. JOSEPH'S GENERAL HOSPITAL
LIBRARY
PO Box 3251
Thunder Bay, ON, Canada P7B 5G7   Phone: (807) 343-2431
Ms. Wright, Libn.
Subjects: Medicine, nursing, management, rehabilitation, ethics. **Holdings:** 800 books. **Subscriptions:** 42 journals and other serials.

★10619★ ACADEMY OF MEDICINE, TORONTO
WILLIAM BOYD LIBRARY
288 Bloor St., W.
Toronto, ON, Canada M5S 1V8   Phone: (416) 964-7088
Sheila Swanson, Libn.
Subjects: Clinical medicine, history of medicine. **Holdings:** 40,000 books; 40,000 bound periodical volumes; 10,000 pamphlets, reports, and reprints. **Subscriptions:** 600 journals and other serials.

★10620★ ADDICTION RESEARCH FOUNDATION
LIBRARY
33 Russell St.
Toronto, ON, Canada M5S 2S1   Phone: (416) 595-6144
Subjects: Alcoholism and drug abuse. **Holdings:** 14,500 books; 12,500 reprints; 250 films. **Subscriptions:** 450 journals.

★10621★   BAYCREST CENTRE FOR GERIATRIC CARE
STAFF LIBRARY
3560 Bathurst Ave.
Toronto, ON, Canada M6A 2E1   Phone: (416) 789-5131
Madeline Grant, Mgr., Lib.Serv.
Subjects: Geriatrics, geriatric psychiatry and nursing, gerontology, medical sciences, hospital administration. **Holdings:** 2000 books; 950 bound periodical volumes; article files; 60 video cassettes; 300 audio cassettes; VF materials; Baycrest publications; government documents. **Subscriptions:** 220 journals and other serials.

★10622★   C.M. HINCKS TREATMENT CENTER
C.M. HINCKS INSTITUTE
JACKMAN LIBRARY
440 Jarvis St.
Toronto, ON, Canada M4Y 2H4   Phone: (416) 972-1935
Mary W. Smith, Libn.
Subjects: Child and adolescent psychiatry and psychology, child development and care, social work, family therapy. **Holdings:** 1600 books; 700 bound periodical volumes; VF drawers; reprints; bibliographies. **Subscriptions:** 69 journals and other serials.

★10623★   CANADIAN DIABETES ASSOCIATION
NATIONAL OFFICE ARCHIVES
78 Bond St.
Toronto, ON, Canada M5B 2J8   Phone: (416) 362-4440
Marian Cooke, Libn.-Archv.
Subjects: Diabetes. **Holdings:** 50 books; association minutes and annual reports; pamphlets; films; cassettes; scrapbooks.

★10624★   CANADIAN FOUNDATION FOR CHILDREN, YOUTH AND THE LAW
JUSTICE FOR CHILDREN AND YOUTH RESOURCE CENTRE
720 Spadina Ave., Ste. 405
Toronto, ON, Canada M5S 2T9   Phone: (416) 920-1633
Marie A. Irvine, Exec.Dir.
Subjects: Children's rights and legal representation, education, child welfare and abuse, medical and foster care, family law. **Holdings:** 2000 books; 355 bound periodical volumes; clipping files; subject files; government reports; organization information files; government documents. **Subscriptions:** 230 journals and other serials.

★10625★   CANADIAN HEARING SOCIETY
LIBRARY
271 Spadina Rd.
Toronto, ON, Canada M5R 2V3   Phone: (416) 964-9595
Marion Baker, Libn.
Subjects: Hearing impairment, education of the deaf, social work and rehabilitation in the field of hearing loss. **Holdings:** 600 books; 3 VF drawers of reports and reprints. **Subscriptions:** 22 journals and other serials.

★10626★   CANADIAN MEMORIAL CHIROPRACTIC COLLEGE
C.C. CLEMMER HEALTH SCIENCES LIBRARY
1900 Bayview Ave.
Toronto, ON, Canada M4G 3E6   Phone: (416) 482-2340
Marilyn E. Schafer, Dir., Lib.Serv.
Subjects: Chiropractic, orthopedics, sports medicine, nutrition, radiology, neurology. **Holdings:** 12,000 books; 5500 bound periodical volumes; 5600 reprints; 25,667 slides; 401 slide-tape presentations; 540 x-ray transparencies; 1098 audio cassettes; 354 video cassettes; 81 videotapes; 69 films; 36 phonograph records; 25 charts; 27 anatomical models; 20 computer assisted instructions (CAI). **Subscriptions:** 419 journals and other serials.

★10627★   CANADIAN NATIONAL INSTITUTE FOR THE BLIND
NATIONAL LIBRARY SERVICES
1929 Bayview Ave.
Toronto, ON, Canada M4G 3E8   Phone: (416) 480-7520
Helen Perry, Exec.Dir.
Subjects: General and scholarly topics. **Holdings:** 10,000 titles in braille; 14,000 titles on audiotape. **Subscriptions:** 62 journals and other serials in braille and on tape.

★10628★   CLARKE INSTITUTE OF PSYCHIATRY
FARRAR LIBRARY
250 College St.
Toronto, ON, Canada M5T 1R8   Phone: (416) 979-6820
Diane Thomas, Hd., Lib.Serv.
Subjects: Psychiatry, psychology, psychiatric nursing, neuroendocrinology, neurochemistry, occupational therapy, social work. **Holdings:** 6500 books; 6500 bound periodical volumes; 10 VF drawers of reprints; 12 VF drawers of staff publications; 2 VF drawers of government documents. **Subscriptions:** 350 journals and other serials.

★10629★   DOCTORS HOSPITAL
HEALTH SCIENCES LIBRARY
340 College St., 6th Fl.
Toronto, ON, Canada M5T 3A9   Phone: (416) 963-5464
Sharon Virtue, Mgr./Libn.
Subjects: Clinical medicine, nursing, hospital administration. **Holdings:** 1500 books; 500 cassettes. **Subscriptions:** 250 journals and other serials; 2 newspapers.

★10630★   GEORGE BROWN COLLEGE OF APPLIED ARTS AND TECHNOLOGY
LIBRARY
Box 1015, Sta. B
Toronto, ON, Canada M5T 2T9   Phone: (416) 944-4632
John L. Hardy, Assoc.Dir., Educ.Rsrcs.
Subjects: Engineering and architectural technology, nursing, business and commerce, food technology, fashion technology, child care, addiction counselling. **Holdings:** 89,969 books; 1600 bound periodical volumes; 900 films; 180 meters of archival materials. **Subscriptions:** 493 journals and other serials; 6 newspapers.

★10631★   GLAXO CANADA, LTD.
LIBRARY INFORMATION CENTRE
1025 The Queensway
Toronto, ON, Canada M8Z 5S6   Phone: (416) 252-2281
Shirley Atha, Info.Ctr.Coord.
Subjects: Pharmacology, medicine, pharmacy, chemistry, microbiology. **Holdings:** 700 books. **Subscriptions:** 120 journals and other serials.

★10632★   HOSPITAL FOR SICK CHILDREN
HOSPITAL LIBRARY
555 University Ave.
Toronto, ON, Canada M5G 1X8   Phone: (416) 598-6693
Deirdre Green, Libn.
Subjects: Pediatrics. **Holdings:** 7500 books; 25,000 periodical volumes. **Subscriptions:** 626 journals and other serials.

★10633★   HUGH MACMILLAN REHABILITATION CENTRE
HEALTH SCIENCES LIBRARY
350 Rumsey Rd.
Toronto, ON, Canada M4G 1R8   Phone: (416) 425-6220
Miss Pui-Ying Wong, Libn.
Subjects: Rehabilitation, disability, pediatrics, biomedical engineering. **Holdings:** 2000 books; 600 bound periodical volumes. **Subscriptions:** 130 journals and other serials.

★10634★   INDUSTRIAL ACCIDENT PREVENTION ASSOCIATION
INFORMATION CENTRE
2 Bloor St., W., 31st Fl.
Toronto, ON, Canada M4W 3N8   Phone: (416) 965-8888
Dolores Harms Penner, Mgr.
Subjects: Accident prevention, occupational health and safety. **Holdings:** 8000 books and reports. **Subscriptions:** 400 journals and other serials.

★10635★   LYNDHURST HOSPITAL
HEALTH SCIENCES LIBRARY
520 Sutherland Dr.
Toronto, ON, Canada M4G 3V9   Phone: (416) 422-5551
Ann Marie Chin, Dir.
Subjects: Spinal cord injuries, neurological disabilities, rehabilitation and physical medicine. **Holdings:** 400 books; 130 bound periodical volumes; 60 staff research publications. **Subscriptions:** 75 journals and other serials.

★10636★ METROPOLITAN TORONTO REFERENCE LIBRARY
AUDIO VISUAL SERVICES DEPARTMENT
789 Yonge St.
Toronto, ON, Canada M4W 2G8   Phone: (416) 393-7110
Laura Murray, Mgr.
Subjects: Disabled. Holdings: 9000 16mm films; 1000 videotapes. Subscriptions: 135 journals and other serials.

★10637★ METROPOLITAN TORONTO REFERENCE LIBRARY
SCIENCE AND TECHNOLOGY DEPARTMENT
789 Yonge St.
Toronto, ON, Canada M4W 2G8   Phone: (416) 393-7090
Jean Forde, Mgr.
Subjects: Physical, biological, and medical sciences; engineering sciences; natural history; horticulture; technology and food technology; cookery; sports and recreation. Holdings: 125,250 books; 5982 volumes of Canadian, American, and British patent abstracts; 12,000 volumes of standards; 4250 volumes of Canadian and American radio, television, and personal computer schematics; 7956 VF folders; 4019 maps; 5000 automotive shop manuals; 1250 cookbooks. Subscriptions: 1256 journals and other serials.

★10638★ MICHENER INSTITUTE FOR APPLIED HEALTH
TECHNOLOGY
LIBRARY
222 St. Patrick St.
Toronto, ON, Canada M5T 1V4   Phone: (416) 596-3123
Ray Banks, Libn.
Subjects: Medical technology - laboratory, radiological, respiratory; nuclear medicine; cytotechnology; cytogenetics; cardiovascular perfusion; neonatology; chiropody. Holdings: 15,000 books; 200 bound periodical volumes; 250 slide/tape programs; 96 slide programs; 30 16mm films; 250 videotapes; 73 filmstrips. Subscriptions: 215 journals and other serials.

★10639★ MOUNT SINAI HOSPITAL
SIDNEY LISWOOD LIBRARY
600 University Ave.
Toronto, ON, Canada M5G 1X5   Phone: (416) 586-4614
Linda Devore, Dir., Lib.Serv.
Subjects: Health sciences. Holdings: 2000 books. Subscriptions: 400 serials.

★10640★ ONTARIO CANCER INSTITUTE
LIBRARY
500 Sherbourne St.
Toronto, ON, Canada M4X 1K9   Phone: (416) 926-4482
Carol A. Morrison, Libn.
Subjects: Cancer, radiotherapy, biophysics. Holdings: 7000 books; 10,000 bound periodical volumes; pamphlets. Subscriptions: 375 journals and other serials.

★10641★ ONTARIO MEDICAL ASSOCIATION
LIBRARY
250 Bloor St., E., Ste. 600
Toronto, ON, Canada M4W 3P8   Phone: (416) 963-9383
Jan Greenwood, Mgr. of Lib.Serv.
Subjects: Canadian medical economics, medico-legal practices and sociomedical affairs, hospital library service. Holdings: 2000 books. Subscriptions: 250 journals and other serials.

★10642★ ONTARIO MINISTRY OF COMMUNITY AND
SOCIAL SERVICES
LIBRARY AND LEARNING RESOURCES
880 Bay St., 5th Fl.
Toronto, ON, Canada M7A 1E9   Phone: (416) 965-2300
Dolly E. Lyn, Mgr., Lib. & LRC
Subjects: Adolescence, adoption, aged, public welfare, developmentally disabled, child abuse, child welfare, physically handicapped, rehabilitation, social problems, social work, juvenile delinquency, personnel management, career development. Holdings: 35,000 books; 1000 bound periodical volumes; 500 reels of microfilm; 18,000 microfiche; 300 audio cassettes; 200 video cassettes; 1500 reprints. Subscriptions: 450 journals and newsletters.

★10643★ ONTARIO MINISTRY OF HEALTH
LIBRARY
15 Overlea Blvd., 1st Fl.
Toronto, ON, Canada M4H 1A9   Phone: (416) 965-7881
Veronica Brunka, Lib.Supv.
Subjects: Public health, preventive medicine, health care services, hospital administration. Holdings: 9000 books; 25 VF drawers; 400 microfiche. Subscriptions: 1100 journals and other serials.

★10644★ ONTARIO MINISTRY OF HEALTH
PUBLIC HEALTH LABORATORIES
LIBRARY
Box 9000, Postal Terminal A
Toronto, ON, Canada M5W 1R5   Phone: (416) 235-5935
Doris A. Standing, Libn.
Subjects: Medical microbiology, medical laboratory technology. Holdings: 3500 volumes; 3 VF drawers of pamphlets. Subscriptions: 135 journals and other serials.

★10645★ ONTARIO NURSES ASSOCIATION
ONA LIBRARY
85 Grenville St., Ste. 600
Toronto, ON, Canada M5S 3A2   Phone: (416) 964-8833
Victoria Scott, Libn.
Subjects: Industrial relations, nursing, occupational health and safety, medical and health care. Holdings: 3000 books; 200 bound periodical volumes; 4 drawers of ONA archives; 15 VF drawers of nursing and industrial relations materials; 1 drawer of news clippings. Subscriptions: 204 journals and other serials.

★10646★ ORTHOPAEDIC AND ARTHRITIC HOSPITAL
HEALTH SCIENCES LIBRARY
43 Wellesley St., E.
Toronto, ON, Canada M4Y 1H1   Phone: (416) 967-8545
Sheila M. Lethbridge, Libn.
Subjects: Orthopedics, arthritis, physical and occupational therapy. Holdings: 1000 books; 550 bound periodical volumes. Subscriptions: 80 journals and other serials.

★10647★ QUEEN STREET MENTAL HEALTH CENTRE
HEALTH SCIENCES LIBRARY
1001 Queen St., W.
Toronto, ON, Canada M6J 1H4   Phone: (416) 535-8501
Mary Ann Georges, Staff Libn.
Subjects: Psychiatry, psychology, nursing, psychopharmacology, sociology, administration, rehabilitation. Holdings: 3000 books; 3000 bound periodical volumes; 50 theses; 150 AV cassettes; 4 VF drawers. Subscriptions: 185 journals and other serials.

★10648★ REGISTERED NURSES' ASSOCIATION OF ONTARIO
RESOURCE CENTRE
33 Price St.
Toronto, ON, Canada M4W 1Z2   Phone: (416) 923-3523
Subjects: Nursing, health. Holdings: 2000 books; 258 bound periodical volumes; 8 VF drawers of reports. Subscriptions: 50 journals and other serials.

★10649★ ST. JOSEPH'S HEALTH CENTRE
GEORGE PENNAL LIBRARY
30 The Queensway
Toronto, ON, Canada M6R 1B5   Phone: (416) 530-6726
Barbara Iwasiuk, Med.Libn.
Subjects: Medicine, nursing, hospital administration, pastoral care. Holdings: 3500 books; 3000 bound periodical volumes. Subscriptions: 172 journals and other serials.

★10650★ ST. MICHAEL'S HOSPITAL
HEALTH SCIENCE LIBRARY/ARCHIVES
30 Bond St.
Toronto, ON, Canada M5B 1W8   Phone: (416) 864-5059
Anita Wong, Dir.
Subjects: Medicine and surgery. Holdings: 8300 books; 12,900 bound periodical volumes; reprints of staff publications. Subscriptions: 500 journals and other serials.

★10651★ TORONTO EAST GENERAL AND ORTHOPAEDIC
HOSPITAL
HEALTH SCIENCES LIBRARY
825 Coxwell Ave.
Toronto, ON, Canada M4C 3E7   Phone: (416) 469-6011
Glenda West, Libn.
Subjects: Medicine, nursing, allied health sciences. Holdings: 1750 books. Subscriptions: 175 journals and other serials.

★10652★   TORONTO GENERAL HOSPITAL
FUDGER MEDICAL LIBRARY
200 Elizabeth St.
Toronto, ON, Canada M5G 2C4
Jennifer Bayne, Chf.Libn.   Phone: (416) 595-3429
Subjects: Cardiovascular surgery, obstetrics and gynecology, psychiatry, dermatology, neurosurgery, family and community medicine. **Holdings:** 8000 books; 15,000 bound periodical volumes; cassettes; tapes. **Subscriptions:** 472 journals and other serials.

★10653★   TORONTO WESTERN HOSPITAL
R.C. LAIRD HEALTH SCIENCES LIBRARY
399 Bathurst St.
Toronto, ON, Canada M5T 2S8
Elizabeth A. Reid, Dir.   Phone: (416) 369-5750
Subjects: Medicine. **Holdings:** 2000 books; 10,000 bound periodical volumes; 100 AV kits. **Subscriptions:** 375 journals and other serials.

★10654★   UNIVERSITY OF TORONTO
A.E. MACDONALD OPHTHALMIC LIBRARY
1 Spadina Crescent, Rm.116
Toronto, ON, Canada M5S 2J5
Elizabeth A. Le Ber   Phone: (416) 978-2635
Subjects: Ophthalmology. **Holdings:** 1250 volumes; 750 bound periodical volumes; reprints of publications by Ophthalmology Department members, 1950 to present. **Subscriptions:** 40 journals and other serials.

★10655★   UNIVERSITY OF TORONTO
BANTING AND BEST DEPARTMENT OF MEDICAL RESEARCH LIBRARY
Best Institute, Rm. 304
112 College St.
Toronto, ON, Canada M5G 1L6
Colin Savage   Phone: (416) 978-2588
Subjects: Medicine, physiology, diabetes, insulin, anticoagulants, lipid metabolism. **Holdings:** 7814 volumes. **Subscriptions:** 32 journals and other serials.

★10656★   UNIVERSITY OF TORONTO
FACULTY OF DENTISTRY LIBRARY
124 Edward St., Rm. 267
Toronto, ON, Canada M5G 1G6
Susan Goddard, Fac.Libn.   Phone: (416) 979-4560
Subjects: Dentistry, medicine, health sciences. **Holdings:** 24,522 books and bound periodical volumes; 403 microforms; 72 videotapes; 128 slide/tape sets; 10.5 linear feet of clippings, pamphlets, and other vertical file materials. **Subscriptions:** 194 journals and other serials.

★10657★   UNIVERSITY OF TORONTO
FACULTY OF PHARMACY
R.O. HURST LIBRARY
25 Russell St.
Toronto, ON, Canada M5S 1A1
Thomasin Adams-Webber, Libn.   Phone: (416) 978-2872
Subjects: Pharmacy, chemistry, history of pharmacy and medicine. **Holdings:** 9775 volumes. **Subscriptions:** 122 journals and other serials.

★10658★   UNIVERSITY OF TORONTO
GENERAL LIBRARY
SCIENCE AND MEDICINE DEPARTMENT
Toronto, ON, Canada M5S 1A5
Ms. G. Heaton, Hd.   Phone: (416) 978-2284
Subjects: Technology (excluding engineering), science, medicine, nursing, anatomy, food sciences, bacteriology, industrial hygiene. **Holdings:** 662,950 volumes; 83,637 microforms. **Subscriptions:** 3231 journals and other serials.

★10659★   UNIVERSITY OF TORONTO
PATHOLOGY LIBRARY
Banting Institute, Rms. 108-109
100 College St.
Toronto, ON, Canada M5G 1L5
Sophia Duda, Libn.   Phone: (416) 978-2558
Subjects: Pathology, immunology, bacteriology. **Holdings:** 4163 volumes. **Subscriptions:** 71 journals and other serials.

★10660★   WELLESLEY HOSPITAL
LIBRARY
160 Wellesley St., E.
Toronto, ON, Canada M4Y 1J3
Verla E. Empey, Dir.   Phone: (416) 926-7071
Subjects: Medicine, nursing, and hospital administration. **Holdings:** 10,000 books; 8000 bound periodical volumes; 1 VF drawer of bibliographies; 2 VF drawers of staff publications; 200 AV programs; 4 VF drawers. **Subscriptions:** 400 journals and other serials.

★10661★   WEST PARK HOSPITAL
HEALTH DISCIPLINES LIBRARY
82 Buttonwood Ave.
Toronto, ON, Canada M6M 2J5
Lois Elliott, Libn.   Phone: (416) 243-3600
Subjects: Medicine, nursing, and allied health sciences, including geriatrics, social services, administration, and rehabilitation. **Holdings:** 600 books; patient records, journals, and other early material on treatment of tuberculosis. **Subscriptions:** 71 journals and other serials.

★10662★   WOMEN'S COLLEGE HOSPITAL
MEDICAL LIBRARY
76 Grenville St.
Toronto, ON, Canada M5S 1B2
Margaret Robins, Dir.   Phone: (416) 323-6078
Subjects: Dermatology, diabetes, perinatal medicine, obstetrics, gynecology, high risk pregnancy. **Holdings:** 4000 books; 4200 periodical volumes; 500 video cassettes. **Subscriptions:** 260 journals and other serials.

★10663★   NIAGARA COLLEGE OF APPLIED ARTS AND TECHNOLOGY
LEARNING RESOURCE CENTRE
Woodlawn Rd.
Box 1005
Welland, ON, Canada L3B 5S2
P. Labonte, Libn.   Phone: (416) 735-2211
Subjects: Applied arts, business, technology, health. **Holdings:** 35,000 books; 3000 AV programs. **Subscriptions:** 440 journals and other serials; 13 newspapers.

★10664★   HUMBER MEMORIAL HOSPITAL
HEALTH SCIENCES LIBRARY
200 Church St.
Weston, ON, Canada M9N 1N8
M. Dorbolo, Libn.   Phone: (416) 243-4597
Subjects: Medicine, nursing, and allied health sciences. **Holdings:** Figures not available.

★10665★   CONNAUGHT LABORATORIES, LTD.
BALMER NEILLY LIBRARY
1755 Steeles Ave., W.
Willowdale, ON, Canada M2R 3T4
Hugh McNaught, Libn.   Phone: (416) 667-2662
Subjects: Immunology, virology, bacteriology. **Holdings:** 23,000 volumes. **Subscriptions:** 250 journals and other serials.

★10666★   NORTH YORK GENERAL HOSPITAL
W. KEITH WELSH LIBRARY
4001 Leslie St.
Willowdale, ON, Canada M2K 1E1
Marjory L. Morphy, Mgr., Lib.Serv.   Phone: (416) 756-6142
Subjects: Medicine, nursing, administration. **Holdings:** 2400 books; 100 audio cassettes; 1 file drawer of government documents. **Subscriptions:** 300 journals and other serials.

★10667★   BULIMIA ANOREXIA NERVOSA ASSOCIATION
LIBRARY
c/o Psychological Services
University of Windsor
401 Sunset Ave.
Windsor, ON, Canada N9B 3P4
Mary Kaye Lucier, M.S.W.   Phone: (519) 253-7545
Subjects: Eating disorders, stress management, assertiveness. **Holdings:** 100 books; 50 AV programs. **Subscriptions:** 2 journals and other serials; 46 newsletters.

★10668★ CANADIAN MENTAL HEALTH ASSOCIATION
WINDSOR-ESSEX COUNTY BRANCH LIBRARY
880 Ouellette Ave., Ste. 901
Windsor, ON, Canada N9A 1C7   Phone: (519) 255-7440
Patricia Hayward, Mgr., Educ. & Prevention
Subjects: Bereavement, mental health, stress. **Holdings:** 500 books; 40 AV programs. **Subscriptions:** 5 journals and other serials.

★10669★ HOTEL-DIEU OF ST. JOSEPH HOSPITAL
MEDICAL LIBRARY
1030 Ouellette Ave.
Windsor, ON, Canada N9A 1E1   Phone: (519) 973-4444
Toni Janik, Libn.
Subjects: Medicine and allied health sciences. **Holdings:** 400 books; 2000 bound periodical volumes; 15 slide/tape programs; 30 video cassettes; 100 vertical files. **Subscriptions:** 300 journals and other serials.

★10670★ METROPOLITAN GENERAL HOSPITAL
MEDICAL LIBRARY
1995 Lens Ave.
Windsor, ON, Canada N8W 1L9   Phone: (519) 254-1661
Patricia Black, Med.Libn.
Subjects: Medicine, nursing. **Holdings:** 600 books. **Subscriptions:** 200.

★10671★ SALVATION ARMY GRACE HOSPITAL
LIBRARY
339 Crawford Ave.
Windsor, ON, Canada N9A 5C6   Phone: (519) 255-2245
Anna Henshaw, Libn.
Subjects: Medicine, nursing. **Holdings:** 2000 books; 880 bound periodical volumes. **Subscriptions:** 200 journals and other serials.

★10672★ ONTARIO MINISTRY OF COMMUNITY AND
SOCIAL SERVICES
RESOURCE LIBRARY
Hwy. 59 N.
PO Box 310
Woodstock, ON, Canada N4S 7X9   Phone: (519) 539-1251
Rita Thompson, Libn.
Subjects: Mental retardation, epilepsy, tuberculosis. **Holdings:** 800 books; tapes, cassettes. **Subscriptions:** 69 journals and other serials.

Prince Edward Island

★10673★ MEDICAL SOCIETY OF PRINCE EDWARD ISLAND
LIBRARY
559 N. River Rd.
Charlottetown, PE, Canada C1E 1J7   Phone: (902) 368-7303
Marilyn Lowther, Exec.Dir.
Subjects: Medicine - practice and politics. **Holdings:** Archives.

★10674★ QUEEN ELIZABETH HOSPITAL
FRANK J. MACDONALD LIBRARY
PO Box 6600
Charlottetown, PE, Canada C1A 8T5   Phone: (902) 566-6371
Marion K. MacArthur, Libn.
Subjects: Medicine, nursing, allied health sciences, hospital administration. **Holdings:** 500 books; 500 bound periodical volumes. **Subscriptions:** 119 journals and other serials.

★10675★ PRINCE COUNTY HOSPITAL
MEDICAL LIBRARY
259 Beattie Ave.
Summerside, PE, Canada C1N 2A9   Phone: (902) 436-9131
Dr. J.P. Schaefer, Dir.
Subjects: Medicine. **Holdings:** 2000 books; 200 bound periodical volumes. **Subscriptions:** 20 journals and other serials.

Quebec

★10676★ HOTEL-DIEU D'ARTHABASKA
MEDICAL LIBRARY-DOCUMENTATION SERVICE
5 des Hospitalieres
Arthabaska, PQ, Canada G6P 6N2   Phone: (819) 357-1151
Micheline LeClair, Lib.Techn.
Subjects: Health sciences, nursing. **Holdings:** 2630 books; 3366 bound periodical volumes. **Subscriptions:** 94 journals and other serials.

★10677★ CENTRE HOSPITALIER ROBERT-GIFFARD
BIBLIOTHEQUE PROFESSIONNELLE
2601, de la Canardiere
Beauport, PQ, Canada G1J 2G3   Phone: (418) 663-5300
Yolande Plamondon, Techn.
Subjects: Psychiatry, neurology, general medicine, psychology, social sciences, nursing. **Holdings:** 9750 books; 5000 bound periodical volumes; 35 magnetic tapes; 150 video cassettes. **Subscriptions:** 110 journals and other serials.

★10678★ HOPITAL DE CHICOUTIMI INC.
BIBLIOTHEQUE
305, rue St-Vallier
C.P. 5006
Chicoutimi, PQ, Canada G7H 5H6   Phone: (418) 509-2195
Angele Tremblay, Biblio.
Subjects: Medicine, public health. **Holdings:** 6300 books; 9100 bound periodical volumes; 15,000 slides and cassettes. **Subscriptions:** 100 journals and other serials.

★10679★ INSTITUT ROLAND-SAUCIER
BIBLIOTHEQUE MEDICALE
150, rue Pinel
C.P. 2250
Chicoutimi, PQ, Canada G7G 3W4   Phone: (418) 549-5474
Danielle Saucier, Biblio.
Subjects: Clinical psychiatry, mental health, psychopharmacology, psychology, psychiatric social work. **Holdings:** 3500 books; 500 bound periodical volumes. **Subscriptions:** 100 journals and other serials; 21 newspapers.

★10680★ SANDOZ CANADA INC.
BIBLIOTHEQUE/LIBRARY
385 Bouchard Blvd.
Dorval, PQ, Canada H9S 1A9   Phone: (514) 631-6775
Lise Langevin
Subjects: Pharmaceuticals, cardiology, immunology, endocrinology, neurology. **Holdings:** 3250 books; 500 bound periodical volumes; 50,000 microfiche. **Subscriptions:** 300 journals and other serials.

★10681★ QUEBEC PROVINCE OFFICE DES PERSONNES
HANDICAPEES DU QUEBEC
CENTRE DE DOCUMENTATION
C.P. 820
Drummondville, PQ, Canada J2B 6X1   Phone: (819) 477-7100
Sophie Janik, Doc.
Subjects: Handicapped persons - social and vocational integration, adaptation and rehabilitation, deinstitutionalization, impairment, disabilities. **Holdings:** 3500 books; 15 bound periodical volumes; 500 audio cassettes; 4000 other documents; ministry reports; AV programs. **Subscriptions:** 200 journals and other serials; 10 newspapers.

★10682★ CENTRE HOSPITALIER HOTEL-DIEU DE GASPE
CENTRE DE DOCUMENTATION
C.P. 120
Havre de Gaspe, PQ, Canada G0C 1R0   Phone: (418) 368-3301
Mathilda Adams, Resp.
Subjects: Medicine, surgery, pharmacy, radiology, cardiology, nursing, obstetrics. **Holdings:** 1000 books. **Subscriptions:** 85 journals and other serials.

★10683★ CENTRE HOSPITALIER REGIONAL DE
LANAUDIERE
BIBLIOTHEQUE MEDICALE
1000 Ste-Anne Blvd.
Joliette, PQ, Canada J6E 6J2   Phone: (514) 759-8222
Francine Garneau, Biblio.
Subjects: Medicine, psychiatry, addictions, psychology, social work, nurs-

ing, hospital administration. **Holdings:** 15,000 volumes; 393 other cataloged items; 400 cassettes. **Subscriptions:** 250 journals and other serials.

★10684★ **BURROUGHS WELLCOME COMPANY**
MEDICAL INFORMATION CENTER
16751 Trans Canada Rd.
Kirkland, PQ, Canada H9H 4J4   Phone: (514) 694-8220
Georgette Pucser, Libn.
Subjects: Medicine, basic sciences, pharmacy. **Holdings:** 250 books; 2500 unbound periodicals; 15,000 microfiche; 700 binders of medical articles; 200 tape cassettes. **Subscriptions:** 300 journals and other serials; 6 newspapers.

★10685★ **CITE DE LA SANTE DE LAVAL**
CENTRE DE DOCUMENTATION
1755, blvd. Rene Laennec
Laval, PQ, Canada H7M 3L9   Phone: (514) 662-5493
France Pontbriand, Libn.
Subjects: Medicine, nursing, community health. **Holdings:** 4300 books; 4000 bound periodical volumes. **Subscriptions:** 275 journals and other serials.

★10686★ **INSTITUT ARMAND-FRAPPIER**
APPLIED MICROBIOLOGY RESEARCH CENTRE
LIBRARY
PO Box 100, LDR Sta.
Laval, PQ, Canada H7N 4Z3   Phone: (514) 687-5010
Monique St. Jean, Libn.
Subjects: Microbiology, preventive medicine, biotechnology, biochemistry, immunology, virology, food sciences. **Holdings:** 13,000 books. **Subscriptions:** 512 journals and other serials.

★10687★ **INSTITUT ARMAND-FRAPPIER**
EPIDEMIOLOGY AND PREVENTIVE MEDICINE RESEARCH
CENTRE
LIBRARY
531 blvd. de Priaries
Laval, PQ, Canada H7V 1B7   Phone: (514) 687-5010
Monique St. Jean, Libn.
Subjects: Bacteriology, immunology, virology, comparative medicine, veterinary medicine, epidemiology, statistics. **Holdings:** 35,000 volumes. **Subscriptions:** 375 journals and other serials.

★10688★ **JEWISH REHABILITATION HOSPITAL**
HEALTH SCIENCES INFORMATION CENTRE
3205 Alton Goldbloom
Laval, PQ, Canada H7V 1R2   Phone: (514) 688-9550
Irene Deborah Shanefield, Med.Libn.
Subjects: Medicine, physical therapy, cognitive rehabilitation, occupational therapy, nuerology, therapeutics. **Holdings:** 1300 books; 800 bound periodical volumes. **Subscriptions:** 90 journals and other serials.

★10689★ **HOTEL-DIEU DE LEVIS**
BIBLIOTHEQUE
143, rue Wolfe
Levis, PQ, Canada G6V 3Z1   Phone: (418) 835-7121
Jocelyne Dufour
Subjects: Medicine. **Holdings:** 5394 books. **Subscriptions:** 278 journals and other serials.

★10690★ **CANADA**
HEALTH AND WELFARE CANADA
HEALTH PROTECTION BRANCH
REGIONAL LIBRARY
1001, Blvd. St. Laurent, W., Ch. 345
Longueuil, PQ, Canada J4K 1C7   Phone: (514) 646-1353
France Lachapelle, Libn.
Subjects: Food and drugs, organic chemistry, forensic chemistry, nutrition, medical devices, pesticides, pharmacology, cosmetics, microbiology. **Holdings:** 2100 books; 600 bound periodical volumes; 3500 pamphlets and other cataloged items. **Subscriptions:** 150 journals and other serials.

★10691★ **INSTITUT NAZARETH ET LOUIS-BRAILLE**
BIBLIOTHEQUE
1111 St. Charles, W.
Longueuil, PQ, Canada J4K 5G4   Phone: (514) 463-1710
Claire Dubois, Chf. of Info.Serv.
Subjects: Humanities. **Holdings:** 40,000 braille books (13,000 titles);

15,000 musical Braille books; 1400 bound periodical volumes. **Subscriptions:** 25 journals and other serials in braille.

★10692★ **HOPITAL DE MONT-JOLI**
BIBLIOTHEQUE
800 Sanatorium
Mont-Joli, PQ, Canada G5H 3L6   Phone: (418) 775-7261
Helene Jean, Biblio.
Subjects: Psychiatry, psychology, medicine, health care, long-term care, physical and geriatric rehabilitation. **Holdings:** 5350 books; 88 periodical volumes.

★10693★ **ABBOTT LABORATORIES, LTD.**
COMPANY LIBRARY
Sta. A, PO Box 6150
Montreal, PQ, Canada H3C 3K6   Phone: (514) 340-7100
Genevieve Heroux, Libn.
Subjects: Medicine, nutrition, pharmacology. **Holdings:** 1000 volumes. **Subscriptions:** 90 journals.

★10694★ **THE ASBESTOS INSTITUTE**
ARCHIVES
1130 Sherbrooke St., W., Ste. 410
Montreal, PQ, Canada H3A 2M8   Phone: (514) 844-3956
Claude deLery, Dir./Adm.
Subjects: Biological effects of asbestos. **Holdings:** 775 books; 7000 documents. **Subscriptions:** 53 journals and other serials.

★10695★ **ASSOCIATION QUEBECOISE POUR ENFANTS AVEC**
PROBLEMES AUDITIFS
CENTRE DE DOCUMENTATION EN DEFICIENCE AUDITIVE
3700 rue Berri, 4th Fl.
Montreal, PQ, Canada H2L 4G9   Phone: (514) 842-8706
Marie Noelle Ducharme, Info.Spec.
Subjects: Deafness, information for parents. **Holdings:** 150 books; 300 bound periodical volumes; 150 other cataloged items; 20 videotapes; 35 films.

★10696★ **BRISTOL-MYERS SQUIBB COMPANY**
MEDICAL LIBRARY
2365 Cote de Liesse Rd.
Montreal, PQ, Canada H4N 2M7   Phone: (514) 333-2057
Donna Gibson, Med.Libn.
Subjects: Medicine, pharmacology, chemistry, pharmaceuticals. **Holdings:** 2500 unbound periodical volumes; 350 monographs. **Subscriptions:** 130 journals; 8 newsletters.

★10697★ **CANADA**
NATIONAL FILM BOARD OF CANADA
FILM PREVIEW LIBRARY
3155 Cote de Liesse Rd.
PO Box 6100, Sta. A
Montreal, PQ, Canada H3C 3H5   Phone: (514) 283-9437
Marielle D. Cartier, Libn./Hd., AV Coll.
Subjects: History, industry, health and medicine, social sciences, sports and recreation, social geography, animation. **Holdings:** 14,217 16mm films; 5252 35mm films; 5550 3/4 and 1/2 inch videotapes.

★10698★ **CANADIAN PSYCHOANALYTIC SOCIETY**
LIBRARY
7000 Cote des Neiges Rd.
Montreal, PQ, Canada H3S 2C1   Phone: (514) 738-6105
Nadia Gargour, Adm.Dir.
Subjects: Psychoanalysis. **Holdings:** 4000 books. **Subscriptions:** 22 journals and other serials.

★10699★ **CANADIAN TOBACCO MANUFACTURERS COUNCIL**
INFORMATION CENTER
1808 Sherbrooke St., W., 2nd Fl.
Montreal, PQ, Canada H3H 1E5   Phone: (514) 937-7428
Selma D. Trevick, Coord., Lib.Serv.
Subjects: Smoking and health, tobacco, environment, pollution, biology, agriculture. **Holdings:** 545 books; 46 bound periodical volumes; 180 binders of clippings; 8 VF drawers of motion pictures and tapes; 80 boxes of reports; 20 boxes of pamphlets. **Subscriptions:** 284 journals and other serials; 20 newspapers.

★10700★ **CENTRE HOSPITALIER COTE-DES-NEIGES**
BIBLIOTHEQUE
4565, chemin de la Reine-Marie
Montreal, PQ, Canada H3W 1W5   Phone: (514) 340-1424
Louise Bourbonnais, Chf.Libn.
Subjects: Geriatrics, chronic care and allied specialties, neurolinguistics, brain disorders. **Holdings:** 2525 books. **Subscriptions:** 185 journals and other serials; 14 newspapers.

★10701★ **CENTRE HOSPITALIER JACQUES-VIGER**
CENTRE DE DOCUMENTATION
1051 St. Hubert St.
Montreal, PQ, Canada H2L 3Y5   Phone: (514) 842-7181
Subjects: Geriatrics, gerontology, medicine, long term care, nursing. **Holdings:** 300 books; 600 bound periodical volumes; 200 brochures. **Subscriptions:** 50 journals and other serials.

★10702★ **CENTRE DE READAPTATION CONSTANCE-**
LETHBRIDGE
MEDICAL LIBRARY
7005, blvd. de Maisonneuve, W.
Montreal, PQ, Canada H4B 1T3   Phone: (514) 487-1770
Jane Petrov, Libn.
Subjects: Rehabilitation medicine, physical and occupational therapy, vocational rehabilitation, psychology, speech. **Holdings:** 2500 books; 1000 bound periodical volumes. **Subscriptions:** 80 journals and other serials.

★10703★ **CENTRE DE SERVICES SOCIAUX DU MONTREAL**
METROPOLITAIN
BIBLIOTHEQUE
1001, blvd. de Maisonneuve, E.
Montreal, PQ, Canada H2L 4R5   Phone: (514) 527-7261
Helene Neilson
Subjects: Social service, child welfare, juvenile delinquency, child abuse, aged, psychotherapy. **Holdings:** 13,500 books; 300 periodical titles; 12 VF drawers of subject files. **Subscriptions:** 75 journals and other serials.

★10704★ **CLINICAL RESEARCH INSTITUTE OF MONTREAL**
MEDICAL LIBRARY
110 Pine Ave., W.
Montreal, PQ, Canada H2W 1R7   Phone: (514) 987-5599
Lorraine Bielmann, Doc.
Subjects: Medicine, allied health sciences. **Holdings:** 2600 books; 1100 bound periodical volumes; 222,421 reprints. **Subscriptions:** 123 journals and other serials.

★10705★ **CORPORATION PROFESSIONNELLE DES**
MEDECINS DU QUEBEC
INFORMATHEQUE
1440, rue Sainte-Catherine, W., Rm. 914
Montreal, PQ, Canada H3G 1S5   Phone: (514) 878-4441
Helene Lefebvre, Lib.Techn.
Subjects: Social medicine, legal medicine, health insurance, medical education, medical ethics, hospital administration, state medicine. **Holdings:** Books; periodicals; federal, provincial, U.S. Government publications. **Subscriptions:** 136 journals and other serials; 19 newspapers.

★10706★ **DOUGLAS HOSPITAL CENTRE**
STAFF LIBRARY
6875 LaSalle Blvd.
Montreal, PQ, Canada H4H 1R3   Phone: (514) 762-3029
Elaine Mancina, Chf.Libn.
Subjects: Psychiatry, psychopharmacology, psychology, child psychiatry, psychiatric nursing, rehabilitation. **Holdings:** 4000 books; 4400 bound periodical volumes; bibliographies. **Subscriptions:** 210 journals and other serials.

★10707★ **FEDERATION DES MEDECINS OMNIPRACTICIENS**
DU QUEBEC
DOCUMENTATION CENTRE
1440 Ouest Ste-Catherine, Ste. 1100
Montreal, PQ, Canada H3G 1R8   Phone: (514) 878-1911
Ghislaine Lincourt, Adm.
Subjects: Medicine - social aspects, unions, law, teaching. **Holdings:** 4000 books; 600 bound periodical volumes; government publications; reports. **Subscriptions:** 192 journals and other serials; 8 newspapers.

★10708★ **FEDERATION DES MEDECINS SPECIALISTES DU**
QUEBEC
BIBLIOTHEQUE
2 Complexe Desjardins
Tour de l'Est, Porte 3000
Montreal, PQ, Canada H5B 1G8   Phone: (514) 288-7277
Ghislaine Lussier, Dir., Archv. & Doc.
Subjects: Legal aspects of health management. **Holdings:** 5000 books; 800 bound periodical volumes; 20,000 archival items; 800 microfiche; statistical reports. **Subscriptions:** 196 journals and other serials; 8 newspapers.

★10709★ **FRANK W. HORNER, INC.**
RESEARCH LIBRARY
PO Box 959
Montreal, PQ, Canada H3C 2W6   Phone: (514) 731-3931
Mr. Yvon Dugas, Libn.
Subjects: Medical sciences, analytical chemistry, biochemistry, pharmacology, sales. **Holdings:** 2000 books; 5000 bound periodical volumes. **Subscriptions:** 125 journals and other serials.

★10710★ **HOPITAL JEAN-TALON**
BIBLIOTHEQUE MEDICALE
1385 E. Jean-Talon
Montreal, PQ, Canada H2E 1S6   Phone: (514) 273-5151
Pierrette Galarneau, Med.Libn.
Subjects: Medicine. **Holdings:** 1800 books. **Subscriptions:** 160 journals and other serials.

★10711★ **HOPITAL LOUIS H. LAFONTAINE**
BIBLIOTHEQUE
7401, rue Hochelaga
Montreal, PQ, Canada H1N 3M5   Phone: (514) 251-4000
Camil Lemire, Biblio.
Subjects: Psychology, psychiatry, psychoanalysis. **Holdings:** 6400 books; 3000 bound periodical volumes. **Subscriptions:** 150 journals and other serials.

★10712★ **HOPITAL MAISONNEUVE-ROSEMONT**
SERVICE DES BIBLIOTHEQUES
5415 de l'Assomption Blvd.
Montreal, PQ, Canada H1T 2M4   Phone: (514) 252-3463
Helene Lauzon, Hd.Libn.
Subjects: Medicine, surgery, psychiatry, pneumology, gynecology, pediatrics, hospital administration, nursing, medical technology, immunology, obstetrics, neurology, cardiology. **Holdings:** 3000 books; 26,854 bound periodical volumes; 153 other cataloged items. **Subscriptions:** 423 journals and other serials.

★10713★ **HOPITAL NOTRE DAME**
MEDICAL LIBRARY
C.P. 1560, Succ. C.
Montreal, PQ, Canada H2L 4K8   Phone: (514) 876-6862
Andre Allard, Chf.Libn.
Subjects: Medicine, allied health sciences. **Holdings:** 10,000 books; 40,000 bound periodical volumes. **Subscriptions:** 600 journals and other serials.

★10714★ **HOPITAL REINE ELIZABETH**
A. HOLLIS MARDEN BIBLIOTHEQUE
2100 Marlowe Ave.
Montreal, PQ, Canada H4A 3L6   Phone: (514) 488-2311
Ms. S.L. Mullan, Lib.Techn.
Subjects: Medicine, nursing. **Holdings:** 12,744 volumes. **Subscriptions:** 200 journals and other serials.

★10715★ **HOPITAL RIVIERE-DES-PRAIRIES**
BIBLIOTHEQUE DU PERSONNEL
7070, blvd. Perras, E.
Montreal, PQ, Canada H1E 1A4   Phone: (514) 323-7260
Robert Aubin, Hd.
Subjects: Child psychiatry, mental retardation. **Holdings:** 9000 books; 3000 bound periodical volumes; 1800 reprints; 100 videotapes; 800 cassettes; 1500 microfiche. **Subscriptions:** 200 journals and other serials.

★10716★ HOPITAL DU SACRE COEUR
PAVILLON ALBERT-PREVOST
BIBLIOTHEQUE
6555 Gouin Blvd., W.
Montreal, PQ, Canada H4K 1B3   Phone: (514) 338-4284
Subjects: Psychiatry, psychoanalysis, child psychiatry, psychology. **Holdings:** 3424 books; 2017 bound periodical volumes; 272 Audio-Digest tapes on psychiatry; 174 other cataloged items. **Subscriptions:** 106 journals and other serials.

★10717★ HOPITAL STE. JEANNE D'ARC
BIBLIOTHEQUE MEDICALE
3570, rue St. Urbain
Montreal, PQ, Canada H2X 2N8   Phone: (514) 282-6951
Louise Lemay, Biblio.
Subjects: Medicine, surgery, psychology, psychiatry. **Holdings:** 1800 books; 1000 bound periodical volumes; 1300 cassettes. **Subscriptions:** 98 journals and other serials; 6 newspapers.

★10718★ HOPITAL STE. JUSTINE
CENTRE D'INFORMATION SUR LA SANTE DE L'ENFANT
3175, chemin Cote Ste-Catherine
Montreal, PQ, Canada H3T 1C5   Phone: (514) 345-4680
Louis-Luc Lecompte, Hd.
Subjects: Pediatrics, obstetrics and gynecology, pediatric nursing, child psychiatry, adolescence. **Holdings:** 11,000 books; 6200 reports, videotapes, other cataloged items. **Subscriptions:** 750 journals and other serials.

★10719★ HOPITAL ST. LUC
BIBLIOTHEQUE MEDICALE
1058 St. Denis St.
Montreal, PQ, Canada H2X 3J4   Phone: (514) 281-6167
Pierre Duchesneau, Hd.
Subjects: Medicine, paramedical sciences, surgery, hospital administration, nursing. **Holdings:** 8400 books; 4000 bound periodical volumes. **Subscriptions:** 450 journals and other serials.

★10720★ HOPITAL SANTA CABRINI
CENTRE DE DOCUMENTATION
5655 E. St-Zotique St.
Montreal, PQ, Canada H1T 1P7   Phone: (514) 252-6488
Diane Seguin, Lib.Techn.
Subjects: Medicine, pathology, surgery, nursing, urology, cardiology. **Holdings:** 2800 books; 1955 bound periodical volumes. **Subscriptions:** 198 journals and other serials.

★10721★ HOTEL-DIEU DE MONTREAL
SERVICE DE DOCUMENTATION
3840 Rue St-Urbain
Montreal, PQ, Canada H2W 1T8   Phone: (514) 843-2638
Ginette Boyer, Chf.Libn.
Subjects: Medicine, nursing. **Holdings:** 3000 books; 26,500 bound periodical volumes; 58,271 slides. **Subscriptions:** 250 journals and other serials.

★10722★ INSTITUT PHILIPPE PINEL DE MONTREAL
CENTRE DE DOCUMENTATION
10905 Henri-Bourassa Blvd., E.
Montreal, PQ, Canada H1C 1H1   Phone: (514) 648-8461
Marc Lamarre, Libn.
Subjects: Forensic psychiatry, mentally ill offenders, criminology, clinical psychology. **Holdings:** 2500 books; 850 bound periodical volumes; 5 VF drawers of reprints and pamphlets. **Subscriptions:** 150 journals and other serials.

★10723★ INSTITUT RAYMOND-DEWAR
CENTRE DE DOCUMENTATION
3600, rue Berri, Ste. 034
Montreal, PQ, Canada H2L 4G9   Phone: (514) 284-2581
Sylvie Laverdiere, Libn.
Subjects: Hearing impairment, audiology, deaf-blindness, rehabilitation, psychology, social sciences. **Holdings:** 4000 books; 210 bound periodical volumes; 290 reprints and reports; 100 dissertations; 135 videotapes; 35 sign language courses on videotape. **Subscriptions:** 85 journals and other serials.

★10724★ INSTITUT DE READAPTATION DE MONTREAL
BIBLIOTHEQUE MEDICALE
6300 Darlington Ave.
Montreal, PQ, Canada H3S 2J4   Phone: (514) 340-2085
Maryse Boyer, Lib.Techn.
Subjects: Rehabilitation, physical medicine, occupational and physical therapy, orthopedics, neurology, prosthetics and orthotics, physically handicapped. **Holdings:** 2000 books; 500 bound periodical volumes. **Subscriptions:** 130 journals and other serials.

★10725★ INSTITUT DE RECHERCHE EN SANTE ET EN
SECURITE DU TRAVAIL
INFORMATHEQUE
505, blvd. de Maisonneuve, W., 11th Fl.
Montreal, PQ, Canada H3A 3C2   Phone: (514) 288-1551
Francois Lemay, Hd.
Subjects: Industrial hygiene and safety, ergonomics. **Holdings:** 6500 books; 19,900 reprints; 700 standards; 120 microfiche; 20 AV programs. **Subscriptions:** 150 journals and other serials.

★10726★ INTER/UNIVERSITY GROUP FOR RESEARCH IN
ETHNOPSYCHIATRY AND MEDICAL ANTHROPOLOGY
LIBRARY
University of Montreal
PO Box 6128, Sta. A
Montreal, PQ, Canada H3C 3J7   Phone: (514) 343-5832
Subjects: Ethnopsychiatry, medical anthropology. **Holdings:** Figures not available.

★10727★ JOHNSON & HIGGINS WILLIS FABER INC.
EMPLOYEE BENEFIT DOCUMENTATION CENTRE
800 Place Victoria, Ste. 2624
Montreal, PQ, Canada H4Z 1E2   Phone: (514) 878-1780
Claire Gendreau, Coord., Doc.Ctr.
Subjects: Employee benefits; insurance - life, health, dental; pensions. **Holdings:** 500 books; 60 government reports; 150 internal reports; 300 single and gazetted laws; 30 volumes of loose-leaf information services; 1000 clippings. **Subscriptions:** 40 journals and other serials; 10 newspapers.

★10728★ MAIMONIDES HOSPITAL GERIATRIC CENTRE
POLLACK LIBRARY
5795 Caldwell Ave.
Montreal, PQ, Canada H4W 1W3   Phone: (514) 483-2121
Sheindel Bresinger, Libn.
Subjects: Geriatrics, gerontology, medicine, social work, nursing, psychiatry. **Holdings:** 2100 books; 1000 bound periodical volumes; 90 reprints of staff articles; 4 drawers of current topics in geriatrics and gerontology. **Subscriptions:** 110 journals and other serials.

★10729★ MCGILL UNIVERSITY
EXPERIMENTAL SURGERY LIBRARY
Donner Bldg.
740 Dr. Penfield Ave.
Montreal, PQ, Canada H3A 1A4   Phone: (514) 398-3980
Irene Sidorenko, Adm.Sec.
Subjects: Immunology, Cancer metastasis. **Holdings:** 1550 volumes; 300 theses. **Subscriptions:** 30 journals and other serials.

★10730★ MCGILL UNIVERSITY
HEALTH SCIENCES LIBRARY
McIntyre Medical Sciences Bldg.
3655 Drummond St.
Montreal, PQ, Canada H3G 1Y6   Phone: (514) 398-4723
David S. Crawford, Life Sci. Area Libn.
Subjects: Medicine, dentistry, and allied health sciences. **Holdings:** 78,648 books; 134,664 bound periodical volumes; 4842 slides. **Subscriptions:** 2323 serials.

★10731★ MCGILL UNIVERSITY
OSLER LIBRARY
McIntyre Medical Sciences Bldg.
3655 Drummond St.
Montreal, PQ, Canada H3G 1Y6   Phone: (514) 398-4718
Faith Wallis, Hist.Med.Libn.
Subjects: History of medicine. **Holdings:** 38,929 books; 2043 bound periodical volumes. **Subscriptions:** 129 journals and other serials.

★10732★ MONTREAL ASSOCIATION FOR THE
INTELLECTUALLY HANDICAPPED
MULTI-MEDIA DOCUMENTATION CENTER
8605, rue Berri, 3rd Fl.
Montreal, PQ, Canada H2P 2G5   Phone: (514) 381-2307
Michelle Jacques, Doc.
Subjects: Intellectual deficiencies. Holdings: 1500 books; 41 bound period-
ical volumes; pamphlets; vertical files; AV programs. Subscriptions: 75
journals and other serials.

★10733★ MONTREAL CANCER INSTITUTE
LIBRARY
1560 Sherbrooke St., E.
Montreal, PQ, Canada H2L 4M1   Phone: (514) 876-7078
Ginette Bujold, Lib.Techn.
Subjects: Cellular biology, virology, genetics, molecular biology, biochemistry, cancer. Holdings: 200 books; 4000 bound periodical volumes; 50
scientific reports; 50 annual reports; 20 theses. Subscriptions: 53 journals
and other serials.

★10734★ MONTREAL CHEST HOSPITAL CENTRE
MEDICAL LIBRARY
3650 St. Urbain St.
Montreal, PQ, Canada H2X 2P4   Phone: (514) 849-5201
Marianne Constantine, Med.Libn.
Subjects: Chest medicine, respiratory diseases. Holdings: 2500 volumes.
Subscriptions: 100 journals and other serials.

★10735★ MONTREAL CHILDREN'S HOSPITAL
MEDICAL LIBRARY
2300 Tupper St.
Montreal, PQ, Canada H3H 1P3   Phone: (514) 934-4401
Joanne Baird, Med.Libn.
Subjects: Pediatrics, pediatric surgery, child psychiatry, nursing. Holdings:
6,000 volumes. Subscriptions: 220 journals and other serials.

★10736★ MONTREAL GENERAL HOSPITAL
MEDICAL LIBRARY
1650 Cedar Ave.
Montreal, PQ, Canada H3G 1A4   Phone: (514) 937-6011
Gary Lee Kober, Chf.Med.Libn.
Subjects: Medicine, surgery, gynecology, pathology, radiology, anesthesia.
Holdings: 2000 books; 7000 bound periodical volumes; 1 VF drawer of
pamphlets. Subscriptions: 300 journals and other serials.

★10737★ MONTREAL GENERAL HOSPITAL
NURSES LIBRARY
1650 Cedar Ave., Rm. 619
Montreal, PQ, Canada H3G 1A4   Phone: (514) 937-6011
Mrs. B.A. Covington, Lib.Techn.
Subjects: Nursing. Holdings: 2500 books; 150 bound periodical volumes.
Subscriptions: 40 journals and other serials.

★10738★ MONTREAL NEUROLOGICAL INSTITUTE
LIBRARY
3801 University St.
Montreal, PQ, Canada H3A 2B4   Phone: (514) 398-1980
Carol L. Wiens, Libn.
Subjects: Neurosciences. Holdings: 3600 books; 3500 bound periodical
volumes; 300 theses and reprints. Subscriptions: 75 journals and other
serials.

★10739★ ORDRE DES INFIRMIERES ET DES INFIRMIERS
DU QUEBEC
CENTRE DE DOCUMENTATION
4200 Dorchester, W.
Montreal, PQ, Canada H3Z 1V4   Phone: (514) 935-2501
Maryse Dumas, Libn.
Subjects: Nursing. Holdings: 10,000 books; 150 bound periodical volumes;
12 films; 8 slide programs; 25 videotapes. Subscriptions: 325 journals and
other serials.

★10740★ QUEBEC PROVINCE COMMISSION DE LA SANTE
ET DE LA SECURITE DU TRAVAIL
CENTRE DE DOCUMENTATION
1199 de Bleury, 4th Fl.
C.P. 6067, Succ. A
Montreal, PQ, Canada H3C 4E1   Phone: (514) 873-3160
Marc Fournier, Chef de Serv.
Subjects: Occupational health and safety. Holdings: 39,300 books; 700
bound periodical volumes; 500 AV programs; 35,000 other cataloged
items. Subscriptions: 500 journals and other serials; 6 newspapers.

★10741★ ROYAL VICTORIA HOSPITAL
ALLAN MEMORIAL INSTITUTE
ERIC D. WITTKOWER LIBRARY
1025 Pine Ave., W.
Montreal, PQ, Canada H3A 1A1   Phone: (514) 842-1231
Barbara Gartner, Libn.
Subjects: Psychiatry, psychology, child psychiatry. Holdings: 3000 books;
2500 bound periodical volumes; 120 unbound journals. Subscriptions: 46
journals and other serials.

★10742★ ROYAL VICTORIA HOSPITAL
MEDICAL LIBRARY
687 Pine Ave., W., Rm. H4.01
Montreal, PQ, Canada H3A 1A1   Phone: (514) 842-1231
Sandra R. Duchow, Chf.Med.Libn.
Subjects: Medicine, surgery, anesthesia, nursing. Holdings: 2000 books;
10,000 bound periodical volumes. Subscriptions: 300 journals and other
serials.

★10743★ ROYAL VICTORIA HOSPITAL
WOMEN'S PAVILION LIBRARY
687 Pine Ave., W.
Montreal, PQ, Canada H3A 1A1   Phone: (514) 842-1231
Lynda Dickson, Libn.
Subjects: Gynecology, obstetrics, newborn physiology, neuroendocrinolo-
gy. Holdings: 500 books; 1000 bound periodical volumes; 4 drawers of
reprints. Subscriptions: 30 journals and other serials.

★10744★ ST. MARY'S HOSPITAL
HEALTH SCIENCES LIBRARY
3830 Lacombe
Montreal, PQ, Canada H3T 1M5   Phone: (514) 345-3317
Jeannine Lawlor, Libn.
Subjects: Medicine, nursing, obstetrics, gynecology, psychiatry, surgery.
Holdings: 3000 books; 5600 bound periodical volumes; 1300 audio
cassettes; 65 video cassettes; 5065 slides; 60 slide/tape sets. Subscriptions:
230 journals and other serials.

★10745★ SIR MORTIMER B. DAVIS JEWISH GENERAL
HOSPITAL
INSTITUTE OF COMMUNITY AND FAMILY PSYCHIATRY
LIBRARY
4333 Cote St. Catherine Rd.
Montreal, PQ, Canada H3T 1E4   Phone: (514) 340-8210
Ruth Stilman, Libn.
Subjects: Psychiatry, psychotherapy, family therapy, community mental
health, psychopharmacology. Holdings: 5200 books; 1600 bound periodi-
cal volumes; 300 VF materials; 450 audiotapes. Subscriptions: 83 journals
and other serials.

★10746★ SIR MORTIMER B. DAVIS JEWISH GENERAL
HOSPITAL
LADY DAVIS INSTITUTE FOR MEDICAL RESEARCH
RESEARCH LIBRARY
3755 Cote St. Catherine Rd.
Montreal, PQ, Canada H3T 1E2   Phone: (514) 340-8260
Arlene Greenberg, Chf.Med.Libn.
Subjects: Biochemistry, molecular biology, cancer research, cell genetics,
medical research, diabetes. Holdings: Books housed at hospital's main
library. Subscriptions: 70 journals and other serials.

★10747★ SIR MORTIMER B. DAVIS JEWISH GENERAL HOSPITAL
MEDICAL LIBRARY
3755 Cote St. Catherine Rd.
Montreal, PQ, Canada H3T 1E2   Phone: (514) 340-8260
Ross C. Gordon, Chf.Med.Libn.
Subjects: Medicine, nursing, allied health sciences, administration. **Holdings:** 30,000 books and bound periodical volumes. **Subscriptions:** 500 journals and other serials.

★10748★ UNIVERSITE DE MONTREAL
BIBLIOTHEQUE PARA-MEDICALE
C.P. 6128, Succursale A
Montreal, PQ, Canada H3C 3J7   Phone: (514) 343-6180
Johanne Hopper, Libn.
Subjects: Nursing, health administration, nutrition, epidemiology, environmental health, audiology, ergotherapy, orthophonics, physiotherapy, social and preventive medicine, gerontology and geriatrics. **Holdings:** 53,916 books; 18,377 bound periodical volumes; 12,576 microforms; 1673 slides; 1322 AV programs. **Subscriptions:** 1563 journals and other serials.

★10749★ UNIVERSITE DE MONTREAL
BIBLIOTHEQUE DE LA SANTE
C.P. 6128, Succursale A
Montreal, PQ, Canada H3C 3J7   Phone: (514) 343-6826
Subjects: Medicine, dentistry, pharmacy. **Holdings:** 85,157 books; 108,243 bound periodical volumes; 3189 microforms; 12,720 slides. **Subscriptions:** 2495 journals and other serials.

★10750★ UNIVERSITE DE MONTREAL
OPTOMETRIE-BIBLIOTHEQUE
C.P. 6128, Succursale A
Montreal, PQ, Canada H3C 3J7   Phone: (514) 343-7674
Diane Clerk, Libn.
Subjects: Optometry. **Holdings:** 4666 books; 5443 bound periodical volumes; 2592 slides. **Subscriptions:** 130 journals and other serials.

★10751★ UNIVERSITE DE MONTREAL
PSYCHO-EDUCATION-BIBLIOTHEQUE
C.P. 6128, Succursale A
Montreal, PQ, Canada H3C 3J7   Phone: (514) 385-2556
Subjects: Child psychology, rehabilitation of maladjusted children. **Holdings:** 10,443 books; 2925 bound periodical volumes; 88 microforms; 135 reports; 110 slides. **Subscriptions:** 143 journals and other serials.

★10752★ UNIVERSITE DU QUEBEC A MONTREAL
AUDIOVIDEOTHEQUE
C.P. 8889, Succursale A
Montreal, PQ, Canada H3C 3P3   Phone: (514) 987-4332
Huguette Tanguay, AV Libn.
Subjects: Sexology, administration, earth sciences, psychology, education. **Holdings:** 3748 films and videotapes.

★10753★ UNIVERSITE DU QUEBEC A MONTREAL
BIBLIOTHEQUE DES SCIENCES DE L'EDUCATION
C.P. 8889, Succursale A
Montreal, PQ, Canada H3C 3P3   Phone: (514) 987-6174
Andre Champagne, Dir.
Subjects: Continuing teacher education, elementary and secondary education, physical education, disadvantaged and exceptional child education, hearing and learning disabilities, professional and vocational information, vocational education, pre-school education, neurokinetics. **Holdings:** 48,000 books; 8000 bound periodical volumes; 275,000 ERIC microfiche; 3900 microcards; 820 reels of microfilm; 125 film loops. **Subscriptions:** 425 journals and other serials.

★10754★ CANADIAN INSTITUTE OF HYPNOTISM
LIBRARY
110 Greystone
Pointe Claire, PQ, Canada H9R 5T6   Phone: (514) 426-1010
Maxine Kershaw, Coord.
Subjects: Hypnosis - medical, dental, historical. **Holdings:** 1100 books; 45 bound periodical volumes. **Subscriptions:** 5 journals and other serials.

★10755★ LAKESHORE GENERAL HOSPITAL
MEDICAL LIBRARY
160 Stillview Rd.
Pointe Claire, PQ, Canada H9R 2Y2   Phone: (514) 630-2101
Aimee Muther, Chf., Lib.Serv.
Subjects: Medicine, surgery, obstetrics, gynecology, pathology, psychiatry, nursing. **Holdings:** 3811 books; 2549 bound periodical volumes; 1233 magnetic tapes; 2294 microfiche. **Subscriptions:** 166 journals and other serials.

★10756★ MERCK FROSST CANADA INC.
RESEARCH LIBRARY
PO Box 1005
Pointe Claire-Dorval, PQ, Canada H9R 4P8   Phone: (514) 695-7920
Claire B. Kelly, Sr.Res.Libn.
Subjects: Medicine, chemistry, pharmacy, general science. **Holdings:** 3000 books; 9000 bound periodical volumes. **Subscriptions:** 300 journals and other serials.

★10757★ PFIZER CANADA INC.
MEDICAL LIBRARY
PO Box 800
Pointe Claire-Dorval, PQ, Canada H9R 4V2   Phone: (514) 695-0500
Miriam Hayward, Sci.Info.Off.
Subjects: Pharmacology, drug therapy, rheumatology, cardiovasology, psychotherapy, microbiology, allergies, dermatology. **Holdings:** 800 books; 100 bound periodical volumes; 50 audio cassettes; 7500 reprints; 125 meeting and symposia proceedings; 90 pieces of product information; journals on microfilm; 80 other cataloged items. **Subscriptions:** 130 journals and other serials.

★10758★ UNIVERSITE DE QUEBEC A POINTE-CLAIRE
INSTITUT NATIONAL DE LA RECHERCHE SCIENTIFIQUE-SANTE
BIBLIOTHEQUE
245 Hymus Blvd.
Pointe-Claire, PQ, Canada H9R 1G6   Phone: (514) 630-8800
Gilbert LeBlanc
Subjects: Pharmacology, biochemistry, environment. **Holdings:** 7000 books. **Subscriptions:** 125 journals and other serials.

★10759★ ASSOCIATION DE PARALYSIE CEREBRALE DU QUEBEC, INC.
CENTRE DE DOCUMENTATION
525, boul. Hamel est, Sous-Sol/Aile A-50
Quebec, PQ, Canada G1M 2S8   Phone: (418) 529-5371
Subjects: Cerebral palsy, handicaps, treatment methods. **Holdings:** Figures not available. **Subscriptions:** 40 journals and other serials.

★10760★ HOPITAL DE L'ENFANT-JESUS
BIBLIOTHEQUE SCIENTIFIQUE CHARLES-AUGUSTE GAUTHIER
1401 18ieme Rue
Quebec, PQ, Canada G1J 1Z4   Phone: (418) 649-5686
Madeleine Dumais, Resp.
Subjects: Medicine. **Holdings:** 1600 books; 4775 bound periodical volumes. **Subscriptions:** 220 journals and other serials.

★10761★ HOPITAL L'HOTEL-DIEU DE QUEBEC
BIBLIOTHEQUE MEDICALE
11, Cote du Palais
Quebec, PQ, Canada G1R 2J6   Phone: (418) 691-5073
Lizette Germain, Libn.
Subjects: Cancer, nephrology. **Holdings:** 3255 books. **Subscriptions:** 356 journals and other serials.

★10762★ HOPITAL ST. FRANCOIS D'ASSISE
BIBLIOTHEQUE MEDICALE ET ADMINISTRATIVE
10, rue de l'Espinay
Quebec, PQ, Canada G1L 3L5   Phone: (418) 525-4408
Ulric Lefebvre, Chief
Subjects: Obstetrics, neonatology, pediatrics, gynecology, internal medicine, surgery, perinatology. **Holdings:** 5200 books; 4650 bound periodical volumes; annual reports; documents. **Subscriptions:** 360 journals and other serials.

★10763★ HOPITAL DU ST-SACREMENT
BIBLIOTHEQUE MEDICALE
1050, chemin Ste-Foy
Quebec, PQ, Canada G1S 4L8   Phone: (418) 682-7730
Diane St-Pierre, Biblio.Techn.
Subjects: Medicine. **Holdings:** 1120 books. **Subscriptions:** 210 journals and
other serials.

★10764★ HOTEL-DIEU DU SACRE-COEUR DE JESUS DE
    QUEBEC
BIBLIOTHEQUE MEDICALE
1, Ave. du Sacre-Coeur
Quebec, PQ, Canada G1N 2W1   Phone: (418) 529-6851
Christian Martel, Lib.Techn.
Subjects: Child psychiatry, neurology. **Holdings:** 4200 books. **Subscriptions:** 100 journals and other serials.

★10765★ QUEBEC PROVINCE MINISTERE DE LA SANTE ET
    DES SERVICES SOCIAUX
SERVICE DE LA DOCUMENTATION
1005, chemin Ste-Foy, R.C.
Quebec, PQ, Canada G1S 4N4   Phone: (418) 643-6392
Yvon Papillon, Hd.Libn.
Subjects: Health and social services, medical economics, aging, occupational and environmental health, family. **Holdings:** 30,000 books. **Subscriptions:** 325 journals and other serials.

★10766★ UNIVERSITE LAVAL
BIBLIOTHEQUE SCIENTIFIQUE
Quebec, PQ, Canada G1K 7P4   Phone: (418) 656-3967
Alain Bourque, Hd.
Subjects: Science, technology, medical and paramedical sciences, agriculture, forestry, food and nutrition, wood science technology and forest ecology (mycories), animal science, soils, phytopathology, electrochemistry and corrosion, noise pollution, wind energy. **Holdings:** 100,000 books; 200,000 bound periodical volumes; 16,153 reels of microfilm; 18,526 microfiches. **Subscriptions:** 2738 journals and other serials; 30 newspapers.

★10767★ CENTRE HOSPITALIER DE L'UNIVERSITE LAVAL
BIBLIOTHEQUE DES SCIENCES DE LA SANTE
2705, blvd. Sir Wilfred Laurier
Ste. Foy, PQ, Canada G1V 4G2   Phone: (418) 656-8188
Beatrice Dionne, Chf.
Subjects: Medicine, allied health sciences. **Holdings:** 5000 books; 1300 bound periodical volumes. **Subscriptions:** 400 journals and other serials.

★10768★ UNIVERSITE DE MONTREAL
MEDECINE VETERINAIRE-BIBLIOTHEQUE
C.P. 5000
St. Hyacinthe, PQ, Canada J2S 7C6   Phone: (514) 773-8521
Jean-Paul Jette, Libn.
Subjects: Veterinary medicine, animal science. **Holdings:** 30,451 books; 14,075 bound periodical volumes; 146 reports; 3455 microforms; 1577 government publications; 302 slides; 238 AV programs. **Subscriptions:** 494 journals and other serials.

★10769★ HOPITAL DU HAUT-RICHELIEU
BIBLIOTHEQUE MEDICALE
920, Blvd. du Seminaire
St. Jean, PQ, Canada J3A 1B7   Phone: (514) 359-5055
Helene Heroux-Bouchard, Biblio.
Subjects: Medicine, psychiatry, pediatrics, obstetrics and gynecology, surgery. **Holdings:** 1900 books; 850 bound periodical volumes. **Subscriptions:** 85 journals and other serials.

★10770★ AYERST, MCKENNA & HARRISON, INC.
LIBRARY
1025 Blvd. Laurentien
St. Laurent, PQ, Canada H4R 1J6   Phone: (514) 744-6771
Nicole Barrette-Pilon, Libn.
Subjects: Chemistry, medicine, pharmaceuticals, veterinary medicine. **Holdings:** 1000 books; 5000 bound periodical volumes; 400 reels of microfilm. **Subscriptions:** 210 journals and other serials.

★10771★ CENTRE HOSPITALIER HOTEL-DIEU DE
    SHERBROOKE
BIBLIOTHEQUE
580 S. Bowen St.
Sherbrooke, PQ, Canada J1G 2E8   Phone: (819) 569-2551
Nicole Fontaine, Doc.Techn.
Subjects: Medicine, medical specialties, hospital administration, nursing.
Holdings: 2700 books; 3800 unbound and bound periodical volumes; 980 cassettes; 30 videotapes. **Subscriptions:** 161 journals and other serials.

★10772★ UNIVERSITE DE SHERBROOKE
FACULTE DE MEDECINE
BIBLIOTHEQUE DES SCIENCES DE LA SANTE
Centre Hospitalier Universitaire
Sherbrooke, PQ, Canada J1H 5N4   Phone: (819) 564-5297
Germain Chouinard, Dir.
Subjects: Health sciences. **Holdings:** 58,571 volumes. **Subscriptions:** 974 journals and other serials.

★10773★ CENTRE HOSPITALIER DE LA REGION DE
    L'AMIANTE
BIBLIOTHEQUE MEDICALE
1717 rue Notre-Dame N.
Thetford Mines, PQ, Canada G6G 2V4   Phone: (418) 338-7777
Jacinthe Ouellet, Biblio.
Subjects: Medicine, nursing, administration. **Holdings:** 2000 books; AV programs. **Subscriptions:** 252 journals and other serials.

★10774★ CENTRE HOSPITALIER COOKE
BIBLIOTHEQUE MEDICALE ET ADMINISTRATIVE
3450, rue Ste-Marguerite
Trois-Rivieres, PQ, Canada G8Z 1X3   Phone: (819) 375-7713
Nicole LaPointe, Biblio.
Subjects: Medicine, allied health sciences, administration. **Holdings:** 3022 volumes. **Subscriptions:** 145 journals and other serials.

★10775★ CENTRE HOSPITALIER ST. JOSEPH
BIBLIOTHEQUE MEDICALE ET ADMINISTRATIVE
731, rue Ste-Julie
Trois-Rivieres, PQ, Canada G9A 1Y1   Phone: (819) 373-2603
Solange De Rouyn, Chf.
Subjects: Medicine, administration. **Holdings:** 4773 books; 1277 bound periodical volumes. **Subscriptions:** 231 journals and other serials.

★10776★ CHRIST-ROI HOSPITAL
LIBRARY
300 blvd. W-Hamel
Vanier, PQ, Canada G1M 2R9   Phone: (418) 682-1711
Gratien Gelinas, Biblio.
Subjects: Medicine, nursing, pharmacy, allied health sciences. **Holdings:** 1000 books. **Subscriptions:** 80 journals and other serials.

★10777★ CENTRE HOSPITALIER DE VERDUN
BIBLIOTHEQUE MEDICALE
4000 Blvd. LaSalle
Verdun, PQ, Canada H4G 2A3   Phone: (514) 765-8121
Mrs. Andree N. Mandeville, Libn.
Subjects: Medicine. **Holdings:** 2000 books; 8200 bound periodical volumes. **Subscriptions:** 150 journals and other serials.

Saskatchewan

★10778★ MOOSE JAW UNION HOSPITAL
MEDICAL LIBRARY
455 Fairford St., E.
Moose Jaw, SK, Canada S6H 1H3   Phone: (306) 694-0377
Isolde Albraum, Dir., Hea.Rec.
Remarks: No further information was supplied by the respondent.

★10779★ VALLEY VIEW CENTRE
HARRISON MEMORIAL LIBRARY
Box 1300
Moose Jaw, SK, Canada S6H 4R2   Phone: (306) 694-3096
Diane McPherson
Subjects: Special training programs, psychology, nursing. **Holdings:** Figures not available. **Subscriptions:** 36 journals and other serials.

★10780★   BATTLEFORD'S UNION HOSPITAL
MEMORIAL LIBRARY
1092 107th St.
North Battleford, SK, Canada S9A 1Z1   Phone: (306) 446-7381
Debbie Iwanchuk, Hosp.Libn.
Subjects: Medicine, nursing, emergency medicine, surgery, pediatrics, pharmacy. **Holdings:** 1100 books; AV programs. **Subscriptions:** 90 journals.

★10781★   SASKATCHEWAN HOSPITAL
DEPARTMENT OF PSYCHIATRIC SERVICES
STAFF LIBRARY
PO Box 39
North Battleford, SK, Canada S9A 2X8   Phone: (306) 446-7913
Doris Allan, Libn.
Subjects: Psychiatry, medicine, psychology, nursing, hospital administration. **Holdings:** 1500 books; 700 bound periodical volumes. **Subscriptions:** 35 journals and other serials; 5 newspapers.

★10782★   VICTORIA UNION HOSPITAL
MEDICAL LIBRARY
1200 24th St., W.
Prince Albert, SK, Canada S6V 5T4   Phone: (306) 764-1551
Joan I. Ryan, Dir.Hea.Rec.
Subjects: Medicine. **Holdings:** 243 books; 350 bound periodical volumes. **Subscriptions:** 14 journals and other serials.

★10783★   PASQUA HOSPITAL
HEALTH SCIENCES LIBRARY
4101 Dewdney Ave.
Regina, SK, Canada S4T 1A5   Phone: (306) 527-9641
Leona Lang, Dir.
Subjects: Medicine, nursing, administration. **Holdings:** 1200 books; 2800 bound periodical volumes; Audio-Digest tapes; videotapes. **Subscriptions:** 72 journals and other serials.

★10784★   PLAINS HEALTH CENTRE
DR. W.A. RIDDELL HEALTH SCIENCES LIBRARY
4500 Wascana Pkwy.
Regina, SK, Canada S4S 5W9   Phone: (306) 584-6426
Beth Silzer, Dir.
Subjects: Medicine, nursing, pharmacy, physiotherapy. **Holdings:** 4764 books; 4500 bound periodical volumes; 800 AV programs. **Subscriptions:** 294 journals and other serials.

★10785★   REGINA GENERAL HOSPITAL
HEALTH SCIENCES LIBRARY
1440 14th Ave.
Regina, SK, Canada S4P 0W5   Phone: (306) 359-4314
Ms. Terry Bouchard-DeVenney, Hea.Sci.Libn.
Subjects: Pediatrics, perinatology, neonatology, obstetrics/gynecology, surgery, medicine, family practice, radiology, psychiatry, nursing, allied health sciences. **Holdings:** 8000 books; bound periodical volumes; VF drawers; AV programs. **Subscriptions:** 425 journals and other serials; 5 newspapers.

★10786★   SASKATCHEWAN ALCOHOL AND DRUG ABUSE
    COMMISSION
LIBRARY
1942 Hamilton St., 3rd Fl.
Regina, SK, Canada S4P 3V7   Phone: (306) 787-4656
Andrew Stirling
Subjects: Alcohol and alcoholism, drugs and other dependencies, health care. **Holdings:** 5000 books; 400 bound periodical volumes; 100 archival items; reports; pamphlets; government publications. **Subscriptions:** 90 journals and other serials.

★10787★   SASKATCHEWAN CANCER FOUNDATION
ALLAN BLAIR MEMORIAL CLINIC
LIBRARY
4101 Dewdney Ave.
Regina, SK, Canada S4T 7T1   Phone: (306) 359-2203
Barbara Karchewski, Libn.
Subjects: Cancer, medical and radiation oncology, physics. **Holdings:** 900 books; 500 bound periodical volumes; 1500 reprint articles on cancer. **Subscriptions:** 100 journals and other serials.

★10788★   SASKATCHEWAN HEALTH
LIBRARY
3475 Albert St.
Regina, SK, Canada S4S 6X6   Phone: (306) 787-8699
Lynn Kozun, Libn.
Subjects: Public health, nutrition, public health nursing, medicine. **Holdings:** 6000 books; 8000 bound periodical volumes; 2000 technical reports. **Subscriptions:** 358 journals and other serials.

★10789★   SASKATCHEWAN REGISTERED NURSES
    ASSOCIATION
L. JANE KNOX RESOURCE CENTRE
2066 Retallack St.
Regina, SK, Canada S4T 2K2   Phone: (306) 757-4643
Alice M.A. Lalonde
Subjects: Nursing. **Holdings:** 4000 books; 140 bound periodical volumes. **Subscriptions:** 100 journals and other serials.

★10790★   WASCANA REHABILITATION CENTRE
HEALTH SCIENCES LIBRARY
Ave. G & 23rd Ave.
Regina, SK, Canada S4S 0A5   Phone: (306) 359-5650
Donna Cargill, Dir.
Subjects: Rehabilitation, gerontology, pediatrics, physically handicapped. **Holdings:** 2400 books; 1300 bound periodical volumes. **Subscriptions:** 100 journals and other serials.

★10791★   CANADA
NATIONAL FILM BOARD OF CANADA
FILM LIBRARY
424 21st St., E.
Saskatoon, SK, Canada S7K 0C2   Phone: (306) 975-4245
Lucie Joyal, AV Supv.
Subjects: Canadian studies, creative arts, social science, health and medicine, recreation. **Holdings:** 3500 films; 900 video cassettes; 20 VF drawers of information sheets.

★10792★   PARKRIDGE CENTRE
STAFF LIBRARY
110 Gropper Crescent
Saskatoon, SK, Canada S7M 5N9   Phone: (306) 978-2333
Kristine Goulding, Dir. of Hea.Rec.
Subjects: Medicine, nursing, gerontology, psychosocial and rehabilitation therapies. **Holdings:** 345 volumes. **Subscriptions:** 21 journals and other serials.

★10793★   ST. PAUL'S HOSPITAL OF SASKATOON, GREY
    NUNS
MEDICAL LIBRARY
1702 20th St., W.
Saskatoon, SK, Canada S7M 0Z9   Phone: (306) 664-5224
Colleen Haichert, Lib.Techn.
Subjects: Medicine, nursing. **Holdings:** 880 books. **Subscriptions:** 64 journals and other serials.

★10794★   SASKATOON CANCER CENTRE
HAROLD E. JOHNS LIBRARY
University of Saskatchewan Campus
20 Campus Dr.
Saskatoon, SK, Canada S7N 4H4   Phone: (306) 966-2662
Mrs. B. Piercy, Libn.
Subjects: Treatment and diagnosis of cancer, radiation therapy, physics, nuclear medicine. **Holdings:** 600 books; 700 bound periodical volumes; 25 tapes. **Subscriptions:** 55 journals and other serials.

★10795★   SASKATOON CITY HOSPITAL
MEDICAL LIBRARY
701 Queen St.
Saskatoon, SK, Canada S7K 0M7   Phone: (306) 934-0228
Shirley Blanchette, Lib.Techn.
Subjects: Medicine. **Holdings:** 300 books; 257 bound periodical volumes. **Subscriptions:** 62 journals and other serials.

★10796★   UNIVERSITY OF SASKATCHEWAN
HEALTH SCIENCES LIBRARY
Saskatoon, SK, Canada S7N 0W0   Phone: (306) 966-5991
Dr. Wilma P. Sweaney, Libn.
Subjects: Medicine, clinical and basic sciences, nursing, dentistry, bio-

chemistry, microbiology, pharmacology, physiology, physical therapy, cancer research. **Holdings:** 95,630 volumes; 11,045 slides; 171 cassettes; 45 kits; 20 realia. **Subscriptions:** 1454 journals and other serials.

★10797★ UNIVERSITY OF SASKATCHEWAN
THORVALDSON LIBRARY
Thorvaldson Bldg.
Saskatoon, SK, Canada S7N 0W0   Phone: (306) 966-6038
G.D. Armstrong, Sci.Libn.
Subjects: Chemistry, pharmacy, chemical engineering, nutrition and dietetics. **Holdings:** 16,000 books; 5000 bound periodical volumes; 100 microforms. **Subscriptions:** 493 journals and other serials.

★10798★ UNIVERSITY OF SASKATCHEWAN
VETERINARY MEDICAL LIBRARY
Western College of Veterinary Medicine
Saskatoon, SK, Canada S7N 0W0   Phone: (306) 966-7206
John V. James, Vet.Med.Libn.
Subjects: Veterinary medicine, animal science. **Holdings:** 32,000 books; 30,000 bound periodical volumes. **Subscriptions:** 556 journals and other serials.

★10799★ SOURIS VALLEY REGIONAL CARE CENTRE
HEALTH SCIENCES LIBRARY
Box 2001
Weyburn, SK, Canada S4H 2L7   Phone: (306) 842-8344
Melva Cooke, Libn.
Subjects: Gerontology, nursing, geriatrics, psychology, nutrition, physical and occupational therapy. **Holdings:** 800 books; 90 bound periodical volumes; 300 articles; 3 VF drawers of clippings. **Subscriptions:** 75 journals and other serials; 7 newspapers.

★10800★ WEYBURN MENTAL HEALTH CENTRE
LIBRARY
Box 1056
Weyburn, SK, Canada S4H 2L4   Phone: (306) 842-5461
Shirley Biliak
Subjects: Psychiatry, psychology, social work, nursing, child and youth services, occupational therapy, vocational guidance. **Holdings:** 1545 volumes. **Subscriptions:** 37 journals and other serials; 6 newspapers.

Master Name and Keyword Index to Volume 2

A

A. Barton Hepburn Hospital • Medical Library **9247**
A.E. Livingston Health Sciences Library - BroMenn Healthcare **8029**
A.E. Macdonald Ophthalmic Library - University of Toronto **10654**
A.F. Parlow Library of the Health Sciences - Los Angeles County/Harbor-UCLA Medical Center **7506**
A. Foster Higgins & Company, Inc. • Research Library **9136**
A.G. Holley State Hospital • Benjamin L. Brock Medical Library **7763**
A Granite Publishers **4901**
A.H. Aaron Health Sciences Library - Buffalo General Hospital **9053**
A. Hollis Marden Bibliotheque - Hopital Reine Elizabeth **10714**
A.M. Best Life/Health Insurance Companies **6734**
A. Stephen Dubois Library - Gowanda Psychiatric Center **9101**
A.T. Still Memorial Library - Kirksville College of Osteopathic Medicine **8742**
A.T. Still Osteopathic Library and Research Center - American Osteopathic Association **7912**
AA Guide for the Disabled Traveller **3777**
AA World Services, Inc. **6139**
AAAD Bulletin **1727**
AABB News Briefs **1728**
AACC Press **4902**
AACP News **1729**
AACPDM News **1730**
AADPA Communicator **1731**
AAHA Provider News **1732**
AALAS Bulletin **1733**
AAMT Newsletter; Tuning In: **3046**
AANA Journal **1**
AAO News **1734**
AAOA News **1735**
AAOA Record **1736**
AAOHN News **1737**
AAOMS Surgical Update **1738**
AAOS Report **1739**
AAP News **1740**
AAPA Newsletter **1741**
AAPSM Newsletter **1742**
AARN Newsletter **1743**
Aaron Health Sciences Library; A.H. - Buffalo General Hospital **9053**
AAROT Newsletter **1744**
AARP Bulletin **1745**
AARP Database **6742**
AAWH—Quarterly **1746**
AAZPA Communique **1747**
The ABA Newsletter **1748**
ABBE Publishers Association of Washington, DC **4903**
Abbott Laboratories
    Abbott Information Services **7891**
    Company Library **10693**

Abbott-Northwestern Hospital Corporation • Library/Media Services **8657**
ABC Distribution Company • Capital Cities/ABC Video Enterprises **6140**
ABC Video Enterprises; Capital Cities/ - ABC Distribution Company **6140**
ABDA-Pharma **6735**
Abdominal Surgeons; American Society of • Donald Collins Memorial Library **8493**
Abdominal Surgery; Journal of **853**
Abigail Smith Timme Library - Ferris State University **8537**
Abilene State School • Special Library **9970**
Ability Testing, Inc.; Institute for Personality and **5498**
Ability Workshop Press **4904**
Abington Memorial Hospital
    School of Nursing Library **9615**
    Wilmer Memorial Medical Library **9616**
ABLEDATA **6736**
Ablex Publishing Corporation **4905**
Ablin Press **4906**
ABMS Compendium of Certified Medical Specialists **3778**
ABMS—Directory of Certified Allergists/Immunologists **3779**
ABMS—Directory of Certified Anesthesiologists **3780**
ABMS—Directory of Certified Colon and Rectal Surgeons **3781**
ABMS—Directory of Certified Dermatologists **3782**
ABMS—Directory of Certified Emergency Physicians **3783**
ABMS—Directory of Certified Family Physicians **3784**
ABMS—Directory of Certified Internists **3785**
ABMS—Directory of Certified Neurological Surgeons **3786**
ABMS—Directory of Certified Neurologists **3787**
ABMS—Directory of Certified Nuclear Medicine Specialists **3788**
ABMS—Directory of Certified Obstetricians and Gynecologists **3789**
ABMS—Directory of Certified Ophthalmologists **3790**
ABMS—Directory of Certified Orthopaedic Surgeons **3791**
ABMS—Directory of Certified Otolaryngologists **3792**
ABMS—Directory of Certified Pathologists **3793**
ABMS—Directory of Certified Pediatricians **3794**
ABMS—Directory of Certified Physical Medicine and Rehabilitation Specialists **3795**
ABMS—Directory of Certified Plastic Surgeons **3796**
ABMS—Directory of Certified Preventive Medicine Physicians **3797**
ABMS—Directory of Certified Psychiatrists **3798**
ABMS—Directory of Certified Radiologists **3799**
ABMS—Directory of Certified Surgeons **3800**
ABMS—Directory of Certified Thoracic Surgeons **3801**
ABMS—Directory of Certified Urologists **3802**
Abnormal Child Psychology; Journal of **854**
Abnormal Psychology; Journal of **855**
Abortion Alternative Organizations Directory **3803**
Abortion Bibliography **3495**
Abortion Federation—Membership Directory; National **4565**
Abortion Federation; National • Library **7692**
Abortion Research Notes **1749**

Alin Foundation Press **4940**

Alinda Press **4941**

Allan Blair Memorial Clinic • Library **10787**

Allan Memorial Institute • Eric D. Wittkower Library **10741**

Allegheny County Health Department • Library **9781**

Allegheny County Pharmacist **1822**

Allegheny General Hospital • Health Sciences Library **9782**

Allen Enterprises; Chaney **5182**

Allen Hospital; Fanny • Health Science Library **10104**

Allen Memorial Hospital • Libraries **8186**

Allen Memorial Library - Cleveland Health Sciences Library **9450**

The Allentown Hospital • Lehigh Valley Hospital Center • Health Sciences Library **9617**

Allentown Osteopathic Medical Center • Learning Resource Center **9618**

Allentown State Hospital • Heim Memorial Library **9619**

Allergan, Inc. **6153**
    Corporate Information Center **7297**

Allergists/Immunologists; ABMS—Directory of Certified **3779**

Allergy **46**

Allergy Advocate; Asthma and **1946**

Allergy Alert **1823**

Allergy, Annals of **129**

Allergy and Antiallergy; CA Selects: **3540**

Allergy and Applied Immunology; *International Archives of* **768**

Allergy Association; American **4951**

Allergy; Clinical and Experimental **409**

Allergy and Clinical Immunology; *Five-Year Cumulative Index to The Journal of* **3660**

Allergy and Clinical Immunology; Journal of **863**

Allergy; Clinical Reviews in **3219**

Allergy Clinics of North America; *Immunology and* **3339**

Allergy and Immunology; American Academy of **4948**

Allergy and Immunology; American College of **6173**

Allergy and Immunology—Membership Directory; American Academy of **3851**

Allergy and Immunology—News & Notes; American Academy of **1841**

Allergy and Infectious Diseases; National Institute of • Rocky Mountain Laboratory Library **8796**

Allergy; Medical Information Systems: **3731**

Allergy; The Newsletter for People With Lactose Intolerance and Milk **2708**

Allergy Products Directory **3843**

Allergy Publications Inc. **4942**

Allergy Research Foundation; Practical **5847**

Alliance Press **4943**

Alliant Health System • Library/Media Services **8236**

Allied and Alternative Medicine **6764**

Allied Health Database; Nursing and **7055**

Allied Health Education Directory **3844**

Allied Health Education Newsletter **1824**

Allied Health; Journal of **864**

Allied Health Literature; *Cumulated Index to Nursing and* **3591**

Allied Health Professions; Sargent College of
    Center for Psychiatric Rehabilitation **6244**
    George K. Makechnie Instructional Resource Center **6245**

Allied Health Professions—Trends; American Society of **1881**

Allied Health Sciences: Books, Journals, Media; Core Collection in Nursing and the **4062**

Allied Health Sciences Library; Schools of Nursing Library/ - Florida A&M University **7804**

Allied Health Sciences; Massachusetts College of Pharmacy and • Sheppard Library **8442**

Allied Sciences; Clinical Otolaryngology and **435**

Allnutt Health Sciences Library - St. Elizabeth Medical Center, Edgewood, KY **8221**

Alm Publishers, Inc. **4944**

Alopecia Areata Newsletter; National **2645**

Aloray, Inc. **4945**

ALPHA Action Reporter **1825**

Alpha Omega Alpha Honor Medical Society **6154**

Alpha Omega International Dental Fraternity—Leadership Newsletter **1826**

ALS Association—Link **1827**

ALS and Neuromuscular Research Foundation • Brian Polsley Memorial Audio/Video Library **7434**

ALS News **1828**

ALS Newsletter **1829**

Alta Bates-Herrick Hospitals
    Alta Bates Hospital • Stuart Memorial Library **7241**
    Herrick Health Sciences Library **7242**
    Vintage Health Library and Resource Center **7243**

Altenheim Adressbuch **3845**

Alternative Birth Services and Consumer Guide; NAPSAC Directory of **4561**

Alternative Futures; Institute for • Library **10121**

Alternative Health Care Services in the U.S.; Directory of Holistic Medicine and **4130**

Alternative Health Therapies **1830**

Alternative Medicine; Allied and **6764**

Alternatives **1831**

Alternatives to Animal Testing—Newsletter; Johns Hopkins Center for **2495**

Alternatives in Cancer Treatment; *Choices: Realistic* **4034**

Alternatives in Childbirth; National Association of Parents and Professionals for Safe **5713**

ALTERNATIVES for the Health Conscious Individual **1832**

Alton Mental Health Center • Professional Library **7892**

Alton Ochsner Medical Foundation • Medical Library **8265**

Altoona Hospital • Glover Memorial Library **9624**

The Altschul Group, Inc. **6155**

Altschul Medical Library - Monmouth Medical Center **8894**

Alza Corporation • Research Library **7388**

Alzheimer Family Program Newsletter **1833**

Alzheimer Society of Metropolitan Toronto—Newsletter **1834**

Alzheimer's Association Newsletter **1835**

Alzheimer's Association—Newsletter; Lexington/Bluegrass **2519**

Alzheimer's Disease Database **6765**

Alzheimer's Disease: A Guide for Families **3846**

Alzheimer's Disease and Related Disorders; Loss of Self: A Family Resource for the Care of **4495**

Alzheimer's Disease and Related Memory Dysfunctions; CA Selects: **3541**

Alzheimer's Disease Treatment Facilities and Home Health Care Programs **3847**

Alzheimer's Patients: A Guide for Family and Health Care Providers; Caring for **4018**

Alzheimer's Research Review **1836**

Amberly Publications **4946**

Ambleside Publishers, Inc. **4947**

Amblyopia and Other Diseases of Ocular Motility; Current Citation on Strabismus, **3595**

Ambrose Video Publishing, Inc. **6156**

Ambulance Association; American • Resource Library **7412**

Ambulance Service Directory **3848**

Ambulatory Anesthesia Newsletter **1837**

Ambulatory Care Management; Journal of **865**

Ambulatory Center Directory; Freestanding **4264**

Ambulatory Foot Surgery—Membership Directory; Academy of **3804**

Ambulatory Health Care Administration; Center for Research in **5174**

Ambulatory Maternal Health Care and Family Planning Services **3849**

Ambulatory Monitoring and Blood Pressure Variability **3186**

Ambulatory Pediatric Association—Membership Directory **3850**

Ambulatory Pediatric Association—Newsletter **1838**

AMC Cancer Research Center • Medical Library **7529**

AMCRA's Managed Care Monitor **1839**

AMECD Newsnotes **1840**

American Academy of Allergy and Immunology **4948**

American Academy of Allergy and Immunology—Membership Directory **3851**

American Academy of Allergy and Immunology—News & Notes **1841**

American Academy of Child and Adolescent Psychiatry **6157**

American Academy of Child and Adolescent Psychiatry; Journal of the **866**

American Academy of Child and Adolescent Psychiatry—Membership Directory **3852**

American Academy of Child and Adolescent Psychiatry—Newsletter **1842**

American Academy of Dermatology **6158**

American Academy of Dermatology; Journal of the **867**

American Academy of Facial Plastic and Reconstructive Surgery **6159**

American Academy of Family Physicians **6160**
    Huffington Library **8725**

American Academy of Forensic Psychology—Directory of Diplomates **3853**

American Academy of Husband-Coached Childbirth **6161**

American Academy of Implant Dentistry—Directory **3854**

American Academy of Implant Dentistry—Newsletter **1843**

American Academy of Natural Family Planning—Directory **3855**

American Academy of Neurological and Orthopaedic Surgery—Directory **3856**

American Academy of Ophthalmology **6162**
    Library **7435**

Annals of Tropical Paediatrics **152**
Annals of Vascular Surgery **153**
Anne Arundel Medical Center • Memorial Library **8315**
Annie Penn Memorial Hospital • Medical Library **9374**
Annuaire CNRS: Sciences de la Vie **3941**
Annual Amyloid **1901**
Annual of Cardiac Surgery **3187**
Annual of Gastrointestinal Endoscopy **3188**
Annual of Opthalmic Laser Surgery **3189**
Annual Progress in Child Psychiatry and Child Development **3190**
Annual Reports in Medicinal Chemistry **3191**
Annual Review of Addictions Research and Treatment **3192**
Annual Review of Biochemistry **3193**
Annual Review of Biophysics and Biomolecular Chemistry **3194**
Annual Review of Cell Biology **3195**
Annual Review of Genetics **3196**
Annual Review of Gerontology and Geriatrics **3197**
Annual Review of Immunology **3198**
Annual Review of Medicine: Selected Topics in the Clinical Sciences **3199**
Annual Review of Microbiology **3200**
Annual Review of Neuroscience **3201**
Annual Review of Nursing Research **3202**
Annual Review of Nutrition **3203**
Annual Review of Pharmacology and Toxicology **3204**
Annual Review of Physiology **3205**
Annual Review of Psychology **3206**
Annual Review of Public Health **3207**
Annual Review of Sociology **3208**
Annual Reviews, Inc. **5020**
Annual Scientific Session News **1902**
Annuals and Review Serials—See Chapter 3
Anoka-Metro Regional Treatment Center • Library **8640**
Anoka Technical College • Media Center **8639**
Anorexia/Bulimia Association—Newsletter, American **1847**
Anorexia Nervosa and Associated Disorders; National Association of • Library **8002**
Anorexia Nervosa Association; Bulimia • Library **10667**
ANR Update **1903**
Anthony C. Pfohl Health Science Library - Mercy Health Center, Dubuque, IA **8175**
Anthony J.D. Marino, M.D. Memorial Library - Underwood-Memorial Hospital **8977**
Anthropology, Embryology and Histology; Excerpta Medica: Anatomy, **3616**
Anthropology; Inter/University Group for Research in Ethnopsychiatry and Medical • Library **10726**
Anthropology; Medical **1286**
Anthroposophic Press Inc. **5021**
Antiallergy; CA Selects: Allergy and **3540**
Antiarrhythmic; CA Selects: **3543**
Antibiotics and Chemotherapy **3209**
Antibodies; CA Selects: Monoclonal **3560**
Antibodies and Hybridomas; Human **714**
Antibodies; Monoclonal **4555**
Antibody and Antisera Buyer's Guide Issue; Biomedical Products Magazine— **3990**
Anticancer Agents; Bioresearch Today: Cancer B— **3531**
Anti-Cancer Drugs **154**
Anticancer Research **155**
Anticonvulsants and Antiepileptics; CA Selects: **3544**
Antiepileptics; CA Selects: Anticonvulsants and **3544**
Antifungal and Antimycotic Agents; CA Selects: **3545**
Anti-Inflammatory Agents and Arthritis; CA Selects: **3546**
Antimicrobial Agents and Chemotherapy **156**
Antimicrobial Chemotherapy; Journal of **891**
The Antimicrobic Newsletter **1904**
Antimycotic Agents; CA Selects: Antifungal and **3545**
Antisera Buyer's Guide Issue; Biomedical Products Magazine— Antibody and **3990**
Antitumor Agents; CA Selects: **3547**
Antitumor and Antiviral Agents—Experimental Therapeutics, Toxicology, Pharmacology; ICRDB Cancergram: **3679**
Antitumor and Antiviral Agents—Mechanism of Action; ICRDB Cancergram: **3680**
Antiviral Agents Bulletin **1905**
Antiviral Agents—Experimental Therapeutics, Toxicology, Pharmacology; ICRDB Cancergram: Antitumor and **3679**
Antiviral Agents—Mechanism of Action; ICRDB Cancergram: Antitumor and **3680**
Antiviral Chemistry and Chemotherapy **157**
Antiviral and Immunomodulatory Therapies for AIDS; Database of **6860**

Antiviral Research **158**
Antler Publishing Company **5022**
Anton Boisen Professional Library - Elgin Mental Health Center **7985**
AODRM Newsletter **1906**
AOE Network **1907**
AOHA **1908**
AORN Journal **159**
AOSA Foresight **1909**
APA Guide to Research Support **3942**
APAGS Newsletter **1910**
Apheresis; Journal of Clinical **943**
Aphra Behn Press **5023**
APLIC-International **5024**
APLICommunicator **1911**
APM-Sterngold **6211**
APMA News **1912**
APMIS **160**
Apnea and Neonatal Monitoring **3943**
Apogee Communications Group **6212**
Apothecaries; American College of **4969**
Apothecaries—Newsletter, American College of **1859**
Apothecary **1913**
Apotheken Telefonregister **3944**
Appalachian Regional Healthcare • Beckley Appalachian Regional Hospital • Medical Library **10241**
Appalshop Films **6213**
Appetite **161**
Apple Creek Developmental Center • Professional Library/Information Center **9408**
Apple Press **5025**
Apple Tree Productions **6214**
Appleton Davies, Inc. **5026, 6215**
Appleton & Lange **5027, 6216**
Appliances; Seibt Directory of Medical **4781**
Applications and Instrumentation, Part B: Nuclear Medicine and Biology; International Journal of Radiation **818**
Applied Bacteriology, Journal of **892**
Applied Biochemistry and Biotechnology **162**
Applied Biochemistry; Biotechnology and **257**
Applied Cardiology; Journal of **893**
Applied Developmental Psychology; Advances in **3121**
Applied and Environmental Microbiology **163**
Applied Genetics News **1914**
Applied Genetics; Theoretical and **1651**
Applied Health Physics Abstracts and Notes **3511**
Applied Immunology; International Archives of Allergy and **768**
Applied Mental Health; Year Book of Psychiatry and **3487**
Applied Microbiology; Advances in **3122**
Applied Microbiology and Biotechnology **164**
Applied Microbiology; Microbiology Abstracts, Section A: Industrial and **3733**
Applied Microbiology; Microbiology Abstracts, Section A: Industrial and **7031**
Applied Neurobiology; Neuropathology and **1380**
Applied Nutrition; Clinics in **450**
Applied Nutrition; Directions in **2186**
Applied Pathology **165**
Applied Pharmacology; Toxicology and **1672**
Applied Physiology; Journal of **894**
Applied Physiology and Occupational Physiology; European Journal of **567**
Applied and Preventive Psychology **166**
Applied Psychology; Journal of **895**
Applied Psychology; PsycSCAN: **3756**
Applied Radiology **167**
Applied Social Sciences Index and Abstracts **6772**
Applied Therapeutics, Inc. **5028**
Applied Toxicology; Fundamental and **632**
Applied Toxicology; Journal of **896**
APPM Update **1915**
Apprentice Academics **5029**
Approved Hospitals and House Officer Posts in the United Kingdom; List of **4486**
Approved Providers of Continuing Pharmaceutical Education **3945**
Aquarian Research Foundation **5030**
Aquinas Medical Library - St. Michael Medical Center **8914**
ARC **168**
ARC Audio-Video Inc. **6217**
Archbold Memorial Hospital; John D. • Ralph Perkins Memorial Library **7863**
Archie R. Dykes Library of the Health Sciences - University of Kansas Medical Center **8192**

Assistive Device Sources; International Directory of Child-Oriented **4410**

Assistive Device Sources; International Directory of Job-Oriented **4413**

Assistive Device Sources; International Directory of Recreation-Oriented **4419**

Assistive Technology Sourcebook **3950**

Assmann Health Sciences Library - Mountainside Hospital **8898**

Associacao Portuguesa da Industria Farmaceutica—Lista de Associados **3951**

Associate Degree Education for Nursing **3952**

Associates in Thanatology **5044**

Association for Advancement of Behavior Therapy—Membership Directory **3953**

Association for the Advancement of Behavior Therapy, Neuropsychology Special Interest Group—Directory **3954**

Association for the Advancement of Health Education **5045**

Association for the Advancement of Medical Instrumentation **5046**

Association for the Advancement of Medical Instrumentation—Membership Directory **3955**

Association of American Medical Colleges **6220**

Association of American Medical Colleges—Curriculum Directory **3956**

Association of American Medical Colleges—Directory of American Medical Education **3957**

Association of American Medical Colleges Group on Public Affairs—Membership Directory **3958**

Association of Biotechnology Companies—Details **1939**

Association of Birth Defect Children—Newsletter **1940**

Association of British Health-Care Industries Directory **3959**

Association of the British Pharmaceutical Industry—Data Sheet Compendium **3960**

Association of the British Pharmaceutical Industry—Directory of Members **3961**

Association of the British Pharmaceutical Industry—Veterinary Data Sheet Compendium **3962**

Association for the Care of Children's Health **5047, 6221**

Association for Child Psychoanalysis—Newsletter **1941**

Association for Children with Down Syndrome • Library **9012**

Association for Death Education and Counseling—The Forum **1942**

Association of Federal Safety and Health Professionals—Directory **3963**

Association for Gerontology in Higher Education **5048**
Resource Library **7663**

Association of Halfway House Alcoholism Programs of North America **5049**

Association of Halfway House Alcoholism Programs of North America—Membership Directory **3964**

Association of Health Facility Survey Agencies—Directory **3965**

Association for the History of Chiropractic—Bulletin **1943**

Association for Humanistic Psychology **5050**

Association of Medical Illustrators—Membership Directory **3966**

Association of Medical Rehabilitation Administrators **5051**

Association of Medical Rehabilitation Administrators—Membership Directory **3967**

Association of Medical Rehabilitation Administrators—Newsletter **1944**

Association of Medical Research Charities—Handbook **3968**

Association of Official Analytical Chemists **5052**

Association of Operating Room Nurses **6222**
Library **7530**

Association of Otolaryngology Administrators—Resource Notebook **3969**

Association de Paralysie Cerebrale du Quebec, Inc. • Centre de Documentation **10759**

The Association for Persons with Severe Handicaps **6223**

Association for Persons With Severe Handicaps—Newsletter **1945**

Association for Persons with Severe Handicaps; TASH: The **6024**

Association of Physician's Assistants in Cardiovascular Surgery—Membership Directory **3970**

Association Quebecoise pour Enfants avec Problemes Auditifs • Centre de Documentation en Deficience Auditive **10695**

Association Register; Medical Meeting/ **4527**

Association for Retarded Citizens • Library **9973**

Association for Retarded Citizens of the U.S. **5053**

Association for the Study of Dreams; Dreaming: The Journal of the **536**

Association of Surgeons of Great Britain and Ireland—Handbook **3971**

Association of Tongue Depressors • Library **8849**

Association of University Programs in Health Administration **5054**
Resource Center for Health Services Administration Education **10127**

Association for Voluntary Surgical Contraception • Library **9145**

Associations of Clinical Toxicology Centers and Poison Control Centers—Membership List; World Federation of **4885**

Associations; Health Sciences Information in Canada: **4327**

Associations and Meetings Issue; Medical Meetings—Directory of Medical **4528**

Associations Section; National Head Injury Foundation Newsletter—NHIF State **4599**

Associations, Self Help Groups, and Hotlines for Mental Health and Human Services...; The Resource Book: Directory of Organizations, **4752**

Ast Resource Collection; Birdie Goldsmith - Barnard Center for Research on Women - Barnard College **9146**

Aster Publishing Corporation **5055**

Asthma and Allergy Advocate **1946**

Asthma; Journal of **899**

Asthma Management **203**

Asthma Resources Directory **3972**

Asthma Update **1947**

Asthmology—Membership Directory; International Association of **4393**

Astor Home for Children • Professional Library **9264**

Astra Pharmaceutical Products, Inc. **6224**

Astre Corporate Group • Library **10120**

Atascadero State Hospital • Professional Library **7235**

ATCC Quarterly Newsletter **1948**

Atcherley Medical Library - Northridge Hospital Medical Center **7371**

Atcom, Inc. **5056**

Athens Mental Health Center • Staff Library **9409**

Atherosclerosis **204**

Atherosclerosis and Heart Disease; CA Selects: **3548**

Athletes; U.S. Association for Blind **6064**

ATIN: AIDS Targeted Information Newsletter **3512**

Atlantic City Medical Center
Atlantic City Division • Health Science Library **8846**
Mainland Division • Health Science Library **8931**

Atlanticare Medical Center • Health Sciences Library **8487**

Atlantis Publishing Company **5057**

Atochem North America • Research Library **9571**

Atomic Veterans Status Information System **6776**

ATS News **1949**

A2LA News **1950**

Auburn House Publishing Company **5058**

Auburn Memorial Hospital • Library/Resource Center **9006**

Auburn University • Veterinary Medical Library **7137**

Audecibel **205**

Audio-Digest Foundation **6225**

Audio-Forum - Jeffrey Norton Publishers, Inc. **6435**

Audio-Learning, Inc. **6226**

Audiologists Directory **3973**

Audiologists; Directory of Bilingual Speech-Language Pathologists and **4098**

Audiologists—Membership Directory; Academy of Dispensing **3807**

Audiology **206**

Audiology; British Journal of **284**

Audiology; Guide to Graduate Education in Speech-Language Pathology and **4279**

Audiology; Guide to Professional Services in Speech-Language Pathology and **4284**

Audiology; Scandinavian **1585**

Audiovisual Center; National • Customer Services **8371**

Audiovisual Center; U.S. National **6642**

Audio-Visual Directory; Behavior Therapy **3982**

Audio-Visual Materials in the Health Sciences; International Guide to Locating **4429**

Audiovisual Media in Medicine; Journal of **900**

Audiovisual Medical Marketing, Inc. **6227**

Audiovisual Producers and Services—See Chapter 7

Audio-Visual Resources Related to Family Interaction with a Handicapped Member: An Annotated Bibliography **3974**

Audiovisuals Catalog; National Library of Medicine **3737, 4611**

Audiovisuals Online **6777**

Augustus C. Long Health Sciences Library - Columbia University **9154**

AUL Newsletter **1951**

Aultman Hospital
Medical Library **9415**
School of Nursing Library **9416**

Aura Publishing Company **5059**

Auricle Press **5060**

Aurora Press **5061**

Aurora Publishing Company **5062**

Austen Fox Riggs Library - Austen Riggs Center, Inc. **8510**

Austen Riggs Center, Inc. • Austen Fox Riggs Library **8510**

Biomedical Communications - School of Veterinary Medicine - North Carolina State University **6527**

Biomedical Communications Center - University Media Services - University of Louisville **6664**

Biomedical Communications Center for Educational Television - School of Medicine - Southern Illinois University **6600**

Biomedical Communications; Department of - M.D. Anderson Cancer Center - University of Texas **6685**

Biomedical Communications Department - Medical Center - University of Nebraska **6675**

Biomedical Communications Department - University of Texas Southwestern Medical Center at Dallas **6687**

Bio-Medical Computing; International Journal of **781**

Biomedical Division Library - Samuel Roberts Noble Foundation **9546**

Biomedical Engineering; Annals of **130**

Biomedical Engineering; Critical Reviews in **3246**

Biomedical Engineering; IEEE Transactions on **727**

Biomedical Engineering; Journal of **917**

Biomedical and Environmental Sciences **246**

Biomedical Ethics—Newsletter; Center for **2058**

Biomedical and Health Care Grants; Directory of **4099**

Biomedical Imaging Computer Resources; Mayo • Library **8676**

Biomedical Index to PHS Supported Research **3988**

Bio-Medical Information Service, Inc.; International **5513**

Biomedical Instrumentation and Technology **247**

Biomedical Library - St. Jude Children's Research Hospital **9944**

Bio-Medical Library - University of Alaska, Fairbanks **7172**

Bio-Medical Library - University of Minnesota **8668**

Biomedical Library - University of Pennsylvania **9773**

Biomedical Library; Dana - Dartmouth College **8838**

Biomedical Library; Woodward - University of British Columbia **10438**

Biomedical Materials and Engineering **248**

Biomedical Materials Research; Journal of **918**

Biomedical Products—Cell Biology Buyer's Guide Issue **3989**

Biomedical Products Magazine—Antibody and Antisera Buyer's Guide Issue **3990**

Biomedical Publications **5103**

Biomedical Research Association; California **6251**

Biomedical Research: The Blue Sheet; DDR Health Policy and **2163**

Biomedical Research; Computers and **468**

Biomedical Research; Foundation for **6354**

Biomedical Research Foundation; National • Library **7693**

Biomedical Research Institute—Messenger; Boston **2001**

Biomedical Research—Newsletter; Foundation for **2268**

Biomedical Research; Resources for Comparative **4757**

Biomedical Research; Southwest Foundation for • Preston G. Northrup Memorial Library **10070**

Biomedical Research Technology Resources—A Research Resources Directory **3991**

Biomedical Research; Undersea **1691**

Biomedical Safety and Standards **1983**

Biomedical Science and Technology **3212**

Biomedical Sciences; College of Veterinary Medicine and - Colorado State University **6283**

Biomedical Sciences, Inc.; Exxon • Library **8871**

Biomedical Sciences Instrumentation **249**

Biomedical Serials in Scandinavian Libraries; List Bio-Med: **3726**

Biomedical Standards; Guide to **4276**

Biomedical Support Program: A Research Resources Directory; Minority **4552**

Biomedical Technology and Human Factors Engineering; Abstract Newsletter: **3497**

Biomedical Technology and Human Factors Engineering: An Abstract Newsletter **1984**

Biomedical Technology Information Service **1985**

Biomedical and Zoological Specimens; Directory of Resources of **4187**

Biomedicine; Computer Methods and Programs in **465**

Biomedicine; Issues in **3345**

Biomembranes **250**

Biomembranes; Journal of Bioenergetics and **912**

Biometric Bulletin **1986**

Biometrics **251**

Biometrika **3528**

Biomolecular Chemistry; Annual Review of Biophysics and **3194**

Bion Publishing **5104**

Bionic and Prosthetic Assistive Device Sources; International Directory of **4409**

Bio-Nouvelles **1987**

Bioorganic and Medicinal Chemistry Letters **252**

Biopharmaceutics; Journal of Pharmacokinetics and **1178**

Biophysical Chemistry **253**

Biophysical Journal **254**

Biophysical Methods; Journal of Biochemical and **909**

Biophysical Research Communications; Biochemical and **227**

Biophysical Society—Directory **3992**

Biophysics; Archives of Biochemistry and **170**

Biophysics, Bioengineering and Medical Instrumentation; Excerpta Medica: **3619**

Biophysics and Biomolecular Chemistry; Annual Review of **3194**

Biophysics; Cancer Biochemistry **347**

Biophysics; Indian Journal of Biochemistry and **739**

Biophysics and Molecular Biology; Progress in **3374**

Biophysics; Radiation and Environmental **1552**

Bio-Probe, Inc. **5105**

BIOREP **6790**

Bioresearch Today: Bioengineering and Instrumentation **3529**

Bioresearch Today: Cancer A—Carcinogenesis **3530**

Bioresearch Today: Cancer B—Anticancer Agents **3531**

Bioresearch Today: Cancer C—Immunology **3532**

Bioresearch Today: Food Microbiology **3533**

Bioresearch Today: Human and Animal Aging **3534**

Bioresearch Today: Human and Animal Parasitology **3535**

Bioresearch Today: Industrial Health and Toxicology **3536**

Biorheology **255**

Bioscience Reports **256**

Biosciences Inc.; Triton • Library **7231**

BIOSIS Previews **6791**

Biosocial Development and Human Health, Inc.; International Foundation for **5518**

Biosocial Research; American Institute for • Library **10229**

Biosocial Research; Huxley Institute for • Library and Resource Center **7735**

Biosocial Science; Journal of **919**

Biotech Business **1988**

Biotechnical Veterinary Consultants **5106**

Biotechnology Abstracts **6792**

Biotechnology Abstracts; Current **3594**

Biotechnology Abstracts; Current **6855**

Biotechnology Advances **3213**

Biotechnology—Analects; Pharmacia LKB **2823**

Biotechnology; Applied Biochemistry and **162**

Biotechnology and Applied Biochemistry **257**

Biotechnology; Applied Microbiology and **164**

Biotechnology Companies—Details; Association of **1939**

Biotechnology Companies in Scotland; Healthcare and **4334**

Biotechnology; Critical Reviews in **3247**

Biotechnology Equipment Suppliers; DECHEMA **6865**

Biotechnology; Frontiers in Immunoassay and **2275**

Biotechnology Information Resources; Directory of **6874**

Biotechnology in Japan Newsservice **1989**

Biotechnology News **1990**

Biotechnology News Watch **1991**

Biotechnology Newsletter **1992**

Biotechnology Newswatch **6793**

Biotechnology Newswatch; McGraw-Hill's **2550**

Biotechnology Report; Olsen's **2759**

Biotechnology Research Abstracts **3537**

Biotechnology Research Abstracts **6794**

Biotechnology; World Journal of Microbiology and **1722**

BioUPDATE **1993**

Bird, III, M.D. Library of Diagnostic Imaging; Gustavus C. - Diagnostic Imaging Department - Temple University Hospital **9766**

Birdie Goldsmith Ast Resource Collection - Barnard Center for Research on Women - Barnard College **9146**

Birth **258**

Birth; Center for the Study of Multiple **5176**

Birth Defect Children—Newsletter; Association of **1940**

Birth Defects Foundation; March of Dimes **6463** Reference Room **9324**

Birth Defects Information System **6795**

Birth Defects Original Article Series **259**

Birth Services and Consumer Guide; NAPSAC Directory of Alternative **4561**

Birthparents, Inc.; Concerned United **5220**

Bishop of Books **5107**

Bishop Clarkson Memorial Hospital • Pathology/Medical Staff Library **8814**

Bishop Lane Library - St. Anthony College of Nursing **8059**

Bissell Hospital; Emily P. • Medical Library **7647**

Bittersweet **5108**

Biviano, M.D., Inc.; Ronald S. **5922**

Bixby Hospital; Emma L. • Patmos/Jones Memorial Library **8522**

BJO's Enterprises **5109**

Canadian Agriculture Library - Agriculture Canada - Canada 10572
Canadian AIDS News 2017
Canadian Association of Anatomists—Newsletter 2018
Canadian Association of Critical Care Nurses—News and Views 2019
Canadian Association on Gerontology—Newsletter 2020
Canadian Association of Pathologists—Newsletter 2021
Canadian Association of Physical Medicine and Rehabilitation News 2022
Canadian Association of Radiologists; Journal of the 922
Canadian Association of Social Work Administration in Health Facilities—Newsletter 2023
Canadian Cancer Society • Library 10450
Canadian Centre for Occupational Health and Safety 10523
Canadian Council on Children and Youth • Resource Centre 10579
Canadian Deaf and Hard of Hearing Forum • Resource Library 10580
Canadian Dental Association • Sydney Wood Bradley Memorial Library 10581
Canadian Dental Association Journal 331
Canadian Diabetes Association • National Office Archives 10623
Canadian Directory of Completed Master's Theses in Nursing 6809
Canadian Film Institute • National Science Film Library 10553
Canadian Forces Medical Services School • Library 10508
Canadian Foundation for Children, Youth and the Law • Justice for Children and Youth Resource Centre 10624
Canadian Hearing Society • Library 10625
Canadian Horticultural Therapy Association—Newsletter 2024
Canadian Hospital Directory 4010
Canadian Hospital Market Directory 4011
Canadian Hospitals; List of 4487
Canadian Institute of Hypnotism • Library 10754
Canadian Journal of Anaesthesia 332
Canadian Journal of Cardiology 333
Canadian Journal of Medical Radiation Technology 334
Canadian Journal of Medical Technology 335
Canadian Journal of Microbiology 336
Canadian Journal of Neurological Sciences 337
Canadian Journal of Ophthalmology 338
Canadian Journal of Physiology and Pharmacology 339
Canadian Journal of Psychiatry/Revue Canadienne de Psychiatrie 340
Canadian Journal of Psychology 341
Canadian Journal of Public Health/Revue Canadienne de Sante Publique 342
Canadian Journal of Surgery 343
Canadian Journal of Veterinary Research 344
Canadian Library of Family Medicine - College of Family Physicians of Canada 10545
Canadian Locations of Journals Indexed for MEDLINE 4012
Canadian Medical Association • Library 10582
Canadian Medical Association Journal 345
Canadian Medical and Biological Engineering Society—Newsletter 2025
Canadian Medical Directory 4013
Canadian Memorial Chiropractic College • C.C. Clemmer Health Sciences Library 10626
Canadian Mental Health Association • Windsor-Essex County Branch Library 10668
Canadian Mental Health Association, Alberta Division • Suicide Information and Education Centre 10373
Canadian National Institute for the Blind • National Library Services 10627
Canadian Nurses Association • Helen K. Mussallem Library 10583
Canadian Organizations Involved in Food and Nutrition; Directory of 4101
Canadian Paediatric Society—News Bulletin 2026
Canadian Paraplegic Association • Library 10512
Canadian Paraplegic Association, Manitoba • Library 10451
Canadian Pharmaceutical Association—Impact 2027
Canadian Programs for Graduate Training in Pharmacology; United States and 4849
Canadian Psychoanalytic Society • Library 10698
Canadian Red Cross Society • National Office • Library 10584
Canadian Rehabilitation Council for the Disabled 6258
Canadian Society of Laboratory Technologists—Bulletin 2028
Canadian Studies/Etudes Canadiennes 6810
Canadian Tobacco Manufacturers Council • Information Center 10699
Canadian Union Catalogue of Library Materials for the Handicapped 6811
Canadian Wholesale Drug Association Newsletter 2029
Canadienne de Psychiatrie; Canadian Journal of Psychiatry/Revue 340

Canadienne de Sante Publique; Canadian Journal of Public Health/Revue 342
Canby Community Health Services • Medical Library 8645
Cancer 346
Cancer A—Carcinogenesis; Bioresearch Today: 3530
Cancer Agency; British Columbia • Library 10423
Cancer B—Anticancer Agents; Bioresearch Today: 3531
Cancer Biochemistry Biophysics 347
Cancer and Blood Research; Institute for • Library 7252
Cancer Book House; Cancer Control Society/ 5152
Cancer, British Journal of 285
Cancer Bulletin; National 2652
Cancer C—Immunology; Bioresearch Today: 3532
Cancer, CA Selects: Nutritional Aspects of 3562
The Cancer Calendar 2030
Cancer Care Center; J.L. and Helen Kellogg • Library 7989
Cancer Care; European Journal of 569
Cancer Care Foundation; National 5717
Cancer Causes and Control 348
CANCER-CD 6812
Cancer Center - Scripps Memorial Hospital 6591
Cancer Center; M.D. Anderson • Research Medical Library 10043
Cancer Center; Memorial Sloan-Kettering • Medical Library • Nathan Cummings Center 9183
Cancer Center—Newsletter; Arizona 1917
Cancer Center—Report; Rush 2927
Cancer Center; Sylvester Comprehensive • The Cancer Information Service 7772
Cancer Centre; London Regional • Library 10547
Cancer Centre; Ottawa Regional • Library 10589
Cancer Centre; Saskatoon • Harold E. Johns Library 10794
Cancer Centre; Tom Baker • Library 10379
The Cancer Challenge 2031
Cancer Chemotherapy and Pharmacology 349
Cancer and Clinical Oncology; European Journal of 570
Cancer Communication 2032
Cancer Control Society/Cancer Book House 5152
Cancer, Current Problems in 3294
Cancer Detection and Management—Biological Markers; ICRDB Cancergram: 3682
Cancer Detection and Management—Diagnostic Radiology; ICRDB Cancergram: 3683
Cancer Detection and Management—Nuclear Medicine; ICRDB Cancergram: 3684
Cancer Detection and Prevention 350
Cancer—Diagnosis, Treatment; ICRDB Cancergram: Lung 3692
Cancer—Diagnosis, Treatment, Preclinical Biology; ICRDB Cancergram: Breast 3681
Cancer on Disc 6813
Cancer Drugs; Anti- 154
Cancer Education; Journal of 923
Cancer Epidemiology Biomarkers and Prevention 351
Cancer Epidemiology; Directory of On-Going Research in 4163
Cancer Epidemiology; Directory of On-going Research in 6877
Cancer; Excerpta Medica: 3620
Cancer Facts and Figures 4014
Cancer Forum 6814
Cancer Foundation; Michigan • Leonard N. Simons Research Library 8553
Cancer Foundation; Ontario • Hamilton Regional Centre • Library 10530
Cancer Foundation; Regional 6570
Cancer Foundation; Saskatchewan • Allan Blair Memorial Clinic • Library 10787
Cancer Foundation; Whedon • Library 10364
Cancer Foundation—Youth Newsletter; Candlelighters Childhood 2036
Cancer Genetics and Cytogenetics 352
Cancer Immunology, Immunotherapy 353
Cancer; Indian Journal of 740
Cancer Information File; Physician Data Query 7075
The Cancer Information Service - Sylvester Comprehensive Cancer Center 7772
Cancer Information and Support; Y-ME National Organization for Breast • Library 8006
Cancer Institute; Cross • Library 10395
Cancer Institute; Dana-Farber
Professional Staff Library 8429
Social Work Oncology Group 6295
Cancer Institute; Journal of the National 1105
Cancer Institute; Montreal • Library 10733
Cancer Institute; National • Frederick Cancer Research and Development Center • Scientific Library 8387
Cancer Institute, Inc.—Newsletter; Walther 3083

Center for Consumer Healthcare Information **5167**
Center for Corporate Health Promotion **5168**
Center for Devices and Radiological Health • Library HFZ-46 **8402**
Center for Emergency Medicine of Western Pennsylvania • Library **9784**
Center for Empirical Medicine **5169**
Center for Food Safety and Applied Nutrition • Library **7725**
Center for Forensic Psychiatry - Michigan Department of Mental Health **6489**
Center for Gestalt Development **5170**
Center for Health Affairs • Greater Cleveland Hospital Association Library **9447**
Center for Health Services—Newsletter **2059**
Center for the History of Foot Care and Footwear - Pennsylvania College of Podiatric Medicine **9748**
Center for Humane Options in Childbirth Experiences • Library **9498**
Center for Interdisciplinary Studies **6269**
Center for Marital and Sexual Studies **6270**
Center for Medical Consumers and Health Information • Consumer's Medical Library **9151**
Center for Mental Health • Library **8088**
Center for Modern Psychoanalytic Studies
   Library **9152**
   Publications Division **5171**
Center for Neural Sciences - Brown University **9863**
Center for Neurodevelopmental Studies, Inc. • Library **7182**
Center News **2060**
Center for Population Options • Library **7666**
Center Press **5172**
Center for Psychiatric Rehabilitation - Sargent College of Allied Health Professions - Boston University **6244**
Center for Public Representation **5173**
Center for Rehabilitation Technology—News Update **2061**
Center for Research in Ambulatory Health Care Administration **5174**
Center for the Rights of the Terminally Ill • Resource Library **9391**
Center for Science in the Public Interest **5175**
Center for Senility Studies • Library **9785**
Center for Sickle Cell Disease—Newsletter **2062**
Center for the Study of Aging • Library **8998**
Center for the Study of Aging and Human Development - Duke University **5281**
Center for the Study of Drug Development—Newsletter **2063**
Center for the Study of the History of Nursing • Special Collections **9714**
Center for the Study of Multiple Birth **5176**
Center for Thanatology Research • Library **9033**
Center for Thanatology Research and Education **5177**
Centinela Hospital Medical Center • Edwin W. Dean Memorial Library **7295**
Central DuPage Hospital • Medical Library **8087**
Central General Hospital • Medical Library **9254**
Central Hospital Services, Inc. **6271**
Central Institute for the Deaf • Professional Library **8755**
Central Institute for the Deaf - Washington University **6100**
Central Islip Psychiatric Center • Health Science Library **9071**
Central Louisiana State Hospital • Medical and Professional Library **8276**
Central Maine Medical Center • Health Science Library **8299**
Central Newfoundland Regional Health Center • Hospital Library **10479**
Central Patents Index **3574**
Central and South American Medical Schools; Directory of North, **4158**
Central Soya Company, Inc.
   Feed Research Library **8097**
   Food Research Library **8107**
Central State Hospital, Indianapolis, IN • Medical Library **8117**
Central State Hospital, Milledgeville, GA • Libraries **7856**
Central State Hospital, Norman, OK • Professional Library **9551**
Central State Hospital, Petersburg, VA • Medical Library **10156**
Central States Institute of Addictions • Addiction Material Center • Library **7915**
Central Suffolk Hospital • Medical Library **9266**
Central Vermont Hospital • Medical Library **10096**
Central Virginia Training Center • Professional Library **10145**
Central Washington Hospital • Heminger Health Sciences Library **10239**
Central Wisconsin Center for Developmentally Disabled • Library Information Center **10285**
Centre Communications **6272**

Centre Community Hospital • Esker W. Cullen Health Sciences Library **9829**
Centre Films, Inc. **6273**
Centre for Gerontology—Newsletter **2064**
Centre Hospitalier Cooke • Bibliotheque Medicale et Administrative **10774**
Centre Hospitalier Cote-des-Neiges • Bibliotheque **10700**
Centre Hospitalier Hotel-Dieu de Gaspe • Centre de Documentation **10682**
Centre Hospitalier Hotel-Dieu de Sherbrooke • Bibliotheque **10771**
Centre Hospitalier Jacques-Viger • Centre de Documentation **10701**
Centre Hospitalier de l'Universite Laval • Bibliotheque des Sciences de la Sante **10767**
Centre Hospitalier de la Region de l'Amiante • Bibliotheque Medicale **10773**
Centre Hospitalier Regional de Lanaudiere • Bibliotheque Medicale **10683**
Centre Hospitalier Robert-Giffard • Bibliotheque Professionnelle **10677**
Centre Hospitalier St. Joseph • Bibliotheque Medicale et Administrative **10775**
Centre Hospitalier de Verdun • Bibliotheque Medicale **10777**
Centre de Readaptation Constance-Lethbridge • Medical Library **10702**
Centre de Services Sociaux du Montreal Metropolitain • Bibliotheque **10703**
Centre for Traditional Acupuncture **5178**
Centron Productions **6274**
Centurion Hospital of Carrollwood • Medical Library **7807**
Century Publisher **5179**
Cerebral Blood Flow and Metabolism; Journal of **935**
Cerebral Circulation; Stroke—A Journal of **1633**
Cerebral Palsy Associations; United **6637**
Cerebral Palsy of New York City; United • Library **9234**
Cerebral Palsy Research and Educational Foundation; United • Library **9235**
Certification Board; Healthcare Safety Professional **5438**
Certification and Licensure Requirements for School Psychologists; Handbook of **4290**
Certified Clinical Electrologists; National Commission for Electrologist Certification—Directory of **4576**
Certified Counselors; National Directory of **4580**
Certified Health Care Engineering Professionals; Directory of **4102**
Certified Healthcare Safety Professionals; Directory of **4103**
Certified Ophthalmic Medical Personnel; Directory of **4104**
Cervical Pathology—Membership List; American Society for Colposcopy and **3928**
CFBS Newsletter **2065**
CGM, Inc. **5180**
CH News **2066**
CHAC Info **2067**
Chain Directory; Home Health Agency **4355**
Chain Directory; Nursing Home **4634**
Chain Drug Store Guide; Hayes **4296**
Chain Drug Stores—Membership Directory; National Association of **4568**
The Chalice **2068**
Challis Resource Centre - Confederation College of Applied Arts and Technology **10615**
Chalmers Hospital; Dr. Everett • Dr. Garfield Moffatt Health Sciences Library **10468**
Champaign Campus Library - Covenant Medical Center **7904**
Champion Press **5181**
A Chance to Grow • Kretsch Brain Injury Resource Library **8658**
Chaney Allen Enterprises **5182**
Change and Exchange **2069**
Changing Medical Markets **2070**
Channel One Video Tape, Inc. **6275**
Channell National EMS Clearinghouse; Sam - National Association of State Emergency Medical Services Directors **8230**
Channing L. Bete Company, Inc. **5183**
Chanute Technical Training Center • Medical Library **7906**
Chapelle Medical Library; Clarence De La - Bellevue Hospital **9147**
Char Inc.; John K. **5553**
Character Laboratory—Newsletter; National **2653**
Charfoos & Christensen, P.C. • Library **8542**
Charities—Handbook; Association of Medical Research **3968**
Charity and Children **2071**
Charity-Delgado School of Nursing • Library **8266**
Charles A. Dana Medical Library - University of Vermont **10103**
Charles C. Thomas, Publisher **5184**
Charles Camsell General Hospital • Peter Wilcock Library **10394**

Current Problems in Surgery **3300**
Current Problems in Urology **3301**
Current Pulmonology **3302**
Current Studies in Hematology and Blood Transfusion **3303**
Current Surgery **3304**
Current Topics in Bioenergetics **3305**
Current Topics in Cellular Regulation **3306**
Current Topics in Developmental Biology **3307**
Current Topics in Experimental Endocrinology **3308**
Current Topics in Eye Research **3309**
Current Topics in Learning Disabilities **490**
Current Topics in Membranes and Transport **3310**
Current Topics in Microbiology and Immunology **3311**
Current Topics in Nutrition and Disease **3312**
Current Topics in Pathology **3313**
Current Work in the History of Medicine **3603**
Curry College • Louis R. Levin Memorial Library • Special Collections **8496**
Curtis Health Science Library; Mary Beth - Elmbrook Memorial Hospital **10265**
Curtis Industries, Inc.; Helene • Corporate Library **7929**
Curtis Memorial Hospital; Charles S. • Medical Library **10480**
Cushing General Hospital; Cardinal • Staff Library **8463**
Cushing/John Hay Whitney Medical Library; Harvey - Yale University **7602**
Cutaneous Pathology; Journal of **979**
Cutis **491**
Cutler Army Hospital • Medical Library **8475**
Cutter Library and Information Services - Miles, Inc. **7245**
CVO Update **2158**
CVPH Medical Center • Medical Library **9255**
Cybele Society **5255**
Cybernetics Foundation; Medical • Library **7754**
Cystic Fibrosis Foundation **6294**
Cystic Fibrosis Foundation—Metro News **2159**
Cytochemistry—Histochemical Society Directory Issue; Journal of Histochemistry and **4462**
Cytochemistry; Journal of Histochemistry and **1037**
Cytochemistry; Progress in Histochemistry and **3384**
Cytogen Corporation • R & D Library **8935**
Cytogenetics; Cancer Genetics and **352**
Cytogenetics and Cell Genetics **492**
Cytologica; Acta **8**
Cytology and Histology; Analytical and Quantitative **120**
Cytology; International Review of **3341**
Cytology; Tutorials of **6635**
Cytometry **493**
Cytopathology **494**
Cytopathology; Diagnostic **517**
Cytoskeleton; Cell Motility and the **377**

D

D.D. Eisenhower Army Medical Center • Medical Library **7852**
D.J. Vincent Medical Library - Riverside Methodist Hospital **9482**
D. Samuel Gottesman Library - Albert Einstein College of Medicine - Yeshiva University **9026**
DA Document Data Base **6883**
D'Agrosa Medical Library; Dr. Joseph - Brookhaven Memorial Hospital Medical Center **9252**
Dahlgren Memorial Library - Medical Center - Georgetown University **7682**
Dakota Hospital • Library **9392**
DALCTRAF **6858**
Dalhousie University • W.K. Kellogg Health Sciences Library **10499**
Dallas; Children's Medical Center of • Lauren Taylor Reardon Family Library **10002**
Dallas-Fort Worth Medical Center • Library **10027**
Dallas Sandt Company **5256**
D'Amico, D.O.; Paul M. **5816**
Damien Dutton Call **2160**
Dana Biomedical Library - Dartmouth College **8838**
Dana-Farber Cancer Institute
    Professional Staff Library **8429**
    Social Work Oncology Group **6295**
Dana Institute for Disease Prevention; Naylor • Library **9314**
Dana Medical Library; Charles A. - University of Vermont **10103**
Dana Productions **6296**
Danbury Hospital • Health Sciences Library **7574**
Dance Therapy Association; American **4979**
Dance Therapy Association—Membership Directory; American **3896**
Daniel Carroll Payson Medical Library - North Shore University Hospital **9122**

Daniel Freeman Hospital • Medical Library & Resource Center **7354**
Daniel Freeman Hospitals • Health Sciences Library **7296**
Daniel T. Banks Health Science Library - St. Vincent's Medical Center **7573**
Danny Foundation • Library **7232**
Darling Biomedical Library; Louise - University of California, Los Angeles **7347**
Darling Memorial Library; Samuel Taylor - Gorgas Army Community Hospital **7731**
Darnall Army Hospital • Medical Library **10015**
Darnall Library; William L. - National Naval Dental Clinic - Naval Dental School - National Naval Medical Command - U.S. Navy **8366**
Dartmouth College • Dana Biomedical Library **8838**
Dartmouth-Hitchcock Medical Center
    Connective Tissue Disease Section **6297**
    Department of Visual Communications **6298**
Dartnell **6299**
Data Archive on Adolescent Pregnancy and Pregnancy Prevention **6859**
Data Bases, 1976-1987; Inventory of U.S. Health Care **4453**
Data Resources in Gerontology: A Directory of Selected Information Vendors, Databases, and Archives **4072**
Database of Antiviral and Immunomodulatory Therapies for AIDS **6860**
Database and Directory of AIDS-Specific Periodicals and Databases **6861**
Database and Directory of Cancer-Specific Periodicals and Databases **6862**
Databases—See Chapter 8, Computer-Readable Databases
Databases; Directory of Online Healthcare **4164**
Databases; Online Medical **4647**
Date Rape; National Clearinghouse on Marital and **7246**
Date Rape—Newsletter; National Clearinghouse on Marital & **2654**
DAV **2161**
Davenport Medical Center • Medical Staff Library **8162**
David A. Amos Health Sciences Library - Mercy Hospital, Muskegon, MI **8615**
David B. Kriser Dental Center - College of Dentistry - New York University **6525**
David B. Kriser Dental Center • John and Bertha E. Waldmann Memorial Library **9214**
David D. Palmer Health Sciences Library - Palmer College of Chiropractic **8164**
David Goldberg Memorial Medical Library - Pascack Valley Hospital **8973**
David Grant Medical Center • Medical Library **7508**
David J. Withersty, M.D. & Associates **6300**
David Knox McKamy Medical Library - Lloyd Noland Hospital **7149**
David L. Reeves Medical Library - Cottage Hospital **7484**
David W. Green Medical Library - Memorial Hospital of Salem County **8950**
Davidson Films **6301**
Davies Medical Center • O.W. Jones Medical Library **7442**
Davis Company; F.A. **5322, 6335**
Davis and Geck Film Library - American Cyanamid Company **6181**
Davis Jewish General Hospital; Sir Mortimer B.
    Institute of Community and Family Psychiatry • Library **10745**
    Lady Davis Institute for Medical Research • Research Library **10746**
    Medical Library **10747**
Davis Library; Stanley K. - Albany General Hospital **9579**
Dawson Technical Institute Library - Chicago City-Wide College **7916**
Daycare Health **2162**
Daystar Publishing Company **5257**
Dayton Lab **6302**
Dayton Mental Health Center • Staff Library **9487**
Dayton Press **5258**
DBS-MDI **6863**
D'Carlin Publishing **5259**
DCI Publishing **5260**
DCM Systems, Inc. • Instructional Systems Division **6303**
DDR Health Policy and Biomedical Research: The Blue Sheet **2163**
De Haen Drug Data **6864**
De Haen International, Inc.; Paul • Drug Information Systems and Services **7557**
De Kalb Medical Center • Health Sciences Library **7848**
De Nonno Pix, Inc. **6304**
De Paul Health Center • Medical Library **8712**
De Paul Medical Center
    Dr. Henry Boone Memorial Library **10153**

675

Elliott E. Carter **5302**
Ellis Hospital • MacMillan Library **9289**
Ellon Bach Newsletter **2217**
Elm Press **5303**
Elmbrook Memorial Hospital • Mary Beth Curtis Health Science
Library **10265**
Elmhurst Hospital Center • Medical Library **9079**
Elmhurst Memorial Hospital • Marquardt Memorial Library **7988**
Elmira Psychiatric Center • Professional Library **9081**
Elsevier Science Publishing Company, Inc. **5304**
Elwyn Institutes • Staff Library **9656**
Elyria Memorial Hospital • Library **9494**
EM Resident **2218**
Emanuel Hospital and Health Center • Library Services **9591**
Emanuel Medical Center • Medical Library **7509**
EMBASE plus **6892**
EMBO Journal **550**
Embryo Transfer, Journal of In Vitro Fertilization and **1049**
Embryology; Anatomy and **122**
Embryology and Cell Biology; Advances in Anatomy, **3119**
*Embryology and Histology; Excerpta Medica: Anatomy,
Anthropology,* **3616**
EMCANCER **6893**
EMDRUGS **6894**
Emergency **551**
Emergency Care Nurses; Technology for **3019**
Emergency Care; Pediatric **1458**
Emergency Care Quarterly **552**
Emergency Department Management **2219**
Emergency Film Group **6326**
Emergency Legal Briefings **2220**
Emergency Management Agency; Federal • National Emergency
Training Center • Learning Resource Center **8382**
Emergency Medical Services **553**
Emergency Medical Services—Buyers Guide Issue **4228**
Emergency Medical Services Directors; National Association of State •
Sam Channell National EMS Clearinghouse **8230**
Emergency Medical and Surgical Service Directory **4229**
Emergency Medicine **554**
Emergency Medicine; American Journal of **65**
Emergency Medicine; Annals of **135**
Emergency Medicine; Archives of **175**
Emergency Medicine Clinics of North America **3322**
Emergency Medicine; Journal of **993**
Emergency Medicine Magazine—List of Poison Control Centers **4230**
Emergency Medicine Reports **2221**
Emergency Medicine; Topics in **1663**
Emergency Medicine of Western Pennsylvania; Center for •
Library **9784**
Emergency Medicine; Year Book of **3465**
Emergency Nursing, JEN: Journal of **850**
Emergency Nursing; Journal of **994**
Emergency Physicians; ABMS—Directory of Certified **3783**
Emergency Response Institute, Inc. **5305**
Emergency Training **5306, 6327**
Emergency Training Center; National • Learning Resource
Center **8382**
Emergindex System **6895**
EMFORENSIC **6896**
Emge Medical Library - Northern California Health Center **7449**
EMHEALTH **6897**
Emil and Lilly Gutheil Memorial Library - Postgraduate Center for
Mental Health **9223**
Emily P. Bissell Hospital • Medical Library **7647**
Emma L. Bixby Hospital • Patmos/Jones Memorial Library **8522**
Emma Pendleton Bradley Hospital • Austin T. and June Rockwell
Levy Library **9858**
Emory University
School of Medicine • Health Sciences Center Library **6328**
School of Medicine • Health Sciences Library **7826**
Science Library **7827**
Emory University; Crawford Long Hospital of • Medical
Library **7825**
*Emotional and Behavioral Disorders; National Directory of
Organizations Serving Parents of Children and Youth with* **4590**
*Emotional Disabilities; A Reader's Guide for Parents of Children with
Mental, Physical, or* **4733**
*Emotional Disabilities; Youth in Transition: A Description of Selected
Programs Serving Adolescents With* **4900**
*Emotionally Handicapped Children and Youth; Directory of Residential
Facilities for* **4184**
Emotive Therapy; Institute for Rational/ **6417**

Empire Blue Cross Blue Shield • Archives and Corporate
Library **9162**
Empire Health Services • Health Information Center **10224**
Empirical Medicine; Center for **5169**
Employee Benefit Documentation Centre - Johnson & Higgins Willis
Faber Inc. **10727**
Employee Health; Hospital **2404**
Employees with Disabilities; Meeting the Needs of **4544**
Employers' Health Benefits Management Letter **2222**
*Employment: A Guide to Postsecondary Vocational Education for
Students with Disabilities; Education for* **4220**
Employment of People with Disabilities; President's Committee
on **5853**
*Employment Programs for Americans with Disabilities; National
Directory: Training and* **4596**
The EMS Leader **2223**
EMS/Rescue Buyers' Guide Issue; Fire Chief— **4260**
EMTOX **6898**
The Encyclopedia of Child Abuse **4231**
Encyclopedia of Drug Abuse **4232**
Encyclopedia of Health Information Sources **4233**
Encyclopedia of Medical Organizations and Agencies **4234**
End-Stage Renal Disease Sourcebook **4235**
The Endeavor **2224**
Endocrine Pathology **555**
Endocrine Research **556**
Endocrine Reviews **3323**
*Endocrine Tumors—Diagnosis, Treatment, Pathophysiology; ICRDB
Cancergram:* **3688**
Endocrinologica; Acta **10**
Endocrinology **557**
Endocrinology Abstracts **3611**
Endocrinology; Advances in Human Fertility and Reproductive **3147**
Endocrinology; Clinical **408**
Endocrinology; Contemporary **3227**
Endocrinology; Current Topics in Experimental **3308**
Endocrinology; Excerpta Medica: **3628**
Endocrinology; General and Comparative **638**
Endocrinology; Journal of **995**
Endocrinology and Metabolism; Advances in **3141**
Endocrinology and Metabolism Clinics of North America **3324**
Endocrinology and Metabolism; Journal of Clinical **945**
Endocrinology and Metabolism; Trends in **1602**
Endocrinology; Molecular **1352**
Endocrinology; Molecular and Cellular **1348**
Endocrinology; Year Book of **3466**
Endodontic Journal; International **773**
Endodontics; Journal of **996**
Endometriosis Association Newsletter **2225**
Endometriosis Association Research Registry **6899**
*Endometriosis: How to Cope with the Physical and Emotional
Challenges; Living with* **4490**
Endoscopy; Annual of Gastrointestinal **3188**
Endoscopy; Gastrointestinal **635**
Endoscopy; Gynaecological **655**
Endoscopy; Surgical **1638**
Endoscopy; Surgical Laparoscopy and **1639**
Energy Publications, Inc. **5307**
*Engineering; Abstract Newsletter: Biomedical Technology and Human
Factors* **3497**
*Engineering: An Abstract Newsletter, Biomedical Technology and
Human Factors* **1984**
Engineering; Annals of Biomedical **130**
Engineering; Biomedical Materials and **248**
Engineering and Computing; Medical and Biological **1289**
Engineering; Critical Reviews in Biomedical **3246**
Engineering; IEEE Transactions on Biomedical **727**
Engineering Information Service; Clinical **2102**
Engineering; Journal of Biomedical **917**
*Engineering Laboratory and Classroom; Access to the Science
and* **3813**
Engineering Letter; Genetic **2283**
Engineering Logistics and Planning, Inc.; Hospital • Library **8937**
*Engineering—Membership Directory; International Federation for
Medical and Biological* **4425**
Engineering; Pritzker Institute of Medical • Library **7933**
Engineering Professionals; Directory of Certified Health Care **4102**
*Engineering Society—Newsletter; Canadian Medical and
Biological* **2025**
Engineering and Technology; Journal of Medical **1079**
Engineers; American Society of Safety **5010**
England; Annals of the Royal College of Surgeons of **148**

England Library; Joseph W. - Philadelphia College of Pharmacy and Science **9755**

England, Wales and Northern Ireland; Directory of Residential Accommodation for the Mentally Handicapped in **4182**

Englewood Hospital
    Learning Center Library **8878**
    School of Nursing Library **8879**

Ensminger Publishing Company/Pegus Press **5308**

ENSR Health Sciences • Library/Information Center **7230**

Enteral Nutrition; JPEN: Journal of Parenteral and **1250**

Entomology; Abstracts of **3502**

Entomology Abstracts **3612**

Entomology; Journal of Medical **1080**

Entomology; Medical and Veterinary **1307**

Entomology; Review of Medical and Veterinary **3763**

Entomology; Review of Medical and Veterinary **7097**

Entrepreneur's Newsletter; Hospital **2405**

Environment and Health; Scandinavian Journal of Work, **1597**

Environment; Indoor **754**

Environmental Biophysics; Radiation and **1552**

Environmental Contamination and Toxicology; Archives of **176**

Environmental Contamination and Toxicology; Bulletin of **316**

Environmental Control; Critical Reviews in **3250**

Environmental Corporation; Concord • Library **10517**

The Environmental Guardian **2226**

Environmental Health; Archives of **177**

Environmental Health Association; National **5724**
    Library **7542**

Environmental Health Association—Newsletter; National **2658**

Environmental Health Foundation; Hanford • Resource Center **10200**

Environmental Health; International Archives of Occupational and **769**

Environmental Health; Journal of **997**

Environmental Health; Journal of Toxicology and **1236**

Environmental Health Library - American Cyanamid Company **8971**

Environmental Health Library; Department of - University of Cincinnati **9436**

Environmental Health News **6900**

Environmental Health Perspectives **558**

Environmental Health and Pollution Control; Excerpta Medica: **3629**

Environmental Health and Safety News **2227**

Environmental Health Sciences; National Institute of • Library **9379**

Environmental Health; Society for Occupational and **5973**

Environmental Medicine; Aviation, Space and **216**

Environmental Medicine; Defence and Civil Institute of • Scientific Information Centre **10516**

Environmental Medicine; Year Book of Occupational and **3478**

Environmental Microbiology; Applied and **163**

Environmental and Molecular Mutagenesis **559**

Environmental Mutagen Information Center - Health and Safety Research Division - Oak Ridge National Laboratory **9968**

Environmental Mutagen Information Center Data Base **6901**

Environmental Nutrition **2228**

Environmental Pathology, Toxicology and Oncology; Journal of **998**

Environmental Physiology; Journal of Comparative Physiology B: Biochemical, Systematic, and **971**

Environmental Pollution and Control: An Abstract Newsletter **3613**

Environmental Press **5309**

Environmental Protection Agency; Illinois • Library **8072**

Environmental Protection; New Jersey Department of • Information Resource Center **8965**

Environmental Research **560**

Environmental Research Institute; Lovelace Biomedical and • Inhalation Toxicology Research Institute • Library **8981**

Environmental Resource Library - Huxley College of Environmental Studies **10184**

Environmental Safety; Ecotoxicology and **547**

Environmental Sciences; Biomedical and **246**

Environmental Sciences; Current Contents/Agriculture, Biology and **3596**

Environmental Studies; Huxley College of • Environmental Resource Library **10184**

Environmental Substances; Carcinogenicity Information Database of **6819**

Environmental Teratology Information Center Data Base **6902**

Environs **2229**

Envision Corporation **6329**

Enzyme **561**

Enzyme Regulation; Advances in **3142**

Enzymology; Advances in Clinical **3134**

Enzymology; Methods in **1322**

Enzymology and Related Areas of Molecular Biology; Advances in **3143**

Epi Notes **2230**

Epidemic **2231**

Epidemiologic Research—Membership Directory; Society for **4801**

Epidemiologic Reviews **3325**

Epidemiology; American Journal of **66**

Epidemiology; Annals of **136**

Epidemiology Biomarkers and Prevention; Cancer **351**

Epidemiology Bulletin **2232**

Epidemiology; Community Dentistry and Oral **456**

Epidemiology and Community Health; Journal of **999**

Epidemiology; Directory of On-Going Research in Cancer **4163**

Epidemiology; Directory of On-going Research in Cancer **6877**

Epidemiology; Excerpta Medica: Public Health, Social Medicine and **3653**

Epidemiology; Genetic **641**

Epidemiology and Infection **562**

Epidemiology; Infection Control and Hospital **756**

Epidemiology; International Journal of **791**

Epidemiology; Journal of Clinical **946**

Epidemiology; Paediatric and Perinatal **1445**

Epidemiology and Public Health Library; Ira V. Hiscock - Yale University **7603**

Epidemiology Resources Inc. **5310**

Epidemiology; Social Psychiatry and Psychiatric **1616**

Epidemiology; Worldwide Serial Reports: **3113**

EPI-Gram **2233**

Epilepsia **563**

Epilepsy Abstracts; Excerpta Medica: **3630**

Epilepsy Foundation of America **5311, 6330**

Epilepsy Library; National **8393**

Epilepsy: A Parents' Guide; Children with **4029**

Epilepsy USA **2234**

Episcopal Facilities for the Elderly; Directory of **4116**

Episcopal Health Services, Inc. • St. John's Episcopal Hospital • Smithtown Medical Library **9290**

Episcopal Health Services of Long Island • St. John's Episcopal Hospital, South Shore Division • Medical Library **9083**

Episcopal Hospital, Philadelphia, PA • Medical Library **9718**

Episcopal Hospital; St. John's
    Interfaith Medical Center • Nursing and Medical Library **9045**
    Smithtown Medical Library **9290**

Episcopal Hospital, South Shore Division; St. John's • Medical Library **9083**

Equipment; Biofeedback **3985**

Equipment Buyers Guide Issues; Medical Electronics—Medical **4513**

Equipment Directory; Oxygen Therapy **4670**

Equipment for Disabled People **4236**

Equipment Markets: United States, Western Europe, and Japan; Blood Pressure **3993**

Equipment Suppliers; DECHEMA Biotechnology **6865**

Equipment and Supplies Directory; Hospital **4366**

Equipment and Supplies Directory; Physicians and Surgeons **4696**

Equipment and Supplies Directory; Veterinarians **4862**

Equipment and Supplies Wholesalers/Manufacturers Directory; Dental **4074**

Equipment and Supply Dealers; Access Guide to Effective Laboratory **3812**

Equipment and Supply Guide; Made in Europe—Medical **4498**

Equipment for Visually Disabled People—An International Guide **4237**

Eric D. Wittkower Library - Allan Memorial Institute - Royal Victoria Hospital **10741**

Eric Miller Company **6331**

Eric W. Hamber Library - University of British Columbia **10436**

Erich Lindemann Mental Health Center • Library **8431**

Erickson Foundation, Inc.; Milton • Archives **7189**

Erickson Foundation—Newsletter; Milton H. **2607**

Erie County Medical Center • Medical Library **9056**

Erlanger Medical Center • Medical Library **9925**

Erlbaum Associates, Inc.; Lawrence **5589**

Erle M. Blunden, M.D. Memorial Library - American River Hospital **7260**

Escambia County Health Department • Library **7788**

ESHA Research, Inc. **5312**

Esker W. Cullen Health Sciences Library - Centre Community Hospital **9829**

Eskualdun Publishers, Ltd. **5313**

Espanolas; Especialidades Farmaceuticas **6904**

Especialidades Consumidas por la Seguridad Social **6903**

Especialidades Farmaceuticas Espanolas **6904**

Especialidades Farmaceuticas en Tramite de Registro **6905**

Essential Fatty Acids; Prostaglandins, Leukotrienes and **1517**

Essential Guide to Generic Drugs **4238**

F

Facilities—Newsletter; Canadian Association of Social Work Administration in Health **2023**

Facilities Obligated to Provide Uncompensated Services; Directory of **4120**

Facilities Offering Vocational Evaluation and Adjustment Training to Hearing Impaired Persons; National Directory of Rehabilitation **4592**

Facilities in Scotland; Directory of Residential **4185**

Facilities and Services for the Learning Disabled; Directory of **4121**

Facilities and Services for Lesbian and Gay Alcoholics; National Directory of **4586**

Facility Directory; Homes—Residential Care **4362**

Facility Survey Agencies—Directory; Association of Health **3965**

Fact Publishing **5325**

Faculty of Dentistry Library - University of Toronto **10656**

Faculty Directory of the Schools and Colleges of Optometry **4252**

Faculty of Ophthalmologists—Annual Report **4253**

FAHS Review **608**

Fair Acres Geriatric Center • Medical Library **9664**

Fair Oaks Hospital • Medical Library **8959**

Fairfax Hospital • Jacob D. Zylman Memorial Library **10136**

Fairfield Hills Hospital • Health Sciences Library **7609**

Fairview Audio-Visuals **6336**

Fairview Developmental Center • Staff Library **7265**

Fairview General Hospital • Medical Library **9456**

Fairview-Ridges Hospital • Medical Staff Library **8644**

Fairview Southdale Hospital • Mary Ann King Health Sciences Library **8650**

Fairview Veterinary Laboratory • Branch Library **10409**

Falk Library of the Health Sciences - University of Pittsburgh **9805**

Falkynor Books **5326**

Fallsview Psychiatric Hospital • Staff Library **9485**

Families: A Reference Handbook; Focus on **4263**

Families: A Resource Guide; Programs to Strengthen **4714**

Family and Children Services; Jewish Board of • Mary and Louis Robinson Library **9175**

Family Communications, Inc. **6337**

Family and Community Health **609**

Family Counselors Directory; Marriage and **4502**

The Family Doctor **6915**

Family Focus; NKF **2718**

Family Foundations; CCL **2051**

Family Guide; Caring for the Mentally Impaired Elderly: A **4019**

Family and Health Care Providers; Caring for Alzheimer's Patients: A Guide for **4018**

Family Health International **5327**
    Library **9377**

Family Health International—Network **2250**

Family Health Media **5328**

Family Health—Membership Roster; International Federation for **4424**

Family Health Sciences Library; Taylor - St. Luke's Hospital, Cleveland, OH **9464**

The Family Institute • Crowley Library **7927**

Family Institute; Boston **6243**

Family Interaction with a Handicapped Member: An Annotated Bibliography; Audio-Visual Resources Related to **3974**

Family Law; National Center on Women and • Information Center **9193**

Family Library; Lauren Taylor Reardon - Children's Medical Center of Dallas **10002**

Family Life Information Exchange **7678**

Family Life Promotion; International Federation of • Library **7690**

Family Medical Library; MacGrath - Cheshire Hospital **8839**

Family Medicine; Canadian Library of - College of Family Physicians of Canada **10545**

Family Medicine Literature Index (FAMLI) **3659**

Family Medicine—Membership Directory; Society of Teachers of **4807**

Family Medicine; Society of Teachers of **5974**

Family Newsletter; Parents/ **2795**

Family Physician; American **50**

Family Physician; American **6766**

Family Physician; Australian **210**

Family Physicians; ABMS—Directory of Certified **3784**

Family Physicians; American Academy of **6160**
    Huffington Library **8725**

Family Physicians of Canada; College of • Canadian Library of Family Medicine **10545**

Family Planning Addresses; World List of **4888**

Family Planning Council; Los Angeles Regional • Library **7336**

Family Planning, Current Literature in **3601**

Family Planning—Directory; American Academy of Natural **3855**

Family Planning Grantees, Delegates, and Clinics; Directory of **4122**

Family Planning Information Centers Directory **4254**

Family Planning, Latest Literature in **3724**

Family Planning, Nongovernmental Organizations in International Population and **4627**

Family Planning Perspectives **610**

Family Planning Perspectives; International and **774**

Family Planning Resource Directory; Fertility Awareness and Natural **4257**

Family Planning Services; Ambulatory Maternal Health Care and **3849**

Family Planning, Studies in **1634**

Family Practice; Journal of **1011**

Family Practice Library at Cheyenne - Family Practice Residency Program at Cheyenne - University of Wyoming **10354**

Family Practice Research Journal **611**

Family Practice Residency Programs; Directory of **4123**

Family Practice; Year Book of **3467**

Family Process **612**

Family Process, Inc. **5329**

Family Program Newsletter; Alzheimer **1833**

Family Publications **5330**

Family Publishing Company **5331**

Family and Social Services; Alberta • Library **10385**

Family Studies; Journal of Child and **938**

Family Support Bulletin **2251**

Family Therapy Letter; The Brown University **2014**

Family Violence Audiovisual Catalog; Child Abuse and Neglect and **4026**

Family Violence Information; Clearinghouse on **7671**

FAMLI **3659**

Fanlight Productions **6338**

Fanny Allen Hospital • Health Science Library **10104**

FANS—Newsletter **2252**

Farb Memorial Medical Library; Jean - Mercy Hospital and Medical Center, San Diego, CA **7428**

Farber Cancer Institute; Dana • Social Work Oncology Group **6295**

Faribault Regional Center • Library **8651**

Farmaceuticas Espanolas; Especialidades **6904**

Farmaceuticas en Tramite de Registro; Especialidades **6905**

Farnham Company, Inc.; Frank C. • Library **9719**

Farquhar Library; Grover C. - Missouri School for the Deaf **8722**

Farquharson Health Sciences Library; C.D. - Centenary Hospital **10606**

Farrar Library - Clarke Institute of Psychiatry **10628**

Farrell Library - Kansas State University **8196**

Fatality Reports **6916**

Fatigue; International Journal of **793**

Fatty Acids; Prostaglandins, Leukotrienes and Essential **1517**

Fauchard Academy—Membership Directory; Pierre **4699**

Faulkner Hospital • Ingersoll Bowditch Library **8433**

Faxton-Children's Hospital • Medical Library **9310**

Fay Library; Oliver J. - Iowa Methodist Medical Center **8171**

Fayetteville Area Health Education Center • Library/Information Services **9354**

FC & A **5332**

FDA Consumer **613**

FDA Drug Bulletin **614**

FDA Drug Bulletin **6917**

FDA Medical Bulletin **2253**

FDA Surveillance Index for Pesticides **2254**

FEBS Letters **615**

Federal Emergency Management Agency • National Emergency Training Center • Learning Resource Center **8382**

Federal Government; Health Information Resources in the **4318**

Federal Hospital Phone Book **4255**

Federal Medical Treatment Facilities Issue; U.S. Medicine—Directory of Major **4852**

Federal Resources in Maternal and Child Health; Starting Early: A Guide to **4820**

Federal Safety and Health Professionals—Directory; Association of **3963**

Federal Veterinarian **2255**

Federally Qualified Report **4256**

Federation of American Health Systems **2256**

Federation of American Health Systems **5334**

Federation des Medecins Omnipracticiens du Quebec • Documentation Centre **10707**

Federation des Medecins Specialistes du Quebec • Bibliotheque **10708**

Federation of State Medical Boards of the United States—Federation Bulletin **2257**

Federlin; Tom **6048**

Feed Research Library - Central Soya Company, Inc. **8097**

H

Infectious Diseases; Current Opinion in **3278**
Infectious Diseases; Journal of **1052**
Infectious Diseases; Medical Research Institute of • Medical
Library **8386**
Infectious Diseases; National Institute of Allergy and • Rocky
Mountain Laboratory Library **8796**
Infectious Diseases Newsletter **2447**
Infectious Diseases; Reviews of **3414**
Infectious Diseases; Scandinavian Journal of **1590**
Infectious Diseases; Year Book of **3471**
Infertility: Medical and Social Choices **4386**
Infertility and Reproductive Medicine Clinics **759**
Infertility; Year Book of **3472**
Infinity Impressions, Ltd. **5486**
Inflammation **760**
Inflammation Research; Advances in **3152**
Inflammatory Bowel Disease; Progress in **2862**
Info ALS **2448**
Infomart Research Services • Library **7485**
InfoMedix **6415**
Information Bureaus Directory; Physicians and Surgeons **4697**
**Information Centers—See Chapter 9, Libraries and Information
Centers**
Information From HEATH **2449**
Information; Global Guide to Medical **4268**
Information Handbook; Health **4317**
Information for Handicapped Travelers **4387**
Information; Index to Health **3702**
Information Management; Healthcare **2360**
*Information and Management Systems Society—Monthly Update;
Healthcare* **2361**
*Information, Prevention, and Early Intervention Programs; Substance
Abuse and Kids: A Directory of Education,* **4828**
Information, Protection, and Advocacy Center for Handicapped
Individuals, Inc. **5487**
Information Resources; Directory of **4141**
Information Resources in the Federal Government; Health **4318**
Information Resources on Victimization of Women; Directory of **4142**
Information Sources; Encyclopedia of Health **4233**
*Information Sources on Handicapping Conditions and Related Services;
Directory of National* **4156**
Information Sources in Paramedical Sciences; Keyguide to **4469**
Information Sources in Pharmacy; Keyguide to **4470**
Information Sources: A Referral Directory; Medical **4520**
*Information Specialists in Disability and Rehabilitation; NARIC
Directory of Librarians and* **4563**
Information System Products; Directory of Hospital **4133**
Information Systems, Inc.; Essential Medical **5314**
Information and Treatment Centers Directory; Smokers **4798**
*Information Vendors, Databases, and Archives; Data Resources in
Gerontology: A Directory of Selected* **4072**
Information Ventures, Inc. • Library **9729**
*Informational Materials on Sexually Transmitted Diseases; Resource
List for* **4756**
*Informationsdienst Krankenhauswesen/Health Care Information
Service* **3713**
InforMED **2450**
InforMed; Medical Society of Nova Scotia— **2577**
Ingalls Memorial Hospital • Medical Library **8000**
Ingeborg S. Kauffman Library - California School of Professional
Psychology **7279**
Ingersoll Bowditch Library - Faulkner Hospital **8433**
Ingham Medical Center Corporation • John W. Chi Memorial
Medical Library **8597**
Ingham Publishing, Inc. **5488**
Inhalation Toxicology **761**
Inhalation Toxicology Research Institute • Library **8981**
Inherited Metabolic Disease; Journal of **1053**
*Inherited Metabolic Diseases; National Survey of Treatment Programs
for PKU and Selected Other* **4616**
Injury: British Journal of Accident Surgery **762**
Injury; Burns, Including Thermal **326**
*Injury Foundation Newsletter—NHIF State Associations Section;
National Head* **4599**
Injury Information Clearinghouse; National **7700**
Injury Prevention Programs **2451**
Injury Rehabilitation Services; National Directory of Head **4588**
Injury Research Foundation of Canada; Traffic • Library **10592**
Injury Resource Library; Kretsch Brain - A Chance to Grow **8658**
Injury Statistical Center Database; National Spinal Cord **7048**
Inlow Clinic • Library **8148**
Inman E. Page Library - Lincoln University of Missouri **8724**
Inner Ear **2452**

Inner Growth Books **5489**
Inner Traditions International Ltd. **5490**
Inner Vision Publishing Company **5491**
Innovations **2453**
Inorganic Biochemistry; Journal of **1054**
Inpharma **3714**
*Inquiry: The Journal of Health Care Organization, Provision, and
Financing* **763**
Inquiry Press **5492**
*Insemination: A Complete Resource Guide; Having Your Baby by
Donor* **4295**
Inside Al-Anon **2454**
Inside MS **2455**
The Insider's Guide to Medical and Dental Schools **4388**
IN-SIGHT • Technical Information Center **9875**
Insight; Healthcare Convention and Exhibitors Association— **2357**
InSight Press **5493**
Insight Press **5494**
Inspiration University • Library **7495**
Insta-Tape, Inc. **6416**
Institut Armand-Frappier
Applied Microbiology Research Centre • Library **10686**
Epidemiology and Preventive Medicine Research Centre •
Library **10687**
Institut National de la Recherche Scientifique-Sante •
Bibliotheque **10758**
Institut Nazareth et Louis-Braille • Bibliotheque **10691**
Institut Philippe Pinel de Montreal • Centre de
Documentation **10722**
Institut Raymond-Dewar • Centre de Documentation **10723**
Institut de Readaptation de Montreal • Bibliotheque Medicale **10724**
Institut de Recherche en Sante et en Securite du Travail •
Informatheque **10725**
Institut Roland-Saucier • Bibliotheque Medicale **10679**
Institute for Advanced Research in Asian Science and Medicine -
Hofstra University **5460**
Institute for Advanced Study of Human Sexuality • Research
Library **7445**
Institute for the Advancement of Health **5495**
Institute on Aging Newsletter **2456**
Institute for Alternative Futures • Library **10121**
Institute for Cancer and Blood Research • Library **7252**
Institute for Cancer Research • Talbot Research Library **9730**
Institute for Clinical Science, Inc. **5496**
Institute for Clinical Social Work • Library **7936**
*Institute for Health, Health Care Policy, and Aging Research—
Newsletter* **2457**
Institute of Living • Medical Library **7587**
Institute of Logopedics • Clyde C. Berger Resource Center **8210**
Institute of Mental Health • Learning Resource Center **9857**
Institute of Mind and Behavior **5497**
Institute of Noetic Sciences • Library **7493**
Institute of the Pennsylvania Hospital • Medical Library **9731**
Institute for Personality and Ability Testing, Inc. **5498**
The Institute for Phobic Awareness **5499**
Institute for Positive Weight Management—Newsletter **2458**
Institute Press **5500**
Institute for Psychoanalysis, Chicago **5501**
Institute for Psychohistory **5502**
Institute for Rational-Emotive Therapy **6417, 5503**
Institute for Rehabilitation and Research **6418**
Information Services Center **10033**
Institute for Research in Hypnosis • Bernard B. Raginsky Research
Library **9170**
Institute of Science and Medicine—Newsletter; Linus Pauling **2530**
Institute for Scientific Information **5504**
Corporate Communications Department Library **9732**
Institute of Social Sciences and Arts, Inc. **5505**
Institute for the Study of Developmental Disabilities - Indiana
University **5483**
Institute for the Study of Human Issues **5506**
Institute for Substance Abuse Research **5507**
Institute of Surgical Research on Burns • Library **10017**
Institutes of Religion and Health • Library **9171**
Instructional Materials Center for the Visually Handicapped -
Colorado Department of Education **7534**
Instructional Technology; Agency for **6145**
Instructional Television Station, Inc.; Milwaukee Regional
Medical **6494**
*Instructors of Alaryngeal Speech; International Association of
Laryngectomees—Directory of* **4395**
Instrumentation; Association for the Advancement of Medical **5046**
Instrumentation; Biomedical Sciences **249**

JAPIC Drugs Data Bank **6986**
JAPICDOC **6987**
Jason Aronson, Inc. **5541**
JB Press **5542**
JBBA Publishing, Inc. **5543**
JBI Points **2487**
JBK Publishing, Inc. **5544**
J.C. Printing Company **5545**
JCAHO Perspectives **2488**
JCU: Journal of Clinical Ultrasound **849**
Jean Crew Deeks Memorial Library - Health Resource Centre - Scarborough City Health Department **10608**
Jean Farb Memorial Medical Library - Mercy Hospital and Medical Center, San Diego, CA **7428**
Jefferson House Gerontology Resource Center - Hartford Hospital **7606**
Jefferson University; Thomas
    Cardeza Foundation • Tocantins Memorial Library **9767**
    Scott Memorial Library **9768**
Jeffrey Norton Publishers, Inc. • Audio-Forum **6435**
Jen House Publishing Company **5546**
JEN: Journal of Emergency Nursing **850**
Jennie Edmundson Memorial Hospital • School of Nursing • Library **8161**
Jepson Memorial Library; Henry G. - Wheeling Hospital **10263**
Jerome Medical Library - St. Joseph's Hospital, St. Paul, MN **8688**
Jerome S. Leopold Health Sciences Library - Lenox Hill Hospital **9177**
Jersey City Medical Center • Medical Library **8892**
Jersey Shore Medical Center
    Ann May School of Nursing Library and Media Center **8905**
    Medical Library **8906**
Jesman Publishing Company **5547**
Jessen Health Science Library; Lloyd W. - Silver Cross Hospital **8013**
Jewish Board of Family and Children Services • Mary and Louis Robinson Library **9175**
Jewish Braille Institute of America, Inc. **5548**
Jewish Center for Immunology and Respiratory Medicine; National • Gerald Tucker Memorial Medical Library **7543**
Jewish General Hospital; Sir Mortimer B. Davis
    Institute of Community and Family Psychiatry • Library **10745**
    Lady Davis Institute for Medical Research • Research Library **10746**
    Medical Library **10747**
Jewish Guild for the Blind • JGB Cassette Library International **9176**
Jewish Guild for the Blind—Newsletter **2489**
Jewish Homes and Housing for the Aged—Perspectives; North American Association of **2723**
Jewish Hospital of Cincinnati • Medical Library **9427**
Jewish Hospital, Louisville, KY • Medical Library **8241**
Jewish Hospital, St. Louis, MO • School of Nursing • Moses Shoenberg Memorial Library **8760**
Jewish Hospital at Washington University Medical Center • Rothschild Medical Library **8761**
Jewish Medical Center; Kingsbrook • Medical Library **9038**
Jewish Medical Center; Long Island
    Health Sciences Library **9133**
    Hillside Hospital • Health Sciences Library **9094**
    Queens Hospital Center • Health Science Library **9110**
Jewish Rehabilitation Hospital • Health Sciences Information Centre **10688**
JGB Cassette Library International - Jewish Guild for the Blind **9176**
JICST File on Medical Science in Japan **6988**
JICST File on Science, Technology and Medicine in Japan **6989**
Jigsaw Publishing House **5549**
Jim Stokes Communications **6436**
Jin Shin Do Acupressure Newsletter **2490**
JMCI: Journal of Molecular and Cellular Immunology **851**
Joan Staats Library - Jackson Laboratory **8288**
Joanne Friedman **5550**
Job-Oriented Assistive Device Sources; International Directory of **4413**
Job Safety Consultant **2491**
Job Safety and Health **2492**
Job Safety and Health **6990**
Job Safety and Health Quarterly **2493**
JOGNN: Journal of Obstetric, Gynecologic, and Neonatal Nursing **852**
Johmax Books, Inc. **5551**
John A. Burns School of Medicine • Pacific Basin Rehabilitation Research and Training Center Library **7878**

John A. Graziano Memorial Library - Merritt Peralta Medical Center **7381**
John A. Prior Health Sciences Library - Ohio State University **9478**
John A. Whyte Medical Library - Delaware Valley Medical Center **9685**
John and Bertha E. Waldmann Memorial Library - David B. Kriser Dental Center - New York University **9214**
John C. Lincoln Hospital • Library **7185**
John C. Rogers Medical Management Advisory **2494**
John C. Whitaker Library - Forsyth Memorial Hospital **9384**
John Crerar Library - University of Chicago **7970**
John Curley & Associates, Inc. **5552**
John D. Archbold Memorial Hospital • Ralph Perkins Memorial Library **7863**
John Davis Williams Library • Austin A. Dodge Pharmacy Library **8709**
John E. Meyer Eye Foundation Library - Eye Foundation Hospital **7141**
John E. Savage Medical Library - Greater Baltimore Medical Center **8321**
John F. Kennedy Medical Center • Medical Library **8874**
John F. Kennedy Memorial Hospital • Medical and Nursing Libraries **7294**
John Hay Whitney Medical Library; Harvey Cushing/ - Yale University **7602**
John J. Dumphy Memorial Library - St. Vincent Hospital, Worcester, MA **8518**
John J. Madden Mental Health Center • Professional Library **8003**
John K. Char Inc. **5553**
John L. McGehee Library - Baptist Memorial Hospital, Memphis, TN **9937**
John M. Wheeler Library - Edward S. Harkness Eye Institute **9161**
John Milton Society for the Blind **5554**
John Moritz Library - Nebraska Methodist Hospital **8817**
John Muir Medical Center • Medical Library **7517**
John N. Shell Library - Nassau Academy of Medicine - Nassau County Medical Society **9091**
John Peter Smith Hospital • Marietta Memorial Medical Library **10021**
John R. Keach Memorial Library - Johnson County Mental Health Center **8198**
John R. Williams, Sr. Health Sciences Library - Highland Hospital, Rochester, NY **9273**
John S. McKee, Jr., M.D. Memorial Library - Broughton Hospital **9365**
John T. Burch, M.D. Memorial Library - San Pedro Peninsula Hospital **7479**
John T. Mather Memorial Hospital • Medical Library **9256**
John Tracy Clinic **5555**
John Umstead Hospital • Learning Resource Center **9338**
John W. Chi Memorial Medical Library - Ingham Medical Center Corporation **8597**
John W. Scott Health Sciences Library - University of Alberta **10408**
John Wiley & Sons, Inc. **5556, 6437**
John Young Brown Memorial Library - St. John's Mercy Medical Center, St. Louis, MO **8770**
Johns Hopkins Center for Alternatives to Animal Testing— Newsletter **2495**
Johns Hopkins Hospital
    Department of Radiology • Library **8324**
    Wilmer Ophthalmological Institute • Jonas S. Friedenwald Library **8325**
The Johns Hopkins Medical Letter—Health After 50 **2496**
Johns Hopkins University
    Johns Hopkins University Press **5557**
    Population Information Program **8326**
    School of Hygiene and Public Health • Abraham M. Lilienfeld Memorial Library **8327**
    School of Hygiene and Public Health • Population Dynamics Library **8328**
    School of Medicine • Department of Pediatrics • Baetjer Memorial Library **8329**
    School of Medicine • Joseph L. Lilienthal Library **8330**
    School of Medicine • Medical Video Production **6438**
    William H. Welch Medical Library **8331**
Johns Hopkins University Press - Johns Hopkins University **5557**
Johns Library; Harold E. - Saskatoon Cancer Centre **10794**
Johnson County Memorial Hospital • Library **8112**
Johnson County Mental Health Center • John R. Keach Memorial Library **8198**
Johnson Foundation; Robert Wood • Library **8942**

L

Microbiology Abstracts, Section C: Algology, Mycology and Protozoology **3735**

Microbiology Abstracts, Section C: Algology, Mycology and Protozoology **7033**

Microbiology; Advances in Applied **3122**

Microbiology; American Society for **6205**

Microbiology; Annual Review of **3200**

Microbiology; Applied and Environmental **163**

Microbiology; Archives of **182**

Microbiology Bacteriology, Mycology and Parasitology; Excerpta Medica: **3640**

Microbiology; BINARY: Computing in **226**

Microbiology; Bioresearch Today: Food **3533**

Microbiology and Biotechnology; Applied **164**

Microbiology and Biotechnology; World Journal of **1722**

Microbiology; Canadian Journal of **336**

Microbiology; Critical Reviews in **3253**

Microbiology; Current **489**

Microbiology and Immunology; Contributions to **3241**

Microbiology and Immunology; Current Topics in **3311**

Microbiology and Immunology; Medical **1301**

Microbiology and Immunology; Progress in Veterinary **3397**

Microbiology; Indian Journal of Pathology and **748**

Microbiology and Infectious Disease; Diagnostic **518**

Microbiology and Infectious Diseases; Comparative Immunology, **461**

Microbiology; Journal of Clinical **953**

Microbiology; Journal of General **1020**

Microbiology; Journal of Medical **1084**

Microbiology; Microbiology Abstracts, Section A: Industrial and Applied **3733**

Microbiology; Microbiology Abstracts, Section A: Industrial and Applied **7031**

Microbiology Newsletter; Clinical **2106**

Microbiology; Research in **1570**

Microbiology; Reviews in Medical **3416**

Microbiology; Veterinary **1704**

Microchemical Journal **1328**

Microscopy Abstracts; Electron **3610**

Microscopy; Journal of **1096**

Microscopy; Scanning **1598**

Microscopy Technique; Journal of Electron **992**

Microsurgery **1329**

Microsurgery; Journal of Reconstructive **1200**

Microvascular Research **1330**

Mid-Atlantic Region; MARHGN Directory: Genetic Services in the **4501**

Mid-Coast Mental Health Center • Vincent Lathbury Library **8307**

Middle East Committee for the Welfare of the Blind—Directory **4550**

Middlesex Memorial Hospital • Health Sciences Library **7595**

Middleton Memorial Veterans Hospital; William S. • Library **10291**

Middletown Psychiatric Center • Medical/Professional Library **9126**

Middletown Regional Hospital • Ada I. Leonard Memorial Library **9512**

Midewiwin Press **5679**

Mid-Maine Medical Center • Clara Hodgkins Memorial Health Sciences Library **8310**

Mid-Manhattan Library • Project Access **9211**

MidMichigan Regional Medical Center • Health Sciences Library **8610**

Mid-Valley Hospital • Physician's Library **9707**

Midway Hospital • Health Sciences Library **8685**

Midwest Alliance in Nursing **5680**

Midwest Health Center for Women **5681**

Midwifery **1331**

Midwifery Practices; Directory of Nurse- **4159**

Midwifery Programs for Registered Nurses; Directory of Primary Care Nurse Practitioner/Specialist Program for Registered Nurses and Nurse **4176**

Midwives; American College of Nurse- **4972**

Migel Memorial Library; M.C. - American Foundation for the Blind **9141**

Migrant Health Centers Directory; 330/329-Funded Community and **4836**

Migrant Health Services Directory **4551**

Milbank Memorial Library - Teachers College **9233**

Miles, Inc.
    Cutter Library and Information Services **7245**
    Diagnostics Division **6492**
    Pharmaceutical Division • Library **7630**
    Research Center • Library **7631**
    Science and Business Information Services **8099**

Milford Hospital • Health Sciences Library **7598**

Milford Memorial Hospital • Medical Library **7638**

Military Medicine **1332**

Milk Allergy; The Newsletter for People With Lactose Intolerance and **2708**

Millard Fillmore Hospitals • Kideney Health Sciences Library **9059**

Miller Company; Eric **6331**

Miller-Dwan Medical Center • Tilderquist Memorial Medical Library **8647**

Miller Memorial Library; Ira - Michigan Psychoanalytic Institute **8629**

Miller Rare Book Room; Hugh Thomas - Irwin Library - Butler University **8115**

Miller Research Corporation; Herman • Library **8525**

Mills-Peninsula Hospitals
    Health Sciences Library **7256**
    Mills Hospital • Medical Library **7477**

Mills Publishing Company **5682**

Mills & Sanderson, Publishers **5683**

Milner-Fenwick, Inc. **6493**

Milton Erickson Foundation, Inc. • Archives **7189**

Milton H. Erickson Foundation—Newsletter **2607**

Milton Helpern Library of Legal Medicine - New York City Office of Chief Medical Examiner **9201**

Milton J. Chatton Medical Library - Santa Clara Valley Medical Center **7473**

Milton S. Hershey Medical Center • Sleep Research and Treatment Center **6551**

Milton Society for the Blind; John **5554**

Milwaukee Academy of Medicine • Library **10317**

Milwaukee County Mental Health Complex • Michael Kasak Library **10318**

Milwaukee; First Call For Help, **10314**

Milwaukee Regional Medical Instructional Television Station, Inc. **6494**

MIMS **3736**

Mind and Behavior; Institute of **5497**

Mind Matters **2608**

Mind and Memory Loss; Aging Myths: Reversible Causes of **3830**

Mind Science Foundation • Library **10064**

Mind Science Foundation—News **2609**

Mindbody Press **5684**

Miner Library; Edward G. - School of Medicine and Dentistry - University of Rochester **9282**

Mineral; Bone and **268**

Mineral and Electrolyte Metabolism **1333**

Mineral Springs Hospital • Medical Library **10366**

Minimally Invasive Therapy **1334**

Ministries; Directory of Health and Welfare **4129**

Minnesota Department of Health • Robert N. Barr Public Health Library **8663**

Minnesota Department of Human Services • DHS Information Center **8673**

Minnesota Medicine **1335**

Minnesota—Network News; Planned Parenthood of **2837**

Minnesota Nursing Accent **2610**

Minnesota; Planned Parenthood of • Phyllis Cooksey Resource Center **8686**

Minority AIDS Council; National • Library **7703**

Minority Biomedical Support Program: A Research Resources Directory **4552**

Minority Health Resources Directory **4553**

Minority Professionals in Psychology; Directory of Ethnic **4117**

Minority Student Opportunities in United States Medical Schools **4554**

Minthorn Memorial Library; Herbert H. - St. John's Medical Center, Longview, WA **10192**

Miracles in Progress **2611**

Miramichi Hospital • Health Sciences Library **10472**

Miriam Hospital • Health Sciences Library **9866**

Miriam Lodge Professional Library - Rosewood Center **8394**

Misericordia General Hospital • Hospital Library **10459**

Misericordia Hospital
    Medical Library **9742**
    Weinlos Medical Library **10403**

Missing Children; North American Directory of Programs for Runaways, Homeless Youth and **4629**

Mississauga Hospital • L.G. Brayley Health Sciences Library **10556**

Mississippi Baptist Medical Center • Library **8699**

Mississippi Department of Health • Audiovisual Library **8700**

Mississippi Department of Mental Health • Library **8701**

Mississippi State Medical Association; Journal of the **1097**

Mississippi State University • College of Veterinary Medicine • Branch Library **8706**

Mothering Magazine **5696**
Mothers and Children **1357**
*Mothers, Healthy Babies—Directory of Educational Materials;
Healthy* **4340**
Mothers; Total Nutrition for Breast-Feeding **4838**
*Motility; Current Citation on Strabismus, Amblyopia and Other
Diseases of Ocular* **3595**
Motility and the Cytoskeleton; Cell **377**
Motility; Journal of Gastrointestinal **1017**
Motility; Journal of Muscle Research and Cell **1103**
Motivational Media, Inc. **6498**
Motor Research; Somatosensory and **1620**
Motoring and Mobility for Disabled People **4557**
Moulton; LeArta **5593**
Mount Auburn Hospital • Health Sciences Library **8470**
Mount Carmel Health, Columbus, OH • Mother M. Constantine
Memorial Library **9470**
Mount Carmel Mercy Hospital • Medical Library **8555**
Mount Clemens General Hospital • Stuck Medical Library **8611**
Mount Pleasant Mental Health Institute • Professional Library **8182**
Mount Sinai Hospital, Hartford, CT • Health Sciences Library **7588**
Mount Sinai Hospital Medical Center • Lewison Memorial
Library **7944**
Mt. Sinai Hospital, Philadelphia, PA • Medical Library **9744**
Mount Sinai Hospital, Toronto, ON, Canada • Sidney Liswood
Library **10639**
Mt. Sinai Journal of Medicine **1358**
Mount Sinai Medical Center of Cleveland • George H. Hays
Memorial Library **9460**
Mount Sinai Medical Center of Greater Miami • Medical
Library **7778**
Mount Sinai School of Medicine of the City University of New York
• Gustave L. and Janet W. Levy Library **9188**
Mount Sinai Services • Elmhurst Hospital Center • Medical
Library **9079**
Mount Vernon Hospital • Library and Information Services **9132**
Mount Zion Medical Center • Harris M. Fishbon Memorial
Library **7465**
Mountain Area Health Education Center • Information and Media
Services **9333**
Mountain Home Publishing **5697**
Mountain Spring Press Ltd. **5698**
Mountainside Hospital
Assmann Health Sciences Library **8898**
School of Nursing Library **8899**
Mountaintop Consciousness Publishing **5699**
Movement; Adventures in **1781**
MP&P Medical Library • Library **7583**
MR; Seminars in Ultrasound, CT, and **3443**
MRC Relay **2620**
MRI Education Foundation, Inc. **6499**
MRI Newsletter **2621**
MS Canada **2622**
MTI Film Video; Coronet/ **6287**
Mueller Health Sciences Library - Lancaster General Hospital **9683**
Muhlenberg Hospital Center • Medical Library **9630**
Muhlenberg Regional Medical Center • E. Gordon Glass, M.D.,
Memorial Library **8930**
Muir Medical Center; John • Medical Library **7517**
Mulford Library; Raymon H. - Medical College of Ohio at
Toledo **9530**
Multi-Fit Publications **5700**
Multi-Focus, Inc. **6500**
*Multi-Hospital Systems and Group Purchasing Organizations
Directory* **4558**
Multiple Birth; Center for the Study of **5176**
*Multiple Myeloma—Diagnosis and Treatment; ICRDB Cancergram:
Leukemia and* **3691**
Multiple Sclerosis Research Projects **7034**
Multiple Sclerosis Society; National • Information Resource Center
and Library **9194**
Multipurpose Arthritis Center Library - Medical University of South
Carolina **9880**
Municipal Insurance Claim Forms and History Data Base; Medical
Malpractice and **7016**
Munro Medical Library; Dr. E.H. **7563**
Muriel C. Clausen Company **5701**
Muriel Ivimey Library **9189**
Murphy Memorial Health Science Library; William K. - Veterans
Home of California **7519**
Murray Developmental Center; Warren G. • Library **7903**
Muscatatuck State Developmental Center • Resident and Staff
Development Library **8096**

Muscle and Nerve **1359**
Muscle Research and Cell Motility; Journal of **1103**
Musculoskeletal Pain; Journal of **1104**
Musculoskeletal Rehabilitation; Journal of Back and **904**
Musculoskeletal and Skin Diseases Database; Arthritis and **6774**
Musculoskeletal and Skin Diseases Information Clearinghouse;
National Arthritis and **8357**
Musculoskeletal and Skin Diseases; National Institute of Arthritis and
• Office of Scientific and Health Communication **8360**
*Museum Directory for Blind and Visually Impaired People; Access to
Art: A* **3811**
Museum of Science and Industry • Library **7945**
Music Medicine Clearinghouse - Medical and Chirurgical Faculty -
Maryland State Medical Society **8340**
Music Therapy Clinical Training Facilities Directory **4559**
*Music Therapy—Membership Directory; American Association
for* **3876**
Music Therapy—Membership Directory; National Association for **4570**
Mussallem Library; Helen K. - Canadian Nurses Association **10583**
Mutagen Information Center Data Base; Environmental **6901**
Mutagen Information Center; Environmental - Health and Safety
Research Division - Oak Ridge National Laboratory **9968**
Mutagenesis **1360**
Mutagenesis; Environmental and Molecular **559**
Mutagenesis; Teratogenesis, Carcinogenesis, and **1648**
Mutagens, and Teratogens; CA Selects: Carcinogens, **3552**
Mutation Research **1361**
Mutual Aid **2623**
Mutual Life Insurance Company of New York • Law Library **9190**
*Mycobacterial Diseases; International Journal of Leprosy and
Other* **804**
Mycology; Abstracts of **3504**
Mycology; Journal of Medical and Veterinary **1088**
*Mycology—Membership List; International Society for Human and
Animal* **4438**
*Mycology and Parasitology; Excerpta Medica: Microbiology
Bacteriology,* **3640**
*Mycology and Protozoology; Microbiology Abstracts, Section C:
Algology,* **3735**
Mycology and Protozoology; Microbiology Abstracts, Section C:
Algology, **7033**
Mycology; Review of Medical and Veterinary **3410**
Mycology; Review of Medical and Veterinary **7098**
Mycoplasmology—Newsletter; International Organization for **2474**
*Myeloma—Diagnosis and Treatment; ICRDB Cancergram: Leukemia
and Multiple* **3691**
Myers Library; Richard O. - Valley Presbyterian Hospital **7515**

N

NAACLS News **2624**
NAACOG Newsletter **2625**
NAACOG: The Organization for Obstetric, Gynecologic, and
Neonatal Nurses **6501**
NAAFA Newsletter **2626**
NABP Newsletter **2627**
NABR Alert **2628**
NABR Update **2629**
The NACA News **2630**
NACDS Legislative Newsletter **2631**
NADAP News/Report **2632**
NAFAC News **2633**
NAHC Report **2634**
NAIC AIDS Education Materials Database **7035**
NAIC Resources and Services Database **7036**
NAMES News **2635**
NAN Directory of AIDS Education and Service Organizations **4560**
NAOSMM Newsline **2636**
Napa State Hospital • Wrenshall A. Oliver Professional Library **7366**
NAPH National Newsletter **2637**
NAPM News Bulletin **2638**
*NAPSAC Directory of Alternative Birth Services and Consumer
Guide* **4561**
NAPSAC International **5702**
NAPSAC News **2639**
NAPT Newsletter **2640**
NARAL Newsletter **2641**
Naramore Library; J.T. - Larned State Hospital **8194**
Narcotic and Drug Research Inc. • Resource Center **9191**
Narcotic Treatment Programs; Directory of **4154**
Narcotics Anonymous, Inc.; World Service Office of **6130**
Narcotics; Bulletin on **321**
Narcotics and Drug Abuse: A-Z **4562**

Newsletter From the Sierra Madre 2706
Newsletter; The Triplet Connection— 3044
Newsletters—See Chapter 2
Newsounds 2710
Newton-Wellesley Hospital • Paul Talbot Babson Memorial Library 8500
Ney Company; J.M. 6433
NFCR Reports 2711
NFPRHA News 2712
NHO NewsLine 2713
NIAAA Research Library - National Institute on Alcohol Abuse and Alcoholism 7701
Niagara Centre for Independent Living Newsletter 2714
Niagara College of Applied Arts and Technology Learning Resource Centre 10599, 10663
NIDA Notes 2715
NIDR ONLINE 7051
NIDR Research Digest 2716
The Nightingale 2717
NIH Guide for Grants and Contracts 4626
The NIJ Drugs and Crime CD-ROM Library 7052
Nisonger Center - Ohio State University 6536
Nitrogen Fixation; CA Selects: 3561
NKF Family Focus 2718
NKI Report 2719
NLM Serial Titles; Index of 3705
NMCD: Nutrition, Metabolism and Cardiovascular 1405
Noble Army Hospital • Medical Library 7150
Noble Foundation; Samuel Roberts • Biomedical Division Library 9546
NOCIRC—Newsletter 2720
Noetic Sciences; Institute of • Library 7493
NOHA News 2721
Nolan D.C. Lewis Library - Carrier Foundation 8847
Noland Hospital; Lloyd • David Knox McKamy Medical Library 7149
Nomis Publications, Inc. 5764
Nongovernmental Organizations in International Population and Family Planning 4627
Noninvasive Cardiology; American Journal of 82
Non-Isotopic Immunoassay 4628
Non-Medical Research Relating to Handicapped People; Directory of 4157
Nonprescription Drug Manufacturers Association • Library 7708
The Nonsmokers' Voice 2722
NORD Services/Rare Disease Database 7053
NORDRUG 7054
Norfolk Regional Center • Staff Library 8811
Norman D. Weiner Professional Library - Friends Hospital 9722
Norman F. Feldheym Library - St. Bernardine Medical Center 7417
Norman Geller 5765
Norman Publishing 5766
Norman Regional Hospital • Health Sciences Library 9552
Normed Verlag, Inc. 5767
Normes et Repertoires; Standards and Directories/ 7115
Norris, Jr. Visual Science Library; Kenneth T. - Estelle Doheny Eye Institute 7323
Norris Medical Library - Health Sciences Campus - University of Southern California 7350
Norristown State Hospital • Professional/Staff Library 9701
North American Association of Jewish Homes and Housing for the Aged—Perspectives 2723
North American Directory of Programs for Runaways, Homeless Youth and Missing Children 4629
North American Society of Adlerian Psychology—Newsletter 2724
North American Society of Pacing and Electrophysiology—Membership Directory 4630
North American Youth Sport Institute • Information Center 9363
North Atlantic Books 5768
North Bay College Education Centre • Library 10562
North Bay Psychiatric Hospital • Library 10563
North Carolina Agricultural and Technical State University • F.D. Bluford Library 9359
North Carolina; Blue Cross and Blue Shield of • Information Center 9349
North Carolina Department of Cultural Resources • Library for the Blind and Physically Handicapped 9368
North Carolina Department of Environment, Health, and Natural Resources • Public Health Pest Management Section • Environmental Health Division • Library 9369
North Carolina Department of Labor • Charles H. Livengood, Jr. Memorial Labor Law Library 9370
North Carolina Medical Journal 1406

North Carolina State University
    School of Veterinary Medicine • Biomedical Communications 6527
    Veterinary Medical Library 9371
North Central Bronx Hospital • J.L. Amster Health Sciences Library 9023
North, Central and South American Medical Schools; Directory of 4158
North Conway Institute • Resource Center • Alcohol and Drugs 8452
North Country Hospital and Health Center • Medical Library 10107
North Dakota Society for Medical Technology—Newsletter 2725
North Dakota State Department of Health • Division of Health Promotion and Education 9388
North Dakota State Hospital • Health Science Library 9401
North Dakota State University • Pharmacy Library 9395
North Detroit General Hospital • Medical Library 8556
North General Hospital • Medical Library 9217
North Hills Passavant Hospital • Medical Library 9797
North Kansas City Hospital • Medical Library 8745
North Memorial Medical Center • Medical Library 8675
North Mississippi Medical Center • Resource Center 8708
North Princeton Developmental Center • Health Services Library 8940
North Shore Medical Center • Medical Library 7771
North Shore University Hospital • Daniel Carroll Payson Medical Library 9122
North Texas Medical Center • Library 10055
North York General Hospital • W. Keith Welsh Library 10666
Northampton Community College • Learning Resources Center • Special Collections 9631
Northeast Alabama Regional Medical Center • Medical Library 7136
Northeast Baptist Hospital • Bates Library 10065
Northeast Georgia Medical Center and Hall School of Nursing/Brenau College • Library 7853
Northeast Georgia Regional Education Service Agency • Northeast Georgia Learning Resource System 7866
Northeast Wisconsin Technical College • Learning Resource Center 10275
Northeastern Hospital • School of Nursing Library 9745
Northeastern Ohio Universities College of Medicine • Oliver Ocasek Regional Medical Information Center 9523
Northeastern Vermont Regional Hospital • Information Center/Library 10112
Northern Alberta Institute of Technology • Learning Resource Centre 10404
Northern California Health Center • Emge Medical Library 7449
Northern Cumberland Memorial Hospital • Frederick W. Skillin Health Sciences Library 8293
Northern Ireland; Directory of Residential Accommodation for the Mentally Handicapped in England, Wales and 4182
Northern New England; Planned Parenthood of • PPNNE Resource Center 10102
Northern Publishing 5769
Northern Westchester Hospital Center • Health Sciences Library 9131
Northridge Hospital Medical Center • Atcherley Medical Library 7371
Northrup Memorial Library; Preston G. - Southwest Foundation for Biomedical Research 10070
Northville Regional Psychiatric Hospital • Professional Library 8616
Northwest Arctic NUNA 2726
Northwest Area Health Education Center, Boone, NC • NW AHEC Library 9336
Northwest Area Health Education Center, Hickory, NC • NW AHEC Library 9362
Northwest Area Health Education Center, Salisbury, NC • NW AHEC Library 9380
Northwest Community Hospital • Medical Library 7895
Northwest General Hospital • Medical Library 10320
Northwest Georgia Regional Hospital at Rome • Medical Library 7859
Northwest Geriatric Education Center • Clearinghouse Resource Center 10206
Northwest Hospital • Effie M. Storey Learning Center 10207
Northwest Learning Associates, Inc. 5770
Northwest Territories Department of Health • Dr. Otto Schaefer Health Resource Centre 10493
Northwest Territories Registered Nurses' Association—Newsletter 2727
Northwest Territories Safety Division • Department of Safety and Public Services • Safety/Education Resource Centre 10494
Northwestern College of Chiropractic • Library 8641
Northwestern Connecticut Community College • Library 7635

Obstetrics and Gynecology; Excerpta Medica: **3643**

Obstetrics and Gynecology and Fertility; Current Problems in **3298**

Obstetrics and Gynecology; Key **3719**

Obstetrics, Gynecology, and Reproductive Biology; European Journal of **580**

Obstetrics and Gynecology; Year Book of **3477**

Obstetrics; International Journal of Gynecology and **798**

Obstetrics; Surgery, Gynecology and **1637**

Ocasek Regional Medical Information Center; Oliver - Northeastern Ohio Universities College of Medicine **9523**

Occupational Diseases; Selected Abstracts on **3766**

Occupational and Environmental Health; International Archives of **769**

Occupational and Environmental Health; Society for **5973**

Occupational and Environmental Medicine; Year Book of **3478**

Occupational Exposure and Hazards; CA Selects: **3563**

Occupational Health and Industrial Medicine; Excerpta Medica: **3644**

Occupational Health Nurses; American Association of • Library **7822**

Occupational Health Nurses Journal; American Association of **49**

Occupational Health Program—Monitor, Labor **2505**

Occupational Health and Safety **1424**

Occupational Health and Safety; Alberta
Library **10369**
Library Services **10391**

Occupational Health and Safety; Canadian Centre for **10523**

Occupational Health and Safety; International Courses in **4405**

Occupational Health and Safety Letter **2752**

Occupational Health and Safety Purchasing Sourcebook **4641**

Occupational Hygiene; Annals of **143**

Occupational Medicine; Journal of **1141**

Occupational Medicine; Journal of the Society of **1218**

Occupational Medicine—Membership Directory; American College of **3893**

Occupational Physiology; European Journal of Applied Physiology and **567**

Occupational Psychology Offering Consultancy Services; British Psychological Society—List of Members of the Division of **4003**

Occupational Safety and Health Daily; BNA **6798**

Occupational Safety and Health Library - Maryland Department of Licensing and Regulation **8336**

Occupational Safety and Health Reference Centre - Library Services - Labour Canada - Canada **10575**

Occupational Safety and Health Reporter **2753**

Occupational Safety and Health Reporter **7059**

Occupational Safety and Health; U.S. National Institute for • Taft Center C-21 • Library **9434**

Occupational Therapists Directory **4642**

Occupational Therapists Register **4643**

Occupational Therapy; American Journal of **85**

Occupational Therapy Association; American **4996, 6194**

Occupational Therapy Association—Federal Report; American **1874**

Occupational Therapy; Department of - San Jose State University **6586**

Occupational Therapy Foundation and Association; American • Wilma L. West Library **8397**

Occupational Therapy in Geriatrics; Physical and **1483**

Occupational Therapy in Health Care **1425**

Occupational Therapy in Mental Health **1426**

Occupational Therapy in Pediatrics; Physical and **1484**

Occupational Therapy Programs; Educational Programs in **4224**

Occupations Center; Health • Library **7492**

Ochsner Medical Foundation; Alton • Medical Library **8265**

O'Connor, Cavanagh, Anderson, Killingsworth & Beshears, P.A. • Law Library **7190**

O'Connor Hospital • Library Media Center **7468**

O'Connor Hospital; Lindsay A. and Olive B. • Library **9076**

OCP Newsletter **2754**

Ocular Motility; Current Citation on Strabismus, Amblyopia and Other Diseases of **3595**

ODN Productions **5786**

O'Donoghue Medical Library - St. Anthony Hospital, Oklahoma City, OK **9561**

Odontologica Scandinavica; Acta **16**

ODPHP National Health Information Center - Office of Disease Prevention and Health Promotion - U.S. Public Health Service **7727**

Of Current Interest **2755**

OFA Hip Dysplasia Registry - Orthopedic Foundation for Animals **8715**

Office Practice; Primary Care: Clinics in **3370**

Officers Association—Newsletter; National Disabled Law **2657**

Officers News; Local Health **2532**

Officers of Schools Association—Rules and List of Members; Medical **4530**

Ohio Bureau of Workers' Compensation • Rehabilitation Division Library **9471**

Ohio College of Podiatric Medicine • Library/Media Center **9461**

Ohio Department of Aging • Resource Center **9472**

Ohio Department of Drug and Alcohol Addiction Services • Regional Alcohol and Drug Awareness • Resource Center **9473**

Ohio Department of Mental Health • Educational Media Center **9474**

Ohio Division of Safety and Hygiene • Resource Center **9475**

Ohio GASP, Inc. Newsletter **2756**

Ohio School for the Deaf • Library **9476**

Ohio State Medical Journal **1427**

Ohio State School for the Blind • Library **9477**

Ohio State University
College of Medicine • Biomedical Communications **6534**
College of Medicine • Continuing Medical Education **6535**
John A. Prior Health Sciences Library **9478**
Nisonger Center **6536**
Pharmacy Library **9479**
Social Work Library **9480**
Veterinary Medicine Library **9481**

Ohio University • Health Sciences Library **9410**

Ohio Valley General Hospital • Professional Library **9693**

Ohio Valley Hospital • Health Sciences Library **9528**

Ohio Valley Medical Center • Hupp Medical Library **10262**

Ohio VMA Newsletter **2757**

OHIS Newsletter **2758**

Ohrstrom Library; Elizabeth J. - Department of Neurology - Medical Center - University of Virginia **10133**

Ohsawa Macrobiotic Foundation; George **5367**

OK Publishing **5787**

O'Kelly Library; C.G. • Special Collections **9387**

Oklahoma; Children's Hospital of
CHO Medical Library **9554**
Family Resource Center **9555**

Oklahoma Department of Health • Information and Referral Healthline **9557**

Oklahoma Regional Library for the Blind and Physically Handicapped **9558**

Oklahoma School for the Blind • Parkview Library **9549**

Oklahoma School for the Deaf • Library **9569**

Oklahoma State Medical Association; Journal of the **1142**

Oklahoma State University
Audiovisual Center **6537**
College of Osteopathic Medicine • Medical Library **9573**
College of Veterinary Medicine • Learning Resources Center **6538**
Veterinary Medicine Library **9568**

Old Age; CPA World Directory of **4067**

Old Age; New Literature on **3739**

Old Age: A Register of Social Research **4644**

Older Adults, People With Disabilities; Focus: Library Service to **2266**

Older People; Resource Directory for **4755**

Oliphant Library; Jacob T. - Indiana Board of Health **8120**

Olive View Medical Health Center; Los Angeles County/ • Health Sciences Library **7505**

Oliver J. Fay Library - Iowa Methodist Medical Center **8171**

Oliver Ocasek Regional Medical Information Center - Northeastern Ohio Universities College of Medicine **9523**

Oliver Professional Library; Wrenshall A. - Napa State Hospital **7366**

Ollie A. Randall Library - The National Council on the Aging **7696**

Olsen's Biotechnology Report **2759**

Olson & Company; C. **5145**

Olympia Fields Osteopathic Medical Center Library - Chicago College of Osteopathic Medicine **8040**

Olympic Resource and Information Center - U.S. Olympic Committee **7528**

Omaha Public Library • Business, Science and Technology Department **8818**

Omni Learning Institute **5788**

OmniComm Publications **5789**

On the Beam **2760**

On the Record **2761**

On the Scene **2762**

On Your Mark **2763**

ONA Newsletter **2764**

OncoDisc **7060**

Oncogenes and Growth Factors Abstracts **7061**

Oncogenesis; Critical Reviews in **3256**

Onco-Logic **2765**

Pediatrics; Advances in Developmental and Behavioral 3138
Pediatrics; American Academy of 4950
    Bakwin Library 7987
Pediatrics; Clinical 436
Pediatrics; Combined Cumulative Index to 3583
Pediatrics; Core Journals in 3589
Pediatrics; Current 3292
Pediatrics; Current Opinion in 3286
Pediatrics; Current Problems in 3299
Pediatrics on Disc 7065
Pediatrics; European Journal of 582
Pediatrics—Fellowship List; American Academy of 3859
Pediatrics; Indian 752
Pediatrics; Indian Journal of 749
Pediatrics; Journal of 1167
Pediatrics; Journal of Developmental and Behavioral 985
Pediatrics for Parents 2809
Pediatrics and Pediatric Surgery; Excerpta Medica: 3648
Pediatrics; Physical and Occupational Therapy in 1484
Pediatrics; Year Book of 3484
Pediculosis Association—Progress; National 2671
Pedipress, Inc. 5819
Pee Dee Area Health Education Center Library 9896
Peer Review; Hospital 2415
Pegus Press; Ensminger Publishing Company/ 5308
Peninsula Center for the Blind 5820
Peninsula Hospital Center • Medical Library 9084
Penn Memorial Hospital; Annie • Medical Library 9374
Pennal Library; George - St. Joseph's Health Centre, Toronto, ON, Canada 10649
Pennant Books 5821
Pennock Hospital • Medical Library 8585
Pennsylvania; Blue Cross of Western • Health Education Center Library 9783
Pennsylvania; Center for Emergency Medicine of Western • Library 9784
Pennsylvania College of Optometry • Albert Fitch Memorial Library 9747
Pennsylvania College of Podiatric Medicine 6548
    Center for the History of Foot Care and Footwear 9748
    Charles E. Krausz Library 9749
Pennsylvania Department of Health • Bureau of Laboratories • Herbert Fox Memorial Library 9691
Pennsylvania Department of Public Welfare
    Mayview State Hospital • Mental Health and Medical Library 9636
    Norristown State Hospital • Professional/Staff Library 9701
    Office of Children, Youth and Families • Research Center 9673
    Philadelphia State Hospital • Staff Library 9702
    Philipsburg State General Hospital • Library 9780
    Somerset State Hospital • Library 9825
    Western Center • Library Services 9642
Pennsylvania Hospital
    Department for Sick and Injured • Historical Library 9750
    Department for Sick and Injured • Medical Library 9751
Pennsylvania; Hospital Association of • Library Services 9672
Pennsylvania Medical Society 6549
Pennsylvania Medicine 1469
Pennsylvania; Planned Parenthood Southeastern • Resource Center 9759
Pennsylvania School for the Deaf • Library 9752
Pennsylvania and Southern New Jersey; Dorland's Medical Directory: Eastern 4208
Pennsylvania State University
    Audio-Visual Services 6550
    College of Medicine • George T. Harrell Library 9677
    Gerontology Center • Human Development Collection 9833
    Laboratory for Human Performance Research • Library 9834
    Life Sciences Library 9835
    Milton S. Hershey Medical Center • Sleep Research and Treatment Center 6551
PennWell Books 5822
Pennypress, Inc. 5823
Penrose Hospital • Webb Memorial Library 7527
People Concerned for the Unborn Child—Newsletter 2810
People-to-People News & Views 2811
People With AIDS Update 2812
Peoplenet 2813
People's Medical Society—Newsletter 2814
PEP Exchange 2815
PEP-USA 6552
Peptide and Protein Research; International Journal of 813
Peptides 1470

Peptides and Proteins; Cambridge Scientific Biochemistry Abstracts, Part 3: Amino Acids, 3573
Peptides and Proteins; Cambridge Scientific Biochemistry Abstracts, Part 3: Amino Acids, 6808
Peptides; Regulatory 1560
Peralta Medical Center; Merritt • John A. Graziano Memorial Library 7381
Perception and Performance; Journal of Experimental Psychology: Human 1009
Percy Howe Memorial Library - Forsyth Dental Center 8434
Perennial Education, Inc. 6155
Performance Elements; Human 2423
Performance; Journal of Experimental Psychology: Human Perception and 1009
Performance Resource Press, Inc. 5824
Pergamon Press, Inc. 5825
Perinatal Addiction Research and Education Update 2816
Perinatal Epidemiology; Paediatric and 1445
Perinatal Loss 5826
Perinatal Medicine; Journal of 1168
Perinatal Medicine; Year Book of Neonatal and 3474
Perinatal and Neonatal Nursing; Journal of 1169
Perinatal Press, Inc.—Newsletter 2817
Perinatology; American Journal of 93
Perinatology; Clinics in 3223
Perinatology; Journal of 1170
Perinatology/Neonatology—Buyers Guide Issue 4676
Perinatology Press 5827
Perinatology; Seminars in 3436
Periodical Literature on Aging; Index to 3706
Periodicals Database; Health 6951
Periodicals; Guide to Health-Oriented 4280
Periodicals; Index to Indian Medical 3703
Periodicals; NARIC Guide to Disability and Rehabilitation 4564
Periodicals Published in the Western Pacific Region of the World Health Organization—A Directory; Current Medical and Health-Related 4071
Periodicals Related to Deafness; International Directory of 4417
Periodontal Research; Journal of 1171
Periodontology; Journal of 1172
Periodontology; Journal of Clinical 959
Perioperative Nursing; Seminars in 3437
Perkins Memorial Library; Ralph - John D. Archbold Memorial Hospital 7863
Perkins School for the Blind • Samuel P. Hayes Research Library 8515
Perrin & Treggett's Review 2818
Perry Memorial Hospital • Dr. Kenneth O. Nelson Library of the Health Sciences 8052
Personal Construct Psychology; International Journal of 814
Personality and Ability Testing, Inc.; Institute for 5498
Personality Assessment; Advances in 3168
Personality Assessment—Directory; Society for 4804
Personality Assessment; Journal of 1174
Personality; Journal of 1173
Personality and Social Psychology; Journal of 1175
Personnel Database; Hospital 6962
Personnel; Directory of Hospital 4134
Personnel Records Center; National - National Archives and Records Administration 8767
Personnel Responsible for Radiological Health Programs; Directory of 4171
Personnes Ressources; Resource People/ 7096
Perspectives in Biology and Medicine 1471
Perspectives on Cats 2819
Perspectives on Dyslexia 2820
Perspectives in Pediatric Pathology 3366
Perspectives in Psychiatric Care 1472
Pestana; Carlos V. 5156
Pesticides; FDA Surveillance Index for 2254
Pesticides; National Coalition Against the Misuse of • Library 7694
Pet Care Update 2821
Pet Medicine; Seminars in Avian and Exotic 3423
Peter Carras Library - Christian Health Care Center 8978
Peter Wilcock Library - Charles Camsell General Hospital 10394
Peters Health Sciences Library - Rhode Island Hospital 9870
Peterson's Guide to Colleges with Programs for Learning-Disabled Students 4677
Peterson's Guide to Graduate Programs in Business, Education, Health, and Law 4678
Pew, Jr. Medical Library; Joseph N. - Bryn Mawr Hospital 9638
Pfeiffer Library; Henry - MacMurray College 8010

Pharmacy Library and Learning Center - University of Connecticut **7624**
Pharmacy Library; Veterinary Medical/ - Washington State University **10196**
Pharmacy Management; Topics in Hospital **1667**
Pharmacy; National Association of Boards of **5708**
 Library **8044**
Pharmacy News **2824**
Pharmacy, Nursing and Health Sciences Library - Purdue University **8152**
Pharmacy and Pharmacology; Journal of **1181**
Pharmacy Reading Room - School of Pharmacy - Ferris State University **8538**
Pharmacy Reading Room; Social and Administrative - University of Minnesota **8672**
Pharmacy Reports—The Green Sheet; Weekly **3090**
Pharmacy—Roster of Teaching Personnel in Colleges and Schools of Pharmacy; American Association of Colleges of **3866**
Pharmacy; St. Louis College of • O.J. Cloughly Alumni Library **8771**
Pharmacy School Admission Requirements **4684**
Pharmacy and Science; Philadelphia College of • Joseph W. England Library **9755**
Pharmacy; Southern College of • H. Custer Naylor Library **7834**
Pharmacy and Therapeutics Forum **2825**
Pharmacy and Therapeutics; Journal of Clinical **961**
Pharmacy Today **2826**
Pharmacy; Who's Who in American **4874**
Pharmaprojects **7071**
Pharmascope **2827**
PharmChem Newsletter **2828**
PharmIndex **2829**
Pharmindex **3747**
Pharmline **7072**
PHARMSEARCH **7073**
Phi Delta Epsilon News and Scientific Journal—Directory Issue **4685**
Philadelphia; AIDS Library of **9708**
Philadelphia Association for Psychoanalysis • Louis Kaplan Memorial Library **9628**
Philadelphia; Child Custody Services of • Resource Center **9665**
Philadelphia Child Guidance Center **6553**
Philadelphia; Children's Hospital of • Medical Library **9716**
Philadelphia College of Osteopathic Medicine
 Hospital • Medical Library **9753**
 O.J. Snyder Memorial Medical Library **9754**
Philadelphia College of Pharmacy and Science • Joseph W. England Library **9755**
Philadelphia; College of Physicians of • Library **9717**
Philadelphia Corporation for Aging • Library **9756**
Philadelphia Geriatric Center • Library **9757**
Philadelphia; Library Company of **9736**
Philadelphia; Marriage Council of • Division of Family Study and Marriage Council Library **9738**
Philadelphia Psychiatric Center • Professional Library **9758**
Philadelphia State Hospital • Staff Library **9702**
Philanthropically Supported Institutions; Guide to Gifts and Bequests: A Directory of **4278**
Philhaven Hospital • Library **9697**
Philip A. Hoover, M.D. Library - York Hospital **9848**
Philip B. Hardymon Library - St. Anthony Medical Center, Columbus, OH **9484**
Philipsburg State General Hospital • Library **9780**
Phillips Health Sciences Library; Seymour J. - Hospital for Joint Diseases Orthopaedic Institute - Beth Israel Medical Center **9149**
Phillips-Neuman Company **5829**
Philosophy; Journal of Medicine and **1092**
PHLS Directory; Public Health Laboratory Service— **4726**
PHN AIDS Network **7074**
Phobic Awareness; The Institute for **5499**
The Phoenix **2830**
Phoenix Children's Hospital • Family Learning Center • Library **7191**
Phoenix Day School for the Deaf • Library/Media Center **7192**
Phoenix Films, Inc. **6554**
Phoenix Indian Medical Center • Library **7193**
Phoenix International **5830**
Phoenix Public Library
 Business & Sciences Department **7194**
 Special Needs Center **7195**
Phoniatrics—List of Individual Members, List of Affiliated Societies; International Association of Logopedics and **4396**
Phosphoprotein Research; Advances in Second Messenger and **3176**
Phosphoproteins; Second Messengers and **1605**
Photobiochemistry; CA Selects: **3565**
Photobiology; Photochemistry and **1481**

Photochemistry and Photobiology **1481**
Photographers; Harwyn Medical **6383**
Photographers' Society—Directory; Ophthalmic **4649**
Photographic Association—Membership Directory; Biological **3987**
Photography; Journal of Biological **914**
PHS Supported Research; Biomedical Index to **3988**
Phyllis Cooksey Resource Center - Planned Parenthood of Minnesota **8686**
The Physiatrist **2831**
Physical Disabilities Special Interest Section—Newsletter **2832**
Physical Education—Calendar of Events; International Council of Sport Science and **4404**
Physical Education Gold Book: Directory of Physical Education in Higher Education **4686**
Physical Education and Health; Cambridge **6256**
Physical Education Index **3748**
Physical Education; National Association for Sport and • Media Resource Center **9884**
Physical Education, Recreation & Dance; American Alliance for Health, **4952**
Physical Education, Recreation, and Dance—Update; American Alliance for Health, **1846**
Physical Education and Recreation Library; Health, - Indiana University **8090**
Physical Education and Recreation Materials; Educators Guide to Free Health, **4225**
Physical Education and Recreation Microform Publications Bulletin; Health, **3671**
Physical, or Emotional Disabilities; A Reader's Guide for Parents of Children with Mental, **4733**
Physical Fitness; Journal of Sports Medicine and **1223**
Physical Fitness Programs Directory; Exercise and **4249**
Physical Fitness/Sports Medicine **3749**
Physical Medicine; Excerpta Medica: Rehabilitation and **3655**
Physical Medicine and Rehabilitation; American Journal of **95**
Physical Medicine and Rehabilitation; Archives of **190**
Physical Medicine and Rehabilitation Clinics **1482**
Physical Medicine and Rehabilitation News; Canadian Association of **2022**
Physical Medicine and Rehabilitation Specialists; ABMS—Directory of Certified **3795**
Physical and Occupational Therapy in Geriatrics **1483**
Physical and Occupational Therapy in Pediatrics **1484**
Physical and Rehabilitation Medicine; Critical Reviews in **3259**
Physical Therapists Directory **4687**
Physical Therapy **1485**
Physical Therapy Association; American **4999, 6196**
 Library **10119**
Physical Therapy Association—Membership Directory; Private Practice Section of the American **4709**
Physical Therapy; Clinical Management in **424**
Physical Therapy Clinics; Orthopaedic **1439**
Physical Therapy; Journal of Orthopaedic and Sports **1149**
Physically Disabled Persons in Canada; CRCD Information Directory: Rehabilitation Treatment Centres for **4068**
Physically Disadvantaged; The First Whole Rehab Catalog: A Comprehensive Guide to Products and Services for the **4262**
Physically Handicapped; Address List, Regional and Subregional Libraries for the Blind **3822**
Physically Handicapped; Arizona State Library for the Blind and **7181**
Physically Handicapped; Bureau of Library Services for the Blind and - Florida Division of Blind Services - Florida Department of Education **7742**
Physically Handicapped; Division for the Blind and - Texas State Library **9984**
Physically Handicapped; Library for the Blind and - District of Columbia Public Library **7676**
Physically Handicapped; Library for the Blind and - Georgia Department of Education **7829**
Physically Handicapped; Library for the Blind and - North Carolina Department of Cultural Resources **9368**
Physically Handicapped; Library for the Blind and - Public Library of Cincinnati and Hamilton County **9431**
Physically Handicapped; Library for the Blind and - Tennessee State Library **9962**
Physically Handicapped; Library and Resource Center for the Blind and - Alabama Institute for the Deaf and Blind **7163**
Physically Handicapped; Library Resources for the Blind and **4484**
Physically Handicapped; Library Services for the - Library System - University of Puerto Rico **9851**
Physically Handicapped; National Library Service for the Blind and - U.S. Library of Congress **6066**

Physically Handicapped; Oklahoma Regional Library for the Blind and **9558**

Physically Handicapped; Reading Material for the Blind and **7088**

Physically Handicapped; Regional Library for the Blind and - Alabama Public Library Service **7158**

Physically Handicapped; Regional Library for the Blind and - Idaho State Library **7883**

Physically Handicapped; Regional Library for the Blind and - New York Public Library **9212**

Physically Handicapped; Services for the Blind and - West Virginia Library Commission **10243**

Physically Handicapped—Update; Manitoba League of the **2546**

Physically Handicapped—Update; National Library Service for the Blind and **2664**

Physically Handicapped; Washington Library for the Blind and **10222**

Physically Handicapped; Wayne County Regional Library for the Blind and **8635**

Physician; American Family **50**

Physician; American Family **6766**

Physician Assistant **1486**

Physician Assistant Programs; National Directory of **4591**

Physician Assistants; American Academy of • Information Center **10117**

Physician Assistants; Journal of the American Academy of **868**

Physician; Australian Family **210**

Physician Data Query Cancer Information File **7075**

Physician Data Query Directory File **7076**

Physician Data Query Protocol File **7077**

Physician Executives; American College of **4974**

Physician Executives—Membership Directory; American College of **3894**

Physician Guide; PC **4674**

Physician Insurers Association of America—Membership Directory **4688**

Physician; New **1400**

Physician Office: Clinical Chemistry Instrumentation **4689**

Physician Office Distribution **4690**

Physician Office Products **4691**

Physician; Resident and Staff **1573**

Physician Resources Alert; St. Anthony's **2933**

Physician Service Opportunities Overseas Issue; Journal of the American Medical Association— **4459**

The Physician and Sportsmedicine **1487**

The Physician and Sportsmedicine **7078**

Physicians; ABMS—Directory of Certified Emergency **3783**

Physicians; ABMS—Directory of Certified Family **3784**

Physicians; ABMS—Directory of Certified Preventive Medicine **3797**

Physicians; American Academy of Family **6160**
  Huffington Library **8725**

Physicians; American College of **6178**

Physicians; American College of Chest **4970, 6175**

Physicians; American Osteopathic Association—Yearbook and Directory of Osteopathic **3916**

Physician's Assistants in Cardiovascular Surgery—Membership Directory; Association of **3970**

Physicians of Canada; College of Family • Canadian Library of Family Medicine **10545**

Physicians' Clinics Directory **4692**

Physicians and Dentists Database **7079**

Physicians' Desk Reference **4693**

Physicians' Desk Reference **7080**

Physicians' Desk Reference for Ophthalmology **4694**

Physicians—Directory; American Society of Bariatric **3924**

Physician's Library - Mid-Valley Hospital **9707**

Physician's Management **1488**

Physician's Marketing and Management **2833**

Physicians and Medical Institutions Abroad; Directory of Participating **4169**

Physicians—Membership Directory; American College of Chest **3889**

Physicians—Membership Directory; American College of International **3891**

Physicians—Membership Directory; American Society of Psychoanalytic **3934**

Physicians—Membership Roster; American Association of Public Health **3879**

Physicians—Newsletter; American Association of Senior **1854**

The Physician's Patient Newsletter **2834**

Physicians of Philadelphia; College of • Library **9717**

Physicians and Scientists Publishing Company **5831**

Physicians and Suppliers that Accept Medicare; Directory of **4173**

Physicians and Surgeons Association—Membership Directory and Concordance; United States of America- **4848**

Physicians and Surgeons of British Columbia; College of • Medical Library Service **10429**

Physicians and Surgeons—Bulletin; International Academy of Chest **2465**

Physicians and Surgeons Directory **4695**

Physicians and Surgeons Equipment and Supplies Directory **4696**

Physicians and Surgeons Information Bureaus Directory **4697**

Physicians and Surgeons; International Academy of Chest **5508**

Physicians and Surgeons of Manitoba—Newsletter; College of **2113**

Physics Abstracts and Notes; Applied Health **3511**

Physics; Advances in Cardiovascular **3130**

Physics Data Base; International Health **6979**

Physics; Health **676**

Physics; International Journal of Radiation Oncology, Biology, **820**

Physics; Journal of the Optical Society of America B, Optical **1144**

Physics; Medical **1304**

Physics and Medical NMR; Physiological Chemistry and **1491**

Physics in Medicine and Biology **1489**

Physics and Physiological Measurement; Clinical **439**

Physics Publishing Corporation; Medical **5663**

Physics Research Abstracts; Health **3672**

Physiologia Bohemoslovaca **1490**

Physiologic Imaging; American Journal of **96**

Physiologica Scandinavica; Acta **21**

Physiological Chemistry and Physics and Medical NMR **1491**

Physiological Measurement; Clinical Physics and **439**

Physiological Optics; Ophthalmic and **1430**

Physiological Psychology; Progress in Psychobiology and **3391**

Physiological Research **1492**

Physiological Reviews **3368**

Physiological Therapeutics; Journal of Manipulative and **1074**

Physiologist **1493**

The Physiologist **2835**

Physiology A: Sensory, Neural, and Behavioral Physiology; Journal of Comparative **970**

Physiology; American Journal of **97**

Physiology; Annual Review of **3205**

Physiology B: Biochemical, Systematic, and Environmental Physiology; Journal of Comparative **971**

Physiology and Behavior **1494**

Physiology and Biochemistry; Clinical **441**

Physiology, Biochemistry and Pharmacology; Reviews of **3417**

Physiology; Clinical **440**

Physiology; Clinical and Experimental Pharmacology and **414**

Physiology; Excerpta Medica: **3650**

Physiology; Experimental **607**

Physiology; Frontiers of Oral **3332**

Physiology; Human **723**

Physiology; Journal of **1182**

Physiology; Journal of Applied **894**

Physiology; Journal of Cellular **934**

Physiology; Journal of Developmental **986**

Physiology; Journal of General **1021**

Physiology; Neuroscience and Behavioral **1391**

Physiology and Occupational Physiology; European Journal of Applied **567**

Physiology, Part A: Comparative Physiology; Comparative Biochemistry and **458**

Physiology, Part B: Comparative Biochemistry; Comparative Biochemistry and **459**

Physiology, Part C: Comparative Pharmacology and Toxicology; Comparative Biochemistry and **460**

Physiology; Pflugers Archiv: European Journal of **1473**

Physiology and Pharmacology; Canadian Journal of **339**

Physiology and Pharmacology; Indian Journal of **750**

Physiology; Progress in Sensory **3395**

Physiology; Renal **1563**

Physiology; Respiration **1575**

Physiology; Society for the Study of Male Psychology and • Library **9513**

Physiotherapists Register **4698**

Physiotherapy Canada **1495**

PIA Press **5833**

Pick Memorial Library; Lawrence Mercer - LaRabida Children's Hospital and Research Center **7939**

Pickett Medical Library; Ralph E. - Licking Memorial Hospital **9515**

Piedmont Hospital • Sauls Memorial Library **7837**

Pierce County; Medical Library of **10231**

Pierose Memorial Health Sciences Library; Dean - Moritz Community Hospital **7890**

Pierre Fauchard Academy—Membership Directory **4699**

Pierson Medical Library; William - Hospital Center at Orange **8919**

Pigment Cell Research **1496**

S

St. John's Mercy Medical Center • John Young Brown Memorial Library **8770**

St. John's Northeast Hospital • Memorial Medical Library **8656**

St. John's Regional Health Center
Medical Library **8786**
School of Nursing Library **8787**

St. John's Regional Medical Center • Health Science Library **7387**

St. John's Riverside Hospital • Library **9330**

St. John's University • College of Pharmacy and Allied Health Professions • Health Education Resource Center **9111**

St. Joseph Community Hospital • Library **10235**

St. Joseph Health Center, Kansas City, MO • Health Science Library **8734**

St. Joseph Health Center, St. Charles, MO • Health Science Library **8747**

St. Joseph Hospital, Bellingham, WA • Library **10185**

St. Joseph Hospital, Cheektowaga, NY • Library **9072**

St. Joseph Hospital, Denver, CO
Health Reach Patient and Community Library **7547**
Health Sciences Library **7548**

St. Joseph Hospital, Flint, MI • Health Sciences Library **8574**

St. Joseph Hospital and Health Care Center, Chicago, IL • Library **7961**

St. Joseph Hospital and Health Care Center, Tacoma, WA • Hospital Library **10232**

St. Joseph Hospital and Health Center • Medical Library **9507**

St. Joseph Hospital, Houston, TX • Health Science Library **10036**

St. Joseph Hospital, Lancaster, PA • William O. Umiker Medical Library **9684**

St. Joseph Hospital, Lexington, KY • Medical Library **8231**

St. Joseph Hospital, Memphis, TN • Health Science Library **9943**

St. Joseph Hospital, North Providence, RI • Fatima Unit • Health Science Library **9861**

St. Joseph Hospital, Orange, CA • Burlew Medical Library **7384**

St. Joseph Hospital, Providence, RI • Our Lady of Providence Unit • Health Science Library **9873**

St. Joseph Hospital, Reading, PA • Health Sciences Library **9816**

St. Joseph Hospital, Towson, MD • Otto C. Brantigan, M.D. Medical Library **8412**

St. Joseph Medical Center, Albuquerque, NM • Medical Library **8984**

St. Joseph Medical Center, Burbank, CA • Health Science Library **7255**

St. Joseph Medical Center, Joliet, IL • Health Science Library **8012**

St. Joseph Medical Center, Stamford, CT • Health Sciences Library **7622**

St. Joseph Memorial Hospital • Health Science Library **8138**

St. Joseph Mercy Hospital, Mason City, IA • Medical Library **8181**

St. Joseph Mercy Hospital, Pontiac, MI • Library **8622**

St. Joseph State Hospital • Professional Library **8750**

St. Joseph's General Hospital • Library **10618**

St. Joseph's Health Centre of London • Library Services **10548**

St. Joseph's Health Centre, Toronto, ON, Canada • George Pennal Library **10649**

St. Joseph's Hospital of Atlanta • Russell Bellman Memorial Library **7838**

St. Joseph's Hospital Centers • Medical Library **8613**

St. Joseph's Hospital, Elmira, NY • Helene Fuld Learning Resource Center **9082**

St. Joseph's Hospital, Flushing, NY • Medical Library **9088**

St. Joseph's Hospital, Hamilton, ON, Canada
Drug Information Centre **10531**
Library Services **10532**

St. Joseph's Hospital Health Center • Medical and School of Nursing Libraries **9300**

St. Joseph's Hospital and Health Center, Dickinson, ND • Medical Library **9390**

St. Joseph's Hospital and Health Center, Tucson, AZ • Bruce M. Cole Memorial Library **7211**

St. Joseph's Hospital, Lowell, MA • Health Science Library **8486**

St. Joseph's Hospital, Marshfield, WI • Learning Resource Center **10307**

St. Joseph's Hospital and Medical Center • Health Sciences Library **8923**

St. Joseph's Hospital, Milwaukee, WI • Samuel Rosenthal Memorial Library **10325**

St. Joseph's Hospital, Phoenix, AZ • Health Sciences Library **7196**

St. Joseph's Hospital, St. Paul, MN • Jerome Medical Library **8688**

St. Joseph's Hospital, Savannah, GA • Medical Library **7862**

St. Joseph's Hospital, Tampa, FL • Medical Library **7810**

St. Joseph's Medical Center, Fort Wayne, IN • Medical Library **8111**

St. Joseph's Medical Center, South Bend, IN • Medical Library **8151**

St. Joseph's Medical Center, Stockton, CA • Library **7500**

St. Joseph's Medical Center, Yonkers, NY • Medical Library **9331**

St. Jude Children's Research Hospital • Biomedical Library **9944**

St. Jude Medical Center • Medical Library **7285**

St. Lawrence Hospital • Medical Library **8603**

St. Lawrence Psychiatric Center • Professional Library **9248**

St. Louis Children's Hospital Library - Washington University Medical Center **8784**

St. Louis College of Pharmacy • O.J. Cloughly Alumni Library **8771**

St. Louis Hearing and Speech Centers • Library **8772**

St. Louis Psychoanalytic Institute • Betty Golde Smith Memorial Library **8773**

St. Louis Regional Medical Center • Medical Library **8774**

St. Louis University • Medical Center Library **8775**

St. Louis University Medical Center • Educational Media Department **6582**

St. Luke Medical Center • William P. Long Medical Library **7400**

St. Luke's Episcopal and Texas Children's Hospitals • Medical Library **10037**

St. Luke's Hospital Association • Medical, Nursing and Allied Help Library **7755**

St. Luke's Hospital of Bethlehem, Pennsylvania
Audiovisual Library **9632**
School of Nursing • Trexler Nurses' Library **9633**
W.L. Estes, Jr. Memorial Library **9634**

St. Luke's Hospital, Cedar Rapids, IA • Health Science Library **8158**

St. Luke's Hospital Center • Richard Walker Bolling Memorial Medical Library **9227**

St. Luke's Hospital, Cleveland, OH • Taylor Family Health Sciences Library **9464**

St. Luke's Hospital, Denver, CO • Health Sciences Library **7549**

St. Luke's Hospital, Duluth, MN • Hilding Medical Library **8648**

St. Luke's Hospital, Fargo, ND • MeritCare Library **9396**

St. Luke's Hospital of Kansas City • Medical Library **8735**

St. Luke's Hospital Medical Center • Education Department **6583**

St. Luke's Hospital of Middleborough • Medical Staff Library **8495**

St. Luke's Hospital, San Francisco, CA • Medical Library **7454**

St. Luke's Medical Center, Milwaukee, WI • Medical Library **10326**

St. Luke's Medical Center, Phoenix, AZ • Rosenzweig Health Sciences Library **7197**

St. Lukes Midland Regional Medical Center • Dr. Paul G. Bunker Memorial Medical Library **9909**

St. Luke's Regional Medical Center, Boise, ID • Medical Library **7885**

St. Luke's Regional Medical Center, Sioux City, IA • Instructional Technology Center **8185**

St. Margaret Hospital • Sallie M. Tyrrell, M.D. Memorial Library **8114**

St. Margaret Memorial Hospital • Paul Titus Memorial Library and School of Nursing Library **9799**

St. Mark's Hospital • Library and Media Services **10092**

St. Martha's Hospital • School of Nursing Library **10495**

St. Mary-Corwin Hospital • Finney Memorial Library **7567**

St. Mary Hospital, Livonia, MI • Medical Library **8606**

St. Mary Hospital, Port Arthur, TX • Health Science Library **10059**

St. Mary Hospital, Quincy, IL • Staff Library **8054**

St. Mary Medical Center • Bellis Medical Library **7313**

St. Mary of Nazareth Hospital Center • Sister Stella Louise Health Sciences Library **7962**

St. Mary's Health Center • Health Sciences Library **8776**

St. Mary's Hospital of Brooklyn • Medical Library **9046**

St. Mary's Hospital, Decatur, IL • Health Sciences Library **7980**

St. Mary's Hospital, Enid, OK • Medical Library **9547**

St. Mary's Hospital, Grand Rapids, MI • Library **8582**

St. Mary's Hospital and Health Center • Ralph Fuller Medical Library **7212**

St. Mary's Hospital, Huntington, WV • Medical Library **10251**

St. Mary's Hospital, Kitchener, ON, Canada • Medical Library **10544**

St. Mary's Hospital, Lewiston, ME • Health Sciences Library **8300**

St. Mary's Hospital and Medical Center • Medical Library **7455**

St. Mary's Hospital, Milwaukee, WI • Health Sciences Library **10327**

St. Mary's Hospital, Montreal, PQ, Canada • Health Sciences Library **10744**

St. Mary's Hospital, Passaic, NJ • Medical Allied Health Library **8922**

St. Mary's Hospital, Pierre, SD • Medical Library **9915**

St. Mary's Hospital, Richmond, VA • Health Sciences Library **10164**

St. Mary's Hospital, Rochester, MN • Library **8679**

St. Mary's Hospital, Troy, NY • Medical Staff Library **9306**

St. Mary's Hospital, Waterbury, CT • Finkelstein Library **7628**

St. Mary's Hospital, West Palm Beach, FL • Health Sciences Library **7818**

St. Mary's of the Lake Hospital • Gibson Medical Resource Centre **10542**

St. Mary's Medical Center, Evansville, IN • Herman M. Baker, M.D. Memorial Library **8105**

St. Mary's Medical Center, Knoxville, TN • Medical Library **9933**

St. Mary's Medical Center, Racine, WI • Library **10337**

St. Mary's Regional Medical Center • Max C. Fleischmann Medical Library **8826**

St. Mary's School for the Deaf • Information Center **9062**

St. Michael Hospital, Milwaukee, WI • Regner Health Sciences Library **10328**

St. Michael Medical Center • Aquinas Medical Library **8914**

St. Michael's Hospital, Stevens Point, WI • Health Sciences Library **10339**

St. Michael's Hospital, Toronto, ON, Canada • Health Science Library/Archives **10650**

St. Nicholas Hospital • Health Sciences Library **10338**

St. Patrick Hospital—Messenger **2934**

St. Patrick Hospital, Missoula, MT • Library **8800**

St. Paul Medical Center • C.B. Sacher Medical Library **10006**

St. Paul Ramsey Medical Center • Medical Library **8689**

St. Paul's Hospital Health Sciences Library, Vancouver, BC, Canada - University of British Columbia **10437**

St. Paul's Hospital of Saskatoon, Grey Nuns • Medical Library **10793**

St. Peter Hospital, Olympia, WA • Library Services **10195**

St. Peter Regional Treatment Center • Burton P. Grimes Staff Library **8692**

St. Peter's Hospital, Albany, NY • Health Sciences Library **9003**

St. Peter's Hospital, Hamilton, ON, Canada • Library **10533**

St. Peter's Medical Center • Library **8909**

St. Rita's Medical Center • Medical Library **9505**

St. Thomas Institute • Library **8219**

St. Thomas Medical Center • Medical Library **9407**

St. Thomas Psychiatric Hospital • Library Services **10602**

St. Vincent Charity Hospital • Library **9465**

St. Vincent Health Center, Erie, PA • Health Science Library **9659**

St. Vincent Hospital, Green Bay, WI • Health Science Library **10276**

St. Vincent Hospital and Medical Center, Portland, OR • Health Sciences Library **9601**

St. Vincent Hospital, Ottawa, ON, Canada • Library/AV Services **10591**

St. Vincent Hospital, Santa Fe, NM • Library **8993**

St. Vincent Hospital, Worcester, MA • John J. Dumphy Memorial Library **8518**

St. Vincent Infirmary • Medical Library **7226**

St. Vincent Medical Center, Los Angeles, CA • Health Sciences Library **7341**

St. Vincent Medical Center, Toledo, OH • Health Science Library **9534**

St. Vincent's Hospital, Birmingham, AL • Cunningham Wilson Library **7142**

St. Vincent's Hospital, Indianapolis, IN • Garceau Library **8132**

St. Vincent's Hospital and Medical Center of New York • Medical Library **9229**

St. Vincent's Hospital and Medical Center of New York, Westchester Branch • Medical Library **9099**

St. Vincent's Hospital, New York, NY • School of Nursing Library **9228**

St. Vincent's Medical Center • Daniel T. Banks Health Science Library **7573**

St. Vincent's Medical Center of Richmond • Medical Library **9293**

Sts. Mary and Elizabeth Hospital • Health Sciences Library **8245**

Salem Hospital, Salem, MA • Health Sciences Library **8504**

Salem Hospital, Salem, OR • Health Sciences Library **9613**

Salenger Films **6584**

Salk Institute for Biological Studies—Newsletters **2935**

Sallie M. Tyrrell, M.D. Memorial Library - St. Margaret Hospital **8114**

Salubritas **2936**

Salvation Army Grace General Hospital, St. John's, NF, Canada • Chesley A. Pippy, Jr. Medical Library **10490**

Salvation Army Grace General Hospital, Winnipeg, MB, Canada • Library **10461**

Salvation Army Grace Hospital, Calgary, AB, Canada • Hospital Library **10377**

Salvation Army Grace Hospital, Windsor, ON, Canada • Library **10671**

Sam Channell National EMS Clearinghouse - National Association of State Emergency Medical Services Directors **8230**

Sam Mitminger Library Resource Centre - Mohawk College of Applied Arts and Technology **10529**

Sam Rayburn Memorial Veterans Center • Medical Library **9989**

Sam and Rose Stein Children's Center • Parent Resource Library **7327**

Samaritan Hospital • Medical Library **9307**

Same-Day Surgery **2937**

Samford University; Baptist Medical Centers- • Ida V. Moffett School of Nursing • L.R. Jordan Library **7139**

Samuel Frank Medical Library - Sinai Hospital of Detroit **8561**

Samuel H. Shapiro Developmental Center • Professional Library **8016**

Samuel J. Stabins, M.D. Medical Library - Genesee Hospital **9272**

Samuel J. Wood Library • C.V. Starr Biomedical Information Center **9159**

Samuel P. Hayes Research Library - Perkins School for the Blind **8515**

Samuel Roberts Noble Foundation • Biomedical Division Library **9546**

Samuel Rosenthal Memorial Library - St. Joseph's Hospital, Milwaukee, WI **10325**

Samuel Taylor Darling Memorial Library - Gorgas Army Community Hospital **7731**

Samuels Library; Bernard - New York Eye and Ear Infirmary **9204**

San Antonio Community Hospital • Weber Memorial Library **7511**

San Antonio and South Central Texas; Planned Parenthood of • Library **10066**

San Antonio State Chest Hospital • Health Science Library **10067**

San Antonio State Hospital **6585**
    Staff Library **10068**

San Bernardino Community Hospital • Medical Library **7418**

San Bernardino County Medical Center • Medical Library **7419**

San Francisco General Hospital Medical Center • Barnett-Briggs Library **7456**

San Gorgonio Memorial Hospital • Medical Library **7238**

San Jose Medical Center • Health Sciences Library **7471**

San Jose State University • Department of Occupational Therapy **6586**

San Pedro Peninsula Hospital • John T. Burch, M.D. Memorial Library **7479**

Sandoz, Inc. • Library **8869**

Sandoz Canada Inc. • Bibliotheque/Library **10680**

Sandoz Pharmaceuticals • Medical Information Services **8870**

Sandpiper Press **5935**

Sandridge Publishing **5936**

Sandt Company; Dallas **5256**

Sanger Center; Margaret • Planned Parenthood New York City • Abraham Stone Library **9179**

Santa Clara County Health Department • Library **7472**

Santa Clara Valley Medical Center • Milton J. Chatton Medical Library **7473**

Santa Monica Hospital Medical Center • Library **7490**

Santa Rosa Health Care Corporation • Health Science Library • Educational Resources Department **10069**

Sanuk, Inc. **5937**

Sarah and Julius Steinberg Memorial Library - Riverside Hospital, Toledo, OH **9533**

Sarasota Memorial Hospital • Medical Library **7802**

Saratoga Community Hospital • Health Science Library **8560**

Saratoga Hospital • Medical Staff Library **9288**

Sarcomas and Related Tumors—Diagnosis, Treatment; ICRDB Cancergram: **3698**

Sargent College of Allied Health Professions
    Center for Psychiatric Rehabilitation **6244**
    George K. Makechnie Instructional Resource Center **6245**

Saskatchewan Abilities Council—Bulletin **2938**

Saskatchewan Alcohol and Drug Abuse Commission • Library **10786**

Saskatchewan—The Bulletin; Chiropractors' Association of **2087**

Saskatchewan Cancer Foundation • Allan Blair Memorial Clinic • Library **10787**

Saskatchewan Health • Library **10788**

Saskatchewan Hospital • Department of Psychiatric Services • Staff Library **10781**

Saskatchewan Medical Journal **2939**

Saskatchewan Registered Nurses Association • L. Jane Knox Resource Centre **10789**

Saskatoon Cancer Centre • Harold E. Johns Library **10794**

Saskatoon City Hospital • Medical Library **10795**

SATH News **2940**

Sauk River Press **5938**

Saul Schwartzbach Memorial Library - Prince George's Hospital Center **8375**

Sauls Memorial Library - Piedmont Hospital **7837**

Sault Ste. Marie General Hospital • Health Sciences Library **10604**

Saunders Company; W.B. **6093, 6714**

Substance Abuse; The National Report on 7046
Substance Abuse Report 3008
Substance Abuse Research; Institute for 5507
Substance Abuse Residential Treatment Centers for Teens 4829
Substance Abuse Trainers and Educators—Directory; National Association of 4574
Substance Abuse Treatment; Journal of 1228
Substances; Carcinogenicity Information Database of Environmental 6819
Substances Data Bank; Hazardous 6936
Sudbury General Hospital • Hospital Library 10614
Sudden Infant Death Syndrome Clearinghouse; National 10150
Sudden Infant Death Syndrome Programs and Resources; Directory of 4196
Suffolk Academy of Medicine • Library 9100
The Sugar Association, Inc. • Library 7713
Suicide Information and Education 7119
Suicide Information and Education Centre - Canadian Mental Health Association, Alberta Division 10373
Suicide and Life-Threatening Behavior 1635
Suicide Prevention/Crisis Intervention Agencies in the United States; Directory of 4197
Suicide Support Groups; Directory of Survivors of 4198
Suicidology—Newslink; American Association of 1855
Sullivan Medical Library - St. Anne's Hospital 8473
Sulzbacher Memorial Library - Spring Grove Hospital Center 8372
Summerville Medical Library; W.W. - Bethany Medical Center 8190
Sumter Regional Hospital • Medical Library 7821
Sun Eagle Publishing 6008
The Sun Group 6613
Sun and Skin News 3009
Sunbelt Medical Publishers 6009
Sunburst Communications 6614
SunHealth, Inc. • SunHealth Resource Center 9348
Sunland Center at Gainesville • Tacachale Library 7747
Sunnybrook Health Science Centre • Health Sciences Library 10565
Sunshine Press 6010
SUNY
    College of Optometry • Harold Kohn Memorial Visual Science Library 9232
    Health Science Center at Brooklyn • Department of Psychiatry Library 9048
    Health Science Center at Brooklyn • Library 9049
SUNY at Buffalo
    Health Sciences Library 9064
    Industry/University Center for Biosurfaces • Library 9065
    School of Pharmacy • Drug Information Service • Library 9066
SUNY at Cortland • Memorial Library 9075
SUNY at Stony Brook • Health Sciences Library 9078
SUNY at Syracuse • Health Science Center • Library 9301
Super G Publishing Company 6011
Supervisor; Health Care 668
Supervisor's Bulletin; Hospital 2418
Suppliers; DECHEMA Biotechnology Equipment 6865
Suppliers; Hospitals and Health Services Yearbook and Directory of Hospital 4373
Suppliers that Accept Medicare; Directory of Physicians and 4173
Supplies; Dental 4077
Supplies Directory; Hospital Equipment and 4366
Supplies Retail Directory; First Aid 4261
Supplies Wholesalers/Manufacturers Directory; Dental Equipment and 4074
Supply Houses; Hayes Directory of Dental 4297
Supply Houses; Hayes Directory of Medical 4298
Support Group Newsletter 3010
Support Groups; Directory of Survivors of Suicide 4198
Support Source 6012
Supportive Care; ICRDB Cancergram: Rehabilitation and 3697
Surgeon; American 115
Surgeons; ABMS—Directory of Certified 3800
Surgeons; ABMS—Directory of Certified Colon and Rectal 3781
Surgeons; ABMS—Directory of Certified Neurological 3786
Surgeons; ABMS—Directory of Certified Orthopaedic 3791
Surgeons; ABMS—Directory of Certified Plastic 3796
Surgeons; ABMS—Directory of Certified Thoracic 3801
Surgeons; American Academy of Orthopaedic 4949, 6163
Surgeons; American Association of Oral and Maxillofacial 6167
Surgeons; American College of 6180
Surgeons; American College of Osteopathic 4973
Surgeons; American Society of Abdominal • Donald Collins Memorial Library 8493
Surgeons; American Society of Plastic and Reconstructive • Plastic Surgery Educational Foundation 6206

Surgeons Association—Membership Directory and Concordance; United States of America-Physicians and 4848
Surgeons of British Columbia—Bulletin; College of Dental 2111
Surgeons of British Columbia; College of Physicians and • Medical Library Service 10429
Surgeons; Bulletin of the American College of 315
Surgeons—Bulletin; International Academy of Chest Physicians and 2465
Surgeons: Collected Letters; Correspondence Society of 2144
Surgeons Directory; Physicians and 4695
Surgeons of Edinburgh; Journal of the Royal College of 1209
Surgeons of England; Annals of the Royal College of 148
Surgeons Equipment and Supplies Directory; Physicians and 4696
Surgeons of Great Britain and Ireland—Handbook; Association of 3971
Surgeons—Handbook; British Association of Urological 4001
Surgeons Information Bureaus Directory; Physicians and 4697
Surgeons; International Academy of Chest Physicians and 5508
Surgeons of Manitoba—Newsletter; College of Physicians and 2113
Surgeons—Members List; West African College of 4867
Surgeons—Membership Directory; American Association of Oral and Maxillofacial 3878
Surgeons—Membership Directory; American Society of Outpatient 3932
Surgeons—Membership Directory; International College of 4402
Surgery 1636
Surgery; Advances in 3178
Surgery; Advances in Cardiac 3128
Surgery; Advances in Ophthalmic Plastic and Reconstructive 3160
Surgery; Advances in Orthopaedic 3161
Surgery; Advances in Otolaryngology: Head and Neck 3162
Surgery; Advances in Plastic and Reconstructive 3171
Surgery; Aesthetic 1784
Surgery; Aesthetic Plastic 30
Surgery; American Academy of Facial Plastic and Reconstructive 6159
Surgery; American Journal of 105
Surgery; American Journal of Proctology, Gastroenterology and Colon and Rectal 98
Surgery and American Society of Ophthalmic Administrators—Membership Roster; American Society of Cataract and Refractive 3925
Surgery; Annals of 149
Surgery; Annals of Plastic 146
Surgery; Annals of Thoracic 150
Surgery; Annals of Vascular 153
Surgery Annual 3447
Surgery; Annual of Opthalmic Laser 3189
Surgery; Archives of 193
Surgery; Archives of Orthopaedic and Traumatic 186
Surgery; Archives of Otolaryngology-Head and Neck 187
Surgery; Australian and New Zealand Journal of 214
Surgery; British Journal of 309
Surgery; British Journal of Oral and Maxillofacial 300
Surgery; British Journal of Plastic 303
Surgery: British Volume; Journal of Hand 1031
Surgery; Canadian Journal of 343
Surgery Center Directory; Freestanding Outpatient 4265
Surgery Clinics of North America; Chest 386
Surgery; Clinics in Plastic 3224
Surgery; Clinics in Podiatric Medicine and 3225
Surgery; Current 3304
Surgery; Current Bibliography of Plastic and Reconstructive 3593
Surgery; Current Practice in 3293
Surgery; Current Problems in 3300
Surgery; Digestive 527
Surgery—Directory; American Academy of Neurological and Orthopaedic 3856
Surgery—Directory of Diplomates; American Board of Orthopaedic 3882
Surgery Educational Foundation; Plastic - American Society of Plastic and Reconstructive Surgeons 6206
Surgery; European Journal of Cardiothoracic 571
Surgery; European Journal of Implant and Refractive 578
Surgery; European Journal of Plastic 584
Surgery; European Journal of Vascular 587
Surgery; Excerpta Medica: 3656
Surgery; Excerpta Medica: Cardiovascular Disease and Cardiovascular 3621
Surgery; Excerpta Medica: Orthopedic 3646
Surgery; Excerpta Medica: Pediatrics and Pediatric 3648
Surgery; Excerpta Medica: Plastic 3651

Tripler Army Medical Center • Medical Library **7877**
The Triplet Connection—Newsletter **3044**
Triton Biosciences Inc. • Library **7231**
Tropical Diseases Bulletin **3773**
Tropical Doctor **1683**
Tropical Medicine Data Base; Public Health and **7086**
Tropical Medicine and Hygiene; American Journal of **107**
Tropical Medicine and Hygiene; Journal of **1238**
Tropical Medicine and Hygiene; Transactions of the Royal Society of **1676**
Tropical Medicine and Hygiene—Year Book; Royal Society of **4770**
Tropical Medicine and Parasitology; Annals of **151**
Tropical Medicine and Public Health; Southeast Asian Journal of **1623**
Tropical Paediatrics; Annals of **152**
Trudeau Institute Immunobiological Research Laboratories • Library **9287**
Trumbull Memorial Hospital • Wean Medical Library **9536**
Trustee **1684**
TSI • Mason Research Institute • Library **8519**
Tuality Community Hospital • Health Sciences Library **9586**
Tuality Healthcare Foundation • Tuality Health Information Resource Center **9587**
Tubercle **1685**
Tuberculosis; Excerpta Medica: Chest Diseases, Thoracic Surgery and **3622**
Tuberous Sclerosis Association; National **5742**
Tuberous Sclerosis Association—Perspective; National **2681**
Tucker Memorial Medical Library; Gerald - National Jewish Center for Immunology and Respiratory Medicine **7543**
Tucker Memorial Medical Library; Mollie Sublett - Memorial Hospital, Nacogdoches, TX **10056**
Tucker Publications, Inc. **6057**
Tucson General Hospital • Medical Library **7213**
Tucson Medical Center • Medical Library **7214**
Tufts University
    Center for the Study of Drug Development • Library **8453**
    Health Sciences Library **8454**
Tufts University Diet & Nutrition Letter **3045**
Tulane University of Louisiana
    Delta Regional Primate Research Center • Science Information Service **8260**
    School of Medicine • Rudolph Matas Medical Library **8273**
Tulsa Regional Medical Center • L.C. Baxter Medical Library **9576**
Tumor Association—Message Line; American Brain **1858**
Tumor Markers in the Clinical Laboratory **4843**
Tumor Pharmacotherapy; Medical Oncology and **1302**
Tumor Research; Progress in Experimental **3380**
Tumors of Children; Renal **7091**
Tumors—Diagnosis, Treatment; ICRDB Cancergram: Gynecological **3690**
Tumors—Diagnosis, Treatment; ICRDB Cancergram: Sarcomas and Related **3698**
Tumors—Diagnosis, Treatment; ICRDB Cancergram: Upper Gastrointestinal **3699**
Tumors—Diagnosis, Treatment, Pathophysiology; ICRDB Cancergram: Endocrine **3688**
Tumour Biology **1686**
Tuning In: AAMT Newsletter **3046**
Turner Memorial Library - Franklin Memorial Hospital **8297**
Turning Point Publications **6058**
Tuskegee University • Veterinary Medicine Library **7166**
Tutorials of Cytology **6635**
The Twelve Step Rag **3047**
Twenty-first Century Publications **6059**
Twin Peaks Press **6060**
Twin Services Reporter **3048**
Twinlab Nutrition Update **3049**
200 Ways to Put Your Talent to Work in the Health Field **4844**
Tyrrell, M.D. Memorial Library; Sallie M. - St. Margaret Hospital **8114**

U

UAB Arthritis Today **3050**
UCLA Cancer Trials **3051**
Uhlmann Medical Library; Robert - Menorah Medical Center **8731**
UICC International Directory of Cancer Institutes and Organizations **4845**
UK National Food Nutrient Databank **7124**
Ukrainian Medical Association of North America • Ukrainian Medical Archives and Library **7966**
Ulcer Inhibitors; CA Selects: **3568**

Ultrasonic Imaging **1687**
Ultrasound, CT, and MR; Seminars in **3443**
Ultrasound; JCU: Journal of Clinical **849**
Ultrasound in Medicine; American Institute of **4991, 6190**
Ultrasound in Medicine and Biology **1688**
Ultrasound in Medicine; Journal of **1239**
Ultrasound in Medicine—Membership Roster; American Institute of **3908**
Ultrasound Quarterly **1689**
Ultrastructural Pathology **1690**
Umbilicus **3052**
UMDNJ and Coriell Research • Library **8860**
Umiker Medical Library; William O. - St. Joseph Hospital, Lancaster, PA **9684**
Umstead Hospital; John • Learning Resource Center **9338**
UNA Newsbulletin **3053**
Unborn Child—Newsletter; People Concerned for the **2810**
Uncompensated Services; Directory of Facilities Obligated to Provide **4120**
Undersea Biomedical Research **1691**
Understanding Arthritis: What It Is, How It's Treated, How to Cope With It **4846**
Underwood-Memorial Hospital • Anthony J.D. Marino, M.D. Memorial Library **8977**
Uniformed Services Medical/Dental Facilities in the U.S.A. **4847**
Unifour Productions, Inc. **6636**
Union Catalogue of Serials in Swiss Libraries **7125**
Union Hospital • Medical Library **8969**
Union Memorial Hospital
    Library and Information Resources **8347**
    Nursing Library **8348**
The Union Signal **3054**
Uniontown Hospital
    Professional Library **9831**
    School of Nursing • Library **9832**
Unitarian Universalist Women's Federation—The Communicator **3055**
United Cerebral Palsy Associations **6637**
United Cerebral Palsy of New York City • Library **9234**
United Cerebral Palsy Research and Educational Foundation • Library **9235**
United Health Services/Binghamton General Hospital • Stuart B. Blakely Memorial Library **9015**
United Health Services/Wilson Hospital • Learning Resources Department **9112**
United Hospital • Nursing Education and Research Department **6638**
United Hospital Center Inc. • Information Center **10246**
United Hospital Fund of New York **6061**
    Reference Library **9236**
United Hospital, Grand Forks, ND • Library **9399**
United Hospitals Medical Center • Library **8915**
United Kingdom; List of Approved Hospitals and House Officer Posts in the **4486**
U.K. Organizations for Visually Disabled People; Guide to **4288**
United Kingdom and Republic of Ireland; Directory of Medical and Health Care Libraries in the **4149**
United Kingdom and Republic of Ireland; Directory of Medical and Health Care Libraries in the **6875**
United Learning **6639**
United Parkinson Foundation—Newsletter **3056**
United Press, Inc. **6062**
United Samaritans Medical Center • Library **7977**
United Scleroderma Foundation **6063**
United Scleroderma Foundation—Newsletter **3057**
U.S. Air Force
    Air Force Systems Command • Human Systems Division • School of Aerospace Medicine • Strughold Aeromedical Library **9991**
    Air Training Command • U.S. Air Force 3790 Medical Service Training Wing • Academic Library **10076**
U.S. Air Force Academy • Medical Library **7568**
U.S. Air Force Base, Luke AFB, AZ • Luke Base Medical Library **7177**
U.S. Air Force Hospital, Carswell AFB, TX • Robert L. Thompson Strategic Hospital • Medical Library/SGEL **9992**
U.S. Air Force Hospital, Chanute AFB, IL • Chanute Technical Training Center • Medical Library **7906**
U.S. Air Force Hospital, Elmendorf AFB, AK • Medical Library **7171**
U.S. Air Force Hospital, Fairchild AFB, WA • Medical Library **10190**
U.S. Air Force Hospital, Griffiss AFB, NY • 416 Strategic Hospital • Medical Library **9096**

U.S. Air Force Hospital, Mather AFB, CA • Medical Library **7356**
U.S. Air Force Hospital Medical Center, Scott AFB, IL • Medical Library **8067**
U.S. Air Force Hospital, Montgomery, AL • Air University Regional Hospital • Health Sciences Library **7161**
U.S. Air Force Hospital, Offutt AFB, NE • Ehrling Bergquist Strategic Hospital • Medical Library **8812**
U.S. Air Force Hospital, Patrick AFB, FL • Medical Library **7786**
U.S. Air Force Hospital, Reese AFB, TX • Medical Library **10060**
U.S. Air Force Hospital, San Antonio, TX • Wilford Hall U.S.A.F. Medical Center • Medical Library **10072**
U.S. Air Force Hospital, Sheppard AFB, TX • Sheppard Technical Training Center Hospital • Health Sciences Library **10077**
U.S. Air Force Hospital, Tinker AFB, OK • Medical Library **9570**
U.S. Air Force Hospital, Travis AFB, CA • David Grant Medical Center • Medical Library **7508**
U.S. Air Force Hospital, Washington, DC • Malcolm Grow Medical Center • Medical Library/SGEL **7715**
U.S. Air Force Medical Center, Keesler AFB, MS • Medical Library **8705**
U.S. Air Force Medical Center, Wright-Patterson AFB, OH • Medical Library **9540**
U.S. Air Force; U.S. Army/ • Offices of the Surgeons General • Joint Medical Library **10137**
United States of America-Physicians and Surgeons Association— Membership Directory and Concordance **4848**
U.S. Armed Forces Institute of Pathology
  Ash Library **7716**
  Media Center **6641**
U.S. Armed Forces Radiobiology Research Institute • Library Services **8362**
U.S. Army
  Health Services Command • Academy of Health Sciences • Stimson Library **10016**
  Health Services Command • Environmental Hygiene Agency • Library **8313**
  Institute of Surgical Research on Burns • Library **10017**
  Letterman Army Institute of Research • Herman Memorial Library **7459**
  Medical Research and Development Command • Aeromedical Research Laboratory • Scientific Information Center **7151**
  Medical Research and Development Command • Biomedical Research and Development Laboratory • Technical Library **8385**
  Medical Research and Development Command • Medical Research Institute of Chemical Defense • Wood Technical Library **8314**
  Medical Research and Development Command • Medical Research Institute of Infectious Diseases • Medical Library **8386**
  Medical Research and Development Command • Walter Reed Army Institute of Research • Library **7717**
U.S. Army Hospitals, Aurora, CO • Fitzsimons Army Medical Center • Medical-Technical Library HSHG-ZBM **7520**
U.S. Army Hospitals, El Paso, TX • William Beaumont Army Medical Center • Medical Library **10014**
U.S. Army Hospitals, Fort Benning, GA • Martin Army Community Hospital • Medical Library **7851**
U.S. Army Hospitals, Fort Bragg, NC • Womack Army Community Hospital • Medical Library **9356**
U.S. Army Hospitals, Fort Campbell, KY • Blanchfield Army Community Hospital • Medical Library **8222**
U.S. Army Hospitals, Fort Carson, CO • Evans Army Community Hospital • Medical Library **7559**
U.S. Army Hospitals, Fort Devens, MA • Cutler Army Hospital • Medical Library **8475**
U.S. Army Hospitals, Fort Dix, NJ • Walson Army Hospital • Medical Library **8882**
U.S. Army Hospitals, Fort Eustis, VA • McDonald Army Community Hospital • Medical Library **10138**
U.S. Army Hospitals, Fort Gordon, GA • D.D. Eisenhower Army Medical Center • Medical Library **7852**
U.S. Army Hospitals, Fort Hood, TX • Darnall Army Hospital • Medical Library **10015**
U.S. Army Hospitals, Fort Huachuca, AZ • Bliss Army Hospital • Medical Library **7176**
U.S. Army Hospitals, Fort Lee, VA • Kenner Army Community Hospital • Medical Library **10139**
U.S. Army Hospitals, Fort Leonard Wood, MO • General Leonard Wood Army Community Hospital • Medical Library **8720**
U.S. Army Hospitals, Fort McClellan, AL • Noble Army Hospital • Medical Library **7150**

U.S. Army Hospitals, Fort Ord, CA • Commander Silas B. Hays Army Community Hospital • Medical Library **7276**
U.S. Army Hospitals, Fort Polk, LA • Bayne-Jones Army Community Hospital • Medical Library **8261**
U.S. Army Hospitals, Fort Riley, KS • Irwin Army Hospital • Medical Library **8188**
U.S. Army Hospitals, Fort Rucker, AL • Lyster Army Community Hospital • Medical Library **7152**
U.S. Army Hospitals, Fort Sam Houston, TX • Brooke Army Medical Center • Medical Library **10018**
U.S. Army Hospitals, Fort Wainwright, AK • Bassett Army Community Hospital • Medical Library **7173**
U.S. Army Hospitals, Honolulu, HI • Tripler Army Medical Center • Medical Library **7877**
U.S. Army Hospitals, San Francisco, CA • Letterman Army Medical Center • Medical Library **7460**
U.S. Army Hospitals, Tacoma, WA • Madigan Army Medical Center • Medical Library **10233**
U.S. Army Hospitals, Washington, DC • Walter Reed Army Medical Center • WRAMC Medical Library **7718**
U.S. Army Hospitals, West Point, NY • Keller Army Community Hospital • MEDDAC Library **9323**
U.S. Army/U.S. Air Force • Offices of the Surgeons General • Joint Medical Library **10137**
U.S. Association for Blind Athletes **6064**
United States and Canadian Programs for Graduate Training in Pharmacology **4849**
U.S. Centers for Disease Control
  CDC Information Center **7839**
  CDC Information Center-Chamblee **7840**
  Office on Smoking and Health • Technical Information Center **8401**
U.S. Defense Logistics Agency • Defense Personnel Support Center • Directorate of Medical Materiel • Medical Information Center **9769**
U.S. Department of Health and Human Services
  Library and Information Center **7719**
  Policy Information Center **7720**
U.S. Department of Labor
  OSHA • Billings Area Office Library **8790**
  OSHA • Office of Training and Education • Library **7982**
  OSHA • Region III Library **9770**
  OSHA • Region X Library **10215**
  OSHA • Technical Data Center **7721**
U.S.D.A.
  Agricultural Research Service • National Animal Disease Center • Library **8155**
  Agricultural Research Service • Plum Island Animal Disease Center • Library **9095**
  Human Nutrition Research Center on Aging • Library **8456**
  National Agricultural Library • Food and Nutrition Information Center **8353**
U.S. Department of Veterans Affairs
  Central Office Film Library **6644**
  Department of Medicine and Surgery • Library Service **9070**
  Office of Technology Transfer • Resource Center **8350**
U.S. Department of Veterans Affairs, Albany, NY • Medical Center Library **9004**
U.S. Department of Veterans Affairs, Albuquerque, NM • Medical Center Library **8985**
U.S. Department of Veterans Affairs, Alexandria, LA • Medical Center Medical Library **8254**
U.S. Department of Veterans Affairs, Allen Park, MI • Medical Center Library Service **8523**
U.S. Department of Veterans Affairs, Altoona, PA • James E. Van Zandt Medical Center • Library Service **9626**
U.S. Department of Veterans Affairs, Amarillo, TX • Hospital Library **9972**
U.S. Department of Veterans Affairs, Ann Arbor, MI • Hospital Library **8527**
U.S. Department of Veterans Affairs, Asheville, NC • Medical Center Library **9334**
U.S. Department of Veterans Affairs, Augusta, GA • Hospital Library **7843**
U.S. Department of Veterans Affairs, Baltimore, MD • Medical Center Library Service **8349**
U.S. Department of Veterans Affairs, Batavia, NY • Medical Center Library **9008**
U.S. Department of Veterans Affairs, Bath, NY • Medical Center Library Service **9009**
U.S. Department of Veterans Affairs, Battle Creek, MI • Medical Center Library **8535**

W

W.A. Budden Memorial Library - Western States Chiropractic College **9606**

W.A. Foote Memorial Hospital • Medical Library **8589**

W. Alton Jones Cell Science Center • George and Margaret Gey Library **9117**

W.B. Patterson **6092**

W.B. Saunders Company **6093, 6714**

W.D. Hoard & Sons Company **6094**

W.K. Kellogg Health Sciences Library - Dalhousie University **10499**

W. Keith Welsh Library - North York General Hospital **10666**

W.L. Estes, Jr. Memorial Library - St. Luke's Hospital of Bethlehem, Pennsylvania **9634**

W.S. Konold Memorial Library - Doctors Hospital, Columbus, OH **9468**

W.W. Summerville Medical Library - Bethany Medical Center **8190**

Wadley Institutes of Molecular Medicine • Research Institute Library **10011**

Wadsworth Center for Laboratories and Research Library - New York State Department of Health **9000**

Wadsworth Medical Library - U.S. Department of Veterans Affairs, Los Angeles, CA **7343**

Wainwright General Hospital • Medical Library **10415**

Wake County Medical Center • Medical Library **9373**

Wake Forest University
  Bowman Gray School of Medicine **6715**
  Bowman Gray School of Medicine • Coy C. Carpenter Library **9386**

Waldmann Memorial Library; John and Bertha E. - David B. Kriser Dental Center - New York University **9214**

Waldo County General Hospital • Marx Library **8290**

Wales and Northern Ireland; Directory of Residential Accommodation for the Mentally Handicapped in England, **4182**

Walker Library - American Council on Alcoholism **8316**

Walker Medical Library; Hastings H. - Hawaii Department of Health **7870**

Walker Memorial Hospital • S.C. Pardee Medical Library **7732**

Walker Staff Library; Elisha - New York Infirmary Beekman Downtown Hospital **9207**

Walking, Inc.; Creative **5246**

WalkWays **3082**

Walla Walla College • School of Nursing Professional Library **9604**

Wallace Library; James A. - Memphis Mental Health Institute **9940**

Wallcur Inc. **6095**

Walson Army Hospital • Medical Library **8882**

Walter Brooks Library - New York Institute for Special Education **9022**

Walter F. Prior Medical Library - Frederick Memorial Hospital **8384**

Walter F. Schaller Memorial Library - St. Francis Memorial Hospital **7453**

Walter J. Klein Company, Ltd. **6716**

Walter L. Wilkins Bio-Medical Library - Naval Health Research Center - U.S. Navy, San Diego, CA **7431**

Walter Lawrence Memorial Library - West Suburban Hospital Medical Center **8037**

Walter Reed Army Institute of Research • Library **7717**

Walter Reed Army Medical Center
  WRAMC Medical Library **7718**
  WRAMC-TV **6717**

Walter Steiner Memorial Library - Hartford Medical Society **7586**

Walters College; Raymond • Library **9440**

Waltham Weston Hospital and Medical Center • Medical Library **8513**

Walther Cancer Institute, Inc.—Newsletter **3083**

Wangensteen Historical Library of Biology and Medicine; Owen H. - Bio-Medical Library - University of Minnesota **8669**

Wann Langston Memorial Library - Baptist Medical Center, Oklahoma City, OK **9553**

War, Medicine and **1314**

Warden Woods Campus Resource Centre - Centennial College of Applied Arts and Technology **10607**

Ward's Natural Science Establishment, Inc. **6718**

Warfield Communications, Inc. **6096**

Warne Clinic; Pottsville Hospital and • Medical Library **9811**

Warner-Lambert Company • Corporate Library **8900**

Warner-Lambert/Parke-Davis • Research Library **8532**

Warren Book Publishing Company **6097**

Warren G. Murray Developmental Center • Library **7903**

Warren General Hospital • Medical Staff Library **9537**

Warren H. Green, Inc. **6098**

Warren Hospital • Medical Library **8925**

Warren State Hospital • Medical Library **9703**

Wascana Rehabilitation Centre • Health Sciences Library **10790**

Washington Adventist Hospital • Health Sciences Library **8411**

Washington Business Information, Inc. **6099**

Washington County Hospital • Wroth Memorial Library **8391**

Washington Drug Letter **3084**

Washington Health Record **3085**

Washington Hospital • Health Sciences Libraries **9836**

Washington Hospital Center • Medical Library **7729**

Washington Hospital; Mary • Gordon W. Jones Medical Library **10140**

Washington Library for the Blind and Physically Handicapped **10222**

Washington News and Document Retrieval Network; DIOGENES: **6873**

Washington Park Zoo • Animal Management Division • Library **9605**

Washington Psychoanalytic Society • Hadley Memorial Library **7730**

Washington Report **3086**

Washington Social Legislation Bulletin **3087**

Washington State Department of Veterans Affairs • Staff & Member Library **10199**

Washington State Library
  Eastern State Hospital Library **10193**
  Lakeland Village Branch Library **10194**
  Rainier School Branch Library **10188**
  Western State Hospital Branch Library **10191**

Washington State School for the Deaf • McGill Library **10237**

Washington State University
  Instructional Media Services **6719**
  Veterinary Medical/Pharmacy Library **10196**

Washington University
  Central Institute for the Deaf **6100**
  George W. Brown School of Social Work • Learning Resources Video Center **6720**
  George W. Brown School of Social Work • Library and Learning Resources Center **8780**
  School of Medicine • Department of Psychiatry Library **8781**
  School of Medicine • Mallinckrodt Institute of Radiology Library **8782**
  School of Medicine Library **8783**

Washington University; George • Medical Center • Paul Himmelfarb Health Sciences Library **7681**

Washington University Medical Center • St. Louis Children's Hospital Library **8784**

Washington University Medical Center; Jewish Hospital at • Rothschild Medical Library **8761**

Washoe Medical Center • Medical Library **8830**

Waste Management Association; JAPCA: The International Journal of the Air and **848**

Waste News; Medical **2583**

Waste News; Medical **7021**

Waterbury Hospital • Health Center Library **7629**

Waterford Hospital • Health Services Library **10491**

Waterville Osteopathic Hospital • M.J. Gerrie, Sr. Medical Library **8311**

Watson Clinic • Medical Library **7762**

Watson Library; Eugene P. • Shreveport Division **8279**

Watson Publishing International **6101**

Watson W. Wise Medical Research Library - University of Texas Health Center, Tyler **10082**

Watts School of Nursing • Library **9351**

Waukesha County Technical College • WCTC Library **10336**

Waukesha Memorial Hospital • Medical Library **10345**

Wayne County Regional Library for the Blind and Physically Handicapped **8635**

Wayne State University
  College of Nursing • DENT Project **6721**
  Media Library **6722**
  Vera Parshall Shiffman Medical Library **8563**

Wean Medical Library - Trumbull Memorial Hospital **9536**

The Web **3088**

Webb Memorial Library - Penrose Hospital **7527**

Webb Memorial Library; Del E. - Loma Linda University **7305**

Webb Memorial Medical Information Center; Del E. - Eisenhower Medical Center **7407**

The Webb Report **3089**

Weber; Charles E. **5185**

Weber Memorial Library - San Antonio Community Hospital **7511**

Webster Library - Evanston Hospital **7990**

Weehawken Book Company **6102**

Weekly Pharmacy Reports—The Green Sheet **3090**

Weight Control Services Directory **4866**

Weight Management—Newsletter; Institute for Positive **2458**

Weinberg Library; Jack - Illinois State Psychiatric Institute **7935**

Z